Orthopedic Rehabilitation

CLINICAL ADVISOR

Orthopedic Rehabilitation
Clinical Advisor

Derrick Sueki, PT, DPT, GCPT, OCS

Adjunct Orthopedic Faculty
Mount St. Mary's College
Los Angeles, California

Clinical Mentor
Orthopedic Residency Program
University of Southern California
Division of Biokinesiology and Physical Therapy at the School of Dentistry
Los Angeles, California

Owner and President
Knight Physical Therapy Inc
Garden Grove, California

Strength and Conditioning Consultant
Chapman University Volleyball
Los Angeles, California

Jacklyn Brechter, PhD, PT

Chair Person and Associate Professor of Orthopedics
Department of Physical Therapy
Chapman University
Los Angeles, California

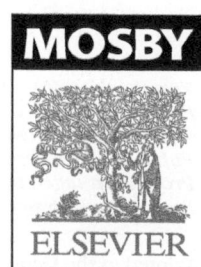

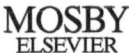

3251 Riverport Lane
Maryland Heights, Missouri 63043

ORTHOPEDIC REHABILITATION CLINICAL ADVISOR ISBN: 978-0-323-05710-3

Notice

Knowledge and best practice in this field are constantly changing. As new research and experience broaden our understanding, changes in research methods, professional practices, or medical treatment may become necessary.

Practitioners and researchers must always rely on their own experience and knowledge in evaluating and using any information, methods, compounds, or experiments described herein. In using such information or methods they should be mindful of their own safety and the safety of others, including parties for whom they have a professional responsibility.

With respect to any drug or pharmaceutical products identified, readers are advised to check the most current information provided (i) on procedures featured or (ii) by the manufacturer of each product to be administered, to verify the recommended dose or formula, the method and duration of administration, and contraindications. It is the responsibility of practitioners, relying on their own experience and knowledge of their patients, to make diagnoses, to determine dosages and the best treatment for each individual patient, and to take all appropriate safety precautions.

To the fullest extent of the law, neither the Publisher nor the authors, contributors, or editors, assume any liability for any injury and/or damage to persons or property as a matter of products liability, negligence or otherwise, or from any use or operation of any methods, products, instructions, or ideas contained in the material herein.

Library of Congress Cataloging-in-Publication Data

Orthopedic rehabilitation clinical advisor / [edited by] Derrick Sueki, Jacklyn Brechter. - 1st ed.
   p. ; cm.
  Includes bibliographical references and index.
  ISBN 978-0-323-05710-3 (hardcover : alk. paper) 1. Orthopedics. 2. Musculoskeletal system–Wounds and injuries–Patients–Rehabilitation.
 I. Sueki, Derrick. II. Brechter, Jacklyn.
  [DNLM: 1. Musculoskeletal Diseases–rehabilitation. 2. Musculoskeletal Diseases–diagnosis.
3. Orthopedic Procedures–methods. 4. Physical Therapy Modalities. WE 140 O775 2010]
  RD795.O78 2010
  616.7–dc22
                                                2009034503

Vice President and Publisher: Linda Duncan
Executive Editor: Kathryn Falk
Senior Developmental Editor: Christie M. Hart
Publishing Services Manager: Pat Joiner-Myers, Hemamalini Rajendrababu
Project Manager: Shereen Jameel
Senior Book Designer: Teresa McBryan

Printed in the United States of America

Last digit is the print number: 9 8 7 6 5

To my wife, Lynne, *and my children,* Summer *and* Jake. *They reveal to me daily the reason for life and the importance of seeking answers to its many questions.*

Also dedicated to my parents, George *and* Beatrice. *They have demonstrated to me from childhood the importance of setting goals, working hard, and keeping my commitments.*

Derrick Sueki

This book is dedicated to Catia *who always inspires me to explain clearly and from whom time was taken in order to complete this project.*

It is also dedicated to those students and medical professionals embarking on careers in the field of orthopedic rehabilitation. There is never enough time to absorb all there is to learn in school. I hope these pages can provide answers and direction as you walk the path to clinical excellence.

Jacklyn Brechter

Contributors

Nancy Adachi, PT, BA
Clinical Specialist and Coordinator
    of Clinical Education
Kaiser Permanente, Los Angeles
University of California, Los Angeles
Part time faculty UCLA Orofacial Pain
Lecturer Kaiser Permanente Orthopaedic
    Residency Program
Lecturer UCLA Orofacial Pain and Dental
    School
Los Angeles, California

Leesha Augustine, PT, DPT
Children's Hospital of Orange County
Orange, California

Audra Ponci Bado, MPT, OCS, CHT
Senior Physical Therapist
Kaiser Permanente
Harbor City, California

Ronald Belczyk, DPM
Assistant Professor
Division of Podiatric Medicine and
    Surgery
Department of Orthopedics
University of Texas Health Center at San
    Antonio
San Antonio, Texas

Ross Biederman, MD, DPM
Professor
Department of Physical Therapy
Chapman University
Orange, California

Jacklyn Brechter, PhD, PT
Chairperson and Associate Professor of
    Orthopedics
Department of Physical Therapy
Chapman University
Orange, California

Robin Burks, DPT, CHT
Hand Therapy
University of Southern California
University Hospital Outpatient
    Rehabilitation
Los Angeles, California

Robert S. Burns, PT, DPT
Co-owner
NUDOC Physical Therapy, LLC
Clinical Director and Co-owner
Novi Doctors of Physical Therapy
Novi, Michigan

Christopher R. Carcia, PhD, PT, SCS
Associate Professor
Department of Physical Therapy
Program Director
Graduate Program in Rehabilitation
    Sciences
John G. Rangos School of Health Sciences
Duquesne University
Pittsburgh, Pennsylvania

Lee Anne Carothers, PT, PhD
Adjunct Faculty
Chapman University
Orange, California
Acute Care Physical Therapist
Alaska Regional Hospital
Anchorage, Alaska

Donna Cespon, MPT, OCS
Owner/Director
Clinical Coordinator/Clinical Instructor
Body Re-Balance Physical Therapy
Irvine, California
Lab Assistant for Sahrmann Movement
    Impairment Syndrome Courses

**Joshua Cleland, DPT, PhD, OCS,
    FAAOMPT**
Associate Professor
Franklin Pierce University
Rindge, New Hampshire

Cynthia Cooper, MFA, MA, OTR/L, CHT
Clinical Specialist in Hand Therapy
Scottsdale Healthcare
Scottsdale, Arizona

Benjamin Cornell, PT, OCS
Adjunct Orthopedic Faculty
Mount St. Mary's College
Clinical Faculty
Orthopedic Residency Program
HealthCare Partners Medical Group
Torrance, California

**Josephine Louise Coulter, BSc (Physio)
    Hons, MSc (Manual Therapy)**
Private Practice
London, England

**Bryan Dennison, PT, DPT, MPT, OCS,
    CSCS**
Affiliate Faculty School of Physical Therapy
Rueckert-Hartman College for Health
    Professions
Regis University
EIM Residency/Fellowship Lead Faculty
Denver, Colorado

**Katina Dimopoulos, B App Sc Physio,
    M Sports Physio**
Titled Sports Physiotherapist
Senior Sports Physiotherapist
Director of Rehabilitation Physiosports
Australian Physiotherapy Association
Brighton, Melbourne Australia

Skye Donovan, PT, PhD, OCS
Assistant Professor
Department of Physical Therapy
Marymount University
Arlington, Virginia

**Sarah Graham, BSc(Hons) Physio,
    BSc(Hons) Spt Sci, PgD Spt Physio**
Clinical Specialist Physiotherapist
London Sports Medicine Centre
London, United Kingdom

Sara Grannis, DPT, OCS, ATC
Physical Therapist
Clinical Instructor
Coordinator of Clinical Education
Orange County, California

Julie Guthrie, PT, DPT, OCS
Davis and De Rosa Physical Therapy
El Segundo, California

Chris Izu, PT, OCS
Part-time Faculty
Mount St. Mary's College
Los Angeles, California
Clinical Faculty
Healthcare Partners Orthopedic Residency
    Program
Torrance, California

**Pamela J. Kikillus, PT, DHSc, OCS,
    COMPT, FAAOMPT**
Clinic Director
Olympic Sports and Spine Rehabilitation
Puyallup, Washington
Adjunct Faculty
University of Puget Sound
Tacoma, Washington
Certified Fellowship Instructor
North American Institute of Manual
    Therapy
Eugene, Oregon

Daniel J. Kirages, PT, DPT, OCS, FAAOMPT
Adjunct Assistant Professor of Clinical Physical Therapy
University of Southern California
Division of Biokinesiology and Physical Therapy
Adjunct Orthopedic Faculty
Mount St. Mary's College
Department of Physical Therapy
Los Angeles, California
Curriculum Coordinator
Kaiser Permanente Los Angeles Orthopaedic Manual Therapy Fellowship
Clinical Faculty
Kaiser Permanente Southern California Orthopaedic Physical Therapy Residency
Clinical Specialist II
Kaiser Permanente Los Angeles Medical Center
Department of Physical Medicine and Rehabilitation
Los Angeles, California
President
Body Solutions Physical Therapy
Arcadia, California

Michael Ko, DPT, OCS, ATC
Director of Physical Therapy
Director of Sports Medicine
Center Coordinator of Clinical Education
Pine Street Physical and Occupational Therapy
Stockton, California

Rhonda K. Kotarinos, PT, MS
Rhonda Kotarinos Physical Therapy, Ltd.
Oakbrook Terrace, Illinois

Mark Kozuki, PT, MA, OCS, CSCS
Adjunct Clinical Faculty, Instructor
Department of Physical Therapy
Chapman University
Orange, California
Co-Owner and Director of Optimum Performance Specialists
Costa Mesa, California
Staff Physical Therapist Orthopedic Specialty Institute
Orange, California

Robert Landel, PT, DPT, OCS, CSCS
Associate Professor of Clinical Physical Therapy
Division of Biokinesiology and Physical Therapy at the School of Dentistry
University of Southern California
Los Angeles, California

Susan Layfield, PT, DPT, MS, OCS
Adjunct Clinical Faculty
Department of Physical Therapy
Los Angeles, California
University of Southern California
President and Director of Physical Therapy
Layfield and Associates Physical Therapy, Inc.
Encino, California

Michael Leal, PT, DPT, MPT, OCS
Affiliate Faculty School of Physical Therapy
Rueckert-Hartman College for Health Professions
Regis University
Adjunct Faculty School of Physical Therapy
Azusa Pacific University
EIM Residency/Fellowship Lead Faculty
Clinical Specialist
Kaiser Permanente Department of Physical Medicine & Rehabilitation
Downey, California

Della Lee, DPT, ATC, OCS
Adjunct Instructor of Clinical Physical Therapy
Department of Biokinesiology and Physical Therapy
University of Southern California
Center Coordinator of Clinical Education
Rehabilitation Department
St. Vincent Medical Center
Los Angeles, California

Bernard Li, DPT, OCS
Adjunct Faculty
Instructor of Clinical Physical Therapy
Clinical Mentor Orthopedic Residency
Division of Biokinesiology and Physical Therapy at the School of Dentistry
University of Southern California
Select Physical Therapy
Los Angeles, California
Harbor Physical Therapy
San Pedro, California

Mildred V. Limcay, DPT, OCS
Adjunct Orthopedic Faculty
Mount St. Mary's College
Adjunct Clinical Faculty
Clinical Mentor, Orthopedic Residency Program
University of Southern California, Division of Physical Therapy
Physical Therapist
Kaiser Permanente
Los Angeles, California

Elaine Lonnemann, DPT, OCS, MTC, FAAOMPT
Assistant Professor
Bellarmine University
Assistant Professor Online Division
Adjunct Instructor Continuing Professional Education Division
University of Saint Augustine
Louisville, Kentucky

Deborah L. Lowe, MA, MPT, PhD
Director and Chair, Department of Physical Therapy
Doctor of Physical Therapy Program
Mount St. Mary's College
Los Angeles, California

Keith Mahler, PT, MPT, CEAS
Keith Mahler Physical Therapy
La Jolla, California
Adjunct Professor of Physical Therapy
Chapman University
Orange, California

Robert C. Manske, PT, DPT, SCS, MEd, ATC, CSCS
Associate Professor
Department of Physical Therapy
Wichita State University
Wichita, Kansas

RobRoy Martin, PhD, PT, CSCS
Associate Professor
Department of Physical Therapy
Duquesne University
Staff Physical Therapist
Centers for Rehabilitation Services
Center for Sports Medicine
University of Pittsburgh
Pittsburgh, Philadelphia

Neil McKenna, DPT, FAAOMPT, OCS, CSCS
Adjunct Faculty
Chapman University
Clinical Specialist Doctors of Physical Therapy
Encinitas, California

Alison L. McKenzie, PT, PhD
Professor of Physical Therapy
Chapman University
Orange, California

John L. Meyer, PT, DPT, OCS, FAFS
Director of Rehabilitation
Department of Athletics
Adjunct Assistant Professor
Division of Biokinesiology and Physical Therapy
University of Southern California
Adjunct Orthopedic Faculty
Mount St. Mary's College
Los Angeles, California

Paul E. Mintken, PT, DPT, OCS, FAAOMPT
Assistant Professor
Denver School of Medicine
Department of Physical Therapy
University of Colorado
Aurora, Colorado
Lead Clinician
Wardenburg Health Center at the University of Colorado
Boulder, Colorado
Primary Faculty
Evidence in Motion
Louisville, Kentucky

Lou Ann Moore, MsAppScPT, PT
Physical Therapist
Orange Park, Florida

William H. O'Grady, PT, DPT, MA, MTC, COMT, OCS, FAAOMPT, DAAPM
Advisory Faculty, Examiner, Clinical Faculty Instructor
Manual Therapy Fellowship Program
North American Institute of Orthopedic Manual Therapy
Eugene, Oregon
Adjunct Faculty
University of Nevada, Las Vegas
Las Vegas, Nevada
Ex CEO
Olympic Sports and Spine Rehabilitation Inc.
Pierce County, Washington

Erica Pablo, PT, DPT, OCS
Clinical Director
Knight Physical Therapy Inc
Garden Grove, California

Stephen Paulseth, PT, DPT, SCS, ATC
President, Foot & Ankle SIG of the APTA's Orthopedic Section
Paulseth & Associates Physical Therapy, Inc.
Los Angeles, California

Amy B. Pomrantz, PT, DPT, OCS, ATC
Adjunct Instructor of Clinical Physical Therapy
Division of Biokinesiology and Physical Therapy
University of Southern California
USC Physical Therapy Associates
Los Angeles, California

Stephanie A. Prendergast, MPT
Co-owner
Pelvic Health and Rehabilitation Center
San Francisco, California

Daniel Prohaska, MD
Orthopedic Surgeon
Advanced Orthopedic Associates
Wichita, Kansas

Akemi Rico, DPT
Staff Physical Therapist
CompletePT
Los Angeles, California

Sarah McPhee Riley
Mount St. Mary's College
Los Angeles, California
Knight Physical Therapy Inc
Garden Grove, California

Suzanne Rowles, PT, DPT
Select Physical Therapy
Atlanta, Georgia

Elizabeth Rummer, MSPT
Co-partner
Pelvic Health and Rehabilitation Center
San Francisco, California

Patricia A. Rudd, PT, DPT, CCTT
Assistant Clinical Professor
Department of Oral and Maxillofacial Surgery
University of California
San Francisco Center for Orofacial Pain
San Fransisco, California

Stephanie S. Saito, DPT, OCS
Adjunct Faculty
Mount St. Mary's College
Staff Physical Therapist
HealthCare Partners Medical Group - Physical Therapy
Los Angeles, California

Alison R. Scheid, DPT, OCS
Adjunct Instructor of Clinical Physical Therapy
Clinical Mentor
Orthopedic Residency Program
University of Southern California
Department of Physical Therapy
Los Angeles, California

Adam Schultz, PT, M Manip Ther
Adjunct Orthopedic Faculty
Mount St. Mary's College
Clinical Mentor Orthopedic Residency Program
Cedars-Sinai Medical Center
Los Angeles, California

Teresa Scully, PT
Physical Therapist
University of North Florida
Jacksonville, Florida

Chris A. Sebelski, PT, DPT, OCS, CSCS
Assistant Professor
Department of Physical Therapy & Athletic Training
Doisy College of Health Sciences
Saint Louis University
St. Louis, Missouri

Michael Shacklock, FACP, MAppSc, DipPhysio, MAPA, MMPA
Adjunct Clinical Faculty
Division of Physical Therapy
Georgia State University
Atlanta, Georgia
Director
Neurodynamic Solutions
Adelaide, Australia
Principal and Director
City Physiotherapy and Sports Injury Clinic
Adelaide, Australia

Derrick Sueki, DPT, GCPT, OCS
Adjunct Orthopedic Faculty
Mount St. Mary's College
Department of Physical Therapy
Los Angeles, California
Clinical Mentor
Orthopedic Residency Program
University of Southern California
Division of Biokinesiology and Physical Therapy at the School of Dentistry
Los Angeles, California
Owner and President
Knight Physical Therapy Inc.
Garden Grove, California

Jason Tonley, DPT, OCS
Adjunct Faculty
Mount St. Mary's College
Program Coordinator for Physical Therapy Residency and Fellowship Programs
Kaiser Permanente Southern California
Los Angeles, California

Son Trinh, DPT
Hallmark Rehabilitation
Garden Park Care Center
Garden Grove, California

Wolfgang Vogel, MS, PhD
Professor Emeritus
Department of Pharmacology
Jefferson Medical College
Thomas Jefferson University
Philadelphia, Pennsylvania
Adjunct Professor
Florida Gulf Coast University
Fort Meyers, Florida

Dane K. Wukich, MD
Associate Professor of Orthopaedic Surgery
Chief, Division of Foot and Ankle Surgery
Assistant Program Director
Orthopaedic Surgery Residency
University of Pittsburgh School of Medicine
Pittsburg, Pennsylvania

Brian Yee, PT, MPhty, OCS, FAAOMPT
Clinical Instructor
Georgia State University
Department of Physical Therapy
Course Instructor
Neurodynamic Solutions
Motion Stability, LLC, Owner
Atlanta, Georgia

Steven M. Yun, PT, DPT, OCS, FAAOMPT (cand.)
Orthopaedic Residency Coordinator
Co-Center Coordinator of Clinical Education
Advanced Practice Physical Therapist
St. Jude Centers for Rehabilitation & Wellness
Brea, California

Preface

As long as people have been injured, people have been trying to return to their preinjury state. The origins of medicine can be dated back to the time of ancient Egypt and probably existed even before this time. It is logical to surmise that efforts to rehabilitate can be dated back to a similar time. In spite of their common origin, the field of rehabilitation has lagged behind that of medicine. In medicine, early theory was closely related to religious practice. Hippocrates has been credited with being the first to separate religion and medicine. He believed that illness and disease had its roots in physical rational explanations and not in religion or superstition. He is credited with greatly advancing the systematic study of clinical medicine. Since that time, the process of research, education, and learning has evolved and become fairly well established in clinical medicine. The same cannot be said for rehabilitative medicine. Although the clinical science of medicine can be dated back to Hipprocrates in 480 BC, the fields of rehabilitation did not exist until the late 1800s. Physical therapy became a profession in 1894, chiropractic in 1890, occupational therapy in 1910, athletic training in 1930, and physiatry in 1938. The field of rehabilitation science is still in its relative infancy. Research, clinical practice, and education are all evolving and changing as new research, technology, or methodology reshapes the field.

Medicine has established and refined its method of education. Although not all medical schools educate the same way, most reflect a similar method of preparing a clinician to practice medicine. Medical knowledge is imparted in academia, whereas clinical experience is gained through an apprenticeship process in the form of residencies and fellowships. Rehabilitation professions such as physical therapy are in the process of developing programs that are modeled after the medical field's system of mentorship. Residencies and fellowships are becoming more commonplace but still are not the norm. Because of space limitations and financial factors, residency programs and clinical mentorships will probably never be available to all clinicians. Many clinicians cannot or choose not to complete residencies for a variety of reasons. From a clinician's standpoint, financial and personal factors often make residency training impossible. From a profession standpoint, the resources and manpower needed to provide advanced training to all graduating clinicians would create a near impossible task. Yet, the need for advanced training is real and necessary. This book was founded out of this need. It is intended to be a clinical resource that can provide the mentorship that may not be available to all clinicians. The title of the series "Clinical Advisor" implies that the purpose of the series is to provide guidance to the clinician. This book is intended to be that resource.

Teaching students to make appropriate clinical decisions or learning to reason through clinical-based problems is a difficult task. Part of the difficulty is due to the fact that no two individuals reason the same. It can also be argued that a person may use different reasoning styles for a similar clinical problem given different settings, experiences, educational backgrounds, or emotional status. With this complexity in mind, this book was developed to help the student or novice clinician think through clinical problems in a variety of manners. It starts by developing propositional or book knowledge. Section I of this book is designed to provide the basic foundational knowledge needed to make decisions in a rehabilitation setting.

How does expert thought differ from novice thought patterns? Novices are often fluently able to recite data, but these data do not always equate to knowledge. Knowledge is achieved only when data become usable. One of the methods our brain uses to store data is within patient-based schema or clinical-based patterns. These patterns are developed so that information can be easily retrieved. It becomes usable. Pattern recognition is one of the characteristics of expert thought. The goal of this book is to provide clinical guidance to students and novice clinicians. It is organized in a manner that facilitates the attainment of clinical expertise and expert thought processes.

Section II of this book allows the student and novice clinician insight into the clinical reasoning and decision-making processes of expert clinicians. Experts in particular body regions from around the nation and world have been asked to provide insight into how they make decisions regarding patient care. The authors have been asked to focus primarily on their decision-making process regarding diagnosis of pathology and tissue impairment. Each expert has written about how they think during a patient-subjective examination, thus taking the novice through the questions typically asked during a subjective examination. With each line of questioning, they share how the line of questioning influences their decision-making processes. In essence, the novice has the opportunity to be mentored by the expert clinician. Most novice clinicians desire mentorship from an experienced clinician. This section allows access to the minds of some of leading clinicians in their field.

The novice is then guided by the clinical reasoning and decision-making chapters to Section III, the pathology section. Here again, experienced clinicians give their insight into specific pathologies. The design of the text has been standardized across pathologies to allow for ease of use. The material has been organized to parallel the clinical decision-making chapters. Each pathology is laid out in a format that follows a subjective examination and provides the clinician with an evolving clinical pattern or schema of a patient who has a particular pathology.

Section IV of this book is the rehabilitation section. It has been formatted in a regional manner. Many of the principles of rehabilitation are similar for different body regions. Instead of repeating information for each body region, many similar regions were combined. For instance, foot, ankle, knee, and hip were all combined to create a section that focuses on rehabilitation of the lower quarter. Once again, experts in their field were asked to write how they made decisions regarding the rehabilitation process.

Many medications can influence the rehabilitative process. It is not the intent of the text to make the rehabilitation clinician an expert in pharmacology, but to give them a reference that will grant them ready access to the common medications that can influence rehabilitation. Section V is designed to provide the clinician with quick information regarding the medications that they will see most commonly in the clinic.

The intent of the text is to be usable. The reader will see efforts throughout the book to make information easily accessible. Chapters have been formatted in a question-and-answer design to allow the clinician quick access to the information they need. Pathology sections have been organized in a bullet-list layout. It is hoped that when a clinician needs quick insight into a patient's pathology, the bulleted format will allow them to find information quickly without getting lost in verbiage. Clinicians and students alike demand quick answers to their questions. This book was designed with this goal in mind. Reasoning requires well-organized data.

ACKNOWLEDGMENTS

Books, like people, are shaped by the individuals that come in contact with it. No book comes to fruition without the combined effort of many people. Sincere thanks go to the authors and experts who have dedicated their valuable time and expertise to the creation of this book. Their knowledge will help shape the minds and thoughts of the future clinicians. Additional thanks go to the faculty and staff of Mount St. Mary's College, Chapman University, and the University of Southern California, all of whom have contributed greatly to the creation of this book. To the staff of Elsevier, Kathy Falk, Christie Hart, Joy Moore, Shereen Jameel, and crew, thanks for the patience and guidance in helping us traverse the road from idea to publication. It's been a fun and educational journey. Thanks and acknowledgement also goes out to Tamiko Murakami for providing us with the her talent. The fruits of her labor are seen in the graphics interspersed throughout the book. Finally, acknowledgment goes to the students and clinicians whose inquisitiveness and passion for knowledge have motivated us to produce a book that would help answer their questions.

Derrick Sueki, PT, DPT, GCPT, OCS

Jacklyn Brechter, PhD, PT

Contents

Foundational Knowledge

AUTHOR: SKYE DONOVAN, JACKLYN BRECHTER, DERRICK SUEKI

INTRODUCTORY INFORMATION

HOMEOSTASIS

Homeostasis is the tendency of the body to maintain a constant state of balance or equilibrium. Normal physiology results in a state of normal homeostasis. A body faced with conditions outside its normal state is forced to adapt to return to its state of equilibrium. Stress equals adaptation. With the study of orthopedic pathology, we are interested in how conditions that exceed or alter a body's normal state affect the musculoskeletal system.

Pathology occurs when physiological, systemic, or mechanical stresses that exceed the limits of tissue result in tissue failure. All injury can be associated with a failure of normal tissue. In orthopedics, injury and pathology occur when stresses exceed the normal limits of the musculoskeletal systems. Proper assessment and treatment of musculoskeletal pathology and tissue injury require a knowledge of tissue capability. Conversely, tissue healing requires an understanding of the inflammatory and healing process.

INFLAMMATION AND REPAIR

An understanding of the inflammatory process plays an important role in the clinical diagnosis of musculoskeletal pathology. Understanding of the repair process aids in the development of rehabilitation programs for a patient's pathology. Repair begins immediately following an injury by attempting to reestablish tissue continuity. In general, humans do not regenerate tissue, they repair it with scar tissue (or dense connective tissue). This quick process reduces the chances of infection and quickly restores tissue function.

WHAT ARE THE PHASES OF TISSUE HEALING?

The healing process involves three phases and several subphases (Table I-1-1). Phase 1 is the inflammatory phase and involves two subphases, vascular and cellular. Phase 2 is the reparative phase, but it has also been called the proliferative, the fibroplastic, or the regenerative phase. These terms, for the most part, can be used interchangeably. Phase 2 includes three subphases, reepithelization, fibroplasia with neovascularization, and wound closure. The final phase, Phase 3, is the remodeling phase. It involves two subphases, the consolidation phase and the maturation phase.

TABLE I-1-1   Phases of Tissue Healing

Phase	Name of Phase	Subphase	Timeframe
Phase 1	Inflammatory	Vascular	0–14 days (greatest at 48 hours)
		Cellular	0–14 days (greatest at 48 hours)
Phase 2	Reparative	Reepithelization	0–2 days
	Proliferative	Fibroplasia with	2–5 days
	Fibroplastic	neovascularization	
	Regenerative	Wound closure	4–21 days
Phase 3	Remodeling	Consolidation	21–60 days
		Maturation	61–360 days

INFLAMMATORY PHASE (PHASE 1)

WHAT IS THE INFLAMMATION PHASE?

The purpose of the inflammatory phase is the removal of all foreign debris along with dying or dead tissue, thereby reducing the likelihood of infection. The inflammatory phase is composed of two tissue responses:
1. Vascular response
2. Cellular response

WHAT IS THE VASCULAR RESPONSE?

The vascular response is hallmarked by heat and redness of the injured tissue. The following physiological responses occur in the injured tissue as a result of tissue injury:
1. Coagulation seals off injured blood vessels and temporarily closes the wound space.
2. Noninjured blood vessels in area dilate.

WHAT IS THE TIMEFRAME OF THE VASCULAR RESPONSE?

It is most active in the first 48 hours and is generally completed by 14 days.

WHAT SYSTEMS ARE INVOLVED IN THE VASCULAR RESPONSE?

1. The Kinin System increases vascular permeability through the release of chemical mediators (i.e., Bradykinins).
2. The Complement System results in release of histamine from mast cells. This in turn increases vascular permeability.
3. The Clotting System is activated in response to injury. Clotting is utilized to stem the loss of blood from injured tissues. Thrombin results in the release of fibrin, which plugs capillaries. Mast cells release hyaluronic acid, which forms a gel to plug capillaries.

WHAT IS THE CELLULAR RESPONSE?

The cellular response involves the proliferation of cells in the region of the injury. These cells are responsible for cleaning debris from the injury site and the prevention of infection.

HOW DOES THIS RESPONSE OCCUR?

Most chemicals released in the inflammatory response process are chemotaxic in nature (migrate along chemical gradients). Polymorphonuclear leukocytes (neutrophils) are attracted to wound sites by the chemicals mediators. Neutrophils act as a first line of defense against foreign antigens. The role of the neutrophil is the prevention or elimination of infection. Macrophages are also drawn to the area to dispose of bacteria and necrotic tissue via phagocytosis. Macrophages sterilize the area via release of hydrogen peroxide.

REPARATIVE OR FIBROPLASTIC PHASE (PHASE 2)

WHAT IS THE PURPOSE OF THE REPARATIVE PHASE?

The purpose of the reparative phase of healing is the formation of scar tissue to restore continuity of damaged tissue. The phase is named for the fibroblasts that form the scar tissue. The reparative phase is composed of three subphases:
1. Reepithelization
2. Fibroplasia with neovascularization
3. Wound contracture

WHAT IS REEPITHELIZATION?

The purpose of the reepithelization phase is to reestablish the epidermis across the surface of the skin, thus preventing infection. To accomplish this task, a fibrin and collagen type IV matrix forms across the wound in the form of a scab. This process is generally completed in 48 hours.

WHAT IS FIBROPLASIA WITH NEOVASCULARIZATION?

The purpose of the fibroplasias with neovascularization phase is to repair the site of injury in order to establish of structural integrity. Fibroplasia involves neutrophils that produce platelet-derived growth factors (PDGF). The PDGF attract fibroblasts to the site of injury. The resultant tissue is called granulation tissue. Once within the injured area, fibroblasts synthesize the construction materials needed for repair. This includes collagen, proteoglycans, glycosaminoglycans (GAGs), and elastin. In addition to fibroplasias, neovascularization occurs. Neovascularization refers to the formation of new blood supplies within the injured area. To accomplish this process, angioblasts are attracted by PDGF. Angioblasts link together and extend toward existing vessels to reestablish vascularization. This process generally begins within 2 to 5 days and continues until vascularity is reestablished.

WHAT IS THE WOUND CONTRACTURE PHASE?

The body is well designed. Rather than heal a large wound the body can decrease the size of the injury through the process of wound contracture. Myofibroblasts attach to the extracellular matrix and draw the matrix together, essentially decreasing the size of the injury that needs to be healed. This process generally begins 4 days postinjury and continues for 21 days.

REMODELING PHASE (PHASE 3)

WHAT OCCURS DURING THE REMODELING PHASE?

In the remodeling phase of healing the main purpose of the body is strengthening of the newly generated tissue not the generation of tissue. The body will strengthen in response to forces applied to it. This phase is composed of two subphases:
1. Consolidation
2. Maturation

WHAT IS THE CONSOLIDATION SUBPHASE?

Initially during the healing process, the injured area is inundated with cells. Some cells will combat infection and other cells will generate new tissue. In the consolidation phase the tissue begins the conversion from cellular to fibrous in nature. Fibroblasts and myofibroblasts are still in the area but slowly begin to leave the injured area. The other event that occurs during this phase is the strengthening of the scar in response to stress. The scar stops growing by 21 days. On average, this phase takes place between 21 and 60 days postinjury.

WHAT OCCURS DURING THE MATURATION SUBPHASE?

During the maturation phase, the scar tissue continues to strengthen while almost all of the cellular components of the healing response have left the tissue. The distinguishing characteristic between the consolidation subphase and the maturation subphase is the reduction in the presence of cells. Because there are fewer cells available in the maturation sub-phase, the amount of activity diminishes. Collagen turnover, however, remains high until approximately 4 to 6 months after injury. At this time the turnover rate diminishes. The timeframe for the maturation subphase is 60 to 360 days after the initial insult.

NORMAL MUSCULOSKELETAL TISSUE

Most tissue in the body is composed of similar structural components. Understanding the basic components of tissue gives the clinician insight into the mechanism of injury and expected recovery potential. Normal musculoskeletal tissue is designed to resist the loading and demands placed upon it throughout the day. Each tissue is designed to resist specific loading. Injury to tissue occurs when loading exceeds the tissue capacity. Knowledge of the types of loads each tissue is capable of resisting is necessary to diagnose pathology. An understanding of a pathology's effect on each of the basic components of tissue will give the clinician insight into morphological and clinical manifestation that are commonly seen in clinical practice.

BASIC COMPONENTS

In reality, injury in the orthopedic setting can be simplified if you know the basic components of tissue, if you understand the physiological properties of these building blocks, and if you understand how each component responds to stress (Table I-1-2). Bodily tissue is composed of several basic components present in differing amounts in each tissue (Table I-1-3):
1. Collagen
2. Elastin
3. Proteoglycans
4. Inorganic components
5. Water
6. Cells

COLLAGEN

Collagen functions to give tensile strength to tissue. Collagen fibrils are composed of a triple helix of three polypeptides. These fibrils are then staggered in a quarternary pattern (a quarter turn from each other). Currently, 20 types have been identified. Of these types, type I and II are the most abundant. Bone, ligaments, tendons, meniscus, the annulus of the intervertebral disc, and skin are all primarily type I collagen.

Articular cartilage and the nucleus pulposus of the intervertebral disc are primarily composed of type II collagen.

ELASTIN

Elastin is primarily composed of the amino acids glycine, valine, alanine, and proline. It is made by linking many soluble tropoelastin protein molecules. Elastin functions to provide elasticity to bodily tissue and when stretched allows the stretched tissue to return to its original length. Elastin is found in varying degrees in most tissues of the body.

PROTEOGLYCANS

Proteoglycans provide the binding properties of tissue. They are composed of aggrecans or GAGs, which are predominantly composed of chondroitin sulfate. The structure of the proteoglycan involves a protein core surrounded by hydranate arms. This structure gives the proteoglycan a "bottlebrush" appearance. The proteoglycan is negatively charged and hydrophilic. The regulation of water in the extracellular matrix is aided by the hydrophilic properties of the proteoglycan. When compressed, proteoglycans in the matrix resist loss of water. When unloaded, proteoglycans draw water back into the matrix.

TABLE I-1-2 Role of Tissue Components

Tissue Type	Function
Collagen	Tensile strength
Proteoglycans	Provides binding properties of tissue
Inorganic components	Compressive strength in bone
Elastin	Provides for tissue elasticity
Cells	Regeneration, repair, and healing
Water	Cushion

TABLE I-1-3 **Percentage of Components**

	Collagen	Water	Proteoglycans	Other
Bone	17% type I	8%	5%	70% Ca/Ph
Tendon	22% type I	70%	1%	7%
Articular cartilage	16% type II	80%	3%	1% proteins
Ligament	21% type I	70%	1%	8%
Meniscus	21% type I	70%	1%	8% Na+
Annulus fibrosis	10% type I	80%	2%	8%
Nucleus pulposa	10% type I/II	80%	10%	6%
Nerve	Present, but amounts unknown			
Artery	Present, but amounts unknown			
Muscle	Present, but amounts unknown			

INORGANIC COMPONENTS

The role of inorganic components in most tissues of the body is dependent upon the tissue type. There are many different inorganic components in tissue and each plays a different role. The tissue in which inorganic materials play the most significant role is in bone. In bone, the inorganic materials are calcium and phosphate. The purpose of these two inorganic materials in bone is to give the tissue strength against compressive loading.

EXTRACELLULAR MATRIX

The extracellular matrix is a component of most body tissues. It is composed of collagen, proteoglycans, elastin, and inorganic material. These structures form the scaffolding or framework of tissue. It has both a solid component and a fluid component, which allow the extracellular matrix to resist both tensile and compressive loads. The solid components of the matrix, collagen and proteoglycans, act to resist tensile forces. The fluid component of the matrix, water, acts to resist compression and provide lubrication. Proteoglycans and collagen fibers work together to resist tensile loads. The electrostatic forces and hydrophilic nature of proteoglycans, when coupled with water, expand articular cartilage. Collagen fibers work to contain this expansion. The mechanical properties of the extracellular matrix of tissue, such as cartilage and the nucleus pulposa, are prime examples of how the extracellular matrix can resist tensile forces while at the same time act to resist vertical compression.

WATER

Water plays a significant role in maintaining the body's homeostasis. In certain tissues, it functions to help resist and cushion body parts from compressive loading. When coupled with the hydrophilic nature of the extracellular matrix in tissue such as articular cartilage, water is bound to the matrix and acts as a cushion.

CELLS

Cells are the living component of tissue. They function to allow regeneration, repair, and healing of bodily tissue. In most musculoskeletal tissue, cells can be divided into several major groupings:
1. Blasts—osteoblast, fibroblast, etc are responsible for tissue formation.
2. Cytes—osteocytes, fibrocytes, etc are responsible for the maintenance of tissue and response of tissue to stress.
3. Clasts—osteoclast, fibroclast, etc are responsible for resorption of tissue.

TISSUE INJURY AND TISSUE HEALING

The innate physiology of the tissue involved dictates the response of that tissue to load and to the healing process that follows. The tissues commonly injured by patients seen for orthopedic

or musculoskeletal rehabilitation include (1) muscle, (2) tendons and ligaments, (3) bone, (4) cartilage, and (5) nerve. Thus, these tissues will be addressed in the following chapter. To understand the healing process, it is necessary to understand the role of a tissue and the structure of that tissue, including the affect of the structural make-up on the ability of the tissue to function. Understanding these factors helps to outline the organization of this chapter. Each tissue type will be presented with the role of the tissue, followed by the implications of the tissue structure on the function, the general types of pathologies that occur, and the mechanism of these injuries.

SKELETAL MUSCLE

The role of skeletal muscle is to coordinate joint motion and participate in metabolic homeostasis and thermal regulation, all while withstanding forces up to 1000 kg.[109-111] Muscle injuries are often the result of high demand activities or from an insult of significant force. These types of injuries constitute 10% to 55% of all sports-related injuries.[16,38,48] The muscles at greatest risk of injury are two joint muscles (e.g., rectus femoris or gastrocnemius). From a physiological standpoint muscle is composed of contractile elements (myofibers) surrounded by three layers of connective tissue (endomysium, perimysium, and epimysium) that is attached to a tendon. Varying nervous inputs and fiber recruitment account for the difference in strength and control needed for gross versus refined movements. Muscle fibers are classified according to metabolic profile and are described as type 1 (slow oxidative), type 2a (fast oxidative/glycolytic), and type 2b (fast glycolytic). Although all muscles are mixed in fiber type, the ratio of each type varies from muscle to muscle. By and large, muscles with more type 1 fibers are used for balance and low-intensity demands whereas those with more type 2 fibers are used for higher intensity activities.

Muscle damage (strain) is characterized by disruption of fibers and impact on contractile strength. Contusions or strains account for 90% of all sports injuries.[48] In skeletal muscle the area at highest risk for injury is the myotendinous junction. Also of note is that contusion injuries are more detrimental to relaxed muscle as compared to contracted muscle.

WHAT IS THE MOLECULAR MAKEUP OF MUSCLE?

The molecular makeup of a muscle is driven by three primary factors, the need to resist tensile loading, the need to contract, and the need to heal and repair. Tensile strength is provided by integrins and the dystrophin–glycoprotein complex that function to connect myofibers to extracellular matrix.[19] Muscle contraction involves the following molecular elements:
• Actin = thin filament
• Myosin = thick filament, cross bridge formation

- Troponin/tropomyosin complex = calcium-binding regulatory molecules
- C protein = maintains thick filament
- M line proteins = centrally located disk-like protein aggregate: acts as an embedding matrix for myosin, which extends on both sides of the M line
- Titin = huge protein preserves the length of the sarcomere; holds actin and myosin in place
- Nebulin = maintains thin filaments

Healing of muscle is accomplished via satellite cells, which are undifferentiated cells capable of regeneration and muscle stem cells that are able to form into myoblasts.

HOW ARE MUSCLE INJURIES CLASSIFIED?

Injuries to muscles occur when forces exceed the muscles structural capability. Muscle injuries are graded on a three-degree system:

- Minor (first-degree strain/contusion) = tearing of a few fibers, minimal loss of strength
- Moderate (second-degree strain/contusion) = more damage to fibers with associated loss of contractile strength
- Severe (third-degree strain/contusion) = cross-sectional rupture with complete loss of contractile strength

WHAT ARE THE MOST COMMON MECHANISMS OF MUSCLE INJURY?

Muscle injuries can be classified into grouping based upon the nature of the tissue damage. The following terms are commonly utilized to define injury to muscle:

- Strain = involves excessive force leading to overstretching of muscle. This result in rupture or tissue injury near the myotendinous junction
- Contusion = usually involves compressive force or direct trauma to the muscle causing injury
- Laceration = involves disruption of muscle continuity

HOW DO MUSCLE INJURIES HEAL?

Jarvinen et al has proposed a three-phase process of healing.[54]

1. The destruction phase (acutely following injury) involves the necrosis of contractile elements, hematoma formation, and inflammation. Within a few days of the formation of the initial hematoma, fibrin and fibronectin form early linkages to provide support against contraction.[45,65-67]
2. The repair phase (after a few days to a few weeks) involves the phagocytosis of necrotic tissue, the regeneration of contractile elements via satellite cell activation, and the release of growth factors and cytokines that stimulate myofiber formatio©n and scar formation. Fibrin and fibronectin form early linkages to provide support against contraction.[45,65-67]
3. Remodeling (4 to 6 weeks) involves the reorganization of tissue integrity and functional maturation.

DOES MUSCLE TISSUE HEAL INTO ITS ORIGINAL FORM?

Very small injuries to muscle can repair with muscle tissue, but in general most muscle injuries heal with dense connective tissue or scar tissue.

HOW DO SMALL MUSCLE INJURIES HEAL?

Small muscle lesions can repair with muscle tissue. It does so through the following process. Injured fiber degenerates back from the injured area. Necrotic tissue is next removed from the area by macrophages and other phagocytic cells. Activation of reserve myoblasts (cell proliferation) is initiated and finally myoblasts fuse together to form myotubules, which become muscle.

HOW DO LARGE MUSCLE INJURIES HEAL?

Large lesions to muscle do not repair with muscle tissue; instead they heal through the formation of dense connective tissue. This tissue is known as scar tissue. Immediately following injury the body begins the following process of scar tissue formation:

1. Macrophages rid the muscle of debris and nonfunctional cells; these macrophages also secrete growth factors that will stimulate satellite cells.
2. Satellite cells and muscle stem cells differentiate into myoblasts.
3. Myoblasts fuse together to form myotubes, which then join with the original injured myofibers and form a scar.[28,46,48]
4. Within the scar, fibroblasts start to form the proteoglycans needed to form the extracellular matrix.
5. Synthesis of elastic proteins (tenascin-C and fibronectin) followed by synthesis of collagen type III and I occurs.[20,40,45,65-67]
6. Small bundles of type I collagen are imbedded in muscle.

WHAT ARE SOME OF THE COMPLICATIONS ASSOCIATED WITH MUSCLE HEALING?

1. Healing myofibers (and blood vessels) need energy to regenerate. This energy is supplied largely through aerobic metabolism; however, growing myotubes have a few mitochondria.[49]
2. The gap formed between avulsed myofibers cannot withstand the contractile force. This weakness will lasts for about 10 days until type I collagen starts to form.
3. Myotubes may not be able to extend all the way through and/or fibroblasts may proliferate excessively resulting in residual scar formation interspersed within muscle.[1,112]
4. Scar tissue formed as a result of tissue damage does not have the same properties as muscle, but continuity of tissue is maintained.
5. With increased age, fewer satellite cells are formed resulting in less tissue regeneration.[47]
6. Rerupture of a muscle leads to excessive fibroblast activity and more dense scar is formed. The formation of dense scar tissue can be potentially disabling as regenerating myotubes cannot penetrate through scar.

WHAT ARE SOME IMPORTANT FACTORS SURROUNDING IMMOBILIZATION AND THE NEED FOR EARLY MUSCLE MOBILIZATION?

Immobilization of muscle should occur for only a few days after injury. If immobilization lasts for more than a few days it can lead to the development of greater interstitial fibrosis.[48,51,65] Prolonged immobilization leads to atrophy of healthy fibers, whereas early mobilization promotes capillary regrowth, enhanced fiber regeneration, better fiber alignment, and earlier return of strength. Strengthening should be completed within the limits of pain tolerance.[49,50-53] If tissue is returned to normal use prematurely there can be an increased risk of scar formation and an increased risk for rerupture of the muscle.

WHAT CAUSES DELAYED ONSET MUSCLE SORENESS?[7,8,99,100]

Delayed onset muscle soreness (DOMS) usually occurs following a combination of high tensile force and eccentric contraction. Eccentric contraction will result in damage at the level of the skeletal muscle Z line[8,32-35,55,79] and stretch-induced damage to connective tissue sheaths surrounding muscle.[103] As a result of these contractions there is a subsequent accumulation of Ca^{2+} and degradative enzyme activation. This further results in an elevation of inflammatory molecules and ultimately nociceptor activation.

CAN DOMS LEAD TO FURTHER MUSCLE INJURY?[25]

Soreness impairs neuromuscular function, joint range of motion, strength, power, and motor control. As a result of this diminished muscle capacity the tissue is unable to absorb shock. The reduction in shock-absorbing capacity can result in structural compensation strategies that can lead to secondary injury of tissues not accustomed to performing activity.

WHAT ARE THE CLINICAL IMPLICATIONS FOR REHABILITATION?

Small injuries will repair with muscle tissue and larger injuries will fill with scar tissue. Initially, rehabilitation should focus on rest that will allow the tissue to form in either normal muscle tissue or with dense connective tissue. Initial interventions may include rest, ice, compression, and elevation of the injured area. Modalities can be utilized to reduce pain, edema, and stiffness. Rehabilitation should include immediate immobilization followed by early activity to optimize flexibility and gains in strength and to prevent the formation of adhesions. Active stretching of the muscle should be avoided for 3 to 7 days postinjury.[54] By 10 days the scar is actually stronger than the intact muscle.[56] Stretching is an important part of rehabilitation in the repair and remodeling phase, at which time the scar is still pliable. Stretching helps prevent scar adhesions. Full strength restoration takes several weeks.[51,53,57] The clinician should also target agility and trunk stabilization as opposed to working only the individual muscle.

TENDONS AND LIGAMENTS

Both tendons and ligaments are composed of dense connective tissue and, unlike muscle tissue, tendons and ligaments lack the ability to contract. Tendons and ligaments are similar in structural composition, but vary in the amount of basic components in each tissue type. Tendons have slightly more collagen than ligaments, reflecting their primary role as tensile structures. Ligaments are designed to resist tensile loads but must do so in multiple planes of motion. As a result, most ligaments are multipennated. Tendons function to transmit forces generated by muscles to bony attachment to facilitate skeletal movement. Ligaments function to provide passive guidance of bone position during normal function and give passive stability to joints. Because of its neural network it also plays a role in joint proprioception. Tendons and ligaments are also different in several other ways:

1. Ligaments are shorter and wider
2. Ligaments connect bone to bone
3. Ligaments contain smaller amounts of collagen
4. Ligaments have a higher concentration of ground substance
5. Ligaments have a broader distribution of fiber orientations.

WHAT IS THE ROLE OF A TENDON?

In general, the role of the tendon is to provide movement of a joint by transmitting force from muscle to bone. It provides a transitional tissue between contractile muscle tissue and bone.

HOW DOES THE STRUCTURE OF THE TENDON AFFECT THIS ROLE?

The molecular makeup of tendon tissue largely consists of cells (tenoblasts, tenocytes, chondrocytes), collagen (type I), elastin, water, and ground substance.[58] The combination of these components leads to the tendon's fibroelastic properties. Because of its elasticity, the tendon is able to withstand larger forces than muscle and to return to its original length when unloaded. In addition, tendons exhibit various shapes and dimensions dependent on their role in the body. Thicker and more collagen-rich tendons demonstrate increased tensile strength.[29,82,95] The collagen is generally arranged in a parallel fashion to allow the transfer of force from the muscle to the bone in the direction of muscle pull or in the direction of the aligned collagen.

WHAT IS THE ROLE OF THE LIGAMENT?

Ligaments are similar to tendons; however, their role is to provide bone-to-bone attachments and to provide joint support. The main function of ligaments is to withstand force in one or more directions, while allowing movement in particular planes of motion.

HOW DOES THE STRUCTURE OF THE LIGAMENT AFFECT THIS ROLE?

Much like tendons, ligaments are made up of cells (fibroblasts), collagen (type I, III, and V), elastin, water, and ground substance. To accommodate their function, ligaments possess greater percentages of GAGs and lower amounts of collagen than tendons.[89] Likewise, ligaments must be able to stretch and shrink in multiple directions, depending on the joint. This leads to another subtle difference between ligaments and tendons: the alignment of collagen fibers. Whereas tendons have collagen arranged in a parallel fashion, ligaments have a more disorganized collagen matrix, again allowing for multiplanar force transduction.[5]

WHAT ARE THE MECHANICAL PROPERTIES OF TENDONS AND LIGAMENTS?[61,80,83]

Tendons and ligaments are designed to resist tensile loading; as a result they must possess the mechanical strength to resist the tensile loads, yet the flexibility and elasticity to allow for deformation of the tissue. Tendons are somewhat different than ligaments in that they are designed to resist loads primarily in one direction, whereas ligaments must resist loads from multiple directions. The structure and properties of both tendons and ligaments reflect these differences.

WHAT IS THE MOLECULAR MAKEUP OF TENDONS?

Tendons are composed of the extracellular matrix that is composed of collagen (primarily type I), elastin, and ground substance. The ground substance is composed of proteoglycans, GAGs, and glycoproteins.[58] Tenoblasts, tenocytes, and chondrocytes are the cellular components of tendons. Water is the final component of tendons.

WHAT IS THE MOLECULAR MAKEUP OF LIGAMENTS?

Ligament have a makeup similar to tendons, but unlike tendons, the extracellular matrix is composed of different types and quantities of collagen. The collagen in ligaments is type I, II, and V. The cellular makeup of the tissue is also different. Fibroblasts constitute the cellular component of ligaments. Like tendons, ligaments contain elastin, ground substance, and water. These components are the same, but the amount of each is different from the tendons.

HOW ARE TENDONS AND LIGAMENTS INJURED?

Although they are thought to be relatively strong tissues, tendons and ligaments are at risk for injury stemming from acute forceful demands or from overuse. Overuse injury results from repetitive motion stress or repetitive overload on the tendon or ligament. Over time, the damage to tissue exceeds the body's ability to repair and failure or injury occurs.

WHO ARE MOST LIKELY TO HAVE THESE INJURIES?

Ligament and tendon injuries have a high prevalence in athletes and those engaging in regular or occasional exercise. Many intrinsic factors can lead to tendon and ligament dysfunction by predisposing the tissue to excessive loading during activities. These include altered biomechanics (e.g., overpronation predisposes some to Achilles tendinopathies), collagen alignment, frictional forces, excessive apoptosis, and compromised healing.

WHAT INJURIES ARE SEEN IN TENDONS AND LIGAMENTS?

Injuries seen in tendons and ligaments include ruptures. Primarily larger forceful motions create tension in the tendon or ligament. As the tensile force increases the tissue fails and the two ends of the tissue are pulled apart. The load needs to be of sufficient magnitude to overcome the structural properties of the tissue.

WHAT DOES THIS MEAN FOR ME AS A HEALTH CARE PRACTITIONER?

The ligament or tendon will be unable to protect the joint as it was designed. External protection (e.g., bracing) and/or surgery will be required (depending on the location and severity of the damage) while healing progresses.

WHAT ARE THE DEFINITIONS OF TENDON INJURIES?

Tendon pathology can be broadly grouped under the term tendinopathy, which is a blanket term used to describe tendon pathology. Tendinopathies are caused primarily by motions that occur repetitively placing load upon the tendon that leads to microtearing of tissue. With insufficient rest time between loading, the tendon is unable to heal, and the microtears enlarge and lead to progressively greater damage. Examples of such repetitive loading include forces from external sources such as biomechanical factors (e.g., overpronation causing Achilles tendinopathies), overload (e.g., tennis elbow, patella tendon), and frictional forces. Damage can also be caused by internal sources such as collagen alignment, excessive apoptosis, and compromised healing. Within this grouping of tendinopathies there are various terms utilized to further define and classify damage to the structure of the tendon:

- Strain = injury to the musculotendinous unit from abrupt contraction or stretch
- Tendinitis = pathology accompanied by inflammation
- Tendinosis = pathology associated with the extracellular matrix[71,85]

WHAT IS THE PHYSIOLOGICAL RESPONSE OF TENDONS TO REPETITIVE AND EXCESSIVE OVERLOADING?[17]

Physiologically, excessive overloading either singly or repetitively will result in the microfailure of the tendon. As a result of the damage to tissue the body will respond acutely with inflammation and/or with tissue degeneration.

WHAT IS THE PHYSIOLOGICAL MECHANISM FOR TENDON PATHOLOGY?

With tensile loading, the tendon will elongate and as the force continues to be applied strain in the tendon will increase and eventually the following sequelae will occur:

1. Strain greater than 4% leads to microscopic failure.[26]
2. Collagen fibers elongate eventually leading to gaps between adjoining molecules.
3. This results in "slippage" of the collagen molecules.[92]
4. Excess slippage leads to complete rupture and fibers recoil into a tangled bud.[9]

WHAT CAUSES TENDINOPATHY?

Tendinopathy can result from one of two processes. Shear stress or high load beyond the tissue capacity leads to ischemia. Reperfusion that occurs when stress is removed generates free radicals leading to tendon damage (which may also induce apoptosis).[9,97] Subsequently, there is a release of inflammatory molecules; this includes prostaglandins and cytokines.[104,106] The lack of oxygen leads to cell death and degeneration.[21,41]

WHAT ARE THE PROPERTIES ASSOCIATED WITH TENDINOPATHY?[96]

Tendinopathy without an inflammatory component is characterized by the lack of inflammatory molecules. In addition, tendons have a less consistent blood supply than that found in ligaments. This low level of blood supply is related to a reduced ability to heal. As the primary tissue resisting stress, the collagen fibers become damaged and general degeneration and thinning of the fibers occur. There is an increase in the number of GAGs. Finally, as the tissue is not utilized in a normal fashion due to the injury, there is a malalignment of collagen fibers. This malalignment of fibers creates abnormal cross-linking and a reduction in the available resistance to tensile forces.

WHAT ARE THE MOST COMMON MECHANISMS OF TENDON RUPTURE?[13–15,37,63,101,102]

There are three common mechanisms for tendon rupture:
1. Quick oblique eccentric contractions
2. Acceleration–deceleration motions
3. Preexisting tendon degeneration

DO TENDONS REPAIR WITH TENDON TISSUE?

Tendon do not repair with tendon tissue, they repair with dense connective scar tissue.

WHAT IS THE HEALING PROCESS FOR TENDONS?

The healing process for tendons begins with an *inflammatory phase*. This acute phase begins immediately following injury and is characterized by a release of vascular and chemical factors to promote an increase in the number of inflammatory cells and angiogenesis. There is a locally increased concentration of erythrocytes and neutrophils. Damaged and necrotic tissue is phagocytized by monocytes and macrophages[96] that are also attracted to the area. Clinically, there is often redness to visual inspection and increased temperature that can often be detected on palpation. The inflammatory phase continues for several days to several weeks.

Following the inflammatory phase is the *proliferative or reparative phase*, which begins within a few days to a few weeks. The proliferative phase is characterized by collagen (type III) synthesis along with increased water and GAG content.[36] The proliferative phase continues for up to 6 weeks.

The *remodeling* phase begins at about 6 weeks and is characterized by the induction of fibrous repair. Collagen fibers align with the direction of stress placed on the new tissue.[43] Strengthening of the tissue begins.

The final phase of tendon healing is *scar formation*, which begins at about 10 weeks and lasts for up to 1 year. This phase shows a decline of tendon metabolism and vascularity. Strengthening in the tissue continues. Normal strength may take 40 to 50 weeks to achieve.[108]

WHAT DOES THIS MEAN FOR ME AS A HEALTH CARE PRACTITIONER?

The repetitive load causing the damage must be identified and reduced or eliminated for healing to occur. Depending on the severity of the damage, external protection and/or surgery may be required for healing. Internal factors, when present, must also be considered (reduced or eliminated) for optimal healing.

HOW ARE INJURIES TO LIGAMENTS GRADED?

Sprain is ligament damage caused by an excessive range of motion or lengthening of the ligament. Ligaments can be partially torn or completely ruptured. To describe the magnitude of the damage to the ligament, a grading scale is utilized:
- Grade I = ligament is stretched, no fiber damage.
  - Test for grade I sprain: pain is experienced by the patient when tension is applied to the ligament, but no excessive range of motion is present.
- Grade II = ligament is stretched with some fibers torn, resulting in moderate joint laxity.
  - Test for grade II sprain: pain and some laxity is found on applying a tensile force to the ligament.
- Grade III = nearly complete ligament disruption, resulting in significant joint laxity.
  - Test for grade III sprain: significant joint laxity is found on applying a tensile load to the ligament.

DO LIGAMENTS REPAIR WITH LIGAMENT TISSUE?

Like muscle and tendons, most ligament injuries do not heal back with their original tissue. Instead a dense connective scar tissue patch forms in the area of damage and takes the place of the original tissue.

WHAT IS THE HEALING PROCESS FOR LIGAMENTS?

The *inflammatory phase* of ligament healing begins within 72 hours of insult with the formation of a hematoma. In addition, there is deposition of ground substance and disorganized collagen during this phase.[116]

The *regenerative phase* of ligament healing begins within a few days and lasts for up to 6 weeks. This phase is characterized by fibroblast proliferation and collagen production (type III). The new collagen together with ground substance fills in the injured areas and becomes more organized, with collagen aligning itself with the direction of force placed on the tissue. Collagen eventually switches to type I.

The *remodeling phase* begins about 6 weeks postinsult and lasts up to 1 year. This phase is characterized by remodeling of tissue and improved collagen alignment but without the same organization as the prior, healthy ligament.

DOES THE MOLECULAR MAKEUP OF THE HEALED LIGAMENT RETURN TO NORMAL?

The molecular makeup of the healed ligament does not return to the same makeup as that present premorbidly. The molecular makeup of the healed tissue reveals a decreased ratio of type I to type V collagen content and an increased amount of collagen fibrils. In addition, the healed ligament shows that the collagen fibril is reduced in diameter with a reduced number of crosslinks. Since the crosslink number and strength are related to the tensile strength of the ligament, this change in molecular makeup may indicate a reduction in the overall tensile strength of the newly healed ligament. In contrast, however, the total thickness of the healed ligament is increased.

WHAT ARE THE TREATMENT OPTIONS FOR LIGAMENT DAMAGE?[116]

Treatment options will be dependent upon the access of the ligament to vascular supply. Intraarticular ligaments, such as the anterior cruciate ligament, have limited access to blood sources, therefore their healing potential is poor. Surgery is often considered for this type of injury. Extraarticular ligaments, such as the tibial collateral ligament, have good access to blood supplies, therefore conservative care for collateral ligaments is generally considered to have similar results to surgical intervention. In comparison, for cruciate ligaments, with a significant amount of laxity present in the joint, surgical repair is recommended.

DO MEDICATIONS HELP WITH TENDON AND LIGAMENT HEALING?

There is conflicting evidence on the influence of nonsteroidal antiinflammatory drugs (NSAIDs) (only *in vitro* studies) on healing in tendons and ligaments. In rabbits, indomethacin and naproxen both slow cell proliferation and GAG synthesis,[39] but indomethacin used for 16 weeks shows healing improvement evidenced by increased tensile strength, but no effect on collagen synthesis.[31] Ibuprofen decreased the rupture strength of repaired tendons in a primate model.[88]

HOW CAN WE IMPROVE TENDON AND LIGAMENT TENSILE STRENGTH?

Training improves tensile strength by inducing an increase in both total collagen network and collagen thickness. In addition, stressing the tissue during the proliferative and remodeling phases leads to a more organized collagen network and improved tissue strength.[44] Furthermore, controlled stretching after the inflammatory phase increases collagen synthesis.[60] Finally, repetitive motion increases DNA and protein synthesis as well as cellular proliferation.[3,118]

WHAT ARE THE BIOPHYSIOLOGICAL LIGAMENT HEALING STRATEGIES?[116]

With advances in technology related to health care, there are some new biophysiological strategies for ligament healing. These strategies include gene transfer, collagen scaffolds, use of growth factors, and mesenchymal stem cell implantation.

WHAT FACTORS MAKE TENDONS AND LIGAMENTS RESISTANT TO HEALING?

In general, tendons and ligaments have a low metabolic rate.[115] In addition, there is a lack of vascularity, especially in tendons with sheaths. Although tendons without sheaths have greater vascularity, the blood supply is not consistent throughout the tissue.[10] Age has a greater impact on ligaments than tendons. Ligament strength begins to weaken at middle age. Ligaments become less viscous, have more crosslinks, and become stiffer. In tendons, there is no significant loss of strength with age. The endocrine system impacts the healing rate of tendons and ligaments as stress results in increased glucocorticoid, which diminishes connective tissue strength via decreased crosslinks and decreased collagen turnover. Chronic compression results in less mature crosslinks, decreased collagen, and decreased blood flow. Poor nutrition can affect healing as vitamin A, vitamin C, copper, and iron are important in collagen synthesis and crosslink formation.

WHAT COMPLICATIONS CAN OCCUR AS A RESULT OF TENDON AND LIGAMENT HEALING?

When rehabilitating a patient, the clinician must be wary of the formation of adhesions for these can limit joint range of motion. Following injury, it is not unusual for the region affected to have altered biomechanical function and therefore the region becomes less resistant to force.

WHAT ARE THE CLINICAL IMPLICATIONS FOR REHABILITATION?

During the rehabilitation process the clinician should allow the knowledge of normal tissue physiology and normal tissue healing to guide the progression of the patient. In general, palliative treatment should be utilized during the inflammatory phase. The clinician should avoid prolonged periods of immobilization as this can lead to the formation of adhesions and ultimately altered tissue mechanics. During the proliferative phase, treatment should focus upon correcting altered biomechanics and compensatory posture and restoring proper tissue gliding and collagen synthesis through the use of early passive movement. Treatment should also focus on improving tensile properties of the tissue through stretching and **controlled** repetitive strengthening exercises. It is important to note that following ligament injuries, despite the type of repair, joint instability increased over time and joint kinematics were ultimately altered.

BONE

Lamellar bone (compact and spongy) makes up most of the adult skeleton. This type of bone is characterized by a calcified matrix containing protein and collagen fibers and vascular spaces throughout. Turnover of bone (remodeling) is a result of the balance between bone formation and resorption and continues through life. Osteoblasts are responsible for bone formation, whereas osteoclasts participate in bone resorption. The activity of each of these cells is controlled by hormonal signals and mechanical strain; if either of these is disrupted bone formation and/or resorption is abnormal.

Bone pathology can arise from trauma, aging, and metabolic abnormalities. The healing process incorporates the actions of bone cortex and marrow, periosteum, and the surrounding vasculature and soft tissues. Here we describe fracture healing from a physiological perspective and offer considerations for physical therapists. Fractures can be caused by direct impact and overuse injuries or arise secondary to underlying pathology (e.g., cancer, osteoporosis). The severity of the fracture (e.g., displaced vs. non-displaced and open vs. closed) will determine the rate of healing and return of function.

HOW ARE FRACTURES CLASSIFIED?

There are multiple methods of classifying bone fractures. One of the more commonly utilized methods is as follows:
1. Complete—the fracture extends through the entire bone.
2. Incomplete (i.e., Greenstick, Torus, or Buckle)—the fracture does not continue through the entire bone.
3. Comminuted—the bone breaks into more than two pieces.
4. Segmental—a piece of bone is floating between two broken segments.

HOW DO FRACTURES HEAL?

Fractures can heal through either direct or indirect healing processes. Direct or primary fracture healing very rarely occurs. For direct fracture healing to occur bone fragments need to be in very close proximity to each other and the pieces need to be completely stable and encounter only minimal strain. In direct fracture healing, cortical bone reestablishes the continuity of the bone by forming a cutting cone.[75] Osteoprogenitor cells in turn transform directly into osteoblasts. As a result, no callus is formed. Indirect or secondary fracture healing is the much more common type of healing process. It involves intramembranous and endochondral ossification to reestablish bone continuity.

WHAT IS ENDOCHONDRAL OSSIFICATION?

Endochondral ossification is the process by which a cartilaginous model is formed before its calcification into bone. This cartilaginous model will eventually mineralize to create the final bone.

WHAT IS INTRAMEMBRANOUS OSSIFICATION?

In intramembranous ossification, no cartilaginous model is created. Bone is formed directly at the fracture site.

WHAT OCCURS AT THE FRACTURE SITE DURING INDIRECT HEALING?

1. Immediately following injury to the bone macrophages enter the area and phagocytize necrotic material.
2. Mesenchymal cells (some from bone marrow) are then transported and activated at the injury site and differentiate into osteoblasts.
3. Growth factors, cytokines, and signaling molecules are released from the hematoma, macrophages, mesenchymal cells, and osteoblasts.
4. An extracellular scaffold is formed to promote cellular activity and interaction.
5. Angiogenesis is initiated.
6. Mesenchymal cells develop into osteoblasts, which begin making osteoid and granulation tissue.
7. Osteoids are configured into a woven bone pattern.
8. Hard and soft callus are formed.
   a. *Hard callus*: occurs in the underlying cortical bone, periosteum, and bone marrow. It is formed through intramembranous ossification of mesenchymal cells and osteoprogenitor cells. These cells are located in the periosteum.
   b. *Soft callus*: occurs in the periosteum and external soft tissues. Mesenchymal cells differentiate into cartilage and eventually ossify to form bone. The primary role is to serve as a quick and temporary bridge to stabilize bone fragments.[70]
9. The fractured bone will remodel over the next few months by replacing the woven (weak, disorganized) bone with compact, organized lamellar bone.

WHAT IS THE TIMEFRAME FOR FRACTURE HEALING?

1. Initial (6 to 12 hours): Bleeding ceases and a clot is formed.
2. Day 1 to 2: There is an acute inflammatory reaction and granulation tissue is formed.
3. Weeks 1 to 3: Osteogenesis, fibrous union, and callus formation occur.
4. Six weeks: There is continuity of the external callus.
5. Four months to 1 year: There is remodeling of the medullary canal and organized lamellar bone.

WHY ARE PATIENTS IMMOBILIZED AFTER A FRACTURE?

Fractured bone ends need to be in close apposition and the fracture needs to be immobilized. If this does not occur, bone healing will be delayed.[11] Surgery is performed when the bones are displaced. Fixation of the bony fragments helps to bring the bone in close proximity to its adjoining fragments. It also functions to limit bone motion. Both surgery and casting are utilized to speed up the healing process.

WHAT FACTORS HINDER PROPER FRACTURE HEALING?

1. Inadequate blood supply
2. Poor general nutritional status
3. Poor apposition of the fractured bone ends
4. Presence of foreign bodies, infection, or necrotic tissue
5. Corticosteroid therapy

WHAT GROWTH FACTORS SHOULD BE PRESENT AT THE FRACTURE SITE?

Growth factors (bone morphogenetic protein, transforming growth factor-beta, fibroblast growth factor, platelet-derived growth factor, and insulin-like growth factor) are proteins secreted by cells that act on the appropriate target cells to carry out a specific action[6]. In bone they can stimulate and enhance bone formation.

WHAT CAN BE DONE SURGICALLY TO AID HEALING?

1. Fixators or metal places can be applied to the bone to bring healing bone ends into closer approximation.
2. Biomaterials can be used to make scaffolds.
3. Allograft of trabecular bone to the site of fracture.
4. Bone void fillers such as calcium based ceramics can be utilized.[12,74,91,105]

WHAT FACTORS IMPACT BONE REMODELING?

Bone remodeling refers to the adaptation of bone in response to tissue stress. Wolff's law states that bone will alter its properties based on external stress placed on bone.[18]

Hormonal and cellular signals, low serum calcium levels, skeletal microdamage, age, and the amount of osteoprogenitor cells are all factors.[84] Weight-bearing exercise can contribute to morphological development.

WHAT CONDITIONS OR FACTORS CAN ACCELERATE THE HEALING RATE?[75,87]

The availability of growth factors, hormones, nutrients, proper pH levels, oxygen tension, the electrical environment, a stable fracture site, and micromotion of the bone can all enhance the healing process.

WHAT TYPES OF ABNORMAL FRACTURE HEALING CAN OCCUR?

1. Malunion
2. Nonunion
3. Delayed union
4. Pseudoarthrosis

WHAT ARE THE IMPLICATIONS FOR REHABILITATION?

Proper treatment of fractures requires a firm knowledge of when the fracture occurred. Initially, fractures will be immobilized until evidence of callus formation is present on x-ray. Once the immobilization is removed, treatment of the edema, pain, and range of motion deficits associated with fractures and bone pathologies are important aspects of bone healing. The clinician should employ controlled weight-bearing exercise during early stages to allow for deposition of cartilage callus and to prevent the formation of deep vein thrombosis. Weight-bearing status should be increased as pain and symptoms allow. Often during immobilization range of motion and joint mobility are lost. The clinician should take care to restore normal joint mobility and attempt to restore normal joint mechanics. Strengthening may commence and be advanced according to the patient's tolerance for pain and the presence of other factors that indicate healing is continuing (e.g., absence of swelling). If fractures are the result of repetitive loading, the bone should be unloaded through immobilization or activity modification to allow for proper healing.

CARTILAGE

The primary role of articular cartilage is to allow for joint movement while redistributing force imposed on the joint. Hyaline cartilage has an incredible load-bearing potential with essentially frictionless properties. The main role of fibrocartilage is to resist compressive force as evidenced by its high collagen content. Because cartilage consists of a solid and fluid phase, the interaction of these layers allows it to exhibit viscoelastic properties. Unlike other tissues that have nutrients supplied by the circulation, cartilage receives nutrients via diffusion provided by compressive joint movement. Cartilage damage can result in pain, loss of movement, and alterations of joint kinematics. Damage to this tissue is often the result of trauma or degeneration from abnormal biomechanics. The lack of vasculature supplying cartilage greatly impedes its regeneration capabilities. Understanding the structure, function, and regeneration capabilities of cartilage can shed light on the pathophysiology of osteoarthritis. In addition, investigation of the basic science of cartilage formation may aid in the development of appropriate rehabilitation programs.

WHAT ARE THE DIFFERENT TYPES OF CARTILAGE?

1. Fibrocartilage is located in intervertebral discs, temporomandibular joint, menisci of knee, and temporarily exists at fracture sites
2. Elastic cartilage is located in eustachian tube of the ears and the epiglottis
3. Hyaline cartilage is located in joint surfaces and in the growth plates of long bones

HOW IS CARTILAGE ORGANIZED?

Cartilage is organized into four zones:
1. *The Superficial Tangential Zone* receives shear stress and serves to protect deeper layers of chondrocytes. It contains relatively small quantities of proteoglycan and large quantities of collagen arranged in a parallel fashion. The secretion of lubricin acts to decrease friction in joints.
2. *The Middle Zone* functions to provide the primary resistance of cartilage to compressive loading. It contains the highest level of proteoglycan among the four zones and a random arrangement of collagen fibers.
3. *The Deep Zone* contains collagen fibrils that are arranged perpendicular to the underlying bone. It also has columns of chondrocytes arrayed along the axis of fibril orientation.
4. *The Calcified Cartilage Zone* is partly mineralized and acts as the transitional zone between cartilage and the underlying subchondral bone.

WHAT ARE THE MOLECULAR COMPONENTS OF HYALINE CARTILAGE?

Unlike most other tissue, cartilage is composed of primary type II collagen instead of type I. Its extracellular matrix combines collagen, proteoglycans, hyaluronic acid, and aggrecan, which all combine to bind and contain water within the structure of the cartilage. When healthy, cartilage is composed of approximately 70% to 80% water. Chondrocytes are present to maintain the structure of cartilage.

WHAT ARE THE MOLECULAR COMPONENTS OF FIBROCARTILAGE?

Fibrocartilage is different from hyaline cartilage. Instead of type II collagen, it is composed of type I collagen, which reflects the tissues need to resist tensile loading. The proteoglycans of the extracellular matrix work to bind water while the collagen in the matrix works to resist the tensile loading. Fibrocartilage is comprised of 60% to 70% water.

WHAT ARE THE CAUSES OF CARTILAGE INJURY?

1. Trauma
2. Limb malalignment
3. Altered biomechanics
4. Ligamentous instability
5. Meniscus deficiency

HOW ARE CARTILAGE INJURIES CLASSIFIED?

According to the International Cartilage Repair Society cartilage can be graded as follows:[22]
- Grade 0—Normal
- Grade 1—Nearly normal: Superficial lesions, soft indentations, and/or fissures and cracks
- Grade 2—Abnormal: lesions extending <50% of the cartilage depth
- Grade 3—Severely abnormal: lesions extending >50% of the cartilage depth
- Grade 4—Severely abnormal: lesions extending down into the subchondral bone; full thickness injury

WHAT ARE SOME UNIQUE ASPECT OF CARTILAGE AND CARTILAGE HEALING?[76]

1. Most cartilage damage cannot heal into its original tissue. Cartilage is ineffective at healing and has a very low potential of regeneration.
2. Cartilage is aneural, avascular, and devoid of immune system recognition. Therefore, it is incapable of generating pain, does not heal well, and will not cause an immune system response.
3. Most injuries heal because of the formation of fibrous cartilage tissue or fibrocartilage. The fibrocartilage is not anything like the original hyaline cartilage.
4. Synovial membrane damage results in an increased number of cells and thickening of the cartilage; this in turn can alter the function of cartilage.

WHAT EVENTS OCCUR WITH A PARTIAL THICKNESS CARTILAGE INJURY?

The following changes occur when mechanical stress is the cause of the cartilage damage:[59,68]

1. Chondrocyte hypertrophy and apoptosis
2. Increased cartilage water content
3. Collagen becomes disorganized
4. Increased osteophyte production
5. Increased chondral ossification
6. Secretion of degradative enzymes that further damaging the articular surface

WHAT EVENTS OCCUR WITH A FULL THICKNESS CARTILAGE INJURY?

The following changes occur when mechanical stress is the cause of the cartilage damage:[68]

1. Subchondral bleeding
2. Hematoma formation
3. Bone marrow mesenchymal cells infiltrates into the damaged area
4. Type I collagen is formed (fibrocartilage)

WHAT CHANGES OCCUR WITH DEGENERATION OR DETERIORATION OF CARTILAGE?[113,114]

Many changes occur in the body with cartilage degeneration. These changes can occur grossly at the tissue level or microscopically at the cellular level (Box I-1-1).

HOW DOES CARTILAGE DEGENERATION OCCUR?

1. Repetitive loading of the cartilage causes microfractures of subchondral bone.
2. This results in increased ossification in response to the microfractures.
3. The thickening of the subchondral bone in turn decreases the overlying cartilage thickness.
4. The reduced thickness of the cartilage increases the shear forces per unit of cartilage.
5. The increased forces cause splitting of the cartilage or fibrillations to occur.
6. Proteoglycans are lost as a result of the fibrillations and chemical factors are released into the synovial fluid.
7. There is a subsequent increase in the release of cartilage degrading substances by synovium that further degrades the surface of the surface cartilage.
8. This results in a loss of lubrication and surface integrity.

WHAT FACTORS CAN IMPACT THE HEALING POTENTIAL OF CARTILAGE?

1. Age—chondrocyte numbers are significantly reduced with age.
2. Immobilization—motion and loading are needed for cartilage integrity.

BOX I-1-1 **Gross and Microscopic Changes in Articular Cartilage**	
Gross Changes	**Microscopic Changes**
Fibrillation of the surface	Increased water content
Fraying/splitting of the surface	Decreased proteoglycans
	Increased tidemarks
Color change from transparent blue to opaque yellow	Degradation of collagen (unwinding of the triple helix)
Decreased ability to withstand forces	Increased collagen cross-bridging
	Increased calcification
Osteophyte formations in subchondral bone	Hypertrophy and clustering of chondrocytes
Decreased blood supply	Subchondral bone sclerosis

---

3. Depth of injury—superficial injuries have a decreased potential of healing.

HOW DOES IMMOBILIZATION AFFECT CARTILAGE INTEGRITY?

Prolonged immobilization or rigid fixation of a joint has been shown to result in decreased amounts of GAGs, uronic acid, proteoglycans, and cartilage thickness.[23] Decreased weight bearing can lead to a loss of cartilage.[23]

WHAT METHODS ARE AVAILABLE TO RESTORE OR REGENERATE CARTILAGE?[81]

There are many methods available to restore cartilage. In reality, the restoration potential is limited due to the body's poor capacity to repair any damage to articular or hyaline cartilage. Surgically, lavage and debridement can clean out debris and irritants within the joint space. Subchondral drilling, abrasion, and microfracture surgery can be performed in hopes of stimulating the formation of fibrocartilage in the damaged region. Stem cells can be implanted within the damaged area with the hope that they will differentiate into cartilage tissue. Cartilage can be removed from the body and grown in laboratory setting and then reimplanted into the body on scaffolds. Growth factors and hyaluronic acid can be injected into the site of damage in hopes of stimulating cartilage growth or cartilage repair. Other methods of surgery include cell transplant (chondrocytes/chondrocyte precursor), an osteochondral graft, and periosteal/perichondral arthroplasty. Clinically, continuous passive movement, electrical stimulation, ultrasound, and lasers all are commonly utilized to treat patients with cartilage injury. Unfortunately, none of the above treatment methods are universally successful at restoring cartilage integrity. Restoring joint biomechanics and controlled loading, short of cartilage damage, should be paramount for rehabilitation of cartilage lesions.

WHAT IS THE ROLE OF NONSTEROIDAL ANTIINFLAMMATORY DRUGS IN THE MANAGEMENT OF CARTILAGE INJURIES?

Physiologically, NSAIDs block the effects of an enzyme called cyclooxygenase, which is critical in the body's production of prostaglandins. Prostaglandins increase cell permeability and inflammation in response to injury. Therefore by interfering with cyclooxygenase, there is a decrease in the production of prostaglandins and a decrease in the pain and swelling associated with these conditions. Prostaglandins aid in anabolic growth of chondrocytes; therefore NSAIDs are not recommended for those with chondrocyte grafts.[4]

WHAT IS THE EFFICACY OF CHONDROITIN SULFATE SUPPLEMENTATION?

Meta-analysis indicates that supplementation has a slight to moderate efficacy in the symptom relief of osteoarthritis.[77]

WHAT ARE THE CLINICAL IMPLICATIONS FOR REHABILITATION?

The focus of rehabilitation should be on restoring normal joint mobility, decreasing inflammation and pain, and removing the factors that contribute to the damage of cartilage tissue such as malalignment and biomechanical abnormalities. Arthritic joints require and respond well to motion and respond poorly to excessive weight-bearing activities.[62] Continuous passive motion machines (CPM) have been shown to improve healing, while immobilization has been shown to have no impact on healing.[90]

NERVE

Peripheral nerve injury primarily alters conduction resulting in motor and/or sensory loss. Ordinarily sensory deficits precede motor loss. Nerve injuries can vary in intensity from demyelination to complete axonal disruption. Although peripheral nerves have the capability to regenerate, the process depends on several factors including severity and conditions of the injury. Axons have inherent plasticity when the proper growth factors and connective tissue are present to provide axonal guidance. Likewise, axons also possess programs for degeneration when injured or not needed.

Return to normal conduction velocity differs with the extent of the injury. Compression and entrapment injuries may return to normal conduction in a few days to weeks, whereas axonal disruption may take months or years. Severe and/or long-term nerve damage can result in skeletal muscle atrophy and weakness and potential loss of excitability.

WHAT IS THE FUNCTION OF NERVES?

Neurons are highly specialized cells designed for the processing and transmission of electrical and chemical signals. The function of the axon of the nerve is to transmit information from the brain to the periphery and from the periphery to the brain. But also, the axon of the nerve functions to transmit nutrients and chemicals down its lumen.

WHAT IS THE ANATOMY OF A NERVE?

Nerves take on many shapes and sizes depending on the function and demands placed on them. All nerves have several basic elements. The soma is the central part of the neuron. It contains the nucleus of the cell. The dendrites of a neuron are the linear extensions of a nerve that receive information from the periphery for transmission and processing at the soma. The axon is a linear extension from the soma, but unlike the dendrite that transmits information to the soma for processing, the axon transmits information away from the soma after processing has occurred. The axon terminal contains the synapses of the nerve where electrical impulses are relayed to adjoining structures.

WHAT ARE NEURIUMS?

Neuriums provide a framework for support of the nerve; they facilitate sliding of the nerve and provide a protective barrier.

WHAT IS AXOPLASM?

The axon is filled with axoplasm. Axoplasm is necessary for nerve healing; when it is disrupted, the nerve will die. Axoplasm is a viscous substance composed primarily of cytoplasm. It is thixotrophic in nature meaning it needs constant agitation or motion or it will gel.

DO NERVES HAVE A LYMPHATIC SYSTEM?

The area surrounding nerves are drained by the body's lymphatic system. The nerve has a blood and nerve barrier that prevents foreign substances from invading the nerve. The amount of drainage is highly dependent upon the region of injury. Inside the blood–nerve barrier there is no lymphatic system. The consequence of this is that if nerves are damaged irritants and inflammation can be allowed within the structure of the nerve. With no lymphatic system, drainage within the nerve can take a long time. The standing edema can result in long-standing pain and it can interfere with endoneural capillary flow. The decreased capillary flow causes hypoxia, electrolyte imbalance, and fibroblast invasion.

CAN NERVE CELLS HEAL?

Mast cells exist in the epineurium, therefore there is a potential for nerve repair. Conversely, mast cells release inflammatory mediators (histamines) that can increase edema in and around the nerve. Neurons are incapable of dividing and migrating, therefore regeneration occurs only through existing neurons.

DO NERVES HAVE A NERVE SUPPLY?

Neural connective tissue is self-innervated by the nervi nervorum. Therefore, nerves themselves can be sources of pain. The vasculature of the nerve is sympathetically regulated.

ARE THERE ANATOMICAL DIFFERENCE THAT MAKE CERTAIN AREAS OF THE NERVE MORE SUSCEPTIBLE TO NERVE INJURY?

Nerves can be trapped at the spinal level by the disc, osteophytes, and stenotic changes.

Entrapment at the nerve root differs from along the nerve in that nerve roots do not have an epineurium. Because they lack an epineurium nerves are more susceptible to injury at the nerve root. Irritation of the nerve roots will result in pain along the length of the nerve or in certain sections of the nerve. With nerve damage, areas of the nerve can be hypersensitive and spontaneously give off impulse along the length of the nerve. These areas of increased sensitivity are called ectopic neural pacemakers (ENP).

WHAT IS RADICULAR PAIN?

Radicular pain refers to pain that originates from damage or irritation at the nerve root. At times the pain can be distributed in a dermatomal pattern, although these dermatomal patterns of nerve root involvement are highly variable, changing from person to person. Double crush or multiple crush may also occur. In double crush syndromes, when one area of a nerve is injured, it leaves the other areas more vulnerable to smaller insults resulting in two or more sites of damage along the nerve.

WHAT IS REFERRED PAIN?

Certain tissues of the body originate from similar embryotic tissue. This is the result of embryotic development. Visceral tissue and limb tissue often originate from the same embryotic tissue; as a result when patients have pain in the visceral organ, they also feel pain in the limb. Visceral afferents also converge at the spinal cord with afferents from other parts of the body. The result of this convergence is referred pain. Heart dysfunction is a common example. When individuals have a heart attack, they often feel pain in the arm.

HOW CAN NERVES BE INJURED?

Nerves can be injured directly or indirectly. Directly, excessive compression or tension can result in nerve damage. Sustained compression can cause injury. Irreversible injury to the nerve can be expected after 8 hours of continuous compression. Tension or elongation of the nerve can also cause nerve damage. A 20% to 30% increase in length will cause the nerve to break. As the nerve stretches, the perineurium tightens, intraneural pressure increases, and intrafascicular capillaries stop flowing. This occurs at 8% elongation.

Nerves do not like to be stretched. Indirectly, chemicals, temperature, hormones, and poor circulation can lead to nerve damage. Crush injuries, nerve avulsion or transection, compression, excessive stretch, and ischemia can all result in long- or short-term damage to a nerve.

WHAT IS THE SEDDON INJURY CLASSIFICATION SYSTEM FOR NERVE INJURY?[94]

Neurapraxia = with neurapraxia: the myelin is usually damaged from compression. The axonal flow through the nerve is temporary disrupted, but the axon and the axon sheath remain intact so there is no distal degeneration. Once the compressive load is removed, nerve function returns.

Axonotmesis = with axonotmesis: the axon of the nerve is disrupted but the connective tissue sheath is spared. Although the conduction of the nerve is disrupted, the maintenance of the sheath allows for quicker nerve regrowth.

Neurotmesis = neurotmesis involves the complete disruption of the nerve. Recovery and regrowth are much slower as there is no sheath to provide nutrients or to act as a guide for the nerve to regrow.

WHAT IS THE SUNDERLAND INJURY CLASSIFICATION SYSTEM FOR NERVE INJURY?[107]

Type 1: There is myelin damage from compression.

Type 2: The axon is disrupted, but the nervous connective tissue (epineurium, perineurium, and endoneurium) is spared.

Type 3: The axon and endoneurium are disrupted; the epineurium and perineurium remain intact.

Type 4: The axon, endoneurium, and perineurium are disrupted; the epineurium remains intact.

Type 5: There is complete disruption of the nerve.

WHAT IS WALLERIAN DEGENERATION?

Wallerian degeneration occurs as a result of injury to the nerve. It involves the degeneration of the nerve distal to the site of injury. After injury, the distal segment of the nerve loses its nutrient flow because the lumen of the nerve not only conducts electrical impulse but is an important route for nutrient transport. Following injury, degeneration commences at the damaged area and continues sequentially to the neighboring nodes of Ranvier. Subsequently, macrophages act to clear necrotic and unwanted material as the nerve tissue dies.

WHAT IS THE HEALING SEQUENCE OF EVENTS AFTER AXON DISRUPTION?[64]

1. Neuronal cell bodies increase the production of growth-associated proteins.
2. The injured area undergoes Wallerian degeneration and all tissue dies where nutrients are not present. Wallerian degeneration of distal axons occurs 2 to 4 days postinjury.
3. Schwann cells and macrophages are recruited to the site of injury to remove unwanted materials. At about 8 days, Schwann cells align (Bungner bands) to form a support system for regenerating nerve (growth cone).[2,30]
4. Neurotrophic, neurite-promoting, and extracellular matrix factors are secreted (Ca^{2+} and cAMP-dependent process) into the region of injury.[72,78,86] As a result, new axonal sprouts are formed and the nerve begins the regeneration process.
5. Endoneurium compromised interstitial fibrosis often occurs and prevents the growth of the nerve. If this happens the potential for full functional recovery diminishes.[64]

WHAT GROWTH FACTORS ARE IMPORTANT FOR NERVE HEALING AND REGENERATION?

Nerve growth factors are small secreted proteins that induce cell differentiation. They are important for the survival of nerve cells. The following is a list of common nerve growth factors:

1. Nerve growth factor
2. Ciliary neurotrophic factor[73]
3. Motor nerve growth factor[98]
4. Neurotrophin 3[117,119,120]
5. Brain-derived neurotrophic factor[117,119,120]

WHAT ARE THE IMPORTANT NEURITE-PROMOTING FACTORS INVOLVED IN NERVE HEALING AND REGENERATION?

A neurite can refers to any immature or developing projection from the cell body of a neuron. It can refer to either an axon or a dendrite. The following factors help promote the formation and growth of neuritis:

1. Laminin[24]
2. Fibronectin[42]
3. Neural cell adhesion molecule[27]
4. N-cadherin[27]

HOW QUICKLY DOES NERVE REGENERATE?

Nerve growth is dependent upon several factors including the health of the tissue, the state of the nerve and nerve sheath, and the region of the injury, but on average nerves regenerate at a rate of 1 to 3 mm per day. If nervous connective tissue (endoneurium) remains intact axons are more likely to regenerate to full function due to guidance provided by the endoneurium. All neurotmesis injuries require surgery if there is any hope of complete recovery.

HOW DOES REGENERATION DIFFER IN PERIPHERAL AND CENTRAL NERVOUS SYSTEMS?

In many ways, regeneration of nerves in the peripheral and central nervous system is similar, although there are several points in which they are different. There are no astrocyte scars formed after injury in the peripheral nervous system; however, they do develop in injuries to the central nervous system. In the peripheral nervous system, Schwann cells work to remove debris and regenerate nerve myelin. In the central nervous system, this task is the responsibility of oligodendrocytes.[93] There are no myelin inhibitory molecules (Nogo-A) in the peripheral nervous system and expression of laminin is present in the peripheral nervous system only following injury.[69]

WHAT ARE THE IMPLICATIONS FOR REHABILITATION?

Rehabilitation of nerves following nerve injury involves a wait and see attitude. The clinician's responsibility is to help provide a favorable environment for the nerves to grow. Initially, rehabilitation involves the reduction of inflammation, the protection of the injured area, and the promotion of circulation and blood flow to the injured area. Nerves will degenerate and then regrow. During this process the clinician should promote the maintenance of range of motion. Once signs that regrowth have progressed to the target muscle, the clinician can initiate motor and sensory reeducation programs. It has been suggested that direct current electrical stimulation can improve the functional recovery of muscle following nerve injury, but currently research results are variable.

SUMMARY

Proper rehabilitation of musculoskeletal and orthopedic injuries requires a sound understanding of the physiological mechanisms behind the injury. Knowledge of what tissues are injured, expected time frames of healing, factors that can influence tissue regeneration, and conversely factors that inhibit tissue healing should aid clinicians as they attempt to develop rehabilitation programs. All tissues heal at different rates and respond to different stimulus, therefore no two rehabilitation programs should be identical. Knowledge of the physiology of injury and healing is the foundation for patient rehabilitation.

REFERENCES

1. Aarimaa V, Kaariainen M, Vaittinen S, et al. Restoration of myofiber continuity after transaction injury in the rat soleus. *Neuromuscul Disord*. 2004;14:421-428.
2. Akassoglou K, Yu WM, Akpinar P, Strickland S. Fibrin inhibits peripheral nerve remyelination by regulating Schwann cell differentiation. *Neuron*. 2002;33:861-875.
3. Almekinders LC, Baynes AJ, Bracey LW. An in vitro investigation into the effects of repetitive motion and nonsteroidal anti-inflammatory medication on human tendon fibroblasts. *Am J Sports Med*. 1995;23:119-123.
4. Amin AR, Dave M, Attur M, et al. Cox-2, NO and cartilage damage and repair. *Curr Rheumatol Rep*. 2000;2(6):447-453.
5. Amis AA. Biomechanics of bone, tendon and ligament. In: Hughes SPF, McCarthy ID, eds. *Sciences Basic to Orthopaedics*. Philadelphia, PA: WB Saunders Company; 1998:221-223.
6. Andrew JG, Hoyland JA, Freemont AJ. Platelet-derived growth factor expression in normally healing human fractures. *Bone*. 1995;16:455-460.
7. Armstrong RB. Initial events in exercise-induced muscular injury. *Med Sci Sports Exerc*. 1990;22:429-435.
8. Armstrong RB. Mechanisms of exercise-induced delayed onset of muscular soreness: a brief review. *Med Sci Sports Exerc*. 1984; 16:529-538.

9. Arnoczky SP, Tian T, Lavagnino M, Gardner K, Schuller P, Morse P. Activation of stress-activated protein kinases (SAPK) in tendon cells following cyclic strain: the effects of strain frequency, strain magnitude, and cytosolic calcium. *J Orthop Res*. 2002;20:947-952.

10. Astrom M. Laser Doppler flowmetry in the assessment of tendon blood flow. *Scand J Med Sci Sports*. 2000;10:365-367.

11. Augat P, Margevicius K, Simon J, et al. Local tissue properties in bone healing: influence of size and stability of the osteotomy gap. *J Orthop Res*. 1998;16:475-481.

12. Babis GC, Soucacos PN. Bone scaffolds: the role of mechanical stability and instrumentation. *Injury*. 2005;36(suppl 4):S38-S44.

13. Barnfred T. Experimental rupture of the Achilles tendon. Comparison of various types of experimental rupture in rats. *Acta Orthop Scand*. 1971;42:528-543.

14. Barnfred T. Experimental rupture of the Achilles tendon. Comparison of various types of experimental rupture in rats of different ages and living under different conditions. *Acta Orthop Scand*. 1971;42:406-428.

15. Barnfred T. Kinesiological comments on subcutaneous ruptures of the Achilles tendon. *Acta Orthop Scand*. 1971;42:397-405.

16. Beiner JM, Joki P. Muscle contusion injuries: current treatment options. *J Am Acad Orthop Surg*. 2001;9:227-237.

17. Benazzo F, Maffulli N. An operative approach to Achilles tendinopathy. *Sports Med Arthroscopy Rev*. 2000;8:96-101.

18. Bertram JEA, Swartz SM. The law of bone transformation: a case of crying Wolff?. *Biol Rev*. 1991;66:245-273.

19. Best TM, Garrett WE. Basic science of soft tissue: muscle and tendon. In: DeLee JC, Drez D Jr, eds. *Orthopaedic Sports Medicine: Principles and Practice*. Philadelphia, PA: WB Saunders; 1994:1.

20. Best TM, Shehadeh SE, Leverson G, Michel JT, Corr DT, Aeschlimann D. Analysis of changes in RNA levels of myoblast and fibroblast-derived gene products in healing skeletal muscle using quantitative reverse transcription-polymerase chain reaction. *J Orthop Res*. 2001;19:565-572.

21. Bestwick CS, Maffulli N. Reactive oxygen species and tendon problems: review and hypothesis. *Sports Med Arthroscopy Rev*. 2000;8:6-16.

22. Brittberg M, Winalski CS. Evaluation of cartilage injuries and repair. *J Bone Joint Surg Am*. 2003;85(2):58-69.

23. Burr DB, Frederickson RG, Pavlinch C, Sickles M, Burkhart S. Intracast muscle stimulation prevents bone and cartilage deterioration in cast-immobilized rabbits. *Clin Orthop*. 1984;19:183-184.

24. Chen ZL, Yu WM, Stickland S. Peripheral regeneration. *Annu Rev Neurosci*. 2007;30:2009-2033.

25. Cheung K, Hume PA, Maxwell L. Delayed onset muscle soreness. Treatment strategies and performance factors. *Sports Med*. 2003.

26. Curwin S, Stanish WD. *Tendinitis; its etiology and treatment*. Lexington, MA: Collamore Press; 1984.

27. Dodd J, Jessel TM. Axonal guidance and the patterning of neuronal projections in vertebrates. *Science*. 1988;242:692-699.

28. Dreyfus PA, Chretien F, Chazaud B, et al. Adult bone marrow-derived stem cells in muscle connective tissue and satellite cell niches. *Am J Pathol*. 2004;164:773-779.

29. Elliot DH. Structure and function of mammalian tendon. *Biol Rev Camb Philos Soc*. 1965;40:392-421.

30. Fawcett JW, Keynes RJ. Peripheral nerve regeneration. *Annu Rev Neurosci*. 1990;13:43-60.

31. Forslund C, Bylander D, Aspenberg P. Indomethacin and celecoxib improve tendon healing in rats. *Acta Orthop Scand*. 2003;74:465-469.

32. Friden J, Kjorell U, Thornell LE. Delayed muscle soreness and cytoskeletal alterations: an immunocytological study in man. *Int J Sports Med*. 1984;5:15-18.

33. Friden J, Seger J, Ekblom B. Sublethal muscle fibre injuries after high-tension anaerobic exercise. *Eur J Appl Physiol*. 1988;57:360-368.

34. Friden J, Sjostrom M, Ekblom B. A morphological study of delayed onset muscle soreness. *Experientia*. 1981;37:506-507.

35. Friden J, Sjostrom M, Ekblom B. Myofibrillar damage following intense eccentric exercise in man. *Int J Sports Med*. 1983;170-176.

36. Fukuda H, Hamada K, Yamanaka K. Pathology and pathogenesis of bursal-side rotator cuff tears viewed from en bloc histologic sections. *Clin Orthop*. 1990;254:75-80.

37. Fyfe I, Stanish WD. The use of eccentric training and stretching in the treatment and prevention of tendon injuries. *Clin Sports Med*. 1992;11:601-624.

38. Garrett WE. Muscle strain injuries. *Am J Sports Med*. 1996;24:S2-S8.

39. Gerstenfeld LC, Thiede M, Siebert K, Mielke C, Phippard D, Svagr B, et al. Differential inhibition of fracture healing by non-selective and cyclooxygenase-2 selective non-steroidal anti-inflammatory drugs. *J Orthop Res*. 2003;21:670-675.

40. Goetsch SC, Hawke TJ, Gallardo TD, Richardson JA, Garry DJ. Transcriptional profiling and regulation of the extracellular matrix during muscle regeneration. *Physiol Genomics*. 2003;14:261-271.

41. Goodship AE, Birch HL, Wilson AM. The pathology and repair of tendon and ligament injury. *Vet Clin North Am Equine Pract*. 1994;10:323-349.

42. Gundersen RW. Response of sensory neurites and growth cones to patterned substrata of laminin and fibronectin in vitro. *Dev Biol*. 1987;121:423-431.

43. Hooley CJ, Cohen RE. A model for the creep behavior of tendon. *Int J Biol Macromol*. 1979;1:123-132.

44. Houghum P. Soft tissue healing and its impact on rehabilitation. *J Sports Rehabil*. 1992;1:19-39.

45. Hume T, Kalimo H, Sandberg M, Lehto M, Vuorio E. Localization of type I and III collagen and fibronectin production in injured gastrocnemius muscle. *Lab Invest*. 1991;64:76-84.

46. Hume T, Kalimo H. Activation of myogenic precursor cells after muscle injury. *Med Sci Sports Exerc*. 1992;24:197-205.

47. Jarvinen M, Aho AJ, Lehto M, Toivonen H. Age dependent repair of muscle rupture: a histological and microangiographical study in rats. *Acta Orthop Scand*. 1983;54:64 74.

48. Jarvinen M, Lehto MUK. The effect of early mobilization and immobilization on the healing process following muscle injuries. *Sports Med*. 1993;15:78-89.

49. Jarvinen M, Sovari T. A histochemical study of the effect of mobilization and immobilization on the metabolism of healing muscle injury. In: Landry F, ed. *Sports Medicine*. Miami, FL: symposium specialists, Orban WAR; 1978:177-181.

50. Jarvinen M, Sovari T. Healing of a crush injury in rat striated muscle, 1: description and testing of a new method of inducing a standard injury to the calf muscles. *Acta Pathol Microbiol Scand*. 1975;83A:259-265.

51. Jarvinen M. Healing of a crush injury in rat striated muscle, 2: a histological study of the effect of early mobilization and immobilization on the repair processes. *Acta Pathol Microbiol Scand*. 1975;83A:269-282.

52. Jarvinen M. Healing of a crush injury in rat striated muscle, 3: a microangiographical study of the effect of early mobilization and immobilization on capillary ingrowth. *Acta Pathol Microbiol Scand*. 1976;84A:85-94.

53. Jarvinen M. Healing of a crush injury in rat striated muscle, 4: effect of early mobilization and immobilization on the tensile properties of gastrocnemius muscle. *Acta Chir Scand*. 1976;142:47-56.

54. Jarvinen TA, Jarvinen TL, Kaariainen M, Kalimo H, Jarvinen M. Muscle injuries: biology and treatment. *Am J Sports Sci*. 2005; 33:745 764.

55. Jones DA, Newham DJ, Round JM, et al. Experimental human muscle damage: morphological changes in relation to other indices of damage. *J Physiol*. 1986;375:435-448.

56. Kaariainen M, Kaariainen J, Jarvinen TL, et al. Integrin and dystrophin associated adhesion protein complexes during regeneration of shearing-type muscle injury. *Neuromuscul Disord*. 2000;10:121-134.

57. Kaariainen M, Kaariainen J, Jarvinen TLN, Sievanen H, Kalimo H, Jarvinen M. Correlation between biomechanical and structural changes during the regeneration of skeletal muscle after laceration injury. *J Orthop Res*. 1998;16:197-206.

58. Kannus P, Josza L, Jarvinnen M. Basic science of tendons. In: Garret WE, Speer KP, Kirkendall DT, eds. *Principles and Practice of Orthopaedic Sports Medicine*. Philadelphia, PA: Lippincott Williams and Wilkins; 2000:21-37.

59. Kawaguchi H. Endochondral ossification signals in cartilage degradation during osteoarthritis progression in experimental mouse models. *Mol Cells*. 2008;25:1-6.

60. Kellet J. Acute soft tissue injuries – a review of the literature. *Med Sci Sports Exerc*. 1986;18:489-400.

61. Kirkendall DT, Garrett WE. Function and biomechanics of tendons. *Scand J Med Sci Sports*. 1997;7:62-66.

62. Kiviranta I, Jurvelin J, Tammi M, et al. Weight bearing controls glycosaminoglycan concentration an articular cartilage thickness in the knee joints of young beagle dogs. *Arthritis Rheum*. 1987;30:801-809.

63. Komi PV. Physiological and biomechanical correlates of muscle function: effects of muscle structure and stretch-shortening cycle on force and speed. *Exerc Sport Sci Rev*. 1984;12:81-121.

64. Lee SK, Wolfe SW. Peripheral nerve injury and repair. *J Am Acad Orthop Surg*. 2000;8:243-252.

65. Lehto M, Duance VC, Restall D. Collagen and fibronectin in a healing skeletal muscle injury: an immunohistochemical study of the effects of physical activity on the repair of injured gastrocnemius muscle in the rat. *J Bone Joint Surg Br*. 1985;67:820-828.

66. Lehto M, Jarvinen M, Nelimarkka O. Scar formation after skeletal muscle injury: a histological and audioradiographical study in rats. *Arch Orthop Trauma Surg*. 1986;104:366-370.

67. Lehto M, Jarvinen M. Collagen and glycosaminoglycan synthesis of injured gastrocnemius muscle in rat. *Eur Surg Res*. 1985;17:179-185.

68. Lewis PB, McCarty LP, Kang RW, Cole BJ. Basic Science and treatment options for articular cartilage injuries. *J Orthop Sports Phys Ther*. 2006;36:717-727.

69. Luckenbill-Edds L. Laminin and the mechanism of neuronal outgrowth. *Brain Res Brain Res Rev*. 1997;23:1-27.

70. Lyritis GP. The history of the walls of the Acropolis of Athens and the natural history of secondary healing process. *J Musculoskelet Neuronal Interact*. 2000;1:1-3.

71. Maffulli N, Khan KM, Puddu G. Overuse tendon conditions: time to change a confusing terminology. *Arthroscopy*. 1998;14:840-843.

72. Makawana M, Raivich G. Molecular mechanisms in successful peripheral regeneration. *FEBS J*. 2005;272:2628-2638.

73. Manthorpe M, Skaper SD, Williams LR, Varon S. Purification of adult rat sciatic nerve ciliary neuronotrophic factor. *Brain Res*. 1986;367:282-286.

74. Matzioliz G, Tuischer J, Kasper G, et al. Simulation of cell differentiation in fracture healing: mechanically loaded composite scaffolds in a novel bioreactor system. *Tissue Eng*. 2006;12:201-208.

75. McKibbin B. The biology of fracture healing in long bones. *J Bone Joint Surg Br*. 1978;60:150-162.

76. Mollenhauer JA. Perspectives on articular cartilage biology and osteoarthritis. *Injury*. 2008;39S1:S5-S12.

77. Monfort J, Matell-Pellitier J, Pellitier JP. Chondroitin sulphate for symptomatic osteoarthritis: critical appraisal of meta-analyses. *Curr Med Res Opin*. 2008;24(5):1303-1308. Epub 2008 Apr 15.

78. Neumann S, Bradke T, Tessier-Lavigne M, Basbaum AI. Regeneration of sensory axons within the injured spinal cord induced by intraganglionic camp elevation. *Neuron*. 2002;34:885-893.

79. Newham DJ, Mills KR, Edwards RHT. Large delayed plasma creatine kinase changes after stepping exercise. *Muscle Nerve*. 1983;6:380-385.

80. O'Brien M. Functional anatomy and physiology of tendons. *Clin Sports Med*. 1992;11:505-520.

81. O'Driscoll SW. The healing and regeneration of articular cartilage. *J Bone Joint Surg AM*. 1998;80-A:1795-1812.

82. Oakes BW, Singleton C, Haut RC. Correlation of collagen fibril morphology and tensile modulus in the repairing of normal rabbit patella tendon. *Trans Orthop Res Soc*. 1998;23-34.

83. Oxlund H. Relationships between the biomechanical properties, composition and molecular structure of connective tissues. *Connect Tissue Res*. 1986;15:65-72.

84. Pearson OM, Liberman DE. The aging of Wolff's "law" ontogeny and responses to mechanical loading in cortical bone. *Yrbk Phys Anthropol*. 2004;47:63-99.

85. Puddu G, Ippolito E, Postacchini F. A classification of Achilles tendon disease. *Am J Sports Med*. 1976;4:145-160.

86. Raivich G, Bohatschek M, Da Costa C, Iwata O, Galiano M, et al. The AP-1 transcription factor c-Jun is required for efficient axonal regeneration. *Neuron*. 2004;43:57-67.

87. Riedel GE, Valentin-Opran A. Clinical evaluation of fhbmp-2/ACS in orthopaedic trauma: a progress report. *Orthopaedics*. 1999;22:663-665.

88. Riley GP, Cox M, Harrall RL, Clements S, Hazelman BL. Inhibition of tendon cell proliferation and matrix glycosaminoglycan synthesis by non-steroidal anti-inflammatory drugs in vitro. *J Hand Surg Br*. 2001;26:224-228.

89. Rumian AP, Wallace AL, Birch HL. Tendons and ligaments are anatomically distinct but overlap in molecular and morphological features: a comparative study in an ovine model *J Orthop Res*. 2007;25:458-464.

90. Salter RB. History of rest and motion and the scientific basis for early continuous passive motion. *Hand Clin*. 1996;12(1):1-11.

91. Sammarco VJ, Change L. Modern issues in bone graft substitutes and advances in bone tissue technology. *Foot Ankle Clin*. 2002;7:19-41.

92. Sasaki N, Shukunami N, Matsushima N, Izumi Y. Time resolved X-ray diffraction from tendon collagen during creep using synchrotron radiation. *J Biomech*. 1999;32:285-292.

93. Schafer M, Fruttiger M, Montag D, Schachner M, Martini R. Disruption of the gene for the myelin-associated glycoprotein improves axonal regrowth along the myelin in C57BL/Wlds mice. *Neuron*. 1996;16:1107-1113.

94. Seddon HJ. *Surgical Disorders of the Peripheral Nerves*. Baltimore, MD: Williams & Wilkins; 1972.

95. Shadwick RE. Elastic energy storage in tendons: mechanical differences related to function and age. *J Appl Physiol*. 1990;68:1033-1040.

96. Sharma P, Maffulli N. Tendon injury and tendinopathy: healing and repair. *J Bone Joint Surg Am*. 2005;87:187-202.

97. Skutek M, van Griensven M, Zeichen J, Brauer N, Bosch U. Cyclic mechanical stretching of human patellar tendon fibroblasts: activation of JNK and modulation of apoptosis. *Knee Surg Sports Traumatol Arthrosc*. 2003;11:122-129.

98. Slack JR, Hopkins WG, Pockett S. Evidence for a motor nerve growth factor. *Muscle Nerve*. 1983;6:243-252.

99. Smith LL. Acute inflammation: the underlying mechanism in delayed onset muscle soreness? *Med Sci Sports Exerc*. 1991;23:542-551.

100. Smith ME, Jackson CGR. Delayed onset muscle soreness (DOMS) serum creatine kinase (SCK) and creatine kinase MB (%CK-MB) related to performance measurements in football [abstract]. *Med Sci Sports Exerc*. 1990;22(suppl 2):S34.

101. Soldatis JJ, Goodfellow DB, Wilber JH. End-to-end operative repair of Achilles tendon rupture. *Am J Sports Med*. 1997;25:90-95.

102. Stanish WD, Curwin S, Rubinovich M. Tendinitis: the analysis and treatment for running. *Clin Sports Med*. 1985;4:593-609.

103. Stauber WT. Eccentric action of muscles: physiology, injury. In: Pandolf KP, ed. *Exercise and Sport Science Reviews*. Baltimore, MD: Williams and Wilkins; 1989:157-186.

104. Stone D, Green C, Rao U, et al. Cytokine-induced tendinitis: a preliminary study in rabbits. *J Orthop Res*. 1999;17:168-177.

105. Stylios G, Wan T, Giannoudis P. Present status and future potential of enhancing bone healing using nanotechnology. *Injury*. 2007;38(suppl 1):S63-S74.

106. Sullo A, Maffulli N, Capasso G, Testa V. The effects of prolonged pretendinous administration of PGE1 to the rat Achilles tendon: a possible animal model of chronic Achilles tendinopathy. *J Orthop Sci*. 2001;6:349-357.

107. Sunderland S. *Nerve Injuries and Their Repair: A Critical Appraisal*. New York, NY: Churchill Livingstone; 1991.

108. Tepper SH, McKeough DM. Injury, inflammation, and healing. In: Goodman, Fuller, Boissonnault, eds. *Pathology: Implications for the Physical Therapist*. 2nd ed. Philadelphia, PA: Saunders; 2003.

109. Tidball JG. Force transmission across muscle membrane. *J Biomech*. 1991;24(suppl 1):43-52.

110. Tidball JG. Inflammatory cell response to acute muscle injury. *Med Sci Sports Exerc*. 1995;27:1022-1032.

111. Tidball JG, Daniel TL. Myotendinous junctions of tonic muscle cells: structure and loading. *Cell Tissue Res*. 1986;245:315-322.

112. Vaittinen S, Hume T, Ratanen J, Kalims H. Transected myofibres may remain permanently divided in two parts. *Neuromuscul Disord*. 2002;12:584-587.

113. Walker JM. Cartilage of human joints and related structures. In: Zachazewski JE, Magee DJ, Quillen WS, eds. *Athletic Injury and Rehabilitation*. Philadelphia, PA: WB Saunders; 1996.

114. Walter JB. *Principles of disease*. 2nd ed. Philadelphia: WB Saunders; 1982.

115. Williams JG. Achilles tendon lesions in sport. *Sports Med*. 1986;3:114-135.

116. Woo SL-Y, Debski RE, Zeminski J, Abramowitch SD, Chan Saw SS, Fenwick JA. Injury and repair and ligaments and tendons. *Annu Rev Biomed Eng*. 2000;2:83-118.

117. Yoshimura T, Kawano Y, Arimura N, Kawabata S, Kikuchi A, Kaibuchi K. GSK-3 beta regulates phosphorylation of CRMP-2 and neuronal polarity. *Cell*. 2005;120:137-149.

118. Zeichen J, van Griensven M, Bosch U. The proliferative response of isolated human tendon fibroblasts to cyclic biaxial mechanical strain. *Am J Sports Med*. 2000;28:888-892.

119. Zhou FQ, Walzer M, Wu YH, Zhou J, Dedhar S, Snider WD. Neurotrophins support regenerative axon assembly over cspgs by an ECM-integrin-independent mechanism. *J Cell Sci*. 2006;119:2787-2796.

120. Zhou FQ, Zhou J, Dedhar S, Wu YH, Snider WD. NGF-induced axon growth is mediated by localized inactivation of GSK-3 beta and functions of the microtubule plus end binding protein APC. *Neuron*. 2004;42:897-912.

AUTHOR: ALISON L. MCKENZIE

WHAT DO I NEED TO KNOW ABOUT PAIN MECHANISMS?

Understanding what causes pain at the tissue level and knowing how the sensation of pain is conveyed will help you isolate and treat the cause of your patients' symptoms more efficiently and accurately. By identifying the specific tissues that are involved and the possible routes of pain transmission, you can determine the best course of action to take. Having a clear picture of the underlying pain mechanisms and pathways will also allow you to understand how certain factors may modify the perception of pain. Relating your patients' symptoms to the known neural circuitry of pain will enhance your ability to make even better clinical decisions. (Section II will help you identify potential types and sources of pain; Section III reviews the circuitry of pain transmission and changes that can occur in the nervous system following injury.)

WHAT ARE POTENTIAL SOURCES OF PAIN?

Pain can be transmitted from most tissues for a variety reasons. Among the tasks of the rehabilitation clinician is to determine the location, source, type, level of irritability, and cause of pain in order to develop an accurate working diagnosis, treatment intervention, and prognosis. First, the clinician must consider information gathered from the subjective examination, including the patient's history, mechanism of injury, and body diagram, to form an initial working hypothesis regarding the source of pain (Table I-2-1). Next, the possible pain sources should be related to the patient's description of pain (Table I-2-2) to refine the list of likely causes. (An alternative approach is to consider the type of reported pain and relate it to suspected pain sources to see if consistencies exist.) The hypothesis can then be confirmed or refuted through the objective examination process (Table I-2-3).

Although the focus of this section is on pain of musculoskeletal or neuromuscular origin, other sources of pain (e.g., visceral, psychological, or emotional) also must be considered and either ruled out or ruled in. (Please also refer to the chapter on Clinical Decision Making: Red Flags of Nonmusculoskeletal Origin in this text as well as to Section III.) Once the clinician has determined that the cause of pain is likely musculoskeletal or neuromuscular in nature, she or he can proceed to the next step of establishing which specific tissues are involved.

HOW DOES MY KNOWLEDGE OF THE NEURAL CIRCUITRY OF PAIN ENHANCE MY ABILITY TO TREAT PATIENTS?

Understanding the mechanisms and neural pathways underlying pain transmission can help clinicians make sense of the pain-related signs and symptoms of patients. Knowing the source and route of pain transmission and modulation can guide the clinician in the processes of performing an appropriate examination, determining a diagnosis and intervention plan, and making an accurate prognosis. By appreciating the neural circuitry of pain and by recognizing the peripheral and central influences on it,[39,42-44] clinicians also can provide better explanations to their patients regarding what they are experiencing and why. In short, being able to translate and incorporate the foundational (basic) science of pain into practice allows clinicians to have a more comprehensive approach as they develop a working diagnosis and plan of care suitable for each patient.

Some of the basics of pain pathways and mechanisms are outlined in Table I-2-4 through I-2-6 and Figures I-2-1 through I-2-3, but the reader is encouraged to consult the references provided for a more thorough understanding.[1,15,17,20-24,28,29,37-39,42-44] Briefly, when carrying out an examination, the clinician should attempt to determine the source, type, and pattern of pain relative to the patient's history. The more precise and specific the pain-related information gleaned from the subjective and objective examinations, the better the therapist is able to proceed.

Likewise, clinicians must be attuned to how psychological and emotional factors may influence pain perception on a neurological level.[17] The changes that can occur in neural circuitry resulting from certain conditions (e.g., depression and anxiety, fear-avoidance behaviors) can have a profound effect on patients' symptoms and response to treatment. Similarly, clinicians should be aware of the central mechanisms and circuitry pertaining to chronic pain to better guide their intervention and to better educate their patients.[2-6,9-11,22,27,33,35,40,46] Lastly, with an understanding of pain mechanisms and transmission, it is possible to understand the mechanisms underlying neuropathic pain and pharmacological interventions for the various types of pain.[2-4,6,9, 22,35,40,46]

OVERVIEW OF PAIN CIRCUITRY AND PATHWAYS

WHAT IS THE NEURAL CIRCUITRY OF PAIN?

In general, the neural circuitry of pain is described in terms of peripheral receptors (receptors in the peripheral tissues that respond to painful stimuli), peripheral afferent fibers (the fibers that convey pain information), dorsal root ganglia (DRG, the location of the cell bodies for the peripheral afferent fibers, located near the intervertebral foramen), dorsal (and sometimes ventral) roots (central processes of the peripheral afferent fibers that project to the spinal cord), lamina of the spinal cord gray matter, long tracts (carrying ascending/descending information through the spinal cord and brainstem), brainstem modulation centers, thalamic nuclei, and cortical and subcortical targets. Primary, secondary, and association cortical areas also may be involved.

WHERE IN THE CIRCUITRY CAN PAIN BE MODULATED?

Table I-2-4 summarizes the types of pain receptors and their associated fiber types by tissue, whereas Table I-2-5 defines the afferent fiber type by their respective conduction velocities. In general, most pain is transmitted by slowly conducting, small-diameter fibers that enter the spinal cord via the dorsal rootlets; approximately 30% of fibers traveling in the ventral root are unmyelinated; of these about 50% are sensory.[28] Both peripheral and central mechanisms and centers for pain modulation are described (Table I-2-6) and will be illustrated (Figures I-2-1 through I-2-3). Indeed, pain can be modulated at every step along the way: receptor, DRG, spinal cord, brainstem, thalamus, subcortical, and cortical structures.

Ascending fibers synapse with interneurons in the brainstem, including those in the reticular formation, the parabrachial nucleus, and the periaqueductal gray (PAG), among others. Ascending fibers from the lateral spinothalamic (neospinothalamic) tract mainly project to the ventroposterolateral (VPL) nucleus, then the somatosensory cortex to facilitate pain localization. Fibers from the paleospinothalamic and other more primitive tracts project to more medial, diffuse thalamic nuclei, then on to subcortical and cortical limbic system areas to process the more affective elements of pain.

CAN THE DESCENDING NEURAL PATHWAYS INFLUENCE THE PERCEPTION OF PAIN?

As one can see from Figure I-2-4, the descending influences on pain perception and modulation are significant and may be helpful

TABLE I-2-1　Potential Sources of Pain[8,15,17,21,24,25,28,29,36–38,44]

Tissue Source	Types of Injury	Source (Refer to Table I-2-5)	Location of Pain	Quality of Pain
Skin	*Mechanical:* Tear/incision	Pain receptors and fibers in the epidermal and dermal layers	Generally well localized to injury site, but may expand with inflammatory changes	Usually acute, sharp initially; may "itch" with healing
	Pressure	Compression of cutaneous nerves, vascular beds (may cause ischemia)	Generally less localized than acute tear, especially in those with sensory loss	Dull, ache; may have prickly or tingling sensations; may be insensate
	Ischemia	Vascular insufficiency to tissues, venous stasis; hypoxia-induced cellular changes	Tissues supplied by ischemic vessels–the site of ischemia and distal peripheral tissues	May initially feel like pins and needles, but become dull over time
	Inflammation	Chemical mediators of inflammation*	May extend beyond the area of inflammation in a diffuse pattern; area may be warm, red, swollen	May be sharp initially; burning, tender
	Referred	May be underlying visceral or somatic structures	Can refer to the same segmental levels as the overlying somatic tissues or in a pattern that reflects embryologic origin	May be sharp, especially if connective tissue coverings are irritated; may be dull ache, cramping
Fascia	*Mechanical:* Tearing/incision	Fiber disruption, damage to pain and mechanoreceptors	May be localized or may refer more diffusely, especially for deep tissues	May be sharp initially, becoming achy
	Overstretch	Fiber elongation, disruption of nerve endings	May be localized or follow myotomal/sclerotomal pattern or trigger points; if visceral coverings, may be referred pain pattern	May be sharp initially, then become more diffuse, dull; if compartment syndrome– very painful
	Adhesions	Binding, cross-linkage of collagen fibers; compression; if compartment syndrome, may cause neurovascular compression		
Muscle	*Mechanical:* Tear	Tear, contusion, or overstretch of muscle fibers, myotendinous junction	Initially localized, but painful area will spread as nerve's receptive fields increase in size	Sharp, acute initially, becoming dull over time; pain with use
	Incision	Laceration or surgical incision		
	Strain	Usually mechanical (first, second, third degree), depending on the number of fibers damaged (third is complete)		
	Inflammation	May be secondary to tissue damage or secondary to systemic disease; inflammatory mediators trigger response	As above; if compartment syndrome, hematoma present: entire muscle compartment and surrounding structures affected	As above; if compartment syndrome– may have numbness and tingling, lack of circulation distally
	Referred	Secondary to soft tissue injury or systemic disease process Myofascial trigger points, underlying viscera, deep somatic structure, somatization of psychological pain	May extend beyond localized area to surrounding tissues, trigger points; may be poorly localized	Varies with acuity and cause
Tendon	Tendinitis Tendinosis	Mechanoreceptors, nociceptors; pain with contraction (painful arc)	Generally well-localized and point tender, but may be difficult to distinguish from related structures; tendinosis: pain with deep palpation and contraction	Varies with acuity: tendinitis: sharper; tendinosis: pain with deep pressure
Ligament	Strain First degree Second degree Third degree	Free nerve endings, nociceptors, mechanoreceptors; worse with joint gapping (especially passive end range)	May have point tenderness with testing at site of damage, if superficial; deeper structures may be poorly localized	If third degree, laxity with pain in surrounding tissues; otherwise, may be sharp when tissues stressed, dull ache at rest
Other joint structures	Cartilage Compression Tearing Erosion	No pain receptors; pain is usually indirect, from surrounding/ neighboring tissues	Indirectly localized through tissue interfaces (e.g., neighboring ligaments, capsule, periosteum)	Pain primarily from surrounding structures
Synovium	Inflammation Disruption	Direct tissue damage, edema, and chemical inflammatory mediators	Periarticular pain, may be warm, red, swollen	Deep, dull ache but may be more acute if recent injury
Disc	Compression, tearing of cartilage and fibers, extrusion of contents	Axial loading, shearing, compression May involve vertebral endplate	Relatively broad, may refer to surrounding tissues; compression may cause nerve impingement and distal, radicular symptoms	Can be sharp, radiating, pinching, cramping (if surrounding nerves and muscles are irritated; ache in static positions)
Facet	Compression, fracture, inflammation of periarticular structures	Pain with approximation/compression of articular surfaces, irritation of sinuvertebral branches of dorsal rami (which also innervate dura)	Should be restricted to joint and overlying articular and soft tissues, not radicular/ peripheral symptoms	Often sharp, pinching, especially if meniscoid pads are compressed

TABLE I-2-1 Potential Sources of Pain (Continued)

Tissue Source	Types of Injury	Source (Refer to Table I-2-5)	Location of Pain	Quality of Pain
Bone	Contusion Fracture Inflammation	Pain with stimulation/damage of periosteum and its nerve endings; may have secondary inflammatory mediators	At injury site, but may refer beyond Sclerotomal distribution	"Exquisite" pain (sharp, acute, stabbing), transitions to dull ache with healing
Nerve	Impingement Overstretch Tear/cut Systemic Sensitization	Damage to axons/peripheral fibers, myelin sheath, dorsal root ganglia, or central modulation and perception centers Hyperalgesia, allodynia, or centralized pain (refer to Section II)	Pain at peripheral neuroma, along nerve path, along radicular pattern (dermatome) May be referred to large area	Burning, stabbing, electrical, tingling May be constant or intermittent, depending on other stimuli
Viscera	Compression Distention Traction Congestion Edema Ischemia Inflammation Chemicals	Pressure from surrounding organs or structures Pressure/irritation from within the organ Elongation/pulling from related structures Physiological processes or systemic infection Compression/occlusion of blood supply Local or systemic Acids, toxins, inflammatory mediators	Diffuse, difficult to localize; often refers to somatic tissues innervated by nerve branches that carry visceral sensory fibers, which enter the cord via ventral roots; may elicit autonomic reflexes; may project to diffuse centers	Can be sharp and stabbing or dull ache, cramping
Visceral connective tissue coverings	Overstretch Compression	Afferent fibers travel through autonomic plexuses; have cell bodies in dorsal root ganglia, project to diffuse interneuronal pools in the CNS	May refer to body wall, overlying musculature and other somatic structures Rebound tenderness	Usually sharp, stabbing, or very tender
Vasculature	Occlusion Compression Ischemia and hypoxia Inflammation Hemorrhage	 Inflammatory mediators	Initially localized, but spreads to larger area May be able to note trophic changes or decreased temperature, blood flow (e.g., capillary refilling, nail bed) Redness, swelling, tenderness; lack of blood in peripheral tissues	Throbbing, cramping; may cause pins and needles; prickly/tingly; ache with activity If cardiac, may have severe (crushing) pain, which may be referred
Emotional	May be related to anxiety, depression, conversion disorder	May be caused by central sensitization from previous injury May be related to increased activity in peripheral receptors, axons, WDR neurons, or brainstem, subcortical, or cortical centers and circuitry	Usually diffuse, but may be localized; does not generally follow expected or known pattern	Horrible, unrelenting, constant, excruciating Descriptions of pain are often exaggerated or heightened

*Arachidonic acid cleavage from the cell membrane is metabolized by the cyclooxygenase (COX) enzyme system to produce eicosanoids [prostaglandin (usually vasodilators and pain mediators that increase receptor sensitivity to mechanical pressure; increase effects of bradykinin) and thromboxanes (COX, COX 2 enzymes)]. Lipoxygenase (LOX) enzymes produce leukotrienes, which act mainly on the respiratory system.[10]

TABLE I-2-2 Pain Descriptors[17,28]

Type of Pain	Potential Source
Aching	Tissue damage or irritation/inflammation; can be related to overuse (including abnormal posture) or tissue injury/reinjury. Deep joint pain/arthritis is a common cause. Possible systemic virus (e.g., flu). Symptoms pertaining to systemic problems will not usually be reproduced by biomechanical testing of tissue integrity. Possible vascular insufficiency that worsens with demand (e.g., intermittent claudication). Possible visceral irritation (e.g., prostatitis).
Burning	May pertain to nerve irritation, but can be visceral (e.g., GERD, appendicitis). Need to localize source of pain and relate symptoms to history. If neuromuscular in nature, symptoms should be reproduced with biomechanical testing (e.g., nerve tension testing, tapping/compression).
Dull	If poorly localized, diffuse, and unrelated to position or movement: probably due to viscera or overlying connective tissues, but pathology of deep somatic structures should be considered.

Continued on following page.

TABLE I-2-2 **Types of Pain** (*Continued*)

Type of Pain	Potential Source
Nagging	May be musculoskeletal if related to position, activity, use, time of day, etc. Determine if symptoms are related to prior or unresolved tissue damage (and/or reinjury of previously damaged tissues). Usually characteristic of subacute to chronic phases of tissue damage and repair. In chronic cases, symptoms may persist in the absence of any remaining tissue damage or pathology, indicating that the pain has become "centralized" or hard-wired in the CNS. If unable to determine any relationship to musculoskeletal or neuromuscular source, may need to refer out.
Point tenderness	Localized skin lesion, bursitis, superficial muscle, tendon, ligamentous/meniscal damage. Should rule out rebound tenderness or visceral involvement through palpation if the symptoms are in an area overlying organs (e.g., abdomen) or if pain is in area to which visceral pain may be referred.
Poorly localized	Visceral, deep joint, or other deep somatic tissues.
Rebound tenderness	Fascial coverings (e.g., peritoneum) surrounding the viscera.
Sharp	Usually direct trauma (e.g., bone fracture), but may be visceral (e.g., gallstones, kidney stones), especially if the connective tissue coverings (e.g., pericardium, pleura, peritoneum) are irritated.
Shooting	Usually nerve or nerve root irritation; may be related to restriction of connective tissue coverings.
Stabbing	Visceral (e.g., kidney stones), ischemia (infarction), nerve.
Throbbing	Usually related to blood flow, vascular involvement; not to be confused with waves of cramping associated with gastrointestinal distress.
Tingling/numbness	Vascular or neural compression or nerve irritation. Do the symptoms follow a radicular or peripheral nerve pattern? If stocking/glove pattern, check peripheral pulses and circulation. Is there any associated muscle fatigue?

TABLE I-2-3 **Pain Patterns (Provocation)**[15,17,21,25,28,29,36–38,44]

Tissue	Stimulus	Observation/Tests	Pattern
Skin	Palpation, pressure, stretch	Check for any lesions, adhesions to underlying tissues	Usually localized to affected area; if dermatomal pattern, check for nerve root compression
Muscle	Active range of motion (ROM) Muscle contraction	Pain with contraction in mid ROM; degree of weakness related to tissue damage Weak but painless	Similar to skin—damage to muscle fibers (localized), but may refer in myotomal distribution (decreased innervation density) Possible complete avulsion Localized to involved muscle or muscles
Joint	Active and passive ROM, weight bearing or compression, end-feel testing	Joint compression (e.g., scour test, axial loading); greater pain with passive motion Weak and painful Repeated motions	Pain with compression/shearing; pain may be deep and poorly localized Gentle repeated motion may increase joint lubrication and ease pain but if capsular damage, edema, and/or effusion are present, motions may increase pain
Ligament	Passively gap joint or elongate ligamentous fibers End range active movements may produce pain if tissue damage or joint laxity is present	Laxity testing, positional deformities	Unstable joint, pain at end range or attachment points Pain may not be well localized with damage to deeper structures
Tendon	Painful arc (active ROM) Overstretch End range contraction	Strong but painful	Generally localized to tendon, myotendinous junction, or bony insertion May refer to sclerotomal pattern
Fascia	Pressure with elongation of fibers	Restrictions in soft tissue mobility	May be point tender or associated with trigger point pain pattern
Arterial	Compression/occlusion Trauma resulting in hemorrhage or bleeding	Check pulses/capillary bed refilling, temperature of tissues supplied; observe for trophic changes (indicates autonomic disturbance) Check for swelling, edema, hematoma, ecchymosis	Throbbing, spasms; may cause numbness, tingling, achiness, fatigue in structures supplied Initially localized to affected area, but may expand as tissue damage continues (Some constituents of blood can cause cell death, necrosis)
Visceral/ referred	Distension, compression, ischemia, position, physiological processes (eating, urination, defecation, etc.)	Refer to chapter on Clinical Decision Making In general, visceral pain will be related to processes that put demands on the tissues, not reproduced through biomechanical testing Pain cycles and time of day likewise will relate to the demands placed on the involved organ; night pain is especially worrisome, since it may be a red flag for cancer	Refer to chapter on Clinical Decision Making: Red Flags and Nonmusculoskeletal Pain and to Section II on referred pain patterns In general, viscera/visceral coverings refer to multiple segmental levels via the spinal nerves; as a result, the patterns of referred pain vary across individuals and may cover broad, poorly localized areas Pain may be sharp/stabbing, dull and aching, intermittent or persistent, depending on the nature of the pathology

TABLE I-2-3   Pain Patterns (Provocation) *(Continued)*

Tissue	Stimulus	Observation/Tests	Pattern
Neuropathic	Nerve damage: trauma, compression, overstretch, metabolic (e.g., diabetic), infection, malnutrition, radiation, neurotoxin (e.g., chemotherapy agents), inflammation, genetic disorders, mutations	Sensory and motor testing Check dermatomes and myotomes for suspected nerve root damage; check peripheral nerve distribution May need to refer for nerve conduction velocity, electromyogram testing	Tingling, numbness, shooting, stabbing, prickly, crushing, hot, "twitchy" Generally follows pattern of the peripheral nerve or nerve root (dermatome/myotome), but may become more centralized in chronic cases Some polyneuropathies/peripheral neuropathies will result in a more stocking-glove distribution of symptoms
Chronic	May be present in the absence of tissue pathology (i.e., musculoskeletal tissues have healed, but pain persists)	Distinguish between centralized pain and possible recurrence/reinjury causing tissue damage Check for hyperalgesia and allodynia Pain cycle: determine if a relationship to position, activity, or use exists If so, are symptoms proportional to activity/demand? May need to administer depression scale or refer for psychological evaluation	Symptoms may be reported as constant, unrelenting, nagging, aching Symptoms may not relate directly to activity, use, biomechanical testing, position, or posture Symptoms may be similar in distribution to acute/subacute injury or may be more diffuse (e.g., trigger points, large body areas)
Emotional	Anxiety, depression, stress, fatigue, irritability, sadness May coexist with tissue damage or may be present in the absence of tissue pathology	Psychological evaluation to help determine cause and effective coping strategies May benefit from exercise program; it is usually best to minimize hands-on treatment	Horrible, agonizing, nauseating, unbearable Heightened response to sensory testing Exaggerated or heightened report/description of pain, response to biomechanical testing Unrelated or inconsistently related to activity, position, posture

TABLE I-2-4   Characteristics of Peripheral Afferent Fibers Conveying Pain[15,24,28,38,44]

Tissue	Receptors	Fiber Type
Skin	Type IA mechano-heat receptors, moderate pressure; low mechanical/high thermal threshold	Aβ/Aδ
	Type IIA mechano-heat nociceptors	Aδ
	Free nerve endings, nociceptors	C
	Mechano-heat, cold, polymodal nociceptors (heat, chemical, mechanical) (Merkel disk, Pacinian Meissner's, Ruffini, may be sensitized)	
Muscle	Free nerve endings [mechanical, algesic chemicals (ATP, capsaicin, GNF), protons]	III, IV
Tendon	Free nerve endings (some intertwined with collagen, periarticular vessels)	III, IV
Joint: capsule, ligament, periosteum, perineurium of articular nerves Absent on cartilage	Mechanosensitive and mechanoinsensitive (can become sensitized), chemical	III, IV
Viscera	Some may have polymodal nociceptive endings (urogenital system), but mainly nonspecific visceral afferents; polymodal nociceptors (urogenital system); rapidly and slowly adapting mechanoreceptors, chemoreceptors (gastrointestinal system); lung irritant and J receptors (respiratory system); visceral nociceptors	Aδ, C

TABLE I-2-5   Sensory Fiber Types[24,28,38,44]

Fiber Type	Conduction Velocity
Aα (Ia and Ib), myelinated	80–120 m/sec
Aβ (II), myelinated	35–75 m/sec
Aδ (III), thinly myelinated	2.5–30 m/sec
C (IV), nonmyelinated	<2.5 m/sec

in mitigating the perception of pain. Activating descending, inhibitory pathways may provide a mechanism for reducing pain; some analgesics work this way (How Can Medication Affect Pain?).[39,42,44]

CLINICAL PEARL

Descending cortical projection fibers can strongly influence pain modulation and perception, therefore, behavioral training (e.g., relaxation training, imagery, cognitive training) can be a powerful tool in helping patients redirect, manage, and control their perceptions of pain. Stimulating large afferent fibers (e.g., through touch, vibration, and rubbing) can "override" noxious input from the smaller pain fibers and attenuate pain perception at the level of the spinal cord and above: recall that this is the basis for the use of TENS. A word of caution: the nervous system can adapt to sensory stimuli, so therapists must vary the timing and type of such nonnoxious stimuli.

TABLE I-2-6 Overview of Pain Pathways[24,28,38,44]

Tissue	Peripheral Nerve	Spinal Cord Tracts*	Brainstem	Higher Centers
Skin	PAF in named peripheral nerves, which help form spinal nerve roots; first-order cell bodies in DRG; first-order in trigeminal ganglion; fibers enter dorsal root			
	Small RFs, localized, short-lasting, monosynaptic fibers; somatotopically organized	Anterolateral system (ALS): *neospinothalamic* (lateral spinothalamic) and	Possible collaterals to NRM, Ret Form, PAG	VPL/Vc, VPM of thalamus to somatosensory cortex
	Large RFs, conveys more affective elements of poorly localized pain, arousal, motor responses to pain; monosynaptic or polysynaptic	*paleospinothalamic* tracts (medial spinoreticular, spinobulbar, spinopontine, spinomesencephalic, spinoreticular-thalamic, spinodiencephalic);	Collateral branches to interneurons at multiple levels (NRM, Ret Form, VLRF, DRN, RVM, PNG, PBN, PAG)	Intralaminar thalamic nuclei, ventrobasal, VL, VPL thalamic nuclei, amygdala, hypothalamus, limbic areas of cortex, sensorimotor, cingulate, prefrontal cortex
	Aβ, Aδ, C, low threshold, WDR mostly for hair, skin; lateral cervical nucleus	Spinocervicothalamic tract Spinotelencephalic tract		Ventrobasal thalamus Some ascending fibers may bypass the thalamus and go straight to the basal ganglia and limbic areas of the cortex
	Nociceptors in face/head have first-order neuron in trigeminal ganglion, which projects to spinotrigeminal nucleus (pars caudalis)	Spinotrigeminal tract		VPM
Muscle, tendon, joint, ligaments	As above, but joint sensory fibers travel in deeper peripheral nerve branches	Typically, mechanoreceptors for proprioception, vibration send PAF in dorsal column/medial lemniscal pathway, but painful input is conveyed by the ALS and other pain tract (above)	As above	
Viscera, vasculature	Autonomic PAF that contribute to ANS plexuses, then travel with spinal nerves; first-order cell bodies in DRG; afferent fibers may enter dorsal or ventral root	Spinobulbar Spinomesencephalic Spinodiencephalic Spinohypothalamic	NTS, PBN, PAG	Ventral thalamus, intralaminar nuclei, hypothalamus, amygdala, septal area Medial thalamic nuclei, limbic areas of the cortex Medial and lateral hypothalamic nuclei
	Visceral distention from spinal cord and pars caudalis			

PAF, peripheral afferent fibers; DRG, dorsal root ganglia; RF, receptive field; NRM, nucleus raphe magnus; Ret Form, reticular formation; VLRF, ventrolateral reticular formation; RVM, rostral ventromedial medulla; PNG, pontine noradrenergic group; DRN, dorsal reticular nuclei; PAG, periaqueductal gray matter; NTS, nucleus tractus solitarii. The PBN (in the pons) and PAG (in the midbrain) are especially important brainstem pain modulation centers. The PAG is also involved in motor responses to pain; the PBN projects to the PAG, paracentral thalamus, prefrontal cortex, and amygdala. Both the PAG and PBN are involved in pain aversion responses; the PAG mediates vasopressor and locomotor (or immobility) responses.

VPL, ventral posterior lateral nucleus (receives input from body); Vc, ventrocaudal; VPM, ventral posterior medial nucleus (receives input from the head); intralaminar nuclei receive poorly localized, diffuse pain input and project to multiple cortical areas, including limbic system structures, for the emotional components of pain.

*In the spinal cord, neospinothalamic PAF can ascend or descend one to three segments in Lissauer's fasciculus before synapsing on second-order neurons in the dorsal horn.[11,12] Wide dynamic range neurons in the dorsal horn may mediate abnormal pain responses.[23] Axons from second-order neurons or interneurons may cross in the anterior commissure and ascend in the ventrolateral fasciculus and up through the lateral brainstem to synapse on thalamic nuclei. Some paleospinothalamic PAF ascend in the ventromedial fasciculus ipsilaterally, some contralaterally, and some bilaterally to reach the thalamus.[11,12] Nociceptive PAF from the head have their first-order cell bodies in the trigeminal ganglion, the central processes of which synapse on second-order neurons in the spinal trigeminal nuclei, including the nucleus caudalis, in the medulla, and upper cervical spinal cord.[11,12] Within the spinal cord gray matter, interneurons, particularly WDR neurons, modulate pain perception.[23]

PAIN TRANSMISSION, HYPERALGESIA, ALLODYNIA, AND NEUROPATHIC PAIN[1,2–6,9–11,15,20–24,27,29,35,37,40,43,44,46]

HOW IS PAIN GENERATED AND PROPAGATED?

Ordinarily, pain receptors (nociceptors) are activated by an environmental stimulus (e.g., mechanical, chemical, thermal), causing transduction that produces a conformational change in the peripheral nerve terminal, triggering opening or closing of ion channels and a resultant change in the membrane potential. If the threshold is reached, an action potential is propagated toward the central terminal of the sensory neuron, causing it to release neurotransmitters at the synapse, which is usually in the gray matter of the spinal cord (primarily the dorsal horn).

The action potential produces both central and peripheral effects. The central effect of pain perception is mediated by the central nervous system as the impulse is transmitted to higher centers (Table I-2-6). The peripheral effect results as the action potential induces changes at the peripheral ending. Since branches from one nociceptor can extend over a large receptive area, stimulation of one receptor can spread to other branches, expanding the area of pain perception.

WHAT IS THE PRIMARY NEUROTRANSMITTER FOR PAIN IN THE CENTRAL NERVOUS SYSTEM (CNS)?

A number of neuropeptides are released at the nociceptor and in the dorsal horn of the spinal cord (Box I-2-1). The primary excitatory amino acid neurotransmitter for pain in the CNS appears to be glutamate.

CAN NONDESTRUCTIVE STIMULI CAUSE PAIN?

Even with nondestructive mechanical excitation of the nociceptor, the peripheral nerve terminal releases neuropeptides into the

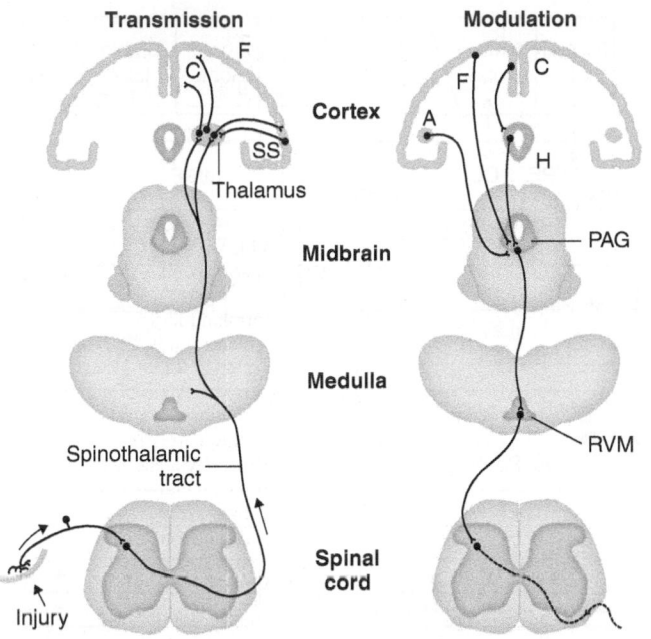

FIGURE I-2-1 Pain transmission and modulation pathways. Left: A noxious stimulus applied to the skin (lower left) elicits a train of impulses beginning in peripheral nociceptors and propagated to the dorsal horn of the spinal cord, where they activate the nerve cells of origin of the spinothalamic tract. The spinothalamic tract activates thalamic neurons, which project to and activate neurons in the cingulate cortex (C), frontal cortex (F), and somatosensory cortex (SS). Right: A variety of stimuli can activate pain modulation circuits. Frontal and cingulate cortex projections and afferents from the amygdala (A) and hypothalamus (H) converge on midbrain periaqueductal gray (PAG) neurons, which, through a relay in the rostral ventromedial medulla (RVM), control spinothalamic pain transmission neurons. (Redrawn from Fields HL: Pain modulation: expectation, opioid analgesia and virtual pain. *Progr Brain Res* 2000;122:245–253. © 2000, with permission from Elsevier Science.)

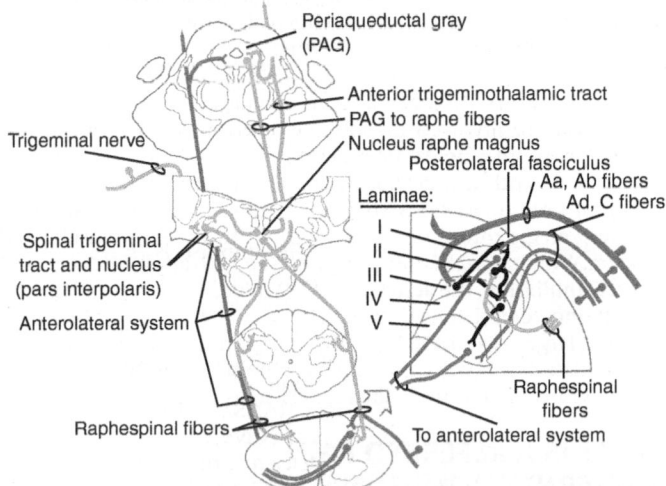

FIGURE I-2-2 Descending brainstem pathways that influence and control pain transmission within the brainstem (for trigeminal pathways) and in the spinal cord (for anterolateral system projections). (From Haines D: Fundamental Neuroscience for Basic and Clinical Applications. Philadelphia, 2006, Elsevier.)

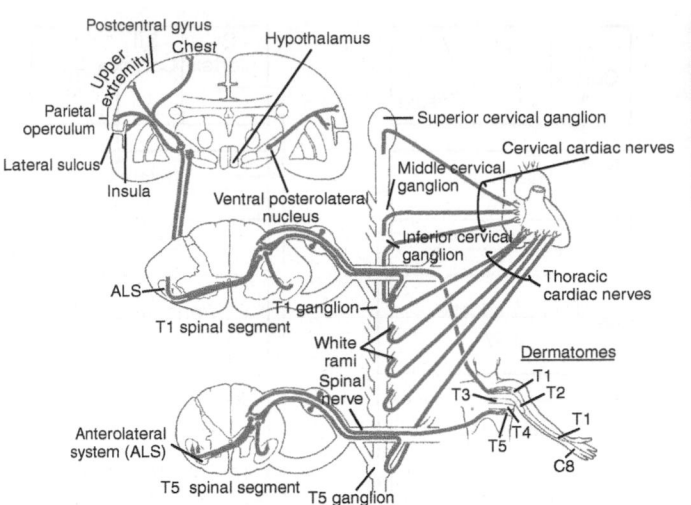

FIGURE I-2-3 The pathways mediating cardiac pain and the circuits through which cardiac pain may be referred to superficial parts of the body wall. (From Haines D: Fundamental Neuroscience for Baisc and Clinical Applications. Philadelphia, 2006, Elsevier.)

interstitial tissues, setting off a sequence of events. For example, substance P (SP) causes mast cells to release histamine; the actions of SP and another neuropeptide, calcitonin gene-related peptide (CGRP), cause vasodilation and increased vascular permeability. In the interstitial space adjacent to blood vessels, bradykinin (BK) is cleaved from kallidin, a plasma protein, and serotonin (5-hydroxytryptamine, 5-HT) and prostaglandins are released from platelets and endothelium, respectively. As a result, a nonnoxious stimulus can result in swelling and increased pain. That is, neurogenic inflammation can be caused by stimulation of nociceptors and the endogenous neuropeptides (SP, CGRP, NK-A) that are released can alter the functions of neighboring immune cells and synovial lining cells. Neurogenic inflammation may be one of the mechanisms involved in neuropathic pain. Likewise, nerve injury or inflammation can induce changes in the nerve and surrounding tissues that can increase our perception of pain (hyperalgesia). When axons are cut, their nociceptors may develop sensitivity to mechanical, chemical, or thermal stimuli. That is, previously nonnoxious stimuli now act as noxious stimuli (allodynia).[28]

WHAT ARE ECTOPIC GENERATORS?

In addition to the changes that can occur at the peripheral nerve terminal with nerve injury, changes can also occur at the dorsal root ganglia, the spinal cord, and higher centers. So-called ectopic generators, which are sites of maladaptive, pathological impulse generation, are most commonly found in the DRG following damage to the axon, soma, or myelin sheath. Ectopia develops over time, resulting in increased neural activity in the endbulbs of cut axons, newly formed sprouts, and the DRG soma. Protein synthesis and delivery are subsequently disrupted. Initially, ectopia develops in large IA (myelinated) fibers (hence the effect of Tinel's sign, characterized by tapping over a nerve and eliciting electric shock-like symptoms, or positive neural tension testing), but eventually C-fibers can be affected. Subsequently, increased central sensitization occurs along with concomitant hyperalgesia and/or allodynia. The ectopic generator neurons begin to fire repetitively and spontaneously; in some cases, increased neuronal firing and an associated pain response is elicited by ischemia, hypoxia, hypoglycemia, temperature, inflammatory mediators (such as prostaglandins, which affect membrane excitability), or simply increasing catecholamine and noradrenergic input, which may be related to the sensory–sympathetic coupling often observed.[11]

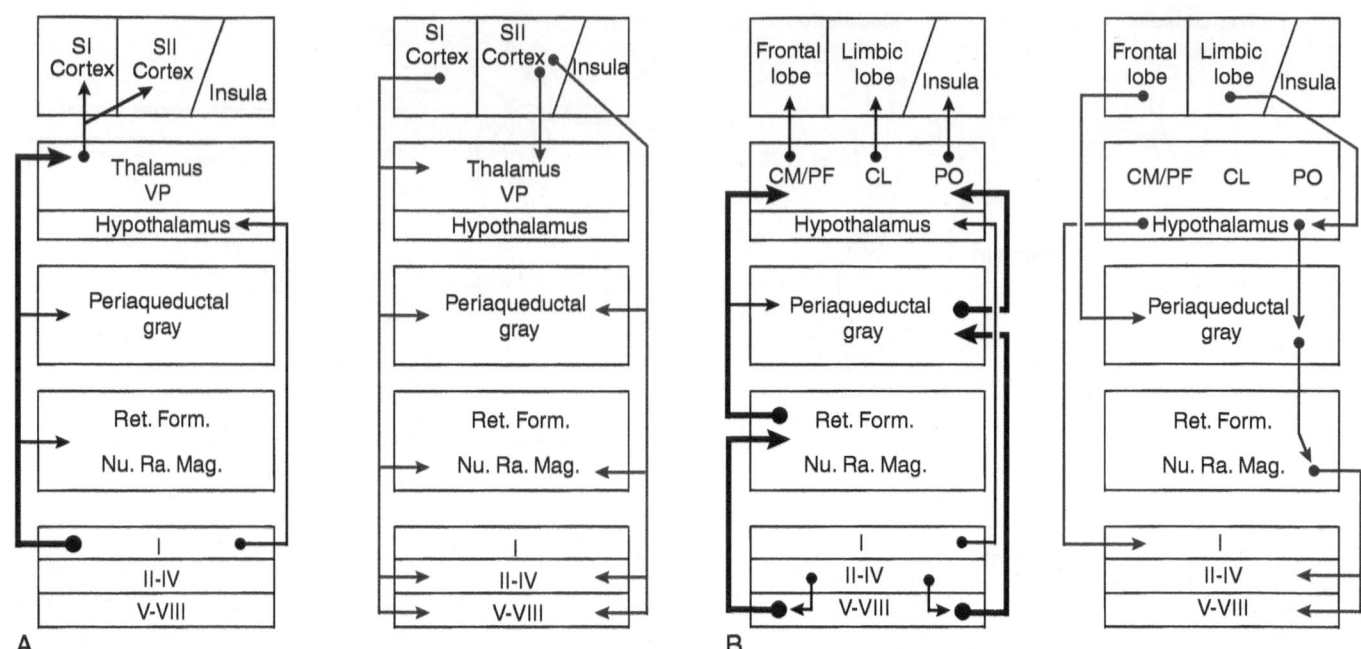

FIGURE I-2-4 Schematic summary of the pathways associated with pain localization (A) and the motivational-affect (B) components of pain perception. Ascending excitatory connections are shown on the left side of each pair of diagrams; descending modulatory connections are shown on the right side of each pair of diagrams. The spinothalamic tract (neospinothalamic tract) inputs influence specific descending modulatory circuits involved with pain localization (A). Spinoreticular and spinomesencephalic tract (paleospinothalamic tract) inputs activate specific descending modulatory circuits involved in motivational-affect components of pain perception (B). CL, central lateral nucleus; CM/PF, centromedian-parafascicular nucleus; Nu. Ra. Mag., nucleus raphe magnus; PO, posterior group of the thalamus; Ret. Form., reticular formation; SI and SII, primary and secondary somatosensory cortices, respectively; VP, ventral posterior nuclei. (From Haines D. *Fundamental Neuroscience for Basic and Clinical Applications.* Philadelphia, PA: Elsevier; 2006.)

> **BOX I-2-1 Neuropeptides Found in Pain Circuitry**[15,28,44]
>
> **Common Neuropeptides**
> Bradykinin (BK), calcitonin gene-related peptide (CGRP), capsaicin, potassium (K+), prostaglandins (PGE_2), serotonin (5-HT), substance P (SP), somatostatin (SOM), neurokinin (NK)-A, galanin, neuropeptide Y, nerve growth factor (NGF), CCK, VIP, bombesin, dyorphin

WHAT ARE OTHER CAUSES OF HYPERALGESIA?

Other causes of hyperalgesia include spinal cord injury, systemic illness, chronic opiate exposure, mechanical stimulation, or tissue injury, which is known to increase the size of sensory receptive fields. With hyperalgesia, levels of glutamate and other excitatory amino acid neurotransmitters may increase whereas levels of inhibitory neurotransmitters (e.g., gamma-aminobutyric acid, GABA) decrease, and changes in levels of several neuropeptides, neurotransmitter transporters, ion channels, scaffolding proteins, receptors, glial cells, and neuroglial interactions are observed.[9]

WHAT CAN CAUSE ALLODYNIA?

Allodynia may be due to decreased response thresholds in C-fibers or less activity in low threshold mechanosensitive Aβ-fibers whose signals are amplified in the spinal cord secondary to central sensitization processes. With sensitization, not only is the perception of painful stimuli increased, but mechanical stimulation of inflamed viscera and deep somatic

tissues can be perceived as painful or joint pain can be increased with weight bearing due to decreased thresholds for mechanoreceptors.[11]

WHAT CAN CAUSE CENTRAL SENSITIZATION?

One factor in the development of central sensitization is the presence of wide dynamic range (WDR) cells in the dorsal horn, predominantly in lamina V, and in the trigeminal nucleus pars caudalis. The WDR cells are considered to be multireceptive and convergent neurons that are activated by both nociceptive and nonnociceptive inputs at sites at which excitatory and inhibitory signals converge. They receive input from Aβ-, Aδ-, and C-fibers and their axons project via spinothalamic and spinoreticular tracts and are involved in polysynaptic reflexes at several levels. The receptive fields for WDR neurons include portions that respond to both nonnoxious stimuli and peripheral areas that respond only to noxious stimuli; in some cases, WDR serve as convergence centers for input coming from skin, muscle, and viscera. With inflammation, peripheral sensitization, or decreased central inhibition, the activity of WDR neurons increases, thereby facilitating central sensitization. The WDR neurons can be inhibited if a large area of the body distant from their receptive fields is stimulated or if descending diffuse noxious inhibitory control (DNIC) fibers from the brainstem are activated.[22]

WHAT IS A REFERRED PAIN PATTERN?[7,14,17,19,33,38,41,44,45]

Clinicians must be familiar with referred pain patterns from the viscera that may initially present as possible musculoskeletal problems. For instance, the shoulder girdle, an area frequently treated in rehabilitation settings, is a common site for referred pain from the viscera and its connective tissue coverings. Some tissues (e.g., muscle, fascia, nerve, disc) may refer pain to surrounding somatic tissues, beyond the area of actual tissue damage. Patients with depression or anxiety disorders may perceive pain in their somatic tissues in the absence of tissue injury or pathology.

The primary focus of this section will be on the mechanisms underlying poorly localized referred pain of visceral origin, with the caveat that much of the phenomenon remains unclear.

WHAT IS THE CAUSE OF REFERRED PAIN?

Difficulty localizing the source of visceral pain may have several causes. Afferent sympathetic autonomic pain fibers, whose cell bodies lie in the thoracic and upper lumbar dorsal root ganglia, travel through rather complex, diffuse routes (e.g., through the cardiac and splanchnic nerves) and the sympathetic ganglia, passing through the gray ramus to reach the spinal cord, hitchhiking along the available segmental spinal nerves, only to enter through both dorsal (lateral fibers) and ventral roots. Central afferent processes may ascend or descend in the cord before synapsing in either laminae I and V or VII and VIII. Inputs from skin, muscle, and viscera can converge on certain WDR interneurons in the spinal cord, thereby blurring the lines between receptive fields. Neuronal pools in the dorsal horn synapse on efferent (presynaptic) sympathetic neurons in the intermediolateral horn and/or give rise to ascending fibers of the ALS/lateral spinothalamic tract (axons from laminae I and V) or the spinoreticular tract (laminae VII and VIII). Generally speaking, the visceral afferents from and visceral efferents to a particular organ enter and exit the cord at the same level. Some ascending fibers project to the VPL of the thalamus, then on to the somatosensory cortex. Others project to brainstem reticular formation nuclei, the PAG of the midbrain, the hypothalamus, the intralaminar thalamic nuclei, then on to diffuse cortical areas. Pelvic viscerosensory information is conveyed via sacral parasympathetic afferents that travel through the pelvic nerve plexuses, sending central processes into the cord via the dorsal and ventral roots to terminate in the dorsal horns, near presynaptic parasympathetic efferent neurons. Ascending information is conveyed much as it is for the ascending sympathetic afferents from the thoracic and abdominal viscera. Additionally, some parasympathetic sensory input from the viscera is conveyed via cranial nerves (VII, IX, X) and their sensory ganglia, where their cell bodies are located, then on to medullary centers (solitary nucleus and tract), and then on to higher centers in the brainstem and cortex.[14,19]

The patterns of referred visceral pain into somatic tissues reflect the use of shared spinal segments (for the affected viscera and overlying somatic tissues); embryological origins of segmental innervations relative to organ development and migration; and convergence of neuronal pools in the spinal cord, brainstem, and higher centers.[14,44,45] Specific visceral pain referral patterns are discussed in the chapter on Clinical Decision Making: Red Flags and Nonmusculoskeletal Pain.

The pathways mediating cardiac pain and the circuits through which cardiac pain travels may be referred to superficial parts of the body walls.

CLINICAL DECISION MAKING CASE STUDY—PATIENT PROFILE **?**

Tiffany is a pleasant, petite, 28-year-old office worker who reports that she has recurring left-sided suboccipital, jaw, neck and thoracic pain (6/10). She has no cardiac risk factors and is an otherwise healthy nonsmoker who exercises at the gym three times per week. Past medical history is positive for a minor cervical hyperflexion/hyperextension (whiplash) injury 1 year ago secondary to a motor vehicle accident. Her current medications

include oral contraceptives, Prozac for depression, and occasional ibuprofen for pain. She drinks two to four alcoholic beverages per week. Her pain is exacerbated by stress, fatigue, and sustained forward head posture with right cervical rotation (the position she sits at her computer). Her pain is at its worst at the end of the day, but decreases with sleep/rest (in a supine position), NSAIDs, and stretching. During the interview, she sits with her head side-bent to the left and rotated right. She denies any radicular signs, peripheral numbness, tingling, or pain into her extremities.

What tissues are the likely sources of her pain? What led you to that conclusion? How might you confirm or refute your hypothesis? Does she have psychological or emotional overlay? Possible central sensitization?

Answer

Musculoskeletal-cervical musculature with possible joint and/or ligamentous involvement; pain is conveyed via the cervical spinal nerves and the trigeminal nerve, the nucleus of which (pars caudalis) is in close proximity to the cervical dorsal gray matter; hence, she may be getting some convergence of signals and referral to her jaw. Gently test active and passive ROM, including accessory or physiological movements and over-pressures, and evaluate soft tissue restrictions, muscle tension/tone, and strength. She may be at risk for developing psychological overlay, but does not seem to be exhibiting worrisome signs of symptom exaggeration or magnification at this point. Her treating psychiatrist should be consulted to determine how well her depression is being controlled and to rule out possible anxiety or fear-avoidance behavior to assist with treatment planning.

WHAT ARE SOME OF THE MECHANISMS OF INJURY (MOI) AND HOW DO THEY RELATE TO PAIN SYMPTOMS?[12,16,17,25,26,31]

Tissues can be injured in many ways. The focus of this section is on injury to musculoskeletal and neuromuscular injuries, rather than injuries to the viscera. Understanding the mechanism of tissue injury can help clinicians determine which tissues are likely damaged, thereby helping direct the processes of making an accurate diagnosis. Many of the musculoskeletal and neuromuscular problems that patients exhibit are the result of some sort of deformation of tissues, either through trauma, overuse, or malalignment. Often, the mechanism of injury may be multifaceted or may change or progress over time. For example, an acute contractile tissue strain (muscle or tendon) may begin as a mechanical deformation, resulting in inflammation, edema, and swelling. The affected individual may subsequently try to find a position of comfort that leads to a secondary postural deformation or may overuse other body parts to compensate for an inability to use the structure that was originally injured. Therefore, the wise clinician will pay attention to which symptoms are primary, secondary, or tertiary and will try to determine cause and effect for the variety of symptoms as they pertain to altered use. As the initially injured tissue heals and transitions to subacute and remodeling phases, new, secondary injuries may surface and present as acute, superimposed on the symptoms specific to the subacute stage of healing.

For long-term symptom resolution, recurrences of tissue injury must be prevented. As a result, clinicians must not only identify and treat their patients' damaged tissues, they must also determine cause and effect to help individuals modify whatever factors contributed to their initial problems. For example, reducing localized inflammation in bursitis may help reduce an individual's symptoms, but unless and until the factors that caused the bursa

TABLE I-2-7   Factors That Contribute to Mechanisms of Injury[16,17,25,26]

Mechanism of Injury	Contributing Factors
Tissue deformation Postural Mechanical Overstretch	Typically involve malalignment or suboptimal alignment of tissues and structures. Fatigue and limited endurance may result in problems even if alignment is adequate. May also be related to abnormal posture or alignment. Can affect either contractile (muscle and/or tendon) or noncontractile tissues (ligament, joint capsule, nerve, connective tissues). Microtrauma to contractile tissues (e.g., sarcomeres and/or surrounding connective tissues; collagen and elastin fibers) or noncontractile tissues (e.g., fascia, nerve, and surrounding connective tissues).
Compression/impingement	Compression of tissues (contractile or noncontractile) can impede localized blood flow and oxygen delivery and/or venous and lymphatic return; can cause direct tissue damage, especially if moving tissues are compressed in a limited space. Edema, swelling, inflammation, and friction may exacerbate this.
Shearing/stress	Load or force and movement applied to tissues may cause tissue damage.
Overuse	May be related to deformation: sustained positions of abnormal alignment may cause some tissues to be overstretched and others shortened or compressed when assuming static postures or carrying out activities (e.g., neck pain secondary to poor ergonomics or body mechanics when sitting at a computer). Repeated motions, particularly in positions of suboptimal length–tension relationships for the involved tissues (e.g., tendinitis/tendinosis resulting from repeated, rapid finger movements while computer keyboarding, particularly if upper extremities are not appropriately positioned or if the movement pattern is suboptimal).
Trauma	Can be direct trauma, such as a sharp blade incising tissue (e.g., lacerations, amputation, incision); blunt trauma/crushing injuries to soft tissues and bone (e.g., motor vehicle accident); sudden mechanical injuries (e.g., spinal hyperextension injury when tackled in football).
Inflammation/edema	Swelling, hemorrhage of affected tissues can lead to secondary tissue injury, including mechanical (e.g., mechanical deformation of joint capsule, pressure from hematoma or blood accumulation in compartment syndrome) and physiological effects (e.g., release of prostaglandins, bradykinins, etc.).

to become inflamed in the first place are identified and corrected, long-term resolution of the symptoms is unlikely. Clinicians whose patients seem to be following a "revolving door" pattern of visits may need to consider altering their approach. Specifically, they should pay more attention to analyzing and correcting the factors that contribute to the development of symptoms and the underlying mechanism of injury (Table I-2-7).

HOW DO I RULE IN/RULE OUT CAUSE OF PAIN?[16,17,25,26]

A key component of the examination process is determining the type and source of pain. Ruling in sources of pain that are beyond the scope of a clinician's practice will help determine the next appropriate step, such as referring to another provider or treating *and* referring. Knowing the acuity, type, and suspected sources of pain will help the clinician determine if the problem is potentially life-threatening (e.g., left shoulder pain due to musculoskeletal problems vs. angina or myocardial infarction).

Using information gleaned from the patient's history (e.g., mechanism of injury, time since symptom onset, comorbidities or history of related problems, sensitivity, 24-hour pain cycle, easing/aggravating factors), a body diagram of pain, and a physical examination (e.g., palpation/localization, biomechanical provocation of pain), the therapist can then generate a working hypothesis for the cause of the symptoms. Follow-up objective testing should confirm the hypothesis, providing that the appropriate tests were selected. In general, normal tissues will not be painful with normal amounts of stress, but pain can be elicited with normal stresses or abnormal stress applied to abnormal tissues or with abnormal, but nondamaging, stress applied to normal tissues.

If the results of a special test are negative when you had hypothesized that a suspected injury would have been ruled in, consider the following factors: (1) Was the test performed correctly? (2) What are the sensitivity and specificity of that particular test? (3) Would a different test be better or more accurate? (4) Did the patient understand and cooperate in a way that would render an accurate outcome? (5) Are the results of the test consistent with the patient's history and mechanism of injury? (6) Was my hypothesis incorrect or should other structures be tested? (Refer to Table I-2-3.)

HOW DOES MY KNOWLEDGE OF THE SOURCE AND TYPE OF PAIN AFFECT TREATMENT?

If the clinician determines that the source and type of pain indicate that treatment is appropriate, the next step is to determine the type, intensity, frequency, and duration of treatment intervention indicated. In the case of pain of musculoskeletal or neuromuscular origin, treatment intervention should target the affected tissue and/or the structures that contribute to the problem. The cause of pain, tissues involved, irritability of the symptoms, and the stage of healing will help determine the appropriate intervention and progression.

When addressing symptoms of pain in the absence of specific tissue pathology (e.g., some chronic pain conditions, pain related to psychogenic or systemic diseases), the focus will be more on the behavioral components of managing pain, while encouraging and facilitating greater function.

As treatment progresses, the clinician must continue to reexamine and reassess the patient's response to intervention, including monitoring signs and symptoms pertaining to pain. Care should be taken to minimize the risk of having acute or subacute pain become chronic or centralized. If the pain is chronic and centralized, focusing on behavioral techniques for pain management (e.g., relaxation training, meditation, guided imagery) and functional gains, rather than overemphasizing pain as the primary indicator of healing or lack thereof, may be necessary.

Some examples of how patients' pain symptoms might influence examination technique and intervention selection include the following:

- Sharp, intense pain associated with recent trauma, such as ligamentous strain: test movements and intervention should be gentle to avoid further irritation/damage; emphasis should be on reducing pain and inflammation.
- Recurring, nagging low back pain secondary to abnormal posture/positioning or certain activities: if the symptoms are latent, test movements may need to be firmer or more sustained to provoke symptoms; if testing provokes referred pain during or after the movement, exercise more caution.
- Radiating shooting pains into the upper extremities, worsening as the work day progresses: this is likely due to nerve compression and/or impingement; it may be related to degeneration of the cervical discs or bony compression of nerve roots and/or poor postural alignment with resultant abnormal muscle shortening or overstretch.
- Diffuse, generalized pain apparently unrelated to (or disproportionate to) tissue injury: relate this to the patient's history [possible central sensitization of chronic pain, neuropathic pain, conversion reaction, psychological (depression, anxiety) or emotional (fear-avoidance behavior) problems?]. It may be necessary to screen with behavioral tests.
- Aches, tingling, and numbness in the feet and legs: check for possible vascular compression or insufficiency or neural compression.

HOW DO HEALING STAGES AFFECT PAIN?[16]

The phases of tissue healing often correspond to changes in pain symptoms—ideally, as healing progresses, pain lessens. In some cases, however, pain may stay constant or intensify. Such a phenomenon is cause for concern, since it may indicate that the pain is becoming centralized and, therefore, at risk for becoming chronic and intractable. Also, the clinician must be mindful of the precautions for the various phases of healing, so as to avoid causing any further tissue damage or disruption, resulting in an unnecessary, unintended increase in the patient's pain. Some guidelines about pain behavior as it pertains to stages of healing are presented below. Keep in mind, however, that the stages of healing overlap.

STAGES OF HEALING

Hemostasis, degeneration, and inflammation (acute) begin within 24 hours of injury and are generally more intense, more easily localized pain for musculoskeletal structures (see Table I-2-8). The pain increases with use or strain on the involved tissues (e.g., pressure, contraction of damaged muscle, elongation of damaged ligament or tendon, movement of fractured bone, compression/shearing of intervertebral discs). The goal is to reduce pain and inflammation and avoid further tissue injury. Under certain circumstances, inflammation can become chronic, which may limit the return of function.

PROLIFERATION AND MIGRATION, REPARATIVE, OR FIBROPLASTIC (ACUTE TO SUBACUTE)

This begins about 2 days postinjury and continues for many weeks (subacute). It helps reestablish the vascular system to damaged tissue, fill gaps, and early scar tissue formation. It is

TABLE I-2-8   Stages of Tissue Healing[16]

Tissue	Timeframe
Muscle	Hemostasis, inflammation (24–48 hours); phagocytosis, myofiber regeneration (6–8 weeks); remodeling, contraction, scar tissue reorganization
Bone (fracture)	Inflammatory phase (1–2 weeks); reparative phase (2–12 weeks); remodeling (months to years)
Peripheral nerve	Approximately 1 mm per day, if sprouting, regeneration occurs
Tendon and ligament	Hemostasis (1–5 days), inflammation (overlaps with hemostasis and proliferative phase); proliferative phase (48 hours–3 weeks); maturation and remodeling (3–16 weeks); may take up to 50 weeks or more to reach full strength
Cartilage	Requires source of matrix, chondrocytes, intact subchondral bone, elimination of joint stresses, otherwise only scar tissue healing

still necessary to protect healing tissues and avoid excessive loads or demands. This is less acutely painful than the hemostasis/inflammatory phases, but can still result in a dull ache. More acute pain is cause for concern and is likely related to tissue damage.

REMODELING PHASE AND MATURATION (CHRONIC)

This can take years. Tissue contraction and regeneration occur and scar tissue is strengthened, remodeled, repaired. If precautions are taken to protect the integrity of the tissue, minimal pain should be evident.

Once tissue damage is healed or the direct source of pain is removed, the perception of pain may persist due to central mechanisms and pathways. The pain pathways involved continue to be stimulated through neural networks (as if "hard wired" for pain sensation). Hyperalgesia (heightened pain perception) or allodynia (pain in the absence of noxious stimuli) may be present in the absence of extrinsic pain-producing factors.

HOW CAN MEDICATION AFFECT PAIN?[8,13,18,30,31,32,34]

Knowing some of the basic pharmacological interventions for pain management and any potential reactions or drug interactions that may be associated with medications for pain or other conditions will assist therapists in their assessment and planning of treatment. The main categories of medications frequently encountered in musculoskeletal rehabilitation are nonsteroidal antiinflammatory drugs NSAIDs, opioid analgesics, muscle relaxants, and local anesthetics. Patients suffering from chronic pain also may be on antidepressants and those with neuropathic pain may be on anticonvulsant medications that facilitate inhibitory (i.e., GABA-ergic) neural circuits. Although a comprehensive review of pharmacology is beyond the scope of this chapter, a few key points can be made (see Table I-2-9).

Most noninflammatory arthritis and deep joint pain can be treated effectively with acetaminophen.

In summary, the clinician should be aware of the patient's medications, medication schedule, and potential drug interactions and potential side effects.

TABLE I-2-9	Common Medications for Musculoskeletal or Neuromuscular Pain[8]	
Condition	**Example**	**Mechanism**
Inflammation	NSAIDs: Aspirin, Ibuprofen, Naproxen	Cyclooxygenase inhibitors block prostaglandin synthesis
Muscle spasm	Sedative-hypnotic (e.g., Diazepam)	GABA agonist
	Cyclobenzaprine (e.g., Flexeril)	Polysynaptic inhibitor
Chronic or neuropathic pain	Anticonvulsants (e.g., Gabapentin/Neurontin)	GABA agonist
	Tricyclic antidepressants	Inhibits 5-HT, NE reuptake
	Barbiturates (e.g., Phenobarbital)	GABA agonist; Cl$^-$ influx
	Benzodiazepines (e.g., Valium)	GABA agonist; Cl$^-$ influx
	Local anesthetics (e.g., Lidocaine)	Decreased membrane Na$^+$ permeability
	Antidepressants	Blocks monoamine reuptake
	Tricyclics (e.g., Elavil)	Blocks biogenic amine metabolism
	MAOI (e.g., Nardil, Parnate)	Inhibits serotonin reuptake
	SSRI (e.g., Prozac, Zoloft, Paxil)	Opiate agonist
	Opioid analgesics (Oxycodone, Fentanyl)	

GABA, gamma-aminobutyric acid; 5-HT, 5-hydroxytryptamine (serotonin); NE, norepinephrine; MAOI, monoamine oxidase inhibitor; SSRI, selective serotonin reuptake inhibitor.

REFERENCES

1. Apkarian A. Human brain mechanism of pain perception and regulation in health and disease. *Eur J of Pain*. 2005;9:464-484.
2. Attal N, Fermanian C, Fermanian J, et al. Neuropathic pain: Are there distinct subtypes depending on the aetiology or anatomical lesion? *Pain*. 2008;Mar 4 (Epub ahead of print).
3. Aurilio C, Pota V, Pace MC, et al. Ionic channels and neuropathic pain: physiopathology and applications. *J Cell Physiol*. 2008;215:8-14.
4. Baron R. Peripheral neuropathic pain: from mechanisms to symptoms. *Clin J Pain*. 2000;16:(suppl): S12-S20.
5. Bird G, Han J, Fu Y, Adwanikar H, et al. Pain-related synaptic plasticity in spinal dorsal horn neurons: role of CGRP. *Mol Pain*. 2006;2:31.
6. Cavero S, Bonicalzi V. Central pain syndrome: elucidation of genesis and treatment. *Expert Rev Neurother*. 2007;7:1485-1497.
7. Cervero F. Pathophysiology of referred pain and hyperalgesia from viscera. In: Vecchiet L, Albe-Fessard D, Lindblom U, Giamberardino M, eds. *New Trends in Referred Pain and Hyperalgesia*. Elsevier; 1993:35-46.
8. Ciccone C. *Pharmacology in Rehabilitation*. 4th ed. Philadelphia, PA:: FA Davis; 2007.
9. Coderre TJ. Spinal cord mechanisms of hyperalgesia and allodynia. In: Basbaum A, Bushnell M, eds. *Science of Pain*. Boston, MA: Elsevier; 2009:339-380.
10. Craig AD. Pain mechanisms: labeled lines vs. convergence in central processing. *Annu Rev Neurosci*. 2003;26:1-30.
11. Devor M. Ectopic generators. In: Basbaum A, Bushnell M, eds. *Science of Pain*. Boston, MA: Elsevier; 2009:83-88.
12. Dhesi S, Hurley R. The neurobiology of pain. In: Satterthwaite J, Tollison J, eds. *Practical Pain Management*. Philadelphia, PA: Williams and Wilkins; 2002:10-25.
13. Dworkin RH, O'Connor AB, Backonja M, Farrar JT, et al. Pharmacologic management of neuropathic pain: evidence-based recommendations. *Pain*. 2007;132:237-251.
14. Gebhart G, Bielefeldt K. Visceral pain. In: Basbaum A, Bushnell M, eds. *Science of Pain*. Boston, MA: Elsevier; 2009:543-569.
15. Gold M, Caterina M. Molecular biology of the nociceptor/transduction. In: Basbaum A, Bushnell M, eds. *Science of Pain*. Boston, MA: Elsevier; 2009:43-75.
16. Goodman C, Boissonnault W, Fuller K, eds. *Pathology: Implications for the Physical Therapist*. 2nd ed. Philadelphia, PA: Saunders; 2003.
17. Goodman C, Snyder T. Pain types and viscerogenic pain patterns. In: *Differential Diagnosis for Physical Therapists: Screening for Referral*. 4th ed. St Louis, MO: Saunders; 2007:110-178.
18. Guindon J, Walczak JS, Beaulieu P. Recent advances in the pharmacological management of pain. *Drugs*. 2007;67:2121-2133.
19. Hardy S, Naftel J. Viscerosensory pathways. In: Haines D, ed. *Fundamental Neuroscience for Basic and Clinical Applications*. 3rd ed. Philadelphia, PA: Churchill Livingstone Elsevier; 2006: 302-310.
20. Julius D. Molecular mechanism of nociception. *Nature*. 2001;413: 203-210.
21. Katz WA, Rothenberg R. Section 3: The nature of pain: pathophysiology. *J Clin Rheumatol*. 2005;11:S11-S15.
22. Le Bars D. What is a wide-dynamic range cell? In: Basbaum A, Bushnell M, eds. *Science of Pain*. Boston, MA: Elsevier; 2009:331-338.
23. Lewin G. Mechanosensation and pain. *J Neurobiol*. 2004;61:30-44.
24. Lima D. Ascending pathways: anatomy and physiology. In: Basbaum A, Bushnell M, eds. *Science of Pain*. Boston, MA: Elsevier; 2009:477-526.
25. Maitland G, Mengeveld E, Banks K, English K. *Maitland's Vertebral Manipulation*. 6th ed. Auckland, NA: Butterworth Heinemann; 2001:112-185.
26. McKenzie RA. *The Lumbar Spine: Mechanical Diagnosis and Therapy*. Spinal Publications; 1981.
27. Melzack R, Coderre T, Katz J, Vaccarino A. Central neuroplasticity and pathological pain. *Ann NY Acad Sci*. 2001;933:157-174.
28. Mense A. Anatomy of nociceptors. In: Basbaum A, Bushnell M, eds. *Science of Pain*. Boston, MA: Elsevier; 2009:11-41.
29. Millan M. The Induction of Pain: An Integrative Review. *Prog Neurobiol*. 1999;57:1-164.
30. Munir MA, Enany N, Zhang JM. Nonopioid analgesics. *Anesthesiol Clin*. 2007;254:761-774.
31. Phillips WJ, Currier BL. Analgesic pharmacology: I. Neurophysiology. *J Am Acad Orthop Surg*. 2004;124:213-220.
32. Raffa R. Pharmacological aspects of successful long-term analgesia. *Clin Rheumatol*. 2006;25:(suppl 1): S9-S15.
33. Schlereth T, Birklein F. The sympathetic nervous system and pain. *Neuromolecular Med*. 2007; Nov 8 (Epub ahead of print).
34. Schnitzer TJ. Update on guidelines for the treatment of chronic musculoskeletal pain. *Clin Rheumatol*. 2006;25:(suppl 1):S22-S29.
35. Shehab S, Al-Marashda K, Al-Zahmi A, et al. Unmyelinated primary afferents from adjacent spinal nerves intermingle in the spinal dorsal horn: possible mechanism contributing to neuropathic pain. *Brain Res*. 2008;Mar 10 (Epub ahead of print).
36. Slipman C, Plastaras C, Patel R. Provocative cervical discography symptom mapping. *Spine J*. 2005;5:381-388.
37. Sorkin LS, Wallace MS. Acute pain mechanisms. *Surg Clin North Am*. 1999;79:213-229.
38. Standing S. *Gray's Anatomy: The Anatomical Basis of Clinical Practice*. 39th ed. New York, NY: Elsevier Churchill Livingstone; 2005.
39. Tavares I, Lima D. From neuroanatomy to gene therapy: searching for new ways to manipulate the supraspinal endogenous pain modulatory system. *J Anat*. 2007;211:261-268.

40. Ueda H. Peripheral mechanisms of neuropathic pain-involvement of lysophosphatidic acid receptor-mediated demyleination. *Mol Pain.* 2008;4(1):11 Ebup ahead of print.

41. Wall P. Neurophysiological mechanisms of referred pain and hyperalgesia. In: Vecchiet L, Albe-Fessard D, Lindblom U, Giamberardino M, eds. *New Trends in Referred Pain and Hyperalgesia.* Elsevier; 1993:3-11.

42. Wang J, Chang J, Woodward D, et al. Corticofugal influences on thalamic neurons during nociceptive transmission in awake rats. *Synapse.* 2007;61:335-342.

43. Wang J, Zhang H, Chang H, et al. Differential modulation of nociceptive neural responses in medial and lateral pain pathways by peripheral electrical stimulation: a multichannel recording study. *Brain Res.* 2004;1014:197-208.

44. Warren S, Yezierski R, Capra N. The somatosensory system II: touch, thermal sense, and pain. In: Haines D, ed. *Fundamental Neuroscience for Basic and Clinical Applications.* 3rd ed. Philadelphia, PA: Churchill Livingstone Elsevier; 2006:280-301.

45. Willis W, Westlund K. Dorsal columns and visceral pain. In: Basbaum A, Bushnell M, eds. *Science of Pain.* Boston, MA: Elsevier; 2009:527-543.

46. Zimmermann M. Pathobiology of neuropathic pain. *Eur J Pharmacol.* 2001;429:23-37.

Section I

FOUNDATIONAL KNOWLEDGE

AUTHOR: ROSS BIEDERMAN

INTRODUCTORY INFORMATION

The need for radiological skills, both to integrate the radiologist's report into therapy planning and to directly read imaging films, has become vital within rehabilitation medicine. It is often simply not possible to completely explore subtleties of various pathologies without visualizing the involved anatomy and pathology. Additionally, the therapist must be aware that misinterpretation of radiographic images is a common source of error in both inpatient and outpatient treatment. In response, analogous to monitoring of pharmacotherapy, it is incumbent upon the clinician to acquire sufficient diagnostic imaging skills to both translate the radiologist's report into clinical planning and confirm findings for integration into the treatment design.

WHAT TYPES OF IMAGING ARE MOST COMMONLY SEEN IN REHABILITATION CLINICS?

Diagnostic imaging now includes a complex array of imaging techniques, any of which may be presented to the practitioner for review and analysis. The most common imaging modalities encountered in private practice are plain film radiography, magnetic resonance imaging, and computerized tomography. Each of these diagnostic techniques has specific indications and protocols for selection based on their relative abilities to display a particular anatomy and pathology.

PLAIN FILM RADIOGRAPHY

WHY AND WHEN IS PLAIN FILM RADIOLOGY UTILIZED?

Due to its broad availability, relative affordability, and wealth of useful information, displayed plain film radiography remains the first-line imaging tool for most patient pathologies treated within rehabilitation clinics. X-ray images are excellent for assessment of
- bone structures and relationships
- biomechanical assessment
- bone deformity
- arthritic disorders
- fractures and staging of fracture healing
- metabolic disorders
- avascular necrosis
- bone tumors

WHEN IS PLAIN FILM RADIOLOGY NOT THE MOST APPROPRIATE IMAGING STUDY TO USE?

X-rays are much less capable of producing contrast and detail in soft tissue structures and are not used for detailed stand-alone studies of muscle, capsule, or ligamentous pathologies. All soft tissues have very similar grayish appearance on x-ray and thin or small structures such as a ligament, tendon, or capsule are generally not visible at all. Caution is advised when assessing soft tissue with plain films due to limited visibility.

ARE THERE ANY SOFT TISSUE STRUCTURES THAT WILL APPEAR ON AN X-RAY?

If the structure is very thick (e.g., heart, liver, muscle) or pathologically calcific (e.g., heterotopic ossification or bone callus), or if substantial edema is present, it may be radiologically visible. The addition of edema or hematoma is frequently seen simply as a vague cloudiness.

CAN X-RAYS DETECT STRESS FRACTURES?

A clinical note regarding the evaluation of stress fractures should be made in light of the limited ability of x-ray images to demonstrate soft tissues. During the inflammatory phase of bone healing only hematoma, fibrous hematoma, and inflammatory products are present within a fracture site, none of which is visible on plain film x-ray. A high index of suspicion must be maintained, even if no osseous abnormality is visible on x-ray, when evaluating a patient with clinical evidence of stress fracture. Histologically, fibrous callus, which is not radiographically visible, begins calcium deposition and ossification at about 10 to 14 days postinjury, then becoming *bone* callus, which is radiographically visible. Bone callus is the confirming, and often the only, evidence of stress fracture. Bone callus formation (also termed *periosteal bone formation*) first appears at 10 to 14 days postinjury with a vague, cloudy, cotton ball-like appearance at the cortical edges of the involved bone. Visible periosteal new bone on x-ray is evidence of reactive bone formation whether related to fracture healing or to pathologies such as infection or bone tumor. The evaluating therapist should request repeat films at about 2 weeks posttrauma to confirm or rule out stress fracture and, based on clinical presentation, rule out red flag findings.

HOW CAN X-RAYS BE UTILIZED TO DIAGNOSE SOFT TISSUE INJURIES?

Commonly a soft tissue injury is diagnosed indirectly by noting if resultant edema displaces adjacent structures rather than by direct observation of the injured structure. Increased visibility of fascial planes produced by spread of edema, altered density produced by hemorrhage, or fat displacement caused by bleeding, are signs that a soft tissue injury may be present. Magnetic resonance imaging (MRI) fills this gap by being almost the opposite in image characteristics. MRI is excellent for detailed observation and the study of soft tissues but is somewhat less adept at revealing bone tissue detail.

HOW ARE X-RAY IMAGES GENERATED?

Plain film x-ray images owe their appearance and diagnostic value to the ability of x-ray particles to differentially penetrate body tissues of varying (molecular) density. The differences in tissue density and resultant x-ray beam penetration produce the most important characteristics of the image: contrast (the difference between densities of adjacent tissues) and recorded detail (clarity and resolution) on x-ray images. X-ray images might be more descriptively termed *densograms* given that the black to white gray scale seen on x-ray is not a photographic feature but a representation of tissue density. Low-density tissues such as lung or fat tend to allow x-ray particles to traverse the body nearly unimpeded and strike the x-ray film plate resulting in high adhesion of the film emulsion to the cellulose plate resulting in a dark or black coloration.

High-density structures such as bone are more likely to attenuate x-ray particles leaving few to strike the film plate. Little or no emulsion therefore adheres to the film plate during processing, leaving clear or nearly clear areas on the cellulose film plate that appear white or whitish in color.

THE GRAY SCALE

WHAT IS TISSUE RADIODENSITY?

It becomes apparent that the black–gray–white color scale observed on an x-ray film is a direct representation of tissue density. Both normal structures and pathological changes are identified by their characteristic tissue density, or in radiological context, *radiodensity*.

Tissue radiodensity is formally defined by the "gray scale," which includes four named tissue densities: air, fat, water/organ or mid-density, and bone density. These terms are properly used nomenclature; the film reader refers to a black region of the film as "low density" or "air density," a mid-gray area as "water density," and white or whitish areas as "high density" or "air density" as

TABLE I-3-1 Gray Scale and Tissue Density

Lowest Density Air Black	Low Density Fat Dark Gray	"Neutral" or Water Density Mid-Gray	Moderate Density Mineral Light Gray	High Density Heavy Metals White
Lungs Trachea Bowel Thin fat Thin connecting tissue Adipose	Thicker adipose, multiple layers of thin tissue, osteoporotic bone	Muscle, tendon, thin bones, overlapping soft tissues, blood, vasculature	Cancellous bone, thin cortical thick muscle, tendon, organ tissues, superimposition of thin soft tissues, large blood vessels	Thick cortical bone, dental fillings, jewelry, orthopedic hardware, zippers and buttons

appropriate. In orthopedic imaging two additional densities are recognized: metal density (orthopaedic hardware) and contrast media, such as used in arthography. Table I-3-1 illustrates tissue densities and their gray scale appearance on x-ray film plates.

WHICH TISSUES APPEAR DARKER IN X-RAYS AND WHICH TISSUES APPEAR WHITER?

On the left side of Table I-3-1 are the less dense tissues: air and fat. Low-density tissues appear as black or dark gray on the film and are referred to as lucent, radiolucent, or demonstrating lucency. The lung field on a chest x-ray, for example, is normally lucent (blackish) with vascular structures and airway walls showing slightly greater density and appearing as light shades of gray. Radiolucent areas of the body appear black or dark gray because many, or most, x-ray photons emitted by the x-ray machine have penetrated the tissue, emerged from the body without deflection or attenuation, and impacted the photosensitive emulsion of the film plate to produce a recorded image. On the right side of the table are the more dense tissues that produce a light gray to white appearance on the film plate.

SUPERIMPOSITION AND DENSITY

HOW IS TISSUE RADIODENSITY PRODUCED?

Radiodensity may be produced in two different ways, either by tissues that actually are dense or by superimposing or stacking multiple structures in the path of the x-ray beam creating the appearance of density. Normal bone, of course, is radiodense and appears so on film. However, multiple soft tissues in the path of the x-ray beam also create the appearance of *density*.[7] This is apparent in a myriad of anatomic regions on any normal film examined: where ever multiple structures are aligned with the x-ray beam the appearance of increased density will be produced on the film. Sufficiently thick air, fat, or water can create the appearance of greater density, at times equal to bone. In each case the film reader must make the distinction between true regions of radiodensity that may be pathological versus illusionary regions of density created by superimposed structures.

CLINICAL PEARL

(!)

A firm understanding and knowledge base of anatomy and structural relationships are vital in the interpretation of any radiographic image.

CLINICAL EXAMPLE – SUPERIMPOSITION

An anterior-to-posterior view of the right shoulder will demonstrate an opaque region in the axilla. Knowledge of anatomy suggests this is superimposition of the anterior and posterior axillary folds composed of mid-density muscle and low-density fat, which together create an area of density equal to that of the medullary humerus and exceeding that seen at the scapular fossa. Such findings must be cor-

rectly identified as the superimposition of normal anatomy and excluded from the differential diagnosis. If no anatomic explanation is available pathology may then be considered.

HOW CAN A TWO-DIMENSIONAL IMAGE REFLECT THREE-DIMENSIONAL STRUCTURES?

Another consideration is that x-ray images depict three-dimensional anatomic structures in two dimensions only. The clinician's knowledge of anatomy serves to reconstruct a three-dimensional impression from the two-dimensional images allowing understanding and interpretation. For example, when studying an anterior-posterior (AP) view of the shoulder, anterior, intermediate, and posterior structures are superimposed and depth—the anterior-posterior anatomic relationships—is not differentiated by the film. The AP view superimposes all structures aligned with the beam direction and therefore presents only coronal plane relationships. Similarly, a lateral view of the knee superimposes the lateral and medial aspects of the femur and tibia and does not allow a medial–lateral orientation.

Additionally, superimposition of three-dimensional structures into a two-dimensional film image can sometimes create odd shapes and forms on the film image. When evaluating the thoracic spine on a PA (or AP) film the anterior ribs are superimposed on the posterior ribs, creating alternating regions of density and opacity seen as boxes and rectangles in a scotch-plaid pattern. The plaid configuration, of course, does not exist anatomically; it is a product of superimposition created by the x-ray image production process. The clinician's knowledge of anatomy is therefore the foundation of the recognition and interpretation of both normal and abnormal findings.

Superimposition has been discussed as the source of radiographic distortion and considerable potential error in film reading. To avoid this, the film reader must consider the effects of superimposition on radiodensity and structural morphology before entertaining the possibility of pathology. If a change in radiodensity or tissue relationships cannot be explained anatomically only then should pathology be considered.

ALGORITHMS OF FILM READING: X-RAY VIEWS

An x-ray film, like a painting or photograph, has a tendency to naturally draw the observer's eyes to specific shapes and regions of interest. An obvious fracture or presence of orthopaedic hardware attracts immediate attention and may so dominate the film that it causes the viewer to miss more subtle findings. Experienced artists develop organized search patterns when observing a painting or photograph. Similarly clinicians with radiological experience tend to employ orderly search patterns or algorithms of film study to avoid missing subtle features that may be obscured by the obvious. Radiologists wryly suggest, "studying the boring stuff first". By training yourself to examine every feature of the film—no matter how tedious—and not allow distraction by points of high interest helps avoid missing a finding or "under-calling" the film. Another search method is the "ABCS" technique. This search pattern employs a step-by-step process of study.

A: alignment and architecture of bones

B: bone density

C: cartilage, joint space thickness and regularity

S: soft tissues, morphology, density, normal or abnormal appearance

The film reader explores every aspect of each bone and soft tissue structure in an ABCS order. Both methods are helpful and the reader is encouraged to practice and employ a thorough search pattern as a means of minimizing the risk of missing important features.

HOW SHOULD A CLINICIAN DETERMINE WHICH X-RAY VIEWS ARE NECESSARY?

Plain film x-ray films are studied on the basis of views or projections. X-ray views are ordered with consideration toward what anatomic region or structure is being studied and what view best demonstrates that structure. As a result, there are advantages and disadvantages associated with each x-ray view depending on the structure or pathology of interest. The entry–exit route of the x-ray beam determines and describes different x-ray views with each view specifically designed to demonstrate particular aspects of anatomy. The x-ray beam angle, area of projection, and final film are defined by radiological convention so that a given view, no matter where obtained, will present the same anatomy from the same perspective. A ready familiarity with common views (including multiple names used for the some views) and the normal anatomy displayed—or not displayed—by a specific x-ray view is of critical importance to the clinician. An understanding of views also allows the therapist to use a myriad of lines, measurements and angles employed in radiography for detailed and quantifiable evaluation of bone relationships.

HOW SHOULD A CLINICIAN ORDER X-RAYS?

Plain film studies may be ordered by individually specifying the desired views or projections, or, more commonly, as a "study." Specific views included within a particular study are fairly standardized and incorporate those views known to best present the anatomic region of interest. The clinician's request for films should include a diagnosis, preliminary diagnosis, or "rule out" and request for a study of the area of concern. In addition to the standard or routine views, "special views" are employed, when needed, by the radiology technician to better exhibit specific areas or potential diagnoses not readily revealed by standard views. There are hundreds of routine and special views employed in plain film radiography. The clinician is best served by focusing attention on the common views included within routine studies, and exploring special views as they are encountered in practice.

WHAT ARE THE MOST COMMON ROUTINE STUDIES AND VIEWS FOR EACH BODY REGION?

- Foot: AP, lateral, oblique (usually medial oblique)
- Leg: AP, lateral, mortise, oblique
- Knee: AP, lateral, sunrise or patellofemoral axial view, tunnel or notch view
- Hip: AP, frog-leg lateral
- Lumbar spine and pelvis: AP, lateral, coned down lateral, right and left posterior oblique
- Sacroiliac joints: AP axial plus lumbar spine projections
- Chest/thoracic spine: PA, lateral
- Shoulder: AP, AP internal rotation, AP external rotation, lateral view of scapula
- Elbow: AP, lateral, oblique, internal or external
- Wrist, hand, or digits: PA, lateral, oblique
- Cervical spine: AP, open-mouth, or dens/odontoid view, lateral, right and left posterior oblique

X-RAY VIEW NOMENCLATURE

AP views (see Figure I-3-1) project the x-ray beam in an anterior-to-posterior direction and are among the most common views of both axial and appendicular structures seen clinically.

DP (dorsal-planta or dorsal-palmar) views of the foot and hand are the same as AP views.

PA views are produced by projecting the x-ray beam in a posterior-to-anterior direction and are less commonly utilized than the AP projection. PA views are, however, the standard projection for study of the hand, wrist, and routine chest films. Hand PA views may also be referred to as dorsal-volar projections. Both AP and PA views present coronal plane relationships and superimpose anterior–posterior structures.

Lateral views (see Figure I-3-2) are obtained by projecting the x-ray beam through the anatomic region of interest either in a lateral-to-medial (e.g., elbow) or medial-to-lateral direction (e.g., knee). In either case the view is simply termed a *lateral view* without the need to identify the beam direction. Lateral views demonstrate sagittal plane relationships but superimpose left and right side structures. When obtaining a lateral view of the trunk, cervical, thoracic, or lumbar spine the patient is usually positioned so that the beam enters the patient's right side and exits the left. This may, as with the extremities, be simply termed a "lateral" view as it is the standard projection or, at times, a *left* lateral view if a *right* lateral view is also being obtained. In large/thick body regions such as the thorax a left or right beam direction will produce a somewhat different appearance due to *enlargement*, the spreading of the x-ray beam in flashlight beam fashion as it traverses the body. The body part nearest the beam source will appear largest on the x-ray film thus giving the left and right lateral views a slightly different appearance that can be helpful in the evaluation of subtle pathology.

Oblique projections (see Figures I-3-4 and I-3-5) are obtained with the body region rotated 45° between an AP/PA and lateral view position. An oblique view of the wrist, for example, positions the patient's wrist, ulnar side down on the film plate, and rotated internally 45°. Some confusion exists regarding oblique views due to the variation in orientation of both the patient and beam angle that may occur when setting up the view. Common variants include the ankle oblique view, most commonly taken with the ankle rotated 15 to 18° internal to reveal the talofibular and talotibial joint surfaces. This view is technically called the *mortise view* but in practice is commonly referred to as an oblique view. Oblique views of the elbow can be obtained either by rotating the arm internally or externally.

Spinal oblique views in particular generate confusion as to what anatomic structures are displayed. Understanding precisely what is being seen on spinal oblique films is of particular importance to physical therapists because each of these views reveals not only relevant clinical and potential "red flag" findings but does so with left or right side specificity. Part of the interpretation problem is that oblique projections of the *cervical* spine use the same naming scheme but demonstrate different structures than do *lumbar* oblique views. Cervical spine oblique views are typically used to evaluate intervertebral foramina whereas lumbar oblique projections evaluate posterior vertebral elements.

Spinal oblique views are named in relation to the body region in contact with the x-ray table, which then corresponds to the left or right side of structures being displayed. If the patient first lies supine, then rotates his or her body 45° to the left so that the right side is rotated up and off the table (supported by a wedged foam positioning pad), the posterior vertebral elements of the left side are nearest the film plate and are demonstrated on the view. The view is therefore termed a left posterior oblique (LPO) view. When shooting a right posterior oblique (RPO) view the patient rotates to the right and the raised left side is supported with a foam wedge. The posterior oblique views demonstrate ipsilateral zygapophysial joints, pedicles, and pars interarticularis. On the film the body of the vertebrae will be appear rotated 45° and face or point to the side, right or left, of the structures being studied. The ala of the ipsilateral side will appear in "broadside" view on the film whereas the contralateral side is seen virtually end-on.

Usually posterior rather than anterior oblique views are performed as part of a routine cervical or lumbar study. If warranted, anterior oblique views (right and left anterior oblique) can also be included in a lumbar study but are much less frequently encountered than posterior oblique views. Oblique projection radiographs must be properly labeled, e.g., RPO, LPO, RAO, and LAO, for a proper study. At times a different labeling nomenclature may be encountered in which oblique projections are termed an AP oblique. This is an anterior-posterior beam direction so is the same as a posterior oblique. The L or R labels assist in discerning which AP oblique view is being viewed. By convention the right or left label (the letter R or L) is placed opposite the side of the spine being studied. A right posterior oblique image will have the "R" placed anterior to the spine whereas a right anterior oblique image will have the "R" place posterior to the spine. It is very difficult if not impossible to distinguish right from left oblique views if they are not labeled. Films labeled or described in texts simply as an "oblique" view are customarily posterior oblique views.

Lumbar spinal oblique views are useful for assessing the facet joints and the posterior spinal elements. Structures revealed by specific oblique views are not intuitive: using a skeletal model to visualize vertebral structures in relation to the x-ray beam angle is helpful. In the RPO position the patient's vertebrae are rotated approximately 45° to the right bringing the right pedicles, facet joints, and pars interarticularis into view. You are in essence looking through the right pedicle and facet joint surfaces. With the patient in the lumbar RPO or LPO position, the posterior elements of the ipsilateral side are studied and in the RAO and LAO position the contralateral posterior elements are studied.[7] Table I-3-2 lists the anatomic structures studied on specific oblique views.

Oblique views visualize the inferior-superior articular facets, pedicles, and pars interarticularis. These are the elements of the celebrated "Scotty dog" sign of Lachapele. The superimposed left and right posterior vertebral structures—with a little imagination—actually do resemble a Scotty dog in side view. The ear, eye, neck, back tail, and legs of the dog are superimposed posterior spinal structures viewed at an oblique angle and creating the likeness. Figure I-3-1 illustrates the Scotty dog appearance created by superimposed vertebral structures. The beauty of the Scotty dog representation is the ease with which it allows study of the lumbar spine posterior elements.

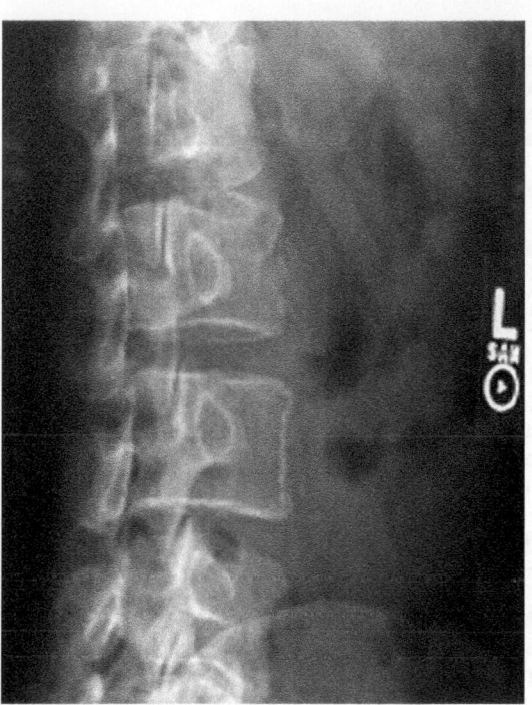

FIGURE I-3-1 Scotty dog fracture.

CLINICAL EXAMPLE – THE ANATOMIC CORRELATIONS OF THE SCOTTY GO SIGN

- Nose: transverse process
- Eye: pedicle
- Ear: superior articulating process
- Neck: pars interarticularis
- Front leg: inferior articular process of the studied vertebral body
- Rear leg: inferior articular process, opposite side, of the vertebral body

Note that on *cervical* spine oblique views the side studied is reversed: a cervical spine RPO demonstrates the left (contralateral) intervertebral foraminal structures whereas anterior oblique views display the right (ipsilateral) foramina junction.[5]

CLINICAL PEARL

Awareness and recognition of common sources of interpretation error, particularly the effects of superimposed structures on radiodensity and image appearance, are essential first steps in film interpretation.

WHAT COMMON SPECIAL VIEWS ARE UTILIZED IN REHABILITATION SETTINGS?

There are numerous *special* views, many of which are rarely seen in private practice. Several, however, are particularly valuable to the clinician and therefore are worth noting and/or requesting as part of the initial evaluation and outcome assessment. For instance, the AP of the cervical spine poorly displays the superior vertebral bodies due to superimposition of the mandible and dentition. An odontoid or "open mouth" view (taken just as it sounds) is normally included in a cervical study to allow clear visualization of the superior vertebrae. Lateral views of the cervical spine may be obtained in flexion or extension to evaluate

TABLE I-3-2 Anatomical Structures Studied on Oblique Views

Lumbar Oblique Projection	Anatomy Studied
Left posterior oblique	Left pars and zygapophysial joints
Right posterior oblique	Right pars and zygapophysial joints
Left anterior oblique	Right pars and zygapophysial joints
Right anterior oblique	Left pars and zygapophysial joints
Cervical Oblique Projection	**Anatomy Studied**
Left posterior oblique	Right foramina
Right posterior oblique	Left foramina
Left anterior oblique	Left foramina
Right anterior oblique	Right foramina

position-related symptoms or boney limitations of motion. The swimmer's view will be seen by therapists, especially post trauma, for visualization of the inferior cervical spine without both shoulders superimposed.

Other shoulder views of note to therapists include the West Point view for visualization of Hill–Sachs lesions. Frog leg views of the hip joint allow evaluation of femoral–acetabular relationships with the femur abducted and externally rotated. A knee view gaining some commentary in the physical therapy literature is the notch or tunnel view. This PA view, obtained with the patient standing and knee flexed 45°, is considered to be of particular value in assessing degenerative arthritic changes of the knee joint. The notch view is an example of weight-bearing, or standing, views. In particular, when assessing spinal and lower extremity structures, weight-bearing films should be considered routine by the physical therapist for assessment of closed chain kinematic relationships that are not displayed by standard non-weight-bearing images.

ARTHROGRAPHY

WHAT IS ARTHOGRAPHY AND WHEN IS IT USED?

Because soft tissues (muscle, tendon, capsule, organs, blood vessels) produce nearly the same radiodensity on plain film x-ray a way of distinguishing these tissues from their surroundings is sometimes necessary. Conventional arthrography is plain film x-ray technology combined with contrast enhancement for a more detailed assessment of joint injury and pathology. Contrast media (iodinated contrast material, a radiopaque dye) with or without air is injected into the joint to be studied. Air may be used alone or in combination with radiopaque dyes to enhance contrast. X-ray images obtained will demonstrate either localization of contrast material within the joint capsule indicating no leakage into adjacent regions, or spread of dye out of the capsule and contiguous structures in which case anatomic features and regions of injury are brought into sharp contrast by the presence of high-density contrast media. Arthrography is useful for the study of capsule, ligament, and tendon pathologies such as rotator cuff tears, meniscus injury of the knee, and ligamentous injury at the wrist, and in the evaluation of painful joint prosthesis. Conventional arthrography has been largely replaced by computerized tomography (CT), MRI, and MR arthrography.[8]

A second type of arthrography is MRI rather than x-ray. MR arthrography is performed by injection of a paramagnetic agent into the joint before MRI examination. MRI arthrography displays tears of cartilage, ligaments, and tendons more clearly than does conventional arthrography technique.[4]

MAGNETIC RESONANCE IMAGING

WHAT IS AN MRI?

Plain film x-ray is poor at revealing distinction or detail within mid-density structures including ligaments, tendons, muscle, and capsule that may be of primary focus to the physical therapist. This is a significant diagnostic weakness of x-ray images and the impetus for the development of imaging technologies such as MRI that are able to reveal mid-density tissues in superb contrast and resolution.

MRI utilizes a magnetic field in combination with a radio wave transmitter and receiver to produce images. MRI images represent a completely different form of image production than either plain film x-ray or CT, both of which are x-ray technologies. The MRI gray scale has no correlation to that of conventional radiography; both the method of film study and nomenclature are quite different. The MR image is produced by recording the response of hydrogen protons to radiofrequency energy within a strong magnetic field. Given that hydrogen is most prevalent within water in the human body, and that the radiographic mid-density

soft tissue structures are in large part composed of water, MRI becomes an ideal tool to visualize these structures.

WHAT ARE THE ADVANTAGES AND INDICATIONS FOR ORDERING MRI STUDIES?

Images may be obtained from any plane allowing the images to be angled to conventional sagittal, axial, or coronal planes allowing better anatomic visualization.
- Good contrast in water density tissues
- Excellent musculoskeletal and neurological anatomic detail
- No known health hazards
- Evaluation of soft tissue injuries of knee, ankle, and shoulder joints
- Evaluation of neurology: spinal nerve, nerve root compression, peripheral nerve compression, and injury
- Does not involve ionizing radiation
- No significant health risks associated with medical use of MRI imaging[2]

WHAT ARE THE DISADVANTAGES OF MRI?
- The high cost of equipment and imaging studies may be prohibitive for smaller hospitals and patients alike.
- MRI is not the modality of choice when studying bone tissue.
- An extended length of time is required for some studies. Early design MR units required 30 to 60 minutes to acquire some body region images. Rapid image acquisition techniques have helped overcome this obstacle.

HOW IS AN MRI GENERATED?

The MRI machine consists of a main magnet and sets of coils used to produce local magnetic field gradients affecting the spatial orientation of protons. Multiple coils in the machine produce different angles and distances between nuclei and magnets. Like visible light, magnetic field strength decreases as the square of distance. So, the further a body part is from a coil, the weaker the magnetic field strength and the slower the corresponding spin frequency.

The MRI main magnet and coils accomplish two results: (1) organized alignment of the axis of proton spin or precession and (2) a gradient of spin frequencies decreasing with the distance from the coils. A computer determines spatial orientation of the protons by their frequency in the same fashion a pianist can determine near, middle, or far key location based on the frequency. By using multiple coils surrounding the patient a three-dimensional image can be created.

MR then generates a radiofrequency (RF) beam that matches the spin frequency of the aligned protons (within the tissue "slice" being studied), which then absorb the radio wave energy and resonate. The strength of the transmitted RF signal is based on the properties of the tissue studied. Nuclei may be "perturbed" by the RF resulting in a shift in their axis of precession. The angle to which protons shift their spin axis is referred to as the "flip angle." Protons may, for example, be perturbed 90° (a 90° pulse) or 180° (180° pulse) from their normal or relaxed axis of motion. The RF signal is stopped and the protons relax to their original axes of spin and emit a RF signal correlating, in our example, to a 90° or 180° shift that is recorded by a radio receiver.

WHY DO THE DIFFERENT TISSUES LOOK DIFFERENT IN MRIs?

The rate at which RF signals are generated, the duration between signals, and the speed at which protons recover to their resting or original frequency is the foundation of MR imaging sequences. Fat tissue protons are capable of very rapid recovery and as a result will send a recordable RF in a short period of time following cessation of transmitted radiofrequency energy from the MRI machine. Water (e.g., synovial fluid, effusions, or edema) protons, in comparison, recover their relaxed spin axis relatively slowly after perturbation by RF. As a result, a pulse sequence characterized by brief intervals allows only rapidly recovering protons sufficient time to release absorbed RF energy and be recorded by the radio receiver. Consequently, short RF interval settings on the machine tend to favor recording and image production of fat tissue rather than water-containing tissues. If the pulse recording intervals are lengthened, allowing sufficient time for slower recovery protons such as water or edema to release absorbed radio energy the recorded image changes in appearance. This is the basis of image contrast and visual tissue differentiation on MRI.

It follows then, that MR images differ in appearance from plain film x-rays because the MRI gray scale image corresponds to the amount and behavior of hydrogen protons in the tissue rather than radiodensity. Correspondingly, a major difference in terminology exists between plain film radiography and MRI. Standard radiographic terms such as *density* and *opacity* are not used. MRI gray scale shades are described in terms of *signal intensity* (SI). Terms used to describe MRI images include *normal signal, abnormal signal,* and *low, intermediate,* or *high signal, isointense signal, homogeneous signal,* or *signal inhomogeneity*.

PULSE SEQUENCES

WHAT ARE PULSE SEQUENCES?

There is a ever expanding and confusing array of MRI pulse sequences or simply "sequences" available to the radiologist. The therapist will discover multiple film sheets, of multiple pulse sequences, when presented with a patient's MRI study. The studies generally include two to three pulse sequences, each obtained in three planes of view (coronal, sagittal, and axial) with 16 to 20 images per plane of study. It is not uncommon for an MRI study to contain well over 100 images.

MRI images or "slices" are similar to the slices in a loaf of bread. If you cut the bread from beginning to end you create a series of slices, each containing a piece of the loaf's anatomy. The slices are viewed in sequential order. The loaf could be slice in each of the 3 anatomic planes. Each plane of study (sagittal, coronal, axial) will show exactly the same anatomy in each sequence obtained. For example, image #3 in the T1 sagittal study of a knee will be exactly the same slice of knee anatomy as seen in image #3 of the T2 or STIR [short T1 (or tau) inversion recovery] sequences. This allows the clinician to view identical anatomic features displayed by different sequences each presenting particular features and pathology in a visually unique way. Acquisition techniques (pulse sequences) may favor visualization of capsular tissue, edema or effusion, tendon tears, or other diagnostic features. The radiologist selects pulse sequences that will best reveal suspected pathology. Multiple images of the same anatomic feature, presented—by virtue of differing pulse sequences—with differing tissue highlights, allow the reader greater accuracy in observation and diagnosis.

The MR image reflects the strength or signal intensity (SI) of the radiofrequency signal received from the tissue sample, which in turn depends on both hydrogen (proton) density (proton density is literally the number of protons present) and two magnetic factors termed T1 and T2. Both T1 and T2 are a measurement of elapsed time. In the early years of MRI development many images were produced entirely with T1, T2, or proton density (PD) weighting as a means of visually accenting specific behavioral characteristics of protons within different tissues. As MRI technology advanced the desire for greater tissue contrast and image resolution led to many variants in machine capability, such as strength of the magnets, instrument settings (e.g., fat suppression and fast acquisition times), and tissue appearance based on "mixtures" of T1, T2, and PD weighting with various radiofrequency pulse sequence modifications. As a result a variety of hybrid sequences are now utilized in MRI studies. An understanding of PD, T1, and T2 pulse sequences helps clarify hybrid sequences and the characteristic appearance and corresponding methods of MRI image interpretation.

WHAT ARE PROTON DENSITY IMAGES?

Proton density (PD) or spin density (SD) is simply a statement of the number of hydrogen nuclei present, per unit volume, in a tissue to create a signal. All MR contrast is created by differing numbers of protons in differing tissues; therefore PD-derived contrast is inherent in all MR image techniques. However a PD image employs that quantity as the principal method of tissue differentiation. To minimize T1- and T2-based differences, PD images use a long repetition time (TR) permitting full recovery for both fat and water, and a short echo time (TE) in which neither fat nor water has had much time to decay (Table I-3-3).

WHICH TISSUES APPEAR DARKER IN PD IMAGES AND WHICH TISSUES APPEAR LIGHTER?

High water content tissues such as synovial fluid and effusions tend to appear as high SI and low water content tissues such as bone or air-filled lung will demonstrate low SI (dark gray or black) in a proton density weighted image.[3] Proton density images are commonly ordered to evaluate orthopedic trauma and pathology in patients (see Figure I-3-2).

WHAT ARE T1-WEIGHTED IMAGES?

T1 time may be briefly described as the rate at which protons realign themselves (after being perturbed or flipped 90° to 180°) with the main magnetic field upon cessation of the RF signal. If RF signals are repeated more quickly (the rate is noted as TR on the film sheets) than the nuclei will not have returned to their original state between successive pulses and will have less opportunity to emit or echo an RF signal. The recovery, or return to prior precessional alignment, after being perturbed by RF (T1), of fat is shorter than that of water so more of the hydrogen nuclei in fat will have recovered and emit an RF signal. T1-weighted images, therefore, favor recording of fatty tissues.

TABLE I-3-3 A Simplified Look at Repetition Time (TR) and Echo Time (TE) and Their Relationship to Image Appearance

Abbreviation	Full Form	Definition
TR	Delay interval repetition time	A short TR favors T1 weighting and a long TR favors T2 weighting of the image.
TE	Delay period echo time	A short TE also favors T1 weighting whereas a longer TE shifts the image toward T2 weighting.

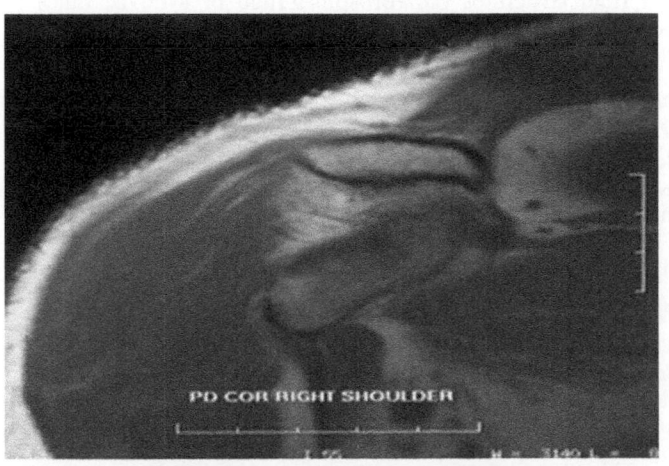

PD COR RIGHT SHOULDER

FIGURE I-3-2   Proton density image.

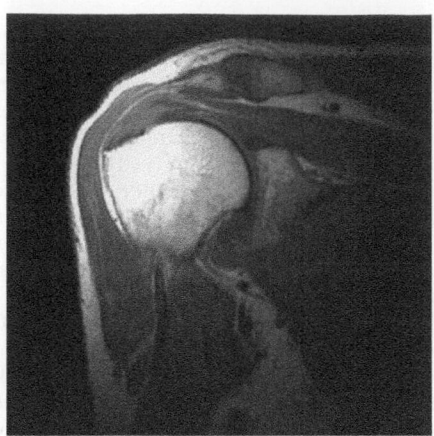

FIGURE I-3-3   MRI T1-weighted image.

WHICH TISSUES APPEAR DARKER IN T1 IMAGES AND WHICH TISSUES APPEAR LIGHTER?

When looking at a T1-weighted MRI study fat tissues will show high signal intensity and appear bright white. When studying an MRI film look to regions known to contain fat for a bright intense signal indicating you are viewing a T1-weighted image. Cortical bone shows very low SI on T1, and all other pulse sequences, simply because it contains little water and therefore few hydrogen nuclei. T1-weighted images are considered to display anatomy and anatomic features more clearly than do T2- or PD-weighted images (see Figure I-3-3).

WHAT ARE T2-WEIGHTED IMAGES?

T2 relaxation time reflects a somewhat different behavior of protons than T1. T2 relaxation occurs more quickly in liquids in which protons are more mobile than in solids in which protons tend to be more fixed.[3] As a result, T2 weighting of an MR image favors the display of water and water-based tissues whereas T1 images do not.

WHICH TISSUES APPEAR DARKER IN T2 IMAGES AND WHICH TISSUES APPEAR LIGHTER?

When looking at T2-weighted MRI images water, synovial fluid, cerebrospinal fluid, and effusions (but not blood) tend to show high signal intensity and appear bright white. Fat, which is bright on T1, appears as mid-signal intensity on T2-weighted images. When studying an MR image look to known fluid-containing anatomic structures for a bright high signal intensity indicating a T2-weighted image. Once high signal intensity is observed in normal fluid structures (cerebrospinal fluid or synovial fluid) to establish a baseline, fluid-based lesions and/or edema can also be identified based on high signal intensity.

WHEN SHOULD T2 IMAGES BE UTILIZED INSTEAD OF T1 IMAGES?

Because most pathology involves water-containing tissues such as edema, tumors, or hematoma formation (not the same as moving blood on MR) T2-weighted images tend to be better than T1-weighted images for evaluating pathology (see Box I-3-1 and Figures I-3-4 and I-3-5).

WHEN ARE FLUID-SENSITIVE SEQUENCES UTILIZED?

Water in the form of joint effusion or edema is most visible in *fluid-sensitive sequences* that include PD, T2, and STIR shown in Figure I-3-6, which shows an STIR image of a tibial plateau fracture. Fluid-sensitive sequences are excellent for viewing trauma, joint effusions, bone edema articular cartilage, joint fluid, and bone or soft tissue tumors.

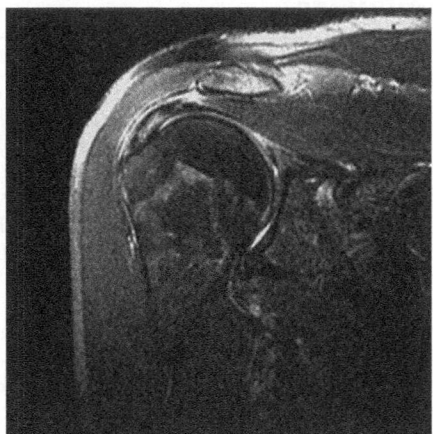

FIGURE I-3-4   MRI T2-weighted image.

WHY ARE HYBRID MRI PULSE SEQUENCES UTILIZED?

Although all acquisition techniques are based on T1, T2, and PD tissue characteristics, modern MR studies are often mixtures of these weighting sequences. The clinician evaluating an MRI is not always presented with "pure" T1, T2, or spin density/PD images but sequences such as T2 SE, T2 FSE, gradient echo, and STIR, all designed to better display suspected pathology. With the continued modification of RF pulse sequences to perturb protons between varied spin axis at assorted rates, intervals, and energy levels, growing numbers of acquisition sequences producing a distinctive tissue appearance are available. Radiologists will consider many pulse sequences to determine those most likely to clearly demonstrate specific tissues, injury, or pathology.

WHAT IS THE FIRST THING A CLINICIAN SHOULD LOOK AT WHEN READING AN MRI SEQUENCE?

The clinician should look at the upper left or lower right portions of the first film sheet of each study. The labeling or "scout film" window is typically seen at these areas. In the label or scout film window will be found information on the type of sequence employed. At times the film is labeled PD, T1, or T2. If not, look for the TR and TE notations on the film. The TR and TE values give information on the nature of the sequence. Unlike the physically defined characteristics of spin density, T1, and T2, the TE and TR are operator controlled settings. TE and TR can be manipulated such that differences between tissues signals can be highlighted by variations in spin density T1, and T2 influences.

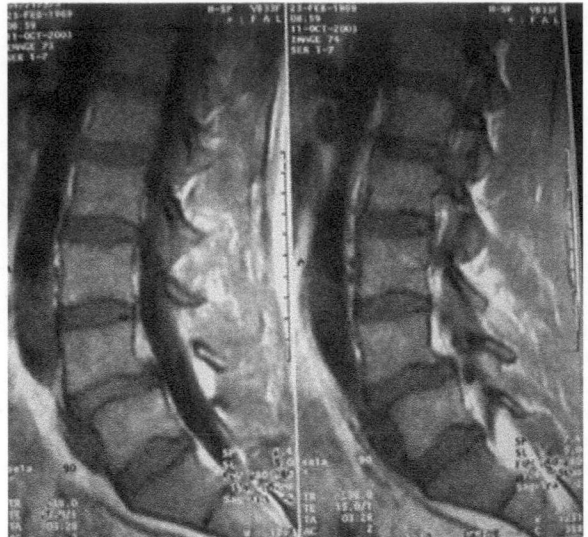

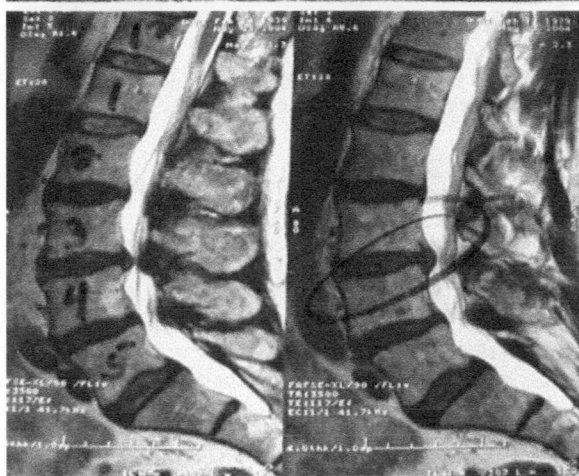

FIGURE I-3-5   MRI T1- and T2-weighted images.

CLINICAL PEARL

When evaluating any MRI sequence the basic search algorithm should be as follows:

Look at the film label window, usually in the upper left corner, and note the TR and TE to get an idea of the relative T1 or T2 weighting of the image.

You do not need to have in depth knowledge of image production physics to understand or apply the radiology report to treatment. Identify the SI of known tissues and compare observed SI patterns to identify additional normal and abnormal features. Knowledge of anatomy plays an extremely important role in MR study. The ability to perceive anatomy three dimensionally is a fundamental to understanding and incorporating MR information into rehabilitation planning, delivery, and outcome study.

The MRI in Figure I-3-7 demonstrates high SI within the subcutaneous fat and bone marrow and intermediate SI at the popliteal

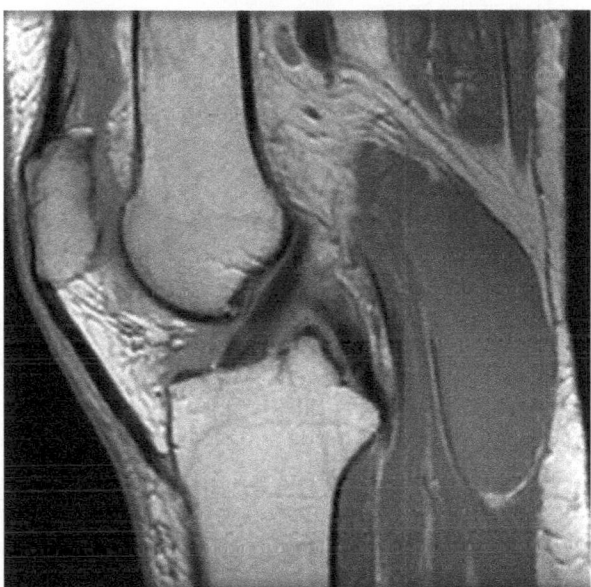

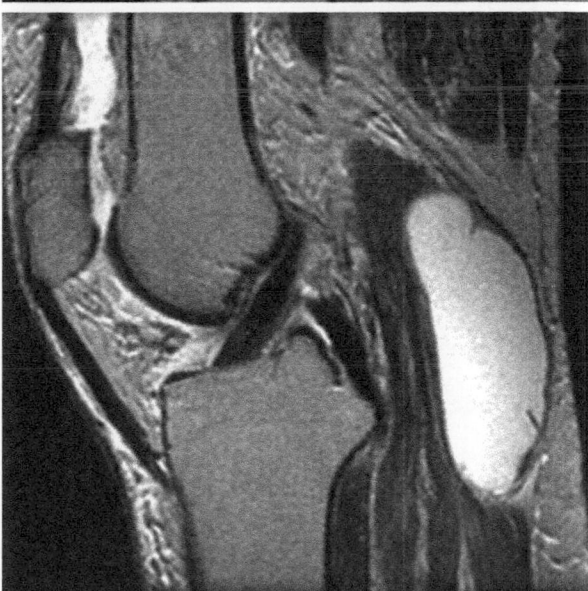

FIGURE I-3-7 T1 coronal image of the knee. This MRI demonstrates high signal intensity (SI) within the subcutaneous fat and bone marrow and intermediate SI at the popliteal cyst. A fluid-sensitive T2 image reveals the cyst as increased SI, consistent with fluid at the popliteal fossa.

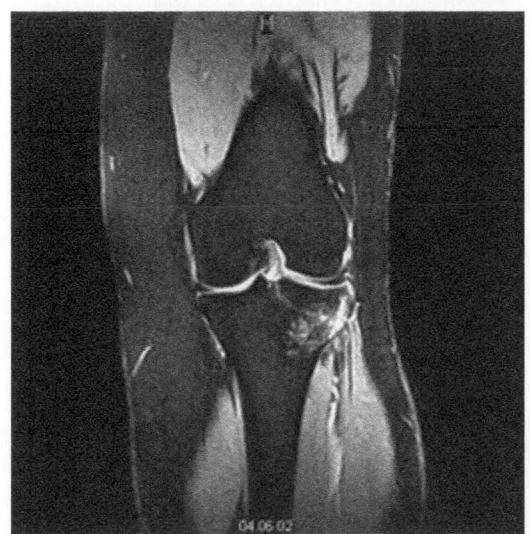

FIGURE I-3-6   STIR image of a tibial plateau fracture.

cyst. A fluid-sensitive T2 image reveals the cyst as increased SI, consistent with fluid at the popliteal fossa.

WHAT ARE SOME OF THE IMAGE ENHANCEMENT TECHNIQUES NOW BEING EMPLOYED?

A few of the many technical modifications available include fast acquisition such as FSE and others designed to speed MR.[1] Another is fat suppression in which otherwise high SI fatty tissues can be presaturated with the RF signal to decrease SI and allow better visualization of adjacent nonadipose tissues.[6] Fat suppression techniques and their acronyms vary with equipment manufacturers but are often abbreviated as "fat sat" in conversation and denoted on films as FS or FATSAT.

The film label FS FSE PD may then be translated as a fat suppressed fast spin echo proton density image. FS FSE PD sequences are fairly common in orthopedic studies. FSE T2 FS sequences are often seen when studying the wrist and FSE PD, FS FSE T2, and T1 for the shoulder. Sequences are also obtained specific to the anatomic plane of the images.

Soft tissue detail may be enhanced by use of gadolinium dye. Gadolinium, or "Gad" in conversation, is injected before acquiring images and serves to highlight subtle details of soft tissue. Gadolinium is used on all MRI patients by some imaging centers and is reserved for specific cases in others. Gadolinium is also used as the contrast media in MRI arthrography.

COMPUTERIZED TOMOGRAPHY SCANS

WHAT ARE CT SCANS?

CT is a major advancement in x-ray-based imaging technology and is particularly useful in rehabilitation settings for the evaluation of bone pathologies.

The study of CT images is quite similar to evaluation of MRI images. CT studies are again presented as sequential slices in the same three planes of study: axial, sagittal, and coronal planes. The viewer arranges the film provided into groups based on image plane, orients via a scout film, and studies the rows of images in the same fashion as reading a page of text: from left to right and top to bottom. As an x-ray-based technology CT images are described in x-ray terms such as density, opacity, or lucency. And as an x-ray technology CT exposes the patient to ionizing radiation, considerably more than does plain film radiography. In response the clinician chooses CT studies with due consideration for radiation exposure. However, CT is capable of revealing invaluable and unique information vital to the diagnosis and treatment of many patients and therefore should be utilized when indicated (see Figures I-3-8 and I-3-9).

WHAT ARE THE CHARACTERISTICS AND INDICATIONS FOR THE USE OF CT?

- X-ray-based technology
- Multiple plane and three-dimensional images are available
- The gray scale is the same as in x-ray interpretation
- CT utilizes a computer to enhance the contrast of mid or water grays to create a much better differentiation of soft tissue densities
- Accurately measures bone density
- Trauma
- Fracture detection and evaluation
- Spine alignment
- Intracranial hemorrhage
- Abdominal injury
- Detection of foreign bodies, especially in joints
- Diagnosis of primary and secondary tumors
- Tumor staging

HOW DO CT SCANS DIFFER FROM NORMAL X-RAYS?

CT provides much greater information than plain film x-rays because it allows multiple plane views and spectacular three-dimensional images in which the region or bone to be studied can be viewed from infinite angles as a freely movable and visually isolated object.

CT images show brilliant computer-enhanced detail and, in soft tissues, greater contrast between very subtle gray shades seen on plain x-ray. The enhanced contrast makes pathologies and trauma obvious that might be visually undetectable with conventional radiography. CT is commonly used to assess

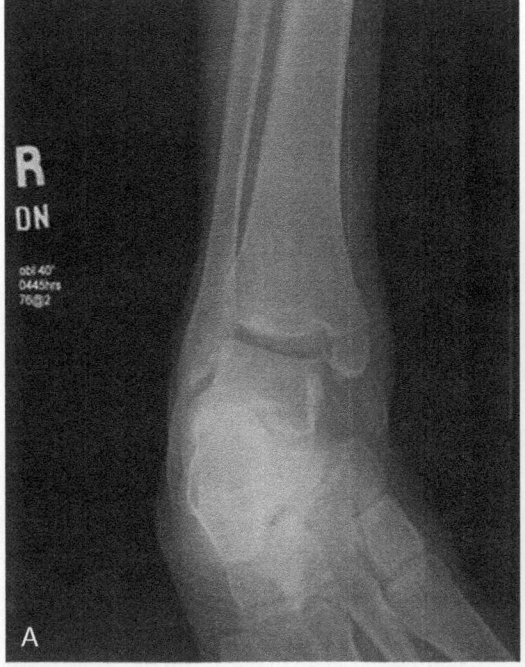
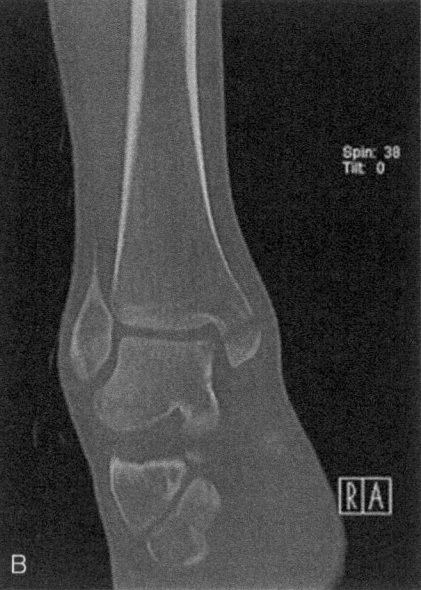

FIGURE I-3-8   A, a plain x-ray view of ankle fracture. B, Coronal plane CT view of same ankle fracture.

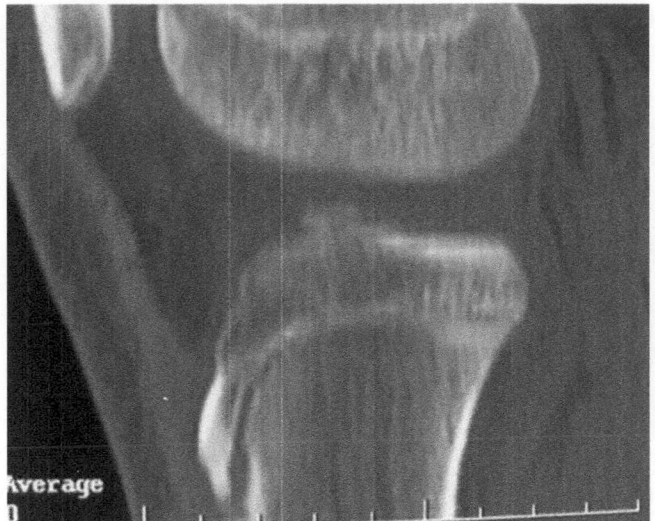

FIGURE I-3-9   Sagittal CT view of Osgood-Schlatter's Disease.

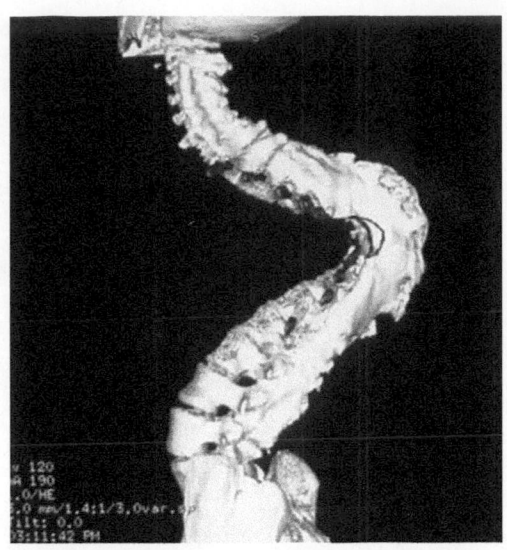

FIGURE I-3-11   3D CT of kyphoscoliosis.

fractures that are either difficult to diagnose on x-ray or to demonstrate three-dimensional relationships important to planning surgical reduction and/or rehabilitation. CT is also an imaging modality of choice for brain pathologies allowing rapid assessment of cranial hemorrhage and cerebrovascular accident. Various CT studies are capable of revealing brain morphology, the extent of tissue damage, and detailed brain vascular perfusion and metabolic uptake status. Orthopedic and neurological specialist physical therapists may incorporate data from CT scans for detailed evaluation of cerebrovascular accidents and other brain pathologies, bone pathologies, and complex fractures with or without joint involvement (see Figures I-3-10, I-3-11, and I-3-12).

WHICH TISSUES APPEAR DARKER WITH CT SCANS AND WHICH TISSUES APPEAR LIGHTER?

Expansion of the gray scale is a key component of CT understanding. The human eye is able to differentiate a limited number (perhaps 30 or so) of gradated gray tones. Soft tissues such as organs, nerve, muscle, joint, and ligamentous structures are seen as homogeneous gray shades on plain film x-rays; therefore the ability to make diagnostically useful conclusions is very limited. CT technology, by artificially exaggerating contrast within specific predetermined ranges of x-ray gray shades, creates an entire black–gray–white scale where only a homogeneous gray had previously been

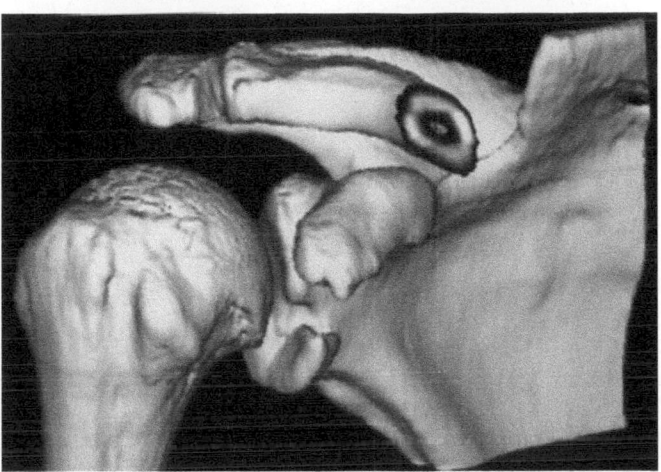

FIGURE I-3-12   3D CT of shoulder.

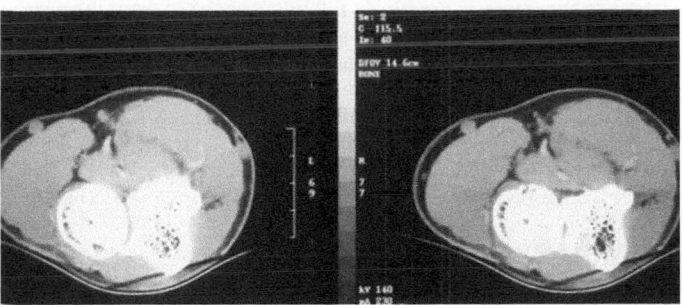

FIGURE I-3-13   CT of elbow utilizing "Bone Window".

visible. Figure I-3-13 demonstrates the contrast amplification and distinction between cortical bone and medullary bone.

Tissues of particular interest fall within CT "windows." A bone window, for example, will exaggerate the white and gray tones produced by bone or bone-like tissues. A lung window does the same by generating high contrast between subtle variations in lung tissue density. The computer exaggerated black–gray–white contrast that can initially be unfamiliar or confusing. Bone viewed in a soft tissue window may be so brilliantly white as to be unreadable

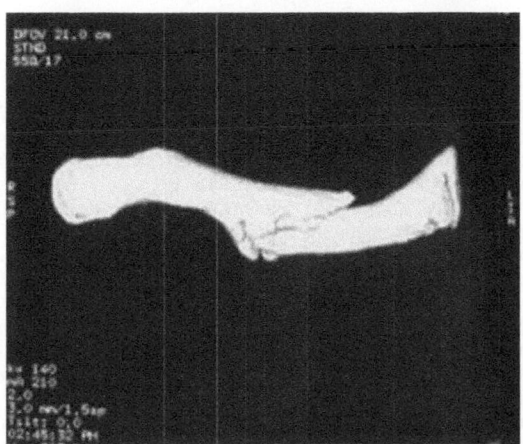

FIGURE I-3-10   3D CT of clavicular fracture.

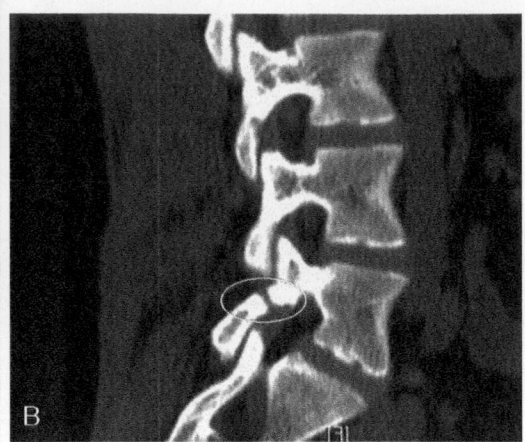

FIGURE I-3-14 A, Lateral x-ray view of lumbar spine demonstrating L5 pars fracture. B, Sagittal CT of lumbar spine demonstrating (same) L5 pars fracture.

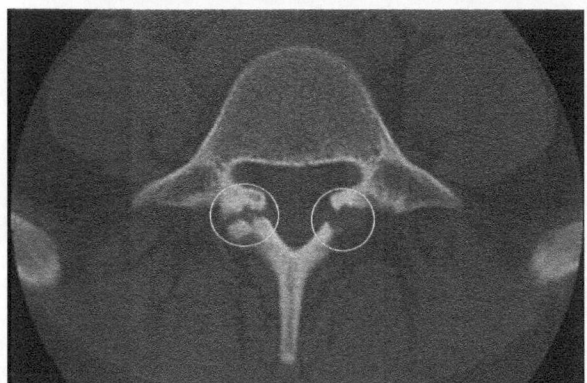

FIGURE I-3-15 Axial CT of lumbar vertebrae demonstrating pars fracture.

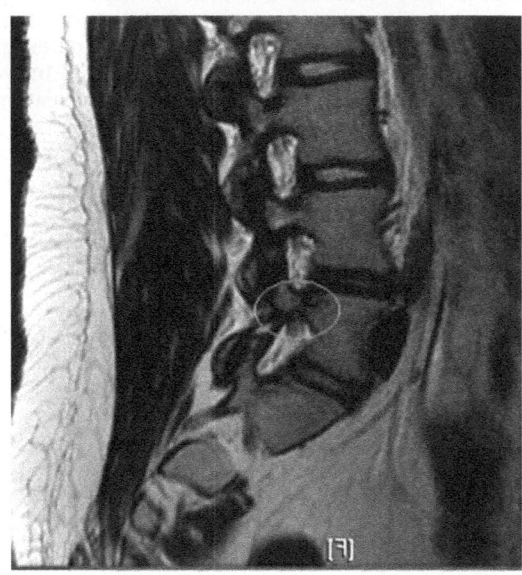

FIGURE I-3-16 Sagittal MRI of L5 pars fracture.

because the image is creating a full gray spectrum from the narrow range of grays associated with soft tissue densities. In this setting bone density is relatively off the scale. In a "bone window" bone will be displayed in its typical plain film appearance, albeit with greater detail, with cortical bone white and cancellous bone light gray. Soft tissues will appear much darker as they are much less radiographically dense than bone and the contrast will be computer exaggerated (see Figures I-3-14 to I-3-16).

SUMMARY

The role of radiology in rehabilitation medicine is evolving. Clinicians are expected to have a solid understanding of the methods utilized with various imaging studies. In most instances, clinicians will not be required to read a radiographic image. Radiologists are the experts in the field and should be deferred to in all matters of image interpretation. Instead, the clinician will be called upon to further explain the results of a radiographic image. In these instances, the rehabilitation clinician should have enough of a knowledge base to view an image, read the radiologist's report, and then educate the patient on the radiologist's findings. The goal of the rehabilitation clinician should not be to become an expert in radiology, but simply a good consumer and educator of radiographic studies.

REFERENCES

1. Berquist T. *MRI of the Musculoskeletal System*. Philadelphia, PA: Lippincott Williams & Wilkins; 2001.
2. Daffner R. *Clinical Radiography*. Philadelphia, PA: Lippincott Williams & Wilkins; 1999.
3. Fleckenstein P, Tranum-Jensen J. *Anatomy in Diagnostic Imaging*. Copenhagen: Blackwell Publishing; 2001.
4. Freitas A. *Knee, Collateral Ligament Injuries*. Retrieved June 4 2006, from http://www.emedicine.com/radio/topic886.htm; 2005.
5. Harvey CJ, Richenberg JL, Saifuddin A, Wolman RL. The radiological investigation of lumbar spondylolysis. *Clin Radiol*. 1998;53(10):723-728.
6. Link T. *MRI of Bone Marrow. Current Concepts in Neuro and Musculoskeletal Imaging*. Kona Hawaii: University of California at San Francisco School of Medicine; 2006.
7. McKinnes L. *Fundamentals of Musculoskeletal Imaging*. Philadelphia, PA: FA Davis; 2005.
8. Steinbach L. *MRI of the Shoulder. Current Concepts in Neuro and Musculoskeletal Imaging*. Kona Hawaii: University of California at San Francisco Medical Center; 2006.

AUTHOR: JACKLYN BRECHTER

INTRODUCTORY INFORMATION

Rehabilitation of patients with musculoskeletal complaints primarily involves five basic types of tissue: bone, cartilage, tendons/ligaments, muscle, and nerve. To make successful rehabilitation decisions, it is important to have an understanding of how the involved tissue responds to stress. The following sections describe these tissues of the body in a fashion that attempts to be clear to the clinician as opposed to the basic scientist. To the basic scientist, the information here may seem extraordinarily simplified. However, the purpose of this information is to impart to the clinician an understanding of how to make rehabilitation decisions based on the tissue involved. The information provides some basic knowledge that may lead to informed decision making regarding the testing and rehabilitation of specific tissues.

BONE

Bone is one tissue that is often involved in injuries of the musculoskeletal system. Although many health care practitioners are not directly involved in the rehabilitation of the fracture or bone injury, knowledge of the bony tissue and its mechanics can aid in the prevention of injury or in protecting the bone from further damage. In addition, a knowledge of the relationship between bone and other tissues (such as muscles) can help in determining when additional testing is necessary based on the presenting.

WHAT IS THE FUNCTION OF BONES OR THE SKELETAL SYSTEM?[35,59,63]

One primary purpose of bone is to protect the internal organs and key soft tissue components of the body. Examples of this protective role can be seen in the skull protecting the brain, the pelvic bowl protecting the digestive and some reproductive organs, the rib cage and chest bone or sternum protecting the heart, and the bones of the spine or vertebrae protecting the spinal cord.

The second purpose of bony tissue is upright support. The skeletal system provides the ability to maintain posture, not only when standing still, but during daily activities. In addition, bone helps to dampen or transmit external forces that are applied to the body to avoid jarring or to control motion.

The third purpose of bony tissue is to provide a point of attachment for muscles or tendons. This anchors the muscle and allows the bone to act as levers for motion. The muscle therefore provides links between bones that then generate body motion.

WHAT IS THE COMPOSITION OF BONE?[41,46,59,65]

Bone is composed of both cells and an organic matrix made by the cells. The cells include osteoblasts, osteocytes, and osteoclasts, which create, support, and reabsorb osteoid. In addition, fibroblasts and fibrocytes are present to help produce and support collagen, a large part of the bone matrix.

The matrix of bone is quite interesting, and it provides bone with its structural integrity and response to load. The extracellular matrix is composed of both fibrillar and interfibrillar components. The fibrillar components are primarily collagen fibrils (type I collagen). This type of collagen has the unique ability to bind together with minerals. These minerals become imbedded in and between the collagen fibrils.

The minerals include calcium, phosphate, and calcium carbonate as well as smaller amounts of sodium, magnesium, and fluoride. The minerals are embedded within collagen fibers and serve to create a resistance to compression or deformation. Collagen, conversely, has the ability to resist stretch and provides bone with its flexibility. It makes up most of the organic material in bone. The ground substance (interfibrillar portion of the matrix) is like the glue or cementing substance between the mineral-coated fibers of collagen. The water found in bony tissue is mostly around the organic matrix, but is also located within the canals that hold the cells.

WHAT IS THE STRUCTURE OF BONE?[46,55,59,63,65]

The osteon (Haversian system) is the functional unit of cortical bone. Each osteon is composed of concentric rings of bone around a central canal that holds the nerve and vessels of the bone tissue. Collagen fibers within a layer (lamella) are parallel with each other, but each lamella has its own fiber direction. Cells have small spaces (lacuna) throughout the osteon and are connected to each other through a series of interconnecting canals (canaliculi).

Trabecular bone is found inside a layer of cortical bone. It is a less dense bone composed of thin plates or trabeculae lined up within the bone to withstand the stress placed on the bone. Trabecular bone also surrounds the bone marrow, the site of blood cell production.

The high porosity in trabecular bone gives it high energy storage and stress distribution during loading. The combination of cortical and trabecular bone makes bone very strong, yet light in weight. Vertebral bodies have a high percentage of trabecular bone and are therefore more likely to succumb to compression fracture than the long bones with higher amounts of cortical bone.

WHAT ARE THE BIOMECHANICAL PROPERTIES OF BONE?[12,40,41,46,55]

The material composition of bone provides some of its mechanical properties. In addition, the shape or size of the bone itself provides some of the mechanical properties of bone.

Water provides bone with a mechanical property called viscosity, which is a resistance to fluid flow. Collagen provides bone with resistance to tension or stretch and a mechanical property called elasticity. Elasticity allows a tissue to return to its resting shape after the removal of a deforming load. The mineral composition of bone provides bone with its strength or resistance to deformation. The combination of material properties results in a product that is greater than each component would provide alone. Bone provides the greatest resistance to stress in the direction of compression. Cortical bone is stiffer and stronger than trabecular bone, but trabecular bone deforms more (stores more energy) before fracture. With both cortical and trabecular bone present the bone has resistance to load and the ability to deform. In addition, the trabecular bone allows the bone to be strong and flexible yet lightweight.

In addition to the material components of bone providing the mechanical properties of bone, bone shape contributes as well. Cross-sectional area (CSA), bone length, and the distribution of bone about a central axis (moment of inertia) all influence the mechanics of the bone. A larger CSA means greater load before failure and the tubular shape of long bones helps resist bending loads.

WHAT IS THE MECHANICAL BEHAVIOR OF BONE?[34,44,62,78]

Mechanical behavior is the response of a structure under the influence of different loads (forces or moments). Mechanical behavior changes in bone with a change in the method of loading, the rate, frequency, and direction of load, as well as the geometric characteristics of the tissue being loaded.

Loading may be in the direction of tension, compression, shear, bending, torsion, or combinations of these (Figure I-4-1). Each type of load creates a characteristic deformation in the bony tissue. Muscle activity has an important influence on bone deformation during loading.

TENSION: A tension load occurs when forces pull a bone apart, with the load applied perpendicular to the cross section of the bone. Tension loads are common at insertion sites of muscles and ligaments. Tension loading causes internal lengthening and narrowing of bone tissue.

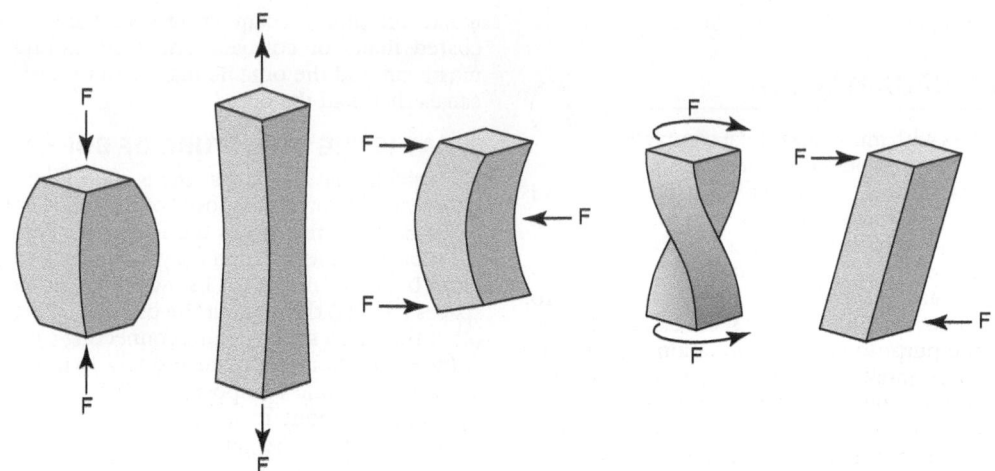

FIGURE I-4-1 Typical types of stress including compression, tension, bending, torsion, and shear.

COMPRESSION: Compression loading occurs during weight bearing for the long bones; again the load is perpendicular to the cross section of the bone and is applied to bring the two ends toward each other. It may also occur during muscle contraction. Compression loading causes an internal shortening and widening of bone tissue.

SHEAR: Shear loading is loading parallel to the cross section of a bone. It causes internal deformation within the bone leaving structures angled with respect to the stress instead of their normal orientation. This change can increase a bone's susceptibility to additional loading.

BENDING: Bending of a structure occurs when forces are applied that cause a bending around an axis (e.g., when you try to break a stick). When a bending load occurs, bone experiences both compression and tension. Compression occurs on one side of the axis and tension occurs on the other side of the axis. The bone most often fails on the side of the tensile force. A common way this force is produced is through a combination of forces at three points. This is usually two forces acting perpendicular to the bone at the ends of the bone and then a force in the opposite direction in the middle of the bone. This can produce fractures, but is also used in bracing, i.e., for scoliosis forces applied at the top and bottom of the spine and then an opposite force applied at the curve.

TORSION: In torsion, a load is applied to a structure that causes it to twist about an axis. Torsional loading causes shear forces as well as compression and tension forces to be distributed over the bony structure. For example, an injury mechanism from torsional load occurs when the foot is planted and the body changes direction.

COMBINATION LOADING: Normally, bone loading is not unidirectional. Within one functional activity such as walking, the lower extremity bones go through alternating periods of compression, tension, shear, and torsion. Often, while one portion of the bone experiences one load, another portion experiences a different sort of load. In general, bone can withstand compression forces better than tension and both better than shear. Breakdown or bone damage during bending and torsional loading is a result of the shear, tension, or compressive loads on the tissue.

WHAT IS THE CLINICAL IMPORTANCE OF LOADING TYPES?

When a bone is damaged, characteristic fractures occur with each type of loading. The insulting load must be removed or significantly reduced for healing. It is up to the clinician to assist the patient in determining what activity or posture is responsible for load. It is also the clinicians who assist the patient in determining what activity is responsible for the tissue damage. Performing observational analysis of the patient moving, or understanding the effect of motion, while considering the biomechanics of bone loading will lead the clinician to determine the activity or activities responsible for bone damage.

DOES MUSCLE ACTIVITY AFFECT THE LOAD OR DEFORMATION OF A BONE DURING LOADING?[59,63]

Muscle activity applies load to bones. At the site of tendon insertion muscle activity results in a tensile load on the bone. At the joint surface or other portions of the bone, muscle activity may cause compression or otherwise change the distribution of forces or stress (force per unit area) on the bone. For example, weight bearing causes a bending force across the femoral neck, which produces tension on the superior side of the neck and compression on the inferior side of the femoral neck (Figure I-4-2). As the gluteus medius contracts, the muscle activity counters the tensile force on the superior neck of the femur. Thus, instead of the detrimental bending load (top half in tension, bottom half in compression) the neck of the femur now experiences only compression forces.[71] Thus, the muscle activity decreases the likelihood of injury due to tension and allows the femoral neck to better resist loads. In the event of reduced or inadequate muscular activity (weak gluteal medius) the neck of the femur may experience increased tensile stress and may be more likely to be damaged.

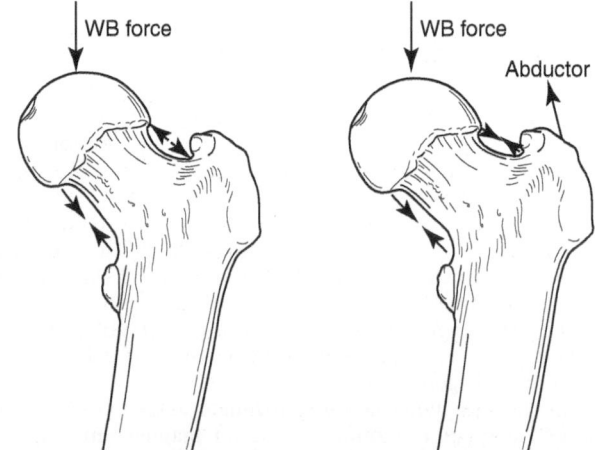

FIGURE I-4-2 Weight bearing (WB) force on the femoral head causes bending in the femoral neck (tension superiorly, compression inferiorly). Abductor muscle contraction alters the force and the femoral neck experiences compression both superiorly and inferiorly.

WHAT IS THE CLINICAL RELEVANCE OF MUSCLE ACTIVITY AND BONE?

The effect of muscle activity altering the type of load on a bone is prevalent throughout daily activities. Muscle activity absorbs loads that otherwise would be transmitted to bone. Thus, it is critical to consider the effect of muscle weakness on overuse injuries that affect the bone tissue. Clinicians should examine muscle strength and/or endurance in surrounding muscles whenever there is evidence of bony involvement with overuse injury.

DOES THE RATE OF LOADING AFFECT BONE RESPONSE?[2,36]

Yes, bone responds differently to loads depending on the rate of the load application as a result of a material property of bone called viscosity. Viscosity is a measure of resistance to fluid flow. A viscous material reacts differently whether the load is applied slowly or rapidly. With faster loading, bone has more resistance to deformation compared to slower loading rates. Additionally, viscous material does not return to its original resting shape on removal of the load. Some of the energy is absorbed in the material, due to a property called hysteresis.

The type of damage that occurs when bone is loaded to excess depends on the rate of loading. Slower loads will generally result in a single crack. At high rates of loading, the energy cannot be dissipated fast enough so multiple fractures usually occur.

DOES REPETITIVE LOADING CHANGE THE BONE RESPONSE TO LOAD?[9,10,64]

Fracture of a bone may occur because of a single excessive load that exceeds the strength of the bone as seen with a car accident, fall, or other traumatic injury. Another way to fracture bone is with multiple smaller loads that build to produce a fracture. This repetitive loading causes the bone to fatigue, which leads to micro-failure of the bone and ultimately fracture. This can be caused by few repetitions at a high load or multiple repetitions at a lower load. If the repetitions occur at a rapid enough frequency, the bone is more likely to fail because it is not allowed to repair itself between loads.

Damage to bone (even microfracture) without sufficient time for repair reduces the ability of bone to withstand normal loads. Therefore, in the presence of bony defects or fractures, the bone will require periods of reduced loading until it is able to repair itself. These bony defects may include the hole from surgical removal of a screw or a bone biopsy. Clinicians treating individuals with damaged bony tissue should include the reduced loading capacity of the bone in the selection of therapeutic activities.

HOW DOES BONE RESPOND TO EXERCISE OR USE OR LACK OF USE?[1,20,51]

When bone undergoes stress or use there is an increase in osteoblast activity and more bone is produced. In cases of reduced or absent load or stress (or in some disease states), there is a decrease in osteoblast activity and an increase in the amount of breakdown of bony material. This process may produce osteoporosis if left unchecked. Bone responds very well to change in function; Julius Wolff (1868) described what has become known as Wolff's Law, which states that "every change in the form or function of a bone is followed by adaptive changes in its internal architecture and its external shape." Another way of saying this is that bone is laid down according to the force that is exerted on it.

HOW DOES BONE RESPOND TO AGING?[54,75,77]

In general, bone is less able to deform with age; it becomes more brittle and thus more susceptible to fracture. In addition, bone has a tendency to become less dense with age, resulting in a reduction in its ability to withstand force. Again this change with age increases the susceptibility of bone to fracture.

CARTILAGE

Cartilage is a difficult tissue to rehabilitate when damaged. Because cartilage has little blood or nervous supply, it is hard to know when it is damaged and is ineffective at healing. Not until the damage involves the periphery of the cartilage or the subchondral bone is there warning that cartilage is involved or damaged. Keeping the joint mechanics normalized and keeping regular activity at moderate levels help to prevent damage to the cartilage tissue. To understand when to examine cartilage for involvement in joint dysfunction or pathology, it is important to know what cartilage does for a joint and what reaction is expected from cartilage when the joint is loaded. Knowledge of what is expected can trigger examination when those functions or responses become abnormal. In addition, the clinical practitioner can select treatment intervention more appropriately based on the response of cartilage tissue to stress.

The following pages are designed to describe a very basic understanding of the function and mechanical aspects of cartilage. The depth and presentation of the information has been adjusted for ease of application to the clinical situation.

WHAT ARE THE FUNCTIONS OF ARTICULAR CARTILAGE?[59,63]

Articular cartilage, also called hyaline cartilage, is found covering the articulating surfaces of bones participating in diarthrodial joints. The functions of the articular cartilage include distributing the joint load over a larger area, to decrease the loading at any single point on the bone. Other functions include absorbing shock or compressive loads and decreasing friction to allow for smooth articulation between the bony surfaces.

WHAT IS THE COMPOSITION OF ARTICULAR CARTILAGE?[11,37,66,67]

Cartilage is composed of cells, primarily chondrocytes, and an extracellular matrix, which includes water and solids. The solid component of the matrix is composed of collagen (type II) and proteoglycan aggrecans.

WHAT IS THE STRUCTURE OF ARTICULAR CARTILAGE?[11,26,67]

In general, articular cartilage is generally arranged in three layers, a superficial tangential zone (10% to 20% of the cells), a middle zone (40% to 60% of the cells), and a deep zone (about 30% of the cells). The deep zone lies over the calcified zone of the cartilage (Figure I-4-3).

In the superficial tangential zone, the chondrocytes are arranged tangential to the surface. The collagen fibers are also arranged similarly. This arrangement of the cells and collagen helps to provide a resistance to shear forces crossing the surface of the cartilage.

The middle zone of the cartilage has chondrocytes arranged in a more haphazard fashion, similar to the arrangement of the collagen fibers. This layer appears to function to resist loads in any direction.

The deep zone of the cartilage has chondrocytes arranged perpendicular to the bony surface, again in a similar fashion to the collagen fibers found in this zone. Such an arrangement favors resistance to compressive and tensile forces.

Under the deep zone of the cartilage is a calcified layer that provides a transition to subchondral bone underlying the cartilage. This transition layer helps provide a more gentle change between the bone and cartilage.

WHAT ARE THE BIOMECHANICAL PROPERTIES OF CARTILAGE?[26,37,43]

Collagen provides tensile strength to cartilage, but collagen has very little resistance to compression. The variations in collagen

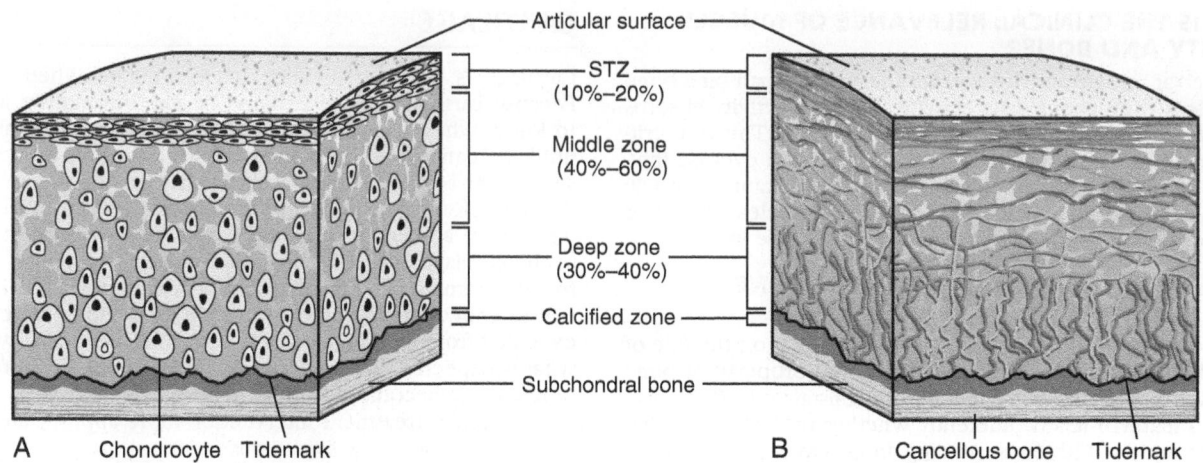

FIGURE I-4-3 **Zones of cartilage showing cellular arrangement (A, B).** Insets indicate the relative diameter and arrangement of collagen fibrils in the different zones. (From Neumann DA. *Kinesiology of the Musculoskeletal System: Foundations for Physical Rehabilitation*. 2nd ed. St. Louis, MO: Mosby, 2010.)

alignment contribute to the ability of cartilage to withstand tensile forces in different directions and return to resting shape.

Proteoglycans (PGs) are proteins containing one or more linked glycosaminoglycans. An aggrecan is the major component of cartilage and is one of the most studied PGs. The PG aggrecan provides the structural stability to the extracellular matrix in cartilage.

Water fills the area between the PGs and contains ions that influence the mechanical behavior of cartilage (Na^+, K^+, Ca^{2+}). The water is key for nutrient exchange and waste disposal within cartilage, as cartilage has little blood supply or lymph vessels. As the cartilage tissue is compressed, the water flows out of the tissue, carrying the waste material with it. As the cartilage is unloaded, the water is attracted back into the tissues carrying the nutrients essential to the cartilage. Thus regular loading and unloading of the cartilage tissue is required for healthy articular cartilage.

The interactions of the collagen, PGs, and water provide much of the mechanical properties of cartilage. The PG aggrecans have negative charges and are arranged to form macromolecules. The negative forces repulse each other and cause a stretching and stiffening of the tissue. These negative forces attract the water and its positive ions. As the water flows in and fills the space, there is a stretching of the collagen fibers. At some point, a natural balance is found and no further water enters. With compression of the cartilage and the outflow of water and ions, there is an increase in the repulsive forces until no further compression occurs. As the load is released, the water is attracted once again and the normal state of tissue tension resumes. PGs also act as cross-links for collagen fibers, providing interfibril connections, so the PGs work with the collagen together to improve the resistance to tensile forces.

WHAT IS THE MECHANICAL BEHAVIOR OF ARTICULAR CARTILAGE?[26,37,43]

Articular cartilage must be able to withstand considerable loading forces, which may exceed 10 times the body weight of the individual.[78,79] In fact, compressive forces in gymnastics may be significantly larger.

COMPRESSION: Under a compressive load, cartilage is viscoelastic, having the fluid property of viscosity or resistance to fluid flow and the solid property of elasticity or the ability to return to a resting length following deformation. Cartilage also exhibits properties of creep stress relaxation, and hysteresis, a result of its viscoelasticity. Creep is a response to a constant load during which the tissue gradually continues to deform. Stress relaxation is a response to a constant deformation.

While holding the constant change in shape (deformation) of the tissue, the amount of stress required to hold the deformation relaxes over time.

For cartilage under a constant load, fluid begins to exit the tissue and the tissue deforms. As the PG solid matrix begins to resist the compression, an equilibrium state is reached and no more deformation occurs. Resistance to deformation is a result of the repulsive forces in the PG aggrecans. The charges repulse each other more with proximity to each other and with the exit of the positive ions with water. Eventually, the repulsive forces increase to a point at which no further compression can occur. Another reason that the deformation eventually stops is the solid material (PGs, collagen, cells, and even water) must have a certain amount of space to exist. The size or thickness of each of these structures presents further resistance to compression in cartilage. Finally, as compression increases, the permeability of cartilage decreases, which causes a resistance to fluid exiting the cartilage. To provide an idea of how long cartilage takes to reach the point at which it will no longer deform (time scale on the creep diagrams), for 2 to 4 mm of cartilage it takes 4 to 16 hours of sustained load to maximally deform.

TENSION: Cartilage also responds to tension forces placed on it. The response of cartilage to tension is not equal in all directions, making cartilage anisotropic. In addition, the response to tension is stiffer and stronger in the superficial tangential zone than in other zones of cartilage. Cartilage and the additional reinforcements caused by PG linkages to the collagen fibers contribute strongly to the resistance to tensile loading. As such, the response of cartilage to tension follows a pattern similar to that of collagen. In particular, when tension is placed on the cartilage tissue, there is a toe region, thought to occur due to the collagen fibers straightening out. The toe region is similar to taking a rubber band and pulling it until the resistance is first felt. If you keep pulling on the rubber band after resistance is felt, it will begin to deform (lengthen); a similar process occurs with cartilage. When the tissue has reached its maximum ability to resist tensile forces, it will fail.

SHEAR: Collagen is responsible for controlling shear forces in cartilage as well as tension. Increased collagen content results in reduced deformation from shear forces.

HOW DOES CARTILAGE DIFFER FROM OTHER TISSUES?[3,11,67]

Hyaline cartilage is unique among tissues since it has very little blood supply. In addition, it lacks lymph vessels. Thus, it is dependent on the daily loading and unloading to obtain nutrition and eliminate waste. Cartilage is also unique in that it lacks a nerve supply. The subchondral bone underneath the cartilage is richly supplied with nerve endings. Thus, when pain is involved as part of the complaint, usually the cartilage should not be suspected as the cause of that pain.

DOES THE RATE OF LOADING AFFECT CARTILAGE RESPONSE?[21,56,68]

Cartilage, having the property of viscosity, does respond with increased stiffness to loads that are applied at a faster rate.

DOES REPETITIVE LOADING CHANGE THE CARTILAGE RESPONSE TO LOAD?[48]

Repetitive loading is a large factor in cartilage breakdown. If repetition occurs faster than regeneration, then the cartilage will not be able to recover between loads and breakdown will accumulate.

HOW DOES CARTILAGE RESPOND TO EXERCISE OR USE OR LACK OF USE?[6,7,16,17,70,76]

Cartilage requires regular activity for healthy tissue. The lack of blood supply into the cartilage necessitates other methods for nutritional intake and waste removal. The flow out of fluid with cartilage compressive loading and flow back in with the removal of the load is the mechanism cartilage utilizes for nutrition and waste removal. With a lack of use, cartilage will break down in a fashion similar to that seen with overuse. In connective tissue matrix, there may be an increase in the production and lysis of collagen. The lack of normal motion causes an absence of stress and therefore no force to assist with alignment of fibers. The collagen lays down in a haphazard fashion. An example may be observed in the patellofemoral joint. Medial facet breakdown has been observed without medial facet contact during loading.

A decrease in glycosaminoglycan content and therefore water content has two affects. One, the collagen fibrils are in closer contact with each other and two, there is a loss of lubrication. Collagen then forms abnormal cross links and exhibits a loss of tissue extensibility.

Clinicians should take note of the factors that may be manipulated during the treatment of patients with joint complaints. For example, the magnitude of the stress, the point loading, and the number of repetitions are all factors under a clinician's influence. Each of these should be considered as factors to be manipulated during treatment to prevent further wear and promote recovery of cartilage from damage.

LIGAMENT AND TENDON

WHAT IS THE FUNCTION OF LIGAMENTS AND TENDONS?

Ligaments are passive structures that connect bone to bone. They help to increase joint stability and function to guide and restrain joint motion.

Tendons are also passive structures, designed to connect muscle to bone. The tendon must then be able to transmit the tensile loads from the muscle to the bone. In addition, the tendon may be able to fit in locations in which the bulk of a muscle may not fit.

WHAT IS THE COMPOSITION OF LIGAMENTS AND TENDONS?[4,58]

Ligaments and tendons are similar in nature and are composed of cells and an extracellular matrix. The cells are primarily fibroblasts. The extracellular matrix is composed of water and solid material, which is, in turn, composed of collagen, elastin, and ground substance. The amount of collagen and elastin differs in tendons when compared to ligaments. In tendons, more collagen is present, whereas ligaments have a greater amount of elastin.

These component materials provide the mechanical properties of ligaments and tendons.

Collagen is mostly of type I and is made by the fibroblasts. In tendons, the alignment of the collagen fibers is organized in the same direction as the tendon. However, in ligaments, while the collagen is largely unidirectional, there are fibers laid down in other directions. This provides the ligament with the ability to resist tension forces in more than one direction. Elastin is a protein with elastic properties, providing the ligaments and tendons with the ability to deform and return to the resting shape when unloaded. Ligaments tend to have greater amounts of elastin than do tendons. Ground substance is made of PGs similar to those in cartilage. The PGs bind the water and form a gel-like fluid in which the collagen fibers are found.

WHAT IS THE STRUCTURE OF LIGAMENTS AND TENDONS?[4,5,59]

Tendons are composed of collagen organized into gradually increasing size of bundles. The bundles are organized together to form the next size bundle (Figure I-4-4). In other words, groups of the collagen fibers at their smallest (tropocollagen) bundle together to form the collagen molecule, the bundles of the collagen organize into microfibers, groups of microfibers form the subfibril, groups of subfibrils form the fibril, groups of fibrils form the fascicles, then groups of fascicles come together to form the tendon itself. These bundles are surrounded by connective tissue sheaths.

Collagen fibers retain a naturally wavy appearance. This relaxed wave responds to load by first straightening out (pulling taut) before tension or stress increases in the collagen. This taking out the slack in the collagen is responsible for the initial toe region in a stress–strain curve for structures with high collagen composition.

Tendons receive their blood supply from vessels in the perimysium (connective tissue covering of a fascicle of skeletal muscle), periosteal insertion, or the paratenon or mesotenon.

Mesotenon is defined as "the delicate connective tissue sheath attaching a tendon to its fibrous sheath,"[14] whereas paratenon is defined as "fatty areolar tissue filling the interstices (space) of the fascial compartment in which a tendon is situated."[14] Tendons with a sheath (example: flexor digitorum profundus) receive less blood supply than those without sheaths.

Ligaments receive a more diffuse and uniform blood supply. This blood supply comes from the ligament insertion into bone. The increased blood supply to ligaments provides for a better healing when compared to sheathed tendons.

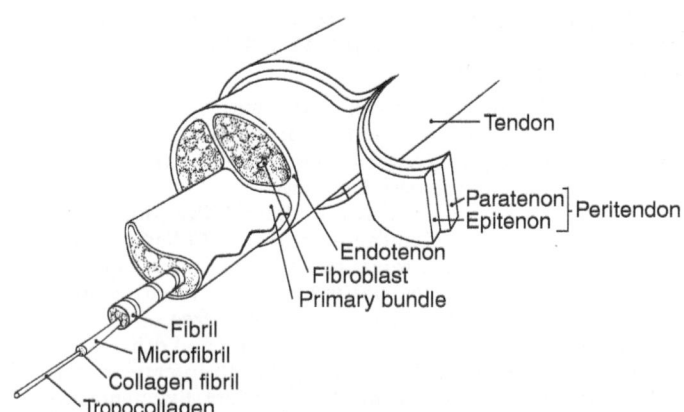

FIGURE I-4-4 Structural organization of tendon. (DeLee JC, *Drez D Jr, eds. DeLee & Drez's Orthopaedic Sports Medicine: Principles and Practice.* 2nd ed. Philadelphia: Saunders, 2003.)

WHAT ARE THE BIOMECHANICAL PROPERTIES OF TENDONS AND LIGAMENTS?[4,5,58]

Ligaments have viscoelastic properties similar to those previously discussed. Therefore tendons and ligaments exhibit rate- and time-dependent responses to loading.

WHAT IS THE MECHANICAL BEHAVIOR OF TENDONS AND LIGAMENTS?[4,5]

Tendons and ligaments respond primarily to unidirectional tensile loads with ligaments resisting load in more than one direction. As a tensile load is applied, the collagen fibers initially straighten out and then show an elastic response. If the load is released during this linear deformation period, the tendon or ligament will return to its original resting length. Should additional tensile load be placed on the tissue, the tendon or ligament will experience microscopic breakdown. When the load is removed, the tissue does not return to its original length but exhibits plastic deformation or retention of the new tissue length resulting from the load. Given sufficient rest, the tendon or ligament is capable of recovery.

In comparison with capacity, normal loading for tendons and ligaments is 25% to 33% of maximum. Strain or deformation during activity is 2% to 5%.[29] The magnitude of this physiological strain is considerably less than that found when testing isolated tendon tissue. The shape and size of the tendon or ligament influence the capacity of the structure with larger structures able to handle larger loads.

Tendons join the contractile tissue at the myotendinous junction (MTJ). The method of insertion into the contractile tissue allows for the force of the muscle contraction to be transmitted to the collagen fibers of the tendons and, thus, muscular force is transmitted to the bone for movement via the tendon. The MTJ is the weakest point of the muscle–tendon unit and the primary site of damage.

DOES THE RATE OR FREQUENCY OF LOADING AFFECT TENDON AND LIGAMENT RESPONSE?[4,5,60]

Rate of loading and frequency of loading do affect the tendon and ligament response. In general, the higher rate of loading causes less strain for a given load (steeper linear region). Tendons and ligaments fail at greater force magnitude under higher rates of loading. Finally, higher rates of loading result in a greater elongation or larger strain before failure when compared to lower rates of loading.

Repetitive loading or cyclical loading causes a change in the tendon and ligament strain response. In general, with repeated loading, there is a greater elongation or strain for a given load (the stress–strain curve is shifted to the right).

HOW DOES TENDON AND LIGAMENT TISSUE RESPOND TO EXERCISE OR USE OR LACK OF USE?[4,5,8,25,31,50,60]

With increased exposure to load, as seen with systematic exercising, the tendon and ligaments tend to become stronger and stiffer. There may also be an increase in the size of the tendon or ligament associated with increased exercise.

Conversely, with a lack of use or immobilization, there is a resultant decrease in strength and stiffness. Collagen turnover is reduced and the tissue tends to lay down more haphazardly rather than in the direction of the load as seen with more normal amounts of loading. The cross-sectional area of the tendon or ligament is reduced with long-term disuse and other mechanical properties exhibit a decreased ability to tolerate load with both short-term and long-term disuse. In fact, ligaments immobilized for a period of time and then reconditioned still show reduced load to failure in comparison with control ligaments after 12 months of reconditioning.[61]

HOW DO TENDONS AND LIGAMENTS RESPOND TO AGING?[15,60]

As tendon and ligament tissue matures, there is an increase in the number and strength of cross-links. This increase has two results: one is limited magnitude of the elongation and the second is increased strength of the tissue. With increased age, there is a tendency toward a reduced diameter and water content, with a resultant reduction in the tensile capacity of the tendon and ligament.

WHAT ARE THE SECONDARY EFFECTS OF DAMAGE TO THE TENDONS AND LIGAMENTS?

Damage to the tendon will affect the muscle–tendon unit (MTU) and may result in a reduction in the force generation of the contractile tissue due to pain. Reduction in the force-generating capacity of an MTU can have implications for the underlying bony tissue, since muscular contractions influence the loads experienced by the bone (see Bone).

Damage to the ligament sufficient to cause ligamentous laxity (a Grade II or III sprain or total rupture) will affect the motion of the joint. Abnormal joint motion will result, which can lead to breakdown of the articular cartilage or the subchondral bone.

It is important that the clinician understands the implication of altered mechanics as a result of damage to or loss of the tendon or ligament in order to minimize the secondary damage that may result.

MUSCLE

There are three muscle types present in the body: cardiac muscle, smooth muscle of the organs and vessels, and skeletal muscle. For the clinical practitioner seeing patients with musculoskeletal complaints, the skeletal muscle is by far the most relevant muscle tissue. The following information will focus on skeletal muscle only.

This depth and presentation of this material is designed for ease of application in clinical situations. To the basic scientist, it may appear to be extraordinarily simplified. This is by design. The intent is to demonstrate the relevance of the basic science to clinicians in terms that she or he may understand better than the normal terminology associated with the relevant basic science research.

WHAT IS THE FUNCTION OF SKELETAL MUSCLE?

Muscle tissue is the only tissue in the body that has the ability to contract; thus its primary purpose is to generate movement. Additional functions of the skeletal muscle include the maintenance of postural alignment and upright position and generally overcoming the normal forces placed on the body such as gravity. Muscles also provide strength to and protection of the skeletal system by helping to redistribute loads and to absorb shock.

WHAT IS THE COMPOSITION OF SKELETAL MUSCLE?[22,24,30,32]

Skeletal muscle is composed of sarcomeres, which are formed from contractile proteins. These contractile proteins include the following:
- Actin, troponin, and tropomyosin function to regulate muscle contraction.
- Myosin generates the contraction.
- Titin attaches myosin to the Z bands (elastic portion) and to the M line or center of the sarcomere (inelastic portion).

These contractile proteins are arranged in a systematic pattern to allow exposure of the actin to myosin and a resultant "sliding of the filament" to generate contraction. The contraction and subsequent relaxation require the presence of calcium and energy to occur.

WHAT IS THE STRUCTURE OF SKELETAL MUSCLE?[22,24,30,32]

Sarcomeres are organized together to create myofibrils. The myofibrils then organize together to form a muscle fiber, which is the basic unit of the muscle. Each myofibril is surrounded by a membrane called the sarcolemma, which is a key factor in the function of muscles and the release of calcium.

The thickness or diameter of a muscle fiber is determined by the number of myofibrils that composes the fiber, which in turn determines its strength. When abnormal muscle fiber diameters are noted in muscle, it is an indication that the level of muscle use has changed.

The muscle itself is composed of groups of muscle fibers arranged into bundles or fascicles. These fascicles have a connective tissue sheath called a perimysium (continuous with the tendon fascicle covering called the endotenon). The muscle itself has a connective tissue sheath called the epimysium.

A motor unit is the smallest portion of a muscle that can be made to contract independently. Motor units are defined as one motor neuron and all the muscle fibers it innervates. When the nerve is stimulated, all of the muscle fibers are activated. *In vivo*, generally smaller motor units are activated first, with an increase in the number of motor units as demand increases. Different muscles have motor units that are larger or smaller dependent of the function of the muscle. Muscles that require precision activity, such as those in the hands, have a smaller number of muscle fibers for each motor unit, allowing for very selective muscle activation. Muscles that have more of a strength and less of a precision demand (such as the quadriceps) have larger numbers of muscle fibers innervated by a single motor unit. Muscle fibers for a particular motor unit are not located in a single spot in the muscle, but are distributed throughout the muscle.[19,57]

WHAT ARE THE MECHANICAL TERMS ASSOCIATED WITH MUSCLE CONTRACTION?

- Muscle tension is the force exerted by the MTU on the bone.
- Load is the force exerted on the muscle by gravity, by an object being lifted, etc.
- Moment or torque is the rotational force of the muscle and is quantified in the literature as (muscle force × lever arm). Lever arm is the perpendicular distance from the center of rotation of the joint to the line of action of the muscle.
- Mechanical work is (force × distance over which it moves).
- Power is (force × velocity) for linear power or (moment × angular velocity) for rotational power.

WHAT ARE THE BASIC TYPES OF MUSCLE CONTRACTION?[23]

Muscle contraction can be either dynamic or static. Dynamic contractions occur when muscle contracts during a change in the joint angle. Dynamic contractions can be either concentric, during which the muscle is shortening in length, or eccentric, during which the muscle is lengthening. Additional terminology that may be associated with dynamic contractions: isokinetic contractions require a constant velocity, isoinertial contractions are defined as a constant external load, and isotonic contractions mean that there is a constant muscle force present throughout the range of motion.

Static contractions are also called isometric contractions. There is no mechanical work done during an isometric contraction, although energy is expended (physiological work is done).

Generally, muscles can generate the greatest amount of force either isometrically or eccentrically. Force production in muscle is also influenced by the mechanical properties of muscles.

WHAT ARE THE MECHANICAL PROPERTIES OF SKELETAL MUSCLE?[47]

The mechanical properties of the muscle include the following:
- Length-tension relationship
- Force-velocity relationship
- Force-time relationship
- Skeletal muscle architecture

LENGTH–TENSION RELATIONSHIP: The force or tension developed within a muscle varies with the length of the muscle at the time of contraction. Each muscle has an optimal length at which it generates greater force than other lengths. This is its ideal length-tension relationship. Usually this ideal length is somewhere in the middle of the range of motion for the muscle, although this is an oversimplification. To fully develop a muscle, training should include all ranges of length at which the muscle will be required to act in the desired function.

FORCE–VELOCITY RELATIONSHIP: The velocity of the contraction or the rate of change of the angle of the joint at the time of the contraction will influence the force generation capacity. For concentric contractions, as the velocity of motion increases, the force producing capacity decreases. For eccentric contraction, there is a small increase in force producing capacity with increased velocity; however, the capacity to produce force appears to peak quickly. For optimal muscular development, muscles should be trained at the velocity required for the desired function.

FORCE–TIME RELATIONSHIP: The ability to generate a contraction in muscle tissue is related to the amount of time available. Larger forces can be generated if more time is available; with shorter time to generate force, the magnitude of the force is reduced.

Note: the connective tissue sheath surrounding the muscle fascicles (perimysium) and the entire muscle (epimysium) has mechanical properties apart from the contractile tissue it surrounds. These sheaths respond in a fashion similar to other structures with collagen as a component. Active muscle contraction is strongest in midrange and tension in these passive structures increases toward end range. Thus passive structures influence total force production.

WHAT IS THE EFFECT OF SKELETAL MUSCLE ARCHITECTURE ON THE ABILITY TO GENERATE FORCE?[27,73]

Muscles that have a larger number of sarcomeres arranged in series (end to end) generally have longer myofibrils. Velocity and excursion of a muscle are proportional to the length of the myofibrils. Longer myofibrils indicate a faster muscle and larger excursion. Conversely, muscles with more sarcomeres in parallel have thicker myofibrils and generally a larger CSA. Force production in a muscle is proportional to the CSA of the muscle. Muscles with fibers that are angled or pennated can pack larger numbers of fibers into a smaller area and so increase the CSA and the force production capacity of the muscle.

The type of muscle fiber also affects the function of the muscle, with muscle type dependent on differing contractile and metabolic processes. The metabolic process is largely the ability to generate ATP and the rate at which the energy is available to the sarcomere.

Type I fibers are slow oxidative muscles, showing low activity of myosin ATPase in the muscle fiber and therefore a slow contraction time coupled with a high potential for oxidative or aerobic activity. These fibers are difficult to fatigue due to a high blood supply. Slow oxidative muscles are used as postural muscles, such as the soleus muscle.

Type 2A muscles are a cross between type I and type IIB. These muscle fibers have a fast contraction time combined with a good capacity for both aerobic (oxidative) and anaerobic (glycolytic) activity. Type 2A muscles can maintain contractions for extended periods of time, but the high frequency of contraction exceeds the ability of the muscle to provide ATP.

Type 2B muscles are fast glycolytic muscles; they depend on anaerobic activity for ATP, have few capillaries, but they contract quickly and the large muscle fibers associated with these muscles produce large amounts of tension (gastrocnemius). Type 2B muscles are generally recruited for high power activities that are more intermittent in nature.

Most muscles have more than one fiber type. Fiber types are generally thought to be genetically determined, but may be trained as well. When training stops or with aging, more of the fibers become slow oxidative.

WHAT FACTORS HELP TO VISUALLY IDENTIFY MUSCLE FATIGUE?

When muscles have depleted the available energy source, the muscle will begin to fatigue. As clinical practitioners, it is our business to determine when the muscle is fatigued and discontinue training. Fatigue of a muscle is noted with a decrease in muscle coordination or ability to shock absorb. There will be a decrease in accuracy or speed of muscle contraction and a general flushing of the area.

HOW DOES MUSCLE RESPOND TO EXERCISE OR USE OR LACK OF USE?[18,27,28,45]

Muscle has a tremendous capacity for remodeling and responds well with recovery from injury or with increased demand. Generally an increase in use or demand is met with an increase in the CSA of the muscle over time. It can take 4 to 6 weeks to increase the CSA of a muscle. Strength changes that occur earlier than the 4- to 6-week time period are generally thought to be a result of learning and improved motor control as contrasted with a true increase in the CSA. Training of a muscle tends to be specific to the demand placed on the muscle. If training occurs at low velocity, then the capacity of the muscle to perform at low velocity increases. The capacity to perform at high velocity is not affected. If high-velocity performance is desired, then high-velocity training is required. Similarly, the entire range of motion should be trained in a muscle. Muscles trained at a specific joint angle improve performance at that joint angle (with some effect at near angles). Muscles trained throughout the available range will demonstrate improved performance throughout the range.

With disuse and/or immobilization, muscles respond with a decrease in endurance capacity and a decrease in strength. Over time, there is a reduction in the number and size of muscle fibers, resulting in a decrease in the CSA of the muscle. Generally, type I fibers tend to atrophy first. If disuse persists, fatty tissue may infiltrate and take over the muscle fibers. With immobilization (as in casting) muscle sarcomeres may be lost if casted in a shortened muscular position.

WHAT IS AN ELECTROMYOGRAM?

An electromyogram (EMG) is the electrical signal associated with the contraction of a muscle. This signal can be recorded and studied. The study of EMG signals is called electromyography. Diagnostic EMG is utilized to assess neuromotor function, whereas kinesiological EMG is utilized to analyze muscle function, including muscle activation patterns. Biofeedback EMG is utilized to provide feedback to the clinician or patient regarding the muscle activation for therapeutic use. It can be utilized to help increase muscle activation or to decrease muscle activation, as seen in patients with excessive activation of the upper trapezius muscles.

NERVE

Although the central nervous system (CNS) is certainly critical, the peripheral nervous system (PNS) contains the nerves that orthopedic practitioners are most likely to address as part of musculoskeletal complaints. Thus, this work will focus on the components of the PNS.

WHAT IS THE FUNCTION OF NERVES?

Nervous tissue is required for control of the body and activation of the muscles. In addition, it is the mechanism by which the body obtains feedback from the environment. Motor nerves take directions from the spinal cord and the brain to the muscles. Sensory nerves take the sensory information from the receptors to the spinal cord and the brain.

WHAT IS THE COMPOSITION AND STRUCTURE OF PERIPHERAL NERVES?[38,49,72]

Nerves fibers are axons or elongated processes that extend from the cell body to the end organ the nerve targets such as a muscle, sensory receptor, etc. Most nerve fibers have a myelin sheath produced by Schwann cells. Fibers are grouped together in bundles called fascicles, which are themselves grouped together in bundles to make up the peripheral nerve. The peripheral nerve begins as the nerve root terminates, which is at the point at which the root splits into the dorsal ramus and the ventral ramus. The ventral ramus becomes the peripheral nerve, which carries both sensory and motor information (Figure I-4-5).

As a protective mechanism for nerves, the nerve fibers have a protective connective tissue layer (endoneurium) that covers the myelin sheath. The fascicles, in turn, have a protective connective tissue covering called the perineurium, which also creates a chemical barrier isolating the fascicles from the surrounding tissue. The entire nerve has an outer covering called the epineurium. The epineurium is also located between the fascicles and serves to protect the nerve. Vascular supply to the nerve is present at all structural levels of the nerve.

WHAT IS THE MECHANICAL BEHAVIOR OF PERIPHERAL NERVES?[38,49,72]

TENSION: Peripheral nerves with their connective tissue sheaths are able to experience considerable deformation before rupture. However, as tension is applied to the nerve, the lumen of the nerve narrows and axonal transport is slowed or interrupted. In addition, similar changes are experienced in the blood vessels supplying the nerves. As the vessel constricts, the blood supply (and nutrient supply) may be reduced or eliminated. Damage to the nerve, then, may occur before the ultimate failure point on a stress–strain curve.

COMPRESSION: Peripheral nerves subject to compression experience damage depending on the magnitude and duration of the compressing force. Compressive forces can slow or eliminate axonal transport in the nerve fiber or may impair or eliminate blood flow to the area of compression. Sustained compression

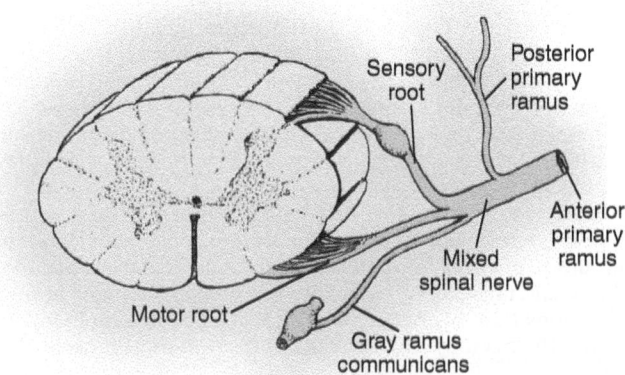

FIGURE I-4-5 Diagram of the arrangement of a spinal nerve. The peripheral nerve is formed after the posterior ramus branches off. The anterior primary ramus becomes the peripheral nerve. (From Jobe MT, Martinez SF. Peripheral nerve injuries. In: *Campbell's Operative Orthopaedics*, 11th ed. Philadelphia, PA: Elsevier Mosby, 2008.)

even at low levels (30 to 40 mm Hg) may cause damage that is irreversible. Compression also causes an increase in vascular permeability and therefore intraneural edema, which may also reduce blood supply and nutrition to the nerve.

The edema may exist after release of the pressure and so affect the function of the nerve more long term, even causing intraneural fibrosing (scarring).

LIMITATION TO GLIDING: Peripheral nerves have functional requirements that may involve considerable change in length as a result of limb motion. For example, median nerve excursion has been measured at greater than 12 mm of motion[80,81] or strain of 7.6%.[82] In the absence of the ability to glide as in the presence of spinal stenosis or osteophytes, or when there is adhesions restricting nerve movement, portions of the nerve may experience tension or compression. Clinicians should be aware of the range limitations for the nervous tissue as well as the single joint motion limitations as they examine patients.

BIOMECHANICS OF THE HUMAN BODY AND JOINTS

WHAT IS BIOMECHANICS?

According to Dorland's *Illustrated Medical Dictionary*, biomechanics is defined as the application of mechanical laws to living structures, specifically to the locomotor system of the human body.[14]

Many people have an interest in the study of biomechanics, including surgeons (especially orthopedic surgeons), physical therapists, coaches and trainers, prosthetists/orthotists, and biomedical engineers. Individuals with an understanding of biomechanics are well suited to collect, analyze, and assess human motion disorders (as seen clinically) or to answer or address questions concerning performance enhancement. With the advance of technology, questions regarding the analysis of human movement are becoming more commonplace and, thus, more information is available for the health care practitioner.

WHAT ARE THE COMPONENTS OF A BIOMECHANICAL ANALYSIS?

Components of a quantitative biomechanical analysis may include the following:

- Kinematics or the study of motion (which forms the basis of the observational analysis performed by many clinicians)
- Kinetics, which is the study of forces causing the motion
- Anthropometry or the study of the size, weight, and measurement of the body
- Electromyography, which is the measurement of the electrical signals generated by muscles during function (see Muscle).

When applied to the entire body, these components of biomechanical analysis can be helpful in understanding the general body movement or may be applied alone or in concert to the level of the individual tissues.

Study of the biomechanical properties of the specific tissue will help to identify how the tissue responds to a single load or what the fatigue characteristics of the tissue are (response to multiple number of loads). In addition, it is possible to determine if there are other factors that influence the response of tissue to load, such as the rate of loading, frequency of loading, and age of the tissue.

Knowledge of the response of tissue to load can help to identify what sort of activity may be causing or influencing the damage to the tissue. Identification of the offending mechanism is imperative for a positive response to treatment of the involved tissue. In addition, knowledge of tissue response to load assists the clinician with selection of appropriate exercise or therapeutic interventions for tissue rehabilitation.

Study of the biomechanics of a particular motion or motions will provide information that includes range of motion necessary for the movement, estimation of the minimum forces required

for the motion to occur both linear and angular, and the on/off patterns of the muscle activity. The magnitude or quantity of muscle activity may also be quantified if normalization has been completed.

KINEMATICS

Kinematics, or the study of motion, may include quantitative analysis and qualitative analysis. Kinematic analysis provides information regarding position, velocity, and acceleration. The movement may be linear (in a line) or angular (about an axis of motion). Most of the motion in the human body is angular motion.

A quantitative motion analysis is conducted utilizing motion capture equipment and computational processes to determine the positional coordinates of each of the body segments either at one point or over time. In this case the practitioner must begin with a defined starting point, the "you are here" point. All other markers on the body are expressed some distance from this starting point so the position of all segments can be defined and recreated. Quantitative methods that may be utilized in the clinic include use of photos (still or motion frames) and measuring tools including rulers (physical or electronic). Velocity may be captured with a stopwatch. More sophisticated motion analysis is usually conducted in a motion analysis laboratory.

Qualitative analysis is more likely what will be completed during the normal patient examination. This is an observational process that begins with a static analysis of the posture of the patient and continues throughout the examination and intervention. In the case of a qualitative analysis, the clinician learns to observe human motion and make a subjective report of what she or he has seen. In the case of qualitative analysis, neither velocity nor acceleration can be quantified.

To communicate with other health care practitioners, it is important that terminology be consistent. Thus, all motion description begins with the starting point called the anatomical position. Motion then occurs in a plane about an axis of rotation at each joint. Three planes of motion are generally described: the sagittal plane (medial/lateral axis) is for flexion and extension (or dorsiflexion/plantar flexion at the ankle). The frontal plane (anterior/posterior axis) holds abduction/adduction (or inversion/eversion in some joints of the foot such as the subtalar joint). Finally, the transverse plane (superior/inferior axis) holds rotations, pronation/supination of the elbow and some joints of the foot, and horizontal abduction/adduction of the shoulder.

WHY IS THE AXIS AND PLANE OF MOTION IMPORTANT TO ME AS A CLINICIAN?[35,59]

When examining joint integrity, as a clinician you should determine whether the quantity and quality of motion are what you expect from that joint. Utilizing terminology that is consistent with other health care practitioners will improve communication and improve understanding between clinicians. If you are exposed to a joint that requires examination with which you are less familiar, knowledge of the principles will assist you in determining the expectations and communicating your findings.

POSTURE AND MOTION ANALYSIS OF THE BODY

The examination of the patient in the orthopedic clinic begins with an examination of posture. Posture should begin with observation of the patient at rest and should proceed to examine one or more motions that are reported to aggravate the complaint.

WHAT IS POSTURE?

Posture is the relative arrangement of the parts of the body. Good posture is that state of muscular and skeletal balance that protects the supporting structures of the body against injury or progressive deformity. The muscles will function most efficiently

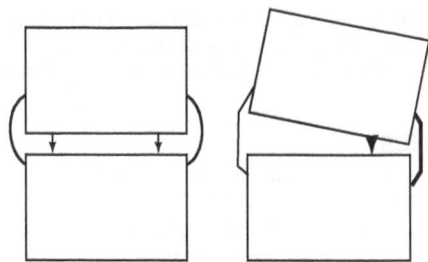

FIGURE I-4-6 Left: Bones in ideal contact, even distribution of load, equal tension in connective tissue on both sides. **Right:** Bones not in ideal contact, increased load on the right, increased tension on connective tissue on the left, and adaptive shortening of connective tissue on the right.

with good posture. Poor posture is a faulty relationship of the various parts of the body that produces increased strain on the supporting structures and in which there is less efficient balance of the body over its base of support. Kendall and McCreary concur with this report, stating that ideal contact between bones in a joint minimizes the stress and strain placed on bones, joints, ligaments, and muscles (Figure I-4-6) and maximizes the efficiency of the muscles.[42]

HOW DO PEOPLE DEVELOP FAULTY POSTURE?

Possible causes include poor postural habits, repetitive movements, sustained sitting, and ergonomics of the work environment. When an individual maintains a certain position for a prolonged period of time, the body will assume this sustained alignment as its normal posture.[42] If this newly adapted posture subjects the body to malalignment of structures, pain may result.[42]

WHY ARE CLINICIANS CONCERNED WITH POSTURE?

With less than ideal posture or poor posture, an increase in strain is placed on some of the tissues (Figure I-4-6: altered posture with an example of the change in length of soft tissue). This results in less than ideal function of the soft tissues and a reduction in the muscular efficiency.

Additionally, joint alignment may be altered causing increased point pressure or increased stress on portions of the joint surface. Such increased stress has been associated with joint surface breakdown and osteoarthritis. In fact, pathological posture has been defined as anatomic or physiological malalignments from normal that result in physical or functional limitations.[69] Resulting neuromusculoskeletal pathology can occur either at the site of the malalignment or at distal areas, which may be referred to as sites of correlated or compensatory motions or postures.[69]

Deviations from ideal resting posture, which may cause a change in length of muscles, ligaments, and joint capsules, as well as uneven distribution of forces between bones, have been associated with pain. Muscles, ligaments, bones, disks, and even nerves themselves are all innervated by nerves that transmit the sensation of pain. Pain may result from compressing or stretching a nerve, muscle fatigue, abnormal stresses on ligaments and joint capsules, and wearing down the cartilage that covers the end of bones.[13,53,74] All of these scenarios may occur when the body deviates from ideal alignment.

Griegel-Morris et al studied the correlation between cervical, shoulder, and thoracic postural abnormalities and the incidence of pain in 88 healthy adults.[33] The results showed that more severe deviations from ideal alignment correlated with a higher incidence of pain; however, cause and effect could not be determined.[12]

Clinicians should examine posture for affect on the area of complaint, carefully examining areas that demonstrate less than ideal alignment in order to guide further testing. On the shortened side

of the postural deviation, length should be assessed (muscle or joint). On the lengthened side of the postural deviation, strength should be assessed. The clinician is ascertaining if the posture is a required position resulting from inadequate available range of motion (ROM) then treat with increasing ROM. If posture is a choice, then treat with change in habit or reeducation.

Following examination of the static posture, one or more specific movements that are known to aggravate the complaint should be analyzed. These functional activities are also examined to see how the activity places stress on the involved area.

For example, if the involved area is the patellofemoral joint, a step down may be analyzed. During the step down, it is possible to see that that the hip lacks control over the thigh, visualizing uncontrolled internal rotation (IR) or external rotation (ER) (or abduction/adduction) of the thigh. Alternately, it is possible to notice that the ankle reaches end range dorsiflexion (DF) rapidly and foot pronation commences early, with concomitant tibial movement causing internal rotation of the hip. Both of these motions may lead to a more laterally directed patella and increased point loading with resulting pain. They also would indicate that further examination is warranted, if not treatment directed at the hip or foot, respectively.

WHAT ARE THE KINEMATICS OF THE JOINTS OF THE BODY?

There are two main types of joints in the body, synarthrodial and diarthrodial joints. While health care professionals may address the motion of synarthrodial joints, it is much more likely that the second type of joint, the diarthrodial joint, is involved in clinical patients since most of the motion in the body arises from the diarthrodial joints.

Diarthrodial joints have an articular cavity and a capsule or a ligamentous bag enclosing the joint lined by a synovial membrane, which secretes synovial fluid. The articulating surfaces are smooth and covered with hyaline cartilage, although some have fibrocartilage at the margins. The shape of the diarthroses determines what physiological motion, and the accompanying accessory motion, is available at each joint.

WHAT ARE THE JOINT SHAPES AND WHAT TYPE OF MOTION IS PRESENT AT EACH?

1. Plane (arthrodial), which allows only a gliding movement; therefore there is no axis of motion. Examples are the carpal or tarsal bones.
2. Hinge (ginglymus), which is like a door opening; motion is in only one direction, about a single axis. An example is the elbow joint. Motion allowed is forward and backward rotation (angular movement) defined as flexion and extension.
3. Pivot (trochoid), which allows a spinning motion (rotation), like a top, as the only motion. Therefore, like the ginglymus joint the pivot joint is uniaxial. Examples include the atlantoaxial joint or the radial-ulnar joint.
4. Condyloid (ovoid, ellipsoidal), which allows motion in two directions, forward and backward rotation, plus side to side (biaxial); these motions are defined as flexion and extension and abduction/adduction. Examples include the wrist joint and metacarpal phalangeal joint.
5. Saddle (sellar) is like two condyloid joints together. It looks like a saddle shape (reciprocally convex and concave). The saddle shape allows motion like a condyloid joint in two directions, or biaxially. It also allows some rotation. An example is the carpometacarpal joint of the thumb.
6. Ball-and-socket (spheroidal), which have the same shape as the condyloid joints; however, it also has muscles that are capable of causing rotation. The extra motion allows for triaxial or triplanar motion. Example are the glenohumeral joint and the hip joint.

WHAT IS THE DIFFERENCE BETWEEN PHYSIOLOGICAL MOTION AND ACCESSORY MOTION?

Physiological motion, also referred to as osteokinematics, is the active motion that is present in the joint. Physiological motions are the angular motions of the bones or the ROM at a joint.

Accessory motions, also known as joint play, are the involuntary motions that occur at the joint surface during physiological motion. Joint play mobility depends on the configuration of the joint surfaces. In general, most of the joints with which health care practitioners work are joints with concave/convex joint pairs, although plane joints and saddle joints may also need examination or intervention.

When examining physiological joint ROM, the practitioner should determine if the ROM is full or if it is limited. If ROM is limited, a determination should be made as to the cause of the limitation. Some examples of reasons for limited ROM include inadequate muscle length, swelling or fluid in the joint, space occupying material, or capsular hypomobility. Capsular mobility is associated with inadequate accessory joint mobility.

WHAT ARE THE TYPES OF ACCESSORY JOINT MOTIONS?

There are three main accessory motions associated with physiological motion of the joint: spin, roll, and glide or slide. Spin is defined as a single point of contact continuously on both of the participating bones. An arc is formed by some points on the moving bone. An example of spin can be seen as the motion of a top. Roll is defined as occurring when new points on one bone meet new points on the other, as occurs with a ball in motion. Slide or glide occurs when the same points on one bone meet new points on the other, as occurs between skates and the ice in ice-skating. For plane synovial joints, this is the only motion available at the joint surface. Normally, accessory movements are combined, with more than one occurring simultaneously.

During normal joint physiological motion, accessory mobility is required. Roll motion always takes place in the same direction as the moving bone. The direction of the glide motion will depend on which bone is moving. When the concave bony partner is moving, the glide motion occurs in the same direction as the bone movement. When the convex partner is moving, glide motion is in the direction opposite to the bone motion (Figure I-4-7). Gliding motion occurs parallel to the concave surface of the joint.

In addition to the accessory motions occurring during physiological motion, two translator motions may be described as accessory motions: compression and distraction or traction. Compression and distraction occur perpendicular to the plane or concave surface of the joint. Compression is the motion of one joint surface toward the other, and is utilized more as an examination tool to determine the integrity of the joint surface. Traction is a gapping motion between the joints and can be utilized for general assessment or improvement of joint surface mobility.

In the presence of inadequate or limited joint mobility at a joint, a clinical practitioner may utilize accessory joint mobilization as a tool to improve joint motion. In this case the glide accessory motion is the primary tool for increasing joint range of motion. When utilizing joint accessory mobilizations, it is important to recall that the mobilizations are normally applied parallel to the concave surface of the joint. This concave surface of the joint describes the treatment plane of the joint.

To determine what direction of glide is appropriate to select for improving joint ROM, you can apply a test glide. Test glides are normally applied at the point in the ROM at which the joint tissues are most lax, defined as the loose pack position. At this point in the ROM, the greatest joint play mobility will be present. Test glides, however, may be applied anywhere in the ROM. The direction of the glide mobilization utilized should be in the direction of the greatest glide restriction. An alternate method is the Convex–Concave Rule.[39]

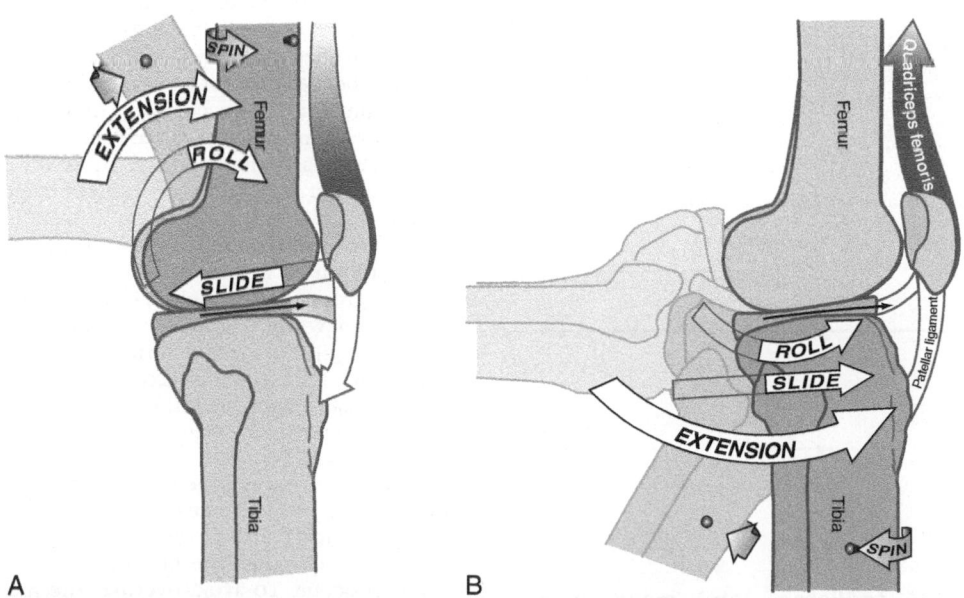

FIGURE I-4-7 (A, B) Roll and glide accessory motions occur at the joint surface during normal flexion and extension of the knee joint. Here the tibia is held still and the femur is moving. (From Newmann DA. *Kinesiology of the Musculoskeletal System: Foundations for Physical Rehabilitation,* 2nd ed. St Louis, MO: Mosby; 2010.)

WHAT IS THE CONVEX–CONCAVE RULE?

The Convex–Concave Rule[39] states that as the convex portion of the joint pair is stabilized, the glide mobilization should be applied in the same direction as the moving concave bone. If the concave bone is stabilized, glide mobility should be opposite to the direction of the moving bone. Regardless of which bony surface is moving, the treatment plane is parallel to the concave surface of the joint. The Convex–Concave Rule is based on the normal accessory motions present during physiological motion. In the presence of shortened tissues that are not part of the joint itself (such as shortened muscle length), the glide mobilization may not be the preferred treatment to improve ROM.

WHAT IS A JOINT OR GLIDE MOBILIZATION?

Joint mobilizations are small translatory motions applied at the joint surface in the direction of the treatment plane (parallel to the concave bony partner). They are intended to improve the accessory mobility of the joint and thus improve physiological ROM at the joint. Joint mobilizations are more likely to be effective if the cause of the limited range is due to joint capsule hypomobility as opposed to limitations in muscle length. Before applying joint mobilizations, the clinical practitioner should be aware of the indications and contraindications, which is not a part of this chapter.

Maitland[52] has described oscillatory joint mobilizations of Grades I–V (Figure I-4-8). Grade I mobilization is a low-velocity, small-amplitude oscillation applied early in the ROM and is used to treat pain or assist with fluid flow in very painful, irritable joints. Grade II mobilization is a low-velocity, large-amplitude oscillation applied early in ROM and is also utilized to treat pain and to assist fluid flow. Grade II mobilizations are more beneficial for less irritable disorders. Both Grade I and II mobilizations are applied in the joint ROM *before* the onset of tissue resistance. Grade III joint mobilization is a low-velocity, large-amplitude oscillation applied toward the end of the available joint ROM. It is normally used with a small amount of traction. Grade III mobilization is used to treat resistance. Larger amplitudes are particularly beneficial with chronic resistance problems or resistance through larger ROMs. Grade IV mobilization is a small-amplitude oscillation applied at the end of the available joint ROM. It is also used with a small amount of traction and is beneficial to treat resistance or lack of ROM.

Oscillatory techniques are usually applied in "bouts" of 30 seconds to 2 minutes at a rate of two to three oscillations per second until a change in the status of the tissue is accomplished.

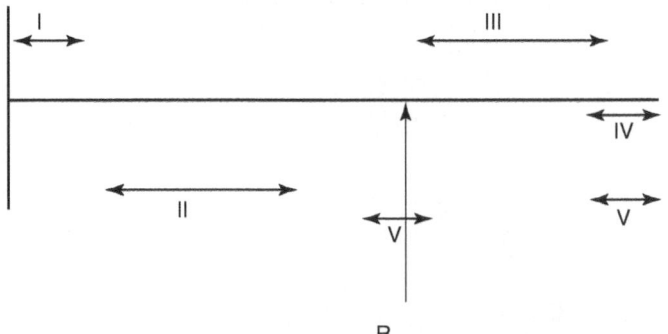

FIGURE I-4-8 Grades of oscillatory joint mobilizations (Grade I–V) designed to improve joint range of motion. R = onset of resistance in the joint. Grades I–IV are low-velocity low-amplitude (I, IV) or high-amplitude (II, III) mobilizations. Grade V is a high-velocity, low-amplitude mobilization.

A Grade V mobilization is a high-velocity, low-amplitude mobilization and may be applied at any point in the available ROM. This mobilization may be utilized when oscillatory techniques have stalled or may be applied according to applicable clinical prediction rules.

Kaltenborn[39] also describes joint mobilizations, but utilizes a different grading system. A Grade I mobilization is a traction force utilized to overcome normal joint compressive forces and reduce friction. A Grade II mobilization is a "tightening" movement designed to move into more resistance. The range of this movement is from a Grade I movement to the beginning of the Grade III point. Grades I and II (before tissue stretch) are utilized for pain relief. A Grade III movement is a "stretching" movement applied at the end of range, at the point resistance begins to increase markedly. Grade II within the resistance and Grade III mobilizations are utilized for increases in mobility.

KINETICS

Kinetics is the study of the forces that cause motion. In the human body, examples of forces that affect motion include external and internal forces. External forces include gravitational force and ground reaction forces; internal forces may include muscle and ligament forces. Recall that force (F) is equal to mass times acceleration ($F = ma$).

Gravitational force is a constant pull on our body toward the earth. The body must exert a constant force at least equal to the pull of gravity to remain upright. Individuals without the ability to generate this force are pulled to the ground. This is what happens in the presence of paralysis. The muscle force that normally opposes the pull of gravity is absent.

The force due to gravity is the mass of the body × 9.8 m/sec². The ability of the muscle to generate force must exceed the force of gravity. To function without overuse to the muscle, the magnitude of the force that is generated by the muscle must be far greater than the force of gravity. In general, muscles that function at less than 20% of maximum capacity can continue to function for extended periods of time before fatigue. The force due to gravity is considered to be an external force.

Ground reaction forces (GRF) are those forces that the body exerts on the ground and the ground exerts back on the body. The GRF acts over the entire part of the system in contact with the ground (whole foot). It may be considered to act at a single point and in that case is referred to as the center of pressure. GRF is another example of an external force. External forces are caused by anything that is not a part of the system or body. These external forces must be measured (i.e., by a force transducer).

Muscle and ligament forces are those forces that are exerted by the tissues of the body as movement occurs. Muscle and ligament forces are internal forces and it is difficult to quantify the magnitude of these contributions. Quantitative motion analysis may be utilized to determine the net force acting in a muscle or muscle group, and modeling can be utilized to predict muscle forces. A few investigators have implanted force transducers into the biological tissue to determine the force present; however, very few such human studies exist.

For the health care practitioner in the average clinical situation, a kinetic analysis is not normally available. Estimations of the kinetics must be made utilizing observational motion analysis. When forces exceed the capacity of the muscle, the activity will not occur. When forces are equal to the muscle capacity, a single repetition may be completed. Only when the muscle forces are greater than the demand on the system can repetitive action occur. To avoid overuse, the muscle capacity must be far in excess of the demand. To observe muscle capacity versus demand, the clinician may observe the activity causing complaints and note any fatigue or abnormal posture or muscle activity over one or more repetitions.

ANTHROPOMETRY

Anthropometry is the study of the size, weight, and measurement of the body. For clinical practitioners, the importance of anthropometry is to provide guidance as to the differences between patients. Patients come in all sizes and body types, some with large trunks, some with strong legs, some with small knee caps, etc. In the selection and application of treatment to musculoskeletal complaints, anthropometric characteristics should be included. Such characteristic analysis should include comparisons with normal.

HOW CAN ANTHROPOMETRY HELP ME IN THE CLINIC?

When the clinician keeps anthropometry in mind during examination and intervention, decision making may be improved. For example, in examining a patient with patellofemoral dysfunction, it is noted that the patient has a very small patella relative to the size of the rest of her body. The patella is still required to absorb and distribute loads from the quadriceps muscle as part of normal function. In the presence of a relatively small patella, the amount of stress on the patella will be larger than it is in the same individual with a larger patella (more area over with the force can be distributed). Thus, it may be determined that the prognosis for this patient is less that ideal.

As another example, individuals with relatively large trunks in comparison to the rest of their body may require increased trunk/hip extensor or abdominal muscle strength to accomplish the same task such as forward bending (extensor strength) or sit-up (abdominal strength). In fact, the individual may never be able to perform an abdominal curl without stabilization at the ankles, since the size differentiation between the trunk and legs is large.

Height and weight characteristics may also lead to an understanding of body fat or obesity characteristics. During weight-bearing activities, the forces present in the lower extremity joints are quantified in multiples of body weight. As an individual's body weight increases, the demand on the joint increases proportionally. Decisions may need to be made to avoid weight-bearing exercises until the joint is capable of bearing the increased load or until the weight is reduced sufficiently for safe weight-bearing activities.

SUMMARY

Biomechanical considerations for tissues are important for the rehabilitation professional. Knowledge of the mechanics of individual tissues leads to increased understanding of tissue examination and treatment. Understanding tissue biomechanics will specifically aid in isolating forces involved in the tissue insult as well as selection of what activities to utilize to unload the tissue or to reload it during the rehabilitation process.

In addition, biomechanical analysis is an integral part of the examination and rehabilitation process. Biomechanical analysis includes quantitative or observational examination of the posture, motion (physiological or accessory), kinetics, muscle activity, and anthropometry of the patient. Thus, biomechanical considerations are fundamental to the expert examination and intervention for rehabilitation of orthopedic or musculoskeletal complaints.

REFERENCES

1. Barry DW, Kohrt WM. Exercise and the preservation of bone health. *J Cardiopulm Rehabil Prev*. 2008;28(3):153-162.
2. Bayraktar HH, Morgan EF, Niebur GL, Morris GE, Wong EK, Keaveny TM. Comparison of the elastic and yield properties of human femoral trabecular and cortical bone tissue. *J Biomech*. 2004;37(1):27-35.
3. Benedek TG. A history of the understanding of cartilage. *Osteoarthritis Cartilage*. 2006;14(3):203-209.
4. Benjamin M, Ralphs JR. Tendons and ligaments–an overview. *Histol Histopathol*. 1997;12(4):1135-1144.
5. Best TM, Kirkendall DT, Almekinders LC, Garrett WE. Basic science and injury of muscle, tendon, and ligaments. Section A: Muscle and Tendon. In: DeLee JC, Drez D Jr, eds. *DeLee & Drez's Orthopaedic Sports Medicine: Principles and Practice*. 2nd ed. Philadelphia, PA: Saunders; 2003.
6. Brandt KD. Response of joint structures to inactivity and to reloading after immobilization. *Arthritis Rheum*. 2003;49(2):267-271.
7. Bray RC, Smith JA, Eng MK, Leonard CA, Sutherland CA, Salo PT. Vascular response of the meniscus to injury: effects of immobilization. *J Orthop Res*. 2001;19(3):384-390.
8. Buckwalter JA, Grodzinsky AJ. Loading of healing bone, fibrous tissue, and muscle: implications for orthopaedic practice. *J Am Acad Orthop Surg*. 1999;7(5):291-299.
9. Carter DR, Caler WE. Cycle-dependent and time-dependent bone fracture with repeated loading. *J Biomech Eng*. 1983;105(2):166-170.
10. Choi K, Goldstein SA. A comparison of the fatigue behavior of human trabecular and cortical bone tissue. *J Biomech*. 1992;25(12):1371-1381.
11. Cohen NP, Foster RJ, Mow VC. Composition and dynamics of articular cartilage: structure, function, and maintaining healthy state. *J Orthop Sports Phys Ther*. 1998;28(4):203-215.
12. Cullen DM, Smith RT, Akhter MP. Bone-loading response varies with strain magnitude and cycle number. *J Appl Physiol*. 2001;91(5):1971-1976.
13. Cunha AC, Burke TN, Franca FJ, Marques AP. Effect of global posture reeducation and of static stretching on pain, range of motion, and quality of life in women with chronic neck pain: a randomized clinical trial. *Clinics*. 2008;63(6):763-770.
14. Dorland. *Dorland's Illustrated Medical Dictionary*. 31st ed. Philadelphia, PA: Saunders; 2007.
15. Dressler MR, Butler DL, Wenstrup R, Awad HA, Smith F, Boivin GP. A potential mechanism for age-related declines in patellar tendon biomechanics. *J Orthop Res*. 2002;20(6):1315-1322.
16. Eckstein F, Lemberger B, Gratzke C, et al. In vivo cartilage deformation after different types of activity and its dependence on physical training status. *Ann Rheum Dis*. 2005;64(2):291-295.
17. Eckstein F, Tieschky M, Faber SC, et al. Effect of physical exercise on cartilage volume and thickness in vivo: MR imaging study. *Radiology*. 1998;207(1):243-248.
18. Edstrom L, Grimby L. Effect of exercise on the motor unit. *Muscle Nerve*. 1986;9(2):104-126.
19. English AW, Wolf SL. The motor unit. Anatomy and physiology. *Phys Ther*. 1982;62(12):1763-1772.
20. Evans RK, Antczak AJ, Lester M, Yanovich R, Israeli E, Moran DS. Effects of a 4-month recruit training program on markers of bone metabolism. *Med Sci Sports Exerc*. 2008;40(11 suppl):S660-S670.
21. Ewers BJ, Dvoracek-Driksna D, Orth MW, Haut RC. The extent of matrix damage and chondrocyte death in mechanically traumatized articular cartilage explants depends on rate of loading. *J Orthop Res*. 2001;19(5):779-784.
22. Faulkner JA, Larkin LM, Claflin DR, Brooks SV. Age-related changes in the structure and function of skeletal muscles. *Clin Exp Pharmacol Physiol*. 2007;34(11):1091-1096.
23. Faulkner JA. Terminology for contractions of muscles during shortening, while isometric, and during lengthening. *J Appl Physiol*. 2003;95(2):455-459.
24. Finni T. Structural and functional features of human muscle-tendon unit. *Scand J Med Sci Sports*. 2006;16(3):147-158.
25. Firth EC. The response of bone, articular cartilage and tendon to exercise in the horse. *J Anat*. 2006;208(4):513-526.
26. Fithian DC, Kelly MA, Mow VC. Material properties and structure-function relationships in the menisci. *Clin Orthop Relat Res*. 1990;252(3):19-31.
27. Fitts RH, McDonald KS, Schluter JM. The determinants of skeletal muscle force and power: their adaptability with changes in activity pattern. *J Biomech*. 1991;24(suppl 1):111-122.
28. Fitts RH. Effects of regular exercise training on skeletal muscle contractile function. *Am J Phys Med Rehabil*. 2003;82(4):320-331.
29. Fung Y. Quasi-linear viscoelasticity of soft tissues. *Biomechanics: Mechanical Properties of Living Tissues*. New York, NY: Springer-Verlag; 1981.
30. Geeves MA, Holmes KC. The molecular mechanism of muscle contraction. *Adv Protein Chem*. 2005;71:161-193.
31. Gondret F, Hernandez P, Remignon H, Combes S. Skeletal muscle adaptations and biomechanical properties of tendons in response to jump exercise in rabbits. *J Anim Sci*. 2009;87(2):544-553.

32. Grefte S, Kuijpers-Jagtman AM, Torensma R, Von den Hoff JW. Skeletal muscle development and regeneration. *Stem Cells Dev.* 2007;16(5):857-868.

33. Griegel-Morris P, Larson K, Mueller-Klaus K, Oatis CA. Incidence of common postural abnormalities in the cervical, shoulder, and thoracic regions and their association with pain in two age groups of healthy subjects. *Phys Ther.* 1992;72(6):425-430.

34. Gupta HS, Zioupos P. Fracture of bone tissue: The 'hows' and the 'whys'. *Med Eng Phys.* 2008;30(10):1209-1226.

35. Hamill J, Knutzen KM. *Biomechanical Basis of Human Movement.* 2nd ed. Baltimore, MD: Lippincott Williams & Wilkins; 2003.

36. Hansen U, Zioupos P, Simpson R, Currey JD, Hynd D. The effect of strain rate on the mechanical properties of human cortical bone. *J Biomech Eng.* 2008;130(1):011011.

37. Hasler EM, Herzog W, Wu JZ, Muller W, Wyss U. Articular cartilage biomechanics: theoretical models, material properties, and biosynthetic response. *Crit Rev Biomed Eng.* 1999;27(6):415-488.

38. Jobe MT, Martinez SF. Peripheral nerve injuries. In: Canale ST, Beaty JH, eds. *Campbell's Operative Orthopaedics.* 11th ed. Philadelphia: Mosby Elsevier; 2008.

39. Kaltenborn FM, Evjenth O, Kaltenborn TB, Morgan D, Vollowitz E. *Manual Mobilization of the Joints.* 4th ed. Oslo, Norway: Norli; 2003.

40. Keaveny TM, Wachtel EF, Ford CM, Hayes WC. Differences between the tensile and compressive strengths of bovine tibial trabecular bone depend on modulus [see comments]. *J Biomech.* 1994;27:1137-1146.

41. Keaveny TM. Strength of trabecular bone. *Bone Mechanics Handbook.* 2001;16:1-42.

42. Kendall FP, McCreary EK, Provance PG, Rodgers MM, Romani WA. Posture. In: *Muscles Testing and Function with Posture and Pain.* 5th ed. Baltimore, MD: Lippincott Williams & Wilkins; 2005:49-118.

43. Knecht S, Vanwanseele B, Stussi E. A review on the mechanical quality of articular cartilage –implications for the diagnosis of osteoarthritis. *Clin Biomech (Bristol, Avon).* 2006;21(10):999-1012.

44. Korecki CL, MacLean JJ, Iatridis JC. Dynamic compression effects on intervertebral disc mechanics and biology. *Spine.* 2008;33(13):1403-1409.

45. Kraemer WJ, Fleck SJ, Evans WJ. Strength and power training: physiological mechanisms of adaptation. *Exerc Sport Sci Rev.* 1996;24:363-397.

46. Li B, Aspden RM. Composition and mechanical properties of cancellous bone from the femoral head of patients with osteoporosis or osteoarthritis. *J Bone Miner Res.* 1997;12:641-651.

47. Lieber RL. *Skeletal muscle structure function & plasticity: The Physiological Basis of Rehabilitation.* 2nd ed. Philadelphia, PA Lippincott Williams & Wilkins; 2002.

48. Lucchinetti E, Adams CS, Horton WE Jr, Torzilli PA. Cartilage viability after repetitive loading: a preliminary report. *Osteoarthritis Cartilage.* 2002;10(1):71-81.

49. Lundborg G. Structure and function of the intraneural microvessels as related to trauma, edema formation, and nerve function. *J Bone Joint Surg Am.* 1975;57(7):938-948.

50. Maffulli N, King JB. Effects of physical activity on some components of the skeletal system. *Sports Med.* 1992;13(6):393-407.

51. Maimoun L, Simar D, Caillaud C, et al. Response of calciotropic hormones and bone turnover to brisk walking according to age and fitness level. *J Sci Med Sport.* 2008;September 1.

52. Maitland GD. Manipulation-mobilization. *Physiotherapy.* 1966;52:382-385.

53. Mannheimer JS, Rosenthal RM. Acute and chronic postural abnormalities as related to craniofacial pain and temporomandibular disorders. *Dent Clin North Am.* 1991;35(1):185-208.

54. McCalden RW, McGeough JA, Court-Brown CM. Age-related changes in the compressive strength of cancellous bone. The relative importance of changes in density and trabecular architecture. *J Bone Joint Surg Am.* 1997;79(3):421-427.

55. McElhaney JH. Dynamic response of bone and muscle tissue. *J Appl Physiol.* 1966;21(4):1231-1236.

56. Milentijevic D, Torzilli PA. Influence of stress rate on water loss, matrix deformation and chondrocyte viability in impacted articular cartilage. *J Biomech.* 2005;38(3):493-502.

57. Miles TS. The control of human motor units. *Clin Exp Pharmacol Physiol.* 1994;21(7):511-520.

58. Milz S, Benjamin M, Putz R. Molecular parameters indicating adaptation to mechanical stress in fibrous connective tissue. *Adv Anat Embryol Cell Biol.* 2005;178:1-71.

59. Nordin M, Frankel VH. *Basic Biomechanics of the Musculoskeletal System.* 3rd ed. Baltimore, MD: Lippincott Williams & Wilkins; 2001.

60. Nordin M, Lorenz T, Campello M. Biomechanics of tendons and ligaments. In: Nordin M, Frankel VH, eds. *Basic Biomechanics of the Musculoskeletal System.* 3rd ed. Philadelphia, PA: Lippincott Williams & Wilkins; 2001:102-125.

61. Noyes FR. Functional properties of knee ligaments and alterations induced by immobilization. *Clin Orthop.* 1977;123:210-242.

62. Nyman JS, Roy A, Reyes MJ, Wang X. Mechanical behavior of human cortical bone in cycles of advancing tensile strain for two age groups. *J Biomed Mater Res A.* 2008;April 24.

63. Oatis C. *Kinesiology: The Mechanics & Pathomechanics of Human Movement.* Philadelphia, PA: Lippincott Williams & Wilkins; 2004.

64. Pattin CA, Caler WE, Carter DR. Cyclic mechanical property degradation during fatigue loading of cortical bone. *J Biomech.* 1996;29(1):69-79.

65. Pidaparti RM, Turner CH. Cancellous bone architecture: advantages of nonorthogonal trabecular alignment under multidirectional joint loading. *J Biomech.* 1997;30:979-983.

66. Plainfosse M, Hatton PV, Crawford A, Jin ZM, Fisher J. Influence of the extracellular matrix on the frictional properties of tissue-engineered cartilage. *Biochem Soc Trans.* 2007;35(Pt 4):677-679.

67. Poole AR, Kojima T, Yasuda T, Mwale F, Kobayashi M, Laverty S. Composition and structure of articular cartilage: a template for tissue repair. *Clin Orthop Relat Res.* 2001;(391 suppl):S26-S33.

68. Quinn TM, Allen RG, Schalet BJ, Perumbuli P, Hunziker EB. Matrix and cell injury due to sub-impact loading of adult bovine articular cartilage explants: effects of strain rate and peak stress. *J Orthop Res.* 2001;19(2):242-249.

69. Riegger-Krugh C, Keysor J. Skeletal malalignments of the lower quarter: correlated and compensatory motions and posture. *J Orthop Sports Phys Ther.* 1996;23:164-170.

70. Roos EM, Dahlberg L. Positive effects of moderate exercise on glycosaminoglycan content in knee cartilage: a four-month, randomized, controlled trial in patients at risk of osteoarthritis. *Arthritis Rheum.* 2005;52(11):3507-3514.

71. Rudman KE, Aspden RM, Meakin JR. Compression or tension? The stress distribution in the proximal femur. *Biomed Eng Online.* 2006;5:12.

72. Rydevik B, Brown MD, Lundborg G. Pathoanatomy and pathophysiology of nerve root compression. *Spine.* 1984;9:7.

73. Squire JM, Al-Khayat HA, Knupp C, Luther PK. Molecular architecture in muscle contractile assemblies. *Adv Protein Chem.* 2005;71:17-87.

74. Straker LM, O'Sullivan PB, Smith AJ, Perry MC. Relationships between prolonged neck/shoulder pain and sitting spinal posture in male and female adolescents. *Man Ther.* 2008;June 12.

75. Strube P, Sentuerk U, Riha T, et al. Influence of age and mechanical stability on bone defect healing: age reverses mechanical effects. *Bone.* 2008;42(4):758-764.

76. Vanwanseele B, Pirnog C, Szekely G, Stussi E. Quantitative analysis of local changes in patellar cartilage in spinal cord injured subjects. *Clin Orthop Relat Res.* 2007;456:98-102.

77. Zioupos P, Currey JD, Hamer AJ. The role of collagen in the declining mechanical properties of aging human cortical bone. *J Biomed Mater Res.* 1999;45(2):108-116.

78. Zioupos P, Hansen U, Currey JD. Microcracking damage and the fracture process in relation to strain rate in human cortical bone tensile failure. *J Biomech.* 2008;41(14):2932-2939.

79. Andriacchi TP, Hurwitz DE. Gait biomechanics and total knee arthroplasty. *Am J Knee Surg.* 1997;10(4).

80. Chockley C. Ground reaction force comparison between jumps landing on the full foot and jumps landing en pointe in ballet dancers. *Journal of Dance Medicine & Science.* 2008;12(1):5.

81. Coppieters MW, Alshami AM. Longitudinal excursion and strain in the median nerve during novel nerve gliding exercises for carpal tunnel syndrome. *J Orthop Res.* 2007;25(7):972-980.

82. Coppieters MW, Hough AD, Dilley A. Different nerve-gliding exercises induce different magnitudes of median nerve longitudinal excursion: an in vivo study using dynamic ultrasound imaging. *J Orthop Sports Phys Ther.* 2009;39(3):164-171.

83. Byl C, Puttlitz C, Byl N, Lotz J, Topp K. Strain in the median and ulnar nerves during upper-extremity positioning. *J Hand Surg Am.* 2002;27(6):1032-1040.

Orthopedic Reasoning

AUTHOR: DERRICK SUEKI

INTRODUCTORY INFORMATION   (*i*)

In recent years, clinical reasoning has taken on increased attention as educators and clinicians strive to help students and novice orthopedic clinicians think and make clinical-based decisions. The landscape of orthopedic rehabilitation and medicine is changing. As a result of these changes, rehabilitation clinicians are being asked to play a greater role in the decision-making processes. Orthopedic rehabilitation clinicians must be able to make accurate and educated decisions about the nature of a patient's injuries and the most beneficial means to bring about healing and recovery.

WHY IS CLINICAL REASONING IMPORTANT?

Studies in medicine have revealed an interesting fact. Doctors make mistakes. For some reason, it has always been expected that medical personnel are supernatural. We believe that our doctors are incapable of error, but in reality, to error is natural, it's human. For a physician to operate on the wrong arm or prescribe the wrong medication is a medical error, and unfortunate as it is, it happens. The problem is that most medical errors are not the result of errors of practice, but are errors of thinking. In a study of 100 medical mistakes, it was found that only four were the result of inadequate knowledge; the remainder were the result of cognitive reasoning processes. In a separate study, it was estimated that 80% of medical errors were the result of errors in thinking or clinical reasoning.[51] Minimizing the number of mistakes is the goal of medicine and of educating medical practitioners. How can the number of errors be diminished? Evidence seems to be pointing to clinical reasoning as the answer.[2,5,6,20,29,32,49]

Kassirer and Kopelman discussed the challenges that needed to be overcome in order to change current medical education. "Instead of learning how diagnostic hypotheses are initiated and refined and how treatment decisions are formulated, teachers of clinical medicine have substituted standardized histories and physicals, book chapters that list myriad causes of individual symptoms, in an apprentice system in which the student is expected to imitate others, formal approaches to recording patient problems, and lock-step algorithmic charts for blind guidance, none of these methods focusing on essential reasoning processes, critical to optimal performance."[34]

WHAT IS CLINICAL REASONING?[27,32,33,39]

Clinical reasoning is the process by which a clinician makes clinical-based decisions regarding a patient's health, status, and care. Often clinical reasoning and clinical decision making are utilized synonymously, but in actuality, they are two portions of the same process. Reasoning is the means by which the clinician computes information. Decision making is the conclusion on which the clinician ultimately decides.

This is an academic definition of clinical reasoning, but in reality clinical reasoning is much more difficult to define than a simple definition would imply. The limitations of many of the models developed to date involve, in part, the fact that they were developed to address mathematical models of logic and thinking. Clinical reasoning is a much more difficult proposition. Clinical reasoning is made difficult in part by several factors.

- The patient—no two people have the exact experiences and no two people have the same past experiences or backgrounds.
- The situation—no two situations have exactly the same parameters, because no two patients or incidences are exactly the same.
- The clinician—no two clinicians have the same past experiences or the same exact mental processes. They bring their own inherent biases to any situation.

All three of these elements have innumerable variations and, therefore, the possible factors that can influence a patient's clinical presentation are also innumerable. Clinical reasoning is a challenge.

WHAT ARE THE COMPONENTS OF CLINICAL DECISION MAKING? [15-18]

There are many theories and views regarding how people think and make decisions. From a simplistic point of view, clinical decision making involves three main components:
- Data Acquisition
- Clinical Reasoning
- Clinical Decision Making

WHAT IS DATA ACQUISITION?

Data acquisition is the method by which a person, or in this instance a clinician, gathers information regarding a patient or situation. How are data gathered? In actuality, the process involves all senses of the clinician. It can involve the subjective interview of a person in which information is verbally and auditorily gathered about the situation. It can take the form of the physical examination in which information is gathered through measures and testing. Information can be gathered visually as a clinician observes movement patterns or body language. It can also be gathered internally as clinicians search their memory bank for information regarding the patient or their situation.

Historically, medical models of reasoning have focused primarily on the physical examination and testing. The average patient interview lasts only 16 minutes. Only a limited amount of information can be gathered about a patient in 16 minutes.[40] One study found that physicians typically wait only 23 seconds after a patient begins describing his or her chief complaint before interrupting and redirecting the discussion. Such premature redirection can lead to late-arising concerns and missed opportunities to gather important data.[37,52] Recent clinical reasoning models have questioned this practice and place a higher primacy on the role that the patient has in the situation.

WHAT IS CLINICAL REASONING? REVISITED

Reasoning is a form of cognitive processing. It is the internal processing that occurs in response to a stimulus. Clinical reasoning is the process utilized to make the choices about a patient's state and care. In the past, discussions regarding clinical reasoning would often involve summaries of basic foundational diagnostic reasoning processes such as inductive (concept formation) and deductive reasoning (logical argument) processes. Recent study and thought regarding the clinical reasoning processes have expanded past this humble beginning.

CLINICAL PEARL

Clinical reasoning involves the interaction of three knowledge systems.
- *Propositional Knowledge—book learning or academic acquired knowledge*
- *Personal Knowledge—knowledge acquired through life learning and experiences*
- *Professional Craft Knowledge—knowledge acquired through clinical learning and experiences*[23,30-33]

WHAT IS CLINICAL DECISION MAKING?

Clinical decision making from a technical aspect is the actual act of coming to a conclusion or judgment, but in reality, it overlaps the reasoning and cognitive process. So, just as clinical reasoning involves decision making, decision making involves aspects of clinical reasoning (see Figure II-1-1).

CLINICAL DECISION MAKING
CASE STUDY—PATIENT PROFILE

Darren was frustrated and anxious. For the past several months, he had been experiencing shoulder pain. This shoulder pain had been preventing him from practicing ultimate Frisbee. He was now only 4 weeks away from an ultimate Frisbee tournament and was fearful that he would not be able to play in it. Over the past month and a half he had seen several doctors and physical therapists each of whom had diagnosed him with various pathologies including shoulder strain and rotator cuff tendinitis. Each time, antiinflammatory medication was prescribed and he was told it should get better in a couple of weeks. Yet he did not improve. What was the matter with him? Would he ever get better? It was with this mindset that he was advised by friends to seek the opinion of one final clinician that specialized in shoulder rehabilitation.

At the clinician's office, an intern began the evaluative process. On questioning, it was learned that Darren had injured his shoulder playing ultimate Frisbee. He had landed awkwardly on his chest with his arm outstretched overhead to catch a Frisbee. He initially had felt a sharp pain in his chest and shoulder, but was able to continue playing. As he continued to play the shoulder began to get achy and by the end of the hour match, he was having difficulty lifting his arm without pain. Since that time, his shoulder symptoms had not changed much. The pain was located primarily in his shoulder. It had gotten a little better over the course of the subsequent weeks, but pain was still noted whenever he played Frisbee. It hurt the most when he brought his arm across his chest and when he bench pressed weights at the gym. Further questioning about other parts of the body such as the neck, middle back, elbow, and hand all came back with the same answer, no pain. The intern proceeded to process the information and like those before him came up with the primary hypothesis of rotator cuff tendinitis secondary to shoulder impingement. This hypothesis appeared to be confirmed by objective testing. Darren was disappointed; the answer was the same as the previous opinions.

The senior clinician began his examination at this point. Rather than asking questions about the shoulder, the clinician began with questions about the injury itself. He learned that the arm never touched the ground. All of the impact was on the upper chest and sternum. Rather than focus the examination on the shoulder, the clinician focused on the chest rather than the shoulder. He asked questions about breathing, pain in the chest, and tenderness in the sternal region. The patient was a little reluctant to answer these questions because he was coming in for shoulder pain not for chest pain. The physical examination began with palpation of the sternum and the sternoclavicular joint. These were both exquisitely tender. The clinician proceeded to mobilize the sternoclavicular joint for several minutes. Following the mobilization the clinician asked the patient to lift his arm overhead and across his body. What had hurt only minutes before was now almost pain free. Later the intern asked the clinician what made him assess the sternoclavicular joint. What had the intern missed?

Answer

Jones and Jensen have done extensive research into the qualities that embody an expert and how they differ from a novice. One of the ways in which they differ is the fact that most experts are very knowledgable and proficient in their chosen

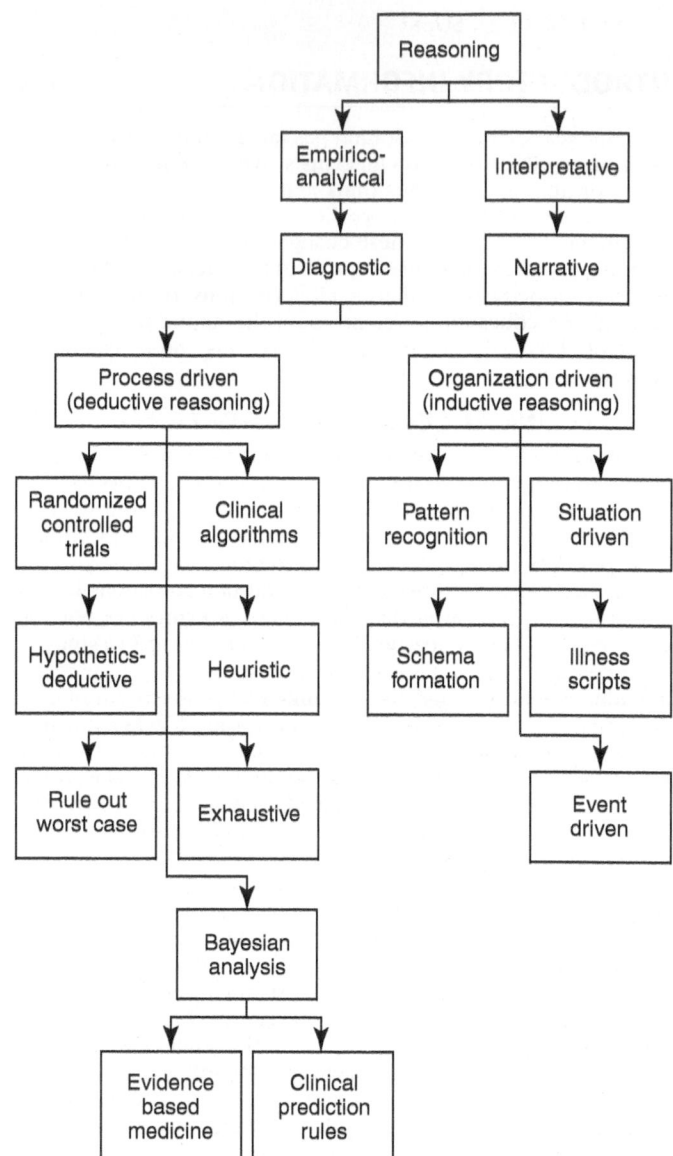

FIGURE II-1-1   Clinical Reasoning Flow Diagram. The figure depicts the clinical reasoning process involved in Rehabilitative Medicine.

area of expertise and not as proficient in other areas. The shoulder specialist had seen many shoulder patients in the past and had come across patients with a similar problem. So he was able to jump toward that diagnosis easily since it was a familiar path for him. The novice clinician and the health care providers before who were not specialists had not seen a similar case in the past. Therefore, they boxed the patient into a pathology they had experienced before, even though the fit was not perfect. Unfortunately, it was not the problem that patient was experiencing. Experts have more clinical schema or patterns developed in their field of expertise and are able to use a different reasoning pattern. Experts utilize a strategy that looks forward to the answer rather than backward. Questioning is geared to validate the hypothesis. Novices must look backward on the data collected before they make a decision. The process is more exhaustive and time consuming.[28-33]

WHAT TYPES OF REASONING STRATEGIES ARE THERE?[10,44,53,54]

Reasoning can be divided into two classifications, empiricoanalytical reasoning and interpretative reasoning. Clinical-based reasoning in medicine has historically focused on a portion of cognitive science called diagnostic reasoning. Diagnostic reasoning is a form of empiricoanalytical analysis. In empiricoanalytical analysis, the driving theory is that truth or answers can always be gleaned from objective and measurable testing and analysis. Logical progression of thought and analysis will ultimately culminate in the one true and only answer. Diagnostic reasoning can be subdivided into two subsets: theories that involve the actual process involved in diagnostic reasoning and theories that involve the organization of information and the thought that results from this organization.

Theories that include the actual process utilized in clinical reasoning address how a clinician logically arrives at a clinical decision. It utilizes testing and measures to develop a cause and effect or causal relationship between findings, hypothesis generation, and decision making. The theory relies on the accumulation of data prior to a decision being made. Examples of the diagnostic processing of information models include hypotheticodeductive reasoning, Bayesian analysis, backward thinking, clinical algorithms, evidence-based medicine, randomized controlled trials, and clinical prediction rules.

Initial research into the reasoning that took place in the health care field revolved around the study of deductive reasoning and its application to the patient model. It was determined that deductive reasoning alone cannot account for the large variability in patient responses to interventions. Deductive reasoning by its nature relies on well-defined rules and laws to define steady and consist responses. Each action should result in a predictable and predetermined response. Logical and linear processing of information is a slow and time consuming process. Many decisions made in clinical situations are quicker and more expedient. This is especially true when clinicians face situations to which they have been exposed in the past. Based on this realization, clinicians developed an organizational model of reasoning. The premise of this model revolves around the concept that the categorical organization of information in the brain allows for faster and easier access. At the center of these reasoning processes is forward thinking or inductive reasoning. The theory relies on instantaneous processing of information in which the clinician gathers data. As the data are acquired, a clinician recognizes certain features of a patient and from this information a picture forms of the patient, the problem, and the solution to the problem. The more frequently the pathway is utilized, the more quickly the information can be processed. Evolving from these thoughts was the development of diagnostic organizational models of reasoning including pattern recognition, illness scripts, and schema formation.

ARE DIAGNOSTIC REASONING PROCESSES THE ONLY PROCESSES UTILIZED IN CLINICAL REASONING?[51]

It was determined that deductive reasoning alone cannot account for the large variability in patient responses to interventions. Newer models have challenged the application of pure hypoteciodeductive strategies to patient care models. Diagnostic reasoning by its nature relies on well-defined rules and laws to define steady and consist responses (see Table II-1-1). Each action should result in predictable and predetermined responses. This is not the case in patient-centered decision making. Decisions made in clinical settings are often determined based on inexact and incomplete data. Few rules or laws can be consistently applied within the realm of clinical decision making. Clinical decisions are based as much on base science as they are on clinician skill in interpreting less objective data. In response to this, interpretive

TABLE II-1-1 Types of Diagnostic Reasoning Processes[1]

Strategy	Variations
Diagnostic process driven	Hypotheticodeductive reasoning
	Bayesian analysis
	Backward thinking
	Clinical algorithms
	Evidence-based medicine
	Randomized controlled trials
	Clinical prediction rules
	Heuristic
	Rule out worse case scenario
	Exhaustive
Diagnostic organization driven	Pattern recognition
	Forward thinking
	Illness scripts
	Schema formation
	Event driven
	Situation driven
Interpretive	Narrative

theories of reasoning developed. These have the patient, situation, context, and clinician at the heart of the reasoning process. It views the reasoning process as a collaboration of clinician and patient. Answers or decisions are based not on set formulas or schemas but answers are free to evolve based on the situation. It realizes that most clinically-based situations have multiple solutions or answers that may change as the situation evolves. Narrative reasoning seeks to understand the unique lived experience of patients—a reasoning activity that could be termed "the construction of meaning." In patients' (or therapists' for that matter) telling of stories or narratives, there is a choice in which some elements are expressed, some elements are emphasized over others, and still other elements may not find expression. For example, the particular "telling" of a story or history by patients represents their interpretation of events over time. Such interpretations (albeit not necessarily consciously constructed) may not be neutral in their effects on the teller.[10,30] In the context of clinical practice, narrative reasoning concerns the understanding of patients' stories in order to gain insight into their experiences of disability or pain and their subsequent beliefs, feelings, and health behaviors.

DEFINE THE DIFFERENT TYPES OF CLINICAL REASONING METHODS[1,10,19,46,49,55]

Empiricoanalytical Research or Scientific—This is the general field of diagnostic reasoning that looks specifically at hypothesis generation and the cognitive processing that accompanies it. It can take the form of processing methodologies such as hypotheticodeductive reasoning or organizational methodologies such as pattern recognition. What separates it from other reasoning theories is its focus on the development of a hypothesis for the situation at hand.

Hypotheticodeductive—Hypotheticodeductive reasoning is probably the most commonly utilized and taught reasoning process in medical field. It involves a clinician collecting data both by verbal and physical examination. Based on the data collected, the clinician proceeds to process the information and then form a decision in the form of a hypothesis. This hypothesis is subsequently tested as new data become available and shaped or modified as warranted.

Bayesian Analysis—The Basyesian model is based on the work of Thomas Bayes. Bayesian logic or reasoning is a branch of logic that is applied to decision making that deals with probability.

It utilizes the knowledge of prior events to predict future events. According to Bayesian logic, the only way to quantify a situation with an uncertain outcome is through determining its probability. It is favored by those who construct algorithms and strictly adhere to evidence-based medicine.

Algorithmic—Algorithmic reasoning is a form of Bayesian analysis. It utilizes flow charts or algorithms to delineate a pathway toward a hypothesis. It is based and founded in probability in which each step leads to a subsequent step, the final answer being a hypothesis.

Pattern Recognition—Pattern recognition is a form of organizational diagnostic reasoning. The clinician is required to generate immediate hypotheses regarding the patient or clinical situation based on past experience and initial data. Through the emerging data, the clinician recognizes a pattern that is familiar and this pattern becomes the hypothesis template from which data analysis begins. The hypothesis template is then altered as new data become available.

Heuristic—Heuristic analysis in its simplest form is a trial-and-error format. With or without much prior cognitive processing, the clinician begins to randomly generate a hypothesis, test its validity, and then move to the next hypothesis. The process is repeated until the correct hypothesis is attained.

Rule Out Worst Case Scenario—The worst case scenario method is a form of diagnostic processing. Instead of starting with an initial hypothesis, the clinician begins with the worst possible hypothesis for the patient. Through testing and examination, it is ruled out and the second worst case scenario is then examined. Through a process of elimination, the working hypothesis is ultimately determined.

Exhaustive—The exhaustive method is a form of hypotheticodeductive reasoning utilized by novice clinicians or experienced clinicians faced with novel situations. In involves collecting all the data possible. The data are then analyzed and a hypothesis is generated.

Event or Situation Driven—Event-driven cognitive processing is a form of organizational diagnostics. Event-driven reasoning proposes that knowledge sets are organized in terms of schema, but unlike schema, situation models can represent unique or novel situations. Situation models are dynamic and continually under the process of revision and modification. New information is continually being added and irrelevant information deleted from situation data sets. The situational or mental model theory provides a framework for a unified approach to thinking, reasoning, and problem solving in the context of real life situations. Situation models are not directly concerned with the representation and organization of general or scientific knowledge; rather every model represents a unique situation. General information in this context is utilized as pointer to help direct the search of long-term memory for the accurate situational model. Even though general knowledge does not directly play a role in the situations, the models construction can depend heavily on the influence of background knowledge.

Narrative—Narrative reasoning is a form of interpretive reasoning. The theory relies on patients narrating or guiding the clinician through their experience. Through the narration the clinician can gain information regarding not only the nature of the injury itself but the psychosocial issues that underlie the situation. The role that these issues play in the situation and ultimate potential for recovery for the patient can then be assessed.[38]

CLINICAL DECISION MAKING CASE STUDY—PATIENT PROFILE

In the case of Darren, how would each of the above reasoning strategies be implemented?

Answer

Hypotheticodeductive—This strategy is similar to the method utilized by the novice; information about Darren would be gathered by the clinician and after the data are gathered a hypothesis is deduced. Therefore, the clinician would ask Darren about his problem and go through a complete physical examination of the shoulder prior to making a hypothesis.

Bayesian Analysis—In Bayesian analysis a clinician would consider the shoulder joint and then based on statistics consider all of the possible pathologies the patient may have. Based on probability he would then rank his hypotheses. With each new piece of information gathered the clinician would rerank the hypotheses based on probability.

Algorithmic—When utilizing an algorithmic approach the clinician would have access to a flow chart of the shoulder. Step by step the clinician would formulate the patient interview around a series of yes or no questions that lead to further questions. Do you have shoulder pain? Does it hurt when you lift your arm to the side? Based on the answer to these questions, the clinician would eventually develop a diagnosis and plan of care.

Pattern Recognition—The clinician would access patients similar to Darren in his memory. The expert clinician utilized this strategy. He had seen a patient similar to Darren in the past. Therefore, he was able to ask a few select questions to confirm his hypothesis.

Heuristic—The heuristic approach would take the approach that most shoulder pain is probably related to some type of inflammation. Clinicians would try antiinflammatories and ice to see if it made it better. If not, they would move on to their next hypothesis and proceed in a similar manner until they found the right approach.

Rule Out Worst Case Scenario—The rule out the worst case scenario would consider a pancoast tumor one of the worse diagnoses that the patient could potentially be experiencing. Therefore, clinicians would order imaging to rule out the diagnosis. If this came back negative, they would proceed to cardiovascular pathology. They would test for this and then move forward until they arrived at the final diagnosis.

Exhaustive—The exhaustive method is utilized by many novices and students. Because they do not have experience or a firm grasp of any hypotheses, they will fully interview and examine the shoulder of the patient and then sit down and develop a hypothesis.

Event Driven or Situational—With the event-driven or situation strategy the clinician would sit down with the patient and ask about the specifics of the injury. How did the patient land, where was the arm, when exactly did the pain begin, how did it progress, how were they feeling immediately? The interview is customized to Darren and the events that surround that particular moment in time.

Narrative—The narrative approach looks at other factors in addition to the biomedical issues surrounding the injury. How does Darren feel about the injury, is he anxious, frustrated, or sad? Is it impacting his work? How about his family life? These questions help to shape factors that may be contributing to the pathology and that keep Darren from getting better.

CLINICAL PEARL

Most clinicians utilize many strategies when they solve a problem.

WHAT ARE THE ADVANTAGES AND DISADVANTAGES OF THE MOST UTILIZED CLINICAL REASONING METHODS?

Table II-1-2 displays the advantages and disadvantages.

TABLE II-1-2 Types of Clinical Reasoning Strategies[51,59,55]

Cognitive Strategy	Key Features	Key Shortcoming	Key Advantage
Hypotheticodeductive	Initial hypothesis generated based on initial assessment Further testing to validate initial hypothesis Modification of hypothesis and repetition of the process	Faulty hypothesis can precipitate dangerous actions Premature closure can result in erroneous conclusions	Flexible
Algorithmic	Preset diagnostic pathways based on preestablished criteria	Inflexible Removes independent thinking	Standardized care Easy to teach
Pattern recognition	Initial hypothesis generated on prior exposure to minimal data Subsequent data collection is performed to validate the initial hypothesis	Clinical experience or clinical case exposure is required to build a library of patterns	Rapid assessment and clinical plan development
Rule out worst case	Beginning with the worst-case scenario, data are collected to eliminate the hypothesis Analysis progresses through a series of critical scenarios	Incomplete differential diagnosis list missing less common disease entities Overtesting Anecdotal practice Value-induced bias	Increased probability of considering/recognizing presentations of critical illness
Exhaustive	Collection of data indiscriminately and analysis of all data to determine a diagnosis	Excessive resource use Time consumption	Thorough evaluations
Event driven	General information in this context is utilized as a pointer to help direct the search of long-term memory for the accurate situational model; testing is utilized to validate the initial model	Dangerous actions possible if faulty hypotheses Potentially inefficient	Flexible Accommodates event-driven environment
Narrative	Seeks to understand the unique lived experience of patients—a reasoning activity that could be termed "the construction of meaning"	Involves good communication skills Time consuming Varies from person to person and event to event	Takes into consideration the patient's view of the pathology

DO CLINICIANS UTILIZE JUST ONE FORM OF CLINICAL REASONING?[8]

Most experts agree that clinicians utilize multiple reasoning processes when making a clinical decision. The processes utilized will depend on the situation, novelty, past experiences, beliefs, and feelings.

HOW IS REASONING IN ORTHOPEDIC REHABILITATION DIFFERENT THAN OTHER FIELDS OF MEDICINE?

In orthopedic rehabilitation, the goal of the reasoning process is not to make a pathological diagnosis. Many times in rehabilitation, the pathology has previously been defined; instead the clinician's clinical reasoning turns to the rehabilitation process. What is a patient's functional or movement dysfunction and what is the most appropriate course of action to return a patient to optimal function or normal movement?

CLINICAL PEARL

The key part of a reasoning strategy is to recognize that therapists must make decisions based on information collected in a number of categories. Information is needed in all these categories for the best understanding of the problem and hence the best management process.[23,30-33]

WHAT ARE THE CLINICAL REASONING METHODOLOGIES BEING IMPLEMENTED IN ORTHOPEDIC PHYSICAL THERAPY EDUCATION?[4,22,23,30,31,32,33,41,42,45,50]

There are several methods being implemented in physical therapy education. Most theories accept the idea that decision making consists of a number of steps or stages such as recognition, formulation, generation of alternatives, information search, selection, and action. It is also well recognized in most of these theories that routine cognitive processes such as memory, reasoning, and concept formation play a primary role in decision making. The difficulty lies in the fact that no two programs educate in the same manner. Some of the basic models being employed currently include the following.

PROCESSING MODELS: Evidence-Based Medicine—Evidence-based medicine is a form of hypotheticodeductive reasoning that relies heavy on the role of empirical evidence to drive hypothesis generation and analysis. Based on a clinician's initial interviews a hypothesis is generated and tested against existing evidence regarding the initial hypothesis. There is a hierarchy of evidence in which specific research methods are held in higher regard than others. Based on a comparison with evidence the hypothesis is accepted or rejected. If it is rejected, additional hypotheses are generated and in turn similarly assessed.

Clinical Prediction Rules—Clinical prediction rules is an emerging method of clinical decision making. It involves the generation of a hypothesis or decision regarding a course of action based on probability. So, in a sense, it is a form of Bayesian analysis in which the hypothesis or decisions will be guided by statistics. Instead of a single test utilized individually to guide decision-making, several tests or data sets are clustered together and utilized as a unit. The probability that they will result in a certain hypothesis is subsequently analyzed. The clinician is asked to assess a cluster of data points and based on the outcome of the testing the probability of a certain decision is determined. Rules are developed for the use of interventions or the diagnosis of pathology based on outcome measures or objective measurements.

Clinical Algorithms—There is another movement afoot to base all clinical decisions on clinical algorithms. Clinical algorithms involve a clinically based set of rules or flow sheets that are followed by the clinician in order to arrive at a clinical decision. The clinician could, in theory, enter in patient data and objective measures and a computer program would produce an algorithm that would have the greatest probability of solving the patient's problem.

ORGANIZATIONAL MODELS: Case-Based Learning—This method utilizes a pattern recognition philosophy to aid a student through the reasoning process. Case-based education is popular in today's physical therapy education. It is known as the cognitive flexibility theory of education. It is the concept that if you teach students to memorize a particular patient case profile, they can in turn recognize the same patients when they encounter them in the future. It relies on several assumptions some of which may not be true for all students. It assumes that all students learn by memorization, there are a finite number of case scenarios, all patients will fit into that finite number of case scenarios, and if a patient does not fit into that case scenario, the student will be able to associate a novel situation to an existing template and make decisions appropriately. Pattern recognition is vital to the success of the case-based learning model. Case based learning fits nicely into the current medical model of algorithms and flow charts. If a patient has A and B, then C is the appropriate course of action. It is easy to teach, easy to research, and easy to standardize across educational institutions.

Hypothesis Categories—Emphasis has recently been placed on the use of categorization systems to allow students easy access to information. This is roughly based on a schema model in which information is stored in folders or categories that can in turn be accessed for use by the clinician. Jones suggests the creation of hypothesis categories in orthopedic therapy to aid in the organization of knowledge.[31] These categories include the source of symptoms, mechanism of the symptoms, contributing factors, precautions and contraindications, management and treatment, and prognosis. The clinician is asked to place patients and their situation into the various categories. Through categorization, the clinician is then able to more readily and easily access the data for review and use in the current patient and in subsequent patients.

Biopsychosocial Model—The biopsychosocial model is an organizational-based model that was developed in response to the failure of medicine to explain many of the orthopedic biomedical pathologies. An example is that there are instances in which the suspected source tissue was surgically removed from the body, yet the patient's symptoms remained. Main and Engel both developed models of processing that addresses issues such as pain, fear, depression, frustration, and anger in addition to the classic tissue and physiology-based processing paradigms. Socioeconomic and occupational factors are also considered in Main's model. The primary definition of the biopsychosocial model lies in its ability to portray the various interactions possible within its elements. The model of disability integrates the influences of biomedical, physiological, psychological, socioeconomic, and iatrogenic factors on disability.[13,35]

Treatment-Based Categorization—Researchers have come to the realization that not all injuries to a specific tissue are created equally. Delitto has advocated the use of subgroupings to narrow down the breadth of a pathology.[7] He has proposed the subgrouping of pathology based on responses to specific interventions. Others have since followed suit and many classification systems are now being developed that look not to define a specific pathology but instead to determine factors that will indicate which patients will benefit from a specific intervention. One of the underlying factors driving the new approach to classification and research is the failure of many traditional interventions, such as exercise, that have been utilized in the rehabilitation field to promote recovery; these have not been proven effective in research. The model was developed with the belief that research fails to substantiate clinical interventions because the breadth of pathology being studied is too wide. Subgrouping is an attempt to narrow the scope of pathology and to identify the patient groups that will most benefit from a particular intervention.

Tissue-Based Assessment—Mueller and Maluf have proposed a model of classification based on the factors that create stress in a tissue.[42] They have named the classification system the Physical Stress Theory. The basic premise of the Physical Stress Theory is that changes in the relative level of physical stress will cause a predictable adaptive response in all biological tissue. They suggest that any hypothesis or diagnosis be based on factors that can contribute to tissue stress and result in tissue adaptation. Interventions are then determined. The choice of the most appropriate intervention is guided by which intervention can normalize the stresses placed on the specific tissue.

Movement-Based Assessment—The foundations of the Movement System Balance theory were developed by Sahrmann. The Movement System Balance theory utilizes the concepts and principles of muscle and movement function to identify and categorize movement impairment syndromes. Normal movement is the foundation of the theory. Classification is based on common abnormal movement patterns observed in each body region. Diagnosis and hypotheses are derived from these observations, and interventions are planned to normalize the abnormal movement patterns.[48] The Case Study below and Table II-1-3 illustrate how each of the above methodologies would address a specific patient problem.

CLINICAL PEARL

- *Pattern recognition is a characteristic of all mature thought*
- *Data do not equal knowledge*
- *Similarly, in our mind, data are stored within patterns so that we can readily retrieve the data housed in these patterns*
- *Reasoning requires well-organized data.*[23,30-33]

CLINICAL DECISION MAKING CASE STUDY—PATIENT PROFILE

Mary is a 48-year-old female who has been experiencing low back pain for the past 6 months. The back pain has come and gone but in the past week it has returned. It limits her ability to sit for prolonged periods of time. The symptoms began insidiously. She has no prior mechanism of injury. How could a clinician learn about or an educator help a clinician reason through this patient?

Answer

Evidence-Based Medicine—A clinician utilizing evidence-based medicine would use the latest research to guide the evaluative and decision-making process. Clinicians would look at the patient's symptoms and complaints, as well as the results of objective testing. They would then compare this with the latest evidence regarding low back pain. A decision would be made using research as the guiding factor.

Clinical Prediction Rules—Clinical prediction rules have been developed for diagnosis in regions such as the ankle where the Ottawa ankle rules help to determine whether a patient should have an x-ray to rule out fracture. No such prediction rule has been developed for the lumbar spine but clinical prediction rules are currently being developed that address which interventions are the most appropriate for low back pain patients regardless of the pathophysiology.

Clinical Algorithms—The clinician would follow established low back flow charts. Based on yes or no answers to various questions, the clinician would follow the flow until a diagnosis is reached.

Case Based Learning—The novice would be presented with cases that represent various patient scenarios. Typical patient presentations for the lumbar spine, such as a herniated disc, lumbar stenosis, lumbar instability, and spondylolithesis, would be presented. Based on these scenarios, the novice would choose the scenario that best represents Mary.

Hypothesis Categories—Mary would be interviewed and based on this interview she would be placed in several categories. Typical categories include activity and participation capabilities, the patient's perspectives on the experience, pathobiological mechanisms behind the symptoms, contributing factors to the pathology, physical impairments, and associated tissue sources. The clinician would then utilize these categories to narrow down a list of hypotheses regarding the patient's symptomology.

Biopsychosocial Model—The clinician would be guided to look at the other factors that could contribute to Mary's low back pain experience. Does Mary have stress in her life; is she working; how does she feel about her injury; how is she adapting to the pain? These questions would help the clinician to look at Mary as a person and not merely a pathology. Her case would take on added dimensions in addition to the physiology behind the pain.

Treatment-Based Categorization—Mary would be interviewed and based on the evaluative process she would be placed into one of several categories. The categorization would then guide the ultimate treatment that she would receive. The categorization and treatment relationship would be determined through research. The research looks at which interventions have the best probability of benefiting a specific patient profile.

Tissue-Based Categorization—Mary would be questioned about how her lower back was injured and further questioned regarding which motions or activities continue to aggravate or stress her. From her responses, she would be categorized and diagnosed based on which bodily tissues were most likely injured.

Movement-Based Categorization—Mary would be assessed through a series of functional movements. From these movements, movement abnormalities would be determined. Her diagnosis would be based on her movement abnormalities and not a tissue. Treatment would be focused on normalizing the movement abnormalities.

CLINICAL PEARL

Expert clinicians utilize a forward thinking reasoning strategy whereas novice clinicians utilize a backward thinking reasoning strategy.

HOW IS REASONING IN AN EXPERT DIFFERENT THAN IN A NOVICE? [12,14,21,28,41,29,51]

Research regarding expertise has become more commonplace in recent years as individuals and organizations strive to develop excellence in their particular field of endeavor. In physical therapy, the question of expertise continues to be studied. These studies reveal that the skills of an expert clinician depend not only on the clinician's knowledge but also on the clinician's ability to think and to reason. Experience alone does not guarantee that a clinician will excel. Nor does knowledge alone equate to clinical competency. Expertise requires a happy marriage of clinical reasoning and base knowledge. Although all clinicians, novice and expert, utilize portions of many cognitive processing theories, research shows that experts utilize organizational paradigms more frequently than process paradigms. In other words, experts can generate a clinical picture for a patient much more readily than a novice. The reasoning process entails the validation of the clinical picture. Novices, however, use a great proportion of procedural paradigms. They have not

Section II

ORTHOPEDIC REASONING

TABLE II-1-3 Types of Clinical Reasoning Strategies Used in Rehabilitation

Cognitive Strategy	Key Features	Key Shortcoming	Key Advantage
Processing			
Evidence-based medicine	Relies on the role of empirical evidence to drive hypothesis generation and analysis	Lack of evidence supporting rehabilitation	Easy to teach Easy to implement
Clinical prediction rules	The generation of a hypothesis or decision regarding course of action based on probability	Lack of research and prediction rules Removes independent thinking	Easy to use and to teach Can be utilized by novices and experts
Clinical algorithms	A clinically based set of rules or flow sheets that are followed by the clinician in order to arrive at a clinical decision	Hard to use and follow Focuses on the average patient not the extremes Removes independent thinking	Easy to teach Standardizes care
Organizational			
Case-based learning	If you teach students to memorize a particular patient case profile, they can recognize the same patient profile when they encounter it in the future	Utilizes standardized patients that represent averages Most patients do not follow the generic pattern	Facilitates learning in novice clinicians with little to no experience
Hypothesis categories	Information is stored in folders or categories in the brain that can, in turn, be accessed for use by the clinician	Difficult to foresee and address all potential hypotheses in patient assessment and care	Allows a broader breadth of thinking Aids in independent thinking
Biopsychosocial model	Integrates the influence of biomedical, physiological, psychological, socioeconomic, and iatrogenic factors on disability	Difficult to quantify Difficult to standardize Varies from patient to patient and time to time	Looks at all aspects of a patient's pain experience
Treatment-based categorization	Subgrouping of pathology based on their response to specific interventions; subgrouping is utilized to make clinical decisions	Lack of research validating system	Allows clinician to pair appropriate invention with specific patient profile
Tissue-based categorization	Diagnosis is based on factors that can contribute to tissue stress and result in tissue adaptation	Can address acute injuries with a specific mechanism of injury but has difficulty with application to a chronic population	Ties physiology to injury Fits into a scientific and medical model Logical progression from basic science coursework to clinical-based coursework
Movement-based categorization	Utilizes the concepts and principles of muscle and movement function to identify and categorize movement impairment syndromes	Several schools of thought that utilize different nomenclature for similar motions Looks at changing motion with minimal emphasis on pathology	Fits well in the rehabilitation model of diagnosis and treatment

generated the clinical pattern library that the expert has accumulated over time and experience. Therefore, they must collect more data before beginning analysis. [3]

HOW DO WE DEVELOP EXPERTISE?[25,28,29,47]

Elstein has proposed that expertise is a combination of four factors. These factors are knowledge, clinical reasoning, virtue, and movement.[11] These four elements are integrated fluidly in the expert clinician's cognitive processing. Experience alone does not guarantee the integration of these elements. Experience must be accompanied by a process of reflection and information organization.

Metacognition is a common theme in the cognitive processing of all experts. Metacognition is the awareness and understanding of our own thought processes. Expertise requires an ability to undertake a process that includes associating experiences and integrating them into recognizable patterns. Experiences allow clinicians to develop patterns of injury and illness. Reflection in the form of metacognition and clinical reasoning processes results in the ability to interpret and utilize these patterns in patient care.

CLINICAL PEARL

Key components of an expert:
- *Experts seek to excel and have a drive to improve*
- *Are able to use patterns to categorize information and speed processing*
- *Reflect on their own thought processes*
- *Are able to think laterally*
- *Are open to feedback and constructive criticism*
- *Are willing to work with others to improve their thought processes*[23,31]

WHAT IS THE DIFFERENCE BETWEEN DATA AND KNOWLEDGE?[24]

Data consist of information, but this information is not valuable until it can be utilized. Knowledge is data that have been well organized and accessible for use by the clinician.

DO WE ALL LEARN AND REASON THE SAME?

There are at least 70 learning style theories that have been developed, all of which educational psychologists criticize in some respect because of the lack of evidence and dubious theoretical grounds. Many experts and research have come to the conclusion that all people have at least two learning styles. Unfortunately, most instructors have only one teaching style.

WHAT IS THE ROLE OF INTUITION IN DECISION MAKING?

Intuition can have numerous definitions but in the context of clinical reasoning it is a form of pattern recognition. It is the ability to process information, not just information in the environment, but also information available internally from past experiences and knowledge, that allows you to make intuitive decisions. Intuition often involves mental pathways that have been accessed multiple times. As the pathways become more familiar, simple cues such as vision, hearing, touch, or memories can trigger the pattern recognition process. Many times a clinician will overprocess information allowing their other cognitive processes to override their intuition, but intuition is just another form of cognitive process that should be analyzed and, when appropriate, utilized.

HOW IS THIS BOOK ORGANIZED TO PROMOTE CLINICAL REASONING?

Teaching students to make appropriate clinical decisions or learning to reason through clinical-based problems is a difficult task.

Part of the difficulty is due to the fact that no two people reason the same. It can also be argued that a person may use different reasoning styles for a similar clinical problem given different settings or emotional status. With this in mind, this book was developed to help the student or novice clinician think through clinical problems in a variety of ways. It starts by developing propositional or book knowledge. It continues on by giving the student or novice access to the reasoning processes of experts in the field. Each expert in a giving body region has written about how he or she thinks during a patient subjective examination. They take the novice through the questions typically asked during a subjective examination. With each line of questioning, they share how the line of questioning influences their decision-making processes. Through this process, the expert mentors the novice. The novice is then guided by the clinical reasoning and decision-making chapters toward the pathology section. Here again, experienced clinicians give their insight into specific pathologies. Finally, the clinician is guided to the rehabilitation and pharmacology sections by the pathology and reasoning sections. In the rehabilitation section, the clinician is given insight, by the expert, on how to rehabilitate the patient. The book is set up to utilize a number of the clinical reasoning strategies mentioned above. In this way, the novice can learn from a variety of methodologies. [5,26,27,43]

WHAT ARE THE LIMITATIONS OF THE BOOK?

Clinicians utilize a variety or reasoning strategies when they solve a clinical problem. The strategies described in this book are by no means exhaustive. This book is able to utilize only a few of the methods commonly seen in clinical settings. It also is able to give a clinician insight only into the average patient with the full realization that many factors besides physiological tissue damage impact a patient's clinical presentation. Narrative reasoning and the psychosocial factors that impact a patient's situation are not addressed in this book, although they do play a major role in shaping patients and their response to the rehabilitation process.

SUMMARY STATEMENT[9,36]

Expertise lies in an individual's ability to organize knowledge into meaningful and logical patterns and to take into consideration the patient's own psychosocial biases into the overall equation. Clinical reasoning provides the avenue for the organization of these data. Clinical reasoning and scientific knowledge are two sides of the same coin. They are independent but interdependent. Expertise cannot exist without both faces of the coin.

Clinical reasoning and decision making are still works in progress. There are many schools of thought regarding how a clinician thinks and processes information. In reality, most clinicians utilize multiple reasoning strategies. They may fall back on a specific strategy in times of confusion, but most clinicians will transition seamlessly from strategy to strategy. They will utilize the best for the particular time or occasion. Instruction regarding clinical reasoning should utilize a number of reasoning strategies as no two clinicians think or process information identically.

REFERENCES

1. Baddeley A. *Essentials of Human Memory*. East Sussex: Psychology Press, Ltd; 1999.
2. Bordage G, Grant J, Marsden P. Quantitative assessment of diagnostic ability. *Med Educ*. 1990;24:413-425.
3. Boshuizen HPA, Schmidt HG. On the role of biomedical knowledge in clinical reasoning by experts, intermediates and novices. *Cognitive Science*. 1992;16:153-184.
4. Carr J, Jones M, Higgs J. Learning reasoning in physiotherapy programs. In: Higgs J, Jones M, eds. *Clinical Reasoning in the Health Professions*. 2nd ed. Oxford: Butterworth-Heinemann; 2000.
5. Crandall B, Wears RL. Expanding Perspectives on Misdiagnosis. *Am J Med*. 2008;121(5A):S30-S33.

6. Croskerry P, Norman G. Overconfidence in Clinical Decision Making. *Am J Med*. 2008;121(5A):S24-S29.

7. Delitto A, Erhard F, Bowling RW. A treatment based classification approach to low back syndrome: identifying and staging patients for conservative treatment. *Phys Ther*. 1995;75:470-485.

8. Doody C, McAteer M. Clinical Reasoning of Expert and Novice Physiotherapists in an Outpatient Orthopaedic Setting. *Physiotherapy*. 2002;88(5):258-268.

9. Downing AM, Hunter DG. Validating clinical reasoning: a question of perspective, but whose perspective? *Man Ther*. 2003;8(2):117-119.

10. Edwards I, Jones M, Carr J, BraunackMayer A, Jensen GM. Clinical Reasoning Strategies in Physical Therapy. *Phys Ther*. 2004;84(4):312-330.

11. Elstein AS. Clinical reasoning in medicine. In: Higgs J, Jones M, eds. *Clinical Reasoning in the Health Professions*. Oxford, U.K.: Butterworth-Heinemann; 1995:49-59.

12. Embrey DG, Guthrie MR, White OR, et al. Clinical decision making by experienced and inexperienced pediatric physical therapist for children with diplegic cerebral palsy. *Phys Ther*. 1996;76:20,00.

13. Engel GL. The need for a new medical model: a challenge for biomedicine. *Science*. 1977;196:129-136. Academy Press, 2001.

14. Eshach H, Bitterman H. From Cased-based Reasoning to Problem-based Learning. *Acad Med*. 2003;78(5):491-496.

15. Fleming MH. The therapist with the three track mind. *Am J Occup Ther*. 1991;45:1007-1014.

16. Fleming MH. The search for tacit knowledge. In: Mattingly C, Fleming MH, eds. *Clinical Reasoning: Forms of Inquiry in a Therapeutic Practice*. Philadelphia: F.A. Davis Company; 1994.

17. Fleming MH, Mattingly C. Giving language to practice. In: Mattingly C, Fleming MH, eds. *Clinical Reasoning: Forms of Inquiry in a Therapeutic Practice*. Philadelphia: F.A. Davis Company; 1994.

18. Gale J. Some cognitive components of the diagnostic thinking process. *Br J Educ Psychol*. 1982;52:64-76.

19. Garnham A. Representing information in mental models. In: Conway MA, ed. *Cognitive Models of Memory*. Cambridge: MIT Press; 1998.

20. Graber ML, Franklin N, Gordon R. Diagnostic Error in Internal Medicine. *Arch Intern Med*. 2005;165:1493-1499.

21. Grant J, Marsden P. The structure of memorized knowledge in students and clinicians: an explanation from diagnostic expertise. *Med Educ*. 1987;21:92-98.

22. Grimmer K, Bialocerkowski A, Kumar S, Milanese S. Implementing evidence in clinical practice: the therapies dilemma. *Physiotherapy*. 2004;90:189-194.

23. Higgs J, Jones MA. Clinical reasoning in the health professions. In: Higgs J, Jones MA, eds. *Clinical Reasoning in the Health Professions*. 2nd ed. Boston, Mass: Butterworth-Heinemann; 2000:3-14.

24. Higgs J, Titchen A. Knowledge and reasoning. In: Higgs J, Jones MA, eds. *Clinical Reasoning in the Health Professions*. 2nd ed. New York, NY: Butterworth-Heinemann; 2000:23-32.

25. Higgs J. Developing knowledge: A process of construction mapping and review. *New Zealand Journal of Physiotherapy*. 1992;20:23-30.

26. Higgs J. Fostering the acquisition of clinical reasoning skills. *New Zealand Journal of Physiotherapy*. 1990;(Dec):13-17.

27. Higgs J, Jones M. Clinical reasoning in the health professions. In: Higgs J, Jones M, eds. *Clinical Reasoning in the Health Professions*. 2nd ed. Oxford: Butterworth-Heinemann; 2000.

28. Jensen GM, Gwyer J, Hack LM, Shepard KF. *Expertise in Physical Therapy Practice*. Boston, Mass: Butterworth-Heinemann; 1999.

29. Jensen GM, Gwyer J, Shepard KF, Hack LM. Expert Practice in Physical Therapy. *Phys Ther*. 2000;80(1):28-43.

30. Jones M, Edwards I, Gifford L. Conceptual models for implementing biopsychosocial theory in clinical practice. *Man Ther*. 2002;7(1):2-9.

31. Jones MA. Clinical reasoning in manual therapy. *Phys Ther*. 1992;72:875-884.

32. Jones M, Jensen G, Edwards I. Clinical Reasoning in Physiotherapy. In: Higgs J, Jones M, eds. *Clinical Reasoning in the Health Professions*. 2nd ed. Oxford: Butterworth-Heinemann; 2000.

33. Jones MA. Clinical reasoning and pain. *Man Ther*. 1995;1(1):17-24.

34. Kassirer JP, Kopelman RL. Cognitive errors in diagnosis: instantiation, classification, and consequences. *Am J Med*. 1989;86:433-441.

35. Main CJ. *Pain Management: Practical applications of the biopsychosocial perspective in clinical and occupational settings*. 2nd ed. Churchill Livingstone; 2007.

36. Mann PJ, Darrah J. Linking research and clinical practice in physical therapy: strategies for integration. *Physiotherapy*. 2006;92:88-94.

37. Marvel MK, Epstein RM, Flowers K, Beckman HB. Soliciting the patient's agenda: have we improved? *JAMA*. 1999;281(3):283-287.

38. Mattingly C. The narrative nature of clinical reasoning. *Am J Occup Ther*. 1991;45:998-1005.

39. Mattingly C. What is clinical reasoning?, *Am J Occup Ther*. 1991;45:998-1005.

40. Mechanic D, McAlpine MA, Rosenthal M. Are Patients' Office Visits with Physicians Getting Shorter? *New J Med*. 2001;344(3):198-204.

41. Mildonis MK, Godges JJ, Jensen GM. Nature of clinical practice for specialist in orthopaedic physical therapy. *J Orthop Sports Phys Ther*. 1999;29(4):240.

42. Mueller MJ, Maluf KS. Tissue Adaptation to Physical Stress: A Proposed "Physical Stress Theory" to Guide Physical Therapist Practice, Education, and Research. *Phys Ther*. 2002;82(4):383-403.

43. Newble C, Norman G, van der Vleuten C. Assessing clinical reasoning. In: Higgs J, Jones M, eds. *Clinical Reasoning in the Health Professions*. 2nd ed. Oxford: Butterworth-Heinemann; 2000.

44. Patel VL, Groen GJ. Knowledge-based solution strategies in medical reasoning. *Cognitive Science*. 1986;10:91-108.

45. Payton OD. Clinical reasoning process in physical therapy. *Phys Ther*. 1985;65:924-928.

46. Radvansky GA, Zachs RT. The retrieval of situation-specific information. In: Conway MA, ed. *Cognitive Models of Memory*. Cambridge: MIT Press; 1997.

47. Rivett D, Higgs J. Experience and Expertise in Clinical Reasoning. *NZ Journal of Physiotherapy*. 1995:16-21.

48. Sahrmann S. *Diagnosis and Treatment of Movement Impairment Syndromes*. Mosby; 2001.

49. Samdhu H, Carpenter C. Clinical Decisionmaking: Opening the Black Box of Cognitive Reasoning. *Ann Emerg Med*. 2006;48(6):713-719.

50. Sevdalis N, McCulloch P. Teaching Evidence-Based Decision Making. *Surg Clin N Am*. 2006;86:59-70.

51. Shacklock MO. The clinical application of central pain mechanisms in manual therapy. *Aust J Physio*. 1999;45:215-221.

52. Travaline JM, Ruchinskas R, D'Alonzo GE. Patient-Physician Communication: Why and How. *AOA*. 2005;105(1):13-18.

53. Wolf SL. Summation: Identification of principles underlying clinical decision. In: Wolf SL, ed. *Clinical Decision Making in Physical Therapy*. Philadelphia: F.A. Davis Company; 1985.

54. Wood DJ. Problem Solving—The Nature and Development of Strategies. In: Underwood G, ed. *Strategies of Information Processing*. New York: Academic Press, Inc.; 1978.

55. Woolever DR. The art and science of clinical decision making. *Fam Pract Manag*. 2008:31-36.

AUTHORS: AMY B. POMRANTZ and ROBERT LANDEL

INTRODUCTORY INFORMATION

WHAT IS THE PREVALENCE OF NECK PAIN?

Neck pain is a common musculoskeletal disorder, with a reported lifetime prevalence of 22% to 67%.[75]

WHAT PORTION OF NECK PAIN CAN BE LINKED TO INJURIES TO THE UPPER CERVICAL REGION?

Injuries to the atlantoaxial complex account for approximately 25% of all cervical spine injuries.[74] Of cervical rotation 50% occurs in the upper cervical spine. Therefore, dysfunction in this region can transfer movement stresses to the lower cervical spine resulting in subsequent injury in that region.

LIST THE MAJOR STRUCTURES THAT COMPRISE THE UPPER CERVICAL SPINE REGION AND ARE TYPICALLY ASSOCIATED WITH PATHOLOGY IN THIS REGION

C1 and C2 vertebrae
Odontoid process on C2
Alar and transverse ligaments
Suboccipital musculature
Trigeminal and occipital nerves
Spinal cord
C1, C2, and C3 spinal nerves
Brainstem
Tectorial membrane
Vertebrobasilar artery

WHAT FACTORS MAKE DIAGNOSIS DIFFICULT IN THE UPPER CERVICAL SPINE?

Because of the complexity of structures and commonly traumatic mechanisms involved, injuries to the upper cervical spine can be difficult to diagnose.[74] Due to the high density of neurological structures in the region, pathologies in the upper cervical region can refer symptoms to areas quite distal, in the trunk and upper and lower extremities.

Conversely, the source of upper cervical spine symptoms may also be far away from this region. Some examples include dysfunction in the temporomandibular joint (TMJ), which can lead to dysfunction in the cervical spine, and vice versa. Postural dysfunction in the lower extremities and trunk can also influence head position, leading to upper cervical spine dysfunction (i.e., postural dysfunction can lead to capital flexion causing hypomobility in the joints and extensor soft tissues).

WHAT IS THE PROGNOSIS FOR RECOVERY?

The prognosis for recovery depends on the source of the symptoms. There are limited data available in the literature for many upper cervical spine pathologies. Available information is presented below.

GENERAL NECK PAIN

- Between 60% and 80% of workers with neck pain report neck pain 1 year after injury. Few workplace or physical job demands were identified as being linked to recovery from neck pain. However, workers with little influence on their own work situation had a slightly poorer prognosis, and white-collar workers had a better prognosis than blue-collar workers. General exercise was associated with better prognosis; prior neck pain and prior sick leave were associated with a poorer prognosis.

WHIPLASH INJURIES

- Between 16% and 71% of those with a whiplash injury go on to develop Late Whiplash Syndrome (the presence of pain, restriction of motion or other symptoms 6 months or more after injury, sufficient to hinder the return to normal activities).[77]
- In 2003, a systematic review of the literature was performed on 29 independent cohort studies to identify prognostic factors associated with delayed functional recovery in patients with whiplash-related disorder.[62]
  - Higher initial levels of pain and disability, older age, cold hyperalgesia, impaired sympathetic vasoconstriction, and moderate posttraumatic stress symptoms have been shown to be associated with poorer outcomes 6 months following whiplash injury.[66-68,77]
  - Older age, female gender, high acute psychological response, angular deformity of the neck, rear end collision, and compensation were found to have no influence on outcomes.
  - There was no evidence found to allow for conclusions on the influence of factors such as coping, anxiety, cognition, educational level, head restraint, and seat belt on prognosis.

ODONTOID FRACTURES

- The classification system for odontoid fractures, described in 1974 by Anderson and D'Alonzo,[6] is based on the anatomic level of the fracture, and has been shown to have a correlation to prognosis for fracture healing.[29]
  - Type I fractures occur at the tip of the odontoid process, superior to the transverse ligament. They are the least common odontoid injury and are generally stable.
  - Type II fractures occur at the junction of the base of the odontoid and the body of the axis. They are the most common fracture type and are least likely to heal with nonsurgical treatment.
  - Type III fractures extend into the body of the axis. They are thought to be more stable than type II fractures and have a higher union rate with nonsurgical treatment.

UPPER CERVICAL RHEUMATOID ARTHRITIS

- The prognosis depends on whether a surgical or conservative treatment approach is used.
- A study using 40 matched control patients with upper cervical instability and myelopathy due to rheumatoid arthritis demonstrated a better prognosis for patients who underwent surgery (occipitocervical fusion associated with C1 laminectomy) versus patients who did not undergo surgery. The survival rate 10 years after surgery was 37%. Ten years after the development of myelopathy, the survival rate for patients who did not undergo surgery was 0%.[42]

TRIGEMINAL NEURALGIA

- Presents with a relapsing or remitting course. More than 50% of individuals have at least a 6-month remission during their lifetime and 24% have a 12-month remission.[54]

OCCIPITAL NEURALGIA AND CERVICOGENIC HEADACHE

- No information about the prognosis for these pathologies has been identified in the literature.

CERVICOGENIC DIZZINESS

- Of people with neck pain due to whiplash 60% to 88% get better and 12% to 40% become chronic. Of that amount, some percentage ends up having dizziness. The prognosis for those is unknown.[55]
- Of patients who received physical therapy directed at cervical impairments 14 of 17 had no or less dizziness at 6 months, and 11 of 17 at 2 years. There was no control group in this study.[41]

HOW SUCCESSFUL ARE PHYSICAL THERAPY INTERVENTIONS IN TREATING PATHOLOGY IN THIS REGION?

The success rate of physical therapy interventions depends on the source of the symptoms. There are limited data available in the literature for many upper cervical spine pathologies. Available information is presented below.

WHIPLASH

- A 2001 systematic review of the literature performed to assess the efficacy of conservative treatment in patients with whiplash injury found the following[47]:
  - The methodological quality of most studies was low.
  - Although it was difficult to draw a valid conclusion on the efficacy of conservative treatment in patients with whiplash injury, available knowledge indicates a beneficial long-term effect of active treatments on at least one primary outcome measure: pain, global perceived effect, and participation in daily activities.
  - They also cautiously conclude that active interventions may have a tendency to be more effective in patients with whiplash injury.

UPPER CERVICAL RHEUMATOID ARTHRITIS

- A recent study by Hakkinen et al[23] demonstrated that isometric exercises toward flexion significantly decreased the atlantoaxial distance in patients with unstable anterior atlantoaxial subluxation. Submaximal resisted extension, even in the neutral position of the cervical spine, led to a decrease in the width of the cervical spine canal and is, therefore, not recommended for patients with unstable anterior atlantoaxial subluxation
  - The authors conclude that resisted isometric flexion exercises might have potential in rheumatoid arthritis (RA) patients; however, further studies are needed before recommending this type of treatment.
- An uncontrolled study by Kauppi et al[33] demonstrated a significant ($p < 0.001$) reduction of cervical spine pain and continued effect for 12 months with conservative treatment including physical therapy, patient education for posture and use of assistive devices, collars, medications for symptom relief, and disease-modifying antirheumatic drugs. Physical therapy consisted of isometric exercises and minimal dynamic motion of the cervical spine and shoulders to facilitate strengthening. Exercises focused on the activation of the deep neck flexors and avoidance of maximal cervical flexion and rotation.
- No studies have been identified demonstrating the benefits of transcutaneous electrical stimulation on the cervical spine in rheumatoid arthritis.[45,49]
- Modalities such as massage and heat therapy have not demonstrated proven benefits.[49]
- Soft cervical collars have been reported to help with local neck pain but have not been shown to limit motion or progression of the disease.[35,45,49]

TRIGEMINAL NEURALGIA

- No studies were identified in the literature demonstrating the benefits of physical therapy interventions for symptoms of trigeminal neuralgia.

OCCIPITAL NEURALGIA AND CERVICOGENIC HEADACHE

- No studies were identified in the literature demonstrating the effects of physical therapy interventions for symptoms of occipital neuralgia.

CERVICOGENIC DIZZINESS

- A review of physical therapy interventions designed specifically to address neck pain and reduce the symptoms of cervicogenic dizziness found uniformly positive outcomes; however, the studies cited were not randomized controlled or blinded, and many did not include functional or objective outcome measures.[50] The interventions included in this review were manual therapy (including mobilization), soft tissue mobilization, manipulation, and stretching.
- Sustained natural apophyseal glides (SNAGs) to the cervical spine have been shown to significantly reduce neck pain, improve range of motion, and have a positive effect on balance.[51]
- The presentation of cervicogenic dizziness includes complaints of imbalance. Soft tissue treatment, stabilization exercises of the trunk and cervical spine, passive and active mobilization, relaxation techniques, home exercise programs, and minor ergonomic changes have been shown to improve postural performance in patients with cervical disorders, despite specifically avoiding interventions aimed at improving balance or vestibular function.[32]
- Some patients with chronic neck pain have been shown to be more susceptible to cervical extensor muscle fatigue, which coincides with increased postural sway. Physical therapy intervention aimed at reducing pain, strengthening the paravertebral musculature, and improving the mobility of the cervical spine resulted in reduced susceptibility to fatigue and improved sway patterns.[65]
- Cervical manipulation has been reported to be superior to acupuncture and nonsteroidal antiinflammatory medication in reducing cervicogenic dizziness, although all interventions resulted in patient benefits.[25]

CERVICOGENIC HEADACHE

- Manipulative therapy and specific exercises resulted in reduced headache frequency and intensity compared to controls, maintained at 12 month follow-up. A combination of the two interventions was not significantly better than either alone.[30]
- There is no consistent pattern of variables that can identify who will or will not achieve success with manipulative therapy or exercise. The absence of light-headedness indicated higher odds of achieving either a 50% to 79% [odds ratio (OR) = 5.45)] or 80% to100% (OR = 5.7) reduction in headache frequency in the long term. Headaches of at least moderate intensity, the patient's age, and chronicity of headache did not mitigate against a successful outcome from physiotherapy intervention.[31]

HOW SUCCESSFUL IS SURGERY IN TREATING PATHOLOGIES IN THIS REGION?

ODONTOID FRACTURES

- A Cochrane review by Shears and Armitstead concluded that there was not adequate evidence to conclude that surgical treatment of odontoid fractures gives a better outcome than conservative treatment.[64]

INSTABILITY DUE TO RHEUMATOID ARTHRITIS

- Studies have suggested that early stabilization of an atlantoaxial subluxation may decrease the chances of developing subaxial instability.[13]
- Nonunion rates have been quoted to be as high as 20% to 30% for attempted surgical fusions.[13]
- In a study of 110 patients with rheumatoid arthritis, a study by Agarwal et al found that the recurrence rate of cervical instability following a previous surgical fusion was 15%.[2]
- For patients presenting with atlantoaxial subluxation, who report pain but no major significant neurological deficit, the mortality rate after atlantoaxial fusion was significantly lower than for conservative treatment.[70]
- A study by Boden et al found the posterior atlantodental interval to be a predictor of surgical outcome. In patients with a preoperative posterior atlantodental interval of <10 mm, no significant neurological recovery was demonstrated. In patients with isolated atlantoaxial subluxation, a posterior atlantodental interval of at least 10 mm predicted some neurological improvement. All patients with a preoperative posterior atlantodental interval and subaxial sagittal canal diameter of at least 14 mm experienced complete motor recovery.[10]

TRIGEMINAL NEURALGIA

- Microvascular decompression has been shown to provide the longest duration of relief for patients with drug-resistant trigeminal neuralgia. Studies have demonstrated improvement in greater than 70% of patients 10 years after surgery.[12]

This technique has been shown to have a low risk of symptom recurrence and sensory loss.[36]

CERVICOGENIC HEADACHE, OCCIPITAL NEURALGIA, AND CERVICOGENIC DIZZINESS

- Surgery is not indicated for these pathologies.

PERSONAL INFORMATION

WHAT INFLUENCE DOES AGE HAVE ON YOUR CLINICAL DECISION-MAKING PROCESS?

- With advancing age, degeneration of spinal discs leads to the accentuation of the normal spinal curve including hyperextension of the cervical spine. This results in the shortening of posterior structures. The loss of mobility in the mid- and lower cervical region will lead to a loss of mobility in the upper cervical spine, which then subsequently causes increased degeneration of the mid-cervical spine as a compensation.
- Hyperkyphosis of the thoracic spine will contribute to hyperlordosis of the cervical spine, which will result in excessive capital extension as a compensation to allow the patient to be able to interact with the world at eye level.

CLINICAL PEARL

Successful intervention in the upper cervical spine often necessitates managing spinal conditions (mobility, strength, endurance, etc.) in a thoracic and lumbar spine, since the position of the head and neck is dictated in large part by the posture of the caudal spinal segments.

Age has also been shown to influence various factors with regard to specific upper cervical spine pathologies. Available information from the literature follows.

- Likelihood and location of injury: fractures
  - In a study by Ryan and Henderson on the epidemiology of cervical spine fractures and fracture dislocations,[56] C2 was the most commonly injured level. Whereas overall fractures and fracture dislocations most commonly occurred at in third decade of life and demonstrated decreasing incidence in advancing age, the incidence of fractures at C1 and C2 increased with age, correlated with falls in the elderly population.
  - Cervical spine fractures have a prevalence of 2.6% to 4.7% in patients older than 65 years old.[21]
  - In patients 65 years and older, fractures to C1 and C2 occur more commonly than at other cervical spine levels.[38,56]
- Mechanism of injury
  - High-velocity trauma, such as motor vehicle accidents, accounts for most odontoid fractures in young adults, while low-velocity injuries, such as falls, account for the majority of injuries in the elderly and children.[29]
- Onset of other factors
  - Onset of rheumatoid arthritis presents a peak in the fifth decade of life according to the majority of epidemiological studies.[4]
  - The onset of trigeminal neuralgia is typically after age 40 in 90% of cases,[16,54] with peak incidence at 60% to 70 years old.[36]
  - The mean age of onset of osteoarthritis is 70 years. The radiological prevalence of degenerative changes at the lateral atlantoaxial joints was found to increase with age, ranging from 5.4% in the sixth decade to 18.2% in the ninth decade of life.[80]
  - Cervicogenic headache and dizziness and occipital neuralgia: No information has been identified in the literature regarding the typical onset of these pathologies.

WHAT INFLUENCE DOES A PATIENT'S OCCUPATION HAVE ON YOUR CLINICAL DECISION-MAKING PROCESS?

- Occupations, which involve repetitive motions such as flexion, extension, lateral flexion, or rotation, will aggravate pathologies of the upper cervical spine.
- Improper posture during sedentary occupations can also lead to dysfunction. Most people maintain a flexed trunk posture during sitting, which leads to hyperextension of the occipitoatlantal (OA) joint so the individual can keep the head level and view the world. Chronic habitual posture of this sort will lead to tightness in the posterior upper cervical structures. The Case Study below illustrates how occupation can influence upper cervical symptoms.

CLINICAL PEARL

Many individuals lack capital flexion because of the generalized and wide-spread tendency to sit in a flexed posture. Therefore upper cervical mobility, particularly into flexion, should be a routine part of a clinical examination.

CLINICAL DECISION MAKING CASE STUDY—PATIENT PROFILE

Your patient is a 36-year-old female data entry operator who complains of neck pain and headaches. The onset was insidious, starting 6 to 8 months ago. Her pain is worse at the end of the day and better on weekends. Her job requires her to sit at a computer all day, with a 30-minute lunch break and a 15-minute break each morning and afternoon. She denies a history of trauma, does not smoke, and is otherwise healthy. What impairments would you expect to find in the upper cervical spine, and what would appropriate management include?

Answer

The upper cervical spine must be examined based on this history, because of the overwhelming tendency of individuals to sit in a flexed posture, which places the upper cervical spine in extension. Prolonged positioning in capital extension can lead to compromise of the structures, including the occipital nerve, which could be a cause of her headaches. Physical examination should attempt to reveal the presence of palpable suboccipital tenderness, restricted capital flexion, shortened capital extensor muscles, and restricted mobility of the upper cervical joints. Appropriate management would include measures to improve upper cervical mobility, particularly flexion.

WHAT INFLUENCE DOES A PATIENT'S GENDER HAVE ON YOUR CLINICAL DECISION-MAKING PROCESS?

Although many pathologies of the upper cervical region are not influenced by gender, the following trends have been identified in the literature.

- Rheumatoid arthritis
  - More likely to affect women than men by a 3:1 ratio.[46]
  - Atlantoaxial subluxation is more likely to affect men than women with rheumatoid arthritis.[37]
- Trigeminal neuralgia is more likely to affect women than men by a 2:1 ratio.[16]
- Upper cervical spine osteoarthritis has been observed to affect women at a higher frequency than men.[19,58]

ETHNICITY

No information was identified in the literature demonstrating the influence of ethnicity on pathology in the upper cervical spine.

SYMPTOM HISTORY

WHAT MECHANISMS OF INJURY MOST COMMONLY LEAD TO INJURY OF THE STRUCTURES OF THE UPPER CERVICAL SPINE?

• High-velocity trauma

Upper cervical spine injuries are generally a result of high-velocity trauma with motor vehicle accidents as the most frequent cause (whiplash). Falls, diving accidents, and gunshot wounds are also common mechanisms.

  ○ High-velocity trauma, such as motor vehicle accidents (whiplash), accounts for most odontoid fractures in young adults.
  ○ The cervical facet joint has been found to be the most common source of chronic neck pain after whiplash injury.[61]
  ○ The most commonly reported cause of sudden-onset vertebrobasilar insufficiency (VBI) is trauma, particularly from high-velocity flexion-distraction and rotational forces that may occur during a whiplash incident.[14]

• Low-velocity trauma

  ○ Low-velocity injuries, such as falls, account for the majority of injuries in the elderly and children.[29]

• Congenital and developmental abnormalities

  ○ Down syndrome
    1. Atlantoaxial instability affects 10% to 20% of individuals with Down syndrome, although it is mostly asymptomatic in this condition.[5]
    2. Instability can occur at the atlantoaxial or occipitocervical joint.
    3. Ligamentous laxity due to abnormal collagen as well as bony abnormalities such as hypoplasia of the odontoid may contribute to the instability.
  ○ Klippel-Feil Syndrome[57]
    1. Uncommon congenital condition characterized as the improper segmentation or fusion of at least two cervical vertebrae.
    2. Can lead to abnormal cervical spine degeneration and canal stenosis.

• Arthritis

  ○ Rheumatoid arthritis
    1. Involves erosive sinovitis, which leads to ligamentous distension and rupture, damage to the articular cartilage and bone erosion, osteoporosis, and cyst formation. The end result is joint laxity and subluxation.[17,37]
    2. The prevalence of cervical spine involvement in rheumatoid arthritis ranges from 25% to 80%. Atlantoaxial instability (AAI) or subluxation is the common deformity seen in this disease process and has been reported to occur in up to 49% of patients with RA.[52]
  ○ Ankylosing spondylitis
    1. Erosion of the odontoid or destruction of the transverse ligament may occur leading to C1 subluxation on C2.[76]

• Improper postural alignment

  ○ Improper posture during sedentary occupations can also lead to dysfunction. Most people maintain a flexed trunk posture during prolonged sitting, which leads to hyperextension of the OA joint.

• Repetitive activities

  ○ Occupations that involve repetitive motions such as flexion, extension, lateral flexion, or rotation will aggravate pathologies of the upper cervical spine.

• Mixed or unknown mechanisms

  ○ Occipital neuralgia
    1. Many mechanisms have been hypothesized:[76]
       a. Damage to the occipital nerve may occur following a compressive blow to the nerve.
       b. Damage to the C2 nerve may occur with whiplash injury or due to degenerative arthritis of the atlantoaxial joint.

    c. Occupations involving excessive hypextension and rotation may cause repeated compression of the C2 nerve root.
  ○ Trigeminal neuralgia
    1. The exact mechanism is unknown. The pathology can be idiopathic or secondary.
    2. Studies have shown a high success rate with microvascular decompression surgery in cases that were resistant to medical therapy.[12] These findings suggest that vascular compression of the sensory roots of the trigeminal nerve may contribute to symptoms.

CLINICAL PEARL

The most common abnormality observed with rheumatoid arthritis of the cervical spine is atlantoaxial subluxation. Two-thirds of rheumatoid cervical subluxations occur in this region.[17]

LOCATION OF SYMPTOMS

WHAT INFLUENCE DOES THE LOCATION OF SYMPTOMS HAVE ON YOUR CLINICAL DECISION-MAKING PROCESS?

Symptoms from the upper cervical spine can present at or near the location of the structures involved, with possible referral into the head and eyes including headache and dizziness, especially when upper cervical hypermobility is present. Symptoms from spinal cord pathology can be referred into the extremities. Upper cervical mechanical dysfunction can lead to TMJ dysfunction and, therefore, result in pain in the jaw, face, and temporal regions.

REFERRAL OF SYMPTOMS

• Muscles/tendons

  ○ Symptoms from the suboccipital musculature can be referred to the ipsilateral occiput, eye, and forehead.[72]

• Ligaments

  ○ Ligamentous instability can result in spinal cord impingement, resulting in distal symptoms. Bilateral extremity symptoms associated with neck movements, especially flexion, would be an indication of upper cervical instability.
  ○ Transverse and alar ligaments: Neck pain due to instability is typically reported in the cervical, suboccipital, occipital regions, and shoulder regions either continuously or episodically. With severe pain, symptoms can extend to the temporal or even frontal regions and to the back of the eye on one or both sides. Symptoms from instability are commonly described as a sensation of the head falling forward.[73]

• Bone

  ○ C1 vertebrae, C2 vertebrae, odontoid process of C2: Symptoms of pain due to fracture can present in the upper cervical, suboccipital, and occipital regions. Symptoms due to instability, which may occur as a result of a fracture, may present as described above.

• Zygapophyseal (facet) joints and cervical dorsal rami

  ○ Research by Fukui et al[20] has identified the following referral patterns from facet joints to the upper cervical spine region (see Figure II-2-1):

C0/1	Upper posterolateral cervical region
C1/2	Upper posterolateral cervical region
C2/3	Occipital region, upper posterolateral cervical region, upper posterior cervical region
C3/4	Upper posterior cervical region

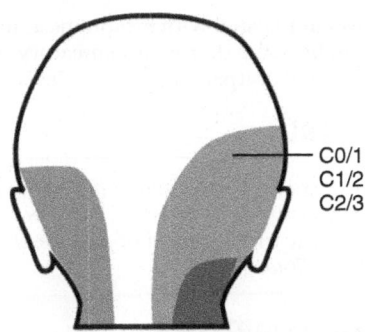

FIGURE II-2-1 Referral patterns from facet joints to the upper cervical spine region. (Adapted from Fukui S, Ohseto K, Shiotani M, et al. Referred pain distribution of the cervical zygapophyseal joints and cervical dorsal rami. *Pain.* 1996;68(1):79–83.)

○ Studies by Lord et al[39] and Bogduk and Marsland[11] have found that C2/3 is one of the most common levels for chronic facet joint pain after a whiplash injury.
• Nerves
  ○ C1 spinal nerve: The first spinal nerve is known as the suboccipital nerve and consists of motor fibers only. It therefore lacks a corresponding sensory field.[63]
  ○ C2 spinal nerve: C2 provides sensory information to the posterior and lateral head (the remainder of the head is not innervated by the trigeminal nerve) via the greater and lesser occipital nerves.[9] Sensation to the upper anterior cervical region is also provided by C2.
  ○ C3 spinal nerve: C3 provides sensory information to the occipital region, upper posterior cervical region, and lower anterior cervical region.
  ○ Occipital nerve (greater and lesser) (see Figure II-2-2)
    1. The occipital nerve provides sensory information to the posterior and lateral head through the greater (C2) and lesser (C2, C3) occipital nerves.[3]
    2. Symptoms due to occipital neuralgia typically affect the suboccipital region, posterior neck, and posterior and lateral scalp, and can lead to headaches.
    3. Symptoms typically occur unilaterally.[1,16]

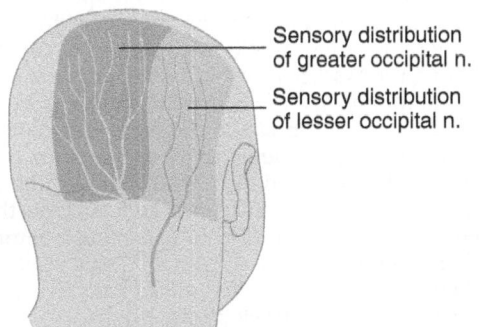

Sensory distribution of greater occipital n.

Sensory distribution of lesser occipital n.

FIGURE II-2-2 Greater and lesser occipital nerve anatomy. The greater occipital nerve pierces the fascia just below the superior nuchal ridge along with the artery. It supplies the medial portion of the posterior scalp. The lesser occipital nerve passes superiorly along the posterior border of the sternocleidomastoid muscle, dividing into the cutaneous branches that innervate the lateral portion of the posterior scalp and the ear. (From Waldman SD. *Atlas of Interventional Pain Management,* 2e. Philadelphia: Saunders; 2004.)

○ Trigeminal nerve
  1. The trigeminal nerve provides sensory innervation to the face through three divisions: the maxillary (skin of the middle third of the face), mandibular (skin of the inferior third of the face), and ophthalmic (skin of the superior third of the face) divisions.
  2. Symptoms due to trigeminal neuralgia occur most commonly in the maxillary and mandibular divisions, and much less frequently in the ophthalmic division.[54]
     a. The right side of the face is affected more than the left. Only 4% of patients experience bilateral symptoms and most have underlying multiple sclerosis.
     b. Trigeminal neuralgia never spreads across the midline and bilateral cases are never synchronous.
○ Spinal cord: Symptoms from spinal cord pathology can be referred into the extremities.
• Vascular systems
  ○ Vertebrobasilar artery insufficiency
    1. This can cause ipsilateral head and neck pain localized to region of vascular disruption.[59]
    2. Vertebrobasilar compromise rarely occurs without being accompanied by neurological signs and symptoms.
    3. Bartels reported on 24 patients with 28 vertebral artery dissections. In all patients, the initial symptom was pain in the occipital or neck region.
  ○ Internal carotid artery dissection[76]
    1. Unilateral neck pain occurs in 19% of cases and can be localized to the upper anterior neck, mastoid region, angle of the jaw, and sternocleidomastoid muscle.
    2. Headache can also result and may be retroorbital, orbital, frontal, temporal, or in the area of the ear and mastoid process.

WHAT STRUCTURES CAN REFER SYMPTOMS INTO THE UPPER CERVICAL SPINE?

• Brain and spinal cord
  ○ Meningitis
    1. Can present with neck stiffness (nuchal rigidity) and pain, especially with cervical flexion and rotation, and severe headache.[76]
  ○ Chiari malformation
    1. Can present with neck pain, headache, and dizziness.
• Mid-cervical zygapophyseal joints
  ○ Can refer symptoms to the upper cervical spine region.
• Temporomandibular joint
  ○ Dysfunction can result in excessive muscular contraction in the upper cervical musculature, compressing the greater occipital nerve and causing pain referred into the upper neck and the posterior head (primarily the occiput).
• Visceral structures
  ○ Myocardial infarction or coronary insufficiency[76]
    1. Pain can radiate into the anterior and/or left-sided neck commonly described as a tightness, ache, choking, or suffocating sensation.

CLINICAL PEARL

Referral of pain, paresthesias or numbness into the upper or lower extremities bilaterally when the neck is flexed suggests instability of the upper cervical spine. Undiagnosed signs of instability necessitate a referral to a physician.

SYMPTOM DESCRIPTORS

QUALITY OF SYMPTOMS

Quality	Possible Tissues Involved
Superficial	Nerve, muscle
Deep ache	Bone, ligament, viscera
Dull ache	Bone, ligament
Sharp pain	Bone, ligament, nerve
Continuous	Bone, viscera
Burning	Nerve, vascular
Tingling	Nerve, vascular
Numbness	Nerve, vascular
Colicky and cramping	Viscera
Woozy, off, dizzy	Muscle, joint, vascular

DEPTH OF SYMPTOMS

WHAT INFLUENCE DOES THE DEPTH OF SYMPTOMS HAVE ON THE CLINICAL DECISION-MAKING PROCESS?

- Superficial symptoms suggest the source may be nerve or muscle pathology that can be more easily localized or reproduced with palpation or other testing.
- Deep symptoms suggest the source may be bone, ligament, or visceral structures that are more difficult to localize or reproduce with testing.

CLINICAL PEARL

!

Pain arising from trigeminal neuralgia is described as superficial with severe burning or "shock-like" quality.[16]

CONSTANCY OF SYMPTOMS

WHAT INFLUENCE DOES CONSTANCY OF SYMPTOMS HAVE ON YOUR CLINICAL DECISION-MAKING PROCESS?

- Intermittent or constant but varying symptoms with identifiable aggravating and easing factors suggest a musculoskeletal or neural source of symptoms.
- Constant symptoms that do not change suggest cancer, visceral structures, or infection as possible sources of symptoms.

TWENTY-FOUR-HOUR SYMPTOM PATTERN

IF A PATIENT HAS SYMPTOMS IN THE MORNING, WHAT PATHOLOGY DOES THIS IMPLICATE?

Pain and stiffness that are worse in the morning can be due to inflammation that becomes stagnant at night due to decreased circulation and decreased muscle activation. Movement in the morning helps to dissipate the inflammation.

IF A PATIENT HAS SYMPTOMS IN THE AFTERNOON, WHAT PATHOLOGY DOES THIS IMPLICATE?

Fatigue and postural influences may be implicated.

IF A PATIENT HAS SYMPTOMS IN THE EVENING, WHAT PATHOLOGY DOES THIS IMPLICATE?

Fatigue, postural influences, and overuse may be implicated.

IF A PATIENT HAS SYMPTOMS WHEN SLEEPING, WHAT PATHOLOGY DOES THIS IMPLICATE?

Pain at night can be due to sleep position. For example, sleeping in a prone position requires cervical extension and rotation. Because 50% of rotation comes from the upper cervical region, dysfunction is this region could cause pain when sleeping in a prone position. Night pain could also be due to a lack of sensory information that may have been masking the pain throughout the day. Cancer is also implicated with symptoms at night. Night pain in extremities can be a sign that an inflammatory process contributes to symptoms (e.g., carpal tunnel syndrome)

CLINICAL PEARL

!

If a patient's pain is aggravated when the patient awakes from sleep, subjective questioning should investigate sleep position, the use and position of pillows, and the age of the mattress and pillows.

STABILITY OF SYMPTOMS

CHANGES IN SYMPTOMS

HOW DOES THE PROGRESSION OF A PATIENT'S SYMPTOMS IMPACT THE CLINICAL DECISION-MAKING PROCESS?

- As always, lack of progress with appropriate interventions and management is an indication to change the plan of care, up to and including discharge from physical therapy and referral to the appropriate health care provider.
- Hypermobility is common in the cervical spine. If the symptomatic segment is a hypermobile one, then reduction in symptoms depends on improving mobility at adjacent segments, and improving dynamic stability through increased muscle strength, endurance, and control. Improving mobility can take from one treatment (e.g., manipulation) to several treatment sessions if the appropriate intervention is applied to the correct location. Increasing neuromuscular control may occur within 2 weeks, but improving muscle strength and endurance may take 6 weeks at minimum under optimal conditions, and 8 to 12 weeks in the presence of pain or other pathology.
- Hypomobility is more common in the upper cervical spine than is hypermobility, due to habitual usage patterns that are typical in Western society (sitting in a flexed posture, causing a forward head position with capital extension). As noted, improvements and mobility should occur within a few treatments. However, gaining length in the capital extensor muscles may take 6 to 8 weeks of consistent stretching, combined with an increase in capital flexion strength.

IF A PATIENT'S SYMPTOMS ARE IMPROVING, WHAT PATHOLOGY DOES THIS IMPLICATE?

- Improvement with the application of traction suggests the pathology lies within structures that are sensitive to compression.
- An overstretched facet joint capsule will improve gradually over a several week period, much as ankle sprain would.
- Muscle strains should improve relatively quickly, on the order of a few days to a few weeks, if the muscles are allowed to rest. Although it has fallen out of fashion, the use of soft and hard collars to mobilize the neck after traumatic injuries such as whiplash is as appropriate in the neck as immobilizing the ankle would be after an acute ankle sprain. Fears of inducing weakness can be mitigated through the application of isometric exercises while in the collar. Research suggests that one of the predictors for acute neck pain becoming a chronic condition is higher initial severity of pain.[62,66] Logic suggests aggressive pain-relieving interventions applied early may prevent the chronic condition from developing.

IF A PATIENT'S SYMPTOMS ARE WORSENING, WHAT PATHOLOGY DOES THIS IMPLICATE?

- Traction should improve most conditions within the cervical spine. The upper cervical spine is no exception. Worsening of symptoms with the application of traction, or the production of central signs, should make us suspicious of a Chiari malformation, or upper cervical hypermobility.
- In the absence of such pathology, the therapist should critically examine his or her application of the traction, looking for errors in direction, amount, or duration of pull.

- Upper cervical hypermobility will not improve on its own. Symptoms are more likely to increase over time.

CLINICAL PEARL

After an acute injury such as a whiplash, there is a high likelihood of ligamentous sprains and muscle tears. Respect should be given to the time it takes for tissues to heal. Appropriate measures early in the acute phase should be directed at alleviating pain, and preventing long-term dysfunction.

FUNCTIONAL OR ACTIVITY PARTICIPATION LIMITATIONS

BEHAVIOR OF SYMPTOMS—AGGRAVATING BEHAVIOR

FLEXION-BASED ACTIVITIES

- Pathologies aggravated by flexion include transverse ligament sprain, alar ligament sprain, fracture, and muscle strain.
  - Flexion will aggravate the structures that work to restrict this motion including the ligaments and bony anatomy, therefore aggravating a sprain of the alar and transverse ligaments and a fracture.
  - As the suboccipital musculature is lengthened by flexion, a strain of this musculature will be aggravated by flexion activities.
  - If there is insufficiency of the transverse ligament or atlan-todens complex, then flexion will be an aggravating movement and symptoms may be felt in the upper and lower extremities.

EXTENSION-BASED ACTIVITIES

- Pathologies aggravated by extension include central canal stenosis, facet joint dysfunction, muscle strain, and spondylolisthesis
  - Extension will decrease the diameter of the spinal canal and intervertebral foramen therefore aggravating pathologies such as stenosis due to increased compression or irritation of the spinal cord.
- The volume of the canal decreases with an increasing extension angle, because of the decrease in length and width of the canal.[26]
  - Extension may aggravate facet joints by increasing compression at the articulating surfaces.
  - Once injured, pain may be elicited in muscle during either concentric or eccentric muscle contraction. Therefore, extension may aggravate symptoms in the suboccipital musculature.
  - Extension can cause further translation of the vertebrae in spondylolisthesis.

LATERAL FLEXION AND ROTATION ACTIVITIES

- Pathologies aggravated by lateral flexion include: alar ligament sprain, fracture, facet joint dysfunction, lateral stenosis, and muscle strain.
  - The volume of the spinal canal decreases with lateral flexion, although less than that seen in flexion–extension.[26] This can result in the aggravation of pathologies such as lateral stenosis due to increased compression or irritation of the neural structures.
  - Because the contralateral alar ligaments restrict rotation and lateral flexion, these motions will put strain on the alar ligaments, potentially leading to symptoms.
  - The action of the suboccipital musculature includes ipsilateral rotation. Rotation may, therefore, aggravate a strain of this musculature.
  - Lateral flexion and rotation may aggravate facet joint conditions by increasing compression of the articulating surfaces.

COMBINED MOTION ACTIVITIES

- Pathologies aggravated by extension and rotation/lateral flexion include alar ligament sprain, facet joint dysfunction, central stenosis, lateral stenosis, muscle strain, and spondylolisthesis.
- Pathologies aggravated by flexion and rotation/lateral flexion include transverse ligament sprain, alar ligament sprain, fracture, lateral stenosis, and muscle strain.

STATIC ACTIVITIES (SITTING AND STANDING)

- Pathologies aggravated by sitting and standing include fracture, transverse ligament sprain, and alar ligament sprain.
  - Static activities will aggravate symptoms that are due to instability. Symptoms from instability are commonly described as a sensation of the head falling forward. When muscle actions are absent, support from passive structures is necessary to prevent excess motion in the spinal segments. Therefore static motions can aggravate symptoms from fractures and ligament sprains.

SUSTAINED POSITIONS

- Complaints of dizziness accompanied by neurological signs while the patient is held in sustained positions could indicate VBI.

BEHAVIOR OF SYMPTOMS—EASING BEHAVIOR

FLEXION-BASED ACTIVITIES

- Pathologies eased by flexion include central stenosis, facet joint dysfunction, and spondylolisthesis.
  - Cervical spine flexion will increase the diameter of the spinal canal therefore easing pathologies such as central stenosis due to decreased compression or irritation of the spinal cord.

EXTENSION-BASED ACTIVITIES

- Pathologies eased by extension include transverse ligament sprain, alar ligament sprain, and muscle strain.

LATERAL FLEXION AND ROTATION ACTIVITIES

- Pathologies eased by lateral flexion and rotation include facet joint dysfunction, lateral stenosis, and muscle strain.

COMBINED MOTION ACTIVITIES

- Pathologies eased by flexion and rotation/lateral flexion include facet joint dysfunction, central stenosis, lateral stenosis, muscle strain, and spondylolisthesis.
- Pathologies eased by extension and rotation/lateral flexion include transverse ligament sprain, alar ligament sprain, lateral stenosis, and muscle strain.

STATIC ACTIVITIES (LYING DOWN WITH SUPPORT FOR THE HEAD AND NECK)

- Pathologies eased by lying down with the head and neck supported include instability, fracture, transverse ligament sprain, alar ligament sprain, and muscle strain.

  Since cervical spine structures rely on support from passive structures to prevent excess motion in the spinal segments, when the passive support is lost through ligamentous sprains or laxity, and fractures, support of the head and neck can help to reduce symptoms. (Table II-2-1 summarizes the relationship between pathology and specific functional and activity limitations.)

MEDICAL HISTORY

WHAT ROLE DOES A PATIENT'S PAST MEDICAL HISTORY PLAY IN THE DIFFERENTIAL DIAGNOSIS OF PATHOLOGY?

- A history of rheumatoid arthritis, advanced ankylosing spondylitis, Down syndrome, and Klippel-Feil syndrome should make us wary of upper cervical instability.
- A history of trauma (whiplash) should make us consider the presence of fractures, or instability due to ligamentous insufficiency.

TABLE II-2-1 Functional or Activity Participation Limitations

Motion	Functional Activities	Pathology if Symptoms Are Aggravated by Activity	Pathology if Symptoms Are Eased by Activity
Flexion	Looking down	Transverse ligament sprain, alar ligament sprain, fracture (particularly dens), muscle strain	Central stenosis, facet joint dysfunction, spondylolisthesis
Extension	Looking up, reaching up, walking	Central stenosis, facet joint dysfunction, muscle strain, spondylolisthesis	Transverse ligament sprain, alar ligament sprain, muscle strain
Lateral flexion and rotation	Tilting head, looking over shoulders	Alar ligament sprain, fracture, facet joint dysfunction, lateral stenosis, muscle strain	Facet joint dysfunction, lateral stenosis, muscle strain
Combined motion	Flexion and rotation or lateral flexion	Transverse ligament sprain, alar ligament sprain, fracture, lateral stenosis, muscle strain	Facet joint dysfunction, central stenosis, lateral stenosis, muscle strain, spondylolisthesis
	Extension and rotation or lateral flexion	Alar ligament sprain, facet joint dysfunction, central stenosis, lateral stenosis, muscle strain, spondylolisthesis	Transverse ligament sprain, alar ligament sprain, lateral stenosis, muscle strain
Static positions	Sitting	Fracture, transverse ligament sprain, alar ligament sprain	
	Lying down with head/neck supported		Fracture, transverse ligament sprain, alar ligament sprain, muscle strain

- A history of cardiovascular disease should make us consider carotid or vertebral artery problems, particularly if there is a complaint of dizziness or other neurological symptoms.
- A history of osteoporosis should make us aware of an increased fracture risk.
- A history of a Chiari malformation should be considered when the patient presents with signs and symptoms of brainstem compression associated with head and neck movements.

CLINICAL DECISION MAKING CASE STUDY—PATIENT PROFILE (?)

Your patient is a 50-year-old female diagnosed with rheumatoid arthritis 2 years ago. She reports neck pain and the inability to keep her head from falling forward. She notes tingling in her hands when she looks down. What are your hypotheses regarding her pathology?

Answer

The most common abnormality observed with rheumatoid arthritis of the cervical spine is atlantoaxial subluxation. Two-thirds of rheumatoid cervical subluxations occur in this region. Common symptoms of instability include a sensation of the head falling forward.[73] Instability can also lead to neurological symptoms including tingling in the extremities.

MEDICAL AND ORTHOPEDIC TESTING

WHAT MEDICAL AND ORTHOPEDIC TESTS INFLUENCE YOUR DIFFERENTIAL DIAGNOSIS PROCESS?

Imaging, including x-rays and magnetic resonance imaging (MRI), special tests, and clinical decision-making rules play roles in the differential diagnosis process.

- Imaging
  - Plain radiographs
    1. Standard versus flexion/extension views for evaluation of fractures and ligamentous injury
       a. A review of 106 cases of blunt trauma by Insko et al[28] found that when there was adequate flexion and extension range of motion present, the flexion and extension radiographic examination of the cervical spine had a very low (zero) false negative rate for ligamentous injuries. However, in the acute setting, where 30% of patients had a limited ability to flex and extend the cervical spine, flexion/extension radiographs were found to have a higher likelihood of yielding false negatives. Because these patients are at increased risk for injury, imaging with other modalities [computed tomography (CT) or MRI] was suggested by the authors.
       b. A study performed in 21 emergency departments participating in the National Emergency X-Radiography Utilization Study (NEXUS) found that three-view radiography of the cervical spine (lateral, AP, and open-mouth odontoid) adequately identified the majority of patients with acute spinal injury. Therefore, the potential benefit of flexion/extension imaging is limited. They concluded that when there is concern about ligamentous instability, MRI is preferable to flexion/extension radiographs and occult fractures are better evaluated with CT.[48]
    2. Instability with rheumatoid arthritis
       a. Of patients with rheumatoid subluxations 40% to 80% demonstrate radiographic progression.[17,35]
       b. An atlantoaxial displacement of greater than 3 mm on flexion–extension films is considered abnormal.
       c. Reported risk factors for cord compression based on radiographic examination measurement include atlantoaxial subluxation of greater than 9 mm, space available for the cord (SAC) of 14 mm or less, and the presence of basilar invagination.[49]
       d. A study by Boden et al found that as measured on the radiographs of the cervical spine, the posterior atlantodens interval (PADI) demonstrates an excellent correlation ($p = 0.000001$) with the severity of paralysis and has been shown to be more reliable than the anterior atlantoodontoid interval in predicting the development of neural compromise. In a study of 73 patients with long-term follow-up, a PADI of 14 mm or less yielded 97% sensitivity for detecting patients with paralysis.[10]
       e. Routine cervical spine radiography of patients with RA should include lateral view radiographs taken in flexion and extension.
       f. In a recent study, neutral position radiographs would have failed to confirm the diagnosis of atlantoaxial subluxation in 31 cases (48%) and would have failed to record its true severity in 43 cases (66%). The diagnostic sensitivity was 52%. The sensitivity of the neutral radiographs in showing the reversibility of atlantoaxial subluxation was 48%.[34]

Section II

ORTHOPEDIC REASONING

∘ Plain radiographs versus CT
  1. Plain radiographs (x-rays) are commonly recommended as initial screening for alert and stable patients, whereas CT is recommended for use in patients with a depressed mental status.
  2. A meta-analysis comparing the two imaging modalities found that in patients with a significantly depressed mental status due to blunt trauma, despite the absence of randomized controlled trials, evidence suggests that CT significantly outperforms plain radiography as a screening tool for patients at very high risk of cervical spine injury. It was concluded that CT should be the initial screening test in patients with a significantly depressed mental status.
     a. However, it was concluded that there was not sufficient evidence to suggest that cervical spine CT should replace plain radiography as the initial screening test for less injured patients who are at low risk for cervical spine injury.[27]
  3. Other recent studies support the use of initial CT for patients with altered mental status due to blunt trauma.
     a. In a study of 367 patients with altered mental status due to blunt trauma, Harris et al found that CT imaging identified all unstable cervical spine injuries. Subsequent upright radiographs did not identify additional injuries.[24]
     b. In a study of 1356 patients with altered mental status after blunt traumatic injury, Schenarts et al found that CT scan of C0 to C3 was superior to plain films in the early identification of upper cervical spine injury. Plain films failed to identify 45% of upper cervical spine injuries.[60]
∘ MRI
  1. CT versus MRI
     a. There is disagreement in the literature regarding the use of CT versus MRI to identify cervical spine injuries due to blunt trauma in patients with altered mental status.
        i. Some studies suggest that newer generation CT can miss cervical spine injuries in unreliable patients and, therefore, recommend continued use of MRI for clearance of the cervical spine in the unreliable patient.[44]
        ii. Other studies suggest that outside of its appropriate use in obtunded patients with a neurological deficit, MRI is unlikely to uncover unstable C-spine injuries in these patients when cervical spine CT using modern imaging protocols is normal.[71]
  2. Trigeminal neuralgia
     a. The primary roles of imaging in trigeminal neuralgia is in the exclusion of other pathologies and the identification of possible causes of secondary trigeminal neuralgia.[22,78,79]
     b. MRI is recommended to assess head and neck pathology and can be supplemented with angiography to identify compression of the nerve by vascular structures.[43,79]
     c. A review of the neuroradiologic literature by Zakrzewska was unable to identify studies from which an accurate sensitivity and specificity could be calculated secondary to a lack of diagnostic criteria provided, lack of blinding of investigators, or a lack of comparison to surgical findings.[79]
• Clinical decision-making rules
  ∘ Canadian C-Spine Rules[69]: Following an algorithm to identify the necessity of radiography for alert and stable patients with trauma is recommended.
    1. The algorithm consists of three questions:
       a. Is there any high-risk factor present that mandates radiography (age ≥65 years, dangerous mechanism, or paresthesias in extremities)? If yes, radiographs are required.

b. If there was no high-risk factor present, is there any low-risk factor present that allows safe assessment of range of motion (i.e., simple rear-end motor vehicle collision, sitting position in emergency department, ambulatory at any time since injury, delayed onset of neck pain, or absence of midline cervical spine tenderness)? If no, radiographs are required. If yes, question c must be answered.
       c. Is the patient able to actively rotate the neck 45° to the left and right? If no, radiographs are required. If yes, no radiographs are required.
    2. Validation: Cross-validation demonstrated a sensitivity of 100% and a specificity of 42.5%.
• Special tests
  ∘ Alar ligament stress test[7,40]
    1. Performed with the patient sitting: The examiner stabilizes the spinous process and lamina of C2 between the thumb and index finger. For this example, passive left lateral flexion of the occiput is performed. Left lateral flexion should increase tension in the left occipital and right atlantal portions of the alar ligament causing left rotation of the axis and, therefore, the spinous process of C2 to move to the right. Because C2 is stabilized at the start of testing, if the ligamentous structures are intact, minimal lateral flexion should occur with a solid capsular end feel.
    2. Because the ligaments are multipennated, the test should be performed in upper cervical flexion, neutral, and upper cervical extension. A positive in all three positions is necessary for the test to be deemed positive.
    3. No information regarding the sensitivity or specificity of this test is available in the literature.
  ∘ Sharp-Purser (transverse ligament test)
    1. Performed with the patient sitting: The patient is asked to relax the neck in a semiflexed position. The examiner places the palm of one hand on the patient's forehead and the index finger of the other hand on the tip of the spinous process of the axis. While pressing backward with the palm, a sliding motion of the head posteriorly in relation to the axis is indicative of atlantoaxial instability due to disruption of the transverse ligament.
    2. In a study by Uitvlugt and Indenbaum,[73] positive findings were compared to radiographic findings and were shown to correlate with an atlantodens interval of greater than 3 mm.
       a. Testing was shown to have a sensitivity of 69% and specificity of 96% if the threshold for an abnormal atlantodens interval was set at greater than or equal to 3 mm.
       b. Testing was shown to have a sensitivity of 88% and specificity of 96% if the threshold for an abnormal atlantodens interval was set at greater than 4 mm.

CLINICAL DECISION MAKING
CASE STUDY—PATIENT PROFILE   (?)

Your patient is a 75-year-old female who reports that she fell from her bed this morning. She reports neck pain. Are radiographs necessary for this patient?

Answer
Research has suggested that patients 70 years or older who report neck pain with a traumatic mechanism of injury should be suspected of having an odontoid fracture, until proven otherwise.[56] The Canadian C-Spine Rules algorithm also considers age 65 years or older a high risk factor necessitating radiography for alert and stable patients with trauma.[69]

MEDICATIONS

HOW DOES A PATIENT'S RESPONSE TO MEDICATION INFLUENCE THE DECISION-MAKING PROCESS?

In general, lack of response to appropriate antiinflammatory medication therapy would suggest that inflammation does not play a role in the patient's presentation.

Chronic use of over-the-counter analgesics for managing headaches can result in a rebound effect (an increase in the frequency and severity of the headaches) when these medications are halted. This may make decisions regarding the appropriate management of cervicogenic headaches more difficult.

HOW DOES PREVIOUS USE OF MEDICATIONS INFLUENCE THE DECISION-MAKING PROCESS?

Previous corticosteroid use may increase the risk of developing osteoporosis and therefore increase the likelihood of a fracture with a low-velocity mechanism of injury.

BIOMECHANICAL

WHAT ROLE DOES BIOMECHANICS PLAY IN THE DECISION-MAKING PROCESS?

The major motion available at the OA joints is capital flexion/extension and capital lateral flexion. The major motion available at the AA joints is rotation. Dysfunctions at either level can be quickly identified by close observation of simple active range of motion of the neck.

- If the patient actively rotates the neck and you observe ipsilateral lateral flexion at the end of their available range, you should suspect the presence of upper cervical hypomobility, specifically, a lack of contralateral lateral flexion at the OA joints.
- If the patient actively laterally flexes their neck and you observe ipsilateral rotation at the end of their available range, you should suspect the presence of upper cervical hypomobility, specifically, a lack of contralateral rotation in the AA joints.

WHAT BIOMECHANICAL ABNORMALITIES IN OTHER REGIONS AFFECT YOUR DECISION-MAKING PROCESS?

- Any condition that results in hypomobility of the lower cervical spine will increase the mechanical stresses in the upper cervical spine, potentially leading to symptoms.
- Upper thoracic hyperkyphosis (as seen in the dowagers hump) will result in an increase in cervical lordosis. For the patient to keep the eyes level and hold the head up, an increase in capital extension will result. This places excessive stress on the upper cervical region.
- Disorders of the temporomandibular joint will result in the dysfunction of the upper cervical spine, due to the closely interrelated mechanics of the two regions.

CLINICAL PEARL

Any patient who presents with a primary complaint that is suggestive of temporomandibular joint dysfunction must be evaluated for upper cervical dysfunctions as well. The converse is also true.

CLINICAL DECISION MAKING CASE STUDY—PATIENT PROFILE

Your patient is a 42-year-old male accountant who complains of headaches and neck pain. It seems to be aggravated by neck movements, and he notices it is difficult for him to look over his shoulder to change lanes or to back the car up out of the driveway. He sits postured in excessive thoracic kyphosis, excessive neck extension, and a forward head. Active range of motion is limited in all planes, and you notice that at the end of right rotation he laterally flexes to the right. What other findings on physical examination would you expect to see, and what would appropriate intervention include?

Answer
The patient's observed posture places increased stress on the upper cervical spine, and is potentially the underlying cause of his symptoms. You might expect to find decreased thoracic mobility, particularly into extension; poor strength and endurance of the thoracic extensors; hypomobility of the upper thoracic spine; hypermobility of the mid-cervical spine, particularly into extension; poor mid-cervical muscle strength and control in endurance; and decreased upper cervical mobility, particularly left lateral flexion at the OA joint. In addition, abnormalities in jaw motion and tooth wear and tenderness in the muscles of mastication may be present. Appropriate management would include local interventions at the upper cervical spine, stabilization exercises for the mid-cervical spine, and interventions to manage the thoracic spine hypomobility. As the patient's mobility, strength, and endurance improve, changes must be made in his daily posture to improve alignment of the head and neck over the thorax and lumbar spine. Appropriate interventions directed to the temporomandibular joint may be necessary.

ENVIRONMENTAL FACTORS

DO PSYCHOSOCIAL ISSUES INFLUENCE CLINICAL DECISION MAKING?

- As in other regions, depression, stress, and other psychosocial factors can impact the autonomic, endocrine, and immune systems, which can heighten or depress the response to injury.
- The physical manifestations of emotional stress are often located in the cervical spine. Muscle tension from increased stress in the upper cervical spine can lead to symptoms such as headache and neck pain.
- Dizziness is a common symptom in psychological conditions such as anxiety. Therefore, psychological conditions must be taken into account during the decision-making process when managing a patient who complains of dizziness with a suspected cervical component.

DO WORK-RELATED INJURIES INFLUENCE CLINICAL DECISION MAKING?

- Always consider the demands of the workplace when designing an appropriate physical therapy plan of care, so that the patient is optimally prepared for a return to work with a resumption of premorbid activities.
- It is commonplace for the clinician to view all work-related injuries with a bit of skepticism. It is advisable to give all patients the benefit of the doubt when examining and treating for upper cervical pathology.

PERSONAL FACTORS

PRIOR SURGERY

WHAT PRIOR SURGERIES INFLUENCE YOUR CLINICAL DECISION MAKING?

Any surgery that limits the mobility of the lower cervical spine (i.e., mid-cervical fusion) has the potential of transmitting motion stresses to the upper cervical spine.

Mounting evidence suggests that distal pathology and dysfunction can impact cervical mobility. Research to date studying this relationship has focused on the effects of thoracic manipulation on the cervical pain.[15] Clinically, changes can be seen in pain and in range of motion. It is difficult to determine whether the changes in motion are due to upper and lower cervical motion increases. Therefore, it is possible that some of the increases in motion were the result of improved upper cervical mobility. With this in mind, surgeries performed in the thoracic region (i.e., cardiac surgery, mastectomies, shoulder surgeries) can all influence the upper cervical region and contribute to pathology in that region.

DOES A FAMILY HISTORY OF PATHOLOGY IN THE REGION INFLUENCE YOUR CLINICAL REASONING PROCESS?

Because certain medical pathologies have shown a familial relationship, a family history of pathologies such as Down syndrome, rheumatoid arthritis, Klippel-Feil syndrome, or other diseases that impact ligament laxity and integrity should be assessed prior to any interventions being performed. Patients should be questioned regarding the presence of these diseases in their immediate family.

CHRONICITY OF PAIN

WHAT CENTRAL PROCESSING CHANGES OCCUR THAT INFLUENCE YOUR DECISION MAKING?

- The upper cervical spine is no different from other regions of the body when it comes to the responses to chronic pain. Chronic pain behaviors, fear avoidance behaviors, and altered central processing of otherwise nonnociceptive stimuli are typical responses to chronic pain.
- Higher initial levels of pain and disability, older age, cold hyperalgesia, impaired sympathetic vasoconstriction, and moderate posttraumatic stress symptoms have been shown to be associated with poorer outcomes 6 months following whiplash injury.[66-68]

DISCUSS HOW CHRONICITY OF SYMPTOMS INFLUENCE YOUR DECISION-MAKING PROCESS

As with chronic pain conditions for any region, the clinician must be aware of the presence of fear avoidance behaviors. The focus of patient management in these cases includes behavior modification, pain management, stress management, reactivation of function, self-management through exercise and lifestyle modifications, and a multidisciplinary approach. Typically, manual interventions should be deemphasized.

DISCUSS HOW AUTONOMIC, ENDOCRINE, AND IMMUNE SYSTEMS INFLUENCE DECISION MAKING IN THE REGION

Many patients with upper cervical symptoms such as headaches, dizziness, and ringing in the ears will notice an increase during stressful situations. Traditionally, these symptoms have been attributed to decreased blood flow to the upper cervical region and brain due to increased muscle tension in the cervical region. Increased evidence is now supporting a relationship between blood flow, stress, autonomic system activity, and endocrine function. Although evidence is still forthcoming, it is possible that stress may impact the autonomic system and subsequently create some of the symptoms experienced by the patient in the upper cervical region.[18,53]

RED FLAGS THAT WARRANT REFERRAL TO A MEDICAL PHYSICIAN

WHAT SYMPTOMS ALERT YOU TO PATHOLOGIES THAT MAY REQUIRE A REFERRAL TO A MEDICAL PHYSICIAN?

- A clinical presentation that includes neck pain in combination with dizziness, diplopia, dysarthria, dysphagia, syncope, diminished papillary light reflex, nystagmus, motor or sensory deficits, especially if correlated with a traumatic mechanism of injury, may suggest fracture, instability, or damage to vascular and neural structures.
- The Canadian C-Spine Rules recommend that radiographs should be performed in patients who present with trauma combined with the presence of a high-risk factor including age greater than 65 years, dangerous mechanism, or paresthesias in the extremities.[69]
- Patients over the age of 70 years, who present with neck pain due to a traumatic mechanism of injury should be suspected of having an odontoid fracture, until proven otherwise.[56]
- Distal symptoms, such as extremity numbness and tingling or weakness, that is bilateral and is exacerbated with neck flexion is suggestive of upper cervical instability that potentially needs surgical fusion.
- Facial neurological symptoms, such as parasthesia or anesthesia, that is aggravated with neck movements should be referred to a physician for possible vertebral artery compromise or upper cervical instability.
- Initial symptoms of pain in the occiput or neck that is temporally related to trauma could be caused by vertebral artery dissection. The additional symptoms of vertigo and nausea should increase the index of suspicion.[8]

WHAT SYMPTOMS IMPLICATE SPECIFIC VISCERAL SYSTEMS?

Symptoms that are unremitting, not correlated with movements, palpation, or testing, described as "deep and gnawing," or that become worse at night are suggestive of a visceral source. The heart structures, including the carotid artery, can refer pain into the cervical region.

SUMMARY STATEMENT

Neck pain is a common musculoskeletal disorder. Due to the complexity of structures in the upper cervical spine and the risk for traumatic injury with dangerous consequences, differential diagnosis of pathology in this region is of vital importance. It is also important to remember that the source of upper cervical spine symptoms may be far away from this region. Conversely, the upper cervical region can also refer symptoms to areas quite distal, in the trunk and the upper and lower extremities. Table II-2-2 summarizes the factors that help a clinician differentiate among different sources of symptoms in the upper cervical region.

TABLE II-2-2 Body Structure and Tissue-Based Pathology (Nociceptive and Peripheral Neurogenic Pain)

	Facet Joint Capsule	Facet Joint	Muscles	Vertebral Bodies	Posterior Vertebral Bodies	Ligament	Nerves	Visceral Tissue
Pathology	Rheumatoid arthritis	Cervicogenic headaches Rheumatoid arthritis	Cervicogenic headaches	Odontoid fracture	Rheumatoid arthritis	Alar and transverse ligament injury	Cervicogenic headaches Occipital neuralgia Trigeminal neuralgia Dizziness	Dizziness
Age		>70 years for degeneration	Any age	20 to 30 years old = age most common for fractures overall, >65 years = C1, C2 fractures most common	>65 years = odontoid fracture the most common	Onset of rheumatoid arthritis peaks in the fifth decade of life	Onset of trigeminal neuralgia is typically after 40 years, with peak incidence at 60 to 70 years	Myocardial infarction typically occurs at >45 years old for men, >55 years old for women
Occupation	Repetitive flexion and/or rotation activities	Repetitive extension, rotation, or lateral flexion activities	Repetitive flexion or rotation activities	Repetitive flexion, rotation activities	Repetitive extension activities	Repetitive flexion or rotation activities	Hyperextension and rotation	Not typically associated with occupation
Gender	Not applicable	Osteoarthritis affects females more than males	Not applicable	Not applicable	Not applicable	Rheumatoid arthritis affects females more than males at a 3:1 ratio overall; however, with a diagnosis of rheumatoid arthritis, atlantoaxial subluxation is more likely to affect men than women	Trigeminal neuralgia affects females more than males at a 2:1 ratio	Coronary heart disease prevalence is slightly higher for males than females
Ethnicity	Not applicable	Not applicable	Not applicable	Not applicable	Not applicable	Not applicable	Not applicable	
History	New onset or history of previous pain	New onset or history of previous pain	New onset or history of previous pain	New onset or history of previous pain	New onset	New onset	New onset or history of previous pain	New onset
Mechanism of injury	Flexion, rotation, lateral flexion	Extension, rotation, lateral flexion	Flexion, rotation	Flexion, rotation, trauma	Repetitive extension, hyperextension, trauma	Repetitive flexion, hyperflexion, trauma	Unknown	Generally no known mechanism
Type of onset	Sudden	Sudden or gradual	Sudden or gradual	Sudden and traumatic	Sudden and traumatic	Sudden, gradual, or traumatic	Sudden or gradual	Sudden
Referral from local tissue	Occipital region, upper posterolateral cervical region, upper posterior cervical region	Occipital region, upper posterolateral cervical region, upper posterior cervical region	Ipsilateral occiput	Upper cervical, suboccipital, and occipital regions	Upper cervical, suboccipital, and occipital regions	Typically symptoms are present in cervical, occipital, and shoulder regions Symptoms can extend to the temporal or even frontal regions and to the back of the eye on one or both sides Distal symptoms into the extremities can occur	Varies depending on pathology	Chest pain

Referral to other regions	Dizziness (not vertigo)	Dizziness (not vertigo)	Eye, and forehead Dizziness (not vertigo)		Can refer to the temporal and frontal regions and back of the eye on one or both sides	Spinal cord can refer symptoms to extremities Suboccipital nerves can refer to the head (headache)	May refer into shoulders, jaw, cervical spine
Changes in symptoms	Improves with traction	Improves with traction					
24-hour pain pattern (morning)	Morning stiffness and pain	Morning stiffness and pain	Morning stiffness and pain	Morning stiffness and pain	Morning stiffness and pain	Pain is typically present on waking	Varies but does not change with mechanical stresses
24-hour pain pattern (afternoon)	Worsens with activity	Worsens with activity	Pain may decrease with movement and worsen with prolonged activity	Worsens with activity	Worsens with activity	May worsen with prolonged aggravating activity	Varies but does not change with mechanical stress
24-hour pain pattern (evening)	Sleep may be difficult	Sleep may be difficult	Sleep may be difficult	Sleep may be difficult	Sleep may be difficult	Sleep may be difficult	May vary but does not change with mechanical stress
Description of symptoms	Sharp pain Dizziness in not spinning	Sharp pain or dull ache Dizziness in not spinning	Stiffness and diffuse ache Dizziness in not spinning	Stiffness and sharp pain or diffuse ache	Stiffness and sharp pain or diffuse ache	Numbness, tingling, burning, sharp, "shock-like"	Sharp pain, deep ache
Depth of symptoms	Deep	Deep	Superficial	Deep	Deep	superficial	Deep, poorly localized
Constancy of symptoms	Intermittent	Intermittent	Intermittent	Constant but varying	Constant but varying	Intermittent and brief with possible persistent ache	Constant
Aggravating factors	Flexion, contralateral rotation, contralateral side bend	Extension, ipsilateral rotation, ipsilateral lateral flexion	Flexion, contralateral rotation; if tight or torn, adding tension to the muscle	Extension, sitting, standing	Flexion, rotation, sitting, standing	Trigeminal Neuralgia: In ~50% of patients, triggers include nonnoxious stimuli touching small areas around the face, nose, and lips Occipital neuralgia: hyperextension and rotation Spinal nerves: extension, rotation, lateral flexion	Not associated with mechanical movements
Easing factors	Extension, ipsilateral rotation, ipsilateral lateral flexion; unweighting or traction	Flexion, contralateral rotation, contralateral lateral flexion; unweighting or traction	Extension, ipsilateral rotation If torn, putting the muscle on slack If tight, gradual lengthening through stretching	Lying supine	Lying supine	Occipital neuralgia: avoidance of hyperextension and rotation Spinal nerves: flexion, contralateral rotation, contralateral lateral flexion	Not associated with mechanical movements

Continued on following page.

TABLE II-2-2 Body Structure and Tissue-Based Pathology (Nociceptive and Peripheral Neurogenic Pain) (Continued)

	Facet Joint Capsule	Facet Joint	Muscles	Vertebral Bodies	Posterior Vertebral Bodies	Ligament	Nerves	Visceral Tissue
Pathology	Rheumatoid arthritis	Cervicogenic headaches Rheumatoid arthritis	Cervicogenic headaches	Odontoid fracture	Rheumatoid arthritis	Alar and transverse ligament injury	Cervicogenic headaches Occipital neuralgia Trigeminal neuralgia Dizziness	Dizziness
Stability of symptoms	Gradual improvement over 6-week period	Slow gradual progression of symptoms	Gradual improvement over 6-week period	Gradual improvement over 8-week period	Gradual improvement over 8-week period for fracture; may continue to worsen for spondylolisthesis	Gradual improvement over 6-week period	Relapsing and remitting	Will worsen over time
Past medical history				Osteoporosis, previous corticosteroid use	Osteoporosis, previous corticosteroid use	Congenital or developmental anomalies		May or may not have history of heart disease
Past surgical history	Any previous surgery that limits the mobility of the lower cervical spine (i.e., mid-cervical fusion) has the potential of transmitting motion stress to the upper cervical spine							May or may not have previous cardiac surgical history
Special questions	For care of dizziness: rule out central and peripheral causes	For care of dizziness: rule out central and peripheral causes	For care of dizziness: rule out central and peripheral causes			Are there extremity neurological symptoms (particularly bilateral) with neck flexion?	Numbness, tingling, burning associated with symptoms?	Is neck pain associated with chest pain, jaw pain, shoulder pain, or shortness of breath?
X-rays	Negative	Can be positive depending on pathology	Negative	Positive	Positive	Positive for instability (ADI > 3 mm)	Can be positive depending on pathology	Negative
Electromyogram	Not commonly performed	Not commonly performed	Not commonly performed	Not commonly performed	Not commonly performed	Not commonly performed	May be performed for trigeminal neuralgia	Not commonly performed
Special laboratory tests	Not commonly performed	Not commonly performed	Not commonly performed	Not commonly performed	Not commonly performed	Testing of rheumatoid factor seropositive status is performed for rheumatoid arthritis	Not commonly performed	Electrocardiogram and blood testing for measurement of cardiac enzymes (serum isozyme levels) can help with diagnosis of myocardial infarction
Red flags				Rule out fracture, instability	Rule out fracture, instability	Rule out instability		Rule out myocardial infarction

REFERENCES

1. Acar F, Miller J, Golshani KJ, Israel ZH, McCartney S, Burchiel KJ. Pain relief after cervical ganglionectomy (C2 and C3) for the treatment of medically intractable occipital neuralgia. *Stereotact Funct Neurosurg.* 2008;86(2):106-112.

2. Agarwal AK, Peppelman WC, Kraus DR, et al. Recurrence of cervical spine instability in rheumatoid arthritis following previous fusion: can disease progression be prevented by early surgery? *J Rheumatol.* 1992;19(9):1364-1370.

3. Agur AMR, Lee MJ. *Grant's Atlas of Anatomy.* 10th ed. Philadelphia: Lippincott Williams & Wilkins; 1999.

4. Alamanos Y, Drosos AA. Epidemiology of adult rheumatoid arthritis. *Autoimmun Rev.* 2005;4(3):130-136.

5. Ali FE, Al-Bustan MA, Al-Busairi WA, Al-Mulla FA, Esbaita EY. Cervical spine abnormalities associated with Down syndrome. *Int Orthop.* 2006;30(4):284-289.

6. Anderson LD, D'Alonzo RT. Fractures of the odontoid process of the axis. *J Bone Joint Surg Am.* 1974;56(8):1663-1674.

7. Aspinall W. Clinical testing for the craniovertebral hypermobility syndrome. *J Orthop Sports Phys Ther.* 1990;12(2):47-54.

8. Bartels. Dissection of the extracranial vertebral artery: Clinical findings and early noninvasive diagnosis in 24 patients. *J Neuroimaging.* 2006;16:24-33.

9. Blumenfeld H. *Neuroanatomy through clinical cases.* Sunderland: Sinauer Associates, Inc.; 2002.

10. Boden SD, Dodge LD, Bohlman HH, Rechtine GR. Rheumatoid arthritis of the cervical spine. A long-term analysis with predictors of paralysis and recovery. *J Bone Joint Surg Am.* 1993;75(9):1282-1297.

11. Bogduk N, Marsland A. The cervical zygapophysial joints as a source of neck pain. *Spine.* 1988;13(6):610-617.

12. Broggi G, Ferroli P, Franzini A. Treatment strategy for trigeminal neuralgia: a thirty years' experience. *Neurol Sci.* 2008;29(suppl 1):S79-S82.

13. Casey AT, Crockard HA, Pringle J, O'Brien MF, Stevens JM. Rheumatoid arthritis of the cervical spine: current techniques for management. *Orthop Clin North Am.* 2002;33(2):291-309.

14. Childs JD, Flynn TW, Fritz JM, et al. Screening for vertebrobasilar insufficiency in patients with neck pain: manual therapy decision-making in the presence of uncertainty. *J Orthop Sports Phys Ther.* 2005;35(5):300-306.

15. Cleland JA, Childs JD, McRae M, Palmer J, Stowell T. Immediate effects of thoracic manipulation in patients with neck pain: a randomized clinical trial. *Man Ther.* 2005;(10):127-135.

16. De Simone R, Ranieri A, Bilo L, Fiorillo C, Bonavita V. Cranial neuralgias: from physiopathology to pharmacological treatment. *Neurol Sci.* 2008;29(suppl 1):S69-S78.

17. Dreyer SJ, Boden SD. Natural history of rheumatoid arthritis of the cervical spine. *Clin Orthop Relat Res.* 1999;(366):98-106.

18. Elenkow IJ, Wilder RL, Chrousos GP, Vizi ES. The Sympathetic Nerve—An Integrative Interface between Two Supersystems: The Brain and the Immune System. *Pharm Reviews.* 2000;52(4):595-638.

19. Finn M, Fassett DR, Apfelbaum RI. Surgical treatment of nonrheumatoid atlantoaxial degenerative arthritis producing pain and myelopathy. *Spine.* 2007;32(26):3067-3073.

20. Fukui S, Ohseto K, Shiotani M, et al. Referred pain distribution of the cervical zygapophyseal joints and cervical dorsal rami. *Pain.* 1996;68(1):79-83.

21. Golob Jr JF, Claridge JA, Yowler CJ, Como JJ, Peerless JR. Isolated cervical spine fractures in the elderly: a deadly injury. *J Trauma.* 2008;64(2):311-315.

22. Goru SJ, Pemberton MN. Trigeminal neuralgia: the role of magnetic resonance imaging. *Br J Oral Maxillofac Surg.* 2008.

23. Hakkinen A, Makinen H, Ylinen J, et al. Stability of the upper neck during isometric neck exercises in rheumatoid arthritis patients with atlantoaxial disorders. *Scand J Rheumatol.* 2008;37(5):343-347.

24. Harris TJ, Blackmore CC, Mirza SK, Jurkovich GJ. Clearing the cervical spine in obtunded patients. *Spine.* 2008;33(14):1547-1553.

25. Heikkila H, Johansson M, Wenngren BI. Effects of acupuncture, cervical manipulation and NSAID therapy on dizziness and impaired head repositioning of suspected cervical origin: a pilot study. *Man Ther.* 2000;5(3):151-157.

26. Holmes A, Han ZH, Dang GT, Chen ZQ, Wang ZG, Fang J. Changes in cervical canal spinal volume during in vitro flexion-extension. *Spine.* 1996;21(11):1313-1319.

27. Holmes JF, Akkinepalli R. Computed tomography versus plain radiography to screen for cervical spine injury: a meta-analysis. *J Trauma.* 2005;58(5):902-905.

28. Insko EK, Gracias VH, Gupta R, Goettler CE, Gaieski DF, Dalinka MK. Utility of flexion and extension radiographs of the cervical spine in the acute evaluation of blunt trauma. *J Trauma.* 2002;53(3):426-429.

29. Jackson RS, Banit DM, Rhyne 3rd AL, Darden 2nd BV. Upper cervical spine injuries. *J Am Acad Orthop Surg.* 2002;10(4):271-280.

30. Jull G, Trott P, Potter H, et al. A randomized controlled trial of exercise and manipulative therapy for cervicogenic headache. *Spine.* 2002;27(17):1835-1843 [discussion 1843].

31. Jull GA, Stanton WR. Predictors of responsiveness to physiotherapy management of cervicogenic headache. *Cephalalgia.* 2005;25(2):101-108.

32. Karlberg M, Magnusson M, Malmstrom E, Melander A, Moritz U. Postural and symptomatic improvement after physiotherapy in patients with dizziness of suspected cervical origin. *Arch Phys Med Rehabil.* 1996;77(9):874-882.

33. Kauppi M, Leppanen L, Heikkila S, Lahtinen T, Kautiainen H. Active conservative treatment of atlantoaxial subluxation in rheumatoid arthritis. *Br J Rheumatol.* 1998;37(4):417-420.

34. Kauppi M, Neva MH. Sensitivity of lateral view cervical spine radiographs taken in the neutral position in atlantoaxial subluxation in rheumatic diseases. *Clin Rheumatol.* 1998;17(6):511-514.

35. Kim DH, Hilibrand AS. Rheumatoid arthritis in the cervical spine. *J Am Acad Orthop Surg.* 2005;13(7):463-474.

36. Krafft RM. Trigeminal neuralgia. *Am Fam Physician.* 2008;77(9):1291-1296.

37. Lipson SJ. Rheumatoid arthritis in the cervical spine. *Clin Orthop Relat Res.* 1989;(239):121-127.

38. Lomoschitz FM, Blackmore CC, Mirza SK, Mann FA. Cervical spine injuries in patients 65 years old and older: epidemiologic analysis regarding the effects of age and injury mechanism on distribution, type, and stability of injuries. *AJR Am J Roentgenol.* 2002;178(3):573-577.

39. Lord SM, Barnsley L, Wallis BJ, Bogduk N. Chronic cervical zygapophysial joint pain after whiplash. A placebo-controlled prevalence study. *Spine.* 1996;21(15):1737-1744 [discussion 1744-1735].

40. Magee DJ. *Orthopedic Physical Assessment.* 4th ed. Philadelphia: Saunders; 1992.

41. Malmstrom E-M, Karlberg M, Melander A, Magnusson M, Moritz U. Cervicogenic dizziness—musculoskeletal findings before and after treatment and long-term outcome. *Disabil Rehabil.* 2007;29(15):1193-1205.

42. Matsunaga S, Sakou T, Onishi T, et al. Prognosis of patients with upper cervical lesions caused by rheumatoid arthritis: comparison of occipitocervical fusion between C1 laminectomy and nonsurgical management. *Spine.* 2003;28(14):1581-1587 [discussion 1587].

43. Meaney JF, Eldridge PR, Dunn LT, Nixon TE, Whitehouse GH, Miles JB. Demonstration of neurovascular compression in trigeminal neuralgia with magnetic resonance imaging. Comparison with surgical findings in 52 consecutive operative cases. *J Neurosurg.* 1995;83(5):799-805.

44. Menaker J, Philp A, Boswell S, Scalea TM. Computed tomography alone for cervical spine clearance in the unreliable patient—are we there yet? *J Trauma.* 2008;64(4):898-903 [discussion 903-894].

45. Moncur C, Williams HJ. Cervical spine management in patients with rheumatoid arthritis. Review of the literature. *Phys Ther.* 1988;68(4):509-515.

46. Nguyen HV, Ludwig SC, Silber J, et al. Rheumatoid arthritis of the cervical spine. *Spine J.* 2004;4(3):329-334.

47. Peeters GG, Verhagen AP, de Bie RA, Oostendorp RA. The efficacy of conservative treatment in patients with whiplash injury: a systematic review of clinical trials. *Spine.* 2001;26(4):E64-E73.

48. Pollack Jr CV, Hendey GW, Martin DR, Hoffman JR, Mower WR. Use of flexion-extension radiographs of the cervical spine in blunt trauma. *Ann Emerg Med.* 2001;38(1):8-11.

49. Rawlins BA, Girardi FP, Boachie-Adjei O. Rheumatoid arthritis of the cervical spine. *Rheum Dis Clin North Am.* 1998;24(1):55-65.

50. Reid SA, Rivett DA. Manual therapy treatment of cervicogenic dizziness: a systematic review. *Man Ther.* 2005;10:4-13.

51. Reid SA, Rivett DA, Katekar MG, Callister R. Sustained natural apophyseal glides (snags) are an effective treatment for cervicogenic dizziness. *Man Ther.* 2008;13(4):357-366.

52. Reiter MF, Boden SD. Inflammatory disorders of the cervical spine. *Spine.* 1998;23(24):2755-2766.

53. Roy-Byrne PP, Kavidson KW, Kessler OC, et al. Anxiety disorders and comorbid medical illness. *Gen Hosp Psych.* 2008;30:208-225.

54. Rozen TD. Trigeminal neuralgia and glossopharyngeal neuralgia. *Neurol Clin.* 2004;22(1):185-206.

55. Rubin AM, Woolley SM, Dailey VM, Goebel JA. Postural stability following mild head or whiplash injuries. *Am J Otol.* 1995;16(2):216-221.

56. Ryan MD, Henderson JJ. The epidemiology of fractures and fracture-dislocations of the cervical spine. *Injury.* 1992;23(1):38-40.

57. Samartzis D, Kalluri P, Herman J, Lubicky JP, Shen FH. 2008 Young Investigator Award: The role of congenitally fused cervical segments upon the space available for the cord and associated symptoms in Klippel-Feil patients. *Spine.* 2008;33(13):1442-1450.

58. Schaeren S, Jeanneret B. Atlantoaxial osteoarthritis: case series and review of the literature. *Eur Spine J.* 2005;14(5):501-506.

59. Schellinger PD, Schwab S, Krieger D, et al. Masking of vertebral artery dissection by severe trauma to the cervical spine. *Spine.* 2001;26(3):314-319.

60. Schenarts PJ, Diaz J, Kaiser C, Carrillo Y, Eddy V, Morris Jr JA. Prospective comparison of admission computed tomographic scan and plain films of the upper cervical spine in trauma patients with altered mental status. *J Trauma.* 2001;51(4):663-668 [discussion 668-669].

61. Schofferman J, Bogduk N, Slosar P. Chronic whiplash and whiplash-associated disorders: an evidence-based approach. *J Am Acad Orthop Surg.* 2007;15(10):596-606.

62. Scholten-Peeters GG, Verhagen AP, Bekkering GE, et al. Prognostic factors of whiplash-associated disorders: a systematic review of prospective cohort studies. *Pain.* 2003;104(1-2):303-322.

63. Schuenke M, Schulte E, Schumacher U. *Thieme: Atlas of Anatomy.* Stuttgart: Thieme; 2006.

64. Shears E, Armitstead CP. Surgical versus conservative management for odontoid fractures. *Cochrane Database Syst Rev.* 2008;(4): CD005078.

65. Stapley PJ, Beretta MV, Dalla Toffola E, Schieppati M. Neck muscle fatigue and postural control in patients with whiplash injury. *Clin Neurophysiol.* 2006;117(3):610-622.

66. Sterling M. Identifying those at risk of developing persistent pain following a motor vehicle collision.[comment]. *J Rheumatol.* 2006;33(5):838-839.

67. Sterling M, Jull G, Kenardy J. Physical and psychological factors maintain long-term predictive capacity post-whiplash injury. *Pain.* 2006;122(1-2):102-108.

68. Sterling M, Jull G, Vicenzino B, Kenardy J. Sensory hypersensitivity occurs soon after whiplash injury and is associated with poor recovery.[see comment]. *Pain.* 2003;104(3):509-517.

69. Stiell IG, Wells GA, Vandemheen KL, et al. The Canadian C-spine rule for radiography in alert and stable trauma patients. *JAMA.* 2001;286(15):1841-1848.

70. Tanaka N, Sakahashi H, Hirose K, Ishima T, Takahashi H, Ishii S. Results after 24 years of prophylactic surgery for rheumatoid atlantoaxial subluxation. *J Bone Joint Surg Br.* 2005;87(7):955-958.

71. Tomycz ND, Chew BG, Chang YF, et al. MRI is unnecessary to clear the cervical spine in obtunded/comatose trauma patients: the four-year experience of a level I trauma center. *J Trauma.* 2008;64(5):1258-1263.

72. Travell JG, Simons DG. *Myofascial Pain and Dysfunction: The Trigger Point Manual.* Baltimore: Williams & Wilkins; 1983.

73. Uitvlugt G, Indenbaum S. Clinical assessment of atlantoaxial instability using the Sharp-Purser test. *Arthritis Rheum.* 1988;31(7):918-922.

74. Vieweg U, Meyer B, Schramm J. Differential treatment in acute upper cervical spine injuries: a critical review of a single-institution series. *Surg Neurol.* 2000;54(3):203-210 [discussion 210-201].

75. Walker MJ, Boyles RE, Young BA, et al. The effectiveness of manual physical therapy and exercise for mechanical neck pain: a randomized clinical trial. *Spine.* 2008;33(22):2371-2378.

76. Wiener SL. *Differential Diagnosis of Acute Pain By Body Region.* New York: McGraw-Hill; 1993.

77. Williams M, Williamson E, Gates S, Lamb S, Cooke M. A systematic literature review of physical prognostic factors for the development of late whiplash syndrome. *Spine.* 2007;32(25):E764-E780.

78. Yang J, Simonson TM, Ruprecht A, Meng D, Vincent SD, Yuh WT. Magnetic resonance imaging used to assess patients with trigeminal neuralgia. *Oral Surg Oral Med Oral Pathol Oral Radiol Endod.* 1996;81(3):343-350.

79. Zakrzewska JM. Diagnosis and differential diagnosis of trigeminal neuralgia. *Clin J Pain.* 2002;18(1):14-21.

80. Zapletal J, de Valois JC. Radiologic prevalence of advanced lateral C1-C2 osteoarthritis. *Spine.* 1997;22(21):2511-2513.

AUTHOR: WILLIAM H. O'GRADY

INTRODUCTORY INFORMATION

WHAT IS THE PREVALENCE OF NECK PAIN?

About two-thirds of the population will experience neck pain during their lifetime.[22,73] The Bone and Joint Decade 2000–2010 Task Force on Neck Pain and its Associated Disorders reported that the 12-month prevalence of neck pain ranged between 30% and 50%; of these people only 1.7% to 11.5% experienced pain that limited activity.[14] In the adolescent population neck pain is not uncommon and is usually related to postural considerations and excessive activity. There is a higher prevalence of neck pain in adolescent females.[2]

WHAT IS THE PROGNOSIS FOR RECOVERY FROM NECK PAIN?

Neck pain usually resolves in days or weeks, but can recur and become chronic. The prognosis is variable but seems to be poorer when the patient has had a previous history of neck pain. Poorer prognosis is also present for patients who are over the age of 40 years and for individuals who have concomitant low back pain.[60]

WHAT IS THE RECURRENCE RATE?

The recurrence of neck pain is highly variable depending on the cause. Many studies have shown that there is a high recurrence rate with neck pain. The results of the studies place the recurrence rate between 22% and 50% depending on the study.[15,23] A major problem with most of the studies regarding neck pain is that the population samples are different and most of the studies are based on questionnaires. Hence, the cause of pain cannot be validated. Also neck, shoulder, and upper extremity pain are considered together, which further obfuscates the statistics.

WHAT FACTORS MAKE DIAGNOSIS OF NECK PAIN DIFFICULT?

Clinicians may experience some challenges when diagnosing the source of neck pain. This may be due to several factors:

- Radiographs do not always correlate with the patient's symptoms.[88] The validity of radiographs, computed tomography (CT), and magnetic resonance imaging (MRI) in nonemergency neck pain without radiculopathy is currently lacking.
- Symptoms from distal sites such as the carpal tunnel and certain red flag conditions can radiate into the neck, which confounds the assessment.[109]
- Dysfunctions in the shoulder girdle and thoracic spine can impact the cervical spine and lead to cervical pain.[19,39,48]
- Diagnosis in the cervical spine can be difficult due to the many different tissues that could potentially become pain generators for the region.
- Postural, emotional, central, and peripheral pain mechanisms have all been shown to directly and indirectly impact cervical pain. In addition, immediate and long-term tissue changes may also affect the primary source of pain.[47,48,103]

CLINICAL PEARL !

Always look to the thoracic spine for loss of motion and posture that affect the motion and head position in the cervical spine. Restoring motion in the thoracic spine will often change the mechanics of cervical spine kinematics.

HOW SUCCESSFUL IS THERAPY IN TREATING NECK PAIN?

Manipulation and patient education, which includes stretching, have shown more success in treating nontraumatic neck pain groups than control groups.[18] There is some evidence that supports the use of strengthening exercises combined with manual therapy for chronic neck pain.[11,16,37,112] Manipulation or exercise alone has not proven to be beneficial and neither was superior to the other.[49,63] In general, current research is mixed regarding the benefits of therapy for the treatment of cervical pain. Fritz and others[18,41] have suggested that a new classification based on impairment of spinal function may be a more useful indicator and may provide better outcomes when treating and researching interventions in the cervical spine.

HOW SUCCESSFUL IS SURGERY IN TREATING NECK PAIN?

The outcomes following cervical surgery are mixed. Recent information from the Bone and Joint Decade 2000–2010 Task Force on Neck Pain and Its Associated Disorders suggests that surgery may be considered in patients who have serious impairment. Moderate success with surgery has been demonstrated in the more serious conditions. However, this success is less favorable in patients who have multiple joint involvements.[24] Surgical treatment for neck pain alone, without radicular symptoms or clear serious pathology, seems to lack scientific support.[31,32]

PERSONAL INFORMATION

WHAT INFLUENCE DOES AGE HAVE ON YOUR CLINICAL DECISION-MAKING PROCESS?

Age can be utilized initially to form preliminary hypotheses regarding a patient's source of pain. In patients below the age of 20 years, neck pain is unusual but not uncommon. The source of the pain varies, but is usually attributed to postural issues such as carrying backpacks. Prolonged static postures, vigorous exercise, and reports of daytime tiredness are also often associated with neck pain in adolescents. The onset of the neck pain usually corresponds to the onset of puberty, but the exact cause of this comorbidity is unclear. It has been hypothesized that the symptoms may be related to rapid changes in body morphology or changes in hormones.[2,33,106]

In adults 20–50 years old, myofascial pain, disc pathology, facet impingement, capsular entrapment, facet dysfunction, uncovertebral dysfunction, hypermobility, instability, and muscle strain should be primary considerations.[65,67]

As adults age, in patients above the age of 50 years, degenerative changes in the cervical spine become of greater concern. Lateral and central stenosis, degenerative disc disease, and occasionally red flag conditions should also be considered as potential sources of pain in the cervical region.[8,113]

WHAT INFLUENCE DOES A PATIENT'S OCCUPATION HAVE ON YOUR CLINICAL DECISION-MAKING PROCESS?

The occupation of a person seems to correlate with neck pain. People with jobs that require repetitive use of the upper extremities such as machine operators, carpenters, and office workers appear to be at greater risk of developing neck pain.[33,64]

Ariens et al[1] indicated that there was positive evidence for the development of neck pain with the following work-related activities: neck flexion, arm force, arm posture, duration of sitting, twisting or bending of the trunk, hand–arm vibration, and workplace design.

WHAT INFLUENCE DOES GENDER HAVE ON YOUR CLINICAL DECISION-MAKING PROCESS?

Although the major pathologies do not seem to have a gender preference, several studies have indicated that neck pain in general is more common in females of all ages. Females appear to suffer more neck injuries in the workplace than males. This may be attributed to conditioning, psychosocial issues, and biomechanical differences.[100,101]

WHAT INFLUENCE DOES ETHNICITY HAVE ON YOUR CLINICAL DECISION-MAKING PROCESS?

Ethnicity is usually not a major factor when diagnosing neck pathology. However, research has suggested some interesting trends:

- Ankylosing spondylitis is less prevalent in blacks than North American Indians and whites.[36,108]
- One UK epidemiological study suggests that South Asian ethnicity was a significant predictor of chronic neck and back pain.[108]

CLINICAL DECISION MAKING CASE STUDY—PATIENT PROFILE (?)

The patient is a 23-year-old female who reported the onset of neck pain about 3 months ago. She states that she is a student and spends long hours at her computer. She also complains of some aching into her right arm and stiffness and soreness in her thoracic spine. She believes her pain and coexisting complaints of fatigue are related to her job. She states that her pain seems worse at night and with inactivity. What are some possible hypotheses regarding her pathology?

Answer

Postural and/or myofascial pain in the neck are common in female office workers and students. However, consider the possibility of ankylosing spondylitis. Females often have a different presentation with symptoms in the peripheral joints and T and C spines not being uncommon as the first symptoms. Further confusing the situation is that symptoms in females initially may be milder, thus making this diagnosis difficult. Her fatigue and pain with inactivity and at night may also further indicate something other than a postural problem. More information will be needed to adequately assess this patient.[10,26,52]

MECHANISM OF INJURY

WHAT INFLUENCE DOES THE MECHANISM OF INJURY HAVE ON YOUR CLINICAL DECISION-MAKING PROCESS?

Knowing the mechanism of injury will help the clinician make a differential diagnoses in patients with acute onset of neck symptoms. Chronic symptoms may require more investigation as pain may not be associated with a single tissue source. Information such as the onset of symptoms, prior history of trauma, and lack of a mechanical cause of injury will provide other clues that will lead to a more accurate examination and to a correct diagnosis.

If the patient's mechanism of injury was traumatic in nature, fractures, disc protrusion/extrusion, ligamentous and capsular injury, myelopathy, muscle strain/sprain, brachial plexus irritation/injury, and vascular injury should be considered as primary hypotheses.

Sudden onset without trauma can often be linked to facet impingement, capsular pathology, acute torticollis, and discogenic causes.

Insidious onset can often be associated with central stenosis, lateral stenosis, degenerative disc disease, or degenerative joint disease visceral pain and pain from distal sources other than viscera.

CLINICAL DECISION MAKING CASE STUDY—PATIENT PROFILE (?)

The patient is a 52-year-old longshoreman who states that he was pulling heavy cable for 2 hours repetitively. He states he started experiencing pain in his right shoulder later that night. He reports that he had increased pain when he had to use his shoulder, especially with over the head usage. He notes that most of his pain was in the right supraspinatus area and upper trapezius region. His pain did not go away over a period of a few weeks. He noted that sometimes the pain went into his upper arm but it was not constant. What is your hypothesis regarding the source of this patient's symptoms?

Answer

It is often assumed by the patients and the referring doctor based on the history that this is a clear case of tendinitis or overuse of the shoulder by virtue of the location of the initial symptoms and history. This patient is at an age at which disc pathology and degenerative changes in the neck become more of a factor. Symptoms from the shoulder can produce neck pain and vice versa. Foraminal entrapment, cervical instability, and thoracic position can all affect the shoulder mechanics. Referred pain and abnormal scapulothoracic muscle mechanics may influence normal spine and shoulder girdle mechanics.

SYMPTOM LOCATION

WHAT INFLUENCE DOES THE LOCATION OF SYMPTOMS HAVE ON YOUR CLINICAL DECISION-MAKING PROCESS?

There are many structures that can refer pain to the neck. Often through palpation and movement of the cervical spine specific pain patterns can be reproduced. The carpal tunnel can refer pain to the neck. In the case of double crush injuries, symptoms may emanate from both proximal and distal origins. A facilitated cervical segment may masquerade as lateral epicondylitis.[28,68] The neck may also refer pain distally. Local structures such as the facets, disc, myofascial structures, and impinged nerves have well-described pain referral patterns.[20]

CLINICAL PEARL (!)

Pain from a cervical disc may be localized, referred, or radicular.

REFERRAL OF SYMPTOMS

Structures in the cervical spine may refer symptoms in the following patterns.

CERVICAL DISC (see Figure II-3-1)

While performing cervical discography, Cloward[20] found that stimulating the anteriolateral cervical disc created pain consistently into the ipsilateral scapular area.

- Pain from C3–C4 was felt in the C7 spinous process and the posterior border to the trapezius muscle.

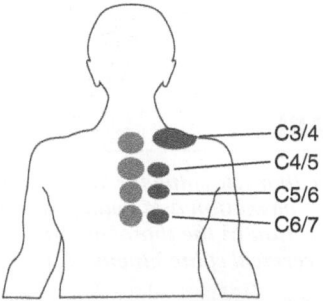

FIGURE II-3-1 Cervical disc pain referral pattern. The pattern of disc referral is from the work of Cloward.[20] Hence, they are often called Cloward Sign's. The darker circles indicate primary referral patterns and the lighter circles secondary referral patterns.

- Pain from C4–C5 was felt in the scapular spine and superior angle.
- Pain from C5–C6 was felt in the medial scapular border.
- Pain from C6–C7 was felt in the inferior angle of the scapula.

Cloward[12] also found that stimulating the midline of the anterior aspect of the cervical disc produced pain between the shoulders in the middle of the back. Pain intensity was greater when stimulating the posterolateral aspect of the cervical disc than when stimulating the anterior aspect of the disc. By stimulating the anterior aspect of the disc the pain spread from the vertebral border of the scapula out to the shoulder and upper arm as distal as the elbow. Midline posterior disc protrusions were found to refer pain to a confined area overlying the fifth cervical to the second thoracic spinous processes near the midline with proximal discs more cephalad and distal discs more caudad. When extensive disc rupture and degeneration were present, a combination of the posterolateral and midline posterior referral patterns was found.[20]

CLINICAL PEARL

What disc is implicated in a C5 nerve root involvement and why is it rare that even a large disc bulge at a single level will not affect multiple levels as in the cervical spine? The disc between the C4 and C5 segment is the likely source of pain. The nerve roots in the cervical spine run horizontally, unlike those in the lumbar spine that traverse more inferiolaterally. The direction of the nerve roots coming out of the intervertebral foramen makes it almost impossible for a disc to affect more than one level. In the presence of multilevel nerve root involvement, suspect a space-occupying lesion, especially in the absence of multilevel foraminal stenosis.

ZYGAPOPHYSEAL JOINTS

Dwyer et al[30] mapped the following cervical zygapophyseal pain patterns (see Figure II-3-2):

C2–C3: The posterior upper cervical region and head
C3–C4: The posterolateral cervical region without extension into the head or shoulder
C4–C5: The posterolateral middle and lower cervical region to the top of the shoulder
C5–C6: Joint refers pain to the posterolateral middle and primarily lower cervical spine and the top and lateral parts of the shoulder and caudally to the spine of the scapula
C6–C7: The top and lateral parts of the shoulder extending caudally to the inferior border of the scapula

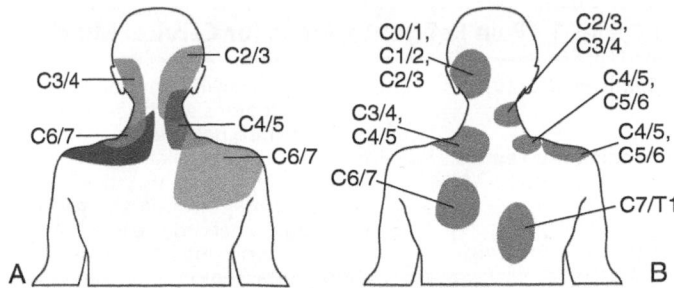

FIGURE II-3-2 Cervical zygapophyseal joint pain referral patterns. Cervical zygapophyseal joints referred pain in the following distributions. **(A)** From the work of Dwyer et al.[30] **(B)** From the work of Fukui et al.[43]

CERVICAL MUSCLES[104]

Although injury to the various muscles of the cervical spine can result in a variety of clinical presentations, the work of Travell and Simon[104] (see Figure II-3-3) has given the clinician insight into how an injury to specific cervical muscles will present (Box II-3-1).

LIGAMENTS

Ligaments have a referred pain pattern similar to the disc and capsules, muscles, and dura mater; these are sclerotomal pain patterns. The difference is that sclerotomal pain is described as deep aching and diffuse while radicular pain is described as sharp, numbing, or tingling and well localized at a specific dermatome.

CLINICAL PEARL

Research has shown that the structures most commonly injured in whiplash-associated injuries (WAD) are the zygapophyseal joints, cervical discs, and upper cervical ligaments. It has been proposed that zygapophyseal joint damage is likely the most common contributor to chronic WAD. The resultant soft tissue injury usually subsides in 3 months.[5]

DERMATOMAL DISTRIBUTION OF SPINAL NERVE ROOTS[62] (see Figure II-3-4)

C3: Lower jaw and neck down to the clavicle
C4: Across the shoulders covering just below the clavicles
C5: Lateral upper arm and shoulder above the elbow

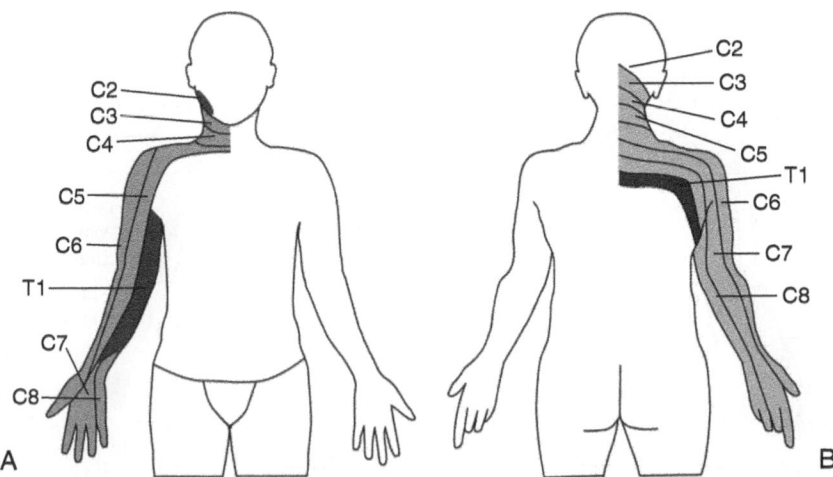

FIGURE II-3-3 Upper extremity dermatomes. A dermatome is an area of skin innervated by a single pair of dorsal nerve roots. Dermatomal patterns of symptoms vary greatly from person to person. The clinician should keep this in mind when utilizing dermatomes for clinical diagnostic purposes. The figures illustrate the anterior **(A)** and posterior **(B)** distribution of the spinal dermatomes.

BOX II-3-1 Pain Reference Areas for Cervical Muscles

Semispinalis capitus	Ipsilateral lateral temporal and occipital regions and over the area of the semispinalis cervicis
Longissimus capitus	Area around the ipsilateral ear and may extend a short way down the neck and may include the periorbital region behind the eye
Semispinalis cervicis	Most commonly into the ipsilateral suboccipital region
Cervical multifidi	Ipsilateral suboccipital region and sometimes down to the upper vertebral border of the scapula
Rotatores	Deep in the muscle at the same segmental level of the affected rotators
Longus colli	Not clearly known—can cause pain and difficulty with swallowing
Scalenes	Pain can be referred into the chest, to the medial border of the scapula, into the shoulder, and down the posterior and lateral sides of the arm to the thumb and index finger
Sternocleidomastoid	Sternal division: Pain is referred upward to the cheek and sinuses, occiput, eye (orbicularis), and top of head; pain referred downward to the sternum Clavicular division: Pain referred bilaterally across the forehead; frontal sinus-like headache, earache

C6: Lateral distal arm down to the thumb radial palm and index finger

C7: Middle finger, ulnar half of the index finger and radial half of the ring finger

C8: Ulnar side of the hand and little finger and ulnar side of the ring finger

MYOTOMAL DISTRIBUTION OF SPINAL NERVE ROOTS[62]

C3: Lateral neck flexion (trapezius, splenus capitis)

C4: Shoulder shrug (trapezius and levator scapula)

C5: Shoulder abduction (deltoid), elbow flexion (biceps)

C6: Elbow flexion (biceps, supinator), wrist extension

C7: Elbow extension (triceps), wrist flexion

C8: Ulnar deviation, thumb extension, finger flexion and abduction

CLINICAL PEARL

What are the distinguishing differences between peripheral nerve and spinal nerve injury? Peripheral nerve compromise involves the muscles that are supplied by a specific nerve. All the muscles supplied by a spinal level nerve will be involved when a spinal nerve root is involved. Sensory loss in a peripheral nerve is very circumscribed whereas dermatomal distribution is not and can vary from patient to patient.

NERVES IMPLICATED WITH REFLEX LOSS[25]

There is some controversy as to the existence of these reflexes and what level they involve. Watson et al found that the deltoid and pectorals reflexes were pathonomic of myelopathies at C3, C4, or C5.[107] Most authors do not feel that there are true deep tendon reflexes above C5 (Box II-3-2).[59,84]

DERMATOMAL DISTRIBUTION OF PERIPHERAL NERVES[81]

Supraclavicular	Over deltoid and upper chest
Medial antebrachial cutaneous (axillary)	Over both lateral shoulder and upper arm
Medial brachial cutaneous (second intercostal)	Inside of arm
Intercostobrachial (second intercostal)	Upper inner posterior arm
Lateral antebrachial cutaneous (musculocutaneous)	Lateral forearm
	Posterior surface of arm
Posterior brachial cutaneous (radial)	Lower lateral aspect of arm
	Posterior surface of forearm
Lower lateral brachial cutaneous (radial)	Radial thumb, proximal half
	Index and middle finger, proximal dorsal radial side of ring finger
Posterior brachial cutaneous (radial)	Palmar surface of thumb, index, middle, and radial half of ring finger, dorsal tips of thumb, index, middle and radial part of ring finger
Radial superficial (radial)	
Palmar digital branch (median)	Anterior and posterior ulnar palm, little finger and ulnar aspect of ring finger
Superficial branch of ulnar nerve (ulnar)	

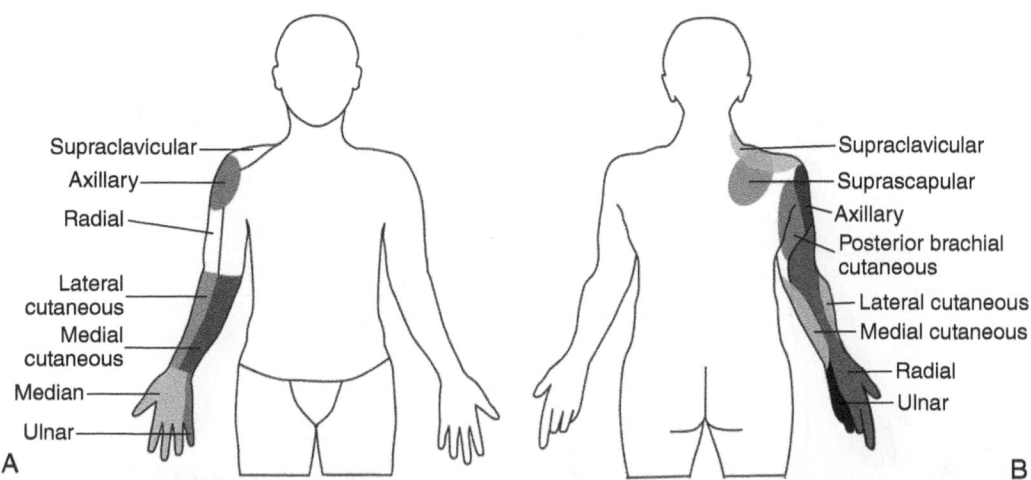

FIGURE II-3-4 Sensory distribution of peripheral nerves. The referral pattern of the sensory nerves is different from the referral pattern of the spinal nerve root. The clinician can utilize the differences to aid in the diagnostic process. The figures illustrate the anterior (**A**) and posterior (**B**) distribution of the upper extremity peripheral nerves.

BOX II-3-2   Deep Tendon Reflexes of the Upper Extremities

Levator scapula reflex	C3, 4, 5
Pectoralis reflex	C4
Deltoid reflex	C4, C5
Biceps reflex	C5
Brachioradialis reflex	C6
Triceps reflex	C7
Pisiform reflex	C8, T1
Finger jerk reflex	C8

MYOTOMAL DISTRIBUTION OF UPPER EXTREMITY PERIPHERAL NERVES[80]

Axillary	Shoulder abduction
Lateral pectoral/ thoracodorsal	Shoulder adduction
Musculocutaneous	Elbow flexion, shoulder flexion (coracobrachialis)
Radial	Elbow extension, forearm supination
Posterior interosseous	Wrist extension with ulnar deviation, digit extension, thumb abduction and extension, index finger extension
Median	
Anterior interosseous	Forearm pronation, wrist flexion with radial deviation
Ulnar	Finger and thumb flexion, metacarpophalangeal (MP) flexion of index and middle finger, abduction and adduction of index and middle fingers, forearm pronation, opposition of thumb
	Thumb flexion, adduction, and opposition, MP flexion, and finger abduction/adduction of ring and little fingers

WHAT OTHER MUSCULOSKELETAL STRUCTURES CAN REFER PAIN TO THE CERVICAL SPINE AND NECK?

The sternoclavicular joint, shoulder pathology, nerve compression neuropathies of the median and ulnar nerves around the elbow, and carpal tunnel syndrome can refer pain to the neck.[71,77,109]

CLINICAL DECISION MAKING CASE STUDY—PATIENT PROFILE   ?

The patient is a 44-year-old female who was involved in a motor vehicle accident. She was wearing a seatbelt. Initially she complained of neck pain and then pain in the lateral base of her right neck anterior to her upper trapezius. A few days later she developed lateral shoulder and arm pain. What is a possible hypothesis for her symptoms?

Answer

There is no prior medical history available. However, she is at the age when degenerative changes are frequently seen in the cervical spine. Her symptoms began with neck pain and then muscle pain in the lateral base of her neck. This is a common referral pattern for both the disc and sternoclavicular joint. Injury to the sternoclavicular joints is common with shoulder restraint belts. Symptoms in the lateral arm and shoulder may be a disc or a stenosis that has been exacerbated. Unfortunately, without knowing the aggravating and relieving factors, investigating the cause of her pain will be difficult.

WHAT VISCERAL STRUCTURES CAN REFER TO THE CERVICAL SPINE AND NECK AREA?[9,45] (see Figure II-3-5)

- Gallbladder, liver, and duodenum (resulting from irritation of the diaphragm) to the right lateral neck and shoulder.

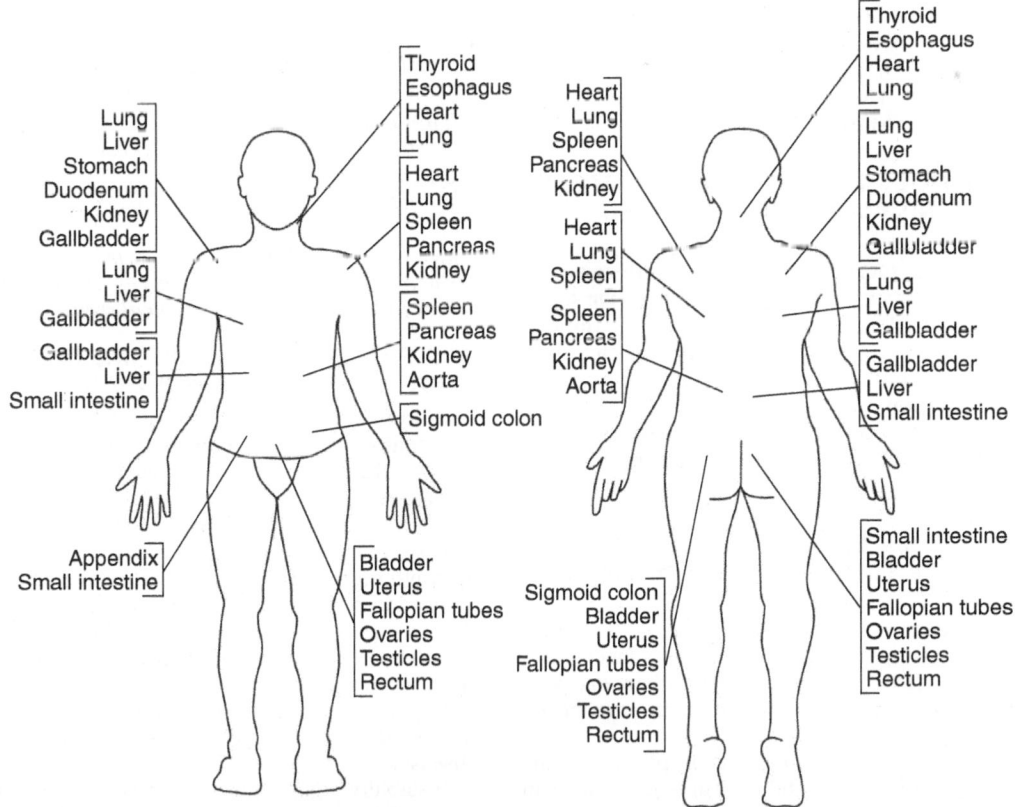

FIGURE II-3-5   Symptom referral pattern of visceral tissue. The figure illustrates the visceral tissues that most commonly refer symptoms to the upper quarter region. Symptoms are generally described as a deep dull ache that is hard to localize. Symptoms may wax and wane in intensity and may not be elicited by motions of the region.

- Heart problems such as angina can refer pain to the neck, shoulder, and jaw.
- Pulmonary tumors can be referred to the lower neck and shoulder.
- Subdiaphragmatic abscesses can cause neck pain.

CLINICAL PEARL

How does a nerve entrapped by a disc differ from a nerve entrapped by a facet? History will partially tell you. Disc problems have a history of previous or current trauma. The referred pain will depend on the structure that is compromised. Extension quadrant testing will close down the facets and intervertebral foramen causing pain down the arm. With a disc problem flexion of the neck away from the involved side may reproduce the symptoms. Valsalva maneuvers exacerbate intradiscal pressure and thus discogenic pain.[59,72]

SYMPTOM DESCRIPTORS[45]

WHAT INFLUENCE DOES THE DEPTH OF SYMPTOMS HAVE ON YOUR CLINICAL DECISION-MAKING PROCESS?

The descriptors that a patient utilizes can often aid a clinician in the differentiation process. The following descriptors have commonly been associated with specific tissues:

Deep ache:	Disc
Dull ache:	Bone, inflammation
Sharp pain:	Capsule, facet joint
Sharp and continuous pain:	Bone
Burning:	Nerves, Inflammation, Vein, Artery, Lymphatics
Tingling:	Nerves
Numbness:	Nerves
Deep boring:	Viscera
Colicky and cramping:	Viscera
Sore stiffness:	Muscle

WHAT INFLUENCE DOES THE DEPTH OF SYMPTOMS HAVE ON YOUR CLINICAL DECISION-MAKING PROCESS?[45]

Deep symptoms appear to incriminate the deeper tissues such as bone, disc, and visceral structures. Deeper tissues have fewer proprioceptors than superficial tissues. This makes it difficult to localize deep-seated pain generators. Deeper tissues have pressure-sensitive pain receptors, further compounding the difficulty of specific localization.

Superficial tissues such as muscle and ligament have more proprioceptors. This makes it somewhat easier to localize a source of pain.

WHAT INFLUENCE DOES CONSTANCY OF SYMPTOMS HAVE ON YOUR CLINICAL DECISION-MAKING PROCESS?[44]

Intermittent presentation of symptoms aggravated by change of position or certain movements suggests more of a mechanical cause. These symptoms also can be relieved by changing positions. Tissues such as joints, muscles, and ligaments can be responsible for producing these symptoms.

Constant symptoms with variable intensity implicate inflammation as the primary cause. Discs and fractures of bones can create this type of symptom.

Constant symptoms unchanged by movement or mechanical deformation suggest a more sinister cause such as cancer or pain from a visceral source.

IF A PATIENT HAS SYMPTOMS IN THE MORNING, WHAT ARE THE DIAGNOSTIC OPTIONS?

It is not uncommon to have neck stiffness in the morning that resolves after 30 minutes. This timing suggests mechanical pain. Osteoarthritis is an example of a problem that usually clears up in a short time. These mechanical disorders can be altered by biomechanical motion. Degenerative joint disease, facet pathology, stenosis, and joint instability will all present with stiffness and are relieved with motion. It is difficult to determine which of these structures is producing the pain as many these conditions are overlapping. Creep, abnormal resting positions, and lack of movement during sleep could conceivably contribute to this stiffness.

Pain and morning stiffness that is longer lasting is suggestive of inflammatory conditions such as rheumatoid arthritis, fibromyositis, and lupus. Fibromyalgia varies somewhat and stiffness and soreness can last for several hours into the afternoon. In the case of rheumatoid arthritis and lupus, stiffness and pain can last for several hours. Inflammation will generally subside once there is increased movement aiding circulation to the region. Resolution of local edema via the lymphatic system requires muscular contractions and movement. Hence, it takes a longer period of time for the pain and stiffness to abate.

Patients will often report stiffness following injury to the cervical spine. When a person is injured there is an immediate inflammatory reaction. The muscles are activated to protect the injured area and prevent further damage. The longer and harder the muscles have to work the more inflammatory byproducts are produced. These irritate the free nerve endings and nociceptors generating a more continuous muscle contraction. If the spine is held stiff by the tight musculature for more than 1 or 2 days collagen cross fibers will develop. Abnormal cross-link alignment across the capsule producing further capsular stiffness then occurs.

CLINICAL PEARL

Which level in the cervical spine has the greatest incidence of disc pathology? The most common site for disc herniation is C6-C7 then C5-C6. However, this is considered somewhat controversial. C5-C6 and C6-C7 are the most anterior to the center of gravity line and most mechanical stress is placed on them. It has also been postulated that the long lever arm of the neck and the weight of the head place the most stress on that part of the cervical spine.

IF A PATIENT HAS SYMPTOMS IN THE AFTERNOON, WHAT ARE THE DIAGNOSTIC OPTIONS?

Pain in the afternoon suggests that the disc, instability, stenosis, ligamentous injury, muscle injury, or degenerative joint disease may be the major source of the symptoms. The ability to differentiate between these will be dependent on what activities were performed earlier in the day.

Disc and degenerative joint disease will be aggravated due to the motion created by the repetitive activities of daily living. Extension or flexion with rotation may irritate the disc depending on the severity of the bulge. Other activities that create a Valsalva effect and static forward head postures will also similarly increase symptoms.

Repeated extension or prolonged forward head postures will exacerbate the pain from underlying degenerative joint disease.

Instability, ligamentous injuries, and the more rare cervical spondylolisthesis will become more symptomatic in the afternoon as the muscle fatigues and stretches highly innervated cervical ligaments. The build-up of lactic acid from poor posture also exacerbates the pain.

IF A PATIENT HAS SYMPTOMS IN THE EVENING WHAT ARE THE DIAGNOSTIC OPTIONS?

Evening symptoms are essentially an extension of the symptoms that occur in the afternoon. Their severity will be dependent on the vigor and irritability of the activities performed earlier in the day. If the activities are discontinued earlier the symptoms should not be as severe in the evening.

IF A PATIENT HAS SYMPTOMS WHEN SLEEPING, WHAT ARE THE DIAGNOSTIC OPTIONS?

Pain that occurs when sleeping can be a result of several factors. Pain due to movement may incriminate disc and stenotic pathology. Pain that arises from being in static positions at night may implicate instabilities and ligamentous problems. Pain that awakens a person without movement or is not relieved with a change of position can be a sign of a visceral pathology.[9,45]

STABILITY OF SYMPTOMS

How does the progression of a patient's symptoms impact your clinical decision-making process?

With acute injuries mechanical symptoms are most severe during the first several days. The symptoms should subsequently subside. If not, it will be necessary to identify the structural, biomechanical, or ergonomic cause.

Bone, muscle, and ligaments are highly vascularized. Injury will create an immediate response. If the patient gets immediate pain but does not improve during the remainder of the day, a structure that has become entrapped or pinched such as a joint capsule or facet may be the culprit.

Cervical discs have a poor blood supply. As a result the inflammatory response is therefore slow. The patient will likely develop pain the following day as enough inflammation occurs.

CLINICAL PEARL

!

Given that there is a poor vascularity and nerve supply why can a disc be so painful? Chemical radiculitis is produced by the release of inflammatory mediators such as proteoglycans, phospholipases, interleukin 6, and nitric oxide.

IF A PATIENT'S SYMPTOMS ARE IMPROVING, WHAT PATHOLOGY DOES THIS IMPLICATE?

The natural course of most neck pain is that of improvement. The speed of recovery will provide clues as to the possible source of symptoms. With a cervical impingement or dysfunction, improvement is rapid as the entrapped or stuck structure is released. Disc irritation will usually subside in 6–8 weeks as swelling and chemical irritation subsides. With more chronic disc situations, there will be a reoccurrence of symptoms because there has been trauma. Activities and certain positions aggravate the injured disc causing an inflammatory reaction. When inflammation subsides so should the symptoms.

CLINICAL DECISION MAKING CASE STUDY—PATIENT PROFILE

?

The patient is a 45-year-old male who has been having recurrent neck pain for the last several years. He feels good some days and other days he has symptoms into his left arm; it feels as if someone has rubbed sandpaper on his radial forearm. He has had a few neck injuries from old motor vehicle accidents each of which resolved after 4–6 weeks of treatment. He occasionally gets "popping" and sometimes a "catch" in his neck with neck rotation. He is frustrated because he feels good for a few days and then feels bad for several days.

Answer

This patient falls into the category in which you start to see more degenerative disc disease. He has a history of at least two motor vehicle accidents from which he previously recovered. His parasthesias and/or distal symptoms suggest that a structure is pressing on one of his nerve roots. This can occur with degenerative joint disease and with degenerative disc disease with the degenerative cascade. Finally, the "catch" and "popping" along with the inconsistency of his symptoms suggest the possibility that he has a hypermobility in the cervical spine. Because the ligaments are highly vascularized, mechanical stress causes a rapid painful inflammatory response that subsides.

IF A PATIENT'S SYMPTOMS ARE WORSENING, WHAT PATHOLOGY DOES THIS INDICATE?

- Typically an acute injury causes a rapid inflammatory response due to nociceptor stimulation. This results in the perception that the arm pain is more severe.
- Symptoms that do not change and seem to gradually worsen are most indicative of a degenerative process. With disc narrowing or osteophytes that produce either a central or lateral stenosis symptoms may subside for a period of time. They will return periodically and get worse as the changes progress. The distal symptoms will gradually get worse over several months to years.
- There are conditions in the neck that are inconsistent in their presentation. Minor insults, positions, and movements may provoke pain. This is suggestive of a hypermobility/instability in the cervical spine. After a short bout, the symptoms may disappear for weeks at a time and then recur. Because of vertebral slippage and poor motor control, tissue compression and ligamentous stress can produce both short- and long-term pain.[21]

CLINICAL PEARL

!

What is the natural progression of central cervical stenosis over time? Cervical stenosis progresses in about a third of affected individuals. It is most commonly seen in males over 55 years old. In the early stages, the condition is more often asymptomatic. It most commonly occurs at the C5–C7 level. Patients commonly become symptomatic when 30% of the spinal cord is compromised. However, this can vary from patient to patient. Many patients have a propensity for initial deterioration followed by a period of stability (often for years) and subsequent progression to a myelopathy. Surgical treatment 1 year postonset of symptom does not have as good an outcome. Up to two-thirds of people with this condition either deteriorate or remain unchanged. These individuals risk a greater chance of spinal cord injury with minor trauma.[27,31,57,78,80,102]

FUNCTIONAL AND ACTIVITY PARTICIPATION LIMITATIONS

WHAT INFLUENCE DOES AGGRAVATING FUNCTIONS HAVE ON YOUR CLINICAL DECISION-MAKING PROCESS?

FLEXION-BASED ACTIVITIES
- When a patient's symptoms are elicited with flexion-based activities the following tissues and pathology should be considered as potential source tissues: posterior muscles, posterior capsule, posterior ligaments, and nerve irritation caused by a posterior disc bulge.

- Activities that require a prolonged forward head posture with the neck in some flexion, as in sitting at a desk, may aggravate the posterior aspect of the disc, posterior ligaments, and posterior muscles. Prolonged cervical flexion could also conceivably produce some dural irritation, especially when there is some pathology in the lumbar and thoracic areas.
- Flexion can also stress the posterior elements such as the ligamentum flavum, the supraspinous and interspinous ligaments, the posterior longitudinal ligament, and the tectorial membrane.

EXTENSION-BASED ACTIVITIES

- Facet, capsule, anterior cervical ligament, anterior muscles, spondylolisthesis, instability, and degenerative changes to the zygapophyseal joint should be primary hypotheses if the patient is experiencing pain with extension-based activities.
- The posterior aspect of the disc may also be symptomatic with extension-based activities due to compression on the disc or compression of local inflammation.
- In the case of muscle strain, posterior muscles may be symptomatic if the extension is active. This pain should be less if the neck is taken into passive extension.
- Prolonged forward position of the head with sitting postures can produce increased muscle strain on several groups of muscles including the sternocleidomastoids, the trapezius, splenius capitis, multifidii, rhomboids, and semispinalis muscles that support the neck. This is commonly seen with office/clerical workers with poor ergonomics.
- The weight of the head is supported both by the spinal column and ligaments and muscles in the neck. The average weight of the head is 4–5 kg. When the head is more forward in the presence of a cervical instability the passive, active, and neural subsystems described by Panjabi are severely tested.[90] The muscles are working hard to stabilize the segment while the ligaments are stressed with the slippage. Because of the slippage the cervical column is not in the optimal position of control. The result is increased neck pain with static forward head positions.

CLINICAL PEARL

Cervical disc bulges and flexion of the neck to the contralateral side may reproduce peripheral symptoms in the ipsilateral upper limb.[35] It has been proposed by McKenzie that in lateral flexion and rotation (coupling movement) of the cervical spine, there is offset loading of the intervertebral disc on the side of the flexion and rotation. Nuclear material moves to the opposite side (the side of the convexity), and the posterolateral annular wall is stretched.[76]

LATERAL FLEXION AND ROTATION ACTIVITIES

- Pathology and tissues aggravated by lateral flexion and rotation activities include the facet joint tissue, radiculopathy, lateral stenosis, muscle strain, and brachial plexus and uncovertebral joint problems.
- Side impact injuries due to motor vehicle accidents appear to be more injurious than rear end impacts. Maak et al[71] have shown that side impact caused multiplanar injuries at C3–C4 through C7–T1 and significantly greater injury at C6–C7, as compared with head-forward rear impact injuries. Carlson et al[14] have concluded that elongation-induced vertebral artery injury is more likely to occur during side impact compared with frontal impact injuries.
- The scalenes can be stretched with side impact injuries resulting in forceful side bending of the neck. This can produce neurogenic thoracic outlet syndrome.
- Muscle and ligamentous strain is often aggravated by poor ergonomics with the head having to be side bent and rotated to one side such as sitting at a desk.

COMBINED MOTION ACTIVITIES

- Activities that are aggravated with combined flexion and rotation/lateral flexion include disc pathology, ligamentous and capsular strain, muscle strain, radiculopathy, and vertebral artery injury.
- Activities that are aggravated with combined extension and rotation/lateral flexion include facet pathology, lateral stenosis, ligamentous strain, and muscle strain.

OTHER ACTIVITIES

- As in the lumbar region, coughing and sneezing will also increase the disc pressure in the cervical spine. Both may cause rapid flexion, which will further increase the disc pressure in the cervical spine.[59] Valsalva maneuvers increase the interdiscal pressure and may produce distal symptoms.[59,72]
- Pain with static positions can be indicative of spinal instability or spondylolysis.
- Wearing a heavy helmet or carrying objects on the head can increase interdiscal pressure.[58] Table II-3-1 summarizes the relationship between cervical pathology and functional or activity limitations.

WHAT INFLUENCE DOES EASING FUNCTIONS HAVE ON YOUR CLINICAL DECISION-MAKING PROCESS?

FLEXION-BASED ACTIVITIES

- Tissues and pathologies eased by flexion include the posterior disc, anterior ligaments, facet joint, lateral stenosis, and radiculopathy (varies with offending structures).
- Flexion-based activities will unload the facets and will increase the diameter of the intervertebral foramen. It will also unload the anterior longitudinal ligaments and posterior disc. With radiculopathy flexion will reduce the pressure on the nerve by either increasing the diameter of the intervertebral foramen or unloading the disc, thereby reducing its incursion onto the nerve. Flexion without a forward head could conceivably ease discomfort in the sternocleidomastoids and scalenes.

EXTENSION-BASED ACTIVITIES

- If symptoms are eased by extension the following tissues and pathologies should be considered as possible sources of symptoms: posterior ligaments, the facet capsule as long as it is not impinged, certain disc pathology (depending on location and severity), and the posterior musculature.

CLINICAL PEARL

A good rule of thumb when examining a patient for exacerbating or remitting of symptoms is to understand anatomy, selective tissue tension signs, the nature and pattern of the pain, and the location of the structures being tested. Selective tissue tension is very specific and will identify a specific tissue by its physiological properties (i.e., muscle, ligamentous, and nerves respond differently when stressed). Additionally, understanding the anatomical characteristics and kinematics of the structure being tested is critical (i.e., facet surfaces will be stressed with compression whereas facet capsules will be stressed with distraction). Understanding how inert structures influence surrounding soft tissues is critical (i.e., closing the intervertebral foramen will affect cervical nerve roots due to its reduced diameter). Finally, different tissues have different pain descriptions and referral patterns (i.e., nerve pain presents with burning while muscle pain with aching).

LATERAL FLEXION AND ROTATION ACTIVITIES: Because of the shape of the facets and ligaments, the facets will close down with both lateral flexion and rotation in the direction of the movement. Hence, lateral flexion and rotation will ease

TABLE II-3-1 Functional or Activity Participation Limitations

Motion	Functional Activities	Pathology if Symptoms Are Aggravated by Activity	Pathology if Symptoms Are Eased by Activity
Flexion	Prolonged sitting with flexed forward head (i.e., working at a computer, driving), reading in bed with neck in too much flexion	Disc pathology, muscle strain, posterior ligamentous strain, radiculopathy, central stenosis, facet capsular strain, anterior end plate, DJD	Facet pathology, radiculopathy, lateral stenosis
Extension	Overhead work that requires looking up, forward head posture with head in extension	Facet pathology, posterior disc pathology, stress on anterior ligaments, stress on scalenes and SCMs, DJD	Some disc pathology, capsular and posterior ligament strain, some posterior muscle strains
Lateral flexion and rotation	Changing lanes while driving, phone activities at office and with driving, sports activities	Lateral stenosis, radiculopathy, muscle strains, contralateral facet capsules, facet and uncovertebral joints, DJD, DDD, instabilities	Some disc pathology, contralateral radiculopathies and lateral stenosis, ipsilateral facet capsules, ipsilateral muscle strains
Combined motion	Extension and rotation/lateral flexion	Facet pathology, radiculopathy, lateral stenosis, contralateral ligament and facet capsule pathology, some disc pathology, contralateral muscle strains, DJD, DDD, instability	Ipsilateral muscle and ligament strains, contralateral facet pathology, contralateral lateral stenosis, ipsilateral facet capsule strain
Combined motion	Flexion and rotation/lateral flexion	Some lower disc pathology, facet capsule and ligament strain, muscle strain, end plate and disc pathologies	Some disc pathology, facet pathology on convex side
Static positions	Sleep, sitting, looking up for long periods	Instability, spondylosis, lateral stenosis, ligamentous strain, muscle strain	Muscle strain, ligamentous strain, some disc pathology, spondylosis, lateral stenosis, disc pathology, central stenosis*
General movement	General motion/movement in neck within pain-free range		DJD and some inactive or noninflammatory arthritic conditions
Other	Coughing, sneezing, straining	Disc pathology, instability, radiculopathy	

DJD, degenerative joint disease; SCM, sternocleidomastoid; DDD, degenerative disk disease.
*These conditions will respond best with semirecumbent sitting or recumbent with these structures unloaded while in a static position.

pathologies on the convex side of the curve such as lateral stenosis, some disc pathology, and radiculopathy (depending on the offending structure). On the concave side or side of rotation, the facet capsules (providing they are not impinged), muscle strain, and ligament strain are placed in a position of ease.

COMBINED MOTION ACTIVITIES: Pathologies eased by extension and rotation/lateral flexion include posterior muscle strains and some capsule and ligamentous strain.

Pathology and tissues eased by flexion and rotation/lateral flexion include some disc pathology, lateral stenosis, facet joints, and some muscle strains (varies with location).

STATIC ACTIVITIES: Most of the static activities that provide relief are those that unload the offending structures and tissues in a position of rest. In the cervical spine this appears to be best accomplished in recumbent or semirecumbent positions with head and neck support.

CLINICAL PEARL

!

Most patients with cervical spine spondylolisthesis are asymptomatic. It is not very common, but has been associated with trauma to the neck and with degenerative cervical changes in the elderly. When it does produce symptoms, it may start as simple neck pain. More serious problems result with unstable segments sliding forward producing myelopathic symptoms. Myelopathic symptoms are usually bilateral.

GENERAL MOVEMENT: General movement of the cervical spine not at end range will provide relief from some instabilities and nonactive arthritic conditions.

MEDICAL HISTORY

WHAT ROLE DOES THE PATIENT'S PRIOR MEDICAL HISTORY PLAY IN THE DIAGNOSIS OF CERVICAL PATHOLOGY?

- Past surgeries, past injuries, especially whiplash injuries, and other medical pathology affect the function and production of pain in the cervical spine. Prior neck laminectomy and fusion will affect the mobility of the spine. Radical neck, mandibular surgery, first rib removal, lateral clavicular excision (Mumford procedure), and thyroidectomy all have the potential of producing scar tissue and increasing the stress on the tissues about the neck.
- Enlargement of lymph nodes from sinusitis, laryngitis, and infections in the salivary ducts can cause neck pain.[45]
- Patients who have a history of heart problems and angina can have pain in the neck and down the arm mimicking radicular symptoms.[45]
- Patients with a history of carpal tunnel surgery may have pain in the neck.[109]
- Certain medications such as long term use of corticosteroids can produce side effects such as osteoporosis and produce fat deposits in the neck and face.
- Although coumadin and some other medications do not produce neck pain directly, patients are at risk to bleed with minor trauma, which in turn could cause pain and limited mobility in the neck.
- Patients who have had subdural injections can often present with neck and back pain when there is a spinal fluid leak.

- Menstruating females commonly complain of headaches and neck and back pain.
- Injuries in the thoracic and lumbar spine can lead to postural adaptations and compensatory movements, which can affect the cervical spine.

MEDICAL AND ORTHOPEDIC TESTING

WHAT MEDICAL AND ORTHOPEDIC TEST INFLUENCES YOUR DIFFERENTIAL DIAGNOSIS PROCESS IN THE CERVICAL SPINE?

MRIs, radiographs, electromyograms (EMGs), discography, CT scans, myelograms, and a less common variety of nuclear medicine studies combined with clinical tests and observations will influence your decision-making process.

HOW DO RADIOGRAPHIC OR OTHER EXAMINATIONS INFLUENCE YOUR DECISION-MAKING PROCESS?

- Cervical radiographs may be helpful in ruling out tumors, fractures, and congenital deformities such as fusions and spondylolisthesis. Degenerative changes and some other findings may not correlate with your clinical findings. Findings on the radiographs will be significant only if they are correlated with your clinical findings.
- The Canadian C Spine Rule suggests that radiographs of the cervical spine should be taken in high-risk cases with persons who
  - ○ are 65 years or older
  - ○ have experienced a dangerous injury mechanism
  - ○ have parasthesias in the extremities
  - ○ have any low-risk injury (simple rear end motor vehicle accidents, etc.) that will not allow safe assessment of active range of motion (AROM).[99]

HOW RELIABLE ARE RADIOGRAPHS IN ASSESSING THE CERVICAL SPINE?

Radiographs are one of the most common methods of ruling out fractures in the cervical spine; unfortunately the reliability of radiographs for assessing nontraumatic neck pain and neck pain without radiculopathy is not supported by the evidence.[88] Vandemark[105] claimed that well-positioned and optimally exposed radiographs of the cervical spine will disclose 95% of clinically significant cervical spine fractures, but lamented that, unfortunately, such high-quality examinations are frequently impossible to obtain. Nuñez et al[89] reported that nearly 40% of cervical spine fractures are missed on conventional radiography but are later revealed on CT.

HOW RELIABLE ARE MRIs IN ASSESSING THE CERVICAL SPINE?

MRI imaging is the most common method of diagnosing cervical disc pathology. Zheng et al[114] found that MRIs had a 51% false-positive rate and 27% false-negative rate in diagnosing cervical herniated discs. Klein et al[66] found that MR imaging was not very effective in identifying cervical fractures. Sengupta et al[95] found that MRI alone was not a very good diagnostic tool in distinguishing between hard and soft disc problems. Factors affecting the quality of the MRI include patient motion, patient size, surface coil technology, and strength of the magnet[64] (see Box II-3-3).

HOW RELIABLE ARE EMGs AND NERVE CONDUCTION STUDIES IN THE CERVICAL SPINE?

There seems to be a lot of controversy about the clinical relevance, reliability, and responsiveness of surface EMG examination methods.[58] Needle EMGs are most useful in diagnosing nerve root and peripheral nerve compressions. These studies can be

---

BOX II-3-3 Sensitivity and Specificity of Magnetic Resonance Imaging on Musculosketal Diagnoses

Sensitivity	
Blunt trauma	97.2%[83]
Stenosis	88.9%[7]
Disc	89% to 95.6%[93,95]
Tumor/infection	94% to 96%[78]
Specificity	
Blunt trauma	98.7%[83]
Stenosis	99.1%[7]
Disc	44%[93,95]
Tumor/infection	92%[78]

---

affected by surrounding tissue being irritated with the nerve still intact. Conversely, estimates as high as 30% to 40% false negatives have been reported. Medications, sampling errors, excess fatty tissue, poor relaxation, the timing of the examination, and age of the patient, and the temperature of the room can affect this outcome.[86,87]

MEDICATIONS

HOW DOES PATIENT MEDICATION INFLUENCE YOUR DECISION-MAKING PROCESSES?[9,45]

- Muscle relaxants and pain and antiinflammatory medications are commonly prescribed for neck and back problems. Muscle relaxants and pain medications taken concurrently with a patient assessment may obscure some of the diagnostic findings. Most patients with symptomatic neck pathology will exhibit pain with muscle guarding.
- If antiinflammatory medication is effective in providing relief then it may help in differentiating some of the following structures affected by the inflammatory process: disc pathology, ligament strain, muscle strains, facet pathologies, and radiculopathies.
- Pathologies that normally do not have an acute inflammatory response are lateral stenosis, spondylolisthesis, degenerative joint disease, instability, and central stenosis.

BIOMECHANICAL FACTORS

WHAT ROLE DOES BIOMECHANICS PLAY IN CERVICAL SPINE PAIN?

- The biomechanics of the mid and low cervical spine have been well established though research. C2-C3 to C7-T1 all have a similar coupling pattern. Sidebend to one sided is accompanied by rotation to the same side. This pattern is controlled by the shape of the facets and ligamentous restraints.[77] These joints allow flexion, extension, side bending, and rotation to occur.
- Injury can impact the biomechanics of the cervical spine. Whiplash injuries are a prime example of how injury can impact spinal mechanics. The forced closing action produced by the whiplash-type injury will produce posterior shear, extension, and axial compression of the spine. This in turn will alter the normal mechanics of the cervical region.[97]
- Arthritic changes and the degenerative cascade will affect the biomechanics by limiting motion in some segments and increasing motion in other segments in an attempt to maintain normal motion.[55,91]
- Surgical procedures such as fusion will alter the biomechanics, also producing undue stress on adjacent segments and other segments attempting normal coupling.[20,30,37,54]

WHAT BIOMECHANICAL ABNORMALITIES IN OTHER REGIONS CAN AFFECT CERVICAL PATHOLOGY?

- Leg length discrepancies, scoliosis, excessive upper thoracic kyphosis, or a flat curve or reversal of that curve can conceivably affect neck pathology by altering the position of the facets and head.
- Excessive kyphosis will cause the head to be more forward and will increase the lordotic curve in the cervical spine. This will close down the facets and intervertebral foramen. The forward head will place more stress on the scalenes, sternocleidomastoids, and upper trapezius muscles. It can conceivably affect respiration by shortening the anterior neck muscles used in upper respiratory breathing.[13]
- The reversal of the kyphotic curve can reduce the lordotic curve in the cervical spine, thus placing more stress on the posterior structures, facet capsules, and discs.
- Leg length discrepancies and scoliosis can travel proximally and conceivably alter the posture of the head and neck, compressing structures on one side of the neck while stretching tissues on the other side.

ENVIRONMENTAL FACTORS

DO PSYCHOSOCIAL ISSUES INFLUENCE CLINICAL DECISION MAKING?

Depression, anxiety, family and job stressors, alcohol, drugs, cigarette usage, and other psychosocial factors can affect both the response and chronicity of symptoms. These psychological issues can also compromise the immune, autonomic, and endocrine systems.[51]

CAN EMOTIONS INFLUENCE NECK PAIN?

The limbic system is of great importance. It processes the emotions and the hypothalamus releases stress hormones. Whitten et al[110] have suggested that the limbic system is stimulated during the acute pain experience. With the onset of acute pain, the limbic system tells the spinal cord to limit the pain signals. The brain does not want to receive these signals temporarily. The limbic system is working hard to repress the pain signals, while the spinal cord, also in the case of stress, is abuzz with activity. The spinal cord can stand only so much stimulation gracefully; after this, the pain threshold is reduced. The result is a chronic pain situation in which the patient is hypersensitive to pain. Research with MRIs show a direct relationship between the amount of focus given to the pain and the amount of pain perceived.[8]

DO WORK-RELATED INJURIES INFLUENCE CLINICAL DECISION MAKING?

This should always be a consideration. Poor ergonomics and continued postural stress and activities will always be a factor in clinical decision making. Job satisfaction will be another factor that needs to be considered in this milieu. Malingering is also always a potential factor with work-related injuries, but the patient should be given the benefit of the doubt unless the patient's symptom patterns do not match recognized symptom patterns[34] (see Box II-3-4).

BOX II-3-4 Contextual Factors[51,108]	
Contextual Factor	**Contributing Factors**
Environmental	Poor ergonomics, repetitive tasks can lead to tissue breakdown and maintain chronicity of the condition
Personal	Job satisfaction, personal and family stressors, personal habits, depression, cultural and religious pressures, and emotional lability can all influence neck pain

PERSONAL FACTORS

PRIOR SURGERIES

WHAT PRIOR SURGERIES INFLUENCE YOUR CLINICAL REASONING IN THE CERVICAL SPINE?

Several prior surgeries in the neck itself will change the biomechanics in the neck. These have been previously mentioned. The Mumford, which involves excision of the distal third of the clavicle, is one of the surgeries that may cause neck pain. This resultant loss of the only boney attachment of the shoulder girdle to the axial skeleton forces the muscles and ligaments supporting the neck and shoulder girdle to work harder to hold up the shoulder girdle and upper extremity. This potentially places excessive stress on the muscles around on the neck resulting in neck pain.[6,85] A good understanding of the kinetic chain relationships can often help the clinician to understand the distal influences on cervical biomechanics.

FAMILY HISTORY

DOES FAMILY HISTORY OF CERVICAL PATHOLOGY INFLUENCE YOUR CLINICAL REASONING PROCESS?

Recent research has suggested that there may be a genetic predisposition with some cervical pathology.[46] Therefore, a family history of conditions such as congenital spinal cord lesions and malformations,[56] instability, a history of temporomandibular joint (TMJ) problems,[17] osteoporosis, stenosis,[27,98] degenerative disc disease, some types of torticollis[96,97] and some other arcane diagnoses should be considered in your clinical assessment.[53,56,111]

CHRONICITY OF PAIN

DOES THE CHRONICITY OF NECK PAIN INFLUENCE YOUR CLINICAL REASONING PROCESS?

Chronic neck pain continues to be an enigma to medicine. Specific conditions that have been hypothesized to account for chronic neck pain are facet pathology, degenerative disc disease, degenerative joint disease, postural considerations, pain perception, cultural considerations, and psychosocial issues.[51,75]

Ferrari and Russell[40] have suggested that despite years of research and increasingly sophisticated radiological assessment techniques few advances have been made in attributing chronic neck pain to specific structural sources.

At present, the general consensus appears to be that most of the chronicity in the cervical spine is related to some type of previous trauma. There also seems to be a greater incidence of chronic neck pain in those persons with concurrent low back pain.

HAS MEDICAL TREATMENT BEEN SUCCESSFUL IN TREATING INDIVIDUALS WITH CHRONIC NECK PAIN?

Recent research has shown that multimodal treatment of chronic neck pain is better than home exercise or advice alone.[103] In a recent review of the literature, Gross et al[49] suggested that mobilization and manipulation with exercise seem to provide the best relief and are superior to either individually or in combination with physical medicine agents. There continues to be an ongoing debate on the benefits of surgical treatment versus conservative management of chronic neck pain.[92]

CLINICAL PEARL

Patients with chronic neck pain have a greater activation of their accessory neck muscles with upper extremity use. This may be due to an altered pattern of motor control to compensate for reduced activation of painful muscles.[38]

CLINICAL DECISION MAKING
CASE STUDY—PATIENT PROFILE **?**

The patient is a 55-year-old male who injured himself in a motor vehicle accident 3 months ago. He had a little soreness in the neck but subsequently started getting referred pain into the right medial scapular region and shoulder. Later pain progressed down to the inside of his arm to the right hand. His triceps reflex was diminished and he has lost some grip strength in his right hand. He reports increased pain with abduction and flexion of the shoulder. He gets some relief of his arm pain when he supports his elbow. He was a long time 1–2 pack a day smoker, but gave it up 2 years earlier.

Answer
The patient does have a history of trauma that could be indicative of a disc injury or an irritation of a preexisting stenotic condition. Other things that need to be ruled out are thoracic outlet, shoulder involvement (rotator cuff or labral tears) because of the painful movements in the shoulder, and possible injury to the brachial plexus. This gentleman was a longtime smoker. His pain pattern and its progression, the loss of the triceps reflex, weakness in the grip, and supporting the elbow to take pressure of the offending neural structures should send up red flags. The early signs of a Pancoast tumor can be confused with thoracic outlet syndrome and disc pathology.

CAN DISCS BE INJURED WITH CHRONIC NECK PAIN?
It is estimated that about 25% of chronic neck pain is generated by the disc and 60% is generated by facet problems.[8] It has been hypothesized that in the case of trauma to the disc, as in whiplash or compression injuries, the facets are more involved, whereas the disc involvement is more of a byproduct of the injury. In degenerative conditions, it is believed that neck pain is produced by pressure in various directions by the annulus aided by the degenerative cascade.

HOW DO THE AUTONOMIC, ENDOCRINE, AND IMMUNE SYSTEMS INFLUENCE DECISION MAKING IN THE CERVICAL REGION?
The three systems work together to help regulate most of the body functions. The endocrine system controls things such as bone growth, inflammation, mood, blood vessels, and both the immune and autonomic systems. Dysfunction in the endocrine system can affect healing in chronic neck pain.[9,45]

The autonomic system affects visceral function, affects blood flow to the skeletal muscle, and can alter mood. With depression the chronicity of neck symptoms will likely be sustained.[70,79]

A depressed immune system has a diminished capacity. Both prolonged stress and depression can affect the body's ability to heal because they impede the immune system's ability to heal. Underlying diseases such as hepatitis C will result in muscle soreness and tightness. Other subclinical conditions that affect the immune system may be obfuscated by the neck pain they produce[4] (see Box II-3-5).

RED FLAGS THAT REQUIRE REFERRAL TO A MEDICAL PHYSICIAN

WHAT SYMPTOMS ALERT YOU TO PATHOLOGY THAT MAY REQUIRE A REFERRAL TO A MEDICAL DOCTOR?[9,45]
- A clear history should be taken in determining the cause of neck pain. Patients in pain and distress do not always describe their pain in a way that unequivocally points to a visceral problem.
- Visceral pain that varies more often than not is poorly localized. It is often described as heaviness, discomfort, deep and boring pain, and occasionally deep and burning pain.

BOX II-3-5   Output Mechanisms

Output Mechanism	Contributing Factors
Autonomic	Recent evidence has suggested that posture induced head and neck pain may be a result of an underlying autonomic disorder. [94]
Endocrine	Dysfunctions in the thyroid can produce sleep disturbances, muscle aches and fatigue, emotional lability all of which can contribute the chronicity of neck pain[29]
Immune	Several studies have shown that infections and diseases in the cervical spine can be the source of neck pain[3,12,44,61,74]

- Positional changes or movements in the neck will not typically alter symptoms. Mechanical treatment will be ineffective in pain relief.
- Pain will not be relieved with rest and will often be worse at night. Patients will typically awaken due to pain without a provoking movement or position.
- Patients with nonmusculoskeletal involvement will describe their pain as constant and nonvarying and often progressive.

CLINICAL DECISION MAKING
CASE STUDY—PATIENT PROFILE **?**

The patient is a 62-year-old male with the primary complaint of neck pain. He reports neck pain, spasm, and decreased range of motion. He states he occasionally gets numbness down into his hands. He complains of night pain relieved by change of position. He also states he has started having night sweats, chills, and a low-grade fever recently. He has a history of diabetes, which he has under control. He had a kidney transplant 3 months previously.

Answer
It is difficult for a clinician to make a definitive diagnosis as to the exact cause of this patient's symptoms. The ominous symptoms at night such as the night pain and sweats, chills, and fever suggest a possible infection. Because he has a history of diabetes and a transplant operation it is possible he is immunodeficient, opening him up to infection. The clinician must also be aware of possible local tumors that could produce these symptoms. A referral back to his primary physician to rule out a possible red flag condition is necessary.

WHAT SYMPTOMS INDICATE A SPECIFIC VISCERAL SYSTEM?
RESPIRATORY SYSTEM
- Symptoms include hoarseness, shortness of breath, and pain in the chest, shoulder, and neck. Horner's syndrome and atrophy in the hand muscles are indicative of Pancoast tumors. Other symptoms include chronic cough with or without blood, difficulty in swallowing, and enlarged lymph nodes or swelling in the neck.[9,45]
CARDIOVASCULAR SYSTEM
- Persons with a possible heart attack will have an uncomfortable fullness, pressure, or heaviness in the center of the chest. Pain can be present in the neck, jaw, and down the arm often mimicking a radicular pain pattern. However, the patient will also have a feeling of lightheadedness, sweating, pallor, nausea, and shortness of breath with an irregular heart rate. Pain is generally on the left, but can occasionally present as symptoms on the right.[9,45]
ENDOCRINE SYSTEM
- This system can produce mood changes, depression, anxiety, blood pressure changes, fatigue, joint pains, excessive or delayed bone growth, loss of hair, temperature sensitivity, muscle aches,

TABLE II-3-2   Body Structures and Tissue-Based Pathology (Nociceptive and Peripheral Neurogenic Pain)

Tissue	Intervertebral Disc	Zygapophyseal Joint Capsule	Zygapophyseal Joint	Muscles	Vertebral Bodies	Posterior Vertebral Elements	Ligaments	Nerves	Visceral Tissue
Pathology	Cervical disc pathology	Whiplash	Cervical facet dysfunction, rheumatoid arthritis, whiplash	Cervical muscle strain, torticollis, whiplash	Whiplash	Whiplash	Rheumatoid arthritis, whiplash	Cervical myelopathy, cervical radiculopathy, whiplash	Vertebral artery injury, whiplash
Age[69]	HNP < 40 DDD > 40	30–70, most common after 50 as it becomes more chronic	30–70, most common after 50 as it becomes more chronic	20–40	Any age for Fx, 60+ for greatest DJD	Any age for Fx. 50+ for DJD	30–70	Disc related < 40, peak incidence 50–55 for stenosis/DJD	Increases after 40
Occupation	Prolonged flexed postures, repetitive overhead work, lifting heavy objects	Prolonged flexed postures, repetitive overhead work, static forward head postures	Prolonged overhead work, or overhead carrying, static forward head postures	Prolonged sitting postures	Carrying loads on head or overhead	Prolonged overhead work and prolonged sitting postures	Varies based on prior history	Varies, see related pathology	Varies based on pathology
Gender Ethnicity	No preference n/n	No preference n/a	No preference n/a	Females n/a	No preference n/a	No preference n/a	No preference n/a	No preference n/a	No preference n/a
History	History of trauma, whiplash	History of trauma, whiplash	History of trauma or repetitive injury	History of trauma but can be from repetitive use or static postures	History of trauma	History of trauma or can be gradual with DJD	History of trauma or gradual onset	Varies related to pathology	History depends on tissue affected
Mechanism of injury	Forced flexion or extension, compression or rotation	Sudden flexion and/or rotation	Sudden extension and/or flexion	Prolonged overuse and sudden extension/flexion	Compression forced extension/flexion	Forced flexion or extension	Trauma	Varies based on pathology	No clear cut mechanism
Type of onset	Sudden	Sudden	Can be sudden with trauma and gradual with repetitive overuse	Can be sudden with trauma and gradual with overuse	Sudden with trauma and gradual with DJD	Sudden with fracture and gradual with DJD	Sudden or traumatic	Gradual mostly but can be sudden with trauma	Sudden to gradual depending on structure
Referral from local tissue	Near midline in neck and down into medial scapula	Neck and upper back	Head, neck, scapula, and shoulder	Skull, suboccipital and neck regions, upper back and chest	Local and general pain in neck and into shoulders	Head, neck, scapula, and shoulders	Head, neck, scapula, and shoulders	Pain in neck and shoulders	Usually more local depending on structure
Referral to other regions	May refer to upper extremity pain	Ipsilateral head, neck, scapula, and shoulder	Ipsilateral head, neck, scapula, and shoulder	Can refer into the arm and forearm with scalene involvement	May refer into upper extremity if nerve is involved	Generally does not refer to other areas	Generally does not refer to other areas	Referral to distinct upper extremity distribution depending on nerve root involved	May refer to surrounding area depending on involved structure
Change in symptoms	More dependent on position of neck; more painful in the next morning	Sudden pain with no relief as the day progresses	Slow progressive worsening over time; sudden pain that subsides initially but returns later	Sudden pain	Sudden pain with no relief as the day progresses	Sudden sharp pain that subsides in 6–8 weeks and becomes more chronic	Sudden relief but no relief as the day progresses	Symptoms increase until the offending structures are addressed	Will not change and perhaps gets worse as the pathology progresses

Continued on following page.

TABLE II-3-2 Body Structures and Tissue-Based Pathology (Nociceptive and Peripheral Neurogenic Pain) (Continued)

Tissue	Intervertebral Disc	Zygapophyseal Joint Capsule	Zygapophyseal Joint	Muscles	Vertebral Bodies	Posterior Vertebral Elements	Ligaments	Nerves	Visceral Tissue
24-hour pain pattern (morning)	Stiff and painful initially due to inability to control neck position while asleep	Stiff for 5 minutes but could be longer if it is more acute	Pain and stiffness most pronounced in the morning	Stiff in the morning until moving around; usually less stiff after 30 minutes	Stiff initially in the morning	Stiff for initial 30 minutes with fracture	Stiff for initial 30 minutes in the morning.	Stiff and painful for first 30 minutes	Varies but does not change with mechanical stresses
24-hour pain pattern (afternoon)	A little less stiff but may worsen depending on head position	Worsens with activity and with flexion activities	Worsens if put in a lot of activities that require extension	Less stiff but may get worse with prolonged sitting with forward head postures	Less stiff during the day with activity but stiff by end of day	Less stiff but may get worse with prolonged sitting and forward head postures	May get worse with prolonged activity and forward head postures	May worsen with prolonged positions and activities	Varies but does not change with mechanical stresses
24-hour pain pattern (evening)	May have difficulty with sleep due to positional discomfort	May interrupt sleep with turning neck in sleep	Less pain as long as not moving around in sleep	May find it difficult to sleep due to getting comfortable; pain will not usually awaken the patient	May be difficult to get to sleep	Initially difficult getting to sleep but usually not impaired	Sleep usually not interrupted except with poor sleeping positions	Sleep may be interrupted with poor positions or neck movements during sleep	May have more night pain
Description of symptoms	Without nerve root involvement it is vague, diffuse, and distributed axially	Sharp when acute; typically unilateral dull and aching	Typically unilateral, dull, and aching when chronic	Achiness and muscle tightness; may be able to localize bands or trigger points	Aching but can be sharp with certain movements such as flexion and side bending	Aching but can get sharp with motions that stress it	Aching and stiffness that get sharp with movements that stress them	Numbness, tingling, and burning	Deep boring pain, gnawing ache that cannot be localized superficially
Depth of symptoms	Deep	Deep	Deep	Superficial	Deep	Deep	Deep	Superficial	Deep and poorly localized
Constancy of symptoms	Intermittent	Intermittent	Intermittent	Intermittent	Constant but varies in intensity	Constant but varying in intensity	Intermittent but can be more constant if affected ligaments are put on stretch for longer periods	Intermittent to constant but varies due to position of offending structures	Constant but may come in waves
Aggravating factors	Extension and flexion away from bulge site, Valsalva	Flexion activities and rotation away from affected joint, axial tractioning	Extension and rotation/side bending into the affected joint, quadrant testing with compression and/or overpressure	Prolonged sitting or activities with forward head postures, resistive extension	Coughing, axial compression	Extension mostly but can be flexion in cases such as clay shoveler's fractures	Any activity or position in the neck that places stretch on the ligaments, flexion and rotation mostly	Coughing, sneezing, and Valsalva depending on structure involved; varies with related pathology	Not provoked by mechanical means
Easing factors	Unloading in supine, axial tractioning	Avoidance of flexion and other positions that will stretch capsules	Unloading joint and avoiding extension activities at the joint	Lying supine or lying semirecumbent with neck support	With fractures limiting motion	Avoidance of extremes of extension and flexion in certain cases	Lying or semirecumbant with some support;. avoidance of extremes of motion that will stress ligaments	Varies with the type of pathology or offending structure	Not eased typically by mechanical means

	1	2	3	4	5	6	7	8	9
Stability of symptoms	Gradual improvement over 8-12 weeks; about 5% will need surgery; with DDD it will become more chronic	Gradual improvement over 4-8 weeks	With acute facet dysfunction; relief is anywhere from 1-7 days depending on treatment; trauma related will get better initially but symptoms will progress slowly	Gradual improvement over 6 weeks if postural and other issues are addressed	Gradual improvement over 8 weeks; may become more chronic with DJD	Gradual improvement with fractures over 8 weeks; may become chronic with an unstable spondylolisthesis	Gradual improvement over 6-8 weeks; if ligamentous laxity is severe it could contribute to recurring chronic symptoms	Gradual improvement over 6-8 if source of irritation is removed	May worsen if pathology progresses
Past medical history	All structures may have previous medical issues that impact on the surrounding tissue		All structures may have previous medical issues that impact on the function of the surrounding tissue		Osteoporosis	All structures may have previous medical issues that impact on the function of the surrounding tissue			May have history of visceral pathology
Past surgeries	All structures may have previous surgeries that impact on the surrounding tissue		All structures may have previous surgeries that impact on the function of the surrounding tissue		May have history of hysterectomy	All structures may have previous surgeries that impact on the function of the surrounding tissue			May have history of surgery for visceral pathology
Special questions	Does the pain stay in your neck or go down your arm?				Are you on corticosteroids and are you a smoker? Excess alcohol use?			Is there anything you can do to change your pain?	
X-Rays	Negative with acute injury but will show disc narrowing later	Negative	Negative acutely but may show degenerative changes as it becomes chronic	Negative	Will show fractures and bony matrix/demineralization and spurring	Positive with fractures and degenerative changes	Usually negative but occasionally positive when there is calcification in the ligaments	Negative for the most part unless there is a lytic lesion on the spine from mets	Positive for pathology
MRI	Positive	Negative	Positive	Positive	Positive	Positive	Positive	May be positive depending on related pathology	Positive for pathology
EMG	Positive if nerve involvement	Not typically done here	Positive if nerves involved	Not done except if palsy is detected	Not done unless neural involvement	Not done unless neural involvement	Not typically done here	Positive	Not typically done
Special laboratory tests					Tests for Ca levels				Varies depending on pathology
Red flags					Current treatment or prior treatment for cancer				Rule out visceral structures

DJD, degenerative joint disease; DDD, degenerative disc disease; HNP, herniated nucleus pulposus; Fx, fracture; MRI, magnetic resonance imaging; EMG, electromyogram.

Section II

ORTHOPEDIC REASONING

water retention, brittle nails and hair loss, weight variations, tremors, sleep disturbances, mental changes (memory problems), and changes in vital signs.[9,45]

HEPATIC SYSTEM

- Pain from the liver and gallbladder can be referred to the right shoulder mimicking pain from a more proximal source. Patients can experience polymyalgias, arthritic symptoms, malaise, spider angiomas, jaundice, cutaneous vasculitis, and fibromyalgia symptoms. Other symptoms include confusion, sleep disturbances, muscle tremors, and pallor.[9,45]

CANCER

- Persons with a prior history of cancer, family history of cancer, history of smoking, and a job history that placed them around toxic substances will be at a greater risk for cancer. The onset of pain in the neck that is getting progressively worse without any prior history of trauma should be evaluated with caution. Hoarseness, Horner's syndrome, unexplained fatigue and malaise, problems with swallowing, shortness of breath, painless swelling of the lymph nodes in the neck, rapid unexplainable weight loss, night pain, and multiple level cervical nerve root involvement are all ominous signs that need to be evaluated by the patient's primary care physician.[9,45]

SUMMARY STATEMENT

The care of cervical spine problems continues to be an area of great concern in the United States, especially with the high incidence of whiplash-associated disorders. Most of the sustained symptoms seem to be related to damage to the facets. There does not seem to be any relationship to neck pain and degenerative joint disease. Many individuals with degenerative joint disease are asymptomatic. Neck pain is a common problem in our society and at any given time affects about 10% of the general population. The actual cause of the problem is frequently difficult to determine. Neck pain in as many as one-third of patients is not self-limiting and may produce moderate long-term disabilities. Table II-3-2 summarizes the factors that help a clinician differentiate among the different sources of symptoms in the cervical spine region.

Successful rehabilitation must involve early intervention before the fibroblastic stage. Except for some success with multimodal treatments of manual therapy, and instruction, combined with exercise, rehabilitation of the chronic neck will continue to be a challenge to the clinician. A further focus in research in the area of less common pain generators in the cervical spine is desperately needed.

REFERENCES

1. Ariens GA, van Mechelen W, Bongers PM, et al. Physical risk factors for neck pain. *Scand J Work Environ Health*. 2000;26(1):7-19 [Review].
2. Auvinen J, Tammelin T, Taimela S, et al. Neck and shoulder pain in relation to physical activity and sedentary activity in adolescents. *Spine*. 2007;32(9):1038-1044.
3. Baker AS, Ojemann RG, Morton NS. Ric. Spinal epidural abscess. *N Engl J Med*. 1975;293(10):463-468.
4. Barkhuizen A, Rosen H, Wolf S, et al. Musculoskeletal pain and fatigue are associated with chronic hepatitis. *Am J Gastroenterol*. 1999;94(5):1355-1360.
5. Barnsley L, Lord SM, Wallis BJ, Bogduk N. The prevalence of chronic cervical zygapophysial joint pain after whiplash. *Spine*. 1995;20(1):20-25 [discussion 26].
6. Berg E, Ciullo J. The SLAP lesion: A cause of failure after distal clavicle resection. *Arthroscopy*. 1997;13(1):85-89.
7. Birchall D, Connelly D, Walker L, Hall K. Evaluation of magnetic resonance myelography in the investigation of cervical spondylotic radiculopathy. *Br J Radiol*. 2003;76(908):525-531.
8. Boden SD, McCowin PR, Davis DO, et al. Abnormal magnetic-resonance scans of the cervical spine in asymptomatic subjects: A prospective investigation. *J Bone Joint Surg Am*. 1990;72(8):1178-1184.
9. Boissonnault WG, ed. *Examination in Physical Therapy Practice: Screening for Medical Disease*. 2nd ed. New York: Churchill Livingstone; 1995.
10. Braunstein EM, Martel W. Moidel Robert. Ankylosing spondylitis in men and women: A clinical and radiological comparison. *Radiology*. 1982;144(1):91-94.
11. Bronfort G, Evans R, Nelson B, et al. A randomized clinical trial of exercise and spinal manipulation for patients with chronic neck pain. *Spine*. 2001;26(7):788-797.
12. Buchelt M, Lack W, Kutschera HP, et al. Comparison of tuberculous and pyogenic spondylitis: An analysis of 122 cases. *Clin Orthop*. 1993;(296):192-199.
13. Cagnie B, Daneels L, Cools A, et al. The influence of breathing type, expiration and cervical posture on the performance of the cranio-cervical flexion test in healthy subjects. *Man Ther*. 2008;13(3):232-238.
14. Carlson EJ, Tominaga Y, Ivancic PC, Punjabi MM. Dynamic vertebral artery elongation during frontal and side impacts. *Spine*. 2007;7(2):222-228.
15. Carroll LJ, Hogg-Johnson S, van der Velde G, Haldeman S, et al. Course and prognostic factors for neck pain in the general population: results of the Bone and Joint Decade 2000-2010 Task Force on Neck Pain and Its Associated Disorders. *Spine*. 2008;33(4 suppl):S75-S82 [Review].
16. Chiu TT, Lam TH, Hedley AJ. A randomized controlled trial on the efficacy of exercise for patients with chronic neck pain. *Spine*. 2005;30(1):E1-E7.
17. Ciancaglini R, Testa M, Radaelli G. Association of neck pain with symptoms of temporomandibular dysfunction in the general adult population. *Scand J Rehabil Med*. 1999;31(1):17-22.
18. Clair DA, Edmonston SJ, Allison GT. Physical therapy treatment dose for nontraumatic neck pain: a comparison between 2 patient groups. *J Orthop Sports Phys Ther*. 2006;36(11):867-875.
19. Cleland JA, Flynn TW, Childs JD, Eberhart S. The Audible Pop from Thoracic Spine Thrust Manipulation and Its Relation to Short-Term Outcomes in Patients with Neck Pain. *J Manipulative Physiol Ther*. 2007;30(4):312-320.
20. Cloward R. Cervical discography. A contribution to the etiology of neck, shoulder, and arm pain. *Ann Surg*. 1959;150:1052-1064.
21. Cook C, Brismee JM, Fleming R, Sizer Jr PS. Identifiers suggestive of clinical cervical spine instability: a Delphi study of physical therapists. *Phys Ther*. 2005;85(9):895-906.
22. Cote P, Cassidy D, Carroll L. The Saskatchewan health and back pain survey: the prevalence of neck pain and related disability in Saskatchewan adults. *Spine*. 1998;23(15):1689-1985.
23. Cote P, Cassidy D, Carrol L, Kristman V. The annual incidence and course of neck pain in the general population: a population-based cohort study. *Pain*. 2004;112(3):267-273.
24. Curregee EJ, Hurwitz EL, Cheng I, et al. Treatment of neck pain: injections and surgical interventions: results of the Bone and Joint Decade 2000-2010 Task Force on Neck Pain and Its Associated Disorders. *Spine*. 2008;33(4 suppl):S153-S169.
25. DeJong RN. *The Neurologic Examination*. 3rd ed. New York: Harper & Row; 1967.
26. Doran MF, Brophy S, MacKay K, Taylor G, Calin A. Predictors of long-term outcome in ankylosing spondylitis. *J Rheum*. 2003;30(2):316-320.
27. Ducker TB. Post Traumatic progressive myelopathy in patient with congenital stenosis. *J Spinal Disord*. 1996;9(1):76 [discussion, 77-81].
28. Dutton M. *Orthopaedic Examination, Evaluation, and Intervention*. New York: McGraw-Hill Professional; 2004.
29. Duyff RF, Van den Bosch J, Martin D, Laman M, et al. Neuromuscular findings in thyroid dysfunction: a prospective clinical and electrodiagnostic study. *J Neurol Neurosurg Psychiatry*. 2000;68(6):750-755.
30. Dwyer A, Aprill C, Bogduk N. Cervical zygapophyseal joint pain patterns. I: A 7 study in normal volunteers. *Spine*. 1990;15(6):453-457.
31. Ebersold M, Pare M, Quast L. Surgical treatment for cervical spondylitic myelopathy. *J Neurosurg*. 1995;82(5):745-751.
32. Eck JC, Humphreys SC, Lim TH, et al. Biomechanical study on the effect of cervical spine fusion on adjacent-level intradiscal pressure and segmental motion. *Spine*. 2002;27(22):2431-2434.
33. Ehrmann-Feldman D, Shier I, Rossignol M, Abenhaim L. Risk factors for the development of neck and upper limb pain in adolescents. *Spine*. 2002;27(5):523-528.
33. El-Metwally A, Salminen JJ, Auvinen A, et al. Risk factors for development of non-specific musculoskeletal pain in preteens and early adolescents: a prospective 1-year follow-up study. *BMC Musculoskelet Disord*. 2007;8:46.
34. Eltayeb S, Staal JB, Kennes J, et al. Prevalence of complaints of arm, neck and shoulder among computer office workers and psychometric

evaluation of a risk factor questionnaire. *BMC Musculoskelet Disord.* 2007;8:68.

35. Erhard R, Bowling R. Treatment of the Cervical Spine. In: *Physical Therapy Home study course.* LaCrosse, WI: Orthopaedic Section American; 1996.

36. Eustace S, Coughlan RJ, McCarthy C. Ankylosing spondylitis. A comparison of clinical and radiographic features in men and women. *Ir Med J.* 1993;86(4):120-122.

37. Evans R, Bronfort G, Nelson B, Goldsmith C. Two-Year Follow-up of a Randomized Clinical Trial of Spinal Manipulation and Two Types of Exercise for Patients With Chronic Neck Pain. 2002;27(21):2383-2389.

38. Falla D, Bilenkij G, Jull G. Patients with chronic neck pain demonstrate altered patterns of muscle activation during performance functional upper limb tasks. 2004;29(13):1436-1440.

39. Fernández-de-las-Peñas C, Palomeque-del-Cerro L, Rodríguez-Blanco C, et al. Changes in neck pain and active range of motion after a single thoracic spine manipulation in subjects presenting with mechanical neck pain: a case series. *J Manipulative Physiol Ther.* 2007;30(4):312-320.

40. Ferrari R, Russell AS. Regional musculoskeletal conditions: neck pain. *Best Pract Res Clin Rheumatol.* 2003;17(1):57-70.

41. Fritz JM, Brennan GP. Preliminary examination of a proposed treatment-based classification system for patients receiving physical therapy interventions for neck pain. *Phys Ther.* 2007;7(5):513-524.

42. Fuller DA, Kirkpatrick JS, Emery SE, et al. A kinematic study of the cervical spine before and after segmental arthrodesis. *Spine.* 1998;23(15):1649-1656.

43. Fukui S, Ohseto K, Shiotani M, et al. Referred pain distribution of the cervical zygapophyseal joints and cervical dorsal rami. *Pain.* 1996;68(1):79-83.

44. Ghanayem AJ, Zdeblick TA. Cervical spine infections. *Orthop Clin North Am.* 1996;27(1):53-67 [Review].

45. Goodman CC, Snyder TEK. *Differential Diagnosis in Physical Therapy: Musculoskeletal and Systemic Conditions.* Philadelphia: WB Saunders; 1990.

46. Govender R, Wieselthalter NA, Ramanjam V, et al. Congenital cervical spinal cord lesions: pathogenesis, management, and outcome. *J Child Neurol.* 2007;22(7):874-879.

47. Graff-Radford SB. Myofascial Pain; diagnosis and management. *Curr Pain Headache Rep.* 2004;8(6):463-467.

48. Griegel-Morris P, Larson K, Mueller-Klaus K, Oatis CA. Incidence of common postural abnormalities in the cervical, shoulder, and thoracic regions and their association with pain in two age groups of healthy subjects. *Phys Ther.* 1992;72(6):425-431.

49. Gross AR, Hoving JL, Haines TA, et al. Manipulation and mobilization for mechanical neck disorders. *Cochrane Database Syst Rev.* 2004;(1):CD004249 [Review].

50. Gross AR, Goldsmith C, Hoving JL, et al. Conservative management of mechanical neck disorders: a systematic review. *J Rheumatol.* 2007;34(5):1083-1102.

51. Guez M. Chronic neck pain, an epidemiological, psychological and SPECT study with emphasis on WAD. *Acta Orthop.* 2006;77(Supp):320.

52. Guillemin F, Briancon S, Pourel J, Gaucher A. Long-term disability and prolonged sick leave as outcome measures in ankylosing spondylitis. *Arthritis Rheum.* 1990;33(7):1001-1006.

53. Gunderson CH, Greenspan RH, Glaser GH, et al. The Klippel-Feil Syndrome: genetic and clinical evaluation of cervical fusion. *Medicine (Baltimore).* 1967;46(6):491-512 [Review].

54. Gurvinder DS, Raghu NN, Andersson GB, et al. *Adjacent-level segmental motion after anterior cervical discectomy and fusion: ramifications for fusion versus disc replacement.* 31st Annual Meeting of the Cervical Spine Research Society, Phoenix, AR; 2003.

55. Haig AJ. Paraspinal denervation and the spinal degenerative cascade. *Spine.* 2002;2(5):372-380.

56. Hennsinger RN. Congenital anomalies of the cervical spine. *Clin Orthop Relat Res.* 1991;(264):16-38 [Review].

57. Hochman M, Tuli S. Cervical spondylotic myelopathy: a review. *Int J Neurol.* 2005;4(1).

58. Hogg-Johnson S, van der Velde G, Carroll LJ, et al. The burden and determinants of neck pain in the general population: results of the Bone and Joint Decade 2000-2010 Task Force on Neck Pain and Its Associated Disorders. 2008;33(4 suppl):S39-S51.

59. Hoppenfeld S, Hutton R, Thomas H. *Orthopaedic Neurology: A Diagnostic Guide to Neurologic Levels.* Philadelphia: Lippincott, Williams & Wilkins; 1977.

60. Hoving JL, de Vet HC, Twisk JW, et al. Prognostic factors for neck pain in general practice. *Pain.* 2006;60(8):839-848.

61. Hsu LCS, Leong JCY. Tuberculosis of the lower cervical spine (C2 to C7). *J Bone Joint Surg Br.* 1984;66(1):1-5.

62. Jones HR. *Netter's Neurology: Cervical Radiculopathy.* Philadelphia: WB Saunders; 2005.

63. Jull G, Trott P, Potter H, et al. A randomized controlled trial of exercise and manipulative therapy for cervicogenic headache. 2002;27(17):1835-1843.

64. Kaiser JA, Holland BA. Imaging of the cervical spine. *Spine.* 1998;23(24):2701-2712 [Review].

65. Kelsey JL, Githens PB, Walter SD, et al. An epidemiological study of acute prolapsed cervical intervertebral disc. *J Bone Joint Surg Am.* 1984;66(6):907-914.

66. Klein GR, Vaccaro AR, Albert TJ, et al. Efficacy of magnetic resonance imaging in the evaluation of posterior cervical spine fractures. *Spine.* 1999;24(8):771-774.

67. Kondo K, Molgaard CA, Kurland LT, et al. Protruded intervertebral cervical disk: Incidence and affected cervical level in Rochester, Minnesota, 1950 through 1974. *Minnesota Med.* 1981;64(12):751-753.

68. Korr IM. *The Neurobiologic Mechanisms In Manipulative Therapy.* New York: Plenum Press; 1978.

69. LeMura LM, Von Duvillard SP. *Clinical Exercise Physiology: Application and Physiological Principles.* Philadelphia: Lippincott, Williams & Wilkins; 2003.

70. Lepine JP, Briley M. The epidemiology of pain in depression. *Hum Psychopharmacol.* 2004;19(suppl 1):S3-S7 [Review].

71. Maak TG, Ivancic PC, Tominaga Y, Panjabi MM. Side impact causes multiplanar cervical spine injuries. *J Trauma.* 2007;63(6):1296-1307.

72. Magee D. *Orthopedic Physical Assessment.* 3rd ed. WB Saunders; 1987.

73. Mäkelä M, Heliövaara M, Sievers K, et al. Prevalence, determinants, and consequences of chronic neck pain in Finland. *J Epidemiol.* 1991;134(11):1356-1367.

74. Malawski SK, Lukawski S. Pyogenic infection of the spine. *Clin Orthop.* 1991;(272):58-66.

75. Manchikanti L, Singh V, Rivera J, Pampati V. Prevalence of cervical facet joint pain in chronic neck pain. *Pain Physician.* 2002;5(3):243-249.

76. McKenzie RA. *The Cervical and Thoracic Spine. Mechanical Diagnosis and Therapy.* Wakainae, New Zealand: Spinal Publications; 1990.

77. McNabb I, McCulloch JA. *Neck Ache and Shoulder Pain.* Philadelphia: Williams & Wilkins; 1994.

78. Modic MT, Feighlin DH, Piraino DW, et al. Vertebral osteomyelitis: assessment using MR. *Radiology.* 1985;157(1):157-166.

79. Mongini F, Ciccone G, Derigibus A, et al. Muscle tenderness in different headache types and its relation to anxiety and depression. *Pain.* 2004;112(1-2):59-64.

80. Montgomery DM, Brower RS. Cervical myelopathy: clinical syndrome and natural history. *Orthop Clin North Am.* 1992;23(3):487-493.

81. Moore K, Dalley AF, Agur AMR. *Clinically Oriented Anatomy.* 5rd ed. Philadelphia: Lippincott Williams & Wilkins; 2006.

82. Morio Y, Teshima R, Naqashima H, et al. Correlation between operative outcomes of cervical compression myelopathy and MRI of the spinal cord. *Spine.* 2001;26(11):1238-1245.

83. Muchrow RD, Resnick DK, Abdel MP, et al. Magnetic resonance imaging (MRI) in the clearance of the cervical spine in blunt trauma: a meta-analysis. *J Trauma.* 2008;64(1):179-189.

84. Murphy DR. *Conservative Management of Cervical Spine Syndromes.* New York: McGraw-Hill Professional; 1999.

85. Naranja RJ, Iannotti JP. Evaluation and Treatment of the Painful Shoulder after Rotator Cuff-Related Surgery. *UPOJ.* Spring 1997;(10):12-17.

86. Nardin RA, Patel MR, Gudas TF, et al. Electromyography and magnetic resonance imaging in the evaluation of radiculopathy. *Muscle Nerve.* 1999;22(2):151-155.

87. Nouwen A, Bush C. The relationship between EMG and chronic low back pain. *Pain.* 1984;20(2):109-123.

88. Nordin M, Carragee EJ, Hogg-Johnson S, et al. Assessment of neck pain and its associated disorders: results of the Bone and Joint Decade 2000-2010 Task Force on Neck Pain and Its Associated Disorders. *Spine.* 2008;33(4 suppl):S101-S122.

89. Nuñez Jr DB, Quencer RM. The role of helical CT in the assessment of cervical spine injuries. *Am J Roentgenol.* 1998;171(4):951-957.

90. Panjabi MM. The stabilizing system of the spine. Part 1. Function, dysfunction, adaptation, and enhancement. *J Spinal Disord.* 1992;5(4):383-389 [discussion 397].

91. Parke W. Correlative anatomy of cervical spondylotic myelopathy. *Spine.* 1988;13(7):831-837.

92. Persson LC, Carlsson CA, Carlsson JY. Long-lasting cervical radicular pain managed with surgery, physiotherapy, or a cervical collar. A prospective, randomized study. *Spine.* 1997;22(7):751-758.

93. Pui MH, Husen YA. Value of magnetic resonance myelography in the diagnosis of disc herniation and spinal stenosis. *Australas Radiol.* 2000;44(3):281-284.

94. Robertson D, Kincaid DW, Haile V, Robertson RM. The head and neck discomfort of autonomic failure: An unrecognized aetiology of headache. *Clin Auton Res.* 1994;4(3):99-103.

95. Sengupta DK, Kirollos R, Findlay GF, et al. The value of MR imaging in differentiating between hard and soft cervical disc disease: a comparison with intraoperative findings. *Eur Spine J.* 1999;8(3):199-204.

96. Shim JS, Noh KC, Park SJ. Treatment of congenital muscular torticollis in patients older than 8 years. *J Pediatr Orthop.* 2004;24(6):683-688.

97. Siegmund GP, Myers BS, Davis MB, et al. Human cervical motion segment flexibility and facet capsular ligament strain under combined posterior shear, extension and axial compression. *Stapp Car Crash J.* 2000;44:159-170.

98. Smith MG, Fulcher M, Shanklin J, Tillet ED. Prevalence of congenital cervical spinal stenosis in 262 college and high school football players. *J Ky Med Assoc.* 1993;91(7):273-275.

99. Steill IG, Wells GA, Vandemheem KL, et al. The Canadian C-spine rule for radiography in alert and stable trauma patients. *JAMA.* 2001;286(15):1841-1848.

100. Stemper BD, Yoganandan N, Pintar FA, et al. Anatomical gender differences in cervical vertebrae of size-matched volunteers. *Spine.* 2008;33(2):E44-E49.

101. Stemper BD, Yoganandan N, Pintar FA. Gender dependent cervical spine kinematics during whiplash. *J Biomech.* 2003;36:(9):1281-1289.

102. Symon L, Lavender P. The surgical treatment of cervical spondylotic myelopathy. *Neurology.* 1967;17(2):117-127.

103. Taimela S, Takala E, Asklof T, et al. Active treatment of neck pain: A prospective randomized intervention. *Spine.* 2000;25(8):1021-1027.

104. Travell JG, Simons DG. *Myofascial Pain and Dysfunction: The Trigger Point Manual: Volume 1, Upper half of body.* 2nd ed. Philadelphia: Lippincott, Williams & Wilkins; 1999.

105. Vandemark RM. Radiology of the cervical spine in trauma patients: practice pitfalls and recommendations for improving efficiency and communication. *Am J Roentgenol.* 1990;155(3):465-472 [Review].

106. van Gent C, Dols JJ, de Rover CM, et al. The weight of schoolbags and the occurrence of neck, shoulder, and back pain in young adolescents. *Spine.* 2003;28(9):916-921.

107. Watson JD, Broaddus WC, Smith MM, Kubal WS. Hyperactive pectoralis reflex as an indicator of upper cervical spinal cord compression. Report of 15 cases. *J Neurosurg.* 1997;86(1):159-161.

108. Webb R, Brammah T, Lunt M, et al. Prevalence and predictors of intense, chronic, and disabling neck and back pain in the UK general population. *Spine.* 2003;28(11):1195-1202.

109. Werner R. Carpal tunnel syndrome: pathophysiology and clinical neurophysiology. *Clin Neurophysiol.* 2002;113(9):1373-1381.

110. Whitten C, Donovan M, Cristobal K. Treating chronic pain: new knowledge, more choices. Clinical contributions. *The Permanente Journal.* Fall 2005;9(4).

111. Yamamoto T, Kurosawa K, Masuno N, et al. Congenital anomaly of cervical vertebrae is a major complication of Rubinstein-Taybi syndrome. *Am J Med Gen A.* 2005;135(2):130-133.

112. Ylinen JJ, Takala EP, Nykanen HJ, et al. Effects of twelve-month strength training subsequent to twelve-month stretching exercise in treatment of chronic neck pain. *J Strength Cond Res.* 2006;20(2):304-308.

113. Young WF. Cervical spondylotic myelopathy: a common cause of spinal cord dysfunction in older persons. *Am Fam Physician.* 2000;62(5):1064-1070, 1073 [Review].

114. Zheng Y, Liew SM, Simmons ED. Value of Magnetic Resonance Imaging and Discography in determining the level of cervical discectomy and fusion. *Spine.* 2004;29(19):2140-2145.

AUTHORS: PAUL E. MINTKEN and JOSHUA CLELAND

INTRODUCTORY INFORMATION

WHAT IS THE PREVALENCE OF THORACIC PATHOLOGY?

The prevalence of spinal pain in people 35 to 45 years of age has been reported to be 66%; however, only 15% reported that their pain was located in the thoracic region.[93] The 1-month prevalence of thoracic pain in adolescents 14 to 16 years of age has been reported to be approximately 20%.[152] In patients with chronic thoracic pain, the prevalence of zygapophyseal pain is estimated to be around 50%.[100] Osteoporotic vertebral fractures of the thoracic spine are relatively common and are estimated to be 5.1 per 1000 in women aged 55 to 64 years and 15 per 1000 in men. As the age increases over 75 years, the prevalence of osteoporosis in both sexes jumps to almost 3 in 100.[129]

WHAT IS THE PROGNOSIS FOR RECOVERY FROM THORACIC PATHOLOGY?

There is a paucity of published data on the natural history of acute thoracic spinal pain. Most acute sprains and strains resolve within 6 weeks. Manchikanti et al[100] found that of 500 patients with chronic spinal pain, only 6% had painful thoracic facet joints, compared to 25% and 28% in the lumbar spine and cervical spine, respectively.

WHAT IS THE REOCCURRENCE RATE FOR THORACIC PATHOLOGY?

To our knowledge, there have not been any studies investigating the recurrence rate of thoracic pathology. Most patients recover, but structural scoliosis may predispose the patient to chronic pain in the thoracic region. As noted, up to 6% of patients with chronic spinal pain have painful thoracic facets.

WHAT FACTORS MAKE DIAGNOSIS IN THE THORACIC AREA DIFFICULT?

Diagnosis of thoracic pain is complicated by the following factors:
- Radiographic findings do not correlate well with patient symptoms.[159,160]
- The cervical spine can refer pain into the thorax and many organ systems—including the gallbladder, stomach, liver, pancreas, appendix, reproductive organs, and intestines—and can cause pain in the thorax.[102]
- Diagnosis is further complicated by the intimate anatomical relationship between the thoracic spine and the autonomic nervous system.
- Finally, physical therapists need to be vigilant for signs and symptoms of neoplastic disease, as the thoracic spine is a common site for metastases.[118]

In general, it should be expected that mechanical thoracic pain can be influenced by movement or changes in posture, while pain from visceral structures and tumors may not.

CLINICAL PEARL

The thoracic spine tends to have less mobility than the cervical and lumbar regions due to the articulations with the rib cage and the fact that the ratio of the height of the disc to the vertebral body is 1:5, compared to 1:3 in the lumbar spine and 2:5 in the cervical spine.[28]

HOW SUCCESSFUL IS THERAPY IN TREATING THORACIC PATHOLOGY?

There is a lack of quality research studies investigating the effects of therapy on thoracic spine pain.

- Schiller[131] compared the use of thrust spinal manipulation with placebo ultrasound in a randomized controlled trial of 30 patients with mechanical thoracic spinal pain and found significantly better short-term reductions in pain ratings and an improvement in range of motion.
- Weiss et al[153] reported that in-patient rehabilitation with an intensive program of passive forces combined with intensive active spinal stabilization resulted in a statistically significant correction of structural kyphosis in patients with clear signs of Scheuermann disease.

CLINICAL DECISION MAKING CASE STUDY—PATIENT PROFILE

Your patient is a 23-year-old male who reports the onset of mid-back pain and rib cage pain after competing in a tug-of-war contest at a company picnic 2 weeks ago. He complains of pain when laying supine and taking a deep breath. He saw his physician, and radiographs were negative for fracture. He appears to have motion impairments, including limited thoracic extension and right rotation. You also note rib asymmetry on the right with palpation and restricted mobility of the rib cage on the right with deep inspirations. What are your hypotheses regarding his pathology? How would you approach intervention?

Answer

This patient most likely sprained a facet joint and/or a costovertebral joint, which is causing the pain with movement and breathing. Some treatment approaches advocate treating the rib impairments first, then focusing on the thoracic spine. We tend to operate in a pragmatic fashion and treat the thoracic spine first and then reassess any rib impairments.

HOW SUCCESSFUL IS SURGERY IN TREATING THORACIC PATHOLOGY?

Surgery is usually indicated only for patients with severe scoliosis or kyphosis, long-term symptomatic Scheuermann disease, or acute thoracic disc herniations or central canal stenosis with signs or symptoms of thoracic spinal cord myelopathy with progressive neurologic deficit.[149] Most patients respond well to conservative management.[149] Brown et al[12] retrospectively reviewed the magnetic resonance imaging (MRI) results of 55 patients with symptomatic thoracic disc herniations. Forty patients did well with conservative management, and 15 ultimately needed surgery. MRI was not useful in distinguishing the disc herniations that ultimately required surgery. In patients managed with conservative care, 80% return to previous activity levels. Palumbo et al[119] reported 2 to 9 year outcomes on 12 patients who underwent operative decompression for symptomatic stenosis of the lower thoracic spine. Although satisfactory short-term results were achieved, one patient lost neural function following surgery, and five patients had recurrent stenosis.

CLINICAL PEARL

The sympathetic innervation of the upper limb comes from T2 to T6, so treating this area may potentially have an effect on arm symptoms.[136]

PERSONAL INFORMATION

AGE

WHAT INFLUENCE DOES AGE HAVE ON YOUR CLINICAL DECISION-MAKING PROCESS IN THE THORACIC REGION? (See Table II-4-1)
- Under the age of 20 years, thoracic pain is as common as low back pain.

TABLE II-4-1 Differential Diagnosis of Back Pain

Condition	Patient Age (Years)	Location of Pain	Quality of Pain	Aggravating or Relieving Factors	Signs and Symptoms
Thoracic strain	20 to 40	Thoracic region	Ache, spasm	Increased with activity or bending	Local tenderness, limited spinal motion
Acute disc herniation	30 to 50	Local pain; may have radicular and/or myelopathic signs and symptoms	Sharp, shooting, or burning pain, paresthesia around chest wall or into legs	Decreased with standing; increased with bending, twisting, or sitting	Rare to have sensory changes; may have weakness and changes in reflexes if central cord is involved
Osteoarthritis	> 50	Thoracic and lumbar spine	Ache; may have sharp pain	Increased with extension; may be aggravated by any weight bearing or motion	Mild decrease in extension of spine
Spinal stenosis	> 50	Thoracic and lumbar spine; may have radiation to lower leg, often bilateral	Ache, shooting pain, "pins and needles" sensation	Increased with extension and walking, especially up an incline; decreased with sitting	Stenosis of the thoracic spine is more likely to directly affect the spinal cord because of the relatively narrow thoracic spinal canal; may have upper motor-neuron signs
Ankylosing spondylitis	15 to 40	Sacroiliac joints, thoracic and lumbar spine	Ache	Morning stiffness	Decreased back motion, tenderness over sacroiliac joints
Infection	Any age	Thoracic and/or lumbar spine, sacrum	Sharp pain, ache	Varies	Fever, percussive tenderness; may have neurological abnormalities or decreased motion
Malignancy	> 50	Affected bone(s)	Dull ache, throbbing pain; slowly progressive	Increased with recumbency or coughing	May have localized tenderness, neurological signs, or fever

Modified from Patel AT, Ogle AA. Diagnosis and management of acute low back pain. *Am Fam Physician* 2000;61:1779-1786, 1789-1790.

- In a study looking at 806 children and adolescents (aged 8 to 10 and 14 to 16 years, respectively), Wedderkopp et al[152] found that the 1-month prevalence of back pain was 39%, and thoracic pain was the most common area of spinal pain in childhood. Thoracic pain and lumbar pain were equally common in adolescence.
- Thoracic pain is also common in younger individuals with scoliosis (females more than males).
- Scheuermann disease most commonly presents between the ages of 13 and 16 years and is the most common cause of excessive kyphosis in adolescents.[96]
- Disc herniations are rare in children and adolescents.
- From 20 to 50 years of age, the incidence of facet and disc problems increases,[12,100] and the peak incidence of ankylosing spondylitis (AS) is 20 to 40 years of age.
  - Goh et al[58] noted that the prevalence of abnormal findings in the annuli, nuclei, and disc margins increased with increasing age.
  - Diffuse idiopathic skeletal hyperostosis (DISH) affects 3% to 6% of the population over 40 years of age and 11% aged over 70 years.[61]
- Over the age of 50 years, degenerative changes are a common source of thoracic pain.
  - In a patient over the age of 60 years presenting with acute thoracic spine pain, osteoporotic fracture must be considered along with central canal stenosis.[129]
  - Spinal stenosis of the thoracic spine is more likely to directly affect the spinal cord because of the relatively narrow thoracic spinal canal.

CLINICAL DECISION MAKING CASE STUDY—PATIENT PROFILE ?

Your patient is a 62-year-old female who presents to your clinic via direct access with a 4-week history of upper back pain. She does not recall any specific injury. She relates a previous history of breast cancer 3 years ago, and she was free of disease at her last checkup 6 months ago. She also states that her pain is worse at night. What are your initial thoughts? Does this patient need to be referred to a physician?

Answer

This patient has two factors that should make you seriously consider a referral to a physician. The fact that she has had cancer previously is a red flag (specificity of 0.98). Combine this with her age (age > 50 = specificity 0.71), and this patient should be redirected to a physician for further workup.[33,71]

OCCUPATION

WHAT INFLUENCE DOES A PATIENT'S OCCUPATION HAVE ON YOUR CLINICAL DECISION-MAKING PROCESS IN THE THORACIC REGION?

In general, any occupation that requires sustained postures, heavy lifting, or repetitive motion may place a patient at risk for developing thoracic pain. If the injury occurred at work, or is exacerbated by work, the clinician should question the patient as to the specific demands of the job. Full recovery may require the patient to alter duties at work to allow tissues to heal. The following repetitive motions may lead to specific pathologies:

- Repetitive flexion: Disc
- Repetitive rotation: Disc, facet, and rib pathologies
- Repetitive extension: Central or foraminal stenosis, facet sprains, injury to the posterior bony structures

From the low back pain literature, it is clear that the longer patients are off work, the less likely they are to return to their jobs. Godges et al[57] found that education and counseling regarding pain management, physical activity, and exercise can reduce the number of days off work in people with elevated fear-avoidance beliefs and acute low back pain. Linton[91] found a clear link between psychological variables and neck and back pain. The prospective studies indicated that psychological variables were related to the onset of pain and to acute, subacute, and chronic pain. Stress, distress, anxiety, mood and emotions, cognitive functioning, and pain behavior all were found to be significant factors.

CLINICAL PEARL

Numerous research articles have linked impairments in the thoracic spine with pain and dysfunction in other regions, including neck pain, whiplash, T4 syndrome, thoracic outlet syndrome,[86] shoulder pain, and arm pain.[7,20,23,43,44,114,127,138-140] The thoracic spine should be considered in all mechanical musculoskeletal upper-quarter dysfunctions.

GENDER

WHAT INFLUENCE DOES GENDER HAVE ON YOUR CLINICAL DECISION-MAKING PROCESS IN THE THORACIC REGION?

- Males are three times more likely to have AS than females.[42]
- Men are equally as likely to herniate a thoracic disc as women, but over time, degenerative changes in the discs are more common in men.[58]
- DISH is twice as common in men.[61]
- Schmorl's nodes are common in middle-aged women and are strongly genetically determined.[156]
- Adolescent girls are more likely than boys to develop scoliosis.[147]
- In a study of over 46,000 twins, Damborg et al[29] reported the prevalence of Scheuermann disease to be 2.8%, and the male-to-female ratio was close to 2:1. They also reported a major genetic contribution to the etiology of Scheuermann disease.

CLINICAL DECISION MAKING CASE STUDY—PATIENT PROFILE

Your patient is a 28-year-old male who complains of a gradual onset of low back and thoracic pain and stiffness that began 4 months ago. Laying supine does not improve his symptoms. He states that he wakes up at night with intense pain and stiffness that is relieved only by a hot shower. Once he wakes up in the morning and starts moving, he feels much better. He actually states that he feels best after 3 hours of hiking. He reports a family history of lupus. What are your initial thoughts regarding this patient? Does this profile sound like mechanical back pain?

Answer

AS must be ruled out in this patient.[34] A classic sign is that the symptoms are made better with movement and worsen with rest or inactivity.

History	Sensitivity	Specificity
1. Age at onset < 40 years	1.00	0.07
2. Pain not relieved by supine position	0.80	0.49
3. Morning back stiffness	0.64	0.59
4. Pain duration > 3 months	0.71	0.54
5. Did the pain begin slowly?		
Four of the five questions above positive	0.23	0.82

ETHNICITY

WHAT INFLUENCE DOES ETHNICITY HAVE ON YOUR CLINICAL DECISION-MAKING PROCESS IN THE THORACIC REGION?

There have been very few studies investigating the role of ethnicity in thoracic conditions. The astute clinician must keep in mind that cultural differences exist in both the attitudes of health care providers and the coping strategies patients utilize to deal with pain and disability.[13,45,132,145] Treatment strategies, patient education, and prognosis may need to be altered in light of this.

- DISH is common in Japanese and Pima Indians but rare in black and Asian races.[61]
- Bauer and Deyo[3] reported that the risk of osteoporotic fractures was substantially lower in Hispanic women compared to non-Hispanic women.

SYMPTOM HISTORY

MECHANISM OF INJURY

WHAT INFLUENCE DOES THE MECHANISM OF INJURY HAVE ON YOUR CLINICAL DECISION-MAKING PROCESS IN THE THORACIC REGION?

It is important to establish both the duration of symptoms and any causative factors.

- Trauma or a specific identifiable mechanism of injury (MOI) usually point toward potential fractures, strains of muscle tissue, or sprains of ligaments and joints (facet, costovertebral, etc.). Discs may be injured via trauma or overuse.[8]
- If the onset is sudden and there is not an identifiable MOI, other causative factors, such as sustained postures and repetitive motions, must be investigated. Potential causes of sudden onset of pain include facet sprain, capsular entrapment, and disc pathology.[10]
- If the onset is insidious and gradual, degenerative changes, stenosis, or potential visceral referral should be considered.[85]

LOCATION OF SYMPTOMS

WHAT INFLUENCE DOES THE LOCATION OF SYMPTOMS HAVE ON YOUR CLINICAL DECISION-MAKING PROCESS IN THE THORACIC REGION?

Mechanical pain in the thoracic spine and rib cage generally presents very close to the source of the symptoms. There may be referral to the anterior chest wall if the intercostal nerves are involved, but it is very rare for pain originating from the thoracic spine to refer more than one or two levels proximal or distal to the source.[38,51]

REFERRAL OF SYMPTOMS

- Thoracic disc: The thoracic disc may be a pain generator. Although there have not been any studies mapping the referral patterns of the thoracic discs, the surgical literature tells us that they may cause either radicular or myelopathic signs and symptoms or a combination of both.[2] Mellion and Ladeira,[105] in a literature review, reported that 63% of symptomatic patients presented with weakness, 60% had sensory complaints, 59% had hyperreflexia, 57% had radicular pain, 48% had back pain, and 25% had bowel or bladder symptoms. Schellhas et al[130] utilized thoracic discography in patients with thoracic pain. When they injected abnormal thoracic discs (identified via MRI) and at least one control level with contrast or saline, they found a reproduction of the familiar pain (defined as clinical concordance) in approximately 50% of the cases. Discs that had tears in the annulus fibrosis, intrinsic degeneration, and/or vertebral body endplate pathology were painful 75% of the time, but control levels were usually painless.

CLINICAL PEARL

Up to 37% of asymptomatic people have thoracic disc protrusions, so the results of imaging should be interpreted with caution and correlated to the physical examination.[160]

- Zygapophyseal joint: Dwyer et al[40] reported that C5 to C7 can refer to the upper thoracic spine and scapular region; therefore, it is essential to screen the cervical spine in any patient presenting with thoracic pain. Dreyfuss et al[38] demonstrated that the thoracic zygapophyseal joints can generate both local and referred pain in asymptomatic subjects. They injected contrast medium into the thoracic zygapophyseal joints from T3 to T11. The most intense area of pain was slightly lateral and one segment inferior to the joint injected. T3 to T5 caused referral to the anterior chest wall in two subjects. Superior referral was rare, but distal referral was up to 2.5 segments below. Fukui et al[51] injected contrast media from C7 to T3 and from T11 to T12 in 15 symptomatic subjects and found that C7 to T3 demonstrated extensive overlap, with symptoms reported in the paravertebral and interscapular region and the superior and inferior angles of the scapula. The T11 to T12 segment produced pain around the site of injection and the area over the iliac crest from T11 to T12. (See Figure II-4-1.)
- Costovertebral joints: The costovertebral and costotransverse joints may also generate pain. Although there have been no mapping studies that we are aware of, Benhamou et al[6] found that injection into the costovertebral joint relieved pseudovisceral pain in a case series of 28 patients. Due to the proximity of the sympathetic chain, dysfunction in the costovertebral joints may cause pseudovisceral pain.

CLINICAL PEARL

Up to 13% of chest pain in a medical setting is referred pain from the thoracic spine and rib cage.[4]

- Muscles and their referral patterns[134] (see Figure II-4-2):
  - Levator scapulae: Posterior shoulder and medial edge of the scapula
  - Latissimi dorsi: Inferior angle of the scapula, posterior shoulder, iliac crest
  - Rhomboids: Medial border of the scapula
  - Trapezius: Upper thoracic spine to the medial border of the scapula
  - Serratus anterior: Locally around the scapula and anterior into the ribs
  - Iliocostalis thoracis: Ipsilateral low back and lower abdominal quadrant
  - Longissimus thoracis: Ipsilateral low back and medial gluteal region
  - Serratus posterior inferior: Lateral to spine in T9 to T12 posterior to the rib area
- Tendons and ligaments: No studies have been performed on tendon or ligament injury. In our experience, ligament sprains can present with severe pain that later can result in stiffness.
- Bone: Bone pain from degenerative changes or spondylosis may present as dull, deep, achy pain. If the degeneration is severe and compresses nerve roots, it may present as radiating symptoms that follow the path of the ribs or may be described as a "through the chest" pain.[98]
- Joint (capsule/cartilage): Facet syndromes typically present as stiffness and local pain.[98] See the section on zygapophyseal joint pain above.
- Nerves: There is a significant overlap of dermatomes in the thoracic spine, so the absence of a single dermatome may not result in sensory loss
  - Dermatomes tend to follow the ribs. Thoracic nerve-root pain can be severe and may refer in a sloping band along the intercostal

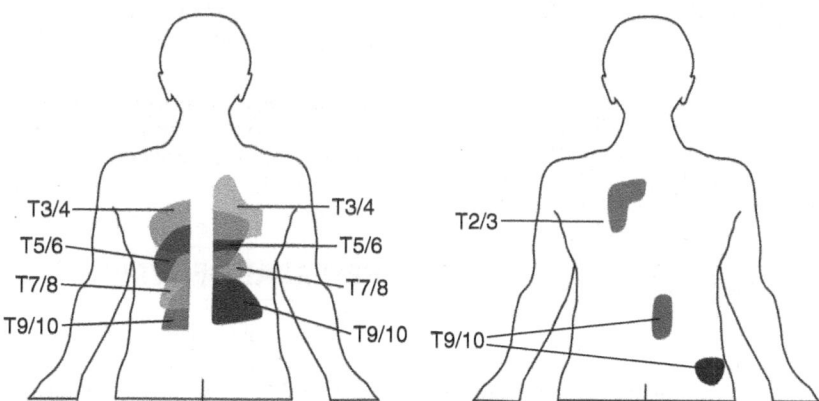

FIGURE II-4-1 Thoracic zygapophyseal facet referral.

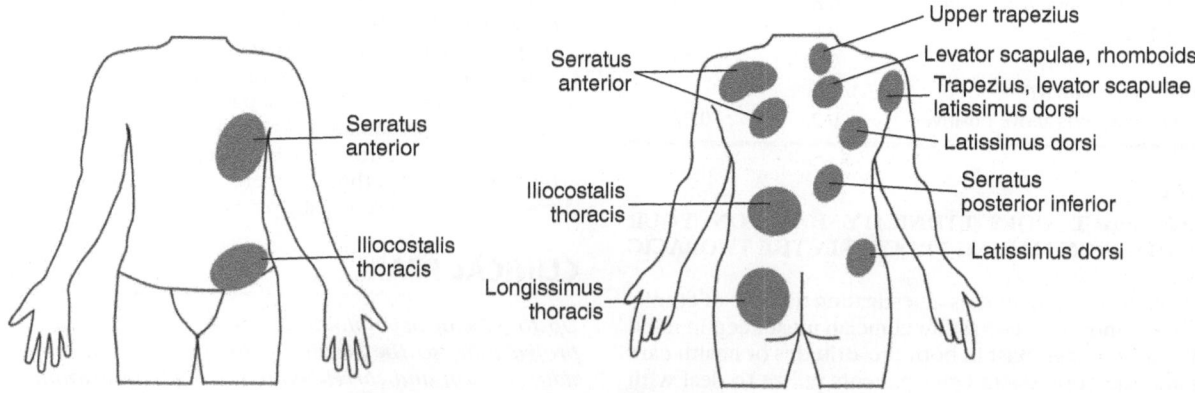

FIGURE II-4-2 Thoracic muscle referral pattern.

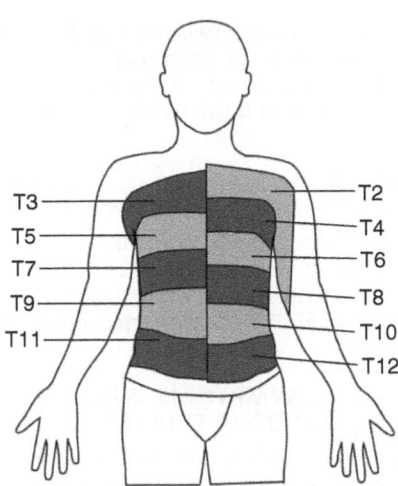

FIGURE II-4-3 Thoracic nerve-root dermatomal referral pattern.

space.[98] Referred pain from thoracic spinal nerve roots may present as follow: (see Figure II-4-3)
1. T5: Pain around the nipple
2. T7: Pain in the epigastric region
3. T10 to T11: Pain in the epigastric or umbilical region
4. T12: Pain in the groin[98]
○ Myotomal distribution of thoracic nerve roots

Rectus abdominis	T6 to T12
External and internal oblique	T7 to T12
Iliocostalis thoracis	T1 to T12
Longissimus thoracis	T1 to T12
Semispinalis thoracis	T1 to T12
Multifidus and rotators	T1 to T12 locally
Serratus posterior inferior	T9 to T12
Serratus posterior superior	Intercostal nerves 2 to 5
Intercostals	Intercostal nerves T1 to T11
Levatores costarum	Dorsal primary rami of spinal nerves C7 to T11
Transversus thoracis	Intercostal nerves 2 to 6
Interspinales	Spinal nerves T1 to T12
Intertransversarii	Spinal nerves T1 to T12 locally
Multifidus and rotators	Spinal nerves T1 to T12 locally

• Vascular systems: Vascular disorders tend to present as throbbing or pounding symptoms, and a thoracic aortic aneurysm may present with pain in the thoracic spine and a palpable pulse in the abdomen.[50]
• Visceral structures: Visceral pain tends to be deep, diffuse, and dull and may include nausea or sweating. It also tends to follow dermatomal patterns; for example, ulcers may refer to T4 to T6, and stomach pain may refer to T6 to T8.[98]

WHAT OTHER MUSCULOSKELETAL STRUCTURES CAN REFER INTO THE THORACIC REGION?
The cervical spine can refer into the thoracic spine and scapular region.[40] Pain between the shoulder blades commonly originates in the cervical spine.[98] It is rare in our clinical experience for lumbar structures to refer proximally into the thoracic spine; however, the thoracolumbar junction is a frequent source of dysfunction in patients with thoracic and lumbar region pain.

WHAT VISCERAL STRUCTURES CAN REFER INTO THE THORACIC REGION?
Visceral structures may manifest as thoracic pain. The stomach, gallbladder, liver, pancreas, intestines, heart, lungs, reproductive

organs, and the appendix may refer pain into the thoracic spine.[102] See Figure II-4-4, which illustrates the referral pattern of visceral structures into the thoracic region.

CLINICAL PEARL

Extension of the thoracic spine is necessary for most overhead functional activities, so impairments in thoracic motion may predispose the patient to injury in the neck and shoulder.[138,140]

SYMPTOM DESCRIPTORS

QUALITY OF SYMPTOMS
• Deep ache: Bone or disc[161]
• Dull ache: Bone, degenerative changes
• Sharp pain: Facet joints, joint capsule, acute ligament sprains
• Sharp and continuous pain: Bone or acute inflammation
• Dull and continuous pain: Viscera
• Burning: Nerves (common with intercostal neuralgia; shingles may also present with an itching sensation)[115]
• Tingling: Nerves
• Numbness: Nerves
• Nausea, colicky, and cramping: Viscera
• Pain with breathing: Ribs versus pulmonary problems

DEPTH OF SYMPTOMS
WHAT INFLUENCE DOES THE DEPTH OF SYMPTOMS HAVE ON YOUR CLINICAL DECISION-MAKING PROCESS IN THE THORACIC REGION (I.E., SUPERFICIAL VERSUS DEEP)?
• Deep symptoms implicate deep structures such as disc, bone, and viscera. There are fewer proprioceptive nerves in deep structures than in more superficial structures, so the ability to localize tissue damage in deep structures is more difficult.
• Superficial symptoms implicate surface structures such as muscles and ligaments. Superficial structures have more proprioceptive nerve fibers, and thus injury to superficial structures is more easily localized.

CONSTANCY OF SYMPTOMS
WHAT INFLUENCE DOES CONSTANCY OF SYMPTOMS HAVE ON YOUR CLINICAL DECISION-MAKING PROCESS IN THE THORACIC REGION?
Constant pain should raise concerns, especially if it does not vary, as it may indicate a systemic cause of the pain. On the other hand, if the symptoms are intermittent or constant but change with movement, this is consistent with mechanical thoracic pain.
• Intermittent symptoms implicate a mechanical source and a structure that is injured and is aggravated only with certain positions or motions.
• Constant but varying symptoms may implicate inflammation as the primary source.
• Constant and unchanging symptoms implicate visceral structures or other pathology such as cancer.

CLINICAL DECISION MAKING CASE STUDY—PATIENT PROFILE

You patient is a 42-year-old male who reports a 3-day history of thoracic back pain and a radiating, burning sensation that courses around his torso to just below his nipple line. On observation, he appears to have skin lesions that follow his right seventh rib. He also complains of an itching sensation that causes him to scratch the area intensely. What is your initial hypothesis regarding this patient's pathology? Would you refer him out?

Answer

The most likely cause of the patient's symptoms is an outbreak of shingles (herpes zoster). This patient should be referred, as antiviral drugs may alter the course of the disease, reducing both pain in the acute phase and the risk of postherpetic neuralgia.[67,115]

TWENTY-FOUR–HOUR SYMPTOM PATTERN

IF A PATIENT HAS SYMPTOMS IN THE MORNING, WHAT PATHOLOGY DOES THIS IMPLICATE?

- If a patient is awakened at night by pain not caused by changes in position, the therapist should investigate a nonmusculoskeletal cause. If a patient wakes up with intense pain and stiffness in the early morning hours (3 to 4 am) that improves with movement or a hot shower, this may be suggestive of AS.
- It is common for a patient with thoracic symptoms to have stiffness in the morning. Stiffness and pain that resolve quickly with movement usually represent a mechanical pathology. Degenerative joint disease, facet pathology, and stenosis may present as stiffness in the morning that resolves quickly with motion.
- Sharp pain and stiffness that persist for greater than 30 minutes may implicate inflammation. Typically these symptoms will improve slowly with movement as circulation is increased in the region and the lymphatic system works to remove edema via muscle contraction and compression.

CLINICAL PEARL

!

Rib fractures are very common (up to 10% of trauma patients may have rib fractures), but up to 50% of rib fractures are missed on standard chest radiographs.[39] The main symptoms with rib fractures include pain on inspiration, palpable tenderness, and possible crepitation. Stress fractures of the first rib are common in overhead activities.[25]

WHAT ROLE DOES MORNING STIFFNESS PLAY IN DIFFERENTIATION?

Morning stiffness is a moderately sensitive and specific finding (0.64 and 0.59, respectively) for AS.[3] The cardinal signs of rheumatoid arthritis are stiffness, swelling, and pain of one or more joints of the body characteristically most severe in the morning.[144]

- As we sleep, the body is in a position of stasis, which can lead to an accumulation of fluid in the area. As stated, the lymphatic system is a passive system that requires muscle contraction and motion to clear fluid, be it from inflammation or metabolic waste processing.
- Stiffness that lasts only minutes and is relieved quickly with motion is more often associated with mechanical factors than with inflammatory factors.
- Following an acute injury to a tissue, the inflammatory response begins to lay down collagen to heal the injured area. If muscle spasm or fear of movement lead to avoidance of movement, stiffness may occur.

IF A PATIENT HAS SYMPTOMS IN THE AFTERNOON, WHAT PATHOLOGY DOES THIS IMPLICATE?

- The pain of osteoarthritis is typically less intense in the morning than in the afternoon or evening. Pain in the afternoon may implicate degenerative changes, disc pathology, stenosis, or soft-tissue injuries. Differentiation is dependent on the postures and activities throughout the day. If patients are sitting in sustained postures, or bending and/or twisting during the day, they may be more symptomatic by the afternoon.
- Soft-tissue injuries to ligaments and muscles may be more symptomatic in the afternoon if the tissues are stressed repeatedly throughout the day.

IF A PATIENT HAS SYMPTOMS IN THE EVENING, WHAT PATHOLOGY DOES THIS IMPLICATE?

- The pain of osteoarthritis is typically more intense in the evening.
- Any soft-tissue injury or degenerative change may be worse in the evening if it is irritated by sustained postures and repetitive movements. Mechanical pathology typically gets worse at the end of the day.

IF A PATIENT HAS SYMPTOMS WHEN SLEEPING, WHAT PATHOLOGY DOES THIS IMPLICATE?

- Pain at night not associated with movement that wakes a patient up is suggestive of visceral pathology including metastatic diseases.[33]
- Bone pain, whether from cancer or trauma, is usually worse at night and presents as an aching, deep, intense pain.
- Mechanical thoracic pain will commonly wake a patient up during the course of normal nocturnal changes of position, so the key question is whether the patient woke up from a dead sleep (without movement) or woke up while rolling over (with movement).[9]

STABILITY OF SYMPTOMS

CHANGES IN SYMPTOMS

HOW DOES THE PROGRESSION OF A PATIENT'S SYMPTOMS IMPACT YOUR CLINICAL DECISION-MAKING PROCESS?

- Maitland[99] popularized an approach to clinical decision making that took into account the severity, irritability, nature, stage, and stability (SINNS) of a patient's symptoms. If a patient's symptoms are unchanging or improving, they are usually considered stable, and examination and treatment can be more aggressive. If a patient's symptoms are getting worse, this would be classified as unstable using the SINSS system; the examination and intervention should then be more conservative, and symptoms should be monitored regularly.

IF A PATIENT'S SYMPTOMS ARE IMPROVING, WHAT PATHOLOGY DOES THIS IMPLICATE?

- Simple sprains and strains typically follow a course of rapid improvement, barring any repetitive motions or sustained postures that impede healing.[103]
- Facet pathology will generally improve in several days to weeks.
- Disc pathology typically improves over the course of 4 to 6 weeks.[135]
- If there is no improvement by 6 weeks, imaging should be considered.[71]

IF A PATIENT'S SYMPTOMS ARE WORSENING, WHAT PATHOLOGY DOES THIS IMPLICATE?

- Symptoms that worsen over a short period of time may implicate inflammation and nociceptive response due to the injury. As the inflammatory process begins, surrounding structures can be irritated by the chemical mediators released due to the inflammatory process. If the process continues unabated, the swelling may begin to compress other structures such as neural tissue.[121]
- Mechanical symptoms that do not change over time are more indicative of degenerative changes. Symptoms may get worse or better episodically, but the baseline symptoms remain

constant. Movement and exercise generally ease symptoms. As the degenerative conditions progress, the symptoms may worsen slowly over time.[121]

- Panjabi[121] theorized that microtrauma to spinal ligaments, facet capsules, and the annulus of the disc may lead to chronic back pain due to muscle control dysfunction via the following sequence:
  - Single trauma or cumulative microtrauma causes microtrauma to the ligaments and embedded mechanoreceptors.
  - The injured mechanoreceptors generate abnormal transducer signals, which lead to changes in muscle response patterns produced by the neuromuscular control unit.
  - Changes then occur in muscle activation and coordination. This results in abnormal stresses and strains in the ligaments, mechanoreceptors, and muscles, along with excessive loading of the facet joints.
  - Due to inherently poor healing of spinal ligaments, accelerated degeneration of the disc and facet joints may occur. The abnormal conditions may persist and, over time, lead to chronic back pain via inflammation of neural tissues.

CLINICAL PEARL

Regional interdependence *is defined as "dysfunction and impairments in distant regions, both extremity and spine, that may affect or contribute to a patient's primary complaint."*[151] *Impairments in the thoracic spine may induce compensatory changes in the shoulder, cervical spine, and lumbar spine.*

FUNCTIONAL AND ACTIVITY PARTICIPATION LIMITATIONS (See Table II-4-2)

BEHAVIOR OF SYMPTOMS: AGGRAVATING BEHAVIOR

WHAT INFLUENCE DO AGGRAVATING FUNCTIONS HAVE ON YOUR CLINICAL DECISION-MAKING PROCESS IN THE THORACIC REGION?

Flexion-based activities

- Pathologies aggravated by flexion include disc pathology, muscle strain, radiculopathy caused by disc pathology, and ligament strain.[121]
- Spinal flexion will lengthen the posterior longitudinal, interspinous, and supraspinous ligaments as well as the ligamentum flavum.[155]
- Flexion of the spine elongates the spinal canal up to 97 mm with the greatest elongation occurring in the lumbar and thoracic regions. Extension shortens the spinal canal 38 mm.[11]

Extension-based activities

- Pathologies aggravated by extension include facet pathology, radiculopathy caused by stenosis, central canal stenosis, and interforaminal stenosis.
- Acute, sharp back pain may be secondary to facet involvement and has been attributed to the entrapment or compression of the joint capsule, degenerative changes, or meniscoid entrapment.[99]
- The main joint of concern in patients with degenerative joint disease is the zygapophyseal or facet joint. The facets limit

TABLE II-4-2 Functional and Activity-Participation Limitations

Motion	Functional Activities	Pathology if Symptoms Are Aggravated by Activity	Pathology if Symptoms Are Eased by Activity
Flexion	Sitting, bending forward, squatting	Disc pathology, muscle strain, posterior ligament sprain, radiculopathy caused by disc herniation	Facet pathology, radiculopathy caused by stenosis, central canal stenosis, interforaminal stenosis, spondylolithesis
Extension	Walking, bending backward, working overhead	Facet pathology, anterior ligament strain, interforaminal stenosis, central stenosis, radiculopathy caused by stenosis, degenerative disc disease	Disc pathology, radiculopathy caused by disc herniation, ligament strain
Lateral flexion and rotation	Bending and twisting, lifting; sports or occupations that require frequent position changes	Facet pathology, radiculopathy, interforaminal stenosis, muscle strain	Disc pathology, muscle strain, radiculopathy, ligament strain, facet joint, interforaminal stenosis
Combined motion	Extension and rotation/lateral flexion	Facet pathology, radiculopathy, ligament strain, central canal stenosis, interforaminal stenosis, muscle strain	Disc pathology, radiculopathy, ligament strain, muscle strain
Combined motion	Flexion and rotation/lateral flexion	Disc pathology, radiculopathy, ligament strain, muscle strain	Facet joint, radiculopathy, ligament strain, interforaminal stenosis, muscle strain
Static positions	Supine, sitting, standing	Prolonged sitting may irritate disc pathology while prolonged standing or lying down may irritate stenotic conditions; ankylosing spondylitis gets worse with inactivity	Disc pathology, muscle strain, ligament strain, facet pathology, central canal stenosis, interforaminal stenosis
General movement	Walking, transfers, activities of daily living	Inflammatory conditions tend to be painful with any movement until the swelling decreases; if everything is painful, it probably signifies an acute inflammatory condition	Ankylosing spondylitis tends to improve with movement
Other	Breathing, coughing, laughing, sneezing, going to the bathroom (Valsalva maneuver)	Rib fractures, chest wall injuries, disc pathology, radiculopathy, spondylosis, muscle strain	None

rotation, protect the disc, and function as load-bearing structures in extension.[155] Consequently, extension-based activities such as walking and working overhead may patients with degenerative joint disease.

- Central canal and intervertebral foraminal stenosis are both impacted by extension. Extension decreases the intervertebral foramen by 20% and also decreases the cross-sectional area of the central canal.[119]

Lateral flexion and rotation activities
- Pathologies aggravated by lateral flexion include facet pathology, radiculopathy, interforaminal stenosis, and muscle strains.
- In muscular injuries, lateral flexion away from the injured tissue may result in pain.
- In facet injuries or cases of foraminal stenosis, lateral flexion or rotation to the same side will close down on the injured tissue and may cause pain.

Combined motion activities
- Pathologies aggravated by extension and rotation/lateral flexion include facet joint, radiculopathy due to stenosis, ligament strain, central canal stenosis, interforaminal stenosis, and muscle strain.
- Pathologies aggravated by flexion and rotation/lateral flexion include disc pathology, radiculopathy due to disc pathology, ligament strain, and muscle strain.

Static activities
- Panjabi conceptualized a model in which joint stability is controlled by the coordinated actions of three subsystems, the passive, active, and neural subsystems. The ligaments, vertebrae, and discs make up the passive subsystem, the muscles and tendons make up the active subsystem, and the nerves and central nervous system make up the neural subsystem.[122] A dysfunction of one of the subsystems may lead to one or more of the following three possibilities: (1) an immediate compensation from another subsystem, (2) a long-term compensation of one or more subsystems, and (3) an injury to the components of subsystem.[122,123]
- If all three subsystems are not working optimally, sustained postures may lead to further pain and injury.[121]
- For example, sustained extension may aggravate facet pathologies, degenerative changes, and stenosis. Sustained flexion may aggravate injuries to the disc, ligaments, and muscles.

Other activities
- The thoracic spine and rib cage work together for respiration. Therefore, pain may be experienced with breathing.[84]
- Any Valsalva maneuver, including coughing and sneezing, may increase disc pressure and aggravate conditions involving the disc and nerve root.[150]

CLINICAL DECISION MAKING CASE STUDY—PATIENT PROFILE ?

Your patient is a 65-year-old male who has had thoracic and low back pain on and off for years. In the past 6 months, he noted the onset of bilateral radiating leg pain, numbness, and tingling. Standing erect and walking make his symptoms worse; sitting in a flexed position completely alleviates his symptoms. His deep tendon reflexes in the lower extremities are hyperactive, and he has a positive Babinski test. What is your hypothesis?

Answer
The most likely cause of his symptoms is central canal stenosis in the thoracic spine. Symptoms of stenosis typically get worse with extension and better with flexion. The fact that the reflexes are elevated and the fact that he has a positive Babinski test suggest that the cord compression is proximal

(above L1 or L2) and most likely represents an upper motor-neuron lesion.

BEHAVIOR OF SYMPTOMS: EASING BEHAVIOR
WHAT INFLUENCE DO EASING FUNCTIONS HAVE ON YOUR CLINICAL DECISION-MAKING PROCESS?
Flexion-based activities
- The cross-sectional area of the spinal canal increases with flexion, and flexion opens the intervertebral foramen. The area of the spinal canal decreases with extension.[155]
- Pathologies eased by flexion include facet pathology, radiculopathy, central canal stenosis, and interforaminal stenosis.
- Radicular symptoms that ease with flexion are associated with stenotic changes.

Extension-based activities
- The cross-sectional area of the spinal canal decreases with extension, and extension closes the intervertebral foramen.[155]
- Pathologies eased by extension include posterior disc herniations, disc-related radiculopathy, and ligament strains.
- Extension-based activities will take the stress off of the posterior spinal ligaments.

Lateral flexion and rotation activities
- Pathologies eased by lateral flexion and rotation include disc pathology, muscle strain, radiculopathy, ligament strain, facet pathology, and interforaminal stenosis.
- Lateral flexion to the contralateral side opens the foramen and the facets while lengthening the muscles and ligaments. Lateral flexion to the same side (ipsilateral) closes the facets on that side and puts slack into the ligaments and muscles.

Combined-motion activities
- Depending on the pathology, combined motion may be aggravating or easing. In general, extension and rotation/lateral flexion may ease posterior and posterolateral disc protrusions while flexion and rotation/lateral flexion may ease symptoms of stenosis. If it is a soft-tissue injury (muscle or ligament), combined motions that put slack on the tissue may decrease symptoms.

Static activities
- Any sustained posture or activity may ease symptoms if it takes pressure off of injured tissue or puts slack into the system. The classic example is spinal stenosis in which extension exacerbates symptoms but a sustained posture, such as sitting, can completely alleviate symptoms.[71] Other pathologies that may benefit from static activities include certain disc pathologies, muscle and ligament strains and sprains, and facet pathology.

General movement
- The thoracic spine is a stable area by nature due to the articulations with the ribs. Generally speaking, the thoracic spine lacks mobility compared to the rest of the spine, so general movement helps most conditions, particularly degenerative changes.

MEDICAL HISTORY

WHAT ROLE DOES A PATIENT'S PAST MEDICAL HISTORY PLAY IN DIFFERENTIAL DIAGNOSIS OF PATHOLOGY?
- Previous injuries and medical problems can influence the normal function of the thoracic spine as well as the degree of disability caused by injuries in this region.
- Slover et al[137] explored the correlation between medical and psychosocial comorbidities in patients with spinal pain (cervical, thoracic, and lumbar) and found that there was an increase in the baseline Oswestry with the addition of each comorbidity. The strongest association was seen with the medical comorbidities of smoking, frequent headaches, osteoarthritis, and osteoporosis.

- In a patient presenting with a new onset of back pain, a past history of cancer is a red flag, and the patient should be screened to rule out cancer as the cause of back pain.[68]
- Pathologies that commonly cause pain in the thoracic region include DISH, AS, osteoporosis, as well as any pathology of the kidneys, lungs, esophagus, gallbladder, heart, and liver.[49]
- Previous musculoskeletal injuries can lead to biomechanical changes in the amount and type of stress placed on the spine. A thorough physical examination should attempt to identify any postural or biomechanical abnormalities.

CLINICAL DECISION MAKING CASE STUDY—PATIENT PROFILE

The patient is a 26-year-old female graduate student who presents with a 2-month history of pain in the right upper back, shoulder, and arm. She also felt paresthesias in all digits of her right hand, glove-like numbness of the hand and forearm, weakness, hand clumsiness, and a deep aching pain in her upper thoracic spine and right shoulder. Springing of the upper thoracic spine was deemed hypomobile and exactly reproduced her symptoms. What is your initial hypothesis?

Answer
T4 syndrome refers to a clinical pattern that involves upper extremity pain and paresthesias with or without symptoms into the neck and/or head.[99] Passive movement of an upper thoracic vertebrae (commonly T4) may reproduce the symptoms.[23] The sympathetic nervous system may provide a pathway for referral from the thoracic spine to the head and arms, so thoracic manual therapy should be considered.

MEDICAL AND ORTHOPEDIC TESTING

WHAT MEDICAL AND ORTHOPEDIC TESTS INFLUENCE YOUR DIFFERENTIAL DIAGNOSIS PROCESS, AND ARE THE TESTS RELIABLE?

- Imaging in the thoracic spine needs to be interpreted with caution. Wood et al[160] found that 73% of 90 asymptomatic individuals had positive anatomical findings on MRI at one level or more.
- In the absence of trauma or red flags, imaging studies are rarely useful in identifying pain generators in the thoracic spine.
- MRI is the most commonly used diagnostic test in the evaluation of thoracic disc problems. It allows the best visualization of the soft-tissue structures. No data are available on the sensitivity or specificity of MRI in the thoracic spine.
- Thoracic discography may pick up disc pathology that is not visible on MRI.[161]
- Severe ligamentous injury of the thoracic spine without bony injury is extremely rare.[36]
- Plain radiography may miss up to 25% of thoracolumbar fractures.[36]
- In a systematic review Diaz et al[36] reported that in conscious patients with normal mental status and no distracting injury, the absence of back pain or tenderness had a 95% negative predictive value for thoracolumbar spinal fractures. They further stated that in asymptomatic trauma patients with normal mental status, no distracting injury, and normal physical examination, no further workup is needed.
- Helical computed tomography (CT) using a reformatted visceral protocol has a sensitivity of 97% for thoracic spine fractures, compared with a sensitivity of 62% for conventional radiographs.[133]
- Spiral CT has been shown to have a sensitivity of 100% in detecting spinal fractures, compared with a 70% sensitivity for plain-film radiographs.[1]
- Moon et al[109] reported that ultrasound appears to be a useful diagnostic tool for posterior ligament complex (PLC) injury in thoracolumbar spine fractures in clinical situations in which MRI is contraindicated.

MEDICATIONS

HOW DOES A PATIENT'S RESPONSE TO MEDICATION INFLUENCE YOUR DECISION-MAKING PROCESS?

- Nonsteroidal antiinflammatory drugs (NSAIDS), often augmented by muscle relaxants, are a standard medical treatment for back pain in primary care.[15]
- Selection criteria for which patients benefit from muscle relaxants and narcotic analgesics are unclear, and these drugs should be prescribed for fixed periods due to the potential for addiction.[32]
- Chronic use of narcotic pain medications may be associated with a centrally mediated pain state that may benefit from a cognitive behavioral approach (graded activity and graded exposure).[94,163]
- Symptom relief with muscle relaxants and pain medications does not aid the diagnostic process. Most patients with symptomatic thoracic spine and rib cage pathology will experience muscle guarding and pain.[27]
- The effectiveness of antiinflammatory medication helps differentiate pathology that has an acute inflammatory process.
  - Pathologies that can have an acute inflammatory process include disc pathology, muscle strain, ligament sprain, facet dysfunction, and radiculopathy.[121]
  - Pathologies that do not normally have an acute inflammatory response include degenerative changes and spinal stenosis.

CLINICAL PEARL

In 1979, Mitchell et al[107] described a "rule of threes," which attempted to predict the location of the level of the thoracic transverse processes (TPs) relative to their corresponding spinous process (SP). A recent study has challenged this paradigm and found that throughout the thoracic spine, the TPs of each thoracic vertebra are generally at the level of the SP of the vertebra one level above.[55]

BIOMECHANICAL

WHAT ROLE DO BIOMECHANICS PLAY IN THE DECISION-MAKING PROCESS IN THE THORACIC REGION?

Posture plays a key role in the prognosis of thoracic spine injuries. Patients with excessive thoracic kyphosis place undue stress on the ligaments and discs, while patients with a flat thoracic spine may overload the posterior elements (facet joints, etc.). Any condition or injury that either increases or decreases the mobility of the region may have pathophysiological ramifications. Additionally, it is imperative to determine the activities and postures the patient engages in on a daily basis. Neglecting these areas may be the difference between clinical success and failure. Injuries to the disc result in changes to sagittal plane movement symmetry, which leads to asymmetric facet joint movements and potential degenerative changes.[125]

WHAT BIOMECHANICAL ABNORMALITIES IN OTHER REGIONS AFFECT YOUR DECISION-MAKING PROCESS?

Wainner et al[151] recently published an editorial discussing the role of regional interdependence in musculoskeletal conditions. Regional interdependence is the concept that seemingly unrelated impairments in a remote anatomical regions may contribute to, or be associated with, the patient's primary complaint. Therefore, our clinical bias is to routinely examine the segments immediately above and below the area of symptoms, and we frequently find impairments that are far removed that may have biomechanical ramifications. Recent research has shown that impairments in the hips can contribute to lower back pain, and impairments in the thoracic spine may contribute to pain in the neck and shoulders.[5,16,19,22,116]

CLINICAL PEARL

Axial rotation and simultaneous lateral flexion of the cervical spine is kinesiologically related to the movements of the upper thoracic spine. The cervical rotation lateral flexion (CRLF) test was developed by Lindgren et al to detect possible restriction of the movement of the first rib in patients with brachialgia. In the presence of a hypomobile first rib, passive lateral flexion is restricted when the cervical spine is maximally rotated passively away from the hypomobile side due to the first thoracic transverse process bumping against the elevated first rib. This test has excellent intertester reliability as well as validity based on cineradiographic examination.[88,89]

ENVIRONMENTAL FACTORS (See Box II-4-1)

DO PSYCHOSOCIAL ISSUES INFLUENCE THE CLINICAL DECISION-MAKING PROCESS?

In patient-centered care, it is imperative that the *whole* person be taken into consideration. Psychosocial issues such as stress, self-perception, job satisfaction, and the individual's psychological status need to be explored. If a patient has significant psychosocial issues that you feel are hindering progress, a referral to another health care provider is warranted. Slover and colleagues[137] explored the correlation between medical and psychosocial comorbidities in patients with spinal pain (cervical, thoracic, and lumbar) and found an increase in the baseline Oswestry with the addition of each comorbidity. Psychosocial comorbidities such as poor job satisfaction, an active compensation case, self-rated health, and low education level have a higher association than traditional medical comorbidities on the SF-36 and the Oswestry Disability Index.

CAN PATIENT EMOTIONS INFLUENCE THE DECISION-MAKING PROCESS?

Patients in pain may be distraught. This needs to be taken into consideration when examining and treating these patients. Additional psychological factors, such as anxiety and depression, may have an effect on the risk of developing back pain as well as the prognosis for recovery.[14] In a recent study investigating the 3-year incidence of back pain in asymptomatic individuals, depression had the largest hazard ratio (2.3) and was an important predictor of back pain.[72] Therapists can easily screen for depression utilizing two questions that have excellent sensitivity:[65]

1. "During the past month, have you often been bothered by feeling down, depressed, or hopeless?" and
2. "During the past month, have you often been bothered by little interest or pleasure in doing things?"

If the patient answers yes to both screening questions, the probability of depression is 59.9%. If the response to one question was positive, the probability is 47.2%. If neither is positive, the probability of depression is 8.6%. So, if the patient answers yes to one or both questions, a referral for psychological screening is warranted.

BOX II-4-1 Environmental and Personal Contextual Factors

Environmental	Work environment, repetitive tasks, and sustained postures can predispose individuals to injury and lead to the breakdown of tissue.[24,26,31,66,70,76-79,81,90,112-114] Although no direct evidence of the effect of the environment was found for patients with thoracic pain, the following research on patients with neck pain may be useful.

Cote et al,[26] in a systematic review, reported that risk factors associated with neck pain in workers included the following:
- Higher age
- Previous musculoskeletal pain
- High quantitative job demands
- Low social support at work
- Job insecurity
- Low physical capacity
- Poor computer workstation design and work posture
- Sedentary work position
- Repetitive work and precision work.

They also found preliminary evidence that the following factors may be associated with neck pain:
- Gender
- Occupation
- Headaches
- Emotional problems
- Smoking
- Poor job satisfaction
- Ethnicity

Johnston et al[79] reported higher rates of neck and upper back pain in subjects who were older, used a computer mouse for more than 6 hours per day, exhibited a negative affect, and worked at an uncomfortable workstation.

Psychosocial	Work-related issues, personal and family factors, depression, and emotional unrest have been shown to influence the prognosis in patients with low back pain, neck pain, and extremity disorders.[14,21,35,37,47,65,73-75,145,148] It is unclear whether the same is true in thoracic pain.

- Johnston and colleagues[77] found that low supervisor support was the only psychosocial risk factor identified with the presence of neck pain.
- It is well documented that fear-avoidance behaviors (avoiding movement because of an unsubstantiated fear of further tissue damage) can lead to a worse prognosis in patients with low back pain.[46-48,56]

DO WORK-RELATED INJURIES INFLUENCE THE CLINICAL DECISION-MAKING PROCESS?

In general, patients with back injuries that occur at work have a poorer prognosis, and approximately 42% of patients who are still off work after 6 months will not return by 12 months.[64] Job satisfaction has both a predictive value for new injuries (patients with poor job satisfaction are more likely to be injured) and for prognosis for recovery (patients with poor job satisfaction are less likely to return to the same job).[26,64] Clinically, the prognosis may need to be modified in light of this information, particularly if there is an active compensation claim.[137]

PERSONAL FACTORS

PREVIOUS SURGERY

WHAT PREVIOUS SURGERIES INFLUENCE THE CLINICAL DECISION-MAKING PROCESS?

In the context of the thoracic spine and rib cage, previous surgeries to the thorax (i.e., heart and lung surgery) may change the biomechanics of the region, which may lead to conditions of hypermobility or hypomobility. Additionally, previous fusions, disc surgeries, or any other surgery that compromises the structural integrity (passive subsystem) or the muscular control (active subsystem) of the thorax should be taken into account.[120]

FAMILY HISTORY

DOES A FAMILY HISTORY OF THORACIC PATHOLOGY INFLUENCE YOUR CLINICAL REASONING PROCESS?

Family history is important for several conditions in the thoracic region, including DISH, AS, idiopathic scoliosis, Schmorl's nodes, childhood-onset arthritis, and Scheuermann disease.[61,82,95,128,154,156] If a patient reports a family history of one of these conditions, the condition should be included in the differential diagnosis.

CHRONICITY OF PAIN

WHAT CENTRAL-PROCESSING CHANGES OCCUR THAT INFLUENCE THE DECISION-MAKING PROCESS?

- When a patient has had symptoms for a long time, central sensitization must be considered.
- *Central sensitization* is defined as a condition in which peripheral noxious inputs into the central nervous system lead to an increased excitability in which the response to normal inputs is greatly enhanced.[162]
- Repeated noxious stimuli lead to the depolarization of low-threshold neurons, with large receptive fields, with "normal" mechanical stimuli.[162]
- Injured neural tissue may actually reorganize synaptic contacts, causing innocuous inputs, to be directed to cells that normally receive only noxious inputs, and the central nervous system becomes hyperexcitable.[164]
- In these situations we shift to an enablement model that encourages the patient to be active, and we utilize a cognitive-behavioral model focused on graded exercise and graded exposure.[92,94,108,117]

CLINICAL PEARL

If a patient's symptoms appear to be more centrally mediated, take a cue from the research in low back pain, and focus your plan of care to an active, cognitive-behavioral approach rather than passive interventions.[94,108,117]

HAS MEDICAL TREATMENT BEEN SUCCESSFUL FOR PATIENTS WITH CHRONIC PATHOLOGY IN THE THORACIC REGION?

Although Manchikanti et al[100] reported that the prevalence of facet joint pain in patients with chronic thoracic spine pain was 42%, there is very little evidence for physical therapy interventions in this region. Manchikanti et al[101] did report on 55 consecutive patients with chronic thoracic facet joint pain treated with thoracic medial branch blocks, and over 70% maintained a 50% reduction in symptoms 2 years later.

DISCUSS HOW CHRONICITY OF SYMPTOMS INFLUENCES YOUR DECISION-MAKING PROCESS

As previously stated, if a patient has chronic symptoms, we shift our focus away from passive therapies toward an active, cognitive-behavioral approach.[108]

DISCUSS HOW AUTONOMIC, ENDOCRINE, AND IMMUNE SYSTEMS INFLUENCE DECISION MAKING IN THE THORACIC REGION (See Box II-4-2)

- The autonomic, endocrine, and immune systems work in unison to maintain homeostasis within the body.
- The autonomic nervous system is comprised of the sympathetic nervous system (SNS) and the parasympathetic nervous system (PNS). The nerves of the SNS arise from the thoracic spinal cord, and the ganglia are located in the paravertebral chain adjacent to the thoracic spine from T1 to L2. Nathan and Schwartz[110] reported that costovertebral joint osteophytes can entrap and stretch the sympathetic trunk. The SNS is involved in several conditions involving the thoracic spine, including T4 syndrome and complex regional pain syndrome (CRPS).[41,53] In patients presenting with symptoms (pain, paresthesias, sweating, vascular changes) that do not follow traditional anatomic distributions, the therapist should perform a careful examination and, in the absence of red flags, consider manual therapy interventions to the thoracic region.[17,23,30,41]
- The hypothalamus controls the autonomic system, adrenal glands produce neural irritants in response to stressors, and the reproductive organs also produce hormones that can act as neural irritants.[69]
- In patients whose immune systems are compromised by medication or disease, the prognosis for recovery must be altered, and timelines for therapeutic interventions should be adjusted accordingly. Moderate bouts of exercise have immunoprotective effects, whereas acute, intense bouts of exercise can lower the immune function for a short period of time.[111]

BOX II-4-2	**Output Mechanisms**
Autonomic	Patients with T4 syndrome, complex regional pain syndrome, thoracic outlet syndrome, whiplash, and numerous other upper-quarter dysfunctions can present with a "sympathetic" pain pattern.[52,54,87,97,104,136,142,143] Thoracic spine hypomobility has been linked to sympathetic symptoms.[23,99] Patients with autonomic symptoms may present with a headache and unilateral or bilateral arm pain and paresthesia. Arm symptoms are usually in a nondermatomal distribution (glovelike). Other symptoms may include weakness, hand clumsiness, upper extremity coldness, fullness or tightness, and a deep aching pain.[104]
Endocrine	The endocrine system is involved in the regulation of body homeostasis. There has not been any research linking the endocrine system to thoracic pathologies, although the prognosis for recovery from musculoskeletal conditions may need to be altered with certain endocrine disorders such as diabetes mellitus and thyroid disorders as healing times may be prolonged.[60]
Immune	Spinal infections are usually acquired through the bloodstream from other sites. Common underlying infections are related to injection drug use, urinary tract infection, or skin infection.[71] Spinal infections typically start at the vertebral endplate and may involve the discs, epidural space, posterior elements, and ultimately soft tissue.[71]

RED FLAGS THAT WARRANT REFERRAL TO A PHYSICIAN

WHAT SYMPTOMS ALERT YOU TO PATHOLOGIES THAT MAY REQUIRE REFERRAL TO A PHYSICIAN?

Symptoms that raise suspicion of a medical condition in a patient with back pain include the following:[83]

- Pain that is unaffected by posture or changes of position
- Abdominal pain
- Colicky pain
- Costovertebral angle tenderness
- Diaphoresis
- Excruciating pain
- Crushing chest pain
- Rapid breathing or tachycardia
- Fever
- Hypertension or hypotension
- Pain at rest or at night

See Table II-4-3 for a list of potential causes of chest pain.

Clinically, if the patient reports a history of cancer, presents with a new onset of spinal pain (cervical, thoracic, or lumbar), and has not had a recent oncology checkup, we advocate referring the patient to see a physician. A previous history of cancer has a specificity of 0.98 in patients presenting with back pain.[32] See Table II-4-4 for clinical findings that may be useful in determining if a patient needs to be referred to a physician for further testing.

CLINICAL DECISION MAKING CASE STUDY—PATIENT PROFILE

(?)

The patient is a 35-year-old male who reports to physical therapy with a 2-week history of thoracic pain and a deep achy pain over the inferior border of his right scapula, particularly after eating a fatty meal. His symptoms are severe at times but appear to be coming in waves. He is unable to find a position of comfort. When the pain is present, no motion or position makes the symptoms better. What would be your leading hypothesis at this point?

Answer

It would be difficult for a clinician to make a definitive diagnosis based on the information given. The fact that the pain is constant, comes in waves, and does not appear to be affected by motion or position would suggest the visceral systems as a source of the symptoms. The increase in symptoms after a fatty meal may implicate the gallbladder or gall stones. This patient's symptoms do not appear to be musculoskeletal in origin. He should be referred to

TABLE II-4-4 Clinical Findings Linking Cancer and Back Pain

Clinical Finding	Sensitivity	Specificity (Range)
History of cancer	0.31	0.98
Weight loss	0.15	0.94
Failure to improve with conservative therapy	0.31	0.90
Age ≥ 50 years	0.77	0.71
Any one or more of the above	0.91	0.59

Modified from Joines JD et al. Finding cancer in primary care outpatients with low back pain: a comparison of diagnostic strategies. *J Gen Intern Med.* 2001;16:14-23.

his primary care physician or to an urgent care setting for further testing and assessment to rule out visceral involvement.

1. Wisniewski A. Taking a closer look at costochondritis. *Nursing* 2006 Nov; 36(11): Critical Care: 64cc1-2 (4 ref).
2. Wisniewski A. Don't worry, it's just chest pain: taking a closer look at costochondritis. *Nursing Made Incredibly Easy!* 2005 Jul-Aug; 3(4):37-39.
3. Deyo RA, Rainville J, Kent DL. What can the history and physical examination tell us about low back pain? *JAMA.* Aug 12 1992;268(6):760-765.

WHAT SYMPTOMS IMPLICATE SPECIFIC VISCERAL SYSTEMS?

See Figure II-4-4 for common pain presentations from visceral structures.

Circulatory: Back pain that is intense, unbearable, and associated with a sensation of "tearing" can be the initial symptom of a dissecting aortic aneurysm.[83] If back pain is present, it is usually localized to the thoracolumbar junction or interscapular area.

Cardiac: Patients experiencing a myocardial infarction may present with midthoracic back pain that may or may not radiate to the arm or axilla. They may also be nauseous, sweating, and have a sense of impending doom. Patients have also reported the following symptoms: anterior chest heaviness, crushing chest pain, diaphoresis, shortness of breath, nausea, vomiting, a sense of impending doom, and pain radiating to the shoulder, neck, arm or arms, or back. Myocardial ischemia may present with substernal and left upper-extremity symptoms as well as with a deep, boring, interscapular pain (usually left sided) or pain across the entire back.[83]

Acute pancreatitis: Abdominal pain with localized, deep-seated mid-back pain and a history of drinking may indicate pancreas dysfunction.[83]

TABLE II-4-3 Causes of Chest Pain

Skeletal	Cardiac	Pulmonary	Gastrointestinal	Metabolic	Hematological
Costochondritis	Angina	Pulmonary embolus	Cholecystitis	Hyperthermia	Anemia
Rib fracture	Myocardial infarction	Pneumothorax	Reflux disease	Hyperthyroidism	Polycythemia
Chest or rib contusion	Pericarditis	Pneumonia	Peptic ulcer		Sickle cell disease
Costovertebral joint sprain	Cardiomyopathy	Asthma	Pancreatitis		
Zygapophyseal joint sprain	Aortic stenosis	Pulmonary hypertension			
	Aortic dissection	Chronic obstructive pulmonary disease			
	Tachycardia				
	Hypertension				

Modified from Wisniewski A. Don't worry, it's just chest pain: taking a closer look at costochondritis. *Nursing Made Incredibly Easy!* 2005;3:37-39; Wisniewski A. Taking a closer look at costochondritis. *Nursing* 2006;36(11): Critical Care: 64cc1-2.

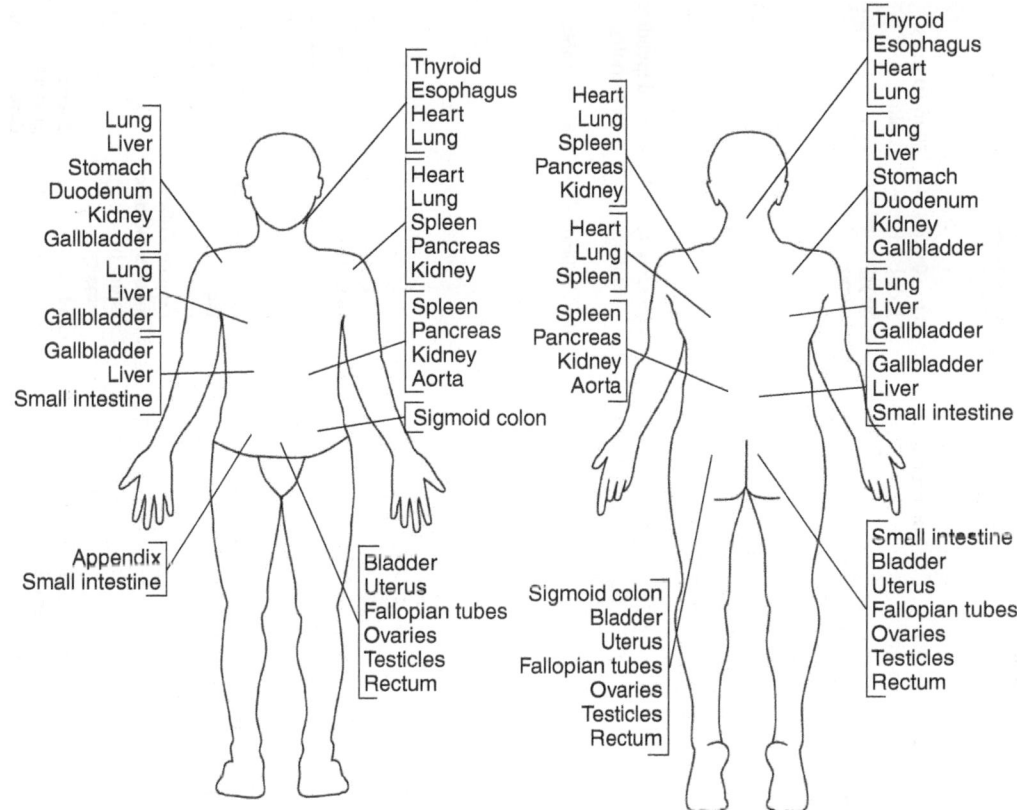

FIGURE II-4-4 Visceral referral into the thoracic region. Many visceral structures can refer pain into the thoracic spine.

Ulcers: Patients presenting with vague back pain and abdominal pain that gets worse with hunger and is relieved by antacids may signify an ulcer. The pain may be located in the middle or upper thoracic spine and may be sharp or stabbing in nature.

Gallstones: Patients with back pain originating in the gallbladder will have episodic colicky, sharp pain that may radiate to the inferior angle of the right scapula. These symptoms are particularly noticeable after fatty meals are eaten.[83]

Kidney stones: A kidney stone may cause colicky, radiating pain from the thoracolumbar and costovertebral region that radiates around to the lower abdomen and groin.[83]

Gastrointestinal (GI) tract: Patients with symptoms arising from the GI tract frequently report changes in symptoms with the ingestion of food and may complain of epigastric pain with radiation to the mid-back.[60] They may also complain of abdominal pain, pain with swallowing, changes in the stools (melena, diarrhea), fecal incontinence, joint pain, and referred shoulder pain.

Hepatic system: Patient with symptoms arising from the liver may present with jaundice (yellowing of the skin and eyes), a sense of fullness of the abdomen, anorexia, nausea, vomiting, bruising of skin, spider angiomas or palmar erythema, dark urine, right shoulder and abdominal pain, confusion, sleep disturbance, muscle tremors, hyperreflexia, and bilateral pallor.[60]

Endocrine system: Disorders of the endocrine system may present with muscle weakness, muscle atrophy, fatigue, arthralgia and myalgia, adhesive capsulitis, hand stiffness, excessive or delayed growth, mental status changes, changes in the hair and skin, changes in vital signs (temperature, heart rate, respiratory rate, blood pressure), increased perspiration, dehydration, or excessive water retention.[60]

Cancer: See Table II-4-4 for clinical findings related to cancer and back pain. Back pain that stems from cancer is generally constant, not relieved by rest, and can be most intense at night.[83] Nonmechanical constant back pain that persists despite activity modifications and medication use should raise a red flag. Risk factors include a previous history of cancer, failure to improve with conservative therapy, recent weight loss, and age ≥ 50 years.[80]

Additionally, cancer should be in the differential diagnosis in women with chest, breast, axillary, or shoulder pain, proximal muscle weakness and changes in reflexes, constant pain, pain at night not related to changing position, development of new neurological deficits, and changes in size, shape, tenderness, and consistency of lymph nodes.[60]

CLINICAL PEARL

A clinical prediction rule was recently derived by Cleland et al[18] that identified patients with neck pain who are likely to benefit from thoracic spine thrust manipulation. Six variables were identified:

1. *Symptom duration of < 30 days*
2. *No symptoms distal to the shoulder*
3. *Extension does not aggravate symptoms*
4. *Cervical extension of < 30°*
5. *Fear-Avoidance Beliefs Questionnaire Physical Activity score of < 12*
6. *Diminished upper thoracic spine kyphosis (T3 to T5)*

If three of the six variables were present (positive likelihood ratio = 5.5), the chance of experiencing a successful outcome based on perceived recovery improved from 54% to 86%.

TABLE II-4-5 Body Structure and Tissue-Based Pathology: Nociceptive and Peripheral Neurogenic Pain Mechanisms

	Intervertebral Disc[39,135,146]	Zygapophyseal Joint Capsule[38,51]	Zygapophyseal Joint[38,100]	Muscles[49,103]	Vertebral Bodies[3,39,129,141]	Rib Fractures[49,63,106]	Ligaments[59,62,109,124]	Nerves	Visceral Tissue[49]
Pathology	Disc pathology	Costochondritis	First rib dysfunction	Muscle strain	Compression fracture Scheuermann disease Scoliosis	Rib fracture	Costochondritis	Thoracic outlet syndrome T4 syndrome	Varies Scoliosis
Age	20 to 50 years old	20 to 50 years old	50 years old and above	20 to 40 years old	Any age for traumatic fracture Over 60 years old for degeneration, compression fracture: age ≥70 years has specificity of 0.9634	Any age for traumatic fracture	Not age related	20 to 50 years old if disc related >50 years old for stenosis	30 to 50 years old
Occupation	Repetitive flexion and lifting activities	Repetitive flexion and lifting activities	Repetitive extension activities	Repetitive flexion and lifting activities, sports	Repetitive flexion and lifting activities		No direct relationship	Varies, see related pathology	Varies depending on pathology
Gender	Men more likely to have degenerative disc changes	Not applicable	Not applicable	Not applicable	Female		Not applicable	Not applicable	Not applicable
Ethnicity					Asian and Caucasian have higher prevalence				
History	May be acute or degenerative over time	History of several bouts of symptoms	History of back pain		May or may not have history of back pain	May or may not have history of back pain		Varies, see related pathology; may have history of herpes zoster (shingles)[67]	Constant pain, unrelieved by positional changes
Mechanism of injury	Flexion with or without rotation	Flexion with or without rotation	Extension	Any motion that exceeds the available range of the muscle involved	Hyperflexion, axial loading, rotation, hyperextension	Trauma, overhead activities	Trauma, lifting	Varies, see related pathology; intercostal neuralgia often follows thoracic injury or surgery	Generally no known mechanism
Type of onset	Sudden	Sudden	Gradual	Sudden	Sudden or traumatic	Sudden in fracture, gradual in stress fracture	Sudden or traumatic	Gradual	Sudden to gradual, depending on structure
Referral from local tissue	Posterior and/or anterior thoracic pain	Most intense area of pain usually lateral and one segment inferior to the joint[38]	Most intense area of pain usually lateral and one segment inferior to the joint[38]	Pain in thoracic region locally around muscle	Pain in thoracic spine	Locally around region of injury	Pain in low back and gluteal region	Burning pain or paresthesias in the thorax that follows the course of a nerve	Pain is generally localized to area adjacent to involved structures

Referral to other regions	May have unilateral or bilateral radicular pain into chest wall; if cord is involved, may refer into lower extremities	May refer into the anterior chest wall or up to 2.5 segments inferior; superior referral is rare[38]	May refer into the anterior chest wall or up to 2.5 segments inferior. Superior referral is rare.[38]	May refer to other regions (see Travell and Simons[136])	May refer around the chest wall	May refer around the chest wall	Generally does not refer to other regions	Referral of symptoms into anterior chest wall	May refer into surrounding areas (see Figures II-4-2 and II-4-3)
Changes in symptoms	Sudden pain decreasing in the remainder of the day; increased pain the next morning	Sudden pain, no relief as day of injury progresses	Slow progressive worsening over time	Acutely there is sudden pain, as inflammatory processes progress, may get very sore and stiff	Sudden pain	Sudden pain, breathing makes pain worse	Sudden pain, no relief as day of injury progresses	Depends on pathology	May worsen as pathology progresses, changes are typically not mechanical in nature
24-hour pain pattern (morning)	Stiff for 30 minutes	Stiff for 5 minutes	Stiff for 5 minutes	Stiff for 30 to 60 minutes	Stiff for 30 minutes	Very sore and stiff for 30 minutes	Stiff for 5 minutes	Varies but does not change with mechanical stresses	Varies but does not change with mechanical stresses
24-hour pain pattern (afternoon)	Less stiff, may be worse with prolonged postures such as sitting	Worsens with activity	Worsens with extension activity	Less stiff, may be worse with prolonged postures	Less stiff, may be worse with prolonged sitting	Achy as day goes on	Less stiff, may be worse with prolonged activity	Depends on pathology	Varies but does not change with mechanical stresses
24-hour pain pattern (evening)	May be difficult to sleep	May be difficult to sleep and turn in bed	Usually not impaired	May be difficult to sleep	May be difficult to sleep	May be difficult to sleep	Sleep should not be impaired	May be difficult to sleep	Increased nocturnal pain
Description of symptoms	Ache and stiffness, poor localization	Sharp pain	Dull ache	Ache and stiffness, may be able to localize	Ache and stiffness, poor localization	Hurts with inspiration; initially sharp and localized, progresses with healing to dull and achy	Ache and stiffness, sharp pain with motions that stress ligament, primarily flexion	Numbness, tingling, burning, itching in cases of shingles	Cramping, peristaltic waves, gnawing ache
Depth of symptoms	Deep	Deep	Deep	Superficial	Deep	Focal, usually superficial pain	Deep	Superficial	Deep, poorly localized
Constancy of symptoms	Intermittent	Intermittent	Intermittent	Intermittent	Constant but varying, may get worse with breathing	Constant, worse with breathing	Intermittent	Intermittent to constant but varying	Constant, may come in waves
Aggravating factors	Sitting, flexion, initial movement after lying down	Extension, lateral flexion and rotation	Extension and walking	Any motion that causes the muscle to contract or be stretched	Sitting, flexion, lifting, coughing, and sneezing	Breathing, coughing, sneezing	Primarily flexion	Varies, see related pathology	Not consistent with mechanical movements
Easing factors	Walking	Sitting	Sitting	Walking, lying	Limited walking, lying	Rest	Extension activities, lying	Varies, see related pathology	Not consistent with mechanical movements

Continued on following page.

Section II

ORTHOPEDIC REASONING

TABLE II-4-5 Body Structure and Tissue-Based Pathology: Nociceptive and Peripheral Neurogenic Pain Mechanisms (*Continued*)

	Intervertebral Disc[39,135,146]	Zygapophyseal Joint Capsule[38,51]	Zygapophyseal Joint[38,100]	Muscles[49,103]	Vertebral Bodies[3,39,129,141]	Rib Fractures[49,63,106]	Ligaments[59,62,109,124]	Nerves	Visceral Tissue[49]
Stability of symptoms	Gradual improvement over a 6- to 12-week period	Gradual improvement over a 2-week period	Slow, gradual progression of symptoms if degenerative	Gradual improvement over a 6-week period	Gradual improvement over an 8- to 12-week period	Gradual improvement over a 6-week period	Gradual improvement over a 6-week period	Gradual improvement over a 6-week period	May worsen if pathology progresses
Past medical history	All structures may have a past history of medical issues that impact the function of the surrounding tissue		Degenerative changes	May have history of visceral pathology	May have history of osteoporosis or osteopenia				Past medical history should be thoroughly explored; may have history of systemic illness or cancer
Past surgeries	Fusions may make the level above or below more susceptible; surgical correction of scoliosis may render the areas above and below the surgery at risk	Fusions may make the level above or below more susceptible	Fusions may make the level above or below more susceptible	May have a history of surgeries related to visceral pathology				Any surgery to the thoracic spine should be investigated	Note any past surgeries for medical problems; may provide a clue for visceral causes
Special questions	Pain with coughing or sneezing, Valsalva maneuver				Corticosteroid use has a specificity of 0.995 in compression fractures[99]	Visceral symptoms, any crepitus with breathing, any blood with coughing			History of cancer, recent weight loss or gain, fever, night pain, changes in pain with eating
X-rays	Negative	Negative	Positive if degenerative changes	Negative	Positive	Positive but missed up to 50% of the time[39]	Negative	Negative, may show degenerative changes	Negative
MRI	Positive	Negative	Positive	Positive	Positive	Positive	Positive	May be positive depending on related pathology	May be positive depending on pathology
EMG	Positive if nerves are involved	Usually not necessary	Usually not necessary	Usually not necessary	Nerve generally not involved	Usually not necessary	Usually not necessary	Positive	Not usually necessary
Special laboratory tests									Erythrocyte sedimentation rate (ESR)[80]
Red flags	Cord signs, bilateral lower-extremity symptoms				Bilateral lower extremity symptoms, rule out cord involvement	Collapsed lung, wheezing, bloody sputum			Rule out visceral structures, previous history of cancer

MRI, magnetic resonance imaging; EMG, electromyogram.

SUMMARY STATEMENT

There has been very little research conducted on mechanical thoracic and rib cage pain. This area should be approached with caution, as numerous visceral structures and systemic disease processes can present as thoracic spine and rib cage pain. In general, thoracic pain is much less common than neck or low back pain in adults. Under the age of 20 years, thoracic pain is as common as low back pain. Wedderkopp et al[152] found that the 1-month prevalence of back pain in children and adolescents aged 8 to 10 and 14 to 16 years was 39%, and thoracic pain was the most common area of spinal pain in childhood. Thoracic pain and lumbar pain were equally common in the adolescence group. Scheuermann disease most commonly presents between the ages of 13 and 16 years and is the most common cause of excessive kyphosis in adolescents.[96] From 20 to 50 years old, the incidence of facet and disc problems increases,[12,100] and the peak incidence of AS is 20 to 40 years of age. Over the age of 50 years, degenerative changes are a common source of thoracic pain. In a patient over the age of 60 years presenting with acute thoracic spine pain, osteoporotic fracture must be considered along with central canal stenosis.[129] Manchikanti et al[100] reported that the prevalence of facet joint pain in patients with chronic cervical spine pain was 55% (95% CI, 49% to 61%); in those with thoracic spine pain, the prevalence was 42% (95% CI, 30% to 53%); and with lumbar spine pain, the rate was 31% (95% CI, 27% to 36%). So clearly, if the pain has been present for more than 6 weeks, the facet joints should be examined for impairments and pain reproduction.

The thoracic spine is a transitional area, and impairments may have ramifications in distant regions. Current research into regional interdependence[151] suggests that the thoracic spine may play a pivotal role in other musculoskeletal pain problems.[7,18] Therefore, we suggest that the thoracic spine be examined in any patient with musculoskeletal complaints adjacent to the thoracic spine, including but not limited to the shoulder, neck, and lower back. Table II-4-5 summarizes the factors that help a clinician differentiate among different sources of symptoms in the thoracic region.

REFERENCES

1. Antevil JL, Sise MJ, Sack DI, Kidder B, Hopper A, Brown CV. Spiral computed tomography for the initial evaluation of spine trauma: a new standard of care? *J Trauma.* 2006;61(2):382-387.
2. Bartels RH, Peul WC. Mini-thoracotomy or thoracoscopic treatment for medially located thoracic herniated disc? *Spine.* 2007;32(20):E581-E584.
3. Bauer RL, Deyo RA. Low risk of vertebral fracture in Mexican American women. *Arch Intern Med.* 1987;147:1437-1439.
4. Bechgaard P. Segmental thoracic pain in patients admitted to a medical department and a coronary unit. *Acta Med Scand Suppl.* 1981;644:87-89.
5. Ben-Galim P, Ben-Galim T, Rand N, et al. Hip-spine syndrome: the effect of total hip replacement surgery on low back pain in severe osteoarthritis of the hip. *Spine.* 2007;32:2099-2102.
6. Benhamou CL, Roux C, Tourliere D, Gervais T, Viala JF, Amor B. Pseudovisceral pain referred from costovertebral arthropathies: twenty-eight cases. *Spine.* 1993;18:790-795.
7. Bergman GJD, Winters JC, Groenier KH, et al. Manipulative therapy in addition to usual medical care for patients with shoulder dysfunction and pain: a randomized, controlled trial [see comment]. *Ann Intern Med.* 2004;141:432-439.
8. Bland JH. Diagnosis of thoracic pain syndromes. In: Giles LGF, Singer KP, eds. *The Clinical Anatomy and Management of Thoracic Spine Pain.* Boston, MA: Butterworth-Heinemann; 2000:145-156.
9. Boissonnault W, Fabio RP. Pain profile of patients with low back pain referred to physical therapy. *J Orthop Sports Phys Ther.* 1996;24:180-191.
10. Bookhout MR. Evaluation of the thoracic spine and rib cage. In: Flynn TW, ed. *The Thoracic Spine and Rib Cage: Musculoskeletal Evaluation and Treatment.* Boston, MA: Butterworth-Heinemann; 1996:147-167.
11. Breig A. *Biomechanics of the Central Nervous System.* Stockholm: Almqvist and Wiksell; 1960.
12. Brown CW, Deffer PA Jr, Akmakjian J, Donaldson DH, Brugman JL. The natural history of thoracic disc herniation. *Spine.* 1992;17:S97-S102.
13. Cano A, Mayo A, Ventimiglia M. Coping, pain severity, interference, and disability: the potential mediating and moderating roles of race and education [corrected; published erratum appears in *J Pain* 2006 Nov;7(11):869-870]. *J Pain.* 2006;7(7):459-468 (43 ref).
14. Cherkin DC, Deyo RA, Street JH, Barlow W. Predicting poor outcomes for back pain seen in primary care using patients' own criteria. *Spine.* 1996;21:2900-2907.
15. Cherkin DC, Wheeler KJ, Barlow W, Deyo RA. Medication use for low back pain in primary care. *Spine.* 1998;23:607-614.
16. Cleland JA, Childs JD, Fritz JM, Whitman JM, Eberhart SL. Development of a clinical prediction rule for guiding treatment of a subgroup of patients with neck pain: use of thoracic spine manipulation, exercise, and patient education. *Phys Ther.* 2007;87(1):9-23.
17. Cleland J, McRae M. Complex regional pain syndrome 1: management through the use of vertebral and sympathetic trunk mobilization. *J Man Manipulative Ther.* 2002;10(4):188-199 (41 ref).
18. Cleland JA, Childs JD, Fritz JM, Whitman JM, Eberhart SL. Development of a clinical prediction rule for guiding treatment of a subgroup of patients with neck pain: use of thoracic spine manipulation, exercise, and patient education. *Phys Ther.* 2007;87:9-23.
19. Cleland JA, Childs JD, McRae M, Palmer JA, Stowell T. Immediate effects of thoracic manipulation in patients with neck pain: a randomized clinical trial [see comment]. *Man Ther.* 2005;10:127-135.
20. Cleland JA, Flynn TW, Palmer JA. Incorporation of manual therapy directed at the cervicothoracic spine in patients with lateral epicondylalgia: a pilot clinical trial. *J Man Manipulative Ther.* 2005;13(3):143-151 (39 ref).
21. Cleland JA, Lee AJ, Hall S. Associations of depression and anxiety with gender, age, health-related quality of life, and symptoms in primary care COPD patients. *Fam Pract.* 2007;24:217-223.
22. Cleland JA, Whitman JM, Fritz JM. Effectiveness of manual physical therapy to the cervical spine in the management of lateral epicondylalgia: a retrospective analysis. *J Orthop Sports Phys Ther.* 2004;34:713-722 [discussion 22-4].
23. Conroy JL, Schneiders AG. Case report: the T4 syndrome. *Man Ther.* 2005;10(4):292-296 (13 ref).
24. Cook TM, Ludewig PM, Rosecrance JC, Zimmermann CL, Gerleman DG. Electromyographic effects of ergonomic modifications in selected meat-packing tasks. *Appl Ergon.* 1999;30:229-233.
25. Coris EE, Higgins IIHW. First rib stress fractures in throwing athletes. *Am J Sports Med.* 2005;33(9):1400-1404 (27 ref).
26. Cote P, van der Velde G, Cassidy JD, et al. The burden and determinants of neck pain in workers: results of the Bone and Joint Decade 2000-2010 Task Force on Neck Pain and Its Associated Disorders. *Spine.* 2008;33:S60-S74.
27. Crisco JJ, Jokl P, Heinen GT, Connell MD, Panjabi MMA. Muscle contusion injury model: biomechanics, physiology, and histology. *Am J Sports Med.* 1994;22:702-710.
28. Cropper JR. Regional anatomy and biomechanics. In: Flynn TW, ed. *The Thoracic Spine and Rib Cage.* Boston, MA: Butterworth-Heinemann; 1996:3-30.
29. Damborg F, Engell V, Andersen M, Kyvik KO, Thomsen K. Prevalence, concordance, and heritability of Scheuermann kyphosis based on a study of twins. *J Bone Joint Surg Am.* 2006;88A(10):2133-2136 (24 ref).
30. DeFranca GG, Levine LJ. The T4 syndrome. *J Manipulative Physiol Ther.* 1995;18(1):34-37 (5 ref).
31. Dekkers-Sanchez PM, Hoving JL, Sluiter JK, Frings-Dresen MHW. Factors associated with long-term sick leave in sick-listed employees: a systematic review. *Occup Environ Med.* 2008;65:153-157.
32. Deyo RA. Drug therapy for back pain: which drugs help which patients? *Spine.* 1996;21:2840-2849 [discussion 49-50].
33. Deyo RA, Diehl AK. Cancer as a cause of back pain: frequency, clinical presentation, and diagnostic strategies. *J Gen Intern Med.* 1988;3:230-238.
34. Deyo RA, Rainville J, Kent DL. What can the history and physical examination tell us about low back pain? *JAMA.* 1992;268:760-765.
35. Deyo RA, Walsh NE, Schoenfeld LS, Ramamurthy S. Studies of the Modified Somatic Perceptions Questionnaire (MSPQ) in patients with back pain: psychometric and predictive properties. *Spine.* 1989;14:507-510.

36. Diaz JJ Jr , Cullinane DC, Altman DT, et al. Practice management guidelines for the screening of thoracolumbar spine fracture. *J Trauma.* 2007;63(3):709-718 (58 ref).

37. Dionne CE, Koepsell TD, Von Korff M, Deyo RA, Barlow WE, Checkoway H. Predicting long-term functional limitations among back pain patients in primary care settings. *J Clin Epidemiol.* 1997;50:31-43.

38. Dreyfuss P, Tibiletti C, Dreyer SJ. Thoracic zygapophyseal joint pain patterns: a study in normal volunteers. *Spine.* 1994;19:807-811.

39. Dutton M. *Orthopaedic Examination, Evaluation, and Intervention.* New York: McGraw Hill; 2004.

40. Dwyer A, Aprill C, Bogduk N. Cervical zygapophyseal joint pain patterns. I: A study in normal volunteers. *Spine.* 1990;15:453-457.

41. Evans P. The T4 syndrome: some basic science aspects. *Physiotherapy.* 1997;83(4):186-189 (9 ref).

42. Fernandez-de-Las-Peñas C, Alonso-Blanco C, Morales-Cabezas M, Miangolarra-Page JC: Two exercise interventions for the management of patients with ankylosing spondylitis: a randomized controlled trial. *Am J Phys Med Rehabil.* 2005;84:407-419.

43. Fernandez-de-las-Peñas C, Cleland JA: Management of whiplash-associated disorder addressing thoracic and cervical spine impairments: a case report [comment]. *J Orthop Sports Phys Ther.* 2005;35: 180-181.

44. Fernandez-de-las-Peñas C, Palomeque del Cerro L, Fernandez Carnero J. Manual treatment of post-whiplash injury. *J Bodyw Mov Ther.* 2005;9(2):109-119 (60 ref).

45. Ferreira PH, Ferreira ML, Latimer J, et al. Attitudes and beliefs of Brazilian and Australian physiotherapy students towards chronic back pain: a cross-cultural comparison. *Physiother Res Int.* 2004;9:13-23.

46. Fritz JM, George SZ. Identifying psychosocial variables in patients with acute work-related low back pain: the importance of fear-avoidance beliefs. *Phys Ther.* 2002;82:973-983.

47. Fritz JM, George SZ, Delitto A. The role of fear-avoidance beliefs in acute low back pain: relationships with current and future disability and work status. *Pain.* 2001;94:7-15.

48. Fritz JM, Whitman JM, Flynn TW, Wainner RS, Childs JD. Factors related to the inability of individuals with low back pain to improve with a spinal manipulation. *Phys Ther.* 2004;84:173-190.

49. Fruth SJ. Differential diagnosis and treatment in a patient with posterior upper thoracic pain. *Phys Ther.* 2006;86(2):254-268 (72 ref).

50. Fukui S, Gigou F, Daneshvar M, et al. Totally laparoscopic assisted thoracic aorta endograft delivery by direct sheath placement into the aorta. *J Vasc Surg.* 2006;43:1274-1277.

51. Fukui S, Ohseto K, Shiotani M. Patterns of pain induced by distending the thoracic zygapophyseal joints. *Reg Anesth.* 1997;22:332-336.

52. Galer BS, Butler S, Jensen MP. Case reports and hypothesis: a neglect-like syndrome may be responsible for the motor disturbance in reflex sympathetic dystrophy (complex regional pain syndrome-1). *J Pain Symptom Manage.* 1995;10:385-391.

53. Galer BS, Henderson J, Perander J, Jensen MP. Course of symptoms and quality of life measurement in complex regional pain syndrome: a pilot survey. *J Pain Symptom Manage.* 2000;20:286-292.

54. Ge H-Y, Fernandez-de-las-Peñas C, Arendt-Nielsen L. Sympathetic facilitation of hyperalgesia evoked from myofascial tender and trigger points in patients with unilateral shoulder pain. *Clin Neurophysiol.* 2006;117:1545-1550.

55. Geelhoed MA, McGaugh J, Brewer PA, Murphy D. A new model to facilitate palpation of the level of the transverse processes of the thoracic spine. *J Orthop Sports Phys Ther.* 2006;36:876-881.

56. George SZ, Bialosky JE, Fritz JM. Physical therapist management of a patient with acute low back pain and elevated fear-avoidance beliefs. *Phys Ther.* 2004;84:538-549.

57. Godges JJ, Anger MA, Zimmerman G, Delitto A. Effects of education on return-to-work status for people with fear-avoidance beliefs and acute low back pain. *Phys Ther.* 2008;88:231-239.

58. Goh S, Tan C, Price RI, et al. Influence of age and gender on thoracic vertebral body shape and disc degeneration: an MR investigation of 169 cases. *J Anat.* 2000;197(Pt 4):647-657.

59. Goldberg AL, Rothfus WE, Deeb ZL, et al. The impact of magnetic resonance on the diagnostic evaluation of acute cervicothoracic spinal trauma. *Skeletal Radiol.* 1988;17:89-95.

60. Goodman CC, Snyder TE. *Differential Diagnosis for Physical Therapists: Screening for Referral.* 4th ed. St. Louis, MO: Elsevier Health Sciences; 2006.

61. Gorman C, Jawad AS, Chikanza I. A family with diffuse idiopathic skeletal hyperostosis. *Ann Rheum Dis.* 2005;64:1794-1795.

62. Gray L, Vandemark R, Hays M. Thoracic and lumbar spine trauma. *Semin Ultrasound CT MR.* 2001;22(2):125-134 (20 ref).

63. Gregory PL, Biswas AC, Batt ME. Musculoskeletal problems of the chest wall in athletes. *Sports Med.* 2002;32(4):235-250 (118 ref).

64. Hagen KB, Thune O. Work incapacity from low back pain in the general population. *Spine.* 1998;23(19):2091-2095 (20 ref).

65. Haggman S, Maher CG, Refshauge KM. Screening for symptoms of depression by physical therapists managing low back pain. *Phys Ther.* 2004;84:1157-1166.

66. Harms-Ringdahl K. On assessment of shoulder exercise and load-elicited pain in the cervical spine: biomechanical analysis of load-EMG—methodological studies of pain provoked by extreme position. *Scand J Rehabil Med* (suppl) 1986;14:1-40.

67. Helgason S, Petursson G, Gudmundsson S, Sigurdsson JA. Prevalence of postherpetic neuralgia after a first episode of herpes zoster: prospective study with long-term follow up. *BMJ.* 2000;321(7264):794-796 (23 ref).

68. Henschke N, Maher CG, Refshauge KM. Screening for malignancy in low back pain patients: a systematic review. *Eur Spine J.* 2007;16:1673-1679.

69. Hurwitz EL, Morgenstern H. Immediate and long-term effects of immune stimulation: hypothesis linking the immune response to subsequent physical and psychological well-being. *Med Hypotheses.* 2001;56:620-624.

70. Hush JM, Maher CG, Refshauge KM. Risk factors for neck pain in office workers: a prospective study. *BMC Musculoskelet Disord.* 2006;7:81.

71. Jarvik JG, Deyo RA. Diagnostic evaluation of low back pain with emphasis on imaging. *Ann Intern Med.* 2002;137:586-597.

72. Jarvik JG, Hollingworth W, Heagerty PJ, Haynor DR, Boyko EJ, Deyo RA. Three-year incidence of low back pain in an initially asymptomatic cohort: clinical and imaging risk factors [see comment]. *Spine.* 2005;30:1541-1548; discussion 49.

73. Jensen MP, Ehde DM, Hoffman AJ, Patterson DR, Czerniecki JM, Robinson LR. Cognitions, coping and social environment predict adjustment to phantom limb pain. *Pain.* 2002;95:133-142.

74. Jensen MP, Nielson WR, Turner JA, Romano JM, Hill ML. Readiness to self-manage pain is associated with coping and with psychological and physical functioning among patients with chronic pain. *Pain.* 2003;104:529-537.

75. Jensen MP, Turner JA, Romano JM. Changes in beliefs, catastrophizing, and coping are associated with improvement in multidisciplinary pain treatment. *J Consult Clin Psychol.* 2001;69:655-662.

76. Johnson EG, Godges JJ, Lohman EB, Stephens JA, Zimmerman GJ, Anderson SP. Disability self-assessment and upper-quarter muscle balance between female dental hygienists and non-dental hygienists. *J Dent Hyg.* 2003;77:217-223.

77. Johnston V, Jimmieson NL, Souvlis T, Jull G. Interaction of psychosocial risk factors explain increased neck problems among female office workers. *Pain.* 2007;129:311-320.

78. Johnston V, Jull G, Souvlis T, Jimmieson NL. Neck movement and muscle activity characteristics in female office workers with neck pain. *Spine.* 2008;33:555-563.

79. Johnston V, Souvlis T, Jimmieson NL, Jull G. Associations between individual and workplace risk factors for self-reported neck pain and disability among female office workers. *Appl Ergon.* 2008;39: 171-182.

80. Joines JD, McNutt RA, Carey TS, Deyo RA, Rouhani R. Finding cancer in primary care outpatients with low back pain: a comparison of diagnostic strategies. *J Gen Intern Med.* 2001;16:14-23.

81. Kaplan RM, Deyo RA. Back pain in health care workers. *Occup Med.* 1988;3:61-73.

82. Khan MA, Ball EJ. Genetic aspects of ankylosing spondylitis. *Best Pract Res Clin Rheumatol.* 2002;16:675-690.

83. Klineberg E, Mazanec D, Orr D, Demicco R, Bell G, McLain R. Masquerade: medical causes of back pain. *Cleve Clin J Med.* 2007;74:905-913.

84. Leong JC, Lu WW, Luk KD, Karlberg EM. Kinematics of the chest cage and spine during breathing in healthy individuals and in patients with adolescent idiopathic scoliosis. *Spine.* 1999;24:1310-1315.

85. Lillegard WA. Medical causes of pain in the thoracic region. In: Flynn TW, ed. *The Thoracic Spine and Rib Cage: Musculoskeletal Evaluation and Treatment.* Boston, MA: Butterworth-Heinemann; 1996:107-120.

86. Lindgren KA. Conservative treatment of thoracic outlet syndrome: a 2-year follow-up. *Arch Phys Med Rehabil.* 1997;78:373-378.

87. Lindgren KA, Leino E. Subluxation of the first rib: a possible thoracic outlet syndrome mechanism. *Arch Phys Med Rehabil.* 1988;69: 692-695.

88. Lindgren KA, Leino E, Hakola M, Hamberg J. Cervical spine rotation and lateral flexion combined motion in the examination of the thoracic outlet. *Arch Phys Med Rehabil.* 1990;71(5):343-344 (5 ref).

89. Lindgren KA, Leino E, Manninen H. Cervical rotation lateral flexion test in brachialgia. *Arch Phys Med Rehabil.* 1992;73:735-737.

90. Linton SJ. Do psychological factors increase the risk for back pain in the general population in both a cross-sectional and prospective analysis? *Eur J Pain: Ejp.* 2005;9:355-361.

91. Linton SJ. A review of psychological risk factors in back and neck pain. *Spine.* 2000;25:1148-1156.

92. Linton SJ, Andersson T. Can chronic disability be prevented? A randomized trial of a cognitive-behavior intervention and two forms of information for patients with spinal pain. *Spine.* 2000;25:2825-2831 [discussion 24].

93. Linton SJ, Hellsing AL, Hallden K. A population-based study of spinal pain among 35- to 45-year-old individuals: prevalence, sick leave, and health care use. *Spine.* 1998;23:1457-1463.

94. Linton SJ, Ryberg M. A cognitive-behavioral group intervention as prevention for persistent neck and back pain in a non-patient population: a randomized controlled trial. *Pain.* 2001;90:83-90.

95. Lupponen T, Korkko J, Lundan T, Seppanen U, Ignatius J, Kaariainen H. Childhood-onset osteoarthritis, tall stature, and sensorineural hearing loss associated with Arg75-Cys mutation in procollagen type II gene (COL2A1). *Arthritis Rheum.* 2004;51:925-932.

96. Lowe TG, Line BG. Evidence-based medicine: analysis of Scheuermann kyphosis. *Spine.* 2007;32(19S):S115-S119 (27 ref).

97. Lowell RC, Gloviczki P, Cherry KJ Jr, et al. Cervicothoracic sympathectomy for Raynaud's syndrome. *Int Angiol.* 1993;12:168-172.

98. Magee DJ. *Orthopedic Physical Assessment.* 5th ed. St. Louis, MO: Saunders Elsevier; 2008.

99. Maitland G. *Vertebral Manipulation.* 5th ed. Sydney, New South Wales, Australia: Butterworths; 1986.

100. Manchikanti L, Boswell MV, Singh V, Pampati V, Damron KS, Beyer CD. Prevalence of facet joint pain in chronic spinal pain of cervical, thoracic, and lumbar regions. *BMC Musculoskelet Disord.* 2004;5:15.

101. Manchikanti L, Manchikanti KN, Manchukonda R, Pampati V, Cash KA. Evaluation of therapeutic thoracic medial branch block effectiveness in chronic thoracic pain: a prospective outcome study with minimum 1-year follow up. *Pain Physician.* 2006;9:97-105.

102. McRae M, Cleland J. Differential diagnosis and treatment of upper thoracic pain: a case study. *J Man Manipulative Ther.* 2003;11(1):43-48 (22 ref).

103. Meleger AL, Krivickas LS. Neck and back pain: musculoskeletal disorders. *Neurol Clin.* 2007;25(2):419-438 (55 ref).

104. Mellick GA, Mellick LB. Clinical presentation, quantitative sensory testing, and therapy of two patients with fourth thoracic syndrome. *J Manipulative Physiol Ther.* 2006;29(5):403-408 (23 ref).

105. Mellion LR, Ladeira C. The herniated thoracic disc: a review of literature. *J Man Manipulative Ther.* 2001;9(3):154-163 (81 ref).

106. Middleton C, Edwards M, Lang N, Elkins J. Management and treatment of patients with fractured ribs. *Nurs Times.* 2003;99(5):30-32 (12 ref).

107. Mitchell FL, Moran PS, Pruzzo NA. *An Evaluation and Treatment Manual of Osteopathic Muscle Energy Procedures.* Valley Park, MO: Mitchell, Moran & Pruzzo and Assoc; 1979.

108. Molton IR, Graham C, Stoelb BL, Jensen MP. Current psychological approaches to the management of chronic pain. *Curr Opin Anaesthesiol.* 2007;20:485-489.

109. Moon S, Park M, Suk K, et al. Feasibility of ultrasound examination in posterior ligament complex injury of thoracolumbar spine fracture. *Spine.* 2002;27(19):2154-2158 (38 ref).

110. Nathan H, Schwartz A. Inverted pattern of development of thoracic vertebral osteophytosis in situs inversus and in other instances of right descending aorta. *Radiol Clin.* 1962;31:150-158.

111. Nieman DC. Current perspective on exercise immunology. *Curr Sports Med Rep.* 2003;2:239-242.

112. Norlander S, Aste-Norlander U, Nordgren B, Sahlstedt B. Mobility in the cervico-thoracic motion segment: an indicative factor of musculoskeletal neck-shoulder pain. *Scand J Rehabil Med.* 1996;28:183-192.

113. Norlander S, Gustavsson BA, Lindell J, Nordgren B. Reduced mobility in the cervico-thoracic motion segment—a risk factor for musculoskeletal neck-shoulder pain: a two-year prospective follow-up study. *Scand J Rehabil Med.* 1997;29:167-174.

114. Norlander S, Nordgren B. Clinical symptoms related to musculoskeletal neck-shoulder pain and mobility in the cervico-thoracic spine. *Scand J Rehabil Med.* 1998;30:243-251.

115. Oaklander AL, Bowsher D, Galer B, Haanpaa M, Jensen MP. Herpes zoster itch: preliminary epidemiologic data. *J Pain.* 2003;4:338-343.

116. Offierski CM, MacNab I. Hip-spine syndrome. *Spine.* 1983;8: 316-321.

117. Osborne TL, Raichle KA, Jensen MP. Psychologic interventions for chronic pain. *Phys Med Rehabil Clin N Am.* 2006;17:415-433.

118. Ozaki T, Halm H, Liljenqvist U, Winkelmann W. Treatment of tumors of the spine. *Hiroshima J Med Sci.* 1997;46:125-131.

119. Palumbo MA, Hilibrand AS, Hart RA, Bohlman HH. Surgical treatment of thoracic spinal stenosis: a 2- to 9-year follow-up. *Spine.* 2001;26:558-566.

120. Panjabi MM. Clinical spinal instability and low back pain. *J Electromyogr Kinesiol.* 2003;13:371-379.

121. Panjabi MM. A hypothesis of chronic back pain: ligament subfailure injuries lead to muscle control dysfunction. *Eur Spine J.* 2006;15:668-676.

122. Panjabi MM. The stabilizing system of the spine. Part I. Function, dysfunction, adaptation, and enhancement. *J Spinal Disord.* 1992;5:383-389 [discussion 97].

123. Panjabi MM. The stabilizing system of the spine. Part II. Neutral zone and instability hypothesis. *J Spinal Disord.* 1992;5:390-396 [discussion 97].

124. Panjabi MM, Hausfeld JN, White AA 3rd. A biomechanical study of the ligamentous stability of the thoracic spine in man. *Acta Orthop Scand.* 1981;52:315-326.

125. Panjabi MM, Krag MH, Chung TQ. Effects of disc injury on mechanical behavior of the human spine. *Spine.* 1984;9:707-713.

126. Patel AT, Ogle AA. Diagnosis and management of acute low back pain. *Am Fam Physician.* 2000;61:1779-1786, 89-90.

127. Pho C, Godges J. Management of whiplash-associated disorder addressing thoracic and cervical spine impairments: a case report [see comment]. *J Orthop Sports Phys Ther.* 2004;34:511-519 [discussion 20-23].

128. Sampaio-Barros PD, Bertolo MB, Kraemer MH, Neto JF, Samara AM. Primary ankylosing spondylitis: patterns of disease in a Brazilian population of 147 patients. *J Rheumatol.* 2001;28:560-565.

129. Santavirta S, Konttinen YT, Heliovaara M, Knekt P, Luthje P, Aromaa A. Determinants of osteoporotic thoracic vertebral fracture: screening of 57,000 Finnish women and men. *Acta Orthop Scand.* 1992;63:198-202.

130. Schellhas KP, Pollei SR, Dorwart RH. Thoracic discography: a safe and reliable technique [see comment]. *Spine.* 1994;19:2103-2109.

131. Schiller L. Effectiveness of spinal manipulative therapy in the treatment of mechanical thoracic spine pain: a pilot randomized clinical trial [see comment]. *J Manipulative Physiol Ther.* 2001;24:394-401.

132. Selim AJ, Fincke G, Ren XS, et al. Racial differences in the use of lumbar spine radiographs: results from the Veterans Health Study. *Spine.* 2001;26:1364-1369.

133. Sheridan R, Peralta R, Rhea J, Ptak T, Novelline R. Reformatted visceral protocol helical computed tomographic scanning allows conventional radiographs of the thoracic and lumbar spine to be eliminated in the evaluation of blunt trauma patients. *J Trauma.* 2003;55(4):665-669 (10 ref).

134. Simons DG, Travell JG, Simons LS. *Travell & Simons' Myofascial Pain and Dysfunction: The Trigger Point Manual.* Vol 1. 2nd ed. Baltimore: Williams & Wilkins; 1999.

135. Singer KP. Pathology of the thoracic spine. In: Giles LGF, Singer KP, eds. *The Clinical Anatomy and Management of Thoracic Spine Pain.* Boston, MA: Butterworth-Heinemann; 2000.

136. Slater H, Vicenzino B, Wright A. "Sympathetic slump": the effect of a novel manual therapy technique on peripheral sympathetic nervous system function. *J Man Manipulative Ther.* 1994;2(4):156-162 (13 ref).

137. Slover J, Abdu WA, Hanscom B, Lurie J, Weinstein JN. Can condition-specific health surveys be specific to spine disease? An analysis of the effect of comorbidities on baseline condition-specific and general health survey scores. *Spine.* 2006;31(11):1265-1271 (29 ref).

138. Sobel JS, Kremer I, Winters JC, Arendzen JH, de Jong BM. The influence of the mobility in the cervicothoracic spine and the upper ribs (shoulder girdle) on the mobility of the scapulohumeral joint. *J Manipulative Physiol Ther.* 1996;19:469-474.

Section II

ORTHOPEDIC REASONING

139. Sobel JS, Kremer I, Winters JC, Arendzen JH, de Jong BM. Reviews of the literature: the influence of the mobility in the cervicothoracic spine and the upper ribs (shoulder girdle) on the mobility of the scapulohumeral joint. *J Manipulative Physiol Ther.* 1996;19(7):469-474 (16 ref).

140. Sobel JS, Winters JC, Groenier K, Arendzen JH, Meyboom de Jong B. Physical examination of the cervical spine and shoulder girdle in patients with shoulder complaints. *J Manipulative Physiol Ther.* 1997;20:257-262.

141. Soreff J, Axdorph G, Bylund P, Odeen I, Olerud S. Treatment of patients with unstable fractures of the thoracic and lumbar spine: a follow-up study of surgical and conservative treatment. *Acta Orthop Scand.* 1982;53:369-381.

142. Sterling M, Jull G, Kenardy J. Physical and psychological factors maintain long-term predictive capacity post-whiplash injury. *Pain.* 2006;122:102-108.

143. Sterling M, Jull G, Vicenzino B, Kenardy J. Sensory hypersensitivity occurs soon after whiplash injury and is associated with poor recovery [see comment]. *Pain.* 2003;104:509-517.

144. Swannell AJ. Biological rhythms and their effect in the assessment of disease activity in rheumatoid arthritis. *Br J Clin Pract.* 1983;38(suppl 33):16-19.

145. Tan G, Jensen MP, Thornby J, Anderson KO. Ethnicity, control appraisal, coping, and adjustment to chronic pain among black and white Americans. *Pain Med.* 2005;6:18-28.

146. Taylor TKF. Thoracic disc lesions. *J Bone Joint Surg Br.* 1964;46:788-794.

147. Troussier B, Marchou-Lopez S, Pironneau S, et al. Back pain and spinal alignment abnormalities in schoolchildren. *Revue du Rhumatisme (English Edition).* 1999;66:370-380.

148. Turner JA, Jensen MP, Romano JM. Do beliefs, coping, and catastrophizing independently predict functioning in patients with chronic pain? *Pain.* 2000;85:115-125.

149. Vanichkachorn JS, Vaccaro AR. Thoracic disk disease: diagnosis and treatment. *J Am Acad Orthop Surg.* 2000;8:159-169.

150. Vroomen PC, de Krom MC, Knottnerus JA. Consistency of history taking and physical examination in patients with suspected lumbar nerve root involvement. *Spine.* 2000;25:91-96 [discussion 97].

151. Wainner RS, Whitman JM, Cleland JA, Flynn TW. Regional interdependence: a musculoskeletal examination model whose time has come. *J Orthop Sports Phys Ther.* 2007;37:658-660.

152. Wedderkopp N, Leboeuf-Yde C, Andersen LB, Froberg K, Hansen HS. Back pain reporting pattern in a Danish population-based sample of children and adolescents. *Spine.* 2001;26:1879-1883.

153. Weiss H, Dieckmann J, Gerner HJ. The practical use of surface topography: following up patients with Scheuermann's disease. *Pediatr Rehabil.* 2003;6(1):39-45 (22 ref).

154. Weiss HR. Idiopathic scoliosis: how much of a genetic disorder? Report of five pairs of monozygotic twins. *Dev Neurorehabil.* 2007;10:67-73.

155. White A, Panjabi M. *Clinical Biomechanics of the Spine.* 2nd ed. New York: Lippincott Raven; 1990.

156. Williams FM, Manek NJ, Sambrook PN, Spector TD, Macgregor AJ. Schmorl's nodes: common, highly heritable, and related to lumbar disc disease. *Arthritis Rheum.* 2007;57:855-860.

157. Wisniewski A. Don't worry, it's just chest pain: taking a closer look at costochondritis. *Nursing Made Incredibly Easy!* 2005;3:37-39.

158. Wisniewski A. Taking a closer look at costochondritis. *Nursing.* 2006;36(11): Crit Care. 64cc1 1-2 (4 ref).

159. Wood KB, Blair JM, Aepple DM, et al. The natural history of asymptomatic thoracic disc herniations. *Spine.* 1997;22:525-529 [discussion 29-30].

160. Wood KB, Garvey TA, Gundry C, Heithoff KB. Magnetic resonance imaging of the thoracic spine: evaluation of asymptomatic individuals. *J Bone Joint Surg Am.* 1995;77:1631-1638.

161. Wood KB, Schellhas KP, Garvey TA, Aeppli D. Thoracic discography in healthy individuals: a controlled prospective study of magnetic resonance imaging and discography in asymptomatic and symptomatic individuals. *Spine.* 1999;24:1548-1555.

162. Woolf CJ. Central sensitization: uncovering the relation between pain and plasticity. *Anesthesiology.* 2007;106:864-867.

163. Woolf CJ. A new strategy for the treatment of inflammatory pain: prevention or elimination of central sensitization. *Drugs.* 1994;47(suppl 5):1-9 [discussion 46-7].

164. Woolf CJ. Pain. *Neurobiol Dis.* 2000;7:504-510.

AUTHORS: DERRICK SUEKI and SUZANNE ROWLES

INTRODUCTORY INFORMATION

WHAT IS THE PREVALENCE OF LOW BACK PAIN?

Pain in the lumbar region is the second leading reason people in the United States visit their doctor. Fifty percent of people experience low back pain by the age of 20 years and this percentage increases to 80% by the age of 60 years.[58]

WHAT IS THE PROGNOSIS FOR RECOVERY FROM LOW BACK PAIN?

Studies in the 1980s and 1990s revealed that 80% to 90% of people with acute low back pain recovered in 6 weeks regardless of the treatment received.[58]

WHAT IS THE REOCCURRENCE RATE?

In a 12-month study of people who experienced low back pain Croft et al found an 82% recurrence rate of low back pain with 60% of people experiencing two or more episodes. These findings indicate that the abatement of pain does not necessarily signify that the lumbar spine structures have healed, simply that they are no longer symptomatic.[17]

WHAT FACTORS MAKE DIAGNOSIS DIFFICULT IN THE LUMBAR SPINE?

Clinicians may experience difficulty when diagnosing the source of lumbar pain due to several factors.
- Radiographic findings do not always correlate with patient symptomology.
- The biomechanics of the lumbar spine are not well defined.
- Dysfunction at the sacrum and thoracic spine can impact the lumbar spine.
- Lumbar spine diagnosis may also be difficult due to the multifaceted aspect of pain itself. Following tissue injury, temporary and long-term changes to the central and peripheral nervous system confound tissue pathology diagnosis.

CLINICAL PEARL !

There are usually numerous factors that contribute to chronic pain symptoms and thus tracing the source of pain to one specific structure is usually not possible. Chronic onset is associated with central processing changes, inflammatory processes, immune reactions, endocrine factors, and fibrosis.

HOW SUCCESSFUL IS THERAPY IN TREATING LOW BACK PAIN?

Manipulation, patient instruction, and exercise are effective therapy treatments with proven satisfactory outcomes for acute low back pain. There is no evidence that therapy treatment for chronic low back pain is more effective than placebo treatment.[4,5,12,19,54]

HOW SUCCESSFUL IS SURGERY IN TREATING LOW BACK PAIN?

Success rates following surgery appear to be no greater than success rates after treatment with more conservative management.
- A 10-year follow-up study of patients with sciatica caused by lumbar disc herniation showed no difference between patients who had surgery and patients who did not have surgery when looking at work rates and disability status.[3]
- Little is known regarding the long-term outcome of lumbar spinal stenosis surgery. Only 60% to 70% of patients report satisfaction 4 to 7 years after surgery.[23,35]

PERSONAL INFORMATION

AGE

WHAT INFLUENCE DOES AGE HAVE ON YOUR CLINICAL DECISION-MAKING PROCESS?

- Below 20 years old, low back pain is fairly rare. Possible sources include: L5/S1 isthmic spondylolithesis, ankylosing spondylitis, and L4/L5 disc pathology.
- Between 20 and 50 years old, pathologies to consider include disc pathology, facet impingement, capsular entrapment, instability, and muscle strains.
- Above 50 years old, degenerative changes to bodily tissue are the primary source of lumbar pain. Consider the following pathologies: interforaminal stenosis, central stenosis, degenerative disc disease, and L4/L5 degenerative spondylolithesis.

OCCUPATION

WHAT INFLUENCE DOES A PATIENT'S OCCUPATION HAVE ON YOUR CLINICAL DECISION-MAKING PROCESS?

Occupation often places a person's lumbar spine in a compromised position and can result in repetitive motions during the course of a workday. The following pathologies are commonly associated with repetitive tasks.
- Repetitive flexion activities: disc pathology
- Repetitive extension activities: interforaminal stenosis, central stenosis, and facet pathology
- Repetitive rotational activities: disc pathology
- Repetitive rotational activities: facet pathology

GENDER

WHAT INFLUENCE DOES GENDER HAVE ON YOUR CLINICAL DECISION-MAKING PROCESS?

Although major pathologies seen in the lumbar spine do not have a gender preference, several less common pathologies do:
- Adolescent disc pathology is more common in females.
- Ankylosing spondylitis is more prevalent in males.
- Spondylolithesis is more prevalent in females between the ages of 15 and 25 years.
- Spondylolysis is more prevalent in males.

CLINICAL DECISION MAKING CASE STUDY—PATIENT PROFILE ?

Your patient is a 16-year-old female who reports low back pain that began 1 month ago. She remembers feeling pain when she bent forward to pick up her book bag. Her pain has been improving over the past month, but still bothers her with sitting and bending forward. What are your hypotheses regarding her pathology?

Answer
Low back pain in adolescents is rare. Ankylosing spondylitis and disc pathology should be considered as sources of the low back pain. Because the patient is a female, disc pathology should be considered primary.

ETHNICITY

WHAT INFLUENCE DOES ETHNICITY HAVE ON YOUR CLINICAL DECISION-MAKING PROCESS?

Ethnicity is generally not considered a major factor when diagnosing pathology; however, research has shown the following trends:
- Spondylolysis occurs more frequently in the white population and Eskimos when compared to the black population.[36]
- Ankylosing spondylitis is less prevalent in blacks and North American Indians.[25]
- Degenerative joint disease has a higher prevalence in the black population.[15,29,30]

Whereas ethnicity is not considered a major factor, inheritance is considered to play a major role in predisposing a person to spondylolithesis. Wynne-Davies and Scott have proposed that a hereditary defect or dysplasia in the cartilaginous model of the posterior neural arch is what predisposes an individual to spondylolithesis.[62]

SYMPTOM HISTORY

MECHANISM OF INJURY

WHAT INFLUENCE DOES THE MECHANISM OF INJURY HAVE ON YOUR CLINICAL DECISION-MAKING PROCESS?
Mechanism of injury plays a large role in the differential diagnosis of patients with acute low back pain and a lesser role for chronic low back pain. Acute traumatic injuries can often be traced back to damage of specific structures.
- Traumatic onset of symptoms: fractures, muscles strains, ligament strains, and facet pathology
- Sudden onset of symptoms without trauma: capsular entrapment, facet pathology, and disc pathology
- Insidious onset: central stenosis, interforaminal stenosis, degenerative disc disease, and visceral pain

CLINICAL DECISION MAKING CASE STUDY—PATIENT PROFILE **（?）**

Your patient is a 42-year-old male who reports low back pain following an injury 2 weeks ago. He reports he injured his back while bending over to lift a box of books from the ground. He initially felt a pain in his back, but it loosened up the remainder of the day. The next day he was unable to get out of bed due to low back pain. The pain has improved over the past several weeks, but continues to limit his ability to sit and bend forward. What are your hypotheses regarding the source of this patient's symptoms?

Answer
The manner in which low back symptoms begin is an important line of questioning when it comes to diagnosing the source of the symptoms. The fact that the patient felt pain indicates tissue injury. Since it took time for the secondary symptoms to appear, the inflammatory process took time to develop. This is typical of a source that has a poor blood supply. The lumbar disc should be considered as the primary source. The direction of injury was flexion based. This could also implicate the disc as a source of symptoms.

LOCATION OF SYMPTOMS

WHAT INFLUENCE DOES THE LOCATION OF SYMPTOMS HAVE ON YOUR CLINICAL DECISION-MAKING PROCESS?
Low back pain generally presents in close proximity to the source of symptoms. Structures in the low back can refer symptoms laterally to the low back region and down into the gluteal region. Less frequently, low back structures refer pain into the lateral thigh, anterior hip, and groin regions. If anterior hip and groin pain are a primary complaint, hip pathology should be the first consideration. Symptoms that are felt down the lower extremity are a result of nerve involvement.

CLINICAL PEARL **（!）**

Forward flexion injuries will cause soft tissue damage to structures in this order: supraspinous ligament, interspinous ligament, facet capsule, and then lumbar disc.

REFERRAL OF SYMPTOMS

LUMBAR DISC
Ohnmeiss et al found a significant relationship between pain location and the level of lumbar disc pathology.[43] Figure II-5-1 illustrates the referral pattern of the lumbar disc.
- No disc pathology referred pain to the low back and buttock pain.
- The L3–L4 disc referred pain into the anterior thigh without pain in the posterior thigh or leg.
- The L4–L5 disc referred pain into the anterior thigh, with or without posterior thigh or leg pain.
- The L5–S1 disc referred pain into the posterior thigh or leg and no pain in the anterior thigh.

CLINICAL PEARL **（!）**

What disc is implicated with L4 nerve root involvement? L3/L4. The spinal cord terminates at the level of L2. Therefore, below L2 in the lumbar region, the nerve roots run in the spinal canal in the form of the cauda equina. The majority of disc pathology occurs in the posterior lateral region of the disc. The L4 spinal nerve root will exit the intervertebral foramen cephalad to the L4/L5 disc. Therefore, if the L4 nerve root is to be entrapped by a disc, the entrapment must occur at the disc of the spinal segment immediately above the L3/L4 disc.

ZYGAPOPHYSEAL JOINT
According to Fukui et al the referral patterns of the lumbar zygapophyseal joint are[24] Figure II-5-2 illustrates the referral pattern of the lumbar zygapophyseal joint.
L1/L2: Lumbar spine
L2/L3: Lumbar spine, greater trocanter
L3/L4: Greater trocanter, lateral thigh, posterior thigh, groin
L4/L5: Lumbar spine, greater trocanter, lateral thigh, posterior thigh, groin
L5/S1: Gluteal, greater trocanter, lateral thigh, posterior thigh, groin

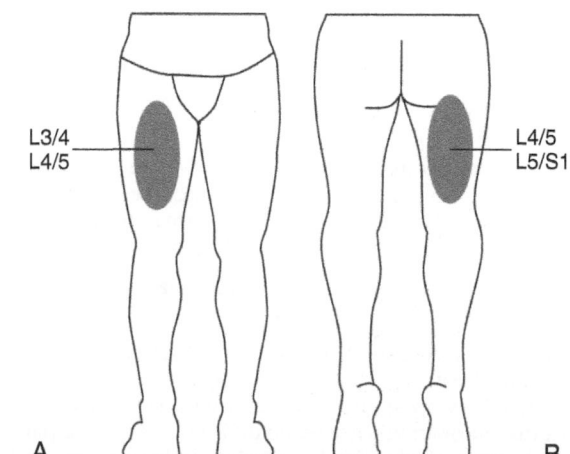

FIGURE II-5-1   Lumbar disc pain referral pattern. The pattern of disc referral is from the work of Ohnmeiss et al.[43] No disc pathology referred pain to the low back and buttock pain. **(A)** The L3/L4 and L4/L5 discs can refer pain into the anterior thigh. **(B)** The L4/L5 and L5/S1 discs can refer pain into the posterior thigh.

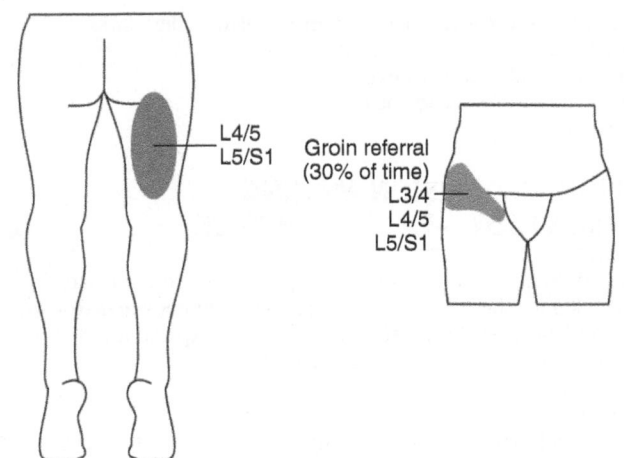

FIGURE II-5-2 Lumbar zygapophyseal joint pain referral patterns. From the work of Fukui et al[24]; cervical zygapophyseal joints referred pain in the following distributions.

CLINICAL PEARL

If a patient presents with L4 nerve root involvement, what intervertebral foramen is implicated? L4/L5. The L4 nerve root exits the spine by passing through the L4/L5 intervertebral foramen. Therefore, pathology such as stenosis or degeneration of the facets of this segment can cause nerve damage to the L4 nerve root.

LUMBAR MUSCLE (see Figure II-5-3)

Iliocostalis thoracis	Ipsilateral low back and lower abdominal quadrant
Iliocostalis lumborum	Ipsilateral low back, T12 ribs down to the gluteal region
Longissimus thoracic	Ipsilateral low back and medial gluteal region
Multifidus	Ipsilateral and adjacent to muscle belly, abdomen, and inner thigh
Abdominal muscles	Ipsilateral into the abdomen and hip or groin region
Serratus posterior inferior	Lateral to spine in T9–T12 posterior to the rib area[53]

BONE AND LIGAMENT INJURY

No studies have been conducted on the referral pattern of bone or ligament pathology in the lumbar spine. Because both tissues are innervated, the likelihood of them being pain generators is high. The pattern in which the pain is referred at this time is unknown.

DERMATOMAL DISTRIBUTION OF SPINAL NERVE ROOTS (see Figure II-5-4)

L1: Inguinal region
L2: Anterior and medial thigh
L3: Anterior thigh and medial knee
L4: Medial leg and medial foot
L5: Lateral leg and dorsum of foot
S1: Posterior thigh and lateral foot
S2: Posterior thigh and medial ankle
S3: Groin and coccyx region
S4: Coccyx region

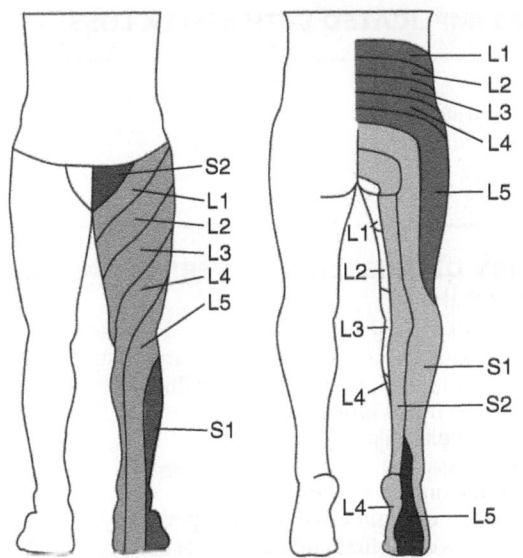

FIGURE II-5-3 Lower extremity dermatomes. A dermatome is an area of skin innervated by a single pair of dorsal nerve roots. Dermatomal patterns of symptoms vary greatly from person to person. The clinician should keep this in mind when utilizing dermatomes for clinical diagnostic purposes.

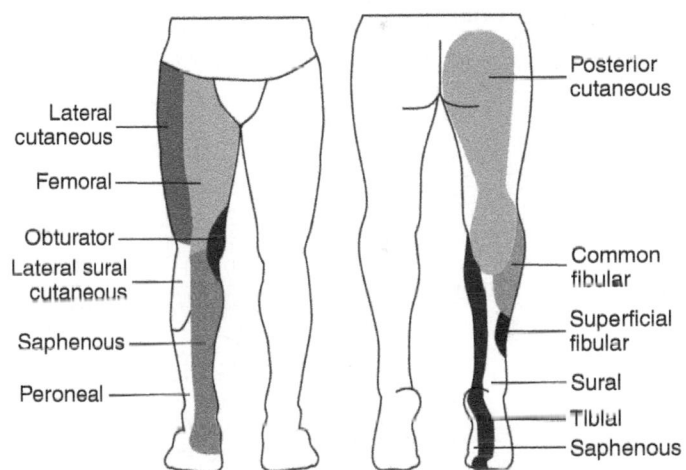

FIGURE II-5-4 Sensory distribution of peripheral nerves. The referral pattern of the sensory nerves is different from the referral pattern of the spinal nerve root. The clinician can utilize the differences to aid in the diagnostic process.

Myotomal distribution of spinal nerve roots
L1: Hip flexion
L2: Hip flexion, hip adduction
L3: Knee extension
L4: Ankle dorsiflexion
L5: Foot/toes dorsiflexion
S1: Plantar flexion foot/toes, ankle eversion, hip extension
S2: Knee flexion
S3: Foot intrinsics

CLINICAL PEARL

How can a clinician differentiate between peripheral and spinal nerve root involvement? Peripheral nerves and nerve roots present symptoms in different sensory distributions as outlined above. In addition, the presence of muscle atrophy and weakness will commonly be seen in myotomal patterns. Diminished reflexes can also be utilized to differentiate nerve involvement.

NERVES IMPLICATED WITH REFLEX LOSS

Patellar reflex	L3/L4
Medial hamstring	L5/S1
Lateral hamstring	S1/S2
Posterior tibial	L4/L5
Achilles reflex	S1/S2

SENSORY DISTRIBUTION OF PERIPHERAL NERVES
(see Figure II-5-5)

Femoral: Medial thigh and calf
Anterior femoral cutaneous: Lateral hip and thigh
Posterior femoral cutaneous: Posterior thigh
Pudendal: Groin and inner thighs
Obturator: Medial thigh
Sciatic: Posterior Leg
Tibial: Plantar surface of foot
Fibular: Lateral calf and dorsolateral aspect of foot
Deep fibular: Web of first and second toes
Sural: Lateral calf and lateral dorsum of foot

MYOTOMAL DISTRIBUTION OF LOWER EXTREMITY PERIPHERAL NERVES

Femoral: Knee extension with/without hip flexion
Lateral femoral cutaneous: None
Posterior femoral cutaneous: None
Saphenous: None
Pudendal: Pelvic floor
Obturator: Thigh adduction

Sciatic: Foot dorsiflexion and inversion, plantar, flexion, knee flexion
Tibial: Plantar flexion and foot inversion
Superficial fibular: Foot eversion
Deep fibular: Foot and toe dorsiflexion
Sural: None

CLINICAL DECISION MAKING CASE STUDY—PATIENT PROFILE

Your patient is a 35-year-old female who injured her back 1 week ago. She initially felt pain in her low back and trocanteric region. The past 2 days she has begun to experience pain in her left lateral leg and dorsum of the foot.

Answer

The initial symptoms of pain in the low back and into the trocanteric region implicate either the disc or facet as the source of the initial pain. Without knowledge of the mechanism of injury, behavior of symptoms, and aggravating factors, it is difficult to differentiate between the potential sources. The inclusion of symptoms into the left lateral leg and dorsum of the foot could implicate an L5 nerve root involvement. The entrapment could occur at either the L5/S1 intervertebral foramen or the L4/L5 disc.

WHAT OTHER MUSCULOSKELETAL STRUCTURES CAN REFER PAIN INTO THE LUMBAR SPINE?

Musculoskeletal structures in the lower thoracic region, the sacroiliac region, and the hip can refer symptoms proximally to the low back.

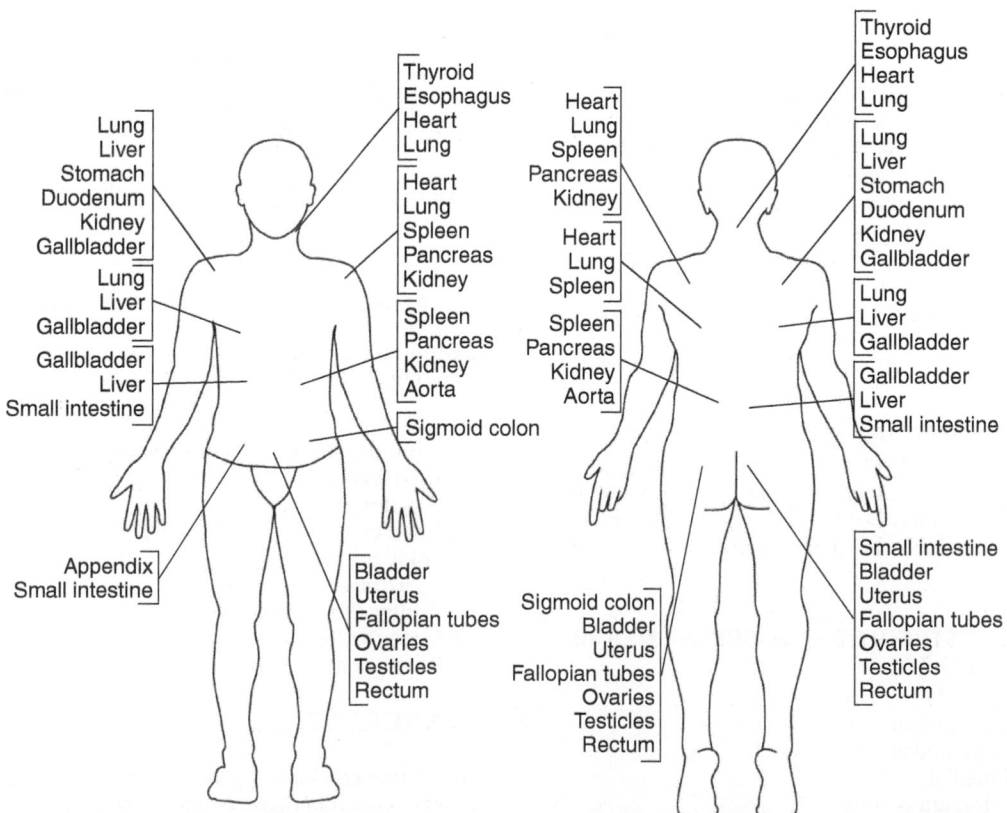

FIGURE II-5-5 Symptom referral pattern of visceral tissue. The visceral tissues that most commonly refer symptoms into the lower quarter region. Symptoms are generally described as a deep dull ache that is hard to localize. Symptoms may wax and wane based on motions of the region.

WHAT VASCULAR TISSUE IN THE LOW BACK CAN RESULT IN PAIN?

There has been no research published regarding vascular tissue such as arteries, veins, and lymphatic systems as sources of low back pain. Preliminary studies suggest that even though vascular tissue is innervated, the innervation is autonomic in origin, the purpose being regulation of smooth muscle in the vessels. There is no evidence to suggest that vascular tissue itself can be the source of pain. Vascular tissue can indirectly result in pain. In response to stress or injury, vascular tissue can vasoconstrict, which will result in diminished blood flow to a region and therefore can result in ischemic pain from tissue being supplied by the vascular tissue. In addition, vasodilation in response to acute injury can result in an influx of chemical mediators, which in turn can sensitize surrounding tissue. This hypersensitivity can result in increased shoulder pain. Preliminary studies into vasodynamics suggests that symptoms related to vascular systems are reported by patients as coldness or heaviness and not as pain.

WHAT VISCERAL STRUCTURES CAN REFER TO THE LUMBAR SPINE? (see Figure II-5-5)

UPPER LUMBAR
- Kidney
- Liver
- Gallbladder
- Stomach
- Small intestine
- Spleen
- Pancreas
- Lung

LOWER LUMBAR
- Bladder
- Ovaries
- Fallopian tubes
- Uterus
- Testes
- Prostate
- Sigmoid colon
- Appendix
- Small intestine[26]

SYMPTOM DESCRIPTORS

QUALITY OF SYMPTOMS

Deep ache: Disc
Dull ache: Bone, inflammation
Sharp pain: Capsule, facet joint
Sharp and continuous: Bone
Burning: Nerves, inflammation, vein, artery, lymphatic system
Tingling: Nerve
Numbness: Nerves
Colicky and cramping: Viscera

DEPTH OF SYMPTOMS

WHAT INFLUENCE DOES THE DEPTH OF SYMPTOMS HAVE ON YOUR CLINICAL DECISION-MAKING PROCESS?

Deep symptoms implicate deep structures such as disc, bone, and visceral structures. There are fewer proprioceptive nerves in deep structures than in more superficial structures so the ability to localize tissue damage in deep structures is more difficult.

Superficial symptoms implicate surface structures such as muscles and ligaments. Superficial structures have more proprioceptive nerve fibers and thus injury to superficial structures is more easily localized.

CONSTANCY OF SYMPTOMS

WHAT INFLUENCE DOES CONSTANCY OF SYMPTOMS HAVE ON YOUR CLINICAL DECISION-MAKING PROCESS?
- Intermittent symptoms implicate a mechanical source and a structure that is injured and is aggravated only with certain positions or motions.
- Constant but varying symptoms implicate inflammation as the primary source.
- Constant and unchanging symptoms implicate visceral structures or other pathology such as cancer.

TWENTY-FOUR-HOUR SYMPTOM PATTERN

IF A PATIENT HAS SYMPTOMS IN THE MORNING, WHAT PATHOLOGY DOES THIS IMPLICATE?

It is common for a patient with low back symptoms to have stiffness in the morning. Generally, stiffness and pain that last for only a short time on awakening corresponds to pathology that is more mechanical in nature. Mechanical disorders are disorders that can be altered by biomechanical motions. Degenerative joint disease, facet pathology, spondylolisthesis, instability, and stenosis will all present as stiffness in the morning that resolves quickly with motion.

Pain and stiffness that persists for a longer period of time, greater than 15 minutes, are common when inflammation is the primary source of the symptoms. Inflammation will abate once movement and circulation is increased in the region. Removal of edema from a region is tied to the lymphatic system. This system is a passive system and requires motion and muscle contractions to move the lymph out of the region. Therefore, symptoms will persist for a longer time frame.

WHAT ROLE DOES MORNING STIFFNESS PLAY IN DIFFERENTIATION?

When the body is in a static position for a prolonged period of time, inflammation can accumulate within a region. Body lymphatic systems are passive systems and require muscle contractions to drain areas. Morning stiffness that lasts for more than 15 minutes indicates that inflammation plays a large role in the feeling of stiffness. Stiffness that lasts only minutes and is relieved quickly with motion is often associated with mechanical factors more than with inflammatory factors.

When injured, an inflammatory reaction occurs. Muscle activation occurs as a protective mechanism to prevent further damage. If the spine is held in this position for more than 1 to 2 days, cross fibers of collagen in the capsule will create a capsular stiffness.

CLINICAL PEARL

Why do disc and joints get injured more frequently at L4/L5? It has been theorized that the higher prevalence of injury at L4/L5 is due to the attachment of the iliolumbar ligament to the L5 transverse process. This ligament functions to stabilize L5 onto the sacrum and is drawn taut when sacral nutation occurs. There is no ligament stabilization at L4 and thus shearing force is greater between these two segments. The end result is more pathology at L4/L5.

IF A PATIENT HAS SYMPTOMS IN THE AFTERNOON, WHAT PATHOLOGY DOES THIS IMPLICATE?
- Pain in the afternoon implicates disc, instability, spondylolisthesis, stenosis, muscle injury, ligament injury, or degenerative joint disease as possible primary sources of symptoms. Differentiation is dependent on the activities that were completed earlier in the day.
- Discs and degenerative joint disease become more aggravated as the day progress. With disc problems, the longer and more

repetitions of flexion-based activities the lumbar region is exposed to, the more symptomatic the low back will become. Therefore, a person sitting or bending forward during the morning will be more symptomatic by the afternoon. If a patient has minimized these activities, then the low back will not be as symptomatic by the afternoon.

- Degenerative joint disease and stenosis will be more irritated with repetitive extension activities.
- Instability, ligament injury, and spondylolithesis will be more symptomatic in the afternoon because the dynamic system of muscles that stabilize the region will become fatigued and slippage will occur.
- Muscles that are injured will also be more symptomatic in the afternoon. An injured muscle will become sore because the muscle is attempting to heal, but has been forced to work rather than rest.

IF A PATIENT HAS SYMPTOMS IN THE EVENING, WHAT PATHOLOGY DOES THIS IMPLICATE?

Evening symptoms can be viewed as an extension of afternoon symptoms. With continual use, the symptoms should continue to worsen if the irritating activities persist. If the activities have ceased for the day, then the symptoms may abate somewhat.

IF A PATIENT HAS SYMPTOMS WHEN SLEEPING, WHAT PATHOLOGY DOES THIS IMPLICATE?

Pain with sleeping can be the result of several factors. If a patient has pain when moving in bed, this can be the result of many types of pathology including disc and stenotic changes. Pain due to static positions may implicate spondylolithesis or instability. Nocturnal pain is also an indicator of visceral pathology and cancer, so red flag pathology should be ruled out.

STABILITY OF SYMPTOMS

CHANGES IN SYMPTOMS

HOW DOES THE PROGRESSION OF A PATIENT'S SYMPTOMS IMPACT YOUR CLINICAL DECISION-MAKING PROCESS?

- Pain and symptoms in the lumbar spine should follow a typical pattern with symptoms remaining severe for the first 3 days. Over the course of the next 2 to 3 weeks the symptoms should begin to resolve with full resolution by week 6. If symptoms do not follow this typical pattern then the preventing factor should be identified.[42]
- The vascularity of a structure will often aid in the differentiation process. Structures that are well vascularized, such as bone, muscle, and ligaments, will have an immediate and significant vascular response. Therefore, if a patient feels immediate pain that does not improve over the remainder of the day of injury, a structure that has become entrapped or pinched such as a joint capsule or a facet joint is implicated.
- Structures that have a poor vascular supply, such as a lumbar disc, will have a slow inflammation process and will be slower to swell. In this case, patients feel pain initially, but the pain quickly resolves for the remainder of the day, and they wake up the next day with excruciating pain.

CLINICAL PEARL

What role does inflammation play in the differentiation of lumbar pathology? The inflammatory process relies on vascularization. Structures that are well vascularized have a rapid inflammatory response and structures with poor vascularity have a delayed or slow inflammatory response. Structures that are well vascularized in the lumbar spine include the lumbar vertebrae, the ligaments, and the muscles of the lumbar spine.

The lumbar disc is more poorly vascularized. Therefore, if a structure stiffens quickly after injury, then more highly vascularized structures are implicated. If stiffness takes overnight or several days to appear, the lumbar disc is implicated. [50]

IF A PATIENT'S SYMPTOMS ARE IMPROVING, WHAT PATHOLOGY DOES THIS IMPLICATE?

Improvement is typical and expected with most pathology. The rate of improvement will help to narrow down the possible source of the symptoms. Facet pathology will generally improve in several days once the entrapment structure is released. Disc pathology will improve in 4 to 6 weeks. The state of the disc will still be impaired, hence the reoccurrence of symptoms with disc pathology, but the inflammatory process will abate within the 4- to 6-week timeframe.

CLINICAL DECISION MAKING CASE STUDY—PATIENT PROFILE

Your patient is a 23-year-old female with complaints of low back pain. Symptoms began insidiously and have been present for the past 2 months. They have become progressive, more frequent, and more intense in nature. Symptoms are worse with standing, sitting, and lying for more than 30 minutes. Symptoms feel better when walking or moving. What are your hypotheses regarding her pathology?

Answer

Typically, most pathology will be aggravated by specific activities or motions. In the first several days after an injury, most activities will aggravate the patient's symptoms. It is not until the initial inflammatory phase has resolved that the true nature of a patient's symptoms can be assessed. The patient has been experiencing pain for the past 2 months and therefore is past the initial inflammatory phase and the pain cannot be considered chronic in nature. The symptoms are worsening, which is not the normal pattern for most lumbar tissue. Most lumbar tissue will be well along the healing continuum by the 2-month mark. The fact that the symptoms are aggravated by static positions and eased by motion implicates instability or spondylolithesis as the primary hypotheses at this time.

IF A PATIENT'S SYMPTOMS ARE WORSENING, WHAT PATHOLOGY DOES THIS IMPLICATE?

- If symptoms worsen over a shorter period of time such as several weeks, inflammation is usually associated with the symptoms. Initially the structure is injured and sharp pain and ache occur. This is the nocioceptive response of the body. As the inflammatory process begins, surrounding structures can be irritated by the chemical mediators released during the inflammatory process. If the process continues then compression of neural structures can occur. Therefore, patients with worsening symptoms secondary to inflammation will report that their symptoms in the back have remained stable, but symptoms in the leg have increased.
- Symptoms that do not change over time are more indicative of stenotic or degenerative changes. These processes are not the result of inflammation and acute processes, therefore resolution in 4 to 6 weeks is not anticipated. Symptoms may decrease for several days, but they will return again. As the stenosis and degenerative processes progress, the symptoms will increase. This process will occur over a period of several months.
- Symptoms that have not changed can implicate instability, spondylolithesis, or disc pathology. Because the symptoms associated with instability and spondylolithesis are the result of spinal slippage and movement, symptoms usually remain unchanged for longer periods.

CLINICAL PEARL !

Will the symptoms of lumbar stenosis worsen over time?
Little is known about the progression of symptoms from lum-
bar stenosis. Preliminary research suggests that decline is not
inevitable and that large percentages of patients can maintain
or improve their symptoms over time.[35]

FUNCTIONAL OR ACTIVITY PARTICIPATION LIMITATIONS

BEHAVIOR OF SYMPTOMS: AGGRAVATING BEHAVIOR (see Table II-5-1)

WHAT INFLUENCE DOES AGGRAVATING FUNCTIONS HAVE ON YOUR CLINICAL DECISION-MAKING PROCESS?

Flexion-based activities
- Pathology aggravated by flexion include disc pathology, muscle strain, radiculopathy, and ligament strain.
- Sitting increases the pressure on the disc 40% and seated flexion will increase the disc pressure 80%.[33]
- Lumbar flexion will aggravate the posterior longitudinal, interspinous, and supraspinous ligaments and the ligamentum flavuum.
- In the case of a sciatic nerve entrapment, a sensitive nerve will be irritated by flexion activities. Within the spine, the nervous system must be allowed to glide. Flexion of the spine elongates the spinal canal up to 97 mm with the greatest elongation occurring in the lumbar and thoracic regions. Extension shortens the spinal canal 38 mm.[52]
- Strain within the dural of the nerve is higher in areas with high segmental mobility. Therefore, strain is highest at L5/S1 and lowest at L1/L2.

CLINICAL PEARL !

Forward flexion and straight leg raising increase ten-
sile loads placed on nerves. Between 0° and 30° of straight leg
raise, slack is taken up in the sciatic nerve. From 35° to 70° the
nerve glides. From 75° to 90° the gliding in the nerve ceases
and a tensile load is placed on the nerve. With straight leg rais-
ing, the nerve will glide toward the hip joint and away from
the foot and knee.

CLINICAL PEARL !

It has been proposed that this occurs because of
a firm dural attachment that exists between the dura and
the posterior longitudinal ligament at the L4 vertebral level.
Dural sleeves of the spinal nerves also tether the spinal cord
at each spinal segment and limit the amount of spinal cord
excursion.

Extension-based activities
- Pathologies aggravated by extension include facet joint, radiculopathy, ligament strain, central canal stenosis, interforaminal stenosis, and spondylolithesis.
- Acute sharp low back pain may be secondary to facet involvement and has been attributed to the entrapment or compression of the joint capsule, free fragments of articular cartilage, roughness of degenerative joint surfaces, or meniscoid involvement.
- The main joint of concern in patients with degenerative joint disease is the zygapophyseal or facet joint. The facets function to limit rotation and therefore protect the disc from torsional damage. They also function as load-bearing structures.

Lumbar extension and lumbar compression place the zygapophyseal joint in a compacted position. The facets carry 25% of the body load in an extended position and this percentage increases to 50% in people with spinal arthritis. Therefore, activities that place an extension force coupled with compressive loading aggravate patients with degenerative joint disease the most.[1,14,27]
- Central canal and intervertebral foramen stenosis are both impacted by extension. Extension decreases the intervertebral foramen by 20% and also decreases the cross-sectional area of the central canal.[13]
- Within the spinal cord, there are two levels of enlargement that correspond to the upper and lower extremity nerves. In the lumbar spine, the level of enlargement occurs at the L2–S3 spinal levels. The reduction of the central foramen and the enlargement of the spinal cord place more pressure on the central cord, the cauda equine, and the spinal nerve root.[13]
- With extension activities, the diameter of the intervertebral foramen is reduced. In the presence of pathology such as stenosis or spondylolithesis the diameter of the foramen is further reduced. This results in nerves being irritated within the smaller foramen.
- Extension of the hip will aggravate the femoral nerve.

CLINICAL PEARL !

Research has shown that this centralization does occur,
but only in cases in which the annulus of the disc is still intact.
When the annulus of the disc is compromised, the centraliza-
tion phenomenon does not occur. Recently, it has been hypoth-
esized that disc-related pain is dependent on the status of the
annulus. When the nucleus pulposa is extruded past the confines
of the annulus, an inflammatory reaction occurs. Therefore,
extension and walking could decrease disc-related pain and
radicular pain by increasing circulation around the disc and
nerve.[48,50]

CLINICAL PEARL !

Disc herniations of the lumbar spine occur most com-
monly at L4/L5 followed, in order, by L5/S1, L3/L4, L2/L3, and
L1/L2. Zygopophyseal joint pathology occurs most often at the
L4/L5 spinal segment.

Lateral flexion and rotation activities
- Pathologies aggravated by lateral flexion include facet joint, radiculopathy, interforaminal stenosis, and muscle strain.
- Maximal force production is often achieved during eccentric muscle contraction. Eccentric muscle contraction in the lumbar region occurs during flexion-based activities such as sitting and bending forward. Lateral flexion contralateral to the injured tissue will result in pain.
- Once injured, pain will be elicited in muscle during muscle contraction. Therefore, eccentric lumbar muscle contraction during forward bending or concentric muscle contraction when returning to an upright position will often produce a patient's symptoms.
- Muscle pain is often aggravated by sitting. During sitting, the muscles of the lumbar region must contract to prevent the patient from slouching. This low-level muscle contraction can produce lumbar pain over prolonged periods of time.

Combined motion activities
- Pathologies aggravated by extension and rotation/lateral flexion include facet joint, radiculopathy, ligament strain, central canal stenosis, interforaminal stenosis, spondylolithesis, and muscle strain.

- Pathologies aggravated by flexion and rotation/lateral flexion include disc pathology, radiculopathy, ligament strain, and muscle strain.

Static activities

- Pathologies aggravated by extension include instability and spondylolithesis.
- Panjabi theorizes that joint stability is achieved by the coordinated actions of three systems: the passive, active, and motor control systems. Disruption or injury to any of these three systems can affect the other systems by forcing them to work harder in order to provide stability to the joint.[18,21,39,46]
- In the case of trauma, ligaments that provide passive support to the spinal vertebra can be strained resulting in joint laxity and instability.
- Motion and activity encourage activation of these active systems; therefore, joint stability is maintained. Static positions or positions of relative rest allow the lumbar musculature to turn off. When the muscles are not activated, lumbar dynamic stability is lost. As the spinal segment loses stability, it slides forward and aggravates pain-producing structures.
- Classically, spondylolithesis will be aggravated by extension-based activities or with static positions.

Other activities

- Coughing and sneezing result in an increase in flexion motion and a 35% increase in disc pressure.
- Laughing produces a 50% increase in disc pressure. The forced contraction of the abdominal muscles coupled with the contraction of the diaphragm increases the compressive forces placed on the lumbar spine in this flexed position.

Table II-5-1 lists the functional and activity limitations commonly seen with lumbar spine pathology

BEHAVIOR OF SYMPTOMS: EASING BEHAVIOR
(see Table II-5-1)

WHAT INFLUENCE DOES EASING FUNCTIONS HAVE ON YOUR CLINICAL DECISION-MAKING PROCESS?

Flexion-based activities

- Pathologies eased by flexion include facet joint, radiculopathy, central canal stenosis, interforaminal stenosis, and spondylolithesis.
- The cross-sectional area of the spinal canal increases with flexion and decreases with extension. The same is true of the intervertebral foramen diameter. Flexion increases the intervertebral foramen by 30%.[13]
- Flexion-based activities will take the load off of the anterior longitudinal ligament.
- Easing activities that will alleviate the symptoms associated with lumbar radiculopathy are dependent on the structures that are creating the nerve irritation. Radicular symptoms that ease with flexion are associated with stenotic changes.
- If fibrosis of the nerve or inflammation surrounding the nerve is the cause of the radicular symptoms, then neither flexion nor extension will alleviate the symptoms.

Extension-based activities

- Pathologies eased by extension include disc pathology, radiculopathy, and ligament strain.
- The mechanism for symptom reduction with disc pathology is still unclear. McKenzie has proposed that the reduction is due to centralization of the disc protrusion.[41]
- Extension-based activities will take the stress off the posterior spinal ligaments.
- Easing activities that will alleviate the symptoms associated with lumbar radiculopathy are dependent on the structures that are creating the nerve irritation. Radicular symptoms that ease with extension are often associated with disc pathology.

TABLE II-5-1 Functional or Activity Participation Limitations

Motion	Functional Activities	Pathology if Symptoms Are Aggravated by Activity	Pathology if Symptoms Are Eased by Activity
Flexion	Sitting, bending forward	Disc pathology, muscle strain, posterior ligament sprain, radiculopathy	Facet joint, radiculopathy, central canal stenosis, interforaminal stenosis, spondylolithesis
Extension	Walking, bending backward	Facet joint, radiculopathy, anterior ligament strain, interforaminal stenosis, central stenosis, spondylolithesis, degenerative disc disease	Disc pathology, radiculopathy, ligament strain
Lateral flexion and rotation	Bending and lifting, sports	Facet joint, radiculopathy, interforaminal stenosis, muscle strain	Disc pathology, muscle strain, radiculopathy, ligament strain, facet joint, interforaminal stenosis
Combined motion	Extension and rotation/ lateral flexion	Facet joint, radiculopathy, ligament strain, central canal stenosis, interforaminal stenosis, spondylolithesis, muscle strain	Disc pathology, radiculopathy, ligament strain, muscle strain
Combined motion	Flexion and rotation/ lateral flexion	Disc pathology, radiculopathy, ligament strain, muscle strain	Facet joint, radiculopathy, ligament strain, interforaminal stenosis, muscle strain
Static positions	Sleep sitting, standing	Instability, spondylolithesis	Disc pathology, muscle strain, ligament strain, facet joint, central canal stenosis, interforaminal stenosis
General movement	Walking and movement		Instability, spondylolithesis
Other	Coughing, laughing, and sneezing	Spondylosis, spondylolithesis, lumbar instability, muscle strain, lumbar disc pathology, lumbar radiculopathy	

CLINICAL PEARL   (!)

Will a disc prolapse heal? Studies indicate that 45% of patients with a disc prolapse will have resorption of the prolapse over time. [48]

Lateral flexion and rotation activities
- Pathologies eased by lateral flexion and rotation include disc pathology, muscle strain, radiculopathy, ligament strain, facet joint, and interforaminal stenosis.
- Ipsilateral lumbar rotation is also believed to open up or gap the zygapophyseal joint. However, based on radiographic studies it is questionable as to whether gapping can or does actually occur at the zygapophyseal joint.

Combined motion activities
- Pathologies eased by extension and rotation/lateral flexion include disc pathology, radiculopathy, ligament strain, and muscle strain.
- Pathologies eased by flexion and rotation/lateral flexion include facet joint, radiculopathy, ligament strain, interforaminal stenosis, and muscle strain.

Static activities
- Pathologies eased by static activities include disc pathology, muscle strain, ligament strain, facet joint, central canal stenosis, and interforaminal stenosis.
- Static activities allow the lumbar muscles to relax and this will alleviate the muscle guarding seen in many pathologies.

CLINICAL PEARL   (!)

Spondylolithesis has been associated with instability, but instability is dependent on the spinal segment affected. Instability rarely occurs at L5/S1 because the segment is stabilized by the iliolumbar ligament. If the spondylolithesis occurs at the L4/L5 spinal segment instability is more likely to occur.

Fifty percent of patients with spondylolithesis report that symptoms began as a result of specific injury.

The degree of vertebral slippage does not directly correlate with the amount of symptoms a patient will experience.

Hypermobility is most likely in the third and fourth decades of life. After the fourth decade, osseous changes in the spine begin to stabilize the spine, but these degenerative changes may eventually lead to degenerative spondylolithesis.

General movement
- Easing activities include motion and movement, which will generally relieve pain due to instability.
- In patients with instability there is a lack of passive stabilizing elements. Active contraction of the lumbar spine muscles is required to stabilize lumbar spinal segments and reduce symptoms.

MEDICAL HISTORY

WHAT ROLE DOES A PATIENT'S PAST MEDICAL HISTORY PLAY IN THE DIFFERENTIAL DIAGNOSIS OF LUMBAR PATHOLOGY?
- Past surgeries, injuries, and other medical pathology can influence the normal function of the lumbar spine. Hernia surgeries, colon surgeries, hysterectomies, and caesarian sections can all result in scar tissue formation, which can influence the normal biomechanics of the region.
- Pathologies such as diverticulitis, Crohn's disease, urinary tract infections, appendicitis, and endometriosis can all result in abnormal biomechanics within the region because

the body may take postures to minimize stress on impacted systems.
- Pregnancy can affect low back pain in several ways. The release of hormones such as relaxin may result in ligament laxity. This laxity can result in symptoms similar to those of instability. It may be difficult for pregnant women to utilize dynamic systems such as the abdominal muscles to stabilize the region. This ligament laxity may also impact the sacroiliac joint and contribute to low back symptoms by changing the mechanics of the region.
- Low back pain that responds to menstrual cycles is a common occurrence. Menstrual cycle body changes, such as cramping, irregular cycles, and difficulty conceiving, can all be symptoms pointing to problems within the reproductive system. The cause of the pain can be related to several factors. Primary dysmenorrheal, or menstrual pain triggered by the release of prostaglandin, will cause strong uterine contractions and muscle spasms within the endometrium of the uterus. Secondary dysmenorrhea is caused by pathological conditions such as endometriosis, uterine fibroids, ovarian cysts, uterine infections, and pelvic inflammatory diseases. In addition to pelvic pain, both primary and secondary dysmenorrhea can cause low back symptoms.
- Reoccurring bladder and kidney infections can also be associated with low back pain. Urinary tract infections account for 8.3 million physician visits per year. A common complaint with these patients is low back pain. [20]
- The gastrointestinal tract runs throughout the lumbar region and pathology within this region can impact the low back in several ways. Symptoms such as diarrhea, constipation, bloating, and cramping can all be signs of gastrointestinal dysfunction. Biomechanically, as the lumen of the tract gets full, it can expand into the lumbar structures and create pressure on nociceptive structures in the low back. The muscle guarding that is associated with gastrointestinal dysfunction can result in abnormal stresses being placed on the lumbar region. Chemically, the colon can leak toxic material from its lumen into the surrounding area and this can irritate the surrounding low back structures.
- Previous musculoskeletal injuries can contribute to biomechanical changes and stresses placed on the lumbar region. Ankle and knee injuries, hip pathology, and sacroiliac dysfunction can all lead to movement compensations, which change the normal mechanics of the lumbar spine. Over time, these changes will result in abnormal wear on lumbar structures leading to deterioration and degeneration.

MEDICAL AND ORTHOPEDIC TESTING

WHAT MEDICAL AND ORTHOPEDIC TESTS INFLUENCE YOUR DIFFERENTIAL DIAGNOSIS PROCESS IN THE LUMBAR SPINE?
- Magnetic resonance imaging (MRI), x-rays, and electromyogram (EMG) tests are used in conjunction with other clinical tests and observations to influence the decision-making process. [8]
- Clinicians often look for the magic assessment tool that will positively diagnose a patient's pathology 100% of the time, but no such test exists. All imaging results should always be correlated with clinical findings.

HOW DO RADIOGRAPHIC OR OTHER EXAMINATIONS INFLUENCE YOUR DECISION-MAKING PROCESS?
Although the existence of and the histological basis for zygapophyseal joint and lumbar disc pain have been scientifically established, their relevance to clinical presentation and their role as pain generators have not been clearly established. There are no

universally common identifying features in the history, physical examination, and radiological imaging of patients with pain originating from the lumbar zygapophyseal joint or lumbar disc. Physicians will diagnose zygapophyseal joint pain based on analgesic response to anesthetic injections directly into the joints or at their nerve supply. MRI imaging will be utilized to diagnose the existence of disc pathology, but the correlation with pain is poor. Therefore, imaging should be utilized as an aid to differential diagnosis, but should not be utilized as the sole source of clinical decisions.[8]

HOW RELIABLE ARE X-RAYS OF THE LUMBAR SPINE?

Abnormalities in x-ray and MRI and the occurrence of non-specific low back pain seem not to be strongly associated.[57] Abnormalities found when imaging people without back pain are just as prevalent as those found in patients with back pain. Van Tulder and Roland reported radiological abnormalities varying from 40% to 50% for degeneration and spondylosis in people without low back pain. Many people with low back pain show no abnormalities.[32,37]

HOW RELIABLE ARE MRIs OF THE LUMBAR SPINE?[6,28]

Sensitivity[28]	
Cancer	0.83-0.93
Infection	0.96
Herniated disc	0.81-0.97
Stenosis	0.81-0.97
Specificity	
Cancer	0.90-0.97
Infection	0.92
Herniated disc	0.89-0.95
Stenosis	Unknown

These numbers can be misleading in regard to herniated discs, because although the specificity and sensitivity of herniated discs are relatively high, there is also evidence to suggest that most disc herniations do not hurt. In asymptomatic patients, MRI studies have demonstrated that 39% to 50% of people had lumbar disc herniations, yet they were asymptomatic. Table II-5-2 further illustrates the reliability of MRI imaging in the lumbar spine. [7,9-11,34,59-61]

HOW RELIABLE ARE EMGs AND NERVE CONDUCTION TESTS OF THE LUMBAR SPINE?

EMG and nerve conduction studies are commonly utilized to help confirm or negate suspected nerve and nerve root involvement. Like any other diagnostic test, the results of the EMG or conduction studies should be correlated with other diagnostic and clinical tests and complaints. EMG and nerve conduction studies test for injury to the nerve, but there are instances in which the nerve is still patent, but irritated by surrounding structures. In these instances EMG and conduction studies may present negatively, while MRI studies reveal entrapment of the nerve. It has been reported that false negatives occur in 30% to 40% of the tests for radiculopathies. This is due to many factors, including the fact that although radiculopathies may be painful, they may actually not cause any nerve damage, sampling or interpretation errors, detection error due to poor relaxation, timing of the examination, age of the patient, or temperature of the room.

MEDICATIONS

HOW DOES PATIENT MEDICATION INFLUENCE YOUR DECISION-MAKING PROCESS?

- Muscle relaxants, pain medications, and antiinflammatory medications are commonly prescribed in association with low back pain.
- Symptom relief with muscle relaxants and pain medications does not aid the diagnostic process. Most patients with symptomatic lumbar pathology will experience muscle guarding and pain.
- The effectiveness of antiinflammatory medication helps differentiate pathology that has an acute inflammatory process.
  - Pathologies that can have an acute inflammatory process include disc pathology, muscle strain, ligament sprain, facet dysfunction, and radiculopathy.
  - Pathologies that do not normally have an acute inflammatory response include stenosis, degenerative joint disease, instability, and spondylolithesis.

BIOMECHANICAL FACTORS

WHAT ROLE DOES BIOMECHANICS PLAY IN LOW BACK PAIN?

- A longtime primary tenet of addressing lumbar pathology is biomechanical assessment and treatment. However, recent studies question this approach due to the fact that the true mechanics of coupled motion of the lumbar spine appear to vary from study to study.[40]
- When structures implicated clinically as sources of pain are surgically removed, the pain is not always eliminated. For this reason, research has begun to extend beyond the scope of biomechanics to other possible sources of pain. These possible sources in chronic lumbar pain include inflammation and circulation, endocrine responses, and immune responses.
- These factors make diagnosing and determining the source of lumbar pain difficult tasks for the clinician.

WHAT BIOMECHANICAL ABNORMALITIES IN OTHER REGIONS AFFECT LUMBAR REGION PATHOLOGY?

- Walking and lumbar extension rely heavily on sacrum mechanics. Therefore, lumbar mechanics are also linked to proper sacral functioning. The sacrum nutates when stability is required to provide a stable base from which the rest of the spine can move.
- Nutation occurs in the stance phase of gait and provides ipsilateral stability to the stance leg.
- Nutation also tightens the iliolumbar ligament. The L5 spinal segment is subsequently pulled caudally onto the sacrum because of its attachments. This is a possible explanation for why the L4/L5 spinal segment has the highest percentage of spondylolithesis and degenerative changes.[38]
- With walking, the increase in compressive forces at L5/S1 and shearing at L4/L5 cause higher interforaminal pressure and stress at these two spinal segments. Symptoms due to

TABLE II-5-2 False-Positive Rates for Lumbar Magnetic Resonance Imaging[7,9-11,34,59-61]

Investigation	Disc Bulge	Disc Protrusion	Disc Extrusion	Root Deviation or Compression
Boden et al[7]		20%		
Jensen et al[34]	52%	27%	1%	
Boos et al[9]		63%	13%	4%
Weishaupt et al[59]	24%	40%	18%	4%
Wood et al[61]	53%	37%		

interforaminal and central canal stenosis are increased with ambulation and backward bending.

- In 64 (62%) of the 104 patients with a leg length discrepancy of 1 mm or more, the pain radiated in the shorter leg.[56]
- Friberg studied patients with low back pain and discovered that patients with a leg length discrepancy of greater than 15 mm were five times more likely to experience low back pain. Hip and sciatic pain occurred in the longer leg 78% of the time. In patients with leg length discrepancies greater than 3 cm, an asymmetrical lateral side bend of the spine occurs on the side of the longer leg. This results in abnormal loading mechanics of the spine. Leg length discrepancies of this magnitude are present in 40% of the general population.[22]

ENVIRONMENAL FACTORS

DO PSYCHOSOCIAL ISSUES INFLUENCE THE CLINICAL DECISION-MAKING PROCESS?

Depression, stress, and other psychosocial factors can impact the autonomic, endocrine, and immune systems. These systems can heighten or depress response to injury.

CAN EMOTIONS INFLUENCE LOW BACK PAIN?

Although empirically the link between emotion and pain has yet to be definitively established, research is beginning to show a strong corelationship between emotions, stress, anxiety, and chronic pain. Inflammation, healing rates, immune response, and visceral responses have all been linked to changes in stress, both physical and emotional. Research has yet to reveal the exact physiology behind this connection, but preliminary data appear to implicate the autonomic system and the hypothalamus–pituitary–adrenal cortex axis as having a significant role in the regulation of inflammation and healing.[49]

DO WORK-RELATED INJURIES INFLUENCE CLINICAL DECISION MAKING?

Other nonmedical-related issues should always be considered as a source of a patient's symptoms. Research is demonstrating that recovery expectation is a major factor predictive of return to work. Patients who have a personal expectation to fully recover return to work more consistently. Other factors such as depression, anxiety, job satisfaction, and job stress are not predictive of return to work potential. Fear avoidance regarding injury has moderate evidence to support the fact that it may be predictive of return to work. There is insufficient evidence to determine whether monetary compensation or feelings of control at work are predictive of work outcomes. Box II-5-1 illustrates other contextual factors that may influence clinical decision making in the lumbar spine.

BOX II-5-1	Contextual Factors
Environmental	Work, environment, and repetitive tasks can lead to breakdown of tissue. Look for activities that required repetitive use of the arm and shoulder.
Personal	Work-related issues, personal and family factors, and depression and emotional unrest can all influence low back pain. Question patients regarding stressors in their life that may influence the ability of the body to heal.

PERSONAL FACTORS

PREVIOUS SURGERIES

WHAT PREVIOUS SURGERIES INFLUENCE YOUR CLINICAL REASONING IN THE LUMBAR SPINE?

- Similar to previous injuries, previous surgeries also change normal biomechanics in the lumbar region and can contribute to low back pain. Previous surgeries result in fibrosis and scar tissue formation. These can impact normal motion in the lumbar region and can result in tethering around the nerves that run through the lumbar region. Surgeries also impact the patient's ability to recruit muscles both locally and globally.
- Anterior surgeries such as hysterectomies, caesarian sections, and hernia surgeries can all impact the low back both from a biomechanical as well as a muscle recruitment standpoint.
- Low extremity surgeries can greatly alter the mechanics and forces applied at the lumbar region.

FAMILY HISTORY

DOES FAMILY HISTORY OF LUMBAR PATHOLOGY INFLUENCE YOUR CLINICAL REASONING PROCESS?

- Although continued research is still required, it appears that there may be some genetic predisposition toward a certain lumbar pathology. These pathologies include degenerative joint and disc disease, spondylolithesis, osteoporosis, and stenosis.[2]

CHRONICITY OF PAIN

WHAT CENTRAL PROCESSING CHANGES ARE PRESENT IN THE LUMBAR SPINE?

Chronic low back pain proves difficult to treat. The difficulty in treating and the continued pain experienced by many low back pain patients are due to the complexity of the region and the many factors that play into chronic pain. Temporary and long-term changes occur immediately on injury of lumbar tissue. Central and peripheral processing changes in the lumbar spine are just one of the factors that play into low back pain.

HAS MEDICAL TREATMENT BEEN SUCCESSFUL FOR PATIENTS WITH CHRONIC LOW BACK PAIN?

Medical progress in the United States has been slow in this area and low back pain continues to be an enigma. It appears that no major strides have been made in the past 20 years in solving the problem. Although the number of surgeries has increased, postsurgical results appear to be no more successful than results of conservative management.[55]

CLINICAL PEARL

Muscle motor control issues appear to occur in chronic low back pain patients as they have an earlier and longer activation of erector spinae muscles.

TO WHAT AREA OF RESEARCH IS MEDICINE TURNING ITS ATTENTION?

In an attempt to discover the cause of chronic low back pain, medical research is currently turning away from biomechanical factors and focusing on systemic factors. There is increasing evidence to support the role of the immune system as a major factor in continued low back pain. Research has demonstrated that the immune system reacts in an inflammatory manner when placed in contact with the nucleus. It has been hypothesized that it is the presence of the nucleus outside the confines of the annulus that results in the chronic inflammation and pain in the low back. Large disc bulges can be asymptomatic whereas small bulges are exquisitely painful. The causative factor is not the size of the bulge but the presence of the nucleus outside of the annulus.[47]

WHY IS MEDICAL RESEARCH FOCUSING ON OTHER CAUSES OF LOW BACK PAIN?

- Biomechanical factors have long been the focus of low back pain for diagnosis and intervention. Little change has been witnessed in the prevalence or incidence of chronic low back pain while utilizing this biomechanical model.
- Biomechanical normalcy can be restored, pain-generating tissue can be removed, and motion can be prevented; yet a patient's pain remains.
- The biomechanical paradigm is effective in treating the mechanical and acute low back pain patient, but factors other than biomechanics must be responsible for pain in patients with chronic low back pain.

CLINICAL DECISION MAKING CASE STUDY—PATIENT PROFILE

Your patient is a 43-year-old female with complaints of low back pain. Symptoms began insidiously and have been present for the past 2 months. They have become progressive, more frequent, and more intense in nature. Symptoms are worse with standing, sitting, and lying for more than 30 minutes. Symptoms feel better when walking or moving. The patient has noticed that her symptoms worsen monthly and it appears to coincide with her menstrual cycles. She has two children and both were born naturally and without complications. She has a history of severe menstrual cramping. What are your hypotheses regarding her pathology?

Answer

The patient's symptoms appear to match those expected with a herniated disc. The factor that complicates the diagnosis is the increase of symptoms that coincides with her menstrual cycles. Pathology such as ovarian cysts and endometriosis can be the source of symptoms or a contributor to disc pain. Cramping and pelvic-related pain can cause biomechanical abnormalities as the body guards and protects irritable regions. Hormones released during menstruation can also result in joint laxity and act on injured tissue, such as a disc or facet, as a tissue irritant.

CAN DISCS BE INJURED WITH CHRONIC LOW BACK PAIN?

- Removal of a disc does not always eliminate pain and many people with disc pathology do not have pain.
- Therefore, the role of discs in chronic low back pain has evolved from being the source of pain to being a contributing factor.

IS THE LUMBAR DISC RESPONSIBLE FOR CHRONIC LOW BACK PAIN?

- In research using cadavers, specimens that had a history of low back pain revealed disc herniation that blocked arterial and venous systems in the region. This vascular congestion results in diminished circulation that slows the healing process and prevents the removal of chemical irritants and waste material from the region.[31,44,45,47]
- Secondarily, long standing inflammation causes fibrosis of tissue and neural structures in the region. Cadaveric research has demonstrated the presence of greater amounts of fibrotic tissue in and around the lumbar region in patients with chronic low back pain. This fibrotic tissue restricts motion in regions that required mobility to eliminate inflammation. In addition, the fibrosis is also present on the nerve, which results in impaired nerve mobility.[31]

HOW ELSE DOES DISC PATHOLOGY CONTRIBUTE TO CHRONIC PAIN?

- The body's immune system is highly reactive to the nucleus pulposa. A disc can bulge without the presence of pain as long as the annulus is intact. When the annulus is disrupted, the nucleus may leak out of the confines of the disc into the surrounding area. The presence of the nuclear material outside of the annulus results in an inflammatory reaction. As long as nuclear material is present outside of the annulus, inflammation will be present. The inflammation will sensitize nerves in the region, which results in the pain.
- Studies of painful discs reveal changes in tissue composition such as the formation of granulation tissue extending from the nucleus pulposus to the outer rings of the annulus fibrosis. These changes result in tears in the annulus and increased immunoreactive nerve fibers in the newly formed granulation tissue.[16,45,48]

WHAT PERIPHERAL CHANGES CAN OCCUR THAT RESULT IN CHRONIC LOW BACK PAIN?

In the periphery, several factors can result in long-standing changes in pain modulation. On injury, inflammation occurs immediately to begin the reparative process to the injured tissue and C-fibers are activated. These previously dormant C-fibers are active long after inflammation resolves. C-fibers transmit nociceptive signals cortically, release chemical mediators that act as irritants to the nerve, and can alter the mechanical and thermal thresholds of nerves. This results in spontaneous impulses from the sensitized periphery.[63]

WHAT CENTRAL CHANGES CAN OCCUR THAT RESULT IN CHRONIC LOW BACK PAIN?

- Increased gene expression. Long-term C-fiber stimulation results in changes that decrease the nociceptive threshold.
- These changes include the expression of transmitters, ions, and neuromodulators.[38]
- Nocioceptor activity triggers the removal of magnesium plugs from the NMDA receptor. This allows for easier activation of pain pathways.
- Phenotypic switching. Long-term C-fiber stimulation results in the production of neuromodulators by A-fibers that are similar to those produced by C-fibers (A-fibers begin to act like C-fibers).
- Denervation (C-fiber loss). Injury can cause the death of inhibitory interneurons in the superficial laminae of the dorsal horn. With less inhibition it is easier to activate nociceptive projection neurons.
- Peripheral nerve injury results in the reorganization of A-fibers. With nerve injury, A-fibers are forced to grow into areas of the dorsal horn (laminae III to laminae II) where there are normally only C-fibers. A-fibers can now activate projection neurons normally triggered only by C-fibers. This is perceived as increased pain.

HOW DO AUTONOMIC, ENDOCRINE, AND IMMUNE SYSTEMS INFLUENCE DECISION MAKING IN THE REGION?

- The autonomic, endocrine, and immune systems are responsible for maintaining a homeostatic environment within the body. In response to an altered environment the three systems work together to return the body to homeostasis. In lumbar patients, the autonomic system reacts to alter blood flow and increase chemical mediators, thus sensitizing the nervous system in the region.[22]
- The endocrine system can also influence pain in many ways. The hypothalamus controls the autonomic system, adrenal glands produce neural irritants in response to stressors, and the reproductive organs also produce hormones that can act as neural irritants.

BOX II-5-2 **Output Mechanisms**

Autonomic	Recent studies explore the relationship of the autonomic system and lumbar pathology. It has been proposed that addressing the autonomic nervous system can alter lumbar symptoms. No conclusive evidence has been provided to date.
Endocrine	The endocrine system is involved in the regulation of body homeostasis. It has been proposed that alteration in endocrine system function can be a source of chronic low back pain.
Immune	Several studies have shown that infections in the tissue of the lumbar spine can be a source of low back pain

HOW IS THE IMMUNE SYSTEM INVOLVED IN LOW BACK PAIN?

Diskitis and osteomyelitis of the vertebra are often the result of infection that has affected the lumbar region. The infection generally does not begin in the lumbar spine but spreads from other regions such as the urinary tract via the circulatory system. Infection can also result from injections or surgery. In the United States the rate is lower, but in developing countries such as Africa, diskitis has been found in 11% of patients with low back pain. The immune system is responsible for defending against these infections. [2] Box II-5-2 illustrates various output mechanisms that may contribute to lumbar pathology.

RED FLAGS THAT REQUIRE REFERRAL TO A MEDICAL PHYSICIAN

WHAT SYMPTOMS ALERT YOU TO PATHOLOGIES THAT MAY REQUIRE A REFERRAL TO A MEDICAL DOCTOR?

- Patient descriptions vary from person to person and should not be the only consideration in the determination of possible visceral involvement.
- Visceral pain has been described on a broad scope from sharp and severe to poorly localized and vague.
- Visceral pain should not be related to positions/movements of lumbar structures and should not respond to appropriate mechanical treatment.
- Rest or position should not relieve visceral pain.
- In patients with visceral or nonmusculoskeletal involvement it is a common complaint that their pain is constant and nonvarying.
- Complaints of increased pain at night is also an indicator of possible visceral involvement. Considerable walking, pacing, and sitting up are commonly required to return to sleep.

CLINICAL DECISION MAKING CASE STUDY—PATIENT PROFILE **(?)**

The patient is a 33-year-old female who reports to physical therapy with complaints of left low back pain. She has been feeling cramping and has had sweats on and off for the past 3 days. Her symptoms are severe at times, but appear to be coming in waves. She is unable to find a position of comfort. No motion seems to increase the symptoms. She seems to feel an increase in symptoms shortly after drinking water. What is your diagnosis?

Answer

It would be difficult for a clinician to make a definitive diagnosis based on the information given. The fact that the pain is constant, comes in waves, and does not appear to be affected by motion or position would suggest the visceral systems as a source of the symptoms. The increase in symptoms when drinking water may implicate urogential involvement. This patient's symptoms do not appear musculoskeletal based. She should be referred to her primary care physician or to an urgent care setting for further testing and assessment to rule out visceral involvement.

WHAT SYMPTOMS IMPLICATE SPECIFIC VISCERAL SYSTEMS?

GASTROINTESTINAL SYSTEM: Symptoms include abdominal pain, pain with swallowing, melena (dark, bloody stool), epigastric pain with radiation to the back, symptoms affected by food, constipation, diarrhea, fecal incontinence, joint pain, and referred shoulder pain.

HEPATIC SYSTEM: Symptoms include a sense of fullness of the abdomen, anorexia, nausea, vomiting, jaundice, bruising of the skin, spider angiomas or palmar erythema, yellow hue in the eyes, dark urine, right shoulder and abdominal pain, confusion, sleep disturbance, muscle tremors, hyperreflexia, bilateral carpal tunnel, and pallor.

UROGENITAL SYSTEM: In men, symptoms include urinary tract, pelvic, low back, or leg pain, painful burning with urination, changes in urinary pattern or urine flow, red urine, penile lesions, swelling or mass in the groin, and impotence.

In women, symptoms include vaginal bleeding, painful menstruation, pelvic mass or lesion, vaginal itch, pain with urination, changes in menstruation, and abdominal, low back, or pelvic pain.

ENDOCRINE SYSTEM: Symptoms include neuromusculoskeletal systems, muscle weakness, muscle atrophy, fatigue, carpal tunnel syndrome, arthralgia and myalgia, adhesive capsulitis, hand stiffness, systemic, excessive, or delayed growth, mental changes, changes in hair, changes in skin, changes in vital signs (body temperature, heart rate, blood pressure), heart palpitations, increased perspiration, dehydration, or excessive water retention.

CANCER: Symptoms include a previous history of cancer, any women with chest, breast, axillary, or shoulder pain, any person with back, pelvic, groin, or hip pain accompanied by vague complaints of abdominal pain, prolonged menstrual bleeding, back injury that does not heal, proximal muscle weakness and changes in reflexes, weight loss of 10 pounds or more in 1 month, constant pain, pain at night, development of new neurological deficits, and changes in size, shape, tenderness, and consistency of lymph nodes, especially painless and hard rubber nodes present in more than one location.

SUMMARY STATEMENT

Very little change has been made over the past 20 years in the battle against low back pain. The number of lumbar surgeries has increased and the success rate following surgery remains poor. Of people in the United States 80% will experience low back pain and regardless of treatment most will have at least one reoccurrence of pain. Successful rehabilitation of low back pain occurs only with pain that is acute in nature. The subjective examination can aid a clinician to determine the source of low back symptoms and with this information, the clinician can effectively and efficiently develop appropriate treatment and intervention plans.

Current rehabilitation protocols for chronic low back pain have not been successful and current interventions have proven ineffective. Attempting to trace chronic symptoms back to a

TABLE II-5-3 Body Structure and Tissue-Based Pathology (Nociceptive and Peripheral Neurogenic Pain)

	Intervertebral Disc	Zygapophyseal Joint Capsule	Zygapophyseal Joint	Muscle	Vertebral Bodies	Posterior Vertebral Elements	Ligaments	Nerves	Visceral Tissue
Pathology	Herniated disc Degenerative disc disease	Degenerative disc disease Lumbar instability	Lumbar spondylosis Lumbar spondylolithesis Degenerative joint disease Lumbar stenosis	Lumbar muscle strain Abdominal strain	Compression fracture Ankylosing spondylitis Osteoporosis	Lumbar spondylolithesis Lumbar instability	Lumbar ligament sprain Lumbar instability	Lumbar radiculopathy Lumbar stenosis Central stenosis	Kidney, liver, gallbladder, stomach, small intestine, spleen, pancreas, lung, ovaries, fallopian tubes, uterus, testes, prostate, sigmoid colon, appendix, small intestines
Age	30 to 40 years old	20 to 40 years old	50 years old and above	20 to 40 years old	Any age for fracture Above 60 years old for degeneration	Any age for fracture 16 to 25 for spondylosis	Not age related	16 to 25 years if spondylolithesis related 30 to 40 years old if disc related 50 years old plus if stenosis related	30 to 50 years old
Occupation	Repetitive flexion and lifting activities	Repetitive flexion and lifting activities	Repetitive extension activities	Repetitive flexion and lifting activities	Repetitive flexion and lifting activities	Repetitive extension activities	No direct relationship	Varies; see related pathology	Varies depending on pathology
Gender Ethnicity	Not applicable Not known	Not applicable	Not applicable	Not applicable	Female Asian and Caucasian higher prevalence	Not applicable Not known	Not applicable	Not applicable	Not applicable
History	History of several bouts of symptoms, progressively worsening	History of several bouts of symptoms	History of low back pain	May or may not have history of low back pain	May or may not have history of low back pain	May or may not have history of low back pain	May or may not have history of low back pain	Varies; see related pathology	
Mechanism of injury	Flexion with or without rotation	Flexion with or without rotation	Extension	Flexion with lifting	Flexion with rotation, flexion-based trauma	Repetitive extension	Trauma	Varies; see related pathology	Generally no known mechanism
Type of onset	Sudden	Sudden	Gradual	Sudden	Sudden or traumatic	Sudden for fracture, gradual for spondylosis	Sudden or traumatic	Gradual	Sudden to gradual depending on structure
Referral from local tissue	Pain in low back and gluteal region	Pain in low back and gluteal region, usually unilateral	Pain in low back and gluteal region	Pain in low back and gluteal region	Pain in low back and gluteal region	Pain in low back and gluteal region	Pain in low back and gluteal region	Pain in low back and gluteal region	Pain is generally localized to an area adjacent to the involved structure

Referral to other regions	May refer unilaterally into lower extremity if the nerve is involved	Very rarely refers distally	May refer unilaterally or bilaterally into legs if nerves are involved	Generally does not refer to other regions	Generally does not refer to other areas	Generally does not refer to other areas	Generally does not refer to other regions	Referral of symptoms into the lower extremity Distribution of symptoms is dependent on nerve root involvement	May refer into surrounding areas depending on the involved structure
Changes in symptoms	Sudden pain decreasing the remainder of the day. Increased pain the next morning	Sudden pain, no relief as day of injury progresses	Slow progressive worsening over time	Sudden pain, no relief as day on injury progresses	Sudden pain	Sudden pain, may improve over 8-week period with fracture, gradual worsening with spondylolisthesis	Sudden pain, no relief as day of injury progresses	Symptoms generally increase gradually over the course of several days to weeks. Symptoms may dissipate as irritating structure is addressed	May worsen as pathology progresses
24-hour pain pattern (morning)	Stiff for 30 minutes	Stiff for 5 minutes	Stiff for 5 minutes	Stiff for 30 minutes	Stiff for 30 minutes	Stiff for 30 minutes with fracture Stiff for several minutes with spondylolisthesis	Stiff for 5 minutes	Stiff for 30 minutes	Varies but does not change with mechanical stresses
24-hour pain pattern (afternoon)	Less stiff, may be worse with prolonged sitting	Worsens with activity	Worsens with extension activity	Less stiff, may be worse with prolonged sitting	Less stiff, may be worse with prolonged sitting	Less stiff, may be worse with prolonged sitting	Less stiff, may be worse with prolonged activity	May worsen with prolonged aggravating activity	Varies but does not change with mechanical stresses
24-hour pain pattern (evening)	May be difficult to sleep	May be difficult to sleep and turn in bed	Usually not impaired	May be difficult to sleep	May be difficult to sleep	May be difficult to sleep	Sleep should not be impaired	May be difficult to sleep	Increased nocturnal pain
Description of symptoms	Aches and stiffness, poor localization	Sharp pain	Dull ache	Aches and stiffness, may be able to localize	Aches and stiffness, poor localization	Aches and stiffness, poor localization, shifting or instability noted	Aches and stiffness, sharp pain with motions that stress ligaments—primarily flexion	Numbness, tingling, burning	Cramping, peristaltic waves, gnawing ache
Depth of symptoms	Deep	Deep	Deep	Superficial	Deep	Deep	Deep	Superficial	Deep, poorly localized
Constancy of symptoms	Intermittent	Intermittent	Intermittent	Intermittent	Constant but varying	Constant but varying	Intermittent	Intermittent to constant but varying	Constant, may come in waves
Aggravating factors	Sitting, flexion, initially movement after lying down	Extension and rotation to side of injury	Extension and walking	Sitting, flexion, contralateral flexion and rotation, resisted extension	Sitting, flexion, lifting, coughing and sneezing	Extension, static positions	Primarily flexion	Varies; see related pathology	Not consistent with mechanical movements

Continued on following page.

Section II

ORTHOPEDIC REASONING

TABLE II-5-3 Body Structure and Tissue-Based Pathology (Nociceptive and Peripheral Neurogenic Pain) (Continued)

	Intervertebral Disc	Zygapophyseal Joint Capsule	Zygapophyseal Joint	Muscle	Vertebral Bodies	Posterior Vertebral Elements	Ligaments	Nerves	Visceral Tissue
Easing factors	Walking	Sitting	Sitting	Walking, lying	Limited walking, lying	Limited walking and motion	Extension activities, lying	Varies; see related pathology	Not consistent with mechanical movements
Stability of symptoms	Gradual improvement over 6-week period	Gradual improvement over 2-week period	Slow gradual progression of symptoms	Gradual improvement over 6-week period	Gradual improvement over 8-week period	Gradual improvement over 8-week period for fracture / Worsening for spondylolithesis	Gradual improvement over 6-week period	Gradual improvement over 6-week period	May worsen if pathology progresses
Past medical history	All structures may have a past history of medical issues that impact the function of surrounding tissue				Osteoporosis	All structures may have a past history of medical issues that impact the function of surrounding tissue			May have a history of visceral pathology
Past surgeries	All structures may have a past history of surgeries that impact the function of surrounding tissue				May have a history of hysterectomy	All structures may have a past history of surgeries that impact the function of surrounding tissue			May have a history of surgeries related to visceral pathology
Special questions	Pain with flexion	Sudden pain with difficulty moving immediately	Pain with extension	Pain with active motion	Osteoporosis, hysterectomy	Instability	Instability	Radicular symptoms	Nocturnal pain / Changes in bowel and bladder / Weight changes / Symptoms not impacted by motion / Gait disturbances
X-rays	Negative	Negative	Positive	Negative	Positive	Positive	Negative	May be positive depending on related pathology	Negative
MRI	Positive	Negative	Positive	Positive	Positive	Positive	Positive	May be positive depending on related pathology	Positive for pathology
EMG	Positive if nerves are involved	Usually not necessary	Positive if nerves are involved	Usually not necessary	Nerves generally not involved	Nerves generally not involved	Usually not necessary	Positive	Not usually necessary
Special laboratory tests	None				Blood test for Rh factors	None			Varies depending on pathology
Red flags	Rule out visceral structures								

MRI, magnetic resonance imaging; EMG, electromyogram.

single tissue source is not possible. Chronic low back pain is multifaceted, attributed in part to changes in the central and peripheral nervous system, autonomic system, endocrine system, and immune system. Table II-5-3 summarizes the factors that help a clinician differentiate among different sources of symptoms in the lumbar region. In the future, low back research should focus on addressing these potential contributors to low back pain.

REFERENCES

1. Adams MA, Hutton WC. The effects of posture on the role of the apophysial joints in resting intervertebral compressive forces. *J Bone Joint Surg.* 1980;62B:358-362.
2. Ala-Kokko L. Genetic risk factors for lumbar disc disease. *Ann Med.* 2002;34(1):42-47(6).
3. Atlas SJ, Keller RB, Wu YA, Deyo RA, Singer DE. Long-term outcomes of surgical and nonsurgical management of sciatica secondary to a lumbar disc herniation: 10 year results from the Maine lumbar spine study. *Spine.* 2005;30:927-935.
4. Badke MB, Boissonnault WG. Changes in Disability Following Physical Therapy Intervention for Patients With Low Back Pain: Dependence on Symptom Duration. *Arch Phys Med Rehab.* 2006;87(6):749-756.
5. Balagué F, Mannion A, Pellisé F, Cedraschi C. Clinical update: Low back pain. *Lancet.* 2007;369(9563):726-728.
6. Bell GR, Ross JS. Diagnosis of nerve root compression. Myelography, computed tomography, and MRI. *Orthop Clin North Am.* 1992;23:405-419.
7. Boden SD, Davis DO, Dina TS, Patronas NJ, Wiesel SW. Abnormal magnetic resonance scans of the lumbar spine in asymptomatic subjects: A prospective investigation. *J Bone Joint Surg Am.* 1990;72A:403-408.
8. Boden SD, Wiesel SW. Lumbar spine imaging: role in clinical decision making. *J Am Acad Orthop Surg.* 1996;4:238-248.
9. Boos N, Rieder R, Schade V, Spratt KF, Semmer N, Aebi M. Volvo Award in clinical science: The diagnostic accuracy of MRI, work perception, and psychosocial factors in identifying symptomatic disc herniations. *Spine.* 1995;20:2613-2625.
10. Boos N, Semmer N, Elfering A, et al. Natural history of individuals with asymptomatic disc abnormalities in MRI: Predictors of low back pain-related medical consultation and work incapacity. *Spine.* 2000;25:1484.
11. Borenstein G, O' Mara JW, Boden SD, et al. The value of magnetic resonance imaging of the lumbar spine to predict low-back pain in asymptomatic individuals: A 7-year follow-up study. *J Bone Joint [Am].* 2001;83:320-334.
12. Bronfort G, Haas M, Evans R, Bouter L. Efficacy of spinal manipulation and mobilization for low back pain and neck pain: a systematic review and best evidence synthesis. *Spine J.* 2004;4(3):335-356.
13. Butler D. *Mobilization of the Nervous System.* Melbourne, Australia: Churchill Livingston; 1991.
14. Cavanaugh J, Ozaktay AC, Yamashita HT, King AI. Lumbar facet pain: Biomechanics, neuroanatomy and neurophysiology. *J Biomech.* 1996;29(9):1117-1129.
15. CDC. Prevalence and impact of arthritis by race and ethnicity—United States, 1989-1991. *MMWR Morb Mortal Wkly Rep.* 1996;45:373-378.
16. Cooper RG, Freemont AJ, Hoyland JA, et al. Herniated intervertebral disc associated periradicular fibrosis and vascular abnormalities occur without inflammatory cell infiltration. *Spine.* 1995;20:591-598.
17. Croft PR, Macfarlane GJ, Papageorgiou AC, Thomas E, Silman AJ. Outcome of low back pain in general practice; a prospective study. *BMJ.* 1998;316:1356-1359.
18. Farfan HF. The pathological anatomy of degenerative spondylolisthesis: a cadaver study. *Spine.* 1980;5:412-418.
19. Flynn T, Fritz J, Whitman J, et al. A Clinical Prediction Rule for Classifying Patients with Low Back Pain Who Demonstrate Short-Term Improvement With Spinal Manipulation. *Spine.* 2002;27:2835-2843.
20. Foxman B. Recurring Urinary Tract Infection: Incidence and Risk Factors. *AJPH.* 1990;80(3):331-333.
21. Fredrickson BE, Baker D, McHolick WJ, Yuan HA, Lubicky JP. The natural history of spondylosis and spondylolisthesis. *J Bone Joint Surg.* 1984;66A:699-707.
22. Friberg O. Clinical symptoms and biomechanics of lumbar spine and hip joint in leg length inequality. *Spine.* 1983;8:643-651.
23. Fritz J, Erhard R, Vignovic M. A nonsurgical treatment approach for patients with lumbar spinal stenosis. *Spine.* 1997;77:962-973.
24. Fukui S, Ohseto K, Shiotani M, Ohno K, Karasawa H, Naganuma Y. Distribution of Referred Pain from the Lumbar Zygapophyseal Joints and Dorsal Rami. *Clin J Pain.* 1997;13(4):303-307.
25. Gofton JP, Bennett PH, Smythe HA, Decker JL. Sacroiliitis and ankylosing spondylitis in North American Indians. *Ann Rheum Dis.* 1972;31:474-481.
26. Goodman CC, Snyder TEK. *Differential Diagnosis in Physical Therapy.* Philadelphia: WB Saunders Co.; 2006.
27. Haher TR, O'Brien M, Dryer JW, Nucci R, Zipnick R, Leone DJ. The role of the lumbar fact joints in spinal stability. *Spine.* 1994;19:2667-2671.
28. Haughton VM. MR imaging of the spine. *Radiology.* 1988;166:297-301.
29. Herkowitz HN. Spine update. Degenerative lumbar spondylolisthesis. *Spine.* 1995;20(9):1084-1090.
30. Hosoe H, Ohmori K. Degenerative lumbosacral spondylolisthesis: Possible factors which predispose the fifth lumbar vertebra to slip. *J Bone Joint Surg Br.* 2008;90(3):356-359.
31. Hoyland J, Freemont A, Jayson M. Intervertebral foramen venous obstruction. *Spine.* 1989;14:558-568.
32. Jarvik JG, Deyo RA. Diagnostic evaluation of low back pain with emphasis on imaging. *Ann Int Med.* 2002;137:586-597.
33. Jensen G. Biomechanics of the Lumbar Intervertebral Disk. A Review. *Phys Ther.* 1980;60(6):765-773.
34. Jenson MC, Brant ZM, Obuchowski N, Modic MT, Malaksian D, Ross JS. MRI imaging of the lumbar spine in people without back pain. *N Engl J Med.* 1994;331:369-373.
35. Johnsson KE, Rosen I, Uden A. The natural course of lumbar spinal stenosis. *Clin Orthop.* 1992;279:82-92.
36. Kettelkamp DB, Wright DG. Spondylolysis in the Alaskan Eskimo. *J Bone Joint Surg (Am).* 1971;53:563.
37. Koes BW, van Tulder MW, Thomas S. Diagnosis and treatment of low back pain. *BMJ.* 2006;332:1430-1434.
38. Lee D, Hodges P. *The Pelvic Girdle: An Approach to the Examination and Treatment of the Lumbopelvic-Hip Region.* Philadelphia: Churchill Livingston; 2004.
39. Love TW, Fagan AB, Fraser RD. Degenerative spondylolisthesis: developmental or acquired? *J Bone Joint Surg.* 1999;81B:670-674.
40. McFadden KD, Taylor JR. Axial Rotation in the Lumbar Spine and Gapping of the Zygapophyseal Joints. *Spine.* 1990;15:04, 295-299.
41. McKenzie RA. *The Lumbar Spine: Mechanical Diagnosis and Therapy.* Waikanae, New Zealand: Spinal Publications; 1981.
42. Nygaard OP, Mellgren SI, Osterud B. The Inflammatory Properties of Contained and Noncontained Lumbar Disc Herniation. *Spine.* 1997;22(21):2484-2488.
43. Ohnmeiss D, Vanharanta H, Ekholm J. Degree of Disc Disruption and Lower Extremity Pain. *Spine.* 1997;22(14):1600-1605.
44. Olmarker K, Rydevik B, Holm S. Edema formation in spinal nerve roots induced by experimental graded compression. *Spine.* 1989;14:569-573.
45. Olmarker K, Rydevik B. Pathophysiology of sciatica. *Orthop Clin North Am.* 1991;22:223-234.
46. Panjabi MM, Abumi K, Duranceau J Oxland T. Spinal stability and intersegmental muscle forces. *Spine.* 1989;14:194-200.
47. Parke WW. The significance of venous return impairment in ischemic radiculopathy and myelopathy. *Orthop Clin North Am.* 1991;22:213-222.
48. Peng B, Wu W, Hou S, Li P, Zhang C, Yang Y. The pathogenesis of discogenic low back pain. *J Bone Joint Surg (BR).* 2005;87B:62.
49. Pincus T, Burton AK, Vogel S, Field AP. A systematic review of psychological factors as predictors of chronicity/disability in prospective cohorts of low back pain. *Spine.* 2002;27:E109-E120.
50. Raoul S, Faure A, Robert R, et al. Role of the sinu-vertebral nerve in low back pain and anatomical basis of therapeutic implications. *Surg Radiol Anat.* 2003;24:366-371.
51. Saal JA. Natural history and nonoperative treatment of lumbar disc herniation. *Spine.* 1996;21(suppl):2S-9S.
52. Shacklock MO, Butler DS, Slater H. The dynamic central nervous system; structure and clinical neurobiomechanics. In: Boyling JD, Palastanga N, eds. *Grieve's Modern Manual Therapy.* 2nd ed. Edinburgh, Scotland: Churchill Livingstone; 1994:21-38.
53. Simon D, Travell J. *Myofascial Pain and Dysfunction: The Trigger Point Manual.* Philadelphia: Lippincott Williams & Williams; 1999.
54. Simotas AC, Dorey FJ, Hansraj KK, Cammisa F. Nonoperative treatment for lumbar spinal stenosis: clinical outcome results and a 3 year survivorship analysis. *Spine.* 2000;25:197-203.

Section II   ORTHOPEDIC REASONING

55. Taylor VM, Deyo RA, Cherkin DC, Kreuter W. Low back pain hospitalization. *Spine*. 1994;19:1207–1213.

56. ten Brinke A, van der Aa HE, van der Palen J, Oosterveld F. Is leg length discrepancy associated with side of radiating pain in patients with a lumbar herniated disc? *Spine*. 1999;24(7):684–686.

57. Van Tulder MW, Assendelft WJ, Koes BW, Bouter LM. Spinal radiographic findings and nonspecific low back pain. A systematic review of observational studies. *Spine*. 1997;22:427–434.

58. Waddell G. A new clinical model for treatment of low back pain. *Spine*. 1987;12:632–643.

59. Weishaupt D, Zanetti M, Hodler J, Boos N. MRI of the lumbar spine: Prevalence of intervertebral disc extrusion and sequestration, nerve root compression and plate abnormalities, and osteoarthritis of the fact joints in Asymptomatic Volunteers. *Radiology*. 1998;209:661–666.

60. Wiesel SW, Tsourmas N, Feffer HL, Citrin CM, Patronas N. A study of computer-associated tomography: I. The incidence of positive CAT scans in asymptomatic group of patients. *Spine*. 1984;9:549–551.

61. Wood KB, Garvey TA, Gundry C, Heithoff KB. 'Magnetic resonance imaging of the thoracic spine. Evaluation of asymptomatic individuals. *J Bone Joint Surg Am*. 1995;77(11):1631–1638.

62. Wynne-Davies R, Scott JHS. Inheritance and spondylolisthesis—a radiographic family survey. *J Bone Joint Surg Br*. 1979;61:301–305.

63. Yoshizawa H, Kobayashi S, Hachiya Y. Blood supply of nerve roots and dorsal root ganglia. *Orthop Clin North Am*. 1991;22:195–211.

AUTHOR: ELAINE LONNEMANN

INTRODUCTORY INFORMATION

WHAT IS THE PREVALENCE OF SACROILIAC JOINT PATHOLOGY?

The prevalence of intraarticular pain arising from the sacroiliac joint has been estimated to be as low as 13% and high as 30%.[45] Maigne et al found the prevalence to be 18.5% when utilizing double diagnostic anesthetic blocks.[34] This fluoroscopically guided process has been advocated as the gold standard to eliminate the need for placebo in joint injections. Laslett et al reportedly found sacroiliac joint-related pain in 33% of their subjects in a study utilizing both single and double blocks.[31] An average number to remember is 20% or one in five.

WHAT IS THE PROGNOSIS FOR RECOVERY FROM SACROILIAC JOINT PATHOLOGY?

The prognosis for recovery from sacroiliac joint pathology depends on the nature of the joint pathology. Joint hypermobility, especially instability, has a less favorable prognosis because of low compliance with the use of sacroiliac binders. The prognosis for patients with displacement seems to be good from a clinical perspective.[2]

WHAT IS THE REOCCURRENCE RATE FOR SACROILIAC JOINT PATHOLOGY?

This has not been studied, most likely because the prevalence rate of sacroiliac joint pathology is fairly low for studies that could measure this accurately.

WHAT FACTORS MAKE DIAGNOSIS DIFFICULT IN THE SACROILIAC JOINT REGION?

Diagnosis in the sacroiliac region is challenging based on a number of factors. First and foremost, the sacroiliac joint is functionally interdependent on the hip, lumbar spine, and pubic symphysis joint. Differential diagnosis of sacroiliac dysfunction versus dysfunction in other areas is difficult because of the transference of forces through the bones of the pelvic ring and the interrelated muscles groups and shared innervation among these regions. The joint mobility is limited and it is difficult to analyze radiographically because of the architectural variations within this joint.

These architectural variations include the orientation of the joint and the size and shape of the sacrum. The joint is oriented in an oblique manner in most cases, but in some it may have a frontal orientation. Gender differences in joint congruity and ligamentous support have also been noted.[53,54] Although there is mobility within the joint, it is limited.[13,48,49,50] Diagnosis based on position, mobility, and classifications systems has very little interrater and intrarater agreement.[16] The lack of definitive horizontal or vertical landmarks to use for mobility testing and positional assessment may factor into this problem.

Provocation testing of this joint has better reliability than other measures and is most indicative of sacroiliac joint (SIJ) diagnosis. However, even provocative maneuvers have limitations because the validity of the gold standard for diagnosis of SIJ pain—the diagnostic block is yet to be proven.[22] There are several factors that impact the sensitivity and specificity of these blocks: placebo effect, convergence and referred pain, neuroplasticity, central sensitization, expectation bias, unintentional sympathetic blockade, systemic absorption of lidocaine, and psychosocial issues.[22] Results of studies examining the radiological findings in patients with SIJ-related pain [bone scan, computed tomography (CT), and radiographic stereophotogrammetry] have also been shown to have poor sensitivity in the diagnosis of SIJ pain.[14,34,45,48]

HOW SUCCESSFUL IS THERAPY IN TREATING SIJ PATHOLOGY?

There has been some evidence to support the management of acute lumbosacral pain with manipulation; however, there was no testing to specify the origin of pain as being from sacroiliac pathology or lumbar pathology.[10,15] In a randomized controlled trial by Stuge et al patients with pelvic pain after pregnancy were treated with specific stabilizing exercises.[47] This was found to be effective in reducing pain, improving functional status, and improving health-related quality of life.

HOW SUCCESSFUL IS SURGERY IN TREATING SIJ PATHOLOGY?

Arthrodesis is the most common surgical treatment for the SIJ. It should be considered only in patients with severe instability or joint destruction from infection or trauma because its effectiveness is controversial.[10] It is typically performed only in patients who are severely disabled by the symptoms and have not responded to conservative care.

PERSONAL INFORMATION

WHAT INFLUENCE DOES AGE HAVE ON YOUR CLINICAL DECISION-MAKING PROCESS?

It is very important to bear in mind the patient's age when considering the SIJ as a potential cause for patient dysfunction. Age-related changes in this joint begin in adolescence and progress throughout life. Fibrous plaques form in the iliac surface of the joint during adolescence; this will make the joint surface less smooth. The plaque formation accelerates during the third and fourth decades causing fibrillation and crevice formation within the joint surface. Changes in the hyaline cartilage of the sacral surface also occur but tend to lag behind the fibrocartilaginous ilial surface by about 10 years. By the sixth decade the joint mobility will be considerably restricted because of fibrous changes in the joint capsule leading to fibrous ankylosis. By the eighth decade the joint surfaces erode and bony ankylosis often occurs.[4,55]

WHAT INFLUENCE DOES A PATIENT'S OCCUPATION HAVE ON YOUR CLINICAL DECISION-MAKING PROCESS?

The occupation is not as much of a consideration as is the consideration of work-related activities such as unilateral stance time and stair climbing, ladder activities, as well as unilateral driving activities. The types of activities are important to determine for return to activity after a joint dysfunction has occurred. There has been some evidence to show an increased incidence in professional athletes who perform unilateral high-velocity, high-force kicking activities and dancers. Occupations or sports that risk a fall onto the ischiotuberosity or gluteal region, such as ice skating or gymnastics, also predispose a patient to sacroiliac pathology.

WHAT INFLUENCE DOES GENDER HAVE ON YOUR CLINICAL DECISION-MAKING PROCESS?

The female SIJ tends to have less stability overall because the ligaments are smaller and weaker to allow for the mobility needed for childbearing. Also the joint surfaces tend to be flatter and less congruent.[6,39] Female's pelvises also go through more trauma than the male pelvis. This is due to the forces exerted during the birthing process. Hormones, such as relaxin, released during pregnancy, result in increased SIJ laxity. Relaxin is released into the body to allow the SIJ and pelvis to widen to accommodate the head and shoulders of the child as it descends out of the birth canal. Relaxin is present in the body as long as the female is nursing. Therefore, laxity of the joint could be present as long as the hormone is present in the system. As a result of the anatomical features, stresses, and hormonal influences, female SIJs are more prone to hypermobility or positional faults then their male counterparts.

WHAT INFLUENCE DOES ETHNICITY HAVE ON YOUR CLINICAL DECISION-MAKING PROCESS?

Ethnicity may affect pelvic type as well as the lumbosacral angle, which affects SIJ position. This in turn could predispose a patient to SIJ dysfunction. To date, this is more of a clinical consideration because research is lacking regarding ethnicity and prevalence of SIJ dysfunction.

The other consideration regarding SIJ dysfunction and ethnicity involves a specific pathology seen in the SIJ. The prevalence of ankylosing spondylitis (AS) varies among different ethnic groups. The prevalence follows the distribution of HLA B27 in populations. HLA-B27 is present in 90% to 95% of patients with AS in the United States and Europe. The prevalence of AS is highest among populations having a high prevalence of HLA-B27. Populations in Germany, Finland, and Norway have reported the following percentages of adults who are diagnosed with AS: 0.86%, 0.15%, and 1.1%, respectively.[5,19,26,27]

CLINICAL DECISION MAKING CASE STUDY—PATIENT PROFILE ❓

A 19-year-old Caucasian male presents with complaints of pinpoint pain in both SIJs and intermittent mid-thoracic pain. He lifts boxes at the local UPS facility for 6 to 8 hours. He states that his pain is a dull ache, worse by the end of his shift, resolves with rest, but is present at night if he wakes. It resolves at night if he gets up and walks for about 5 minutes. His pain was gradual in onset. What are your hypotheses regarding the source of his symptoms?

Answer
Bilateral pain in the SIJs of a young male should be a red flag for potential rheumatic conditions such as AS. This patient did report a family history of AS with two uncles diagnosed with the disease. It is not unusual for patients to report associated thoracic pain present at night. This suggests an inflammatory process causing increased levels of discomfort that are improved with movement.

MECHANISM OF INJURY

WHAT INFLUENCE DOES THE MECHANISM OF INJURY HAVE ON YOUR CLINICAL DECISION-MAKING PROCESS?

It is very common for there to be a mechanism of injury such as trauma or childbirth associated with sacroiliac dysfunction. Instability of the pelvis and SIJ has been demonstrated after child birth. Other causes that have been reported include falls onto the ischial tuberosity, landing hard onto one side of the gluteal region, falls from a bicycle with the foot clipped in, which would result in a unilateral tractional force being applied to the pelvis, stepping into a pothole with the leg fully extended, or motor vehicle accidents with the foot braced against the brake pedal. All of these mechanisms involve a unilateral force being applied either directly or indirectly to one side of the pelvis.

Athletic activities such as skating, golfing, or bowling may also contribute to torsional stresses on this joint.[12] The mechanism of injury may contribute to a direction of force that will influence rotation of the joint, thereby affecting joint position, mobility, and varied ligaments and muscles within the pelvic girdle system.

SYMPTOM LOCATION

WHAT INFLUENCE DOES THE LOCATION OF SYMPTOMS HAVE ON YOUR CLINICAL DECISION-MAKING PROCESS?

Location of symptoms has been found to be a significant indicator of SIJ dysfunction. The pain pattern most frequently seen in

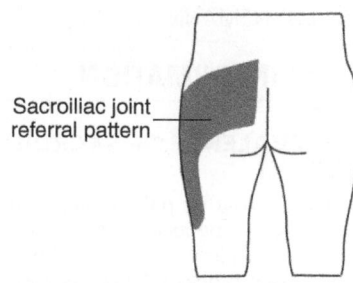

FIGURE II-6-1 Sacroiliac joint pain referral pattern. The illustration is a compilation of the work of several researchers. When injured or the source of patient symptoms, the patient will often describe pain in the following pattern. Symptoms may be experienced in all or a few of the regions indicated.

the clinical situation is at the posterior sacroiliac spine (PSIS) and just inferior to it in an area 3 cm wide and 10 cm long (see Figure II-6-1). This was supported by Fortin and April's work through fluoroscopically guided provocation arthrography in which the SIJ was injected and pain referral patterns were noted. Anterior groin pain has also been found as an area of pain referral. This seems to be most prevalent clinically in clients with sacroiliac or pubic instability. This area of pain referral was found to be a statistically significant indicator of SIJ dysfunction by Schwarzer et al.[18,43,45] In summary, areas of pain in these clients are the unilateral lower lumbar area, buttock, and occasionally reference into the thigh.

REFERRAL OF SYMPTOMS

MUSCLE

Gluteus maximus and minimus:	Ipsilateral buttock and greater trocanter
Obturator:	Central sacrum, coccyx, and ipsilateral posterior thigh
Piriformis:	Buttock, greater trocanter, and posterior thigh
Iliopsoas:	Ipsilateral lower abdomen, groin, anterior thigh, low back, and lateral trunk
Quadratus lumborum	Lower abdomen, anterior lateral trunk, anterior thigh, buttock, greater trocanter, and SIJ

BONE AND LIGAMENT INJURY

No studies have been conducted on the referral pattern of bone or ligament pathology in the lumbar spine.

DERMATOMAL DISTRIBUTION OF SPINAL NERVE ROOTS (See Figure II-6-2)

L1: Inguinal region
L2: Anterior and medial thigh
L3: Anterior thigh and medial knee
L4: Medial leg and medial foot
L5: Lateral leg and dorsum of foot
S1: Posterior thigh and lateral foot
S2: Posterior thigh and medial ankle
S3: Groin and coccyx region
S4: Coccyx region

MYOTOMAL DISTRIBUTION OF SPINAL NERVE ROOTS

L1: Hip flexion
L2: Hip flexion, hip adduction
L3: Knee extension

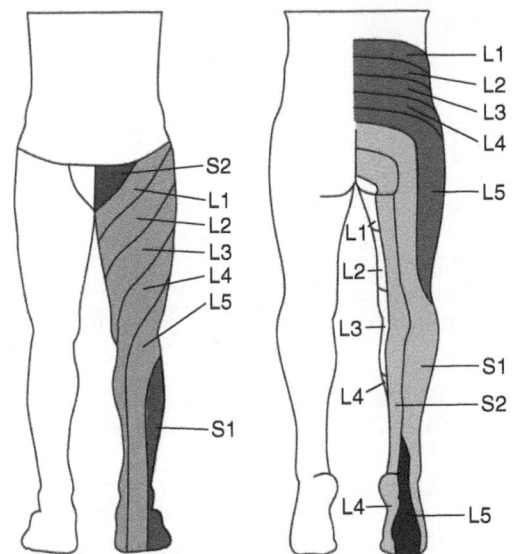

FIGURE II-6-2 Lower extremity dermatomes. A dermatome is an area of skin innervated by a single pair of dorsal nerve roots. Dermatomal patterns of symptoms vary greatly from person to person. The clinician should keep this in mind when utilizing dermatomes for clinical diagnostic purposes.

L4: Ankle dorsiflexion
L5: Foot/toes dorsiflexion
S1: Plantar flexion foot/toes, ankle eversion, hip extension
S2: Knee flexion
S3: Foot intrinsics

NERVES IMPLICATED WITH REFLEX LOSS

Patellar reflex: L3/L4
Medial hamstring: L5/S1
Lateral hamstring: S1/S2
Posterior tibial: L4/L5
Achilles reflex: S1/S2

DERMATOMAL DISTRIBUTION OF PERIPHERAL NERVES (See Figure II-6-3)

Femoral:	Medial thigh and calf
Anterior femoral cutaneous:	Lateral hip and thigh
Posterior femoral cutaneous:	Posterior thigh
Pudendal:	Groin and inner thighs
Obturator:	Medial thigh
Sciatic:	Posterior leg
Tibial:	Plantar surface of foot
Fibular:	Lateral calf and dorsolateral aspect of foot
Deep fibular:	Web of first and second toes
Sural:	Lateral calf and lateral dorsum of foot

MYOTOMAL DISTRIBUTION OF LOWER EXTREMITY PERIPHERAL NERVES

Femoral:	Knee extension with/without hip flexion
Lateral femoral cutaneous:	None
Posterior femoral cutaneous:	None
Saphenous:	None
Pudendal:	Pelvic floor

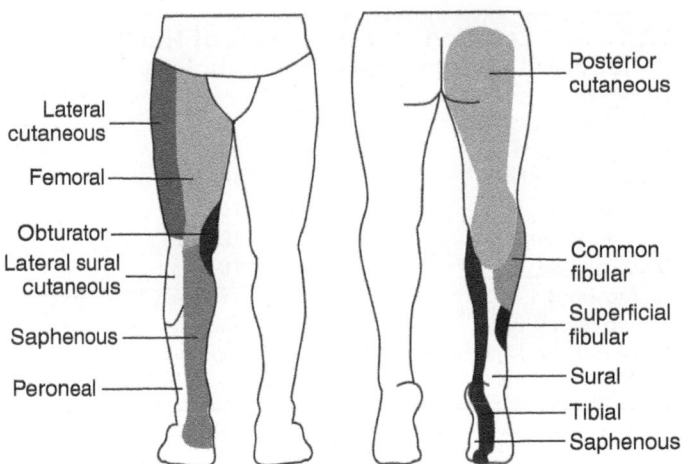

FIGURE II-6-3 Sensory distribution of peripheral nerves. The referral pattern of the sensory nerves is different from the referral pattern of the spinal nerve root. The clinician can utilize the differences to aid in the diagnostic process.

Obturator:	Thigh adduction
Sciatic:	Foot dorsiflexion and inversion, plantar flexion, knee flexion
Tibial:	Plantar flexion and foot inversion
Superficial fibular:	Foot eversion
Deep fibular:	Foot and toe dorsiflexion
Sural:	None

VASCULAR SYSTEMS

There are no published data regarding the referral patterns of arteries and veins in the sacroiliac region.

WHAT STRUCTURES CAN REFER INTO THE SIJ REGION?

- Muscles—The iliocostalis lumborum and longissums thoracic can both refer pain into the gluteal region. Multifidus and the abdominal muscles refer pain into the anterior aspect of the hip and groin.
- Hamstrings
- Quadriceps
- Lumbar disc—Ohnmeiss et al found that no disc pathology referred pain to the low back and buttock. The lower discs referred pain into the thigh. L3/L4 referred to the anterior thigh, L4/L5 referred to the anterior and posterior thigh, and L5/S1 referred to the posterior thigh.[37]
- Zygapophyseal Joint—According to Fukui and Nosaka[18] the L5/S1 facet joint can refer pain into the gluteal region. All other pathology referred pain into the hip, great trocanter, groin, or thigh.
- Hip Joint—The referral pattern of hip pain has been recently summarized by Khan and Woolson. The referral pattern occurs through radiation to portions of the sensory distribution of the femoral, obturator, and sciatic nerves. Pain in the low back and SIJ area is not a positive response because hip joint discomfort does not radiate to these areas[28] (Box II-6-1).
- Pubic symphysis—The pubic symphysis should be included in the discussion regarding the SIJ because it forms the anterior connection of the pelvis. The symphysis pubis has been designed to dissipate and cushion the impaction forces imposed on the pelvis during gait. In healthy individuals, gait results in the rapid weight transfer from one side of the pelvis to the other with the associated forces centered on and applied to the symphysis. Injuries to the region are possible. Examples include

BOX II-6-1 Location and Frequency of Hip Pain in Patients with Intraarticular Hip Pathology	
Location Frequency	%
Groin only	43
Trochanter only	18
Gluteal only	15
Groin/trochanter	12
Groin/gluteal	16
All locations	13
No hip pain	13
Groin only or groin with other locations	73

oseitis pubis and groin strains. Despite the occurrence of the pathology, the referral patterns related to the pubic symphysis have not been studied to date.[25]

- Coccyx—Although fractures and injuries to the coccyx bone are fairly common in clinical settings, the nature and pain presentation patterns of the bone have not been researched in the literature. Clinically, the patient's symptoms are generally local in nature. Pain can expand into the sacroiliac region, but it appears to be the result of inflammation and not due to referral from the coccyx itself.

WHAT VISCERAL STRUCTURES CAN REFER TO THE LUMBAR SPINE (See Figure II-6-4)?

Bladder
Ovaries

Fallopian tubes
Uterus
Testes
Prostate
Descending aorta
Sigmoid colon
Appendix
Small intestine

SYMPTOM DESCRIPTORS

Typically the pain from sacroiliac dysfunction is unilateral and dull in character.[23]

WHAT INFLUENCE DOES THE DEPTH OF SYMPTOMS HAVE ON YOUR CLINICAL DECISION-MAKING PROCESS IN THE SIJ REGION?

The depth of symptoms (i.e., superficial or deep) has little influence in the clinical decision making related to intervention at the SIJ because of the nature of the referred pain as previously discussed. Anterior pelvic pain or pain in the pubic symphysis area should be noted if it is present and a screen of the visceral systems as well as examination of the hip and pubic symphysis joints should be performed.

CLINICAL PEARL

The muscles that cross the SIJ contribute to the stability of the SIJ but are not prime movers. They are designed to be prime movers of the spine or hip. Muscles most closely associated with the joint are the erector spinae, multifidus,

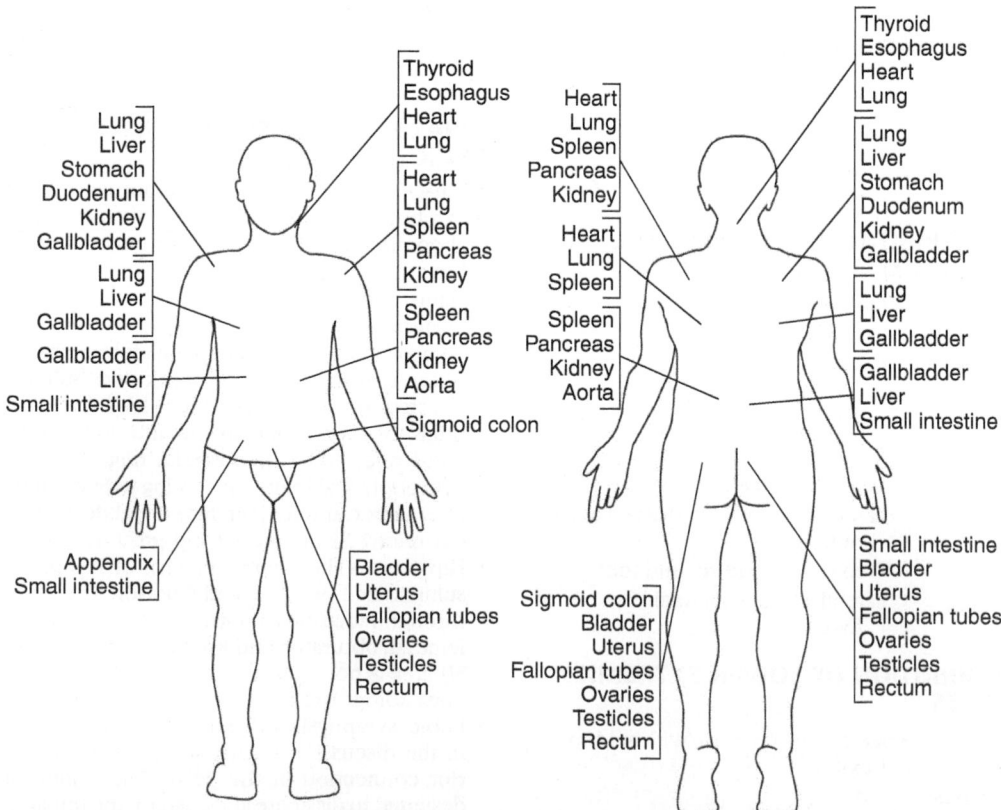

FIGURE II-6-4 Symptom referral pattern of visceral tissue. The figure illustrates the most visceral tissues that most commonly refer symptoms into the upper quarter region. Symptoms are generally described as a deep dull ache that is hard to localize. Symptoms may wax and wane in intensity and may not be elicited by motions of the region.

gluteals, and piriformis. More global muscles that affect its stability include the latissimus dorsi, quadratus lumborum, and abdominal muscles. Palpation of the piriformis and gluteals for muscle tone and during contraction is an important component of the physical examination. The ligaments that provide stability for the SIJ are the anterior sacroiliac ligament, iliolumbar ligament, sacrospinous ligament, sacrotuberous ligament, and the long and short posterior sacroiliac ligaments. To palpate the joint, palpate the joint margin just medial to the PSIS through the skin and gluteal musculature. You will most likely palpate the short and long ligaments overlying the joint.

WHAT INFLUENCE DOES CONSTANCY OF SYMPTOMS HAVE ON YOUR CLINICAL DECISION-MAKING PROCESS IN THE SIJ REGION?

Constant symptoms at the SIJ may indicate an acute inflammatory process either from an acute injury or a viral cause. Most constant symptoms that are related to inflammation may initially be reported by the patient as constant, but on further questioning, the constancy of symptoms will vary. True constant symptoms should be a warning sign to the clinician to rule out visceral involvement. The visceral systems of the lower lumbar and pelvic region should be ruled out. Generally, the symptoms will be worse in the morning or with inactivity, improving slightly with motion. In most cases the symptoms vary related to an activity or position. This variation of symptoms may lead the clinician toward a direction of treatment for exercise or manipulation.

CLINICAL DECISION MAKING CASE STUDY—PATIENT PROFILE **?**

A 34-year-old female presents with complaints of pain in the right lumbosacral region mainly localized in the PSIS area with occasional referral into the buttock. Onset of symptoms began the week before, immediately after she stepped off a curb that was steeper than she realized. The pain was pinpoint at the PSIS immediately after injury. Her pain is made worse by walking for prolonged periods of time, flexing the hip and knee up to negotiate stairs, and lying in a flexed position. She normally sleeps on her side curled up in a fetal position but states that the only relief she can find is by lying in the prone position. What are your hypotheses for the changes in her symptoms based on position?

Answer

Some have theorized that the SIJ, because of its irregular surfaces (concave and convex), can become "locked" or stuck at the end range of a position.[35,36,39] In this case the patient's mechanism of injury occurred while an innominate was rotated in a posterior direction (stepping off the curb with an extended knee). If indeed the joint can become stuck at its end range, it may be stuck in posterior ilial rotation. Therefore any position that creates further posterior ilial rotation (i.e., hip flexion) may induce symptoms, whereas any position that promotes anterior ilial rotation (i.e., hip extension in prone lying) may ease the patient's symptoms.

IF A PATIENT HAS SYMPTOMS IN THE MORNING, WHAT PATHOLOGY DOES THIS IMPLICATE?

Morning symptoms such as stiffness may indicate premature arthritic changes in the SIJ or a state of inflammation within the joint.

WHAT ROLE DOES MORNING STIFFNESS PLAY IN DIFFERENTIATION?

As in the lumbar spine section, any time the body is in a static position for a prolonged period of time, inflammation can accumulate within a region. When injured, an inflammatory reaction occurs. Acute injury may cause inflammation for up to 10 days in the normal healing process. The SIJ has no direct muscle attachment, but muscles cross the joint to create motion.

Morning stiffness that lasts for more than 15 minutes may indicate that inflammation is the cause for stiffness as a symptom. Stiffness that lasts only minutes and is relieved quickly with motion is often more associated with mechanical factors than with inflammatory factors.

IF A PATIENT HAS SYMPTOMS IN THE AFTERNOON, WHAT PATHOLOGY DOES THIS IMPLICATE?

None. Patients will often report an increase in symptoms in the afternoon. These symptoms can be misleading because the symptoms are more related to use or overuse than to the time of day. The patient should be questioned as to whether aggravating activities preceded the afternoon pain.

IF A PATIENT HAS SYMPTOMS IN THE EVENING, WHAT PATHOLOGY DOES THIS IMPLICATE?

Like afternoon pain ligament injury and instability may be more symptomatic in the afternoon because of the dynamic system of muscles that stabilize the region and the demands placed on them during the day.

IF A PATIENT HAS SYMPTOMS WHEN SLEEPING, WHAT PATHOLOGY DOES THIS IMPLICATE?

Night pain in the SIJ that wakes a patient and is nonremittent based on positional changes may indicate a more serious pathology such as a malignant tumor or pathological fracture. Although primary sacroiliac tumors are rare, giant cell tumors, chondrosarcomas, are common neoplasms that can affect the SIJ. Rheumatic diseases such as AS or Reiter's syndrome may present with night symptoms due to inflammatory conditions within the joint. These are diagnosed through radiographs and laboratory findings including a positive HLA-B27 test and an elevated erythrocyte sedimentation rate.

This being said, nocturnal pain from the SIJ is not uncommon. Usually the pain is elicited as the patient turns from side to side, or as the patient's leg drops into adduction when sleeping on the side. A patient may place a pillow between the legs to prevent leg adduction. If this reduces the pain, then the symptoms are more likely musculoskeletal in nature.

CLINICAL DECISION MAKING CASE STUDY—PATIENT PROFILE **?**

A 25-year-old male presents with both central buttock pain and pain in both PSIS areas. He reports his pain is constant and does not change with position. Even rest does not ease the buttock pain. He states his pain stays at a constant level from the minute he wakes until he lies down, regardless of activity. At night it wakes him around 3:00 am with increased deep aching. The onset of pain was gradual in the last month and in the past few days he has noticed he feels weak when negotiating stairs and has also noted symptoms of impotency. What are the red flags that can be identified from this case? What type of pathology might these symptoms implicate?

Answer

The red flags are (1) constant nonremittent pain, (2) pain not influenced by mechanical behaviors, (3) bilateral pain that is worse at night, and (4) potential progressive and multilevel neurological deficit. These symptoms may implicate an inflammatory condition but are more likely to implicate a space-occupying lesion in the sacral region causing neurological deficit. This patient was diagnosed with chondrosarcoma of the sacrum.

STABILITY OF SYMPTOMS

IF A PATIENT'S SYMPTOMS ARE IMPROVING, WHAT PATHOLOGY DOES THIS IMPLICATE?

If the patient's symptoms improve, then the dysfunction is most likely musculoskeletal in nature. The clinician must watch for patterns of improvement and worsening. For example, symptoms that improve and then begin again during or after menstrual flow may indicate a gynecological cause of symptoms.

IF A PATIENT'S SYMPTOMS ARE WORSENING, WHAT PATHOLOGY DOES THIS IMPLICATE?

If a patient's symptoms worsen and the therapist has modified the treatment regimen, consideration should be taken for a visceral cause of pain referred to the sacroiliac region and appropriate measures for referral should be made.

FUNCTIONAL AND ACTIVITY PARTICIPATION LIMITATIONS

WHAT INFLUENCE DO AGGRAVATING ACTIVITIES HAVE ON YOUR CLINICAL DECISION-MAKING PROCESS (Table II-6-1)?

Two studies looked at the validity of history items in subjects who were questioned as to whether pain was made worse or relieved by sitting, standing, or walking. Schwarzer et al and Dreyfuss et al concluded that no aggravating or relieving factor was valuable for the diagnosis of SIJ-related pain.[12,43] One factor noted was that when the patient reported pain relief with standing the specificity was 0.98 although the likelihood ratio was 3.9.

There may be some value in the history of patients who have no lumbar pain and no pain when rising from sitting. When this was coupled with three positive SIJ pain provocation tests Young et al found the likelihood that the SIJ was the source of pain (identified by diagnostic injection) was increased 28 times.[57]

FLEXION-BASED ACTIVITIES

- Pathologies aggravated by flexion include sacral extension dysfunction and the long and short dorsal sacroiliac ligaments.
- Lumbosacral flexion may aggravate symptoms at the SIJ if there is a restriction in sacral extension. Sacral extension is coupled with lumbar flexion. Lumbosacral flexion will also place tension on the long and short dorsal sacroiliac ligaments. In the case of sprained ligaments, these movements may result in pain.

EXTENSION-BASED ACTIVITIES

- Pathologies aggravated by extension include sacral flexion dysfunction and iliolumbar and anterior sacroiliac ligament sprain.
- Lumbosacral extension may aggravate symptoms at the SIJ if there is a restriction in sacral flexion. Sacral flexion is coupled with lumbar extension. Lumbosacral extension will also place tension on the iliolumbar and anterior sacroiliac ligaments. In the case of sprained ligaments, these movements may result in pain.

LATERAL FLEXION AND ROTATION ACTIVITIES

- Ipsilateral lumbosacral sidebending and contralateral lumbosacral rotation will compress the SIJ surfaces, which may cause pain from within the joint surface itself. Pain from gapping the joint may occur with contralateral sidebending and ipsilateral rotation when the ligaments are sprained.

COMBINED MOTION ACTIVITIES

- Pathologies eased by extension and rotation/lateral flexion include sacral flexion dysfunction, posterior innominate derangement, or positional fault, joint hypermobility.

STATIC ACTIVITIES

- Pathologies eased by static activities include joint dysfunction and ligament sprain.

WHAT INFLUENCE DOES EASING ACTIVITIES HAVE ON YOUR CLINICAL DECISION-MAKING PROCESS?

When the joint surfaces are displaced, a position of ease may be attained in the position opposite the displacement (see Table II-6-1). So, for example, if the joint is stuck in an anterior displacement, the client may find relief in a prone position.

TABLE II-6-1   Functional and Activity Participation Limitations

Motion	Functional Activities	Pathology if Symptoms Are Aggravated by Activity	Pathology if Symptoms Are Eased by Activity
Flexion	Sitting, bending forward	Sacroiliac joint (SIJ) sprain, muscle strain, posterior ligament sprain, SIJ dysfunction, pelvic girdle syndrome	SIJ dysfunction—posterior innominate rotation or sacral extension, anterior ligament sprain
Extension	Walking, bending backward	SIJ sprain, SIJ dysfunction, pelvic girdle syndrome, anterior ligament strain	SIJ dysfunction—anterior innominate rotation or sacral flexion, posterior ligament sprain, iliolumbar ligament sprain
Lateral flexion and rotation		SIJ sprain, muscle strain, ligament sprain, SIJ dysfunction, pelvic girdle syndrome	One-sided SIJ dysfunction, muscle strain, ligament strain,
Combined motion	Extension and rotation/lateral flexion	SIJ sprain, muscle strain, ligament sprain, SIJ dysfunction, pelvic girdle syndrome	One-sided SIJ dysfunction, muscle strain, ligament strain
Combined motion	Flexion and rotation/lateral flexion	SIJ sprain, muscle strain, ligament sprain, SIJ dysfunction	One-sided SIJ dysfunction, muscle strain, ligament strain
Static positions	Sleep, sitting, standing	SIJ instability	Muscle strain, ligament strain, one-sided SIJ dysfunction, two-sided SIJ dysfunction, symphysiolysis, pelvic girdle syndrome
General movement	Walking, stair climbing, and movement	SIJ sprain, muscle strain, ligament sprain, SIJ dysfunction, pelvic girdle syndrome, symphysiolysis	Instability
Other	Coughing, laughing, sneezing, valsalva, intercourse, childbirth	SIJ instability	

CLINICAL PEARL ⓘ

How is movement of the SIJ defined based on the osteo-
pathic model? In the sagittal plane, the ilium may move in
anterior and posterior rotation, in the frontal plane, the ilium
may translate superiorly and inferiorly, and in the transverse
plane, the ilium may rotate to the right or left. The sacrum flexes
(nutates) and extends (counternutates) in the sagittal plane.
The sacrum side bends and rotates in a combined motion dur-
ing gait and pelvic rotation

FLEXION-BASED ACTIVITIES
- Pathologies eased by flexion include SIJ dysfunction, posterior innominate rotation or sacral extension positional faults, and anterior ligament sprain.
- Flexion-based activities will take the load off the anterior sacroiliac ligaments.

EXTENSION-BASED ACTIVITIES
- Pathologies eased by extension include SIJ dysfunction, anterior innominate rotation or sacral flexion, and posterior ligament sprain and strain.
- Extension-based activities will take the stress off the posterior joint ligaments.

LATERAL FLEXION AND ROTATION ACTIVITIES
- Pathologies eased by lateral flexion and rotation include one-sided SIJ dysfunction, muscle strain, and ligament strain.
- Ipsilateral lumbar rotation will rotate the sacrum toward the direction of rotation.

COMBINED MOTION ACTIVITIES
- Pathologies eased by extension and rotation/lateral flexion include one-sided SIJ dysfunction, muscle strain, and ligament strain.
- Pathologies eased by flexion and rotation/lateral flexion include SIJ sprain, muscle strain, ligament sprain, and SIJ dysfunction.

STATIC ACTIVITIES
- Pathology eased by static activities include muscle strain, as this will alleviate the muscle guarding seen in many pathologies.

GENERAL MOVEMENT
Pathologies eased by general movement include muscle strain, ligament strain, one-sided SIJ dysfunction, two-sided SIJ dysfunction, symphysiolysis, and pelvic girdle syndrome.

MEDICAL HISTORY

WHAT ROLE DOES A PATIENT'S PAST MEDICAL HISTORY PLAY IN THE DIFFERENTIAL DIAGNOSIS OF PATHOLOGY?

It is important to screen the patient's past medical history for AS, cancer, or trauma that might affect the SIJ. Past history of hip pathology or past injuries to the lower extremity may also alter the loading of the SI joint. These factors may contribute to SIJ dysfunction. The gastrointestinal and urogenital systems may also refer into the lower pelvis and sacral regions; therefore, a past history of pathology in these regions may alert the clinician to possible contributions from these systems.

MEDICAL AND ORTHOPEDIC TESTING

WHAT MEDICAL AND ORTHOPEDIC TESTS INFLUENCE YOUR DIFFERENTIAL DIAGNOSIS PROCESS?

Active movement tests lack reliability as do positional palpation tests. Clinicians who utilize these tests to guide manual physical therapy interventions should do so with the understanding that these tests are reliable on any rating scale.[33]

In Table II-6-2 sensitivity and specificity values are indicated for the sacroiliac tests that appear to have sufficient diagnostic accuracy. The active straight-leg raising (ASLR) test and thigh thrust have good predictive validity for patients with SIJ pain postpartum.

The lunge, ASLR, and thigh thrust provided the most useful evidence in a study performed by Cooke et al.[7] They found these tests were moderately discriminatory in detecting pelvic girdle pain. Clustering provocation tests utilized in Laslett's study[31] and manual muscle testing of the hip improved the diagnostic value of these tests. They also found that when clustering the SIJ tests with the performance of a comprehensive evaluation to assess for radicular signs, the level of diagnostic accuracy was excellent for pain from SIJ dysfunction. Clinicians typically use groups of tests to confirm findings; clustering has been especially useful with testing the SIJ.[29]

CLINICAL PEARL ⓘ

Whereas provocation tests are useful to indicate where a
sacroiliac dysfunction is present, passive mobility testing with
assessment of provocation or alleviation of symptoms during
testing can be helpful in identifying a preferential direction of
treatment. For example, if a patient's pain is provoked with pas-
sive anterior ilial rotation and the pain eases with posterior ilial
rotation, the direction of preference for manipulation (thrust or
nonthrust) would most likely be posterior ilial rotation.

MEDICATIONS

HOW DOES A PATIENT'S RESPONSE TO MEDICATION INFLUENCE YOUR DECISION-MAKING PROCESS?

If a patient does not respond to antiinflammatory medication, there may be a mechanical derangement that continues to provoke the inflammatory process. Typical medications used for the management of SIJ dysfunction or disease are nonsteroidal antiinflammatory drugs, nonopiate analgesics, opiates, antidepressants, and protease inhibitors for inflammatory spondyloarthropathy.[10]

TABLE II-6-2 Special Tests for the Sacroiliac Joint

ORTHOPEDIC TESTS	SENSITIVITY			SPECIFICITY		
	Laslett[30]	Albert[1]	Cook[8]	Laslett[30]	Albert[1]	Cook[8]
ASIS distraction	0.60	0.40	0.53	0.81	1.00	0.67
Thigh thrust	0.88	0.90	0.76	0.60	0.98	0.67
Gaenslen's test	0.75		0.47	0.76		1.0
ASIS compression	0.69	0.70	0.59	0.69	1.00	0.50
FABER		0.70			0.99	
ASLR	0.76 (Damen)		0.53	0.55 (Damen)		0.83

ASIS, anterior sacroiliac spine; FABER, flexion, abduction, and external rotation test; ASLR, active straight-leg-raising test.

BIOMECHANICAL FACTORS

WHAT ROLE DOES BIOMECHANICS PLAY IN THE DECISION-MAKING PROCESS IN THE SIJ REGION?

- Biomechanical assessment and treatment approaches have varied based on descriptions of movement and questionable accuracy in testing the true mechanics of this region.
- Sacral mechanics have been described most functionally during gait by Inman. Inman described posterior iliac rotation during hip flexion through the swing phase, which is accentuated by heel contact and initial loading. During the loading response, the ipsilateral ilium begins to rotate anteriorly. The sacrum seems to rotate forward about a diagonal axis creating torsion via nutation on the side of loading at midstance.
- After about the first 60° of trunk forward bending the pelvis rotates anteriorly around the hip joints. The sacrum initially follows the lumbar spine in flexion; however, near the middle to end range of lumbar flexion, sacral extension or counternutation may occur. During trunk hyperextension of the spine, sacral flexion or nutation occurs. Theoretically, this movement relationship between the spine and sacrum has been described as working like a hinge. Envision a hinge between the lumbar spine and sacrum; when the lumbar spine flexes the sacrum will move in the opposite direction, i.e., extension, and vice versa with lumbar extension.
- No studies have verified these theoretical movements, which make the diagnosis based on mechanics and position a difficult task for the clinician.

CLINICAL PEARL

Self-locking mechanisms of the SIJ can be understood through the principles of form and force closure. Although clinicians cannot affect change in form closure (the close fit of joint surfaces of the SIJ to resist shear forces), they can affect force closure (additional compressive force needed to maintain stability of the pelvis). Specific training of the transversely oriented abdominal muscles (transverse abdominis, internal oblique) with coactivation of the multifidus is a first step in successful stabilization of this region. Additionally, retraining of the gluteals, latissimus dorsi, erector spinae, quadratus lumborum, and hip abductors/adductors should be performed as necessary.[40,41,51,52]

WHAT BIOMECHANICAL ABNORMALITIES IN OTHER REGIONS AFFECT YOUR DECISION-MAKING PROCESS?

- Biomechanical abnormalities in the lumbar region, pubic symphysis, and hip play a significant role in the function of the SIJ.
- Hypomobility or fusion in the lumbar region or hip may result in the need for the SIJ to increase mobility and become hypermobile or unstable.
- The incidence of sacralization is higher than lumbarization and has been indicated to range from 15% to 30%. The association between sacralization and sacroiliac dysfunction has not been established; however, there is a weak association with low back pain.
- Spondylolisthesis in the lower lumbar levels may affect the stability of the sacrum overall because of the interrelationship of the iliolumbar ligaments and lumbosacral ligaments.

CLINICAL PEARL

What diagnoses are utilized to describe impairment in the SIJ?
Many classification systems have evolved for this joint. The earliest model has been described by osteopathic physicians and has been modified for more recent use. This model utilizes a positional approach indicating that the joint is dysfunctional because the sacrum or ilium is out of position.[20,36]
Sacral: nutation, counternutation, torsion
Ilial: anterior rotation, posterior rotation, inflare, outflare, upslip, downslip
Clinicians have also described a mobility-based classification system that utilized positional assessment, but impairments were diagnosed only if mobility was impaired[32,38] (Table II-6-3). Paris has suggested a progressive classification system that includes both systems, but the terminology is based on the impairment model[38]:
1. SIJ sprain
2. Sacroiliac hypermobility
3. Sacroiliac displacement
Lee also distinguishes three types of pelvic girdle disorders[31]:
1. Hypomobility with or without pain
2. Hypermobility with or without pain
3. Normal mobility with pain
More recently Albert et al have described it as a syndrome with four classifications plus one for outliers that do not fit the other four classifications[3]:

TABLE II-6-3	**Classifications Systems for the Sacroiliac Joint**		
Osteopathic Classification	**Paris Classification**	**Lee Classification**	**Albert Classification** **Classification of Pregnant Women with Pelvic Pain**
Sacral nutation	Sacroiliac sprain	Hypomobility with or without pain	One-sided sacroiliac joint (SIJ): pain on one side
Sacral counternutation	Sacroiliac hypermobility	Hypermobility with or without pain	Two-sided SIJ: pain on both sides
Sacral torsion	Sacroiliac derangement: ilial and sacral positional faults	Normal mobility with pain	Symphysiolysis: daily pain in the pubic symphysis confirmed only by objective findings
Ilial anterior rotation	Not applicable	Not applicable	Pelvic girdle syndrome: daily pain in all three pelvic joints confirmed by objective findings
Ilial posterior rotation	Not applicable	Not applicable	Mixed: daily pain from one or more pelvic joints but inconsistent Objective findings from the pelvic joints
Ilial upslip	Not applicable	Not applicable	Not applicable
Ilial downslip	Not applicable	Not applicable	Not applicable
Ilial outflare	Not applicable	Not applicable	Not applicable
Ilial inflare	Not applicable	Not applicable	Not applicable

1. One-sided SIJ
2. Two-sided SIJ
3. Symphysiolysis
4. Pelvic girdle syndrome
5. Mixed

It is difficult to state which system is the best to describe this syndrome, but it is important to note the various manners in which it has been described. The Paris classification system was used and was found to be useful clinically. Albert's classification has been tested for reliability with good results.[1,7]

CLINICAL PEARL !

Pain in the pubic symphysis usually increases with unilateral standing activities. Palpation of this joint will result in increased tenderness if it is dysfunctional. Instability of the pubic symphysis is suggested by radiographic findings of pubic symphysis separation >10 mm and vertical displacement >2 mm in the single leg stance.[46]

CLINICAL DECISION MAKING CASE STUDY—PATIENT PROFILE ?

The patient is a 22-year-old male with complaints of pain in the right posterior SIJ area. Injury occurred 1 week ago when he was playing ice hockey and fell directly on the right buttock. He reports sitting is more comfortable than walking or standing. The patient ambulates with decreased weight bearing on the right lower extremity. The structural assessment (sitting and standing) includes the following:

Iliac crest: Lower on the right
PSIS: Lower on the right
Anterior sacroiliac spine (ASIS): Superior on the right
Active range of motion (AROM): Within normal limits; the lumbar area is painful into extension
Neurological screen: Within normal limits
Special tests: Positive iliac distraction and provocation tests and positive posterior ilial torsion test
Passive mobility: Painful and decreased posterior ilial rotation mobility; anterior ilial rotation eased symptoms

What is your hypothesis regarding this patient's diagnosis/classification?

Answer

This patient presents with one-sided SIJ dysfunction or sacroiliac displacement with a posterior ilial rotation positional fault. The diagnostic indicators are positional assessment, provocation testing with alleviation of symptoms with anterior ilial rotation, and decreased posterior ilial rotation mobility.

CLINICAL DECISION MAKING CASE STUDY—PATIENT PROFILE ?

A 36-year-old female presents with dull aching pain in the left SIJ area. She reports gradual onset of symptoms over the past 3 weeks. Past medical history is negative. Present medical history: gravida para three with the most recent vaginal childbirth 6 months ago. Aggravating positions include standing for prolonged periods of time and lifting her 6-month-old child from the floor. Positions of ease include walking and lying down. Based on her history what is your hypothesis for a diagnosis?

Answer

The patient presented with sacroiliac hypermobility. She most likely continued to sprain the joint with inappropriate lifting techniques. She was still nursing her baby, which may increase the period of laxity of the pelvic ligaments. She was treated with a sacroiliac binder, stabilization exercises, and patient education to reduce stress while lifting and with other functional activities.[9]

ENVIRONMENTAL FACTORS

DO PSYCHOSOCIAL ISSUES INFLUENCE CLINICAL DECISION MAKING?

Psychosocial issues may influence a patient's ability to heal because of the effect on the immune system. They should be assessed as indicated in the lumbar section of this chapter. If the patient's fear avoidance is high the clinician should utilize a graded exercise program to reintroduce movement gradually in a functional manner.

CAN EMOTIONS INFLUENCE THE DECISION-MAKING PROCESS?

A patient who is highly emotional may not be ready for manual therapy/joint manipulation, but may need gradual exposure to the therapeutic regimen.

DO WORK-RELATED INJURIES INFLUENCE CLINICAL DECISION MAKING?

When an injury is work related it is important to consider several factors: perception of fault, duration of pain, physical requirements of the job, if the job performance is affected by symptoms/physical limitations, and the employer's attitude toward limited duty. It is important to note the potential effect of psychosocial factors contributing to disability in the work environment[17,21] (Table II-6-4).

PERSONAL FACTORS

PREVIOUS SURGERIES

WHAT PREVIOUS SURGERIES INFLUENCE YOUR CLINICAL DECISION MAKING?

A previous history of lumbar fusion may be associated with sacroiliac hypermobility or instability because of the biomechanical stresses placed on it. Past surgeries that impact the lower abdominal region may also influence the ability of the abdominal muscles to effectively stabilize the pelvis. These surgeries include caesarian sections, colon resections, hysterectomies, and hernia surgeries. Hip replacement surgeries may also impact the ability of the hip to flex to end range. Therefore with forward flexion, greater contributions from the lumbar and sacral regions are required to make up for the lack of hip mobility. Any lower extremity surgery could also lead to weakness and biomechanic changes at the injured region. Long-term compensations could result in abnormal stresses at the SIJ.

TABLE II-6-4 **Environmental and Personal Contextual Factors**

Contextual Factors

Environmental	Work environment requiring sudden lifting activities, repetitive rotation, and unilateral standing can lead to breakdown of tissue
Psychosocial	Work-related issues, personal and family factors, depression, and emotional unrest can all influence sacroiliac and low back pain

FAMILY HISTORY

DOES A FAMILY HISTORY OF PATHOLOGY IN THE REGION INFLUENCE YOUR CLINICAL REASONING PROCESS?

A family history of rheumatic or metabolic diseases such as AS, Reiter's syndrome, psoriatic arthritis, or Paget's disease would influence clinical reasoning in the area of sacroiliac dysfunction as all of these would influence the mobility and integrity of the SIJ.

CHRONICITY OF PAIN

WHAT CENTRAL PROCESSING CHANGES INFLUENCE DECISION MAKING?

Chronic sacroiliac dysfunction is typically related to hypermobile conditions. Central processing that occurs with these patients can affect the ability to retrain the musculature surrounding the joint. Chronic pain can inhibit musculature and over time these tissues change neurologically and morphologically.

CLINICAL PEARL

(!)

Hypermobility or instability of the SIJ has been correlated clinically with a positional diagnosis of a posteriorly rotated ilium. A clinician who suspects instability can attempt to stabilize the joint utilizing a sacroiliac binder. Reassessment of the pelvic landmarks often shows improved symmetry in landmarks.

HAS MEDICAL TREATMENT BEEN SUCCESSFUL FOR PATIENTS WITH CHRONIC PATHOLOGY IN THE REGION?

The benefit of injection of the SIJ has been demonstrated in controlled studies in patients with spondyloarthropathy, but no controlled studies have been performed for patients with sacroiliac pain from other causes.[10] Uncontrolled studies have suggested some benefit may occur with joint injection followed by manual physical therapy.[11] The efficacy of prolotherapy has not been established, but it may strengthen the ligamentous support because of collagen proliferation from an inflammatory response created by specific agents such as dextrose, glycerine, phenol, and lidocaine. Radiofrequency neurotomy of the dorsal ramus of L5 and the lateral branches from S1-S3 may be effective, but more studies are needed to support this method of treatment.[56]

DOES THE CHRONICITY OF SYMPTOMS INFLUENCE YOUR DECISION-MAKING PROCESS?

A chronic condition may require more time to rehabilitate because of the effect chronic pain has on varied systems over time.

HOW DO THE AUTONOMIC, ENDOCRINE, AND IMMUNE SYSTEMS INFLUENCE DECISION MAKING IN THE SACROILIAC REGION?

Traditionally, assessment and interventions in the sacroiliac region have revolved around biomechanical paradigms. Patients with chronic pain in the sacroiliac region often do not respond favorably or quickly to biomechanical approaches. Recently, medical research has turned to inflammation and the autonomic, endocrine, and immune systems as potential sources for the chronic pain seen in the low back and sacral regions. These paradigms are still evolving and their impact on rehabilitation at this time is unclear (Table II-6-5).

CLINICAL PEARL

(!)

A patient who presents with sacral pain and has had a history of trauma, demonstrates inflammation over the

TABLE II-6-5 **Output Mechanisms**

Output Mechanism	
Autonomic	Recent studies explore the relationship between the autonomic system and lumbar pathology. It has been proposed that addressing the autonomic nervous system can alter lumbosacral symptoms. No conclusive evidence has been provided to date.
Endocrine	The endocrine system is involved in the regulation of body homeostasis. It has been proposed that alteration in the endocrine system function can be a source of chronic lumbosacral back pain.
Immune	Infections in the sacroiliac joint caused by osteomelitis, septic arthritis, and postsurgical infection can be a source of sacroiliac pain. Pelvic pain in general can be caused by appendicitis, diverticulitis, sexually transmitted disease, pelvic inflammatory disease, and salpingitis, all of which are influenced by the immune system.

sacrum, and has pain with hip range of motion and with manual compression should be referred to a physician to rule out a pelvic/sacral fracture.[42]

RED FLAGS THAT REQUIRE REFERRAL TO A MEDICAL PHYSICIAN

WHAT SYMPTOMS ALERT YOU TO PATHOLOGIES THAT MAY REQUIRE A REFERRAL TO A MEDICAL PHYSICIAN?[7,44]

- Pain without trauma or overuse
- Previous history of cancer
- History of ulcerative colitis, Crohn's disease, irritable bowel syndrome
- Bowel and bladder dysfunction
- Severe nonmechanical pain
- Progressive neurological deficit
- Fever
- History of metabolic bone disorder
- Unexplained weight loss

WHAT SYMPTOMS IMPLICATE SPECIFIC VISCERAL SYSTEMS?

BOWEL AND BLADDER DYSFUNCTION

- Pain during, immediately before, or after menses
- Associated signs and symptoms
  - Vaginal discharge
  - Discharge from the penis
  - Rectal pain or bleeding
  - Urological signs or symptoms
  - Unreported abdominal pain
  - Dyspareunia
  - Constitutional symptoms
  - Missed menses
  - Headache, fatigue, irritability
  - Vaginal spotting
  - Bursts of bleeding
  - Abdominal cramping
  - Pelvic pain and pressure—shoulder pain
  - Hypotension or shock if hemorrhage is rapid as in the case of tubal rupture.
  - Simultaneous gastrointestinal symptoms
  - Pain relief with passing gas or bowel movement
  - Colicky pain, or constant pain with waves
  - Risk factors

TABLE II-6-6   Body Structure and Tissue-Based Pathology (Nociceptive and Peripheral Neurogenic Pain Mechanisms)

	Muscles	Sacrum	Innominates	Coccyx	Pubic Symphysis	Joint Capsule	Ligaments	Nerves	Visceral Tissue
Pathology	Piriformis syndrome Hip or adductor strain Avulsion fractures	Sacroiliac joint dysfunction	Sacroiliac joint dysfunction Avulsion fractures	Coccyx fracture	Osteitis pubis	Sacroiliac joint dysfunction Ankylosing spondylitis	Iliolumbar ligament sprain	Obturator nerve Pudendal nerve	Bladder Ovaries Fallopian tubes Uterus Testes Prostate Descending aorta Sigmoid colon Appendix Small intestine
Age Occupation	20 to 50 years Sudden lifting	20 to 60 years Sudden lifting or torsional activities	20 to 40 years Sudden lifting or torsional activities	20 to 50 years Fall on buttocks or sustained direct pressure	20 to 40 years Frequent unilateral activities	Not age related No direct relationship	Not age related Sudden or repetitive lifting	20 to 70 years No direct relationship	20 to 70 years Chemical exposure related to testicular cancer and other cancers
Gender	No direct relationship	No direct relationship	No direct relationship	More common in females than males	Most common in females	No direct relationship	No direct relationship except during pregnancy when ligaments become lax after the first trimester	No direct relationship, pudendal nerve in cyclists; lateral femoral cutaneous with hypermobility of ilium	No direct relationship
Ethnicity	Unknown								
History	May or may not have a history of lumbosacral pain	May or may not have a history of lumbosacral pain, sensitivity = 0.40	May or may not have a history of lumbosacral pain, sensitivity = 0.40	History of a fall or trauma to the buttocks	History of previous pain in the pubic symphysis area	May or may not have a history of lumbosacral pain	History of lumbosacral pain	May or may not have a history of lumbosacral pain	Varies related to the pathology
Mechanism of injury	Flexion with or without rotation	Flexion or extension with or without rotation	Flexion or extension with or without rotation	Compression	Forced hip abduction	No direct relationship	Depends on the individual ligaments Flexion for posterior, extension for anterior, and rotation for either ligaments	Extension with rotation	No direct relationship

Continued on following page.

TABLE II-6-6   Body Structure and Tissue-Based Pathology (Nociceptive and Peripheral Neurogenic Pain Mechanisms) *(Continued)*

	Muscles	Sacrum	Innominates	Coccyx	Pubic Symphysis	Joint Capsule	Ligaments	Nerves	Visceral Tissue
Type of onset	Sudden	Sudden or gradual	Sudden or gradual	Sudden	Sudden or gradual	Sudden or gradual	Sudden or gradual	Gradual	Sudden or gradual depending on structure
Referral from local tissue	Pain in lumbosacral and/or gluteal region, anterior hip, groin, lateral thigh	Pain in lumbosacral and/or gluteal region	Pain in lumbosacral region, anterior hip, groin, lateral thigh	Sacral or coccygeal region	Central pubic region, groin, anterior hip	Pain in lumbosacral or buttock regions occasionally posterior thigh	Dependent on structure involved	May refer into lower extremity Distribution of symptoms is dependent on nerve involved	Distribution of symptoms is local to the visceral structure involved
Referral to other regions	May refer unilaterally into the region just distal to the muscle	May refer unilaterally into buttock, groin, thigh, and lower leg	May refer unilaterally into buttock, groin, thigh, and lower leg	May refer into buttock and posterior thigh	May refer into anterior hip, groin, and anterior thigh	May refer unilaterally into buttock, groin, thigh, and lower leg	Dependent on structure involved	May refer into lower extremity Distribution of symptoms is dependent on nerve root involvement	Distribution of symptoms is dependent on visceral structure involved
Changes in symptoms	Sudden pain decreasing for the remainder of the day Increased pain the next morning	Sudden pain, no relief as day of injury progresses	Sudden pain, no relief as day of injury progresses	Sudden pain, no relief on injury progresses	Sudden pain, no relief as injury progresses	Sudden pain, may improve over 8-week period	Sudden pain, no relief as day of injury progresses	Symptoms generally increase gradually over the course of several days to weeks Symptoms may dissipate as irritating structure is addressed	May worsen as pathology progresses
24-hour pain pattern (morning)	Stiff for 30 minutes	Stiff for 30 minutes	Stiff for 30 minutes	Stiff for 30 minutes	Stiff for 30 minutes	Stiff for 30 minutes	Stiff for 30 minutes	Stiff for 30 minutes	Varies but does not change with mechanical stresses
24-hour pain pattern (afternoon)	Less stiff, may be worse with contractile or stretching	Worsens with aggravating activity	Worsens with aggravating activity	Less stiff, may be worse with prolonged sitting and stair climbing	Less stiff, may be worse with ambulation or unilateral activities	Less stiff, may be worse with lumbar flexion	Less stiff, may be worse with aggravating activity	May worsen with prolonged aggravating activity	Varies but does not change with mechanical stresses
24-hour pain pattern (evening)	May be difficult to sleep	May be difficult to sleep and turn in bed	May be difficult to sleep, turn in bed, or lie in certain positions	May be difficult to sleep in supine position or turn in bed	May be difficult to sleep or turn in bed	May be difficult to sleep	May be difficult to sleep	May be difficult to sleep	Increased nocturnal pain

Description of symptoms	Ache and stiffness, poor localization	Sharp pain if stuck, dull ache if hypermobile	Sharp pain if stuck, dull ache if hypermobile	Sharp or dull ache, often able to localize	Sharp or dull ache, often able to localize	Ache and stiffness, poor localization	Ache and stiffness, sharp pain with motions that stress ligament–primarily flexion	Numbness, tingling, burning, weakness	Cramping, peristaltic waves, gnawing ache
Depth of symptoms	Deep	Deep	Deep	Superficial and sometimes deep	Deep	Deep	Superficial or deep depending on ligament	Superficial	Deep, poorly localized
Constancy of symptoms	Intermittent	Intermittent	Intermittent	Intermittent	Intermittent	Intermittent	Intermittent	Intermittent to constant but varying	Typically constant, may come in waves
Aggravating factors	Lumbosacral flexion, stair climbing, initially with movement, after lying down	Sit to stand, single leg stance, lunge, deep squat Flexion and rotation away from the side of injury, extension and rotation to the side of injury	Sit to stand, single leg stance, lunge, deep squat Flexion, extension, rotation depending on direction of involvement	Sitting, flexion, contralateral flexion and rotation, resisted hip extension	Standing, hip PROM, lifting, coughing and sneezing, isometric hip adduction	Lumbar flexion, sitting to standing, transfer, lunge, deep squat, isometric hip abduction	Primarily flexion	Varies according to structure	Not consistent with mechanical movements
Easing factors	Walking, rest	Walking, sitting	Sitting	Walking, lying prone	Lying down	Limited walking and motion, sitting	Extension positioning, lying, joint support/compression	Varies according to structure	Not consistent with mechanical movements
Stability of symptoms	Gradual improvement over 6-week period	Gradual improvement over 6-week period	Gradual improvement over 6-week period	Gradual improvement over 8-week period	Gradual improvement over 8-week period	Gradual improvement over 6-week period, can take up to 6 months for complete improvement	Gradual improvement over 6-week period	Gradual improvement over 6-week period	May worsen if pathology progresses
Past medical history	All structures may have a past history of medical issues that impact the function of the surrounding tissue	Osteoporosis, ankylosing spondylitis	Osteoporosis, ankylosing spondylitis	None	Multiparae, traumatic birth	Ankylosing spondylitis, Reiter's syndrome, psoriatic arthritis, fever	Multiparae	None	History of pathology in the relevant visceral tissue

Continued on following page.

TABLE II-6-6 Body Structure and Tissue-Based Pathology (Nociceptive and Peripheral Neurogenic Pain Mechanisms) (Continued)

	Muscles	Sacrum	Innominates	Coccyx	Pubic Symphysis	Joint Capsule	Ligaments	Nerves	Visceral Tissue
Past surgeries	All structures may have a past history of surgeries that impact the function of the surrounding tissue	All structures may have a past history of surgeries that impact the function of the surrounding tissue / Lumbar fusion may cause associated sacroiliac dysfunction	All structures may have a past history of surgeries that impact the function of the surrounding tissue / Lumbar fusion may cause associated sacroiliac dysfunction	None	All structures may have a past history of surgeries that impact the function of the surrounding tissue / Lumbar fusion may cause associated sacroiliac dysfunction	All structures may have a past history of surgeries that impact the function of the surrounding tissue / Lumbar fusion may cause associated sacroiliac dysfunction	All structures may have a past history of surgeries that impact the function of the surrounding tissue / Lumbar fusion may cause associated sacroiliac dysfunction	May have a history of surgeries to the pelvic floor	May have a history of surgeries related to visceral pathology
Special questions		Fever, malaise, previous trauma, history of cancer, multiparae, weight before pregnancy (sn = 0.63)	Fever, malaise, previous trauma, history of cancer, multiparae, weight before pregnancy (sn = 0.63)	Fever, malaise, previous trauma, history of cancer	Number of pregnancies? Bowel/bladder symptoms, normal menses, vaginal discharge or bleeding	Fever, malaise, previous trauma, history of cancer, multiparae, weight before pregnancy (sn = 0.63)	Fever, malaise, trauma	Weakness	Saddle paresthesias Bilateral lower extremity weakness Changes in bowel or bladder function Gait difficulties
X-rays	Negative	Usually negative unless sacral fracture is present	Negative unless fracture is present	Negative	Positive	Negative	Negative	Negative	Negative
MRI	Positive	Negative	Negative	Positive	Positive	Positive	Positive	May be positive depending on related pathology	Positive for pathology
EMG	Positive if nerves involved	Usually not necessary						Positive	Usually not necessary
Special laboratory tests	None					ERS	None		Varies depending on pathology
Red flags	Fever Nocturnal pain Pain that is not influenced by motion Bleeding Weight loss Rule out specific visceral structures								

PROM, passive range of motion; MRI, magnetic resonance imaging; EMG, electromyogram; ERS, erythrocyte sedimentation rate.

- ○ Osteoporosis
- ○ Sexually transmitted infection
- ○ Long-term use of antibiotics (colitis)

SUMMARY STATEMENT

Sacroiliac dysfunction should be considered a syndrome. A syndrome is defined as an abnormal condition that is identified by an established group of signs and symptoms. Classifications within this syndrome are varied, but a clinical approach that identifies impairments and treats the impairment, not just the symptom, will be most useful for clinical management of the SIJ. Utilizing the Paris classification has been useful as it combines the osteopathic classification with an impairment and mobility-based measuring system. There is a plethora of tests utilized for examination of this joint, so using the evidence to discriminate the tests that are the best indicators of this syndrome is essential.

Most of the research related to the SIJ has been focused on diagnosing it as a causative factor and methods for diagnosis. Future research should focus on testing the reliability of classification systems and the efficacy of interventions for the classifications. Table II-6-6 summarizes the factors that help a clinician differentiate among the different sources of symptoms in the sacroiliac region.

REFERENCES

1. Albert H, Godskesen M, Westergaard J. Evaluation of clinical tests used in classification procedures in pregnancy-related pelvic joint pain. *Eur Spine J.* 2000;9:161-166.
2. Albert H, Godskesen M, Westergaard J. Prognosis in four syndromes of pregnancy-related pelvic pain. *Acta Obstet Gynecol Scand.* 2001;80:505-510.
3. Albert H, et al. Prognosis in four syndromes of pregnancy-related pelvic pain. *Acta Obstet Gynecol Scand.* 2006;85:1320-1326.
4. Bowen V, Cassidy JD. Macroscopic and microscopic anatomy of the sacroiliac joint from embryonic life until the eight decade. *Spine.* 1981;6:620-628.
5. Braun J, Bollow M, Remlinger G, et al. Prevalence of spondylarthropathies in HLA-B27 positive and negative blood donors. *Arthritis Rheum.* 1998;41:58-67.
6. Cohen SP. Sacroiliac Joint Pain: A Comprehensive Review of Anatomy, Diagnosis, and Treatment. *Anesth Analg.* 2005;101:1440-1453.
7. Cook C. *Orthopedic Manual Therapy. An Evidence Based Approach.* Upper Saddle River, NJ: Prentice Hall; 2007.
8. Cook, et al. Interrater Reliability and Diagnostic Accuracy of Pelvic Girdle Pain Classification. *JMPT.* 2007:252-258.
9. Damen L, Spoor CW, Snijders CJ, Stam HJ. Does a pelvic belt influence sacroiliac joint laxity? *Clin Biomech.* 2002;17(7):495.
10. Dreyfuss P, Dreyer S, Cole A, Mayo K. Sacroiliac Joint Pain. *J Am Acad Orthop Surg.* 2004;12:255-265.
11. Dreyfuss P, Michaelsen M, Horne M. MUJA Manipulation under joint anesthesia/analgesia. A treatment approach for recalcitrant low back pain of synovial joint origin. *J Manipulative Physiol Ther.* 1995;18:537-546.
12. Dreyfuss P, Michaelson M, Pauza M, McLarty J, Bogduk N. The value of medical history and physical examination in diagnosing sacroiliac joint pain. *Spine.* 1996;21:2594-2602.
13. Egund N, Olsson TH, Schmid H, Selvik G. Movements in the sacroiliac joints demonstrated with roentgen stereophotogrammetry. *Acta Radiol Diagn (Stockh).* 1978;19:833-846.
14. Elgafy H, Semaan HB, Ebraheim NA, Coombs RJ. Computed tomography findings in patients with sacroiliac pain. *Clin Orthop.* 2001;382:112-118.
15. Flynn T, Fritz J, Whitman J, Wainner R, Magel J, Rendeiro D, et al. A clinical prediction rule for classifying patients with low back pain who demonstrate short-term improvement with spinal manipulation. *Spine.* 2002;27:2835-2843.
16. Freburger JK, Riddle DL. Using published evidence to guide the examination of the sacroiliac joint region. *Phys Ther.* 2001;81:1135-1143.
17. Frymoyer JW. Predicting Disability from Low Back Pain. *Clin Orthop Relat Res.* 1992;279:101-109.
18. Fukui S, Nosaka S. Pain patterns originating from the sacroiliac joints. *J Anesth.* 2002;16:245-247.
19. Gran JT, Husby G, Hordvik M. Prevalence of ankylosing spondylitis in males and females in a young middle-aged population of Tromso, northern Norway. *Ann Rheum Dis.* 1985;44:359-367.
20. Greenman P. *Principles of manual medicine.* 2nd ed. Philadelphia: Williams & Wilkins; 1996.
21. Hadad GH. Analysis of 2932 Workers' Compensation Back Injury Cases. The Impact on the Cost to the System. *Spine.* 1987;12:765.
22. Hogan QH, Abram SE. Neural Blockade for diagnosis and prognosis: a review. *Anesthesiology.* 1997;86:216-241.
23. Huijbregts P. Sacroiliac joint dysfunction: Evidence-based diagnosis. *Orthopaedic Division Review.* 2004;(May/June):18-44.
24. Inman VT, Ralston HJ, Todd F. *Human walking.* Baltimore (MD): Williams & Wilkins; 1981.
25. Mens J, Inklaar H, Koes BW, Stam HJ. A New View on Adduction-Related Groin Pain. *Clin J Sport Med.* 2006;16(1):16-19.
26. Kaipiainen-Seppanen O, Aho K, Heliovaara M. Incidence and prevalence of ankylosing spondylitis in Finland. *J Rheumatol.* 1997;24:496-499.
27. Khan MA, Braun WE, Kushner I, Grecek DE, Muir WA, Steinberg AG. HLA B27 in ankylosing spondylitis: differences in frequency and relative risk in American Blacks and Caucasians. *J Rheumatol Suppl.* 1977;3:39-43.
28. Khan NQ, Woolson ST. Referral patterns of hip pain in patients undergoing total hip replacement. *Orthopedics.* 1998;21:123-126.
29. Kokmeyer DJ, van der WP, Aufdemkampe G, Fickenscher TCM. The reliability of multitest regimens with sacroiliac pain provocation tests. *J Manipulative Physiol Ther.* 2002;25:42-48.
30. Laslett M, Williams M. The reliability of selected pain provocation tests for sacroiliac joint pathology. *Spine.* 1994;19:1243-1249.
31. Laslett M, Young SB, Aprill CN, McDonald B. Diagnosing sacroiliac joints: A validity study of McKenzie evaluation and sacroiliac provocation tests. *Aust J Physiotherapy.* 2003;49:89-97.
32. Lee D. *The pelvic girdle: an approach to the examination and treatment of the lumbo-pelvic-hip region.* Edinburgh: Churchill Livingstone; 1989.
33. Maigne JY, Aivaliklis A, Pfefere F. Results of sacroiliac joint double block and value of sacroiliac pain provocation tests in 54 patients with low back pain. *Spine.* 1996;21(16):1889-1892.
34. Maigne JY, Boulahdour H, Chatellier G. Value of quantitative radionuclide bone scanning in the diagnosis of sacroiliac joint syndrome in 32 patients with low back pain. *Eur Spine J.* 1998;7:328-331.
35. Mennell JM. *Back Pain: Diagnosis and Treatment using Manipulative Techniques.* USA: Little Brown & Company; 1960.
36. Mitchell Jr FL, Moran PS, Pruzzo NA. *An Evaluation and Treatment Manual of Osteopathic Muscle Energy Techniques.* Valley Park, MO: Mitchell, Moran, and Pruzzo Associates; 1979.
37. Ohnmeiss DD, Vanharanta H, Ekholm J. Degree of disc disruption and lower extremity pain. *Spine.* 1997;22(14):1600-5.
38. Paris S, Loubert P. *Foundation of Clinical Orthopaedics.* St. Augustine, Florida: Institute Press; 1999.
39. Paris SV. Anatomy as related to function and pain. *Orthop Clin North Am.* 1983;14:475-489.
40. Pool-Goudzwaard AL, Vleeming A, Stoeckart R, Snijders CJ, Mens JM. Insufficient lumbopelvic stability: a clinical, anatomical and biomechanical approach to 'a-specific' low back pain. *Man Ther.* 1998;3:12-20.
41. Richardson C, Snijders C, Hides J, et al. The relation between the transverse abdominis muscles, sacroiliac joint mechanics, and low back pain. *Spine.* 2002;27:399-405.
42. Sauerland, et al. Reliability of clinical examination in detecting pelvic fractures in blunt trauma patients: a meta-analysis. *Arch Orthop Trauma Surg.* 2004;124:123-128.
43. Schwarzer AC, Aprill CN, Bogduk M. The sacroiliac joint in chronic low back pain. *Spine.* 1995;20:31-37.
44. Sizer P, Brismee JM, Cook C. Medical screening for red flags in the diagnosis and management of musculoskeletal spine pain. *Pain Pract.* 2007;7(1):53-71.
45. Slipman CW, Jackson HB, Lipetz JS, Chan KT, Lenrow D, Vresilovic EJ. Sacroiliac joint pain referral zones. *Arch Phys Med Rehabil.* 2000;81:334-338.
46. Slipman CW, Sterenfeld EB, Chou LH, et al. The value of radionuclide imaging in the diagnosis of sacroiliac joint syndrome. *Spine.* 1996;21:2251-2254.
47. Stuge B, Laerum E, Kirkesola G, Bollestad N. The Efficacy of a Treatment Program Focusing on Specific Stabilizing Exercises for Pelvic Girdle Pain After Pregnancy: A Randomized Controlled Trial. *Spine.* 2004;29(4):351-359.

48. Sturesson B, Selvik G, Uden A. Movements of the sacroiliac joint: a roentgen stereophotogrammetric analysis. *Spine.* 1989;14:162-165.

49. Sturesson B, Uden A, Vleeming A. A radiostereometric analysis of movements of the sacroiliac joints during the standing hip flexion test. *Spine.* 2000;25:364-368.

50. Sturesson B, Uden A, Vleeming A. A radiostereometric analysis of the movements of the sacroiliac joints in the reciprocal straddle position. *Spine.* 2000;25:214-217.

51. Vleeming A, Albert H, Ostgaard H, Stuge B, Sturesson B. European guidelines on the diagnosis and treatment of pelvic girdle pain. *Eur Spine J.* 2008;17(6):794-819.

52. Vleeming A, Pool-Goudzwaard AL, Hammudoghlu D, et al. The function of the long dorsal sacroiliac ligament: its implication for understanding low back pain. *Spine.* 1996;21:556-562.

53. Vleeming A, Stochart R, Vokers ACW, et al. The sacroiliac joint—anatomical, biomechanical and radiological aspects. *J Man Med.* 1999;5:100-102.

54. Vleeming A, Vokers ACW, Snijders CJ, et al. Relation between form and function in the sacroiliac joint. Part II. Biomechanical Aspects. *Spine.* 1990;15:(2):133-136.

55. Walker JM. The sacroiliac joint; a critical review. *Phys Ther.* 1992;72:903-916.

56. Yin W, Willard F, Carreiro J, Dreyfuss P. Sensory stimulation-guided sacroiliac joint radiofrequency neurotomy: Technique based on neuroanatomy of the dorsal sacral plexus. *Spine.* 2003;28:2419-2425.

57. Young S, Aprill C, Laslett M. Correlation of clinical characteristics with three sources of chronic low back pain. *Spine J.* 2003:460-465.

AUTHORS: SUSAN LAYFIELD and PATRICIA A. RUDD

INTRODUCTORY INFORMATION

Temporomandibular dysfunction (TMD) is a group of related disorders associated with the temporomandibular joint (TMJ) and muscles of mastication. Although a frequent misconception exists that TMD involves only the TMJ, muscles, the cervical spine, the nervous system, and referred pain to the sinuses and teeth are included in TMD. Other possible contributing factors include psychological issues, posture, and parafunctional habits (clenching, bruxism, etc.). Previous terms used to describe TMD include temporomandibular joint dysfunction, myofascial pain-dysfunction syndrome, and temporomandibular pain-dysfunction syndrome. TMD is a major cause of orofacial pain of nondental origin. The most common complaint is pain located at the TMJ or nearby structures (ear, teeth, masseter, and temporalis muscles) responsible for jaw function such as chewing and yawning. Other symptoms include interruption of jaw movement, difficulty with jaw opening or closing, locking, spontaneous changes in occlusion, asymmetrical jaw movement, and joint sounds (crepitus, clicking, popping).

WHAT IS THE PREVALENCE OF TMD?

- Muscle pain disorders are the most common cause of persistent pain in the head and neck, with 20% to 50% of the population presenting with at least one TMD symptom (i.e., jaw pain, ear pain).[20,37]
- The prevalence of at least one sign of TMD dysfunction (i.e., joint clicking, joint crepitus) may be as high as 56%.[2] However, only 6% to 10% of this group had symptoms that were severe enough to seek treatment.[20,37]
- Carlsson[11] reported that as many as 93% of the population may show at least one sign or symptom of TMD during their lifetime. Females are five to nine times more likely to experience symptoms than males.[27]
- Among females, symptoms are most frequent between the ages of 15 and 45 years.[25,42]
- Few studies have examined the prevalence of TMD among children; however, it appears relatively uncommon before puberty, and symptoms are similar for girls and boys.
- TMD symptoms appear to decline in frequency after middle age.[25]

WHAT IS THE PROGNOSIS FOR TMD?

- Treatment effectiveness for TMD varies in the literature. One study reported that articular TMD appears to be self-limiting and nonprogressive in the absence of systemic disease. Because biochemical and biomechanical adaptive mechanisms appear to be important aspects of articular TMD, the initial intervention should be conservative, reversible, and directed toward promoting a joint condition optimal for repair.[16]
- The presence of chronic, unchanging, asymptomatic joint sounds suggests that articular disorders are not always progressive.
- TMD symptoms are typically fluctuating, self-limiting, and remitting over time.[28,32]
- Appropriate physical therapy intervention is crucial in the successful outcome of intervention. Box II-7-1 lists the short-term and long-term intervention goals for TMD.

WHAT FACTORS MAKE TMD DIAGNOSIS DIFFICULT?

TMD may be difficult to diagnose due to the various factors that can contribute to symptoms:

- Trauma
- Dental work
- Emotional stress
- Repetitive loading that causes microtrauma from parafunctional habits

---

BOX II-7-1 Physical Therapy Intervention Goals

Short-Term Goals	Long-Term Goals
Reduce pain	Restore normal lifestyle activities
Restore range of motion	Reduce contributing factors
Restore posture	Regular stretching, postural, and conditioning exercises
Reduce sustained muscle activity	Return to normal function

Adapted from Fricton J. Myogenous temporomandibular disorders: diagnostic and management considerations. *Dent Clin N Am.* 2007; 51:61–83.

- Forward posturing of the head, neck, and mandible
- Articular anomalies
- Occlusal anomalies
- Myofascial pain; referred pain from myofascial trigger points

To add to the complexity of diagnosing TMD, patients may also present with the following signs and symptoms:

- Headaches
- Neck and back pain
- Vision changes
- Hearing changes: hypoacousia and/or stuffiness; ear infection–type pain
- Tingling/numbness in the cheek area
- Upper extremity symptoms
- Motor weakness
- Tinnitus
- Vertigo
- Sharp, stabbing, burning pain
- Jaw locking
- Jaw clicking
- Tooth pain

Figure II-7-1 describes the complexity of TMD.

CLINICAL PEARL

The are five cardinal signs of a TMD disorder: (1) limited or restricted jaw opening or excursion movements; (2) pain with jaw movement; (3) TMJ sounds, such as clicking and crepitus; (4) TMJ tenderness with palpation; and (5) jaw muscle tenderness with palpation.

CLINICAL PEARL

The main qualities of musculoskeletal pain include the following: (1) dull ache; (2) localized, diffuse, or generalized (local myalgia vs. head and neck involvement vs. fibromyalgia); (3) worse with function, use, or loading; (4) may have background resting pain if the tissue is inflamed; (5) may involve muscles, joints, or both; (6) myofascial pain can cause referred pain to adjacent or distant structures; (7) widespread pain may be due to chronic pain changes in the central nervous system; and (8) can be associated with localized headaches in the region of muscle findings (trigger-point tenderness).

HOW SUCCESSFUL IS PHYSICAL THERAPY IN TREATING TMD?

- Physical therapy is an essential component of the successful management of TMD and is in a unique position to provide the most efficacious combination of education, instruction, procedures, and modalities for patients with TMD.
- Accurately diagnosing and treating TMD can be difficult because the patient's symptoms often do not fit into one classification. In many patients one disorder contributes to another; therefore, several classifications may be appropriate. Successful management

1 Local muscle soreness may result in increased intraarticular pressure:

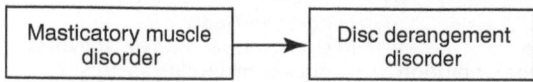

2 Early disc derangement may be accompanied with pain and muscle co-contraction, resulting in masticatory muscle disorder:

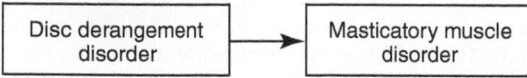

3 If disc derangement progresses, articular surfaces may be affected and result in inflammation:

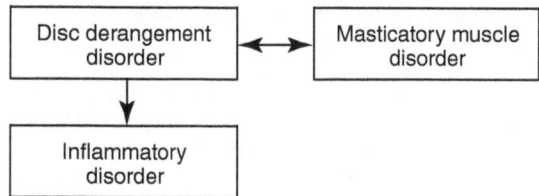

4 If the masticatory muscle disorder persists, limited mandibular movement can result and lead to hypomobility. In addition, inflammatory disorders can result in mandibular hypomobility:

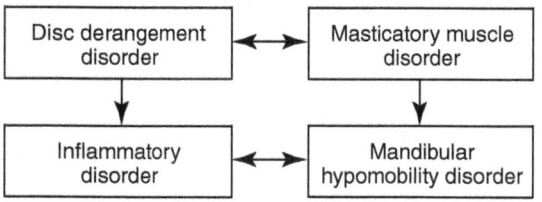

5 Trauma to any element of the masticatory system can cause or contribute to existing TMDs:

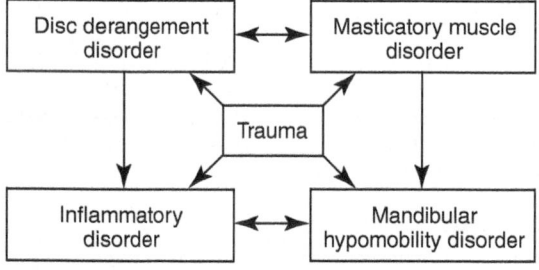

FIGURE II-7-1 The examples illustrate the complex relationships in temporomandibular dysfunction (TMD), why patients may have symptoms associated with more than one TMD, and how these interactions can make diagnosis and intervention decisions difficult. (From Okeson J: Causes of functional disturbances in the masticatory system. In: *Management of Temporomandibular Disorders and Occlusion*, ed. 5, St. Louis, MO: Mosby; 2003, p. 368.)

is dependent on accurately matching the intervention complexity with the patient complexity.

- Although no present evidence-based reviews have been conducted on physical therapy intervention specifically for TMD, a review article by Feine and Lund concluded that there was no good evidence that any intervention reviewed (heat, cold, ultrasound, low intensity laser, TENS, mobilization/manipulation, and exercise) significantly reduced the symptoms associated with TMD.[19] However, we believe that the clinical emphasis for TMD patients must be on education: awareness of correct posture, awareness and correction of parafunctional habits, awareness

> **BOX II-7-2** **Example of Physical Therapy Education and Instruction**
>
> **Initial Home Instruction for Temporomandibular Dysfunction**
> Eat a soft diet
> Check resting jaw position
> Chew on both sides at the same time, or on the least painful side, to minimize muscle strain
> Avoid parafunctional habits such as clenching, bruxing, gum chewing
> Avoid excessive or prolonged mouth opening
> Use over-the-counter analgesics or nonsteroidal antiinflammatory drugs as needed
> Practice relaxation breathing
> Posture correction

of the importance of exercise, and less emphasis on modalities. Credible research must be performed to test this hypothesis. Box II-7-2 gives examples of patient education and instruction.

- De Bont et al[16] reported that conservative management such as education, training to avoid joint loading, control of contributing parafunctional factors (e.g., clenching, bruxing), antiinflammatory medication, and at times jaw exercises can be very successful.
- Having noted that TMD intervention varies greatly, certain considerations are helpful in understanding the variability and controversy surrounding it: (1) there is a paucity of adequate, sound evidence that relates therapy to intervention effects, (2) there is a lack of substantial research regarding comprehensive physical therapy intervention, (3) there is lack of agreement on specific diagnostic categories, (4) some causative factors that contribute to TMD are difficult to control or eliminate (e.g., emotional stress), and (5) several factors contributing to TMD have yet to be identified and may not be influenced by present treatment interventions. However, a review of a group of long-term studies indicates that a logical approach to patient management would be to provide conservative (i.e., reversible) intervention first and consider nonconservative (i.e., irreversible) intervention only when conservative intervention fails.
- Nonsurgical intervention should include some combination of physical therapy, medication, occlusal appliance, and possibly counseling. Box II-7-3 lists criteria that suggest a complex case that will benefit from multidisciplinary intervention.
- Broussard[8] reports that in most studies in which multimodal physical medicine therapy [e.g., occlusal appliances, exercise, short-term use of nonsteroidal antiinflammatory drugs (NSAIDs), patient education] was provided, a positive response was reported in 75% of patients.

> **BOX II-7-3** **Criteria Suggesting Complex Presentation and Need for Team Intervention**
>
> Pain longer than 6 months in duration
> Significant lifestyle disturbances such as loss of work, social activities, home activities
> High use of past health care, including medications for temporomandibular dysfunction (TMD) symptoms
> Emotional difficulties related to TMD symptoms including depression, anxiety, anger
> Daily parafunctional habits such as clenching, bruxing
> Significant stressful life events such as pacing problems, divorce, or recent death in family

From Fricton J. Myogenous temporomandibular disorder: diagnostic and management considerations. *Dent Clin N Am.* 2007;51:61–83.

HOW SUCCESSFUL IS SURGERY IN TREATING TMD?

- Surgery of the TMJ offers a small, but important, option in the management of TMD. Approximately 5% of TMD patients require surgical intervention.[18]
- Surgery should be considered only after conservative efforts have failed and the patient's quality of life is significantly affected.[42]
- Patient selection is the most important consideration in determining surgical outcome. The more localized the pain and dysfunction to the TMJ, the better the surgical prognosis. The most important diagnostic finding is pain and dysfunction within the TMJ (internal derangement).
- When surgery is unsuccessful, it is usually a result of failure to recognize and manage parafunctional factors (clenching, bruxing, etc.).
- There are no randomized controlled studies on TMJ surgery; therefore, the decision to operate and the choice of procedure are based on clinical experience.
- There are three surgical procedures performed on the TMJ: athrocentesis, arthroscopy, and arthrotomy. Occasionally, orthognathic surgery is performed if repositioning of the jaw is necessary.
- Arthrocentesis is the simplest and least invasive procedure and consists of upper-joint TMJ lavage, delivery of medication into the joint (steroids or sodium hyaluronate to alleviate intracapsular inflammation), and manual manipulation of the joint under anesthesia. Multiple studies have reported success with arthrocentesis for the management of painful limited mouth opening.[17,18,36,37] Sembronio et al[39] evaluated the effectiveness of arthrocentesis in releasing acute and chronic TMJ closed lock, reducing pain, and recapturing the displaced disc. Better results in maximum mouth opening and pain reduction were found in the acute closed-lock group. Recapturing the displaced disc was also possible, but only in the acute closed-lock group (less than 6 months).
- The advantages of arthrocentesis are that it is simple, cost-effective, and can be performed with only local anesthesia and in the dental office, it has few complications, and it is minimally invasive.
- Arthroscopy consists of upper-joint examination, lavage, debridement, and sampling of joint tissues if needed. It does not correct the disc position but can improve disc mobility via the release of existing adhesions. Multiple studies report success with arthroscopic lysis and lavage for painful limited mouth opening. Murakami and colleagues reported in studies of 5- and 10-year follow-up that arthroscopy surgery was successful for all stages of internal derangement, and that results were comparable to those obtained with arthrotomy (open-joint surgery).[33,34] The results of disc repositioning via arthroscopy do not appear better than those obtained with simple lysis and lavage.[29,30]
- Arthrotomy (open-joint surgery), although performed much less often than arthrocentesis or arthroscopy, still has a small but important role in TMJ surgical management. Open-joint surgery is reserved for joint ankylosis, neoplasia, chronic dislocations, and severe osteoarthritis that has failed conservative intervention. Inspection for adhesions, articular eminence contour, and disc integrity, position, shape, and mobility is also available with open-joint surgery.[18]
- Orthognathic surgery involves the surgical repositioning of the maxilla and/or mandible to restore the proper anatomic and functional relationship in patients with dentofacial skeletal anomalies. Orthognathic surgery does not address coexisting TMJ pathology and symptoms, therefore, TMJ pathology must be treated before the correction of the associated jaw deformity.[50] Evidence for orthognathic surgery for patients with TMD varies. In a 20-year study following subjects from childhood to adulthood, Carlsson et al[12] concluded that orthognathic surgery with orthodontics is indicated for the correction of skeletal malocclusion or for aesthetics (retruded mandible, facial asymmetry).

HOW SUCCESSFUL IS COMPLEMENTARY AND ALTERNATIVE MEDICINE FOR TMD?

- Complementary and alternative medicine (CAM) is described by the National Institutes of Health (NIH) National Center of Complementary and Alternative Medicine (NCCAM) as a group of unconventional medical systems, practices, and products not presently considered part of the conventional biomedical care provided by physicians and other conventionally trained health professionals.
- CAM therapies consist of five categories: (1) mind–body interventions (i.e., biofeedback, relaxation, hypnosis, Yoga), (2) manipulative and body-based therapies (i.e., massage, chiropractic/osteopathic adjustments), (3) biologically based therapies (i.e., foods, vitamins), (4) energy therapies (i.e., use of electromagnetic fields), and (5) alternative medical systems (i.e., homeopathy, Chinese medicine).
- National data suggest that more than one third of the adult population in the United States uses CAM and that musculoskeletal pain is the leading reason for CAM use.
- The results of preliminary scientific studies on biofeedback, relaxation, and acupuncture indicate the superiority of these three interventions relative to placebo or control, and generally comparable results to other conservative interventions, for persistent facial pain.[35] Scientific studies have not been performed on the other CAM therapies.

PERSONAL INFORMATION

AGE

- Children and young adults demonstrate an increase in signs of TMD as they age; however, they rarely complain of symptoms.
- Adults over the age of 60 years rarely complain of symptoms; however, they demonstrate an increased prevalence of clinical and radiological signs.
- Most TMD symptoms are reported in women between 15 and 45 years of age.[25,42]
- A postmortem study of elderly cadavers found 91% of joints examined had morphological changes, including osteoarthritic changes.[8]

GENDER

- TMD is most prevalent among the female population ranging from 2:1 to 9:1.[10]
- The role of female reproductive hormones, the higher sensitivity of women to painful stimuli, higher scores of stress among women, and differences in care-seeking behavior, as well as in coping and emotions have been proposed as factors contributing to TMD.[5,9,15,26] However, these frequently suggested gender-linked behaviors do not fully explain female susceptibility to TMD nor are these behaviors fully accepted by the professionals who treat TMD.[16]
- TMD has been found to sometimes coexist with other symptoms such as sleep disorder, headache, fatigue, and depression.

CLINICAL DECISION MAKING CASE STUDY—PATIENT PROFILE

Your patient is a 35-year-old female who complains of unilateral facial pain and TMJ clicking with mouth opening. What are your hypotheses regarding her pathology?

Answer

Temporomandibular dysfunction is most common in females between the ages of 15 and 45 years. Sources of her symptoms most likely include myofascial pain and TMJ disc derangement with reduction (ADDR).

SYMPTOM HISTORY

MECHANISM OF INJURY

- The mechanism of injury is an important element in the differential diagnosis of TMD.
- Each area of the masticatory system can tolerate a certain amount of functional change. When functional changes exceed the system's tolerance for adaptation, tissue alteration results.
- Symptoms will develop in the structures least able to adapt. Potential sites are the muscles, joints, and teeth.
- The two most common masticatory problems (other than odontalgia) are masticatory muscle disorders and intracapsular joint disorders. It is very important to differentiate between these two problems because the treatment is different.
- TMD has been described by some as a result of trauma. Traumatic onset of symptoms are divided into two categories: (1) macrotrauma refers to a sudden force that results in structural alterations such as a blow to the face or local tissue trauma caused by dental injection, ligament strain supporting the joint, muscles, or both following prolonged mouth opening; (2) microtrauma refers to repeated, excessive forces that are applied to the masticatory structures over a long period of time such as chewing hard foods, clenching, chewing fingernails, chewing on the lips/inside of mouth, chewing on pencil tips, and chewing gum.
- Intracapsular joint disorders consist of osteoarthritides, anterior disc displacement with reduction (ADDwR), and anterior disc displacement without reduction (ADDw/oR).
- The most common disorders that physical therapists treat include masticatory muscle disorders, disc derangement disorders, osteoarthrosis, inflammatory disorders, and fractures.

CLINICAL DECISION MAKING
CASE STUDY—PATIENT PROFILE (?)

Your patient is a 50-year-old male who complains of dull, unilateral facial pain that began 1 week ago following a root canal. His jaw was sore following the procedure, and the next morning he experienced pain when he opened his mouth to brush his teeth. He subsequently has experienced pain with mouth opening, especially when he yawns, and with chewing. The mandibular opening is 35 mm and painful. What are your hypotheses regarding the source of his symptoms?

Answer

The onset history is always helpful in distinguishing between muscle and joint disorders. The first response to an event such as prolonged mouth opening is protective myospasm (trismus). The key to identifying myospasm is that it almost always immediately follows an event (in this case, prolonged mouth opening). Patients most often experience pain but only mild limitation in opening (10% to 20%). Local muscle soreness is due to inflammation and the release of certain substances, such as bradykinin, substance P, and histamine, produces pain. The patient's history and presentation implicate a masticatory muscle, or extracapsular, source of symptoms.

LOCATION OF SYMPTOMS

- Common sites of TMD pain include jaw pain; facial pain; temple, frontal, or occipital headaches; preauricular pain or earache; and neck pain. Symptoms may be a constant or intermittent dull ache that varies in intensity and ranges from acute to chronic.
- Acute TMD symptoms include some or all of the following: (1) limited jaw opening or excursion, (2) pain with jaw movement, (3) TMJ clicking or crepitation, (4) TMJ tenderness with palpation, and (5) jaw muscle tenderness with palpation.
- Global symptoms include tingling/numbness, tinnitus, vertigo, vision changes, hearing loss, and sharp, stabbing, burning pain. The duration may vary from hours to days.
- The cranial nerves should be screened for neurological disorders of the orofacial region. Cranial nerve dysfunctions present through alterations in smell, movement, vision, hearing, equilibrium, or taste. Table II-7-1 summarizes the cranial nerves and tests.

TABLE II-7-1 Cranial Nerves and Tests*

Cranial Nerve Number	Nerve	Test
I	Olfactory	Sense of smell
II	Optic	Visual acuity, visual fields, ophthalmoscopy
III	Oculomotor	Pupillary symmetry, pupillary light, near reflexes, and lateral and vertical gaze
IV	Trochlear	Looking down and in
V	Trigeminal	Observation of facial expressions; voluntary strength of facial muscles of expression; taste to anterior two-thirds of tongue; pain in ear
VI	Abducens	Sensation of light touch to face in all three divisions; motor innervation of muscles of mastication; corneal reflex (V1 to CN VII)
VII	Facial	Observation of palpebral fissures; position and alignment of eyes on straight-ahead gaze; looking laterally
VIII	Acoustic vestibular	Hearing; Weber and Rinne tests; observation for nystagmus on extraocular muscle testing; caloric testing
IX	Glossopharyngeal	Listen to patient's voice; observation of palate rise when patient says "ah"
X	Vagus	Gag reflex
XI	Accessory	Examination of sternocleidomastoid and trapezius muscles for bulk and strength
XII	Hypoglossal	Tongue bulk and movement

Adapted and reprinted from Ikeson J. *Orofacial Pain: Guidelines for Assessment, Diagnosis and Management.* Chicago: Quintessence Publishing Co. Inc.; 1996.
*Cranial nerves should be screened for neurological involvement of the orofacial region. Physical therapists can rule out gross neurological involvement and make an appropriate referral if needed.

CLINICAL PEARL !

Oral parafunctional habits that produce muscle tension such as clenching, jaw thrusting, gum chewing, and jaw tensing, can add repetitive strain to the masticatory muscles and cause soreness and pain. Postural strain caused by a forward head posture and poor positioning of the head and tongue has been implicated in myofascial pain. Psychological stressors such as relationship conflicts, monetary problems, and poor pacing skills can also play a role. Depression and anxiety are additional behavioral factors that may accompany TMD.

Qualities of musculoskeletal pain include dull ache that is localized, diffuse, or generalized; aggravated with function, use, or loading; which may be constant if inflamed and can be myofascial, arthrogenous, or both.

REFERRAL OF SYMPTOMS

Muscle pain disorders, commonly referred to as *myalgia*, are the most common complaints of patients with masticatory muscle pain.

REFERRAL PATTERN OF MUSCLES[41]

Masseter	Ear, jaw, and around the orbit of the ipsilateral eye
Temporalis	Ipsilateral temporal and zygomatic arch
Lateral pterygoid	Ipsilateral ear and zygomatic arch
Medial pterygoid	Ipsilateral ear and posterior aspect of the jaw
Digastric	Inferior aspect of the jaw
Sternocleidomastoid	Ipsilateral sternum, ear, top of the head, occipital region, and around the orbit of the eye
Trapezius	Lateral neck, posterior aspect of the jaw, and temporal and retroorbital regions

Since pain originates in the muscle, the restriction in mandibular movement is a result of extracapsular muscle pain. There are several types of masticatory muscle pain.

- Muscle splinting (protective cocontraction) is the initial response to altered sensory input or injury. It is common in TMD and consists of increased masticatory muscle activity during jaw opening and closing in an effort to protect the area from further aggravation.[37]
- Myofascial pain is the most common muscle pain disorder and is commonly found in TMD patients.[21] It consists of dull, achy regional pain associated with tender areas called *trigger points*. Myofascial trigger points are taut bands within skeletal muscles that produce a characteristic pattern of referred pain (temporalis muscles refer to teeth; masseter refers into the ear) and/or autonomic symptoms (vasoconstriction, coldness, sweating,

ptosis, and/or hypersecretion) caused by activity of a trigger point in a region separate from the trigger point. It has been suggested that myofascial trigger points begin with muscular strain that progresses to nerve sensitization, an increase in local metabolism, and a decrease in local circulation, resulting in pain and decreased range of motion.[45]
- Earache is reported by approximately 30% of TMD patients. Ear symptoms (e.g., intermittent, sudden, sharp pain, stuffiness, or fullness)[14] are most commonly referred from myofascial trigger points. Most patients will have had ear involvement, such as otitis media, ruled out before referral for physical therapy.

CLINICAL PEARL !

Myofascial trigger points can refer pain in a reproducible and predictable pattern. Trigger-point referred pain is common in TMD and can mimic other TMD symptoms. Knowledge of trigger-point referral patterns is helpful in assessing common patient complaints (e.g., ear pain referred from the deep masseter, toothache referred from the temporalis muscle).

- Myospasm (trismus) is characterized by pain when the affected muscle is stretched. It can result from trauma, biting into hard foods, coexisting disc displacement, parafunctional habits, and dental work.
- Myositis is characterized by constant, significant pain, swelling, and increased temperature, generally following a direct trauma to the muscle or infection. Box II-7-4 describes the categories of muscle disorders.
- Disc displacement of the TMJ is the result of an abnormal relationship between the articular disc and mandibular condyle. Most often the disc displaces anteriorly and medially and generally occurs over a period of time. Two common categories of disc displacement are ADDwR and ADDw/oR.
- ADDwR presents as a clicking or popping joint. The joint sound is a result of the condyle "reducing" onto the disc, most often when translation begins. A closing click may or may not occur. As disc displacement progresses, clicking may progress to momentary locking, in which the patient is unable to fully open (translate) the joint for a short period of time. Patients often discover that they can unlock the joint by relaxing or "wiggling" their mandible to the opposite side. Box II-7-5 describes the categories of articular disc derangements.

CLINICAL PEARL !

ADDwR is thought to result from disc-articular surface adherence; synovial fluid degradation; articular surface irregularity; disc/condyle incoordination resulting from abnormal muscle function; increased muscle activity, and/or disc deformation.

BOX II-7-4   Categories of Muscle Disorders

Muscle Splinting	Myofascial Pain	Myospasm (Trismus)	Myositis
Local, dull pain	Regional, dull, aching pain	Pain at rest	Pain at rest
Minimal/no pain at rest	Trigger points present; pain local and/or referred	Muscle tender to palpation	Diffuse tenderness over muscle
Pain with jaw movement	Pain with jaw movement	Increased pain with jaw movement	Increased pain with jaw movement
Range of motion within normal limits but painful	Mild decrease in ROM (10% to 20%)	Significant ROM limitation (> 50%)	Significant ROM limitation due to pain and edema (>50%)

BOX II-7-5 Categories of Articular Disc Derangements

Disc Displacement with Reduction (ADDwR)	Disc Displacement without Reduction (ADDw/oR)
Click occurs at variable positions during opening and closing but most often at transition from rotation to translation	In acute phase: marked limited opening (25 to 30 mm)
Once click occurs, opening is pain free and complete (40 mm); laterotrusion and protrusion pain-free and unrestricted	History of temporomandibular joint clicking that suddenly stopped resulting in ADDw/oR
	Movement pattern: deflection to ipsilateral side with opening; limited laterotrusion to contralateral side/unrestricted movement to ipsilateral side; deflection to ipsilateral side with protrusion

CLINICAL PEARL

Joint sounds are common and are not necessarily associated with pain or limited range of motion (ROM). Wabeke and Spruijt[46] reported that at least one-third of the population has nonpainful joint sounds. Soft clicking may be thought of as a physiological accommodation without clinical significance.

- ADDRw/oR, or closed lock, is a result of a permanent displacement of the disc. The disc is displaced anteriorly/medially, the condyle cannot translate, and therefore the mouth cannot fully open. The patient will most often report a history of clicking, followed by catching and unlocking, followed by an inability to unlock and open wide (translate). Initially, opening is very painful and is felt locally near the TMJ and often in the ear. Myospasm (trismus) is also common and will further restrict movement.
- When an ADDw/oR becomes chronic, pain diminishes and jaw opening may increase to functional opening (~35 mm).

CLINICAL PEARL

ADDw/oR will present with the following pattern: jaw opening is limited to rotation (25 to 30 mm), the mandible will deflect to the ipsilateral side with opening, laterotrusion will be unrestricted to the ipsilateral side and restricted to the contralateral side, and protrusion will be restricted and deflect to the ipsilateral side.

CLINICAL DECISION MAKING CASE STUDY—PATIENT PROFILE

Your patient is a 17-year-old female complaining of right TMJ pain and limited opening. She reports a history of right joint clicking and intermittent locking, most often in the morning, that she was able to overcome with relaxing her jaw or moving her jaw to the left. One week ago she awoke and could not unlock her jaw. She is able to open her jaw 27 mm with deflection right and painful, 6 mm laterotrusion right pain free and 3 mm laterotrusion left and painful, and protrusion 4 mm with deflection right and painful. Chewing is more comfortable on the ipsilateral side. What is your hypothesis regarding her pathology?

Answer
This patient is demonstrating an ADDw/oR. A history of intermittent locking followed by closed lock, movement pattern, and chewing-side preference supports the presence of an ADDw/oR.

HYPERMOBILITY (SUBLUXATION)

- Hypermobility, or subluxation, describes the position of the condyle anterior to the articular eminence at full opening.
- Subluxation is a result of the disc maximally rotating on the condyle before full translation. At the end range of opening, the condyle suddenly moves forward, causing a "jump" sensation.[37]

CLINICAL PEARL

Patients with hypermobility should be given instruction to avoid end-range opening to prevent irritation of the ligaments and local soft tissue.

TMJ DISLOCATION (OPEN LOCK)

TMJ dislocation, or open lock, refers to a spontaneous dislocation of the condyle and disc anterior to the articular eminence. Most commonly, TMJ dislocation occurs in individuals with hypermobility when the mouth is opened too wide. Spontaneous reduction is possible but can be aggravated by lateral pterygoid myospasm.

CLINICAL PEARL

Patients presenting with a TMJ open lock should be given the same instruction as patients presenting with hypermobility: avoid end-range movement.

RETRODISCAL IRRITATION

- Retrodiscal tissue is a highly innervated, vascular complex that fills with blood as the condyle translates anteriorly (e.g., full mouth opening).
- Retrodiscal irritation, or retrodiscitis, is usually the result of trauma.
- Retrodiscal irritation may result from two types of trauma: extrinsic and intrinsic. Extrinsic trauma is described as a sudden movement of the condyles into the retrodiscal tissues such as with a blow to the chin. Intrinsic trauma results from an anterior displaced disc.
- As the disc becomes anteriorly displaced the condyle comes in contact with the retrodiscal tissues, causing abnormal forces to be placed on these densely innervated and vascularized tissues.
- Retrodiscitis may produce constant periauricular pain and is aggravated with jaw movement and clenching.

HEADACHES

- Headache is one of the most prevalent health problems: the lifetime prevalence of headache is 93% for men and 99% for women.[38]
- In addition, many patients with headache do not seek medical care, and, for those who do, many are misdiagnosed or mismanaged.
- The three large headache groups are cervicogenic (15% to 35% of all chronic and recurrent headaches), tension-type headaches, and common migraine.
- Diagnosis is often difficult as patients often experience several headache types concurrently.
- It is important for physical therapists to be aware of the variety of headaches, the various presentations, and the most efficacious interventions for each.
- Table II-7-2 describes headache signs and symptoms.
- Table II-7-3 describes headache location and common headache etiology.

TABLE II-7-2 Headache Signs and Symptoms

Pain Element/Pattern	Type
Pulsing, pounding	Migraines
Sharp jabs and jolts	Hemicrania continua, cluster, trigeminal neuralgia
Builds up	Tension type
Instantaneous	Neuralgia, "thunderclap" headaches due to aneurysm, subarachnoid hemorrhage
Dull ache	Muscular
Ice pick, multifocal	Migraine, jabs, and joints
Refractory period	Neuralgia
Acute continuous, increasing in intensity and unrelenting	Subarachnoid hemorrhage or tumor
Trigger zones (touch lips, teeth)	Trigeminal neuralgia
Swollen, tender temporal arteries	Temporal arteritis (GSA), pain with chewing that stops when resting jaw
Swallowing or taste anomalies	Glossopharyngeal neuralgia
Throbbing pain in upper posterior teeth of nondental origin	Facial migraine

From Adachi N, Wilmarth MA, Merrill R. *Current Concepts of Orthopaedic Physical Therapy.* 2nd ed. American Physical Therapy Association, 2006. Independent Study Course 16.2.12.

TABLE II-7-3 Location of Headaches and Usual Causes*

Location	Common Causes
Forehead	Sinusitis, eye or nose disorder, muscle spasm of occipital or suboccipital region
Side of head	Migraine, eye or ear disorder, auriculotemporal neuralgia
Occipital	Myofascial problems, herniated disc, eye strain, hypertension, occipital neuralgia
Parietal	Hysteria (viselike), meningitis, constipation, tumor
Face	Maxillary sinusitis, trigeminal neuralgia, dental problems, tumor

Data from Magee D. Cervical spine. In: Magee D, ed. *Orthopedic Physical Assessment.* Philadelphia, PA: W.B. Saunders, 1992, p. 36.
*Knowledge of the common causes of headache is helpful in the differential diagnosis of TMD.

FIBROMYALGIA

- Differential diagnosis of myofascial pain includes fibromyalgia, which presents with widespread regional myalgia, fatigue, stiffness, and sleep disorders.
- Fibromyalgia has a 9:1 female–male ratio, with peak onset of symptoms between ages 45 and 60 years.
- Further diagnosis of fibromyalgia is based on pain in three out of four body quadrants and tenderness of more that 11 of 18 predefined sites.[49]
- Fibromyalgia is not a masticatory pain disorder per se but may coexist with other clinical conditions including TMD.
- Optimal intervention is provided by a combination of education, pharmacological therapy, exercise (i.e., strengthening, endurance, pool), and cognitive-behavioral therapy.[4]

BENIGN PAROXYSMAL POSITIONAL VERTIGO

- Benign paroxysmal positional vertigo (BPPV) is the most common form of vertigo.
- Classic symptoms are brief episodes of vertigo associated with changes in head position relative to gravity.
- Precipitating symptoms include getting up or lying down, rolling, bending over, or looking up.
- Differential diagnosis (BPPV, neuritis, Menière disease, labyrinthitis) consists of the patient's history and testing using the Hall-Pike Dix maneuver.
- Dizziness can be a result of a number of conditions such as an acoustic neuroma, orthostatic hypotension, vestibular disorders, and cervicogenic dizziness.
- Migraine, disequilibrium secondary to aging, anxiety/panic disorders, and central nervous system disorders may cause other forms of dizziness.[1]

BELL'S PALSY[44]

- Idiopathic facial palsy, also called Bell's Palsy, is an acute disorder of the facial nerve (CN VII) that results in full or partial paralysis of movement of one side of the face.
- Increasing evidence suggests that the main cause is reactivation of latent herpes simplex virus type 1 in the cranial nerve ganglia. How the virus damages the facial nerve is uncertain.
- The annual incidence of Bell's Palsy varies between 11.5 and 40.2 cases per 100,000 population. There are peaks of incidence in ages 30 to 50 and 60 to 70 years.
- Prognosis depends on the time which recovery begins. Eighty-eight percent obtain full recovery if recovery begins within the first week; within 1 to 2 weeks, recovery is 83%; and within 2 to 3 weeks, recovery is 61%. Ninety-four per cent of patients with incomplete paralysis and 61% of patients with complete paralysis made a complete recovery.

TRIGEMINAL NEURALGIA

- Trigeminal neuralgia is a neuropathic orofacial condition originating from one or more sensory branches of the trigeminal nerve (CN V).
- Symptoms of trigeminal neuralgia are sudden, severe, episodic, burning, stabbing pain (described as electric shocks).
- The pain is aggravated by nonpainful stimuli such as lightly touching the face, shaving, washing, and/or brushing the teeth.
- The duration of the pain is usually seconds.
- The onset is most commonly found in females over 40 years of age and most commonly in divisions V2 and V3.
- Eighty to ninety percent of trigeminal neuralgia cases have been associated with vascular compression of the trigeminal sensory root by the superior cerebellar artery.[43]

TEMPORAL ARTERITIS

- Temporal arteritis, giant cell arteritis (GCA), is a result of temporal artery inflammation.
- The primary symptom is temporal area headache, but pain with chewing and palpation tenderness of the temporal area are also common.
- Symptoms generally begin insidiously and are found most often after 50 years of age.
- Because sudden blindness is an irreversible complication of GCA, immediate medical attention is imperative.

CLINICAL PEARL

All patients who present with facial pain, nonodontalgic (tooth) pain, nonauricular (ear) pain, headache, or postwhiplash injury should be screened for TMD.

TABLE II-7-4 Dermatome, Myotome, and Reflex Testing for the Upper Cervical Spine and Head

Nerve Root	Dermatome	Myotome	Reflex
C1	Top of head	Contributes to cervical flexion	None
C2	Temporal, occipital regions of head	Cervical flexion (longus colli, sternocleidomastoid, rectus capitis)	None
C3	Posterior cheek, neck	Lateral neck flexion (trapezius, splenius capitis)	None

From Cyriax J. *Text of Orthopaedic Medicine*. London: Bailliere Tindall; 1978: 34-35.

WHAT OTHER MUSCULOSKELETAL STRUCTURES CAN REFER TO THE TMJ AREA?

Musculoskeletal structures in the upper cervical spine and head can refer symptoms to the TMJ area. Table II-7-4 describes the dermatome and myotome distribution from the upper cervical spine. There are no reflex tests for the upper cervical spine nerve roots.

CLINICAL PEARL

Headaches are very common among patients with TMD. Although physical therapy intervention is important, headache treatment often responds optimally with a combination of medical and physical therapy interventions.

WHAT VISCERAL STRUCTURES CAN REFER TO THE TMJ AREA?[48]

- The heart (myocardial infarction/coronary insufficiency, dissecting aneurysm) will refer pain into the lower jaw and face.
- Anterior cervical lymph nodes (cervical lymphadenitis) can also refer pain.
- The parotid gland will refer pain into the preauricular area/angle of the jaw.
- The temporal artery will refer pain into the temporal and periarticular area.

SYMPTOM DESCRIPTORS

Table II-7-5 describes the quality of symptoms related to the type of pain and structure related to the pain type.

CONSTANCY OF SYMPTOMS

- Intermittent pain suggests a mechanical source and is aggravated by movement, prolonged poor posture, abnormal joint loading, and/or muscle fatigue.

TABLE II-7-5 Pain Descriptions and Related Structures*

Type of Pain	Structure
Cramping, dull, aching	Muscle
Sharp, shooting	Nerve root
Sharp, bright, lightning like	Nerve
Burning, pressure stinging, aching	Sympathetic nerve
Deep, nagging, dull	Bone
Sharp, severe, intolerable	Fracture
Throbbing, diffuse	Vasculature

*Determining the type of pain assists in identifying the tissue type responsible for symptoms.

TABLE II-7-6 Joint and Muscle Pain Descriptors*

	Joint Pain	Muscle Pain
Quality	Dull or sharp Constant if acute Intermittent if subacute or chronic	Dull ache Constant if acute Intermittent if subacute or chronic
Location	TMJ or inside ear (localized to TMJ area)	Masticatory muscles (more generalized compared to joint pain) Pain can be referred from myofascial trigger points
Incidence	Chewing on contralateral side Lying on ipsilateral side if acute Restricted translatory ROM	Chewing on ipsilateral side During or subsequent to stress Lying on ipsilateral side if acute Moderate to significant loss of ROM

TMJ, temporomandibular joint; ROM, range of motion.
*It is important to observe the differences between joint and muscle pain. Intervention will differ depending on the structure involved.

- Constant, varying symptoms suggests inflammation.
- Constant, nonvarying symptoms suggest visceral or systemic involvement or other pathology such as cancer.
- Table II-7-6 describes the variations in the quality, location, and incidence between joint and muscle pain.

TWENTY-FOUR-HOUR SYMPTOMS PATTERN

IF A PATIENT HAS SYMPTOMS IN THE MORNING, WHAT PATHOLOGY DOES THIS IMPLICATE?

- TMJ/jaw stiffness and/or soreness in the morning are generally indicative of osteoarthrosis or bruxism and resolve within a short time.
- Pain and stiffness that do not resolve within a short time indicate an inflammatory source of the symptoms.
- Abnormal sleep habits such as sleeping prone with the head turned toward the painful side or the hand placed under the face may cause symptoms on waking.

WHAT ROLE DOES MORNING STIFFNESS PLAY IN DIFFERENTIATION?

- Osteoarthrosis often causes morning stiffness, but the stiffness will subside with movement.
- Bruxism (teeth grinding) can fatigue the muscles of mastication resulting in muscle stiffness and pain on waking (myofascial pain). Pain may subside shortly after waking, but bruxism can contribute to lingering symptoms.
- Internal derangement of the TMJ can also present with stiffness and pain on waking. Stiffness and flexibility will improve within a couple of hours, but full ROM will be limited with a displaced disc without reduction.

CLINICAL DECISION MAKING
CASE STUDY—PATIENT PROFILE

Your patient is a 50-year-old female who is complaining of soreness and stiffness in the left TMJ on waking and soreness with yawning and after eating. The mandibular opening is 35 mm, and guarded and mild pain are reported. Your examination reveals grating sounds in the left TMJ. What is your hypothesis regarding her pathology?

Answer

Considerations that support osteoarthrosis include the patient's age, stiffness on waking, soreness with wide opening and after eating (chewing), mild restriction in opening, and grating sounds in the joint. Grating sounds (crepitis) are characteristic of osteoarthrosis.

IF THE PATIENT HAS SYMPTOMS AS THE DAY PROGRESSES, WHAT PATHOLOGY DOES THIS SUGGEST?

- Myofascial symptoms are most often minimal or nonexistent on waking but increase as the day progresses.
- Myofascial upper back and cervical symptoms are often present with facial myofascial symptoms.
- Symptoms that increase as the day progresses suggest repeated parafunctional habits that overload the tissue's ability to adapt. Examples include poor posture, clenching (isometric contraction of the jaw closing muscles), chewing hard foods, chewing gum, opening wide, biting on fingernails and/or pencil tips, resting the chin on the hands, and cradling the phone between the mandible and shoulder.
- Poor response to stressful tasks or events also contributes to increased symptoms as the day progresses.
- Symptoms secondary to specific articular involvement generally are present during a specific activity that loads the joint, such as eating, clenching, or wide opening.

CLINICAL DECISION MAKING CASE STUDY—PATIENT PROFILE   (?)

Your patient is a 27-year-old female office manager who complains of jaw muscle tightness and temporal headaches. The mandibular opening is limited to 24 mm due to tightness and pain. Palpation of masticatory, cervical, and upper back muscles reveals multiple trigger points and referral of pain into the temporal area. What is your hypothesis regarding her symptoms?

Answer

Upper trapezius active trigger points (myofascial trigger-point referred pain) can refer pain to the temporal area as well as irritate local tissue. Limited opening is a result of muscle splinting and/or trigger-point activity.

IF THE PATIENT HAS SYMPTOMS WHILE SLEEPING, WHAT PATHOLOGY DOES THIS SUGGEST?

- Nocturnal bruxism, if severe, can wake a patient from sleep.
- Inflammation in the TMJ and/or surrounding soft tissue may prevent the patient from sleeping on the ipsilateral side.
- An improperly placed pillow may aggravate neck symptoms as well as exert pressure on the TMJ and surrounding soft tissue.
- Nocturnal pain may also suggest visceral pathology, which must be ruled out.

CLINICAL PEARL   (!)

Bruxism (teeth grinding) exerts extraordinary pressure on the teeth and muscles of mastication. In addition to muscle fatigue and pain, excessive bruxism can result in periodontal irritation, wearing down of teeth, and cracking of teeth (resulting in the need for a root canal, crown, or both). Wearing a night guard will decrease the pressure exerted on the teeth. The night guard should be of hard acrylic, fit without rocking on the teeth, and be carefully adjusted to provide bilateral posterior support when the mouth is closed. With excursive movements (protrusion and laterotrusion), only the anterior teeth should touch.

STABILITY OF SYMPTOMS

CHANGES IN SYMPTOMS

- Both muscular and articular symptoms should respond to intervention that unloads the joint and soft tissue and allows for relaxation and healing.
- Muscular symptoms are often related to parafunctional habits and stress.
- Articular symptoms generally are related to functions such as yawning and chewing (specific joint loading).
- Inflammatory conditions can involve the joint and/or soft tissue, and constant symptoms will subside as the inflammation resolves.

IF A PATIENT'S SYMPTOMS ARE IMPROVING, WHAT PATHOLOGY IS IMPLICATED?

- Improvement of TMD symptoms is typical, although the length of time and speed of improvement will differ, depending on the cause of TMD.
- Myofascial symptoms will respond rather quickly with patient education and intervention designed to restore soft-tissue stability and eliminate or control abnormal parafunctional habits.
- Inflammatory conditions will improve over a longer period of time, allowing the inflammation to resolve.
- Psychosocial symptoms, such as depression, have been shown to respond favorably if intervention is provided early.

IF THE PATIENT'S SYMPTOMS ARE WORSENING, WHAT PATHOLOGY IS IMPLICATED?

- If TMD symptoms do not improve or continue to worsen, continued irritation from a variety of sources must be suspected.
- Inflammation, from an acute injury or myositis, can cause pain to linger, but it should respond steadily to medication and intervention designed to decrease activity of the muscles and/or joints.
- If myofascial symptoms persist or worsen, continued mechanical or emotional contributions must be reviewed. Parafunctional habits must be reviewed, and counseling for psychological issues may be required.
- Symptoms that continue to worsen and do not fit into the above categories may require further evaluation to ensure that the correct diagnosis was made.
- Communication with the patient's dentist or physician is recommended if an explanation for worsening symptoms is unclear.

FUNCTIONAL OR ACTIVITY-PARTICIPATION LIMITATIONS

BEHAVIOR OF SYMPTOMS: AGGRAVATING FACTORS

- Common aggravating factors involve jaw motion such as with chewing hard foods, chewing gum, opening wide, and yawning.
- Poor posture
- Parafunctional habits such as biting fingernails, chewing on pencil tips, biting lips, clenching, and bruxing
- Emotional stress, anxiety, depression, poor coping skills

BEHAVIOR OF SYMPTOMS: EASING FACTORS

- Rest position of jaw, submaximize opening, soft diet, cutting up all food into bite-sized pieces
- Correction of sitting and standing posture
- Relaxation/awareness of stress level; hobbies, exercise
- Use of phone headset

- Proper position of a pillow during sleep
- Soft-tissue mobilization, stretching
- Properly organized work station
- Use of night splint for bruxism
- Moist heat/cold pack
- Medication

MEDICAL HISTORY

WHAT ROLE DOES A PATIENT'S MEDICAL HISTORY PLAY IN THE DIFFERENTIAL DIAGNOSIS OF TMD?

- The medical history of a TMD patient is often lengthy due to the potential complexity of the symptoms and limited knowledge of the evaluation and treatment options for symptoms for TMD in the medical and dental communities. Many patients have been evaluated by multiple physicians and dentists before being referred for physical therapy.
- It is important to create a timeline of professionals consulted and the intervention received as part of the physical therapy evaluation. The timeline should include a chronological history of symptoms, professionals seen, diagnostic tests received, diagnoses made, effectiveness of interventions received (medical, dental, physical therapy, psychological), and effectiveness of medication prescribed.

MEDICAL AND ORTHOPEDIC TESTING

WHAT MEDICAL AND ORTHOPEDIC TESTS INFLUENCE YOUR DIFFERENTIAL DIAGNOSIS PROCESS WITH TMD?

- The information from imaging studies must be correlated with the clinical findings.
- Radiographs can be used to confirm observations of osseous articular involvement.
- Magnetic resonance imaging (MRI) can be used to confirm intracapsular soft-tissue and effusion conditions.
- A dentist may include, as part of the diagnostic examination, testing of the teeth to rule out tooth involvement and diagnostic anesthetic blocks, laboratory work to rule out a hypothyroid condition (can cause muscle pain and/or fatigue), rheumatological problems or temporal arteritis.
- Psychological tests are also available if deemed necessary to accurately assess the psychological contribution to symptoms.

HOW DO RADIOGRAPHIC OR OTHER EXAMINATIONS INFLUENCE YOUR DECISION-MAKING PROCESSES?

- Radiographs can provide information on teeth, tumors, bone loss, and TMJ arthritis.
- Panorex radiographs are commonly found in dental offices and are helpful in identifying jaw fractures, mandibular asymmetries, general tooth problems, position of the teeth, and advanced arthritic changes in the TMJ. However, a clear and unobstructed view of the TMJ is not possible with a panoramic radiograph.
- Tomography (a tomogram) provides the best lateral and anteroposterior views of the TMJ to identify arthritic changes.[37,47]
- Computed tomography images both hard and soft tissues; therefore, the disc–condyle relationship can be observed. Disadvantages to computed tomography include cost and patient exposure to high doses of radiation.
- Bone scanning is helpful to determine whether an inflammatory process is active (i.e., osteoarthritis) or dormant (i.e., osteoarthrosis). However, bone scanning cannot discriminate between bone remodeling and degeneration, so the information must be combined with clinical findings to have meaning.

HOW RELIABLE IS MRI OF THE TMJ?

- MRI has become the gold standard for evaluating the soft tissue and TMJ disc position.
- It does not expose the patient to radiation and thus far has not shown harmful side effects.
- It is important to note that the presence of a displaced disc does not suggest aggressive intervention. Studies have shown that between 26% and 38% of normal, asymptomatic subjects demonstrated disc position abnormalities on MRI.[37]

HOW RELIABLE IS AN ELECTROMYOGRAM (EMG) IN THE DIAGNOSIS OF TMD?

Currently, EMG recordings are not a reliable source for TMD diagnosis.

MEDICATION

HOW DOES MEDICATION INFLUENCE YOUR DECISION-MAKING PROCESSES?

- Medication selection is based on whether the patient has acute pain or chronic pain.
- Analgesics are given for acute TMD pain.
- NSAIDs and muscle relaxants are given for both acute and chronic TMD pain.
- Tricyclic antidepressants are given for chronic TMD pain.
- Injection and stretch consists of an injection of a local anesthetic (1% procaine without a vasoconstrictor) into a myofascial trigger point to eliminate pain. Immediately following the injection, the muscle is passively stretched. Injection and stretch is also diagnostic in that the injection and stretch should eliminate both the local pain and trigger-point referred pain.[45]
- Hyalyronan injections are a promising therapy for reducing friction and promoting joint-healing adaptation. Several studies have found hyaluronan injections helpful with painful clicking, catching joints, and with some cases of painful osteoarthrosis.[2,6,22]
- Injections can be given up to four times, every 3 weeks, in a 1-year period and have been shown to provide symptomatic relief for several months.[19]

BIOMECHANICAL FACTORS

WHAT ROLE DOES BIOMECHANICS PLAY IN TMD?

- The TMJ is a synovial joint that is divided into two joint spaces. The joint spaces are separated by the articular disc, which is attached to the mandibular condyle via ligaments medially and laterally, to the superior head of the lateral pterygoid anteriorly, and to the flexible connective tissue posteriorly.
- The disc–condyle complex allows a combination of hinge movement and gliding in the lower joint space.
- The TMJ remodels as a result of increased loading on the articular surfaces. The intraarticular disc does not undergo active remodeling but passively remodels in response to abnormal compressive forces. If the abnormal forces exceed the joint protective mechanisms, articular tissue begins to break down, resulting in the formation of adhesions, disc displacement, and/or arthrosis. These changes may result in inflammation and pain; however, if the TMJ is able to adapt to these changes, the nonarticular tissues may not become inflamed and painful. Disc displacement most often occurs in an anteromedial direction resulting in an abnormal relationship between the disc and mandibular condyle.

- Disc displacement consists of three stages: (1) early displacement demonstrated by painless clicking (ADDwR), (2) intermittent locking (ADDwR), and (3) an inability to fully open (closed lock or ADDw/oR).
- The most common etiological factor associated with disc-condyle disorders is trauma, either macrotrauma or microtrauma. Macrotrauma is most often a result of a single, sudden, episode of trauma such as a blow to the jaw. Microtrauma is a result of mild, frequent forces over a long period such as chronic muscle hyperactivity from bruxism.

CLINICAL PEARL

Why is an opening TMJ click more evident than a closing TMJ click? Kuboki et al[24] reported that mandibular opening forces were compressive in nature and increase as the jaw opened from 10 to 40 mm. The joint reaction force at a 20-mm opening increased nine times with only a 20% activation of the closing muscles.

WHAT BIOMECHANICAL ABNORMALITIES IN OTHER REGIONS AFFECT TMD?

- The presence of neck pain associated with TMD is a common finding, both in the clinic and in the literature.[15,23,40]
- Clinically, patients with TMD report neck symptoms more frequently than patients who do not have TMD; patients who have neck pain report more signs and symptoms of TMD than do healthy controls.
- The literature is clear that cervical spine tissues refer pain to the head and orofacial areas.[23,40] One study reported a 70% frequency of neck pain associated with TMD. Another study of postural problems in 164 patients with TMD reported poor sitting/standing posture in 96%, forward head in 84.7%, rounded shoulders in 82.3%, and lower tongue position in 67.7%.[20]
- The neuroanatomic explanation of this association is the convergence of the trigeminal afferents and afferents of C1, C2, and C3 in the upper cervical spinal cord within the pars caudalis portion of the spinal nucleus of the trigeminal nerve (trigeminocervical nucleus). Primary sources of head and orofacial pain that are referred from the cervical spine are located in the structures innervated by the C1 to C3 spinal nerves. Box II-7-6 lists the tissues that receive sensory innervation from the upper cervical nerves that may refer symptoms to the head and orofacial areas.[23]
- The greater occipital nerve is a branch from the C2 nerve root. Occipital neuralgia may result from trauma or suboccipital muscle tightness and may refer symptoms to the occipital area, top of the head, TMJ area, and in or around the ear.

CLINICAL PEARL

Neck and shoulder pain is more prevalent in patients who have TMD with a muscle component than in patients who have TMD with an articular component.

CLINICAL PEARL

Although some dentists postulate a relationship between malocclusion and TMD, scientific evidence does not validate this connection.

ENVIRONMENTAL FACTORS

DO PSYCHOSOCIAL ISSUES INFLUENCE THE CLINICAL DECISION-MAKING PROCESS?

- Patients with myofascial pain and arthralgia differ psychologically from those with disc displacement. In a study by

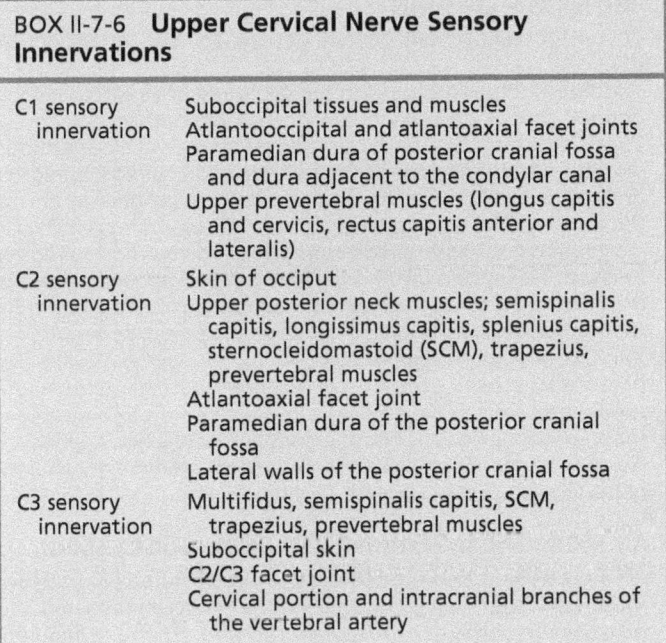

BOX II-7-6 **Upper Cervical Nerve Sensory Innervations**

C1 sensory innervation	Suboccipital tissues and muscles Atlantooccipital and atlantoaxial facet joints Paramedian dura of posterior cranial fossa and dura adjacent to the condylar canal Upper prevertebral muscles (longus capitis and cervicis, rectus capitis anterior and lateralis)
C2 sensory innervation	Skin of occiput Upper posterior neck muscles; semispinalis capitis, longissimus capitis, splenius capitis, sternocleidomastoid (SCM), trapezius, prevertebral muscles Atlantoaxial facet joint Paramedian dura of the posterior cranial fossa Lateral walls of the posterior cranial fossa
C3 sensory innervation	Multifidus, semispinalis capitis, SCM, trapezius, prevertebral muscles Suboccipital skin C2/C3 facet joint Cervical portion and intracranial branches of the vertebral artery

From Kraus S. Temporomandibular disorders, head and orofacial pain: cervical spine considerations. *Dent Clin N Am.* 2007;51:76.

Galon et al,[21] psychological variables (behavioral, emotional, and cognitive) between muscular and articular TMD subjects were compared. The muscular group demonstrated a higher proportion of parafunctional habits (biting lips, hangnails, fingernails), a higher level of anxiety and somatization of symptoms, and less humor, which may lessen the ability to minimize their condition.
- Callahan[10] suggests TMD patients possess a "negative stress coping mechanism which may make a TMD patient more vulnerable to anxiety, anger, and sadness."

CAN EMOTIONS INFLUENCE TMD?

- Pain is strongly affected by emotions. An injury may be essentially painless in the presence of anger, fear, or elation. Conversely, when pain is anticipated or in situations associated with dysphoria, pain is often reported without additional noxious stimulation.
- Psychological factors affect the firing of dorsal horn pain-transmission neurons.[13]
- The hypothalamus–pituitary–adrenal (HPA) axis is known to assist in the coordination of the physiological response to physical and emotional stressors.[31]
- Chronic pain may be considered a form of chronic stress. An increased incidence of depression, anxiety, and stress-related disorders is reported by chronic pain patients.

PERSONAL FACTORS

PAST SURGERIES
DO PAST SURGERIES INFLUENCE YOUR CLINICAL REASONING IN TMD?
- Past TMJ surgeries may change the biomechanics of the TMJ and contribute to TMD.
- Surgery may alter the relationship between the joint, soft tissue, and teeth, which may also contribute to TMD.

FAMILY HISTORY
DOES A FAMILY HISTORY OF TMD INFLUENCE YOUR CLINICAL REASONING PROCESS?
A genetic predisposition for TMD has not been demonstrated.

Section II

ORTHOPEDIC REASONING

CHRONICITY OF PAIN

WHAT CENTRAL-PROCESSING CHANGES ARE PRESENT IN TMD?

- The International Association for the Study of Pain has defined chronic pain as pain lasting longer than 6 months.[3]
- The pain pathway may be divided into two systems. One system, the discriminative system travels through the midbrain and terminates in the thalamus. This system allows the brain to properly locate the site and source of pain. The other system, the motivational/effective system, travels through the thalamus to the hypothalamus and limbic forebrain. This system involves the emotional component of painful experiences. As time progresses, the motivational/effective system gains in strength and begins to dominate the pain experience.[3]
- The most common symptoms of acute pain are headaches, jaw pain, earache, neck pain, muscle soreness, muscle tightness, and tooth pain.
- Common symptoms of chronic pain are headaches, depression, chronic fatigue, sleep disorders, decreased productivity, feelings of inadequacy, low self-esteem, withdrawal, and mood disorders.[3]

HAS MEDICAL INTERVENTION BEEN SUCCESSFUL FOR PATIENTS WITH CHRONIC TMD?

- Although chronic pain continues to be poorly understood and managed, research has broadened the understanding and contributed valuable insight into the management of chronic pain associated with TMD.
- An organized medical approach to the management of chronic pain has been divided into six steps: (1) rule out the presence of diagnosable medical disease, (2) search for psychiatric disorders, (3) build a supportive relationship with the patient, (4) make restoration of function the treatment goal, (5) provide realistic reassurance, and (6) prescribe cognitive behavior therapy for patients who did not respond to steps 1 to 5.[3]
- The intervention goal for chronic TMD becomes the identification and alleviation of factors that amplify and perpetuate symptoms and cause functional impairment. The focus of management should be on coping, rather than curing, and on improving function rather than relieving symptoms.

CLINICAL DECISION MAKING
CASE STUDY—PATIENT PROFILE **?**

Your patient is a 45-year-old female with complaints of chronic daily headaches, neck soreness, and bilateral pain in the temple area, ears, and TMJs. She admits to frequent jaw clenching while at work, and her symptoms worsen as the day progresses. Her symptoms began several months ago during a stressful time at work. What is your clinical assessment?

Answer
The patient's presentation—global symptoms, clenching habit, progressive symptoms throughout the day, and stressful work environment—supports a complex case involving multiple factors, largely stress related. In addition to the physical therapy evaluation, a referral for a psychological evaluation is appropriate.

WHAT AREA OF RESEARCH FOR TMD IS MEDICINE TURNING TOWARD?

The concept of central sensitization (nociceptors activity induced, neuronal changes) has important clinical implications in the development of new approaches to the management of chronic pain.

CLINICAL PEARL **!**

The National Institutes of Health recently suggested that depression is based on central sensitization. Most cases of depression follow stressful events, primarily psychosocial

in nature, that initiate various biological processes. With continued exposure to stress, a progressive sensitization of the central nervous system occurs. Neuronal hyperexcitability then becomes self-sustained so that depression becomes chronic, even without discernible stress.

WHY IS MEDICAL RESEARCH FOCUSING ON OTHER CAUSES OF TMD?

- TMD is rarely the result of a single causative event but, rather, most often involves multiple, complex factors.
- If symptoms are chronic, conventional medical intervention is often ineffective, resulting in frustrated professionals and patients, as well as the unnecessary expenditure of time, money, and energy.

WHAT PERIPHERAL CHANGES CAN OCCUR THAT RESULT IN CHRONIC TMD?

Studies indicate that traumatized C-fiber nociceptors can develop α_1 receptors that react to sympathetic fiber release of norepinephrine, activating nociceptors. It is expected that this reaction will resolve within a reasonable time due to the decreasing activity of the nociceptors and consequent decrease in afferent activity. If these changes are addressed early, they are reversible. If these changes become chronic, modifications in neuroprocessing can develop into permanent central changes that result in chronic neuropathic pain.[37]

WHAT CENTRAL CHANGES CAN OCCUR THAT RESULT IN CHRONIC TMD?

- If acute TMD symptoms are allowed to persist, the symptoms may become chronic and may decrease the patient's threshold for pain.
- The symptoms may include secondary central excitatory effects such as referred pain, localized autonomic symptoms, and skeletal effects.
- Pain from joints and muscles can cause central sensitization, resulting in symptoms in the absence of a local cause.
- Spinal cord reflexes can activate muscles to tighten, thereby producing pain as a protection to guard against further muscle trauma.

HOW DO AUTONOMIC, ENDOCRINE, AND IMMUNE SYSTEMS INFLUENCE DECISION MAKING IN TMD?

- Prevalence patterns of TMD among women (rise in prevalence after puberty, lower prevalence in postmenopausal women) are consistent with a possible etiological role for female reproductive hormones in TMD.
- Several peripheral and central mechanisms through which estrogen could operate to increase pain have been proposed: increased joint laxity, enhanced inflammatory responses in joints, and action on prostaglandin release or serotonin receptors. Gender differences in pain modulation systems, some of which may be estrogen based, have also been suggested.[25]
- In a study on sleep deprivation, Born and Fehm[7] suggested that hippocampal dysregulation of sleep alters the production of hormonal activity that is prominent during early sleep and does not allow for replenishing of the immune system, making it difficult to manage stress the following day.
- Insufficient glucocorticoid (antiinflammatory hormone) signaling by genetic predisposition factors, stress, and endocrine and neurotransmitter systems prevents stress-response systems, including the immune system, from exercising inhibitory control, which leads to unrestrained stress hyperreactivity and a weakened immune system.[3]

CLINICAL PEARL **!**

Estrogen receptors are present in the TMJ capsule.

BOX II-7-7   **Symptoms and Conditions that Require Outside Consultation***

Dentist	Medical Doctor (Internist/Family Practice, Otolaryngologist, Rheumatologist, Neurologist)	Maxillofacial Surgeon	Mental Health Specialist
Constant, nonvarying pain that does not respond to physical therapy intervention	Constant, nonvarying pain that does not respond to physical therapy intervention	Trauma	Depression
Bite changes	Severe headache	Suspected tumor	Anxiety
Significant movement restriction	Facial muscle weakness	Jaw relationship anomalies	Stress
Suspected tooth decay	Increased pain at night		
	Suspected cardiac disease		

*It is important for physical therapists to develop relationships with a variety of medical professionals. Patients with temporomandibular dysfunction will often benefit from multidisciplinary intervention.

HOW IS THE IMMUNE SYSTEM INVOLVED IN TMD?

- All stressors, including infection, physical trauma, and psychological events, are associated with immune activation and release of proinflammatory cytokines.
- Glucocorticoids are the most potent antiinflammatory hormones in the body and serve to suppress the activity of proinflammatory cytokines during exposure to stress and return the body to homeostasis. With repeated and/or prolonged exposure to stress, the return to homeostasis is disrupted, which affects the immune system.

RED FLAGS THAT REQUIRE REFERRAL TO A DENTIST OR PHYSICIAN

WHAT SYMPTOMS AND/OR CONDITIONS PROMPT YOU TO REFER A PATIENT TO A DENTIST OR PHYSICIAN?

- Symptoms that continue to worsen or do not respond to intervention techniques require a review of the physical therapy evaluation findings and intervention techniques to ensure that the assessment and intervention choices were correct. Communication with the patient's dentist or physician is recommended if an explanation for unchanging or worsening symptoms is unclear.
- Additional reasons for requesting a consultation include medication trial, trigger-point injections, further diagnostic testing, and unsuccessful response to physical therapy intervention.
- Box II-7-7 lists symptoms and conditions that may require a referral from physical therapy.

CLINICAL DECISION MAKING
CASE STUDY—PATIENT PROFILE   (?)

Your patient is a 65-year-old male complaining of constant left TMJ pain for 2 weeks. The pain appears worse at night and he complains of constant fatigue. Ipsilateral and contralateral chewing exacerbates left TMJ pain. What are your hypotheses regarding his pathology?

Answer
Although it appears that there may be a myofascial component to the symptoms, pain that worsens at night and constant fatigue are symptoms that should be evaluated by the patient's physician.

SUMMARY STATEMENT

Temporomandibular dysfunction is a common pain problem, occurring in approximately 10% of the population over 18 years of age. It is primarily a condition of young and middle-aged adults rather than of children or of the elderly, and is significantly more common in women than in men. Psychosocial risk factors include stress, depression, and somatic distress. In the past 30 years a better understanding of pain mechanisms and muscle physiology has contributed significantly to the understanding of TMD. More uniform terminology, improved classifications of orofacial pain syndromes, more accurate categorization of TMD, and improved evaluation techniques have resulted in more accurate identification of TMD. The development and expansion of multidisciplinary teamwork (dentists, physical therapists, physicians, maxillofacial surgeons, and psychologists) have been invaluable in the delivery of improved intervention techniques for patients with TMD.

Intervention for TMD has been largely based on clinical results and not on substantial evidence-based research. It is clear that TMD is a multifaceted disorder; therefore it is important for dental and medical professionals, including physical therapists, to continue TMD research. The contribution of hormones in central pain processing, contributing emotional components, etiological factors associated with TMJ signs and symptoms, and the efficacy of physical therapy intervention techniques will all be better understood with continued and persistent research.

REFERENCES

1. Adachi N, Wilmarth MA, Merrill R. *The temporomandibular joint: physical therapy patient management utilizing current evidence.* APTA; 2006.
2. Alpaslan G, Alpaslan C. Efficacy of temporomandibular joint arthrocentesis with and without injection of sodium hyaluronate in treatment of internal derangements. *J Oral Maxillofac Surg.* 2001;59(6):613-618.
3. Auvenshine R. Temporomandibular disorders: associated features. *Dent Clin N Am.* 2007;51:105-127.
4. Balasubramaniam R, Laudenbach J, Stoopler E. Fibromyalgia: an update for oral health care providers. *Oral Surg Oral Med Oral Rad Endo.* 2007;104(5):589-597.
5. Bassols A, Bosch F, Campillo M, et al. An epidemiological comparison of pain complaints in the general population of Catalonia (Spain). *Pain.* 1999;83(1):9-16.
6. Bertolami C, Gay T, Clark G, et al. Use of sodium hyaluronate in treating temporomandibular joint disorders: a randomized, double-blind, placebo-controlled clinical trial. *J Oral Maxillofac Surg.* 1993;51(3):232-242.
7. Born J, Fehm H. Hypothalamus-pituitary-adrenal activity during human sleep: a coordinating role for the limbic hippocampal system. *Exp Clin Endocrinol Diabetes.* 1998;106(3):153-163.
8. Broussard J. Derangement, osteoarthritis, and rheumatoid arthritis of the temporomandibular joint: implications, diagnosis, and management. *Dent Clin N Am.* 2005;49:327-342.
9. Bush F, Harkins S, Harrington W, Price D. Analysis of gender effects on pain perception and symptom presentation in temporomandibular pain. *Pain.* 1993;53:73-80.
10. Callahan C. Stress, coping, and personality hardiness in patients with temporomandibular disorders. *Rehab Psych.* 2000;45(1):38-48.
11. Carlsson C. Epidemiology and treatment need for temporomandibular disorders. *J Orofac Pain.* 1999;13:232-237.
12. Carlsson G, Egermark I, Magnusson T. Predictors of signs and symptoms of temporomandibular disorders: a 20-year follow-up study from childhood to adulthood. *Acta Odontol Scand.* 2002;60:180-185.

13. Ciancaglini R, Testa M, Radaelli G. Association of neck pain with symptoms of temporomandibular dysfunction in the general adult population. *J Rehab Med.* 1999;31(1):17-22.
14. Cuffari L, deSiqueira J, Nemur K. Pain complaint as the first symptom of oral cancer: a descriptive study. *Oral Surg Oral Med Oral Pathol Oral Radiol Endod.* 2006;102:56-61.
15. Dao T, Knight K, Ton-That V. Modulation of myofascial pain by the reproductive hormones: a preliminary report. *J Pros Dent.* 1998;79(6):663-670.
16. De Bont L, Dijkgraaf L, Stegenga B. Epidemiology and natural progression of articular temporomandibular disorders. *Oral Surg Oral Med Oral Pathol Oral Radiol Endod.* 1997;83(1):72.
17. Dimitoulis G, Dolwick M, Martinez A. Temporomandibular joint arthrocentesis and lavage for the treatment of closed lock; a follow-up study. *Br J Oral Maxillofac Surg.* 1995;33:23-27.
18. Dolwick M. Temporomandibular joint surgery for internal derangement. *Dent Clin N Am.* 2007;51:195-208.
19. Feine J, Lund J. An assessment of the efficacy of physical therapy and physical modalities for the control of chronic musculoskeletal pain. *Pain.* 1997;5-23.
20. Fricton J. Myogenous temporomandibular disorders: diagnostic and management considerations. *Dent Clin N Am.* 2007;51:61-83.
21. Galon M, Dura E, Andrew Y, Ferrando M, et al. Multidimensional approach to the differences between muscular and articular temporomandibular patients: coping, distress, and pain characteristics. *Oral Surg Oral Med Oral Pathol Oral Radiol Endod.* 2006;102:40-46.
22. Hepguler S, Akkoc Y, Pehlivan M, et al. The efficacy of intra-articular sodium hyaluronate in patients with reducing displaced disc of the temporomandibular joint. *J Oral Rehabil.* 2002;29(1):80-86.
23. Kraus S. Temporomandibular disorders, head and orofacial pain: cervical spine considerations. *Dent Clin N Am.* 2007;51:161-193.
24. Kuboki T, Takenami Y, Maekawa K, et al. Biomechanical calculation of human TM joint loading with jaw opening. *J Oral Rehabil.* 2000;27:940-951.
25. LeResche L. Epidemiology of temporomandibular disorders: implications for the investigation of etiologic factors. *Crit Rev Oral Biol Med.* 1997;8(3):291-305.
26. LeResche L, Saunders K, Vonkorff M. Use of exogenous hormones and risk of temporomandibular disorder pain. *Pain.* 1997;69:153-160.
27. Levitt S, McKinney M. Validating the TMJ scale in a national sample of 10,000 patients: demographic and epidemiologic characteristics. *J Orofac Pain.* 1994;8:25-35.
28. Magnusson T, Egermark I, Carlsson G. A longitudinal epidemiologic study of signs and symptoms of temporomandibular disorders from 15 to 35 years of age. *J Orofac Pain.* 2000;14(4):310-319.
29. McCain J, DeLaRua H. Principles and practice of operative arthroscopy of the human temporomandibular joint. *Oral Maxillofac Clin North Am.* 1989;135-152.
30. McCain J, Podrasky A, Zabiegalski N. Arthroscopic disc repositioning and suturing: a preliminary report. *J Oral Maxillofac Surg.* 1992;50:568-573.
31. Merrill R. Central mechanism of orofacial pain. *Dent Clin N Am.* 2007;51:45-59.
32. Murakami K, Kaneshita S, Kanoh C, Yamamura I. Ten-year outcome of nonsurgical treatment for the internal derangement of the temporomandibular joint with closed lock. *Oral Surg Oral Med Oral Pathol.* 2002;94(5):572-575.
33. Murakami K, Segami N, Okamoto M, et al. Outcome of arthroscopic surgery for internal derangement of the temporomandibular joint: long-term results covering 10 years. *J Cranio-maxillofac Surg.* 2000;5:264-271.
34. Murakami K, Tsuboi Y, Bessho, et al. Outcome of arthroscopic surgery to the temporomandibular joint correlates with stage of internal derangement: five-year follow-up study. *Br J Oral Maxillofac Surg.* 1998;36:30-34.
35. Myers C. Complementary and alternative medicine for persistent facial pain. *Dent Clin N Am.* 2007;51:263-274. New York: McGraw-Hill; 1993:76-85.
36. Nitzan D, Dolwick M, Martinez G. Temporomandibular joint arthrocentesis. A simplified treatment for severe limited mouth opening. *J Oral Maxillofac Surg.* 1991;49:1163-1167.
37. Okeson J. Causes of functional disturbances in the masticatory system. In: *Management of Temporomandibular Disorders and Occlusion.* 5th ed. St. Louis, MO: Mosby; 2003.
38. Rasmussen B, Jensen R, Olesen J. A population-based analysis of the diagnostic criteria of the international headache society. *Cephalgia.* 1991;11:129.
39. Sembronio S, Albiero A, Toro C, et al. Is there a role for arthrocentesis in recapturing the displaced disc in patients with closed lock of the temporomandibular joint? *Oral Surg Oral Med Oral Pathol Oral Radiol Endod.* 2008;105:(3):274-279.
40. Sessle B, Hu J, Amino M, et al. Convergence of cutaneous, tooth pulp, visceral, neck, and muscle afferents onto nociceptive and nonnociceptive neurons in trigeminal subnucleus caudalis and its implication for referred pain. *Pain.* 1986;27:219-235.
41. Simons DG, Travell JG, Simons LS. *Travell and Simons' Myofascial Pain and Dysfunction: The Trigger Point Manual.* 2nd ed. Baltimore, Md: Williams & Wilkins; 1999.
42. Solberg W. Temporomandibular disorders. *Br Dent J.* 1986;3:1-14.
43. Spencer C, Gremillion H. Neuropathic orofacial pain: proposed mechanism, diagnosis, and treatment considerations. *Dent Clin N Am.* 2007;51:209-224.
44. Teixeira L, Soares B, Vieira V, Prado G. The Cochrane database of systematic reviews: physical therapy for Bell's Palsy. 2008;(3):1-47.
45. Travell J, Simons D. Apropos of all muscles. In: *Myofascial Pain and Dysfunction: The Trigger Point Manual.* Baltimore, MD: Williams & Wilkins; 1983:74-78.
46. Wabeke D, Spruijt R. *Temporomandibular joint sounds: dental and psychological studies [thesis].* Amsterdam: University of Amsterdam; 1994.
47. White W, Heslop E, Hollender L, Mosier K. Parameters of radiologic care: an official report of the American Academy of Oral and Maxillofacial Radiology. *Oral Surg Oral Med Oral Pathol.* 2001;91(5):498-510.
48. Wiener S. Acute lower and midfacial pain. In: *Differential Diagnosis of Acute Pain.*
49. Wolfe F, Smythe H, Yunus N, et al. The American College of Rheumatology 1990 criteria for the classification of fibromyalgia; report of the multicenter criteria committee. *Arthritis Rheum.* 1990;33:160-172.
50. Wolford L. Clinical indications for simultaneous TMJ and orthognathic surgery. *Cranio.* 2007;10:273-287.

AUTHORS: DERRICK SUEKI and SARAH MCPHEE RILEY

INTRODUCTORY INFORMATION   ⓘ

The shoulder is a difficult region to treat. Patients' symptoms often will not correlate to normal tissue patterns and patients' progress is often slow. One reason for this is the fact that the shoulder is different than all other major joints in the body. Unlike other major joints, the shoulder joint relies on the coordinated action of muscles and other active elements to stabilize the joint. The passive structures such as osseous congruence and ligament tension provide far less stabilizing action in the shoulder than in other joints in the body. In the knee and hip, osseous and ligamentous structures work to stabilize the joint. These structures coupled with weight placed axially into the joint result in joint stability. In the shoulder, there is no weight bearing through the joint with many normal daily activities. Any motion of the shoulder in an open chain manner results in a tractional force through the joint that must be offset by the shoulder muscles for joint stability to be achieved. This fact coupled with the small size of the glenoid fossa in comparison to the humeral head results in a joint teetering on the verge of instability.[72]

WHAT IS THE PREVALENCE OF THE PATHOLOGY? [3,70,71]

Shoulder pain is the third most common musculoskeletal complaint in the United States, accounting for between 5% and 16% of all general practitioner musculoskeletal consults. A study on the demographics of shoulder pain presenting to primary care found rotator cuff tendinopathy in 85%, subacromial impingement in 74%, acromioclavicular joint disease in 24%, adhesive capsulitis in 15%, and referred pain in 7% of patients.

WHAT IS THE PROGNOSIS FOR RECOVERY FROM THIS PATHOLOGY? [4,35,69,70,71]

Unfortunately, only about 50% of patients reporting shoulder pain to primary care fully recover within 6 months. After 12 months, only about 60% of these patients report complete recovery. Unfavorable prognosis is associated with a longer duration of symptoms at initial examination, high pain intensity, recurrent symptoms, concomitant neck pain, and gradual onset of shoulder pain. Trauma, overuse before the onset of symptoms, and acute onset are associated with a better outcome.

WHAT IS THE RECURRENCE RATE? [7,8,69]

Research shows about 41% of patients experience recurrent or persistent shoulder pain after 1 year. In particular, shoulder instability has a high rate of recurrence. Recurrence of shoulder dislocation is indirectly correlated with age. Patients who experience an initial dislocation before the age of 20 years have nearly a 90% chance of recurrent dislocations. Patients experiencing an initial dislocation after the age of 20 years have a significantly decreased risk of recurrence.

WHAT FACTORS MAKE DIAGNOSIS DIFFICULT IN THE PATHOLOGY?

- Many structures in the shoulder, such as muscle and bone, will refer pain into a similar pattern.
- Many structures, such as the brachial plexus and arterial venous system, run through the shoulder and can complicate the clinical picture.
- Many structures, such as the neck and viscera, can refer pain into the shoulder region.

- Shoulder function is heavily reliant on stability gained at the thoracic spine and scapulothoracic regions. Dysfunction at these regions will often result in shoulder compensations.
- Shoulder structures are not as well vascularized as other regions; therefore, symptoms often take longer to resolve.

CLINICAL PEARL   ⓘ

Panjabi has proposed the following model for stability in the spine, but in reality it can apply to any joint in the body. Alterations in any one of these three elements will have a chain reaction effect and alter the other two.

Panjabi suggests that three components are required for a joint to be stable:
1. *Passive restraints—joint congruence and ligament stability*
2. *Active restraint—rotator cuff musculature*
3. *Neuromuscular control—control and coordinated action of the rotator cuff and scapulothoracic muscles*

Therefore, if passive restraints (i.e., joint stability) are altered, the active and neuromuscular systems will have to compensate to maintain shoulder function.

HOW SUCCESSFUL IS THERAPY IN TREATING THE PATHOLOGY? [9,13,17,63]

Successful interventions for shoulder pain include activity modification, such as reducing overhead activity, joint mobilization, electrophysical modalities, and stretching and strengthening exercises. Currently, research does not support the use of ultrasound for most disorders in the shoulder region; however, Edenbichler et al[9] found that ultrasound was effective in treating calcific tendinitis of the shoulder.

HOW SUCCESSFUL IS SURGERY IN TREATING THE PATHOLOGY? [2,6,11,12,28,40]

In general, surgical intervention in the shoulder region has a favorable outcome; however, surgery should be considered only after conservative management has failed.
- Rotator cuff repair produces good results, particularly in the reduction of pain. The recurrence of rotator cuff tear has been reported to range from 13% to as high as 68%. The best indicator of tear recurrence is the size of the initial tear. Larger rotator cuff tears have a much higher rate of recurrence after repair.
- Surgical intervention for anterior instability produces a good outcome and a very low recurrence rate. Bankart repair is the treatment of choice for anterior instability and has a high rate of patient satisfaction. Studies report the recurrence rate to be 1% to 10% with open Bankart repair and 15% to 20% with arthroscopic Bankart repair.
- Both total shoulder arthroplasty and hemiarthroplasty have a high rate of patient satisfaction; however, total shoulder arthroplasty demonstrates a better functional outcome. Further degeneration of the glenoid after hemiarthroplasty may result in continued pain and decreased range of motion.
- Controversy surrounds the use of manipulation under anesthesia and anterior inferior release for adhesive capsulitis. Because adhesive capsulitis is a self-limiting disorder many medical professionals do not believe surgery is necessary. Studies show that although these procedures do not decrease recovery time they do decrease pain and increase functional range of motion.
- Most surgical interventions of the acromioclavicular joint involve stabilization of the distal clavicle. Early surgical intervention (within 3 weeks of injury) yields the best results after acromioclaviclar joint separation.

- Surgical intervention for sternoclavicular joint instability is not recommended unless closed treatment has failed and instability persists. This type of surgery is associated with a poor surgical outcome and high risk due to nearby visceral structures.

PERSONAL INFORMATION[58,67,70]

AGE

HOW DOES AGE INFLUENCE YOUR DECISION-MAKING PROCESS?
Age will influence the decision-making process in several ways.

Younger adult patients (18–30 years old) usually present with symptoms secondary to acute trauma. Patients can usually indicate a specific activity that caused their symptoms and this makes the diagnostic process a little easier. Rotator cuff injuries, subacromial impingement, labral tears, bicepital tendon pathology, ligament injuries, and fractures should all be considered as potential primary hypotheses.

As a person progresses into their 30s and 40s activity levels begin to decrease and therefore the injuries associated with sports and acute trauma begin to diminish. Work-related overuse injuries increase. Therefore, overuse shoulder injuries increase with this age group. Tendinosis, subacromial bursitis, and referral from nerve irritation should be considered as primary hypotheses.

As patients continue the aging process, acute injuries begin to occur more frequently. Unlike the acute trauma that occurs in younger patients, the acute trauma that occurs in the elderly is related more to falls. In the case of a fall, rotator cuff injury and fractures should be primary considerations. Degenerative overuse also occurs most frequently in the elderly age group. This is due in part to diminished vascularity to the area that occurs with aging and in part to repetitive wear and tear on the structures of the shoulder. Osteoarthritis, rotator cuff pathology, and nerve pathology should all be considered primary hypotheses.

OCCUPATION

DOES A PATIENT'S OCCUPATION INFLUENCE YOUR DECISION-MAKING PROCESS?
Occupations or sports that require repetitive movement result in more shoulder injuries. Adults engaged in baseball, swimming, cricket, volleyball, and tennis have a higher likelihood of shoulder pathology than normal sedentary adults. Athletes engaged in overhead activities are prone to repetitive use injuries. In baseball internal impingements occur during the late cocking phase of pitching. Anterior impingement will occur during the follow through and deceleration phase of pitching. In swimming, it is the catch phase of freestyle swimming that results in shoulder pathology. Work-related activities can also be very taxing to a patient's shoulder and can result in overuse shoulder injuries. String players in an orchestra, house painters, construction workers, flight attendants, or individuals engaged in any occupation that requires repetitive lifting upward or overhead are at risk for shoulder injuries. As with any repetitive use injury in the shoulder, initial hypotheses regarding source tissue should include shoulder bursitis and impingement. As the pathology progresses, bicepital and rotator cuff tears should also be added to the tissues that may be the source of the patient's symptoms.

GENDER

WHAT INFLUENCE DOES GENDER HAVE ON YOUR CLINICAL DECISION-MAKING PROCESS?
Overall, shoulder complaints tend to be more common in females. The incidence of shoulder complaints in females is 11.1/1000 per year compared with 8.4/1000 per year in males. In addition, males are more likely to experience shoulder pain resulting from trauma. It is reasonable to assume that many of these injuries go unreported if the injured individual does not seek medical attention.

Therefore, the actual ratio of male to female may be different as these statistics reflect individuals who seek medical attention.

ETHNICITY

WHAT INFLUENCE DOES ETHNICITY HAVE ON YOUR CLINICAL DECISION-MAKING PROCESS?
Most pathologies in the shoulder region do not have an ethnicity prevalence; however, there are a higher number of fall-related proximal humerus fractures in Caucasian and Asian women over 50 years of age. Evidence shows a higher percentage of osteoporosis and osteopenia in Caucasian and Asian women compared to African American and Hispanic women.[23]

SYMPTOM HISTORY

MECHANISM OF INJURY

HOW DOES THE MECHANISM OF INJURY INFLUENCE YOUR DECISION-MAKING PROCESS?
The mechanism of injury reveals a lot about the structures that may be involved in the injury. So, careful questioning about the shoulder position and direction of force at the time of injury will help greatly in the differentiation process (Box II-8-1).

Acute trauma such as falls should be distinguished from trauma occurring secondary to overuse. Acute trauma to the shoulder could be the result of falls or direct blows to the shoulder. Therefore, rotator cuff injuries, dislocations, and fractures should be primary considerations. Falls directly on the lateral aspect of the shoulder will result in acromioclavicular (AC) joint separations and clavicle fractures. Falls onto an outstretched arm can potentially result in any number of pathologies including rotator cuff injury, subacromial impingement, bicep tendon tears, labral tears, subacromial bursitis, and labral tears. The direction of the forces, speed of the force, health of the tissue, and stability of the joint will all help determine which specific tissue fails in response to the fall.

CLINICAL DECISION MAKING
CASE STUDY—PATIENT PROFILE

John is a 27-year-old male who presents to you with complaints of right shoulder pain. Symptoms began 6 month ago following an injury while playing football. He reports that while going up to catch a football with his arm extended overhead his arm was hit by another player. As a result, his shoulder dislocated. His friend, who had dislocated his own shoulder in the past, knew how to put his shoulder into place. After a couple minutes of trying, he was able to relocate his shoulder. His shoulder has improved since that initial injury, but he continues to experience pain with overhead activities and is still not able to play any sports involving overhead motion. What potential structures should the clinician be concerned about when evaluating this patient?

Answer

Shoulder dislocation typically occurs with the arm in 90° of flexion, 90° of abduction, and 90° of external rotation. The most typical direction of dislocation is anterior. Posterior dislocations do occur, but the mechanism of injury is generally with a posterior-directed force through the arm when it is flexed to 90° and slightly internally rotated. Because the shoulder was relocated on the field and no radiographs were obtained, there is a chance that there was a fracture of the glenoid or humeral head. Generally, dislocations should have a completed x-ray before relocation to rule out fractures and to reduce the chance of nerve damage. Injuries common with anterior shoulder dislocations include Bankart lesions, Hill-Sachs lesions, labral tears, biceps tendinopathy, rotator cuff tendinopathy, and axillary nerve injury. The fact that the shoulder was reduced quickly lends itself to a better prognosis for recovery and

---

BOX II-8-1   Mechanisms of Injury for Select Shoulder Pathologies

Pathology	Mechanism of Injury
Acromioclavicular joint separation	The two most common causes of an acromioclavicular joint separation are either a direct blow to the shoulder (often seen in football or falling off a bicycle) or a fall onto an outstretched hand (commonly seen after a fall).
Adhesive capsulitis	Minor trauma or surgery will often be the trigger event, but just as often insidious onset will be reported.
Bankart lesions	The pathology is damage to the attachment of the labrum to the anterior glenoid margin. This often occurs in conjunction with an anterior shoulder dislocation.
Biceps tendon pathology	Injury to the biceps tendon can involve tendinosis from repetitive overhead use or repetitive activities such as rowing or bench pressing, which cause the humeral head to translate anteriorly and superiorly therefore impinging the biceps tendon. Biceps tendon ruptures will result from a forced eccentric contraction of the biceps. Often this is with the shoulder partially flexed. Examples of mechanisms would be trying to catch a falling object or lifting a heavy weight.
Clavicular fracture	Clavicular fractures can occur when a patient falls on an outstretched hand or fall and hit the outside of their shoulder. Clavicular fractures can also occur from a direct hit to the clavicle as in football or from a seatbelt during a motor vehicle accident. In newborns, clavicle fractures occur at birth during passage through the birth canal.
Hill-Sachs lesion	A Hill-Sachs lesion is a compression fracture of the superior and posterior head of the humerus. The fracture most commonly occurs in conjunction with an anterior shoulder dislocation. The humeral head travels out of the glenoid fossa and on its return it contacts the posterior rim of the glenoid and impacts with such force that a fracture occurs.
Humeral fracture	Humeral fractures can be caused by direct trauma to the arm such as a fall onto the outside of the shoulder or by axial loading transmitted through the elbow or hand such as a fall onto an outstretched hand. Attachments from pectoralis major, deltoid, and rotator cuff muscles influence the amount of displacement of proximal humerus fractures.
Impingement syndromes	Impingement is a catch basin term. It refers to some structure being pinched. The inciting event can be traumatic, such as a fall, or insidious, such as overuse. The term itself does not specify a specific structure.
Labral tears	Labral tears can occur as a result of acute or chronic traction and/or compression (carrying or catching a heavy object), lifting of or stabilizing overhead objects , a fall onto an outstretched arm, or anterior dislocations.
Pectoral muscle strain	Pectoralis major muscle tears are relatively rare injuries that primarily occur while lifting weights, particularly when doing a bench press. Complete ruptures are most commonly avulsions at or near the humeral insertion. Ruptures at the musculotendinous junction and intramuscular tears usually are caused by a direct blow.
Rotator cuff tears	Rotator cuff tears can be the result of a direct trauma such as a fall, but generally they are the result of a slow degenerative process. Overuse of impingement results in initial tissue injury. Continued use results in further tissue injury. Scar tissue forms and weakens the muscle. Eventually, with continued use, the muscle tears when forces exceed its diminished capacities.
Rotator cuff tendinitis/ tendinosis	Rotator cuff tendon pathologies are an extension of rotator cuff tears. The failure often occurs at the myotendinous junction. Tendinosis and tendinitis can be the result of direct trauma or repetitive use.
Shoulder dislocations/ subluxations	Anterior dislocations that occur with mechanism of injury usually involve forced shoulder horizontal abduction with external rotation. The mechanism of injury is usually shoulder flexion, internal rotation, or adduction coupled with a fall onto an outstretched arm.
Shoulder instability	Shoulder instability can be multidirectional, in which case the instability is generally congenital and laxity will be seen bilaterally and in other joints as well. The instability can be unidirectional, in which case the instability is the result of trauma and is usually a sequelae of shoulder dislocations.
Subacromial bursitis	Subacromial bursitis is inflammation of the bursa sac under the acromion. The mechanism of injury is similar to that seen with impingement syndromes.

---

decreases the likelihood of another dislocation, but glenohumeral instability is still common following shoulder dislocation.

LOCATION OF SYMPTOMS

DOES THE LOCATION OF A PATIENT'S SYMPTOMS AID IN THE DECISION-MAKING PROCESS?

As in any other region, the location of a patient's symptoms will help narrow down the potential sources of pain. Acute symptoms are generally localized to the region of injury; as the inflammatory response progresses, pain and achiness will spread. This is due in part to peripheral sensitization of nerves and in part to the spread of inflammation in the surrounding regions. Therefore,

the best time to assess the shoulder is usually immediately after injury and before the inflammatory response begins to impact joint mobility and muscle guarding. Careful questioning regarding the exact location of the current symptoms and a description of how the symptoms have spread will allow the clinician to narrow down the list of source tissue.

REFERRAL OF SYMPTOMS

WHAT ARE THE REFERRAL PATTERNS OF THE DIFFERENT TISSUE TYPES IN THE SHOULDER?
(Box II-8-1 and Figure II-8-1)

• Muscles[61,68]

BOX II-8-2	**Referral Patterns of Muscles in the Shoulder Region**
Supraspinatus	Refers pain above the spine of the scapulae, the lateral aspect of the shoulder, and may extend down the lateral aspect of the upper arm and forearm. Pain does not progress into the hand.
Infraspinatus	Refers pain on the lateral and anterior aspect of the shoulder. Pain may extend down the lateral and anterior side of the arm. Pain can extend into the anterior and posterior aspect of the lateral three fingers.
Subscapularis	Refers pain into the posterior aspect of the shoulder and posterior medial aspect of the upper arm. Pain can refer into the wrist.
Teres major	Refers pain to the lateral shoulder over the region of the posterior deltoid and into the posterior aspect of the forearm.
Teres minor	Refers pain to the posterior aspect of the shoulder and upper arm.
Upper trapezius	Refers pain into the suboccipital region and along the posterior aspect of the scapula.
Mid and lower trapezius	Refers pain into the upper back and the medial edge of the scapula.
Latissimus dorsi	Refers pain to the posterior aspect of the scapula and into the posterior aspect of the upper arm and forearm. Symptoms are generally in a medial distribution and can refer pain into the medial two fingers of the hand.
Scalene	Pain may extend into the ipsilateral chest, shoulder, the area medial to the scapula, and down the arm to the dorsal index finger and thumb.
Levator scapulae	Refers pain into the posterior aspect of the neck and scapula. Can also produce pain down the medial border of the scapula.
Deltoid	Refers pain into the lateral aspect of the shoulder and upper arm. Pain may be felt more intensely in the posterior aspect of the shoulder.
Rhomboids	Refers pain into the medial aspect of the scapula. Symptoms remain relatively localized to the region around the muscle.
Biceps brachii	Refers pain into the anterior aspect of the shoulder and down the length of the biceps muscle to the elbow.
Brachialis	Refers in a weaker version of the biceps pain pattern with the addition of pain at the base of the thumb.
Coracobrachialis	Refers pain into the lateral aspect of the shoulder and the posterior aspect of the upper arm and forearm. Pain may progress into the dorsal aspect of the hand and fingers.
Triceps brachii	Refers pain into the posterior shoulder extending as far up as the angle of the neck, down the posterior aspect of the arm and forearm. Pain generally does not refer into the hand.
Serratus anterior	Refers pain into the axillary region and down the medial aspect of the arm and down into the medial aspect of the hand.
Subclavius	Refers pain locally to the front of the clavicle and anterior shoulder, down the anterior arm along the biceps, and the lateral (thumb) side of the arm as far as the thumb, index, and middle fingers.
Pectoralis major	Refers pain into the chest and anterior shoulder. Can refer pain down the medial aspect of the upper arm into the medial elbow.
Pectoralis minor	Refers pain in a weaker version of pectoralis major. Pain is noted over the chest and anterior shoulder, extending down the medial side of the arm as far as the medial three fingers.

CLINICAL PEARL

Normal muscle strength for the shoulder is as follows:
- *Internal rotation is stronger than external rotation by a 3:2 ratio*
- *Adduction is stronger than abduction by a 2:1 ratio*
- *Extension is stronger than flexion by a 5:4 ratio*
- *Joint (capsule/cartilage)*
  - *Cervical facet joints can refer pain into the shoulder region, but pain is generally localized more axially and does not progress laterally to the shoulder.*

- Tendons
  - Studies that explore the pain referral pattern of tendons alone have not been conducted. From a hypothetical standpoint, the tendons are extensions of muscles and therefore most have the same innervation and fetal tissue origins. Therefore, tendon referral patterns should mimic the muscles to which they are attached.
- Ligaments
  - Although shoulder ligaments are richly innervated and should be considered as a source of pain, no studies have specifically looked at the referral pattern of ligaments in the shoulder.

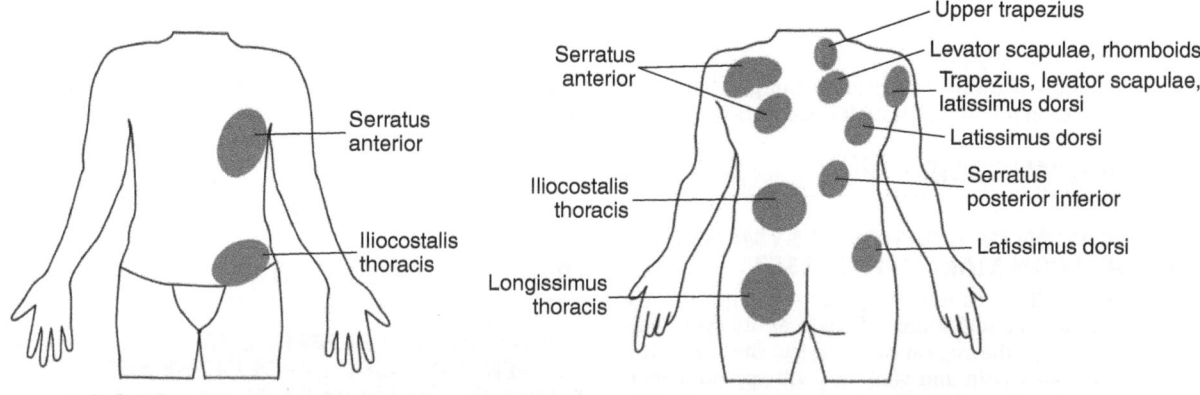

FIGURE II-8-1 Shoulder muscle referral pattern. Muscles can refer pain both locally and remotely. The figure illustrates the referral pattern of the thoracic spine. The illustration is adapted from the work of Travell and Simons[68] and shows some of the muscle referral patterns of the shoulder.

CLINICAL PEARL !

Tears of the long head of the biceps can decrease both shoulder and elbow strength. Elbow flexion can decrease by 30%, abduction of the shoulder can decrease by 20%, and forearm supination can decrease by 20%.

- Bone
  - To date, no studies have specifically looked at the referral pattern of bone. Clinically, a patient with a fractured bone will initially report a sharp pain local to the site of injury. As time progresses, the region of pain will expand due to inflammation. The site of pain will expand, but will continue to be centered around the site of injury. The patient will experience the pain as a deeper achiness. Pain can also be referred down the shaft of the injured bone. Nerves can also refer pain in a bone pattern. This pattern is referred to as a sclerotome.
  - Sclerotome pain patterns are as follows:[43]
    1. C4 refers pain into the clavicle
    2. C5 refers pain into the upper two-thirds of the scapula and the lateral aspect of the humerus
    3. C6 refers pain into the lower third of the scapula, the medial aspect of the humerus, the radius, and the first ray of the hand
    4. C7 refers pain into the lateral border of the scapula, the medial humerus, the medial epicondyle, the ulna, and the index and middle finger of the hand

5. C8 refers pain to the elbow and the medial aspect of the ulna and fourth and fifth fingers of the hand

CLINICAL DECISION MAKING CASE STUDY—PATIENT PROFILE[33] ?

Summer is a 24-year-old female who presents to you with complaints of left shoulder pain. The pain began 2 months ago. She cannot remember a specific incident that caused the pain. She is in her second year of medical school and has remarked that the books have gotten progressively heavier. She carries her books in a backpack and has a tendency to carry it over the left shoulder. Physical examination reveal significant scapular dyskinesia with scapular winging present. What is your hypothesis regarding the cause of the shoulder pain?

Answer

Hester et al[20] studied six fresh cadaveric shoulders to look at the potential dynamic causes of long thoracic nerve palsy. They discovered that a combined shoulder abduction and external rotation coupled with scapular medial and upward migration cause the most bowstringing and tension on the long thoracic nerve. Previous studies have suggested that long thoracic nerve palsy is due in part to compression of the medial scalene muscle. They suggested that the combination of medial scalene muscle

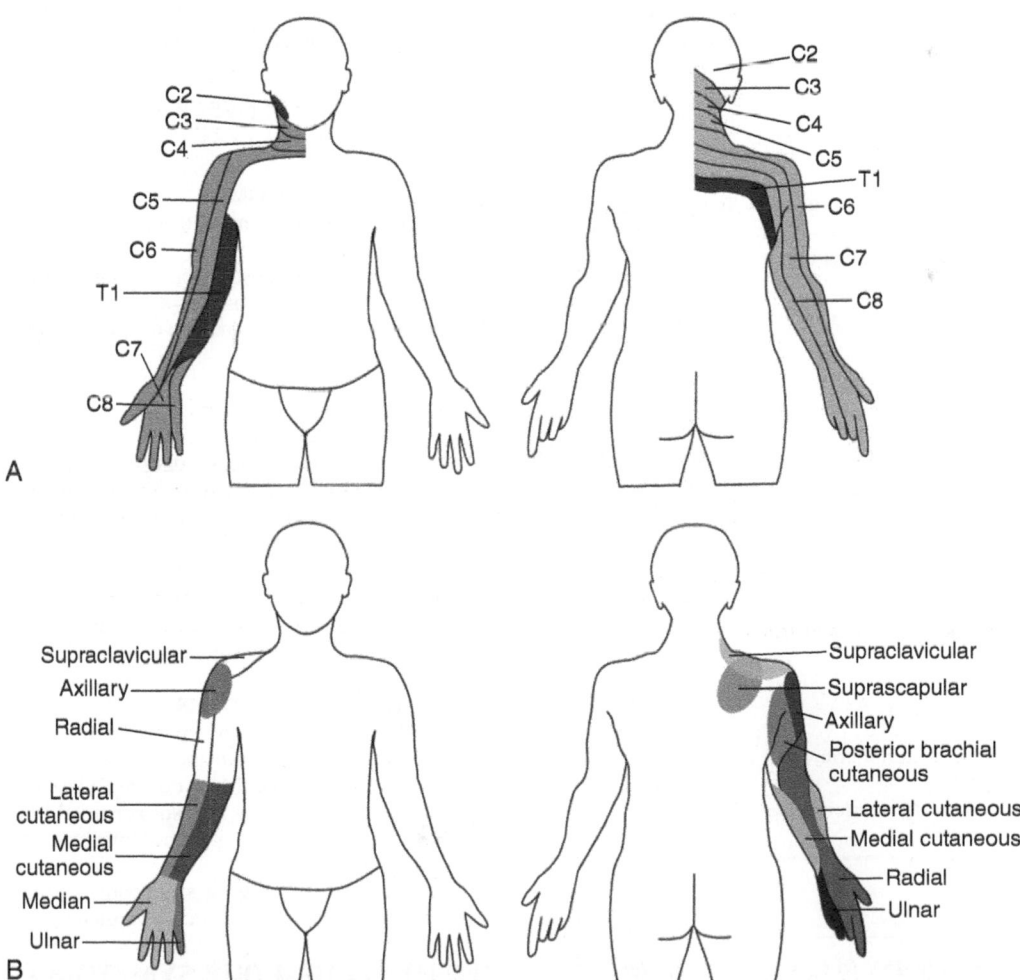

FIGURE II-8-2 **(A)** Upper extremity dermatomes. A dermatome is an area of skin innervated by a single pair of dorsal nerve roots. Dermatomal patterns of symptoms vary greatly from person to person. The clinician should keep this in mind when utilizing dermatomes for clinical diagnostic purposes. **(B)** Sensory distribution of peripheral nerves. The referral pattern of the sensory nerves is different from the referral pattern of the spinal nerve root. The clinician can utilize the differences to aid in the diagnostic process.

contraction and shoulder abduction, shoulder external rotation, scapular upward migration, and scapular medial migration may cause tethering of the long thoracic nerve over the tight fascial bands of the scalene muscle. They postulated that the scapular hiking commonly seen in patients with shoulder pain or with weakness and fatigue of the scapular stabilizer may result in the tethering affect of the long thoracic nerve.

- Peripheral and spinal nerves (Figure II-8-2 on page 173)

Nerve	Sensory Innervation	Motor Innervation
Axillary	Deltoid region Anterior shoulder	Deltoid Teres minor
Supraclavicular	Lower cervical and upper shoulder	None
Suprascapular	Top of shoulder from the clavicle to scapular spine	Supraspinatus Infraspinatus
Long thoracic	None	Serratus anterior
Dorsal scapular	None	Levator scapulae Rhomboids
Musculocutaneous	Lateral forearm	Biceps Brachialis Coracobrachialis
Spinal accessory	Brachial plexus symptoms	Trapezius
Subscapular	None	Subscapularis Teres major
Lateral pectoral	None	Pectoralis major Pectoralis minor
Thoracodorsal	None	Latissimus dorsi
Posterior brachial cutaneous	Posterior upper arm	None
Lower lateral brachial cutaneous	Lower upper arm	None
C4 spinal nerve	Shoulder and lower neck	Trapezius Levator scapulae
C5 spinal nerve	Shoulder and lateral upper arm	Deltoid Pectoralis major Rotator cuff Rhomboids Biceps Brachioradialis Brachialis
C6 spinal nerve	Shoulder and lateral upper and lower arm	Deltoid Pectoralis major Rotator cuff Rhomboids Biceps Brachioradialis Brachialis Pronator teres
C7 spinal nerve	Anterior shoulder and arm	Biceps Triceps Latissimus Pronator teres Flexor carpi ulnaris
T2 spinal nerve	Axilla, posterior arm, and chest	None
T3 spinal nerve	Axilla and posterior upper arm	None

CLINICAL PEARL

Women have approximately 45% to 65% of the shoulder strength of men.

- Vascular systems
  - There has been no research published on vascular tissue such as arteries, veins, and lymphatic systems as sources of shoulder pain. Preliminary studies suggest that although vascular tissue is

innervated, the innervation is autonomic in origin, the purpose being regulation of smooth muscle in the vessels. There is no evidence to suggest that vascular tissue itself can be the source of pain. Vascular tissue can indirectly result in pain. In response to stress or injury, vascular tissue can vasoconstrict, which will result in diminished blood flow to a region and therefore can result in ischemic pain from tissue being supplied by the vascular tissue. In addition, vasodilation in response to acute injury can result in an influx of chemical mediators, which in turn can sensitize surrounding tissue. This hypersensitivity can result in increased shoulder pain. Preliminary studies into vasodynamics suggest that symptoms related to vascular systems are reported by patients as coldness or heaviness and not as pain.

- Visceral structures (Figure II-8-3)
  - Heart: Left chest, shoulder, neck, and upper back pain; can refer down the medial aspect in an ulnar nerve distribution
  - Lung: Pain referred into the upper trapezius, chest, axilla, or anterior lower ribs; pain may refer in an ulnar nerve distribution
  - Stomach and duodenum: Right shoulder and mid-sternum at the xiphoid
  - Pancreas: Left shoulder and mid-sternum at the xiphoid
  - Kidneys: Can refer into the shoulder; pain is usually ipsilateral to the involved kidney
  - Liver and gallbladder: Can refer pain into the right shoulder, upper back, and right abdomen
  - Spleen: Left shoulder

SYMPTOM DESCRIPTORS

WHICH SYMPTOM DESCRIPTORS ARE THE MOST HELPFUL IN DIAGNOSING A PATIENT'S PATHOLOGY?
QUALITY OF SYMPTOMS
Deep ache: Cartilage, labrum, bone
Dull ache: Bone, inflammation
Sharp pain: Capsule, muscle, tendon, ligament
Sharp and continuous: Bone
Burning: Nerves, inflammation, vein, artery, lymphatic system
Tingling: Nerve
Numbness: Nerves
Colicky and cramping: Viscera
DEPTH OF SYMPTOMS
- Deep symptoms implicate deep structures such as cartilage, bone, and visceral structures. There are fewer proprioceptive nerves in deep structures than in more superficial structures, so the ability to localize tissue damage in deep structures is more difficult.
- Superficial symptoms implicate surface structures such as muscles, tendons, and ligaments. They have more proprioceptive nerve fibers and thus injury to superficial structures is more easily localized.
CONSTANCY OF SYMPTOMS
- Intermittent symptoms implicate a mechanical source and a structure that is injured and is aggravated only with certain positions or motions. This is common in rotator cuff pathology, tendinopathies, bursitis, and subacromial impingement.
- Constant but varying symptoms implicate inflammation as the primary source.
- Constant and unchanging symptoms implicate visceral structures or other pathology such as cancer.

TWENTY-FOUR-HOUR SYMPTOM PATTERN

IF A PATIENT HAS SYMPTOMS IN THE MORNING, WHAT PATHOLOGY DOES THIS IMPLICATE?
- It is common for a patient with shoulder symptoms to have stiffness in the morning. Generally, stiffness and pain that last

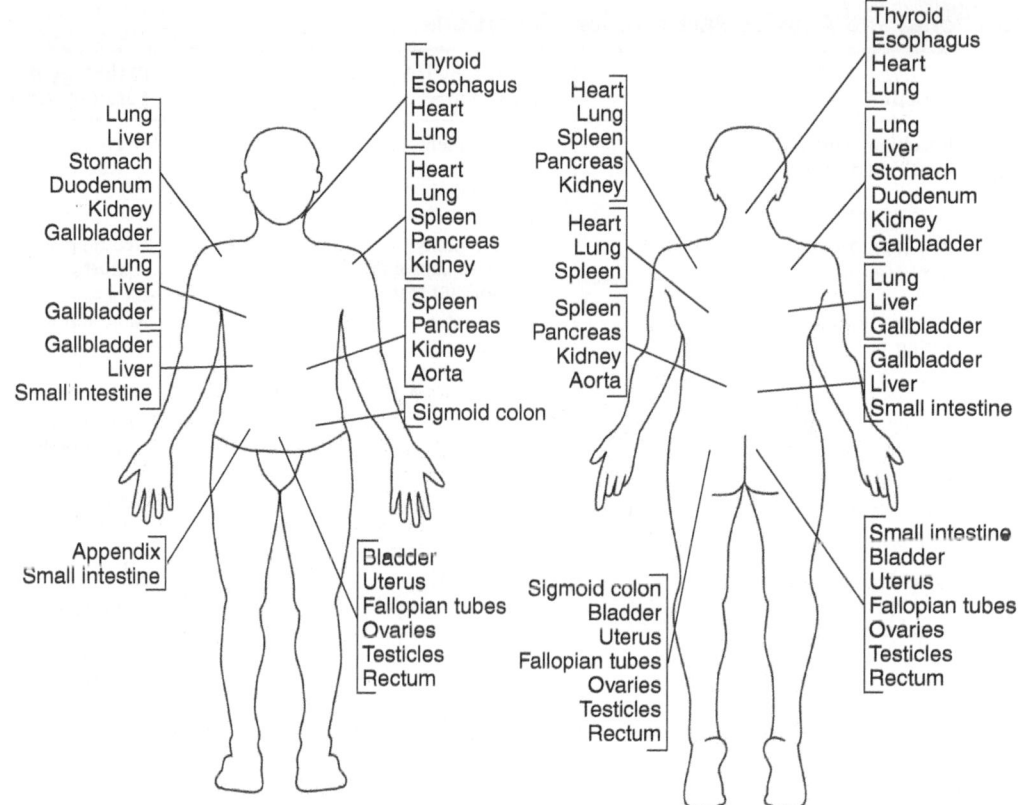

FIGURE II-8-3 Symptom referral pattern of visceral tissue. The figure shows the visceral tissues that most commonly refer symptoms into the upper quarter and shoulder region. Symptoms are generally described as a deep dull ache that is hard to localize. Symptoms may wax and wane in intensity and may not be elicited by motions of the region.

for only a short time on awakening correspond to pathology that is more mechanical in nature. Mechanical disorders can be altered by biomechanical motions. Degenerative joint disease, AC joint pathology, and shoulder instability will all present as stiffness in the morning that resolves quickly with motion.

- Pain and stiffness that persist for a longer period of time, greater than 15 minutes, are common when inflammation is the primary source of the symptoms. Inflammation will abate once movement and circulation are increased in the region. Removal of edema from a region is tied to the lymphatic system. This system is passive and requires motion and muscle contractions to move the lymph out of the region. Therefore, symptoms will persist for a longer time frame. Bursitis and tendinitis are prime examples of this response.

STABILITY OF SYMPTOMS

CHANGES IN SYMPTOMS

- Pain and symptoms in the shoulder should follow a typical pattern with symptoms remaining severe the first 3 days. Over the course of the next 2 to 3 weeks the symptoms should begin to resolve with full resolution by week 6. If symptoms do not follow this typical pattern than the exacerbating factor should be identified.
- The vascularity of a structure will often aid in the differentiation process. Structures that are well vascularized, such as bone and muscle, will have an immediate and significant vascular response. Therefore, if a patient feels immediate pain that does not improve over the remainder of the day of injury, a structure that has become entrapped or pinched such as a joint capsule or a facet joint is implicated.
- Structures that have a poor vascular supply, such as the supraspinatus tendon, cartilage, and labrum, will have a slow inflammation process and will be slower to swell. In this case, patients feel

pain initially, but the pain quickly resolves for the remainder of the day and they wake up the next day with excruciating pain.

FUNCTIONAL AND ACTIVITY PARTICIPATION LIMITATIONS (Table II-8-1)

BEHAVIOR OF SYMPTOMS: AGGRAVATING BEHAVIOR

WHICH AGGRAVATING ACTIVITIES HELP IN THE CLINICAL REASONING PROCESS?

It is difficult to diagnose a specific tissue source of symptoms based solely on activities that aggravate a patient's symptoms. This is because many shoulder pathologies exhibit a continuum of shoulder pain, all with the same mechanism. That mechanism is subacromial impingement. As the structures beneath the acromion are impinged, symptoms will progress from inflammation to muscle damage to muscle failure. As a result, the pathologies will progress from bursitis to tendinitis to tendinosis to partial rotator cuff tear to full thickness rotator cuff tears.

The following aggravating activities will exemplify this cycle of pathology.

Flexion: impingement, bursitis, tendinopathy, rotator cuff tear
Extension: tendinopathy, adhesive capsulitis, rotator cuff tear
Abduction: impingement, bursitis, tendinopathy, rotator cuff tear
Adduction: AC joint pathology, SC joint pathology, clavicle fracture
Internal rotation: tendinopathy, adhesive capsulitis, rotator cuff tear
External rotation: tendinopathy, adhesive capsulitis, rotator cuff tear
Aggravating activities should be used as an aid in the diagnostic process and not be the only factor on which a clinician makes a decision. It should be combined with all other subjective and objective data gained during the patient examination.

TABLE II-8-1 Functional and Activity Participation Limitations

Motion	Functional Activities	Pathology if Symptoms Are Aggravated by Activity	Pathology if Symptoms Are Eased by Activity
Flexion	Reaching overhead Combing or washing hair	Impingement Bursitis Tendinopathy Rotator cuff tear	Nerve pathology
Extension	Reaching backward	Tendinopathy Adhesive capsulitis Rotator cuff tear	Neutral position will decrease most pathologies
Abduction	Lifting out to the side Eating	Impingement Bursitis Tendinopathy Rotator cuff tear	Neutral position will decrease most pathologies
Adduction	Putting on seatbelt Reaching across the body Sleeping	AC joint pathology SC joint pathology Clavicle fracture	Neutral position will decrease most pathologies
External rotation	Reaching out to the side	Tendinopathy Adhesive capsulitis Rotator cuff tear	Neutral position will decrease most pathologies
Internal rotation	Reaching behind your back Tucking in shirt Fastening brassiere	Tendinopathy Adhesive capsulitis Rotator cuff tear	Neutral position will decrease most pathologies
Static positions	Sleep	Visceral pathology Inflammation Bone fracture	Neutral position will decrease most pathologies

AC, acromioclavicular; SC, sternoclavicular.

CLINICAL PEARL

The supraspinatus muscle has two muscle bellies, the anterior and the posterior sections. Of the two, the anterior portion is larger, but has a smaller tendon. Therefore stress is much greater through the anterior tendon than the posterior supraspinatus tendon. Consequently, the anterior section may be more prone to earlier failure.

BEHAVIOR OF SYMPTOMS: EASING BEHAVIOR

WHICH EASING ACTIVITIES HELP IN THE CLINICAL REASONING PROCESS?

In response to many shoulder pathologies, the patient will take similar protective postures to protect and offload the irritated structures. The most common position of ease for patients with shoulder pain is the arm in a position internally rotated across the abdomen and supported by the other hand. This position off-loads the rotator cuff muscles as well as the joint itself. The patient's position of ease cannot definitively point to a specific pathology, but suggests rotator cuff pathology, tendinpathy, bursitis, or fracture.

Another pattern of pain relief is relief when the hand is placed overhead, such as on the head. If this pattern is noted in a patient, then nerve pathology should be considered as a potential source of symptoms.

MEDICAL HISTORY

WHAT ARE THE IMPLICATIONS OF A PATIENT'S PAST MEDICAL HISTORY ON SHOULDER PATHOLOGY?

As medical research advances, research is demonstrating that most pathologies do not occur in isolation. Consequently, all aspects of medical history should be considered, because all medical issues could potentially influence shoulder pain. Acute pain, for the most part, can be traced back to a specific

mechanism of injury. Determining this mechanism can allow the clinician to determine a tissue source. Many patients seen in the clinic, however, have either chronic shoulder pain or pain that began insidiously. In these cases, the mechanism of injury is often not as valuable as knowledge of a patient's past medical history.

Thyroid pathology has been linked to shoulder and neck pain. The heart, lung, pancreas, liver, gallbladder, and stomach can all refer pain into the shoulder region. Hormones and menopause have been loosely tied to adhesive capsulitis. Breast and lung cancer can result in shoulder pain. All of these illustrations demonstrate how shoulder pain can either be directly or indirectly linked to past or present medical pathology. It is critical for a clinician to question all aspects of a patient's past medical history.

MEDICAL AND ORTHOPEDIC TESTING

WHICH ORTHOPEDIC AND MEDICAL TESTS ARE THE MOST IMPORTANT IN THE CLINICAL REASONING PROCESS?

There are an overwhelming number of clinical tests utilized by clinicians to rule in or rule out shoulder pathology. [15,21,25,27,48,65] The following tests are most commonly utilized in clinical situations (Tables II-8-2 and II-8-3).

Park et al[60] found that a combination of the drop arm test, painful arc and infraspinatus test, or lag sign test yielded the best posttest probability (91%) for full thickness rotator cuff tears (Tables II-8-4 and II-8-5).

MAGNETIC RESONANCE IMAGING (MRI)[23,49,64,66]

MRI aids in diagnosing soft tissue abnormalities in the shoulder region. Studies show MRI in the shoulder region is very accurate with sensitivities ranging from 91% to 100% and specificities ranging from 75% to 95% for rotator cuff pathology, labral pathology, and glenohumeral instability.

TABLE II-8-2 Results of Tests Used to Diagnose Superior Labrum or Labrum Lesions

Test	Study	Finding	Sensitivity (%)	Specificity (%)	PPV (%)	NPV (%)
Active compression	O'Brien et al[55]	Labral tear	100	98.5	94.6	100
	Guanche and Jones[16]	Labral tear	63	73	87	40
	McFarland et al[45]	SLAP	47	55	10	91
	Morgan et al[51]	Anterior type II SLAP	88	42		
		Posterior type II SLAP	32	13		
		Combined type II SLAP	85	41		
	Myers et al[52]	Unstable SLAP	77.8	11.1	70	14.3
	Stetson and Templin[66]	Labral tear	54	31	34	50
	Nakagawa et al[53]	SLAP	54	60	52	62
	Oh et al[57]	SLAP type II	63	53	55	61
	Parentis et al[59]	SLAP type I and II	62.5	50	35.5	75.4
Anterior apprehension	Oh et al[57]	SLAP type II	62	42	56	49
Anterior slide	Kibler[30]	SLAP	78.4	91.5	66.7	80.8
	McFarland et al[45]	SLAP	8	84	5	90
	McFarland[46]	Partial biceps tendon tear	23	84	9	94
	Parentis et al[59]	SLAP type I and II	10	81.5	19	67.6
	Oh et al[57]	SLAP type II	21	70	38	50
Belly press	McFarland[46]	Partial biceps tendon tear	17	92	24	88
Biceps palpation	McFarland[46]	Partial biceps tendon tear	53	54	6	95
Biceps load I	Kim et al[33]	SLAP	90.9	96.9	83	98
Biceps load II	Kim et al[32]	SLAP	89.7	96.9	92.1	95.5
	Oh et al[57]	SLAP type II	30	78	59	52
Passive compression	Kim et al[34]	SLAP	81.8	85.7	87.1	80
Compression rotation	McFarland et al[45]	SLAP	24	76	9	90
	Nakagawa et al[53]	SLAP	25	100	100	58
	Oh et al[57]	SLAP type II	61	54	55	61
Crank test	Liu et al[38]	Labral tear	91	93	94	90
	McFarland[46]	Partial biceps tendon tear	34	77	11	93
	Myers et al[52]	Unstable SLAP	34.6	70	75	29.2
	Mimori et al[50]	SLAP	83	100	100	57
	Nakagawa et al[53]	SLAP	58	72	63	68
	Parentis et al[59]	SLAP type I and II	12.5	82.6	23.8	68.4
	Stetson and Templin[66]	Labral tear	46	56	41	61
Forced abduction	Nakagawa et al[53]	SLAP	67	67	62	71
Fulcrum	Nakagawa et al[53]	SLAP	83	40	53	75
Hawkins[19]	McFarland[46]	Partial biceps tendon tear	55	38	5	94
	Parentis et al[59]	SLAP type I and II	67.5	30.4	29.7	68.3
Lift-off test	McFarland[46]	Partial biceps tendon tear	28	89	15	95
Neer	McFarland[46]	Partial biceps tendon tear	64	41	5	96
	Parentis et al[59]	SLAP type I and II	50	52.2	31.3	70.6
Pain provocation	Mimori et al[50]	SLAP	100	90	95	100
	Parentis et al[59]	SLAP type I and II	15	90.2	40	70.9
Resisted supination external rotation	Myers et al[52]	Unstable SLAP	82.8	81.8	92.3	64.3
Relocation (Jobe)[26]	Guanche and Jones[16]	Labral tear	44	87	91	34
	Morgan et al[51]	Anterior type II SLAP	4	27		
		Combined type II SLAP	59	54		
		Posterior type II SLAP	85	68		
	Oh et al[57]	SLAP type II	44	54	52	47
	Parentis et al[59]	SLAP type I and II	50	53.3	31.7	71
Speed	McFarland[46]	SLAP type II	28	72	12	91
		Partial biceps tendon tear	50	67	8	96

Continued on following page.

Section II

ORTHOPEDIC REASONING

TABLE II-8-2   **Results of Tests Used to Diagnose Superior Labrum or Labrum Lesions** (Continued)

Test	Study	Finding	Sensitivity (%)	Specificity (%)	PPV (%)	NPV (%)
	Morgan et al[51]	Posterior type II SLAP	29	11		
		Anterior type II SLAP	100	70		
		Combined type II SLAP	78	37		
	Oh et al[57]	SLAP type II	32	66	46	53
	Parentis et al[59]	SLAP type I and II	47.8	67.7	34.8	72.1
Whipple	Oh et al[57]	SLAP type II	65	42	50	57
Yergason	Nakagawa et al[53]	SLAP	13	100	100	59
	Parentis et al[59]	SLAP type I and II	12.5	93.5	45.5	71.1
	Oh et al[57]	SLAP type II	12	87	44	53

From McFarland EG, Tanaka MJ, Papp DF: Examination of the shoulder in the overhead and throwing athlete. *Clinics Sports Med.* 2008;27(4):553–78.
NPV, negative predictive value; PPV, positive predictive value; SLAP, superior labrum anterior to posterior.

TABLE II-8-3   **Summary of the Literature on Examination for Rotator Cuff Disease**

Study	Diagnosis	Test Studied	Sensitivity (%)	Specificity (%)	PPV (%)	NPV (%)
Park et al[60]	Bursitis	Neer	86	49	21	96
		Kennedy-Hawkins	76	45	17	92
		Painful arc	71	47	12	94
		Supraspinatus muscle test	25	67	9	87
		Speed test	33	70	14	88
		Cross-body adduction test	25	80	15	89
		Drop-arm test	14	77	8	86
		Infraspinatus muscle test	25	69	9	88
	Partial-thickness rotator cuff tear	Neer	75	48	18	93
		Kennedy-Hawkins	75	44	17	92
		Painful arc	67	47	15	91
		Supraspinatus muscle test	32	68	11	88
		Speed test	33	71	16	89
		Cross-body adduction test	17	79	10	87
		Drop-arm test	14	78	8	87
		Infraspinatus muscle test	19	69	10	88
	Full-thickness rotator cuff tear	Neer	59	47	41	65
		Kennedy-Hawkins	69	48	45	71
		Painful arc	76	62	61	76
		Supraspinatus muscle test	53	82	68	71
		Speed test	40	75	50	67
		Cross-body adduction test	23	81	45	62
		Drop-arm test	14	78	8	87
		Infraspinatus muscle test	19	69	10	88
Leroux et al[36]	Impingement syndrome	Neer	89			
		Kennedy-Hawkins	87			
		Yocum	78			
Calis et al[5]	Impingement syndrome	Neer	89	31	76	52
		Kennedy-Hawkins	92	25	75	56
		Speed	69	56	79	42
		Yergason	37	86	87	36
		Painful arc	33	81	81	33
		Drop-arm test	8	97	88	30
MacDonald et al[41]	Bursitis	Neer	75	48	36	83
		Kennedy-Hawkins	92	44	39	93
		Neer or Kennedy-Hawkins	96	41	39	96
		Neer and Kennedy-Hawkins	71	51	36	82
	Rotator cuff pathosis	Neer	83	51	40	89
		Kennedy-Hawkins	88	43	38	90
		Neer or Kennedy-Hawkins	88	38	36	89
		Neer and Kennedy-Hawkins	83	56	43	58
	Bursitis or rotator cuff tear	Neer	77	63	70	71
		Kennedy-Hawkins	89	60	71	83

TABLE II-8-3 Summary of the Literature on Examination for Rotator Cuff Disease *(Continued)*

Study	Diagnosis	Test Studied	Sensitivity (%)	Specificity (%)	PPV (%)	NPV (%)
Holtby and Razmjou[22]	Supraspinatus tendinitis or partial rotator cuff tear	Supraspinatus test	62	54		
	Full-thickness rotator cuff tear		41	70		
	Large to massive rotator cuff tear		88	70		

From McFarland EG, Tanaka MJ, Papp DF: Examination of the shoulder in the overhead and throwing athlete. *Clinics Sports Med.* 2008;27(4):553-78.
NPV, negative predictive value; PPV, positive predictive value.

TABLE II-8-4 Results of Tests for Anterior Shoulder Instability

Test	Criteria	Study	Sensitivity (%)	Specificity (%)	PPV (%)	NPV (%)
Apprehension	Pain or apprehension	Lo et al[39]	53	99	98	73
	Relief of pain	Farber et al[10]	50	56	14	88
	Relief of apprehension	Farber et al[10]	72	96	75	96
Relocation	Relief of pain	Speer et al[65]	30	58	38	49
		Lo et al[39]	40	43	15	73
		Farber et al[10]	30	90	19	94
	Relief of apprehension	Speer et al[65]	57	100	100	73
		Lo et al[39]	32	100	100	65
		Farber et al[10]	81	92	53	98
Surprise	Pain or apprehension	Lo et al[39]	64	99	98	78

From McFarland EG, Tanaka MJ, Papp DF: Examination of the shoulder in the overhead and throwing athlete. *Clinics Sports Med.* 2008;27(4):553-78.
NPV, negative predictive value; PPV, positive predictive value.

TABLE II-8-5 Results of Tests for Scapulothoracic Motion

Test	Specificity of Tests (%)	Sensitivity of Tests (%)	Likelihood Ratios
Kibler[29,31]	Not reported	Not reported	42/not reported
Lateral scapular slide[56]	Not reported	Not reported	52-66/45-79

MR arthography for SLAP lesions:
  Reliability: 0.77
  Specificity: 0.78
  Sensitivity: 0.89
  Positive likelihood ratio (LR): 4.04
  Negative LR: 0.014
MRI for labral tear:
  Specificity: 0.92
  Sensitivity: 0.42
  Positive LR: 5.25
  Negative LR: 0.63
MRI for rotator cuff tear:
  Specificity: 0.67
  Sensitivity: 1.0
  Positive LR: 4.35
  Negative LR: 0

X-RAYS[14]

Radiographs are used as the first line of imaging for the shoulder joint. Radiographic images allow the clinician to visualize the glenohumeral joint and other surrounding bony structures. Many radiographic projections exist to evaluate specific pathologies; however, a typical series includes anteroposterior, axillary, and scapular Y views.

The following radiographic projections are commonly used to evaluate the shoulder:
- Anteroposterior: General assessment of the glenohumeral joint, acromioclavicular joint, and distal clavicle
- Axillary: Subluxation, dislocation, cartilage space, Bankart lesion
- Grashey: Glenohumeral cartilage space
- Rockwood: Subacromial space
- Scapular Y: Dislocation, Hill-Sachs lesion, scapular fracture, acromion, and coracoid process
- Stryker notch: Posterosuperior humeral head, Hill-Sachs lesion
- Supraspinatus outlet: Subacromial space
- West Point: Anteroinferior glenoid rim, Bankart lesion

ELECTROMYOGRAPHY (EMG)

EMG is typically utilized to evaluate nerve pathology. It will be covered in more depth in other upper extremity and nerve sections. Its use for the shoulder exclusively is generally limited to ruling out spinal nerve pathology (C3 to C5) and damage to a few peripheral nerves such as the long thoracic, suprascapular, dorsal thoracic, musculocutaneous, and axillary nerve. Most other nerves will run through the shoulder region and most likely do not manifest themselves as shoulder pain. Hence, they will be addressed as part of other sections.

It is essential that the clinician realize that no one test or piece of information provided by interview or examination can definitively diagnose a shoulder pathology. It is the compilation of all aspects of the patient examination combined with clinical experience that allows the clinician to make the best informed decision possible. Even then, the clinician will never be 100% certain that the assumptions made are completely accurate. With this in mind, the objective tests noted above should be used to assist the decision-making process and not define it.

MEDICATIONS

HOW DOES A PATIENT'S RESPONSE TO MEDICATIONS INFLUENCE YOUR DECISION-MAKING PROCESSES?

- Muscle relaxants, pain medications, and antiinflammatory medications are commonly prescribed in association with shoulder pain.
- Symptom relief with the use of muscle relaxants and pain medications does not aid the diagnostic process. Most patients with symptomatic shoulder pathology will experience muscle guarding and pain.
- The effectiveness of antiinflammatory medication helps differentiate pathology that has an acute inflammatory process.
  - Pathologies that can have an acute inflammatory process include humeral fractures, clavicular fractures, rotator cuff muscle strains, bicep tendinitis, rotator cuff tendinitis, ligament sprains, labral tears, and radiculopathies.
  - Pathologies that do not normally have an acute inflammatory response include tendinosis, degenerative joint disease, and instability.

BIOMECHANICAL

WHAT ARE THE NORMAL BIOMECHANICS OF THE SHOULDER?[29,44,47]

The biomechanics of the shoulder are relatively well established and provide a solid framework for diagnosis and assessment of shoulder pathology and dysfunction. Scapulohumeral rhythm refers to the coordination of the scapula and humerus during shoulder elevation. Normal scapular motion varies, but as a whole, the scapula in relationship to the humerus should move in a two-to-one rhythm. The humerus is responsible for 120° of elevation whereas the scapular will rotate upward 60° with shoulder flexion. The timing of this motion is as follows:

- During the first 30° of motion, the humerus will move upward but the scapula will remain stationary, setting itself onto the thoracic spine to provide a relatively solid base from which the arm can move.
- Between 30° and 90° of shoulder flexion there is a 2 to 1 ratio of humeral elevation to scapular protraction and upward rotation.
- From 90° to 170° degrees of shoulder flexion there is a 1 to 1 ratio of humeral elevation to scapular protraction and upward rotation.
- The final 10° of motion is accomplished through thoracic extension.

HOW DOES THE CLAVICLE MOVE DURING SHOULDER FLEXION?[1,42,54]

The clavicle is the main connection of the shoulder to the thoracic spine. The sternoclavicular joint is the only true joint connecting the shoulder girdle to the body. The clavicle elevates approximately 40° and rotates posteriorly 10° during shoulder flexion.

HOW DOES THE SHOULDER TRANSLATE DURING SHOULDER FLEXION?[37,54]

When the shoulder moves, anterior and posterior translation of the humeral head results in tightening and loosening of the capsuloligamentous structures. When the shoulder flexes over 55°, the humeral head will translate anteriorly. When the shoulder extends greater than 35°, the humeral head posteriorly translates. When the shoulder flexes, the humeral head will slide superiorly 3 mm. Following the initial superior translation, the humeral head will rotate in place with very little translation.

CLINICAL PEARL   (!)

Which ligament is tightest with adhesive capsulitis?[18] The coracohumeral ligament functions to limit shoulder external rotation when the shoulder is at the side. It is often implicated as a limiting structure with adhesive capsulitis.

WHAT IS THE ROLE OF THE BICEPS TENDON IN STABILIZING THE SHOULDER?[1,12]

The exact contribution that the long head of the biceps makes on shoulder stability is still not well defined. It has been hypothesized that the long head of the biceps may function to provide anterior stability to the shoulder. It does so by decreasing anterior and superior translation of the humeral head.

CLINICAL DECISION MAKING CASE STUDY—PATIENT PROFILE   (?)

Jake is a 23-year-old professional tennis player who began to experience shoulder pain half way through the season. Over the past month the symptoms have begun to get progressively worse to a point at which he cannot lift his arm overhead without significant shoulder pain. His physician ordered an MRI, which revealed a full thickness tear through his supraspinatus muscle. What are the implications of this tear on normal glenohumeral joint biomechanics during upward motion of the shoulder?

Answer
The center of rotation in the normal glenohumeral joint is at the center of the humeral head at the mid-glenoid level. In severe rotator cuff deficiency of the glenohumeral joint the head of the humerus migrates superiorly and medially secondary to the unopposed pull of the deltoid and the loss of the humeral head depressing function of the rotator cuff. As a result, the center of rotation moves superiorly and leads to impingement.

WHAT BIOMECHANICAL ABNORMALITIES IN OTHER REGIONS AFFECT YOUR DECISION-MAKING PROCESS?

The most obvious abnormality that could directly impact the shoulder would be the thoracic spine. Because thoracic extension accounts for 10° of motion, increased thoracic kyphosis or lack of thoracic extension could lead to early shoulder impingement and all the shoulder pathologies commonly seen as a result of this impingement. For this reason, one of the easiest ways to off-load or decompress subacromial structures is to improve a patient's posture.

The cervical spine also directly impacts the shoulder region. Many of the muscles responsible for cervical function are also movers or stabilizers of the shoulder. Pathology in the neck could result in guarding and increased global muscle activity in the trapezius, sternocleidomastoid, and levator scapulae, all of which function to move and stabilize the shoulder.

Medical and biomechanical alterations in any body region could potentially impact the shoulder region. A foot injury in a baseball pitcher could prevent him from properly transferring weight onto the injured foot. This would throw off the mechanics of his delivery and ultimately result in shoulder injury. Therefore, a thorough evaluation of any athlete who uses overhead motion should also include a screen of the lower extremity, thoracic spine, cervical spine, and low back.

CLINICAL PEARL

The dynamic stabilizers of the shoulder make the greatest contribution to stability by keeping the humeral head centered in the glenoid fossa. The anterior band of the inferior glenohumeral ligament is the principal static restraint of the anterior translation of the humeral head with the arm in the 90° abducted and externally rotated position

The middle glenohumeral ligament is a significant restraint to anterior translation of the mid-range of shoulder elevation. The superior glenohumeral ligament appears to prevent excessive external rotation and inferior translation with the arm at the side.

ENVIRONMENTAL FACTORS

DO PSYCHOSOCIAL ISSUES INFLUENCE THE CLINICAL DECISION-MAKING PROCESS?[24]

Depression, stress, and other psychosocial factors can impact the autonomic, endocrine, and immune systems. These systems can be heightened or depressed in response to injury.

CAN EMOTIONS INFLUENCE SHOULDER PAIN?[62]

- Medical research is demonstrating that there is a relationship between emotions and pain. Pain is a multifaceted experience. When tissue is injured, the injury does not occur in isolation. There are memories and emotions that accompany the injury. The connection was previously not well established. Medical research is now providing experimental and clinical studies that show serial interactions between emotions and pain sensation intensity. The connection between pain and emotions appears to be related to a central network of brain structures that processes nociceptive information. Physiologically, spinal pathways to limbic structures and medial thalamic nuclei provide direct input to brain areas involved in emotion. A secondary source of cortical processing involves integration of information from spinal pathways to the somatosensory thalamic area. Processing then continues to cortical areas and then through a corticolimbic pathway. The corticolimbic pathway integrates nociceptive input with contextual information and memory to provide cognitive mediation of pain affect. Corticolimbic pathways terminate at the anterior cingulated structures, which may be responsible for modulating the impact of emotions on pain and response to pain.
- Although most clinicians believe that emotion can alter pain, little well-controlled research has been conducted to examine this issue. Current research suggests that positive emotions can lead to pain reduction as long as a minimal threshold of arousal is attained and negative emotions lead to pain inhibition only when emotions are highly arousing. Negative emotions coupled with low-to-moderate arousal appear to facilitate pain.

DO WORK-RELATED INJURIES INFLUENCE CLINICAL DECISION MAKING?[24]

Other nonmedical-related issues should always be considered as a source of a patient's symptoms. Research is demonstrating that expectation of recovery is a major factor predictive of return to

---

BOX II-8-3 Contextual Factors

Environmental	Work, environment, and repetitive tasks can lead to breakdown of tissue. Look for activities that require repetitive use of the arm and shoulder.
Personal	Work-related issues, personal and family factors, depression, and emotional unrest can all influence shoulder pain. Question patients regarding stressors in their life that may influence the body's ability to heal.

---

work. Patients who expect to fully recover return to work more consistently. Other factors such as depression, anxiety, job satisfaction, and job stress are not predictive of return to work potential. Fear avoidance regarding injury has moderate evidence to support the fact that it may be predictive of return to work. There is insufficient evidence to determine whether monetary compensation or feelings of control at work are predictive of work outcomes (Box II-8-3).

PERSONAL FACTORS

PREVIOUS SURGERY

WHAT PREVIOUS SURGERIES INFLUENCE CLINICAL DECISION MAKING?

Previous surgeries can directly and indirectly impact your clinical decision-making processes. Directly, previous surgeries to the shoulder such as the Mumford procedure, which removes the lateral portion of the clavicle, can impact shoulder biomechanics.

Indirectly, many surgeries, both locally and remotely, can impact shoulder function. Locally, surgery to remove cancerous tissue from the chest or breast can result in pain and motion limitations. Even radiation therapy following breast cancer can result in tissue damage, pain, and limited range of motion both acutely and long after surgery.

Abdominal and chest surgery can limit the result in tissue restriction and limit trunk extension. Lack of thoracic extension can prevent a patient from achieving full extension since the last 10° of shoulder flexion can actually be the result of trunk extension.

Remotely, hysterectomies can impact the production of hormones. Hormone imbalances have been cited as a potential contributing factor impacting adhesive capsulitis.

Like past medical history, a carefully interview that includes questioning regarding past surgeries is critical to gain a full appreciation of all the factors that influence a patient's shoulder symptoms and function.

FAMILY HISTORY

DOES A FAMILY HISTORY OF PATHOLOGY IN THE REGION INFLUENCE YOUR CLINICAL REASONING PROCESS?

A family history of shoulder pain and general medical comorbidities are important information to gather from the patient. Although research is limited, there appears to be a genetic predisposition in some patients with shoulder instability. In addition, studies have shown an increased prevalence of adhesive capsulitis in patients with diabetes mellitus and thyroid disease, which are commonly inherited diseases.

A family or personal history of liver, gallbladder, pancreas, kidney, spleen, lung, and heart disease should also be taken from the patient as these visceral structures can refer pain into the shoulder region.

CHRONICITY OF PAIN

WHAT CENTRAL PROCESSING CHANGES OCCUR THAT INFLUENCE YOUR DECISION MAKING?

Chronic pain in the shoulder region is commonplace. As previously noted, the rate of acute pain that turns into chronic is high. Of patients, 40% will not recovery fully from their shoulder pain and 40% of those who do recover will experience a reoccurrence of shoulder symptoms. Part of the problem lies in the inherent instability of the shoulder region and its relatively poor blood supply, both of which lead to increased susceptibility to injury and poor healing rates. Additionally, alterations in pain perceptions and the body's ability to modulate pain could ultimately impact shoulder mechanics. This is devastating in a region that relies heavily on proper muscle activation and biomechanics to prevent shoulder injury.

HAS MEDICAL TREATMENT BEEN SUCCESSFUL FOR PATIENTS WITH CHRONIC PATHOLOGY IN THE REGION?

The statistics would suggest that conservative medicine has been somewhat ineffective in treating shoulder pain. Surgical outcomes have produced better results and may be a viable alterative for those patients who continue to experience shoulder dysfunction and pain.

DISCUSS HOW CHRONICITY OF SYMPTOMS INFLUENCE YOUR DECISION-MAKING PROCESS.

Initial treatment should focus on reducing inflammation since inflammation alters muscle recruitment. Treatment should then focus on normalizing muscle activation and shoulder biomechanics as quickly as possible. The identification of the source of pain (i.e., rotator cuff tear) is important, but when the symptoms become chronic other factors are preventing proper tissue healing and these must be addressed before the shoulder will fully recover. These factors could include posture, altered muscle recruitment, inflammation, muscle guarding, and biomechanical alterations in remote areas of the body.

DISCUSS HOW THE AUTONOMIC, ENDOCRINE, AND IMMUNE SYSTEMS INFLUENCE DECISION MAKING IN THE REGION

Medicine is now linking the autonomic, endocrine, and immune systems to chronic pain. The shoulder is no different. Pancreas function, thyroid function, and sexual hormone alterations all have been linked to or listed as comorbidities for shoulder adhesive capsulitis. If this is true, then in the future, links may be established tying these functions to other shoulder pathologies as well. The clinician should keep abreast of the findings in other fields of medicine and consider how they relate to orthopedics (Box II-8-4).

BOX II-8-4	**Output Mechanisms**
Autonomic	Recent studies explore the relationship of the autonomic system and shoulder pathology. No conclusive evidence has been provided to date.
Endocrine	The endocrine system is involved in the regulation of body homeostasis. In theory, alterations in endocrine function in the form of changes in thyroid, pancreas, and reproductive hormones can be loosely tied to shoulder pathology such as adhesive capsulitis.
Immune	Lymph nodes are part of the immune system and their removal as a result of breast cancer can indirectly limit shoulder motion and result in altered shoulder biomechanics.

CLINICAL DECISION MAKING CASE STUDY—PATIENT PROFILE

Jeff is a 54-year-old male who comes to you with complaints of right shoulder pain and weakness. These symptoms began insidiously and have been present for the past week. They have been increasing in intensity and in frequency. He complains of a deep diffuse pain in the right shoulder region that comes and goes in waves and with no particular pattern. In addition, he has been complaining of nausea, fatigue, and occasional right pelvic pain. Shoulder motions do not appear to increase or decrease pain, but shoulder pain is his primary complaint at this time and is the reason he is seeking your evaluation. He has no previous history of shoulder symptoms. What are the potential sources of his right shoulder pain.

Answer

The patient is coming to you for shoulder pain, but the shoulder evaluation may come back negative. This is because most normal mechanical motions do not seem to aggravate the symptoms. As part of the reasoning process, the clinician should also consider visceral sources for the cause of the patient's symptoms. For right-sided shoulder pain, the clinician should also consider the liver, lung, and gallbladder as potential visceral sources for the patient's pain. Liver and gallbladder are probably higher on your ranking list due to the location of the symptoms and the connection with nausea. You can rule out lung by asking questions concerning breathing, colds, respiratory disorders, etc. Differentiation between liver and gallbladder can often be made through palpation, a yellow hue in the eyes, and reactions to fatty foods. Fatty foods are problematic for patients with gallbladder problems and the yellow hue in the eyes and skin can be indicative of liver disorders. In any case, the patient should be referred back to his physician to rule out the presence of other visceral pathology.

RED FLAGS THAT REQUIRE REFERRAL TO A MEDICAL PHYSICIAN

WHAT SYMPTOMS ALERT YOU TO PATHOLOGIES THAT MAY REQUIRE A REFERRAL TO A MEDICAL DOCTOR?

- Patient descriptions vary from person to person and should not be the only consideration in the determination of possible visceral involvement.
- Visceral pain has a wide range from sharp and severe to poorly localized and vague.
- Visceral pain should not be related to positions/movements of shoulder structures and should not respond to appropriate mechanical treatment.
- Rest or position should not relieve visceral pain.
- In patients with visceral or nonmusculoskeletal involvement it is a common complaint that their pain is constant and nonvarying.
- Complaints of increased pain at night is also an indicator of possible visceral involvement. Considerable walking, pacing, and sitting up are commonly required to return to sleep.

SUMMARY STATEMENT

The shoulder region is often a difficult region for rehabilitation clinicians to assess and subsequently treat. The reasons for this difficulty are in part the result of inherent the instability in the region, the poor vascularity, the dependence on the coordinated activity of muscles and tendons, and the number of structures that can refer into the region or pass through the region. The complexity of the region is apparent when you look at the

TABLE II-8-6 Body Structure and Tissue-Based Pathology (Nociceptive and Peripheral Neurogenic Pain)

	Muscles	Bones	Cartilage	Labrum	Capsule	Tendons	Ligaments	Nerves	Visceral Tissues
Pathologies	Pectoral strain Rotator cuff tear	Hill-Sachs lesion Humeral fracture Clavicular fracture	Glenohumeral osteoarthritis	Labral tear SLAP lesion Bankart lesion	Adhesive capsulitis	Bicep tendinopathy Rotator cuff tendinopathy	AC joint separation Shoulder dislocation/subluxation Shoulder instability	Long thoracic Suprascapular Brachial plexus Thoracic outlet Axillary	Heart Lungs Liver Gallbladder Pancreas Spleen
Age	Trauma: 20 to 30 years old Degenerative: over 60 years old	Fractures: Older than 60 years old Contusions: any age	Older than 60 years	Trauma: 20 to 30 years old Degenerative: over 60 years old	Trauma: 20 to 30 years old Adhesive capsulitis: over 50 years old	Trauma: 20 to 30 years old Degenerative: over 60 years old	20 to 30 years old	Any age	Any age
Occupation	Trauma: sports or activity related Degenerative: occupations requiring repetitive overhead activities	May be but not necessarily related to sports or activity related	Years of shoulder and upper extremity use	Trauma: sports or activity related Degenerative: years of overuse	Overhead sports or activity related	Overhead sports or activity related	Overhead sports or activity related	No correlation established although occupations that required repetitive cervical extension may predispose for nerve irritation	No correlation established
Gender	No correlation noted	Females are more prone due to osteoporosis	No correlation noted	No correlation noted	Females are more prone to adhesive capsulitis	No correlation noted	No correlation noted	No correlation noted	
Ethnicity	No correlation noted	Caucasian and Asians are more prone	No correlation noted	No correlation noted	No correlation noted	No correlation noted	No correlation noted	No correlation noted	
History	May have history of previous muscle strains or shoulder pain	May have history of osteopenia	May have history of upper extremity surgery or injury	Trauma: no previous history Degenerative: may have history of upper extremity surgery or injury	Females may have history of hysterectomy or hormone imbalances	May have history of slowly increasing shoulder pain associated with increase in activity	Usually related to trauma, no previous history is necessary	May have previous history of neck or upper extremity injury	May have history of cardiac, pulmonary, or thyroid pathology
Mechanism of injury	Usually related to forced eccentric contraction of the injured muscle, but can be related to repetitive overuse	Usually related to trauma such as a fall onto the shoulder or outstretched arm	May be related to trauma such as a fall, but generally related to repetitive overuse	Usually related to trauma such as a fall onto the outstretched arm or forced contraction of the biceps	May be insidious but will often report surgery or injury to the shoulder that triggered a capsular response	Generally related to repetitive overhead activities	Usually related to trauma such as a fall onto the shoulder or outstretched arm	May be related to trauma to an outstretched arm, can be related to repetitive overuse	Not correlated to a particular mechanism

Continued on following page.

Section II

ORTHOPEDIC REASONING

TABLE II-8-6 Body Structure and Tissue-Based Pathology (Nociceptive and Peripheral Neurogenic Pain) *(Continued)*

	Muscles	Bones	Cartilage	Labrum	Capsule	Tendons	Ligaments	Nerves	Visceral Tissues
Type of onset	Generally sudden onset	Generally sudden onset	Generally, slow gradual onset	Sudden or gradual onset	Generally, slow gradual onset	Generally, slow gradual onset	Generally sudden onset	Generally, slow gradual onset	May be sudden or gradual
Referral to local tissue	May refer into shoulder, neck, or thoracic spine	Generally localized to the shoulder	Generally localized to the shoulder	Generally localized to the anterior shoulder	Generally localized to the shoulder	Generally localized to the shoulder, neck, or thoracic spine	Generally localized to the shoulder	Nerves entrapped at the shoulder can refer pain proximally or distally	Can be localized to the region adjacent to injured tissue
Referral to other regions	May refer into the upper extremity depending on muscle	May refer into the upper arm	May refer into the upper arm	May refer into the biceps muscle	May refer into the upper arm	May refer into the upper or lower arm	Generally does not refer past the shoulder	Can refer into the upper extremity or neck depending on the involved nerve	May refer into the shoulder, arm, neck, thoracic spine, or head depending on tissue
Changes in symptoms	Immediate pain and inability to use muscle	Fractures: immediate pain and inability to use arm Contusion: immediate pain and difficulty using arm	Gradual increase in symptoms over several weeks or months	Trauma: immediate pain and difficulty using arm Degenerative: slow increase in symptoms over weeks or months	Slow increase in symptoms over weeks or months	Slow increase in symptoms over weeks or months Tendon ruptures will result in immediate loss of function	Immediate pain and instability noted; some loss of function may be noted	Trauma: immediate pain, numbness, and burning with eventual return of function over several minutes to hours Nontraumatic: slow increase in symptoms over weeks or months	May be slow increase or sudden onset with gradual increase May be episodic in nature
24-hour pain pattern (morning)	Pain throughout the day; activity dependent	Pain throughout the day; activity dependent	Stiff for several minutes on awakening	Stiff for several minutes on awakening	Stiff for a long time in the morning	Stiff for several minutes on awakening	May or may not be painful in the morning	May be numb in the morning depending on sleep position	May or may not be better depending on tissue
24-hour pain pattern (afternoon)	Pain throughout day; activity dependent	Pain throughout day; activity dependent	Better with use but sore with overuse	Symptoms are activity dependent	May be better with use but worsen with overuse	May be better with use but worsen with overuse	Symptoms are activity dependent	May be better with use but worsen with overuse	May or may not be better depending on the tissue

24-hour pain pattern (evening)	Pain throughout day; activity dependent	Pain throughout day; activity dependent Throbbing at night	May be painful at night	Symptoms are activity dependent	May be painful and throbbing at night	Symptoms are activity dependent	Symptoms are activity dependent	Symptoms may worsen at night
Description of symptoms	Sharp pain	Achiness	Achiness, grinding, and crepitus	Sharp pain and catching	Achiness	Sharp pain	Sharp pain	Numbness, tingling, weakness
Depth of symptoms	Superficial or deep	Deep	Deep	Superficial	Deep	Superficial or deep	Superficial or deep	Superficial or deep
Constancy of symptoms	Intermittent	Constant but varying	Intermittent	Intermittent	Constant but varying or intermittent	Intermittent	Intermittent	Intermittent or constant but varying
Aggravating factors	Use of injured muscle	Activities that put pressure on injured bone	Overhead activities and weight-bearing activities	Use of biceps for carrying, reaching behind back, or reaching overhead	Overhead activities, reaching behind back	Overhead activities	Overhead or weight-bearing activities	Repetitive use of the arm or hand
Easing factors	Rest Antiinflammatories Ice	Rest Antiinflammatories Ice	Rest Antiinflammatories Gentle range of motion exercises	Rest Antiinflammatories Ice	Rest Antiinflammatories Gentle range of motion exercises	Rest Antiinflammatories Ice	Rest Antiinflammatories Ice	Rest Gentle range of motion exercises Splinting to prevent overuse
Stability of symptoms	Pain increases for first 3 days and slow improvement over 6-week period	Pain increases for first 3 days and slow improvement over 8-week period	Symptoms will wax and wane depending on use Slow increase in symptoms over time	Depends on size of injury Small injuries should improve over 6-week period Larger defects will not get better	May take weeks to over a year to improve Symptoms will wax and wane over that period	Depends on size of injury Pain increases for first 3 days and slow improvement over 6-week period Larger injuries may not improve	Should improve over the course of 6 to 8 weeks	Should improve over the course of 6 to 8 weeks
Past medical history	Usually on dominant hand	Osteoporosis, osteopenia, steroid use	Rheumatoid arthritis, autoimmune disorders	Usually on dominant hand	Hormone imbalances, autoimmune disorders	Steroid use	Steroid use	Cervical or arm pathology, cancer, radiation, or chemotherapy

Additional rightmost column:

24-hour pain pattern (evening)	Symptoms may worsen at night
Description of symptoms	Achiness, cramping, heaviness, difficulty breathing
Depth of symptoms	Deep
Constancy of symptoms	Constant, unremitting, or episodic
Aggravating factors	Not activity dependent
Easing factors	Not activity dependent
Stability of symptoms	Waxes and wanes with no particular time frame
Past medical history	Cardiac, pulmonary, or thyroid pathology, cancer, radiation, or chemotherapy

TABLE II-8-6 **Body Structure and Tissue-Based Pathology (Nociceptive and Peripheral Neurogenic Pain)** (*Continued*)

	Muscles	Bones	Cartilage	Labrum	Capsule	Tendons	Ligaments	Nerves	Visceral Tissues
Past surgeries	Not directly related	Not directly related	Not directly related	Not directly related	Hysterectomy	Not directly related	Not directly related	Shoulder, neck, or thoracic surgery	Not directly related
Special questions	Strength loss Bruising	Deep Ache Bruising	Crepitus	Catching	Hysterectomy Hormones	Strength loss Repetitive use	Traumatic injury	Numbness and tingling	Deep unremitting pain
X-rays	Negative	Positive for fracture Negative for contusion	Negative	Negative	Negative	Negative	Negative	Negative	Negative
MRI	Positive	Positive	Positive	Positive	Negative	Positive	Positive	May or may not be positive	May or may not be positive
EMG	Negative	Negative	Negative	Negative	Negative	Negative	Negative	Positive	Negative
Special laboratory tests	Not applicable	Not applicable	Blood work to rule out rheumatoid factors	Not applicable	Blood work to rule out rheumatoid factors	Not applicable	Not applicable	Not applicable	Varies and is dependent on suspected pathology
Red flags	Unremitting pain, weight loss, nocturnal pain								

MRI, magnetic resonance imaging; EMG, electromyogram.

number of patients who fail conservative treatment. Often discovering the source of tissue symptoms, such as the supraspinatus tendon, is not as important as discovering the factors that prevent it from proper healing, such as scapular dyskinesia. A tissue-based assessment is often the driving diagnosis behind the evaluative process. The failure of rehabilitation regarding shoulder pathology may signal the need to focus more on the contributing factors behind shoulder pain and less on the actual tissue source of pain. Table II-8-6 summarizes the factors that help a clinician differentiate among different sources of symptoms in the shoulder region.

REFERENCES

1. Bradley JP, Elkousy H. Decision making: operative versus nonoperative treatment of acromioclavicular joint injuries. *Clin Sports Med*. 2003;22:277-290.
2. Bryant D, Litchfield R, Sandow M, et al. A Comparison of Pain, Strength, Range of Motion, and Functional Outcomes After Hemiarthroplasty and Total Shoulder Arthroplasty in Patients with Osteoarthritis of the Shoulder. A Systematic Review and Meta-Analysis. *J Bone Joint Surg*. 2005;87:1947-1956.
3. Burbank KM, Stevenson JH, Czarnecki GR, et al. Chronic Shoulder Pain: Part I. Evaluation. *Am Fam Physician*. 2008;77(4):453-460.
4. Burbank KM, Stevenson JH, Czarnecki GR, Dorfman J. Chronic Shoulder Pain: Part II: Treatment. *Am Fam Physician*. 2008;77(4):493-497.
5. Calis M, Akgun K, Birtane M, et al. Diagnostic values of clinical diagnostic tests in subacromial impingement syndrome. *Ann Rheum Dis*. 2000;59(1):44-47.
6. Chambler AFW, Carr AJ. The role of surgery in frozen shoulder. *J Bone Joint Surg*. 2003;85(6):789-795.
7. Dodson CC, Cordasco FA. Anterior glenohumeral joint dislocations. *Orthop Clin N Am*. 2008;39:507-518.
8. Dowdy PA, O'Driscoll SW. Shoulder Instability: An analysis of family history. *J Bone Joint Surg (Br)*. 1993;75-B:782-784.
9. Edenbichler GR, Erdogmus CB, Resch KL, et al. Ultrasound therapy for calcific tendonitis of the shoulder. *N Engl J Med*. 1999;340:1533-1538.
10. Farber AJ, Castillo RC, Clough M, et al. Clinical assessment of three common tests for traumatic anterior shoulder instability. *J Bone Joint Surg Am*. 2006;88(7):1467-1474.
11. Favard L, Bacle G, Berhouet J. Rotator cuff repair. *Joint Bone Spine*. 2007;74:551-557.
12. Gill TJ, Micheli LJ, Gebhard F, et al. Bankart repair for anterior instability of the shoulder. *J Bone Joint Surg*. 1997;79(6):850-857.
13. Ginn KA, Cohen ML. Conservative treatment for shoulder pain: prognostic indicators of outcome. *Arch Phys Med Rehabil*. 2004;85:1231-1235.
14. Goud A, Segal D, Hedayati P, et al. Radiographic evaluation of the shoulder. *Eur J Radiol*. 2008;68:2-15.
15. Greis PE, Kuhn JE, Schultheis J, et al. Validation of the lift-off test and analysis of subscapularis activity during maximal internal rotation. *Am J Sports Med*. 1996;24(5):589-593.
16. Guanche CA, Jones DC. Clinical testing for tears of the glenoid labrum. *Arthroscopy*. 2003;19(5):517-523.
17. Gursel YK, Ulus Y, Bilgic A, et al. Adding ultrasound in the management of soft tissue disorders of the shoulder: a randomized placebo-controlled trial. *Phys Ther*. 2004;84:336-343.
18. Hand C, Clipsham K, Rees JL, et al. Long-term outcome of frozen shoulder. *J Shoulder Elbow Surg*. 2008;17:231-235.
19. Hawkins RJ, Kennedy JC. Impingement syndrome in athletes. *Am J Sports Med*. 1980;8(3):151-158.
20. Hester P, Caborn DN, Nyland J. Causes of long thoracic nerve palsy: a possible dynamic fascial sling cause. *J Shoulder Elbow Surg*. 2000;9(1):31-35.
21. Holtby R, Razmjou H. Accuracy of the Speed's and Yergason's tests in detecting biceps pathology and SLAP lesions: comparison with arthroscopic findings. *Arthroscopy*. 2004;20:231-232.
22. Holtby R, Razmjou H. Validity of the supraspinatus test as a single clinical test in diagnosing patients with rotator cuff pathology. *J Orthop Sports Phys Ther*. 2004;34(4):194-200.
23. Iannotti JP, Zlatkin MB, Esterhai JL, et al. Magnetic resonance imaging of the shoulder. Sensitivity, specificity, and predictive value. *J Bone Joint Surg*. 1991;73-A:17-29.
24. Iles RA, Davidson M, Taylor NF. Psychosocial predictors of failure to return to work in non-chronic non-specific low back pain: a systematic review. *Occup Environ Med*. 2008;65:507-517.
25. Itoi E, Kido T, Sano A, et al. Which is more useful, the "full can test" or the "empty can test," in detecting the torn supraspinatus tendon? *Am J Sports Med*. 1999;27(1):65-68.
26. Jobe CM. Superior glenoid impingement. Current concepts. *Clin Orthop Relat Res*. 1996;330:98-107.
27. Jones GL, Galluch DB. Clinical assessment of superior glenoid labral lesions: a systematic review. *Clin Orthop Relat Res*. 2007;455:45-51.
28. Jost B, Pfirrmann CWA, Gerber C, et al. Clinical outcome after structural failure of rotator cuff repairs. *J Bone Joint Surg*. 2000;82(3):304-314.
29. Kibler WB, McMullen J. Scapular dyskinesias and its relation to shoulder pain. *J Am Acad Orthop Surg*. 2003;11(2):142-151.
30. Kibler WB. Specificity and sensitivity of the anterior slide test in throwing athletes with superior glenoid labral tears. *Arthroscopy*. 1995;11(3):296-300.
31. Kibler WB, Andrews JR, Morgan CD. *The painful throwing shoulder anterior instability versus posterior tightness*. Presented at the Annual Meeting of The American Orthopaedic Society for Sports Medicine, Quebec, Canada, June 24-27, 2004.
32. Kim SH, Ha KI, Ahn JH, et al. Biceps load test II: a clinical test for SLAP lesions of the shoulder. *Arthroscopy*. 2001;17(2):160-164.
33. Kim SH, Ha KI, Han KY. Biceps load test: a clinical test for superior labrum anterior and posterior lesions in shoulders with recurrent anterior dislocations. *Am J Sports Med*. 1999;27(3):300-303.
34. Kim YS, Kim JM, Ha KY, et al. The passive compression test. A new clinical test for superior labral tears of the shoulder. *Am J Sports Med*. 2007;35(9):1489-1494.
35. Kuijpers T, van der Windt DAWM, Boeke AJP, Twisk JWR, et al. Clinical prediction rules for the prognosis of shoulder pain in general practice. *Pain*. 2006;120:276-285.
36. Leroux JL, Thomas E, Bonnel F, et al. Diagnostic value of clinical tests for shoulder impingement syndrome. *Rev Rheum Engl Ed*. 1995;62(6):423-428.
37. Lintner SA, Levy A, Kenter K, et al. Glenohumeral translation in the asymptomatic athlete's shoulder and its relationship to other clinically measurable anthropometric variables. *Am J Sports Med*. 1996;24(6):716-720.
38. Liu SH, Henry MH, Nuccion SL. A prospective evaluation of a new physical examination in predicting glenoid labral tears. *Am J Sports Med*. 1996;24(6):721-725.
39. Lo IK, Nonweiler B, Woolfrey M, Litchfield R, Kirkley A. An evaluation of the apprehension, relocation, and surprise tests for anterior shoulder instability. *Am J Sports Med*. 2004;32(3):301-307.
40. Lo IKY, Litchfield RB, Griffin S, et al. Quality-of-Life Outcome Following Hemiarthroplasty or Total Shoulder Arthroplasty in Patients with Osteoarthritis. A Prospective, Randomized Trial. *J Bone Joint Surg*. 2005;87:2178-2185.
41. MacDonald PB, Clark P, Sutherland K. An analysis of the diagnostic accuracy of the Hawkins and Neer subacromial impingement signs. *J Shoulder Elbow Surg*. 2000;9(4):299-301.
42. MacDonald PB, Lapointe P. Acromioclavicular and sternoclavicular joint injuries. *Orthop Clin N Am*. 2008;39:535-545.
43. McCredie J, Willert HG. Longitudinal limb deficiencies and sclerotomes. *J Bone Joint Surg (Br)*. 1999;81 B:9-23.
44. McFarland EG, Campbell G, McDowell J. Posterior shoulder laxity in asymptomatic athletes. *Am J Sports Med*. 1996;24(4):468-471.
45. McFarland EG, Kim TK, Savino RM. Clinical assessment of three common tests for superior labral anterior-posterior lesions. *Am J Sports Med*. 2002;30(6):810-815.
46. McFarland EG. *Examination of the shoulder: the complete guide*. New York: Thieme; 2006.
47. McFarland EG. Instability and laxity. In: Kim TK, Park HB, El Rassi G, et al., eds. *Examination of the shoulder: the complete guide*. New York: Thieme; 2006:162-212.
48. McFarland EF, Kim TK, Savino RM. Clinical assessment of three common tests for superior labral tears of the shoulder. *Am J Sports Med*. 2002;30:810-815.
49. McMenamin D, Koulouris G, Morrison WB. Imaging of the shoulder after surgery. *Eur J Radiol*. 2008;68:106-119.
50. Mimori K, Muneta T, Nakagawa T, et al. A new pain provocation test for superior labral tears of the shoulder. *Am J Sports Med*. 1999;27(2):137-142.

51. Morgan CD, Burkhart SS, Palmeri M, et al. Type II SLAP lesions: three subtypes and their relationships to superior instability and rotator cuff tears. *Arthroscopy*. 1998;14(6):553-565.

52. Myers TH, Zemanovic JR, Andrews JR. The resisted supination external rotation test: a new test for the diagnosis of superior labral anterior posterior lesions. *Am J Sports Med*. 2005;33(9):1315-1320.

53. Nakagawa S, Yoneda M, Hayashida K, et al. Forced shoulder abduction and elbow flexion test: a new simple clinical test to detect superior labral injury in the throwing shoulder. *Arthroscopy*. 2005;21(11):1290-1295.

54. Norkin CC, Levangie PK. *The shoulder complex. Joint Structure and Function: A Comprehensive Analysis*. 2nd ed. Philadelphia: F.A. Davis Company; 1992.

55. O'Brien SJ, Pagnani MJ, Fealy S, et al. The active compression test: a new and effective test for diagnosing labral tears and acromioclavicular joint abnormality. *Am J Sports Med*. 1998;26(5):610-613.

56. Odom CJ, Taylor AB, Hurd CE, Denegar CR. Measurement of scapular asymmetry and assessment of shoulder dysfunction using the Lateral Scapular Slide Test: a reliability and validity study. *Phys Ther*. 2001;81:799-809.

57. Oh JH, Kim JY, Kim WS, et al. The evaluation of various physical examinations for the diagnosis of type II superior labrum anterior and posterior lesion. *Am J Sports Med*. 2008;36(2):353-359.

58. Ostor AJK, Richards CA, Prevost TA, et al. Diagnosis and relation to general health of shoulder disorders presenting to primary care. *Rheumatology*. 2005;44:800-805.

59. Parentis MA, Glousman RE, Mohr KS, et al. An evaluation of the provocative tests for superior labral anterior posterior lesions. *Am J Sports Med*. 2006;34(2):265-268.

60. Park HB, Yokota A, Gill HS, et al. Diagnostic accuracy of clinical tests for the different degrees of subacromial impingement syndrome. *J Bone Joint Surg Am*. 2005;87(7):1446-1455.

61. Petilon J, Carr DR, Sekiya JK, Unger DV. Pectoralis Major Muscle Injuries: Evaluation and Management. *J Am Acad Orthop Surg*. 2005;13(1):59-68.

62. Rhudy JL, Meagher MW. The role of emotion in pain modulation. Review Article. *Curr Opin Psychiatry*. 2001;14(3):241-245.

63. Robertson VJ, Baker KG. A review of therapeutic ultrasound: effectiveness studies. *Phys Ther*. 2001;81:1339-1350.

64. Sher JS, Iannotti JP, Williams GR, et al. The effect of shoulder magnetic resonance imaging on clinical decision making. *J Shoulder Elbow Surg*. 1998;7:205-209.

65. Speer KP, Hannafin JA, Altchek DW, et al. An evaluation of the shoulder relocation test. *Am J Sports Med*. 1994;22(2):177-183.

66. Stetson WB, Templin K. The crank test, the O'Brien test, and routine magnetic resonance imaging scans in the diagnosis of labral tears. *Am J Sports Med*. 2002;30(6):806-809.

67. Stevenson JH, Trojian T. Evaluation of shoulder pain. *J Fam Pract*. 2002;51:605-611.

68. Travell JG, Simons DG. *Myofascial Pain and Dysfunction: The Trigger Point Manual*. Baltimore: The Upper Extremities. Williams & Wilkins; 1983.

69. Van der Windt DAWM, Koes BW, Boeke AJP, Deville W, de Jong BA, Bouter LM. Shoulder disorders in general practice: prognostic indicators of outcome. *Br J Gen Prac*. 1996;46:519-523.

70. Van der Windt DAWM, Koes BWK, de Jong BAD, et al. Shoulder disorders in general practice: incidence, patient characteristics, and management. *Ann Rheum Dis*. 1995;54:959-964.

71. Wofford JL, Mansfield RJ, Watkins RS. Patient characteristics and clinical management of patients with shoulder pain in US primary care settings: Secondary data analysis of the National Ambulatory Medical Care Survey. *BMC*. 2005;6:4-9.

72. Panjabi MM, Lydon C, Vasavada A, Grob D, Crisco JJ, Dvorak J. On the understanding of clinical instability. *Spine*. 1994;19:2642-2650.

AUTHOR: CHRIS A. SEBELSKI

INTRODUCTORY INFORMATION

The elbow region is often overlooked in terms of pathology. Clinically, it is seen far less frequently than other regions of the body such as the shoulder, knee, or spine. From a diagnostic and rehabilitation standpoint, it is often a difficult region to treat. Overuse injuries are often resistant to rehabilitation efforts and recovery from fractures often requires long rehabilitation timeframes. Small injuries to the elbow will often result in long-term loss of motion and function. The key to rehabilitation and recovery is a firm understanding of the tissue pathology underlying the symptoms.

WHAT IS THE PREVALENCE OF ELBOW PATHOLOGY?

- The elbow is the second most common dislocated joint in adults, with posterior dislocation being the most common.[60] It is the most commonly dislocated joint in the pediatric age group.[38] Associated injuries such as fractures occur in the young and or with advanced age whereas noncomplex dislocations most commonly occur in younger, athletic populations.[48]
- The incidence of elbow fractures is from 10% to 14% in children 16 years and under.[40] The specific prevalence of all types of elbow fractures in adults is unknown, although 50% of upper extremity injuries in adults admitted to the hospital are fractures of some type.[9]
  - ○ Specifically, fractures of the radial head and neck are estimated to account for 1.7% to 5.4% of all fractures representing approximately 33% of the fractures involving the elbow. They represent one third of all fractures involving the elbow.[8,26,44]
- Epicondylar injury has been suggested to occur in 50% of athletes participating in overhead sports.[32] Lateral epicondylar pain, in particular, has been seen in 1% to 3% of the general population and up to 15% for those in an at-risk profession.[3,4] Medial epicondylar pain is less common than lateral epicondylar pain (up to 20% of cases reported) with the majority of cases occurring during the fourth and fifth decades.[10]
- The upper extremity is at high risk for neural injury. Injury to the ulnar nerve as it travels through the cubital tunnel (cubital tunnel syndrome) is the second most common nerve injury of the upper extremity, especially with overhead athletes.[50]
- Primary degenerative arthritis of the elbow is relatively uncommon.[1]
- Olecranon septic bursitis is considered to be "not rare," with 0.6 to 1.2 per 1000 admissions.[31]
- Forearm compartment syndrome has been reported with distal radius fractures at 0.25% and 3.1% for diaphyseal fractures of the forearm.[47]

WHAT IS THE PROGNOSIS FOR RECOVERY FROM ELBOW PATHOLOGY?

According to the study by Bot et al,[6] "not much is known about the prognosis of elbow complaints after presentation in general practice." Overall, the greatest risk to full recovery is residual discomfort and limitation to range of motion.

Based on the diagnosis, the following information was found.
- Simple elbow dislocations have a good prognosis with up to 95% of persons affected returning to their previous level of activity.[30]
- Outcomes for neural injury of the elbow are dependent on the staging of the injury before instituting treatment.[50] Such staging systems are still evolving, with current treatments a mixture of nonoperative and operative managements.

- The prognosis for epicondylar injuries includes resolution of symptoms from this potentially self-limiting disorder within 3 months with or without intervention.[3] Complicating factors and therefore a potentially poorer prognosis include concomitant neck and shoulder pain, high occupational physical work, high baseline pain,[24] and/or a longer duration of elbow symptoms.[65]
- In a single study by Rettig et al,[58] throwers with chronic medial instability were treated nonoperatively. They achieved a 42% success rate in returning the athlete to sport. None of the subjective or physical examination measures taken could successfully predict with any significance which patient would benefit from nonoperative therapy.
- Harrington et al[27] tracked patients for 12 years following postsurgical repair of complex radial head fractures with an 80% good to excellent rate overall. The average range of motion was an arc of 17° to 120° of flexion, 74° of pronation, and 65° of supination. There was an overall reduction in muscle strength of up to 20%.

CLINICAL PEARL

Specific prognostic data for each fracture type of the elbow are difficult. Communication with the surgeon and/or orthopedist, imaging, and surgical reports are essential for optimizing prognosis. Consideration for prognosis should include the complexity of the injury, presence of intraarticular fracture, concomitant injuries along the ipsilateral extremity, type of surgical approach, and the length of immobilization.

CLINICAL PEARL

Radial fractures are classified with the Mason Johnston classification system. Type I is a nondisplaced fracture. Type II is a displaced fracture with an impact of the articular cartilage. Type III is a comminuted fracture type involving the entire radial head and Type IV is associated with ulnohumeral dislocation and is now considered part of the spectrum for complex elbow instability. Simple radial fractures are treated according to the Mason Johnston classification; however, treatment of the more complex injuries are guided by the associated injuries.[33]

WHAT IS THE RECURRENCE RATE FOR ELBOW PATHOLOGY?

- Recurring instability following a simple dislocation is rare.[30] Instability following a more complex dislocation occurs in up to 17% of cases.[34]
- It has been suggested that of the overhead athletes with lateral epicondylalgia, 90% will have no further recurrence.[35] However, Binder and Hazleman[2] reported a recurrence rate of 26% with over 40% of the patients have lingering minor discomfort.
- In a study by Mowlavi et al,[50] "minimal to moderate stage" patients with cubital tunnel syndrome who were treated nonoperatively had the greatest rate of recurrence.

CLINICAL PEARL

Despite the apparent success of treatment of lateral epicondylar pain, this is one of the most difficult disorders to treat due to challenges in identifying the structural source of the complaint and the contributing cause. Causes may be related to structural deficits such as an underlying instability or neural compression or it may be related more to interregional dependence issues such as inadequate proximal flexibility or stability.

Section II ORTHOPEDIC REASONING

WHAT FACTORS MAKE DIAGNOSIS DIFFICULT IN THE ELBOW REGION?

- Elbow dysfunction rarely occurs in isolation.[72] The clinician must determine the role of interregional dependence and referred pain in determining the diagnosis.
- Epicondylar symptoms are common in the elbow; however, the underlying mechanism by which the tendinous attachment becomes inflamed or degenerates needs to be explored by the clinician with considerations for local instability and interregional dependence.
- Due to the structural proximity and the ambiguity of the symptoms, it is frequently difficult to assess the true structure that is the source of the symptoms.

HOW SUCCESSFUL IS THERAPY IN TREATING ELBOW PATHOLOGY?

- It has been reported that nonoperative intervention for epicondylar pain may be successful in 88% to 96% of cases.[17] Binder and Hazleman[2] reported a recurrence rate of 26% and report that over 40% of the patients continue to demonstrate minor discomfort. An in-depth systematic review found less than promising results when attempting to determine the success of specific interventions for the treatment of epicondylar pain and determined the evidence is inconclusive even when compared to a "wait and see" approach to care.[3,4]
- Nonoperative management of patients with cubital tunnel syndrome whose presentations include intermittent paresthesias and subjective complaints of weakness/clumsiness among other physical signs will respond to therapy with 65% achieving total relief.[50]
- Radial head elbow fractures of Mason Type II, III, and IV demonstrate degenerative changes without joint space reduction over time. This was regardless of treatment and did not correlate well with symptoms.[29]

CLINICAL PEARL

Even patients with trivial elbow traumas are at risk for loss of motion. With articular trauma at the elbow there will be a loss of motion. A loss of extension greater than flexion is a risk whether the condition is congenital or acquired, inflammatory or noninflammatory. Rehabilitation of the elbow must be uniquely balanced between early mobilization and the risk of aggravating the injured area.

HOW SUCCESSFUL IS SURGERY IN TREATING ELBOW PATHOLOGY?

- Olecranon fractures are typically addressed via open repair internal fixation. As with all fractures, the more complex the injury, the less favorable the outcome. The fracture pattern influences the timing of the repair, the quality of healing, and the risk of future arthrosis. The presence of any additional ipsilateral upper extremity injuries directly affects elbow function with the patient at a five to six times greater risk for elbow range of motion deficits into flexion and extension, respectively.[59]
- Gabel and Morrey[17] reported that surgical intervention was 87% successful for patients with medial epicondylar pain and mild ulnar nerve compression
- With appropriate preoperative staging based on sensory, motor, and physical examinations, surgical intervention of cubital tunnel via medial epicondylectomy, anterior subcutaneous transposition, or submuscular transposition surgeries is reported to produce the greatest relief for patients. However, patients demonstrating severe symptoms including persistent sensory loss and/or loss of grip/pinch test measures recovered only 78% of normal strength with the best outcomes from surgical decompression.[17,50]

CLINICAL DECISION MAKING CASE STUDY—PATIENT PROFILE

JR is a 38-year-old male who has had elbow surgery for an olecranon fracture following a slip and fall on an icy stairwell. The surgery was performed 1 week ago. During your patient interview, what questions should be included to assist with prognosticating recovery?

Answer
The clinician should request the surgical report from the referring physician and request updated images and/or radiograph reports as they become available. In addition, questions should be asked regarding the amount of time from injury to repair as well as the classification of the injury to determine the complexity of the injury and to assess for any additional ipsilateral extremity injuries.

PERSONAL INFORMATION

WHAT INFLUENCE DOES AGE HAVE ON YOUR CLINICAL DECISION-MAKING PROCESS IN THE ELBOW REGION?

- Below the age of 5 years: nursemaid elbow is the most common of congenital disorders.
- Below the age of 20 years: Panner's disease (ages 6 to 12) osteochondritis dissecans (adolescents), instability, elbow dislocation, and fractures are more common. Epicondylar pain is fairly rare.
- Between 20 and 50 years: instability, epicondylar pain, olecranon bursitis, radial head fractures, forearm compartment syndrome, and rheumatoid arthritis are common.
- Over the age of 50 years: Degenerative conditions are more common as age advances. Consider degenerative joint disease and olecranon bursitis.

WHAT INFLUENCE DOES A PATIENT'S OCCUPATION HAVE ON YOUR CLINICAL DECISION-MAKING PROCESS IN THE ELBOW REGION?

- With lateral epicondylar pain, the focus should not be only on the classification of the occupation as highly strenuous, manual, and/or repetitive, but also consideration should be given to the psychosocial factors within the occupational setting. Psychosocial risk factors at work including organizational issues were found to be of greater importance when the level of physical work risk was greater than if the physical work was considered less of a risk.[13,23]
- Predisposition to injury such as exposure to repeated weight bearing on the elbow has been identified as a risk factor for the development of bursitis.[31]
- Medial instability rarely affects the nonathletic population within their activities of daily living; however, it has a great effect on the performance of the overhead athlete.[21]
- Posterior impingement syndrome is most frequently seen in overhead athletes.[63]

WHAT INFLUENCE DOES GENDER HAVE ON YOUR CLINICAL DECISION-MAKING PROCESS IN THE ELBOW REGION?

- Lateral epicondylar pain: females with poor support within the organizational structure and manual jobs have been implicated as having a higher risk.[23]
- Olecranon bursitis: slight predisposition to males.[31]
- Forearm compartment syndrome: males under 35 years.[47]

WHAT INFLUENCE DOES ETHNICITY HAVE ON YOUR CLINICAL DECISION-MAKING PROCESS IN THE ELBOW REGION?

Specific data regarding ethnicity could not be found related to various elbow pathologies, and ethnicity is generally not considered a major factor when determining the diagnosis at the elbow.

CLINICAL DECISION MAKING CASE STUDY—PATIENT PROFILE

CM is a 48-year-old female who has had lateral elbow pain for the past 2 months. She cannot recall a specific incident, but the onset was at work. She is a machinist at a factory. What are your hypotheses regarding her pathology?

Answer

The information given concerning the location of the pain, gender, and occupation should be the focus of the primary diagnostic list. These three factors should indicate lateral epicondylitis and lateral epicondylalgia as the probable primary diagnoses. Others should include underlying instability and the neural compression syndromes. Further questioning should include an exploration of job tasks and the support network at work.

SYMPTOM HISTORY

WHAT INFLUENCE DOES THE MECHANISM OF INJURY HAVE ON YOUR CLINICAL DECISION-MAKING PROCESS IN THE ELBOW REGION?

- Trauma: In an acute episode, direct trauma would implicate the structures in the region injured, such as fracture, muscular strains, and ligament strains.
- Overuse/repetition: Though these injuries may have acute episodes of pain, they also may have a long history of recurring episodes. The mechanism may be a single episode of short duration with intense activity or long duration of repetitive low-grade intensity.
- Insidious onset: The clinician should consider systemic disease such as infection, arthritic disorders or gout, cervical spine referral, or the initial phases of an overuse injury from long duration activities with low-grade repetitive loads.

LOCATION OF SYMPTOMS

WHAT INFLUENCE DOES THE LOCATION OF SYMPTOMS HAVE ON YOUR CLINICAL DECISION-MAKING PROCESS IN THE ELBOW REGION?

The location of symptoms may be directly related to the anatomical structures in the region under consideration.
- Medial: medial collateral ligament sprain/tear, medial epicondylar pain from the common flexor tendon, flexor/pronator strain, ulnar neuritis within the cubital tunnel
- Lateral: lateral collateral ligament sprain/tear, lateral epicondylar pain from the common extensor tendon, extensor muscle strain, radial head fracture
- Posterior: olecranon bursitis, distal triceps tendinitis, olecranon fracture
- Anterior (cubital fossa): distal biceps tendinitis, distal biceps tendon tear, tear of the brachialis, median nerve compression in the proximal forearm, posterior interosseous nerve compression, coronoid fracture

REFERRAL OF SYMPTOMS

WHAT IS THE REFERRAL PATTERN OF DIFFERENT STRUCTURES IN THE ELBOW REGION?

- Muscles
  - Trigger points within the muscles of the brachioradialis, extensor carpi radialis brevis/longus, and extensor digitorum communis have been shown to produce pain locally within the dorsolateral aspect of the forearm. For patients who present with lateral epicondylalgia, the referral pattern is larger with potential extension into the dorsum of the hand.[16]
  - The supinator may refer pain to the lateral epicondyle.[69]
  - The triceps may refer pain to the medial or lateral epicondyle, depending on which aspect of the muscle is irritated.[69]
- Nerves (Figure II-9-1 for peripheral nerve distribution pattern)
  - Medial cutaneous nerve of the forearm: from the medial cord of the brachial plexus. It gives sensory innervation to the anterior and posterior medial forearm from slightly proximal of the medial epicondyle to the distal radioulnar joint.
  - Musculocutaneous nerve: It gives branches to the lateral cutaneous nerve, which is the sensory innervation from the mid cubital fossa to the lateral, anterior, distal forearm.

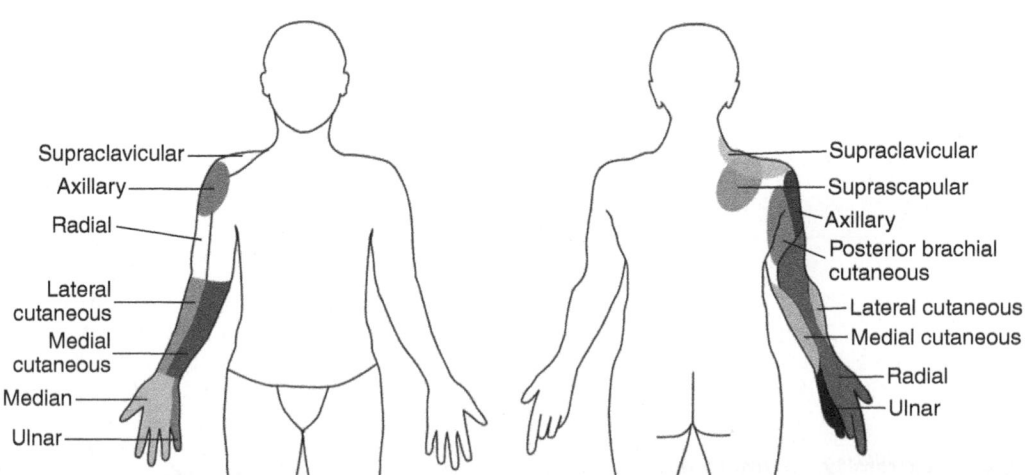

FIGURE II-9-1   Upper extremity peripheral nerve distribution of symptoms. Peripheral nerves, when entrapped or irritated, will commonly refer pain in the following patterns.

○ Median nerve: Entrapment of this nerve and its branches within the forearm as it courses toward the wrist can generate deep forearm aching.

○ Radial nerve: It give branches to the inferior lateral cutaneous nerve and the posterior cutaneous nerve. This is the sensory innervation to a wide area extending from the lateral mid-brachium distally to the mid-lateral forearm to the posterior aspect of the forearm to the distal radius.

○ Posterior interosseous nerve: Impingement of this structure creates localized pain in the region of the extensor mechanism of the forearm.

○ Ulnar nerve: It does not give branches for sensory innervation before its entry into the hand. However, the ulnar nerve may give localized elbow pain and pain into the ulnar nerve distribution via irritation within the cubital tunnel.

- Vessels of the upper extremity: Referral patterns from the individual vessels of the upper extremity were not found in the literature. However, patients diagnosed with aneurysms of the upper extremity vessels presented with a variety of signs and symptoms including the presence of a mass, pain/paresthesia, and/or cold intolerance. The size of the thrombus did not correlate with the presenting signs/symptoms. Symptoms were not attributed directly to the vessel as the pain-producing structure.[22]

- Joint (capsule/cartilage)/ligament: Articular cartilage is aneural; however, the ligaments and the joint capsule are innervated with both myelinated and unmyelinated fibers generating localized pain with injury.[43]

- Bone: No studies have been conducted on the referral pattern of specific bone pathology in the elbow.

- Tendon: It is theorized that there is a biochemical element that may irritate the free endings within the tendon producing pain in the immediate area associated with tendon injury. The specific biochemical factor at this time is unknown.[36]

WHAT STRUCTURES CAN REFER INTO THE ELBOW REGION?

- Cervical spine referral is from nerve roots C5, C6, C8, and T1 (Figure II-9-2).

- Injections into the paravertebral muscles of the neck have induced deep aching pain into various aspects of the upper extremity that extends beyond dermatomal patterns.[15]

- Cardiac referral is potentially into the medial elbow region (Figure II-9-3).

- Rotator cuff pathology typically presents with aching in the anterolateral portion of the brachium that may extend to the level of the elbow.[11]

- In a small study by Hassett and Barnsley,[28] injection of the sternoclavicular joint with saline produced ipsilateral deep elbow pain within 60 seconds of injection.

- In rare instances, somatic pain patterns from the acromioclavicular joint and the subacromial space include the radial and ulnar aspect of the forearm.[19]

SYMPTOM DESCRIPTORS

QUALITY OF SYMPTOMS

Deep ache: Cervical spine[15]
Dull ache: Bone, inflammation
Sharp pain: Capsule, ligament
Sharp and continuous: Bone
Burning: Nerves, inflammation, vein, artery, lymphatic system
Tingling: Nerve
Numbness: Nerve
Colicky and cramping: Viscera
Catching/locking: Loose body, instability

WHAT INFLUENCE DOES THE DEPTH OF SYMPTOMS HAVE ON YOUR CLINICAL DECISION-MAKING PROCESS IN THE ELBOW REGION?

- Deep symptoms implicate structures such as the cervical spine (disc, muscular, or ligamentous structures), deep structures such as bone within the local region, and/or visceral structures. The symptoms felt from these structures are three dimensional in nature, which limits the ability to localize the sensation to a single tissue.[15]

- Superficial symptoms are typically directly correlated to the local structure such as the muscle, ligament, and skin.

WHAT INFLUENCE DOES THE CONSTANCY OF SYMPTOMS HAVE ON YOUR CLINICAL DECISION-MAKING PROCESS IN THE ELBOW REGION (I.E., CONSTANT VERSUS INTERMITTENT VERSUS CONSTANT BUT VARYING)?

- Intermittent symptoms may be associated with a specific position or activity. This typically implies a mechanical source. True intermittent symptoms are unlikely to be generated by a chemical irritant.

- Constant but varying symptoms: The constancy of the symptom implicates a chemical irritant (inflammation). The variability in intensity of the symptoms indicates a mixture of both

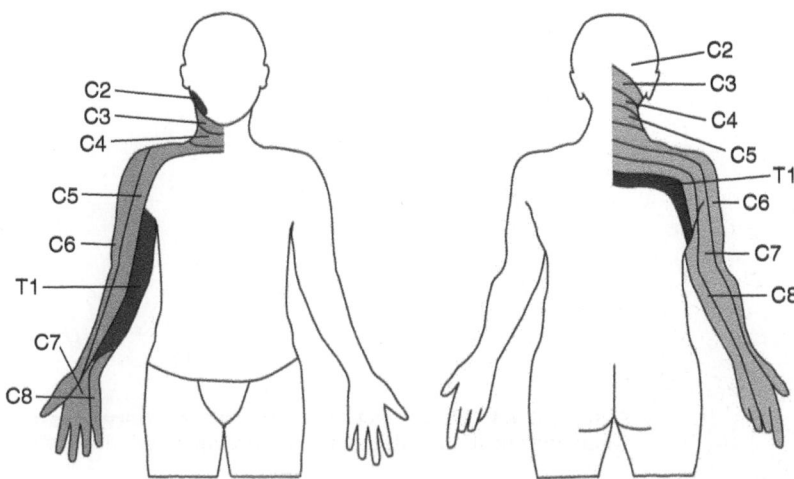

FIGURE II-9-2 Upper extremity dermatomes. Cervical spinal nerves when entrapped or irritated will commonly refer pain in the following pattern. It is important to note that many of the dermatomes overlap distributions.

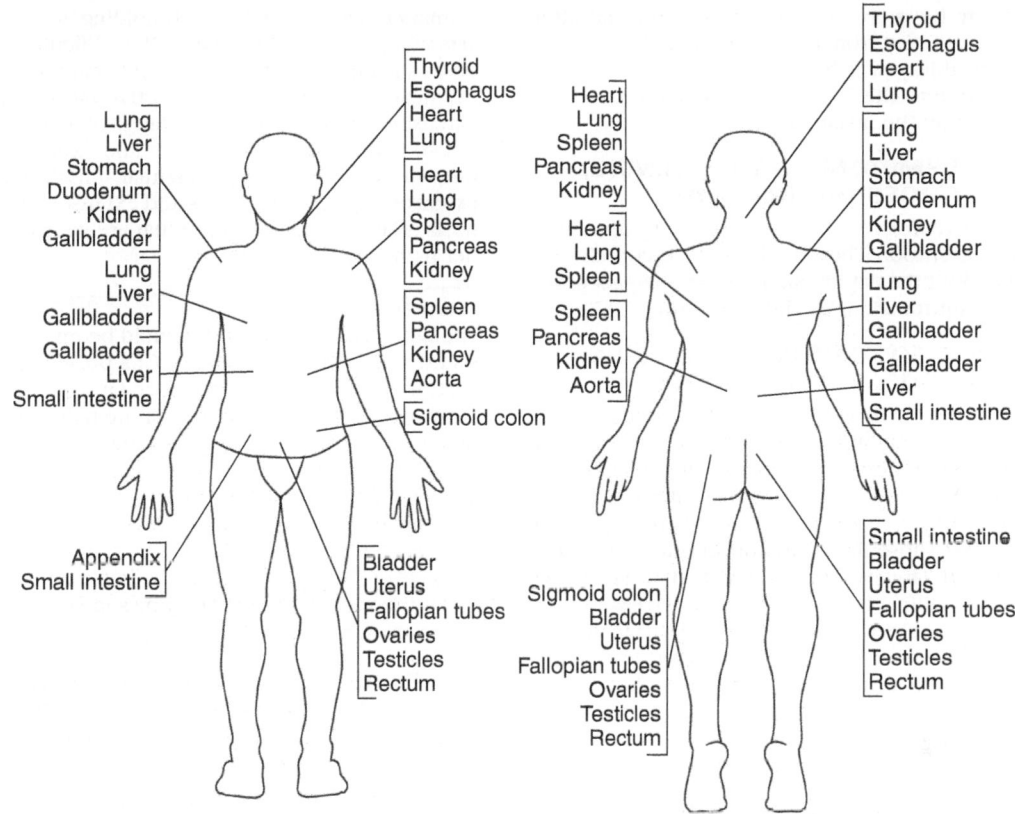

FIGURE II-9-3 Visceral referral pattern. Visceral structures can refer pain into distal regions of the body. Cardiac and pulmonary systems will commonly refer pain into the elbow and forearm region.

mechanical and chemical irritants. The contribution of the mechanical sources gives the appearance of aggravation with specific positions or activity.

- Constant and unchanging symptoms: Again, the constancy of the symptoms implicates an underlying chemical irritant. The unchanging intensity of the symptoms does not implicate a mechanical cause and typically visceral structures or other systemic pathology such as cancer should be considered.

TWENTY-FOUR-HOUR SYMPTOM PATTERN

IF A PATIENT HAS SYMPTOMS IN THE MORNING, WHAT PATHOLOGY DOES THIS IMPLICATE?

- Morning symptoms are not uncommon for patients with musculoskeletal conditions, especially if a chemical irritant is present within the source of the symptoms. During prolonged inactivity such as positioning throughout the night, stasis of the inflammatory condition occurs due to the inactivity of the muscle pump. The muscle pump system assists in moving fluid throughout the body via the vascular system, especially the lymph system. If the condition has a mechanical component then motion will change the symptoms. During the activity or motions of the morning, the muscle pump system is reactivated moving the inflammatory factors out of the region. The symptoms should therefore decrease relatively quickly if generated from mechanical and inflammatory conditions. Instability, epicondylitis, and degenerative disorders should be considered.
- Symptoms of a longer duration (60 minutes) are a sign of a systemic inflammatory condition such as rheumatoid arthritis.

WHAT ROLE DOES MORNING STIFFNESS PLAY IN DIFFERENTIATION?

- Stiffness is typically indicative of an inflammatory condition. Stasis of the fluids of the body may occur any time the body is in a static position for a prolonged period of time. Therefore, to differentiate between the potential diagnoses to which the symptom "stiffness" is attributed, the clinician must clarify the amount of time the stiffness is present. Stiffness that is alleviated relatively quickly is typically attributed to a mechanical irritant. Comments that the stiffness lasts for approximately 15 minutes indicate a chemical irritant where inflammation plays a role. If the symptoms in the morning are protracted and last closer to 60 minutes then the clinician should consider rheumatological disorders.
- Cross-linking of the nonligamentous periarticular tissues following injury or with aging can generate the symptom of stiffness. This will contribute to a reduction in joint range of motion. Engagement in activity or motion reduces this type of stiffness.

IF A PATIENT HAS SYMPTOMS IN THE AFTERNOON, WHAT PATHOLOGY DOES THIS IMPLICATE?

- Symptoms in the afternoon are highly dependent on the activities that were completed throughout the day. Potential sources include muscle, ligament, tendinopathies, and arthrosis.
- Repetitive activities will generate increased aggravation of epicondylar pain. If the symptoms are generated due to a tendinitis, which has an inflammatory component, the activity that stresses the musculotendinous junction will generate symptoms. Symptoms may be prolonged following termination of the activity but they will resolve within a maximum of 48 hours. However, tendinosis may be painful during the activity such that it forces an alteration of the activity. Symptoms of tendinosis will be intermittent in nature and therefore occur during rest without aggravation from a prior activity.[51]

- Muscular injury may be more symptomatic during the afternoon based on the activities from earlier in the day.
- Symptoms from instability will become more pronounced as the day progresses due to the fatigue of the dynamic stabilization system surrounding the instability.

IF A PATIENT HAS SYMPTOMS IN THE EVENING, WHAT PATHOLOGY DOES THIS IMPLICATE?

No particular elbow pathology will generate more symptoms in the evening than the afternoon. The clinician should consider the activities from throughout the day, similar to when the patient has a greater amount of symptoms during the afternoon.

IF A PATIENT HAS SYMPTOMS WHEN SLEEPING, WHAT PATHOLOGY DOES THIS IMPLICATE?

Several factors play a role in the generation of symptoms while sleeping. The position the person assumes may stress the injured segment causing an interruption of the sleep cycle while the person changes positions. If there is a chemical irritant related to the symptoms then the relative inactivity of the sleeping position may cause irritation and subsequent disruption due to the pooling of the inflammation. The patient again will typically awake and change positions, falling back to sleep relatively quickly. However, disruption of the sleep cycle may also be due to visceral or systemic pathology and must be considered, especially if symptoms do not allow for a quick return to sleep.

STABILITY OF SYMPTOMS

HOW DOES THE PROGRESSION OF A PATIENT'S SYMPTOMS IMPACT YOUR CLINICAL DECISION-MAKING PROCESS?

- Muscles, ligaments, and bones have well defined, though complex, phases of healing following injury. The immediate response is inflammation with an observable response such as pain, swelling, redness, and warmth, which is associated with the chemical response of the body and the tissue's vascularity. Structures that are well vascularized have a different and more efficient rate of healing than structures that do not. In clinical presentation, the patient should have an immediate pain response to these injuries that continues throughout the day.
- Tendons and vascularity are being studied. As evidenced in the patellar tendon, areas of the tendon that are nearest to the musculotendinous junction and the insertion into the bone appear to have the greatest vascularity.[74] It is theorized that mid substance injuries will have a different response to injury and healing due to the lack of vascularity.
  - As these mid substance injuries begin to heal, the patient will demonstrate a protracted duration of pain and sensitivity to motion beyond what is expected from a well-vascularized region. Examination of these injuries reveals neovascularization, which is associated with the pain response.[75]
  - Within the clinical examination, the patient should demonstrate a delay in the inflammatory response if the injury is in the mid substance of the tendon. Patients may feel discomfort initially, which then resolves and reoccurs at a later time.
- In the absence of acute trauma, symptoms of peripheral nerve injury typically manifest from irritation to the nerve along its course. As the irritation continues, there may be development into loss of range of motion.[7]

CLINICAL DECISION MAKING CASE STUDY—PATIENT PROFILE

CL is a 36-year-old female with intermittent right cubital crease and lateral forearm pain for the past several months. Her primary functional limitation is holding her infant son in her right arm while feeding him a bottle. It is difficult for her to specify the onset and duration of her pain. Significant findings of the physical examination include a loss of active range of motion with wrist extension and a loss of passive range of motion with wrist flexion. Active end range elbow flexion and extension are both painful but within normal ranges. Manual muscle testing reveals: 3+/5 extensor carpi radialis brevis and extensor carpi ulnaris. The diagnosis is lateral epicondylitis. What are your hypotheses regarding her pathology?

Answer

Though lateral epicondylitis should be on the differential diagnosis list, this is less likely due to CL's presentation. Specifically, the protracted duration of pain (several months) and the lack of specificity regarding the irritability of the pain generate a longer diagnoses list. Lateral epicondylosis and a mid substance muscular strain of the extensors are possible. However, the clinician must also include the radial nerve as a potential source of pathology, not only because of the pathway of the nerve (radial tunnel syndrome and posterior interosseous nerve syndrome) but also because of the innervation of the brachialis and the brachioradialis. Furthermore, the cervical spine should be examined for pathology at the C5 to C6 segment.

IF A PATIENT'S SYMPTOMS ARE IMPROVING, WHAT PATHOLOGY DOES THIS IMPLICATE?

Improvement of symptoms and function are expected with musculoskeletal disorders. The constant pain that follows an acute trauma should demonstrate declining but variable intensity of symptoms when moving through the healing phases.

IF A PATIENT'S SYMPTOMS ARE WORSENING, WHAT PATHOLOGY DOES THIS IMPLICATE?

- Neural injury may initially manifest as symptoms only from irritation to the nerve along its course. If the initial insult is not identified, then loss of range of motion may occur as the dysfunction progresses and changes the nerve pathomechanics.
- Degenerative disorders may demonstrate initial improvement; however, as the disease process progresses, the symptoms will return. This may continue for many months.

IF A PATIENT'S SYMPTOMS ARE NOT CHANGING, WHAT PATHOLOGY DOES THIS IMPLICATE?

- Medial and lateral epicondylar pain often see immediate improvement with intervention for the inflammation of the soft tissues; however, if the underlying cause of the dysfunction goes untreated the patient's progress will often plateau and eventually return to the initial status.
- Lack of change of symptoms may be seen with articular cartilage injury.
- Long duration of symptoms before entering into therapy forces the clinician to investigate episodic pain of a chronic disorder. Tendinopathies and neural pathology should be considered.

FUNCTIONAL AND ACTIVITY PARTICIPATION LIMITATIONS (Table II-9-1)

BEHAVIOR OF SYMPTOMS: AGGRAVATING BEHAVIOR

WHAT INFLUENCE DOES AGGRAVATING FUNCTIONS HAVE ON YOUR CLINICAL DECISION-MAKING PROCESS IN THE ELBOW REGION?

Flexion-based activities

- Pathologies implicated by elbow flexion-based activities include biceps brachialis, brachialis, and brachioradialis strain, capsulitis,

TABLE II-9-1　Functional and Activity Participation Limitations

Motion	Functional Activities	Pathology if Symptoms Are Aggravated by Activity	Pathology if Symptoms Are Eased by Activity
Elbow flexion	Eating, grooming, using telephone	Capsulitis, medial collateral ligament sprain, lateral collateral ligament sprain, muscle strain	Rheumatoid arthritis, muscle strain, ligament sprain
Elbow extension	Hygiene, dressing	Capsulitis, lateral collateral ligament sprain, medial collateral ligament sprain, muscle strain	Rheumatoid arthritis, muscle strain, ligament sprain
Pronation	Opening doors, driving, grasping, gripping, using telephone	Lateral epicondylitis/losis, muscle strain, pronator syndrome, radial tunnel syndrome	Muscle strain, ligament sprain
Supination	Reaching, eating	Lateral collateral ligament sprain, muscle strain	Muscle strain, ligament sprain
General movements	Pushing up from a chair	Degenerative joint disease, posterolateral rotatory instability, lateral epicondylitis	
	Weight bearing	Olecranon bursitis, ulnar neuritis, degenerative joint disease	
	Repetitive wrist extension	Lateral epicondylitis/epicondylosis	
	Repetitive wrist flexion	Medial epicondylitis/epicondylosis	
Throwing		Ulnar collateral ligament strain	
		Late cocking and early acceleration phase: ulnar neuritis, medial instability, valgus extension overload, posteriomedial impingement	
		Acceleration phase: flexor-pronator muscle strain	

medial collateral ligament sprain, lateral collateral ligament sprain, and ulnar neuritis or cubital tunnel syndrome.
• Pathologies implicated by wrist flexion-based activities include medial epicondylalgia and radial tunnel syndrome.

Extension-based activities
• Pathologies implicated by elbow extension-based activities include triceps strain, capsulitis, lateral collateral ligament sprain, and median neuritis.
• Pathologies implicated by wrist extension-based activities include lateral epicondylalgia and posterior interosseous nerve syndrome.

Pronation-based activities
• Pathologies implicated include lateral epicondylalgia, radial tunnel syndrome, posterior interosseous nerve syndrome, pronator syndrome, pronator or brachioradialis strain, and lateral collateral ligament strain.

Supination-based activities
• Pathologies implicated include medial epicondylalgia, supinator syndrome, radial tunnel syndrome, and supinator, brachioradialis, or biceps brachii strain.

CLINICAL PEARL

There are three ligaments of the medial collateral ligament (MCL) complex: the anterior oblique or bundle, the posterior oblique/band, and the transverse ligament/band. The origin of the MCL is slightly posterior to the elbow joint; thereby increasing tension is generated by greater degrees of flexion. The anterior portion of the anterior oblique is primarily taut from full extension to 60° of flexion. The posterior portion of the anterior oblique is taut from 60° to 120° of flexion. The posterior oblique is a thickening of the capsule that has the greatest restraint at 90° of elbow flexion.[12,61]

BEHAVIOR OF SYMPTOMS: EASING BEHAVIOR
WHAT INFLUENCE DO EASING FUNCTIONS HAVE ON YOUR CLINICAL DECISION-MAKING PROCESS?
Flexion-based activities
• Pathologies eased by elbow flexion-based activities include median neuritis and radial tunnel syndrome.
• Pathologies implicated by wrist flexion-based activities include radial tunnel syndrome and posterior interosseous nerve syndrome.

Extension-based activities
• Pathologies eased by elbow extension-based activities include cubital tunnel syndrome.

CLINICAL PEARL

Functional arc of motion of the elbow is 100° of total motion in the transverse plane (50° pronation to 50° supination) and 100° of total motion in the sagittal plane (30° to 130° of flexion).[49]

MEDICAL HISTORY

WHAT ROLE DOES A PATIENT'S PAST MEDICAL HISTORY PLAY IN THE DIFFERENTIAL DIAGNOSIS OF PATHOLOGY?
• Past injuries and the surgical history of the cervical spine and the upper extremity can have an affect on the normal biomechanics of the elbow through the development of scar tissue, limited tissue extensibility, and motor compensation.
• A past medical history of primary malignancy should be thoroughly explored to rule out less likely metastatic disease as a possible diagnosis. A history of corticosteroid use contributes to osteoporosis and tendon atrophy and affects wound healing.[11]
• A diagnosis of rheumatoid arthritis (RA) or a family history of RA in combination with the early signs and symptoms of RA will influence the differential diagnosis. The wrist, knee, and joints of the fingers are typically affected; however, as the disease progresses approximately 50% of people with RA will have symptoms and bone destruction at the elbow.[41]
• Current or recent pregnancy generates an increased risk of compressive neuropathies in the upper extremity from pregnancy-related edema or prolonged positioning. Hormone fluctuations may result in ligament laxity, which can result in symptoms similar to instability and/or tendinitis.[5]
• Though reported less frequently than the hip, the elbow joint has a greater risk for the development of heterotopic ossification following significant trauma with the peak incidence occurring at 2 months.[18] It is recommended that patients having elbow trauma plus one or more of the risk factors for ectopic bone development be treated with prophylactics. Risk

factors include neural axis trauma, burns, diffuse idiopathic skeletal hyperostosis, hypertrophic osteoarthrosis, ankylosis spondylitis, Paget's disease, and a history of ectopic ossification.[71]

CLINICAL PEARL (!)

Signs and symptoms of RA include joint stiffness, pain, fatigue, weakness, joint swelling, erythema, muscular atrophy, limitation in extension of joints, and the presence of nodules. Joint stiffness and pain are found in the majority of patients lasting up to 60 minutes following periods of sedentary activities or rest such as sleeping.

MEDICAL AND ORTHOPEDIC TESTING

WHAT MEDICAL AND ORTHOPEDIC TESTS INFLUENCE YOUR DIFFERENTIAL DIAGNOSIS PROCESS?

The presence of elbow trauma, no evidence of fracture on plain radiographs, and the "fat pad sign" were almost always (95%) indicative of boney trauma and 75% predictive of occult fracture found via magnetic resonance imaging (MRI).[55]

WHICH TYPE OF IMAGING SHOULD BE USED FOR THE VARIOUS ELBOW PATHOLOGIES?

In the elbow, the complexity of the injury needs to be fully understood. Fractures are often misdiagnosed or the extent of the injury and associated injuries is not recognized. Use of plain radiographs, MRI, magnetic resonance arthrography (MRA), ultrasound (US), and computed tomography (CT) arthrograms are common tools when assessing the extent of trauma or instability. In a comparison review by Shahahpour et al,[64] the following recommendations were made regarding imaging: MRI and MRA are advantageous to detect occult bone injuries, MR arthrogram is the best to directly visualize structures including associated capuloligamentous injuries, CT arthrogram assesses the cartilage of the elbow, and US or MRI can be used to detect chronic epicondylitis, biceps tendon injuries, and bursitis.

HOW RELIABLE ARE RADIOGRAPHS FOR DIAGNOSING ELBOW PATHOLOGY?

In a study by McGinley et al,[46] the sensitivity of lateral and AP x-rays for diagnosing small nondisplaced fractures was 21%.

HOW RELIABLE ARE NERVE CONDUCTION STUDIES (NCS) OF THE UPPER EXTREMITY?

In the diagnosis of radiculopathies and peripheral nerve disorders, nerve conduction studies are conducted with the results compared to normative data to determine pathology. NCS information should be utilized in combination with subjective and other physical examination findings versus reliance on the NCS results alone. In mild cases of neuropathic pain with or without objective sensory loss, NCS will frequently be inconclusive or give normal results.[39] It has been shown that 21% to 51% of the variance in values during testing of the upper extremity in the normal population are due to gender, age, hand temperature, and anthropometric measures, which are believed to affect diagnostic accuracy.[62]

WHAT IS THE DIAGNOSTIC ACCURACY OF ORTHOPEDIC TESTS AT THE ELBOW?

There are a multitude of special tests utilized by clinicians to differentiate elbow pathology. See Table II-9-2 for additional diagnostic information regarding common elbow special tests and their reliability.

CLINICAL DECISION MAKING CASE STUDY—PATIENT PROFILE (?)

Your next patient is a 12-year-old male baseball pitcher with constant but vague reports of pain deep within the elbow with clicking on his dominant extremity. His history is positive for previous episodes of elbow pain over the past 2 years that resolved with a short rest, some trials of physical therapy, and nonsteroidal antiinflammatory drugs. Images have not been completed and the preliminary diagnosis is instability. In consideration of the differential diagnoses list, what tests and measures should be completed?

Answer

As for medical tests, for consideration of instability, a clinician may consider an MR arthrogram. However, though instability is possible due to the activity of the patient, the combination of age, involvement of the dominant arm, and the activity should prioritize Panner's disease and osteochondritis dissecans onto the differential diagnosis list. These two diagnoses require radiographs.

As for orthopedic tests, once bony pathology has been ruled less likely, instability of the medial elbow should be considered due to the valgus stress of the upper extremity during throwing. The moving valgus stress test would be recommended.

TABLE II-9-2 Elbow Special Tests

Orthopedic Test	Diagnosis	Positive Test	Sensitivity	Specificity
Ulnar nerve compression test	Cubital tunnel syndrome	Patient feels numbness and tingling in the ulnar distribution	0.89	0.98[52]
Varus stress test	Lateral joint laxity	Greater laxity is felt by therapist in comparison to contralateral side	None reported	None reported
Posterolateral rotary instability test of elbow	Posterolateral rotary instability	Posterolateral displacement of radius occurs followed by reduction as elbow flexes and progresses to 90°[53]	None reported	None reported
Valgus stress test	Medial joint laxity	Greater laxity is felt by therapist in comparison to contralateral side	None reported	None reported
Milking test[21]	Medial ulnar collateral ligament laxity	A valgus force is applied by the patient with the elbow flexed; medial elbow pain with this maneuver indicates a positive result	None reported	None reported
Moving valgus stress test[54]	Medial collateral ligament laxity	The test is positive if the medial elbow pain is reproduced at the medial collateral ligament and is at maximum between 120° and 70°	1.0	0.75
Grip strength test	Lateral epicondylalgia	8% decrease from grip strength in flexed elbow position versus grip strength in elbow extended position	0.80	0.85[14]

HOW DOES A PATIENT'S RESPONSE TO MEDICATION INFLUENCE YOUR DECISION-MAKING PROCESSES?

- The effectiveness of antiinflammatory medication helps differentiate pathology that has an acute inflammatory process.
  - Pathologies that can have an acute inflammatory process include medial and lateral epicondylitis, muscle strain, and ligament sprain. At the cervical spine, relief may be felt from a radiculopathy.
  - Pathologies that do not normally have an acute inflammatory response include medial and lateral epicondylosis, degenerative joint disease, and instability.
  - Neural compression injuries may or may not be relieved by the use of antiinflammatory medications due to the irritation of the surrounding tissues.

BIOMECHANICAL

WHAT ROLE DOES BIOMECHANICS PLAY IN THE DECISION-MAKING PROCESS IN THE ELBOW REGION?

- The articular capsule of the elbow encompasses all three joints: the proximal radioulnar, the humeroradial, and the humeroulnar.
- Any motion at the elbow and forearm requires mobility at the humeroradial joint.
- Pronation and supination require simultaneous motions at both the proximal and distal radioulnar joints. Therefore, a limitation in one joint will limit motion in the other.

CLINICAL PEARL

The combination of shoulder rotation with pronation or supination allows the hand to rotate nearly 360° versus only 180° with only pronation or supination. Shoulder internal rotation typically occurs with pronation and shoulder external rotation with supination.

WHAT BIOMECHANICAL ABNORMALITIES IN OTHER REGIONS AFFECT YOUR DECISION-MAKING PROCESS?

- Neural compression within the upper extremity is commonly complicated by proximal impingement at the level of the nerve root also known as double crush syndrome. Associated diagnoses that have been acknowledged within certain populations include neck pain/radiculopathy, elevated first ribs, and thoracic outlet syndrome.[67]
- From the study of the interactive nature of the upper extremity during very dynamic activities such as throwing, Putnam[57] suggested that inadequate internal rotation of the shoulder would generate a causal effect for elbow symptoms in pitchers. In a small study of professional pitchers, 20 of 20 achieved relief of their symptoms by addressing the lack of glenohumeral joint internal rotation range of motion.[37]
- Distally, the biomechanics at the wrist need to be considered for a causal effect of symptoms at the elbow.[45,68]

ENVIRONMENTAL FACTORS (Box II-9-1)

DO PSYCHOSOCIAL ISSUES INFLUENCE THE CLINICAL DECISION-MAKING PROCESS?

- Psychosocial issues such as depression, stress, or a lack or change of social support can affect the healing response of the body.[73]

BOX II-9-1	**Contextual Factors**
Environmental/ personal	With the diagnosis of lateral epicondylalgia, psychosocial risk factors at work including organizational issues were found to be of greater importance when the level of physical work risk was greater than if the physical work was considered less of a risk.[13,23]
Environmental	Repetitive tasks and overuse have a role in tissue breakdown, especially with the diagnosis of instability, epicondylalgia, and neural dysfunction.
Personal	An unhealthy lifestyle, lack of social support, depressive illness, and substance abuse are predisposing factors for chronic pain. Further considerations that influence chronic pain include legal, psychological, medication, and family issues.[25]

- Psychosocial skills such as a patient's belief about their pain, self-efficacy, coping, and investment in their care all impact a patient's pain scale.[25]

CAN EMOTIONS INFLUENCE THE DECISION-MAKING PROCESS?

- The portion of the brain that controls depression and social rejection is influential in the emotional response to pain.[70]
- Fear, anxiety, and context can change the patient's perception of acute pain. Fear and anxiety, if elevated, may increase the perception of pain; however, the context may actually dampen the pain response such as a soldier in the midst of a battle.[25]

DO WORK-RELATED INJURIES INFLUENCE THE CLINICAL DECISION-MAKING PROCESS?

Injuries sustained in the workplace add another layer to the psychosocial influences discussed and should be explored by the clinician.

CLINICAL PEARL

The following two questions can be used to screen for depression: "During the past month, have you often been bothered by feeling down, depressed, or hopeless?" and "During the past month, have you often been bothered by little interest or pleasure in doing things?" If the patient responds in the negative to both questions, then it is very unlikely depression is present. These questions have been found to have a sensitivity of 96%.[74]

PERSONAL FACTORS

WHAT PREVIOUS SURGERIES INFLUENCE YOUR CLINICAL DECISION-MAKING PROCESS?

- Past injuries and a surgical history involving the cervical spine and the upper extremities can have an effect on the normal biomechanics of the elbow through the development of scar tissue, limited tissue extensibility, and motor compensation.
- A biometal implant in general increases the risk of infection during the immediate postoperative phase.
- Past surgeries or injuries to the lower extremity or spine in overhead athletes will often result in compensations at the elbow during throwing or overhead motions. Proper mechanics of the elbow require proper function throughout the kinetic chain.

DOES A FAMILY HISTORY OF PATHOLOGY IN THE ELBOW REGION INFLUENCE YOUR CLINICAL REASONING PROCESS?

Careful questioning concerning personal and family medical history is imperative to determine the local, referred, or systemic sources of the symptoms in the elbow region. Family history should be explored for consideration of rheumatoid arthritis, endocrine or metabolic disorders, and cardiopulmonary disorders.

CHRONICITY OF PAIN

HAS MEDICAL TREATMENT BEEN SUCCESSFUL FOR PATIENTS WITH CHRONIC PATHOLOGY IN THE REGION?

Where nonoperative interventions may fail, surgery has shown success for the resolution of the majority of disorders at the elbow. Residual effects of intervention, especially of the most complicated diagnosis, include limitation of motion and mild discomfort.

HOW DO THE AUTONOMIC, ENDOCRINE, AND IMMUNE SYSTEMS INFLUENCE DECISION MAKING IN THE ELBOW REGION? (Box II-9-2)

- Acute pain typically triggers anxiety, which may result in stimulation of the autonomic system in the flight-or-fight response. Increased muscle tension, changes in blood pressure, and an increased heart rate are associated with this response.
- Some diagnoses at the elbow, such as epicondylar pain, have been linked to organizational and workplace stress. Stress has an affect on all three systems. The response of the central nervous system is to activate cytokines that are proinflammatory. The autonomic nervous system signals the release of corticosteroids that disrupt the balance of the body's fluid. The secretion of catecholamine contributes to vasoconstriction, thereby decreasing the delivery of nutrients to muscle and tendons. As muscles and tendons undergo loading, microlesions are naturally generated; vasoconstriction prevents appropriate healing of these lesions.
- The immune system deserves consideration regarding the potential for septic olecranon bursitis, osteomyelitis, cellulitis, and lymphangitis at the elbow. This may occur following surgery, use of an external fixating device, or an underlying infection that began in another region of the body.

RED FLAGS THAT WARRANT REFERRAL TO A MEDICAL PHYSICIAN

WHAT SYMPTOMS ALERT YOU TO PATHOLOGIES THAT MAY REQUIRE A REFERRAL TO A MEDICAL PHYSICIAN?

It is strongly recommended that each situation be assessed individually and symptoms be considered in conjunction with the signs examined during the physical examination. The clinician must consider referral to a medical physician with the following symptoms:
- Fever in combination with swelling, redness, and/or warmth of the upper extremity
- Nondermatomal changes in sensation, especially in combination with cardiac and/or respiratory changes
- Change in pulses

WHAT SYMPTOMS IMPLICATE SPECIFIC VISCERAL SYSTEMS?

It is rare that the various visceral systems would produce symptoms within the elbow region only.
- Pulmonary system: Disease or dysfunction of the pulmonary system may produce suprascapular, mid thoracic, and/or shoulder pain. The mid to distal portion of the upper extremity is rarely affected except in advanced disease states. A history of smoking, pulmonary symptoms, and neurological changes, especially within the C8 to T1 dermatome pattern, may be a sign of the advancement of a Pancoast tumor into the brachial plexus.[20]
- Cardiac system: Referred pain from the cardiac system may include pain into the upper back, neck, jaw, either shoulder (though the left is the most common), and into the upper extremity. Upper extremity symptoms may extend to the elbow and are typically within the ulnar nerve distribution. Not necessarily correlated with localized motion, these symptoms are typically accompanied by "crushing" chest pain, fever, pallor, shortness of breath, or potential nausea. Not all of the symptoms/signs may be present. Symptoms of angina pectoris may be similar but are not as severe and are relieved by termination of activity, rest, or nitroglycerin medication.[20]
- Endocrine system: The patient may present to the clinic with a nonassociated musculoskeletal complaint. However, the presence of an additional constellation of neuromusculoskeletal and/or systemic symptoms may indicate an underlying metabolic or endocrine system influence. These symptoms may include fatigue, weakness, muscle atrophy, muscle and joint pain, stiffness or systemic symptoms such as mental changes, changes in hair or skin pigmentation, changes in vital signs, heart palpitations, and/or increased perspiration.[20]

SUMMARY STATEMENT

There have been significant changes in the diagnosis and treatment of pathologies of the elbow as a result of the study of the ergonomics of the workplace, consideration of the social

BOX II-9-2	**Output Mechanisms**
Autonomic	Recent interventional studies have suggested a relationship between specific mobilization techniques and the sympathetic nervous system during treatment of lateral epicondylalgia.[56] Examination of sympathetic and sensory systems in healthy, human samples of the extensor carpi radialis brevis found an imbalance between the vasoconstrictor and vasodilator innervation of the arteries. The relationship of these findings to the degeneration and vascular proliferation of tendinosis of medial and lateral epicondylalgia needs to be examined further.[42] Studies have shown an abnormal sympathetic vasomotor response in patients with lateral epicondylitis.[66]
Endocrine	Stress is known to activate the endocrine system and organizational stress has been linked to epicondylar pain. It is theorized that compromise of this system is related to the pain patterns of epicondylalgia. Successful treatment of epicondylar pain includes limited research with the use of acupuncture points.
Immune	Stress is known to suppress the immune system and organizational stress has been linked to epicondylar pain. It is theorized that compromise of this system is related to the pain patterns of epicondylalgia.

TABLE II-9-3   Body Structure and Tissue-Based Pathology (Nociceptive and Peripheral Neurogenic Pain Mechanisms)

	Muscles	Tendon/Epicondylar Pain	Bone	Joint/Cartilage	Ligaments	Nerves	Visceral Tissue
Pathology	Biceps or triceps strain	Lateral epicondylopathy Medial epicondylopathy	Elbow fractures	Elbow dislocation Elbow bursitis Posterior impingement syndrome Nursemaid elbow	Nursemaid elbow Elbow dislocation	Cubital tunnel syndrome Forearm compartment syndrome	Cardiac and pulmonary systems
Age	20 to 50 years old	20 to 50 years old	Any age for fracture, above 50 years old for degeneration	Any age	20 to 50 years old	20 to 50 years old	40 years and older
Occupation	Repetitive activities Athletes	Repetitive activities, manual labor	Not applicable	In children—typically athletes In adults—not applicable	Repetitive activities Athletes	Trauma or repetitive activities	Not applicable
Gender	Not applicable	Females may be slightly more at risk	Not applicable	Not applicable	Not applicable	Not applicable	Not applicable
Ethnicity	Not applicable	Not applicable	Not applicable	Not applicable	Not applicable	Not applicable	Not applicable
History	May or may not have history of overuse	May or may not have history of overuse or trauma	Traumatic	May or may not have history of overuse or trauma		May or may not have history of overuse or trauma	May have a history of autonomic symptoms
Mechanism of injury	Overuse	Overuse	Traumatic		Trauma		Generally no known mechanism
Type of onset	Sudden	Insidious	Sudden Insidious for degenerative	Sudden	Insidious or traumatic	Insidious or traumatic	Sudden to gradual depending on structure
Referral from local tissue	Volar or dorsal forearm pain	May refer distally toward the mid forearm	Pain is generally localized to involved structure	Pain is generally localized to area adjacent to involved structure	Localized to the medial or lateral elbow	Distribution of symptoms is dependent on peripheral nerve involvement	Pain is generally localized to area adjacent to involved structure
Referral to other regions	Generally does not refer to other regions		Generally does not refer to other regions	Generally does not refer to other regions	Generally does not refer to other regions	Distribution of symptoms is dependent on nerve root involvement	May refer into surrounding areas depending on involved structure
Changes in symptoms	Sudden pain, no relief as day of injury progresses	Waxes and wanes with changes in activities	Sudden pain, no relief as day of injury progresses	Sudden	Sudden pain, quicker to irritate with repetitive motions or as dynamic system fatigues	Symptoms may dissipate as irritating structure is addressed	May worsen as pathology progresses
24-hour pain pattern (morning)	Stiff for less than 30 minutes	Stiff for less than 30 minutes		Stiff for 30 minutes	Stiff for less than 30 minutes		Varies but does not change with mechanical stresses
24-hour pain pattern (afternoon)	Less stiff, may worsen with prolonged inactivity	Less stiff, may worsen with prolonged inactivity	Less stiff, may worsen with prolonged inactivity	May be worse with prolonged activity	Less stiff, may be worse with prolonged activity	May worsen with prolonged activity	Varies but does not change with mechanical stresses
24-hour pain pattern (evening)	May be difficult to sleep	Sleep should not be impaired	May be difficult to sleep	Sleep should not be impaired	Sleep should not be impaired	May be difficult to sleep	May have increased night pain

Continued on following page.

Section II

ORTHOPEDIC REASONING

TABLE II-9-3 Body Structure and Tissue-Based Pathology (Nociceptive and Peripheral Neurogenic Pain Mechanisms) *(Continued)*

	Muscles	Tendon/Epicondylar Pain	Bone	Joint/Cartilage	Ligaments	Nerves	Visceral Tissue
Description of symptoms	Aches and stiffness, may be able to localize	Aches	Aches and stiffness, may be difficult to localize	Aches and stiffness, sharp pain	Aches and stiffness, sharp pain with motions that stress ligament	Aching, numbness, tingling, deep pain	Cramping, peristaltic waves, gnawing ache
Depth of symptoms	Superficial	Superficial to deep	Deep	Deep	Deep	Superficial to deep depending on affected structure	Deep, poorly localized
Constancy of symptoms	Intermittent	Intermittent to constant	Constant but varies	Intermittent	Intermittent	Constant but varies	Constant, may come in waves
Aggravating factors	Concentric activation of passive stretching	Concentric activation of the muscle affected or passive stretching	Prolonged motion	Weight-bearing stresses	Combined motions of sagittal plane with varus or valgus stresses	Prolonged activity or sustained position	Not consistent with mechanical movements
Easing factors	Resting, ice	Avoidance of activities		Protective rest	Avoidance of those motions	Limited motion	Not consistent with mechanical movements
Stability of symptoms	Gradual improvement over 4- to 6-week period	If inflammatory, gradual improvement over 4- to 6-week period If more chronic, improvement may not be seen for several weeks	Improvement over 8 to 12 weeks If degenerative, may be episodic with more frequent episodes as disease progresses	Improvement over 8 to 12 weeks	If traumatic, possible gradual improvement over 4- to 6-week period. If due to overuse, improvement may not be seen	Improvement over 8 to 12 weeks if any underlying irritating structures are also addressed	May worsen if pathology progresses
Past medical history	All structures may have a past history of medical issues that impact the function of the surrounding tissue	All structures may have a past history of medical issues that impact the function of the surrounding tissue	For degenerative, typical history of trauma in the area	For degenerative, typical history of trauma in the area	All structures may have a past history of medical issues that impact the function of the surrounding tissue		May have a history of visceral pathology
Past surgeries	All structures may have a past history of surgeries that impact the function of the surrounding tissue	All structures may have a past history of surgeries that impact the function of the surrounding tissue	For degenerative, typical history of trauma in the area	For degenerative, typical history of trauma in the area	All structures may have a past history of surgeries that impact the function of the surrounding tissue		May have history of surgeries related to visceral pathology
Special questions				History of RA		History of neck pathology	
X-rays	Negative	Negative	Positive	Positive	Negative	May be significant at the C-spine	Negative
MRI	Positive	Negative	Negative	Negative	Positive	Usually not necessary	Positive for pathology
EMG	Not necessary	May be necessary for unresolving pain	Negative	Negative	Usually not necessary	Recommended	Not usually necessary
Special laboratory tests	Not necessary	Not necessary	May test for rheumatoid factors		Not necessary	Not necessary	Varies depending on pathology
Red flags							Rule out visceral structures

RA, rheumatoid arthritis; MRI, magnetic resonance imaging; EMG, electromyogram.

structure to the development of orthopedic tests, attention to interregional dependence, and new surgical techniques. Despite all of this progress, residual limitations of range of motion and mild discomfort may remain following intervention. Current rehabilitation protocols are multifaceted, with few identifying a single successful approach with strong research support. Table II-9-3 summarizes the factors that help a clinician differentiate among different sources of symptoms in the elbow region.

REFERENCES

1. Antuna SA, Morrey BF, Adams RA, O'Driscoll SW. Ulnohumeral arthroplasty for primary degenerative arthritis of the elbow: Long term outcome and complications. *J Bone Joint Surg Am.* 2002;84:2168-2173.

2. Binder AI, Hazleman BL. Lateral humeral epicondylitis: a study of natural history and the effect of conservative therapy. *Br J Rheumatol.* 1983;22:73-76.

3. Bisset L, Beller E, Jull G, Brooks P, Darnell R, Vicenzino B. Mobilisation with movement and exercise, corticosteroid injection, or wait and see for tennis elbow: randomized trial. *BMJ.* 2006;333:939.

4. Bisset L, Paungmali A, Vicenzino B, Beller E. A systematic review and meta analysis of clinical trials on physical interventions for lateral epicondylalgia. *Br J Sports Med.* 2005;39:411-422.

5. Borg-Stein J, Dugan SA. Musculoskeletal disorders of pregnancy, delivery and postpartum. *Phys Med Rehabil Clin N Am.* 2007;18(3): 459-476,ix.

6. Bot SDM, van der Waal JM, Terwee CB, van der Windt DAWM, Bouter LM, Dekker J. Course and prognosis of elbow complaints: a cohort study in general practice. *Ann Reum Dis.* 2005;64:1331-1336.

7. Butler DS. *Mobilisation of the Nervous System.* Melborne: Churchill; 1991.

8. Calfee R, Madom I, Weiss AP. Radial head arthroplasty. *J Hand Surg [Am].* 2006;31(2):314-321.

9. Chung KC, Spilson SV. The frequency and epidemiology of hand and forearm fractures in the United States. *J Hand Surg.* 2001;26A:908-915.

10. Ciccotti MC, Schwarz MA, Ciccotti MA. Diagnosis and treatment of medial epicondylitis of the elbow. *Clin Sports Med.* 2004;23:693-705.

11. Clarnette RG, Miniaci A. Clinical Exam of the shoulder. *Med Sci Sports Exer.* 1998;30(4 suppl 1):1-6.

12. Cohen MS, Bruno RJ. The collateral ligaments of the elbow. *Clin Orthop Relat Res.* 2001;383:123-130.

13. Devereux JJ, Vlachonikolis IG, Buckle PW. Epidemiological study to investigate potential interaction between physical and psychosocial factors at work that may increase the risk of symptoms of musculoskeletal disorder of the neck and upper limb. *Occup Environ Med.* 2002;59(4):269-277.

14. Dorf ER, Chhabra AB, Golish SR, McGinty JL, Pannunzio ME. Effect of elbow position on grip strength in the evaluation of lateral epicondylitis. *J Hand Surg [Am].* 2007;32(6):882-886.

15. Feinstein B, Langton JNK, Jameson RM, Schiller F. Experiments on pain referred from deep somatic tissues. *J Bone Joint Surg Am.* 1954;36:981-997.

16. Fernández-Carnero J, Fernández-de-las-Peñas C, de la Llave-Rincón AI, Ge HY, Arendt-Nielsen L. Prevalence of and referred pain from myofascial trigger points in the forearm muscles in patients with lateral epicondylalgia. *Clin J Pain.* 2007;23:353-360.

17. Gabel GT, Morrey BF. Operative treatment of medial epicondylitis. Influence of concomitant ulnar neuropathy at the elbow. *J Bone Joint Surg Am.* 1995;77-A(7):1065-1069.

18. Garland DE. A clinical perspective on common forms of acquired heterotopic ossification. *Clin Orthop Relat Res.* 1991;(263):13-29.

19. Gerber C, Galantay RV, Hersche O. The pattern of pain produced by irritation of the acromioclavicular joint and the subacromial space. *J Shoulder Elbow Surg.* 1998;7(4):352-355.

20. Goodman CC, Boissonnault WG. *Pathology: Implications for the Physical Therapist.* Philadelphia; WB Saunders: 1998.

21. Grace SP, Field LD. Chronic medial elbow instability. *Orthop Clin North Am.* 2008;39(2):213-219,vi.

22. Gray RJ, Stone WM, Fowl RJ, Cherry KJ, Bower TC. Management of true aneurysms distal to the axillary artery. *J Vasc Surg.* 1998;28:606-610.

23. Haahr JP, Andersen JH. Physical and psychosocial risk factors for lateral epicondylitis: a population based case-referent study. *Occup Environ Med.* 2003;60:322-329.

24. Haahr JP, Andersen JH. Prognostic factors in lateral epicondylitis: a randomized trial with one year follow up in 266 new cases treated with minimal occupational intervention or the usual approach in general practice. *Rheumatology.* 2003;42:1216-1225.

25. Hansen GR, Streltzer J. The psychology of pain. *Emerg Med Clin North Am.* 2005;23(2):339-348.

26. Harrington IJ, Tountas AA. Replacement of the radial head in the treatment of unstable elbow fractures. *Injury.* 1981;12:405-412.

27. Harrington IJ, Sekyi-Otu A, Barrington TW, Evans DC, Tuli V. The functional outcome with metallic radial head implants in the treatment of unstable elbow fractures: a long-term review. *Journal of Trauma-Injury Infection & Critical Care.* 2001;50(1):46-52.

28. Hassett G, Barnsley L. Pain referral from SCJ: a study in normal volunteers. *Rheumatology.* 2001;40:859-862.

29. Herbertsson P, Josefsson PO, Hasserius R, Besjakov J, Nyqvist F, Karlsson MK. Fractures of the radial head and neck treated with radial head excision. *J Bone Joint Surg.* 2004;86A(9):1925-1930.

30. Hidebrand KA, Patterson SD, King GJW. Acute elbow dislocations. simple and complex. *Orthop Clin North Am.* 1999;30(1):63-79.

31. Ho G, Tice AD, Kaplan SR. Septic bursitis in the prepatellar and olecranon bursae: An analysis of 25 cases. *Ann Intern Med.* 1978;89(1): 21-27.

32. Hume PA, Reid D, Edwards T. Epicondylar injury in sport: epidemiology, type, mechanisms, assessment, management and prevention. *Sports Med.* 2006;36(2):151-170.

33. Johnston GW. A follow up of one hundred cases of fracture of the head of the radius with a review of the literature. *Ulster Med J.* 1962;31:51-56.

34. Josefsson PO, Gentz CF, Johnell O, Wendeberg B. Dislocations of the elbow and intraarticular fractures. *Clin Orthop Relat Res.* 1989;(246):126-130.

35. Kamien M. A rational management of tennis elbow. *Sports Med.* 1990;9(3):173-191.

36. Khan KM, Cook JL, Maffulli N, et al. Where is the pain coming from in tendinopathy? It may be biochemical, not only structural, in origin. *Br J Sports Med.* 2000;34:81-83.

37. Kibler WB, Sciascia A. Kinetic chain contributions to elbow function and dysfunction in sports. *Clin Sports Med.* 2004;23:545-552.

38. Kuhn MA, Ross G. Acute elbow dislocations. *Orthop Clin N Am.* 2008;39:155-161.

39. Kwon HK, Lee HJ, Hwang M, Lee SH. Amplitude ratio of ulnar sensory nerve action potentials in segmental conduction study: reference values in healthy subjects and diagnostic usefulness in patients with ulnar neuropathy at the elbow. *Am J Phys Med Rehabil.* 2008;87(8):642-646.

40. Landin LA, Danielsson LG. Elbow fractures in children. An epidemiological analysis of 589 cases. *Acta Orthop Scand.* 1986;57(4):309-312.

41. Lehtinen JT, Kaarela K, Kauppi MJ, Belt EA, Mäenpää HM, Lehto MU. Bone destruction patterns of the rheumatoid elbow: a radiographic assessment of 148 elbows at 15 years. *J Shoulder Elbow Surg.* 2002;11(3):253-258.

42. Ljung BO, Forsgren S, Fridén J. Sympathetic and sensory innervations are heterogeneously distributed in relation to the blood vessels at the extensor carpi radialis brevis muscle origin of man. *Cells Tissues Organs.* 1999;165(1):45-54.

43. Mapp PI. Innervation of the synovium. *Ann Rheum Dis.* 1995;54:398-403.

44. Mason ML. Some observations on fracture of the head of the radius with a review of one hundred cases. *Br J Surg.* 1954;42:123-132.

45. May-Lisowski TL, King PM. Effect of wearing a static wrist orthosis on shoulder movement during feeding. *Am J Occup Ther.* 2008;62:438-445.

46. McGinley JC, Roach N, Hopgood BC, Kozin SH. Nondisplaced elbow fractures: A commonly occurring and difficult diagnosis. *Am J Emerg Med.* 2006;24(5):560-566.

47. McQueen MM, Gaston P, Court-Brown CM. Acute compartment syndrome. Who is at risk. *J Bone Joint Surg Br.* 2000;82(2):200-203.

48. Mehta JA, Bain GI. Elbow dislocations in adults and children. *Clin Sports Med.* 2004;23(4):609-627,ix.

49. Morrey BF, Askew LJ, Chao EYS. A biomechanical study of normal elbow motion. *J Bone Joint Surg.* 1981;63A:872-877.

50. Mowlavi A, Andrews K, Lille S, Verhulst S, Zook EG, Milner S. The management of cubital tunnel syndrome: A meta-analysis of clinical studies. *Plast Reconstr Surg.* 2000;106:327.

51. Nirschl RP, Ashman ES. Elbow Tendinopathy: tennis elbow. *Clin Sports Med*. 2003;22:813-836.
52. Novak CB, Lee GW, Mackinnon SE, Lay L. Provocative testing for cubital tunnel syndrome. *J Hand Surg [Am]*. 1994;19(5):817-820.
53. O'Driscoll SW, Bell DF, Morrey BF. Posterolateral rotatory instability of the elbow. *J Bone Joint Surg Am*. 1991;73(3):440-446.
54. O'Driscoll SW, Lawton RL, Smith AM. The "moving valgus stress test" for medial collateral ligament tears of the elbow. *Am J Sports Med*. 2005;33(2):231-239.
55. O'Dwyer H, O'Sullivan P, Fitzgerald D, Lee MJ, McGrath F, Logan PM. The fat pad sign following elbow trauma in adults: its usefulness and reliability in suspecting occult fracture. *J Comput Assist Tomogr*. 2004;28(4):562-565.
56. Paungmali A, O'Leary S, Souvlis T, Vicenzino B. Hypoalgesic and sympathoexcitatory effects of mobilization with movement for lateral epicondylalgia. *Phys Ther*. 2003;83(4):374-383.
57. Putnam CA. Sequential motions of body segments in striking and throwing skills. *J Biomech*. 1993;26:125-135.
58. Rettig AC, Sherrill C, Snead DS, Mendler J, Mieling P. Nonoperative treatment of ulnar collateral ligament injuries in throwing athletes. *Am Orthop Soc Sports Med*. 2001;29(1):15-17.
59. Rommens PM, Küchle R, Schneider RU, Reuter M. Olecranon fractures in adults: factors influencing outcome. *Injury Int J Care Injured*. 2004;35:1149-1157.
60. Royle SG. Posterior dislocation of the elbow. *Clin Orthop*. 1991;269:201-204.
61. Safran MR, Baillargeon D. Soft tissue stabilizers of the elbow. *J Shoulder Elbow Surg*. 2005;14:179S-185S.
62. Salerno DF, Franzblau A, Werner RA, Bromberg MB, Armstrong TJ, Albers JW. Median and ulnar nerve conduction studies among workers: normative values. *Muscle Nerve*. 1998;21(8):999-1005.
63. Sellards R, Kuebrich C. The elbow: Diagnosis and treatment of common injuries. *Prim Care Clin Office Pract*. 2005;32:1-16.
64. Shahabpour M, Kichouh M, Laridon E, Gielen JL, De Mey J. The effectiveness of diagnostic imaging methods for the assessment of soft tissue and articular disorders of the shoulder and elbow. *Eur J Radiol*. 2008;65(2):194-200.
65. Smidt N, Lewis M, van der Windt DA, Hay EM, Bouter LM, Croft P. Lateral epicondylitis in general practice: course and prognostic indicators of outcome. *J Rheumatol*. 2006;33(10):2053-2059.
66. Smith RW, Papadopolous E, Mani R, Cawley MI. Abnormal microvascular responses in a lateral epicondylitis. *Br J Rheumatol*. 1994;33(12):1166-1168.
67. Smith TM, Sawyer SF, Sizer PS, Brismee JM. The double crush syndrome: a common occurrence in cyclists with ulnar nerve neuropathy—a case-control study. *Clin J Sport Med*. 2008;18:55-61.
68. Sturgis PAA, Damen PJ, Bakker EWP, et al. Manipulation of the wrist for management of lateral epicondylitis: a randomized pilot study. *Phys Ther*. 2003;83:608-616.
69. Travell JG, Simons DG. *Myofascial pain and Dysfunction—the trigger point annual*. Baltimore: Williams & Wilkins; 1983.
70. Vastag B. Scientists find connections in the brain between physical and emotional pain. *JAMA*. 2003;290(18):2389-2390.
71. Viola RW, Hastings H. Treatment of ectopic ossification about the elbow. *Clin Orthop Relat Res*. 2000;370:65-86.
72. Walker-Bone K, Readin I, Coggon D, Cooper C, Palmer KT. The anatomical pattern and determinants of pain in the neck and upper limbs: an epidemiologic study. *Pain*. 2004;109(1-2):45-51.
73. Whooley MA, Avins AL, Miranda J, Browner WS. Case-finding instruments for depression. Two questions are as good as many. *J Gen Intern Med*. 1997;12(7):439-445.
74. Yepes H, Tang M, Morris SF, Stanish WD. Relationship between hypovascular zones and patterns of ruptures of the quadriceps tendon. *J Bone Joint Surg Am*. 2008;90(10):2135-2141.
75. Zeisig E, Ohberg L, Alfredson H. Extensor origin vascularity related to pain in patients with tennis elbow. *Knee Surg Sports Traumatol Arthrosc*. 2006;14(7):659-663.

AUTHOR: CYNTHIA COOPER

INTRODUCTORY INFORMATION

The hand and wrist can be complex. They are extremely mobile structures that can coordinate a multitude of motions in relation to each of its components. Proper function requires the interaction of multiple structures. Small alterations in structures can result in large implications for the use of the hand and wrist for daily function. Because of the complexity and intricacies of the region, diagnoses involving the wrist and hand are extremely varied and just as plentiful. Problems of the wrist and hand are unique because there are many multiarticulate structures positioned intimately anatomically with no room to accommodate edema or scarring. The multiple structures that interact within the region and refer to the region can result in problems that are musculotendinous, skeletal, neuropathic, or systemic in nature. A firm understanding of the anatomy, physiology, and biomechanics of the hand and wrist is a critical foundation for diagnosis within the region.

CLINICAL PEARL

The quadriga effect is demonstrated by an inability to flex, especially the distal interphalangeal (DIP) joints of the fingers adjacent to the injured finger. It occurs because of the shared muscle belly of the flexor digitorum profundus (FDP). For this reason it is very important to check the FDP glide of each digit, not just the injured digit, and to promote active DIP flexion of the adjacent digits.

WHAT IS THE PREVALENCE OF WRIST AND/OR HAND FRACTURE?[12,15]

- Colles' and Smith's fractures account for 50% of distal radius fractures.
- Carpal fractures have one-tenth the incidence of distal radius fractures.
- Scaphoid fractures represent 60% to 70% of carpal fractures.
- Metacarpal fractures represent 30% to 50% of hand fractures.
- Sports injuries are the leading cause of proximal phalanx fractures.
- Distal phalanx fractures occur most often in the long finger, followed by the thumb.

WHAT IS THE PROGNOSIS FOR RECOVERY FROM HAND AND WRIST INJURY?

- Prognosis for recovery varies greatly, depending on the particular diagnosis. There is no research that looks at the recovery prognosis for the region as a whole, but specific pathology responds in the following manner.
- A closed stable metacarpal fracture will be associated with fewer problems than a more complicated scenario such as a crush injury with a complex metacarpal fracture requiring fixation. In this instance, there is concern that extensor tendon adherence and joint stiffness may occur.
- If a fracture is intraarticular, there is more likelihood of problems and a poorer prognosis for recovery than if a fracture does not involve the articular surface.

CLINICAL PEARL

Prognosis is always worse if edema persists, if pain persists, and/or if there are medical comorbidities.

WHAT FACTORS MAKE DIAGNOSIS DIFFICULT IN THE HAND AND WRIST?

- Several factors make the hand unique, but it is this uniqueness that makes diagnosis challenging.

- The hand involves the coordinated workings of 27 bones and associated articulations.
- Each bone-to-bone interface requires ligamentous structures to secure and stabilize the articulation.
- Tendons have specially designed pulley and sheathing systems to provide for proper hand and wrist function. These result in mechanical advantages for function, but also provide additional regions for tissue breakdown and pathology.
- Special views may be required to accurately diagnose certain fractures.
- Some fractures such as scaphoid fractures may not show up on x-ray for a few weeks following injury.

CLINICAL PEARL

Depending on the mechanism of injury and the physical examination, when a scaphoid fracture is suspected, physicians may immobilize or cast the patient as a precaution while following up diagnostically.

CLINICAL PEARL

When there are signs of nerve compression as in carpal tunnel syndrome or cubital tunnel syndrome, the problem may be coming from a more proximal area such as the cervical region. Diagnostic tests are important so that unnecessary surgery is avoided and the actual source of the problem can be corrected.

- In cases of tendinitis/tendinosis, symptoms may be dynamic and may fluctuate. In some cases it may be necessary to have the patient perform provoking activities before or as part of the evaluation in order to accurately elicit and identify the problem.

HOW SUCCESSFUL IS THERAPY IN TREATING THE HAND AND WRIST?

The success of rehabilitation varies greatly. Certain problems can respond very favorably to hand therapy intervention. These include osteoarthritis, rheumatoid arthritis, tendinopathies, pain syndromes, early carpal tunnel syndrome, early cubital tunnel syndrome, and residual stiffness following fracture, especially if addressed early. Other traumatic injuries such as wrist fractures are greatly dependent on the ability to restore normal alignment and mechanics of the bones and joints involved.

CLINICAL PEARL

Therapy is more successful if edema is prevented/treated successfully.

CLINICAL PEARL

Overzealous hand therapy that is painful can cause complex regional pain syndrome (RSD). Therapists must respect patients' tissue tolerances and should not create or compound pain if therapy is to be successful.

HOW SUCCESSFUL IS SURGERY IN TREATING THE HAND AND WRIST?

Interventions in hand surgery have progressed dramatically in recent years, with advances in fixation of fractures and improved suture techniques in tendon and nerve.[9,17]

PERSONAL INFORMATION

AGE

WHAT INFLUENCE DOES AGE HAVE ON YOUR CLINICAL DECISION-MAKING PROCESS?
- Body structures will always fail at their weakest point when forces are placed on them. In children and the elderly, this weak point is often the bone.
- Fractures in children and teenagers may involve the growth plate. These fractures are categorized as Salter fractures, with numeric designations that describe the severity of growth plate involvement.[11] If these fractures are not managed well medically there could be some disturbance to the growth of the bone.
- Fractures should also be suspected in the elderly as bones become more brittle.
- Injuries to the wrist and hand in the normal adult can involve the bone, but other structures such as tendons and ligaments should also be a consideration as the bone is stronger than in children or the elderly. Avulsions may occur more frequently.
- From an intervention standpoint, it is difficult to splint children and to keep splints on them. For this reason, casts are often used instead.

CLINICAL PEARL

When a splint is required on a child, it is a good idea to cross more proximal (and possibly more distal) parts of the extremity and to add extra securing straps.

- A child with a tendon repair is usually treated with immobilization rather than a standard postoperative tendon protocol that requires strict adherence to protective guidelines, splint use, and particular protective exercises.
- Some elderly patients may have difficulty manipulating small components on dynamic splints. In addition, older people may have fragile skin, especially if they have a history of steroid use. Extra gentle steps are needed with dressing changes and splint edges and straps should not be rough.[8]

CLINICAL DECISION MAKING CASE STUDY—PATIENT PROFILE

Your patient is an 86-year-old female with a history of respiratory and cardiac illness. She has been treated with steroids in the past. She demonstrates memory problems and asks the same questions repeatedly in hand therapy. She has sustained a distal radius fracture and presents with diffuse edema and stiffness of the wrist and hand. What can you do to maximize the success of her hand therapy program?

Answer
This patient's skin is probably fragile from her history of steroid use. Pad the edges of splints and select extra soft straps. Emphasize elevation and pain-free active motions. Simplify the therapy program and observe the patient practice it. Include the patient's spouse or another supportive person. Write all the instructions and have the patient read them out loud, as this reinforces learning. If the patient is able to write the instructions herself, this is even more conducive to learning. Provide encouragement and keep the home program simple.

OCCUPATION

WHAT INFLUENCE DOES A PATIENT'S OCCUPATION HAVE ON YOUR CLINICAL DECISION-MAKING PROCESS?
- Care should be taken during the interview process to determine the nature of a patient's work. Many times demonstration

of the patient's aggravating activities is necessary to understand the mechanics of the injury and the forces that are contributing to the pain and pathology.
- Unsupported or overhead upper extremity use and awkward or prolonged repetitive motions of the hand and wrist may contribute to tendinopathies. Therefore, therapists should instruct patients in upper extremity biomechanical guidelines and ergonomics, pacing, task rotation, and an appropriate exercise regimen with attention to proximal conditioning and postural issues at work and at home.

GENDER

WHAT INFLUENCE DOES GENDER HAVE ON YOUR CLINICAL DECISION-MAKING PROCESS?
- More men than women develop Dupuytren's disease (also called palmar fasciitis), which is a thickening and shortening of palmar fascia leading to digital flexion contractures. In men, it tends to arise in their 50s. When Dupuytren's disease does occur in women, they are usually older and the progression of the disease may not be as severe.[13]
- Pregnant women will often experience carpal tunnel symptoms as their pregnancy progresses.
- Following pregnancy, the woman may experience de Quervain's syndrome or intersection syndrome as they lift and carry their child. This is sometime exacerbated by the ligament laxity present due to increased relaxin in the system.

ETHNICITY

WHAT INFLUENCE DOES ETHNICITY HAVE ON YOUR CLINICAL DECISION-MAKING PROCESS?
Research is limited regarding the role that ethnicity plays in common hand pathologies. Certain pathologies have known ethnicity predispositions. Dupuytren's disease has also been called Viking disease because it occurs most frequently in regions that had Viking history, including Scandinavia and northern Europe. In Australia, 26% of males and 20% of females older than 60 years are affected and the incidence of Dupuytren's is less than 3% in blacks and Asians. Other disease processes such as rheumatoid arthritis can affect all ethnicities.

CLINICAL DECISION MAKING CASE STUDY—PATIENT PROFILE

Your patient is a 65-year-old male with a family history of Dupuytren's disease. He is developing flexion contractures of the ring and small fingers, with palpable thickening of the palmar fascia. His family doctor has sent him to hand therapy to correct this problem. What should you do?

Answer
There is no evidence that splinting, stretching, or exercise will correct the Dupuytren's disease. Explain this to the patient in a supportive manner and help coordinate a referral to a hand surgeon.

SYMPTOM HISTORY

MECHANISM OF INJURY

WHAT INFLUENCE DOES THE MECHANISM OF INJURY HAVE ON YOUR CLINICAL DECISION-MAKING PROCESS?
- Determining the patient's mechanism of injury is important in all areas of the body, but in the hand and wrist, careful questioning can guide the clinician to the source of symptoms.
- In acute trauma such as a fall or laceration, questioning regarding the position of the injury and the forces placed on the hand and wrist will help determine where the tissue failure occurred. In the

case of lacerations, knowledge of where and how the laceration occurred gives insight into which structures were impacted.

- A fall on an outstretched hand (FOOSH) will direct different forces depending on whether the arm was pronated or supinated at the time of the fall. Landing with the wrist extended as opposed to flexed also impacts the diagnostic process. Landing with the wrist extended will often result in a Colles fracture, whereas landing with the wrist flexed will result in a Smith fracture.
- Tendinitis that is traumatic in origin and if treated acutely often recovers more quickly than a tendinopathy that has become chronic. Tendinitis can easily progress to tendinosis if the causative factors are not addressed. Causative factors can involve intrinsic factors such as decreased blood flow to the region or extrinsic factors such as compression or friction on the tendon itself.

CLINICAL PEARL

If a proximal interphalangeal (PIP) digit is hyperextended with the injury, the volar plate may be involved. A PIP joint with volar plate injury should be positioned in 20° to 30° of flexion for the first few weeks in order to recover joint stability.[3]

LOCATION OF SYMPTOMS

WHAT INFLUENCE DOES THE LOCATION OF SYMPTOMS HAVE ON YOUR CLINICAL DECISION-MAKING PROCESS?

Location of the symptoms in the hand and wrist can provide a good indicator as to the structures involved in creating the pain or discomfort. In general, pain within the hand and wrist is localized to the immediate region of injury. Edema and inflammation can confuse the diagnosis by spreading pain outward and remotely from the source of the inflammatory response.

There have been several systems developed to aide in the classification and treatment of hand pathology.

The dorsum of the hand, wrist, and forearm can be divided into eight anatomic zones to facilitate classification and treatment of extensor tendon injuries.

Dorsal Zones of the Hand

Zone 1	DIP joint
Zone 2	Middle phalanx
Zone 3	PIP joint
Zone 4	Proximal phalanx
Zone 5	Metacarpophalangeal (MCP) joint
Zone 6	Dorsum of hand
Zone 7	Wrist
Zone 8	Dorsal forearm

There are six compartments in the dorsal aspect of the wrist. Each compartment contains the tendons of specific structures.

The Tendons in the Six Dorsal Compartments of the Hand

First compartment	Extensor and abductor pollicis brevis
Second compartment	Extensor carpi radialis brevis and longus
Third compartment	Extensor pollicis longus
Fourth compartment	Extensor digitorum communis and extensor indicis
Fifth compartment	Extensor digiti minimi
Sixth compartment	Extensor carpi ulnaris

The flexors of the hand and wrist have been divided into five zones. The following zones apply only to the index through the small fingers. Separate zone boundaries exist for the thumb flexor tendon.

Flexor Zones of the Hand

Zone I	Consists of the profundus tendon only and is bounded proximally by the insertion of the superficialis tendons and distally by the insertion of the FDP tendon into the distal phalanx.
Zone II	Proximal to zone II, the flexor digitorum superficialis (FDS) tendons lie superficial to the FDP tendons. Within zone II and at the level of the proximal third of the proximal phalanx, the FDS tendons split into two slips, collectively known as Camper chiasma. These slips then divide around the FDP tendon and reunite on the dorsal aspect of the FDP, inserting into the distal end of the middle phalanx.
Zone III	Extends from the distal edge of the carpal ligament to the proximal edge of the A1 pulley, which is the entrance of the tendon sheath. Within zone III, the lumbrical muscles originate from the FDP tendons. The distal palmar crease superficially marks the termination of zone III and the beginning of zone II.
Zone IV	Includes the carpal tunnel and its contents (i.e., the nine digital flexors and the median nerve).
Zone V	Extends from the origin of the flexor tendons at their respective muscle bellies to the proximal edge of the carpal tunnel.

- Pain at the base of the thumb could be caused by thumb carpometacarpal (CMC) osteoarthritis or de Quervain's tenosynovitis. The CMC grind test is indicative of CMC osteoarthritis. A positive Finkelstein's test is indicative of de Quervain's tenosynovitis (Table II-10-1).
- If there is swelling and pain in the muscular area on the dorsoradial distal forearm, proximal to the first dorsal compartment [where the adductor pollicis longus (APL) and extensor pollicis brevis (EPB) are palpable over the distal radius], this suggests intersection syndrome rather than de Quervain's disease.
- Tenderness over the pisiform implicates the flexor carpi ulnaris (FCU).

CLINICAL PEARL

Fullness and tenderness at the ulnar wrist may be associated with repetitive ulnar deviation activities. Small finger abduction can also aggravate this area. In this instance, a buddy strap between the small and ring fingers may actually help with the ulnar wrist pain.

- Tenderness over the A1 pulley (in the palm near the distal palmar crease) along with crepitation at this site or locking in digital composite flexion is indicative of flexor tenosynovitis, also called trigger finger.
- A Tinel sign at the volar wrist is associated with carpal tunnel syndrome. Sensory complaints are on the palmar aspect of the thumb, index, long fingers, and the radial aspect of the ring finger. In advanced carpal tunnel syndrome, there may be atrophy of the thenar eminence limiting thumb abduction or opposition.
- A Tinel sign at the cubital tunnel (the funny bone area) is associated with ulnar neuropathy. Sensory complaints occur in the palmar aspect of the ulnar digits, typically the small finger and the ulnar aspect of the ring finger. There might be atrophy of the first dorsal interosseous, noticed on the dorsal hand between the thumb and index finger, and there may be visible hollowing between the metacarpal heads.

TABLE II-10-1 Wrist/Hand Tendinitis/Tendinosis

Diagnosis	Structures Involved	Provoking Tests, Motions, or Functional Activities
de Quervain's tenosynovitis	APL and EPB tendons at first dorsal compartment	Finkelstein's test Resisted thumb radial abduction or extension Thickening or pain at the first dorsal compartment
Intersection syndrome	APL and EPB muscle bellies, approximately 4 cm proximal to wrist, where they intersect with ECRB and ECRL	Localized swelling and pain at APL and EB muscle bellies Resisted wrist extension Same as in de Quervain's tenosynovitis
EPL tendinopathy	EPL at Lister's tubercle	Pain at Lister's tubercle Resisted composite thumb extension Passive composite thumb flexion
ECU tendinopathy	ECU	Pain at ulnar wrist Forearm supination with wrist ulnar deviation
FCR tendinopathy	FCR	Resisted wrist flexion and radial deviation Pain with passive wrist extension Pain over proximal wrist crease at the scaphoid tubercle
FCU tendinopathy	FCU	Pain with palpation over the pisiform Resisted wrist flexion and ulnar deviation Passive wrist extension and radial deviation
Digital flexor tenosynovitis	Digital flexor tendon at the A1 pulley	Tenderness at the A1 pulley Palpable nodule Crepitus with active digital flexion Snapping or locking with active composite digital flexion

Modified from Cooper C, Martin HA: Common forms of tendinitis/tendinosis. In Cooper C, editor: *Fundamentals of Hand Therapy: Clinical Reasoning and Treatment Guidelines for Common Diagnoses of the Upper Extremity,* 1st ed. St. Louis: Elsevier; 2007.
APL, abductor pollicis longus; EPB, extensor pollicis brevis; ECRB, extensor carpi radialis longus; EB, esophageal body; EXL, extensor pollicis longus; ECU, extensor carpi ulnaris; FCR, flexor carpi radialis; FCU, flexor carpi ulnaris.

CLINICAL DECISION MAKING CASE STUDY—PATIENT PROFILE (?)

Your patient is a 43-year-old female who complains of numbness of the dominant ring and small fingers. She does not have any atrophy or weakness noted. Ring and small finger FDP is intact and there is no clawing of the digits. What should her evaluation include and what should her home program consist of?

Answer

Perform a cervical screening and thoracic screening to rule out proximal causes. If these are negative, perform the elbow flexion test and check for a Tinel sign at the cubital tunnel (test for a Tinel sign distal to proximal for more accuracy). Perform a manual muscle test of the lumbricals, the interossei, and the ring and small finger FDP. Observe for intermetacarpal hollowing or subtle signs of clawing of the ring and small fingers. In terms of therapy, emphasize the importance of avoiding elbow flexion at night while sleeping. Demonstrate a towel wrapped around the arm, be creative with pillow positioning, and consider a more rigid elbow splint if needed. Instruct the patient to avoid elbow-intensive activities such as hammering, and explain that it is very important to avoid resting on the posterior elbow. An elbow pad or pillow should be used to protect the posterior elbow from resting on desks or table tops.

REFERRAL OF SYMPTOMS

Nerve—Sensory Distribution (FIGURE II-10-1)

Radial	Radial thumb, proximal half index and middle finger, proximal dorsal radial side of ring finger
Median	Palmar surface of thumb, index, middle, and radial half of ring finger, dorsal tips of thumb, index, middle, and radial part of ring finger
Ulnar	Anterior and posterior ulnar palm, little finger, and ulnar aspect of ring finger
C6 spinal nerve	Lateral distal arm down to thumb radial palm and index finger
C7 spinal nerve	Middle finger, ulnar half of index finger, and radial half of ring finger
C8 spinal nerve	Ulnar side of hand and little finger and ulnar side of ring finger

Nerve—Motor Distribution

Radial	Elbow extension, forearm supination
Posterior interosseous	Wrist extension with ulnar deviation, digit extension, thumb abduction and extension, index finger extension
Median	Forearm pronation, wrist flexion with radial deviation
Anterior interosseous	Finger and thumb flexion, metacarpophalangeal (MP) flexion of index and middle finger, abduction and adduction of index and middle fingers, forearm pronation, opposition of thumb
Ulnar	Thumb flexion, adduction, and opposition, MP flexion, and finger abduction/adduction of ring and little fingers
C6	Elbow flexion (biceps, supinator), wrist extension
C7	Elbow extension (triceps), wrist flexion
C8	Ulnar deviation, thumb extension, finger flexion and abduction

- When sensory symptoms do not follow a peripheral nerve distribution, the cause may be at the level of the brachial plexus.[2]

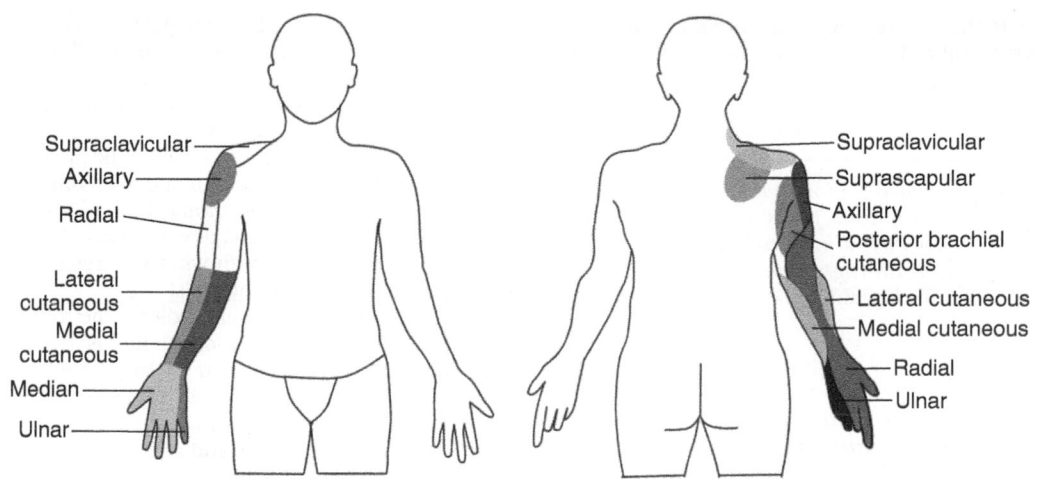

FIGURE II-10-1 Sensory distribution of peripheral nerves. All peripheral nerves innervate different portions of the wrist and hand. Sensory loss or pain distribution in a specific pattern can aid in the differentiation process.

VISCERAL

Visceral structures typically do not refer into the hand or wrist. The few exceptions would be the heart, which can refer into the left hand, and the pulmonary system, which can refer into the ipsilateral hand. Pancoast tumors in the lung can also place pressure on the lower cords of the brachial plexus and cause pain into the ulnar aspect of the hand. Long-term diseases of the pancreas can also result in nerve damage. This usually occurs at the distal aspects of the extremities such as the hand and feet. The symptoms are not directly referred into the hand by the pancreas, but the pancreas contributes to degeneration of the nerves in the distal hand.

CLINICAL PEARL

Peripheralization or worsening of distal upper extremity symptoms with repeated cervical motion is indicative of a problem at the cervical level.

SYMPTOM DESCRIPTORS

QUALITY OF SYMPTOMS

- Sharp burning pain or a Tinel sign is suggestive of nerve irritation.
- Numbness and paresthesia are indicative of possible entrapment.
- Deep or dull ache may be seen with muscle soreness or bone fracture.
- Coldness or weakness can be indicative of vascular pathology.
- Clicking or catching is common with carpal instability.

DEPTH OF SYMPTOMS

WHAT INFLUENCE DOES THE DEPTH OF SYMPTOMS HAVE ON YOUR CLINICAL DECISION-MAKING PROCESS?

- Osteoarthritis of the thumb CMC causes pain with pinching activities. A hand-based thumb spica splint provides support and reduces pain with pinch.
- Most structures in the hand are relatively superficial and therefore can be palpated.
- Pain that cannot be palpated or reproduced through hand and wrist motion may indicate referral of symptoms from remote sites.

CLINICAL PEARL

In osteoarthritis of the upper extremity, the DIP and the first CMC joints are the most typically involved.

CLINICAL PEARL

The larger and more padded an item is, the less joint strain there is. Enlarging the girth of writing utensils and kitchen implements helps protect small joints of the hand.

TWENTY-FOUR–HOUR SYMPTOM PATTERN

IF A PATIENT HAS SYMPTOMS AT A CERTAIN TIME OF DAY, WHAT PATHOLOGY DOES THIS IMPLICATE?

- Morning stiffness is common following wrist fracture and can take many months to resolve.
- Night numbness may be due to sleeping positions, such as flexed wrists, flexed elbows, and sleeping on the arm. This is a common complaint for patients with carpal tunnel syndrome.
- Nighttime hand edema may cause sensory symptoms as well.
- Throbbing at night is often common with fractures.
- Symptoms usually increase throughout the day when repetitive stress disorders such as carpal tunnel and tendinopathies are involved.

STABILITY OF SYMPTOMS

- The normal progression of tissue is increased pain and swelling for the first 3 to 5 days; as the acute inflammatory phase resolves, edema will decrease over the course of the next 2 weeks. With this reduction of edema, pain and stiffness should also decrease. It is not uncommon for persistent swelling to be present in the hand for several months following the injury.
- The normal progression of symptoms following hand and wrist injury should be increased pain and stiffness for the first 5 days, decreasing pain and stiffness over a 3-week time frame, and return to most daily activities by 6 weeks; full recovery of strength and function may take up to a year depending on the nature of the patient's injury.

CHANGES IN SYMPTOMS

- In the case of acute trauma, it is not unusual for the patient's symptoms to increase over the first 1 to 2 weeks. As the inflammation spreads, it begins to hypersensitize the surrounding tissue. Nerve compression secondary to inflammation is also common. Both of these symptoms should dissipate as the edema resolves.
- Worsening symptoms is not common. If they occur, the clinician should determine if the increase in symptoms is due to

a change in use. If the worsening is insidious in nature, the clinician should rule out red flags to determine if referral to the physician is warranted.

CLINICAL PEARL

If the exercise program is causing more edema or pain, modify the exercise program and focus on elevation, pain-free active range of motion including proximal and reciprocal motions, edema mobilization, and light compression. As the edema resolves, range of motion can be restored more successfully.

CLINICAL PEARL

Swollen or inflamed joints or tissues cannot tolerate passive range of motion. Use caution and treat the swelling and inflammation as a priority.

FUNCTIONAL AND ACTIVITY PARTICIPATION LIMITATIONS (Tables II-10-2 and II-10-3)

BEHAVIOR OF SYMPTOMS: AGGRAVATING BEHAVIOR

What influence do aggravating functions have on your clinical decision-making process? (see Table II-10-2)

- It is difficult to definitively differentiate hand and wrist pathology based solely on aggravating activities. In spite of this fact, several trends can be seen clinically regarding wrist and hand pathology.
- Promoting pain-free arcs of motion and identifying and avoiding aggravating motions will speed up recovery.
- Pain with extension of the wrist or hand can be indicative of several pathologies.
  - A strain of any of the extensor muscles would result in pain as the muscle contracts.
  - Mallet finger or disruption of the distal extensor tendon from the distal phalanx can prevent extension of the distal phalanx.
  - Mallet finger can turn into a boutonniere deformity if the lateral bands are allowed to migrate volarly.
  - Trigger finger occurs when the finger can flex but difficulty arises when extension is attempted from the flexed position.
  - Osteoarthritis or rheumatoid arthritis in any finger, hand, or wrist joint would make attainment of full extension difficult.
  - Any of the distal radius fractures (Colles, Smith, or Barton) could result in difficulty with wrist extension.
- Pain or difficulty with palmar flexion of the wrist of hand could indicate the following:
  - Flexor tendon lacerations will present following trauma. If completely disrupted the patient will be unable to flex the involved finger. If it is partially lacerated, motion may be possible.
  - Flexor muscle strains will present with the ability to flex the finger or wrist, but use of the involved muscle will be painful.
  - Wrist fractures will be painful with most motions including flexion.
  - Arthritis, osteo and rheumatoid, will limit joint flexion. Arthritis will often result in swelling of the joint. These are classic signs of finger arthritis. When at the middle joint of one or more fingers, the swellings are called Bouchard's nodes. When located at the fingertip, they are called Heberden's nodes.
  - Wrist flexion will be limited and present with elbow pain if lateral epicondylitis is involved.
- Pain with ulnar deviation could indicate the following:
  - The triangular fibrocartilage complex (TFCC) is a ligamentous and cartilaginous structure that separates the distal ulna from the proximal row of carpals. Pain with ulnar deviation often indicates damage to this structure. Acute injuries, repetitive use, or a history of wrist fracture can all be associated with pathology in this tissue.
  - Intersection syndrome and de Quervain's tenosynovitis will both present with pain during ulnar deviation of the wrist. Unlike

TFCC injuries in which the pain is located on the ulnar side of the wrist, intersection syndrome and de Quervain's tenosynovitis will present with pain on the radial aspect of the wrist.
  - Radial nerve irritation can also present with pain during ulnar deviation of the wrist.
- Pain with radial deviation could indicate the following:
  - Wrist fracture will often result in changes in wrist anatomical alignment and wrist biomechanics. When these alterations occur, pain with radial deviation may be present.
  - de Quervain's tenosynovitis will result in pain with active radial deviation of the wrist.
- Pain with pronation could indicate the following:
  - Like radial deviation, distal radius fractures can result in changes in normal ulnar variance. This could limit the forearm's ability to attain full pronation as impact at the ulnar aspect of wrist blocks full motion. The TFCC can get injured due to these changes and altered forces.
- Pain with supination could indicate the following:
  - Distal radius fractures can also impact a patient's ability to attain full supination, but generally problems at the radial head can be a large source of problems with supination. Proper examination should also explore problems at the radial head.
- Gripping pain could implicate the following:
  - It is difficult to diagnose pathology based solely on pain with gripping. Many pathologies will manifest themselves as pain or weakness with gripping activities.
  - To attain full grip strength 35° of extension and 7° of ulnar deviation are needed. Only 25% of grip strength can be achieved in full wrist flexion.
  - Distal radius fracture impacts gripping because wrist extension is required to grip an object.
  - Carpal instability will not allow the wrist to provide a solid base for gripping to occur.
  - Muscle strain or lacerations will alter grip strength and may cause pain when gripping is attempted.
  - Ulnar nerve injuries will weaken the muscles required for power gripping.
- Pinching pain is indicative of the following:
  - Gripping requires proper function of the ulnar nerve. The fine motor skills required for pinching requires proper function of the median nerve.
  - CMC arthritis will also be painful with pinching activities.

TABLE II-10-2 **Risk Factors**[7]	
Problem	**Risk Factors**
de Quervain's tenosynovitis	Golf
	Knitting
	Lifting baby
	Racquet sports
	Mail sorting
	File handling
Intersection syndrome	Weight lifting
	Rowing
	Canoe
EPL	Drummers
ECU	Scanning at checkout
	Computer postures
FCR	Wrist-intensive activity
FCU	Scanning at checkout
	Computer postures
Flexor tenosynovitis	Sustained gripping
	Using palm as a hammer

EPL, extensor pollicis longus; ECU, extensor carpi ulnaris; FCR, flexor carpi radialis; FCU, flexor carpi ulnaris.

TABLE II-10-3   Functional and Activity Participation Limitations

Motion	Functional Activities	Pathology if Symptoms Are Aggravated by Activity	Pathology if Symptoms Are Eased by Activity
Wrist flexion	Computer use Cooking	Flexor tendon lacerations Flexor muscle strains Wrist fractures Osteoarthritis Rheumatoid arthritis Lateral epicondylitis	Most hand and wrist pathologies are eased with rest and protection
Wrist extension	Gripping Computer use	Extensor muscle strain Osteoarthritis Rheumatoid arthritis Distal radius fractures (Colles, Smith, or Barton)	
Finger flexion	Gripping Writing	Flexor tendon lacerations Flexor muscle strains Osteoarthritis Rheumatoid arthritis Lateral epicondylitis	
Finger extension	Miscellaneous	Extensor muscle strain Mallet finger Boutonniere deformity Trigger finger Osteoarthritis Rheumatoid arthritis	
Ulnar deviation	Hammering Opening jars	Triangular fibrocartilage complex (TFCC) Intersection syndrome de Quervain's tenosynovitis Radial nerve irritation	
Radial deviation	Fishing	Wrist fracture de Quervain's tenosynovitis	
Pronation	Turning door knobs	Distal radius fractures TFCC	
Supination	Carrying objects	Distal radius fractures Radial head pathology	
Gripping	Daily activities	Many pathologies Distal radius fracture Carpal instability Muscle strain or lacerations Ulnar nerve injuries	
Pinching	Daily activities	Median nerve injuries Carpometacarpal arthritis	

BEHAVIOR OF SYMPTOMS: EASING BEHAVIOR

WHAT INFLUENCE DO EASING FUNCTIONS HAVE ON YOUR CLINICAL DECISION-MAKING PROCESS?

- Most wrist and hand pathologies are eased by similar methods. As a result, it is difficult to utilize them in the diagnostic process.
- Generally speaking, joint pain, as in osteoarthritis, is eased by heat and may be aggravated by ice, which can cause a stiffening response.
- Nerve pain also typically worsens with ice and is relieved with heat.
- In contrast, sore or inflamed muscles or tendons may benefit from ice or splinting.

CLINICAL PEARL

Sustained grip and pinch, particularly with extremes of wrist motion, can cause carpal tunnel symptoms due to flexor tendon inflammation. Momentarily changing hand positions, enlarging the handles of tools, wearing padded gloves, and using good posture can help minimize these symptoms.

MEDICAL HISTORY

WHAT ROLE DOES A PATIENT'S PAST MEDICAL HISTORY PLAY IN DIFFERENTIAL DIAGNOSIS OF WRIST AND HAND PATHOLOGY?

- Diabetes is associated with slower healing of incisions and reduced tissue tolerances.
- Diabetes also predisposes a patient to increased risk of ulcerations, fractures, and nerve pathology.
- In patients with cancer, talk to their oncologist before using any electrical modalities because electrical modalities may be contraindicated.
- If there has been any involvement of the lymphatic system such as removal of lymph nodes, massage techniques to reduce the edema should be performed only by a lymphedema-trained therapist.
- Patients with fibromyalgia have decreased tissue tolerance, pain that is often multifocal, and disturbance of sleep.
- Osteoporosis and osteopenia predispose the patient to wrist and hand fractures.
- Long-time corticosteroid use will also result in weakened bone and soft tissue structures. Therefore, injury to these tissues can occur more readily.

- Kidney disease will often result in foot manifestations. Gout is common in the foot and ankle.
- Autoimmune disorders such as rheumatoid arthritis and lupus will also often attack peripheral joints such as the foot and ankle. Therefore, a careful history should include screening for autoimmune disorders in the individual and in their immediate family.

CLINICAL PEARL

Patients with asthma or other respiratory conditions should not be treated with fluidotherapy and may experience respiratory distress if they are in the same room as the fluidotherapy unit when it is running.

MEDICAL AND ORTHOPEDIC TESTING

WHAT MEDICAL TESTS INFLUENCE YOUR DIFFERENTIAL DIAGNOSIS PROCESS?

- For patients with carpal tunnel syndrome (CTS), Semmes Weinstein monofilament testing is highly sensitive (91% in one study) but not highly specific.[10]
- Compression testing with a commercial device is reported to have 87% sensitivity and 90% specificity in diagnosing CTS.[10]

WHAT ORTHOPEDIC TESTS INFLUENCE YOUR DIFFERENTIAL DIAGNOSIS PROCESS?

Table II-10-4, Table II-10-5, Table II-10-6, Table II-10-7, and Table II-10-8 are all orthopedic tests commonly utilized in the assessment and treatment of hand pathology. See tables for futher information.

Waimmer et al developed a clinical prediction rule for the diagnosis of CTS. If the following five variables are present, the positive likelihood ratio is 18.3. If the variables are present, there is a posttest probability of 90% that the patient has CTS.[18]
1. Brigham and Women's Hospital Hand Severity Scale score great than 1.9
2. Wrist ratio index greater than 67
3. Patient reports that shaking the hand decreases symptoms
4. Decreased sensation on the thumb pad
5. Greater than 45 years old

TABLE II-10-4 Lag versus Contracture[6]

Problem	Finding
Lag	PROM greater than AROM
Joint contracture	Passive limitation of joint motion

PROM, passive range of motion; AROM, active range of motion.

TABLE II-10-5 Joint versus Musculotendinous Tightness[5]

Problem	Finding
Joint tightness	PROM of joint does not change with repositioning of the proximal or distal joints
Musculotendinous tightness	PROM of joint changes with repositioning of the adjacent joints that are crossed by the particular musculotendinous unit

PROM, passive range of motion.

TABLE II-10-6 Intrinsic or Extrinsic Tightness[5]

Problem	Finding	Treatment
Interosseous muscle tightness	Passive PIP and DIP flexion is limited when the MP joint is passively extended or hyperextended but not when the MP joint is passively flexed	Perform PIP and DIP flexion with MP hyperextension
Extrinsic extensor tightness	Passive PIP and DIP flexion is limited when the MP joint is passively flexed but not when the MP joint is passively extended. Also passive composite digital flexion is more limited with the wrist flexed than with the wrist extended	Perform composite motions such as combined flexion of the wrist, MPs, CTFg, and IPs
Extrinsic flexor tightness	Passive composite digital extension is more limited with the wrist extended than with the wrist flexed	Perform composite motion s such as combined extension of the wrist, MPs, and IPs

PIP, proximal interphalangeal; DIP, distal interphalangeal; MP, metacarpophalangeal; IP, interphalangeal; CTFg, contralateral trunk flexion group.

TABLE II-10-7 Peripheral Nerve Problems and Functional Splinting[14]

Problem	Functional Splint
Radial nerve	Dynamic MP extension
Median nerve	Thumb abduction
Ulnar nerve	Ring and small finger anticlaw

MP, metacarpophalangeal.

TABLE II-10-8 Special Tests for the Hand and Wrist[4]

Name of Test (Pathology)	Specificity of Tests (%)	Sensitivity of Tests (%)	Likelihood Ratios
Tinels (carpal tunnel)	58 to 97	23 to 62	+ LR: 11.0 − LR: .69
Phalens (carpal tunnel)	47 to 92	34 to 88	+ LR: 9.88 − LR: .89
Watson (carpal instability)	66	69	+ LR: 2.03 − LR: .47
Ballottement (carpal instability)	44	64	+ LR: 1.14 − LR: .82

CLINICAL DECISION MAKING CASE STUDY—PATIENT PROFILE

Your patient is a 27-year-old woman who has just had a baby. She presents with bilateral pain over the dorsal-radial wrists and this is interfering with her ability to lift and hold her baby. What tests and recommendations are appropriate?

Answer

Ask the patient to demonstrate what position her arms and hands are in when she lifts her baby. Perform a Finkelstein test and also a manual muscle test for the extensor pollicis brevis (EPB) and the abductor pollicis longus (APL). Many mothers lift their babies with extreme wrist ulnar deviation and hold and feed their babies with wrist and thumb flexion, positions that are provoking of the EPB and the APL, the structures of the first dorsal compartment. Instruct the patient in maintaining a neutral wrist with activities of daily living including lifting and holding her baby. Promote pain relief and pain-free active arcs of motion of the involved structures. Enlarge the girth of writing implements and kitchen utensils.

CLINICAL PEARL

If passive range of motion (PROM) is equal to active range of motion (AROM), work on AROM and PROM. If PROM is greater than AROM, work on AROM to promote tendon pull-through. If intrinsics are tight, place MPs in hyperextension and work on PIP/DIP flexion.[6]

MEDICATIONS

HOW DOES A PATIENT'S RESPONSE TO MEDICATION INFLUENCE YOUR DECISION-MAKING PROCESSES?

- Blood thinners increase the risk of bruising.
- A history of steroid use contributes to skin fragility.
- Steroid use (as in iontophoresis) may raise the sugar level of patients with diabetes.
- Steroids may cause hypopigmentation of the skin in people of color.
- Steroids weaken bone and soft tissue.

BIOMECHANICAL

WHAT ROLE DOES BIOMECHANICS PLAY IN YOUR DECISION-MAKING PROCESS?

- Functionally, the radiocarpal, ulnocarpal, mid-carpal, and intercarpal joints work together to allow the wrist to function properly. Alterations in any of these structures could result in any of the numerous hand pathologies. Careful examination should be performed to rule out biomechanical alterations that may contribute to the ultimate pathology.
- Teach patients with wrist fracture to isolate the extensor carpi radialis brevis (ECRB) so they do not substitute the extensor digitorum communis (EDC) when trying to extend the wrist. This will also help them improve their digital flexion.

CLINICAL PEARL

Do not have patients work on digital flexion with the wrist in a flexed position unless there is already good wrist active extension and there is evidence of extrinsic extensor tightness. Instead, teach the patient to self-support the wrist in extension or use a wrist cock-up splint while performing digital flexion or grasping activities.

CLINICAL PEARL

It is extremely important for the patient to learn to extend the wrist with the ECRB and not substitute the EDC. For this reason, have the patient hold something such as a tennis ball with the MPs flexed, while actively extending the wrist. Be sure the MPs stay flexed.

- Teach patients to avoid unsupported upper extremity positions for distal symptoms of tendinopathy.
- Teach patients with arthritis about joint protection principles.

WHAT BIOMECHANICAL ABNORMALITIES IN OTHER REGIONS AFFECT YOUR DECISION-MAKING PROCESS?

Proximal weakness, deconditioning, and poor scapular stabilization cause more stress and load on distal structures of the wrist and hand.

ENVIRONMENTAL FACTORS

DO PSYCHOSOCIAL ISSUES INFLUENCE YOUR CLINICAL DECISION-MAKING PROCESS?

Pain and functional limitations of the wrist and hand negatively affect all aspects of a person's daily routine. From self-care to earning an income, the quality of life can be compromised. This can cause stress among family members at a time when psychological support is needed. Autonomic, immune and endocrine systems have all been implicated as potential sources of pain for patients. See Table II-10-9 for additional information.

CAN EMOTIONS INFLUENCE THE DECISION-MAKING PROCESS?

Patients may be embarrassed about their wrist or hand injury, or they may be angry and could possibly be embroiled in litigation related to it. All these factors influence their ability to focus positively on their recovery process.

DO WORK-RELATED INJURIES INFLUENCE CLINICAL DECISION MAKING?

Patients may be afraid to pursue a worker's compensation claim for fear of jeopardizing their job, or they may be angry over employer liability issues. These factors can also interfere with recovery.

CLINICAL DECISION MAKING
CASE STUDY—PATIENT PROFILE

A 31-year-old male engineer works at his computer 10 hours a day and also plays the guitar in a group during his free time. He developed bilateral ulnar wrist pain that worsens through the day and is interfering with his ability to play the guitar. What are your recommendations to improve his ergonomics at work?

Answer

Observe the patient's posture and initiate a proximal stabilization home program. Also explore alternative keyboards such as a split keyboard that will minimize the amount of repetitive ulnar deviation at the wrists. Consider a buddy strap between the ring and small fingers if small finger hyperextension/hyperabduction at the keyboard appears to be provoking. Emphasize pacing and task rotation, and advise the patient to momentarily change positions, stretch, and take some deep breaths every 20 minutes or so.

PERSONAL FACTORS

PRIOR SURGERY
WHAT PRIOR SURGERIES INFLUENCE YOUR CLINICAL DECISION MAKING?
Preexisting range of motion limitations from scar or tendon adherence make it harder to recover maximal clinical gains.

CHRONICITY OF PAIN

HAS MEDICAL TREATMENT BEEN SUCCESSFUL FOR PATIENTS WITH CHRONIC PATHOLOGY IN THE REGION?

- Recurrence of tendinopathy can be discouraging to patients, but it also gives them knowledge of preventive or corrective measures to implement.
- Longstanding joint tightness with decreased tendon excursion (e.g., after distal radius fracture) may be extremely challenging to treat. Abnormal responses are commonplace following wrist or hand pathology. See Table II-10-10 for terminology utilized for different types of pain seen following hand pathology.

CLINICAL PEARL

!

It is very important to document in the initial evaluation whether the joints are tight and if there is hard end-range feel. In these instances, be realistic but hopeful and encouraging with the patient.

CLINICAL PEARL

!

PIP joint sprains can be slow to recover and edema and pain can linger. Permanent limitations in function and range of motion are possible.

RED FLAGS THAT WARRANT REFERRAL TO A MEDICAL PHYSICIAN

WHAT SYMPTOMS ALERT YOU TO PATHOLOGIES THAT MAY REQUIRE A REFERRAL TO A MEDICAL PHYSICIAN?

- Pain in the anatomical snuffbox might indicate a scaphoid fracture.
- The inability to extend the MPs may be indicative of extensor tendon rupture in rheumatoid patients.
- The inability to isolate the FDS or FDP may be indicative of flexor tendon rupture in rheumatoid patients.
- Wrist drop may be indicative of radial nerve involvement.
- First dorsal interosseous atrophy is indicative of ulnar nerve involvement, but could also occur due to an upper motor neuron disease.
- An inability to extend the thumb may be indicative of thumb extensor tendon rupture in patients with distal radius fracture or rheumatoid arthritis.
- Redness, swelling, heat, and pain are objective signs of inflammation and possibly infection.
- Vasomotor instability (blotchiness or discoloration in the palm), hyperhydrosis (dramatic increase in sweating), and pain that is disproportionate to the injury are signs of possible complex regional pain syndrome (Table II-10-11).

CLINICAL PEARL

!

Kanavel's cardinal signs of flexor tenosynovitis are (1) posture in slight digital flexion, (2) uniform volar swelling of the digit, (3) tenderness along the tendon sheath, and (4) pain with passive extension.[16]

TABLE II-10-9 Output Mechanisms

Output Mechanism	Effect on Wrist/Hand
Autonomic	Complex regional pain syndrome (CRPS) (RSD)
Endocrine	May affect healing and can be associated with peripheral neuropathy
Immune	Rheumatoid arthritis and scleroderma are autoimmune disorders

---

TABLE II-10-10 Pain Terminology[1]

Pain Terminology	Description
Allodynia	Pain from sources that do not typically cause pain
Hyperalgia	Increased response to a painful stimulus
Hyperpathia	Pain that continues after the painful stimulus is removed

---

TABLE II-10-11 Symptoms of Complex Regional Pain Syndrome (CRPS)

Symptom	Description
Pain	Disproportionate to the injury, burning quality
Stiffness	Joint tightness, contractures, palmar thickening or nodules
Discoloration	Bluish, mottled, or redness
Trophic changes	Abnormal hair and fingernail growth and texture
Hyperhydrosis	Abnormal sweating along nerve distribution or in an atypical place
Motor dysfunction	Tremor, dystonia, increased tone, muscle spasms, loss of strength and endurance

Modified from Astifidis RP: Pain-related syndromes: complex regional pain syndrome and fibromyalgia. In Cooper C, editor: *Fundamentals of Hand Therapy: Clinical Reasoning and Treatment Guidelines for Common Diagnoses of the Upper Extremity,* 1st ed. St. Louis: Elsevier, 2007.

SUMMARY STATEMENT

Wrist and hand problems limit people's ability to function and can have a devastating effect on their quality of life. Patients often comment that before injury, they did not appreciate what an impact their wrist or hand problem could have on the ordinary and meaningful activities of their day. Good clinical decision making is necessary to expedite their recovery and help improve their quality of life. Table II-10-12 summarizes the factors that help a clinician differentiate among different sources of symptoms in the wrist and hand regions.

TABLE II-10-12   Body Structure and Tissue-Based Pathology

	Muscle	Tendon	Ligament	Bone	Cartilage	Joint	Other	Nerves	Visceral Tissue
Pathology	Muscle strains	Flexor and extensor tendon pathology, Trigger finger, Mallet finger, de Quervain's syndrome, FCU Tendinopathy, Jersey finger, intersection syndrome, Flexor tendon laceration, Dupuytren's contracture	UCL tear, Swan neck deformity, Boutiniere deformity, Scaphoid dislocation/fracture	Barton fractures, Boxer's fracture, Colles fracture, Smith fractures, Finger fractures, Chauffeur's fracture	TFCC irritation, Osteoarthritis, Rheumatoid arthritis	Finger dislocations, Thumb CMC osteoarthritis, Rheumatoid arthritis	Ganglionic cyst	Carpal tunnel syndrome	Cardiac, Pulmonary
Age	20 to 50 years old	20 to 50 years old	20 to 50 years old	60 years old +	60 years old +	60 years old +	Any age	20 to 50 years old	Any age
Occupation	Secondary to trauma	Repetitive use	Secondary to trauma	Secondary to trauma	Secondary to trauma or disease	Repetitive use	No relation to occupation or use	Repetitive use	No correlation established
Gender	No correlation	No correlation	No correlation	No correlation	No correlation	No correlation	No correlation	No correlation	Depends on pathology
Ethnicity	No correlation	No correlation	No correlation	No correlation	No correlation	No correlation	No correlation	No correlation	Depends on pathology
History	May have prior history of muscle strains	No prior history needed	May have history of rheumatoid arthritis	No prior history needed	May have history of trauma to region	May have history of trauma to region	No correlation	May have history of cervical pathology	May have history of cardiac, pulmonary, or thyroid pathology
Mechanism of injury	Trauma	Trauma or overuse	Trauma or overuse	Trauma	Trauma or overuse	Trauma or overuse	No correlation	Overuse	Not correlated to a particular mechanism
Type of onset	Sudden	Sudden or insidious	Sudden or insidious	Sudden	Sudden or insidious	Sudden or insidious	Insidious	Insidious	May be sudden or gradual
Referral from local tissue	May refer down length of the muscle	Generally localized to immediate region	Generally localized to immediate region	May refer down shaft of the bone	Generally localized to immediate region	Generally localized to immediate region	Symptoms are localized to area around the cyst	May refer down length of the involved nerve	Can be localized to region adjacent to the injured tissue
Referral to other regions	May refer down length of the muscle	Generally localized to immediate region	Generally localized to immediate region	May refer down length of the bone	Generally localized to immediate region	Generally localized to immediate region	None	May refer down length of the involved nerve	May refer into shoulder, arm, neck, thoracic spine, or head depending on tissue

Continued on following page.

Section II

ORTHOPEDIC REASONING

TABLE II-10-12 Body Structure and Tissue-Based Pathology (*Continued*)

	Muscle	Tendon	Ligament	Bone	Cartilage	Joint	Other	Nerves	Visceral Tissue
Changes in symptoms	Immediate pain	Immediate pain	Immediate pain	Immediate pain	Gradual increase in symptoms over several weeks or months	Gradual increase in symptoms over several weeks or months	Gradual increase in symptoms over several weeks or months	Generally, slow gradual onset	May be slow increase or sudden onset with gradual increase. May be episodic in nature
24-hour pain pattern (morning)	Pain throughout day Activity dependent	Pain throughout day Activity dependent	Pain throughout day Activity dependent	Stiff for several minutes on awakening	Stiff for several minutes on awakening	Stiff for several minutes on awakening	Symptoms not related to time of day	Stiff for several minutes on awakening due to inflammation	May or may not be better depending on tissue
24-hour pain pattern (afternoon)	Pain throughout day Activity dependent	Pain throughout day Activity dependent	Pain throughout day Activity dependent	Pain occurs with use	Pain increases throughout the day and increases with use	Pain increases throughout the day and increases with use	Symptoms not related to time of day	Worsening in the afternoon if aggravated	May or may not be better depending on tissue
24-hour pain pattern (evening)	Pain throughout day Activity dependent	Pain throughout day Activity dependent	Pain throughout day Activity dependent	Increased pain with sleep	May be achy at night	May be achy at nigh	Symptoms not related to time of day	May have difficulty sleeping	Symptoms may worsen at night
Description of symptoms	Sharp pain	Sharp pain	Sharp pain	Dull ache	Dull ache Crepitus	Dull ache Crepitus	Tight and may be painful to palpation	Numbness, tingling, weakness	Achiness, cramping, heaviness, difficulty breathing
Depth of symptoms	Superficial	Superficial	Superficial	Deep	Deep	Deep	Superficial	Superficial or deep	Deep
Constancy of symptoms	Intermittent	Intermittent	Intermittent	Constant varying	Intermittent	Intermittent	Intermittent	Intermittent	Constant unremitting or episodic
Aggravating factors	Contraction of the muscle	Contraction of the muscle or stretch of the muscle	Stretch of the ligament	Motion	Weight bearing or closed pack position	Weight bearing or closed pack position	Direct pressure onto cyst	Activities that require stretching of the nerve or compression onto the nerve	Not activity dependent
Easing factors	Rest or splinting	Rest or splinting	Rest or splinting	Rest or splinting	Rest or splinting	Rest or splinting	None	Rest or splinting	Not activity dependent

Stability of symptoms	Pain increases for first 3 days and slow improvement over 6-week period	Pain increases for first 3 days and slow improvement over 6-week period	Pain increases for first 3 days and slow improvement over 6-week period	Pain increases for first 3 days and slow improvement over 8-week period	Worsening with time and overuse	Worsening with time and overuse	Stable	Symptom may worsen with time or overuse	Waxes and wanes with no particular time frame
Past medical history	Usually on dominant hand	May have history of steroid use	May have history of steroid use	May have osteopenia or osteoporosis	Autoimmune disorders	Autoimmune disorders	None	May have history of cervical dysfunction	Cardiac, pulmonary, or thyroid pathology, cancer, radiation or chemotherapy
Past surgeries	Not directly related	Not directly related	Not directly related	Not directly related	May have prior history of surgery to the upper extremity	May have prior history of surgery to the upper extremity	None	May have history of upper quarter surgery	Not directly related
Special questions	Strength loss Bruising	Strength loss Repetitive use	Traumatic injury	Deep ache Bruising	Crepitus	Crepitus	None	Numbness and tingling	Deep unremitting pain
X-rays	Negative	Negative	Negative	Positive	Positive	Positive	Negative	Negative	Negative
MRI	Positive	Positive	Positive	Positive	Positive	Positive	Positive	Positive	May or may not be positive
EMG	Negative	Negative	Negative	Negative	Negative	Negative	Negative	Positive	Varies and is dependent on suspected pathology
Special laboratory tests	Not applicable	Not applicable	Not applicable	Not applicable	Not applicable	Not applicable	Not applicable	Not applicable	Not applicable
Red flags	Unremitting pain, weight loss, nocturnal pain								

UCL, ulnar collateral ligament; TFCC, triangular fibrocartilage complex; FCU, flexor carpi ulnaris; MRI, magnetic resonance imaging; EMG, electromyogram.

REFERENCES

1. Astifidis RP. Pain-Related Syndromes: Complex Regional pain Syndrome and Fibromyalgia. In: Cooper C, ed. *Fundamentals of Hand Therapy: Clinical Reasoning and Treatment Guidelines for Common Diagnoses of the Upper Extremity*. 1st ed. St. Louis: Mosby; 2007:376-387.

2. Butler MW. Common Shoulder Diagnoses. In: Cooper C, ed. *Fundamentals of Hand Therapy: Clinical Reasoning and Treatment Guidelines for Common Diagnoses of the Upper Extremity*. 1st ed. St. Louis: Mosby; 2007:151-182.

3. Campbell PJ, Wilson RL. Management of Joint Injuries and Intraarticular Fractures. In: Mackin EJ, Callahan AD, Skirven TM, Schneider LH, Osterman AL, eds. *Rehabilitation of the Hand and Upper Extremity*. 5th ed. St. Louis: Mosby; 2002:396-411.

4. Cleland J. Wrist and Hand. In: Cleland J, ed. *Orthopaedic Clinical Examination: An Evidence-Based Approach for Physical Therapists*. 1st ed. Carlstadt, New Jersey: Icon Learning Systems; 2005:445-500.

5. Colditz JC. Therapist's Management of the Stiff Hand. In: Mackin EJ, Callinan N, Skirven TM, Schneider LH, Osterman AL, eds. *Rehabilitation of the Hand and Upper Extremity*. 5th ed. St. Louis: Mosby; 2002:1021-1049.

6. Cooper C. Fundamentals of Clinical Reasoning: Hand Therapy Concepts and Treatment Techniques. In: Cooper C, ed. *Fundamentals of Hand Therapy: Clinical Reasoning and Treatment Guidelines for Common Diagnoses of the Upper Extremity*. 1st ed. St. Louis: Mosby; 2007:3-21.

7. Cooper C. Hand Impairments. In: Trombly CA, Radomski MV, eds. *Occupational Therapy for Physical Dysfunction*. 5th ed. Philadelphia: Lippincott Williams & Wilkins; 2002:927-963.

8. Cooper C. The Geriatric Hand Patient: Special Treatment Considerations. In: Mackin EJ, Callahan AD, Skirven T, Schneider LH, Osterman AL, eds. *Rehabilitation of the Hand and Upper Extremity*. 5th ed. St. Louis: Mosby; 2002:1949-1958.

9. Culp RW, Taras JS. Primary Care of Flexor Tendon Injuries. In: Mackin EJ, Callahan AD, Skirven TM, Schneider LH, Osterman AL, eds. *Rehabilitation of the Hand and Upper Extremity*. 5th ed. St. Louis: Mosby; 2002:415-430.

10. Hayes EP, Carney K, Wolf J, Smith JM, Akelman E. Carpal Tunnel Syndrome. In: Mackin EJ, Callahan AD, Skirven TM, Schneider LH, Osterman AL, eds. *Rehabilitation of the Hand and Upper Extremity*. 5th ed. St. Louis: Mosby; 2002:643-659.

11. Krop PN. Fractures: General Principles of Surgical Management. In: Mackin EJ, Callahan AD, Skirven T, Schneider LH, Osterman AL, eds. *Rehabilitation of the Hand and Upper Extremity*. 5th ed. St. Louis: Mosby; 2002:371-381.

12. Laseter GF, Carter PR. Management of distal radius fractures. *J Hand Ther*. 1996;9(2):114-128.

13. McFarlane RM, MacDermid JC. Dupuytren's Disease. In: Mackin EJ, Callahan AD, Skirven T, Schneider LH, Osterman AL, eds. *Rehabilitation of the Hand and Upper Extremity*. 5th ed. St. Louis: Mosby; 2002:971-988.

14. Moscony AMB. Common Peripheral Nerve Problems. In: Cooper C, ed. *Fundamentals of Hand Therapy: Clinical Reasoning and Treatment Guidelines for Common Diagnoses of the Upper Extremity*. 1st ed. St. Louis: Mosby; 2007:201-250.

15. Moscony AMB. Common Wrist and Hand Fractures. In: Cooper C, ed. *Fundamentals of Hand Therapy: Clinical Reasoning and Treatment Guidelines for Common Diagnoses of the Upper Extremity*. 1st ed. St. Louis: Mosby; 2007:251-285.

16. Nathan R, Taras JS. Common Infections in the Hand. In: Mackin EJ, Callahan AD, Skirven TM, Schneider LH, Osterman AL, eds. *Rehabilitation of the Hand and Upper Extremity*. 5th ed. St. Louis: Mosby; 2002:359-368.

17. Smith KL. Nerve Response to Injury and Repair. In: Mackin EJ, Callahan AD, Skirven TM, Schneider LH, Osterman AL, eds. *Rehabilitation of the Hand and Upper Extremity*. 5th ed. St. Louis: Mosby; 2002:583-598.

18. Waimmer RS, Fritz JM, Irrgang JJ, Delitto A, Allison S, Boninger MI. Development of a clinical prediction rule for the diagnosis of carpal tunnel syndrome. *Arch Phys Med Rehabil*. 2005;86:609-618.

AUTHOR: JOHN L. MEYER

INTRODUCTORY INFORMATION

Until recently, the diagnosis of hip pathology has grouped hip pain into bursitis, arthritis, or genetic dysplasias. With the advent of new imaging and surgical techniques, pathology of the labrum and other structures around the hip has become potential sources of symptoms. The broader scope of pathologies has made the diagnosis of hip pathology more challenging for the clinician.

WHAT IS THE PREVALENCE OF HIP AND THIGH PATHOLOGY?

The prevalence of hip and thigh pathology varies in different aged populations.

The hip is a common sight for osteoarthritis, affecting 10% to 25% of the population over the age of 55 years.[26,77] Osteonecrosis can occur in people of any age, but it is most common in people in their thirties, forties, and fifties. An estimated 20,000 to 30,000 new cases of osteonecrosis are diagnosed annually.[36] Acute hip pain in children is a very common finding. Most often the cause of the pain is acute transient synovitis of the hip. The incidence of slipped capital femoral epiphysis is about 6.1 per 10,000 in boys and 3.0 per 10,000 in girls.[34] The incidence of Legg-Calvé-Perthes disease is about the same range of 1.5 to 5 per 10,000.[49] In the newborn, the prevalence of developmental dysplasia of the hip (DDH) has been reported in screened populations at rates of 2.5 to 20 per 1000 births, but reaches 40 to 90 per 1000 births in some communities. Differences in reported prevalence may be due to genetic differences and differences in clinical skills and methods used in the detection as well as the definition of the condition.[57]

WHAT IS THE PROGNOSIS FOR RECOVERY FROM HIP AND THIGH PATHOLOGY?

In general, predicting the prognosis in patients with hip pain is difficult. Risk factors for worsening status include increased age, increased body mass index, proprioceptive deficit, and pain intensity, whereas greater muscle strength, mental health, self-efficiency, social support, and anaerobic exercise are associated with better outcomes.[80,81]

WHAT FACTORS MAKE DIAGNOSIS DIFFICULT IN THE HIP AND THIGH REGION?

- The differential diagnosis of hip and thigh pain may require assistance from many health-care specialties from gynecology to general surgery to musculoskeletal medicine and orthopedic surgery.
- Referred pain may arise from lesions or disease in the urogenital or gastrointestinal systems.
- Dysfunction at the foot, knee, and lumbar spine can impact the hip joint.
- Radiographic findings do not always correlate with patient symptomology.

HOW SUCCESSFUL IS THERAPY IN TREATING HIP AND THIGH PATHOLOGY?

Physical therapy has been shown to be effective in the treatment of soft tissue injuries around the hip.[4,83] Several nonpharmacological modalities that can be provided through physical therapy have been shown to be beneficial in the treatment of hip osteoarthritis. These include education, aerobic exercise, muscle strengthening and water-based exercises, weight reduction, walking aids, footwear and insoles, thermal modalities, and transcutaneous electrical nerve stimulation.[92]

CLINICAL PEARL

Hip fracture is a common trauma in the elderly population and is associated with a high risk for death and disability. Of those surviving 6 months past the fracture, less than half regain prefracture physical function. Among them, the muscle strength and power deficit on the fractured side typically impairs mobility.[66]

HOW SUCCESSFUL IS SURGERY IN TREATING HIP AND THIGH PATHOLOGY?

Hip surgery has been shown to be effective in treating a wide variety of pathologies and in helping individuals return to their previous level of function across the lifespan.[21,22,42,45,59,64,69,75,86]

CLINICAL PEARL

Between the ages of 65 and 89 years, explosive lower-limb extensor power has been reported to decline at 3.5% per year compared to a 1% to 2% per year decrease in strength.[72] Older patients must be shown ways to rehabilitate and train for power as well as strength in order to be more independent and recover from injury.

PERSONAL INFORMATION

WHAT INFLUENCE DOES AGE HAVE ON YOUR CLINICAL DECISION-MAKING PROCESS IN THE HIP AND THIGH REGION?

The identification of a given structural disorder of the hip and thigh can be suggested by the patient's age.
- Developmental dysplasia is usually found in infants.[73]
- Legg-Calvé-Perthes disease is found in children 4 to 10 years old.[73]
- Slipped capital femoral epiphysis and apophyseal injuries are found in somewhat older children.[47]
- Young active individuals are more likely to suffer from strains, stress fractures, femoroacetabular impingement, labral pathology, osteitis pubis, and athletic pubalgia.
- Osteonecrosis is common in young to middle-aged adults.
- Degenerative joint disease, trochanteric bursitis, and hip fracture are more common in older adults.

WHAT INFLUENCE DOES A PATIENT'S OCCUPATION HAVE ON YOUR CLINICAL DECISION-MAKING PROCESS IN THE HIP AND THIGH REGION?

Occupation can place a person's hip and thigh in a compromised position leading to excessive stress, wear, or injury.
- A statistically significant association between occupational lifting and hip osteoarthritis has been shown.[65,91]
- However, being employed for more than 20 years in a job that requires heavy activity reduces the risk of hip fracture in postmenopausal women.
- Individuals with labral tears and/or femoroacetabular impingement do not often tolerate occupations that require prolonged sitting.[39]
- Athletes who are currently participating or have recently participated in competitive athletic activity as a livelihood or integral way of life are often at risk for soft tissue injuries, hernias, impingement, and labral tears about the hip.[51]

WHAT INFLUENCE DOES GENDER HAVE ON YOUR CLINICAL DECISION-MAKING PROCESS IN THE HIP AND THIGH REGION?

Some of the major pathologies seen in the hip and thigh have a gender preference.
- Developmental dysplasia is more prevalent in infants of female gender.

Section II   ORTHOPEDIC REASONING

- Legg-Calvé-Perthes disease is more common in males at about a 5:1 ratio.
- Males have a two times greater incidence of slipped capital femoral epiphysis.
- Hip dysplasia and labral tears are more common in women.[37]
- Osteitis pubis tends to be more common in the male athlete.
- Women represent approximately 8.2% of patients with athletic pubalgia.[51]
- Tendinopathy, muscle strains, and osteonecrosis tend to be non-gender specific.
- Hip pain from menstrual conditions and endometriosis would be specific to females.

CLINICAL DECISION MAKING CASE STUDY—PATIENT PROFILE ?

An 11-year-old boy presents with a chief complaint of severe pain at the knee and anterior/medial thigh that was insidious in onset 2 weeks ago. He is unable to bear full weight on the affected lower extremity and walks with a limp and external rotation of the lower leg. What are your hypotheses regarding the source of this patient's symptoms?

Answer
The age and gender of the patient and the manner in which thigh symptoms began are important lines of questioning when it comes to diagnosing the source of the symptoms. The patient is an adolescent male with an acute insidious onset of knee and thigh pain. The fact that the patient felt pain indicates tissue injury; however, there is no specific mechanism. This could implicate slipped capital femoral epiphysis as a source of the symptoms as it is the most common hip disorder observed in adolescent males and is of unknown etiology. If the physical examination finds that active hip range of motion is restricted in abduction, flexion, and internal rotation, the patient should be referred to a pediatric orthopedist for further workup.

SYMPTOM HISTORY

WHAT INFLUENCE DOES THE MECHANISM OF INJURY HAVE ON YOUR CLINICAL DECISION-MAKING PROCESS IN THE HIP AND THIGH REGION?
Mechanism of injury plays a large role in the differential diagnosis of patients with acute hip and thigh pain and less of a role in patients with chronic pain. Acute traumatic injuries can often be traced back to the movement or motion occurring at the time of injury. Muscle strains around the hip and thigh region often occur during eccentric deceleration movements.
- Traumatic onset of symptoms: fractures, subluxation, dislocation, compartment syndromes, muscle strains, contusions, and labral tears
- Gradual onset of symptoms with microtrauma: tendinopathy, bursitis, hernias, osteitis pubis, femoroacetabular impingement, and stress fractures
- Insidious onset: degenerative joint disease and referred pain

CLINICAL DECISION MAKING CASE STUDY—PATIENT PROFILE ?

Your patient is a 23-year-old male who reports anterior hip pain following an injury 5 weeks ago. He reports that he injured his hip after falling during a soccer game. He recalls reaching back for the ball (extension, external rotation) with his right leg and then getting knocked to the ground during the game. He initially felt a pain in the front of his hip but completed the remainder of the game. The next day he had difficulty walking and was uncomfortable when sitting for greater than 15 minutes. The pain has improved over the past several weeks, but continues to limit his ability to sit, bend forward, and run. What are your hypotheses regarding the source of this patient's symptoms?

Answer
The mechanism of injury and the aggravating factors are important lines of questioning when it comes to diagnosing the source of the symptoms. The direction of injury was extension and external rotation. This could implicate the anterior hip capsule, labrum, and/or anterior soft tissues as a source of the symptoms. Because the patient continues to have symptoms that are aggravated by hip flexion, sitting, and axial loading, intraarticular hip pathology and/or hip impingement should be considered as the primary source of symptoms.

LOCATION OF SYMPTOMS

WHAT INFLUENCE DOES THE LOCATION OF SYMPTOMS HAVE ON YOUR CLINICAL DECISION-MAKING PROCESS IN THE HIP AND THIGH REGION?
Pain in the hip joint can indicate various hip conditions. True hip joint pain is actually often felt as groin pain, and needs to be distinguished from thigh pain, particularly upper thigh pain, buttock pain, and side/lateral pain.
   ANTERIOR: Hip flexor strain, snapping hip syndrome, and quadriceps contusion are found.[87]
   ANTERIOR MEDIAL GROIN: Adductor tendinopathy, avascular necrosis, hernia, impingement/labral tear, degenerative joint disease, osteitis pubis, Perthes' disease, slipped capital femoral epiphysis, stress fracture of the femur or pubic ramus, and referred back pain are found.[87]
   LATERAL: Iliotibial band (ITB) friction syndrome, greater trochanteric bursitis, and referred back pain are found.[87]
   POSTERIOR: Hamstring strain, hamstring tendinopathy, piriformis syndrome, posterior thigh compartment syndrome, ischiogluteal bursitis, sacroiliac pain, sciatica, and referred back pain are found.[87]

CLINICAL PEARL !

Lateral hip pain is a common complaint that frequently results in a diagnosis of trochanteric bursitis.[1,7] Injection of a long-acting local anesthetic and corticosteroids into the site of maximal tenderness can provide long-lasting relief; however, recurrence of symptoms after injection can occur. A correlation between lumbar degenerative disease, gluteus medius tendinopathy, and trochanteric bursitis has been demonstrated in the literature. The major predictor of relapse of pain after injection is the presence of moderate to severe lumbar degenerative disease.[84] Therefore, it is necessary to effectively screen the lumbar spine for dysfunction in patient's who present with lateral hip pain.

REFERRAL OF SYMPTOMS

WHAT STRUCTURES CAN REFER INTO THE HIP AND THIGH AND SACROILIAC JOINT REGION?
MUSCLE INJURY
The sacroiliac joint is unable to function in isolation; anatomically and biomechanically it shares all of its muscles with the hip joint. All of the following muscles have connections or an intimate relationship to the various sacroiliac ligaments and can be a source of pain of dysfunction.

Piriformis

- It is in close proximity to the sacroiliac joint.
- Injury to or pathology affecting the sacroiliac joint may result in dysfunction of the piriformis.
- The sciatic nerve, which passes immediately beneath or traverses through the piriformis, may become irritated leading to buttock and lower extremity complaints.[68]
- Trigger points in the piriformis muscle refer pain to the sacroiliac region, to the buttock, and over the hip joint posteriorly. The pain sometimes also extends over the proximal two-thirds of the posterior thigh.[79]

Biceps femoris, semitendinosus, and semimembranosus

- Trigger points in the semitendinosus and semimembranosus refer pain upward to the gluteal fold, downward to the medial region of the posterior thigh, the back medial side of the knee, and the medial calf.
- Trigger points in the biceps femoris project distal to the lateral aspect of the knee and may also extend upward in the posterior thigh to the crease of the buttock.[79]

Gluteus maximus: Trigger points refer pain locally in the buttock region adjacent to the sacrum, at the ischial tuberosity, and to the sacroiliac joint. There can be mild referral into the posterior thigh.[79]

Gluteus medius: It refers pain along the posterior crest of the ilium, to the sacrum, and to the posterior and lateral aspects of the buttock. Trigger points in the muscle can also refer pain to the lower lumbar spine.[79]

Gluteus minimus

- Anterior portion: projects pain and tenderness to the lower lateral part of the buttock, the lateral aspect of the thigh and knee, and to the peroneal region of the leg
- Posterior portion: refers pain to most of the buttock, posterior thigh, and back of the knee and calf[79]

Quadratus lumborum: Referred pain is projected posteriorly to the region of the sacroiliac joint and the lower buttock. Sometimes it can refer anteriorly along the crest of the ilium to the adjacent lower quadrant of the abdomen and groin.[79]

Iliocostalis lumborum: Projects pain from an area lateral to the lumbar spine to the sacral and gluteal area.

Longissimus thoracic: Refers pain from the lower thoracic spine to the posterior iliac crest and gluteal area.

Multifidi: Projects pain from the vertebral level to the sacral area.

External oblique: Refers pain from the lower lateral abdominal wall to the anterior medial groin.[79]

CLINICAL PEARL

Pain and dysfunction in the gluteus minimus can be persistent and severe. It has been referred to as "pseudo-sciatica" because of its referral pattern in the sciatic distribution. Kellgren found that in 55 of 70 patients seen for sciatica the pain was of ligamentous or muscular origin, commonly from the gluteal musculature.[40]

BONE AND LIGAMENT INJURY: No studies have been conducted on the referral pattern of bone or ligament pathology in the hip and thigh regions.

JOINT (CAPSULE/CARTILAGE)

Hip: True hip pain is usually referred to the groin, but it may also be referred to the ankle, knee, lumbar spine, and sacroiliac joints.

Sacroiliac: According to Slipman et al[74] the referral patterns of the sacroiliac joint are quite variable due to the joint's complex innervation. They have established 18 potential pain referral zones throughout the lumbar spine, pelvis, hip, thigh, and lower leg.

LUMBAR ZYGAPOPHYSIAL: Pain from these joints is referred down and very rarely upward. Pain is referred to the lumbosacral spine, sacroiliac joint, gluteal area, iliac crest, anterior thigh, and groin.[23]

CLINICAL DECISION MAKING CASE STUDY—PATIENT PROFILE

Your patient is a 33-year-old female professional dancer with complaints of anterior hip pain. Symptoms began insidiously and have been present for the past 6 months. They have become progressive, more frequent, and more intense in nature. Symptoms are worse with standing, walking, dancing, and running. Symptoms feel better when she limits her activity level. The patient has noticed that her symptoms worsen monthly and it appears to coincide with her menstrual cycles. She has a history of ovarian cysts. What are your hypotheses regarding her pathology?

Answer

The patient's symptoms appear to match those expected with chronic hip instability; the factor that complicates the diagnosis is an increase in symptoms that coincides with her menstrual cycles. Pathology such as ovarian cysts and endometriosis can be the source of symptoms or a contributor to hip pain. Cramping and pelvic-related pain can cause biomechanical abnormalities as the body guards and protects irritable regions. Hormones released during menstruation can also result in joint laxity and act on injured tissue.

CLINICAL PEARL

Individuals who perform repetitive activities involving axial loading and hip rotation may develop atraumatic hip instability and resultant hip pain. Patients with more chronic hip instability may be able to voluntarily sublux their hip. Stretch of the capsular structures can cause anterior hip pain and is tested with prone passive extension and external rotation.[60,71]

CLINICAL PEARL

With capsular laxity, the iliopsoas may become a more important dynamic stabilizer, resulting in stiffness, localized pain, or even flexion contracture.

NERVES

Dermatomal Distribution of Spinal nerve roots relevant to the sacroiliac joint, hip, and thigh (Figure II-11-1)

L1: Inguinal and posterior lateral buttock region
L2: Anterior and medial thigh, sacroiliac, and iliac crest region
L3: Anterior thigh and medial knee
L4: Medial leg and medial foot
L5: Lateral leg and dorsum of foot
S1: Posterior thigh and lateral foot
S2: Posterior thigh and medial ankle
S3: Groin and coccyx region
S4: Coccyx region

Myotomal Distribution of Spinal nerve roots relevant to the sacroiliac joint, hip, and thigh

L1: Hip flexion
L2: Hip flexion, hip adduction
L5: Hip abduction
S1: Hip extension

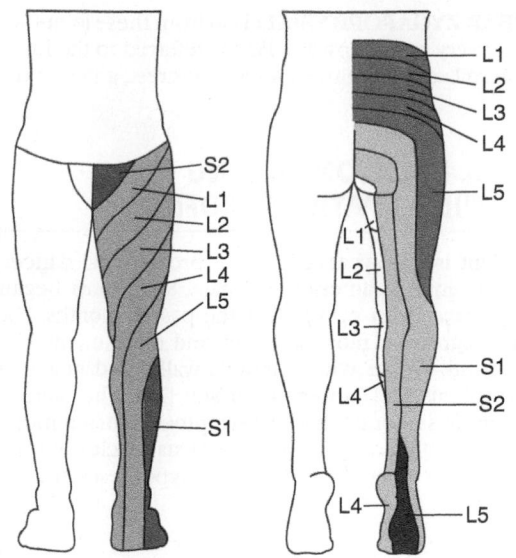

FIGURE II-11-1 Lower extremity dermatome distribution.

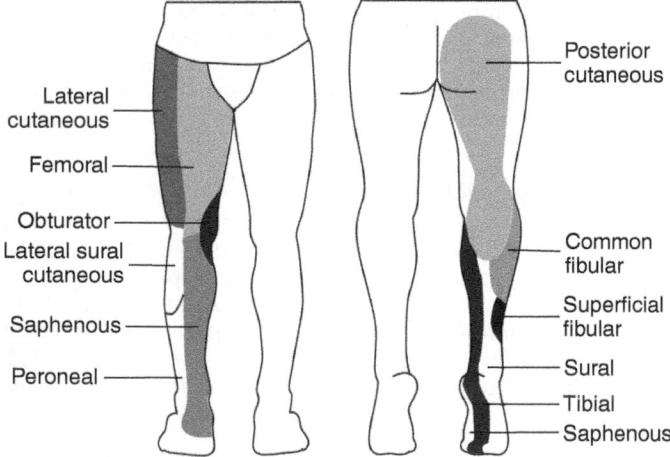

FIGURE II-11-2 Lower extremity peripheral nerve sensory distribution.

Nerves implicated with reflex loss
L3/L4: Patellar reflex
L5/S1: Medial hamstring
S1/S2: Lateral hamstring
Sensory Distribution of Peripheral nerves relevant to the sacroiliac joint, hip, and thigh (Figure II-11-2)
Femoral: medial thigh and calf
Anterior femoral cutaneous: Lateral hip and thigh
Posterior femoral cutaneous: Posterior thigh
Lateral femoral cutaneous: Lateral thigh
Pudendal: Groin and inner thighs
Obturator: Medial thigh
Sciatic: Posterior leg

CLINICAL PEARL

Meralgia paresthetica is a compression injury of the lateral femoral cutaneous nerve near the anterior superior spine of the ilium. Patients usually complain of pain and tingling paresthesias in the lower third of the lateral thigh. Pressure and tapping over this area may provoke lower lateral thigh

paresthesias and pain. The pain and paresthesias may be provoked or intensified by standing, walking, or extension and adduction of the leg.

VISCERAL STRUCTURES (Figure II-11-3)

Liver: Trochanteric and lateral thigh pain can result from osteonecrosis of the hip. Chronic liver disease has been shown to be one of the associated conditions with nontraumatic osteonecrosis of the femoral head.[87]

Pancreas: Inguinal and anteromedial thigh pain can also result from osteonecrosis of the hip. Pancreatitis has been shown to be one of the associated conditions with nontramatic osteonecrosis of the femoral head.[87]

Abdomen
- Inguinal or femoral hernias can refer pain to the anterior medial thigh and inguinal region.
- Abdominal aneurysm can refer pain to the low back or groin.[87]

Kidney/bladder: Ureteral colic is a paroxysm of pain due to abrupt obstruction of ureter from a calculus or blood clot. This condition can cause referred pain to the medial thigh.[87]

Colon: Generalized thigh pain can occur from retroperitoneal perforation of the colon.[87]

Female reproductive system: Tuboovarian lesions can lead to referred medial thigh pain.[87]

SYMPTOM DESCRIPTORS

QUALITY OF SYMPTOMS

Deep ache: Hip joint dysfunction
Dull ache: Hip joint dysfunction, inflammation, muscle strain
Sharp pain: Hip joint dysfunction, muscle strain
Sharp and continuous: Bone
Burning: Nerves, inflammation, vein, artery, lymphatic system
Tingling: Nerve
Numbness: Nerves
Colicky and cramping: Viscera

CLINICAL PEARL

Hawker et al[35] found that people with hip osteoarthritis experience two distinct types of pain: a dull, aching pain, which became more constant over time, punctuated increasingly with short episodes of a more intense, often unpredictable, emotionally draining pain. The latter, but not the former, resulted in significant avoidance of social and recreational activities.

DEPTH OF SYMPTOMS

Deep symptoms implicate deep structures such as the joint, articular cartilage, bone, and visceral structures. There are fewer proprioceptive nerves in deep structures than in more superficial structures so the ability to localize tissue damage in deep structures is more difficult.

Superficial symptoms implicate surface structures such as muscles and ligaments. Superficial structures have more proprioceptive nerve fibers and thus injury to superficial structures is more easily localized.

CONSTANCY OF SYMPTOMS

Intermittent symptoms implicate a mechanical source of pain. They indicate a structure that is injured and is aggravated only with certain positions or motions. Constant but varying symptoms implicate inflammation as the primary source. Constant and unchanging symptoms implicate visceral structures or other pathology such as cancer.

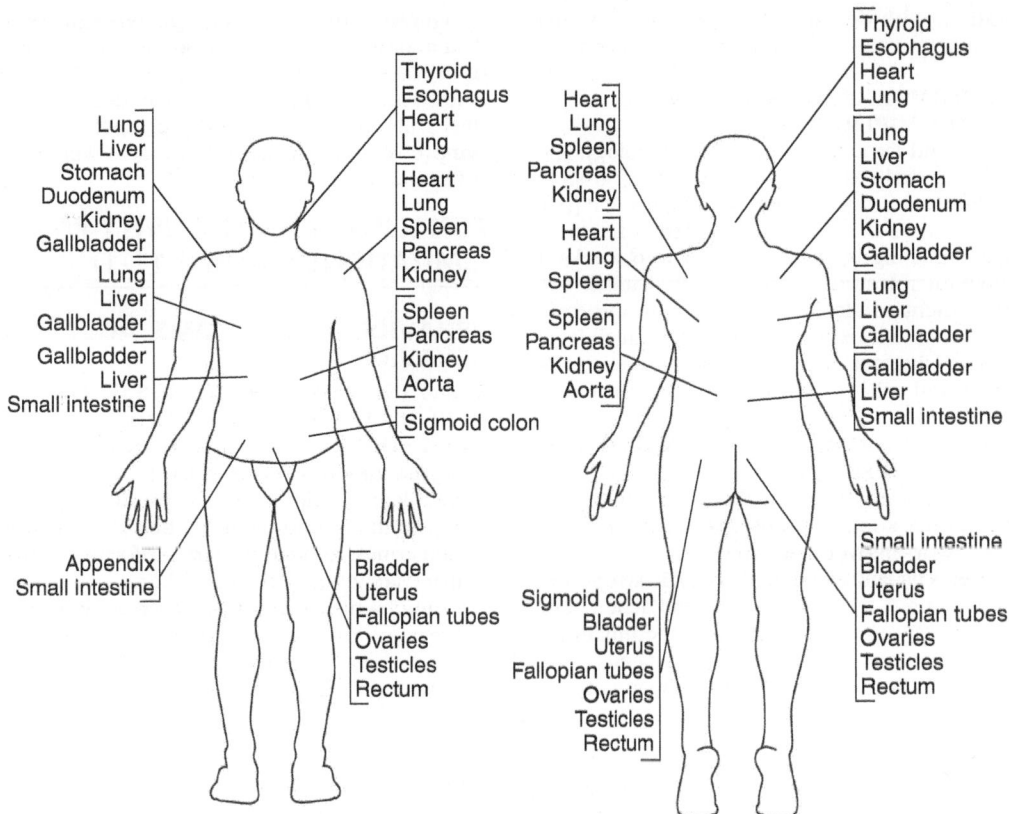

FIGURE II-11-3   Visceral referral pattern.

TWENTY-FOUR–HOUR SYMPTOM PATTERN

IF A PATIENT HAS SYMPTOMS IN THE MORNING, WHAT PATHOLOGY DOES THIS IMPLICATE?

It is common for a patient with hip symptoms to have stiffness in the morning. Generally, stiffness and pain that last for only a short time on awakening correspond to a pathology that is more mechanical in nature. Mechanical disorders are disorders that can be altered by biomechanical motions. Degenerative joint disease, impingement, and labral pathology will all present as stiffness in the morning that resolves quickly with motion.

Pain and stiffness that persist for a longer period of time, greater than 15 minutes, is common when inflammation is the primary source of the symptoms. Inflammation will abate once movement and circulation are increased in the region. Removal of edema from a region is tied to the lymphatic system. This system is a passive system and requires motion and muscle contractions to move the lymph out of the region. Therefore, symptoms will persist for a longer time frame.

WHAT ROLE DOES MORNING STIFFNESS PLAY IN DIFFERENTIATION?

Any time the body is in a static position for a prolonged period of time, inflammation can accumulate within a region. Body lymphatic systems are passive systems and require muscle contractions to drain areas. Morning stiffness that lasts for more than 15 minutes indicates that inflammation plays a large role in the feeling of stiffness. Stiffness that lasts only minutes and is relieved quickly with motion is often associated with mechanical factors more than with inflammatory factors.

When injured, an inflammatory reaction occurs. Muscle activation occurs as a protective mechanism to prevent further damage. If the hip joint is held in this position for more than 1 to 2 days, cross-fibers of collagen in the capsule will create a capsular stiffness.

IF A PATIENT HAS SYMPTOMS IN THE AFTERNOON, WHAT PATHOLOGY DOES THIS IMPLICATE?

Pain in the afternoon does not directly implicate a specific hip or thigh pathology. Differentiation is dependent on the activities and motions that the hip and thigh were exposed to earlier in the day.

IF A PATIENT HAS SYMPTOMS IN THE EVENING, WHAT PATHOLOGY DOES THIS IMPLICATE?

Evening symptoms can be viewed as an extension of afternoon symptoms. With continual use, the symptoms should continue to worsen if the irritating activities persist. If they have ceased for the day, then the symptoms may abate somewhat.

IF A PATIENT HAS SYMPTOMS WHILE SLEEPING, WHAT PATHOLOGY DOES THIS IMPLICATE?

Pain with sleeping can be the result of several factors. If a patient has pain when moving in bed, this can be the result of many types of pathology including degenerative joint disease, hip impingement, labral tears, and muscle strains. Pain due to static positions may implicate contusions and trochanteric or ischiogluteal bursitis. Nocturnal pain is also an indicator of visceral pathology and cancer, so red flag pathology should be ruled out.

STABILITY OF SYMPTOMS

CHANGES IN SYMPTOMS
HOW DOES THE PROGRESSION OF A PATIENT'S SYMPTOMS IMPACT YOUR CLINICAL DECISION-MAKING PROCESS?
Pain and symptoms in the hip and thigh can be variable depending on the patient's activity level and stress placed on the joint and surrounding structures. Muscular strains, tendinopathy, stress fractures, and compartment syndromes should worsen with significant activity and/or overuse. Activity and movement may

initially improve a patient with degenerative joint disease symptoms; however, as the degenerative processes progress, the symptoms will increase.

IF A PATIENT'S SYMPTOMS ARE IMPROVING, WHAT PATHOLOGY DOES THIS IMPLICATE?

Improvement is typical and expected with most pathology. The rate of improvement will help to narrow down the possible source of the symptoms. Muscle strains and contusions will generally improve in several days or 1 to 3 weeks. Stress fractures and tendinopathy will show signs of healing in 4 to 6 weeks if the source of repetitive microtrauma is removed. Individuals suffering from hip impingement and labral tears can show improvement with activity limitation and treatment. However, if high-level athletic competition involving cutting and twisting maneuvers is required of the patient, full relief of symptoms may not occur without surgical intervention.

IF A PATIENT'S SYMPTOMS ARE WORSENING, WHAT PATHOLOGY DOES THIS IMPLICATE?

Severe acute symptoms that are either traumatic or nontraumatic can be associated with muscle strains, contusions, or compartment syndromes. If symptoms worsen over a period of time such as several weeks, inflammation is usually associated with the symptoms. Initially the structure is injured and a sharp pain and ache occur. This is the nocioceptive response of the body. As the inflammatory process begins, surrounding structures can be irritated by the chemical mediators released due to the inflammatory process.

Symptoms that do not change over time are more indicative of degenerative changes. Because these processes are not the result of inflammation and acute processes, resolution in 4 to 6 weeks is not anticipated. Symptoms may decrease for several days, but they will return again. As the degenerative processes progress, the symptoms will increase. This process will occur over a period of several months.

FUNCTIONAL AND ACTIVITY PARTICIPATION LIMITATIONS (Table II-11-1)

BEHAVIOR OF SYMPTOMS: AGGRAVATING BEHAVIOR

WHAT INFLUENCE DOES AGGRAVATING FUNCTIONS HAVE ON YOUR CLINICAL DECISION-MAKING PROCESS IN THE HIP AND THIGH REGION?

Hip flexion-based activities

- Pathologies aggravated by passive hip flexion include hip impingement and labral pathology and muscle strains of the hamstrings, adductors, and piriformis. Active hip flexion can aggravate injuries to the quadriceps, adductors, and hip flexors.
- Sitting increases the pressure on the ischiogluteal bursa as well as the piriformis and may lead to aggravation.
- Hip flexion will stress the sacroiliac ligaments as well as the posterior hip capsule.

| TABLE II-11-1 | **Functional and Activity Participation Limitations** |

Motion	Functional Activities	Pathology if Symptoms Are Aggravated by Passive Activity	Pathology if Symptoms Are Aggravated by Active Activity
Flexion	Bending forward Tying shoes Squatting down Sit to stand	Hip impingement Labral pathology Muscle strains of the hamstrings, adductors, and piriformis Sciatic nerve pathology	Injuries to the quadriceps, adductors, and hip flexors
Extension	Terminal stance phase of gait Bending backward	Hip flexor and quadriceps strains Labral tears Degenerative joint disease Hip capsule laxity Hernias Osteitis pubis	Hamstring and adductor magnus injuries
Abduction	Crossing legs Getting out of car Sports	Hip osteoarthritis Adductor tendinopathy Pudendal or obturator neuralgia	Gluteal muscle injuries
Adduction	Crossing legs Sleeping on side	Greater trocanteric bursitis Piriformis syndrome Hip labral tear	Hip adductor strain
External rotation	Crossing legs Tying shoes Getting out of car Sports	Hip capsular laxity Greater trochanteric bursitis Piriformis syndrome	Piriformis syndrome
Internal rotation	Sleeping on side	Sacroiliac dysfunction Hip impingement Labral tears Degenerative joint disease Hernias Osteitis pubis	Adductor strain
Static positions	Sleep Prolonged sitting	Hip osteoarthritis Visceral pathology Inflammation Bone fracture	Not applicable
General movements	Walking and running	Avascular necrosis Degenerative joint disease Stress fracture of the femur or pubic ramis Greater trochanteric bursitis	Not applicable

- Athletic pubalgia is a set of pelvic injuries involving the abdominal and pelvic musculature outside the ball-and-socket hip joint and on both sides of the pubic symphysis.[51] Patients with this syndrome will often demonstrate significant weakness and/or pain with active hip flexion.
- Hip flexion can also aggravate the sciatic nerve.

Extension-based activities

- Pathologies aggravated by passive hip extension include hip flexor and quadriceps strains, labral tears, degenerative joint disease, hip capsule laxity, hernias, and osteitis pubis. Active extension can aggravate hamstring and adductor magnus injuries as well.
- Hip extension can also increase joint compressive forces in patients with hip degenerative joint disease and generate symptoms.
- With lumbar extension activities, the diameter of the intervertebral foramen is reduced. In the presence of lumbar pathology such as stenosis or spondylolisthesis the diameter of the foramen is further reduced. This results in nerves being irritated within the smaller foramen, which can lead to lumbar spine pain as well as referred hip pain.
- Extension of the hip will aggravate the femoral nerve.

Hip internal and external rotation-based activities

- These motions rarely occur in the hip and thigh region in isolation. They are often combined with sagittal and frontal plane motions in order to complete a functional task.
- Pathologies aggravated by passive hip internal rotation include sacroiliac dysfunction, hip impingement, labral tears, degenerative joint disease, hernias, and osteitis pubis.
- Pathologies aggravated by passive hip external rotation include hip capsular laxity, greater trochanteric bursitis, and piriformis syndrome.

CLINICAL PEARL

Assessment of hip internal rotation can be very valuable in the differential diagnosis of various musculoskeletal disorders. Studies have shown the relationship between limited hip internal rotation and hip impingement, groin injuries, sacroiliac dysfunction, slipped capital femoral epiphysis, degenerative hip joint disease, lumbar dysfunction, patellofemoral pain, and anterior cruciate ligament injuries.[11-14,20,30,32,82,89]

MEDICAL HISTORY

WHAT ROLE DOES A PATIENT'S PAST MEDICAL HISTORY PLAY IN THE DIFFERENTIAL DIAGNOSIS OF HIP AND THIGH PATHOLOGY?

Past injuries, surgeries, and other medical pathology can influence the normal biomechanics and function of the hip joint.

Previous musculoskeletal injuries can contribute to biomechanical changes and stresses placed on the hip region. Ankle, knee, abdominal, groin, thoracic, and lumbar spine injuries can all lead to movement compensations, which change the normal mechanics of the hip. Over time, these changes will result in abnormal wear on hip joint structures leading to deterioration and degeneration.

- Up to 31% of hamstring injuries are reinjuries.[15] Many explanations have been put forward for hamstring muscle strains. Factors thought to be involved include muscle weakness, lack of flexibility, fatigue, inadequate warm-up, and poor lumbar posture. Every muscle has an optimum length of force development. Optimum lengths of previously injured hamstrings are shorter and therefore more prone to eccentric damage than previously uninjured muscles.[9]
- Quadriceps strains often occur because of previous underlying limitations in hip extension and weakness of the iliopsoas.

- Patients who suffer from athletic pubalgia will often describe a history of previous groin injury. The groin injury gradually progressed into a painful lower abdomen. This often overlooked fact may be the real key to solving or understanding the problem. Sports hernias are not traumatic. There is no singular incident but rather a gradual progression.
- Chronic low back pain and stenosis can cause alterations in patient's walking patterns. These alterations often lead to decreases in hip range of motion.[46]
- Limitations and ankle dorsiflexion can lead to increased degenerative changes in the proximal joints of the lower extremity.[5]

CLINICAL DECISION MAKING CASE STUDY—PATIENT PROFILE

(?)

Your patient is a 19-year-old male student athlete with complaints of mild groin and abdominal pain. Symptoms began insidiously and have been present for the past 5 months. They are worse with cutting and twisting movements. The patient has noticed that coughing aggravates his symptoms. He has a history of groin injuries. What are your hypotheses regarding his pathology?

Answer

The patient's symptoms appear to match those expected with athletic pubalgia or osteitis pubis. Pathology such L1 to L2 disc lesion should be ruled out with an appropriate physical examination. Urological diseases including prostatitis and urethritis can cause obscure groin pain and need to be effectively ruled out.

- Pathologies such as chronic liver disease, pancreatitis, kidney dysfunction, urinary tract infection, colitis, and endometriosis can all result in referred pain or abnormal biomechanics within the region because the body may assume postures to minimize stress on impacted systems.
- Pregnancy can affect the hip and sacroiliac joints in several ways. The release of hormones such as relaxin may result in ligament laxity. This laxity can result in symptoms of instability. It may be difficult for pregnant women to utilize dynamic systems such as the lumbopelvic muscles to stabilize the hip region. This ligament laxity may also impact the patient's single leg stability and walking tolerance. Changes in the dynamic shape of the pelvis that occurred during pregnancy may also impair hip muscle function.

MEDICAL AND ORTHOPEDIC TESTING

WHAT MEDICAL AND ORTHOPEDIC TESTS INFLUENCE YOUR DIFFERENTIAL DIAGNOSIS PROCESS?

The differential diagnosis of hip pain is broad and includes intraarticular pathology, extraarticular pathology, and referred pain. Magnetic resonance imaging (MRI) and x-rays are used in conjunction with other clinical tests and observations to influence the decision-making process.

OSTEOARTHRITIS: Plain film x-rays are usually the first imaging modality ordered to assess for the presence of hip osteoarthritis. Radiographs are often examined for the following items: joint space narrowing (superior, axial, and medial), femoral and acetabular osteophytes, femoral and acetabular sclerosis, femoral and acetabular cyst formation, femoral head remodeling, protrusio acetabuli, avascular necrosis (AVN) of the femoral head, and congenital or developmental hip abnormality.[3]

Sutlive et al[76] developed a preliminary clinical prediction rule for diagnosing hip osteoarthritis in individuals with unilateral hip pain. The following five variables form the rule: (1) self-reported squatting as an aggravating factor; (2) active hip flexion causing lateral hip pain; (3) scour test with adduction causing lateral hip or groin pain; (4) active hip extension causing pain; and (5) passive internal rotation of less than or equal to 25°. Having at least three of the five predictor variables resulted in a positive likelihood ratio equal to 5.2 (95% CI: 2.6–10.9), increasing the likelihood of having hip osteoarthritis from a pretest probability of 29% to a posttest probability of 68%. If at least four of five variables were present, the positive likelihood ratio was equal to 24.3 (95% CI: 4.4–142.1), increasing the posttest probability of having hip osteoarthritis to 91%.

LABRAL TEARS: The most reliable study for the diagnosis of labral tears appears to be small-field magnetic resonance arthrography (MRA), which has shown upward of 90% sensitivity and 100% specificity in diagnosing labral tears.[29,78] For patients who cannot undergo MRA, contrast-enhanced computed tomography (CT) has shown similar sensitivity and specificity.[90]

OSTEOCHONDRAL LOOSE BODIES: These are most easily identified on plain radiographs or CT scans because they are radiopaque.[44,53] MRI with gadolinium contrast and MRA are more useful for identifying cartilaginous loose bodies and are useful for characterizing associated synovial or soft tissue pathology.[55]

FEMOROACETABULAR IMPINGEMENT: Patients with suspected femoroacetabular impingement (FAI) should undergo anteroposterior pelvis and cross-table lateral radiographs to assess for the characteristic "pistol-grip" femoral head in cam impingement, or for acetabular retroversion and crossover in pincer impingement.[33,62] MRI and MRA are also indicated for measurement of the alpha angle, quantifying the asphericity of the femoral head, and for the evaluation of resultant labral tears, cartilage damage, and fibrocystic change at the femoral head–neck junction.[32,62,63]

Philippon et al[61] and Meyer (unpublished data) have observed an increased vertical distance between the lateral edge of the knee and the examination table in FAI patients during the flexion in abduction and external rotation (FABER) examination when compared with the contralateral limb.

Martin and Sekiya[50] found that an acceptable level of interrater reliability can be achieved for the FABER test, log roll test, and assessment for greater trochanteric tenderness during the examination of patients with musculoskeletal hip pain. Other work has suggested that the FABER and impingement tests have high sensitivity but low specificity in detecting a labral tear.[52,54]

CLINICAL DECISION MAKING CASE STUDY—PATIENT PROFILE ❓

Your patient is a 54-year-old female with complaints of significant right lateral hip pain and difficulty squatting and walking. Symptoms began insidiously, have been present for the past 8 months, and are getting worse. She also notes difficulty sleeping on her right side. A physical examination reveals limited passive right hip internal rotation, flexion, and abduction with a capsular end feel. What are your hypotheses regarding her pathology?

Answer
The patient's symptoms appear to match those expected with hip osteoarthritis or trochanteric bursitis. The pattern of hip motion restriction, however, is in a capsular pattern suggestive of osteoarthritis as previously described by Cyriax.[17]

GLUTEUS MINIMUS AND MEDIUS INJURY: Although patients should have plain radiographs taken of the affected side, these are generally negative, and only occasionally show calcification at the tendon insertion.

MRI can distinguish between partial and complete tears and evaluate fatty atrophy of the gluteal muscles and calcification

at the tendon insertion. Ultrasound can also be used for evaluation, particularly as tendon thickening and increased fluid can be directly correlated to the site of pain.[43]

ILIOTIBIAL BAND/GREATER TROCHANTER BURSITIS: For the evaluation of iliotibial band/greater trochanter bursitis plain radiographs can be obtained to evaluate any suspected intraarticular pathology. They occasionally show calcifications within the bursa, but are generally negative.[6,84] Dynamic ultrasound is useful, because the iliotibial band can be seen snapping over the greater trochanter. Associated bursitis or gluteal tendinopathy can be assessed at the same time.[38,88] Small-field MRI has been used as the gold standard, but is not necessary to make the diagnosis of trochanteric bursitis.[6,25,84]

ILIOPSOAS TENDINITIS AND INTERNAL/EXTERNAL SNAPPING HIP: These pathologies can be identified via ultrasound examination by a trained musculoskeletal examiner. The ultrasound may show tendinopathy with thickening or hypoechogenicity within the tendon, bursitis with fluid surrounding the tendon, or increased blood flow with color Doppler imaging.[8,28] Dynamic ultrasound is also diagnostic as the tendon can be seen snapping over the iliopectineal eminence.[8,28,88]

ADDUCTOR STRAIN: The diagnosis can be made with focal findings on examination. However, MRI with gadolinium may be useful to confirm the diagnosis or differentiate among adductor strain, osteitis pubis, and sports hernia.[16,70]

CLINICAL PEARL ❗

Adductor magnus has a strong hip extension function during upright activity. Complete rehabilitation of the injury to this muscle must focus on restoring hip extension range of motion, strength, and power.

PIRIFORMIS SYNDROME: Patients with piriformis syndrome have often been evaluated for possible nerve root impingement. An MRI of the lumbar spine will fail to show any disk herniation, whereas an MRI of the pelvis may show piriformis muscle atrophy or hypertrophy and edema surrounding the sciatic nerve at the level of the piriformis.[27,41]

SACROILIAC JOINT PAIN: Plain anteroposterior, inlet, and outlet radiographs of the pelvis should be obtained. If sacroiliac joint instability is suspected, single-leg stance views should be obtained, looking for displacement. CT scan, MRI, and bone scans can be obtained to evaluate specific etiologies of sacroiliac joint pain, although these are not specific for idiopathic pain.[10,18,85]

In patients with low back pain Cibulka and Koldehoff[11] found that utilizing a cluster of tests appears to be a clinically useful method to determine who has and who does not have sacroiliac joint dysfunction. The four sacroiliac joint tests included the standing flexion test, palpation of the posterior-superior iliac spine heights while sitting, the supine long-sitting test, and the prone knee flexion test.

ATHLETIC PUBALGIA: Before 2005 MRI was occasionally helpful in the diagnosis of these injuries and it was possible with some predictability to identify a number of minimal findings in these patients.[2] Studying the various attachments to the pubic bone and refining the MRI technique held the key to specific diagnoses more recently.[58,93] In one study, MRI was found to be sensitive and specific for both rectus abdominus and adductor tendon injuries.[93] Other studies, including radiographs, ultrasound, or bone scan, should be used as necessary to rule out other etiologies of chronic groin pain.[24]

OSTEITIS PUBIS: Bone edema spanning the symphysis with cystic or other degenerative changes or adductor microtears may be visible on MRI.[16,93] Bone scan may show increased uptake at the symphysis, although it can take months to become positive in some athletes.[56,67]

CLINICAL DECISION MAKING CASE STUDY—PATIENT PROFILE ?

Your patient is a 28-year-old female with complaints of the gradual onset of groin and thigh pain that limits her ability to run. She is unable to stand and support her full weight on her involved leg. Symptoms began insidiously 4 weeks ago and radiographs of her thigh and pelvis are negative. What are your hypotheses regarding her pathology?

Answer

The patient's symptoms could be referred from the lumbar spine or sacroiliac joint and should be ruled out with an appropriate physical examination. There is a high incidence of pelvic stress fractures in female runners and radiographs are often normal early in the disease process with only 38% of fractures shown radiologically. When palpation reveals tenderness at the pubic ramus, a bone scan should be ordered and when combined with radiography has been shown to increase the accurate diagnosis of stress fracture to 62%.[19]

MEDICATIONS

HOW DOES A PATIENT'S RESPONSE TO MEDICATION INFLUENCE YOUR DECISION-MAKING PROCESSES?

Pain medications and antiinflammatory medications are commonly prescribed in association with hip and thigh pain. The effectiveness of antiinflammatory medication helps differentiate pathology that has an acute inflammatory process.

CLINICAL PEARL !

Indomethacin is the "gold standard" for heterotopic ossification prophylaxis following total hip arthroplasty and is the only drug proven to be effective against heterotopic ossification following acetabular surgery. It can also be utilized to prevent this condition in muscle contusions of the lower extremity.[48]

BIOMECHANICAL

WHAT BIOMECHANICAL ABNORMALITIES IN OTHER REGIONS AFFECT YOUR DECISION-MAKING PROCESS?

- Chronic low back pain and stenosis can cause alterations in patient's walking patterns. These alterations often lead to decreases in hip range motion.[46]
- Limitations and ankle dorsiflexion can lead to increased degenerative changes in the proximal joints of the lower extremity.[5]
- Giles et al[31] studied patients with low back pain and discovered that patients with a leg length discrepancy of greater than 15 mm were five times more likely to experience low back pain. Hip and sciatic pain occurred in the longer leg 78% of the time.

CLINICAL PEARL !

Patients with lumbar stenosis often develop a flexed hip and spine posture while walking. This posture can increase the demand on the lumbar paraspinals and gluteal muscles leading to fatigue. Treatment focused on restoring hip extension can decrease some of this postural stress and improve upright function.

ENVIRONMENTAL AND PERSONAL CONTEXTUAL FACTORS

DO PSYCHOSOCIAL ISSUES INFLUENCE CLINICAL DECISION MAKING?

Depression, stress, and other psychosocial factors can impact the autonomic, endocrine, and immune systems. These systems can heighten or depress response to injury.

CAN EMOTIONS INFLUENCE THE DECISION-MAKING PROCESS?

You should always consider the possibility of other nonmedical-related issues as the source of a patient's symptoms.

DO WORK-RELATED INJURIES INFLUENCE CLINICAL DECISION MAKING?

Work environment and repetitive tasks can lead to breakdown of tissue (Box II-11-1).

DO AUTONOMIC, ENDOCRINE, AND IMMUNE SYSTEMS INFLUENCE DECISION-MAKING IN THE HIP AND THIGH REGION? (BOX II-11-2)

The autonomic, endocrine, and immune systems are responsible for maintaining a homeostatic environment within the body. In response to an altered environment the three systems work together to return the body to homeostasis. The autonomic system reacts to alter blood flow and increase chemical mediators, which may have an effect on the tissues of the hip and thigh region.

The endocrine system can also influence pain in many ways. The hypothalamus controls the autonomic system, adrenal glands produce neural irritants in response to stressors, and the reproductive organs also produce hormones that can act as neural irritants.

BOX II-11-1	Contextual Factors
Environmental	Work, environment, and repetitive tasks can lead to breakdown of tissue. Look for activities that required repetitive hip flexion, such as kneeling or bending forward.
Personal	Work-related issues, personal and family factors, depression, and emotional unrest can all influence hip pain. Question patients regarding stressors in their life that may influence the body's ability to heal.

BOX II-11-2	Output Mechanisms
Autonomic	No conclusive evidence has been provided to date linking autonomic dysfunction and hip pain.
Endocrine	The endocrine system is involved in the regulation of body homeostasis. In theory, alterations in endocrine function in the form of changes in reproductive hormones can be loosely tied to hip pain in terms of pathology such as endometriosis or ovarian cysts. Cramping during menstruation has been tied to alterations in the balance of reproductive hormones.
Immune	Lymph nodes are part of the immune system and swollen or irritated inguinal lymph nodes could potentially result in hip dysfunction.

TABLE II-11-2 Body Structure and Tissue-Based Pathology (Nociceptive and Peripheral Neurogenic Pain)

	Muscles and Tendons	Bone	Cartilage	Joint	Labrum	Ligaments	Nerves	Visceral Tissue
Pathologies	Hip flexor/adductor strain Posterior thigh compartment syndrome Piriformis syndrome Quadriceps strain Quadriceps contusion Adductor tendinopathy Hamstring tendinopathy Snapping hip syndrome ITB friction syndrome Osteitis pubis Ischiogluteal bursitis	Avascular necrosis Hallux valgus Stress fracture of the femur Stress fracture of the pubic ramus Hip fractures	Hip osteoarthritis	Hip joint laxity	Labral tear	Hip joint laxity Greater trocanteric bursitis	Pudendal Obturator Sciatic Femoral Lateral femoral Cutaneous	Bladder Prostate Large intestines Hernia Appendix Small intestines Uterus Fallopian tubes Ovaries
Age	Not age related	Varies, see related pathology sections	50 years old and above for osteoarthritis or 13 to 50 years old in cases of femoroacetabular impingement	Any age	Any age; 14 to 50 years more common	Not age related	Any age if related to meralgia paresthetica 30 to 50 years old plus if referred from the spine	30 to 50 years old
Occupation	Athletic occupation tends to lead to increased injury rates	Possible repetitive flexion and lifting activities	Repetitive flexion activities	Varies, see related pathology	Repetitive cutting and twisting activities	No direct relationship	Varies, see related pathology	Varies depending on pathology
Gender	Not applicable	Variable depending on the pathology	Not applicable	Not applicable	More common in women	Not applicable	Not applicable	Not applicable
History	May or may not have a history of previous entry	Gradual or sudden onset of pain	Gradual onset of hip pain	May or may not have a history of hip pain	Gradual or sudden onset of hip pain	May or may not have a history of hip pain	Varies, see related pathology	
Mechanism of injury	Varies depending on the muscle injured	Trauma or insidious	Extension or flexion	Varies, see related pathology	Extension and external rotation	Trauma or insidious	Varies, see related pathology	Generally no known mechanism
Type of onset	Sudden	Gradual or sudden	Gradual	Gradual or sudden	Gradual or sudden	Sudden or traumatic	Gradual	Sudden to gradual depending on structure
Referral from local tissue	Pain along the firer orientation of the muscle or any of the referred pain sites	Pain in low back, gluteal region, thigh, and knee usually unilateral	Pain in the groin and anterior thigh region	Pain in the groin and anterior thigh region	Pain in the hip, groin, and anterior thigh region	Pain in the anterior hip and in the groin	Pain in the anterior thigh, lateral hip, and or low back region	Pain is generally localized to area adjacent to involved structure

Referral to other regions	May refer into lower extremity or spine; see related pathology	May refer to the knee or lumbar spine	May refer unilaterally into the leg if the nerve is involved	Generally does not refer to other regions	Generally does not refer to other regions	Generally does not refer to other regions	Referral of symptoms into the lower extremity Distribution of symptoms is dependent on nerve involvement	May refer into the surrounding areas depending on the involved structure
Changes in symptoms	Sudden pain, no relief on day of injury Increased stiffness the next morning	May worsen as pathology progresses	Slow progressive worsening over time	Slow progressive worsening over time	Increased pain with cutting, twisting, and loading activities	Increased pain with walking, running, and cutting	Symptoms generally increase gradually over the course of several days to weeks Symptoms may dissipate as irritating structure is addressed	May worsen as pathology progresses
24-hour pain pattern (morning)	Stiff for 30 minutes or longer, improves as the tissue heals	Stiff for 5 minutes	Stiff for 10 minutes	Stiff for 30 minutes	Stiff for 10 minutes	Stiff for 10 minutes	Stiff for 30 minutes	Varies but does not change with mechanical stresses
24-hour pain pattern (afternoon)	Less stiff, may be worse with prolonged activity	Worsens with activity	Worsens with extension or flexion activity	Less stiff, may be worse with prolonged sitting	Less stiff, may be worse with prolonged sitting	Less stiff, may be worse with prolonged activity	May worsen with prolonged aggravating activity	Varies but does not change with mechanical stresses
24-hour pain pattern (evening)	Usually not impaired	May be difficult to sleep and turn in bed	May be difficult to sleep	May be difficult to sleep	May be difficult to sleep	May be difficult if sleeps on stomach	May be difficult to sleep	Increased nocturnal pain
Description of symptoms	Localized pain/ache in the muscle tissue and stiffness	Sharp pain	Dull ache, sharp pain with motions that stress or impact the cartilage	Ache and stiffness, may be able to localize	Ache and stiffness, occasional clicking and locking	Ache and stiffness, sharp pain with motions that stress the ligament—primarily extension	Numbness, tingling, burning	Cramping, peristaltic waves, gnawing ache
Depth of symptoms	Deep	Deep	Deep	Deep	Deep	Deep	Superficial	Deep, poorly localized
Constancy of symptoms	Intermittent	Intermittent	Intermittent	Intermittent	Intermittent	Intermittent	Intermittent to constant but varying	Constant, may come in waves
Aggravating factors	Any activity that stresses the muscle in a concentric or eccentric function	Loading and repetitive weight bearing	Walking, extension, internal rotation, running, cutting, twisting, flexion, abduction, and internal rotation	Sitting, flexion, internal rotation, extension	Sitting, flexion, internal rotation, cutting and twisting movements	Primarily extension and external rotation	Varies, see related pathology	Not consistent with mechanical movements
Easing factors	Rest	Lying	Lying	Walking, lying	Lying	Lying	Varies, see related pathology	Not consistent with mechanical movements

Continued on following page.

Section II

ORTHOPEDIC REASONING

TABLE II-11-2   Body Structure and Tissue-Based Pathology (Nociceptive and Peripheral Neurogenic Pain) (*Continued*)

	Muscles and Tendons	Bone	Cartilage	Joint	Labrum	Ligaments	Nerves	Visceral Tissue
Stability of symptoms	Gradual improvement over 2- to 4-week period	May worsen if pathology progresses	Slow gradual progression of symptoms	May worsen as pathology progresses	Gradual improvement if activities are significantly limited	Gradual improvement over 6-week period	Gradual improvement over 6-week period	May worsen if pathology progresses
Past medical history	All structures may have a past history of injury that impacts the function of the surrounding tissue				None			May have a history of visceral pathology
Past surgeries	All structures may have a past history of surgeries that impacts the function of the surrounding tissue				Lumbar spine, hernia			May have a history of surgeries related to visceral pathology
Special questions								
X-rays	Negative	Positive	Positive	Positive	Positive for abnormal bone morphology	Negative	May be positive depending on related pathology	Negative
MRI	Positive	Positive	Positive	Positive	Positive	Positive	May be positive depending on related pathology	Positive for pathology
EMG		Usually not necessary		Usually not necessary			Positive	Not usually necessary
Red flags		History of cancer				Female reproductive symptoms		Rule out visceral structures

ITB, iliotibial band; MRI, magnetic resonance imaging; EMG, electromyogram.

RED FLAGS THAT WARRANT REFERRAL TO A MEDICAL PHYSICIAN

WHAT SYMPTOMS ALERT YOU TO PATHOLOGIES THAT MAY REQUIRE A REFERRAL TO A MEDICAL PHYSICIAN?

- Patient descriptions vary from person to person and should not be the only consideration in the determination of possible visceral involvement.
- Visceral pain has been described on a broad scope from sharp and severe to poorly localized and vague.
- Visceral pain should not be related to positions and movements of lumbar structures and should not respond to appropriate mechanical treatment.
- Rest or position should not relieve visceral pain.
- In patients with visceral or nonmusculoskeletal involvement it is a common complaint that their pain is constant and nonvarying.
- Complaints of increased pain at night are also an indicator of possible visceral involvement. Considerable walking, pacing, and sitting up are commonly required to return to sleep.

WHAT SYMPTOMS IMPLICATE SPECIFIC VISCERAL SYSTEMS?

ENDOCRINE SYSTEM: Symptoms include neuromusculoskeletal symptoms, muscle weakness, muscle atrophy, fatigue, carpal tunnel syndrome, arthralgia and myalgia, adhesive capsulitis, hand stiffness, systemic, excessive, or delayed growth, mental changes, changes in hair, changes in skin, changes in vital signs (body temperature, heart rate, blood pressure), heart palpitations, increased perspiration, dehydration, and excessive water retention.

HEPATIC SYSTEM: Symptoms include a sense of fullness of the abdomen, anorexia, nausea, vomiting, jaundice, bruising of the skin, spider angiomas or palmar erythema, yellow hue in the eyes, dark urine, right shoulder and abdominal pain, confusion, sleep disturbance, muscle tremors, hyperreflexia, bilateral carpal tunnel, and pallor.

GASTROINTESTINAL SYSTEM: Symptoms include abdominal pain, pain with swallowing, melena (dark, bloody stool), epigastric pain with radiation to the back, symptoms affected by food, constipation, diarrhea, fecal incontinence, joint pain, and referred shoulder pain.

UROGENITAL SYSTEM: In men symptoms include urinary tract, pelvic, and low back or leg pain, painful burning with urination, changes in urinary pattern or urine flow, red urine, penile lesions, swelling or mass in the groin, and impotence. In women symptoms include abdominal vaginal bleeding, painful menstruation, pelvic mass or lesion, vaginal itch, pain with urination, changes in menstruation, and abdominal, low back, or pelvic pain.

CANCER: Red flags include a previous history of cancer, any women with chest, breast, axillary, or shoulder pain, any person with back, pelvic, groin, or hip pain accompanied by vague complaints of abdominal pain, prolonged menstrual bleeding, a back injury that does not heal, proximal muscle weakness and changes in deep tendon reflex, a weight loss of 10 pounds or more in 1 month, constant pain, pain at night, development of new neurological deficits, and changes in the size, shape, tenderness, and consistency of the lymph nodes, especially painless and hard rubber nodes present in more than one location.

SUMMARY STATEMENT

The differential diagnosis of pain around the hip, groin, and thigh is broad and includes intraarticular pathology, extraarticular soft tissue and tendon pathology, as well as referred pain. Many potential causes of hip pain have overlapping symptoms or physical examination findings. A careful history and physical examination in combination with appropriate imaging and diagnostic or therapeutic injections generally leads to the correct diagnosis. Table II-11-2 summarizes the factors that help a clinician differentiate among different sources of symptoms in the hip and thigh regions.

Appropriate physical therapy centers on restoring gait symmetry, hip range of motion, and functional strength while reestablishing activities of daily living, work, and sports performance.

REFERENCES

1. Adkins 3rd SB. Figler RA. Hip pain in athletes. *Am Fam Physician.* 2000;61(7):2109-2118.
2. Albers SL, Spritzer CE, Garrett Jr WE, Meyers WC. MR findings in athletes with pubalgia. *Skeletal Radiol.* 2001;30(5):270-277.
3. Altman R, Alarcon G, Appelrouth D, et al. The American College of Rheumatology criteria for the classification and reporting of osteoarthritis of the hip. *Arthritis Rheum.* 1991;34(5):505-514.
4. Anderson SJ. Lower extremity injuries in youth sports. *Pediatr Clin North Am.* 2002;49(3):627-641.
5. Astephen JL, Deluzio KJ, Caldwell GE, Dunbar MJ. Biomechanical changes at the hip, knee, and ankle joints during gait are associated with knee osteoarthritis severity. *J Orthop Res.* 2008;26(3):332-341.
6. Baker CJ, Massie R, Hurt W, Savory C. Arthroscopic bursectomy for recalcitrant trochanteric bursitis. *Arthroscopy.* 2007;23(8):827-832.
7. Bewyer DC, Bewyer KJ. Rationale for treatment of hip abductor pain syndrome. *Iowa Orthop J.* 2003;23:57-60.
8. Blankenbaker DG, De Smet AA, Keene JS. Sonography of the iliopsoas tendon and injection of the iliopsoas bursa for diagnosis and management of the painful snapping hip. *Skeletal Radiol.* 2006;35(8):565-571.
9. Brockett CL, Morgan DL, Proske U. Predicting hamstring strain injury in elite athletes. *Med Sci Sports Exerc.* 2004;36(3):379-387.
10. Buijs E, Visser L, Groen G. Sciatica and the sacroiliac joint: a forgotten concept. *Br J Anaesth.* 2007;99(5):713-716.
11. Cibulka MT, Koldehoff R. Clinical usefulness of a cluster of sacroiliac joint tests in patients with and without low back pain. *J Orthop Sports Phys Ther.* 1999;29(2):83-89 [discussion 90-2].
12. Cibulka MT, Sinacore DR, Cromer GS. Delitto A. Unilateral hip rotation range of motion asymmetry in patients with sacroiliac joint regional pain. *Spine.* 1998;23(9):1009-1015.
13. Cibulka MT, Threlkeld J. The early clinical diagnosis of osteoarthritis of the hip. *J Orthop Sports Phys Ther.* 2004;34(8):461-467.
14. Cibulka MT, Threlkeld-Watkins J. Patellofemoral pain and asymmetrical hip rotation. *Phys Ther.* 2005;85(11):1201-1207.
15. Croisier JL. Factors associated with recurrent hamstring injuries. *Sports Med.* 2004;34(10):681-695.
16. Cunningham P, Brennan D, O'Connell M, MacMahon P, O'Neill P, Eustace S. Patterns of bone and soft-tissue injury at the symphysis pubis in soccer players: observations at MRI. *AJR Am J Roentgenol.* 2007;188(3):W291-W296.
17. Cyriax J. *Textbook of Orthopedic Medicine.* Vol 1. London: Bailliere Tindall; 1982.
18. Dreyfuss P, Dreyer S, Cole A, Mayo K. Sacroiliac joint pain. J Am Acad Orthop Surg. 12(4):255-265.
19. Ekberg O, Persson N, Abrahamsson P, Westlin N, Lilja B. Longstanding groin pain in athletes. A multidisciplinary approach. *Sports Med.* 1988;6(1):56-61.
20. Ellison JB, Rose SJ, Sahrmann SA. Patterns of hip rotation range of motion: a comparison between healthy subjects and patients with low back pain. *Phys Ther.* 1990;70(9):537-541.
21. Ethgen O, Bruyère O, Richy F, Dardennes C, Reginster J. Health-related quality of life in total hip and total knee arthroplasty. A qualitative and systematic review of the literature. *J Bone Joint Surg Am.* 2004;86-A(5):963-974.
22. Ethgen O, Vanparijs P, Delhalle S, Rosant S, Bruyère O, Reginster J. Social support and health-related quality of life in hip and knee osteoarthritis. *Qual Life Res.* 2004;13(2):321-330.
23. Fairbank JC, Park WM, McCall IW. O'Brien JP. Apophyseal injection of local anesthetic as a diagnostic aid in primary low-back pain syndromes. *Spine.* 1981;6(6):598-605.
24. Farber AJ, Wilckens JH. Sports hernia: diagnosis and therapeutic approach. *J Am Acad Orthop Surg.* 2007;15(8):507-514.

25. Farr D, Selesnick H, Janecki C, Cordas D. Arthroscopic bursectomy with concomitant iliotibial band release for the treatment of recalcitrant trochanteric bursitis. *Arthroscopy.* 2007;23(8):905, e1-e5.

26. Felson D. Epidemiology of hip and knee osteoarthritis. *Epidemiol Rev.* 1988;10:1-28.

27. Filler A, Haynes J, Jordan S, et al. Sciatica of nondisc origin and piriformis syndrome: diagnosis by magnetic resonance neurography and interventional magnetic resonance imaging with outcome study of resulting treatment. *J Neurosurg Spine.* 2005;2(2):99-115.

28. Flanum ME, Keene JS, Blankenbaker DG, Desmet AA. Arthroscopic treatment of the painful "internal" snapping hip: results of a new endoscopic technique and imaging protocol. *Am J Sports Med.* 2007;35(5):770-779.

29. Freedman BA, Potter BK, Dinauer PA, Giuliani JR, Kuklo TR, Murphy KP. Prognostic value of magnetic resonance arthrography for Czerny stage II and III acetabular labral tears. *Arthroscopy.* 2006;22(7):742-747.

30. Gelberman RH, Cohen MS, Shaw BA, Kasser JR, Griffin PP, Wilkinson RH. The association of femoral retroversion with slipped capital femoral epiphysis. *J Bone Joint Surg Am.* 1986;68(7):1000-1007.

31. Giles LG, Taylor JR. Low-back pain associated with leg length inequality. *Spine.* 1981;6(5):510-521.

32. Gomes JL, de Castro JV, Becker R. Decreased hip range of motion and noncontact injuries of the anterior cruciate ligament. *Arthroscopy.* 2008;24(9):1034-1037.

33. Guanche CA. Bare AA. Arthroscopic treatment of femoroacetabular impingement. *Arthroscopy.* 2006;22(1):95-106.

34. Hägglund G, Hansson L, Ordeberg G. Epidemiology of slipped capital femoral epiphysis in southern Sweden. *Clin Orthop Relat Res.* 1984;(191):82-94.

35. Hawker GA, Stewart L, French MR, et al. Understanding the pain experience in hip and knee osteoarthritis—an OARSI/OMERACT initiative. *Osteoarthritis Cartilage.* 2008;16(4):415-422.

36. Hungerford D, Jones L. Asymptomatic osteonecrosis: should it be treated? *Clin Orthop Relat Res.* 2004;(429):124-130.

37. Hunt D, Clohisy J, Prather H. Acetabular labral tears of the hip in women. *Phys Med Rehabil Clin N Am.* 2007;18(3):497-520, ix-x.

38. Ilizaliturri VJ, Villalobos FJ, Chaidez P, Valero F, Aguilera J. Internal snapping hip syndrome: treatment by endoscopic release of the iliopsoas tendon. *Arthroscopy.* 2005;21(11):1375-1380.

39. Jaglal SB, Kreiger N, Darlington GA. Lifetime occupational physical activity and risk of hip fracture in women. *Ann Epidemiol.* 1995;5(4):321-324.

40. Kellgren J. Sciatica. *Lancet.* 1941;1:561-564.

41. Kobbe P, Zelle B, Gruen G. Case report: recurrent piriformis syndrome after surgical release. *Clin Orthop Relat Res.* 2008;466(7):1745-1748.

42. Kocher MS, Kim YJ, Millis MB, et al. Hip arthroscopy in children and adolescents. *J Pediatr Orthop.* 2005;25(5):680-686.

43. Kong A, Van der Vliet A, Zadow S. MRI and US of gluteal tendinopathy in greater trochanteric pain syndrome. *Eur Radiol.* 2007;17(7):1772-1783.

44. Krebs VE. The role of hip arthroscopy in the treatment of synovial disorders and loose bodies. *Clin Orthop Relat Res.* 2003;(406):48-59.

45. Larson CM, Giveans MR. Arthroscopic management of femoroacetabular impingement: early outcomes measures. *Arthroscopy.* 2008;24(5):540-546.

46. Lee LW, Zavarei K, Evans J, Lelas JJ, Riley PO, Kerrigan DC. Reduced hip extension in the elderly: dynamic or postural? *Arch Phys Med Rehabil.* 2005;86(9):1851-1854.

47. Lehmann C, Arons R, Loder R, Vitale M. The epidemiology of slipped capital femoral epiphysis: an update. *J Pediatr Orthop.* 2006;26(3):286-290.

48. Macfarlane RJ, Ng BH, Gamie Z, et al. Pharmacological treatment of heterotopic ossification following hip and acetabular surgery. *Expert Opin Pharmacother.* 2008;9(5):767-786.

49. Margetts B, Perry C, Taylor J, Dangerfield P. The incidence and distribution of Legg-Calvé-Perthes' disease in Liverpool, 1982-95. *Arch Dis Child.* 2001;84(4):351-354.

50. Martin RL, Sekiya JK. The interrater reliability of 4 clinical tests used to assess individuals with musculoskeletal hip pain. *J Orthop Sports Phys Ther.* 2008;38(2):71-77.

51. Meyers WC, McKechnie A, Philippon MJ, Horner MA, Zoga AC, Devon ON. Experience with "sports hernia" spanning two decades. *Ann Surg.* 2008;248(4):656-665.

52. Mitchell B, McCrory P, Brukner P, O'Donnell J, Colson E, Howells R. Hip joint pathology: clinical presentation and correlation between magnetic resonance arthrography, ultrasound, and arthroscopic findings in 25 consecutive cases. *Clin J Sport Med.* 2003;13(3):152-156.

53. Mullis BH, Dahners LE. Hip arthroscopy to remove loose bodies after traumatic dislocation. *J Orthop Trauma.* 2006;20(1):22-26.

54. Narvani AA, Tsiridis E, Kendall S, Chaudhuri R, Thomas P. A preliminary report on prevalence of acetabular labrum tears in sports patients with groin pain. *Knee Surg Sports Traumatol Arthrosc.* 2003;11(6):403-408.

55. Neckers AC, Polster JM, Winalski CS, Krebs VE, Sundaram M. Comparison of MR arthrography with arthroscopy of the hip for the assessment of intra-articular loose bodies. *Skeletal Radiol.* 2007;36(10):963-967.

56. Paajanen H, Hermunen H, Karonen J. Pubic magnetic resonance imaging findings in surgically and conservatively treated athletes with osteitis pubis compared to asymptomatic athletes during heavy training. *Am J Sports Med.* 2008;36(1):117-121.

57. Peled E, Eidelman M, Katzman A, Bialik V. Neonatal incidence of hip dysplasia: ten years of experience. *Clin Orthop Relat Res.* 2008;466(4):771-775.

58. Petersilge C. Imaging of the acetabular labrum. *Magn Reson Imaging Clin N Am.* 2005;13(4):641-652, vi.

59. Petrigliano F, Lieberman J. Osteonecrosis of the hip: novel approaches to evaluation and treatment. *Clin Orthop Relat Res.* 2007;465:53-62.

60. Philippon M. The role of arthroscopic thermal capsulorrhaphy in the hip. *Clin Sports Med.* 2001;20(4):817-829.

61. Philippon MJ, Maxwell RB, Johnston TL, Schenker M. Briggs KK. Clinical presentation of femoroacetabular impingement. *Knee Surg Sports Traumatol Arthrosc.* 2007;15(8):1041-1047.

62. Philippon MJ, Schenker ML. Arthroscopy for the treatment of femoroacetabular impingement in the athlete. *Clin Sports Med.* 2006;25(2):299-308, ix.

63. Philippon MJ, Stubbs AJ, Schenker ML, Maxwell RB, Ganz R, Leunig M. Arthroscopic management of femoroacetabular impingement: osteoplasty technique and literature review. *Am J Sports Med.* 2007;35(9):1571-1580.

64. Philippon MJ, Yen YM, Briggs KK, Kuppersmith DA, Maxwell RB. Early outcomes after hip arthroscopy for femoroacetabular impingement in the athletic adolescent patient: a preliminary report. *J Pediatr Orthop.* 2008;28(7):705-710.

65. Pope DP, Hunt IM, Birrell FN, Silman AJ, Macfarlane GJ. Hip pain onset in relation to cumulative workplace and leisure time mechanical load: a population based case-control study. *Ann Rheum Dis.* 2003;62(4):322-326.

66. Portegijs E, Kallinen M, Rantanen T, et al. Effects of resistance training on lower-extremity impairments in older people with hip fracture. *Arch Phys Med Rehabil.* 2008;89(9):1667-1674.

67. Radic R, Annear P. Use of pubic symphysis curettage for treatment-resistant osteitis pubis in athletes. *Am J Sports Med.* 2008;36(1):122-128.

68. Sayson SC, Ducey JP, Maybrey JB, Wesley RL, Vermilion D. Sciatic entrapment neuropathy associated with an anomalous piriformis muscle. *Pain.* 1994;59(1):149-152.

69. Schai PA, Exner GU. [Indication for and results of intertrochanteric osteotomy in slipped capital femoral epiphysis]. *Orthopade.* 2002;31(9):900-907.

70. Schilders E, Bismil Q, Robinson P, O'Connor P, Gibbon W, Talbot J. Adductor-related groin pain in competitive athletes. Role of adductor enthesis, magnetic resonance imaging, and entheseal pubic cleft injections. *J Bone Joint Surg Am.* 2007;89(10):2173-2178.

71. Shindle M, Ranawat A, Kelly B. Diagnosis and management of traumatic and atraumatic hip instability in the athletic patient. *Clin Sports Med.* 2006;25(2):309-326, ix-x.

72. Skelton D, Greig C, Davies J, Young A. Strength, power and related functional ability of healthy people aged 65-89 years. *Age Ageing* 1994;23(5):371-377.

73. Skinner HB, Scherger JE. Identifying structural hip and knee problems. Patient age, history, and limited examination may be all that's needed. *Postgrad Med.* 1999;106(7):51-52. 5-6, 61-4 passim.

74. Slipman CW, Jackson HB, Lipetz JS, Chan KT, Lenrow D, Vresilovic EJ. Sacroiliac joint pain referral zones. *Arch Phys Med Rehabil.* 2000;81(3):334-338.

75. Stein-Zamir C, Volovik I, Rishpon S, Sabi R. Developmental dysplasia of the hip: risk markers, clinical screening and outcome. *Pediatr Int.* 2008;50(3):341-345.

76. Sutlive T, Lopez H, Schnitker D, et al. Development of a clinical prediction rule for diagnosing hip osteoarthritis in individuals with unilateral hip pain. *J Orthop Sports Phys Ther.* 2008;38(9):542-550.

77. Tepper S, Hochberg M. Factors associated with hip osteoarthritis: data from the First National Health and Nutrition Examination Survey (NHANES-I). *Am J Epidemiol.* 1993;137(10):1081-1088.

78. Toomayan GA, Holman WR, Major NM, Kozlowicz SM, Vail TP. Sensitivity of MR arthrography in the evaluation of acetabular labral tears. *AJR Am J Roentgenol.* 2006;186(2):449-453.

79. Travell J, Simons D. *Myofascial Pain and Dysfunction: The Trigger Point Manual.* Vol 2. Baltimore, Maryland: Williams & Wilkins; 1992.

80. van der Waal JM, Bot SD, Terwee CB, van der Windt DA, Bouter LM, Dekker J. The course and prognosis of hip complaints in general practice. *Ann Behav Med.* 2006;31(3):297-308.

81. van Dijk GM, Dekker J, Veenhof C, van den Ende CH. Course of functional status and pain in osteoarthritis of the hip or knee: a systematic review of the literature. *Arthritis Rheum.* 2006;55(5):779-785.

82. Verrall GM, Slavotinek JP, Barnes PG, Esterman A, Oakeshott RD, Spriggins AJ. Hip joint range of motion restriction precedes athletic chronic groin injury. *J Sci Med Sport.* 2007;10(6):463-466.

83. Verrall GM, Slavotinek JP, Fon GT, Barnes PG. Outcome of conservative management of athletic chronic groin injury diagnosed as pubic bone stress injury. *Am J Sports Med.* 2007;35(3):467-474.

84. Walker P, Kannangara S, Bruce W, Michael D, Van der Wall H. Lateral hip pain: does imaging predict response to localized injection? *Clin Orthop Relat Res.* 2007;457:144-149.

85. Weksler N, Velan G, Semionov M, et al. The role of sacroiliac joint dysfunction in the genesis of low back pain: the obvious is not always right. *Arch Orthop Trauma Surg.* 2007;127(10):885-888.

86. Wichlacz W, Sotirow B, Sionek A. Czop A. Surgical outcome for children in the early phase of Perthes' disease. *Ortop Traumatol Rehabil.* 2004;6(6):712-717.

87. Wiener S. *Differential Diagnosis of Acute Pain.* Vol 1. New York: McGraw-Hill Inc; 1993.

88. Winston P, Awan R, Cassidy JD, Bleakney RK. Clinical examination and ultrasound of self-reported snapping hip syndrome in elite ballet dancers. *Am J Sports Med.* 2007;35(1):118-126.

89. Wyss TF, Clark JM, Weishaupt D, Notzli HP. Correlation between internal rotation and bony anatomy in the hip. *Clin Orthop Relat Res.* 2007;460:152-158.

90. Yamamoto Y, Tonotsuka H, Ueda T, Hamada Y. Usefulness of radial contrast-enhanced computed tomography for the diagnosis of acetabular labrum injury. *Arthroscopy.* 2007;23(12):1290-1294.

91. Yoshimura N, Sasaki S, Iwasaki K, et al. Occupational lifting is associated with hip osteoarthritis: a Japanese case-control study. *J Rheumatol.* 2000;27(2):434-440.

92. Zhang W, Moskowitz RW, Nuki G, et al. OARSI recommendations for the management of hip and knee osteoarthritis, Part II: OARSI evidence-based, expert consensus guidelines. *Osteoarthritis Cartilage.* 2008;16(2):137-162.

93. Zoga A, Kavanagh E, Omar I, et al. Athletic pubalgia and the "sports hernia": MR imaging findings. *Radiology.* 2008;247(3):797-807.

Section II

ORTHOPEDIC REASONING

AUTHORS: ROBERT C. MANSKE and DANIEL PROHASKA

INTRODUCTORY INFORMATION

WHAT IS THE PREVALENCE OF KNEE PATHOLOGY?

The prevalence of knee pain is very different for the various forms of knee pathology. For example, some knee injuries are very rare—knee dislocations accounted for only two of 700,000 injuries reported to the Workman's Compensation Board of Ontario between the years of 1955 and 1957.[17] Of more than 2 million admissions to the Mayo Clinic from 1911 to 1960, only 14 cases of knee dislocation were found.[12] Other knee injuries are much more common.

Anywhere from 75,000 to over 250,000 individuals in the United States will suffer a new injury to the anterior cruciate ligament (ACL) of the knee each year.[10] One of the larger anterior cruciate injury incidence studies has come from Switzerland. De Loes and colleagues[6] studied ACL and posterior cruciate ligament (PCL) injuries and reported a single ACL or PCL injury per 5000 participants. Males encountered for 76% of the ACL/PCL injuries.

Although there are no statistics to document, one of the more common knee problems seen clinically has to be that of patellofemoral pain,[9,16,21,28] which accounts for approximately 25.6% of knee problems seen.[18]

General knee pain is present in about 20% of the population and accounts for 1 million emergency room visits per year annually and 1.9 million primary care visits in the United States.[15] Osteoarthritis of the knee is the most common cause of disability for those over the age of 65 years (Figure II-12-1).[3]

WHAT FACTORS MAKE DIAGNOSIS DIFFICULT IN THE KNEE REGION?

Although it would seem by appearance that the knee is a simple anatomical specimen, it is actually very complex. The tibiofemoral joint moves in all three planes and injury to the ligamentous structures often alters those patterns of motion. Additionally, it has been recently noted that some forms of knee pain indeed come from alterations of joints either proximal (hip) or distal (ankle/foot) to the knee. Furthermore, diagnostic imaging is not always 100% accurate in determining the pathology contributing to symptoms. All of this makes examination of the knee a difficult task.

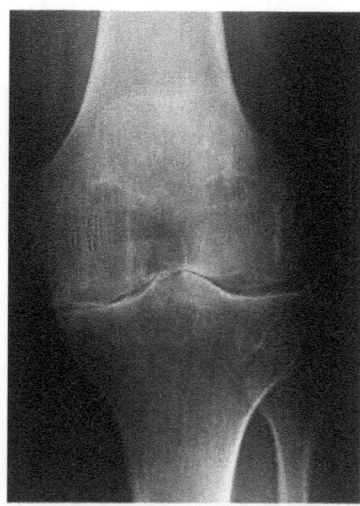

FIGURE II-12-1 Osteoarthritis of the knee. (From Magee D: *Orthopedic Physical Assessment.* 5th ed. St. Louis: Saunders, Elsevier; 2008, Figure 12-146.)

HOW SUCCESSFUL IS THERAPY AND SURGERY IN TREATING KNEE PATHOLOGY?

Success in treating knee pathology is mostly dependent on an accurate diagnosis. It seems reasonable and prudent to assume that a problem such as Legg-Calvé-Perthe's disease cannot be treated with ultrasound to the anterior knee where symptoms of this condition may be felt. Additionally, a lateral retinacular release for a person who exhibits patterns of patellar lateral instability may not be beneficial for the athlete who has excessive foot pronation and falls into a valgus collapse due to proximal hip musculature weakness. Conservative treatment for many causes of knee pathology when accurately diagnosed is very high.

PERSONAL INFORMATION

WHAT INFLUENCE DOES AGE HAVE ON YOUR CLINICAL DECISION-MAKING PROCESS IN THE KNEE REGION?

Age is an important factor as many conditions are typically more common in those of various age groups. For example, adolescents will more often present with pathologies such as Osgood Schlatter's disease (apophysitis at the tibial tubercle), ACL injuries, meniscal pathology, ligamentous pathology,[29] or Legg-Perthe's disease, which, although a hip condition, is a common referral of pain to the knee. The elderly population has a much greater incidence of osteoarthritis of the knee joint. Osteoarthritis significantly affects nearly 10% of adults aged 60 years and above,[19] and may affect more than 10% of adults who are overweight.[7,11]

WHAT INFLUENCE DOES A PATIENT'S OCCUPATION HAVE ON YOUR CLINICAL DECISION-MAKING PROCESS IN THE KNEE REGION?

Occupation is always important as it can give clues to the knee pathology and allow the examiner to better understand the function needed to return patients to their premorbid level of activity. Typically laborers are stronger than their sedentary counterparts, which may predispose them to either overuse or degenerative conditions due to the repetitiveness of many jobs; however, because of increased strength they rarely have muscle strains. Manual laborers such as carpet layers and carpenters who are required to work in deeply flexed knee postures may have higher incidences of anterior knee pain. Laborers and those working in agricultural regions are also thought to have more actual joint damage leading to a higher incidence of osteoarthritis of the knee.

WHAT INFLUENCE DOES GENDER HAVE ON YOUR CLINICAL DECISION-MAKING PROCESS IN THE KNEE REGION?

Patellofemoral pain and knee instability typically occur more often in adolescent females. Elderly men and in particular elderly women exhibit knee pain due to osteoarthritis, with female-to-male ratios that vary from 1.5 to 4.0 among studies.[1]

SYMPTOM HISTORY

The subjective medical history is critical to the success of any evaluation of musculoskeletal injuries and this is never more important than in the knee.[24] The medical history should be done in a consistent and orderly fashion with all patients in order to obtain all important information. In most cases patients will tell you what their problem is if you listen closely and ask the appropriate questions.

MECHANISM OF INJURY

WHAT INFLUENCE DOES THE MECHANISM OF INJURY HAVE ON YOUR CLINICAL DECISION-MAKING PROCESS IN THE KNEE REGION?

The mechanism of injury is generally described as either acute traumatic or nontraumatic.

In the acute nontraumatic injury the examiner must consider various problems such as a septic joint, osteoarthritis, patellofemoral pain, overuse syndromes, calcium pyrophosphate deposition, or tumors.[29] Of major concern here is a septic joint due to multiple causes such as previous surgery, lacerations, intraarticular joint injections, systemic illness, or sexually transmitted diseases.[29] The infected knee will present with all the classic signs of inflammation including swelling, heat, and erythematic discoloration. This is a medical emergency that requires immediate referral to a physician to determine appropriate, treatment which may include oral antibiotics, intravenous antibiotics, or surgical debridement and washout.

The mechanism can be further described by the direction of force or forces exerted on the knee. These include a varus and valgus force, with our without rotation. Additionally hyperextension (Figure II-12-2) and hyperflexion (Figure II-12-3), compression, and distraction can all be causes of potential injury. Magee has described potential mechanisms of knee injury and the structures possibly injured (Table II-12-1).[22]

Ligaments that can be injured in the knee include the anterior cruciate, posterior cruciate, lateral collateral, and medial collateral ligaments. These ligaments provide support for tibial

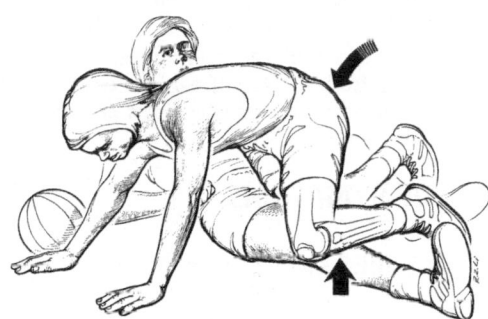

FIGURE II-12-2   Direct trauma onto the proximal tibia can lead to posterior cruciate ligament or anterior cruciate ligament/posterior cruciate ligament disruption. (From Scott WN, ed. *Ligament and Extensor Mechanism Injuries in the Knee: Diagnosis and Management.* St. Louis: Mosby; 1991, Figure 7-2.)

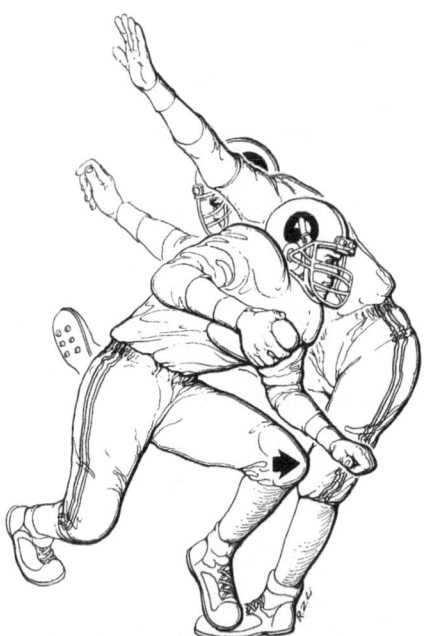

FIGURE II-12-3   A hyperextension injury can lead to anterior cruciate ligament or anterior cruciate ligament/posterior cruciate ligament disruption. (From Scott WN, ed. *Ligament and Extensor Mechanism Injuries in the Knee: Diagnosis and Management.* St. Louis: Mosby; 1991, Figure 7-3.)

TABLE II-12-1 Mechanisms of Injury to the Knee and Structures Possibly Injured

Mechanism of Injury	Structures Possibly Injured
Varus or valgus contact without rotation	Collateral ligament Epiphyseal fracture Patellar dislocation or subluxation
Varus or valgus contact with rotation	Collateral and cruciate ligaments Collateral ligaments and patellar dislocation or subluxation Meniscus tear
Blow to patellofemoral joint, or fall on flexed knee, foot dorsiflexed	Patellar articular injury or osteochondral fracture
Blow to tibial tubercle, or fall on flexed knee, foot plantar flexed	Posterior cruciate ligament
Anterior blow to tibia, resulting in knee hyperextension (contact hypertension)	Anterior cruciate ligament Anterior and posterior cruciate ligament
Noncontact hyperextension	Anterior cruciate ligament Posterior capsule
Noncontact deceleration	Anterior cruciate ligament
Noncontact deceleration, with tibial medial rotation or femoral lateral rotation on fixed tibia	Anterior cruciate ligament
Noncontact, quickly turning one way with tibia rotated in the opposite direction	Patellar dislocation or subluxation
Noncontact, rotation with varus or valgus loading	Meniscus injury
Noncontact, compressive rotation	Meniscus injury Osteochondral fracture
Hyperflexion	Meniscus (posterior horn) Anterior cruciate ligament
Forced medial rotation	Meniscus injury (lateral meniscus)
Forced lateral rotation	Meniscus injury (medial meniscus) Medial collateral ligament and possibly anterior cruciate ligament Patellar dislocation
Flexion-varus-medial rotation	Anterolateral instability
Flexion-valgus-lateral rotation	Anteromedial instability
Dashboard injury	Isolated posterior cruciate ligament Posterior cruciate ligament and posterior capsule Posterolateral instability Posteromedial instability Patellar fracture Tibial fracture (proximal) Tibial plateau fracture Acetabular and pelvic fracture

Adapted from Clancy W: Evaluation of acute knee injuries. In: *American Association of Orthopaedic Surgeons, Symposium on Sports Medicine: The Knee.* St. Louis: Mosby; 1985; Strobel M, Stedtfeld HW. *Diagnostic Evaluation of the Knee.* Berlin: Springer-Verlag; 1990.

TABLE II-12-2 **Primary and Secondary Ligamentous Restraint to Knee Movement**

Tibial Motion	Primary Restraint	Secondary Restraint
Anterior translation	ACL	MCL, LCL, middle third of medial and lateral capsule and iliotibial band
Posterior translation	PCL	MCL, LCL, posterior third of medial and lateral capsule, popliteus tendon, anterior and posterior meniscofemoral ligaments
Valgus rotation	MCL	ACL, PCL, posterior capsule when knee is fully extended
Varus rotation	LCL	ACL, PCL, posterior capsule when knee is fully extended
External rotation	MCL, LCL	
Internal rotation	ACL, PCL	Anterior and posterior meniscofemoral ligaments

From Zachazewski JE, Magee DJ, Quillen WS, eds. *Athletic Injuries and Rehabilitation*. Philadelphia: WB Saunders; 1996, Table 30-1.
ACL, anterior cruciate ligament; PCL, posterior cruciate ligament, LCL, lateral collateral ligament; MCL, medial collateral ligament.

movements. Each ligament has a primary and secondary action at the knee. Primary and secondary ligament restraints for the knee are described in Table II-12-2.

CLINICAL PEARL

It is important to understand the osteokinematics and arthrokinematics of the knee. Knee flexion range of motion (ROM) is normally around 130° to 135°, whereas knee extension is usually about 0° to 10° of hyperextension or genu recurvatum. Knee flexion and extension are the largest knee motions and occur in the sagittal plane. These are generalizations as there is substantial variability depending on weight, age, and history of previous pathology. Rotation of the knee, also known as internal or external tibial rotation, is approximately 10° in each direction. Normal osteokinematics dictate that the last 10° to 15° of extension requires external tibial rotation (screw-home mechanism). Following knee injury, ROM may be limited due to capsular or muscular restrictions or internal derangements. The capsular pattern of the knee is knee flexion limited more than knee extension.

CLINICAL DECISION MAKING CASE STUDY—PATIENT PROFILE

An 18-year-old patient comes into the Saturday morning clinic unable to bear weight and in pain and distress. He was injured last night during a football game. He was hit from the side and his knee was driven forcefully into the ground. He was unable to bear weight and was taken to the emergency room, put in a knee immobilizer, and given pain medication due to "knee sprain." Because of pain that was not relieved, his mother brought him to the Saturday morning clinic for evaluation. The patient presents 12 hours after injury with significant knee joint effusion, a high-riding patella, and non-weight-bearing status due to pain. What is your first clinical concern/impression? Active quadriceps contraction causes extreme pain and the patella exhibits excessive elevation. The patient is unable to perform straight leg rise due to symptoms of pain in the anterior knee.

Answer
The patient is found to have an avulsed tibial tubercle and tibial plateau fracture. It requires surgical intervention to stabilize.

LOCATION OF SYMPTOMS

WHAT INFLUENCE DOES THE LOCATION OF SYMPTOMS HAVE ON YOUR CLINICAL DECISION-MAKING PROCESS IN THE KNEE REGION?
Although location of symptoms is important, at times the location of the pain is distant from the site of pain generation. Box II-12-1 lists general structures that are usually palpable around the various locations at the knee.

REFERRAL OF SYMPTOMS

WHAT STRUCTURES CAN REFER INTO THE KNEE REGION?
Muscles, tendons, and ligaments emit pain somewhat near the region of injury in the knee. Pain from muscles, tendons, and ligaments rarely refers pain to other parts of the body. However, other parts of the body often refer pain to the knee, such as bone/cartilage pathology involving slipped capital femoral epiphysis (SCFE) or adolescent coxa vara, which is one of the most significant lower limb epiphyseal-plate disorders seen in adolescents.[2] In this condition mild hip pain is commonly referred to the medial aspect of the knee.[2] Legg-Calvé-Perthe's disease, an idiopathic avascular necrosis of the hip that occurs predominantly in young boys, may present with nonspecific pain in the hip, thigh, or leg.[27] For a young male with hip and knee pain, the astute clinician should always rule out proximal contributions such as these before continuing treatments directed at the tibiofemoral joint alone. Hip conditions such as these may necessitate a return to the referring physician to rule out these potentially debilitating hip pathologies. Lumbar segmental nerves can be another potential source of referral pain into the leg and knee (Table II-12-3).

Vascular injury to the lower leg will not typically cause generalized knee pain, although any vascular insult to the lower extremity may cause a vague cramping or pain sensation of the area distal to the injury site, which is not being perfused adequately.

BOX II-12-1 **Knee Palpation Sites**

Anterior	Medial	Posterior	Lateral
Patella	Medial joint line	Gastrocnemius tendons	Lateral joint line
Patellar facets	Medial collateral ligament	Popliteal fossa	Lateral meniscus
Patellar tendon	Medial meniscus	Baker's cyst	Lateral collateral ligament
Patellar plica	Semimembranosus tendon	Popliteal artery	Iliotibial band
Medial patellofemoral ligament	Pes anserinus bursa		Biceps femoris tendon
Quadriceps tendon	Medial tibial plateau		
Fat pads			

TABLE II-12-3 **Lumbar Segmental Nerves**			
Nerves	**Segmental Level**	**Sensory**	**Motor Function**
Femoral	L2, L3, L4	Thigh via cutaneous	Iliacus, sartorius, quadriceps, articularis genu, pectineus
Obturator	L2, L3, L4	Medial thigh	Adductor (longus, brevis, and magnus), gracilis, obturator externus
Saphenous	L2, L3, L4	Medial leg and foot	None
Tibial	L4, L5, S1, S2, S3	Posterior heel and plantar surface of foot	Semitendinosus, semimembranosus, biceps femoris, adductor magnus, gastrocnemius, soleus, plantaris, flexor hallucis longus, flexor digitorum longus, tibialis posterior
Common fibular	L4, L5, S1, S2	Lateral posterior leg	Biceps femoris

From Cleland J. *Orthopedic Clinical Examination: An Evidence-Based Approach for Physical Therapists.* Carlstadt, NJ: Icon Learning Systems; 2005.

SYMPTOM DESCRIPTORS

QUALITY OF SYMPTOMS

Deep ache: Indicates an inflammatory condition, osteoarthritis, and degenerative changes

Dull ache: Same as above but can also be used to describe bone pathology

Sharp pain: Mechanical joint pain, tendon tear, ligament tear

Burning: Overuse or neurological involvement

Numbness and tingling: Neurological, compressive neuropathy

Cramping: Fatigue, muscle weakness, dehydration

Constant pain: Pain with no relief of symptoms would indicate a red flag situation, which may necessitate referral back to a physician.

TWENTY-FOUR-HOUR SYMPTOM PATTERN

IF A PATIENT HAS SYMPTOMS IN THE MORNING, WHAT PATHOLOGY DOES THIS IMPLICATE?

Morning stiffness usually indicates some form of joint effusion or congestion. This effusion could be due to degeneration of the joint structures. Pain that is worse during the first few steps, but decreases as time goes on, may suggest arthritis or tendinitis.

WHAT ROLE DOES MORNING STIFFNESS PLAY IN DIFFERENTIATION?

Joint stiffness in the morning generally indicates arthritis, or an effusion.

If a patient has symptoms in the afternoon, what pathology does this implicate?

Symptoms in the afternoon could indicate pathology that is induced by fatigue resulting from activities earlier in the day, or by a gradual progression of swelling in the knee often from a mechanical process or degeneration.

IF A PATIENT HAS SYMPTOMS IN THE EVENING, WHAT PATHOLOGY DOES THIS IMPLICATE?

Symptoms that occur in the evening are more than likely the result of gout. Symptoms in the evening could also be the result of a continuation of the problems that created symptoms earlier in the day or afternoon. Sleep disturbances can also occur due to arthritic symptoms in patients who sleep with a pillow under their knees to put the knee in a position of maximal capsular volume due to swelling.

IF A PATIENT HAS SYMPTOMS WHEN SLEEPING, WHAT PATHOLOGY DOES THIS IMPLICATE?

Unresponsive knee pain at rest can indicate several problems that may need special care. These can include active infection, complex regional pain syndrome, fracture, or tumors. It is advisable to refer a patient with unresponsive knee pain to an orthopedic surgeon for a more enhanced medical evaluation.

STABILITY OF SYMPTOMS

CHANGES IN SYMPTOMS

HOW DOES THE PROGRESSION OF A PATIENT'S SYMPTOMS IMPACT YOUR CLINICAL DECISION-MAKING PROCESS? IF A PATIENT'S SYMPTOMS ARE IMPROVING, WHAT PATHOLOGY DOES THIS IMPLICATE?

Improving symptoms do not necessarily correlate with any specific condition in the knee. Improvement in symptoms can indicate many things including but not limited to resting the offending structures, soft tissue healing, decreased inflammatory response, or simply resolution over time.

IF A PATIENT'S SYMPTOMS ARE WORSENING, WHAT PATHOLOGY DOES THIS IMPLICATE?

Just as improvement of symptoms does not correlate with a specific condition, neither does a general progressing symptom in the knee. A worsening condition generally implicates a more irritable condition or a condition that may require surgical intervention. A worsening of symptoms despite conservative treatment on the other hand could indicate a more severe situation. All soft tissues and structures around the knee should demonstrate a decrease in pain or symptoms when mechanical stress is removed. If a patient continues to have worsening pain despite decreased activity levels and appropriate conservative treatment, a referral back to the physician is necessary. This worsening of symptoms, especially if over a short period of time, is extremely atypical and should not be taken lightly.

CLINICAL DECISION MAKING CASE STUDY—PATIENT PROFILE   **?**

Your patient is a 24-year-old male that you are seeing status postarthroscopic ACL reconstruction with bone-patellar tendon-one autograft 4 weeks previous. He is coming to your clinic, although his surgeon is in another town across the state. The patient is progressing as tolerated, although he continues to have generalized aching in the knee throughout the day. This has increased as he has returned to work as a uniform delivery person. You notice that the inferior portion of his tibial incision is still open, although there is no history of drainage and the incision looks clean.

Is there anything unusual about the case described above? If so what is causing suspicion?

The patient returns later that week still complaining of aching and "stiffness." He does not complain of any illness, fever, nausea, or unusual symptoms other than the persistent knee aching and swelling. What is your next recourse?

Finally at the end of that same week he returns one more time. This time he has another problem. His tibial incision now has some light brownish colored drainage that has leaked. What is your next step?

Hopefully it is an immediate referral to an orthopedic surgeon for evaluation of suspected sepsis.

Answer

Do not always assume that infection will show up in full force immediately after surgery. Although it is important to understand the cardinal signs of infection including pain, heat, redness, and swelling, they are not always clearly presented as such. In this case the infection remained silent for several weeks continuing to fester inside the knee. It was not until the pus was forced out of the tibial incision from inside the joint through the tibial tunnel that any presenting symptoms readily appeared. This case required immediate removal of the graft and hardware and debridement of the synovial membrane. In addition, this patient was placed on intravenous antibiotics to control this septic condition. This was a tragic ending to what appeared to be a normal postoperative progression.

FUNCTIONAL AND ACTIVITY PARTICIPATION LIMITATIONS

BEHAVIOR OF SYMPTOMS: AGGRAVATING BEHAVIOR

WHAT INFLUENCE DOES AGGRAVATING FUNCTIONS HAVE ON YOUR CLINICAL DECISION-MAKING PROCESS IN THE KNEE REGION?

An aggravation to knee flexion can be caused by many conditions including chondromalacia, anterior capsular restrictions, loose bodies, meniscus and cartilage injuries, a torn ACL causing locking of the knee, quadriceps flexibility deficits, hamstring weakness, hamstring muscle spasm, fracture, patellar dislocation, large tense effusion, osteophytes, or a malpositioned graft following ACL reconstruction.

An aggravation to knee extension can be caused by a reduction in quadriceps muscle force production, posterior capsule restriction, hamstring tightness, lack of a "screw home" mechanism or lateral tibial torsion, loose bodies, a large tense effusion, osteophytes, meniscus or articular cartilage injury, or a malpositioned graft following ACL reconstruction. Table II-12-4 lists functional and activity participation limitations.

CLINICAL DECISION MAKING CASE STUDY—PATIENT PROFILE ?

Your 19-year-old male patient is being seen status post-ACL reconstruction with hamstring tendon autograft and partial medial meniscectomy. He is now 5 weeks out of surgery and still lacks about 7° of terminal knee extension. His involved knee measures 2° of knee flexion and the uninvolved knee reveals 5° of hyperextension. The end feel to an anterior tibial glide appears firm bilaterally although in a decreased range on the involved side. What accessory motion can be potentially missed with this patient?

Answer

Remember that to achieve full terminal extension the tibia must also externally rotate as part of what is known as the screw home mechanism. Although the anterior tibial glide appears restricted it may simply be that the lateral rotation portion of normal tibiofemoral arthrokinematics is not occurring appropriately. An assessment of lateral tibial rotation should be checked to ensure that normal amount of motion and appropriate end feel are obtained. This is best done with the knee in 90° of flexion, which is where the tibiofemoral joint exhibits the most internal and external rotation range of motion. Treatment should include external tibial rotation joint mobilization techniques to regain normal motion at this joint.

BEHAVIOR OF SYMPTOMS: EASING BEHAVIOR

WHAT INFLUENCE DOES EASING FUNCTIONS HAVE ON YOUR CLINICAL DECISION-MAKING PROCESS IN THE KNEE REGION?

Ambulating with knee fully extended: Many times patients will ambulate with their knee fully extended. In some respects it seems counterintuitive because of the increased compressive loads and decreased shock absorption occurring at the tibiofemoral joint. This pattern of ambulation is known as a quadriceps avoidance pattern of gait. In the presence of swelling or injury, muscles around the edematous region are neurologically inhibited. Normal gait requires approximately

---

TABLE II-12-4 Functional and Activity Participation Limitations

Motion	Functional Activities	Pathology if Symptoms Are Aggravated by Activity	Pathology if Symptoms Are Eased by Activity
Flexion	Kneeling, squatting, stooping	Pain with passive flexion could include degenerative joint conditions, meniscus tears, instability, patellofemoral pain from chondromalacia, excessive lateral pressure syndrome	
Extension	Walking	Degenerative joint disease, flexion contractures, anterior horn degenerative tears	Knee locked in extension can indicate quadriceps weakness or quadriceps guarding
Combined motions	Planting, cutting	Knee instabilities, degenerative joint conditions, meniscus tears	
General movements	Bicycle riding		The motion bathes the joint and could indicate the presence of inflammation or arthritis Motion in weight bearing could indicate patellofemoral dysfunction
Static positions—positioned in resting position of the knee	Resting, sleeping	Fractures, tumor, edema	Meniscus, osteoarthritis, edema

15° of knee flexion at the initial contact of the foot to the ground. To prevent the knee from buckling into flexion, the quadriceps are recruited. If the quadriceps are weakened or it is painful to contract the muscle, individuals will instinctively lock their knee into extension to prevent buckling of the knee.

Knee positioned in slight flexion: The resting position of the knee is approximately 25° of knee flexion. For many patients this will be the most comfortable position and the patient's position of ease. When this is the case, it is often indicative of edema within the knee. When the tibiofemoral joint is swollen or engorged with fluid, it will take the position that allows the most fluid to accumulate. This occurs at a resting position. Patients will also take this position if there is injury to the meniscus or cartilage within the tibiofemoral joint. The resting position places the least amount of pressure and load on potentially sensitive tissues.

Motion of the knee: Ease of or alterations of ROM of the knee can indicate several forms of pathology. Non-weight-bearing ROM will often ease pain in arthritic knees or knees with inflammation. Knee movement allows spreading of synovial fluid that bathes the injured tissues. The non-weight-bearing aspect of ROM decreases the loading on irritated structures. Motion of the knee regardless of weight-bearing status will often implicate the patellofemoral joint as the source of the symptoms.

MEDICAL HISTORY

The patient's past medical history is of critical importance. The history may be riddled with previous medical and surgical problems or can be completely free of past intervention. Knowing the types of problems related to the entire lower extremity can be very insightful in determining what condition may be bothering them presently. For example, a past history of patellar dislocation would indicate a definite need to rule out patellar disorders as a source of the present pain and symptoms. Additionally a history of previous ACL reconstruction may necessitate a quick screen to rule out the need for revision surgery to replace a torn reconstructed ligament.

CLINICAL PEARL

Synovial joints such as the knee commonly have normal or abnormal end feels. End feels are the sensation imparted to the examiner's hand as the knee is taken gently into passive overpressure and the end of available ROM. Normal end feels for the knee are described as follows:
- *Flexion (tissue approximation)*
- *Extension (tissue stretch)*
- *Medial rotation of the tibia on the femur (tissue stretch)*
- *Lateral rotation of the tibia on the femur (tissue stretch)*
- *Patellar movements (tissue stretch—all directions) See Figure II-12-4 for assessment of medial and lateral patellar mobility.*

All of these end feels are considered normal in their typical locations. Each of these end feels though can be abnormal. For example, a firm or hard end feel at 5° from full extension on the involved extremity, with an uninvolved end feel that exhibits tissue stretch at 5° of hyperextension, is definitely abnormal. A common abnormal end feel that is often missed in the patient who has lost full terminal knee extension is the lateral tibial rotation end feel. This end feel may be abnormal, meaning firm, or hard, or may simply be earlier in the ROM than normal. If this is the case, this patient with knee dysfunction may not be able to gain full extension until their lateral tibial rotation is returned to normal to allow the normal screw home mechanism to occur unimpeded.

MEDICAL AND ORTHOPEDIC TESTING

WHAT MEDICAL AND ORTHOPEDIC TESTS INFLUENCE YOUR DIFFERENTIAL DIAGNOSIS PROCESS?

When performing a thorough knee examination, it is critical to evaluate numerous structures in and around the knee to determine your differential diagnosis. Special tests are performed to implicate or rule out various injuries seen in the knee during this process. To do this in the most expedient manner an algorithm type process is best.[24,25] Because numerous tests exist for the knee complex it is often hard to determine which test works best for various structures. Evidence-based medicine is slowly evolving quality of test procedures via sensitivity and specificity. This shift to evidence-based medicine for examinations allows a clinician to be more selective when identifying which tests should be performed on various patients.[5,22,23] It is for this reason that the use of a special testing algorithm such as the Davies knee special testing algorithm is helpful. The following algorithm utilizes several special testing procedures for most knee pathologies that will be seen in the typical outpatient physical therapy clinic.

KNEE ALGORITHM EXAMINATION

Knee Effusion

Critical Pathways (Clusters, Signs, and Symptoms)	Position	Special Tests	Sensitivity/ Specificity	Tissues Implicated
History of macrotrauma	Supine: knee—0° to 30°	Milking test and fluid wave	Not determined	Intraarticular effusion
Patient complaints of stiffness	Supine: knee—0° to 30°	Ballotment test	Not determined	Intraarticular effusion
Observation of swelling				
Increased anthropometric measurements				

Notes on Special Tests:
Milking Test: The sensitivity and specificity have not been established in any studies.
Ballotment Test: The sensitivity and specificity have not been established in any studies.

Patellofemoral

Test Category (Algorithm)	Critical Pathways (Clusters, Signs, and Symptoms)	Position	Special Tests	Sensitivity/ Specificity	Tissues Implicated
Patellofemoral	All patients	Supine: knee flexed 30°	Medial/lateral glides (see Figure II-12-3) (two quadrants-N)	Not determined	Medial/lateral retinaculum (superficial fibers)
		Supine: knee flexed 30°	Cephalic glides caudal glides (10 mm)	Not determined	Retinaculum, patellar tendon
		Supine: knee 0°	Medial/lateral tilts (15°)	Not determined	Medial/lateral retinaculum (deep fibers)
		Sitting: knee 90° to 0°	Passive tracking ("C"/reverse "C")	Not determined	Noncontractile tissue, femoral groove
		Sitting: knee 90° to 0°	Active tracking Open kinetic chain ("C"/reverse "C")	Not determined	Contractile tissue, femoral groove
		Standing	Active tracking Closed kinetic chain	Not determined	Contractile and noncontractile tissue

Notes on Special Tests:
Medial/lateral glides: The sensitivity and specificity have not been established in any studies.
Cephalic/caudal glides: The sensitivity and specificity have not been established in any studies.
Medial/lateral tilts: The sensitivity and specificity have not been established in any studies.
Passive tracking: The sensitivity and specificity have not been established in any studies.
Active tracking OCK: The sensitivity and specificity have not been established in any studies.
Active tracking CKC: The sensitivity and specificity have not been established in any studies.

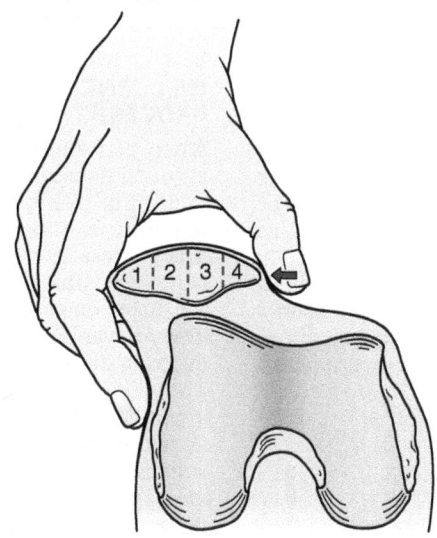

FIGURE II-12-4 Passive patellar medial and lateral glide assessment. (From Magee D. *Orthopedic Physical Assessment.* 5th ed. St. Louis: Saunders, Elsevier; 2008, Figure 12-31.)

Posterior Cruciate Ligament (PCL)

Test Category (Algorithm)	Critical Pathways (Clusters, Signs, and Symptoms)	Position	Special Tests	Sensitivity/ Specificity	Tissues Implicated
PCL	History of macrotrauma	Supine: knee 0°	Recurvatum	Not determined	PCL
	Blunt—dashboard injury Hyperextension injury	Supine: knee flexed 80°	Sag test[37]	Sens = 0.79 Spec = 1.0	PCL
	Fall on anterior tibia with ankle in plantar flexion	Supine: knee flexed 80°	Clancy step-up (10 mm) (Figure II-12-5)	Not determined	PCL
	Intraarticular effusion Suspected anterior cruciate ligament	Supine: knee flexed 80°	Posterior drawer[38-44] (acute versus chronic)	Sens = 0.51 to 1.0 Spec = 0.99	PCL

Notes on Special Tests:
Recurvatum: The sensitivity and specificity have not been established in any studies.
References for studies about the sensitivity and specificity of the Sag Test and the Posterior Drawer Test can be found on pages 249–250.
Clancy Step-up: The sensitivity and specificity have not been established in any studies.

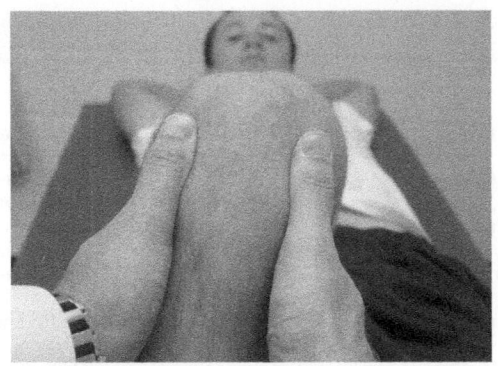

FIGURE II-12-5 The Clancy step-up test for posterior cruciate ligament deficiency. (From Manske RC, ed. *Postsurgical Orthopedic Sports Rehabilitation. Knee and Shoulder.* St. Louis: Mosby; 2006, Figure 3-20.)

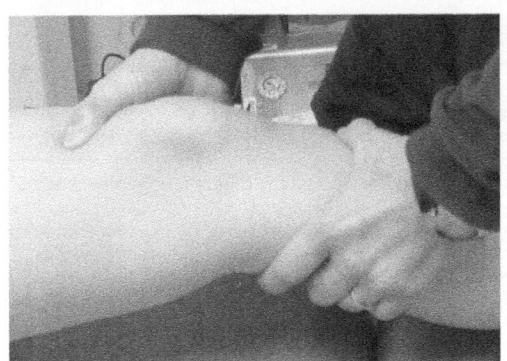

FIGURE II-12-6 The lachman test for anterior cruciate ligament deficiency. (From Manske RC, ed. *Postsurgical Orthopedic Sports Rehabilitation. Knee and Shoulder.* St. Louis: Mosby; 2006, Figure 3-23.)

Anterior Cruciate Ligament (ACL)

Test Category (Algorithm)	Critical Pathways (Clusters, Signs, and Symptoms)	Position	Special Tests	Sensitivity/ Specificity	Tissues Implicated
ACL	History of macrotrauma including twisting, deceleration	Supine: knee flexed 80°	Anterior drawer[45-58]	Sens = 0.18 to 0.98 Spec = 0.78 to 1.0	ACL (AMB)
		Supine: knee flexed 80°	Rotary instability: ALRI, PLRI, AMRI, PMRI	Not determined	ACL, posterior lateral corner, posterior medial corner (several structures)
	History of giving way History of hearing "pop" Rapid accumulation of intraarticular effusion				
		Supine: knee flexed 30°	Lachman's[59-72] (>3 mm) (Figure II-12-6)	Sens = 0.63 to 1.0 Spec = 0.42 to 1.0	ACL
		Supine: knee 0° to 80°	Pivot shift[73-83]	Sens = 0.27 to 0.95 Spec = 0.89 to 1.0	ACL, lateral capsule
		Supine: knee 80° to 0°	Jerk	Not determined	ACL, lateral capsule
		Supine: knee 0° to 60°	Flexion rotation drawer (FRD)	Not determined	ACL, lateral capsule

ALRI, anterolateral rotatory instability; PLRI, posterolateral rotatory instability; AMRI, anteromedial rotatory instability; PMRI, posteromedial rotatory instability; AMB, anteromedial bundle.
Notes on Special Tests:
References for studies about the sensitivity and specificity of the Anterior Drawer Test, the Lachman's Test, and the Pivot Shift can be found on page 250.
Rotary Instabilities: The sensitivity and specificity have not been established in any studies.
Jerk: The sensitivity and specificity have not been established in any studies.
Flexion Rotation Drawer: The sensitivity and specificity have not been established in any studies.

Collateral Ligaments

Test Category (Algorithm)	Critical Pathways (Clusters, Signs, and Symptoms)	Position	Special Tests	Sensitivity/ specificity	Tissues Implicated
Collaterals	MOI: macrotraumatic injury with twisting	Supine: knee 0°	Valgus stress[84,85] (0)	Sens = 0.86 to 0.96	MCL, ACL, PCL, PMOL
	MOI: history of frontal plane macrotrauma	Supine: knee flexed 30°	Valgus stress[84,85] (30)	Spec = not reported	MCL
	Localized edema without intraarticular effusion	Supine: knee 0°	Varus stress[86] (0)	Sens = 0.25 Spec = not reported	LCL, ACL, PCL, PLC
	Localized pain over collateral ligaments	Supine: knee flexed 30°	Varus stress[86] (30)	Sens = 0.25 Spec = not reported	LCL
		Prone: knee flexed 90°	Apley's distraction (ER/IR)	Not determined	MCL/LCL
		Prone	Apley's distraction with DDV (ER/IR)	Not determined	MCL/LCL

MOI, mechanism of injury; MCL, medial collateral ligament; ACL, anterior cruciate ligament; PCL, posterior cruciate ligament; LCL, lateral collateral ligament; ER, external rotation; IR, internal rotation.
Notes on Special Tests: References for studies about the sensitivity and specificity of the Valgus Stress Test and the Varus Stress Test can be found on page 250.

Meniscus

Test Category (Algorithm)	Critical Pathways (Clusters, Signs, and Symptoms)	Position	Special Tests	Sensitivity/ Specificity	Tissues Implicated
Meniscus	History of macrotrauma Twisting MOI	Supine: knee 0°	Recurvatum	Not determined	Meniscus— anterior horns
	Delayed effusion (over 12 hours)	Supine: knee maximum flexion	Steinman's test	Not determined	Meniscus— posterior horns
	Reproducible click/clunk Pseudolocking	Supine: knee flexed 90°	McMurray's [87-95] (Figure II-12-7)	Sens = 0.16 to 0.95 Spec = 0.25 to 0.98	Meniscus— posterior horns
	Joint line pain	Supine: knee flexed or extended	Joint line tenderness[96-99]	Sens = 0.28 to 0.92 Spec = 0.29 to 0.97	Medial and lateral
		Supine: knee 90° to 0°	Dynamic McMurray's[100-101] (ER/IR)	Not determined	Meniscus
		Prone: knee flexed 90°	Apley's compression (ER/IR)	Sens = 0.13 to 0.16 Spec = 0.80 to 0.90	Meniscus— posterior horns
		Prone: knee flexed 90° to 0°	Apley's dynamic compression/DDV (ER/IR)	Not determined	Meniscus
		Standing: 20° knee flexion; weight-bearing internal and external rotation	Thessaly test	Sens at 20° med = 0.89 lat = 0.92 Spec at 20° med = 0.97 lat = 0.96	Meniscus

MOI, mechanism of injury; ER, external rotation; IR, internal rotation.
Notes on Special Tests:
Recurvatum: The sensitivity and specificity have not been established in any studies.
Steinman's Test: The sensitivity and specificity have not been established in any studies.
References for studies about the sensitivity and specificity of McMurray's, Joint Line Tenderness and Apley's Compression can be found on pages 250–251.
Dynamic McMurray's: The sensitivity and specificity have not been established in any studies.

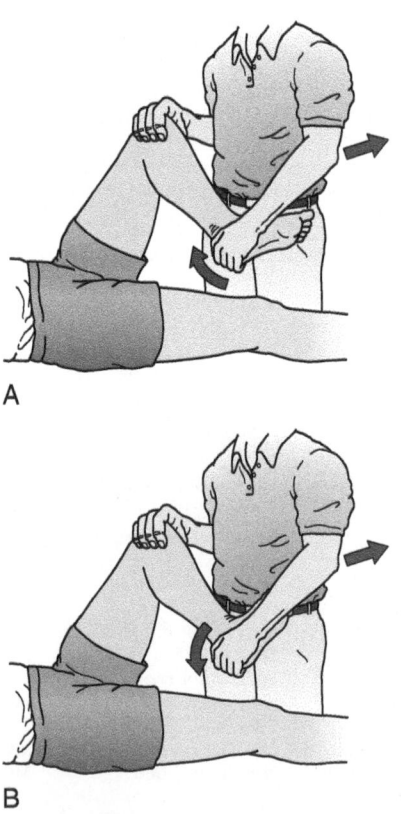

FIGURE 12-2-7 (A,B) McMurray test for meniscus injury. (From Magee D. *Orthopedic Physical Assessment.* 5th ed. St. Louis: Saunders, Elsevier; 2008, Figure 12-100.)

BIOMECHANICAL

WHAT ROLE DOES BIOMECHANICS PLAY IN THE DECISION-MAKING PROCESS IN THE KNEE REGION?

Knee biomechanics are used to assess normal arthrokinematic motions of flexion, extension, and internal or external rotation. Assessment of both passive and active knee extension ROM and end feel provide insight into various pathological entities. The capsular pattern of the knee is that of knee flexion being more limited than knee extension. When this capsular pattern exists an inflammatory condition of the capsule is probable. With this in mind, a knee that has extension more limited than flexion would indicate a problem other than a capsular condition. This may include pathologies such as meniscus tears, mechanical irritation of the medial synovial fold, or even patellofemoral conditions. Both the proximal tibiofibular joint and the patellofemoral joint are plane synovial joints but lack a known capsular pattern. It is thought that a limitation of inferior patellar glide may cause a restriction of knee flexion mobility, whereas a limitation of superior patellar glide can limit knee extension motion.

WHAT BIOMECHANICAL ABNORMALITIES IN OTHER REGIONS AFFECT YOUR DECISION-MAKING PROCESS?

Any biomechanical abnormality, especially below or above the knee, can affect decision making when evaluating conditions in the knee.[20] It is well known that biomechanical abnormalities in the hip and the ankle and foot can cause knee pain and dysfunction. For example, a patient who lacks dorsiflexion ankle ROM may compensate for this restriction in mobility through excessive subtalar joint pronation, which causes the talus to move through a sustained position of extreme adduction and plantar flexion, resulting in an increased amount of tibial internal rotation with weight bearing. This abnormal motion at the tibia can create excessive torsion at the proximal knee resulting in tracking patterns. This is especially true if the femur then compensates with excessive internal rotation during weight bearing as it attempts to achieve full knee extension via the screw home mechanism based on the theory described by Tiberio.[34] Multiple studies have recently proven that proximal hip weakness can result in or contribute to anterior knee pain.[4,14,26,28,31,35]

PERSONAL FACTORS

WHAT PRIOR SURGERIES INFLUENCE YOUR CLINICAL DECISION MAKING?

Any prior surgery must be reviewed and could potentially affect present knee pathology. Mounting evidence indicates that surgery alters normal knee mechanics. Examples of this relationship include the removal of portions of the meniscus. The removal of the meniscus increases the likelihood of developing osteoarthritis later in life. Prior surgeries to the ankle, foot, or hip can also impact the loading and forces seen at the knee. These changes can also increase the chances of subsequent knee injuries.

DOES A FAMILY HISTORY OF PATHOLOGY IN THE REGION INFLUENCE YOUR CLINICAL REASONING PROCESS?

An accurate description of a family history is important to determine the potential risk factors for pathologies that can be carried from first-degree relatives. These include osteoarthritis or rheumatoid arthritis and the development of deep-vein thrombosis. There may even be a familial predisposition to ACL injury.[8]

RED FLAGS THAT WARRANT REFERRAL TO A MEDICAL PHYSICIAN

WHAT SYMPTOMS ALERT YOU TO PATHOLOGIES THAT MAY REQUIRE A REFERRAL TO A MEDICAL PHYSICIAN?

Knee symptoms that would require a referral to a medical physician would include those that could cause immediate physical damage. Generalized symptoms that would indicate referral to a medical physician are typically those that may require further diagnostic testing that physical therapists are unable to perform. These include the following:
- Severe unremitting pain
- Pain unaffected by medication or position
- Severe night pain
- Severe pain with no history of injury
- Severe spasm
- Elevated temperature
- Muscle wasting

  Signs and symptoms consistent with upper motor neuron lesions include the following:
- Spasticity
- Hypertonicity
- Hyperreflexia (deep tendon reflexes)
- Positive pathological reflexes (Babinski, Hoffman)
- Absent or reduced superficial reflexes
- Extensor plantar response (bilateral)

  More specific red flags in the knee include the following:
- Bone or soft tissue tumors or infection may consistently produce night pain that is not altered by position or rest.

- Cellulitis may present with a history of recent superficial skin laceration or trauma, pain, swelling, and increased temperature, discoloration, reddish streaks, and chills or fever.
- Deep venous thrombosis (DVT) will present with multiple symptoms that unfortunately are commonly seen in rehabilitation. A keen eye can differentiate a DVT from simple postoperative discomfort. Symptoms to look for with DVT include leg discomfort and tenderness, an increase in leg (thigh or calf) circumference (swelling or edema), warmth, firmness to palpation, Homan's sign, and pedal edema.
- Gout may present with redness, swelling, pain with ROM, and sensitivity to light touch.
- Other less serious conditions that would necessitate referral are a locked knee that may be held in flexion due to a dislodged meniscal fragment or loose osteochondral defect.

Clinical decision rules have been developed for use to determine the possible risk of having a DVT. Wells et al clinically assessed patients before receiving ultrasound and venography.[36] In 529 patients, their clinical model predicted a prevalence of DVT in three categories: 85% in the high pretest probability category, 33% in the moderate category, and 5% in the low category (Box II-12-2).

The simplicity of this method of evaluation makes it extremely useful as a screening tool for those treating patients complaining of knee pain that may have a DVT. The number of risk factors can indicate the clinical probability that a patient may have a potentially life threatening DVT.

BOX II-12-2 Clinical Model for Predicting Pretest Probability for Deep-Vein Thrombosis

Major Considerations
Active cancer* (treatment ongoing or within previous 6 months or palliative)
Paralysis, paresis, or recent plaster immobilization of the lower extremities
Recently bedridden more than 3 days and/or major surgery within 4 weeks
Localized tenderness along the distribution of the deep venous system
Thigh and calf swollen (should be measured)
Calf swelling 3 cm greater than symptomless side (measured 10 cm below tibial tuberosity)
Strong family history of DVT (two or more first degree relatives with history of DVT)

Minor Considerations
History of recent trauma (≥60 days) to the symptomatic leg
Pitting edema; symptomatic leg only
Dilated superficial veins (nonvaricose) in symptomatic leg only
Hospitalization within previous 6 months
Erythema

Clinical Probability
High
Three or more major points and no alternative diagnosis
Two or more major points and two or more minor points and no other alternative diagnosis
Low
One major point and two or more minor points and has an alternative diagnosis
One major point and one or more minor points and no alternative diagnosis
No major points and three or more minor points + has an alternative diagnosis
No major points + two or more minor points and no alternative diagnosis
Moderate
All other combinations

---

*Active cancer did not include nonmelanomatous skin cancer; deep-vein tenderness had to be elicited either in the calf or thigh in the anatomical distribution of the deep venous system.

CLINICAL DECISION MAKING
CASE STUDY—PATIENT PROFILE

Your 60-year-old female patient is now 4 weeks status post-total knee replacement and is complaining of diffuse calf pain and tenderness. She had an uneventful early recovery and was ambulating with a walker independently several days after her replacement. She was not required to use anticoagulant therapy after surgery but was instructed to wear TED hose for 3 weeks after the surgical procedure. She reports that her calf began to bother her several days ago with an insidious onset. She states she has been doing more around the house lately but does not specifically remember doing anything to hurt her calf. Her involved extremity has pitting edema distal to the knee with mild swelling at the same location. You perform a Homan's test, which is negative, yet she does have tenderness in the region of the gastrocnemius and soleus muscles. She is otherwise healthy. What is the risk that she has a DVT, and should she be sent for further testing?

Answer

She is definitely at high risk according to the CPT developed by Wells and colleagues. She is immediately put into the high-risk group because she has had a major orthopedic surgical procedure, the procedure was performed in the past 4 weeks, and it required some limited bed rest. She also garners a score of +3 points because of each of the following: pitting edema in the lower leg, lower extremity mild swelling, and calf tenderness. Immediate referral is necessary to decrease the risk of developing a pulmonary embolism!

WHAT IS THE DIFFERENCE BETWEEN SINGLE PLANE AND ROTARY INSTABILITY?

CLINICAL PEARL

To begin, the terms laxity and instability, although used interchangeably, are two completely separate entities. Laxity is generally thought to be a looseness of a joint, whereas instability is used to describe the symptoms of giving out. It is theoretically possible to have very lax joints, yet maintain a completely stable knee.

Single-plane instability at the knee occurs when there is translation of the tibia in one direction. Straight plane instabilities may be anterior, posterior, medial, or lateral.[13] Rotary instabilities involve movements in more than one direction and are typically described as anteromedial, anterolateral, posteromedial, and posterolateral. Usually rotary instabilities require a more significant injury to multiple ligament or capsular structures. This occurs due to a larger amount of stress or force causing the injury.

WHEN IS A RADIOGRAPH NECESSARY DUE TO KNEE PATHOLOGY?

CLINICAL PEARL

Radiographs of the knee should be done anytime that significant trauma has occurred. If significant pain is occurring a radiograph can be used to rule out occult fracture before aggressive manipulation of the limb. When viewing radiographs, obvious fractures are easily noted. Other forms of injury that can be viewed on radiograph include intraarticular (Figure II-12-8) or osteochondral fractures, calcifications, joint space narrowing, epiphyseal damage, osteophytes or lipping, loose bodies, tumors, accessory ossification centers, alignment deformity (varus or valgus), patellar alta (Figure II-12-9) (due to tibial tubercle fracture and patellar tendon rupture), patellar baja, asymmetry of femoral condyles, and dislocations.[30]

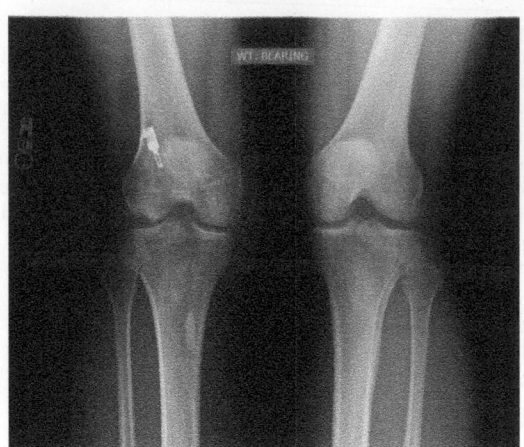

FIGURE II-12-8 Radiograph demonstrating intraarticular knee fracture.

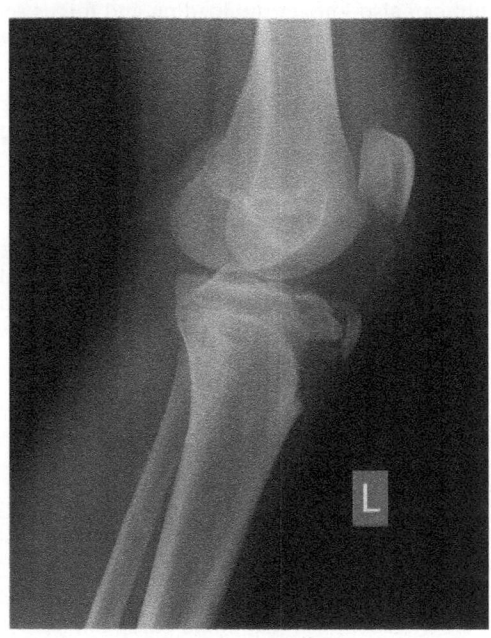

FIGURE II-12-9 Radiograph demonstrating tibial tubercle fracture and patellar tendon rupture.

WHAT ARE CLINICAL DECISION RULES?

Clinical decision rules (CDRs) have been developed in an attempt to increase the accuracy of clinicians' diagnostic and prognostic assessments. Several knee-specific CDRs have been developed including the Ottawa knee rules and the Pittsburgh decision rules.[32]

OTTAWA KNEE DECISION RULES FOR RADIOGRAPHY
INDICATIONS FOR A RADIOGRAPH:
1. Patient older than 55 years of age
2. Tenderness at the head of the fibula
3. Isolated tenderness of the patella
4. Inability to flex knee to 90°
5. Inability to weight bear four steps immediately after the injury and in the emergency department

Exclusion criteria:
1. Age younger than 18 years
2. Isolated superficial skin injuries

TABLE II-12-5   Environmental and Personal Contextual Factors

Pathology	Mechanism of Injury	Signs/Symptoms	Diagnostic Imaging
Anterior cruciate ligament injury: ligament rupture	Twisting, plant and cut, change of direction, deceleration, valgus knee position	Hear and feel "pop" Effusion immediately Giving way, shifting Lachman's test positive Pivot shift tests abnormal Signs of other concomitant pathology (other ligaments, meniscus, etc.)	Radiograph to rule out associated fx MRI
Baker's cyst: capsular defect in posterior knee	Herniation of the posterior capsule due to chronic effusion from meniscal or cartilage damage	Posterior knee pain Discomfort with knee motion Tender to palpation Rule out DVT	MRI Rule out DVT or soft tissue tumor
Bursitis: inflammation of the bursal soft tissue at various locations around the knee Most common over the anterior patella	Mechanical friction and irritation, overuse, repetitive kneeling	Localized swelling Tenderness to palpation Crepitus Discomfort with knee motion May have localized warmth May have discoloration	MRI if symptoms suggest other pathology
Chondromalacia (patellofemoral): softening of articular cartilage on the posterior surface of the patella	Repetitive activity causing mechanical irritation Possibly due to poor biomechanical alignment and/or lower extremity weakness	Generalized anterior knee pain Pain with stairs/steps Weakness of proximal (hip) muscles Genu valgum	MRI—high quality Diagnostic arthroscopy
Compartment syndrome: loss of circulation to the lower extremities	Repetitive overuse Trauma (medical emergency when due to trauma)	Paresthesia, paresis, pain, pallor, pulse less, cramping, aching Compartment pressures: Preexercise ≥15 mm Hg 1 minute postexercise ≥ 30 mm Hg 5 minute postexercise ≥ 20 mm Hg	Radiographs to rule out stress fx Bone scan if symptoms <6 weeks MRI to rule out lumbar spine Nerve conduction studies to rule out nerve entrapment
Degenerative joint disease (DJD): degeneration of the tibiofemoral joint	Aging Repetitive overuse Posttrauma	Pain, loss of motion, swelling, crepitus, stiffness Joint line tenderness at the tibiofemoral joint (medial most common) Patellofemoral joint tenderness (if affected) Stiffness, especially in the morning Angular deformity (most commonly varus more than valgus) May have visible osteophytes	Radiographs—weight bearing preferred to show joint space collapse, both in extension and 45° of flexion
Heterotopic ossification: bone deposited in soft tissues between muscles rather than in muscles like myositis ossificans	Post-blunt trauma to knee (quadriceps most common)	Pain, stiffness, swelling, limited range of motion	Radiographs
IT band friction syndrome: pain in lateral knee due to excessive friction between IT band and lateral femoral condyle	Excessive friction between the IT band and lateral femoral condyle Repetitive overuse Biomechanical factors such as pronation, genu varum	Lateral knee pain Tenderness to palpation of IT band Ambulation with stiff knee to decrease movement of the IT band across the lateral femoral condyle	Radiographs MRI—if diagnosis in question with other lateral pain source Diagnostic ultrasound
Jumpers knee: patellar tendinitis	Repetitive overuse	Anterior knee pain Tender to palpate patellar tendon, distal pole of patella Swelling Crepitus	Radiographs MRI—if conservative treatment fails

Continued on following page.

TABLE II-12-5 Environmental and Personal Contextual Factors (Continued)

Pathology	Mechanism of Injury	Signs/Symptoms	Diagnostic Imaging
Lateral collateral ligament sprain: varus stress injury causing ligament sprain or rupture	Acute injury to lateral side of the knee due to varus force placed on the knee	Pain, swelling, instability, tender to palpate ligament on the lateral joint, range of motion may or may not be limited Range of motion may or may not be limited Varus stress test positive	MRI Radiographs to rule out fracture/avulsion
Medial collateral ligament sprain: valgus stress injury causing ligament sprain or rupture	Acute injury to the medial side of the knee due to a valgus force placed on the knee	Pain, swelling, instability, tender to palpate ligament on medial joint Range of motion may or may not be limited Valgus stress test positive	MRI Radiograph to rule out fractures/avulsion
Meniscus tear: compression/rotation type injury to the knee causing disruption of the meniscus cartilage	Rotary force while weight bearing Knee hyperextension with weight bearing	Joint line tenderness Range of motion may or may not be limited Joint swelling/effusion McMurray's test positive Pain limited motion (flexion more common) Flexion contracture if meniscus displaced	Radiograph to rule out fx, tumors or bony loose bodies MRI
Myositis ossificans: calcification in muscle due to trauma	Most commonly due to trauma Known to occur in spinal cord injuries or head trauma patients	Warmth Tenderness to palpate Firmness felt in muscle Painful hematoma Decreased range of motion Pain with active contraction of muscles	Radiographs
Osteochondritis dissecans: a pathology of the subchondral bone that occurs with insidious onset May be traumatic in nature More common in adolescent aged males than females	Repetitive overuse to subchondral bone that causes disruption of blood supply	Pain Swelling Tenderness to palpation of lesion Most common at the lateral side of the medial femoral condyle Wilson test positive Pain with weight bearing	Radiographs MRI
Osteonecrosis of femoral condyle: microfracture of the subchondral bone that occurs with a segmental collapse	Unknown—may be trauma or stress fracture causing altered blood supply	Pain Swelling Painful range of motion	Radiograph MRI Bone scan
Patellar instability: can be either acute instability, chronic subluxations, or dislocations	Trauma, repetitive microtrauma	Pain Swelling Sensations or instability	None
Patellar tendinitis	Repetitive overuse or muscle-tendon inflexibility issues	Pain Tenderness to palpation of the patellar tendon	None
Patellar tendon rupture	Forceful eccentric contraction of the quadriceps	Weakness of quadriceps Deformity with active quadriceps contraction Pain with knee flexion activity Palpation pain	Radiographs MRI
Plica syndrome: an irritation of the synovial fold usually caused by mechanical abrasion	Direct trauma Repetitive overuse Dramatic increased level of activity	Pain along the medial femoral condyle and medial joint line Clicking, snapping, giving way	Arthroscopy

Popliteal cyst: a herniation of the posterior capsule of the knee	Intraarticular pathology causing swelling/effusion	Posterior knee pain Pain to palpate the popliteal fossa Posterior knee swelling Limited range of motion due to swelling	MRI
Posterior cruciate ligament rupture: injury occurring due to posterior force on the anterior tibia	Landing on knee flexed at 90° Dashboard injury	Swelling and instability Pain with kneeling or use of hamstrings May still be able to tolerate moderate activity	Radiograph to rule out fractures MRI
Superior tibia/fibula joint dysfunction	Cutting Landing awkwardly Twisting motions	Pain with activity Still able to tolerate light to moderate activity Posterolateral knee pain	Physical examination Radiograph to rule out fractures
Tibial plateau fracture	Compression injury Landing from height	Severe pain Limited range of motion due to pain Severe swelling Inability to weight bearing	Radiograph Computed tomography

MRI, magnetic resonance imaging; fx, fracture; DVT, deep vein thrombosis; IT, iliotibial.

TABLE II-12-6 Body Structure and Tissue-Based Pathology (Nociceptive and Peripheral Neurogenic Pain Mechanisms)

	Muscles and Tendons	Bone	Cartilage	Meniscus	Joint	Joint Capsule	Ligaments	Nerves	Visceral Tissue
Pathology	ITB friction syndrome, Pez anserinus Tendinopathy, Patellar tendinopathy/rupture	Tibial plateau fracture, Patellar fracture	Rheumatoid arthritis, Articular cartilage damage, Knee osteoarthritis	Meniscal injury	Superior tibiofibular joint injury, Rheumatoid arthritis, Patellar dislocation, Anterior knee pain	Synovial plica syndrome, Prepatellar bursitis, Baker's cyst	ACL, PCL, LCL, MCL sprains	Femoral, Lateral femoral Cutaneous, Tibial fibular, Sciatic	Not applicable
Age	Any	No correlation with age	Trauma: younger than 18 to 35 years; Degenerative: older than 60 years	Younger than 18 to 35 years of age for traumatic; older than 35 years for degenerative	Trauma: younger than 18 to 35 years; Degenerative: older than 60 years	Trauma: younger than 18 to 35 years	Any: if younger adolescent rule out avulsion fractures	No correlation with age	Not applicable
Occupation		No correlation to occupation	Laborers and sports involvement	Laborers and sports involvement	Laborers and sports involvement	No correlation to occupation	Trauma, sports	Trauma, sports, knee dislocations	Not applicable
Gender	Both	Both		Both	Both	Both	Both	Both	Not applicable
Ethnicity	No correlation noted	No correlation noted	No correlation noted	No correlation noted	No correlation noted	No correlation noted	No correlation noted	No correlation noted	Not applicable
History	Acute trauma or overuse	Acute trauma "Fracture" Overuse "Stress fracture"	Acute trauma "Fracture" Overuse (DJD)	Knee flexion, twisting, acceleration injuries	Knee flexion, twisting, virus, valgus	Overuse adaptive lengthening; trauma—dislocation	Sensation of "pop" Large, quick effusion	Overuse repetitive; trauma; postsurgical	Not applicable
Mechanism of injury	Traction, Overuse, Tension, Trauma	Trauma, Repetitive overuse (stress fix)	Valgus or valgus with rotation (isolated lesion) versus repetitive overuse (DJD)	Virus, valgus, weight bearing with rotation	Valgus or valgus with rotation Repetitive overuse (DJD)	Tension at end of range of motion Dislocation	Virus, valgus, contact, noncontact, rotation, deceleration	Trauma, dislocation, postsurgical	Not applicable
Type of onset	Acute or chronic	Acute or chronic	Trauma: acute Degenerative: chronic	Acute or chronic	Acute or chronic	Acute or chronic	Acute or chronic	Acute or chronic	Not applicable
Referral from local tissue	May be referred proximal or distal	Generally localized	Generally localized	May have joint capsule irritation	Not applicable	Not applicable	Generally localized	Nerves in knee may refer pain either proximally or distally	Not applicable
Referral to other regions	May be referred proximal or distal	Generally localized	Generally localized to knee	Not applicable	Not applicable	Not applicable	Not applicable	Typically in a distal direction	Not applicable
Changes in symptoms	Increased with active motion	Increased with movement or stress	Usually increased symptoms with weight bearing and shearing activities	Activity dependent	Increased with twisting, stairs, squatting	Usually increased pain with end range of motion stress	Usually increased pain with end range of motion stress	Varies; motion dependent	Not applicable

24-hour pain pattern (morning)	Activity dependent	Constant, yet intermittent intensity with loading	Constant, yet intermittent intensity with loading	Activity dependent	Activity dependent	Activity dependent	Activity dependent	Morning stiffness typically indicative of OA	Not applicable
24-hour pain pattern (afternoon)	Activity dependent	Constant, yet intermittent intensity with loading	Constant, yet intermittent intensity with loading	Activity dependent	Activity dependent	Activity dependent	Activity dependent	Pain and stiffness worsening as the day progresses; sign of inflammatory response	Not applicable
24-hour pain pattern (evening)	Activity dependent	Constant, yet intermittent intensity with loading	Constant, yet intermittent intensity with loading	Activity dependent	Activity dependent	Activity dependent	Activity dependent	Positional dependent	Not applicable
Description of symptoms	Sharp pain, acute tear, aching chronic	Deep, intense pain, pain with weight bearing	Sharp, aching, grinding, crepitus	Sharp, popping, grinding, crepitus	Deep, sharp, aching	Sharp pain when stressed, otherwise aching	Sharp when stressed, otherwise aching	Sharp shooting pain, numbness and tingling	Not applicable
Depth of symptoms	Superficial to deep	Deep in knee	Deep in knee	Typically deep, but may be superficial at coronary ligament attachments	Deep or superficial	Deep or superficial	Deep or superficial	Deep or superficial	Not applicable
Constancy of symptoms	Dependent on activity	Fractures may be constant	Acute, may be intermittent; DJD/OA constant	Intermittent with loading and twisting	Intermittent	Intermittent	Intermittent	Intermittent	Not applicable
Aggravating factors	Activity-related pain	Weight bearing, loading, twisting	Weight bearing or shearing stress to knee	Weight bearing or shearing stress to knee	Excessive translation, or immobilization	Excessive translation or immobilization	Excessive translation or immobilization	Repetitive use or direct trauma	Not applicable
Easing factors	Rest, NSAIDs, cold	Rest, NSAIDs, unloading	Rest, NSAIDs, therapeutic exercises	Rest, NSAIDs, unloading	Rest, NSAIDs, unloading, increasing, or limiting motion	Rest, NSAIDs, unloading, increasing or limiting motion	Rest, NSAIDs, unloading	Rest, NSAIDs, unloading	Not applicable
Stability of symptoms	Constant but worse with weight bearing or loading	Constant but can be intermittent in intensity	Constant, but can be intermittent in intensity	When stressed	Constant when mechanically stressed	Constant when mechanically stressed	Constant when mechanically stressed	Constant when mechanically stressed	Not applicable
Past medical history	Past prolonged use of steroids	History of cancer, systemic diseases, osteoporosis, osteopenia, hx of prolonged steroid use	Prior hx of injury, minor OA, past instability, RA	Prior hx of RA or other systemic or autoimmune disorders	Prior hx of prolonged steroid use or autoimmune disorders	Prior hx of prolonged steroid use	Prior hx of prolonged steroid use	History of lumbar or hip pathology	Not applicable

Continued on following page.

TABLE II-12-6 Body Structure and Tissue-Based Pathology (Nociceptive and Peripheral Neurogenic Pain Mechanisms) (*Continued*)

	Muscles and Tendons	Bone	Cartilage	Meniscus	Joint	Joint Capsule	Ligaments	Nerves	Visceral Tissue
Past surgeries	No correlation	No correlation	Hx of prior ligament or cartilage injury	No correlation	Hx of prior ligament or cartilage injury	No correlation	No correlation	No correlation	Not applicable
Special questions	Strength loss, hearing pop with injury, gross loss of motion at knee	Pain with weight bearing or loading Hear pop, crack	Crepitus, catching, locking, swelling	Crepitus, catching, locking, swelling	Hx of giving way, swelling, locking, catching, popping	Hx of giving way or instability	Hx of giving way and instability	Hx of sharp shooting, lancinating pain, numbness, and or tingling	Not applicable
X-rays	Negative for soft tissue pathology	Positive for fractures	Demonstrate joint space narrowing, osteophyte formation, or sclerosis	Negative unless just general joint space loss	Negative	Negative unless still dislocated	Negative unless still dislocated	Negative	Normal
MRI	Demonstrates soft tissue quality very well	Negative for bony pathology	Demonstrates positive findings	Demonstrates soft tissue quality very well	Demonstrates soft tissue quality very well	Demonstrates soft tissue quality very well	Demonstrates soft tissue quality very well	Demonstrates soft tissue quality very well	Normal
EMG	Altered response	Normal	Normal	Normal	Normal	Normal	Normal	Altered response	Normal
Special laboratory tests	Not applicable	Not applicable	Not applicable	Not applicable	Not applicable	Not applicable	Not applicable	Not applicable	Not applicable
Red flags	Inability to bear weight	Inability to bear weight Acute swelling Night pain	Inability to bear weight Acute swelling Night pain	Inability to bear weight Acute swelling Night pain	Inability to bear weight Acute swelling Night pain	Inability to bear weight Acute swelling Night pain	Inability to bear weight Acute swelling Night pain	Numbness and tingling, no active movement available, flaccid limb	Acute swelling Night pain

ITB, iliotibial band; ACL, anterior cruciate ligament; PCL, posterior cruciate ligament; LCL, lateral collateral ligament; MCL, medial collateral ligament; DJD, degenerative joint disease; OA, osteoarthritis; NSAIDs, nonsteroidal anti-inflammatory drugs; hx, history; RA, rheumatoid arthritis; MRI, magnetic resonance imaging; EMG, electromyogram.

3. Injuries more than 7 days old, recent injuries being reevaluated
4. Patients with altered levels of consciousness
5. Paraplegia or multiple injuries

These rules were found to demonstrate near 100% sensitivity for knee fractures and reduced the need for radiographs by 28%.[33]

PITTSBURG KNEE DECISION RULES FOR RADIOGRAPHY

Indications for a radiograph:
1. The mechanism of injury is either blunt trauma or a fall.
2. The patient is younger than 12 years or older than 50 years of age.
3. The injury causes an inability to walk more than four weight-bearing steps in the emergency department.

Exclusion criteria:
1. Knee injuries sustained more than 6 days before presentation
2. Patients with only superficial lacerations and abrasions
3. History of previous surgeries or fractures on the affected knee
4. Patients being reassessed for the same injury

According to a study by Seaberg and colleagues[32] utilization of these rules yields 99% sensitivity and 60% specificity for knee fractures.

From these studies it appears that both the Ottawa and Pittsburgh knee CDRs are very useful in the diagnosis of knee fractures with little difference in sensitivity, although the Ottawa rules appear to be more specific.

SUMMARY STATEMENT

For a seemingly simplistic anatomical bicondylar joint, it requires great skill and practice to master the art of a detailed physical examination of the knee. It is best to use a specific examination format so that nothing is left to chance (Table II-12-5). The difficulty lies within the fact that numerous structures inside or outside of the knee can cause pain or symptoms (Table II-12-6).

REFERENCES

1. Argen N. Osteoarthritis: epidemiology. *Best Practice Res Clin Rheumatol.* 20(1):3-25.
2. Boissonnault WG, ed. *Primary Care for the Physical Therapist. Examination and Triage.* St. Louis: Elsevier Saunders; 2005.
3. Buckwalter JA. Articular cartilage injuries. *Clin Orthop.* 2002;21-37.
4. Cichanowski HR, et al. Hip strength in collegiate female athletes with patellofemoral pain. *Med Sci Sports Exerc.* 2007; 39:1227-1232.
5. Cleland J. *Orthopedic Clinical Examination: An Evidence-Based Approach for Physical Therapists.* Philadelphia, PA: Mosby; 2006.
6. De Loes M, Dahlstedt LJ, Thome R. A 7-year study on the risks and costs of knee injuries in male and female youth participant in 12 sports. *Scand J Med Science Sports.* 2000;10:90-97.
7. Englund M, Lohmander LS. Risk factors for symptomatic knee osteoarthritis fifteen to twenty-two years after meniscectomy. *Arthritis Rheum.* 2004;50:2811-2819.
8. Flynn RK, Pedersen CL, Birmingham TB, Kirkley A, Jackowski D, Fowler PF. The familial predisposition toward tearing the anterior cruciate ligament: A case control study. *Am J Sports Med.* 2005;33:23-28.
9. Fulkerson J, Hungerford D. *Disorders of the Patellofemoral Joint.* 2nd ed. Baltimore: Williams & Wilkins; 1990.
10. Hewett TE. An introduction to understanding and preventing ACL injury. *Understanding and Preventing Noncontact ACL Injuries.* In: Hewett TE, Shultz SJ, Griffin LY, eds. Champaign, IL: American Orthopaedic Society for Sports Medicine, Human Kinetics; 2007.
11. Holmberg S, Thelin A, Thelin N. Knee osteoarthritis and body mass index: A population-based case control study. *Scand J Rheumatol.* 2005;34:59-64.
12. Hoover NW. Injuries of the popliteal artery associated with fractures and dislocations. *Surg Clin North Am.* 1961;41:1099-1124.
13. Hughston JC, Andrews JR, Cross MJ, Moschi A. Classification of knee ligament instabilities. I. The medial compartment and cruciate ligaments. *J Bone Joint Surg.* 1976;58A:159-172.
14. Ireland ML, et al. Hip strength in females with and without patellofemoral pain. *J Orthop Sports Phys Ther.* 2003;33:671-676.
15. Jackson JL, O'Malley PG, Kroenke K. Evaluation of acute knee pain in primary care. *Ann Intern Med.* 2003;139:575-588.
16. Jacobson K, Falndry F. Diagnosis of anterior knee pain. *Clin Sports Med.* 1989;8:179-195.
17. Kennedy JC. Complete dislocation of the knee joint. *J Bone Joint Surg.* 1963;45A:889-904.
18. Laprade J, Lee R. Real-time measurement of patellofemoral kinematics in asymptomatic subjects. *Knee.* 2005;12:63-72.
19. Larsen R, Grana W. *The Knee: Form, Function, Pathology, and Treatment.* Philadelphia: WB Saunders Co; 1992.
20. Leetun DT, et al. Core stability measures as risk factors for LE injury in athletes. *Med Sci Sports Exerc.* 2004;36(6):926-934.
21. Lutter L. The knee and running. *Clin Sports Med.* 1985;4:685-698.
22. Magee D, ed. *Orthopedic Physical Assessment.* 5th ed. Philadelphia: Saunders; 2008.
23. Malanga GA, Nadler SF. *Musculoskeletal Physical Examination: An Evidence-Based Approach.* Philadelphia, PA: Elsevier Mosby; 2006.
24. Manske RC, Stovak M. Preoperative and postsurgical musculoskeletal examination of the knee. In: Manske RC, ed. *Postsurgical Orthopedic Sports Rehabilitation: Knee and Shoulder.* Elsevier, Mosby; 2006:31-54.
25. Manske RC, Vequist S. *Examination of the knee with special and functional testing.* Orthopedic Section of APTA Home Study Course Series. LaCrosse, WI: 2001.
26. Mascal CL, Landel R, Powers C. Management of patellofemoral pain targeting hip, pelvis, and trunk muscle function: 2 case reports. *J Orthop Sports Phys Ther.* 2003;33:642-660.
27. McKinnis LN. *Fundamentals of Musculoskeletal Imaging.* 2nd ed. Philadelphia: FA Davis; 2005.
28. Molnar T, Fox J. Overuse injuries of the knee in basketball. *Clin Sports Med.* 1993;12:349-362.
29. Orndorff DG, Hart JA, Miller MD. Physical examination of the knee. *Curr Sports Med Reports.* 2005;4:243-248.
30. Reinold MR, Berkson EM, Asnis P, Irrgang JJ, Safran MR, Fu FH. Knee: Ligamentous and Patellar Tendon Injuries. In: Magee DJ, Zachazewski JW, Quillen WS, eds. *Pathology and Intervention in Musculoskeletal Rehabilitation.* Philadelphia: Saunders; 2008.
31. Robinson RL, Nee RJ. Analysis of hip strength in females seeking physical therapy treatment of unilateral patellofemoral pain syndrome. *J Orthop Sports Phys Ther.* 2007;37:232-238.
32. Seaberg D, Yealy M, Lukens T, et al. Multicenter comparison of two clinical decision rules for the use of radiography in acute, high-risk knee injuries. *Ann Emerg Med.* 1998;32:8-13.
33. Stiell I, Greenberg G, McKnight R, et al. Prospective validation of a decision rule for the use of radiography in acute knee injuries. *JAMA.* 1996;275:611-615.
34. Tiberio D. The effect of subtalar joint pronation on patellofemoral mechanics. A theoretical model. *J Orthop Sports Phys Ther.* 1987;9:160-165.
35. Tyler TF, et al. The role of hip muscle function in the treatment of patellofemoral pain syndrome. *Am J Sports Med.* 2006;34:630-636.
36. Wells PS, Hirsch J, Anderson DR, et al. Accuracy of clinical assessment of deep-vein thrombosis. *Lancet.* 1995;345:1326-1330.

SPECIAL TESTS REFERENCES

Sag Test

1. Rubinstein RA, Shelbourne KD, McCarroll JR, Van Meter CD, Rettig AC. The accuracy of the clinical examination in the setting of posterior cruciate ligament injuries. *Am J Sports Med.* 1994;22:550-557.

Posterior Drawer Test

1. Clendenin MB, DeLee JC, Hechman JD. Interstitial tears of the posterior cruciate ligament of the knee. *Orthopedics.* 1980;3:764-772.
2. Harilainen A. Evaluation of knee instability in acute ligamentous injuries. *Ann Chir Gynaecol.* 1987;76:269-273.
3. Hughston JC, Andrews JR, Cross MJ, Moschi A. Classification of knee ligament instabilities II: the lateral compartment and cruciate ligaments. *J Bone Joint Surg Am.* 1976;58:173-179.
4. Hughston JC, Andrews JR, Cross MJ, Moschi A. Classification of knee ligament instabilities I: the medial compartment and cruciate ligaments. *J Bone Joint Surg Am.* 1976;58:159-172.

5. Loos WC, Fox JM, Blazina ME, Del Pizzo W, Friedman MJ. Acute posterior cruciate ligament injuries. *Am J Sports Med.* 1981;9:86-92.
6. Moore HA, Larson RL. Posterior cruciate ligament injuries: results of early surgical repair. *Am J Sports Med.* 1980;8:68-78.
7. Rubinstein RA, Shelbourne KD, McCarroll JR, Van Meter CD, Rettig AC. The accuracy of the clinical examination in the setting of posterior cruciate ligament injuries. *Am J Sports Med.* 1994;22:550-557.

Anterior Drawer Test

1. Boeree NR, Ackroyd CE. Assessment of the menisci and cruciate ligaments: an audit of clinical practice. *Injury.* 1991;22:291-294.
2. Braunstein EM. Anterior cruciate ligament injuries: a comparison of arthrographic and physical diagnosis. *Am J Roentgenol.* 1982;138:423-425.
3. DeHaven KE. Arthroscopy in the diagnosis and management of the anterior cruciate ligament deficient knee. *Clin Orthop.* 1983;172:52-56.
4. Donaldson WF, Warren RF, Wickiewicz TG. A comparison of acute anterior cruciate ligament examinations: initial versus examination under anesthesia. *Am J Sports Med.* 1985;13:5-10.
5. Hardaker WT, Garrett WE, Bassett FH. Evaluation of acute traumatic hemarthrosis of the knee joint. *South Med J.* 1990;83:640-644.
6. Jonsson T, Althoff B, Peterson L, Renstrom P. Clinical diagnosis of ruptures of the anterior drawer sign. *Am J Sports Med.* 1982;10:100-102.
7. Katz JW, Fingeroth RJ. The diagnostic accuracy of ruptures of the anterior cruciate ligament comparing the Lachman test, the anterior drawer sign, and the pivot shift test in acute and chronic knee injuries. *Am J Sports Med.* 1986;14:88-91.
8. Kim SJ, Kim HK. Reliability of the anterior drawer test, the pivot shift test and the Lachman test. *Clin Orthop.* 1995;317:237-242.
9. Lee JK, Yao L, Phelps CT, Wirth CR, Czajka J, Lozman J. Anterior cruciate ligament tears: MR imaging compared with arthroscopy and clinical tests. *Radiology.* 1988;166:861-864.
10. Liu SH, Osti L, Henry M, Bocchi L. The diagnosis of acute complete tears of the anterior cruciate ligament. *J Bone Joint Surg Br.* 1995;77:586-588.
11. Mitsou A, Vallianatos P. Clinical diagnosis of ruptures of the anterior cruciate ligament: a comparison between the Lachman test and the anterior drawer sign. *Injury.* 1988;19:427-428.
12. Rubinstein RA, Shelbourne KD, McCarroll JR, Van Meter CD, Rettig AC. The accuracy of the clinical examination in the setting of posterior cruciate ligament injuries. *Am J Sports Med.* 1994;22:550-557.
13. Sandberg R, Balkfors B, Henricson A, Westlin N. Stability tests in knee ligament injuries. *Arch Orthop Trauma Surg.* 1986;106:5-7.
14. Tonino AJ, Huy J, Schaafsma J. The diagnostic accuracy of knee testing in the acutely injured knee. Initial examination versus examination under anesthesia with arthroscopy. *Acta Orthop Belg.* 1986;52:479-487.

Lachman's

1. Boeree NR, Ackroyd CE. Assessment of the menisci and cruciate ligaments: an audit of clinical practice. *Injury.* 1991;22:291-294.
2. Cooperman JM, Riddle DL, Rothstein J. Reliability and validity of judgments of the integrity of the anterior cruciate ligament of the knee using the Lachman test. *Phys Ther.* 1990;70:225-233.
3. Donaldson WF, Warren RF, Wickiewicz TG. A comparison of acute anterior cruciate ligament examinations: initial versus examination under anesthesia. *Am J Sports Med.* 1985;13:5-10.
4. Gurtler RA, Stine R, Torg JS. Lachman test evaluated. Quantification of a clinical observation. *Clin Orthop Relat Res.* 1987;216:141-150.
5. Hardaker WT, Garrett WE, Bassett FH. Evaluation of acute traumatic hemarthrosis of the knee joint. *South Med J.* 1990;83:640-644.
6. Jonsson T, Althoff B, Peterson L, Renstrom P. Clinical diagnosis of ruptures of the anterior drawer sign. *Am J Sports Med.* 1982;10:100-102.
7. Katz JW, Fingeroth RJ. The diagnostic accuracy of ruptures of the anterior cruciate ligament comparing the Lachman test, the anterior drawer sign, and the pivot shift test in acute and chronic knee injuries. *Am J Sports Med.* 1986;14:88-91.
8. Kim SJ, Kim HK. Reliability of the anterior drawer test, the pivot shift test and the Lachman test. *Clin Orthop.* 1995;317:237-242.
9. Lee JK, Yao L, Phelps CT, Wirth CR, Czajka J, Lozman J. Anterior cruciate ligament tears: MR imaging compared with arthroscopy and clinical tests. *Radiology.* 1988;166:861-864.

10. Liu SH, Osti L, Henry M, Bocchi L. The diagnosis of acute complete tears of the anterior cruciate ligament. *J Bone Joint Surg Br.* 1995;77:586-588.
11. Mitsou A, Vallianatos P. Clinical diagnosis of ruptures of the anterior cruciate ligament: a comparison between the Lachman test and the anterior drawer sign. *Injury.* 1988;19:427-428.
12. Rubinstein RA Jr, Shelbourne KD, McCarroll JR, Van Meter CD, Rettig AC. The accuracy of the clinical examination in the setting of posterior cruciate ligament injuries. *Am J Sports Med.* 1994;22:550-557.
13. Torg JS, Conrad W, Kalen V. Clinical diagnosis of anterior cruciate ligament instability in the athlete. *Am J Sports Med.* 1976;4:84-93.
14. Tonino AJ, Huy J, Schaafsma J. The diagnostic accuracy of knee testing in the acutely injured knee. Initial examination versus examination under anesthesia with arthroscopy. *Acta Orthop Belg.* 1986;52:479-487.

Pivot Shift

1. Boeree NR, Ackroyd CE. Assessment of the menisci and cruciate ligaments: an audit of clinical practice. *Injury.* 1991;22:291-294.
2. Dahlstedt LJ, Dalen N. Knee laxity in cruciate ligament injury. Value of examination under anesthesia. *Acta Orthop Scand.* 1989;60:181-184.
3. DeHaven KE. Arthroscopy in the diagnosis and management of the anterior cruciate ligament deficient knee. *Clin Orthop.* 1983;172:52-56.
4. Donaldson WF, Warren RF, Wickiewicz TG. A comparison of acute anterior cruciate ligament examinations: initial versus examination under anesthesia. *Am J Sports Med.* 1985;13:5-10.
5. Hardaker WT, Garrett WE, Bassett FH. Evaluation of acute traumatic hemarthrosis of the knee joint. *South Med J.* 1990;83:640-644.
6. Katz JW, Fingeroth RJ. The diagnostic accuracy of ruptures of the anterior cruciate ligament comparing the Lachman test, the anterior drawer sign, and the pivot shift test in acute and chronic knee injuries. *Am J Sports Med.* 1986;14:88-91.
7. Kim SJ, Kim HK. Reliability of the anterior drawer test, the pivot shift test and the Lachman test. *Clin Orthop.* 1995;317:237-242.
8. Liu SH, Osti L, Henry M, Bocchi L. The diagnosis of acute complete tears of the anterior cruciate ligament. *J Bone Joint Surg Br.* 1995;77:586-588.
9. Lucie RS, Wiedel JD, Messner DG. The acute pivot shift: clinical correlation. *Am J Sports Med.* 1984;12:189-191.
10. Rubinstein Jr RA, Shelbourne KD, McCarroll JR, Van Meter CD, Rettig AC. The accuracy of the clinical examination in the setting of posterior cruciate ligament injuries. *Am J Sports Med.* 1994;22:550-557.
11. Tonino AJ, Huy J, Schaafsma J. The diagnostic accuracy of knee testing in the acutely injured knee. Initial examination versus examination under anesthesia with arthroscopy. *Acta Orthop Belg.* 1986;52:479-487.

Valgus Stress Test

1. Garvin GJ, Munk P, Vellet A. Tears of the medial collateral ligament: magnetic resonance imaging findings and associated injuries. *Can Assoc Radiol J.* 1993;44:199-204.
2. Harilainen A. Evaluation of knee instability in acute ligamentous injuries. *Ann Chir Gynaecol.* 1987;76:269-273.
3. Harilainen A. Evaluation of knee instability in acute ligamentous injuries. *Ann Chir Gynaecol.* 1987;76:269-273.

McMurry's

1. Anderson AF, Lipscomb AB. Clinical diagnosis of meniscal tears: description of a new manipulative test. *Am J Sports Med.* 1986;14:291-293.
2. Akeseki D, Ozcan O, Boya H, Pinar H. A new weight-bearing meniscal test and a comparison with McMurray's test and joint line tenderness. *Arthroscopy.* 2004;20:951-958.
3. Boeree NR, Ackroyd CE. Assessment of the menisci and cruciate ligaments: an audit of clinical practice. *Injury.* 1991;22:291-294.
4. Evans PJ, Bell GD, Frank C. Prospective evaluation of the McMurray test. *Am J Sports Med.* 1993;21:604-608.
5. Fowler PJ, Lubliner JA. The predictive value of 5 clinical signs in the evaluation of meniscal pathology. *Arthroscopy.* 1989;5:184-186.
6. Karahalios T Hanes M, Zibis AH, Zachos V, Karantanas AH, Malizos KN. Diagnostic accuracy of a new clinical test (the Thessaly test) for early detection of meniscal tears. *J Bone Joint Surg.* 2005;87:955-962.
7. Kurosaka M, Yagi M, Yoshiya S, Muratsu H, Mizuno K. Efficacy of the axially loaded pivot shift test for the diagnosis of a meniscal tear. *Int Orthop.* 1999;23:271-274.

8. Noble J, Erat K. In defense of the meniscus: a prospective study of 200 meniscectomy patients. *J Bone Joint Surg.* 1980;62:7-11.
9. Saengnipanthkul S, Sirichativapee W, Kowsuwon W, Rojviroj S. The effects of medial patellar plica on clinical diagnosis of medial meniscal lesion. *J Med Assoc Thai.* 1992;75:704-708.

Joint Line Tenderness
1. Boeree NR, Ackroyd CE. Assessment of the menisci and cruciate ligaments: an audit of clinical practice. *Injury.* 1991;22:291-294.
2. Eren OT. The accuracy of joint line tenderness by physical examination in diagnosis of meniscal tears. *Arthroscopy.* 2003;19:850-854.
3. Fowler PJ, Lubliner JA. The predictive value of 5 clinical signs in the evaluation of meniscal pathology. *Arthroscopy.* 1989;5:184-186.

4. Shelbourne KD, Martini DJ, McCarroll JR, VanMeter DC. Correlation of joint line tenderness and meniscal lesions in patients with acute anterior cruciate ligament tears. *Am J Sports Med.* 1995;23:166-169.

Apley's Compression
1. Fowler PJ, Lubliner JA. The predictive value of 5 clinical signs in the evaluation of meniscal pathology. *Arthroscopy.* 1989;5:184-186.
2. Kurosaka M, Yagi M, Yoshiya S, Muratsu H, Mizuno K. Efficacy of the axially loaded pivot shift test for the diagnosis of a meniscal tear. *Int Orthop.* 1999;23:271-274.

Section II

ORTHOPEDIC REASONING

AUTHORS: ROB ROY MARTIN, CHRISTOPHER R. CARCIA, RONALD BELCZYK, and DANE K. WUKICH

INTRODUCTORY INFORMATION

The foot and the ankle are the body's first connection to the ground. Therefore, pathology or abnormal mechanics can often lead to compensations in joints and structures up the kinetic chain. Ankle and foot dysfunction can result in problems as far away as the neck and the shoulder. Couple this with the relative complexity of the region and the clinician is faced daunting challenge. The body region demands dynamic stability and mobility. When it is not functioning correctly, pathology often results.

WHAT IS THE PREVALENCE OF FOOT AND ANKLE PAIN?

The prevalence of foot and ankle pain will vary greatly depending on age, activity level, and body type. Studies have found that approximately 20% to 25% of individuals have foot and ankle-related complaints,[17,18,20] with ankle injuries being the most common of all athletic injuries.[6,17] Foot pain was found to be associated with increased age, female sex, obesity, and pain in other body regions.[20]

Common causes of foot and ankle pain in younger active individuals are ankle sprains, plantar fasciitis, and Achilles tendinopathy. Ankle sprains were found to occur at a rate of one injury per 10,000 people per day. Approximately 10% of all emergency room visits are due to ankle injuries, with 90% being lateral ankle sprains.[31] Basketball, football, soccer, and volleyball are the sports in which ankle sprains most commonly occur.[49] Plantar fasciitis is another common cause of foot pain affecting approximately 2 million Americans each year and as much as 10% of the population.[41] It accounts for 8% to 15% of all adult foot complaints requiring professional care.[50] Achilles tendinopathy is most prevalent among runners, with an annual incidence reported between 7% and 9%.[22,27]

WHAT IS THE PROGNOSIS FOR RECOVERY FROM FOOT AND ANKLE PAIN?

The prognosis for recovery from foot and ankle pain will depend on severity of injury, age, general health, comorbidity, previous injury, and biomechanical factors. Additionally, the activity level that individuals need to regain will affect the prognosis.

Although recovery from ankle sprains, plantar faciitis, and Achilles tendinopathy is generally good, symptoms can persist. Concurrent injuries such as syndesmotic disruption, articular cartilage lesion, and/or peroneal tendon damage can negatively affect the prognosis after a lateral ankle sprain. It is not uncommon for patients who sustained a sports-related inversion ankle injury to have persistent symptoms for 2 years or more after their injury.[4] Full recovery was reported by 36% to 85% of individuals within a 3-year period.[53] With respect to plantar fasciitis, 80% of individuals who seek treatment have resolution of symptoms within a 12-month period.[29,57] Similar results are observed following intervention for Achilles tendinopathy. Long-term follow-up ranging between 2 and 8 years suggests that between 71% and 100% of patients with Achilles tendinopathy are able to return to their prior level of activity with minimal or no complaints.[1,37,38]

WHAT IS THE RECURRENCE RATE?

After a lateral ankle sprain up to 34% of individuals suffer chronic ankle instability.[23,53] These individuals, described as either having mechanical or functional instability, can have permanent limitations. Generally, however, the recurrence rate of foot and ankle injuries has not been established.

WHAT FACTORS MAKE DIAGNOSIS IN THE FOOT AND ANKLE DIFFICULT?

The interrelation and close proximity of potential sources of pathology in the foot and ankle may make diagnosis difficult. Reproduction of a patient's symptoms is the key to making a correct diagnosis.[58] Chronic conditions can be difficult to diagnose as the symptoms in these individuals are often diffuse and not well localized.

CLINICAL PEARL

There are usually numerous factors that contribute to chronic pain symptoms and thus tracing the source of pain to one specific structure may not be possible. When the onset of symptoms is insidious inflammatory processes, immune reactions, endocrine factors, and posttraumatic arthrosis should be considered. Patients with inflammatory arthropathy typically have symptoms in adjacent joints, including metatarsal phalangeal joints and the subtalar joint. Also symptoms may not be isolated to the foot and ankle.

HOW SUCCESSFUL IS NONOPERATIVE THERAPY IN TREATING FOOT AND ANKLE PAIN?

Nonsurgical treatment of common disorders, such as plantar fasciitis, lateral ankle sprain, and Achilles tendinitis, has been defined. Conservative treatment of plantar fasciitis has a reported success rate of 85% to 95%, but may require 6 to 12 months to resolve.[29,57] Recommended interventions included iontophoresis with dexamethasone or acetic acid, calf and plantar fascia stretching, calcaneal or low-dye taping, and orthotics for short-term improvements.[33] When comparing custom and prefabricated orthoses, there appears to be no difference in pain reduction or functional improvement. Night splints should be considered as an intervention for patients with symptoms greater than 6 months in duration. The recommended length of time for wearing the night splint is 1 to 3 months.[33]

Individuals with first-time grade I and II ankle ligament sprains may best return to preinjury status when treated with an Air-Stirrup brace combined with an elastic wrap.[7] Functional intervention is favorable to immobilization when treating acute ankle sprains.[25] Also there is evidence to support the benefit of a supervised exercise program over home program for the treatment of acute lateral ankle sprains.[52]

For Achilles tendinopathy, significant decreases in pain and improvement in function have been reported following 6 to 12 weeks of an intervention program that focused on eccentric exercise.[2,42] Recent evidence suggests the addition of low-level laser therapy to an eccentric program further accelerates the recovery process[8,47]

HOW SUCCESSFUL IS SURGERY IN TREATING FOOT AND ANKLE PAIN?

Success rates following surgery vary depending on the treating condition and selected procedure. For instance an arthrodesis of ankle, which is considered the gold standard for posttraumatic arthritis, can achieve 80% to 85% successful outcomes.[30] As a guideline, 85% of patients are satisfied, 10% satisfied with reservations, and 5% not improved or dissatisfied with their surgical outcome.

PERSONAL INFORMATION

WHAT INFLUENCE DOES AGE HAVE ON YOUR CLINICAL DECISION-MAKING PROCESS?

Young individuals who are active in sports are more likely to have overuse type injuries including stress fractures and tendinitis.

Older individuals are more likely to have tendinosis and arthritic conditions.

The adolescent patient can have an injury pattern different from those who have achieved skeletal maturity. When growth plates are not yet closed they are susceptible to injury.[35] Common foot and ankle pathology to consider in patients who have unfused growth plates includes osteochondrosis, accessory ossicles, tarsal coalition, apophysitis, and epiphyseal fractures.[28] Osteochondrosis is epiphyseal ischemic necrosis followed by regeneration or recalcification. This can occur at several locations in the foot and ankle region (Table II-13-1). An accessory ossicle (accessory bone) is an ossification center that has not fused. This occurs in 10% of the population. Common locations include the lateral malleolus, medial malleolus, navicular, and talus.[24] A tarsal coalition is a congenital union between two tarsal bones, most commonly at the calcaneonavicular or talocalcaneal joints. Epiphyseal fractures are fractures that involve the growth plate.[28]

The elderly present with pathologies distinctly different from those previously mentioned. The five most common conditions for the elderly are toenail disorders (74.9%), lesser toe deformities (60%), corns and calluses (58.2%), bunions (37.1%), and signs of fungal infection, cracks and fissures, or macerations between toes (36.3%).[11]

WHAT INFLUENCE DOES A PATIENT'S OCCUPATION HAVE ON YOUR CLINICAL DECISION-MAKING PROCESS?

Occupations that involve a considerable amount of weight-bearing activity may put patients at risk for overuse injuries. Heavy labor jobs may also put a patient at risk for traumatic injuries such as fractures and sprains. A patient's job description can be important in guiding treatment to focus on specific job-related activities.

WHAT INFLUENCE DOES GENDER HAVE ON YOUR CLINICAL DECISION-MAKING PROCESS?

Foot and ankle pathology related to gender may be most closely associated with shoe wear issues. Females have a tendency to wear ill-fitting shoes with a narrow toe-box. A narrow toe-box may lead to Morton's neuroma, bunion, bunionette, corns, and calluses. Also females have a tendency to choose shoes with a low heel counter. This type of shoe design may rub the posterior aspect of the heel and may lead to posterior heel pathologies. Males have a higher incidence of Achilles ruptures, particularly middle-aged males who engage in jumping activities.

WHAT INFLUENCE DOES ETHNICITY HAVE ON YOUR CLINICAL DECISION-MAKING PROCESS?

There is little information regarding ethnicity and its relation to foot and ankle pathology. African-Americans may have a higher incident of Achilles ruptures.

DOES BODY WEIGHT AFFECT YOUR DECISION-MAKING PROCESS?

The effect of being overweight or obese can increase the likelihood of many foot and ankle conditions, including tendinopathy, plantar fasciitis, and arthritis.[14]

CLINICAL PEARL

If conservative treatment is to be successful weight loss for individuals who are overweight can be an important component of treatment. For each pound of weight loss there is a fourfold reduction in the load exerted per step during daily activities.[34] Therefore to decrease stress on the foot and ankle, even the loss of a few pounds could potentially be clinically meaningful.

SYMPTOM HISTORY

Symptom location can provide valuable information. However, for individuals with chronic conditions the location of symptoms may provide less information compared to those with more acute or subacute conditions. Generally those with chronic conditions can complain of general pain and have difficulty isolating a specific source of pain.

CLINICAL PEARL

Palpation can provide valuable information in identifying the source of symptoms. Metatarsalgia and metatarsal stress fracture can be distinguished by identifying the most painful area as either the metatarsal head or the shaft, respectively. Palpation can also help to identify sinus tarsi syndrome over lateral ankle impingement. Frequently, symptoms of chronic problems present with diffuse pain. Having the patient point to the most painful spot can help identify the origin of symptoms.

MECHANISM OF INJURY

WHAT INFLUENCE DOES THE MECHANISM OF INJURY HAVE ON YOUR CLINICAL DECISION-MAKING PROCESS?

TRAUMATIC INJURIES: The direction of force in a traumatic injury provides useful diagnostic information. Injuries that involve inversion with the foot in a plantar flexed position usually involve the anterior talofibular ligament (ATFL). Injury to the ATFL accounts for 85% of all ankle sprains.[13] More severe ankle inversion sprains can involve the calcaneal fibular ligament (CFL) as well as the ATFL. Additionally, inversion injuries with the foot in neutral dorsiflexion can cause isolated injury to the CFL. External rotation or forced dorsiflexion of the ankle can involve syndesmotic or distal tibia-fibula injuries (i.e., high ankle sprains). An Achilles rupture should be suspected when the injuries involve landing from a jump. Traumatic injures that involve the forefoot should suggestz a Lisfranc facture (tarsometatarsal sprain) in the differential diagnosis.

Although the ATFL is the most common ligament injured in ankle sprains, the practitioner should maintain a working differential diagnosis and carefully examine the foot and ankle for other less common injuries. The differential diagnosis of an ankle sprain in the acute setting should include a number of potential pathologies as outlined in Box II-13-1. It should be noted that multiple pathologies can occur currently, especially in injuries that involve high force.

TABLE II-13-1	**Common Locations of Osteochondrosis in Children**		
Pathology	Location	Age of Presentation	Gender
Freiberg's infarction	Metatarsal head (second metatarsal most common)	10 to 18 years, but also can occur as adult	F > M
Köhler's disease	Navicular	3 to 6 years	M > F
Sever's disease	Calcaneus	6 to 12 years	Both

BOX II-13-1 **Differential Diagnosis of Traumatic Injury**

Syndesmosis disruption
Ankle dislocation
Malleolar fracture
Lateral talar process fracture
Talar neck fracture
Anterior calcaneal process fracture
Osteochondral lesion of the talar dome
Lateral collateral ankle ligament injury
Medial collateral ankle ligament injury
Subtalar joint dislocation/pathology
Sinus tarsus injury
Peroneal tendon pathology
Achilles pathology
Extensor digitorum brevis strain
Cuboid fracture
Lisfranc fracture
Fifth metatarsal fracture (Jones fracture)

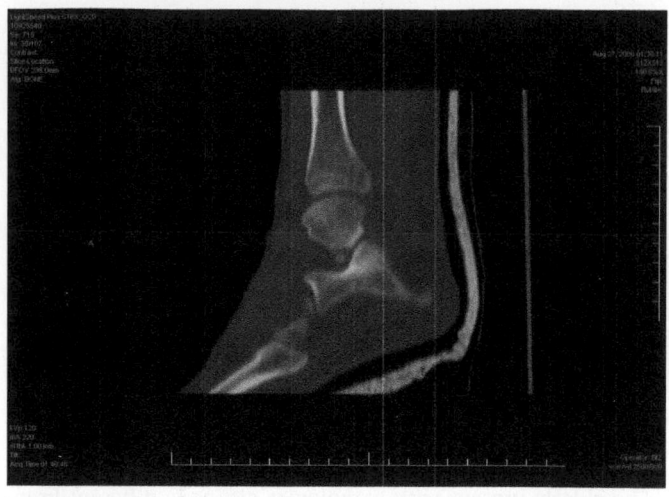

FIGURE II-13-2   Lateral view of foot with talar fracture.

CLINICAL DECISION MAKING CASE STUDY—PATIENT PROFILE **?**

A 21-year-old female injured her foot while playing rugby. She reported twisting her ankle and is having lateral ankle and foot pain. Point tenderness was noted over the sinus tarsi and pain is elicited with passive inversion of the subtalar joint. What do you think is the source of this patient's pain?

Answer
Radiographs (Figure II-13-1) and computed tomography (CT) (Figure II-13-2) demonstrated a fracture of the lateral talar process.

SYMPTOM LOCATION

WHAT INFLUENCE DOES THE LOCATION OF SYMPTOMS HAVE ON YOUR CLINICAL DECISION-MAKING PROCESS?

Differential diagnoses for plantar heel, posterior heel, and forefoot are listed in Box II-13-2. Although plantar fasciitis is the

---

BOX II-13-2 **Differential Diagnoses Based on Region**

Differential Diagnoses for Posterior Heel Pain	Differential Diagnoses for Plantar Heel Pain	Differential Diagnoses for Forefoot Pain
Haglund's deformity	Plantar fasciitis	Neuroma
Retrocalcaneal bursitis	Calcaneal stress fracture	Stress fractures
Achilles tendinosis or rupture	Fat pad atrophy	Metatarsalgia
Posterior impingement syndrome	Tarsal tunnel syndrome	Hallux rigidus
Systemic arthritides	Baxter's neuritis	Hallux valgus
		Turf toe
		Sesamoiditis
		Digital deformities
		Plantar plate rupture
		Tarsal coalition

---

most common etiology of heel pain, other sources of heel pain should also be considered in the differential diagnosis. Nerve entrapment, specifically the first branch of the lateral plantar nerve, can be a source of plantar heel pain. This is known as Baxter's neuritis or neuritis of the nerve to the abductor digiti minimi. This nerve can get impinged at the fascia of the abductor hallucis, which is frequently misdiagnosed as plantar fasciitis.

CLINICAL DECISION MAKING CASE STUDY—PATIENT PROFILE **?**

An 18-year-old female presents with persistent pain of the left ankle of 11 months duration. She states that the pain developed while she was participating in recreational dance. She denies any history of direct trauma to the area. Pain in the posterior ankle was elicited with both active and passive plantar flexion. Severe pain was present on palpation between the Achilles tendon and the peroneal tendons posterolateral to the subtalar joint. What is the likely diagnosis of this patient's persistent ankle pain?

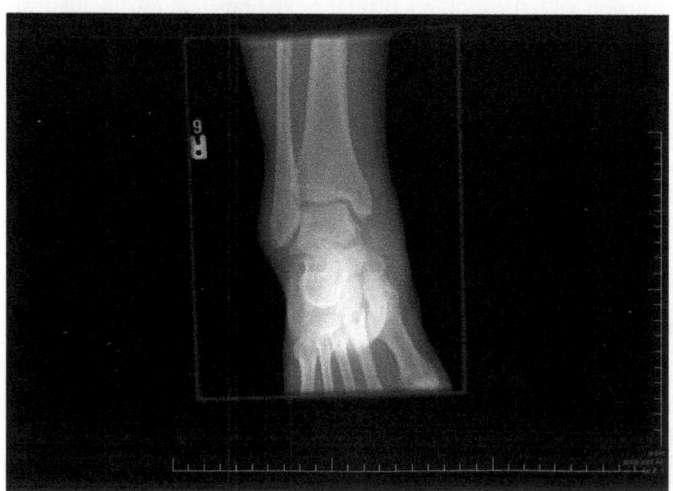

FIGURE II-13-1   AP view of foot with talar fracture.

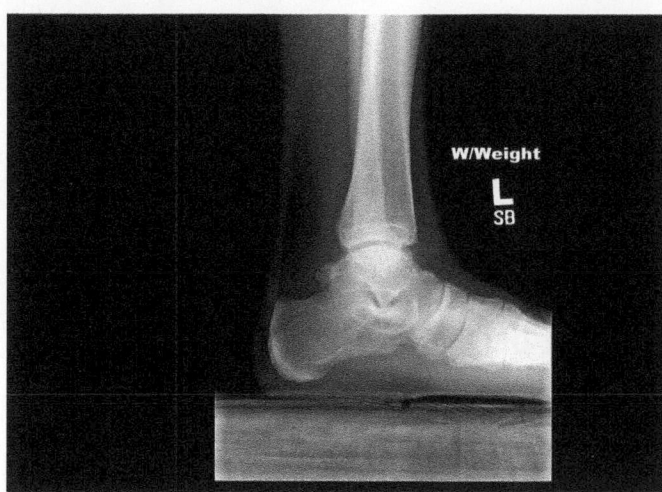

FIGURE II-13-3 Lateral view of foot with well-rounded accessory bone on posterolateral talus.

<table>
<tr><td colspan="2">BOX II-13-3   **Symptom Descriptors of Foot and Ankle Pathology**</td></tr>
</table>

Patient complaint	Pathology
Sharp stabbing pains associated with weight-bearing activities	Cartilage lesions (i.e., talar dome lesions)
Instability	Ligament injury
Dull aching in bone	Stress fracture
Anterior pinching pain with end range dorsiflexion	Anterior impingement
Posterior pinching associated with end range planter flexion	Posterior impingement
Lateral snapping	Subluxing peroneal tendons
Complaint of a painful lump in the forefoot	Forefoot neuroma
A "pop" in the calf when landing from a jump	Achilles rupture
Progressive loss of arch height	Posterior tibial tendon dysfunction

Answer

Radiographs (Figure II-13-3) reveal a well-rounded accessory bone on the posterolateral talus (os trigonum) causing a posterior impingement syndrome.

REFERRAL OF SYMPTOMS

Symptoms can be referred from the lumbar spine with involvement of L4 to S1 nerve roots. Most commonly, pathology at L5 to S1 can mimic plantar heel pathologies. A peripheral nerve entrapment of the sciatic nerve, or one of its branches, could also cause symptoms to radiate in the foot and ankle.

SYMPTOM DESCRIPTORS

QUALITY OF SYMPTOMS

Burning pain and numbness are usually from nerve pathology. Common sources of nerve irritation include the tibial nerve being compressed by the flexor retinaculum around the medial malleolus. This is referred to as tarsal tunnel syndrome and can cause pain in the plantar aspect of the heel. A forefoot neuroma is compression neuropathy of the plantar digital nerve and commonly occurs at the third digital nerve. When this nerve is involved patients complain of burning or tingling in the third and fourth webspace. Numbness can also be associated with compartment syndrome. However, this numbness is in the pattern of the involved peripheral nerve and is associated with a sensation of tightness in the posterior, anterior, and/or lateral leg. These symptoms of numbness and tightness are also activity related and typically occur as the individual exercises. Diabetes can cause symptoms of burning pain and numbness associated with neuropathy. The decreased sensation that can result presents in a "stocking" distribution. Symptoms related to neuropathy generally occur in an older population with a history of diabetes and do not change relative to activity.

Other symptoms that are useful in the diagnostic process are shown in Box II-13-3.

WHAT INFLUENCE DOES THE DEPTH OF SYMPTOMS HAVE ON YOUR CLINICAL DECISION-MAKING PROCESS?

Deep ankle symptoms are usually from ankle cartilage injuries, including arthritis. The three major categories of arthritis are inflammatory, osteo-, and posttraumatic arthritis, with posttraumatic arthritis being most common.[30] Although rheumatoid arthritis is the most common form of inflammatory arthritis, it affects the ankle only 10% to 50% of the time.[21,30] Posttraumatic arthritis and osteoarthritis accounted for 12% and 70% of ankle arthritis cases, respectively.[43] Deep posterior calf pain can be associated with deep vein thrombosis (DVT) and is usually associated with swelling, warmth, and redness in the calf. Another sign of a DVT is increased pain in passive dorsiflexion (Homan's sign).

WHAT INFLUENCE DOES A PATIENT'S DAILY PAIN PATTERN HAVE ON YOUR DECISION-MAKING PROCESS?

When pain is worse at night a nonmusculoskeletal cause, such as neoplasm, should be considered, particularly if symptoms are difficult to reproduce. When symptoms of a red, warm, swollen, and painful joint occur related to eating certain foods, gout should be considered. Although gout can occur in any joint it commonly occurs at the first metatarsal phalangeal joint. Gout is associated with an abnormal metabolism of uric acid and can occur after consuming red meats, yeast, oily fish, and alcoholic beverages.

STABILITY OF SYMPTOMS

HOW DOES THE PROGRESSION OF A PATIENT'S SYMPTOMS IMPACT YOUR CLINICAL DECISION-MAKING PROCESS?

As conditions become chronic the symptoms progress from being intermittent to constant. When the patient's history suggests a chronic condition, with associated constant pain, the overall prognosis for full recovery is poorer.

Plantar fasciitis is thought to be caused by irritation of the proximal plantar fascia near the insertion of the calcaneal tuberosity. Therefore patients complain of "start-up pain" as pain occurs with the first steps in the morning or after sitting for a lengthy period of time as the healing tissue is stretched. It is thought that with prolonged rest the plantar fascia tightens up. A sudden stretch with standing causes pain and possibly microtears in the plantar fascia. Baxter's neuritis causes heel pain that is generally present after activity compared to pain after the first steps as with plantar fasciitis.

FUNCTIONAL AND ACTIVITY PARTICIPATION LIMITATIONS

WHAT INFLUENCE DO AGGRAVATING AND EASING FUNCTIONS HAVE ON YOUR CLINICAL DECISION-MAKING PROCESS?

As with all musculoskeletal overuse conditions, the symptoms should be reproducible. Muscle and tendon conditions should be aggravated when stress is applied by activities or movements that cause the muscle–tendon unit to stretch or contract. Peroneal tendinopathy and flexor hallucis longus tendinopathy would be painful with resisted eversion and great toe flexion, respectively.

Specific behavior of symptoms can help lead to the diagnosis.

Pain in the posterior heel when coming up on the toes with contraction can indicate Achilles tendon pathology (tendinitis/tendinosis). When active movements do not aggravate the symptoms, retrocalcaneal bursitis should be considered.

An inability to rise up on the toes suggests Achilles rupture, posterior tendon dysfunction, or degenerative tear.

Stress fractures and tendon conditions commonly occur in athletes participating in sports that require jumping, long distance marching, and running. Patients with stress fractures complain of pain that is better at rest and worse with prolonged weight bearing. This pain can at first be intermittent but can progress to being constant as the condition becomes chronic.

Neuroma pain is worse at the end of the day and is aggravated by poorly fitting shoe wear such as pointed shoes or high heeled shoes or by activities that hyperextend the metatarsal phalangeal joints such as walking, running, or squatting.

Turf toe and hallux rigidus cause pain and stiffness of the first metatarsal phalangeal joint and are also aggravated by activities that hyperextend the metatarsal phalangeal joint. Turf toe generally occurs after a traumatic hyperextension injury in a young active population. Hallux rigidus is more insidious and occurs in an older population (Table II-13-2).

CLINICAL DECISION MAKING CASE STUDY—PATIENT PROFILE (?)

A 20-year-old male presents with pain in the shin area related to overtraining for a marathon. How do you differentially diagnose the potential sources of pain?

Answer

Posterior tibialis periostitis (posterior shin splints) should be associated with tenderness at the origin of the posterior tibialis. Tenderness at the origin of the anterior tibialis would most likely be anterior tibialis periostitis (anterior shin splints). Tenderness directly on the tibia would likely be a tibial stress fracture. If tightness and numbness were associated with activity, compartment syndrome should be suspected.

TABLE II-13-2 **Functional or Activity Participation Limitations**

Motion	Functional Activities	Pathology if Symptoms Are Aggravated by Activity	Pathology If Symptoms Are Eased by Activity
Dorsiflexion	Walking—mid to terminal stance Squatting Descending stairs	Posterior tendon pathology—if passive stretch Posterior muscle pathology—if passive Posterior tibialis pathology Tibial and peroneal nerve Anterior talocrural joint pathology Turf toe Sesamoid bone injury Tibiofibular syndesmosis pathology Deep vein thrombosis Malleolar fracture Anterior lateral impingement	Anterior talofibular (ATF) ligament pathology Cuboid dysfunction Posterior impingement Retrocalcaneal bursitis Peroneal pathology
Plantar flexion	Walking—terminal stance Driving car Coming up onto toes	ATF ligament pathology Cuboid dysfunction Posterior tendon or muscle pathology—if active Posterior impingement Retrocalcaneal bursitis Deep vein thrombosis—if active Malleolar fracture Peroneal pathology	Posterior tibialis pathology Tibial and peroneal nerve Anterior talocrural joint pathology Turf toe Sesamoid bone injury Tibiofibular syndesmosis pathology Anterior lateral impingement
Inversion and supination	Walking—initial contact Twisting ipsilaterally	Cuboid dysfunction Fracture of the fifth metatarsal Forefoot fracture	Tarsal tunnel syndrome Syndesmosis injury Plantar fasciitis
Eversion and pronation	Walking—mid-stance Twisting contralateral	Plantar fascia Mid-foot laxity Tarsal tunnel nerve entrapment Nerve entrapment at foot Sinus tarsi syndrome	Peroneal tendon pathology
Static positions	Sleep Sitting	Plantar fascia Inflammatory disorders	Fractures Tendon pathology Muscle pathology
Other	Running	Fracture Compartment syndrome Most pathologies	None

MEDICAL HISTORY

WHAT ROLE DOES A PATIENT'S PAST MEDICAL HISTORY PLAY IN THE DIFFERENTIAL DIAGNOSIS OF FOOT AND ANKLE PATHOLOGY?

When an individual has a history of diabetes, Charcot neuroarthropathy should be considered, particularly if trauma is involved. Charcot arthropathy is a chronic and progressive disease of bone and joints commonly found in the feet and ankles of neuropathic patients. The acute Charcot foot manifests as a relatively painless, warm, erythematous, and edematous foot.[15,59] The patient will usually have a good pulse and sensory neuropathy on examination. Patients usually do not have significant pain despite the presence of intense synovitis, fracture, and instability of single or multiple joints.[19,44] Stress fractures can occur and are infrequently diagnosed in patients with peripheral neuropathy as pain is absent and there is no apparent loss of function.[9] The most important factor in potentially altering the outcome of patients with Charcot neuroarthropathy is to have a high clinical suspicion in patients who are "at risk."

CLINICAL DECISION MAKING CASE STUDY—PATIENT PROFILE **?**

A 50-year-old female with a history of insulin-dependent diabetes and peripheral neuropathy presented to the emergency room with an acute ankle sprain. At that time, non-weight-bearing x-ray films were taken and were negative for fracture dislocation (Figure II-13-4). The patient was diagnosed as having a sprain of the right ankle.

She continued to ambulate without any protective bracing. Despite any significant pain she presented 3 months later to a foot and ankle specialist with complaints of swelling and an inability to wear shoes. She states that she twisted her ankle earlier that day and felt something shift. Protective sensation was absent when tested with a monofilament and tuning fork. An obvious valgus deformity of the ankle was present. What disease state needs to be ruled out?

Answer

Charcot neuroarthropathy needs to be ruled out. Figures II-13-5 and II-13-6 show the radiograph taken 3 months after

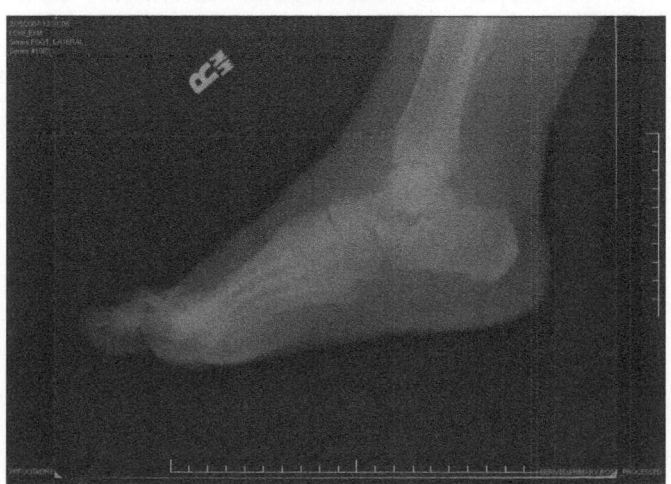

FIGURE II-13-4 Lateral non-weight-bearing view of foot and ankle.

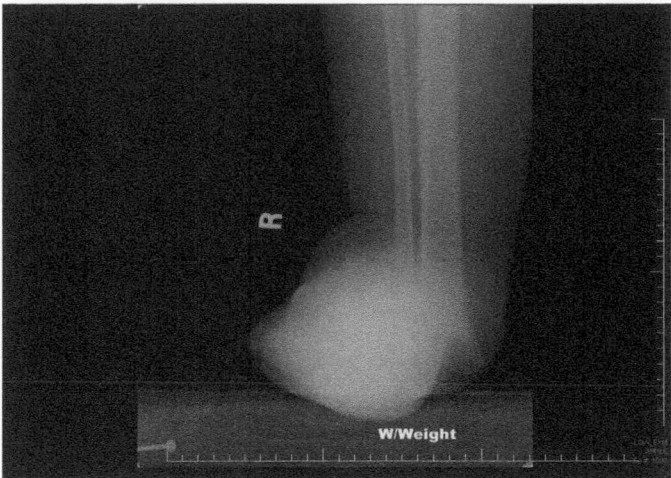

FIGURE II-13-5 AP weight-bearing view of foot and ankle with Charcot neuroarthropathy.

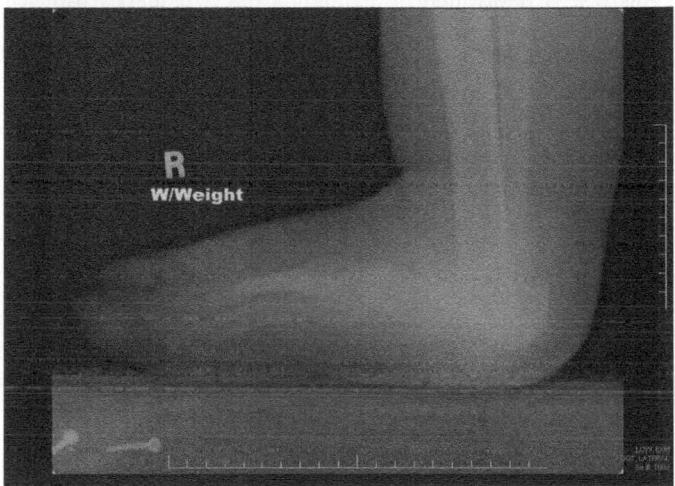

FIGURE II-13-6 Lateral weight-bearing view of foot and ankle with Charcot neuroarthropathy.

injury and reveal extensive collapse of the ankle, hindfoot, and midfoot.

Systemic disorders that can cause foot and ankle pain include osteomylitis, gout, pseudogout, sickle cell disease, complex region pain syndrome, and peripheral vascular disease. Systemic arthritic conditions generally have pain in multiple joints outside of the foot and ankle region.

A medical history of generalized ligamentous laxity, malalignment issues, recent illness, or other musculoskeletal injuries may also help give a prognosis of injury.[5]

MEDICAL AND ORTHOPEDIC TESTING

WHAT MEDICAL AND ORTHOPEDIC TESTS INFLUENCE YOUR DIFFERENTIAL DIAGNOSIS PROCESS IN THE FOOT AND ANKLE?

There are a large number of tests clinicians can use to assess the foot and ankle region; however, the tests we have outlined are the ones we use most frequently. When the origin of symptoms is traumatic in nature, a series of tests is performed to assist in the differential diagnosis process as shown in Table II-13-3.

TABLE II-13-3	**Special Tests of the Foot and Ankle**	
Test	**Structures Assessed**	**Test Reproducibility**
Anterior drawer	Anterior talofibular ligament	Poor interrater reliability[16]
Talar tilt into inversion	Calcaneal fibular ligament	Poor interrater reliability in the absence of pain[16]
Talar tilt into eversion	Deltoid ligament	N/A
Dorsiflexion external Rotation test	Distal tibia-fibula syndesmosis and deltoid ligament	Substantial interrater reliability[3]
Squeeze test	Distal tibia-fibula syndesmosis	Moderate interrater reliability[3]
Thompson test	Achilles tendon	N/A

Tinel's and Morton's tests are commonly done to assess for tarsal tunnel and Morton's neuroma, respectively. The Windlass test can also be performed and is used to assess for plantar fasciitis. This test is performed by extending the first metatarsophalangeal (MTP) joint, in both weight bearing and non-weight bearing, in an attempt to reproduce the patient's heel pain. Although the Windlass test had a high specificity (100%), its sensitivity was poor (<32%).[10]

MEDICATIONS

HOW DOES PATIENT MEDICATION INFLUENCE YOUR DECISION-MAKING PROCESS?

Opiate dependence may indicate an increased severity of pain. Fat pad atrophy is another source of chronic heel pain. The adipose plantar to the calcaneus helps absorb shock that regularly occurs during the gait cycle. Age, trauma, and corticosteroid injections can cause fat pad atrophy.

BIOMECHANICAL FACTORS

WHAT ROLE DOES BIOMECHANICS PLAY IN FOOT AND ANKLE PAIN?

Abnormal biomechanics has been implicated in overuse injuries of the foot and ankle. The literature is inconclusive related to abnormal biomechanics as a risk factor for foot and ankle-related running overuse injuries, including shin splints and plantar fasciitis.[33,56] Biomechanical abnormalities have been identified in up to 60% of athletes with Achilles tendinopathy.[26] Static measures suggest that a forefoot varus deformity is associated with an increased prevalance of Achilles tendinopathy.[26] Dynamically, athletes with Achilles tendinopathy are more inverted at contact, display greater pronation, and take less time to achieve maximal pronation when compared to controls.[32] Related to ankle instability we have found forefoot or rearfoot abnormalities, such as forefoot valgus, plantar-flexed first ray, and rearfoot varus, can result in a laterally directed force. This lateral force can contribute to lateral ankle instability.

Orthotic intervention in many cases produces positive outcomes and therefore we believe it is appropriate to assess individuals for potential biomechanical abnormalities. This is particularly true for individuals with overuse and chronic conditions. Biomechanics plays a larger role when a person is more active. For instance, subtle abnormalities can lead to problems in someone training for a marathon, whereas obvious abnormalities can be well tolerated if someone is less active.

Our assessment includes evaluating individuals standing, walking, and, when necessary, running with a focus on calcaneal position, arch height, and great toe extension. A more thorough biomechanical examination, looking at rearfoot and forefoot abnormalities, can be performed. However, the reliability of this "biomechanical examination" is poor and does not predict dynamic foot function.[12,39,40,51] Navicular drop can be measured to assess the change in arch height from subtalar neutral to the normal comfortable standing position. This measurement has been found to have good reliability.[36,45] In addition to a biomechanical assessment a trial of arch support taping (treatment-directed test[54,55]) can be used to help determine if orthotic intervention should be considered.[46]

WHAT BIOMECHANICAL ABNORMALITIES IN OTHER REGIONS AFFECT FOOT AND ANKLE PATHOLOGY?

Abnormalities in the spine, hip, and knee can potentially affect foot and ankle biomechanics because of the need to maintain a plantigrade foot position when weight bearing. Specifically, leg length discrepancies, coxa valgum and varum, hip anteversion and retroversion, genu valgum and varum, and/or tibial torsion are deformities that can affect foot and ankle biomechanics. Additionally, hip and knee flexion contractures can also affect foot and ankle biomechanics.

ENVIRONMENTAL AND PERSONAL CONTEXTUAL FACTORS (Box II-13-4)

ENVIRONMENTAL FACTORS

Home and job environmental issues such as the need to negotiate stairs, uneven terrain, and hills can be important and may need to be considered in the individual's overall management, including diagnosis, prognosis, and intervention strategies.

PERSONAL FACTORS

SOCIAL HISTORY: The social history can provide valuable information when assessing the patient's present complaint. It provides information on the patient's habits such as use of alcohol, tobacco, or recreational activities and provides insight on the patient's home condition, occupation, and health care resources. Other issues may include recent termination of a significant relationship such as death, divorce, or occupation, physical or emotion illness in family members, and school problems.

PRIOR SURGERIES: Prior surgeries can influence clinical reasoning in the foot and ankle, particularly when these surgeries potentially affect lower extremity biomechanics. Additionally, when previous surgeries have not been successful the clinician should determine why. There might be potential risk factors for complication, such as poor healing ability, that can affect the treat-

BOX II-13-4	**Contextual Factors**
Environmental	Repetitive tasks such as stairclimbing, walking hills, or walking on uneven terrain. Need to wear nonsupportive shoes for work or walking on hard surfaces.
Personal	Smoking, depression, emotional stressors, job satisfaction, and cultural and religious pressures can all influence foot and ankle pain.

TABLE II-13-4 Nociceptive and Peripheral Neurogenic Pain

	Tendon	Tendon	Ligament	Ligament	Bone
Pathology	Achilles tendinitis/tendinosis	Achilles rupture	Lateral ankle sprains	High ankle sprain	Anterolateral impingement
Age (years)	20 to 50	40 to 60	All ages are susceptible	20 to 30	20 to 30
Activity/occupation	Primarily athletic individuals	Weekend warrior	Most common in athletes: soccer, basketball, football, volleyball, and cross-country runners	Primary athletic individuals	Primarily athletic individuals
Gender	M > F	M > F	M = F	M = F	M = F
Ethnicity	Not applicable	Higher incidence in African-Americans	Not applicable	Not applicable	Not applicable
History/mechanism of injury	Typically associated with overuse; repetitive microscopic tensile overload	Chronic tendinosis with or without symptoms; tendency to occur during vigorous eccentric contraction	Trauma; 80% to 85% result from a combination of inversion and plantar flexion	Trauma; results from external rotation of the talus or forced dorsiflexion	History of lateral ankle sprains
Symptoms	Stiffness/pain	Acute pain, significant calf weakness	Instability and pain confined to the anterolateral	Pain just above the ankle	Pain, stiffness, and swelling in the anterolateral ankle region
Aggravating/relieving factors	Pain/stiffness often present upon awakening; decreases with activity; increases after activity	Unable to perform normal activities	Symptoms are often increased with cutting, pivoting, and twisting	Symptoms are often increased with cutting, pivoting, and twisting	Symptoms are often increased with cutting, pivoting and twisting
Clinical findings	Decreased active passive dorsiflexion with knee extended; pain with unilateral heel rise; tender to palpation 2 to 6 cm proximal to insertion; pes planus	Thompson test (+); palpable gap; inability to perform unilateral heel rise	Anterior drawer (+): ATFL; Talar tilt (+): CFL; Tender lateral ankle joint; Ecchymosis and swelling	Squeeze test (+); Dorsiflexion; External rotation test(+); Tender distal tibiafibular articulation	Pain, "pinching" with dorsiflexion; end range inversion is often painful as well
Past medical history	Previous overuse injuries	Fluoroquinolone antibiotic use; prior intratendinous injection, retrocalcaneal spurs or chronic tendinosis	Up to 40% experience recurrence		Recent lateral ankle sprain
Diagnostic tests	X-rays can detect retrocalcaneal spur; MRI and US may be ordered	MRI and US may be ordered	X-rays to rule out fracture	X-rays to rule out fracture	MRI or US is beneficial to visualize soft tissues
Red flags	Inability to perform plantar flexion versus gravity; soft tissue deficit may indicate rupture	If rupture is suspected patient should be referred to a physician	Skeletally immature: avulsion fractures; Ottawa Ankle Rules (+): fracture	Ottawa Ankle Rules (+): fracture	Unremarkable

	Bone	Tendon	Tendon	Tendon	Bone	Bone	Nerve
Diagnosis	Malleolar fractures	Peroneal tendinopathy	Posterior impingement syndrome	Posterior tibial tendinopathy/dysfunction	Anterior/posterior periostitis	Stress fractures	Tarsal tunnel
Age (years)	All ages are susceptible	18 to 40	18 to 40	50 to 80	18 to 40	18 to 40	25 to 50
Activity/occupation	Can occur across all activity levels	Sports—basketball, football, gymnastics, ice skating	Sports—ballet dancing, gymnastics, or downhill running	Repetitive/prolonged weight bearing	Common with repetitive weight bearing (i.e., running)	Repetitive weight bearing	Repetitive/prolonged weight bearing

Continued on following page.

TABLE II-13-4 Nociceptive and Peripheral Neurogenic Pain (Continued)

	Bone	Tendon	Tendon	Tendon	Tendon	Bone	Bone	Nerve
Gender	Age <50 M	M = F	M = F	M = F	M = F	M = F	F > M	M = F
Ethnicity	Not applicable	Not applicable	Not applicable	Not applicable	Not applicable	Not applicable	Not applicable	Not applicable
History/mechanism of injury	Traumatic	Repetitive trauma Complication following an ankle sprian	Isolated lesions rare; can occur with lateral ankle sprain	Gradual	Gradual	Overuse, improper training and/or footwear	Gradual, related to over training or improper training	Gradual
Symptoms	Inability to bear weight, pain, instability	Pain posterior-lateral ankle "Snapping" with tendon instability	Pain posterior-lateral ankle "Snapping" with tendon instability	Posterior ankle pain, local swelling, and at times reports of "catching"	Medial ankle pain Progressive loss of arch height General foot pain from stress on supportive ligaments	Pain related to prolonged activity	Vague poorly localized pain	Pain, burning, and numbness in medial arch and/or the plantar surface of the foot and toes
Aggravating/relieving factors	Weight bearing increases symptoms	Activities that cause strong contraction of evertors; i.e., "cutting and pivoting"	Movement into plantar flexion (active or passive)	Movement into plantar flexion Pain with resisted inversion and plantar flexion	Prolonged weight bearing Pain with resisted inversion and plantar flexion	Worse with repetitive weigh-bearing activities	Excessive weight bearing	Worse with prolonged standing or walking
Clinical findings	Tenderness over the involved bony region Pain with movement, swelling, and ecchymosis	Tenderness over the peroneal tendons Pain with resisted eversion in plantar flexion	Local tenderness Reproduction of symptoms with passive or resisted plantar flexion	Local tenderness Reproduction of symptoms with passive or resisted plantar flexion	Tender posterior tibialis tendon Unable to perform single-leg heel raise	Pain with palpation; pain with stretching or contraction of muscle-tendon that attaches to the affected area of the bone	Tenderness over the involved bony region	Tenderness just posterior to the medial malleolus Positive Tinel sign over the tarsal tunnel
Past medical history	Osteoporosis	Ankle sprain	Ankle sprain	Unremarkable	Unremarkable	Previous overuse injuries	Previous stress fractures	Carpel tunnel
Diagnostic tests	X-rays—routine	MRI	MRI	MRI	MRI	Not applicable	CT or bone scan	NCV and EMG
Red flags	Neurovascular complications and acute compartment syndrome	Persistent symptoms may require surgical intervention	Unremarkable	Unremarkable	Unremarkable	Bone scan to r/o stress fracture for persistent symptoms	Check dietary history	r/o lumbar radiculopathy

Tissue	Ligaments	Bursa	Bone	Bone/Cartilage	Cartilage	Bone
Diagnosis	Turf toe	Retrocalcaneal bursitis	Sesamoid injuries	Sinus tarsi syndrome	Talar dome damage	Cuboid dysfunction
Age (years)	18 to 30	20 to 60	20 to 50	20 to 50	18 to 30	18 to 30
Activity/occupation	Sports with explosive movements	Repetitive/prolonged weight bearing	Repetitive weigh bearing	Sports with explosive movements	Sports with explosive movements	Given the stability of the joint, the condition is rare Most commonly reported in ballet dancers
Gender	M > F	M = F	F > M	M > F	M > F	F > M
Ethnicity	Not applicable	Not applicable	Not applicable	Not applicable	Not applicable	Not applicable
History/mechanism of injury	Traumatic first MTP overload (Hyperextension occurring with explosive push-off or change in direction is most common)	Repetitive (cumulative) trauma Recent change in footwear (e.g., tight athletic shoes or transition from flats to high heels)	Overuse or direct trauma	Traumatic inversion injury of the foot	Occurs with traumatic ankle injuries	Acute or repetitive microtraumatic injury

Clinical presentation (continued from previous page)

Symptoms	Stiffness and pain at the first MTP	Posterior heel pain aggravated by pressure	Local pain with weight bearing	Recurrent instability/giving way, pain inferior/anterior to the ankle, swelling, and stiffness	Ankle pain along with intermittent swelling, weakness, stiffness, catching or locking, and/or instability/giving way	Lateral mid-foot pain	Localized pain and swelling
Aggravating/relieving factors	Pushing-off	Worse when beginning an activity or after resting	Pain when force is transmitted through the great toe (i.e., push-off)	Weight-bearing activity that inverts the foot (e.g., walking on uneven ground)	Weight-bearing activities, particularly pivoting, increase symptoms	Sport activities. Landing from a jump may increase pain. Axial loading of the lateral column of the foot	Pain increasing with weight bearing
Clinical findings	Tenderness around the first MTP joint. Instability, mechanical block, or hypermobility of the first MTP with ROM	Tenderness superficial to the Achilles tendon (subcutaneous bursa) or deep to the Achilles tendon (subtendinous bursa). Swelling; "pump bump"	Tenderness over the sesmoids	Tenderness over the sinus tarsi. Deep pain in the subtalar area with forced inversion of the foot	Palpation: tenderness behind the medial malleolus when the ankle is dorsiflexed and/or anterolateral ankle joint tenderness in maximal plantar flexion	Pressure over the plantar surface of the cuboid in a dorsal direction reproduces symptoms	Palpation: localized tenderness at the involved bones(s)
Past medical history	Unremarkable	Unremarkable	Unremarkable	Unremarkable	Unremarkable	Prior history of ankle sprain	Unremarkable
Diagnostic tests	X-rays positive: compare the sesamoid-to-joint distance	X-ray may reveal a Haglund deformity	X-ray may be positive but MRI is typically used	Diagnostic injection of lidocain	X-ray may be positive but MRI is typically used. Diagnostic injection of lidocaine	Stress and/or weight-bearing radiographs may assist with diagnosis	X-ray is positive
Red flags	r/o fracture	Unremarkable	r/o fracture	Unremarkable	Unremarkable	Injury to peroneal nerve	Unremarkable

	Fascia	Cartilage	Ligament	Fascia	Visceral	Nerve
Diagnosis	Plantar fasciitis	Post traumatic arthrosis	Lisfranc ligament tear	Chronic compartment syndrome	Deep vein thrombosis	Morton's neuroma
Age (years)	20 to 60	40 to 70	All ages, but most common in 20s	20 to 40	Greater incidence with increasing age	40 to 60
Activity/occupation	Prolonged weight bearing	Repetitive/prolonged weight bearing	Specific athletes at elevated risk include gymnasts, ballet, football, and track/field athletes	Long distance runners, skiers, soccer and basketball players	Sedentary, obese individuals are at greater risk	Repetitive/prolonged weight bearing
Gender	F > M	M > F	M > F	M = F	Increased risk for females during and following pregnancy	F > M
Ethnicity	Not applicable	Not applicable	Not applicable	Not applicable	Not applicable	Not applicable
History/mechanism of injury	Graudual	Generally gradual onset, although trauma may precipitate symptoms	Athletics/MVA. Axial loading with plantar flexed mid-foot	Overuse or trauma	Recent surgery with general anesthesia, immobility, recent airline travel	Gradual; related to ill-fitting/narrow shoes

Continued on following page.

TABLE II-13-4 Nociceptive and Peripheral Neurogenic Pain (Continued)

	Fascia	Cartilage	Ligament	Fascia	Visceral	Nerve
Symptoms	Plantar heel pain	Pain, stiffness, catching, locking, clicking or painful giving way episodes	Pain, mid-foot instability	Local pain in affected compartment is primary complaint. Decreased ability to control the foot during exercise	Pain, swelling, and redness in calf	Forefoot pain, numbness, and/or paresthesias in the digital nerve distribution commonly between the third and fourth toes
Aggravating/relieving factors	Pain with the first few steps in the morning or after sitting for long periods: "start-up pain"	Prolonged weight bearing	Pain with weight bearing	Exercise/activity-induced symptoms	Symptomas may be increased with dorsiflexion of the ankle	Excessive pressure from poorly fitting shoes
Clinical findings	Tenderness in the medial calcaneal tubercle. Positive Windlass test	Tender ankle joint. Limited and painful ankle motion	Ecchymosis in the plantar aspect of the mid-foot. Tenderness over TMT joints, particularly over the base of the second metatarsal	Physical examination findings are typically normal	Calf is often tender to palpation; a "cord" may be noted with palpation. Homan's sign may or may not be positive	Webspace tenderness. Positive Morton's sign
Past medical history	Unremarkable	Previous ankle trauma (i.e., fracture)	Unremarkable	Recent increase in activity	Previous venous thromboembolism	Unremarkable
Diagnostic tests	None needed	X-rays are positive for asymmetric joint space narrowing with signs of arthritis (sclerosis and osteophytes)	X-ray and MRI	Measurement of compartmental pressure at rest and during exercise	Ultrasound, MRI, and/or venography	MRI or US can help visualize an enlarged nerve
Red flags	Unremarkable	Unremarkable	Displaced/unstable injuries require surgery	Acute compartment syndrome: pain out of proportion, absence of pulse, pain with stretching or weakness of the affected compartment	Symptoms that migrate proximally. Shortness of breath may indicate a pulmonary embolism	Unremarkable

ATFL, anterior talofibular ligament; CFL, calcaneal fibular ligament; MRI, magnetic resonance imaging; US, ultrasound; CT, computed tomography; NCV, nerve conduction velocity; EMG, electromyogram; MTP, metatarsophalangeal; r/o, rule out; ROM, range of motion; MVA, motor vehicle accident; TMT, tarsometatarsal.

ment outcome. The dates of surgery, hospital location, treating diagnosis, and perioperative complications should be recorded.

FAMILY HISTORY: Family history may establish whether there is a history of bleeding, blood clots, rheumatoid arthritis, vascular disease, cancer, or problems with anesthesia such as malignant hyperthermia. Inflammatory arthropathies such as rheumatoid arthritis, seronegative spondyloarthropathies, systemic lupus erythematosus, crystalline arthropathies, and psoriatic arthropathy have been implicated in foot and ankle pain.

RED FLAGS THAT REQUIRE REFERRAL TO A MEDICAL PHYSICIAN

WHAT SYMPTOMS ALERT YOU TO PATHOLOGIES THAT MAY REQUIRE A REFERRAL TO A MEDICAL DOCTOR?

For individuals who present with inversion ankle injuries the Ottawa Ankle Rules can be used to help in the decision-making process. Referral to a medical doctor for radiographs is indicated if the individual has pain in the malleolar zone and one or more of the following: (1) is unable to bear weight (walk four steps), (2) has tenderness at the posterior tip of the medial malleolus, and (3) has tenderness at the posterior tip of the lateral malleolus or tenderness in the malleolar zone.[48] Radiographs are also indicated if the individual has pain in the mid-foot zone and one or more of the following: (1) is unable to bear weight (walk four steps), (2) has tenderness at the base of the fifth metatarsal, and (3) has navicular tenderness.[48]

Generally, the inability to bear weight, nocturnal pain, calf pain, and/or tenderness, swelling with pitting edema, increased skin temperature, superficial venous dilation, thrombosis, and an abnormally cold foot should raise the suspicion for potential systemic conditions. Diabetic patients should be under the care of a physician because of the potential for Charcot neuropathy and other diabetic-related problems. A patient should be referred to a medical physician when DVT, compartment syndrome, or stress fractures are suspected. Patients with swelling and inflammation in the joints of the foot, especially the big toe, who also have a history of kidney disease, should be referred to their physician to rule out gout as a potential source of their symptoms. Additionally, if conditions have not improved after 4 weeks of physical therapy the patient should be referred to a physician.

SUMMARY STATEMENT

The foot and ankle region has the potential to be a complicated and frustrating region to assess and treat (Table II-13-4). The difficulty results from the fact that the foot and ankle have many articulation, ligament, and muscular attachments. The region has a complex biomechanical arrangement that relies on the proper functioning of multiple joints and structures. It is a weight-bearing region and must support large forces. It is also the most distal part of the body from the heart. Therefore, it is prone to poor circulation. All of these factors make the foot and ankle a challenge for the clinician to rehabilitate and equally challenging for the patient to heal. Table II-13-4 summarizes the factors that help a clinician differentiate among different sources of symptoms in the foot and ankle regions.

REFERENCES

1. Alfredson H, Lorentzon R. Chronic Achilles tendinosis: recommendations for treatment and prevention. *Sports Med.* 2000;29:135.
2. Alfredson H, Pietila T, Jonsson P, et al. Heavy-load eccentric calf muscle training for the treatment of chronic Achilles tendinosis. *Am J Sports Med.* 1998;26:360.
3. Alonso A, Khoury L, Adams R. Clinical tests for ankle syndesmosis injury: reliability and prediction of return to function. *J Orthop Sports Phys Ther.* 1998;27:276.
4. Anandacoomarasamy A, Barnsley L. Long term outcomes of inversion ankle injuries. *Br J Sports Med.* 2005;39:e14 [discussion e14].
5. Baumhauer J, Nawoczenski D, DiGiovanni B, et al. Ankle pain and peroneal tendon pathology. *Clin Sports Med.* 2004;23:21.
6. Beynnon BD, Murphy DF, Alosa DM. Predictive factors for lateral ankle sprains: a literature review. *J Athl Train.* 2002;37:376.
7. Beynnon BD, Renstrom PA, Haugh L, et al. A prospective, randomized clinical investigation of the treatment of first-time ankle sprains. *Am J Sports Med.* 2006;34:1401.
8. Bjordal JM, Lopes-Martins RA, Iversen VV. A randomised, placebo controlled trial of low level laser therapy for activated Achilles tendinitis with microdialysis measurement of peritendinous prostaglandin E2 concentrations. *Br J Sports Med.* 2006;40:76.
9. Chantelau E, Richter A, Ghassem-Zadeh P. "Silent" bone stress injuries in the feet of diabetic patients with polyneuropathy: a report on 12 cases. *Arch Orthop Trauma Surg.* 2007;127:171.
10. De Garceau D, Dean D, Requejo SM, et al. The association between diagnosis of plantar fasciitis and Windlass test results. *Foot Ankle Int.* 2003;24:251.
11. Dunn J, Link C, Felson D, et al. Prevalence of foot and ankle conditions in multiethnic community sample of older adults. *Am J Epidemiol.* 2004;159:491.
12. Elveru RA, Rothstein JM, Lamb RL. Goniometric reliability in a clinical setting. Subtalar and ankle joint measurements. *Phys Ther.* 1988;68:672.
13. Ferran NA, Maffulli N. Epidemiology of sprains of the lateral ankle ligament complex. *Foot Ankle Clin.* 2006;11:659.
14. Frey C, Zamora J. The effects of obesity on orthopaedic foot and ankle pathology. *Foot Ankle Int.* 2007;28:996.
15. Frykberg RG, Armstrong DG, Giurini J, et al. Diabetic foot disorders: a clinical practice guideline. American College of Foot and Ankle Surgeons. *J Foot Ankle Surg.* 2000;39:S1.
16. Fujii T, Luo ZP, Kitaoka HB, et al. The manual stress test may not be sufficient to differentiate ankle ligament injuries. *Clin Biomech (Bristol, Avon).* 2000;15:619.
17. Garrick JG, Requa RK. The epidemiology of foot and ankle injuries in sports. *Clin Sports Med.* 1988;7:29.
18. Greenberg L, Davis H. Foot problems in the US. The 1990 National Health Interview Survey. *J Am Podiatr Med Assoc.* 1993;83:475.
19. Hedlund LMD, Griffiths H. Calcaneal Fractures in Diabetic Patients. *J Diab Comp.* 1998;12:81.
20. Hill CL, Gill TK, Menz HB, et al. Prevalence and correlates of foot pain in a population-based study: the North West Adelaide health study. *J Foot Ankle Res.* 2008;1:2.
21. Jaakkola JI, Mann RA. A review of rheumatoid arthritis affecting the foot and ankle. *Foot Ankle Int.* 2004;25:866.
22. Johansson C. Injuries in elite orienteers. *Am J Sports Med.* 1986;14:410.
23. Karlsson J, Lansinger O. Chronic lateral instability of the ankle in athletes. *Sports Med.* 1993;16:355.
24. Kay RM, Tang CW. Pediatric foot fractures: evaluation and treatment. *J Am Acad Orthop Surg.* 2001;9:308.
25. Kerkhoffs GM, Rowe BH, Assendelft WJ, et al. Immobilisation and functional treatment for acute lateral ankle ligament injuries in adults. *Cochrane Database Syst Rev.* 2002;CD003762.
26. Kvist M. Achilles tendon injuries in athletes. *Ann Chir Gynaecol.* 1991;80:188.
27. Lysholm J, Wiklander J. Injuries in runners. *Am J Sports Med.* 1987;15:168.
28. Martin R. Considerations for differential diagnosis of an ankle sprain in the adolescent. *Orthopaedic Practice.* 2004;16:21.
29. Martin RL, Irrgang JJ, Conti SF. Outcome study of subjects with insertional plantar fasciitis. *Foot Ankle Int.* 1998;19:803.
30. Martin RL, Stewart GW, Conti SF. Posttraumatic ankle arthritis: an update on conservative and surgical management. *J Orthop Sports Phys Ther.* 2007;37:253.
31. Mayeda D. *Ankle and foot.* 3rd ed. St. Louis: Mosby; 1992.
32. McCrory JL, Martin DF, Lowery RB, et al. Etiologic factors associated with Achilles tendinitis in runners. *Med Sci Sports Exerc.* 1999;31:1374.
33. McPoil TG, Martin RL, Cornwall MW, et al. Heel pain--plantar fasciitis: clinical practice guildelines linked to the international classification

of function, disability, and health from the orthopaedic section of the American Physical Therapy Association. *J Orthop Sports Phys Ther.* 2008;38:A1.

34. Messier SP, Gutekunst DJ, Davis C, et al. Weight loss reduces knee-joint loads in overweight and obese older adults with knee osteoarthritis. *Arthritis Rheum.* 2005;52:2026.

35. Micheli L. Overuse injuries in children's sports. *Orthop Clin North Am.* 1983;14:339.

36. Mueller MJ, Host JV, Norton BJ. Navicular drop as a composite measure of excessive pronation. *J Am Podiatr Med Assoc.* 1993;83:198.

37. Ohberg L, Lorentzon R, Alfredson H. Eccentric training in patients with chronic Achilles tendinosis: normalised tendon structure and decreased thickness at follow up. *Br J Sports Med.* 2004;38:8.

38. Paavola M, Kannus P, Paakkala T, et al. Long-term prognosis of patients with Achilles tendinopathy. An observational 8-year follow-up study. *Am J Sports Med.* 2000;28:634.

39. Pierrynowski MR, Smith SB. Rear foot inversion/eversion during gait relative to the subtalar joint neutral position. *Foot Ankle Int.* 1996;17:406.

40. Pierrynowski MR, Smith SB, Mlynarczyk JH. Proficiency of foot care specialists to place the rearfoot at subtalar neutral. *J Am Podiatr Med Assoc.* 1996;86:217.

41. Riddle DL, Pulisic M, Pidcoe P, et al. Risk factors for plantar fasciitis: a matched case-control study. *J Bone Joint Surg Am.* 2003;85-A:872.

42. Roos EM, Engstrom M, Lagerquist A, et al. Clinical improvement after 6 weeks of eccentric exercise in patients with mid-portion Achilles tendinopathy—a randomized trial with 1-year follow-up. *Scand J Med Sci Sports.* 2004;14:286.

43. Saltzman CL, Salamon ML, Blanchard GM, et al. Epidemiology of ankle arthritis: report of a consecutive series of 639 patients from a tertiary orthopaedic center. *Iowa Orthop J.* 2005;25:44.

44. Schon LC, Marks RM. The management of neuroarthropathic fracture-dislocations in the diabetic patient. *Orthop Clin North Am.* 1995;26:375.

45. Shrader JA, Popovich JM, Gracey GC, et al. Navicular drop measurement in people with rheumatoid arthritis: interrater and intrarater reliability. *Phys Ther.* 2005;85:656.

46. Smith M, Brooker S, Vicenzino B, et al. Use of anti-pronation taping to assess suitability of orthotic prescription: case report. *Aust J Physiother.* 2004;50:111.

47. Stergioulas A, Stergioula M, Aarskog R, et al. Effects of low-level laser therapy and eccentric exercises in the treatment of recreational athletes with chronic achilles tendinopathy. *Am J Sports Med.* 2008;36:881.

48. Stiell IG, Greenberg GH, McKnight RD, et al. Ottawa Ankle Rules for radiography of acute injuries. *N Z Med J.* 1995;108:111.

49. Struijs P, Kerkhoffs G. Ankle Sprain, in BMJ. *Clin Evid.* 2008;1.

50. Taunton JE, Ryan MB, Clement DB, et al. A retrospective case-control analysis of 2002 running injuries. *Br J Sports Med.* 2002;36:95.

51. Van Gheluwe B, Kirby KA, Roosen P, et al. Reliability and accuracy of biomechanical measurements of the lower extremities. *J Am Podiatr Med Assoc.* 2002;92:317.

52. van Os AG, Bierma-Zeinstra SM, Verhagen AP, et al. Comparison of conventional treatment and supervised rehabilitation for treatment of acute lateral ankle sprains: a systematic review of the literature. *J Orthop Sports Phys Ther.* 2005;35:95.

53. van Rijn RM, van Os AG, Bernsen RM, et al. What is the clinical course of acute ankle sprains? A systematic literature review. *Am J Med.* 2008;121:324.

54. Vicenzino B. Foot orthotics in the treatment of lower limb conditions: a musculoskeletal physiotherapy perspective. *Man Ther.* 2004;9:185.

55. Vicenzino B, Griffiths SR, Griffiths LA, et al. Effect of antipronation tape and temporary orthotic on vertical navicular height before and after exercise. *J Orthop Sports Phys Ther.* 2000;30:333.

56. Wen DY. Risk factors for overuse injuries in runners. *Curr Sports Med Rep.* 2007;6:307.

57. Wolgin M, Cook C, Graham C, et al. Conservative treatment of plantar heel pain: long-term follow-up. *Foot Ankle Int.* 1994;15:97.

58. Young CC, Niedfeldt MW, Morris GA, et al. Clinical examination of the foot and ankle. *Prim Care.* 2005;32:105.

59. Yu G, Hudson J. Evaluation and Treatment of Stage 0 Charcot's Neuroarthropathy. *J Am Podiatr Med Assoc.* 2002;94:210.

AUTHORS: DANIEL J. KIRAGES, STEPHANIE A. PRENDERGAST, ELIZABETH RUMMER, and RHONDA K. KOTARINOS

INTRODUCTORY INFORMATION

In comparison to other regions of the body, the pelvic region has often been forgotten or disregarded as a source of pain. Recently, increased emphasis has been placed on its role in rehabilitation as a primary source of pain as well as on its role as an important contributor to many of the issues that commonly plague the clinician in orthopedic settings.[47] Low back pain, lower extremity symptoms, and even pathology as remote as the shoulders have been tied to dysfunctions that occur within the pelvic region. A proper understanding of the pelvic floor and its role within the orthopedic field is crucial to all clinicians and to the patients they treat.

WHAT IS THE PREVALENCE OF PELVIC PAIN?

Broadly speaking, the prevalence of pelvic pain ranges from 18% to 21% in women and 8% to 15% in men.[3,5,14,29,30,44,54]

WHAT IS THE PROGNOSIS FOR RECOVERY FROM PELVIC PAIN?

Pelvic pain syndromes often develop from multiple pathophysiological components. Proper identification of the components will result in an effective treatment plan leading to a favorable prognosis. Chronic pelvic pain syndromes will resolve with proper intervention; however, it is important to note the syndromes are often worsened by therapies directed at the symptoms rather than the cause. For example, a patient may report vulvar itching in the absence of an infection. Reasonably, a gynecologist may prescribe an antifungal topical agent to decrease the itching. Pelvic floor dysfunction can cause vulvar itching and the tight muscles can reflexively cause allodynia of the vulvar tissue. Application of a topical agent to the tissues with heightened sensitivity can result in an increase, rather than a decrease in symptoms. In contrast, therapy directed at the impairments will improve the symptoms. Myofascial release to the pelvic floor muscles will decrease hypertonus, removing the stimulus for vulvar allodynia and itching.

WHAT IS THE RECURRENCE RATE?

Clinically speaking, patients with pelvic pain are susceptible to reoccurrences. Most pelvic pain syndromes result from a combination of numerous etiological factors and pathophysiological mechanisms. Causes may include excessive bike riding, chronic constipation, repetitive urinary tract or yeast infections, pregnancy and delivery, and core weakness and structural abnormalities. Collectively and independently, these events can cause myofascial trigger points (MtrPs), pelvic floor dysfunction, connective tissue restrictions, adverse neural tension, and joint dysfunction. The result is often a complex pelvic pain syndrome that will resolve when the impairments are treated but can easily recur based on the high number of events that can lead to the impairments.

CLINICAL PEARL

The pelvic floor is intimately related to the lower urinary and bowel tracts and is very important in sexual functioning. When pelvic floor muscles become hypertonic and/or develop MTrPs, the patient with pelvic pain will also commonly present with urinary, bowel, and sexual dysfunction. Examples of urinary dysfunction include dysuria and urinary urgency, frequency, and hesitancy. These patients commonly present with hypertonus of the levator ani muscle group where it attaches to the pubic bone by the urethra. They also may have MTrPs in the rectus abdominus muscle or the adductors. Patients may also report constipation, incomplete

emptying, and dyschezia. These symptoms may be caused by hypertonus of the puborectalis muscle or a MTrP in the external anal sphincter. An orgasm is a rapid muscle contraction that involves the bulbospongiosis and ischiocavernosis muscles. Patients who report aorgasmia or pain with orgasm may have MTrPs in these muscles.

WHAT FACTORS MAKE DIAGNOSIS DIFFICULT IN PELVIC PAIN?

Accurately diagnosing pelvic pain syndromes may be one the greatest challenges a clinician faces for multiple reasons:

Symptoms of pelvic pain span several disciplines: primary care, dermatology, urology, obstetrics and gynecology, colorectal, physical medicine, neurology, orthopedics and pain management.

- Most pelvic pain syndromes have been studied only since the 1980s.
- Multiple etiologies contribute to pelvic pain syndromes.
- Multiple, complex pathophysiological mechanisms cause the symptoms.
- NIH diagnostic criteria change roughly every 3 years.[12,43,48]
- Research is difficult due to ever-changing diagnostic criteria.
- Few practitioners specialize in pelvic pain and general clinicians are often unfamiliar with the diagnoses.
- Most clinicians receive their education on the syndromes in postgraduate rather than primary educational settings.
- Imaging techniques do not exist to diagnose the syndromes or musculoskeletal dysfunction.
- Electrophysiological testing provides limited information about pelvic pain.
- A tremendously high comorbidity rate exists between pelvic pain syndromes such as vulvodynia, painful bladder syndrome, pudendal neuralgia, chronic pelvic pain syndrome, and irritable bowel syndrome.
- Patients underreport symptoms secondary to embarrassment.
- Clinicians unfamiliar with pelvic pain are likely to be dismissive of the complaints due to the nature of the symptoms and the general anxiety of the patients.
- Viscerosomatic and somatovisceral reflexes and referred pain cause confusion when trying to identify pain generators.
- Patients with pelvic pain may not realize symptoms they experience are related to each other and therefore they may not provide the clinician with all of the necessary information for diagnosis.

CLINICAL PEARL

Pelvic pain syndromes are best managed with a multidisciplinary approach that includes physical therapy, pain management, and cognitive-behavioral therapy. Rather than focusing on diagnosis (such as painful bladder syndrome or pudendal neuralgia), treatments are more effective when the practitioners focus on a working list of underlying impairments. For patients with pelvic pain, the impairments usually include pelvic floor dysfunction, connective tissue restrictions, MTrPs, adverse neural tension, strength, range of motion, and biomechanical issues, depression, and central sensitization. Conservative physical therapy techniques should be implemented first and can include myofascial release, MTrP therapy, connective tissue manipulation, neural mobilizations, muscle energy techniques, biofeedback, and a home exercise program. In the event a patient is not progressing in physical therapy, a pain management physician can assist with more aggressive therapies directed at the impairments that are not resolving. Examples include MTrP injections, peripheral nerve blocks, and pharmaceutical management. Cognitive-behavioral therapists specialize in helping patients cope with their syndrome by changing their thought processes, which can aid tremendously in the therapeutic process.

HOW SUCCESSFUL IS THERAPY IN TREATING PELVIC PAIN?

Several studies have shown that patients with pelvic floor dysfunction as a source of the pelvic pain syndrome will respond to physical therapy with a success rate of 72% to 83%. Physical therapy techniques used include myofascial release, joint mobilization, muscles energy techniques, connective tissue manipulation, and biofeedback.[1,20,31,59]

HOW SUCCESSFUL IS SURGERY IN TREATING PELVIC PAIN?

The most recent studies published on the efficacy of partial pelvic surgeries report surgery can be an effective treatment option; however, results are better when surgery is combined with proper rehabilitation.

- A study reported a 93% patient satisfaction rate among women who underwent a complete vestibulectomy with vaginal advancement to treat vestibulodynia. Additionally, 72% of the women reported apareunia before the procedure and only 11% reported apareunia following it.[27]
- Of women who underwent a partial vestibulectomy to treat dysparenuea 87% reported they would have the procedure again. In the group treated, 68% reported being cured, 24% reported a decrease in their symptoms, and 22% reported muscular pain following surgery.[25]
- In a long-term study, 56% of women with secondary vestibulodynia who were treated with a vestibulectomy reported complete or major improvement 1 year following the procedure. Among women with primary vestibulodynia, 17% reported complete or major improvement.[9]
- A study was conducted to explore the dual importance of treating vestibuloallodynia and pelvic floor myalgia in correcting dyspareunea associated with severe vulvar vestibulitis. The study showed that patients who did not respond to (vestibulectomy) surgery had persistent pelvic floor dysfunction that responded to physical therapy. The study concluded that superficial surgery can correct vulvar vestibulitis, but without treatment for pelvic floor myalgia, women may continue to have dyspareunia. Rehabilitation is an important adjunct to achieve comfort.[26]

Several studies have been published on the outcomes of pudendal nerve decompression procedures.

- A retrospective study concluded that two-thirds of patients with pudendal nerve entrapment improved after a transgluteal pudendal nerve decompression and transposition surgical procedure.[49]
- A case series of 58 patients who underwent pudendal nerve decompression surgery reported a 60% response rate to the procedure. A patient was considered to be a responder if there was a greater than 50% reduction in a VAS score, a greater than 50% improvement in global assessment of pain, or a greater than 50% improvement in overall quality of life.[45]
- Of 104 patients who underwent transischial-rectal pudendal nerve decompression surgery 86% reported being symptom free 1 year following surgery.[6]

PERSONAL INFORMATION

WHAT INFLUENCE DOES AGE HAVE ON YOUR CLINICAL DECISION-MAKING PROCESS?

- Adolescent females reporting severe dysmenorrhea could have endometriosis, fibroids, or ovarian cysts.
- Menopausal women reporting dyspareunea may be estrogen deficient.

WHAT INFLUENCE DOES A PATIENT'S OCCUPATION HAVE ON YOUR CLINICAL DECISION-MAKING PROCESS?

Activities such as prolonged sitting, heavy lifting, prolonged standing in static postures, professions with limited restroom breaks (for example, teachers and nurses), and long commute times in a car can exacerbate and contribute to pelvic pain.

- Prolonged sitting can compress the pudendal nerve and also decrease blood flow to pelvic floor muscles.
- Heavy lifting requires an increase in intraabdominal pressure. This causes the pelvic floor muscles to contract. If this is done either too frequently or forcefully hypertonicity and MTrPs can result.
- Prolonged standing in static postures can exacerbate MTrP in the stabilizing musculature and result in an increase in symptoms.
- Professionals who are unable to void for periods longer than 4 hours in duration can develop pelvic floor hypertonus.
- Long-distance driving may put a person in biomechanical positions that are less than ideal and pelvic pain can result.

WHAT INFLUENCE DOES GENDER HAVE ON YOUR CLINICAL DECISION-MAKING PROCESS?

Certain pelvic pain syndromes affect only women (vulvodynia, vaginismus, endometriosis). Nonbacterial chronic prostatitis affects only men. Syndromes that affect both sexes, such as interstitial cystitis, pudendal neuralgia, levator ani syndrome, and coccygodynia, are reportedly more prevalent in women.

WHAT INFLUENCE DOES ETHNICITY HAVE ON YOUR CLINICAL DECISION-MAKING PROCESS?

Studies show ethnicity may play a role in characteristics of pelvic pain syndromes.

- A total of 4915 women living in diverse Boston suburbs were asked to fill out a self-report questionnaire about lower genital tract discomfort. White and African-American women reported a similar lifetime prevalence of vulvodynia. Hispanic women were 80% more likely than white and African-American women to experience vulvar pain.[30]
- A study reported that Hispanic people were less likely than African-American or white people to visit a physician about pain.[46]
- A study concluded that the prevalence of vulvar pain was similar among women of different racial/ethnic groups.[36]

MECHANISM OF INJURY

WHAT INFLUENCE DOES THE MECHANISM OF INJURY HAVE ON YOUR CLINICAL DECISION-MAKING PROCESS?

Mechanism of injury plays a large role in the differential diagnosis of pelvic pain syndromes. Commonly, a syndrome will develop as a result of a combination of factors that fall into six general categories:

- Viscerosomatic: Visceral disturbances cause somatic dysfunction. Endometriosis, interstitial cystitis, irritable bowel syndrome, vaginal or urinary tract infections, prostate infections, or reproductive disorders can cause pelvic floor dysfunction, MTrPs, nerve irritation, and connective tissue restrictions, which in turn cause pelvic pain.
- Compression: Prolonged sitting, horseback riding, and cycling can cause pudendal nerve irritation and pelvic floor dysfunction.
- Tension: Chronic constipation, vaginal deliveries, high frequency or load of squats, which can lead to pudendal nerve irritation, levator ani avulsion, and MTrPs.

- Structure and biomechanics: Pelvic obliquity, leg length discrepancy, sciatica, and hip, low back, and sacroiliac joint dysfunction can cause pelvic pain.
- Trauma: Surgery, motor vehicle accidents, and athletic injuries can cause pelvic pain.
- Insidious onset: In a small number of cases the etiology appears completely idiopathic.

CLINICAL DECISION MAKING CASE STUDY—PATIENT PROFILE ⑦

The patient is an 18-year-old female athlete who reports burning with urination, vaginal itching, and suprapubic pain. Her symptoms are always worse in the evening after she has worked out in the gym. The results of her cultures are negative for urinary tract and vaginal infections. What are the possible causes of her symptoms and underlying impairments?

Answer
Gym equipment such as the sitting adduction machine and abdominal machine can overload the adductors and rectus abdominus muscles leading to MTrPs in these muscle groups. The trigger points can cause the urinary and vaginal symptoms as well as the suprapubic pain. Additionally, these muscles act as synergists to the pelvic floor muscles and can lead to the development of hypertonus, further contributing to the pelvic pain syndrome.

SYMPTOM LOCATION

WHAT INFLUENCE DOES THE LOCATION OF SYMPTOMS HAVE ON YOUR CLINICAL DECISION-MAKING PROCESS?

The location of pelvic pain is often considered to be anywhere between the umbilicus and the mid-thigh circumferentially around the body (Figure II-14-1).[20] There may be only one small, specific area that is affected, as in the perineum or suprapubic region, or there may be a more diffuse spread of pain symptoms over the entire abdomen, buttocks, or even genital region. Due to the location of symptoms potentially being spread over several body areas, consideration of local structures as well as remote structures is imperative to determine the tissue in peril in an attempt to identify the true pain generator.

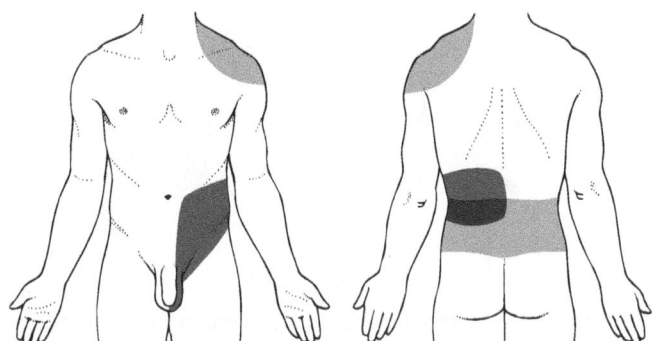

FIGURE II-14-1 Renal pain is typically felt in the posterior subcostal and costovertebral region (dark gray). It can radiate across the low back (light gray) and/or forward around the flank into the lower abdominal quadrant. Ipsilateral groin and testicular pain may also accompany renal pain. Pressure from the kidney on the diaphragm may cause ipsilateral shoulder pain. (From Goodman CC. *Differential Diagnosis for Physical Therapists: Screening for Referral.* 4th ed. Philadelphia: Saunders; 2007.)

REFERRAL OF SYMPTOMS

CONNECTIVE TISSUE CONTRIBUTION
The layer of connective tissue overlying the muscles has an opportunity to play a major role in pelvic pain. Due to the numerous nocioceptors, nerves, and vascular vessels, this tissue layer can experience dysfunction and pain during everyday activities that generate mechanical stress such as sitting or wearing tight clothing. Like all tissues the cutaneous and subcutaneous connective tissue layers may encounter both acute and chronic changes. Some of the alterations noted may be abnormalities in tissue contour, temperature, elasticity, color, turgor, and bulk.[20] The most common zones for these changes to occur are shown in Figure II-14-1. Another potential reason for this tissue layer to become problematic is the result of afferent stimuli arising from dysfunction of a visceral nature.[7] This concept will be discussed further in the visceral contribution section of this chapter.

Subcutaneous connective tissue abnormalities and trigger points can commonly be noted in the abdominal wall, proximal and lateral thighs, inguinal region, buttocks, and perineum.

MUSCULAR CONTRIBUTION
Travell and Simons have shown that muscle can be a direct source of pain symptoms. The concept stems from an MTrP being a hyperirritable spot in skeletal muscle that is associated with a hypersensitive palpable nodule in a taut band. The spot is painful on compression and can give rise to characteristic referred pain, referred tenderness, motor dysfunction, and autonomic phenomena.[56] The population suffering from pelvic pain may have MTrPs in a variety of muscles. Extensive muscular evaluation of the trunk, lumbar spine, pelvic girdle, hips, perineum, and proximal lower extremities must take place when looking for musculoskeletal impairments contributing to pelvic pain. See Table II-14-1 for pelvic muscular referral patterns.

JOINT (CAPSULE/CARTILAGE) CONTRIBUTION
Due to the referral patterns of the lumbar spine, pelvic girdle, and hip regions, these joint structures must be taken into consideration since they may overlap the distribution of pelvic pain.
- According to Fukui et al the following patterns refer to the lumbar zygapophyseal joint:[23]
  L1/2: Lumbar spine
  L2/3: Lumbar spine, greater trocanter
  L3/4: Greater trocanter, lateral thigh, posterior thigh, groin
  L4/5: Lumbar spine, greater trocanter, lateral thigh, posterior thigh, groin
  L5/S1: Gluteal, greater trocanter, lateral thigh, posterior thigh, groin
- The most common referral patterns of the sacroiliac joint (pelvic girdle) are as follows:[21,22,53]
  Posterior sacroiliac spine
  Buttock
  Low back
  Posterior thigh
  Lateral hip
  Groin
- The most common referral patterns of the hip joint are as follows:[34,62]
  Groin
  Lateral hip
  Medial thigh
  Anterior thigh
  Buttock

BONE AND LIGAMENT CONTRIBUTION
No studies have been conducted on the referral pattern of bone or ligament pathology in pelvic pain.

TABLE II-14-1 Muscular Causes of Pelvic Pain

Muscle	Referred Pain Area	Symptoms
Iliopsoas	Ipsilateral spine (thoracic, upper buttock), anterior thigh, groin, lower abdomen	Pain with weight-bearing or hip extension
Piriformis	Low back, buttock, pelvic floor	Pain in referred areas worsening with sitting, standing, walking; sciatica
Quadratus lumborum	Sacroiliac joint and buttock, anterior ilium, lower abdominal region, groin, greater trochanter	Pain in low back with walking, coughing, or sneezing
Abdominal muscles		
Transverse	Groin, inguinal ligament, detrusor, and urinary sphincter spasm	Urinary frequency or retention, groin pain, bladder pain
Rectus	Across the thoracolumbar back, xiphoid process, sacroiliac joints, and low back	Somatovisceral response, projectile vomiting, anorexia, nausea, intestinal colic, diarrhea, dysmenorrhea
Gluteus maximus	Buttock region	Pain with prolonged sitting, walking uphill, or swimming the crawl stroke
Gluteus medius	Posterior crest of the ilium, the sacrum, posterior and lateral buttock	Pain with walking, lying on one's side, and sitting
Sphincter ani, superficial transverse perinea, levator ani, coccygeus	Coccyx, anal area, lower sacrum, vagina	Tailbone, hip and back pain, painful bowel movements, perineal pain with sitting
Ischiocavernous and bulbospongiosus	Genital structures	Dyspareunia, perineal ache
Obturator internus	Vagina, anococcygeal, posterior thigh	Rectal fullness, posterior thigh pain

Prendergast SA, Weiss JM. Screening for musculoskeletal causes of pelvic pain. *Clin Obstet Gynecol* 2003;46(4):773-82.

TABLE II-14-2 Peripheral Nerve Causes of Pelvic Pain

Nerve	Sensory Innervation	Visceral Field of Referred Pain
Iliohypogastric	Posterior superior gluteal region, anterior suprapubic area	Ovary and distal fallopian tube
Ilioinguinal	Medial thigh and lateral labia majora, below inguinal ligament	Proximal tube and uterine fundus
Genitofemoral	Proximal anterior thigh	Proximal tube and uterine fundus
Lateral or femoral cutaneous	Lateral anterior thigh	Fundus and lower uterine segment
Pudendal	Dermatomes S2 to S4, perineum, perianal area	Lower uterine segment, cervix, bladder, distal ureter, upper vagina, rectum

Prendergast SA, Weiss JM. Screening for musculoskeletal causes of pelvic pain. *Clin Obstet Gynecol* 2003;46(4):773-82.

NERVE CONTRIBUTION[15,64,65]

Iliohypogastric nerve (Table II-14-2)
    Ilioinguinal nerve (see Table II-14-2)
    Genitofemoral nerve (see Table II-14-2)
Pudendal nerve (see Table II-14-2) branches below the innervate perineum and genital region
    Inferior rectal branch
    Perineal branch
    Dorsal branch to penis or clitoris
    Lateral femoral cutaneous nerve (see Table II-14-2)
Posterior femoral cutaneous nerve
    Inferior cluneal nerves

VISCERAL STRUCTURES[28]

Bladder/urethra: Suprapubic region, lower abdomen (Figure II-14-2)
    Ureter: Lower abdomen, ipsilateral testis or labium (Figure II-14-3)
    Prostate gland: Pelvis, perineum, testes (Figure II-14-4)
    Uterus: Deep pelvis, lower abdomen
    Appendix: Pelvis
    Small bowel, colon, sigmoid, rectum: Deep pelvis, lower abdomen

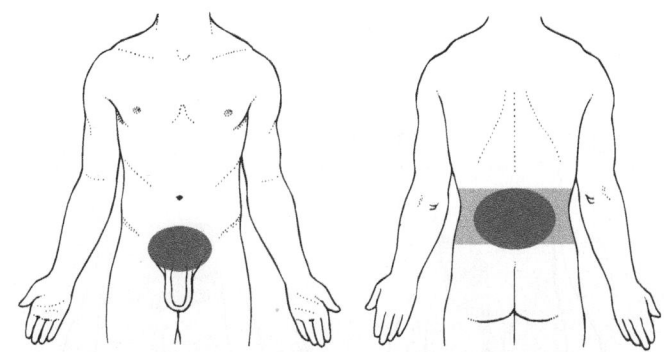

FIGURE II-14-2 (Left) Bladder or urethral pain is usually felt suprapubically or ipsilaterally in the lower abdomen. This is the same pattern for gas pain from the lower gastrointestinal tract for some people. (Right) Bladder or urethral pain may also be perceived in the low back area (dark gray: primary pain center; light gray: referred pain). Low back pain may occur as the first and only symptom associated with bladder/urethral pain, or it may occur along with suprapubic or abdominal pain or both. (From Goodman CC. *Differential Diagnosis for Physical Therapists: Screening for Referral.* 4th ed. Philadelphia: Saunders; 2007.)

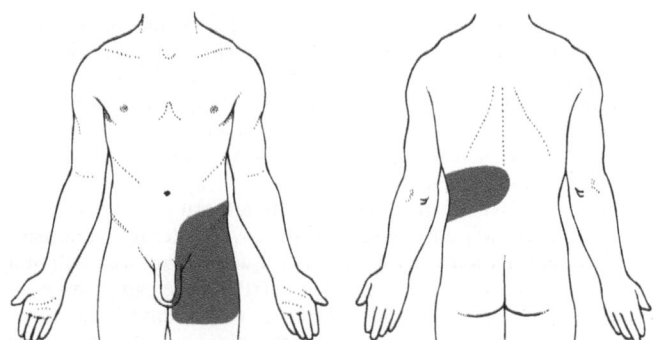

FIGURE II-14-3 Ureteral pain may begin posteriorly in the costovertebral angle. It may then radiate anteriorly to the ipsilateral lower abdomen, upper thigh, testes, or labium. (From Goodman CC. *Differential Diagnosis for Physical Therapists: Screening for Referral.* 4th ed. Philadelphia: Saunders; 2007.)

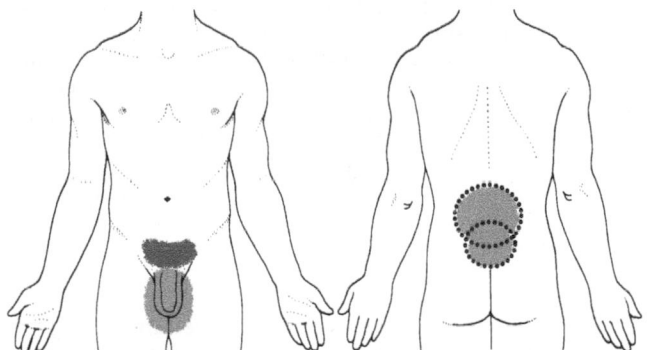

FIGURE II-14-4 The prostate is segmentally innervated from T11 to L1 and S2 to S4. Prostate problems can be painless. When pain occurs, the primary pain pattern is in the lower abdomen, suprapubic region (dark gray), and perineum (between the rectum and testes; not pictured). Pain can be referred to the low back, sacrum, testes, and inner thighs (light gray). (From Goodman CC. *Differential Diagnosis for Physical Therapists: Screening for Referral.* 4th ed. Philadelphia: Saunders; 2007.)

VASCULAR STRUCTURES[28]

Iliac arteries/veins with occlusion
Ovarian veins with varicosities
Abdominal aorta with aneurysm (rare)

SYMPTOM DESCRIPTORS[16]

QUALITY OF SYMPTOMS

Deep ache: Muscle, viscera
Dull ache: Muscle, viscera, skin
Sharp pain: Muscle, skin
Burning: Nerve, vascular, skin
Tingling: Nerve, muscle
Numbness: Nerve, muscle
Throbbing: Vascular
Colicky and cramping: Viscera, muscle
Pressure: Muscle, viscera

The conditions under which the patient feels the particular pain will help direct the clinician as to which tissue to address. This may be one or all of the various tissues. If there is an MTrP present the description may be of a poorly localized deep ache in the referral zone associated with the trigger point.[56]

WHAT INFLUENCE DOES THE DEPTH OF SYMPTOMS HAVE ON YOUR CLINICAL DECISION-MAKING PROCESS?

- Pain complaints described as deep can be of a muscular or visceral origin. A previous pathology in an organ can activate an MTrP that continues to refer pain that is similar to the pain present when the organ was dysfunctional.[56] Similarly, MTrPs can provoke a functional disturbance of an organ.[19] Abdominal trigger points can cause projectile vomiting, diarrhea, urinary bladder and sphincter spasm producing urinary frequency, urinary retention, groin pain, and/or testicular pain.
- Superficial pain complaints may be the result of changes in the cutaneous tissues as a result of the neural reflexes altering the vascularity in the referral zones associated with a trigger point or with a dysfunctional viscus.[11] Trophic changes in the referral zones associated with a trigger point or with a dysfunctional viscus include vasoconstriction, increased thickening of the skin, increased thickening of the subcutaneous tissue, and localized muscular changes.[32] The muscular changes can include hardening, increased tension, and hypersensitivity.[61] Trigger points can develop in the muscles that are within the referral zone of a dysfunctional organ. Mechanical compression of the microvasculature in the referral zone causes additional vascular compromise to the tissues that could cause burning and stinging pain complaints.

WHAT INFLUENCE DOES CONSTANCY OF SYMPTOMS HAVE ON YOUR CLINICAL DECISION-MAKING PROCESS?

- Intermittent symptoms are characteristic of an active MTrP.[56] Activity can aggravate a latent trigger point converting it to an active trigger point. Elimination of perpetuating factors and adequate rest can spontaneously reverse an active trigger point to a latent condition.[56]
- Intermittent symptoms such as those associated with localized provoked vulvar pain would indicate a sensitization of the neural structures.
- Constant pain symptoms such as with unprovoked generalized vulvar pain or the persistent sense of urge associated with painful bladder syndrome would indicate neural sensitization as a result of the trophic changes of a viscerosomatic/somatovisceral reflex.[60] The medical management would have ruled out any acute visceral pathology such as an acute bacterial cystitis or a vaginal fungal or bacterial infection.
- Constant but varying symptoms such as urge with varying degrees of urgency would indicate a neural source. Urgency with urge incontinence can be a consequence of a parasympathetic discharge when there are strong emotional circumstances associated with a generalized sympathetic response.[24]

TWENTY-FOUR-HOUR SYMPTOM PATTERN

IF A PATIENT HAS SYMPTOMS IN THE MORNING WHAT PATHOLOGY DOES THIS IMPLICATE?

- Patients with painful bladder syndrome/interstitial cystitis may wake up with an intense sense of urge, pressure, and suprapubic pain that will be relieved once they void. If they are one of the unfortunate painful bladder syndrome patients who experiences nocturia they may not experience increased symptoms in the morning.
- Vulvar pain syndromes may be increased on awakening depending on the sleep attire.

CLINICAL PEARL

Pelvic pain syndromes are very responsive to the vascular condition of the tissues. Generalized vasoconstriction is present in the connective tissues of the referral zone of an MTrP or a viscerosomatic reflex promoting allodynia.[32] Under extreme allodynic conditions very light movement of bed clothing or sheets can increase pain. Wearing underwear or pajamas with binding elastic around the thigh crease can cause mechanical compression of the microvasculature furthering the vascular compromise in the tissues.

WHAT ROLE DOES MORNING STIFFNESS PLAY IN DIFFERENTIATION?

- Stiffness in the pelvic pain population is primarily related to the soft tissue structures of muscle and connective tissue.
- Stiffness of the pelvic floor musculature is usually present on awakening in patients who have frequency and urge symptoms but who do not have nocturia. Complaints of worsening sensations of urge resulting in frequency after the first void in the morning lasting several hours is very common in this patient population.
- Patients with chronic pelvic pain of an extremely long duration will complain of a sensation of strangulation in the tissues of the lower trunk. It is also described as a sense of "shrink-wrapping." This form of stiffness is not joint related, but is secondary to the trophic changes in the muscle and connective tissue of the referral zones associated with their specific pain syndrome.

IF A PATIENT HAS SYMPTOMS IN THE AFTERNOON, WHAT PELVIC PAIN DOES THIS IMPLICATE?

- Pain symptoms through the day will of course vary depending on the type of activity in which the patient is involved. Obviously, pain in the saddle area worsens with sitting.

CLINICAL PEARL

Rather than have a patient buy cushions to decrease their pain in sitting, have the patient not sit beyond their tolerance level. If they can sit for 15 minutes pain free, at minute 16 they should stand up and do some form of upright aerobic activity such as walking, running, stairs, or jumping jacks. The purpose is to increase the vascular condition of the weight-bearing tissues of the saddle area. Desensitization of the area will be achieved by direct stress loading.

IF A PATIENT HAS SYMPTOMS IN THE EVENING, WHAT PATHOLOGY DOES THIS IMPLICATE?

- Urinary complaints may worsen in the evening once patients are at home as a result of fewer cognitive distractions.
- Pain conditions as a result of MTrPs may worsen at night as a result of the increased activity of patient's workday activating MTrPs.[56]

IF A PATIENT HAS SYMPTOMS WHEN SLEEPING, WHAT PATHOLOGY DOES THIS IMPLICATE?

- Chronic pain syndromes with urinary complaints can cause patients to wake frequently to void. This may be caused by a highly sensitized bladder, activation of acute abdominal MTrPs with bed mobility, or by mechanical irritation of the bladder by adherent scar tissue.
- Falling asleep may be more of a problem secondary to the patient feeling a constant sense of urge, which makes them get up to void four to six times before they even fall asleep. This may be caused by the stretch to the abdominal wall while supine irritating MTrPs that refer to the bladder.
- Pressure to a trigger point with sleep positions will also aggravate symptoms.

STABILITY OF SYMPTOMS

CHANGES IN SYMPTOMS

- There are many pelvic pain syndromes. They include vulvodynia, painful bladder syndrome/interstitial cystitis, chronic prostatitis/chronic pelvic pain syndrome, penile pain, orchialgia, proctalgia fugax, and levator ani syndrome. Variations in their presentations can occur. Some may have no pain, with just bladder or bowel symptoms, or pain with only one or both areas involved. A treatment approach addressing the connective, muscular, and neural tissue involves reflex and direct mechanisms of symptom management.
- Connective tissue manipulation to the referral zones associated with the specific pelvic pain syndrome will reflexively decrease symptoms.[16] Patients with urinary frequency and urge will first notice that their nocturia resolves. MTrP release can provide an immediate decrease in both symptoms of pain and frequency.
- Reflex desensitization that occurs with connective tissue manipulation and trigger point release will provide gradual resolution of extreme allodynia that is present with vulvar pain syndromes.

CLINICAL DECISION MAKING CASE STUDY—PATIENT PROFILE

A 25-year-old female presents to you with grade 4 dyspareunia that has been present since she married a year ago. A medical work-up has resulted in a diagnosis of localized provoked vulvodynia that is eventually going to require a vestibulectomy. The patient wanted to try therapy before surgery. After a year of therapy with many different therapists her symptoms have worsened to the point that the internal treatment exacerbates her symptoms from provoked to unprovoked for several days after therapy. Would you do an internal examination initially and would you start with internal treatment?

Answer

In a case this severe there is no reason to immediately do a pelvic examination. At this time you want to avoid increasing her symptoms so that you can start the desensitization process. Treating the trophic changes of the connective tissue in the muscle and visceral referral zones first will gradually, reflexively desensitize the vulvar tissues.

CLINICAL PEARL

Many female patients with pelvic pain need to be under general anesthesia to have an internal pelvic examination. Physical therapy will not enable an internal evaluation to be done until the allodynia has decreased. External connective tissue manipulation and trigger point release performed over the course of 6 to 8 weeks can reflexively decrease the allodynia. Once an internal examination can be tolerated, direct stress loading can be added to the reflexive therapeutic techniques. As desensitization progresses, directed myofascial manipulation can be done to address the trigger points in the pelvic floor and urogenital musculature.

A steady decrease in symptoms as a result of an integrated soft tissue approach would indicate that the pelvic pain syndrome being treated is associated with a viscerosomatic/somatovisceral reflex.

When symptoms seem to worsen or there is a sudden change in the character of the symptoms the clinician needs to rule out a new onset infectious pathology. This would include acute cystitis, acute prostatitis, and bacterial or fungal vaginal infections.

CLINICAL PEARL

Experiencing long-term pelvic pain can make it difficult for a patient to know that they may actually be experiencing a new infectious process. Painful bladder syndrome/

interstitial cystitis or chronic prostatitis/chronic pelvic pain syndrome patients usually complain of acute infectious symptoms all the time. Over the years all of their cultures have been negative. But during treatment if there has been a steady improvement and then things suddenly change this needs to be checked. This should include a urinalysis and culture and sensitivity. If the office urinalysis is positive the physician will give the patient 3 days of antibiotics and a pain reliever specific to the lower urinary tract such as phenazopyridine. Once the culture results are received the physician will adjust and continue antibiotic management or discontinue it if the culture is negative. If the culture was positive the patient should have a cure culture done 1 week after the last antibiotic is taken.

When treating an acute vaginal infection in patients with vulvar pain syndromes intravaginal cream or suppository medications should be avoided. Migration of the medication out of the vagina will increase their pain through mechanical allodynia.

FUNCTIONAL AND ACTIVITY PARTICIPATION LIMITATIONS

BEHAVIOR OF SYMPTOMS: AGGRAVATING BEHAVIOR

- Most patients with chronic pain stop moving because they feel that there is increased discomfort from all movement. The patient should be encouraged to maintain as high a level of activity as possible. Aerobic activity is especially important to facilitate and maintain the changes in vascular reflex that are being made as a result of the connective tissue manipulation. Walking is the easiest form of aerobic activity to initiate. The patient and clinician should determine the maximum tolerance level that can be performed. It may be only several minutes, but the patient then repeats that level of activity many times a day. The goal for the patient would be a 30-minute brisk walk daily.
- Aggravating behavior for muscles with trigger points would include strenuous use of the muscle, especially in a shortened position, prolonged shortening, a quick stretch to the muscle, repeated or sustained contraction, or pressure to the trigger point.[56]
- Prolonged sitting can have a negative impact on many muscles that may be involved in the various pelvic pain syndromes. Iliopsoas trigger points, which can be aggravated by sitting, can refer pain to the testicle giving rise to the diagnosis of orchialgia.
- The pressure of weight bearing while sitting can aggravate trigger points in the urogenital diaphragm. The lengthening contraction and relaxation of the urogenital diaphragm during voiding and defecation can also aggravate the trigger points of these muscles. Urethral pain is the most common pain complaint in both men and women when there are acute trigger points in the urogenital diaphragm musculature. Levator ani and urogenital diaphragm trigger points in both sexes are activated by the maximal contraction of the muscles during orgasm.

BEHAVIOR OF SYMPTOMS: EASING BEHAVIOR

- Mechanical compression of the microvasculature of the referral zone can increase the symptoms. Releasing the mechanical compression and increasing the vascularity of the tissues will ease the symptoms. This can be accomplished by manual manipulation of the tissues and/or easy repetitive contractions of the large muscles of the area such as when climbing stairs or walking.

CLINICAL DECISION MAKING CASE STUDY—PATIENT PROFILE   (?)

Your patient is a 41-year-old male who presents with a 3-1/2 year history of pain when sitting. The location of the pain is in the area that is "not touched by the toilet seat." It is localized to the outside anal opening, into the cheeks of the buttocks, and at the ischial tuberosities. He is much more comfortable sitting on a hard than a soft surface. Sitting tolerance is 5 to 10 minutes. The onset began after he started a job that required 4+ hours of uninterrupted sitting. He is not a cyclist and had been active in health-related sports before his pain. What is your first impression as to what is the pathological tissue involved?

Answer

Most therapists would initially say that it was probably pudendal neuralgia. He did have a pudendal block that was inconclusive. He had no risk factors for pudendal insult and he had no injuries that he could recall, falls, or motor vehicle accidents. His only report of significance was a new job with prolonged sitting. The average person will sit for a while and then will adjust themselves to unweight the tissues that have been vascularly compromised from compression. This is referred to as ideomotor activities. Many people can get so engrossed in their work that they ignore their body's signals. A prolonged decreased blood supply to the saddle area can compromise the health of the connective tissues and the neural tissues. Some of the areas that he described as having pain are not innervated by the pudendal nerve. There are other nerves in the area that should be considered such as the posterior femoral cutaneous nerve and its branches.

Symptoms from an activated trigger point can be decreased by slow, steady, passive stretching of the muscle, active contraction of the antagonist, or a short period of rest. Levator ani or urogenital diaphragm trigger points activated by orgasm, voiding, or defecation may be decreased by actively lengthening the pelvic floor musculature. This can be done reflexively by squatting. Active lengthening of the pelvic floor while in a squat can also be done to decrease symptoms.

MEDICAL HISTORY

WHAT ROLE DOES THE PATIENT'S PREVIOUS MEDICAL HISTORY PLAY IN THE DIAGNOSIS OF PELVIC PAIN?

Previous surgeries, injuries, and other medical pathology can have an impact on the viscera, muscles, connective tissue, and nerves of the pelvis causing or contributing to the etiology of various pelvic pain syndromes.

- Chronic gynecological or urological infections such as yeast infections, urinary tract infections, bacterial vaginosis, or bacterial prostatitis can cause visceral and/or neural irritation, pelvic floor muscle hypertonus, and/or connective tissue dysfunction.[11,56] This can result in pelvic floor dysfunction and pudendal neuralgia.
- Any gynecological, urological, or colorectal surgical procedure such as a hysterectomy, pelvic reconstruction, sphincterotomy, hemorrhoidectomy, Cesarean section, laparoscopy, and laparotomy can cause scar tissue formation, pelvic floor muscle trauma, and peripheral nerve injury. Scar tissue causes connective tissue dysfunction, which can cause visceral disturbances, such as bladder irritation, via the somatovisceral reflex.[11,56] When pelvic floor muscles are traumatized, MTrPs are likely to develop resulting in decreased motor function, such as urinary or bowel dysfunction, and referred pain. Nerve injury will affect muscle tone and motor control and may cause pain in

its territory. For example, an injury to the pudendal nerve may cause penile pain and erectile dysfunction.

- Pregnancy can cause pelvic pain in several ways. During pregnancy, ligamentous laxity occurs in response to progesterone and relaxin. This laxity can cause sacroiliac joint dysfunction, which may result in adverse neural tension on the pudendal nerve, and/or cause pelvic girdle muscle imbalances leading to muscle hypertonus and MTrPs resulting in pelvic pain. In addition, the mechanical strain of pregnancy posture frequently causes pelvic pain.[4] Vaginal childbirth can cause a pudendal nerve tension injury and/or pelvic floor muscle trauma, particularly the levator ani muscle group, resulting in pelvic pain.[17] Cesarean sections cause suprapubic scar tissue formation and traumatize the abdominal musculature often resulting in abdominal muscle MTrPs that can cause referred pain to the pubic symphysis, groin, and vagina. Lastly, during pregnancy a woman can develop a diastasis recti, which is a midline separation of the rectus abdominus musculature or a defect in the linea alba. A diastasis recti decreases the ability of the rectus muscles to stabilize the core, which results in the formation of MTrPs in the abdominal musculature, which can cause pelvic pain and dysfunction.
- Diseases such as endometriosis commonly cause pelvic pain and dyspareunia. Endometriosis itself and the laparoscopic procedure to remove it will cause scar tissue formation in the pelvis, which can negatively affect muscle and connective tissue.
- Excessive straining from chronic constipation creates adverse neural tension on the pudendal nerve causing pudendal neuralgia and pelvic pain.
- Previous pelvic girdle musculoskeletal injuries, such as an adductor strain, may result in unresolved MTrPs in those muscles, causing referred pain to the pelvis and/or causing biomechanical changes to the pelvis.[56]

CLINICAL PEARL

Chronic constipation can cause adverse neural tension on the pudendal nerve. Symptoms such as chronic constipation coupled with sharp burning pain in the rectum or anus may indicate a diagnosis of pudendal neuralgia. During the internal evaluation, tenderness on palpating the pudendal nerve or a positive Tinel's sign may further indicate a diagnosis of pudendal neuralgia.

CLINICAL PEARL

A diastasis recti is a common disorder in pregnant and postpartum women. In the postpartum woman it decreases core stability causing the other abdominal muscles to overcompensate. MTrPs will often form in these abdominal muscles and may be the cause of pain at the pubic symphysis and vagina and urinary dysfunction such as incontinence and urinary urgency and/or frequency.

MEDICAL AND ORTHOPEDIC TESTING

WHAT MEDICAL AND ORTHOPEDIC TEST INFLUENCES YOUR DIFFERENTIAL DIAGNOSIS PROCESS?

Culture and sensitivity tests, magnetic resonance imaging (MRI), and electroneuromyographic (ENMG) tests have limited use in diagnosing pelvic pain. A comprehensive history and thorough physical examination will provide the most information with which to make your differential diagnosis.

- Lefaucheur et al stated that "perineal ENMG has a limited sensitivity and specificity in the diagnosis of pudendal nerve entrapment and does not give direct information about pain mechanisms."[38]
- Le Tallec de Certaines reported that pudendal nerve terminal motor latency test values can be elevated in patients without pudendal nerve entrapment.[37]
- Urine dip-sticks in the diagnosis of urinary infections have an extremely poor sensitivity and specificity of 36.3% and 57.8%, respectively. Urine culture, with documented efficacy, remains the gold standard.[39]
- Pap smear and vaginal culture test results had a sensitivity of 43.1% and 77.8%, specificity of 93.6% and 97.7%, positive predictive value of 73.8% and 93.3%, negative predictive value of 79.8% and 91.4%, and diagnostic value of 78.8% and 91.8%, respectively, for the diagnosis of bacterial vaginosis. Compared to microbiological test results, a Pap smear is not sensitive enough for screening of bacterial vaginosis.[55]

MEDICATIONS

HOW DOES A PATIENT'S RESPONSE TO MEDICATION INFLUENCE YOUR DECISION-MAKING PROCESS?

Muscle relaxants, pain medications, anticonvulsants, antiinflammatories, antibiotics, and antidepressants are commonly prescribed for patients with pelvic pain depending on the impairments.

- Symptom relief with muscle relaxants, such as valium, suggests that the pain is of musculoskeletal rather than neuropathic origin; however, most patients with pelvic pain, regardless of its etiology, will have muscle hypertonus and therefore may respond to valium.
- Symptom relief from antibiotics is very helpful in the differential diagnosis, suggesting that at least some of the pain is secondary to a bacterial infection. Conversely, the absence of symptomatic relief from antibiotic therapy suggests misdiagnosis and indicates that the symptoms may be due to a myofascial pain syndrome and/or neuropathic pain.
- Although uncommon in pelvic pain, symptom relief with anti-inflammatory medications suggests that the pathology has an acute inflammatory process. A pelvic pain pathology with an acute inflammatory process would involve muscle trauma that occurred during vaginal childbirth.[17]
- Symptom relief with anticonvulsants, such as Neurontin or Lyrica, and antidepressants, such as amyltriptoline and Cymbalta, indicates that the pain is likely of neuropathic origin, which will facilitate the differential diagnosis.[18,63]
- The effectiveness of pain medications is minimal in differentially diagnosing pelvic pain because they decrease pain of various origins.
- Topical analgesics (i.e., lidocaine, Lidoderm® patch) can work as an adjunct with anticonvulsants, antidepressants, and pain medications to effectively decrease neuropathic pain, but a positive response does not facilitate the decision-making process.

BIOMECHANICAL

WHAT ROLE DOES BIOMECHANICS PLAY IN THE DECISION-MAKING PROCESS?

Evaluating the biomechanics of the pelvic girdle is one component of a multifaceted comprehensive evaluation of a patient with pelvic pain. Therefore, biomechanical objective findings should be considered in conjunction with other clinical findings during the decision-making process.

WHAT BIOMECHANICAL ABNORMALITIES IN OTHER REGIONS AFFECT YOUR DECISION-MAKING PROCESS?

Abnormalities in the biomechanics of the spine, lumbosacral junction, and sacroiliac joints can affect the muscle tone, joint stability, and neural mobility of the pelvic girdle causing pelvic pain.

- Baker identified a lumbar lordosis, kyphosis of the thoracic spine, and anterior pelvic tilt posture in 75% of patients with chronic pelvic pain.[4]
- Hunter and Zihlman related the anterior pelvic tilt posture to stretching of the coccygeus and shortening of the piriformis in response to the biomechanical forces generated in that posture.[33] The anterior pelvic tilt posture is also known to shorten the iliopsoas muscle, which was associated with patients with pelvic pain.[4]
- Hypermobile upper lumbar/low thoracic segments may become inflamed and refer pain to the lower abdominal quadrant.
- Lower quadrant symptoms can cause traction on the abdominal, paravertebral, and gluteal muscles; these occur with the asymmetric pelvic posture associated with an anatomic short leg.[52]

ENVIRONMENTAL FACTORS

DO PSYCHOSOCIAL ISSUES INFLUENCE THE CLINICAL DECISION-MAKING PROCESS?

Depression, anxiety, and panic are common psychiatric comorbidities in patients with chronic pelvic pain.[2,13,57] Referral to the proper mental health specialist is a vital component in a successful treatment plan.

CAN EMOTIONS INFLUENCE THE DECISION-MAKING PROCESS?

Due to the high frequency of all psychosocial variables in the patient with chronic pelvic pain, many patients are highly concerned about their pain, current functional state, their relationships, and their prognosis. If patients are continuously focusing on their pain, proper referral to a mental health specialist is indicated.

DO WORK-RELATED INJURIES INFLUENCE THE CLINICAL DECISION-MAKING PROCESS?

All injuries, including those work related, must be taken into consideration when making clinical decisions regarding a patient with pelvic pain since they may have an effect on the patient's symptoms (Box II-14-1).

PERSONAL FACTORS

Personal factors including occupation, personal relationships, and psychological health can all affect pelvic pain.

BOX II-14-1	Contextual Factors
Environmental	Prolonged sitting during work, driving, or recreation (cyclists), frequent urine retention, vigorous sexual activity, or long distance running are all potential factors for the development of trigger points within the pelvic floor musculature.
Personal	Chronic pelvic pain may be a physical manifestation of personal internal stressors from anxiety, personality disorders, depression, and emotional unrest.

WHAT PREVIOUS SURGERIES INFLUENCE YOUR CLINICAL DECISION MAKING?

Gynecological, urological, and colorectal surgical procedures can all exacerbate or cause pelvic pain.

- Some pelvic reconstruction surgical procedures hitch the bladder to the sacrospinous ligament, which can entrap the pudendal nerve; surgical decompression of the pudendal nerve may therefore be indicated.
- Hysterectomies create scar tissue in the pelvis as well as cause pelvic floor muscle trauma that will require manual soft tissue and muscle mobilization to normalize.

CLINICAL PEARL

The presence of sharp, shooting, burning pain in the territory of the pudendal nerve immediately following a hysterectomy or pelvic reconstruction procedure may indicate a pudendal nerve entrapment secondary to the surgical procedure itself. Referring this patient for a consult with a surgeon who performs a surgical decompression of the pudendal nerve is warranted.

DOES A FAMILY HISTORY OF PELVIC PAIN IN THE REGION INFLUENCE YOUR CLINICAL REASONING PROCESS?

There is no literature indicating a genetic predisposition to most pelvic pain syndromes. Although more research is indicated, studies have shown that heritability accounts for the development of endometriosis to an extent similar to other complex genetic diseases.[58]

CLINICAL PEARL

An 18-year-old female reporting severe abdominal and/or pelvic pain and dyspareunia coupled with dysmenorrhea and a family history of endometriosis may have undiagnosed endometriosis. This patient should be referred to her gynecologist for further evaluation.

CHRONICITY OF PAIN

WHAT CENTRAL PROCESSING CHANGES OCCUR THAT INFLUENCE YOUR DECISION MAKING?

Chronic pelvic pain continues to be difficult to diagnose as well as treat. Unfortunately, many patients with chronic pelvic pain are misdiagnosed and therefore receive ineffective treatment. By the time this patient population obtains a correct diagnosis and finds the appropriate clinician, central processing changes have occurred making their case even more complex and challenging to treat. These changes can include central sensitization of the nervous system, which occurs in patients with chronic neuropathic pain and causes the patient to be hypersensitive to all pain stimuli. A patient who has undergone central sensitization will typically require a longer duration of treatment and will likely benefit from pain management.

HAS MEDICAL TREATMENT BEEN SUCCESSFUL FOR PATIENTS WITH CHRONIC PELVIC PAIN IN THE REGION?

Medical interventions for pelvic pain can include manual physical therapy, surgery, pharmaceutical therapy, trigger point injections, nerve blocks, and/or neuromodulation. There has been minimal consensus in studies published on the effectiveness of these interventions on pelvic pain.

- Manual physical therapy to the pelvic floor was found to be effective in patients with interstitial cystitis and urethral syndrome. Of the 42 patients with urethral syndrome, 83% had moderate to marked improvement or complete resolution and 70% of those with interstitial cystitis had moderate to marked improvement.[59]
- A study found that 20% of patients who underwent various laparoscopic procedures for their pelvic pain had unsatisfactory results.[10]
- A recent study showed that approximately 80% of women with vulvodynia treated with 2% to 6% gabapentin demonstrated at least a 50% improvement in pain scores.[8] A qualitative study of women with vulvodynia showed that 27 of 29 women reported a significant benefit from a multidisciplinary management program consisting of medial evaluation and treatment, psychotherapy, physiotherapy, and dietary advice.[41]
- A critical review of published studies concerning the treatment of provoked vestibulodynia showed that surgical treatment had the best success rates, between 61% and 94%; medical treatment had success rates of 13% to 67% and behavioral treatments had success rates of 35% to 83%. However, only 5 of the 38 studies reviewed were randomized clinical trials; therefore the studies have several methodological weaknesses.[35]

DOES THE CHRONICITY OF SYMPTOMS INFLUENCE YOUR DECISION-MAKING PROCESS?

Pelvic pain due to a chronic nerve injury or compression may cause irreversible nerve damage and may be relieved only partially with therapy. This must be considered when creating realistic functional goals. Chronic pelvic floor muscle hypertonicity and/or the presence of MTrPs will require greater frequency and longer duration of treatment. Chronic neuropathic pain causes central sensitization of the nervous system, which may require pharmaceutical management and a longer duration of treatment.

HOW DOES AUTONOMIC, ENDOCRINE, AND IMMUNE SYSTEMS INFLUENCE DECISION MAKING IN THE CERVICAL REGION?

Chronic pelvic pain is typically a multifaceted disorder, simultaneously involving the psychological, peripheral nerve, autonomic, central nervous, visceral, connective tissue, endocrine, and immune systems. Therefore, a single practitioner is often ill-equipped to provide a comprehensive, multidisciplinary treatment.[40] To correctly diagnose and treat this patient population, the patient will likely require a diagnostic work-up from various medical specialists. Although much more research is needed, some diseases/syndromes that commonly cause pelvic pain involve specific systems and therefore may influence a clinician's decision-making progress (Box II-14-2).

- Interstitial cystitis is a syndrome of bladder hypersensitivity with symptoms of urgency, frequency, and chronic pelvic pain. Research has shown that neural upregulation plays a role in

BOX II-14-2	**Output Mechanisms**
Autonomic	Increased sympathetic nervous system output may cause increased tone in pelvic musculature, reduced ability to void, and vasoconstriction to superficial connective tissues. All these tissue changes may be present in chronic pelvic pain.
Endocrine	Endometriosis commonly causes pelvic pain. Although its genesis remains unknown, one common theory involves the interaction of the endocrine system.
Immune	Endometriosis may also involve the interaction of the immune system.

these symptoms.[42] In addition, research has shown that mast cell-derived histamine mediates cystitis pain in patients with interstitial cystitis.[50]

- Endometriosis, a gynecological disorder, commonly causes pelvic pain. Although its genesis remains unknown, one common theory involves the interaction of the immune and endocrine systems.[51]

RED FLAGS THAT REQUIRE REFERRAL TO A MEDICAL PHYSICIAN

WHAT SYMPTOMS ALERT YOU TO PATHOLOGY THAT MAY REQUIRE A REFERRAL TO A MEDICAL DOCTOR?

Many pelvic pain symptoms mimic common gynecological and/or urological conditions; however, when coupled with the following factors, further evaluation is indicated by a physician:

- Vaginal or vulvar itching coupled with an unusual vaginal discharge with or without a foul odor
- Dysuria and urinary frequency coupled with a foul odor and/or darkened color of urine
- Unexplained vaginal, rectal, or urethral bleeding
- Presence of a mass found during internal examination/treatment

WHAT SYMPTOMS IMPLICATE SPECIFIC VISCERAL SYSTEMS?

- The presence of blood, an unusual discharge with or without a foul odor, and unprovoked vaginal pain that does not respond to physical therapy implicate infection or disease in the vagina.
- Abdominal or suprapubic pain (especially cyclical), a change in menses, or severe dysmenorrheal implicates the female reproductive system.
- Hematuria, dysuria, or urinary urgency, frequency, or hesitancy that does not respond to physical therapy implicates the urinary system.
- The presence of blood in the stool, rectal bleeding, a change in the bowel or digestive system, or rectal/anal pain that does not respond to physical therapy implicates the gastrointestinal system.

CLINICAL DECISION MAKING CASE STUDY—PATIENT PROFILE ?

Your patient is a 35-year-old postpartum female reporting sharp, shooting, burning pain in the vagina, perineum, and rectum that began immediately following vaginal childbirth 2 months ago. She reports she "had to push for an unusually long time" during labor. She states that the pain is worse on sitting and deep squatting. What are your hypotheses regarding her pathology?

Answer
Sharp, shooting, burning pain is indicative of neuropathic pain. Pudendal nerve tension injuries can occur during vaginal childbirth, especially during long labors. Pudendal neuralgia typically increases with sitting due to compression of the nerve and increases with deep squatting due to further neural tension over the ischial spine.

CLINICAL DECISION MAKING CASE STUDY—PATIENT PROFILE ?

Your patient is a 25-year-old male who reports continued urinary frequency, weak urine stream, and postejaculatory pain. He has taken 8 weeks of antibiotics after a diagnosis of chronic prostatitis by his urologist even though his prostatic secretions are negative for bacteria and he has had no relief of his symptoms. What are your hypotheses regarding his pathology?

Answer

It is fairly rare for a 25-year-old male to have chronic prostatitis. He was likely misdiagnosed with chronic prostatitis since his prostatic secretions are negative for bacteria and the antibiotics have not decreased his symptoms. His symptoms are likely due to pelvic floor dysfunction (hypertonus), more specifically, in the urogenital diaphragm. The muscles of the urogenital diaphragm are responsible for urinary and sexual function.

SUMMARY STATEMENT

Similar to many other pain conditions, pelvic pain is usually a multifactorial disorder. The evaluation performed by a skilled physical therapist will attempt to identify mechanical changes found in the neuromusculoskeletal system. The initial focus relies heavily on the subjective examination to reveal appropriate pain regions associated with symptom behavior that may build relationships between local muscle and superficial connective tissue sources versus remote referrals from bony structures such as the lumbar spine, hip, or pelvic girdle. What complicates matters in this body region is the influence of the viscera, which can be a source of pain symptoms directly or reflexively referring changes to local somatic tissues that can then generate their own pain response. The inclusion of the viscera, as well as local pelvic muscles, allows pelvic pain conditions to influence bladder, bowel, and sexual function.

It is of paramount importance in treating pelvic pain to objectively identify impairments within the soft tissues of key regions including the superficial connective tissues, urogenital diaphragm, levator ani, and global muscle groups around the pelvis. Once an appropriate pain generator has been identified, intervention can begin. However, many cases of pelvic pain require a multidisciplinary approach to achieve positive outcomes due to the multifactorial contributions associated with this disorder.

REFERENCES

1. Anderson R, Wise D, et al. Integration of MTrP release and paradoxical relaxation training treatment of chronic pelvic pain in men. *J Urol.* 2005;174(1):155-160.

2. Anderson RU, Orenberg ED, Chan CA, Morey A, Flores V. Psychometric profiles and hypothalamic-pituitary-adrenal axis function in men with chronic prostatitis/chronic pelvic pain syndrome. *J Urol.* 2008;179(3):956-960.

3. Bachmann GA, et al. Chronic vulvar and other gynecologic pain: prevalence and characteristics in a self-reported survey. *J Reprod Med.* 2006;51(1):3-9.

4. Baker PK. Musculoskeletal origins of chronic pelvic pain diagnosis and treatment. *Obstet Gynecol Clin North Am.* 1993;20(4):719-742.

5. Bartoletti R, et al. Prevalence, incidence estimation, risk factors and characterization of chronic prostatitis/chronic pelvic pain syndrome in urological hospital outpatients in Italy: results of a multicenter case-control observational study. *J Urol.* 2007;178(6):2411-2415.

6. Bautrant E, de Bisschop E, et al. Modern algorithm for treating pudendal neuralgia: 212 cases and 104 decompressions. *J Gynecol Obstet Biol Reprod.* 2003;32(8):705-712.

7. Beal M. Viscerosomatic reflexes: a review. *J Am Osteopath Assoc.* 85(12):786-801.

8. Boardman LA, et al. Topical gabapentin in the treatment of localized and generalized vulvodynia. *Obstet Gynecol.* 2008;112(3):579-585.

9. Bohm-Starke N, Rylander E. Surgery for localized, provoked vestibulodynia: a long-term follow-up study. *J Reprod Med.* 2008;53(2):83-89.

10. Carter JE. Surgical treatment for chronic pelvic pain. *JSLS.* 1998;2(2):129-139.

11. Chaitow L. *Soft-tissue manipulation: a practitioner's guide to the diagnosis and treatment of soft tissue dysfunction and reflex activity.* New York: Healing Arts Press; 1988.

12. Chronic Prostatitis Scientific Workshop. Baltimore, MD: 2005.

13. Clemens JQ, Brown SO, Calhoun EA. Mental health diagnoses in patients with interstitial cystitis/painful bladder syndrome and chronic prostatitis/chronic pelvic pain syndrome: a case/control study. *J Urol.* 2008;180(4):1378-1382.

14. Clemens JQ. Male chronic pelvic pain syndrome: prevalence, risk factors, treatment patterns, and socioeconomic impact. *Current Prostate Reports.* 2008;6(2):81-85.

15. Darnis B, Robert R, Labat JJ, et al. Perineal pain and inferior cluneal nerves: anatomy and surgery. *Surg Radiol Anat.* 2008;30(3):177-183. Epub 2008 Feb 28.

16. Dicke E, Schliack H, Wolf A. *A Manual of Reflexive Therapy of the Connective Tissue.* Scarsdale: Sidney S. Simon; 1978.

17. Dietz HP, Lanzarone V. Levator trauma after vaginal delivery. *Obstet Gynecol.* 2005;106(4):707-712.

18. Dobecki DA, Schocket SM, Wallace MS. Update on pharmacotherapy guidelines for the treatment of neuropathic pain. *Curr Pain Headache Rep.* 2006;10(3):185-190.

19. Doggweiler R, Jasmin L, Schmidt RA. Neurogenically mediated cystitis in rats: an animal model. *J Urol.* 1998;160:1551-1556.

20. Fitgerald MP, Kotarinos R. Rehabilitation of the short pelvic floor I and II. Background and patient evaluation and treatment. *Int Urogynecol J Pelvic Floor Dysfunct.* 2003;14(4):261-268.

21. Fortin J, Aprill C, Ponthiex B, Pier J. Sacroiliac joint: pain referral maps on applying a new injection/arthrography technique: Part II: Clinical Evaluation. *Spine.* 1994;19(13):1483-1489.

22. Fortin J, Dwyer A, West S, Pier J. Sacroiliac joint: pain referral maps on applying a new injection/arthrography technique. *Spine.* 1994;19:1475-1482.

23. Fukui S, Kiyoshige O, Masahiro S, Ohno K, Karasawa H, Naganuma Y. Distribution of referred pain from the lumbar zygoapophyseal joints and dorsal rami. *Clin J Pain.* 1997;13:303-307.

24. Gatz A. *Manter's Essentials of Clinical Neuroanatomy and Neurophysiology.* Philadelphia: F.A. Davis Company; 1972.

25. Goetsch MF. Patients' assessments of a superficial modified vestibulectomy for vestibulodynia. *J Reprod Med.* 2008;53(6):407-412.

26. Goetsch MF. Surgery combined with muscle therapy for dyspareunea from vulvar vestibulitis: an observational study. *J Reprod Med.* 2007;52(7):597-603.

27. Goldstein AT, Klingman D, et al. Surgical treatment of vulvar vestibulitis syndrome: outcome assessment derived from a postoperative questionnaire. *J Sex Med.* 2006;3(50):923-931.

28. Goodman C, Snyder T. *Differential Diagnosis for Physical Therapists: Screening for Referral.* St. Louis: Saunders-Elsevier; 2007.

29. Gumus II, et al. Vulvodynia: case report and review of literature. *Gynecol Obstet Invest.* 2008;65(3):155-161.

30. Harlow BL, Stewart EG. A population-based assessment of chronic unexplained vulvar pain: have we underestimated the prevalence of vulvodynia? *J Am Med Women's Assoc.* 2003;58(2):82-88.

31. Hartmann EH, Nelson CA. Perceived effectiveness of physical therapy treatment on women with chronic vulvar pain and diagnosed with either vulvar vestibulitis syndrome or dysethetic vulvodynia. *J Sect Women's Health, APTA.* 2001;25:13-18.

32. Head H. On disturbances of sensation with especial reference to the pain. *Brain.* 1893;16:1.

33. Hunter W, Zihlman AL. Abdominal pain from strain of intrapelvic muscles [letter]. *Clin Orthop Relat Res.* 1970;279-280.

34. Khan AM, McLoughlin E, Giannakas K, Hutchinson C, Andrew JG. Hip osteoarthritis: where is the pain? *Ann R Coll Surg Engl.* 2004;86(2):119-121.

35. Landry T, et al. The treatment of provoked vestibulodynia: a critical review. *Clin J Pain.* 2008;24(2):155-171.

36. Lavy RJ, Hynan LS, Harley RW. Prevalence of vulvar pain in an urban, minority population. *J Reprod Med.* 2007;52(1):59-62.

37. Le T, et al. Comparison between the terminal motor pudendal nerve terminal motor latency, the localization of perineal neuralgia and the result of infiltrations. *Ann Readapt Med Phys.* 2007;50(2):65-69. Epub 2006 Aug 30.

38. Leufaucher JP, et al. What is the place of electroneuromyographic studies in the diagnosis and management of pudendal neuralgia related to entrapment syndrome? *Neurophysiol Clin.* 2007;37(4):223-228. Epub 2007 Aug 2.

39. Milcent S, et al. Value and justification of urine dip-sticks in the diagnosis of postoperative urinary infections in urology. *Prog Urol.* 2003;12(2):234-237.

Section II

ORTHOPEDIC REASONING

40. Moise G, Capodice JL, Winfree CJ. Treatment of chronic pelvic pain in men and women. *Expert Rev Neurother.* 2007;7(5):507-520.

41. Munday P, et al. A qualitative study of women with vulvodynia: II. Response to a multidisciplinary approach to management. *J Reprod Med.* 2007;52(1):19-22.

42. Nazif O, Teichman JM, Gebhart GF. Neural upregulation in Interstitial Cystitis. *Urology.* 2007;69(4 suppl):24-33.

43. *NIH Vulvodynia Scientific Meeting and Research Symposium.* Washington, DC: 2003.

44. Parsons JK, Kurth K, Sant GR. Epidemiologic issues in interstitial cystitis. *Urology.* 2007;69(4 suppl):5-8.

45. Popeney C, Ansell V, Renny K. Pudendal Entrapment as an etiology of chronic perineal pain: Diagnosis and treatment. *Neurourol Urodyn.* 2007;26(6):820-827.

46. Portenoy, RK, Ugarte C, et al. *Population-based survey of pain in the United States: differences among white, African American, and Hispanic subjects.*

47. Prendergast SA, Weiss JM. Screening for Musculoskeletal Causes of Pelvic Pain. *Clin Obstet Gynecol.* 2003;46(4):773-782.

48. *Research Insights into Interstitial Cystitis.* Washington, DC: 2003.

49. Robert R, Labat JJ, et al. Neurosurgical treatment of perineal neuralgias. *Adv Tech Stand Neurosurg.* 2007;32:41-59.

50. Rudick CN, et al. Mast cell-derived histamine mediates cystitis pain. *PLoS.* 2008;3(5).

51. Seli E, Arici A. Endometriosis: Interaction of immune and endocrine systems. *Semin Reprod Med.* 2003;21(2):135-144.

52. Sicuranze BJ, Richards J, Tisdal LH. The short leg syndrome in obstetrics and gynecology. *Am J Obstet Gynecol.* 1970;10:217-218.

53. Slipman C, Jackson H, Lipetz J, Chan K, Lenrow D, Vresilovic E. Sacroiliac joint pain referral zones. *Arch Phys Med Rehabil.* 2000;81:334-338.

54. Sutton JT, Bachmann GA et al. Assessment of vulvodynia symptoms in a sample of US women: a follow-up national incidence study. *J Women's Health.* 2008;17(8):1285-1292.

55. Tokyol C, et al. Bacterial vaginosis: comparison of Pap smear and microbiological test results. *Mod Pathol.* 2004;17(7):857-860.

56. Travell J, Simons D. *Myofascial Pain and Dysfunction: The Trigger Point Manual.* Vols I & II. Baltimore: Williams & Wilkins; 1992, 1999.

57. Tribo MJ, et al. Clinical characteristics and psychopathological profile of patients with vulvodynia: an observational and descriptive study. *Dermatology.* 2008;216(1):24-30.

58. Vigano P, Somigliana E, Vignali M, Busacca M, Blasio AM. Genetics of endometriosis: current status and prospects. *Front Biosci.* 2007;12:3247-3255.

59. Weiss JM. Pelvic floor MTrPs: treatment for interstitial cystitis and the urgency-frequency syndrome. *J Urol.* 2001;166(6):2226-2231.

60. Wesselman U. Interstitial cystitis: a chronic visceral pain syndrome. *Urology.* 2001;57(suppl 6A).

61. Wesselman U, Lai J. Mechanisms of referred pain: uterine inflammation in the adult virgin rat results in neurogenic plasma extravasation in the skin. *Pain.* 1997;73:309-317.

62. Wroblewski BM. Pain in osteoarthrosis of the hip. *Practitioner.* 1978;220:140-141.

63. Yamamoto T. Mechanisms of the development of neuropathic pain and its treatment. *Nihon Hansenbyo Gakkai Zasshi.* 2008;77(3):215-218.

64. Yucel S, Baskin LS. Neuroanatomy of the male urethra and perineum. *BJU Int.* 2003;92(6):624-630.

65. Yucel S, De Souza Jr A, Baskin LS. Neuroanatomy of the human female lower urogenital tract. *J Urol.* 2004;172(1):191-195.

AUTHORS: BRIAN YEE and MICHAEL SHACKLOCK

INTRODUCTORY INFORMATION

WHAT IS THE PREVALENCE OF NERVE PATHOLOGY?

- The prevalence of peripheral nerve injuries varies. One study found nerve injuries in 1.64% of patients reporting limb trauma, with 1.9% of those diagnosed by crush injuries, and in 1.46% of nerve injuries due to dislocations.[35]
- Nerve injuries due to stretch mechanisms are the most common in civilian trauma, particularly injuries resulting from motor vehicle accidents, while lacerations, by knife, glass, or fan, comprise 30% of serious nerve injuries.[7,33]
- In a comparison of upper and lower extremity nerve injuries, 73.5% of injuries occur in the upper limb, with the ulnar nerve being the most injured.[22]
- What is the prognosis for recovery from nerve pathology?
- The prognosis for recovery from nerve pathology greatly depends on the classification of the nerve injury (neurapraxia, axonotmesis, neurotmesis).[7,30,34]
- Recovery time
  - Neurapraxia (focal demyelination): ranges from hours to a few months
  - Axonotmesis (axon disrupted/wallerian degeneration): depends on the degree of wallerian degeneration. There is a direct correlation between recovery and the distance from the nerve to its innervated tissue.
  - Neurotmesis (nerve completely severed): poor prognosis; possibly incomplete without surgery

CLINICAL PEARL

- *Nerve repair and recovery occur through three different mechanisms*[7]
  - *Remyelination*
  - *Collateral sprouting of axons*
- *They occur with nerve lesions <20% to 30% of axonal damage.*
  - *Regeneration from the site of the injury*
- *They occur with >90% of nerve injury.*[45]
- *The peripheral nervous system is designed to repair itself.*[5,13]
- *However, the central nervous system does not repair itself; rather it utilizes plasticity, using intact areas to take over the function of damaged areas. This can be a major contributor to chronic pain cycles through central pain processing mechanisms.*

WHAT IS THE RECURRENCE RATE FOR NERVE PATHOLOGY?

- Recurrence rates vary; one study following subjects who had a first-time lumbar discectomy for disc herniation at 6-month follow-up quantified pain rating scores and peridural scar tissue formation. The results showed that patients with extensive peridural scar tissue formation were 3.2 times more likely to experience recurrent radicular pain than those with less scarring.[29]

CLINICAL PEARL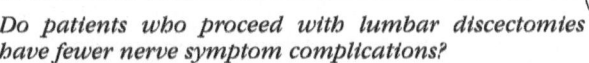

Do patients who proceed with lumbar discectomies have fewer nerve symptom complications?
- *The benefits of surgery versus conservative treatment are highly debated.*
- *In a 13-year follow-up study of 342 patients after lumbar discectomy, recurrence of the same level and side herniation occurred in 8%. Nearly 70% of the patients still reported sciatica.*[26]

- *However, in a 10-year follow-up study of surgical versus conservative treatment for patients with sciatica resulting from a lumbar disc herniation, surgically treated patients had more complete relief of leg pain and improved function compared with nonsurgically treated patients (71% versus 56%).*[2]
- *Regardless of differing statistics, it is important in our rehabilitation assessment to take into consideration the postsurgical effects of tissue inflammation and healing, potentially leading to neural scarring, increased sensitivity to tissues, and altered mechanics and joint stability.*

WHAT FACTORS MAKE DIAGNOSIS DIFFICULT IN NERVE PATHOLOGY?

- The difficulty in diagnosing nerve pathology is based on the tendency of clinicians to focus on the neural symptoms, such as pain, paresthesias, and sensory or motor changes, rather than assessing the full extent of how nerves affect the neuromusculoskeletal system. Keep the following in mind:
  - Electromyographic (EMGs) and nerve conduction velocity (NCV) testing are not the sole indicators of nerve pathology.
  - Assessment and rehabilitation of nerve pathology, also known as clinical neurodynamics, involve "essentially the clinical application of mechanics and physiology of the nervous system as they relate to each other and are integrated with musculoskeletal functions."[31]
  - It is important to understand the interaction between pathomechanics and pathophysiology of the nervous system to fully understand how nerve pathology affects the human body.
  - Pathomechanics includes tension, sliding, and compression abnormalities.
  - Pathophysiology includes changes in intraneural blood flow, increased inflammation, and increased tissue sensitization.[31]

CLINICAL PEARL

Assessment and treatment of nerve pathology and clinical neurodynamics should focus not only on the nerve itself, but rather on a three-part integrated system.[31]
- *Mechanical interface*
  - *This involves any structure that resides next to and thus affects the nervous system, such as tendon, muscle, bone, intervertebral discs, ligaments, fascia, and blood vessels.*
- *Neural structures*
  - *This involves structures that constitute the nervous system, including the brain, cranial nerves and spinal cord, nerve rootlets, nerve roots, and peripheral nerves (including the sympathetic trunks) and all their related connective tissues.*
- *Innervated tissues*
  This involves any tissue that is innervated by the nervous system, including muscle, tendon, and ligaments.

HOW SUCCESSFUL IS THERAPY IN TREATING NERVE PATHOLOGY?

- Studies on the use of electrical stimulation to treat nerve pathology vary; little evidence supports the sole use of this modality for the treatment of nerve pathlogy.[4,16]
- The use of mechanical traction has been shown to improve symptoms in a subgroup of patients characterized by the presence of leg symptoms, signs of nerve root compression, and either peripheralization with extension movements or a crossed straight leg rise.[14]
- There is no large cohort study on the use of manual therapy interventions for nerve pathology; however, a group of cases or small population studies demonstrates the effectiveness of neural mobilization techniques in improving neural pain and dysfunction.[8,17,18,24]

HOW SUCCESSFUL IS SURGERY IN TREATING NERVE PATHOLOGY?

- There are four primary surgical interventions:
  - External neurolysis
  - End-to-end repair
  - Nerve grafting[9,28]
  - Nerve transfer[32]
- The success and selection of a surgery technique depend on the degree of injury and the time interval of injury.
- Immediate reconstruction is done for complete nerve sections such as glass/knife wounds.
- End-to-end repairs are performed preferably with minimal local tissue trauma and healthy nerve ends compared to nerve grafting.
- Other prognostic indicators for surgical success include youth, distal injuries, and operations performed soon after injury onset.[7]

PERSONAL INFORMATION

WHAT INFLUENCE DOES AGE HAVE ON YOUR CLINICAL DECISION-MAKING PROCESS?

- Aging factors can affect nerve healing processes, particularly if there are other health-related factors such as diabetes or previous neural injuries. Any pathology that decreases blood flow to the nerve will ultimately slow the nerve's ability to heal.
- Surgical healing is better in younger than in older patients.
- Traumatic peripheral nerve injuries are more prevalent in the younger population ranging from 16 to 38 years old.[22]

WHAT INFLUENCE DOES A PATIENT'S OCCUPATION HAVE ON YOUR CLINICAL DECISION-MAKING PROCESS?

- Occupation can be a primary contributor to nerve pathology due to the extent of time spent performing either sustained, repetitive, or traumatic activities.
- Consider occupations that require the following:
  - Reaching activities: repetitive tension to the nervous system
  - Prolonged positions: sustained compression of the nervous system
  - Heavy impact: promotes inflammation and nociceptive input

CLINICAL PEARL

- *Peripheral nerves have the capacity to withstand elongation or tension. The perineurium of the nerve sheath has elastic properties that allow the nerve to withstand strain. At 8% elongation, venous blood flow from the nerves begins to diminish, whereas at 15% elongation, all circulation in the nerve is obstructed.[23,27]*
- *Peripheral nerves also have the capacity to be distorted or compressed. The epineurium has spongy qualities that act as the padding of the nerve, protecting the axons from excessive compression. At pressures of 30 to 55 mm Hg, hypoxia and impairment of nerve blood flow, conduction, and axonal transport occur.[15,27]*

WHAT INFLUENCE DOES GENDER HAVE ON YOUR CLINICAL DECISION-MAKING PROCESS?

- Large general studies on peripheral nerve injuries are few, but most studies have found that nerve injuries are more prevalent in men than women, ranging from 74.2% to 96% of cases.[22,25,33]
- There may be a correlation to the findings that the most common mechanism of nerve injury was involved motor vehicle accidents, gunshot wounds, and sports injuries, as these types of traumatic injuries are more common in men.

WHAT INFLUENCE DOES ETHNICITY HAVE ON YOUR CLINICAL DECISION-MAKING PROCESS?

- Factors of ethnicity in nerve pathology should be considered, particularly with specific nerve-related pathologies. For example, in Ethiopia there is a large prevalence of leprosy, which has a significant effect in neural tissue disorders.[11]
- Ethnicities that have a greater risk for diabetes or cardiovascular disorders are at greater risk for nerve pathology and delayed nerve healing.[3] Type 2 diabetes is more prevalent among Hispanics, Native Americans, African-Americans, and Asians/Pacific Islanders.

MECHANISM OF INJURY

WHAT INFLUENCE DOES THE MECHANISM OF INJURY HAVE ON YOUR CLINICAL DECISION-MAKING PROCESS?

Understanding the mechanism of nerve injury can help determine the type of pathology and prognosis for recovery.
- Traumatic: Considerations with incomplete or complete nerve lesions could occur
- Repetitive: Strain of neural tissues causing neural sensitivity through tensioning capacities
- Prolonged: Compression of neural tissues causing a decrease in intraneural blood flow
- Insidious: Possible consideration of central pain, autonomic, or psychosocial driven pain mechanisms; red and yellow flags require further medical examination

SYMPTOM LOCATION

WHAT INFLUENCE DOES THE LOCATION OF SYMPTOMS HAVE ON YOUR CLINICAL DECISION-MAKING PROCESS?

- The location of symptoms can provide possible indications of the peripheral nerve involvement or dermatomal referral pattern.
- It may also indicate the type of pain mechanism occurring: nociceptive, peripheral neurogenic, central pain, autonomic, or psychosocial.[6,43]

REFERRAL OF SYMPTOMS

The peripheral nerves of the upper and lower extremity have specific referral patterns.

UPPER EXTREMITY NERVES (Figures II-15-1 and II-15-2)

- Long thoracic: None
- Suprascapular: None
- Radial: Medial posterior portion of the arm, radial portion of the forearm, and dorsum of the hand
- Median: Skin over the radial side of the palm and palmar and dorsal aspects of the lateral three and a half digits
- Ulnar: Medial dorsal aspect of hand, the dorsal and volar aspect of half of the fourth and fifth digits, and the proximal hypothenar region

LOWER EXTREMITY NERVES (Figures II-15-3 and II-15-4)

- Sciatic: Branches of the tibial and peroneal nerve supply cutaneous innervation
- Common peroneal: Lateral upper leg and the anterior portion of the leg with the exception of the space between the first and second toes
- Deep peroneal: Space between the first and second toes
- Sural: Posterolateral leg and heel

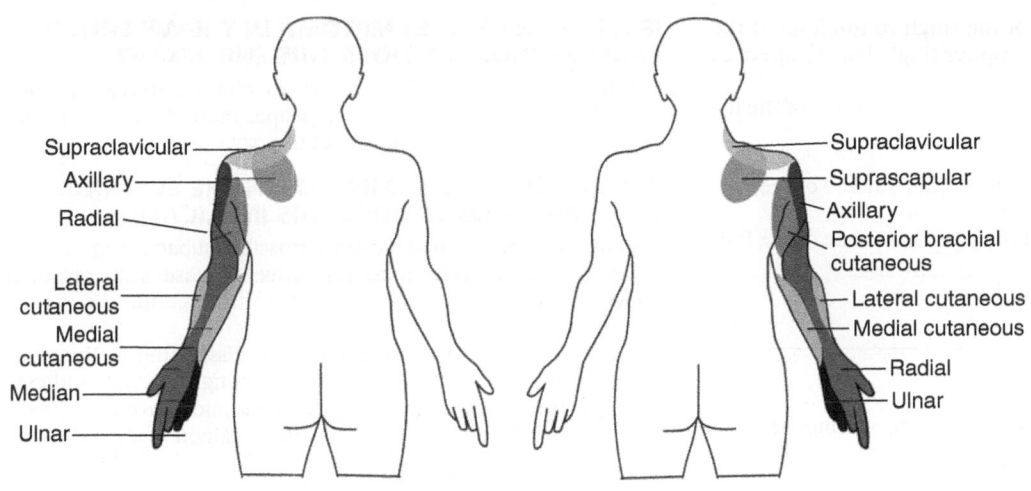

FIGURE II-15-1 Sensory distribution of upper extremity peripheral nerves. The referral pattern of the sensory nerves is different from the referral pattern of the spinal nerve root. The clinician can utilize the differences to aid in the diagnostic process.

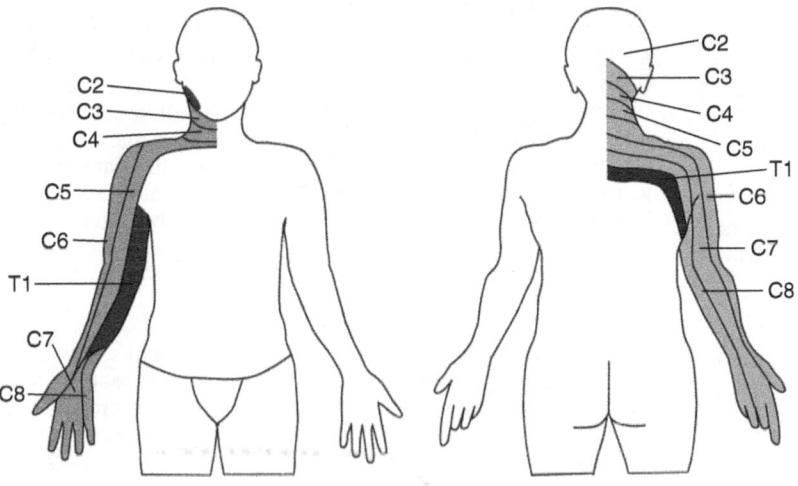

FIGURE II-15-2 Upper extremity dermatomes. A dermatome is an area of skin innervated by a single pair of dorsal nerve roots. Dermatomal patterns of symptoms vary greatly from person to person. The clinician should keep this in mind when utilizing dermatomes for clinical diagnostic purposes.

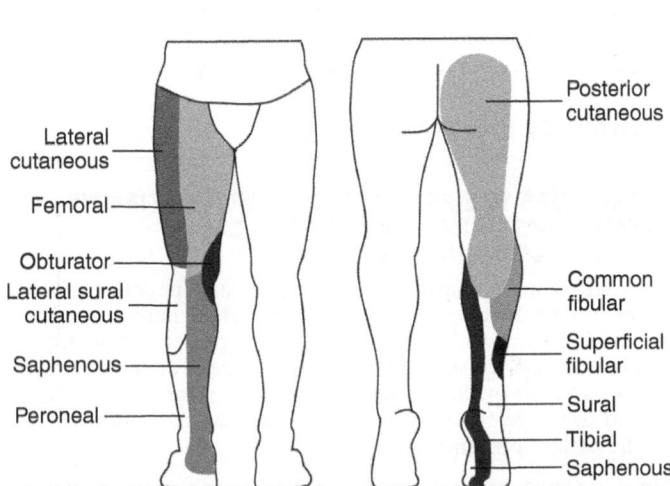

FIGURE II-15-3 Sensory distribution of lower extremity peripheral nerves. The referral pattern of the sensory nerves is different from the referral pattern of the spinal nerve root. The clinician can utilize the differences to aid in the diagnostic process.

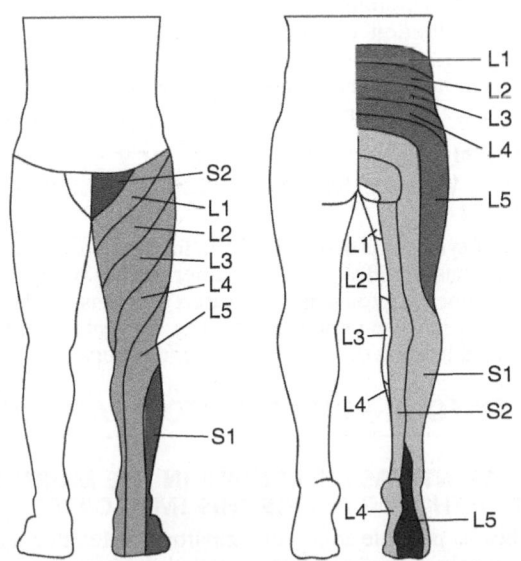

FIGURE II-15-4 Lower extremity dermatomes. A dermatome is an area of skin innervated by a single pair of dorsal nerve roots. Dermatomal patterns of symptoms vary greatly from person to person. The clinician should keep this in mind when utilizing dermatomes for clinical diagnostic purposes.

Section II ORTHOPEDIC REASONING

- Lateral femoral: Anterior aspect of the thigh to the level of the knee and lateral two-thirds of the upper thigh; lateral aspect of the buttocks below the greater trochanter
- Femoral: Anterior portion of the thigh and medial side of the leg and foot
- Tibial: Back of the leg
- Medial plantar: Medial portion of the plantar surface of the foot and medial three and a half digits
- Lateral plantar: Lateral portion of the plantar surface of the foot and lateral one and a half toes

SYMPTOM DESCRIPTORS

QUALITY OF SYMPTOMS

- Neuropathic: Burning, pain, tingling, numb, itching, searing, knifing, lancinating
- Deep ache: Joint, bone, capsule, muscle
- Viscera: Colicky, cramping
- Mechanical: Sharp

CLINICAL DECISION MAKING
CASE STUDY—PATIENT PROFILE (?)

A 32-year-old male presents to physical therapy with complaints of left-sided low back pain and mid-back stiffness; he also notes that "for some reason, my stomach always cramps, no physician has been able to determine where it comes from, I can't eat a lot of types of foods that I used to because it makes my abdomen cramp." How would you deduce that the patient's back pain, mid-back stiffness, and abdominal cramping are interrelated?

Answer
This patient presents with visceral pain and cramping due to restrictions in the thoracic spine, causing a sympathetic nervous response that innervates and causes the internal organ symptoms such as cramping.

WHAT INFLUENCE DOES THE DEPTH OF SYMPTOMS HAVE ON YOUR CLINICAL DECISION-MAKING PROCESS?

- Superficial symptoms could suggest cutaneous/dermatomal nerve distribution or superficial musculoskeletal structural involvement.
- Deep symptoms could suggest underlying structures such as disc, bone, and viscera, and internal joint derangements.

WHAT INFLUENCE DOES CONSTANCY OF SYMPTOMS HAVE ON YOUR CLINICAL DECISION-MAKING PROCESS?

- Constant symptoms may indicate an inflammatory cycle or process that has significantly affected nerve physiology.
- Intermittent symptoms may indicate a less sensitized or healing nerve that may be dependent on the amount of repetitive or prolonged loading or strain placed on the nerve.

TWENTY-FOUR-HOUR SYMPTOM PATTERN

IF A PATIENT HAS SYMPTOMS IN THE MORNING, WHAT PATHOLOGY DOES THIS IMPLICATE?

- It indicates possible acute inflammatory cycle in neural tissues causing pain, paresthesias, and restriction in motion.

WHAT ROLE DOES MORNING STIFFNESS PLAY IN DIFFERENTIATION?

- It indicates a less acute inflammatory cycle in neural tissues and more chronic restricted neural and musculoskeletal immobility.

IF A PATIENT HAS SYMPTOMS IN THE AFTERNOON, WHAT PATHOLOGY DOES THIS IMPLICATE?

- It indicates a possible subacute to chronic nerve irritation related to repetitive overuse, improper motor control, and sustained postures held throughout the day.

IF A PATIENT HAS SYMPTOMS IN THE EVENING, WHAT PATHOLOGY DOES THIS IMPLICATE?

- Similar to afternoon symptoms, possible subacute to chronic nerve irritation related to repetitive overuse and improper motor and sustained postures held throughout the day is implicated.
- If a patient notes that symptoms are dissipating in the afternoon and are occurring later in the evening, this could indicate improvements in neural tissue healing and movement based on less irritability with repetitive or sustained loading through the day.

CLINICAL DECISION MAKING
CASE STUDY—PATIENT PROFILE (?)

A 35-year-old male complains of low back pain and right-sided sciatica that worsens primarily in the later afternoon "around 3 to 4 o'clock" after prolonged standing and walking. Reports of symptoms in the morning are variable, and pain in the evening subsides if the patient rests. Based on the patient's subjective complaints, would the priority in treatment techniques be based on treating the nerve itself through passive interventions such as mechanical traction or active interventions such as neuromuscular reeducation and posture reeducation?

Answer
Focus should be placed on improving the patient's movement patterns, muscular endurance, and postural correction. With poor mechanics and stability in repetitive loading, increased pain occurs. By improving the neuromuscular control, stability, and endurance of the patient, the patient's symptoms should improve and not become aggravated until the evening.

IF A PATIENT HAS SYMPTOMS WHEN SLEEPING, WHAT PATHOLOGY DOES THIS IMPLICATE?

- It implicates possible nerve entrapment due to an altered sleeping posture that compresses or strains the nerve and that is relieved with changing position. Constant pain during sleeping could indicate a medical pathology suggesting referral for medical examination, such as a metastatic tumor.

STABILITY OF SYMPTOMS

HOW DOES THE PROGRESSION OF A PATIENT'S SYMPTOMS IMPACT YOUR CLINICAL DECISION-MAKING PROCESS?

- Progression in improvements in pain and neural symptoms should be matched with the appropriate neural rehabilitation intervention that fits the patient's presenting symptoms. Shacklock proposes a classification system of neurodynamic levels based on the patient's presenting signs and symptoms, and has a treatment progression based on the level in which the patient presents.[31]

IF A PATIENT'S SYMPTOMS ARE IMPROVING, WHAT PATHOLOGY DOES THIS IMPLICATE?

- Improvements in the patient's neural symptoms indicate physiological improvement in sensitivity of neural tissues, changes in blood flow, intraneural inflammation and conduction, as well as mechanical sliding and tensioning of the nervous system.

Improvement of symptoms by therapeutic interventions indicates correct selection of techniques and that progression of techniques is warranted.

IF A PATIENT'S SYMPTOMS ARE WORSENING, WHAT PATHOLOGY DOES THIS IMPLICATE?

- Any recent worsening of neurological symptoms or signs should be considered precautionary with possible referral for medical examination. Increased neural sensitivity, compression leading to sensory, motor, and reflex loss, as well as central pain processing could be happening. Worsening of symptoms after therapeutic intervention indicates improper selection of techniques, and reassessment and reselection of proper treatment should be considered.

FUNCTIONAL AND ACTIVITY PARTICIPATION LIMITATIONS

WHAT INFLUENCE DOES AGGRAVATING ACTIVITIES HAVE ON YOUR CLINICAL DECISION-MAKING PROCESS?

GENERAL AGGRAVATING/EASING FACTORS OF NEURAL TISSUE

- Nerves can be aggravated by lengthening them past their mechanical or physiological threshold.
- The threshold length of nerves that are injured or sensitized may be less than normal and can reproduce the symptoms about which patients complain.
- Each nerve has a different path and each terminates at a different location.
- Specific movements of each joint can result in a mechanical lengthening or shortening of a specific nerve based on the path in which the nerve courses.
- Therefore, aggravating and easing factors are determined by understanding the course of each nerve and the mechanical forces that can further lengthen or shorten the nerve.

STRUCTURAL DIFFERENTIATION

- It is also important to understand that multiple structures can be involved in producing a patient's symptoms during a specific joint movement, such as muscle, ligament, and nerve. To determine whether neural tissue is aggravating the symptoms, it is necessary to use a "structural differentiating" maneuver.
- "Structural differentiation" is performed with all neurodynamic tests to obtain information on whether neurodynamic events participate in the mechanism of symptoms. Differentiation is achieved when the therapist moves the neural structures in the area of question without moving the musculoskeletal tissues in the same region. Any changes in symptoms with the differentiating maneuver may indicate neural involvement.[31]

NEURODYNAMIC TESTING (Table II-15-1)

- Standard neurodynamic testing for each major nerve indicates how each nerve is mechanically sensitized, and thus how the nerve can be aggravated or eased.
- A distal end maneuver along the course of the nerve can be used to structurally differentiate the movement to confirm neural involvement.[31]

MEDIAN NEURODYNAMIC TEST (MNT)
(Figure II-15-5)

STANDARD MOVEMENTS
1. Glenohumeral abduction
2. Glenohumeral external rotation
3. Forearm supination, wrist and finger extension
4. Elbow extension

STRUCTURAL DIFFERENTIATION: If the patient complains of the reproduction of proximal symptoms with the MNT, a change in symptoms by releasing wrist extension can be used to determine if the median nerve is involved. If the symptoms are in a distal location, a change in symptoms by contralateral cervical lateral flexion can be used to determine median nerve involvement.

TABLE II-15-1 Neurodynamic Tests

Neurodynamic Test	Standard Movement	Structural Differentiation	Aggravating Movements	Easing Movements
Median (MNT)	Glenohumeral abduction Glenohumeral external rotation Forearm supination, wrist and finger extension Elbow extension	Proximal symptoms: release wrist extension Distal symptoms: cervical contralateral lateral flexion	Repetitive or sustained arm reaching, combined with contralateral cervical lateral flexion	Involved arm held by side, scapular elevation, ipsilateral cervical lateral flexion
Ulnar (UNT)	Scapular depression Wrist and finger extension/forearm pronation Elbow flexion Glenohumeral external rotation Glenohumeral abduction	Release scapular depression	Repetitive or sustained arm reaching combined with contralateral cervical lateral flexion	Involved arm held by side, scapular elevation, ipsilateral cervical lateral flexion
Radial (RNT)	Scapular depression Elbow extension Glenohumeral internal rotation/forearm pronation Wrist and finger flexion Glenohumeral abduction	Proximal symptoms: release wrist flexion Distal symptoms: release scapular depression	Repetitive or sustained arm reaching, combined contralateral cervical lateral flexion	Involved arm held by side, scapular elevation, ipsilateral cervical lateral flexion
Straight leg raise (SLR)	Hip flexion with knee straight	Proximal symptoms: ankle dorsiflexion Distal symptoms: hip flexion	Kicking, trunk flexion with knees straight, "hamstring" stretching, slouched sitting	Knee bending, trunk neutral/extension
Slump test	Sitting thoracic and lumbar flexion Cervical flexion Knee extension Ankle dorsiflexion	Release ankle dorsiflexion or cervical flexion	Slouched sitting combined with leg extension or cervical flexion	Knee bending, trunk and neck neutral/extension

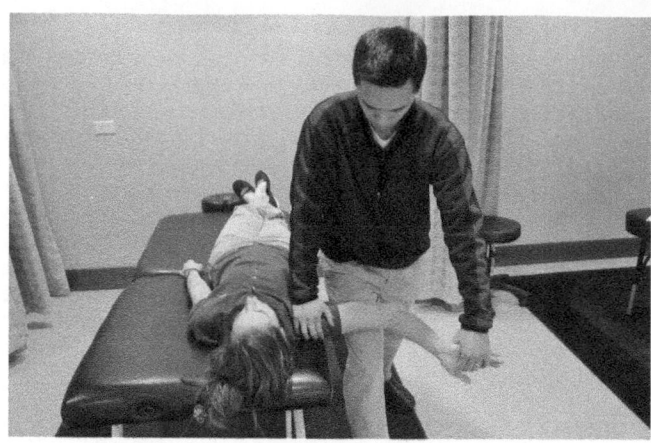

FIGURE II-15-5   Median neurodynamic test.

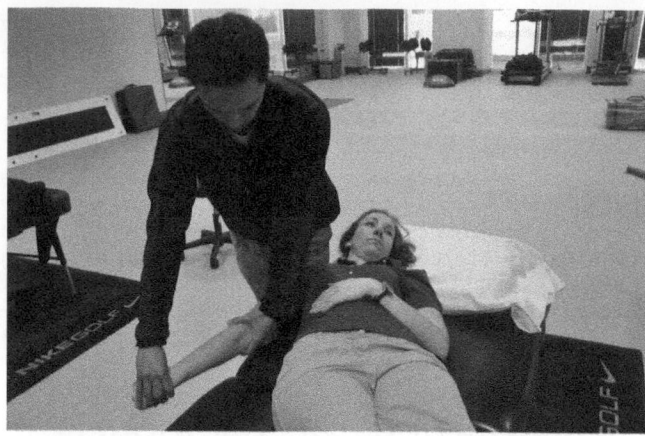

FIGURE II-15-7   Radial neurodynamic test.

AGGRAVATING MOVEMENTS: These include repetitive or sustained arm reaching combined with contralateral cervical lateral flexion.

EASING MOVEMENTS: These include holding the involved arm by the side, scapular elevation, and ipsilateral cervical lateral flexion.

ULNAR NEURODYNAMIC TEST (UNT) (Figure II-15-6)

STANDARD MOVEMENTS
1. Scapular depression
2. Wrist and finger extension/forearm pronation
3. Elbow flexion
4. Glenohumeral external rotation
5. Glenohumeral abduction

STRUCTURAL DIFFERENTIATION: If the patient complains of a reproduction of symptoms with the UNT, a change in symptoms by releasing scapular depression can be used to determine ulnar nerve involvement.

AGGRAVATING MOVEMENTS: These include repetitive or sustained arm reaching combined with contralateral cervical lateral flexion.

EASING MOVEMENTS: These include holding the involved arm by the side, scapular elevation, and ipsilateral cervical lateral flexion.

RADIAL NEURODYNAMIC TEST (RNT)
(Figure II-15-7)

STANDARD MOVEMENTS
1. Scapular depression
2. Elbow extension

3. Glenohumeral internal rotation/forearm pronation
4. Wrist and finger flexion
5. Glenohumeral abduction

STRUCTURAL DIFFERENTIATION: If the patient complains of the reproduction of proximal symptoms with the RNT, a change in symptoms by releasing wrist flexion can be used to determine if the radial nerve is involved. If the symptoms were in a distal location, a change in symptoms by releasing scapular depression can be used to determine radial nerve involvement.

AGGRAVATING MOVEMENTS: These include repetitive or sustained arm reaching combined with contralateral cervical lateral flexion.

EASING MOVEMENTS: These include holding the involved arm by the side, scapular elevation, and ipsilateral cervical lateral flexion.

STRAIGHT-LEG RAISE (SLR): SCIATIC NERVE
(Figure II-15-8)

STANDARD MOVEMENTS: Hip flexion with knee straight

STRUCTURAL DIFFERENTIATION: If the patient complains of the reproduction of proximal symptoms with the SLR, a change in symptoms by ankle dorsiflexion can be used to determine if the sciatic nerve is involved. If the symptoms were in a distal location, the use of further hip flexion can be used to determine sciatic nerve involvement.

AGGRAVATING MOVEMENTS: These include kicking, trunk flexion with knees straight, "hamstring" stretching, and slouched sitting.

EASING MOVEMENTS: These include knee bending and trunk neutral/extension.

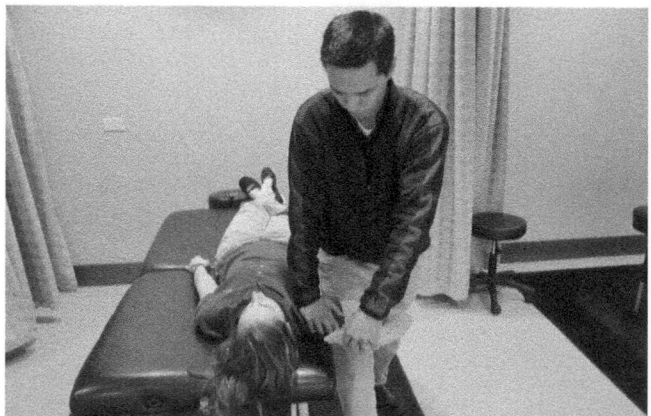

FIGURE II-15-6   Ulnar neurodynamic test.

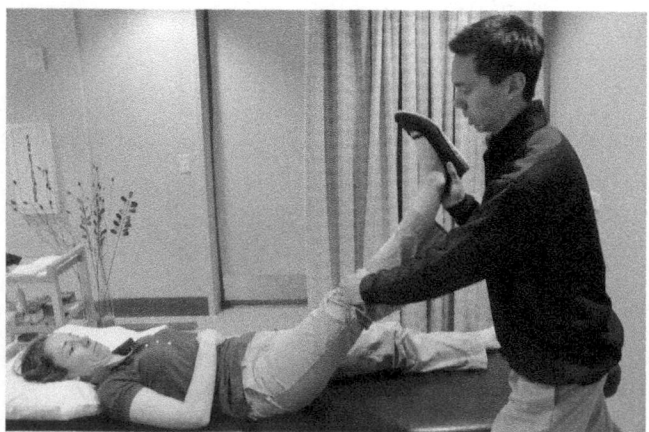

FIGURE II-15-8   Straight-leg test.

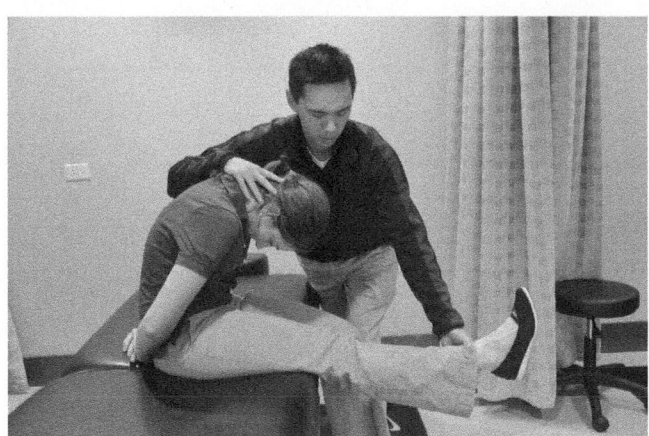

FIGURE II-15-9   Seated slump test.

SLUMP TEST: SPINAL CORD/SCIATIC NERVE
(Figure II-15-9)

STANDARD MOVEMENTS
1. Sitting thoracic and lumbar flexion
2. Cervical flexion
3. Knee extension
4. Ankle dorsiflexion

STRUCTURAL DIFFERENTIATION: If the patient complains of the reproduction of symptoms with the slump test, a change in symptoms by increasing ankle dorsiflexion or releasing cervical flexion can be used to determine if the spinal cord and sciatic nerve are involved.

AGGRAVATING MOVEMENTS: These include slouched sitting combined with leg extension or cervical flexion.

EASING MOVEMENTS: These include knee bending and trunk and neck neutral/extension.

CLINICAL PEARL

Shacklock[31] proposes a physical examination algorithm to determine if a neurodynamic issue is the cause of a patient's symptoms:

- *Neurodynamic tests can be positive in normal asymptomatic patients, so a positive test alone does not indicate that nerve is a contributing factor.*
- *Structural differentiation needs to be established first. The symptoms, range of motion, and resistance to alterations in movement change with the differentiating maneuver.*
- *For the neurodynamic test to be relevant, there must also be asymmetry between the affected and unaffected sides in the reproduction of symptoms, range of motion, and resistance to changes in movement.*
- *Symptoms that are reproduced precisely through neurodynamic testing are considered "overt" response, and treatment should commence with proper neurodynamic interventions.*
- *Symptoms that are produced that are not identical to their complaints, although the patient reports a change in the difference in the quality of symptoms compared with the normal side, are considered a "covert" response, and further advanced neurodynamic testing should be done.[31]*

MEDICAL HISTORY

WHAT ROLE DOES A PATIENT'S PAST MEDICAL HISTORY PLAY IN THE DIFFERENTIAL DIAGNOSIS OF PATHOLOGY?

- Medical diagnoses such as diabetes, AIDS, multiple sclerosis, and leprosy are some examples of medical pathology that can affect the mechanics and physiology of the nervous system. Consideration should be given to the type of effects each pathology has on the nervous system.
- Previous surgeries or trauma injuries such as lumbar fusions or motor vehicle accidents can lead to increased neural mechanosensitivity, intraneural edema, or scarring, possibly predisposing patients to neural pathologies

MEDICAL AND ORTHOPEDIC TESTING

WHAT MEDICAL AND ORTHOPEDIC TESTS INFLUENCE YOUR DIFFERENTIAL DIAGNOSIS PROCESS?

- Medical guidelines suggest that referral for electrodiagnostic consultations should be done within a 6-month period after peripheral nerve injuries occur, not so early that severe axonal degeneration is missed or so late that possible surgical benefits are minimal.[22]
- Guidelines for optimal timing for electrodiagnostic testing:[7]
  1. Immediate to 7 days for localization; differentiating complete from incomplete nerve lesions
  2. One to two weeks for differentiating complete from incomplete nerve lesions; sorting axonotmesis or neurotmesis from neurapraxia
  3. Three to four weeks for most diagnostic information from a single study
  4. Three to four months for detecting reinnervation

MEDICATIONS

HOW DOES A PATIENT'S RESPONSE TO MEDICATION INFLUENCE YOUR DECISION-MAKING PROCESSES?

Medication intake to manage nerve injuries attempts to control pain through the reduction of neural sensitivity. This can include neuropathic medications such as tricyclic antidepressants, serotonin reuptake inhibitors, and anticonvulsants (carbamazepine, phenytoin, lamotrigine, gabapentin, pregabalin, antiarrhythmics, baclofen).[7,12,21]

- If patients respond to such medications, clinicians should progress into neurodynamic interventions to improve nerve mobility and physiology and the interfaces in which the nerves interact (i.e., intervertebral foramen, muscle, ligament, capsule).

BIOMECHANICAL FACTORS

WHAT ROLE DOES BIOMECHANICS PLAY IN THE DECISION-MAKING PROCESS?

- Peripheral nerves interact with multiple joints interdependently. The biomechanics of the nervous system are dependent on the sequencing in which joints are moved.
- "Neurodynamic sequencing" is the performance of a set of particular component body movements so as to produce specific mechanical events in the nervous system based on that sequence or order of component movements.[31]
- Greater strain in the nerve occurs at the site that is moved first.[36]
- There is a greater likelihood of producing a response that is localized to the region that is moved first or more strongly.[31,46]
- For example, in a median neurodynamic test more strain will be placed at the carpal tunnel if the wrist is extended first as opposed to shoulder abduction.

CLINICAL PEARL ⚠

The diagnosis of plantar fasciitis may be caused by nerve pathology. The plantar nerve, a branch of the tibial and sciatic nerve, innervates the plantar surface of the foot. By biasing the sequence of the plantar/tibial nerve first during a straight leg raise neurodynamic test, a patient's foot pain may be reproduced. Treatment plans, thus, need to prioritize the mobility and physiological improvements of the sciatic/tibial nerve for effective rehabilitation.

WHAT BIOMECHANICAL ABNORMALITIES IN OTHER REGIONS AFFECT YOUR DECISION-MAKING PROCESS?

- Alterations in distal or proximal extremities can cause repetitive strain due to altered biomechanics and cause increased strain or compression to neural tissues remote to the altered joint.
- For example, chronic ankle sprains can lead to limited ankle dorsiflexion. With limited ankle mobility in gait cycles, associated restricted hip extension occurs causing increased axial loading to the hip and lumbopelvic region and loss of motor recruitment of primary stabilizers. With repetitious mechanical changes, the sciatic nerve can be injured due to increased shearing, compression, or tensile loading through the lumbopelvic region.

CLINICAL DECISION MAKING CASE STUDY—PATIENT PROFILE ❓

A 25-year-old female complains of right shoulder pain extending into her right arm. She previously was a competitive tennis player. Four years ago, she underwent a right shoulder subacromial decompression due to her complaints of pain; she was diagnosed with a grade III acromial spur. The patient reported relief of symptoms after surgery. After 8 months she returned to tennis, but reported a recurrence of her shoulder pain; she has continued to play, although with range of motion restrictions and pain. She has altered her tennis serve to a side arm position, as an overhead swing aggravates her symptoms. She particularly notices aggravation when she is fatigued and has to turn her head harder when she serves to get more power as her leg strength diminishes. What altered biomechanics suggests that the patient's injury is not only neurodynamic related, but triggered by faulty biomechanics?

Answer
Based on the patient's subjective complaints, head movement away from an abducted arm in her modified tennis serve can cause a neurodynamic response in her right brachial plexus. This is driven from poor leg and core strength to provide proper force transmission to use her right shoulder and neck efficiently. With repetitive faulty mechanics, the patient strains her brachial plexus, which becomes a potential cause of her shoulder pain.

ENVIRONMENTAL FACTORS (Box II-15-1)

DO PSYCHOSOCIAL ISSUES INFLUENCE CLINICAL DECISION MAKING?

- Psychosocial issues such as stress and depression have a direct effect on the autonomic, endocrine, and immune systems. These three systems can play a role in nerve physiology and pathology.

DO WORK-RELATED INJURIES INFLUENCE CLINICAL DECISION MAKING?

- With the amount of time spent in work-related tasks, repetitive, prolonged, or traumatic activities can all lead to tissue injury, nerve strain, and compression.
- Careful attention should be placed on static postures in standing and sitting, as well as movement dynamics with repetitious

BOX II-15-1 **Contextual Factors**	
Environmental	Work activities, especially related to repetitive, prolonged, or traumatic stress, can lead to neural pathology.
Personal	Personal stress or depression can affect the autonomic, endocrine, and immune systems that can affect nerve physiology.

or traumatic work-related activities. Duration of time of these postures or activities should also be taken into account.

CLINICAL DECISION MAKING CASE STUDY—PATIENT PROFILE ❓

A 33-year-old female working as a veterinary surgeon complains of right radial wrist pain. She has been diagnosed with de Quervain's syndrome and reports no improvement with traditional rehabilitation for tendon pain. The pain is aggravated when she performs surgery as she is required to operate with her hands in a wrist-flexed and slight ulnar deviation position. What other positions or movements can you test to determine if her symptoms are musculoskeletal or nerve based?

Answer
Have the patient in a work-related position that aggravates her symptoms, and instruct her to either contralaterally later flex her neck or add scapular depression. If symptoms in her wrist are increased with either movement, the patient has an irritation of the radial sensory nerve that innervates the radial side of the wrist, rather than a standard de Quervain's syndrome tendon injury. Treatment interventions should focus on improving radial nerve mobility and physiology, as well as joint and soft tissue integrity of the wrist and upper quarter.

PERSONAL FACTORS

WHAT PREVIOUS SURGERIES INFLUENCE YOUR CLINICAL DECISION MAKING?

- Any previous surgery should be taken into account when considering potential nerve injuries.
- This could be due to direct surgeries such as lumbar discectomy or fusion that would cause inflammation and possible scar tissue around the lumbosacral nerve roots.
- Or it could be due to indirect surgeries, such as an ankle fusion, that alter gait mechanics and thus indirectly alter the motor control patterns of the lower extremity and lumbopelvic region potentially disrupting the mechanical loading of the sciatic nerve.

DOES A FAMILY HISTORY OF PATHOLOGY IN THE REGION INFLUENCE YOUR CLINICAL REASONING PROCESS?

- Considerations should be made for family histories such as back pain, diabetes, rheumatoid arthritis that can affect the nervous system.

CHRONICITY OF PAIN

WHAT CENTRAL PROCESSING CHANGES OCCUR THAT INFLUENCE YOUR DECISION MAKING?

- Patients presenting with central pain mechanisms will most likely not respond to peripheral neurogenic interventions alone.

- As wide dynamic range (WDR) cells are sensitized in the dorsal root ganglion, peripheral symptoms are altered.
- Patients may present with symptoms not expected along the peripheral nerve's expected cutaneous or dermatomal referral patterns, but rather present with allodynia or even symptoms on the contralateral side may be involved.[10,31,44]
- False positives with normal neurodynamic testing may occur, along with changes to the autonomic, endocrine, and immune systems.
- Clinical decision making should focus on central pain changes rather than on peripheral symptoms alone.

HAS MEDICAL TREATMENT BEEN SUCCESSFUL FOR PATIENTS WITH CHRONIC PATHOLOGY IN THE REGION?

- Neuropathic medications have been found to cause more side effects than significant improvement in treating chronic sciatica.[19,20]
- Weber showed that the results of surgical treatment were superior to conservative treatment at 1 year follow-up, but not significantly better at 4 years; at 10 year follow-up outcomes of surgery and conservative treatment were similar.[41]
- The use of epidural injections provides short-term pain relief, with some studies showing relief lasting 3 to 6 weeks, but does not show differences when compared to saline injections on 1 year follow-ups for patients with sciatica.[1,37]

DOES THE CHRONICITY OF SYMPTOMS INFLUENCE YOUR DECISION-MAKING PROCESS?

- As nerve pathology continues to persist chronic changes to the nerve occur such as scar tissue formation, restriction of movement, decreased intraneural blood flow/conduction, and central pain changes. More importantly, multiple structures as well can be altered such as muscle, ligament, and tendons.
- As nerves are sensitized, the nerve itself is innervated, as a structure called the nervi nervorum releases inflammatory mediators such as substance P and calcitonin gene-related peptide (CGRP) into the nerve causing the nerve to develop intraneural edema.
- Evidence shows that such chemical mediators can travel distally (antidromic impulses) or proximally (retrograde impulses) along the course of the nerve to their termination sites causing inflammatory changes in the target tissues.
- Research has shown degenerative changes in the radiohumeral joint with chronic neck and radicular pain as well as trigger point formation in muscular tissues.[38]
- The diagnosis of "double-crush" syndrome can be validated through evidence of retrograde impulses, such that a wrist injury could ultimately lead to cervical neck dysfunction.
- Ultimately, with chronic symptoms, a multistructural intervention plan should be taken as multiple structures are affected, as well as alterations in movement patterns and psychosocial aspects to pain and dysfunction.

HOW DO THE AUTONOMIC, ENDOCRINE, AND IMMUNE SYSTEMS INFLUENCE DECISION MAKING?

The autonomic, endocrine, and immune systems interactively maintain homeostasis in the body; irregularities in any of the systems can physiologically alter the nervous system.
- The hypothalamus controls secretions such as cortisol from the cortex to maintain cardiovascular and metabolic homeostasis. Diagnoses such as Cushing's syndrome, chronic hypercortisolism, can cause immunosuppression, depression, and tissue degeneration and can slow tissue healing.[6,36,42]
- The sympathetic nervous system through the release of substances such as adrenaline and noradrenaline can contribute to increased sensitivity of inflamed neural tissues.
- Cytokines of the immune system can promote antiinflammatory or proinflammatory conditions. Substance P can activate

the proinflammatory cytokine interleukin-1 (IL-1), resulting in an increased stress response by the ability of IL-1 to promote the secretion of corticotropin-releasing factor.[6,39,40]

RED FLAGS THAT REQUIRE REFERRAL TO A MEDICAL PHYSICIAN

WHAT SYMPTOMS ALERT YOU TO PATHOLOGIES THAT MAY REQUIRE A REFERRAL TO A MEDICAL PHYSICIAN?

- Constant pain or increased pain at night suggesting visceral involvement or pain from a pain-generating source not involving neuromusculoskeletal tissues
- Pain that is not alleviated with rest of unloading positions
- Traumatic injuries, presenting with symptoms of vertebrobasilar artery insufficiency such as dizziness, blurred vision, difficulty swallowing, nausea, and vomiting
- Loss of motor strength, deep tendon reflexes, or sensory alterations

HOW CAN VISCERAL SYMPTOMS BE RELATED TO NEURAL PATHOLOGY?

- In regard to visceral symptoms related to neural pathology, recall that the autonomic nervous system is composed of two major divisions, the parasympathetic and sympathetic divisions. The autonomic regulation of visceral function is controlled in a dualistic fashion as parasympathetic and sympathetic fibers regulate each other.
- The parasympathetic division originates in the brainstem and sacral segments of the spinal cord. The sympathetic division originates in the lateral horn of the spinal cord between the first thoracic spinal vertebrae and the second to third lumbar spinal vertebrae.
- Similar to a nerve root injury affecting the sciatic nerve or brachial plexus due to injury to the lumbar or cervicothoracic region, the sympathetic fibers can be sensitized through dysfunction of the first thoracic to third lumbar spinal vertebrae. Therefore the changes in neural pathology of the sympathetic fibers can cause changes in visceral symptoms.
- In our physical examination, clinicians need to perform a thorough spinal assessment when patients complain of visceral symptoms, particularly with the autonomic nervous system. Although standard neurodynamic testing exists for peripheral nerves of the upper and lower extremities, there is also specific neurodynamic testing for the sympathetic nervous system.

SUMMARY STATEMENT

- Assessment of nerve-related pathologies is essential in orthopedic rehabilitation. Neural tissue can be injured as frequently as other connective tissues, such as muscle, ligament, and capsule. Understanding the pathomechanics and pathophysiology of nerve tissue provides direction on how to properly assess and treat nerve dysfunction. Nerve pathology not only affects the nerve itself, but more importantly affects the mechanical interfaces in which the nerve courses as well as the tissues that it innervates. Table II-15-2 summarizes the factors that help a clinician diagnose nerve pathology.
- Therefore, nerve dysfunction can be a missing link in our orthopedic assessment as it is the "circuitry" that connects everything together. Altered mechanics and physiology of the nerve can alter movement patterns and prolong chronic pain patterns, potentially changing the psychosocial aspects of a patient's pain and function.
- In the future treatment of chronic and recurring injuries should focus on research related to neural interactions with the rest of the neuromusculoskeletal system.

TABLE II-15-2 **Body Structure and Tissue-Based Pathology (Nociceptive and Peripheral Neurogenic Pain Mechanisms)**

Factor	Nerves
Age	Can occur at any age, but healing time is increased in the elderly and those with poor circulation Younger patients are more prone to traumatic injury
Occupation	No specific pattern, but repetitive use occupations or sports predispose to nerve pathology secondary to repetitive tension or compression onto the nerve
Gender	No specific gender correlation although males are more prone to traumatic injuries; females can have nerve pathology due to pregnancy
Ethnicity	No specific ethnic prevalence noted
History	Trauma: consider mechanism of injury and whether nerve was tensioned or compressed Insidious onset: consider systemic pathology that could impede circulation and points at which the nerve can be tensioned or compressed
Mechanism of injury	Traumatic: considerations with incomplete or complete nerve lesions could occur Repetitive: strain of neural tissues causing neural sensitivity through tensioning capacities Prolonged: compression of neural tissues causing a decrease in intraneural blood flow
Type of onset	Traumatic injury can occur suddenly Repetitive strain injuries will develop over a period of days to weeks to months
Referral from local tissue	Nerve pain can be difficult to differentiate because other body tissue can refer in patterns similar to nerve
Referral to other regions	See peripheral nerve distribution
Changes in symptoms	If symptoms are inflammatory in nature, symptoms should peak at 72 hours and dissipate over the course of 14 to 21 days
24-hour pain pattern (morning)	Possible acute inflammatory cycle in neural tissues causing pain, paresthesias, and restriction in motion
24-hour pain pattern (afternoon)	Possible subacute to chronic nerve irritation related to repetitive overuse, improper motor control, and sustained postures held throughout the day
24-hour pain pattern (evening)	Possible subacute to chronic nerve irritation related to repetitive overuse, improper motor control, and sustained postures held throughout the day
Description of symptoms	Burning Tingling Numb Itching Searing Knifing Lancinating
Depth of symptoms	Superficial: cutaneous/dermatomal nerve distribution, or superficial musculoskeletal structural involvement Deep: disc, bone, and viscera, internal joint derangements
Constancy of symptoms	Constant: inflammatory cycle Intermittent: less sensitized or healing nerve that is dependent on the amount of repetitive or prolonged loading or strain placed on the nerve
Aggravating factors	Nerves can be aggravated by lengthening past their mechanical or physiological thresholds or compression that impedes their ability to conduct neural impulses
Easing factors	Nerves are thixotropic; they like motion and dislike compression or tension
Stability of symptoms	Like other tissue, nerves should improve and heal; any worsening of symptoms may indicate possibilities of increased neural sensitivity, compression leading to sensory, motor, and reflex loss, as well as central pain processing
Past medical history	Consideration should be given to pathologies that impair the nerve itself or the ability of the nerve to heal (i.e., diabetes, AIDS, multiple sclerosis, and leprosy)
Past surgeries	Previous surgeries or trauma injuries can lead to increased neural mechanosensitivity, intraneural edema, or scarring, possibly predisposing patients to neural pathologies
Special questions	Visceral tissue can refer in patterns similar to nerve, therefore patients should be screened for associated systemic pathology
X-rays	Can be utilized to locate the site of entrapment but does not show nerve
MRI	Can be used to hypothesize about the site of entrapment and can show nerve interfaces with surrounding tissue
EMG	Is utilized to determine sites of entrapment as well as muscle involvement; serial tests can reveal the state of degeneration/regeneration
Special laboratory tests	Rh tests can rule out autoimmune diseases that impact nerves
Red flags	Increasing neurological symptoms Unexplained weight changes Fevers Unremitting nocturnal pain

MRI, magnetic resonance imaging; EMG, electromyogram.

REFERENCES

1. Arden NK, Price C, Reading I, et al. A multicentre randomized controlled trial of epidural corticosteroid injections for sciatica: the WEST study. *Rheumatology*. 2005;44:1399-1406.
2. Atlas SJ, Keller RB, Wu YA, Deyo RA, Singer DE. Long-term outcomes of surgical and nonsurgical management of sciatica secondary to a lumbar disc herniation: 10 year results from the Maine Lumbar Spine Study. *Spine*. 2005;15, 30(8):927-935.
3. Barbar SM. Peripheral nerve injuries in a Third World country. *Cent Afr J Med*. 1993;39:120-125.
4. Boonstra AM, van Weerden TW, Eisma WH, Pahlpatz VB, Oosterhuis HJ. The effect of low-frequency electrical stimulation on denervation atrophy in man. *Scand J Rehabil Med*. 1987;19:127-134.
5. Burnett MG, Zager EL. Pathophysiology of peripheral nerve injury: a brief review. *Neurosurg Focus*. 2004;16:1-7.
6. Butler DS. *The Sensitive Nervous System*. Australia: Noigroup Publications; 2000.
7. Campbell WW. Evaluation and management of peripheral nerve injury. *Clin Neurophysiol*. 2008;119:1951-1965.
8. Cleland JA, Childs JD, Palmer JA, Eberhart S. Slump stretching in the management of non-radicular low back pain: A pilot clinical trial. *Man Ther*. 2006;11:279-286.
9. Diao E, Vannuyen T. Techniques for primary nerve repair. *Hand Clin*. 2000;16:53-66.
10. Doubell TP, Mannion R, Woolf CJ. The dorsal horn: state dependent sensory processing, plasticity and the generation of pain. In: Wall PD, Melzack R, eds. *Textbook of Pain*. 4th ed. Edinburgh: Churchill Livingstone; 1999.
11. Duncan ME, Hansen S, Tadesse T, et al. Peripheral nerves and nerve function in highland Ethiopians. *Ethiop Med J*. 2007;45(1):61-72.
12. Dworkin RH, Backonja M, Rowbotham MC, et al. Advances in neuropathic pain: diagnosis, mechanisms, and treatment recommendations. *Arch Neurol*. 2003;60:1524-1534.
13. Fenrich K, Gordon T. Canadian association of neuroscience review: axonal regeneration in the peripheral and central nervous systems—current issues and advances. *Can J Neurol Sci*. 2004;31:142-156.
14. Fritz JM, Linday W, Matheson JW, et al. Is there a subgroup of patients with low back pain likely to benefit from mechanical traction? Results of a randomized clinical trial and subgrouping analysis. *Spine*. 2007;15, 32(36):E793-E800.
15. Gelberman RH, Szabo RM, Williamson RV. Tissue pressure threshold for peripheral nerve viability. *Clin Ortho Rel Res*. 1983;178:285-291.
16. Gordon T, Brushart TM, Amirjani N, Chan KM. The potential of electrical stimulation to promote functional recovery after peripheral nerve injury—comparisons between rats and humans. *Acta Neurochir Suppl*. 2007;100:3-11.
17. Haddick E. Management of a patient with shoulder pain and disability: A manual physical therapy approach addressing impairments of the cervical spine and upper limb neural tissue. *J Ortho Sports Phys Ther*. 2007;37(6):342-350.
18. Hall TM, Elvey RL. Nerve trunk pain: physical diagnosis and treatment. *Man Ther*. 1999;4(2):63-73.
19. Khoromi S, Cui L, Nackers L, Max MB. Morphine, nortriptyline and their combination vs. placebo in patients with chronic lumbar root pain. *Pain*. 2007;130:66-75.
20. Khoromi S, Patsalides A, Parada S, Salehi V, Meegan JM, Max MB. Topiramate in chronic lumbar radicular pain. *J Pain*. 2005;6(12):929-836.
21. Kingery WS. A critical review of controlled clinical trials for peripheral neuropathic pain and complex regional pain syndromes. *Pain*. 1997;73:123-139.
22. Kouyoumdjian JA. Peripheral nerve injuries: a retrospective survey of 456 cases. *Muscle Nerve*. 2006;34:785-788.
23. Lundborg G, Rydevik B. Effects of stretching the tibial nerve of the rabbit; a preliminary study of the intraneural circulation and the barrier function of the perineurium. *J Bone J Surg*. 1973;55b:390-401.
24. Nee R, Butler D. Management of peripheral neuropathic pain: Integrating neurobiology, neurodynamics, and clinical evidence. *Physical Therapy in Sport*. 2006;7:36-49.
25. Noble J, Munro CA, Prasad VS, Midha R. Analysis of upper and lower extremity peripheral nerve injuries in a population of patients with multiple injuries. *J Trauma*. 1998;45:116-122.
26. Nykvist F, Hurme M, Alaranta H, Kaitsaari M. Severe sciatica: a 13-year follow up of 342 patients. *Eur Spine J*. 1995;4:335-338.
27. Ogata K, Naito M. Blood flow of peripheral nerve, effects of dissection, stretching and compression. *J Hand Surg*. 1986;11b:10-14.
28. Roganovic Z, Pavlicevic G. Difference in recovery potential of peripheral nerves after graft repairs. *Neurosurgery*. 2006;59:621-633.
29. Ross JS, Robertson JT, Frederickson RC, Petrie JL, et al. Association between peridural scar and recurrent radicular pain after lumbar discectomy: magnetic resonance evaluation, ADCON-L European Study Group. *Neurosurgery*. 1996;38(4):855-861.
30. Seddon H. Three types of nerve injury. *Brain*. 1943;66:237-288.
31. Shacklock M. *Clinical Neurodynamics*. London: Elsevier; 2005.
32. Spinner RJ, Kline DG. Surgery for peripheral nerve and brachial plexus injuries or other nerve lesions. *Muscle Nerve*. 2000;23:680-695.
33. Stanec S, Tonkovic I, Stanec Z, Tonkovic D, Dzepina I. Treatment of upper limb nerve war injuries associated with vascular trauma. *Injury*. 1997;28:463-468.
34. Sunderland S. The anatomy and physiology of nerve injury. *Muscle Nerve*. 1990;13:771-784.
35. Taylor CA, Braza D, Rice JB, Dillingham T. The incidence of peripheral nerve injury in extremity trauma. *Am J Phys Med Rehab*. 2008;87(5):381-385.
36. Tsai Y-Y. *Tension changes in the ulnar nerve by different order of upper limb tension test. Master of Science Thesis*. Chicago: Northwestern University; 1995.
37. Valat JP, Rozenber S. Local corticosteroid injections for low back pain and sciatica. *Joint Bone Spine*. 2008;75:403-407.
38. Vicenzino B, Collins D, Wright A. The initial effects of a cervical spine manipulative physiotherapy treatment on the pain and dysfunction of lateral epicondylalgia. *Pain*. 1996;68:69-74.
39. Watkins LR, Wiertelak EP, Gochler LE, et al. Characterization of cytokine-induced hyperalgesia. *Brain Res*. 1994;654:15-26.
40. Watkins LR, Maier SF. The pain of being sick: implications of immune-to-brain communication for understanding pain. *Annu Rev Psychol*. 2000;51:20-57.
41. Weber H. Lumbar disc herniation: a controlled, prospective study with ten years of observation. *Spine*. 1983;8:131-140.
42. Whitehouse BJ. Adrenal cortex. In: Fink G, ed. *Encyclopedia of Stress*. San Diego: Academic Press; 2000.
43. Woolf CJ, Bennett GJ, Doherty M, et al. Towards a mechanism-based classification of pain. *Pain*. 1998;77:227-229.
44. Woolf CJ. The dorsal horn: state dependent sensory processing and the generation of pain. In: Wall PD, Melzack R, eds. *Textbook of Pain*. 3rd ed. Edinburgh: Churchill Livingstone; 1994.
45. Zochodne DW, Levy D. Nitric oxide in damage, disease and repair of the peripheral nervous system. *Cell Mol Biol*. 2005;51:255-267.
46. Zorn P, Shacklock M, Trott P, Hall R. The effect of sequencing the movements of the upper limb tension test on the area of symptom production. In: *Proceedings of the 9th biennial conference of the Manipulative Physiotherapists' Association of Australia*. 1995:166-167.

Section II

ORTHOPEDIC REASONING

AUTHOR: DERRICK SUEKI

INTRODUCTORY INFORMATION

The study of chronic pain is an evolving science. New discoveries about the cause and nature of pain are occurring yearly. Chronic pain provides an interesting paradox in rehabilitation. Most tissues in the body have specific referral patterns and time frames for healing. When these patterns go astray, recovery and rehabilitation become more challenging and patient outcomes become less optimistic. In general, most tissue will heal in 6 to 8 weeks. The younger and more healthy a person is, the more quickly injuries heal. The older a person is, or the less healthy, the longer tissue recovery takes. Other factors also influence a person's ability to heal and these will be addressed throughout this chapter. But regardless of a person's age, factors occur physically, chemically, or emotionally that prevent or delay healing. These factors will be the focus of this chapter.

WHAT IS THE PREVALENCE OF CHRONIC PAIN?

The prevalence of chronic pain is not a simple question to answer. Chronic pain can refer to long-standing pain in a body region or long-standing pain generalized throughout the entire body. Both have different prevalence rates.

WHAT IS THE PROGNOSIS FOR RECOVERY FROM CHRONIC PAIN?

Because chronic pain encompasses such a wide spectrum of conditions, the prognosis for recovery is very diverse. In the United States, Hardt et al reported the statistics shown in Box II-16-1 regarding the prognoses of recovery for many regions of the body.[24]

WHAT IS PAIN?

Pain can be broadly defined as the suffering or discomfort caused by tissue damage. In reality, pain is a very individual experience and varies from person to person. A specific injury to tissue may be mildly discomforting to one person, but may be debilitating to another. The wide variability and subjectivity of pain make the diagnosis and treatment of it clinically challenging. Physiologically, pain is perceived by the brain when it realizes that a danger to body tissue exists and that action is required. From a purpose standpoint, the body utilizes pain to help avoid dangerous and potentially life-threatening events.

WHAT IS NOCICEPTION?

Nociception is different from pain. Nociception is the actual transmission of neural impulses from damaged tissue to the brain via nociceptive neurons. Pain, on the other hand, is the interpretation of these signals by the brain or other structures. So in a simplified form, nociception is a physiological response to tissue damage and pain is an interpretive response. It is the interpretation of pain that can lead to some of the problems seen clinically in patients. It is also this interpretation that results in the highly subjective nature of pain. It varies from person to person and from moment to moment.

CLINICAL PEARL

The great variability in human pain suggests that the synthesis of pain is not a simple process and that modulation of the transmission of pain is possible.[15]

WHAT OCCURS PHYSIOLOGICALLY WITH ACUTE PAIN?[10,28,29,44]

The physiology behind acute pain is well documented in the literature. Since the time of the Greeks, the biomedical model of pain has been developed and refined. Although the process is not totally complete, here is what we know to date regarding acute pain. Acute pain is a normal and necessary physiological response to tissue injury. The pain itself occurs as a result of the following processes:

1. Stresses outside of the normal limits of tissue result in tissue damage.
2. Injury to tissue will activate free nerve endings that respond to the noxious stimuli.
3. Most of these nerve endings are polymodal and will respond to different stimuli such as mechanical, thermal, or chemical.
4. As a result of the mechanical, thermal, or chemical stimulation of peripheral nociceptive neurons, nociceptive impulses are transmitted to the dorsal horn of the spinal cord.
5. At the dorsal horn, the primary somatosensory neuron will synapse with a secondary or projection neuron.
6. These secondary neurons will project the nociceptive impulses cortically via the spinothalamic (lateral) and spinoreticular (medial) tracts.
7. A large proportion of these secondary neurons belong to the spinothalamic tract and will make additional synapses at the lateral and medial nuclei of the thalamus.
8. At the thalamus these neurons will synapse with tertiary neurons.
9. It is important to note that the secondary neurons may also synapse with neurons in several other nuclei of the brainstem including the periaqueductal gray (PAG) and nucleus raphe magnus (NRM).
10. Tertiary neurons from the thalamus, PAG, and NRM will then project neurons to the primary and secondary somatosensory cortices (SI, SII). The SI and SII are involved in the sensory quality of pain, which includes location, duration, and intensity.
11. Tertiary neurons may also project to areas responsible for emotions such as the anterior cingulate cortex (ACC) and the insula, which are involved in the limbic or emotional component of pain.

CLINICAL PEARL

In the sixteenth century, René Descartes proposed one of the earliest theories on pain. His theory has been called the specificity theory. The specificity theory states that the body has a separate sensory system for perceiving pain, just as it does for hearing, touch, and vision. This system has its own receptors, spinal pathways, and region of the brain that are all designed to transmit and process information about pain. A nociceptive stimulus in the periphery will result in a neural signal propagating to the brain by the same route and to the same cortical destination. Descartes believed that there was one pain center in the brain that processed and interpreted all painful stimuli.[44]

BOX II-16-1 **Chronic Pain Estimates for Body Region**	
Body Region	**Percentage of Patients Polled**
Back pain	10.1%
Pain in the legs/feet	7.1%
Pain in the arms/hands	4.1%
Headache	3.5%
Regional	11.0%
Wide spread pain	3.6%

WHAT IS THE PURPOSE OF PAIN?

Pain is good. It notifies the body that tissue is damaged, activates protective measures to prevent further damage to the tissue, and initiates healing and immune responses to repair the damage and prevent infection. Some of these responses are engaged locally by the release of chemical mediators at the site of injury. Others are engaged systemically. Pain is an important part of the body's prime mission or goal, which is to maintain a state of homeostasis. When circumstances force the body outside of its normal limits, the body must adapt to return it to its normal state. Whether it is an acute injury or a chronic illness, the body has the ability to self-correct. Persistent pain and illness occur when the body cannot return to normal conditions. Chronic pain is an example of how the body cannot return to its normal state.

WHY DO WE GET INFLAMMATION AFTER AN INJURY?[10,42]

After an injury, the following events occur:

1. Pronociceptive inflammatory molecules such as bradykinins, prostaglandins, histamine, serotonin, and adenosine triphosphate are released by various blood cells such as mastocytes, polymorphonuclear leukocytes, and platelets in the tissue immediately adjacent to the site of injury.
2. The release of molecules will result in a local increase in pain known as peripheral hyperalgesia.
3. The injury also triggers immune cells to release interleukins, interferon, and tumor necrosis factors, all of which act to increase localized inflammation.
4. Substance P and calcitonin gene-related protein (CGRP), which act as neurotransmitters in the central nervous system, are also released into the periphery in response to tissue injury and act as proinflammatory factors in the periphery, which produces inflammation in regions outside the immediate area of tissue damage. This process is known as *neurogenic inflammation*.

MEDICATIONS

Table II-16-1 lists various common medications and modalities prescribed for pain and their mechanism of action.

SYSTEMICALLY, WHAT EVENTS OCCUR IN RESPONSE TO ACUTE INJURY?

Injury leads to inflammation. Inflammation is normal and healthy. When the inflammatory process is unable to downregulate inflammation or the body is unable to return to its previous state of homeostasis further tissue injury or disease can occur. Chronic inflammation is being linked to many of the chronic problems associated with health care in the United States. Examples include neck pain, fibromyalgia, congestive heart failure, asthma, arthritis, and the "itis" (bursitis, tendinitis, epicondylitis).

CLINICAL PEARL

Chronic pain varies from person to person. It is always individual and always unique. What has been unclear in the past is whether there is an ethnic or a genetic component to pain. Clinically, different cultures appear to respond to pain differently. Similarly, in the clinic, there appeared to be a genetic component because families would often experience similar chronic pain symptoms. What has always been the problem in the past was the validation of these finding through studies and research. The past decade has begun to reveal that both ethnicity and genetics may play a role in the formation and maintenance of chronic pain.

TABLE II-16-1	Sites and Mechanisms of Analgesia
Modality	**Mechanisms of Action**
Opioid analgesic agents	Bind to opiate receptors in the central nervous system and possibly the periphery
Nonsteroidal antiinflammatory agents	Block the production of prostaglandins
Local anesthetic agents	Block the transmission of nerve impulses
Transcutaneous nerve stimulation	Closes the "gate" in the dorsal horn of the spinal cord; may also have some endorphin component
Acupuncture	Same as transcutaneous nerve stimulation
Nitrous oxide	Blunts the emotional reaction to pain; the endogenous opioid system may play a role
Ketamine	Dissociates the thalamocortical and limbic systems
Hypnosis	Causes the cognitive reinterpretation of pain stimulus
Biofeedback	Decreases muscle tension
Music	Decreases anxiety and allows a cognitive focus on stimuli other than pain
Placebo	Activates descending pain inhibitory paths; also possibly endorphins
Distraction	Allows a cognitive focus on stimuli other than pain

Adapted from Paris PM, Yealy DM. Pain management. In: Marx JA. *Rosen's Emergency Medicine: Concepts and Clinical Practice*. 6th ed. St. Louis: Mosby; 2006.

ETHNICITY AND GENETICS[3,28]

In 2002, in a study of adults, age-adjusted estimates indicated that blacks had a prevalence of arthritis similar to that of whites, but a higher proportion had activity and work limitations attributable to arthritis and thus a higher prevalence of arthritis-attributable activity and work limitations. Overall, blacks with doctor-diagnosed arthritis had a higher prevalence of severe pain attributable to arthritis, compared to whites.[5] In the same study, compared to whites, Hispanics had a lower prevalence of doctor-diagnosed arthritis, but a similar proportion with activity limitations attributed to arthritis, resulting in a lower prevalence of arthritis-attributable activity limitations. Hispanics had a higher proportion of work limitations than whites. A higher proportion of Hispanics with doctor-diagnosed arthritis reported severe joint pain, compared to whites.

In a separate study by Hardt et al, Mexican-Americans, compared to non-Hispanic whites and blacks, were less likely to have chronic back pain, legs/feet pain, arms/hands pain, and regional and widespread pain.[24]

Ethnicity aside, there is now mounting evidence to suggest that there is a genetic component to chronic pain. Genetic predispositions to the development and continued maintenance of pain are well documented in the literature.[8,39] It has been suggested that chronic pain and pain syndromes that appear to have no physiological basis may be influenced by genetic factors. It is recognized by clinicians that no two patients respond identically to a specific treatment regime. The reason for the differed response may have it roots in genetics.[22]

HOW HAS ILLNESS AND DISEASE CHANGED OVER THE PAST 100 YEARS?

Disease and illness rates are difficult to tabulate due to inaccuracies in hospital and physician records. The trends shown in Box II-16-2 have become evident from data compiled by the Centers for Disease Control and Prevention (CDC).

Section II

ORTHOPEDIC REASONING

MOST COMMON MEDICAL PROBLEMS

1. Back or neck problems
2. Allergies
3. Arthritis or rheumatism
4. Difficulty walking
5. Frequent headaches
6. Lung problems
7. Digestive problems
8. Gynecological problems
9. Anxiety attacks
10. Heart problems or chest pain

The take home message of the above statistics is that death and illness are examples of the body's inability to maintain a state of homeostasis. The question plaguing medicine these days is whether there is a common thread that links all of these pathologies. It has been suggested that chronic inflammation may be one of the major common links.

WHY IS INFLAMMATION IMPORTANT AND WHAT HAPPENS WHEN IT GOES AWRY?

Inflammation (Latin, inflammatio, to set on fire) is the complex biological response of vascular tissues to harmful stimuli. In actuality, inflammation has two purposes. It is a protective attempt by the organism to remove the injurious stimuli and it initiates the healing process for the tissue.

One of the most important roles of inflammation is that it protects of the body from foreign substances. This is accomplished through a coordinated effort of the immune and inflammatory systems. In response to psychological or physiological stressors, the acute inflammatory response described earlier is activated. In addition, a systemic stress mobilization response is activated. The response includes the sympathetic nervous system, the hypothalamic-pituitary axis, and the renin-angiotensin system. This activation results in the release of stress hormones (catecholamines, corticosteroids, growth hormone, glucagon, and renin), which, together with cytokines induced by stress, participate in the protective response of inflammation. The response is designed to remove and protect against foreign debris, prevent infection, and restore the normal barriers that protect the body.

Many of the inflammatory cells serve two purposes: they protect and they help in the healing process. Approximately 2 days after the initial injury, neutrophils produce platelet-derived growth factors (PDGF), which attract fibroblasts to the wound. Fibroblasts synthesize the construction materials for repair—collagen, proteoglycans, and elastin. The resultant tissue is called *granulation tissue*. Angioblasts are also attracted by PDGF. They link together and extend toward existing vessels to reestablish vascularization.

WHAT IS THE DIFFERENCE BETWEEN ACUTE AND CHRONIC INFLAMMATION?

Acute inflammation is the initial response of the body to harmful stimuli and is achieved by the movement of plasma and leukocytes from the blood into the injured tissues. Chronic inflammation

TABLE II-16-2 **Physiological Differences between Acute and Chronic Inflammation**

	Acute	Chronic
Cause	Pathogen or injured tissue	Persistent nondegradable pathogens Persistent foreign bodies Autoimmune reaction
Major cells	Neutrophils Monocytes Macrophages	Monocytes Macrophages Lymphocytes Fibroblasts
Primary mediator	Vasoactive amines	Cytokines Growth factors Hydrolytic enzymes
Onset	Immediate	Delayed
Duration	21 days	Many months or years
Physiological Events	Healing Chronic inflammation	Tissue destruction Fibrosis

leads to a shift in the types of cells that are present at the site of inflammation (Table II-16-2).

HOW DO YOU REGULATE THE INFLAMMATORY RESPONSE?

Removal of the injurious stimuli is the key to stopping the inflammatory process. The injurious stimuli can be many things. In infection it is the pathogen, in allergies it is the allergen, and in muscle strains it is the healing of tissue. In all of these cases, once the injurious stimuli are removed, inflammation ceases and tissue regains it state of homeostasis. Many inflammatory mediators have short half-lives and are quickly degraded in the tissue, helping to cease the inflammatory response once the stimulus has been removed.

WHAT HAPPENS WITH CHRONIC INFLAMMATION? WHY IS IT NOT DOWNREGULATED?

In chronically inflamed tissue, the stimulus is persistent, and therefore recruitment of monocytes is maintained. Existing macrophages are tethered in place, and proliferation of macrophages is stimulated. Tissue becomes fibrosed with the entrance of fibroblasts.

DOES CHRONIC INFLAMMATION EQUATE TO CHRONIC PAIN?

It may equate. It is not so simple as to state that inflammation is the only source of chronic pain. We know clinically that removal of inflammation will reduce pain in a large percentage of patients. But many of these patients return with the same inflammation and same pain a short time later. So, is inflammation the culprit or merely a symptom? To answer this we have to look at the some of the previous theories regarding pain.

CLINICAL PEARL

It is very difficult to utilize a patient's symptom history to derive the cause of a patient's symptoms. Most of the time the pain began insidiously, is not well localized, and can be aggravated by factors that do not make biomechanical sense.

SYMPTOM HISTORY

The symptom history does very little to influence the decision-making process. People with chronic pain may or may not have a specific mechanism of injury. The mechanism of injury is not a good predictor of the patient who will eventually progress to chronic pain. Some patients with chronic pain will have a very specific mechanism of injury and in others symptoms will begin more insidiously. The location of symptoms is not a good indicator of chronicity as symptoms may be very similar to those in the acute patient. Symptoms may be a little more wide spread and not so localized, but this cannot be applied universally. Other normal pain descriptors such as depth of symptoms, quality of symptoms, and constancy of symptoms are all similar to the acute patient. No one descriptor can be utilized to predict a patient whose symptoms will become more chronic in nature. Certain specific chronic pain syndromes such as complex regional pain syndrome and fibromyalgia may have a heightened response to stimuli. Normally nonpainful stimuli will now be painful to the patient. This response, however, is not indicative of all patients with chronic pain. The 24-hour pattern of pain that a patient experiences with chronic pain may or may not be different from the acute patient's pain. Many times the patient's symptoms will improve only to be reaggravated. The aggravating activity may be physical, chemical, or emotional in nature. Very rarely do patients have continuous unchanging pain. The pain will wax and wane during the day and over the course of time. There may be times when the patient is nearly pain free only to find that the pain is triggered once again and the whole pain cycle commences once more. Functional activities alone should not be used as an indicator of chronicity as the activities that aggravate and ease a patient's symptoms will be the same as those that are more acute. Symptoms may begin more easily with the chronic pain. This is because patients with chronic pain may become more deconditioned, predisposing them to further injury and further stages of deconditioning.

THE BIOMEDICAL THEORY AND SPECIFICITY THEORY OF PAIN

The biomedical model of pain was created by the ancient Greeks and expanded on by Descartes. The concepts are built on simplicity and logic. Injury to a specific tissue will result in specific pathologies in a predictable and consistent manner. Descartes viewed the body as *healthy* if, like a properly functioning machine, that body was in good working order. Conversely, a body was classified as *diseased* if an impairment of its function could be detected. For many years, even to today, medicine approaches pathology in a biomedical manner. Descartes proposed that the amount of pain a person experienced is directly related to the amount of tissue damage incurred by the body. For example, a paper cut causes very little tissue damage and as a result very little pain should be experienced. For a broken bone, the amount of tissue damage incurred is much larger, therefore the amount of pain experienced is much greater. This theory, the "specificity theory," is generally accurate when applied to certain types of injuries and the acute pain associated with them. This is very appropriate for many pathologies; unfortunately, chronic pain is not one of them. Clinicians know from practice that patients with chronic pain do not follow established rules regarding tissue injury. Injury will result in a completely different pain experience from person to person. Sometimes mild injuries will result in significant pain and other times pain will be present in the absence of any tissue injury.[25]

THE GATE CONTROL THEORY OF PAIN[9,10,29]

In 1962, Melzack and Wall developed a theory on pain that is now known as the Gate control theory of pain.[29] The theory asserts that activation of nonnociceptive nerves, which do not transmit pain signals, can interfere with signals from nociceptive pain fibers, thereby inhibiting or modulating pain. The theory that pain can be modulated or altered was a large step away from the biomedical approach, which viewed pain as being a concrete manifestation of the tissue damaged. Modulation of pain could occur from the periphery in the form of sensory stimulation or cortically from the brain in the form of descending neural inhibition. This was medicine's first attempt at integrating the physiology and psychology of pain. The Gate control theory proposes that environmental and emotional factors can shape the pain experience. In this way, each individual brings unique attributes that can vary the experience of pain. The Descartes biomedical model viewed the mind and the body as separate entities that operated independently of each other. The Gate theory is an important step in the evolution of pain science because it allowed medical science to have a solid testable foundation of neurophysiology while still allowed integration of the less testable psychological components.

THE NEUROMATRIX THEORY

In 1999, Melzack expanded on his Gate control theory.[31] The Gate theory focused primarily on the peripheral nervous system and its interaction at the spinal cord level. Nociception could be modulated at this level by both peripheral and cortical influences. Testing of peripheral modulations has been studied extensively mostly due to its accessibility for testing purposes, but Melzack realized that a large portion of the pain picture was still ill defined. The cortical influences on the Gate theory continue to be a mystery within pain science. It is well established that cortical pathways can modulate nociception. The control and regulation of these pathways are the parts of the puzzle still missing. Without knowledge of the cortical influences on pain, diagnosing the source of pain is similar to trying to find out why your computer is not working. The Gate theory would be equivalent to doing diagnostics on the computer's wiring and connections. To solve the problem of pain Melzack realized that he needed to address what was going on within the computer itself.

WHAT IS THE NEUROMATRIX?[31,32]

The neuromatrix is the processing and decision-making center of the body. It involves the cortex, limbic system, thalamus, and all the structures that support and influence these regions. In the past, it was believed that only one pain center existed in the brain; Melzack stated that the cortex is not the pain center, and neither is the thalamus.[30] The areas of the brain involved in pain experience and behavior are very extensive. They must include the limbic system as well as somatosensory projections. Furthermore, because our body perceptions include visual and vestibular mechanisms as well as cognitive processes, widespread areas of the brain must be involved in pain. The neuromatrix is the anatomical and physiological hardware that controls all activity within the body including the interpretation of pain.

WHAT INFLUENCED THE DEVELOPMENT OF THE NEUROMATRIX?

Melzack was motivated to expand his Gate theory through the realization of its shortcomings. Additionally, he was influenced by the work of Hans Selye. The term *stress*, as it is currently used, was coined by Hans Selye in 1936. He defined stress as "the non-specific response of the body to any demand for change." Selye noted in numerous experiments that laboratory animals subjected to acute but different noxious physical and emotional stimuli (blaring light, deafening noise, extremes of heat or cold, perpetual frustration) all exhibited the same pathological changes of stomach ulcerations, shrinkage of lymphoid tissue, and enlargement of the adrenals. He later demonstrated that persistent stress could cause these animals to develop various diseases similar to those seen in humans, such as heart attacks, stroke, kidney disease, and rheumatoid arthritis. At the time, it was believed that most diseases were caused by specific but different pathogens. Tuberculosis was caused by the tubercle bacillus, anthrax by the anthrax bacillus, syphilis by a spirochete, etc. What Selye proposed was just the opposite, namely that many different insults could cause the same disease, not only in animals, but in humans as well.

HOW DOES STRESS PLAY INTO THE NEUROMATRIX?

When an organism is injured there is an alteration and disruption of homeostatic regulation. This deviation from the body's normal state initiates a complex of neural, hormonal, and behavioral mechanisms designed to restore homeostasis. Melzack hypothesizes that prolonged stress and ongoing efforts to restore homeostasis can suppress the immune system and activate the limbic system. The limbic system has an important role in emotion, motivation, and cognitive processes. As originally proposed by Selye, prolonged activation of the stress regulation system can lead to a predisposition for the development of different states of chronic pain.

CLINICAL PEARL ⚠

A good example of different responses to stress is afforded by observing passengers on a steep roller coaster ride. Some are hunched down in the back seats, eyes shut, jaws clenched, and white knuckled with an iron grip on the retaining bar. They can't wait for the ride in the torture chamber to end so they can get back on solid ground and scamper away.

But up front are the wide-eyed thrill seekers, yelling and relishing each steep plunge, all of whom race to get on the very next ride. In between you may find a few with an air of nonchalance that borders on boredom. So, was the roller coaster ride stressful?

WHAT IS STRESS?

The answer is not known, but we do know that there is good stress or *eustress* and that there is also bad stress or *distress*. If you were to ask a dozen people to define stress, or explain what stresses them, or how stress affects them, you would likely get 12 different answers to each of these requests. The reason for this is that there is no one definition of stress on which everyone agrees. What is stressful for one person may be pleasurable or have little effect on others, and we all react to stress differently. In general, stress is related to both external and internal factors. External factors include the physical environment, including your job, your relationships with others, your home, and all the situations, challenges, difficulties, and expectations with which you are confronted on a daily basis.

Internal factors determine your body's ability to respond to, and deal with, the external stress-inducing factors.

WHY IS STRESS IMPORTANT?[38]

Robert Sapolsky is a neuroendocrinologist who has focused his research on issues of stress and neuron degeneration, as well as on the possibilities of gene therapy strategies for help in protecting susceptible neurons from disease.[38] Sapolsky spends time annually in Kenya studying a population of wild baboons in order to identify the sources of stress in their environment and the relationship between personality and patterns of stress-related disease in these animals. More specifically, Sapolsky studies the cortisol levels between the alpha male and female and the subordinates to determine stress level.

CLINICAL PEARL ⚠

Psychological and emotional factors are important predictors of chronic pain.[2,13,18,35]

WHAT IS THE LONG-TERM IMPACT OF STRESS?

Sapolsky, through his research, has discovered a major role that cortisol, or hydrocortisone, plays in stress responses. The adrenal gland produces cortisol in response to stress. Repeated stress, infections, or chronic illness can deplete the body's adrenal reserves, and the ability to produce adequate amounts of cortisol is affected. People with low adrenal reserve experience rapid drops in blood sugar (hypoglycemia) during stress because there is not enough cortisol to maintain sugar levels. In response, the body starts producing and secreting adrenaline, which raises blood sugar but also causes anxiety. Therefore, people with low adrenal cortisol are more prone to signs of temper, nervousness or shaking, palpitations, irritability, difficulty concentrating, salt cravings, sleep disturbances, and fear of situations that are even moderately stressful; they can have panic attacks, experience fatigue, feel cold, and may have depression.

COMMON SIGNS OF STRESS

Box II-16-3 lists common signs of stress.

STRESS AND ILLNESS

During infections, the adrenal glands normally increase their output to double or triple the amount of cortisol in the blood to help fight the infection. During a viral infection, adrenal hormone

---

BOX II-16-3 Common Signs of Stress

1. Frequent headaches, jaw clenching, or pain
2. Gritting, grinding teeth
3. Stuttering or stammering
4. Tremors, trembling of lips, hands
5. Neck ache, back pain, muscle spasms
6. Light headedness, faintness, dizziness
7. Ringing, buzzing, or "popping" sounds
8. Frequent blushing, sweating
9. Cold or sweaty hands, feet
10. Dry mouth, problems swallowing
11. Frequent colds, infections, herpes sores
12. Rashes, itching, hives, "goose bumps"
13. Unexplained or frequent "allergy" attacks
14. Heartburn, stomach pain, nausea
15. Excess belching, flatulence
16. Constipation, diarrhea
17. Difficulty breathing, sighing
18. Sudden attacks of panic
19. Chest pain, palpitations
20. Frequent urination
21. Poor sexual desire or performance
22. Excess anxiety, worry, guilt, nervousness
23. Increased anger, frustration, hostility
24. Depression, frequent or wild mood swings
25. Increased or decreased appetite
26. Insomnia, nightmares, disturbing dreams
27. Difficulty concentrating, racing thoughts
28. Trouble learning new information
29. Forgetfulness, disorganization, confusion
30. Difficulty in making decisions
31. Feeling overloaded or overwhelmed
32. Frequent crying spells or suicidal thoughts
33. Feelings of loneliness or worthlessness
34. Little interest in appearance, punctuality
35. Nervous habits, fidgeting, feet tapping
36. Increased frustration, irritability, edginess
37. Overreaction to petty annoyances
38. Increased number of minor accidents
39. Obsessive or compulsive behavior
40. Reduced work efficiency or productivity
41. Lies or excuses to cover up poor work
42. Rapid or mumbled speech
43. Excessive defensiveness or suspiciousness
44. Problems in communication, sharing
45. Social withdrawal and isolation
46. Constant tiredness, weakness, fatigue
47. Frequent use of over-the-counter drugs
48. Weight gain or loss without diet
49. Increased smoking, alcohol, or drug use
50. Excessive gambling or impulse buying

is necessary to suppress inflammation. People with low reserves are more prone to higher fever and body aches. Therefore, people with low adrenal reserves may have increased susceptibility to colds and infections, more prolonged infections, and are more prone to allergies and arthritis. The hypothalamus, pituitary, adrenal (HPA) axis is also a prime regulator of the body's response to stress. It also interacts with the immune system, making you more vulnerable to colds and flu, fatigue, and infections. In response to an infection or an inflammatory disorder such as rheumatoid arthritis, cells of the immune system produce three substances that cause inflammation: interleukin 1 (IL-1), interleukin 6 (IL-6), and tumor necrosis factor (TNF).[11]

CLINICAL PEARL

There is a strong link between chronic pain and chronic inflammation. Therefore, the patient may have a past history of medical conditions that results in inflammation. A prime example of these conditions is autoimmune disorders, which result in chronic inflammation as the body fights against itself. The fact that the self is always present results in inflammation that never resolves and pain that never ceases.

MEDICAL HISTORY

STRESS AND GROWTH

The hormones of the HPA axis also influence hormones needed for growth. Prolonged HPA activation (or stress activation) will hinder the release of growth hormone and insulin-like growth factor 1 (IGF-1), both of which are essential for normal growth. Glucocorticoids released during prolonged stress also cause Cushing's syndrome, which results in high glucocorticoid levels. The result is a loss of about 7.5 to 8.0 cm from their adult height. Similarly, premature infants are at an increased risk for growth retardation.

The stress of surviving in an environment for which they are not yet suited, combined with the prolonged stress of hospitalization in the intensive care unit, presumably activates the HPA axis. Growth-retarded fetuses also have higher levels of cortisol releasing hormone (CRH), adrenocorticotropic hormone (ACTH), and cortisol, probably resulting from stress in the womb or exposure to maternal stress hormones. Other research has also shown that the stress from emotional deprivation or psychological harassment may result in the short stature and delayed physical maturity of the condition known as *psychosocial short stature (PSS)*. PSS was first discovered in orphanages, in infants who failed to thrive and grow. When these children were placed in caring environments in which they received sufficient attention, their growth resumed. The children's cortisol levels were abnormally low.[22]

CLINICAL PEARL

External stressors and a history of previous pain or trauma have been shown to be good predictors for the development of chronic pain in patients. Children born prematurely, who as infants receive painful clinical interventions, will be more sensitive to pain later in life. The mechanism by which these children may be sensitized to pain can be partly explained by deficits in pain inhibitory mechanisms.[7,20,22,27,28,41]

ENVIRONMENTAL AND PSYCHOLOGICAL FACTORS

STRESS AND GASTROINTESTINAL DISORDERS

The stress circuit influences the stomach and intestines in several ways. First, CRH directly hinders the release of stomach acid

---

BOX II-16-4   Common Stress-Related Diseases

Chronic pain
Migraines
Ulcers
Heartburn
High blood pressure
Heart disease
Diabetes
Asthma
Allergies
Premenstrual Syndrome (PMS)
Obesity
Infertility
Autoimmune diseases
Irritable bowel syndrome
Skin problems
Fibromyalgia

---

and emptying of the stomach. Moreover, it also directly stimulates the colon, speeding up the emptying of its contents. In addition to the effects of CRH alone on the stomach, the entire HPA axis, through the autonomic nervous system, also hinders stomach acid secretion and emptying and increases the movement of the colon. Also, continual, high levels of cortisol, as occur in some forms of depression, or during chronic psychological stress, can increase appetite and lead to weight gain. Rats given high doses of cortisol for long periods had increased appetites and had larger stores of abdominal fat. The rats also ate heavily when they would normally have been inactive. Overeating at night is also common among people who are under stress.

COMMON STRESS-RELATED DISEASES

Box II-16-4 lists common stress-related diseases.

STRESS AND DEPRESSION

Rather than producing higher amounts of ACTH in response to CRH, depressed people produce smaller amounts of this substance, presumably because their hippocampuses have become less sensitive to the higher amounts of CRH. In an apparent attempt to switch off excess CRH production, the systems of people with melancholic depression also produce high levels of cortisol. However, by-products of cortisol, produced in response to high levels of the substance, also depress brain cell activity. These by-products serve as sedatives, and perhaps contribute to the overall feeling of depression.

STRESS AND LONGEVITY

Patients under stress may also experience suppression of thyroid hormones and of the immune system. Because they are at higher risk for these health problems, such patients are likely to have their life spans shortened by 15 to 20 years if they remain untreated.

CLINICAL PEARL

Age affects pain. The older one gets, the greater the likelihood of experiencing chronic pain.

AGE

It has been well established in the literature that age impacts pain. The prevalence of chronic pain increases with age.[3,5,24,28] Perguin et al discovered the following statistics in their research regarding the prevalence of pain in Dutch children aged 0 to 18 years. Of the over 5000 respondents, 54% had experienced pain within the previous 3 months and 25% had experienced chronic pain. Several interesting trends were noticed. The prevalence of chronic pain increased with age, with the greatest increase occurring in the 12- to 14-year-old age bracket. Chronic pain rates were significantly higher in girls, with the highest rates occurring around puberty. The most frequent regions of pain were the limbs, the head, and the abdominal area. Half of the respondents who had experienced pain reported multiple pain, and one-third of the chronic pain sufferers experienced frequent and intense pain.[34] In a study conducted in adults in Australia by Blyth, chronic pain was reported by 17.1% of the males and 20.0% of the females. Chronic pain was defined as pain experienced every day for 3 months in the 6 months before the interview. For males, prevalence peaked at 27.0% in the 65 to 69 year age group and for females prevalence peaked at 31.0% in the oldest age group, between 80 and 84 years old. Once again, several interesting trends were noted. Chronic pain was significantly higher in the following patient groupings: patients who are older, female, and have lower educational levels, patients with poor self-related health and higher psychological distress, patients receiving disability benefits, and patients without private health insurance.[3]

STRESS AND POSTPARTUM DEPRESSION

Chrousos and his team showed that a sudden cessation of CRH production may also result in the symptoms of postpartum depression. In response to CRH produced by the placenta, the mother's system stops manufacturing its own CRH. When the baby is born, the sudden loss of CRH may result in feelings of sadness or even severe depression for some women.[12]

STRESS AND FERTILITY

The adrenal glands also play a key role in reproductive function. Women with low adrenal output can have skipped or irregular menstrual periods and unusual menstrual bleeding, and are at greater risk for miscarriage or infertility. Because of changes in the functions of the ovaries, women can also have increased facial hair or acne.

STRESS AND HORMONES

The hypothalamus stimulates the pituitary gland to release two other hormones: oxytocin and vasopressin (antidiuretic hormone). These hormones are responsible for keeping the blood pressure elevated, so that the heart, muscles, and brain can obtain the oxygen needed for optimal functioning in the face of danger. Saliva may dry up in the mouth as fluids are transferred to more essential areas, such as the brain and muscles. The blood's clotting ability is also increased, so that the body will lose less blood and fluids in the event of an injury.

STRESS AND THE THYROID

The hypothalamus releases thyrotropic hormone releasing factor (TRF), which stimulates the pituitary gland to release thyrotropic hormone (TTH). As this hormone travels through the bloodstream, it stimulates the thyroid gland (located in the neck) to produce two chemicals: thyroxine and triiodothyronine. These two chemicals are responsible for speeding up the body's metabolism, resulting in the acceleration of the following processes: blood pressure, breathing, heart rate, thinking processes, and perspiration. The liver produces sugar from its stores of glycogen (composed of excess sugars, proteins, and fat) and releases it into the bloodstream to provide extra energy for the body.

STRESS AND INSOMNIA

Recently, Chrousos and Gold uncovered evidence that frequent insomnia involves more than just having difficulty falling asleep. They found that when compared to a group of people who did not have difficulty falling asleep, the insomniacs had higher levels of ACTH and cortisol both in the evening and in the first half of the night. Moreover, insomniacs with the highest cortisol levels tended to have the greatest difficulty falling asleep. It was theorized that in many cases, persistent insomnia may be a disorder of the stress system. Based on their levels of ACTH and cortisol, it appears that the insomniacs have nervous systems that are on overdrive, alert and ready to deal with a threat, when they should be quieting down.[11]

WHAT IS THE OTHER FACTOR THAT INFLUENCES CHRONIC PAIN?

One of the functions of the immune system is to protect the body by responding to invading microorganisms, such as viruses or bacteria, by producing antibodies or sensitized lymphocytes (types of white blood cells). Under normal conditions, an immune response cannot be triggered against the cells of our own body. In certain cases, however, immune cells make a mistake and attack the very cells that they are meant to protect. This can lead to a variety of autoimmune diseases. Unlike some diseases, autoimmune diseases do not generally have a simple, single cause. There are usually two major categories of factors that are involved in causing autoimmune diseases: genetics and environment. Most autoimmune diseases combine these two.

GENDER AND AUTOIMMUNITY: A person's sex also seems to have a major role in the development of autoimmunity.

Most of the known autoimmune diseases tend to show a female preponderance, the most important exceptions being ankylosing spondylitis, which has a male preponderance, and Crohn's disease, which has a roughly equal prevalence in males and females. The reasons for this are unclear. Apart from inherent genetic susceptibility, several animal models suggest a role for sex steroids. It has also been suggested that the slight exchange of cells between mothers and their children during pregnancy may induce autoimmunity. This would tip the gender balance in the direction of the female. It is also very interesting to note that both chronic pain and autoimmunity have a higher prevalence in females and that both autoimmunity and chronic pain increase in prevalence as women age. A positive link has not been established between these facts, but the relationship has been proposed by numerous researchers.

CLINICAL PEARL

Chronic pain rates are higher in females than in males.[16]

WHAT INFLUENCE DOES GENDER HAVE ON YOUR CLINICAL DECISION-MAKING PROCESS?[3,5,16,17,24,28,36,43]

Statistics on gender can be somewhat misleading when it comes to pain. The reason for the confusion rests in the nature of reporting pain. Genders respond to and report pain and injury differently. Women have a tendency to report pain and seek medical attention more readily and frequently than men. Therefore, even though women were more likely to experience headache, abdominal pain, and chronic widespread pain than men, it is difficult to determine if this is a true reflection of the actual picture.

There have been some interesting hypotheses put forth to explain the gender inequity regarding pain. The actual reason for this disparity has not been determined, but the reason for this predisposition is probably multifactorial. Hormonal differences have been proposed as a major factor in the difference experienced between the sexes. Part of the reason for the role of hormones in pain comes from the trends seen in chronic pain prevalence. Spikes in pain prevalence can be seen in two groups of people: girls between 12 and 14 years old and women over 50 years of age. Females experience major fluctuations in hormone balance at both times, at puberty and at menopause. Animal research supports differential responses between the sexes and supports the effect of sex hormones on pain. For instance, females show greater nociceptive responses than males do for the same stimulus, but this difference disappears after gonadectomy. Moreover, if gonadectomized rats receive replacement hormones of the opposite sex, females receiving testosterone and males receiving estrogen and progesterone, they demonstrate the same nociceptive behavior attributable to the sex hormone status. Interestingly, this influence of sex hormones also seems to be true in human beings, as differences in response to pain between men and women appear only after puberty and disappear after menopause or andropause.

RADICULAR PAIN, INFLAMMATION, AND THE DISC: It has been proposed that lumbar radiculopathy secondary to a disc protrusion is not only the result of mechanical compression of a spinal nerve or nerve root. Significant evidence indicates that it is inflammation, which underlies the radicular pain, that is associated with symptomatic lumbar disc herniation. The inflammatory process is believed to sensitize the dorsal root ganglion (DRG) to all incoming stimuli. In such a state, even minor mechanical stimulation of the DRG could evoke severe pain. Autoimmunity has been suggested as a cause of the chronic inflammation that surrounds the nerve. In a follow-up study by Olmarker et al, electron microscopic analyses of normal appearing neural tissue under light microscopy revealed axonal injury and Schwann cell damage. These results demonstrate that nuclear material can cause morphological damage to neural tissue without a concurrent mechanical process such as compression.

THE IMMUNE SYSTEM AND LOW BACK PAIN: With increased evidence that chronic low back pain may involve an autoimmune reaction to the disc, a review of the immune system and low back pain appears warranted.

The nucleus pulposus has been shown to elicit an immune response. It has been reported that disc material can incite a leukocyte cell reaction, cytokine, and immunoglobulin response. Several studies have also suggested that bacterial infection may be a source of pain and inflammation in disc pathology.

- Gronblad et al demonstrated the presence of an abundant number of macrophages (innate immunity) in human disc herniation specimens removed at the time of surgery. Control discs contained only a few macrophages. They also identified inflammatory cytokine (adaptive immunity), interleukin-β immunoreactive cells in herniated disc tissue.[21]
- Another hypothesis regarding the basis for an autoimmune response to the lumbar disc was based on the lack of blood supply to the nucleus pulposus. Following embryological formation, the nuclear proteins do not come in contact with systemic circulation; therefore, it is postulated that a focal protrusion can lead to exposure of nuclear material to the immune system. Because it will be detected as a foreign body, an autoimmune response may be mounted.
- Bobechko and Hirsch demonstrated the inflammation-inducing potential of nuclear material using a rabbit model.[4]
- Olmarker et al showed that the epidural application of autologous nuclear material without mechanical compression in pigs may induce pronounced changes in nerve root structure and function. An epidural inflammatory reaction occurred following application of the nucleus pulposus.

HOW IS THE IMMUNE RESPONSE REGULATED?

It was once believed that the immune system was a completely autonomous system that functioned completely independently of other systems. It is now being discovered that other systems such as the autonomic nervous system and the HPA system can modulate the effects of the immune system. Both of these systems are stress response systems.

HOW DOES THIS ALL TIE INTO MELZACK'S NEUROMATRIX THEORY?

The following is being established through scientific research:
- Science is evolving that demonstrates a link between stress and disease.
- Stress has also been linked to increases in autoimmunity.

- Stress has been linked to diminished immune responses.
- Both stress and the immune response produce inflammation.
- Chronic inflammation has been linked to many of the diseases that currently plague humans.

Stressors are regulated by two systems, the HPA axis and the autonomic nervous system. If we could find means to alter stress, inflammation, and immune responses to the triggers of pathology, then we could make changes to the means by which the body heals and adapts. For this reason, Melzack realized that the key to unlocking the mystery of pain lies not in the peripheral circuitry, but in the processing of information. The neuromatrix is the hardware for those decisions.

WHAT OTHER THEORIES OF PAIN SUPPORT THIS VIEW?

The biopsychosocial model of health postulates that health and function are intimately linked with a patient's psychological and social status. Factors such as emotions, social support, and individual impressions of their health greatly influence people's ability to heal and their response to tissue damage. Psychological and social factors influence biological functions. This theory precedes Melzack's theory by over a decade and was first postulated by the psychiatrist George L. Engel in 1977. Melzack's neuromatrix theory is an integration of the biopsychosocial theory, Selye's stress research, and the Gate theory of pain.[14, 19, 23, 26]

WHAT ROLE DOES BIOMECHANICS PLAY IN THE DECISION-MAKING PROCESS?

In the past, clinical decision making regarding interventions for rehabilitation have traditionally been based on a biomechanical paradigm. Although evidence for the effectiveness of rehabilitation techniques continues to expand, mounting evidence has emerged challenging the usefulness of many tenets of the biomechanical model. That is not to say that biomechanics is not an important part of medicine and rehabilitation, just that medicine and rehabilitation need to expand beyond biomechanics. Biomechanical analysis fits nicely into a biomedical model. It is testable and explainable. Pain is not always testable or explainable. Biomechanics applies nicely to acute conditions in which tissue damage is known and the mechanism of injury justifies the tissue damage. Chronic pain does not follow biomechanical or biomedical principles. Biomechanics should form the basis for assessment and diagnosis, but if the symptoms do not match normal biomechanical principles, alternative theories should be considered.[14]

MECHANISM OF INJURY AND AGGRAVATING ACTIVITIES

Unlike acute injuries, chronic pain injuries do not follow the normal biomechanical model. Aggravating activities, easing activities, and mechanism of injury cannot be utilized to diagnose specific tissue injury.

SUMMARY STATEMENT

Normally, when tissue is damaged, the brain perceives pain. But due to the interactions among psychological, environmental, and normal physiological factors this is not always the case. These factors are a normal but variable part of our everyday life and our personal history. The idea of pain as purely physiological or purely psychological is invalid. All pain is a mixture of these factors. Rehabilitation of patients requires clinicians who can blend these factors together.

A new paradigm: "The structural paradigm has not met the challenge. A paradigm shift is clearly necessary to fill in the blanks and move forward. Immunology, biochemistry, and neurophysiology have the capability of filling this void."[40]

REFERENCES

1. Armitage CJ, Conner M. Social cognition models and health behavior: A structured review. *Psychology and Health.* 2000;15:173–189.
2. Auerbach SM, Laskin DM, Frantsve LM, et al. Depression, pain, exposure to stressful life events, and long-term outcomes in temporomandibular disorder patients. *J Oral Maxillofac Surg.* 2001;59(6):628–633.
3. Blyth FM. Chronic pain in Australia: a prevalence study. *Pain.* 2001;89(2–3):127–134.
4. Bobechko WP, Hirsch C. Auto-immune response to nucleus pulposus in the rabbit. *J Bone Joint Surg Br* 1965;47:574–580.
5. Bolen J, Sniezek J, Theis K, et al. *Racial/Ethnic Differences in the Prevalence and Impact of Doctor-Diagnosed Arthritis.* Morbidity & Mortality Weekly Report; Arthritis National Center for Chronic Disease Prevention and Health Promotion, CDC; 2005.
6. Bruns D, Disorbio JM. Chronic pain and biopsychosocial disorders. *Practical Pain Management.* 2006;6(2).
7. Buskila D, Neumann L, Zmora E, et al. Pain sensitivity in prematurely born adolescents. *Arch Pediatr Adolesc Med.* 2003;157(11):1079–1082.
8. Buskila D. Genetics of chronic pain states. *Best Pract Res Clin Rheumatol.* 2007;21(3):535–547.
9. Butler DS. *The sensitive nervous system.* Adelaide: Noigroup Publications; 2000.
10. Butler DS, Moseley LS. *Explain pain.* Adelaide: Noigroup Publications; 2003.
11. Chrousos GP, Gold PW. The concepts of stress and stress system disorders. Overview of physical and behavioral homeostasis. *JAMA.* 1992;267(9):1244–1252.
12. Chrousos GP, Torpy DJ, Gold PW. Interactions between the hypothalamus-pituitary-adrenal axis and the female reproductive system: clinical implications. *Ann Intern Med.* 1998;129(3):299–240.
13. Currie SR, Wang J. Chronic back pain and major depression in the general Canadian population. *Pain.* 2004;107(1–2):54–60.
14. Engel GL. The need for a new medical model: a challenge of biomedicine. *Science.* 1977;196:129–136.
15. Flor H. The functional organization of the brain in chronic pain. In: Sandkühler J, Bromm B, Gebhart GF, eds. *Progress in brain research.* Vol 129. Amsterdam: Elsevier; 2000.
16. Gaumond I, Arsenault P, Marchand S. Specificity of female and male sex hormones on excitatory and inhibitory phases of formalin-induced nociceptive responses. *Brain Res.* 2005;1052(1):105–111.
17. Gaumond I, Arsenault P, Marchand S. The role of sex hormones on formalin-induced nociceptive responses. *Brain Res.* 2002;958(1):139–145.
18. Gauthier N, Sullivan MJ, Adams H, et al. Investigating risk factors for chronicity: the importance of distinguishing between return-to-work status and self-report measures of disability. *J Occup Environ Med.* 2006;48(3):312–318.
19. Gifford LS, ed. *Topical Issues in Pain 2. Biopsychosocial assessment. Relationships and pain.* Falmouth: CNS Press; 2000.
20. Goffaux P, Lafrenaye S, Morin M, et al. Preterm births: can neonatal pain alter the development of endogenous gating systems? *Eur J Pain.* 2008;130(1–2):137–143.
21. Gronblad M, Virri J, Tolonen J, et al. A controlled immunohistochemical study of inflammatory cells in disc herniation tissue. *Spine.* 1994;19:2744–2751.
22. Grunau RE, Holsti L, Peters JW. Long-term consequences of pain in human neonates. *Semin Fetal Neonatal Med.* 2006;11(4):268–275.
23. Halligan PW, Aylward M, eds. *The Power of Belief: Psychosocial influence on illness, disability and medicine.* UK: Oxford University Press; 2006.
24. Hardt J, Jacobsen C, Goldberg J, Nickel R, Bushwald D. Prevalence of chronic pain in a representative sample in the United States. *Pain Med.* 2008;9(7):803–812.
25. Hutchinson JSO. Health, health education and physiotherapy practice. In: French S, Sims J, eds. *Physiotherapy: a psychosocial approach.* 3rd ed. Elsevier; 2004.
26. Jones MA, Edwards I, Gifford LS. Conceptual models for implementing biopsychosocial theory in clinical practice. *Man Ther.* 2002;7(1):2–9.
27. Linton SJ. A population-based study of the relationship between sexual abuse and back pain: establishing a link. *Pain.* 1997;73(1):47–53.
28. Marchand S. The physiology of pain mechanisms: from the periphery to the brain. *Rheum Dis Clin N Am.* 2008;(34):285–309.
29. Melzack R, Wall PD. *The challenge of pain.* 2nd ed. London: Penguin Books; 1996.
30. Melzack R. Pain and the neuromatrix in the brain. *J Dent Educ.* 2001;65(12):1378–1382.
31. Melzack R. From the gate to the neuromatrix. *Pain.* 1999;(suppl 6):S121–S126.
32. Melzack R. Pain and stress: A new perspective. In: Gatchel RJ, Turk DC, eds. *Psychosocial factors in pain.* New York: Guilford Press; 1999.
33. Olmarker K, Rydevik B, Nordborg C. Autologous nucleus pulposus induces neurophysiologic and histologic changes in porcine cauda equina nerve roots. *Spine.* 1993;18(11):1425–1432.
34. Perguin CW, Hazebroek-Kampschreur AA, Hunfeld JA, et al. Pain in children and adolescents: a common experience. *Pain.* 2000;87:51–58.
35. Pincus T, Burton AK, Vogel S, et al. A systematic review of psychological factors as predictors of chronicity/disability in prospective cohorts of low back pain. *Spine.* 2002;27(5):E109–E120.
36. Robinson JE, Short RV. Changes in breast sensitivity at puberty, during the menstrual cycle, and at parturition. *Br Med J.* 1977;1(6070):1188–1191.
37. Saal J. The pathophysiology of Painful Lumbar Disorder Symposium. *Spine.* 1995;20(16):1803.
38. Sapolsky R. *Why zebras don't get ulcers.* 3rd ed. New York: Holt Paperbacks; 2004.
39. Stamer UM, Stuber F. Genetic factors in pain and its treatment. *Curr Opin Anaesthesiol.* 2007;20(5):478–484.
40. Turk DC, Monarch ES. Biopsychosocial perspective on chronic pain. In: Gatchel RJ, Turk DC, eds. *Psychosocial Factors in Pain.* New York: Guilford Press; 1999.
41. Turner JA, Dworkin SF. Screening for psychosocial risk factors in patients with chronic orofacial pain: recent advances. *J Am Dent Assoc.* 2004;135(8):1119–1125.
42. Vanderah TW. Pathophysiology of Pain. *Med Clin North Am.* 2007;91(1):1–12.
43. Von Kor M, Dworkin SF, Le Resche L, et al. An epidemiologic comparison of pain complaints. *Pain.* 1988;32:173–183.
44. Wall PD, Melzack R, eds. *Textbook of Pain.* 4th ed. Edinburgh: Churchill Livingstone; 1999.

AUTHOR: LEE ANNE CAROTHERS

INTRODUCTORY INFORMATION *i*

WHAT IS THE ROLE OF THE ALLIED HEALTH PROFESSIONAL IN THE DIAGNOSIS OF PATHOLOGY?

Rehabilitation of any patient requires the collaboration of many healthcare professionals. Rehabilitation clinicians must work with other healthcare professionals to provide the best and most accurate care to the patient. Their role, therefore, is not to make a medical diagnosis, but to perform a differential diagnostic process that enables them to determine the potential origin of symptoms and take one of three potential courses of action: *treat, refer*, or *treat and refer*. If the origin of the pathology is within the scope of the clinician's practice (e.g., of musculoskeletal, neuromuscular, or cardiovascular and/or pulmonary origin), the clinician is free to initiate treatment if the condition can be remediated by the chosen treatment or intervention. If the presentation of symptoms and the behavior of the symptoms indicate that the origin of the symptoms is *not* within the scope of the clinician's practice (e.g., pain that indicates a primary gastrointestinal pathology), the patient must be referred to a physician for further workup. This also holds true for conditions that could potentially be treated by the clinician, but require further medical workup via imaging, laboratory or other studies before safely proceeding (e.g., a new onset of low back pain in a patient with a past history of cancer).[1] If the patient's presentation of symptoms indicates two separate conditions, one within the clinician's practice act and one from another system, the clinician can initiate treatment for the appropriate condition *and* refer the patient for the symptoms representing pathologies whose intervention is not within his or her practice act.

WHAT FACTORS MAKE DIFFERENTIATION OF MUSCULOSKELETAL AND NONMUSCULOSKELETAL SYMPTOMS DIFFICULT?

One of the factors that may interfere with a clinician's ability to distinguish which system is responsible for the patient's presentation of symptoms is the tendency to become comfortable in one treatment setting (e.g., outpatient orthopedics or outpatient neurology). When a clinician works in a single treatment setting and primarily sees patients with pathologies from those systems, it is easy to fall into a clinical "rut" and interpret patient findings through the lenses of habit and probability.

The patient's primary complaint may often be pain in a joint or other musculoskeletal structure that may appear at first glance to result from pathology within the musculoskeletal or nervous system. It is only on completion of a thorough examination that includes an interview (to include personal and family medical history), systems review, and physical examination that the nonmuscular source of pain is revealed. The ability to make this differentiation is a critical skill for the clinician because inappropriate attribution of pain to the musculoskeletal system and a delay in appropriate diagnosis or intervention can be detrimental to the patient and put the clinician at risk for litigation. The risk for misattribution of the system that is responsible for the patient's complaint can be a source of angst for clinicians, ranging from new graduates with little clinical experience to seasoned clinicians who have not had the benefit of the didactic material taught in school. This angst can result in a timidity in clinical practice for clinicians who must either have or learn the skills required to distinguish musculoskeletal from nonmusculoskeletal pain.

In many cases, musculoskeletal pain is associated with a clear mechanism of injury. In some cases, as in overuse syndromes, the onset of pain is insidious and not clearly related to a single event or injury. A thorough interview and physical examination, however, can make the process of differentiating the origin of pain a manageable process. It may require learning some new skills and refining the questions utilized either in the health screening form, systems review, or the patient/client interview/examination, but I believe these skills and adaptations are well within the grasp of the average clinician.

PERSONAL INFORMATION *i*

A thorough medical history is essential to screening for nonmusculoskeletal causes of pain, and can easily be accomplished with the use of a medical history form. Given the information in the medical history, the clinician can then ask more pointed questions to identify "red flags" or symptoms that require immediate follow-up, with either further questions or tests and/or a referral for further immediate attention. Additionally, information identified in the medical history can reveal risk factors for the development of medical conditions or comorbidities that may manifest as musculoskeletal pain.

WHAT INFLUENCE DOES AGE HAVE ON YOUR CLINICAL DECISION-MAKING PROCESS WHEN DIFFERENTIATING MUSCULOSKELETAL AND NONMUSCULOSKELETAL SYMPTOMS?

Musculoskeletal symptoms due to sports injuries are often confined to individuals of younger ages, whereas musculoskeletal symptoms due to chronic degenerative diseases of the joints and/or falls are common in older adults. Older adults are also at risk for symptoms that originate in many different medical systems (i.e., cardiovascular, pulmonary, and renal). Although age may increase the risk for both musculoskeletal and nonmusculoskeletal symptoms, it is important to know disease-specific risk factors associated with age.

WHAT INFLUENCE DOES A PATIENT'S OCCUPATION HAVE ON YOUR CLINICAL DECISION-MAKING PROCESS IN DIFFERENTIATING MUSCULOSKELETAL AND NONMUSCULOSKELETAL SYMPTOMS?

Occupational history plays a large role in the development of many diseases. Knowledge of the kinds of diseases associated with different classes of occupations is critical. Some are more obvious than others.

- Occupations that require manual labor or repetitive movement are more likely to result in orthopedic and overuse syndromes.
- Occupations in which workers are exposed to inhaled particles can result in chronic pulmonary diseases or some lung cancers.
- Occupations in which workers are exposed to toxic substances (e.g., pesticides, dyes) can result in visceral cancers.

Unless the symptoms are associated with a clear mechanism of injury (e.g., low back strain associated with incorrect lifting strategies), occupational history will often not be the first piece of information that leads the clinician to the system responsible for the patient's symptoms. It is typically after failure to confirm the system responsible via the usual means that further investigation may reveal an association with an occupational source.

WHAT INFLUENCE DOES GENDER HAVE ON YOUR CLINICAL DECISION-MAKING PROCESS IN DEALING WITH MUSCULOSKELETAL AND NONMUSCULOSKELETAL SYMPTOMS?

Gender may have an effect on the manifestation of or risk for different patterns of visceral pain. Cardiogenic pain is a classic example. According to the American Heart Association: "*As with men, women's most common heart attack symptom is chest pain or discomfort. But women are somewhat more likely than men to experience some of the other common symptoms, particularly shortness of breath, nausea/vomiting, and back or jaw pain.*[2] In addition, the development of symptomatic ischemic cardiac disease in men precedes the development in women by approximately 10 years, or until the onset of menopause.[31] After the completion of menopause, women lose the cardioprotective effect of estrogen, and thus experience an increased incidence of atherosclerotic diseases (coronary artery disease, peripheral vascular disease, and cerebrovascular disease).

Other diseases are more likely to develop in women than in men and vice versa. Gallbladder disease, for example, which can manifest as abdominal, thoracic, or shoulder pain, tends to occur in overweight females of childbearing years. In addition, diseases associated with reproductive organs are confined to individuals of the respective genders, with the exception of breast cancer, which is present in both males and females. The clinician need not know the epidemiology (etiology, prevalence, signs/symptoms, etc.) for every disease, as the medical profession is an open book profession. However, the clinician must know how to access the resources necessary to tease out the risk factors and manifestation of different visceral disorders. More important than knowing the details about individual diseases, therefore, is the ability to identify common patterns of pain associated with different visceral organs and to distinguish visceral from nonvisceral pain.

WHAT INFLUENCE DOES ETHNICITY HAVE ON YOUR CLINICAL DECISION-MAKING PROCESS?

As with gender, some disorders are more likely to occur in different ethnic groups. In the examination process, it is imperative that the clinician knows which diseases and disorders occur more frequently in certain ethnic groups (e.g., sickle cell disease and granulomatosis in people of African descent). Many cancers occur more frequently in people from ethnic minorities,[17] including breast, colorectal, prostate, and lung cancers. People from ethnic minorities experience a higher incidence and mortality from cancers, die at a 40% higher rate from cancers, and die at a 30% higher rate from coronary artery disease compared to Americans in the general population.[8] Knowledge about the unequal incidence and mortality of diseases in different ethnic groups can assist the clinician in his or her clinical reasoning process and in the identification of risk factors while gathering information about a patient.

SYMPTOM HISTORY

WHAT INFLUENCE DOES THE MECHANISM OF INJURY HAVE ON YOUR CLINICAL DECISION-MAKING PROCESS WHEN DIFFERENTIATING MUSCULOSKELETAL AND NONMUSCULOSKELETAL SYMPTOMS?

The mechanism of injury plays a large role in the process of differentiating musculoskeletal from nonmusculoskeletal symptoms. A clear mechanism of injury related to the onset of pain is a major indicator that the pain is likely musculoskeletal in origin. Nonmusculoskeletal (i.e., visceral pain) is rarely, if at all related to a specific action or injury. Individuals may experience pain that is related to movement, but that in itself is not adequate to conclude that the pain is musculoskeletal in nature. For example, the individual with peripheral artery disease (PAD) may experience lower extremity (LE) pain associated with walking that decreases with rest, and this pain is not reproducible with palpation of movement through the range of motion (ROM). This particular manifestation of pain is associated with the ischemia sustained by the LEs due to atherosclerotic lesions in the arteries of the LE, and not due to issues within the muscles or joints. A careful

interview about a potential mechanism of injury in this case will likely reveal no injury; it is more likely that the patient will talk about a progressive decrease in his or her ability to walk without pain and that the patient's medical history will reveal risk factors for the development of atherosclerosis that is, hypertension, diabetes, smoking, sedentary lifestyle, high cholesterol, family history, age, and male gender.

LOCATION OF SYMPTOMS

WHAT INFLUENCE DOES THE LOCATION OF SYMPTOMS HAVE ON YOUR CLINICAL DECISION-MAKING PROCESS?

The location of symptoms is the starting point for the clinical interview, when used in combination with the data collected from the Health Information form. If, for example, the patient's primary complaint is shoulder pain, the clinician should create a list of *all* of the possible systems that could possibly create symptoms in the shoulder, and then proceed to rule in or rule out those systems. This is done by asking the appropriate questions about the location *and* behavior of the pain (including aggravating/alleviating factors, timing of pain, nature of pain, etc.) and then proceeding with a careful and focused physical examination.

REFERRAL OF SYMPTOMS

WHAT IS THE REFERRAL PATTERN OF THE DIFFERENT VISCERAL OR NONMUSCULOSKELETAL TISSUES? (see also Figure II-17-4)

Visceral structures refer pain depending on the location and type of organ involved. The pain produced corresponds to dermatomes from which the organ is innervated.[14]

CARDIOVASCULAR STRUCTURES

THE HEART

The heart is innervated by nerves originating from C3 to T4 spinal nerves and can therefore refer pain to multiple locations above the waist that are also innervated by these nerve roots in the case of ischemia. Myocardial ischemia occurs when there is an imbalance between myocardial supply and demand. Ischemic myocardium refers pain to the skin locations above the waist that were developing at the same time as the sympathetic nervous system,[14] which classically presents as chest pain of some sort, but may occur in the upper extremities, shoulders, neck, jaw, abdomen, or back (Figures II-17-1 and II-17-2). The embryological link between the sympathetic nervous system and the heart accounts for the significant variations observed between individuals of myocardial ischemia.[14]

Valuable information about ischemic myocardial pain and the required clinician response can be gleaned by an examination of the behavior of that pain (i.e., worse with activity, better with rest, relieved by nitroglycerine [NTG]). For example, by definition, stable angina occurs at a predictable workload, is worsened by activity, and is relieved by rest and/or administration of NTG. Unstable angina, on the other hand, occurs at a level of activity that was previously tolerated or even while resting, but still responds favorably to the administration of NTG. Printzmetal's (variant) angina has a behavior different from that of "typical" angina. It typically occurs at rest (vs. with activity), usually in the early morning, and is caused by coronary artery spasm. It is not associated with significant occlusion of coronary arteries by atherosclerosis, but rather with risk factors for the development of it.

Myocardial infarction (MI), or heart attack, occurs due to either prolonged mild ischemia or to complete occlusion of one of the

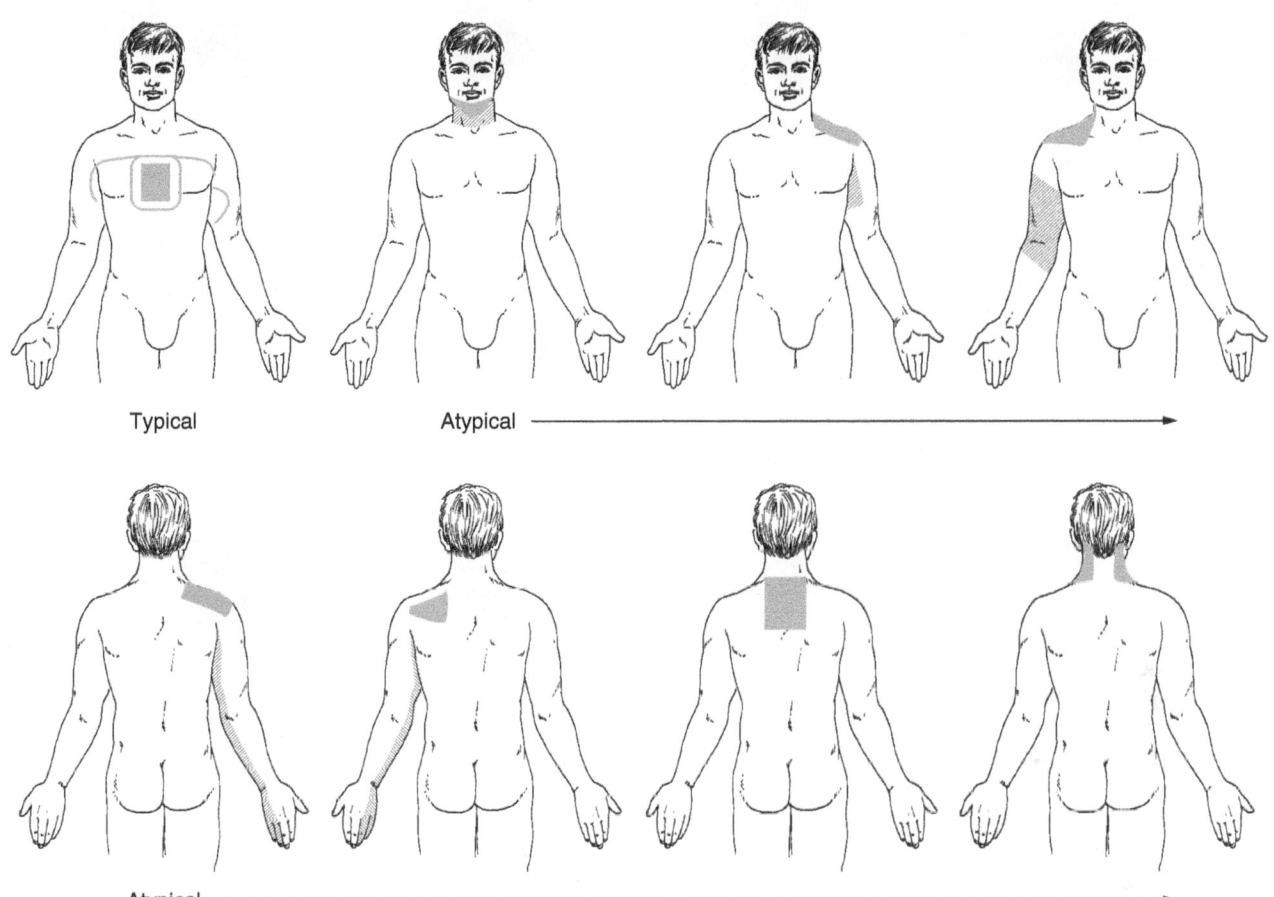

Typical   Atypical ⟶

Atypical ⟶

FIGURE II-17-1 Typical and atypical presentation of angina in men. (From Irwin S, Tecklin J, eds. *Cardiopulmonary Physical Therapy—A Guide to Practice.* St. Louis: Mosby; 2004.)

coronary arteries supplying the heart. The pain produced by MI is different in nature from that produced by stable or unstable angina. Individuals who are having a heart attack frequently report pain that is described as "crushing" substernal pain or the "worst pain ever." It is frequently accompanied by diaphoresis, nausea, or pallor, and is not relieved by NTG.

The pericardium, the sac around the heart that stabilizes the heart in the mediastinum and provides lubrication so the heart can relax and fill during diastole, is richly innervated with sensory nerves. In addition to the primary pain, which is experienced substernally and is described as "sharp, stabbing, or knife-like,"[16] the pericardium refers pain to the anterior and posterior surfaces of the left shoulder and periscapular area, the anterior ribs on the left side, and along the medial border of the left upper extremity and medial two fingers (Figure II-17-3).

In further contrast to the pain that is produced by an ischemic myocardium, pericardial pain is aggravated by movement that causes a stretch of the pericardium, specifically deep breathing, side-bending, or trunk rotation. Alleviating factors include forward leaning, kneeling on all fours, and taking small breaths. Pericardial pain is not reproducible with palpation, and is accompanied by constitutional signs such as fever; chills and malaise can be confirmed by auscultating for the presence of a pericardial friction rub.

CLINICAL DECISION MAKING CASE STUDY—PATIENT PROFILE   **(?)**

Your patient is a 45-year-old man who was referred to you for treatment of neck pain. He is a pack-a-day smoker who is sedentary and overweight. He is currently being treated for hypertension and hypercholesterolemia. How can you be sure that his pain is musculoskeletal in nature and is not caused by an ischemic myocardium?

Answer

If this man's pain were of cardiac origin, it would worsen with activity and remit with rest. True musculoskeletal pain will be exacerbated by movement or palpation and will be associated with a clear mechanism of injury. The pain will be unrelated to activity. Despite this man's history and personal risk factors for the development of heart disease, his current symptoms point to a musculoskeletal problem. Because of his risk for the development of heart disease, however, he could benefit from a program of aerobic exercise and risk factor reduction once his neck pain has resolved.

THE AORTA

The aorta, the first blood vessel to leave the left ventricle of the heart, is the major supplier of oxygenated blood to the body. Because of the high pressure in the arterial system, the aorta is at risk for the development of aneurysms, defined as a "pathologic dilatation of a segment of a blood vessel."[9] Common sites for aortic aneurysms (AAs) are thoracic or abdominal. Thoracic aneurysms typically occur in the ascending, transverse, or descending aorta, and occur in only 5% of AAs. The more common form of AA, however, occurs in the abdominal aorta, typically below the junction of the aorta and the renal arteries.[9] The most important risk factor for the development of AAs is the presence of atherosclerosis, so clinicians must consider the presence of an AA when

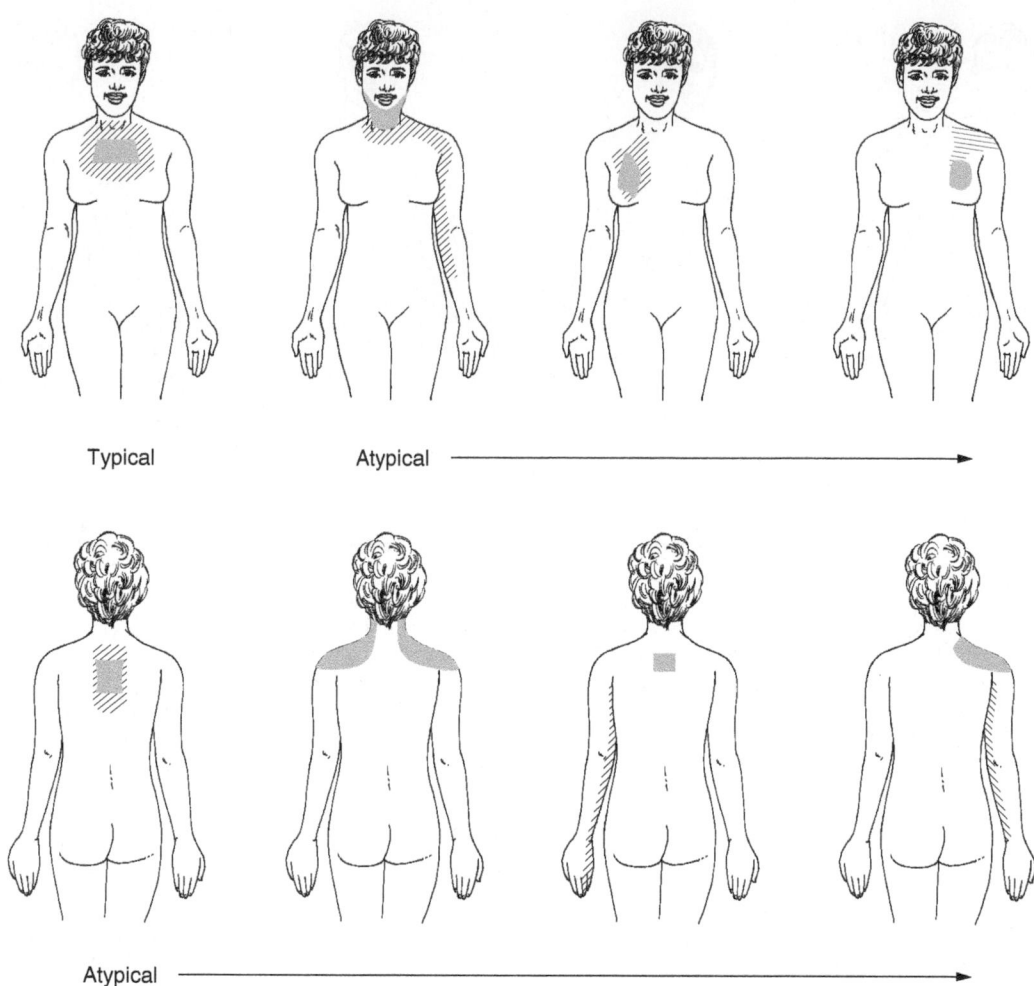

FIGURE II-17-2 Typical and atypical presentation of angina in women. (From Irwin S, Tecklin J, eds. *Cardiopulmonary Physical Therapy—A Guide to Practice.* St. Louis: Mosby; 2004.)

treating patients with known vascular disease and atypical presentation of back pain.

Additionally, AAs can be caused by infection, congenital weakness, or trauma associated with weight lifting, so clinicians treating athletes who use weight lifting as part of their exercise regime (especially older athletes) should be alert for signs and symptoms of aneurysms as well.

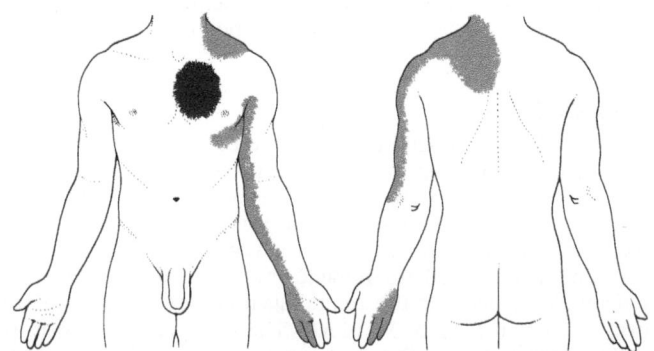

FIGURE II-17-3 Primary pain site (black) and locations of referral (gray) in pericarditis. (From Goodman CC. *Differential Diagnosis in Physical Therapy.* 4th ed. Philadelphia: Saunders; 2007.)

Symptoms associated with an AA vary depending on the stage of the aneurysm. Although most individuals with AAs are asymptomatic, some individuals with AAs that have not ruptured (dissected) will complain of dull pain in the chest (thoracic), abdomen or back (abdominal), and an awareness of a pulsating mass in the abdomen when lying down. A clinician who suspects the presence of an AA based on patient presentation may confirm his or her findings by assessing the width of the aortic pulse. Assessment of an aortic pulse width greater than the average of 2.5 cm associated with the presence of the above symptoms, especially after ruling out orthopedic causes for pain, should result in referral to a physician.

When an AA dissects, it will produce signs and symptoms that are distinctly different from those produced by a stable aneurysm. The peak incidence of aortic dissection occurs in the sixth and seventh decades, and men are twice as likely to be affected by this condition as women.[9] Individuals who are experiencing aortic dissection will complain of a sudden onset of excruciating pain that is sharp, tearing, or knifelike. Associated symptoms include a drop in blood pressure, absent pulses in the lower extremities, abdominal distention, tachycardia, diaphoresis, and an exacerbation of symptoms while lying down. Aortic dissection is a medical emergency. Clinicians who suspect that aortic dissection is occurring, therefore, should call 911 and activate the emergency medical system immediately, as death from aortic dissection can occur very rapidly.

CLINICAL DECISION MAKING CASE STUDY—PATIENT PROFILE

Your patient is a 60-year-old male who you are seeing for bilateral knee pain. He was referred to you by his family physician, who, although he suspects osteoarthritis, would like to attempt conservative management of the pain with therapy before ordering imaging studies and referral to an orthopedic surgeon. Your interview reveals that his pain is intermittent, burning in nature, and is worsened by ambulation and ceases with rest. It is unchanged by the use of NSAIDs. His family history includes atherosclerotic disease, and his personal history is positive for smoking, hypertension, and high cholesterol. Your physical examination reveals no narrowing of joint spaces and no tenderness to palpation over the knee joints. What is the cause of this man's knee pain and what can you do to confirm your suspicions?

Answer

This man's pain is likely caused by peripheral arterial disease, based on the behavior of the pain (worse with activity, better with rest) and his personal and family history. Your findings are further confirmed by the fact that you note no narrowing of the joint spaces and palpation of the joint causes no pain, as well as by the behavior of the pain and its response to medications. The following tests can confirm your suspicions: (1) palpate for peripheral pulses, (2) observe the LEs for loss of hair or pallor, and (3) measure the ankle-brachial index (ABI) [systolic blood pressure (SBP) of the ankle/SBP of the upper esophagus (UE)]. If your suspicions are correct you would note decreased peripheral pulses and an ABI of <0.8. You should refer this patient to his physician with a note explaining your objective and subjective findings. Although this patient may benefit from exercise to increase the efficiency of his LE muscles, you should not proceed with exercise until the patient has had a thorough workup of the patency of his LE arteries.

LOWER EXTREMITY ARTERIES

Peripheral arterial disease results from the formation of atherosclerotic plaques in the arteries of the lower extremities. It is associated with the same risk factors for the development of coronary artery disease (hypertension, diabetes, high cholesterol, age, male gender, obesity, and sedentary lifestyle). It is characterized by intermittent claudication, or LE pain that increases with activity and decreases with rest. The pain results from ischemia that occurs when demand of oxygen to the lower extremities is less than arterial supply. Table II-17-1 summarizes cardiovascular pain.

PULMONARY STRUCTURES

The pulmonary system produces pain in the presence of disease or disorder, although unlike cardiac pain, pulmonary pain is typically localized to the structures overlying the involved lung fields. Pulmonary pain can also radiate to the upper back, neck, shoulder, ribs, or scapulae. The location and behavior of the pain depend on which structures are involved. Referred pain from tracheal or bronchial structures is experienced in the anterior neck and chest at the levels of pathology. Potential pathologies that can produce this type of pain include infection and inflammation, irritation by foreign bodies, and cancer.

The pleural sacs, which encase the lungs, are analogous structures to the pericardium; they produce pain in a very similar way. As with the pericardium, the pleura are densely innervated with sensory nerves, and irritation of the pleura can result in severe pain. This pain is associated with trauma (rib fractures/soft tissue/

Section II

ORTHOPEDIC REASONING

TABLE II-17-1 Summary of Cardiovascular Pain

	Location of Pain	Behavior of Pain	Associated Signs
Stable angina	Anything above the waist: Men: substernal Women: vague GI-like distress	Worse with activity Better with rest Relieved by NTG	ST depression on 12-lead Arrhythmias Abnormal response to exercise
Unstable angina	Anything above the waist: Men: substernal Women: vague GI-like distress	Worse with activity Better with rest Relieved by NTG Increase in frequency/ severity when compared to stable angina	ST depression on 12-lead Arrhythmias Abnormal response to exercise
Printzmetal's angina	Anything above the waist: Men: substernal Women: vague GI-like distress	Occurs at rest in the early morning Not associated with increase in demand	ST elevation on 12-lead
MI	Anything above the waist: Men: substernal Women: vague GI-like distress	Lasts for >30 minutes Not relieved by NTG "Worst pain ever"	Positive enzymes 12-lead ECG changes Cardiogenic shock CHF
Pericarditis	Typically substernal May radiate to upper back or left shoulder	Aggravating: Deep breathing Trunk rotation, side bending Alleviating: All fours Leaning forward	Fever Malaise Pericardial rub
Aortic pain	Chest, abdomen, or back	Aggravating: Supine position Alleviating: Sitting up	Pulsatile mass in abdomen Loss of pulses in LEs Widened aortic pulse
Peripheral arteries	Lower extremities	Aggravating: Walking Alleviating: Rest	Decreased or absent LE pulses Ankle brachial index (SBP in ankle/SBP in arm) < 0.8 Color and hair changes in LEs

GI, gastrointestinal; NTG, nitroglycerine; LEs, lower extremities; MI, myocardial infarction; ECG, electrocardiogram; CHF, congestive heart failure; SBP, systolic blood pressure.

lung parenchymal damage that extends to the pleura), disorders that cause irritation (e.g., pneumothorax or tumor), and inflammation and infection (pleurisy, pneumonia, pleural effusion). Pleural pain is usually not experienced until the disease or disorder causes stretch on or irritation of the parietal pleura.

Pleural pain is typically described as sharp or knifelike, and the onset can be either sudden or gradual, depending on the nature of the disease disorder. Spontaneous pneumothorax or pain caused by trauma causes immediate sharp pain, whereas the pain from inflammation, infection, or tumor has a more gradual onset. In either case, pleural pain is exacerbated by anything that causes stretch to the parietal pleura, including deep breathing, trunk rotation, or side bending. It may also refer to the upper trapezius or lower trunk. Associated signs and symptoms include a dry, hacking, nonproductive cough, tachypnea (rapid breathing), auscultation of a pleural friction rub, and dyspnea (subjective sensation of difficulty breathing). Alleviating factors include taking rapid, small breaths, auto-splinting (lying on the affected side to minimize movement and thus pain), and side-bending toward the side of irritation to put the irritated pleura on slack.

Pulmonary pain produced by tumors can present an interesting challenge for clinicians, as it may manifest in a manner that is similar to musculoskeletal conditions. In addition to the tracheobronchial pain produced by bronchial tumors, tumors located in the apices of the lungs (Pancoast tumors) are also responsible for pain of pulmonary origin. Pancoast tumors can extend to impinge on the lower segments of the brachial plexus (C8 to T2), causing shoulder pain and numbness and weakness in the C8 to T2 distribution. When evaluating the patient with shoulder pain, the clinician should consider nonmusculoskeletal causes of pain, especially if movement, palpation, or other special tests of the shoulder cannot reproduce the pain. History and systems review questions that may point to a pulmonary cause of shoulder pain include positive answers to questions about smoking history, recent unplanned weight loss, chronic cough, hoarseness, or hemoptysis (blood in the sputum). Suspicion by the clinician that the patient's symptoms may be due to a Pancoast tumor is cause for immediate but not emergent referral to a physician for imaging studies and further workup.

Location of Pleural Pain	Behavior of Pleural Pain	Associated Signs
Over location of inflammation/ infection May refer to lower trunk, upper traps Intense stabbing, knifelike	Aggravating: Deep breaths Trunk/pleural stretch Alleviating: Side bending toward the involved side Small rapid breathing	Fever Pleural rub Dyspnea Dry cough Tachypnea

CLINICAL DECISION MAKING CASE STUDY—PATIENT PROFILE (?)

Your patient is a 50-year-old woman whom you are seeing for management of low back pain. She was referred to your office with the diagnosis of "low back pain." The patient interview reveals that her pain had an insidious onset and that there was no clear mechanism of injury. You have been treating her for 3 weeks without a change in her symptoms. She has a history of breast cancer when she was 30 years old that was treated with a mastectomy. Regular mammograms and clinical breast examinations have revealed no recurrence to date, but it has been 1 year since her last physical. You are unable to reproduce her pain with movement or palpation, and she displays no limitations in strength or ROM. What could be responsible for this woman's back pain and should you continue to treat her?

Answer

This woman's history, absence of a mechanism of injury, and failure to respond to treatment indicate a nonmusculoskeletal cause for her pain. You should be particularly concerned about metastasis of her breast cancer, and she should be seen by a physician for further workup, including imaging studies.

ABDOMINAL ORGANS[13]

As with other visceral organs, pain associated with abdominal organs is experienced both in the somatic structures innervated by the nerves that also innervate the organs. It may also be referred to sites distant to the organ in question, and can often be reproduced with palpation over the suspected organ. Pain associated with abdominal organs may be exacerbated by or relieved by food consumption and may be accompanied by nausea, vomiting, or changes in the color, frequency, consistency, amount, or shape of bowel movements.

Several organs produce pain that may initially seem to originate from musculoskeletal sources. Rather than a detailed discussion of the details associated with each organ, see Tables II-17-2, II-17-3, and II-17-4 for a summary of abdominal, pelvic, and urological organ pain sites, referral patterns, and aggravating and alleviating factors.

SYMPTOM DESCRIPTORS

QUALITY OF SYMPTOMS

A patient's description of symptoms can reveal valuable information about the source of the pain, therefore reinforcing the need for a thorough and careful interview. McGill, in his original work on the assessment of pain published in 1975, provided guidelines for discerning the origin of pain based on patient descriptors.[24]

Source of Pain	Pain Descriptors
Neurogenic	Sharp, crushing, pinching, hot, searing, itchy, stinging, pulling, jumping, shooting, pricking, gnawing, electrical
Musculoskeletal	Aching, sore, deep, cramping, dull, hurting, heavy
Vascular	Pulsing, pounding, beating, throbbing
Emotional	Tiring, vicious, agonizing, nauseating, exhausting, cruel, sickening, annoying, unbearable, torturing, dreadful, piercing, punishing, frightful, miserable, killing

Visceral pain, by contrast, is poorly localized, unpleasant, and is often associated with nausea and autonomic symptoms.[12]

WHAT INFLUENCE DOES THE DEPTH OF SYMPTOMS HAVE ON YOUR CLINICAL DECISION-MAKING PROCESS?

The main difference between pain experienced as superficial or deep is likely due to the different nature of the pain evoked by noxious stimuli. This may be due in part to the relative deficiency of A nerve fibers in deep structures. Ganong reports that individuals with irritation or damage to deep structures will experience little rapid, bright pain.[12] He further states that deep pain and visceral pain are poorly localized, nauseating, and frequently associated with autonomic symptoms, such as sweating and changes in blood pressure.[12] Pain in deep structures such as periosteum and ligaments can be elicited by experimental injection of hypertonic saline. The pain thus produced stimulates reflex contraction of nearby skeletal muscles, similar to the muscle spasm experienced by individuals who injure bones, tendons, or joints. The steadily

TABLE II-17-2   Abdominal Organs

Organ	Primary Pain Site	Description	Referral Site	Aggravating Factors	Alleviating Factors	Associated Signs
Esophagus	Substernal at the level of the lesion Radiating pain around the ribs at the site of the lesion	Knifelike, stabbing, sticking Burning (esophagitis) "Heartburn"	Mid T-spine (may be first and only sign of esophageal cancer)	Lying flat Overeating Late-night meals	Sitting up Proton pump inhibitors Antacids	Difficulty swallowing Painful swallowing Melena (black, tarry stool) Hoarseness Frequent belching
Stomach/duodenum	Epigastric Left upper quadrant of the abdomen	Aching Burning Gnawing, cramp-like pain	Mid to low T-spine (T6 to T10) Right shoulder (rare)	Food (especially spicy) (gastric ulcer)	Food (milk) Antacids Vomiting (duodenal ulcer)	Nausea and vomiting (N/V) Decreased appetite Weight loss Melena
Small intestine	Umbilical	Cramping	Low-spine (T9 to T11)		Passing stool or flatus	Nausea Fever Diarrhea Migratory arthritis
Large intestine	Lower abdomen across the right and left lower quadrants	Dull Cramping	Sacrum	Defecation Stress Smoking	Defecation completion Flatus	Bright red blood in stools Diarrhea Change in caliber of stools Weight loss
Pancreas	Epigastric	Burning Gnawing	Upper T-spine (T5 to T9) Left shoulder	Walking Lying supine Chronic alcoholism Large meals	Sitting Leaning forward	Sudden weight loss Jaundice N/V Flatulence Tachycardia Light colored stools Weakness due to changes in digestive enzymes Fever Malaise
Gallbladder	Epigastric Right upper quadrant (RUQ)	Dull ache Deep pain Steady	Right shoulder Periscapular back pain Anterior ribs (T10 to T12)	Deep inspiration Eating fatty foods Upper esophageal movement Lying down		Muscle guarding and tenderness Nausea Fever Malaise Chills Flatulence
Liver	Mid-epigastric RUQ	Dull ache Sense of fullness Progressive	Periscapular back pain (T7 to T10) Right shoulder			Jaundice Itching Fatigue Malaise Nausea Spider angioma Palmar erythema Neurological changes
Appendix	Right lower quadrant (RLQ) Over McBurney's point (halfway between the ASIS and umbilicus)	Aching Comes in waves Progressive over time	Epigastric Periumbilical Right groin			Anorexia N/V Fever Positive rebound tenderness (pain is worse when palpation pressure is released than when it is applied) Positive obturator sign (pain with passive flexion and internal rotation of the right hip) Positive psoas sign (pain with passive extension of the right hip)

ASIS, anterior superior iliac spine.

TABLE II-17-3 Reproductive Organs[8]

Organ	Primary Pain Site	Description	Referral Site	Aggravating Factors	Alleviating Factors	Associated Signs
Ovary	Lower abdomen	Vague pressure Dull pain	Sacrum	Painful during ovulation (2 weeks into the cycle)	Cessation of ovarian activity and the release of the egg into the fallopian tube	Positive rebound tenderness
Uterine corus	Lower abdomen Pelvis	Crampy Deep	Sacrum T-L junction	Painful after ovulation and at the end of the ovulation cycle	Cessation of the menstral cycle	Dyspareunia Unexpected vaginal bleeding Abnormal vaginal discharge
Fallopian tube (ectopic pregnancy)	Lower abdomen Pelvis	Unilateral Progressive	Low back Shoulder	Painful during ovulation (2 weeks into the cycle)	Passage of the egg into the uterus from the fallopian tubes	Positive rebound tenderness Hypotension Shock Unexplained vaginal bleeding Missed period
Testes	Lower abdomen Scrotum	Dull ache	Sacrum Ipsilateral groin	None noted	None noted	Breast tenderness Gynecomastia

TABLE II-17-4 Urological Organs[8]

Organ	Primary Pain Site	Description	Referral Site	Aggravating Factors	Alleviating Factors	Associated Signs
Kidney	Ipsilateral flank	Dull Aching Boring Poorly localized	May radiate to the lower back, groin, upper thigh, testes, or labia Ipsilateral shoulder	Pain is unrelated to position or movement	None noted	Change in urination Positive Murphy's (fist) percussion Constitutional symptoms
Ureter	Ipsilateral flank	Colicky Comes in waves	May radiate to the lower abdomen, groin, upper thigh, testes, or labia	Pain is unrelated to position or movement	None noted	Nausea and vomiting Hyperesthesia of T10 to L1 dermatomes Rectal spasm
Bladder/urethra	Suprapubic Low abdomen Low back	Intermittent	Pelvis	Full bladder	Emptying the bladder	Urinary urgency Rectal spasm Dysuria Burning with urination
Prostate	Suprapubic Low abdomen	Persistent Aching	Low back Pelvis Sacrum Perineum Inner thigh T-L spine	Rectal examination	None noted	Constitutional symptoms Urinary urgency, hesitancy Nocturia Incomplete bladder emptying Arthralgia Myalgia Pain with ejaculation

contracting muscles become ischemic, and ischemia stimulates the pain receptors in the muscles (see below). The pain in turn initiates more spasm, setting up a vicious cycle. Deep somatic pain may also be referred, but superficial pain is not. Visceral pain, however, can be either local or referred. When visceral pain is both local and referred, it may radiate from the original site to a distant site.[12] It is also more likely to produce autonomic symptoms (diaphoresis, changes in heart rate or blood pressure) and nausea, rather than localized muscle contraction and pain.

WHAT INFLUENCE DOES CONSTANCY OF SYMPTOMS HAVE ON YOUR CLINICAL DECISION-MAKING PROCESS?

In general, pain associated with systemic diseases presents as progressive or cyclical, that is, pain that is described as being better or worse at different times or worse over a prolonged period of time. Pain associated with musculoskeletal conditions typically presents with symptoms that are more constant during the day. This may be due, in part, to the fact that people are generally more active during the day, and unlike nonmusculoskeletal pain, movement exacerbates musculoskeletal conditions.

TWENTY-FOUR-HOUR SYMPTOM PATTERN

Symptoms characteristic of different pathologies are associated with the appearance of pain at different times of the day. For example, morning pain is associated with cardiac dysfunction (including stable and unstable angina and MI),[7,26] osteoarthritis (OA) of the hand,[5] renal colic,[22] migraine,[30,32] rheumatoid arthritis,[10,20] and fibromyalgia.[6] Peak pain experienced in the afternoon or evening is associated with OA of the knee,[5,18,21] whereas night pain is associated most frequently with biliary colic,[29] gastroesophageal reflux disease (GERD),[27] onset of labor pains,[4] toothache,[28] and cancer.[15] Of note is the fact that night pain is often the presenting symptom for many cancers.[15]

MEDICAL HISTORY

WHAT ROLE DOES A PATIENT'S PAST MEDICAL HISTORY PLAY IN THE DIFFERENTIAL DIAGNOSIS OF PATHOLOGY?

A patient's past medical history can serve as a roadmap in the differential diagnosis process, thus reinforcing the need for a careful history and systems review. The presence of risk factors for atherosclerosis (hypertension, high cholesterol, diabetes, sedentary lifestyle, smoking, obesity, male gender, and age) can assist the clinician in determining the cause of pain, for example, is LE, shoulder, or back pain being experienced by a patient musculoskeletal in origin, or could it be due to myocardial/LE ischemia or an aortic aneurysm? A history of smoking can assist the clinician in determining whether shoulder pain is due to musculoskeletal injury or a cancerous tumor. Careful inclusion of the medical history in the medical screening process is a vital tool in differentiating the cause or source of pain.

MEDICAL AND ORTHOPEDIC TESTING

WHAT MEDICAL AND ORTHOPEDIC TESTS INFLUENCE YOUR DIFFERENTIAL DIAGNOSIS PROCESS?

At times, patient presentation of symptoms may necessitate the use of traditional "medical" tests to discern the cause of pain. After the clinician has exhausted the possibility of a musculoskeletal origin of pain via attempts to reproduce the patient's pain with movement, palpation, or special orthopedic tests, the use of these "medical" tests can be used to confirm the clinician's findings and provide a language with which to communicate with the physician. For example, the clinician may perform abdominal palpation to test for local and referred pain associated with visceral organs. In the case of right groin pain, the clinician can test for rebound tenderness (pain that is worse after withdrawal of pressure than with application) and for an obturator or psoas sign (pain that is worse with flexion and internal rotation of the right hip or pain that is worse with right hip extension, respectively). In the case of flank pain that is not clearly associated with musculoskeletal structures, the clinician can perform Murphy's percussion over the kidney to confirm that the patient's pain is renal in origin. These traditional "medical" tests are not done for diagnostic purposes, but to determine whether the patient's presentation of symptoms indicates a pathology that falls within the clinician's scope of practice.

CLINICAL DECISION MAKING
CASE STUDY—PATIENT PROFILE

Your patient is a 16-year-old female who was referred to you for treatment of an acute groin strain. She first noticed her pain today while at volleyball practice, and attributes the onset of pain to beginning her volleyball workout without adequate warmup or stretching. Flexion and internal rotation as well as extension of her right hip exacerbate her pain, which she describes as deep and crampy. What further tests can you do and what questions can you ask to confirm that her pain is truly a result of a groin strain and is not from a visceral source.

Answer

There are several systems that could be potentially responsible for this young lady's pain, including musculoskeletal, gynecological, and digestive. Although her symptoms suggest a musculoskeletal origin, further investigation is required. Questions about whether she is sexually active or about the regularity of her menstrual cycle can elucidate a potential gynecological cause (i.e., an ectopic pregnancy or ruptured ovarian cyst). The presence of fever, nausea, or vomiting may point to appendicitis. A good follow-up test to confirm your findings would be to test for rebound tenderness (pain that is worse with release of pressure than with application of pressure). If the test for rebound tenderness is positive, it indicates peritoneal irritation, most likely caused by bleeding into the peritoneal space, consistent with a ruptured appendix, ectopic pregnancy, or ovarian cyst. Regardless of the cause, her pain and associated symptoms are cause for urgent referral to a physician.

MEDICATIONS

HOW DOES A PATIENT'S RESPONSE TO MEDICATION INFLUENCE YOUR DECISION-MAKING PROCESSES?

Whether and how a patient responds to medication can guide the clinician in determining the cause of pain. In the case of cardiogenic chest pain, for example, whether the patient responds to NTG or not can indicate the severity of symptoms and assist the clinician in deciding on the need for or urgency of referral. When attempting to discern viscerogenic from musculoskeletal pain, it is helpful to note the patient's response to nonsteroidal antiinflammatory drugs (NSAIDs), as visceral pain does not usually subside with NSAIDs as musculoskeletal pain does.

ENVIRONMENTAL AND PERSONAL CONTEXTUAL FACTORS

ENVIRONMENTAL FACTORS

Environmental factors may increase the risk for the development of certain visceral disorders. Individuals who are chronically exposed to smoke, be it second-hand cigarette smoke or industrial smoke from factories, are at risk for the development of lung cancers. Smoking increases a person's risk for a variety of cancers, most frequently lung. Exposure to asbestos fibers may result in lung cancer, or mesothelioma, a neoplasm that arises from the cells of the pleura or peritoneal cavities. Long-term exposure to coal particles can result in the development of coal-workers pneumoconiosis, a progressive fibrotic disease of the lung. Hairdressers who are chronically exposed to dyes and gels are at risk for the development of a number of cancers.[11] Although this list is not exhaustive, it serves as an example that reinforces the need to include a thorough occupational history as part of the interview process.

DO PSYCHOSOCIAL OR EMOTIONAL ISSUES INFLUENCE THE CLINICAL DECISION-MAKING PROCESS?

All pain has a psychological or emotional component, as the mere presence of pain can be taxing emotionally. There is an intimate relationship between chronic pain and depression, as the presence of chronic pain greatly increases the risk for depression and vice versa.[25] Pain can also lead to impaired sleep and sleep deprivation, which in turn decrease an individual's coping ability. The presence of psychological or emotional disorders may exacerbate the patient's symptoms or decrease his or her ability to participate in and benefit from treatment. The patient with an anxiety disorder may experience an exaggerated response to symptom provocation tests due to an overall heightened general arousal; he or she may also be more likely to experience psychological symptoms as physical pain due to a decreased ability to access or deal with his or her fears directly. Chronic anxiety is also associated with chronic stress, which has been demonstrated to decrease immune function[19,23] and increase an individual's susceptibility to disease.

The patient with depressive symptoms may have difficulty participating in and complying with therapy treatments, resulting in a longer duration of symptoms than necessary. People with depression often experience a sense of emotional exhaustion and overwhelming inertia that limit their ability to perform even the simplest tasks.[3] In addition, some people with depression suffer from insomnia, resulting in overwhelming fatigue. They also suffer from a distinct lack of coping skills, and may have little or no tolerance for pain or discomfort.

Individuals with panic disorder experience episodes of acute terror or anxiety, often accompanied by a sense of impending doom and the appearance of numerous physical symptoms consistent with autonomic activation, including tachycardia, tachypnea, palpitations, dyspnea, and dizziness. In the presence of these symptoms, the person experiencing a panic attack often believes that he or she is having a heart attack. It is therefore critical that the clinician is able to distinguish between the signs and symptoms of a panic attack and that of an MI. Individuals with panic disorder may or may not have a history of risk factors for atherosclerosis, and the symptoms associated with panic disorder are often unrelated to activity. A general rule of thumb for the clinician whose patient believes that he or she is having a heart attack is to believe them and call 911 to activate the emergency medical system. Because of the overlap of symptoms between these two disorders, the determination of the actual diagnosis is best left to the physician. A clinician who knows that the patient has a history of panic disorder can employ relaxation strategies to assist the patient in regaining control of his or her emotions.

WHAT PRIOR SURGERIES INFLUENCE THE CLINICAL DECISION-MAKING PROCESS?

A history of prior surgery to treat pathology in a given system should alert the clinician to the possibility of recurrence. For example, if a patient has a history of surgery to treat cancer, the clinician should consider metastasis if the patient presents with a new onset of back pain. Other examples include coronary artery bypass surgery or percutaneous transluminal coronary angioplasty to treat atherosclerotic heart disease. A patient with a history of surgical intervention to revascularize ischemic myocardium is at risk for reocclusion, and therefore repeated onset of ischemic myocardial pain (angina). Individuals who have had previous abdominal surgery are at risk for the formation of adhesions, which limit normal organ function, and can result in the development of symptoms consistent with organ pathology. The history of such surgeries should therefore be a factor that the clinician considers when attempting to discern the origin of pain.

DOES A FAMILY HISTORY OF PATHOLOGY INFLUENCE YOUR CLINICAL REASONING PROCESS?

A risk factor for the development of myriad disorders is a family history of the disorder, which can assist the clinician in the screening process. Thus a careful family history should include questions about pathology and the health of family members.

CLINICAL DECISION MAKING CASE STUDY—PATIENT PROFILE

Your patient is a 45-year-old female who you are seeing for shoulder pain that is accompanied by weakness in the hand muscles and paresthesias. Your initial inclination was that her symptoms are cervicogenic in nature and you have been treating her for a month without a significant change in her symptoms.

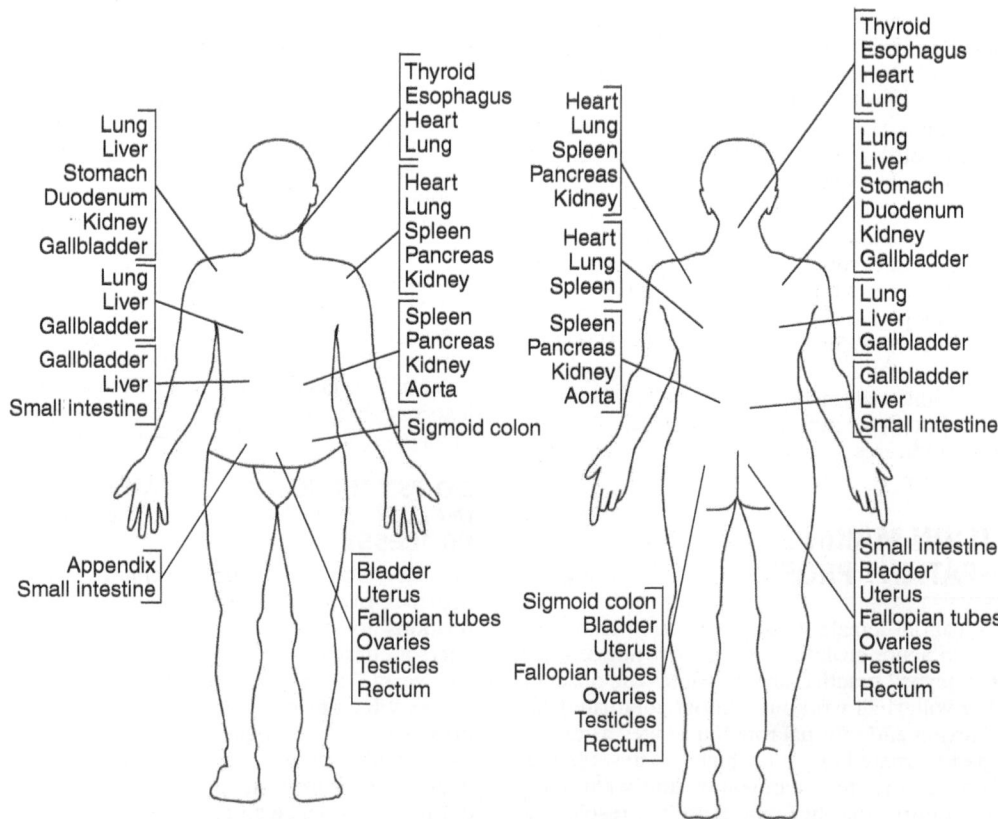

FIGURE II-17-4 Common referral sites for visceral tissue.

One day during your treatment she remarks, "I can't seem to get rid of this cough! I never bring anything up, but this cough is starting to drive me crazy!" This arouses your suspicions, and further questioning reveals that she is a former smoker and has lost 15 pounds over the last several months without really trying. What are your concerns?

Answer

This woman's symptoms may in fact be cervicogenic in nature, but several red flags raise your suspicion for a visceral cause of pain. First, her recent weight loss (without dieting) is suspicious for cancer, especially when coupled with her history of smoking. Her dry, nonproductive cough is suggestive of pleural irritation. Imaging tests will reveal if this pain is truly cervicogenic in nature or if it is caused by impingement of the brachial plexus by a Pancoast tumor of the lung.

RED FLAGS THAT WARRANT REFERRAL TO A MEDICAL PHYSICIAN

WHAT SYMPTOMS ALERT YOU TO PATHOLOGIES THAT MAY REQUIRE A REFERRAL TO A MEDICAL PHYSICIAN? (Figure II-17-4)

Red flag symptoms are symptoms that alert the clinician to the possibility that the patient's symptoms may be viscerogenic or systemic in nature, and thus require interventions that are outside his or her practice act. Red flag symptoms fall into several categories: past personal or family history, the presence of risk factors, the presence of constitutional signs, and clinical presentation, including pain pattern and associated signs and symptoms. These symptoms are summarized in Box II-17-1.

BOX II-17-1　Red Flag Symptoms[10]

Personal or family history	History of any cancer Recent infection Recurrent infection or illnesses History of immunosuppression (HIV/AIDS, chemotherapy, chronic alcoholism, corticosteroid or other immunosuppressant drugs) Intravenous drug use History of trauma
Risk factors	Obesity [body mass index (BMI) > 25] Smoking Substance use/abuse Gender Radiation exposure Sedentary lifestyle Ethnicity Occupation Hysterectomy/oophorectomy Domestic violence
Clinical presentation	Unclear mechanism of injury Insidious, gradual onset, and progression of symptoms Initial resolution of symptoms after treatment, followed by recurrence of symptoms Unexplained weight gain/loss (>10% of body weight in a month) Persistent symptoms despite clinical intervention Symptoms unrelieved by rest Failure of treatment to mitigate symptoms after previous remittance Prolonged experience of symptoms given pathology Symptoms out of proportion to the injury Inability to alter the symptoms during the examination Symptoms do not match "typical" presentation of injury or disorder No discernible pattern of symptoms A growing mass Vaginal bleeding after menopause Bilateral symptoms: 　Edema 　Clubbing 　Paresthesias

	Skin pigmentation changes Skin rash Nail bed changes Change in range of motion and muscle tone in people with neurological conditions
Pain pattern	Pain that is worse with activity and better with rest Pain that is not reproducible with range of motion or movement Night pain Pain that is accompanied by psychological symptoms, e.g., exhaustion, fatigue Constant pain Pain that is described as throbbing, knifelike, boring, or deep Poorly localized/diffuse pain (the patient is unable to point to the area of pain with two fingers) Intermittent, colicky pain Change in symptoms with food or after medication Pain associated with a specific visceral system
Associated signs and symptoms	New onset of neurological symptoms, e.g., confusion Constitutional symptoms: 　Fever 　Chills 　Fatigue 　Malaise 　Night sweats 　Diaphoresis 　Nausea and vomiting 　Diarrhea 　Pallor 　Weight loss 　Dizziness/syncope Abnormal vital signs or abnormal vital sign response to activity Proximal muscle weakness, especially in the presence of decreased deep tendon reflexes Change in bowel or bladder patterns Change in menstruation Rebound tenderness (sign of peritoneal irritation)

SUMMARY STATEMENT

Although the task of differentiating musculoskeletal from nonmusculoskeletal pain may seem daunting at first, it is well within the ability of the clinician who performs a thorough history, physical examination, and systems review. To screen for nonmusculoskeletal conditions the clinician need not memorize all of the intimate details pertaining to every medical condition that produces nonmusculoskeletal pain; rather he or she should be able to identify pain patterns, red flags, and abnormal presentations of signs and symptoms.

REFERENCES

1. American College of Radiology. *ACR Appropriateness Criteria: Expert Panel on Neuroimaging—Low Back Pain.* 2008. http://www.acr.org/SecondaryMainMenuCategories/quality_safety/app_criteria/pdf/ExpertPanelonNeurologicImaging/LowBackPainDoc7.aspx. Accessed January 30, 2009.
2. American Heart Association. *Heart Attack, Stroke and Cardiac Arrest Warning Signs.* 2008. http://americanheart.org/presenter.jhtml?identifier=3053. Accessed January 4, 2009, 2009.
3. American Psychiatric Association. *Diagnostic and Statistical Manual of Mental Disorders: DSM-IV.* Washington, DC: American Psychiatric Association; 1994.
4. Aya A, Vialles N, Mangin R, et al. Chronobiology of labour pain perception: an observational study. *Br J Anaesth.* 2004;93:451-453.
5. Bellamy N, Sothern R, Campbell J, Buchanan W. Rhythmic variations in pain, stiffness, and manual dexterity in hand osteoarthritis. *Ann Rheum Dis.* 2002;61:1075.
6. Bellamy N, Sothern R, Campbell J. Aspects of diurnal rhythmicity in pain, stiffness, and fatigue in patients with fibromyalgia. *J Rheumatol.* 2004;31:379-389.
7. Cannon C, McCabo C, Stone P, et al. Circadian variation in the onset of unstable angina and non-Q-wave acute myocardial infarction (the TIMI III Registry and TIMI IIIB). *Am J Cardiol.* 1997;79:253-258.
8. Committee on Understanding and Eliminating Racial and Ethnic Disparities in Health Care BoHSP. *Unequal Treatment: Confronting Racial and Ethnic Disparities in Health Care.* Institute of Medicine; 2003.
9. Creger M, Loscalzo J. Chapter 242. Diseases of the aorta. In: Fauci AS, Braunwald E, Kasper DL, et al., eds. *Harrison's Principles of Internal Medicine.* 17th ed. http://www.accessmedicine.com/content.aspx?aID=2880207. Accessed February 1, 2009.
10. Cutolo M, Masi A. Circadian rhythms and arthritis. *Rheum Dis Clin North Am.* 2005;31:115-129.
11. Czene K, Tikkja S, Hemminki K. Cancer risks in hairdressers: Assessment of carcinogenicity of hair dyes and gels. *Int J Cancer.* 2003;105(1):108-112.
12. Ganong W. Chapter 7. Cutaneous, deep and visceral sensation. In: Ganong W, ed. *Review of Medical Physiology.* 22nd ed. New York: McGraw-Hill; 2005. http://www.accessmedicine.com/content.aspx?aID=707741.
13. Goodman C, Snyder T. *Differential Diagnosis for Physical Therapists: Screening for Referral.* St. Louis: Saunders; 2007.
14. Goodman C, Snyder T. Pain Types and Viscerogenic Pain Patterns. In: *Differential Diagnosis for Physical Therapists: Screening for Referral.* 4th ed. St. Louis: Saunders; 2007.
15. Goodman C, Snyder T. Screening for cancer. In: *Differential Diagnosis for Physical Therapists: Screening for Referral.* St. Louis: Saunders; 2007.
16. Goodman C, Snyder T. Screening for cardiovascular disease. In: *Differential Diagnosis for Physical Therapists: Screening for Referral.* St. Louis: Saunders; 2007.
17. Jemal A, Murray T, Ward E, Samuels A. Cancer statistics, 2005. *CA Cancer J Clin.* 2005;55:10-30.
18. Job-Deslandre C, Reinberg A, Delbarre F. Chronoeffectiveness of indomethacin in four patients suffering from an evolutive osteoarthritis of hip or knee. *Chronobiologia.* 1983;10:245-254.
19. Kiecolt-Glaser J, Marucha P, Malarkey W, Mercado A, Glaser R. Slowing of wound healing by psychological stress. *Lancet.* 1995;346:1194-1196.
20. Kowanko I, Pownall R, Knapp M, Swannel E, Mahoney P. Circadian variations in the signs and symptoms of rheumatoid arthritis and in the therapeutic effectiveness of flurbiprofen at different times of the day. *Br J Clin Pharmacol.* 1981;11:477-484.
21. Lévi F, Le Louarn C, Reinberg A. Timing optimizes sustained-release indomethacin treatment of osteoarthritis. *Clin Pharmacol Ther.* 1985;37:77-84.
22. Manfredini R, Gallerani M, Cecilia O, Boari B, Fersini C, Portaluppi F. Circadian pattern in occurrence of renal colic in an emergency department: analysis of patients' notes. *Br Med J.* 2002;324:767.
23. McEwen B. Protective and damaging effects of stress mediators. *N Engl J Med.* 1998;338:171-179.
24. Melzac R. The McGill Pain Questionnaire: Major properties and scoring methods. *Pain.* 1975;1(3):277-299.
25. Miller M. Depression and pain. *Harv Ment Health Lett.* 2004;21(3):4.
26. Muller J, Stone P, Turin Z. The Millis Study Group: circadian variation in the frequency of onset of acute myocardial infarction. *N Engl J Med.* 1985;313:1315-1322.
27. Orr W. Night-time gastro-oesophageal reflux disease: prevalence, hazards, and management. *Eur J Gastroenterol Hepatol.* 2005;17:113-120.
28. Pöllman L. Circadian changes in the duration of local anaesthesia. *J Interdiscip Cycle Res.* 1981;12:187-191.
29. Rigas B, Torosis J, McDougall C, Vener K, Spiro H. The circadian rhythm of biliary colic. *J Clin Gastroenterol.* 1990;12:409-414.
30. Solomon G. Circadian rhythms and migraine. *Clevel Clin J Med.* 1992;(59):326-329.
31. Vitale C, Miceli M, Rosano GM. Gender-specific characteristics of atherosclerosis in menopausal women: risk factors, clinical course and strategies for prevention. *Climacteric.* 2007;10(suppl 2):16-20.
32. Waters W, O'Connors P. Epidemiology of headache and migraine in women. *J Neurol Neurosurg Psychiatry.* 1971;34:148-153.

Orthopedic Pathology

BASIC INFORMATION

DEFINITION

The alar and transverse ligaments of the upper cervical spine stabilize the head on the neck. Injury to one or both of these structures can result in instability and risk compromise of the brainstem and spinal cord.

SYNONYMS

- Upper cervical sprain
- Upper cervical ligament tear

ICD-9CM CODES
848.9 Unspecified site of sprain and strain
721.0 Cervical spondylosis without myelopathy
723.8 Other syndromes affecting cervical region

OPTIMAL NUMBER OF VISITS

Will vary based on extent of injury. Mild ligament strains may recover within several weeks, whereas more extensive ligament damage may take up to a year to fully recover.

MAXIMAL NUMBER OF VISITS

Will vary based on extend of injury.

ETIOLOGY

- Damage to the ligaments of the upper cervical region is a serious pathology. The ligaments stabilize the head on the neck and allow the head to move. They also protect the brainstem, as well as the spinal cord as it runs through the region.
- The role of these ligaments is made difficult by the anatomy of the region. Unlike the other segments of the cervical spine, the upper cervical spine (C0-C3) lacks the articular stability of the segments below.
- Cadaveric studies by Wortzman and Dewar show that the C1/2 facet joints are nearly horizontal in alignment. The positioning of the facets allows for maximal rotation but sacrifices stability in return. Passive structures, such as the alar and transverse ligaments, are largely responsible for the stability of the region.
- The transverse ligament is the stronger of the two ligaments. Its function is to prevent anterior to posterior sliding of the head on the neck with cervical flexion and extension. Rupture of the transverse ligament allows the head to slide forward on the neck with cervical flexion. The anterior slippage causes entrapment of the brainstem and can result in spinal cord damage.

- Radiographic studies show that the transverse ligament can fail in the midsubstance of the ligament or avulse from the bone.
- It has been estimated that a force of about 85 kg is required to rupture the transverse ligament.
- The alar ligament functions to limit rotation of the upper cervical region at C1/2.
- Goel et al reported that when rotation exceeds 63 degrees (normal rotation is 45 degrees), there may be rupture of the alar ligament and capsular ligaments.
- Robertson and Swan demonstrated that both alar ligaments must be ruptured before dislocation of the C1/2 segment is possible.

EPIDEMIOLOGY AND DEMOGRAPHICS

- Cervical spine subluxations are observed in 43% to 86% of patients who have rheumatoid arthritis (RA) and occur more frequently in males, despite the greater propensity of RA in women.
- Atlantoaxial subluxation occurs in up to 39% of patients with rheumatoid arthritis.

MECHANISM OF INJURY

- The mechanism of injury is typically trauma, although some disease processes, such as RA or Down syndrome can weaken the ligaments to a point of failure or increased laxity.
- Research by Kaale et al studied patients an average of 6 years after whiplash injury as a result of motor vehicle accidents (MVA). When compared to control patients, the following findings were reported:
  - For all the neck structures considered, the chronic whiplash patients had significantly more magnetic resonance imaging (MRI) pathologic changes than the controls.
  - The alar ligament was the most commonly injured structure; 66% of the whiplash patients showed significant damage to the ligament.
  - The patients who had the head rotated at the instant of collision had more evidence of pathologic changes on MRI than those with the head in a neutral position. A total of 61.7% of the patients with rotated neck position had alar ligament grade 3 lesions as opposed to only 4.4% in the patient group with neutral neck position.
  - The association between head position and high-grade lesions (grade 2-3) of the alar ligaments was more pronounced in rear-end than in front-end collisions.
  - High-grade lesions to the transverse ligament were also more common

among patients with the head turned at the instant of the collision.
  - Severe MRI changes in the transverse ligament and the posterior atlantooccipital membrane were considerably more common in front-end than in rear-end collisions.

COMMON SIGNS AND SYMPTOMS

- Patient will commonly be very hesitant to move their head or neck in any direction.
- When the patient moves the head, the following symptoms may be experienced:
  - Diplopia: Double vision
  - Dysarthria: Difficulty speaking
  - Dysphasia: Difficulty swallowing
  - Dizziness
  - Drop attacks
  - Tinnitus
  - Headaches
  - Blurry vision
  - Nausea
  - Lump in the throat
  - Difficulty concentrating
  - Bilateral paresthesias in the hands and feet

AGGRAVATING ACTIVITY

Cervical motion

EASING ACTIVITIES

- Rest
- Cervical collar
- Supporting head with hands

24-HOUR SYMPTOM PATTERN

- Neck, arms, and legs may feel tired at the end of the day.
- Headaches may increase throughout the day.
- Vision and difficulty concentrating are common complaints.

PAST HISTORY FOR THE REGION

- In trauma, no past history need be present.
- With instability caused by disease, history of diseases that impact ligaments, such as Down syndrome and RA, may be present.

PHYSICAL EXAMINATION

- Physical examination should be undertaken with caution. Further injury to the region is possible if the patient is forced to go beyond their physiological limitations.
- Active and passive ranges of motion will be limited.
- Comparing right and left axial rotations, after transection of the left alar ligament, showed greater percentage increases for the right, as compared to the left, axial rotation, at both C0/1 and C1/2 joints.
- Neurological signs may or may not be present.

Section III

ORTHOPEDIC PATHOLOGY

- Depending on the severity of the injury, cranial nerve symptoms may be present and the clinician should perform a full neurological and cranial nerve test.
  - Unsteady gait
  - Positive Hoffmann's reflex
  - Hyperreflexia
  - Bowel and bladder disturbances

IMPORTANT OBJECTIVE TESTS

- Alar ligament testing is used to test the integrity of the alar ligament. When either sitting or lying supine, the head is laterally flexed on the stabilized C2 of the neck. During lateral flexion of the head on the neck, the ipsilateral occipital portion of the alar ligament becomes slack and the ipsilateral atlantal portion is stretched. This is believed to cause the atlas to move laterally in the direction of the side flexion. With increased side flexion, the occipital portion of the contralateral alar ligament is placed under tensile stress and limits any further side flexion. Under normal conditions, the stretched occipital portion of the ligament also induces forced rotation of the axis in the direction of the side flexion. Immediate rotation should occur at the C2 segment. Laxity in this response would indicate damage to the alar ligament. Research has yet to confirm the specificity or sensitivity of this test.
- Transverse ligament testing requires the patient's head to be passively flexed forward on the neck. If the transverse ligament is not intact, the head will slide forward and produce the symptoms noted above. Placing an anterior to posterior pressure on the head will help to reposition the head on the neck and should reduce the patient's symptoms. Sensitivity 0.69, specificity 0.96 for RA. No testing has been conducted to validate its use on traumatic patients.
- Open-mouth plain radiographs can be taken to rule out the possibility of an odontoid fracture.
- Anterior widening of the atlantodens interval of more than 5 mm on the flexion view suggests that the transverse ligament is incompetent.
- MRI testing should be utilized to confirm the diagnosis of alar or transverse ligament damage.

DIFFERENTIAL DIAGNOSIS

- Odontoid fracture
- Benign positional paroxysmal vertigo
- Cervical pathology
- Chiari malformation
- Concussion
- Cerebrovascular accident
- Cardiac pathology

CONTRIBUTING FACTORS

- Prior trauma to the head or prior whiplash injuries
- RA
- Long-time steroid use
- Down syndrome

TREATMENT

SURGICAL OPTIONS

Dislocations

- Many patients die immediately as a result of complete respiratory arrest caused by brainstem compression in severe upper cervical dislocations. Treatment consists of reduction of the dislocation and stabilization of the atlantooccipital joint. Cervical traction is contraindicated because of severe instability. Immediate application of a halo vest is recommended to stabilize the joint.
- Stabilization is obtained by posterior cervical arthrodesis using large cortical cancellous bone grafts with stabilization by dual plates screwed to the posterior occiput and attached to lateral mass screws.

Rupture of the Transverse Ligament

- Dickman, Greene, and Sonntag classified injuries of the transverse atlantal ligament or its osseous insertions into the following types:
  - Type I injuries involve disruption of the ligament substance. These injuries are unable to heal without internal fixation.
  - Type II injuries involve avulsion of the ligament from its bony attachment. These injuries should be treated initially with a rigid cervical orthosis. Dickman et al had a 74% success rate with nonoperative treatment of type II injuries, reserving surgery for patients who had a nonunion and persistent instability after 3 to 4 months with immobilization.

SURGICAL OUTCOMES

Reports by Anderson et al showed good results without severe complications when plates and screw fixation are used to achieve occipital cervical fusion.

REHABILITATION

- Upper cervical ligament damage is a medical emergency. Any patient who is suspected of having damage to the alar or transverse ligaments should be referred directly to their medical physician or the emergency room for further testing to rule out the presence of these pathologies.
- A collar should be placed on the patient to limit cervical motions.
- Rehabilitation is contraindicated in patients who have upper cervical ligament damage. A patient should be cleared by their physician prior to beginning rehabilitation.

PROGNOSIS

- Prognosis depends on the nature of the injury or pathology.
- Surgical intervention is required in many of the upper cervical instabilities. Even if the patients survive, cervical motion and function is likely to be impaired because of loss of upper cervical mobility.

SIGNS AND SYMPTOMS INDICATING REFERRAL TO PHYSICIAN

Any of the signs and symptoms noted above in association with trauma or diseases that affect ligament integrity.

SUGGESTED READINGS

Anderson PA, Bohlman HH. Anterior decompression and arthrodesis of the cervical spine: long-term motor improvement (two parts). *J Bone Joint Surg Am*. 1992;74A:671.

Canale ST, Beaty JH. Cervical spine injuries. In: Canale ST, Beaty JH: *Campbell's Operative Orthopaedics*. 11th ed. Philadelphia: Mosby Elsevier; 2008.

Craig E. *Rheumatoid arthritis of the spine. Cervical spine trauma: upper and lower cervical spine injury. Clinical Orthopaedics*. New York, NY: Lippincott Williams & Wilkins; 1999.

Derrick IJ, Chesworth BM. Post-motor vehicle accident alar ligament laxity. *J Orthop Sports Phys Ther*. 1992;16(1):6–11.

Dickman CA, Greene KA, Sonntag VK. Injuries involving the transverse atlantal ligament: classification and treatment guidelines based upon experience with 39 injuries. *Neurosurgery*. 1996;38(1):44–59.

Dickman CA, Zabramski JM, Hadley MN, et al. Pediatric spinal cord injury without radiographic abnormalities: report of 26 cases and review of the literature. *J Spinal Disord*. 1991;4:296.

Dvorak J, Schneider E, Saldinger P, Rahn B. Biomechanics of the craniocervical region: the alar and transverse ligaments. *J Orthop Res*. 1988;6:452–461.

Goel VK, Winterbottom JM, Schulte KR, et al. Ligamentous laxity across C0-C1-C2 complex. Axial torque-rotation characteristics until failure. *Spine*. 1990;15:990–996.

Kaale BR, Krakenes J, Albrektsen G, Wester K. Head position and impact direction in whiplash injuries: associations with MRI-verified lesions of ligaments and membranes in the upper cervical spine. *J Neurotrauma*. 2005;22(11):1294–1302.

Krakenes J, Kaale BR, Nordli H, Moen G, Rorvik J, Gilhus NE. MR analysis of the transverse ligament in the late stage of whiplash injury. *Acta Radiol*. 2003;44:637–644.

Lincoln J. Case report: Clinical instability of the upper cervical spine. *Man Ther*. 2000;5(1):41–46.

Panjabi M, Dvorak J, Crisco JJ, Oda T, Wang P, Grob D. Effects of alar ligament transection on upper cervical spine rotation. *J Orthop Res*. 1991;9(4):584–593.

Robertson PA, Swan HA. Traumatic bilateral rotatory facet dislocation of the atlas on the axis. *Spine*. 1992;17:1252–1254.

Wortzman G, Dewar FP. Rotatory fixation of the atlantoaxial joint: rotational atlantoaxial subluxation. *Radiology*. 1968;90:479–487.

AUTHOR: DERRICK SUEKI

BASIC INFORMATION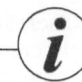

DEFINITION

Headache in the true sense of the definition cannot be considered a pathology, rather it is a symptom of an underlying pathology. Symptomatically, the patient will complain of a pain in the head or facial regions. Headaches can be caused by a number of factors including neuralgia, vascular compromise, tension, and brain trauma. In many cases the true cause of the head pain is unknown.

SYNONYMS

- Cephalalgia
- Cervicogenic headache
- Migraine headache
- Occipital neuralgia
- Horton's neuralgia
- Tension headache
- Cluster headache

ICD-9CM CODES

307.81 Tension headache
784.0 Headache
346.1 Migraine without aura
346.2 Variants of migraine, not
       elsewhere classified

OPTIMAL NUMBER OF VISITS

6 visits

MAXIMAL NUMBER OF VISITS

18 visits

ETIOLOGY

- The cerebral cortex of the brain does not have nociceptors, so technically, it cannot in itself be a source of pain. Other structures, such as nerves, meninges, and dura mater, do have nociceptors, therefore any injury or irritation of these structures could potentially be a pathological source of head pain.
- Many categories of headaches are defined by the International Headache Society; however, defining all types of headaches is beyond the scope of this book. Here, the categories have been generalized into the following four main classifications commonly seen in orthopedic settings:
  - Migraine or vascular headaches
  - Tension or muscular headaches
  - Cluster or inflammatory headaches
  - Cervicogenic headaches
- It is important to note that there is considerable overlap between these classifications.
  - *Migraine headaches:* There are many hypotheses regarding the source of the head pains experienced with a migraine. The true source of the symptoms has yet to be discovered and may be related to several triggers or

there may be several independent subsets within the general classification of migraine headaches. The most frequently associated causes of migraine headaches include vascular changes and diminished blood flow to the cortex, hormones, cortical dysfunction, serotonin, and nerve irritation. There appears to be a genetic component because many patients with migraine headaches have a familial history of migraine headaches.

- *Tension headache* is a generalized term used to define a grouping of headaches related to muscle or myofascial tension and the postural changes that accompany these changes. The source of the headaches may be related to decreased blood flow to the cortex secondary to tonic muscle contraction or irritation of the occipital nerves as a result of either increased capital extension, which may compress the occipital nerves or muscle tension. The greater occipital nerve pierces either through the tendon of the trapezius or between the trapezius and the semispinalis muscle to reach the occipital area. The lesser occipital nerve ascends along the posterior margin of the sternocleidomastoid muscle where it provides sensory fibers to the area of the scalp lateral to the greater occipital nerve. Thus muscle tension in any of these muscles could potentially compress the nerve and result in nerve irritation. Like migraine headaches, there may be a familial history associated with the symptoms. There are additional theories that hypothesize chemical changes in serotonin and endorphins may play a role in muscle tension.
- *Cluster headaches* have been known as suicide headaches because of the intense pain associated with them. They are characterized by excruciating pain, lack of aura, unilateral location, and rapid onset. They come in bouts of 15 minutes to 3 hours and then may resolve again for weeks to months. Currently, the causes are still unknown, but it has been hypothesized that abnormalities of the hypothalamus may play a role. Pathologically, it is believed that dilation of the blood vessels create pressure on the trigeminal nerve. There is no familial history associated with this type of headache.
- *Cervicogenic headaches* are also known as occipital neuralgia. Neuralgia is a word usually used to define pain generated from injury to a nerve. Typically, this nerve is located in the head or facial region. Occipital neuralgia refers to pain along the course of the greater or lesser occipital nerves. Clinically, this nerve irritation will present as pain in the posterior aspect of the head and may refer into

the temples or retroorbitally. The greater occipital nerve is the largest purely afferent nerve in the body. It innervates the posterior skull from the suboccipital area to the vertex and is formed by the posterior division of the second cervical nerve. The afferent fibers from this nerve lie in close approximation to the nucleus and spinal tract of the trigeminal nerve. Rather than exiting through a discrete spinal foramen, the nerve leaves the spinal column between the arch of the atlas and the axis. It travels inferiorly and laterally toward the area of the C2/3 facet joint and then curves around the inferior oblique capitis muscle to ascend toward the occiput deep to the semispinalis capitis muscle. It pierces either through the tendon of the trapezius or between the trapezius and the semispinalis muscle to reach the occipital area. Since the trigeminal nerve nucleus and the greater occipital nerve run in close proximity, it is hypothesized that convergence of the occipital nerve and the trigeminal nerve may occur to produce the pain pattern commonly seen in headache patients.

The lesser occipital nerve forms from the anterior division of the second and third cervical nerves. It ascends along the posterior margin of the sternocleidomastoid muscle, where it provides sensory fibers to the area of the scalp lateral to the greater occipital nerve.

EPIDEMIOLOGY AND DEMOGRAPHICS

- Two-thirds of the population will suffer from headaches.
- 15% to 20% of headaches can be attributed to vascular origins; the remainder are attributed to a wide variety of other causes, including tension, posture, hormones, psychological factors, and trauma (concussion/whiplash).
- Women have a greater prevalence than men as a whole by a 3:1 ratio.
- White collar workers have a higher incidence of headaches than blue collar workers.
- Migraine headache occurs more frequently in women than men at a 2:1 to 3:1 ratio.
- Tension headache occurs more frequently in women than men.
- Cluster headache occurs more frequently in men than women in a 7:1 ratio.
- Cervicogenic headache occurs more frequently in women than men.

MECHANISM OF INJURY

- Migraine headaches
  - Stress
  - Exertion
  - Food, alcohol, nitrates, caffeine withdrawal

- ○ Bright lights
- ○ Noise
- ○ Menstruation
- Tension headaches
  - ○ Neck movements may trigger headaches
  - ○ Stress
  - ○ Tension
  - ○ Sustained capital flexion or extension
  - ○ Poor posture
- Cluster headaches
  - ○ Head position or neck movement may play a role
  - ○ Nitroglycerin, alcohol, chocolate, smoke, or perfumes may trigger attacks
  - ○ Stress or tension
- Cervicogenic headaches
  - ○ Head position or neck movement
  - ○ Sustained capital flexion or extension

COMMON SIGNS AND SYMPTOMS

Migraine Headaches

- Frequency and duration:
  - ○ Can happen several times per week or less frequently and can last 4 to 72 hours but generally lasts less than 24 hours
- Mode of onset:
  - ○ Very rapid onset
  - ○ Warning signs, such as aura, can precede headache
- Area of symptoms:
  - ○ Unilateral temporal, frontal, or retroorbital regions
  - ○ Symptoms may change sides from occurrence to occurrence or day to day
- Quality of symptoms:
  - ○ Throbbing
  - ○ Pounding
  - ○ Moderate-to-severe intensity
- Associated symptoms:
  - ○ Nausea
  - ○ Vomiting
  - ○ Photophobia
  - ○ Phonophobia

Tension Headaches

- Frequency and duration:
  - ○ May occur daily for several hours a day and may be chronic.
  - ○ May last from 30 minutes to an entire week.
- Mode of onset:
  - ○ Onset builds up during the course of the day and with stress or tension.
  - ○ No warning signs, such as aura, will precede the headache.
- Area of symptoms:
  - ○ Bilateral symptoms are felt in the muscles of head, periorbital, temporal, and occipital regions.
- Quality of symptoms:
  - ○ Dull ache
  - ○ Tight band or heavy weight on head
  - ○ Moderate-to-severe intensity
- Associated symptoms:
  - ○ Cervical pain

- ○ Nausea
- ○ Vomiting
- ○ Photophobia

Cluster Headaches

- Frequency and duration:
  - ○ Can happen for several weeks at a time and then remit for years. Episodes can last 15 minutes to 2 hours.
- Mode of onset:
  - ○ No warning signs, such as aura, will precede the headache.
  - ○ Some people will feel a shadow or dull ache in the area preceding an episode.
- Area of symptoms:
  - ○ Unilateral symptoms located in the temporal, frontal, or retroorbital regions.
  - ○ Symptoms may change sides from occurrence to occurrence.
- Quality of symptoms:
  - ○ Severe burning
  - ○ Piercing retroorbital pain
  - ○ Worse pain ever felt, suicidal type of pain
- Associated symptoms:
  - ○ Drooping eye
  - ○ Red eyes
  - ○ Tearing of the eyes
  - ○ Running nose
  - ○ Nausea
  - ○ Vomiting
  - ○ Bradycardia
  - ○ Photophobia
  - ○ Flushed face
  - ○ Possible mild neck symptoms

Cervicogenic Headaches

- Frequency and duration:
  - ○ Occurs daily or at least 2 to 3 times per week.
- Mode of onset:
  - ○ Patient may awaken with headache.
  - ○ Slow increase in symptoms as the day progresses.
- Area of symptoms:
  - ○ Symptoms may be unilateral or bilateral.
  - ○ Pain generally starts in the suboccipital region.
  - ○ As symptoms progress, they may radiate into temporal, frontal, or retroorbital regions.
  - ○ Symptoms generally do not change sides.
- Quality of symptoms:
  - ○ Dull ache or boring pain.
  - ○ May have stabbing, deep pain.
  - ○ Can reach moderate-to-severe intensities.
- Associated symptoms:
  - ○ Nausea and vomiting
  - ○ Blurred vision
  - ○ Difficulty swallowing
  - ○ Photophobia or phonophobia may or may not be present

AGGRAVATING ACTIVITIES

- Many of the categories of headaches will present with similar aggravating factors.

Therefore it is difficult to use them as differentiators. Sustained head positions, stress, and head motions will aggravate most headaches. Most headaches may also be sensitive to light and sound.

- Migraine headaches can be aggravated by other environmental and physiological factors, such as foods and menstruation, whereas the other types of headaches will not be affected by these factors.

EASING ACTIVITIES

- Position and sleep may ease many of the headaches.
- Patients with migraines will need darkened and quiet areas to keep the symptoms to a minimum.
- Prescription hormones will often decrease the frequency and intensity of headaches.
- If a food trigger can be identified, refraining from these foods will ease the headaches symptoms.

24-HOUR SYMPTOM PATTERN

- Migraine headaches
  - ○ Patient may awaken with headache.
- Tension headaches
  - ○ Onset builds up during the course of the day and with stress or tension.
  - ○ Patient generally does not awaken with a headache.
  - ○ No warning signs, such as aura, will precede the headache.
- Cluster headaches
  - ○ Symptoms are very regular and will occur at the same time everyday.
  - ○ Patients may awaken because of headache.
- Cervicogenic headaches
  - ○ Patient may awaken with headache.
  - ○ Symptoms increase as the day progresses.
  - ○ Symptoms are influenced by daily activities.

PAST HISTORY FOR THE REGION

- The past history may include progressive head and neck pain.
- There may be associated trauma or a specific injury in certain instances involving head and/or neck trauma with associated neurological complaints (motor weakness and/or sensation changes).
- There may be a history of concussion, whiplash, or MVAs.

PHYSICAL EXAMINATION

- Observation may include a head or neck posture that is side bent toward the area of pain, if the problem is caused by tension or nerve entrapment. The head posture may also be side bent toward the painful area and extended to unload the nervous system, if nerve mobility is an issue. Commonly, there will also be posture abnormalities in the thoracic spine and the scapulothoracic area as well.

- Cervical range of motion (ROM) is usually limited in a pattern or direction that would either compress the nerve or mechanically challenge the nervous system in terms of mobility.
- There are generally no upper extremity neurological deficits.
- Other associated findings may include pain with palpation over the local neck musculature, shortened anterior chest wall musculature, as well as decreased scapulothoracic muscle strength (lower trapezius, middle trapezius, and serratus anterior). Decreased motor control in the deep neck flexors may also be present combined with overactive superficial muscle control.
- Tenderness and limited mobility in the suboccipital region is also a very common finding.

IMPORTANT OBJECTIVE TESTS

Zito et al examined the presence of cervical musculoskeletal impairment in 77 subjects, 27 with cervicogenic headache, 25 with migraine with aura, and 25 control subjects. Their physical assessments included a photographic measure of posture, range of movement, cervical manual examination, pressure pain thresholds, muscle length, performance in the craniocervical flexion test and cervical kinesthetic sense. Of these physical assessments, they found that diminished cervical flexion and extension, upper cervical joint dysfunction assessment, and increased sternocleidomastoid muscle activity with the craniocervical flexion test could be used to help differentiate cervicogenic headaches from migraine headaches. All other measures showed no differences between the test groups. Analysis revealed that manual examination could discriminate the cervicogenic headache group from the other subjects (migraine with aura and control subjects combined) with an 80% sensitivity.

DIFFERENTIAL DIAGNOSIS

- Stroke
- Concussion
- Cervical strain or sprain
- Upper cervical instability
- Brain tumor
- Encephalitis
- Meningitis
- Cerebral aneurysms
- High blood pressure
- Medications
- Cervical spondylosis
- Cervical stenosis (central or foraminal stenosis)
- Cervical spondylolisthesis
- Cervical myelopathy
- T4 syndrome

CONTRIBUTING FACTORS

- Posture
- Occupation (sitting, lifting, or manual labor)
- Age
- Gender
- Medication
- Diet
- Genetics
- Stress levels

TREATMENT

SURGICAL OPTIONS

- Surgical options are generally not warranted for the general classification of headaches listed above.
- Medically, the following treatments are common for headaches:
  - Migraine: The first line of treatment is prevention. Food avoidance, lifestyle changes, beta blockers, anticonvulsants, antidepressants, and exercise have all been used with varying results. Once a migraine occurs, nonsteroidal antiinflammatory drugs (NSAIDs), serotonin agonists, ergot alkaloids, antidepressants, and steroids have all been used to treat the pain.
  - Tension: Most tension headaches will resolve with the use of NSAIDs. Exercise, stress management, stretching, postural and ergonomic awareness, and biofeedback can all be used to help decrease the frequency and prevent tension headaches.
  - Cluster: Many of the treatment regimes are geared toward prevention of the headaches. Calcium channel blockers, steroids, lithium, muscle relaxants, antipsychotics, magnesium, and melatonin have all been utilized to varying success. When the headaches occur, increasing oxygen to the brain will often help to decrease the length of symptoms so oxygen treatment, exercise, sexual intercourse, caffeine, and hot showers have all been used with varying results.
  - Cervicogenic: As with tension headaches, NSAIDs will alleviate many of the headaches associated with cervical dysfunction. Rehabilitation has proved effective at preventing and reducing the frequency of headaches.

REHABILITATION

- Because of the uncertainty regarding headaches and the multiple potential sources of headaches rehabilitation studies, there have been few research studies investigating the outcomes of rehabilitation on headaches. The studies that have been conducted have focused primarily on cervicogenic headaches.

- In a study by Jull et al, 200 patients with chronic headaches were treated with manual therapy, exercise, and manual therapy with exercise; a control group had no treatment. After 8 to 12 visits over the course of 6 weeks, all treatment groups had decreased headaches 1-year after treatment. Of the 200 patients, 76% were 50% better, 35% had complete relief, and 10% had better outcomes with manual therapy combined with exercise. Improved upper cervical flexion was seen in those groups whose treatment included exercise.
- A systematic review by Vernon concluded that for headaches that are of tension or cervical origin, spinal manipulation is an effective treatment for the reduction of these symptoms.
- Jull suggests that a rehabilitation program designed to treat cervicogenic headaches must address all factors that contribute and directly relate to the headache. Therefore she suggests a program that includes mobilization or manipulation of the involved spinal segments to address the joint component, soft tissue stretching or massage to address the tissue component, and exercises that involve stretching and retraining of the muscle in the cervical and upper cervical region to address the motor recruitment component of the dysfunction.
- A Cochrane review article determined that manipulation of the spine may be effective for migraine and tension headache and that manipulation combined with neck exercises may be effective for cervicogenic headache.

PROGNOSIS

Because of the wide breadth of diagnoses, prognosis will vary greatly. Cluster and migraine headaches have poorer prognosis than cervicogenic and tension headaches. This is due in part to the lack of knowledge regarding the exact cause of the headaches symptoms.

SIGNS AND SYMPTOMS INDICATING REFERRAL TO PHYSICIAN

- Fainting
- Headaches that increase in intensity or frequency
- Loss of limb function
- Sensory disturbances of the hands
- Muscle wasting of the hand intrinsic musculature
- Unsteady gait
- Bowel and bladder disturbances
- Severe limitation during neck active ROM (AROM) in all directions
- Dysphasia
- Dysarthria
- Diplopia
- Blood pressure >165/95 mm Hg
- Resting pulse >100 bpm

SUGGESTED READINGS

Bronfort G, Nilsson N, Haas M, et al. Non-invasive physical treatments for chronic/recurrent headache. *Cochrane Database Syst Rev.* 2004;(3):CD001878.

Bogaards MC, ter Kuile MM. Treatment of recurrent tension headache: a meta-analytic review. *Clin J Pain.* 1994;10(3):174-190.

Capobianco DJ, Dodick DW. Diagnosis and treatment of cluster headache. *Semin Neurol.* 2006;26(2):242-259.

Carlsson J, Augustinsson LE, Blomstrand C, et al. Health status in patients with tension headache treated with acupuncture or physiotherapy. *Headache.* 1990;30(9):593-599.

Guidelines for all healthcare professionals in the diagnosis and management of migraine, tension-type, cluster and medication-overuse headache. British Association for the Study of Headache. 2007.

Jull G. Management of cervicogenic headaches. *Man Ther.* 1997;2(4):182-190.

Vernon H. Spinal manipulation in the management of tension-type migraine and cervicogenic headaches: the state of evidence. *Topics in Clinical Chiropractic.* 2002; 9(1):14-20.

Zito G, Jull G, Story I. Clinical tests of musculoskeletal dysfunction in the diagnosis of cervicogenic headache. *Man Ther.* 2006;11:118-129.

AUTHOR: DERRICK SUEKI

BASIC INFORMATION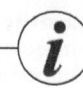

DEFINITION

The odontoid process is a vertical extension of the C2 spinal segment that projects cranially to articulate with the C1 spinal segment. Its role is to provide stability and allow for mobility of the C1 spinal segment on the C2 spinal segment. Fractures of the odontoid process can vary from a small hairline fracture to a total loss of bone continuity. Complete breaks of the bone can result in instability and risk compromise of the brainstem and spinal cord.

SYNONYMS

- Dens fracture
- Upper cervical fracture
- Broken neck

ICD-9CM CODES
805.0   Closed fracture of cervical
        vertebra without mention of
        spinal cord injury
805.00 Closed fracture of cervical
        vertebra unspecified level
805.02 Closed fracture closed of
        second cervical vertebra

OPTIMAL NUMBER OF VISITS

Will vary based on extend of injury. Hairline fractures or partial fractures of the odontoid may heal within six to eight weeks. Severe displaced fractures may require surgical intervention to restore bone function.

MAXIMAL NUMBER OF VISITS

Will vary based on extend of injury.

ETIOLOGY

- Damage to the odontoid process of the upper cervical region is a serious pathology. The bony process in concert with the ligaments of the region function to stabilize the head on the neck. While doing so, they allow head motions but protect the brainstem and spinal cord as it runs through the region.
- Functionally, the transverse ligament runs posterior to the process and stabilizes it against the anterior arch of C1. It prevents anterior translation of the head and C1 of the neck during cervical flexion. The alar ligaments are attached to the superior aspect of the process and act to resist and restrain excessive rotation of C1 on C2.
- The pathology is generally not related to repetitive use or disease processes. Fracture of the odontoid process usually requires significant force; therefore trauma is usually involved.
- Fracture of the odontoid process would result in several secondary effects.

With cervical flexion, the head and C1 would be allowed to translate anteriorly. Excessive translation could result in entrapment or damage to either the brainstem or the spinal cord. Loss of odontoid process integrity would also result in increased cervical rotation at C1/2 because of loss of restraint from the alar ligaments.

- Anderson and D'Alonzo have proposed a three type classification system for odontoid fractures based off of anatomical location:
  - *Type I* is an oblique fracture located in the upper part of the odontoid process. This type of fracture may involve loss of rotational stability and may also impact the alar ligaments. Anterior to posterior stability may not be impacted, depending on the integrity of the transverse ligament. Frequently, the tip of the odontoid is avulsed with the alar ligament. It occurs in approximately 5% of odontoid fractures.
  - *Type II* is a fracture located at the base of the odontoid process. Type II fractures are the most frequent odontoid fractures occurring in approximately 60% of the cases. Anterior posterior stability is generally compromised with this type of fracture. Blood supply is often compromised in type II fractures.
  - *Type III* is a fracture located in the body of the odontoid process. This fracture is less common, occurring in 30% of the cases; similar to type II fractures the anterior to posterior stability of the regions is generally compromised.

EPIDEMIOLOGY AND DEMOGRAPHICS

15% of all cervical spine fractures involve the odontoid process in adults and 75% of cervical spine fractures involve the odontoid in children under 7 years of age.

MECHANISM OF INJURY

- The exact mechanism of injury is unknown. It has been hypothesized that type II and III odontoid fractures occurs as a result of trauma that involves a combination of flexion, extension, and rotation.
- Type I injuries are believed to be the result of a combination of rotation and axial traction.
- Common means of injury include MVAs or falls that involve head trauma.

COMMON SIGNS AND SYMPTOMS

- Patient will commonly be hesitant to move their head or neck in any direction.
- When the patient moves, the following symptoms may be experienced:
  - Diplopia: Double vision
  - Dysarthria: Difficulty speaking

  - Dysphasia: Difficulty swallowing
  - Dizziness
  - Drop attacks
  - Tinnitus
  - Headaches
  - Blurred vision
  - Nausea
  - Lump in the throat
  - Difficulty concentrating
  - Bilateral paresthesias in the hands and feet

AGGRAVATING ACTIVITIES

Cervical motion, especially cervical flexion.

EASING ACTIVITIES

- Rest
- Cervical collar
- Supporting head with hands

24-HOUR SYMPTOM PATTERN

- Neck, arms, and legs may feel for tired at the end of the day.
- Headaches may increase throughout the day.
- Vision and difficulty concentrating are common complaints.

PAST HISTORY FOR THE REGION

- In trauma, no past history need be present.
- With instability caused by disease, history of diseases that impact bone integrity may be present. Examples are osteoporosis and Cushing's disease.

PHYSICAL EXAMINATION

- Physical examination should be undertaken with caution. Further injury to the region is possible if patients are forced to go beyond their physiological limitations.
- Active and passive ranges of motion will be limited.
- Physical findings may range from quadriplegia with respiratory center involvement if the brainstem and spinal cord are injured to minimal upper extremity motor and sensory deficits.
- Comparing right and left axial rotations, type I fractures may have greater rotation ROM caused by loss of alar ligament restraint, but this is highly variable because muscles will generally guard to protect the region and limit rotation. Passive motion in rotation may be greater than active motion.
- Neurological signs may or may not be present.
- Depending on the severity of the injury, cranial nerve symptoms may be present and the clinician should perform a full neurological and cranial nerve test.
- Unsteady gait
- Positive Hoffmann's reflex
- Hyperreflexia
- Bowel and bladder disturbances

IMPORTANT OBJECTIVE TESTS

- Open mouth plain radiographs should be taken to rule out the possibility of an odontoid fracture.
- Alar ligament testing is used to test the integrity of the alar ligament. When either sitting or lying supine, the head is laterally flexed on the stabilized C2 of the neck. During lateral flexion of the head on the neck, the ipsilateral occipital portion of the alar ligament becomes slack and the ipsilateral atlantal portion is stretched. This is believed to cause the atlas to move laterally in the direction of the side flexion. With increased side flexion, the occipital portion of the contralateral alar ligament is placed under tensile stress and limits any further side flexion. Under normal conditions, the stretched occipital portion of the ligament also induces forced rotation of the axis in the direction of the side flexion. Immediate rotation should occur at the C2 segment. Laxity in this response would indicate damage to the alar ligament. Research has yet to confirm the specificity or sensitivity of this test.
- Transverse ligament testing requires the patient's head to be passively flexed forward on the neck. If the transverse ligament is not intact, the head will slide forward and produce the symptoms noted above. Placing an anterior to posterior pressure on the head will help reposition the head on the neck and should reduce the patient's symptoms. Sensitivity is 0.69 and specificity is 0.96 for RA. No testing has been conducted to validate its use on traumatic patients.
- Anterior widening of the atlantodens interval of more than 5 mm on the flexion view suggests that the transverse ligament is incompetent.
- Plain films are generally done first. If pathology is found, computed tomography (CT) is usually performed to help define the extent of the injury.
- MRI testing may be utilized to confirm the involvement of the alar or transverse ligament.

DIFFERENTIAL DIAGNOSIS

- Alar ligament damage
- Transverse ligament damage
- C1 fracture
- C2/3 fracture/dislocation (hangman's fracture)
- Benign positional paroxysmal vertigo
- Cervical pathology
- Chiari malformation
- Concussion
- Cerebrovascular accident
- Cardiac pathology

CONTRIBUTING FACTORS

- Prior trauma to the head or prior whiplash injuries
- RA
- Long-time steroid use
- Down syndrome
- Osteoporosis or osteopenia

TREATMENT

SURGICAL OPTIONS

- Type I: Conservative treatment with hard-collar immobilization.
- Type II and III: Halo immobilization, odontoid screw fixation, anterior fixation, C1/2 posterior transarticular screw fixation, or posterior interlaminar clamps or wiring may be utilized. Halo immobilization is usually considered if the odontoid displacement is <5 mm and the patient is younger than 60 years of age.

SURGICAL OUTCOMES

- Type I will have good success rates after 6 to 8 weeks of immobilization.
- Type II and III: Halo fusion rate is over 90% after 16 weeks of immobilization. Wiring techniques have excellent outcomes with the fusion rate being approximately 95%.
- Many patients die immediately as a result of complete respiratory arrest caused by brainstem compression in severe upper cervical dislocations. Treatment consists of reduction of the dislocation and stabilization of the atlantooccipital joint. Cervical traction is contraindicated because of severe instability. Immediate application of a halo vest is recommended to stabilize the joint.

REHABILITATION

- Odontoid fractures are a medical emergency. Any patient who is suspected of having damage to the odontoid should be referred directly to their medical physician or the emergency room for further testing to rule out the presence of these pathologies.
- A collar should be placed on the patient to limit cervical motions.
- Rehabilitation is contraindicated in patients who have upper cervical fracture.
- Future rehabilitation may begin after fusion of the bone.
- Initially, treatment involves restoring cervical mobility. Full ROM will not be achieved if fusion of C1/2 was performed.
- Once mobility has been restored, strengthening of the deep cervical muscles and then coordinating the

activity of these muscles with large muscle groups, such as the trapezius, is important.

PROGNOSIS

- Prognosis depends on the nature of the injury or pathology.
- Surgical intervention is required in many of the upper cervical instabilities. Even if the patients survive, their cervical motion and function is likely to be impaired because of loss of upper cervical mobility.
- Posterior surgical fusion techniques provide high fusion success rates, but they do so at the expense of cervical rotation. Generally, up to 50% of rotation is lost with these techniques.

SIGNS AND SYMPTOMS INDICATING REFERRAL TO PHYSICIAN

- Any of the signs and symptoms noted above in association with trauma or diseases that affect upper cervical instability.
- Nonunion, malunion, and pseudarthrosis formation are potential major complications.
- Risk factors for nonunion:
  ○ Comminution at the base of the odontoid
  ○ Older age
- Initial fracture displacement amount >2 mm (especially if >4 mm)
- Initial fracture displacement direction (posterior worse than anterior)
- Delays in diagnosis

SUGGESTED READINGS

Anderson LD, D'Alonzo RT. Fractures of the odontoid process of the axis. *J Bone Joint Surg Am.* 1974;56(8):1663-1674.

Aydinli U, Kara GK, Ozturk C, Serifoglu R. Surgical treatment of odontoid fractures with C1 hook and C2 pedicle screw construct. *Acta Orthop Belg.* 2008;74(2):276-281.

Frangen TM, Zilkens C, Muhr G, Schinkel C. Odontoid fractures in the elderly: dorsal C1/C2 fusion is superior to halo-vest immobilization. *J Trauma.* 2007;63(1):83-89.

Levine AM, Edwards CC. Traumatic lesions of the occipitoatlantoaxial complex. *Clin Orthop Relat Res.* 1989;53-68.

Moon MS, Moon JL, Sun DH, Moon YW. Treatment of dens fractures in adults: a report of thirty-two cases. *Bull Hosp Joint Dis.* 2006;63(3):108-112.

Shilpakar S, McLaughlin MR, Haid Jr RW, Rodts Jr GE, Subach BR. Management of acute odontoid fractures: operative techniques and complication avoidance. *Neurosurg Focus.* 2000;8(6):e3.

Ying Z, Wen Y, Xinwei W, et al. Anterior cervical discectomy and fusion for unstable traumatic spondylolisthesis of the axis. *Spine.* 2008;33(3):255-258.

AUTHOR: DERRICK SUEKI

BASIC INFORMATION

DEFINITION

Neuralgia is usually used to define pain generated from injury to a nerve. Typically, this nerve is located in the head or facial region. Trigeminal neuralgia refers to pain along the course of the trigeminal nerve. Clinically, nerve irritation will present as pain in the facial region, including the eye, cheek, and jaw. In many cases, the true cause of the nerve injury is unknown.

SYNONYMS

- Trigeminal neuropathy
- Tic douloureux
- Trifacial neuralgia

ICD-9CM CODE
350.1 Trigeminal neuralgia

OPTIMAL NUMBER OF VISITS

6 visits

MAXIMAL NUMBER OF VISITS

12 visits

ETIOLOGY

- The trigeminal nerve, or cranial nerve V, is the largest of the cranial nerves. It has three major branches; the ophthalmic nerve (V_1), the maxillary nerve (V_2), and the mandibular nerve (V_3). The ophthalmic and maxillary nerves are purely sensory. The mandibular nerve has both sensory and motor functions and also carries touch/position and pain/temperature sensation from the mouth.
- Sensations from the trigeminal nerve are different than those from the peripheral nerves in that sensory distribution or dermatomes have very little overlap. The ophthalmic nerve carries sensory information from the scalp and forehead, the upper eyelid, the conjunctiva and cornea of the eye, the nose, the nasal mucosa, the frontal sinuses, and parts of the meninges. The maxillary nerve carries sensory information from the lower eyelid, cheek, nares, upper lip, upper teeth, gums, nasal mucosa, palate, roof of the pharynx, the maxillary, sinuses, and parts of the meninges. The mandibular nerve carries sensory information from the lower lip, lower teeth, gums, chin, external ear, meninges, and jaw (except the angle of the jaw, which is supplied by C2/3).
- Muscles innervated by the trigeminal nerve include the muscles of mastication (masseter, temporalis, medial pterygoid, and lateral pterygoid), tensor veli palatini, mylohyoid, anterior belly of digastric, and tensor tympani.

- Although the cause of the neuralgia may still be unknown, usually no structural lesion is present. Many investigators agree that vascular compression, typically venous or arterial loops at the trigeminal nerve entry into the pons, is critical to the pathogenesis of the idiopathic variety. This compression results in focal trigeminal nerve demyelination.
- Tumors, swelling in the brain, or viral infections of the nerve have all been hypothesized as potential sources of nerve dysfunction.
- It has been hypothesized that the source of the pain is due to aberrant neural impulses stemming from an inflamed or damaged trigeminal nerve. Central inhibitory control of the nerve may also be impaired. The pathology resulting in the nerve injury or inflammation is still unclear.

EPIDEMIOLOGY AND DEMOGRAPHICS

- The prevalence of trigeminal neuralgia is approximately 107 men and 200 women per 1 million people.
- Approximately 40,000 patients in the United States suffer from this condition at any particular time.
- The incidence is 4 to 5 cases per 100,000.
- Approximately 1% to 2% of patients with multiple sclerosis (MS) develop trigeminal neuralgia.
- Trigeminal neuralgia occurs more frequently in females than males at a 3:2 ratio.
- Trigeminal neuralgia affects the elderly more than other patient populations; the average age of onset is between 60 and 70 years of age.

MECHANISM OF INJURY

- The initial mechanism of injury is unknown, but symptoms can be triggered by brushing the teeth, putting on makeup, or sometimes even a gentle touch.
- Trigeminal neuralgia has been known to occur more frequently in the spring and the fall.

COMMON SIGNS AND SYMPTOMS

- The patient will experience short bouts of intense, stabbing, electric, and shock-like pain in the areas of the face in which the branches of the nerve are distributed.
- Bouts usually last from 1 to 2 minutes and can occur repeatedly or several times a day. No pain is experienced between bouts.
- Sometimes, patients will experience a less intense form of symptoms. If this occurs, it is considered an atypical trigeminal neuralgia.

- Usually the maxillary and mandibular branches are involved. If damage occurs centrally at the pons, loss of function of all three branches of the trigeminal nerve will be seen.
- Symptoms are generally unilateral, although bilateral symptoms can occur on occasion.

AGGRAVATING ACTIVITIES

- Triggers usually involve some type of vibration or light touch.
- Triggers can involve many normal daily activities such as shaving, talking, eating, drinking, or brushing teeth.
- Occasionally, innocuous activities, such as a breeze or gentle touch, can trigger the symptoms.

EASING ACTIVITIES

Once nerve irritation is elicited, few activities can reduce the symptoms.

24-HOUR SYMPTOM PATTERN

Symptoms may occur several times throughout the course of the day but do not appear to be directly impacted by the time of day.

PAST HISTORY FOR THE REGION

The past history may include history of tumor or MS.

PHYSICAL EXAMINATION

- The diagnosis of trigeminal neuralgia is a diagnosis of exclusion. Diagnosis is made by ruling out other possible pathologies. The classic trigeminal neuralgia will have a completely normal physical examination.
- Cranial nerve examinations should be completed and loss of sensation or motor strength in a trigeminal pattern may be noted, but this is not always the case since nerve patency is normal between bouts of symptoms.
- On occasion, symptoms may be elicited through palpation along the course of the trigeminal nerve
- There are generally no upper extremity neurological deficits.

IMPORTANT OBJECTIVE TESTS

MRIs might be ordered by the physician to rule out other pathologies, such as brain tumor, but in classic trigeminal neuralgia, MRI examinations are normal.

DIFFERENTIAL DIAGNOSIS

- Temporomandibular joint (TMJ) syndrome
- Bell's palsy
- MS
- Stroke
- Glossopharyngeal neuralgia

- Concussion
- Cervical strain or sprain
- Upper cervical instability
- Brain tumor
- Encephalitis
- Meningitis
- Cerebral aneurysms
- High blood pressure
- Medications
- Cervical spondylosis
- Cervical stenosis (central or foraminal stenosis)

CONTRIBUTING FACTORS

- Age
- MS
- Gender
- Brain tumor

TREATMENT

SURGICAL OPTIONS

- Surgical options are generally not warranted as a first-line treatment, but if conservative care fails, surgery can be performed to stop the blood vessel from compressing the trigeminal nerve, or to damage the trigeminal nerve to keep it from malfunctioning. Surgical options include the following:
  - Microvascular decompression (MVD) involves relocating or removing blood vessels that are in contact with the trigeminal root.
  - In percutaneous glycerol rhizotomy (PGR), a needle is passed through the face and into the trigeminal cistern and then a small amount of sterile glycerol is injected. After 3 or 4 hours, the glycerol damages the trigeminal nerve and blocks pain signals.
  - In percutaneous balloon compression of the trigeminal nerve (PBCTN),

a hollow needle is passed through the face and into an opening in the base of the skull. A thin, flexible tube (catheter) with a balloon on the end is threaded through the needle. The balloon is inflated with enough pressure to damage the nerve and block pain signals.
  - Percutaneous stereotactic radiofrequency thermal rhizotomy (PSRTR) uses an electric current to selectively destroy nerve fibers associated with pain.
  - A partial sensory rhizotomy (PSR) involves cutting part of the trigeminal nerve at the base of the brain.
  - Gamma-knife radiosurgery (GKR) involves delivering a focused, high dose of radiation to the root of the trigeminal nerve. The radiation damages the trigeminal nerve and reduces or eliminates the pain.

SURGICAL OUTCOMES

Most people undergoing surgery experience some facial numbness and temporary or permanent weakness of the muscles used to chew. In many cases, pain relief from the surgery is only temporary.

MEDICAL OPTIONS

- Medically, the following treatments are common for trigeminal neuralgia:
  - Medications, such as anticonvulsant drugs (carbamazepine or gabapentin), are usually the initial treatment. Some antidepressant drugs also have significant pain-relieving effects. Muscle-relaxing agents, such as baclofen, may be used alone or in combination with other medications.
  - Alcohol injections provide temporary pain relief by numbing the affected areas.

REHABILITATION

Typically, trigeminal neuralgia is not managed in rehabilitation settings.

PROGNOSIS

Symptoms generally relapse and then remit. Recurrence of symptoms is common.

SIGNS AND SYMPTOMS INDICATING REFERRAL TO PHYSICIAN

- Fainting
- Headaches that increase in intensity or frequency
- Loss of limb function
- Sensory disturbances of the hands
- Muscle wasting of the hand intrinsic musculature
- Unsteady gait
- Bowel and bladder disturbances
- Severe limitation during neck AROM in all directions
- Dysphasia
- Dysarthria
- Diplopia
- Temperature >100° F
- Blood pressure >165/95 mm Hg
- Resting pulse >100 bpm
- Resting respiration >25 bpm

SUGGESTED READINGS

Bennetto L, Patel NK, Fuller G. Trigeminal neuralgia and its management. *BMJ.* 2007;334(7586):201-205.

Chole R, Patil R, Degwekar SS, Bhowate RR. Drug treatment of trigeminal neuralgia: a systematic review of the literature. *J Oral Maxillofac Surg.* 2007;65(1):40-45.

Liu JK, Apfelbaum RI. Treatment of trigeminal neuralgia. *Neurosurg Clin N Am.* 2004;15(3):319-334.

AUTHOR: DERRICK SUEKI

BASIC INFORMATION

DEFINITION

- Cervical disc pathology arises from a number of anatomical sources. The primary causes are degenerative processes and space-occupying lesions involving the annulus fibrosis or the nucleus pulposus.
- Cervical degenerative disc disease (DDD) can include annular tears, nuclear disc material degradation, and loss of disc height. A cervical spine herniated nucleus pulposus (HNP) can occur when disc material extends beyond the posterior margin of the vertebral body. A cervical spine HNP can be further grouped into the following four common classes:
  - Disc *bulge* occurs when the nucleus pulposus bulges into the annulus fibrosis and the disc margin extends beyond the endplates of adjacent vertebral levels.
  - Disc *protrusion* occurs when the nuclear pulposus from the disc tears through a small portion of the annulus fibrosis.
  - Disc *extrusion* occurs when the nucleus pulposus breaks past the outer lamina of the annulus fibrosis and into the space beyond.
  - Disc *sequestration* occurs when the nucleus pulposus becomes detached from the annulus and then usually resides within the spinal cord canal.
- Both cervical DDDs and HNPs can cause anatomical changes, but clinical correlation is needed because asymptomatic individuals can show degenerative changes with imaging within the cervical spine.

SYNONYMS

- Cervical degenerative disc disease (DDD)
- Herniated nucleus pulposus (HNP)

ICD-9CM CODES

722.0 Displacement of intervertebral disc without myelopathy
722.4 Degeneration of cervical intervertebral disc
719.48 Arthralgia of cervical spine

OPTIMAL NUMBER OF VISITS

8 visits or less

MAXIMAL NUMBER OF VISITS

16 visits

ETIOLOGY

- Cervical disc pathology rarely occurs as a result of a direct trauma alone and often is attributed to a slow, progressive degenerative process.
- The pathology can include annular tears or nuclear disc material degradation or herniation, as well as a loss of overall disc height.
- Most of these changes are related to aging, with the disc degradation occurring in the second decade of life.
- Circumferential tears involving the annulus may occur with repetitive movements or activities.

EPIDEMIOLOGY AND DEMOGRAPHICS

- Cervical spine HNPs on magnetic resonance imaging (MRI) have been reported as high as 10% in the asymptomatic population younger than 40 years old; this decreases to 5% in individuals older than 40.
- Degenerative disc disease on MRI has been reported as high as 25% in the asymptomatic population younger than 40 years old; this increases to 60% in individuals older than 40.
- It has been reported that between 14% and 18% of people without neck pain have abnormalities on imaging studies.
- Individuals older than 40 are more likely to experience cervical pain caused by DDD, whereas individuals younger than 40 are more likely to experience neck pain caused by cervical spine HNPs.
- There is no current literature that has linked a specific gender or culture to a higher prevalence of cervical disc pathology.

MECHANISM OF INJURY

- Onset is insidious for most cases of DDD because it occurs with natural aging.
- HNP in the cervical spine can occur from repetitive cervical spine loading or stress and is usually not related to a singular traumatic event or episode.

COMMON SIGNS AND SYMPTOMS

- Pain with cervical spine DDD is commonly diffuse, sometimes vague, and located over the cervical spine region and in a nondermatomal pattern.
- Range of motion (ROM) limitations may clinically appear as a "closing" pattern or position of the spine (e.g. cervical spine extension, left lateral rotation, and left rotation), which hypothetically is causing compression at the site of the suspected DDD level.
- A cervical spine HNP involves pain that is diffuse and located over the cervical spine region and at times may or may not radiate to the arm in a dermatomal distribution. Pain that extends past the acromioclavicular joint should be screened with a thorough neurological examination. If the patient has any upper or lower motor neuron signs, spinal nerve root involvement and referred peripheral neurogenic symptoms should be investigated.
- Activities that increase disc pressure, such as a Valsalva maneuver, coughing, sneezing, and/or lifting, may increase symptoms.
- The somatic referral pattern for the cervical spine disc and its related structures commonly refer pain into the neck and intrascapular area, but symptoms may also extend down the arm past the acromioclavicular joint.

AGGRAVATING ACTIVITIES

- Sitting for prolonged periods of time
- Specific neck motions
- Driving
- Sleeping prone or sidelying
- Coughing or sneezing

EASING ACTIVITIES

- Lying down
- Pain medications
- Cervical spine support
- Sleeping with the head supported either sidelying or supine
- Walking
- Modalities such as moist heat and/or ice

24-HOUR SYMPTOM PATTERN

- Cervical DDD symptoms follow a typical pattern of morning stiffness for >30 minutes followed by improved mobility and decreased pain throughout the day with end of day increasing stiffness and pain returning. Sleeping may or may not be problematic.
- Cervical HNP symptoms follow a pattern of morning stiffness and pain, although not as intense as cervical DDD, and become worse throughout the day with prolonged sitting and/or static activities. Sleeping may or may not be problematic.

PAST HISTORY FOR THE REGION

Because of the degenerative process of this condition, usually the patient will have had a history of neck pain episodes that eventually resolved on their own over the past few years. Usually, each bout of neck pain tends to be worse than the previous bout as symptoms magnify over the course of the episodes.

PHYSICAL EXAMINATION

- Tenderness over the surrounding upper cervical spine musculature via palpation testing.
- Decreased cervical spine ROM, most often demonstrating a pattern into either flexion or extension.

- A posture analysis suggesting poor static posture between the upper and lower cervical spine with contributions from the cervicothoracic and scapulothoracic regions.
- Limited joint mobility via posteroanterior mobility testing as described by Maitland and Jull.
- Decreased motor control and deep neck flexor recruitment with increased superficial muscle activity.
- Muscular imbalances found in the cervical and scapulothoracic regions such as the suboccipitals, upper trapezius, middle trapezius, lower trapezius levator scapulae, scalenes, and pectoralis minor and major muscle groups.

IMPORTANT OBJECTIVE TESTS

- Cervical spine ROM testing
  - Test procedure: Patient is seated in an upright position. Flexion and extension are measured with the bubble inclinometer placed on top of the head perpendicular to a bisected line through the external auditory meatus. Sidebending is measured with the bubble inclinometer placed in line with an imaginary line drawn through the auditory meatus. Rotation is measured by placing the goniometer on top of the patient's head and measuring the amount of rotation left and right with the fixed arm bisecting the head.
- Manual examination
  - Test procedure: Patient is examined via central posteroanterior glides, as well as passive physiological intervertebral movements into flexion, extension, sidebending, and rotation.
  - Positive: The level of joint dysfunction was determined by the examiner's ability to assess end-feel, resistance, and pain provocation at that joint level.
  - Sensitivity: 1.0; specificity: 1.0
- Palpation over cervical spine facet joints
  - Test procedure: Palpation was performed on the cervical spine assessing the articular structures of each cervical level.
  - Positive: The patient reported pain with palpation as the therapist was assessing the articular structures.
  - Sensitivity: 0.82; specificity: 0.79
  - Positive likelihood ratio (LR): 3.9; negative LR: 0.23
- Valsalva test
  - Test procedure: The patient is instructed to bear down without exhaling and is assessed if any upper quarter symptoms are reproduced.
  - Positive: Symptoms are reproduced with the maneuver.
  - Sensitivity: 0.22; specificity: 0.94
  - Positive LR: 3.5; negative LR: 0.83

DIFFERENTIAL DIAGNOSIS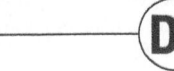

- Muscle strain
- Ligament sprain
- Radiculopathy
- Instability
- Myelopathy
- Spondylolysis

CONTRIBUTING FACTORS

- Heavy lifting
- Prolonged static or sedentary positions
- Previous motor vehicle accidents (MVAs) or head and/or neck injuries

TREATMENT

SURGICAL INDICATORS

- Worsening neurological symptoms, with increased upper extremity pain or weakness
- Pain in the cervical region that is not altered by conservative management

SURGICAL OPTIONS

- Discectomy/microdiscectomy
- Anterior or posterior fusion

SURGICAL OUTCOME

- In a study by Farzannia et al, outcomes of patients who underwent single level anterior cervical discectomy without interbody fusion were assessed. Of these patients, the outcomes were as follows: 61% patients had excellent, 31.5% good, 5% satisfactory, and 2.5% poor.
- A retrospective by Cauthen et al assessed the outcome of 348 patients receiving noninstrumented cervical fusion. The following results were attained: The mean fusion rate for 348 patients in the current study ranged from 75% (multilevel) to 88%. The overall fusion rate was 83%. The persistent complication rate was 0.1%, and patient self-assessments showed that 78% were satisfied with the outcome and that 83% returned to work.

REHABILITATION

- Current best evidence for treating neck pain without any significant medical and/or psychosocial variables has focused on the use of a treatment-based classification schema in providing care.
- This classification system focuses on individuals with cervical spine ROM limitations, headaches of cervical nature, and/or radiating symptoms down the extremity.
- A recent article by Childs et al summarized the current best evidence for individuals presenting with neck pain.

- Cervical mobilization and/or manipulation has shown strong evidence in treating mechanical neck pain.
- Strengthening exercises in the cervical spine, as well as the scapulohumeral area, have shown strong evidence for treating mechanical neck pain.
- Thoracic spine manipulation has shown some evidence in treating mechanical neck pain with early development of a clinical prediction rule for patients that would benefit from manipulation in the thoracic spine for cervical spine pain.
- Exercises based on stretching and flexibility have shown weaker evidence, although they are valuable in treating anterior chest musculature (pectoralis major and minor) and local cervical spine musculature such as the scalenes, upper trapezius, and the levator scapulae.
- Neurodynamic mobilization procedures have shown moderate evidence in patients with neck and arm pain.

PROGNOSIS

No research has been found that addresses specifically the prognosis for patient with cervical disc pathology. As a whole, studies have shown that there is a high recurrence rate with neck pain. The results of the studies place the recurrence rate between 22% and 50%, depending on the study.

SIGNS AND SYMPTOMS INDICATING REFERRAL TO PHYSICIAN

Spinal Fractures
- Major trauma (e.g., MVA, fall, or blow to the head) without proper imaging or the necessity for the Canadian Cervical Spine (C-Spine) Rules
  - Severe limitations during neck active ROM (AROM) in all directions
  - Cervical myelopathy
- Sensory disturbances of the hands
  - Muscle wasting of the hand's intrinsic musculature
  - Unsteady gait
  - Positive Hoffmann's reflex
  - Hyperreflexia
  - Bowel and bladder disturbances
  - Multiple segmental weakness, sensory changes, or both

Neoplastic Conditions
- Age >50 years with a previous history of cancer
  - Unexplained weight loss
  - Constant pain with no relief with bed rest
  - Night pain
  - Upper cervical ligamentous instability
- Occipital headache and numbness
- Severe limitation during neck AROM in all directions
- Signs of cervical myelopathy

Vertebral Artery Insufficiency
- Drop attacks
- Dizziness or lightheadedness related to neck movement
- Dysphasia
- Dysarthria
- Diplopia
- Positive cranial nerve signs

Inflammatory or Systemic Disease
- Temperature >100° F
- Blood pressure >165/95 mm Hg
- Resting pulse >100 bpm
- Resting respiration >25 bpm
- Fatigue

SUGGESTED READINGS

Barnsley L, Lord SM, Wallis BJ, Bogduk N. The prevalence of chronic cervical zygapophysial joint pain after whiplash. *Spine*. 1995;20(1):20-25; discussion 26.

Cauthen JC, Kinard RE, Vogler JB, et al. Outcome analysis of noninstrumented anterior cervical discectomy and interbody fusion in 348 patients. *Spine*. 1998;23(2):188-192.

Childs J, Cleland J, Elliott J, et al. Neck pain: clinical practice guidelines linked to the internal classification of functioning, disability, and health from the orthopaedic section of the american phyiscal therapy association. *J Orthop Sports Phys Ther*. 2008;38(9):A1-A34.

Childs J, Fritz J, Piva S, Whitman J. Proposal of a classification system for patients with neck pain. *J Orthop Sports Phys Ther*. 2004;34:686-696.

Cleland J, Childs J, Fritz J, Whitman J, Eberhart S. Development of a clinical prediction rule for guiding treatment of a subgroup of patients with neck pain: use of thoracic spine manipulation, exercise and patient eduction. *Phys Ther*. 2007;87:9-23.

Cleland JA, Flynn TW, Childs JD, Eberhart S. The audible pop from thoracic spine thrust manipulation and its relation to short-term outcomes in patients with neck pain. *J Manipulative Physiol Ther*. 2007;30(4):312-320.

Cloward R. Cervical discography. A contribution to the etiology and mechanism of neck, shoulder, and arm pain. *Ann Surg*. 1959;150:1052-1064.

Farzannia A, Hadidchi S, Forouzanfar MH. Single level anterior cervical discectomy without interbody fusion: A prospective analysis of outcome. *Kuwait Medical Journal*. 2005;37(4):271-276.

Fritz JM, Brennan GP. Preliminary examination of a proposed treatment-based classification system for patients receiving physical therapy interventions for neck pain. *Phys Ther*. 2007;87(5):513-524.

Jull G, Trott P, Potter H, et al. A randomized controlled trial of exercise and manipulative therapy for cervicogenic headache. *Spine*. 2002;27(17):1835-1843.

Maitland GD. *Vertebral manipulation*. 5th ed. Boston, MA: Butterworth; 1986.

AUTHOR: MICHAEL LEAL

BASIC INFORMATION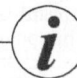

DEFINITION

- Cervical facet dysfunction most commonly involves a pain-generating source located toward the posterior elements of the spine behind the intervertebral foramen and associated nerve roots.
- The facets can act as potential pain generators, but it has also been shown that degenerative changes found within the spine can also be a cause of a patient's pain and discomfort.
- Cervical facet dysfunction can be a primary issue or source of pain (e.g., after a motor vehicle collision or sports injury) or a secondary issue resulting from a primary degenerative process or injury to the intervertebral disc and/or associated ligaments or muscular structures.

SYNONYMS

- Cervical facet arthropathy
- Cervical spine spondylolysis
- Cervical spine facet joint syndrome

ICD-9CM CODES

719.48 Arthralgia of cervical spine
719.08 Edema of cervical facet joint
847.0 Neck sprain

OPTIMAL NUMBER OF VISITS

6 visits or less

MAXIMAL NUMBER OF VISITS

12 visits

ETIOLOGY

- Cervical facet dysfunction is hypothesized as a result of degeneration of the cervical facet joints through normal aging or through a traumatic event.
- Traumatic events can include fractures and/or dislocation injuries, as well as whiplash type events in which either the excessive compression acting on the facet joint or excessive capsular ligament strains beyond physiological limits.

EPIDEMIOLOGY AND DEMOGRAPHICS

- Neck pain is a common complaint with annual prevalence rates as high as 15% in the general population, with 54% of individuals experiencing a neck pain episode within the last 6 months and 34.4% of the population within the last year.
- Cervical facet joint pathology as a potential source of pain has been estimated as high as 55% in a group of patients with chronic nonspecific neck pain.
- An additional study looked at 318 patients with intractable neck pain. Of these

patients, 25% of the sample had pain that was the result of a symptomatic facet.
- It has been shown that cervical spine facet changes are similar among all age groups.

MECHANISM OF INJURY

- In the younger adult patient population, <40 years of age, the most likely mechanism creating facet pain is secondary facet pathology. Secondary refers to the fact that the facet pathology is the result of other factors such as trauma. Whiplash injuries, blows to the head, or falls are all potential events that would cause damage to the cervical facets.
- In the older population, primary facet pathology is the more likely source of pain. In this case, the mechanism is degeneration or change in the joint itself. As a result of the degenerative process, it is common for osteophytes or bone spurs to intrude into the zygapophyseal joint causing pain and biomechanical abnormalities at the facets.

COMMON SIGNS AND SYMPTOMS

- The patient will report diffuse nonspecific neck pain in the posterior neck and/or scapular area, which is usually exacerbated by specific neck motions that may mimic a "closing" pattern of the spine (e.g., extension, left rotation for a left-sided neck problem).
- Cervical spine ROM is limited and there is usually an absence of neurological clinical findings.
- Radiographic evidence of cervical spondylosis, narrowing of the intervertebral foramina, or any other signs of degeneration that may lead to the cervical facet issue as a secondary cause of pain may also be present. It is important to recall even asymptomatic individuals have positive radiograph findings; therefore clinical correlation is always warranted.
- A study by Fukui et al reviewed the relative pain distribution of the cervical zygapophyseal joints using a contrast medium. The findings are listed below:
  - C0/1, C1/2, and C2/3 = Upper posterolateral cervical region
  - C2/C3 = Occipital region
  - C2/3, C3/4, and C3 = Upper posterior cervical region
  - C3/4, C4/5, and C4 = Middle posterior cervical region
  - C4/5, C5/6, and C4 and C5 = Lower posterior cervical region
  - C4/5, C5/6, and C4 = Suprascapular region
  - C6/7, C6, and C7 = Superior angle of the scapulae
  - C7/T1 and C7 = Midscapular region
  - Although the segmental origin of pain through the use of a contrast medium

was found, these patterns are not diagnostic of cervical zygapophyseal joint pain.

AGGRAVATING ACTIVITIES

- Looking in specific directions involving a "closing" pattern (e.g., extension, left sidebend, or left rotation for a symptomatic left-sided neck complaint)
- Sustained or prolonged positions without movement
- Different sleeping positions such as prone or sidelying

EASING ACTIVITIES

- Lying down or gravity eliminated positions
- Positions that involve an "opening" pattern of the cervical spine (e.g., flexion, left sidebend, or left rotation for a symptomatic right-sided neck complaint)
- Modalities such as moist heat and/or ice

24-HOUR SYMPTOM PATTERN

Symptoms follow a typical pattern of morning stiffness with improved mobility and decreased pain throughout the day, depending on the individual's job or daily routine, with end of day increasing stiffness and pain returning. Sleeping may or may not be problematic. Repetitive motions and/or prolonged positions may be bothersome throughout the day.

PAST HISTORY FOR THE REGION

- As a primary problem, cervical facet issues may arise from a variety of acute injuries involving most commonly an acceleration/deceleration injury such as seen in a motor vehicle collision or a sports injury involving a hyperextension injury.
- As a secondary problem arising from degenerative structures in the posterior aspect of the cervical spine, past medical history may include previous bouts of neck pain that have now increased in frequency or duration or may take twice as long to subside. It is not uncommon for a patient to report a history of trauma to the neck in the past that may account for some of the abnormal mechanics and subsequent wear and tear at the facet joint.

PHYSICAL EXAMINATION

- Tenderness over the surrounding upper cervical spine musculature via palpation testing
- Decreased cervical spine ROM most often demonstrating a pattern suggesting a "closing" type of restriction
- A posture analysis suggesting poor static posture between upper and lower cervical spine with contributions from the cervicothoracic and scapulothoracic regions

- Limited joint mobility via posteroanterior mobility testing as described by Maitland and Jull
- Decreased motor control and deep neck flexor recruitment with increased superficial muscle activity
- Muscular imbalances found in the cervical and scapulothoracic regions such as the suboccipitals, upper trapezius, middle trapezius, lower trapezius levator scapulae, scalenes, and pectoralis minor and major muscle groups

IMPORTANT OBJECTIVE TESTS

- Cervical spine ROM testing
  - Test procedure: Patient is seated in an upright position. Flexion and extension are measured with the bubble goniometer placed on top of the head perpendicular to a bisected line through the external auditory meatus. Sidebending is measured with the bubble inclinometer placed in line with an imaginary line drawn through the auditory meatus. Rotation is measured by placing the goniometer on top of the patient's head and measuring the amount of rotation left and right with the fixed arm bisecting the head.
- Manual examination
  - Test procedure: Patient is examined via central posteroanterior glides as well as passive physiological intervertebral movements into flexion, extension, sidebending, and rotation.
  - Positive: The level of joint dysfunction was determined based on the examiner's ability to assess end-feel, resistance, and pain provocation at that joint level.
  - Sensitivity: 1.0; specificity: 1.0
- Palpation over cervical spine facet joints
  - Test procedure: Palpation was performed on the cervical spine assessing the articular structures of each cervical level.
  - Positive: If the patient reported pain with palpation as the therapist was assessing the articular structures.
  - Sensitivity: 0.82; specificity: 0.79
  - Positive LR: 3.9; negative LR: 0.23

DIFFERENTIAL DIAGNOSIS

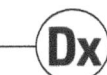

- Cervical disc herniation
- Cervical spondylosis
- Cervical stenosis (central or foraminal stenosis)[†]
- Cervical spondylolisthesis
- Muscular strain
- Ligamentous sprain
- Myofascial pain syndromes
- Instability

[†] See Lumbar section

CONTRIBUTING FACTORS

- Poor posture
- Occupations that require repetitive activities of the neck such a house painter or violinist
- Past history of MVA or trauma

TREATMENT

SURGICAL OPTIONS

There are no current studies that have specifically looked at surgical management of cervical joint dysfunction.

REHABILITATION

- Current best evidence for treating neck pain without any significant medical and/or psychosocial variables has focused on the use of a treatment-based classification schema in providing care.
- This classification system focuses on individuals with cervical spine ROM limitations, headaches of cervical nature, and/or radiating symptoms down the extremity.
- A recent article by Childs et al. summarized the current best evidence for individuals presenting with neck pain.
- Cervical mobilization and/or manipulation has shown strong evidence in treating mechanical neck pain.
- A preliminary clinical prediction rule for individuals who had a favorable response to cervical manipulation demonstrated an 89% success rate if they met at least 4 of 6 variables. The variables were as follows:
  - Pain with at least four of the following variables: Initial scores on the Neck Disability Index <11.50 points, having a bilateral pattern involvement, not performing sedentary work longer than 5 hours a day, feeling better while moving the neck, without feeling worse while extending the neck, and the diagnosis of spondylosis without radiculopathy.
- Strengthening exercises in the cervical spine, as well as the scapulohumeral area, have shown to strong evidence for treating mechanical neck pain.
- Thoracic spine manipulation has shown to have some evidence in treating mechanical neck pain with early development of a clinical prediction rule for patients that would benefit from manipulation in the thoracic spine for cervical spine pain.
- Exercises based on stretching and flexibility have shown weaker evidence, although they are valuable in treating anterior chest musculature (pectoralis major and minor) and local cervical spine musculature such as the scalenes, upper trapezius, and the levator scapulae.

PROGNOSIS

No research has been found that addresses specifically the prognosis for patient with cervical facet pathology. As a whole, studies have shown that there is a high recurrence rate with neck pain. The results of the studies place the recurrence rate between 22% and 50%, depending on the study.

SIGNS AND SYMPTOMS INDICATING REFERRAL TO PHYSICIAN

Spinal Fractures
- Major trauma (e.g. MVA, fall, or blow to the head) without proper imaging or the necessity for the Canadian C-Spine Rules
  - Severe limitations during neck active ROM in all directions

Cervical Myelopathy
- Sensory disturbances of the hands
  - Muscle wasting of the hand's intrinsic musculature
  - Unsteady gait
  - Positive Hoffmann's reflex
  - Hyperreflexia
  - Bowel and bladder disturbances
  - Multiple disc segmental weakness, sensory changes, or both

Neoplastic Conditions
- Age >50 years with a previous history of cancer
  - Unexplained weight loss
  - Constant pain with no relief with bed rest
  - Night pain

Upper Cervical Ligamentous Instability
- Occipital headache and numbness
- Severe limitation during neck active ROM in all directions
- Signs of cervical myelopathy

Vertebral Artery Insufficiency
- Drop attacks
- Dizziness or lightheadedness related to neck movement
- Dysphasia
- Dysarthria
- Diplopia
- Positive cranial nerve signs

Inflammatory or Systemic Disease
- Temperature >100° F
- Blood pressure >165/95 mm Hg
- Resting pulse >100 bpm
- Resting respiration >25 bpm
- Fatigue

SUGGESTED READINGS

Childs J, Cleland J, Elliott J, et al. Neck pain: clinical practice guidelines linked to the internal classification of functioning, disability, and health from the orthopaedic section of the american phyiscal therapy association. *J Orthop Sports Phys Ther.* 2008;38(9):A1–A34.

Childs J, Fritz J, Piva S, Whitman J. Proposal of a classification system for patients with neck pain. *J Orthop Sports Phys Ther.* 2004;34:686–696.

Cleland J, Childs J, Fritz J, Whitman J, Eberhart S. Development of a clinical prediction rule for guiding treatment of a subgroup of patients with neck pain: use of thoracic spine manipulation, exercise and patient eduction. *Phys Ther.* 2007;87:9-23.

Cleland JA, Flynn TW, Childs JD, Eberhart S. The audible pop from thoracic spine thrust manipulation and its relation to short-term outcomes in patients with neck pain. *J Manipulative Physiol Ther.* 2007;30(4):312-320.

Fritz JM, Brennan GP. Preliminary examination of a proposed treatment-based classification system for patients receiving physical therapy interventions for neck pain. *Phys Ther.* 2007;87(5):513-524.

Fukui S, Ohseto K, Shiotani M, et al. Referred pain distribution of the cervical zygapophysial joints and cervical dorsal rami. *Pain.* 1996;68:79-83.

Jull G, Trott P, Potter H, et al. A randomized controlled trial of exercise and manipulative therapy for cervicogenic headache. *Spine.* 2002;27(17):1835-1843.

Maitland GD. *Vertebral manipulation.* 5th ed. Boston, MA: Butterworth; 1986.

Wainner RS, Fritz JM, Boninger M, Irrgang JJ, Delitto T, Allison SC. Reliability and diagnostic accuracy of the clinical examination and patient self-report measures for cervical radiculopathy. *Spine.* 2003;28(1):52-62.

Wainner RS, Gill HM. Diagnosis and non-operative management of cervical radiculopathy. *J Orthop Sports Phys Ther.* 2000;30:728-744.

AUTHOR: MICHAEL LEAL

BASIC INFORMATION

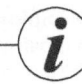

DEFINITION

Cervical muscle strain is a soft tissue injury to the surrounding musculature of the cervical spine that can be caused by a variety of incidents such as a fall, a motor vehicle collision, blow to the head of any type, or any form of trauma that may cause muscle or ligamentous (cervical sprain) disruption via an excessive stretch or compressive force through the cervical spine.

SYNONYMS

- Cervical strain
- Cervical sprain (ligamentous)
- Mechanical neck pain

ICD-9CM CODE
847.0 Neck sprain

OPTIMAL NUMBER OF VISITS

6 visits or less

MAXIMAL NUMBER OF VISITS

12 visits

ETIOLOGY

Cervical strain can occur from a variety of mechanisms such as a motor vehicle collision, a fall, or a blow to the head. Individuals may have insidious episodes with progressive pain and immobility from sleeping awkwardly or having their head and/or neck in prolonged positions, which would add a compressive force on the muscle or ligamentous structures in the cervical spine.

EPIDEMIOLOGY AND DEMOGRAPHICS

The prevalence rate of neck pain for the general population has been estimated to be as high as 30% to 50% of these people during a 12-month period. Only 1.7% to 11.5% experienced pain that limited activity.

MECHANISM OF INJURY

The mechanism of injury is usually a mechanical fall, motor vehicle collision, blow to the head, or any other type of injury in which the muscle and ligamentous structures were exposed to excessive stretch or compressive forces.

COMMON SIGNS AND SYMPTOMS

- Neck pain (posterior upper spine, as well as lower spine or shoulder area)
- Limited cervical spine ROM
- Tenderness on palpation
- Muscle spasms

AGGRAVATING ACTIVITIES

- Cervical spine ROM in positions that stretch or elongate the tissue in question (e.g., while driving, being able to turn to look behind you or in the rearview mirror)
- Prolonged periods of sitting or driving (axial compression)
- Specific sleeping positions that aggravate the neck area

EASING ACTIVITIES

- Supine or lying down, depending on the stage of tissue injury
- Not performing activities in which the cervical spine is placed in excessive stretched or compressive loads
- Modalities, such as ice and/or heat, depending on the stage of tissue healing (e.g., may be more appropriate in the acute phase of injury)

24-HOUR SYMPTOM PATTERN

- Patient will often experience pain and stiffness in the morning. This will decrease as the muscle heals.
- As with many mechanical type injuries, the patient will experience increased pain with usage.
- Night pain may or may not aggravate patient, depending on position of sleep and severity of symptoms.

PAST HISTORY FOR THE REGION

- Past history may or may not be significant based on the patient's presentation.
- Past history of muscle strain may predispose a patient to subsequent muscle strains because of the muscles weakened state.

PHYSICAL EXAMINATION

- An upper quarter posture that alleviates pressure or load of specific muscle tissues, as well as decreasing excessive stress on the muscle or ligament in question
- Potential muscle hypertrophy around the posterior cervical musculature or upper trapezius areas
- Decreased cervical spine ROM
- Decreased strength in global cervical spine muscular structures
- Decreased anterior chest wall mobility
- Decreased motor control of local cervical spine muscular structures
- Decreased muscle length of upper quarter muscular structures

IMPORTANT OBJECTIVE TESTS

- A thorough red flag screening should be completed before the objective component of the physical examination. The Canadian C-Spine Rules should be applied to the patient cohort and appropriate referral made if the patient is found to be positive with the rules. If the patient has had previous imaging for this condition, the practitioner should confirm the results with the patient or referring health care provider.
- The Canadian C-Spine Rule suggests that radiographs of the cervical spine should be performed in cases with the following high-risk factors:
  - Patient is 65 years of age or older.
  - Patient has experienced a dangerous injury mechanism.
  - Patient has paresthesia in the extremities.
  - Patient has any low-risk injury (simple rear-end MVAs, etc.) that will not allow safe assessment of AROM.
- Cervical spine ROM testing
  - Test procedure: Patient is seated in an upright position. Flexion and extension are measured with the bubble inclinometer placed on top of the head perpendicular to a bisected line through the external auditory meatus. Sidebending is measured with the bubble goniometer placed in line with an imaginary line drawn through the auditory meatus. Rotation is measured by placing the goniometer on top of the patient's head and measuring the amount of rotation left and right with the fixed arm bisecting the head.
- Manual examination
  - Test procedure: Patient is examined via central posteroanterior glides, as well as passive physiological intervertebral movements into flexion, extension, sidebending, and rotation.
  - Positive: The level of joint dysfunction was determined based on the examiner's ability to assess end-feel, resistance, and pain provocation at that joint level.
  - Sensitivity: 1.0; specificity: 1.0
- Palpation over cervical spine facet joints
  - Test procedure: Palpation was performed on the cervical spine assessing the articular structures of each cervical level.
  - Positive: If the patient reported pain with palpation as the therapist was assessing the articular structures.
  - Sensitivity: 0.82; specificity: 0.79
  - Positive LR: 3.9; negative LR: 0.23

DIFFERENTIAL DIAGNOSIS

- Cervical disc herniation
- Myofascial pain syndromes
- Instability

CONTRIBUTING FACTORS

- Prior history of muscle injury
- Poor posture
- Long-term use of corticosteroids

TREATMENT

SURGICAL OPTIONS

There is no current evidence to suggest surgical options within this patient cohort.

REHABILITATION

- Current best evidence for treating neck pain without any significant medical and/or psychosocial variables has focused on the use of a treatment-based classification schema in providing care.
- This classification system focuses on individuals with cervical spine ROM limitations, headaches of a cervical nature, and/or radiating symptoms down the extremity.
- A recent article by Childs et al summarized the current best evidence for individuals presenting with neck pain.
- Cervical mobilization and/or manipulation has shown to have strong evidence in the use of treating mechanical neck pain.
- Strengthening exercises in the cervical spine, as well as the scapulohumeral area, have shown strong evidence for treating mechanical neck pain.
- Thoracic spine manipulation has shown some evidence in treating mechanical neck pain with early development of a clinical prediction rule for patients that would benefit from manipulation in the thoracic spine for cervical spine pain.
- Exercises based on stretching and flexibility have shown weaker evidence, although exercises are valuable in treating anterior chest musculature (pectoralis major and minor) and local cervical spine musculature such as the scalenes, upper trapezius, and the levator scapulae.

PROGNOSIS

- No studies have been conducted that look specifically at the long-term rehabilitation prognosis for patients with cervical muscle strains.

- Clinically, muscle strains will heal in 6 to 8 weeks.

SIGNS AND SYMPTOMS INDICATING REFERRAL TO PHYSICIAN

Spinal Fractures
- Major trauma (e.g. MVA, fall, blow to the head) without proper imaging or the necessity for the Canadian C-Spine rules
  - Severe limitations during neck active ROM in all directions

Cervical Myelopathy
- Sensory disturbances of the hands
  - Muscle wasting of the hand's intrinsic musculature
  - Unsteady gait
  - Positive Hoffmann's reflex
  - Hyperreflexia
  - Bowel and bladder disturbances
  - Multiple disc segmental weakness, sensory changes, or both

Neoplastic Conditions
- Age >50 years of age with a previous history of cancer
  - Unexplained weight loss
  - Constant pain with no relief with bed rest
  - Night pain

Upper Cervical Ligamentous Instability
- Occipital headache and numbness
- Severe limitation during neck active ROM in all directions
- Signs of cervical myelopathy

Vertebral Artery Insufficiency
- Drop attacks
- Dizziness or lightheadedness related to neck movement
- Dysphasia
- Dysarthria

- Diplopia
- Positive cranial nerve signs

Inflammatory or Systemic Disease
  - Temperature >100° F
  - Blood pressure >165/95 mm Hg
  - Resting pulse >100 bpm
  - Resting respiration >25 bpm
  - Fatigue

SUGGESTED READINGS

Cleland JA, Flynn TW, Childs JD, Eberhart S. The audible pop from thoracic spine thrust manipulation and its relation to short-term outcomes in patients with neck pain. *J Manipulative Physiol Ther.* 2007;30(4):312-320.

Cleland JA, Markowski AM, Childs JD. *The Cervical Spine: Physical Therapy Patient Management Utilizing Current Best Evidence.* American Physical Therapy Association, Orthopaedic Section; 2006.

Fritz JM, Brennan GP. Preliminary examination of a proposed treatment-based classification system for patients receiving physical therapy interventions for neck pain. *Phys Ther.* 2007;87(5):513-524.

Fukui S, Ohseto K, Shiotani M, et al. Referred pain distribution of the cervical zygapophysial joints and cervical dorsal rami. *Pain.* 1996;68:79-83.

Jull G, Trott P, Potter H, et al. A randomized controlled trial of exercise and manipulative therapy for cervicogenic headache. *Spine.* 2002;27(17):1835-1843.

Wainner RS, Fritz JM, Boninger M, Irrgang JJ, Delitto T, Allison SC. Reliability and diagnostic accuracy of the clinical examination and patient self-report measures for cervical radiculopathy. *Spine.* 2003;28(1):52-62.

Wainner RS, Gill HM. Diagnosis and non-operative management of cervical radiculopathy. *J Orthop Sports Phys Ther.* 2000;30:728-744.

AUTHOR: MICHAEL LEAL

BASIC INFORMATION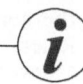

DEFINITION

- Cervical myelopathy is the most prevalent spinal cord compression pathology in individuals over the age of 55 and one of the most common acquired causes of spinal cord dysfunction.
- The natural history of this disorder includes a progressive degeneration of various components within the cervical spine, including the facet joints, intervertebral discs, ligaments, and associated connective tissue, which results in cervical spondylosis.
- These degenerative changes within the cervical spine cause a narrowing or reduced diameter of the spinal canal, thus potentially impacting the spinal cord and neurological function.

SYNONYMS

- Cervical spondylotic myelopathy
- Cervical compressive myelopathy
- Cord compressive myelopathy

ICD-9CM CODES
721.1   Cervical spondylosis with myelopathy
721.91   Spondylosis of unspecified site with myelopathy

OPTIMAL NUMBER OF VISITS

8 visits

MAXIMAL NUMBER OF VISITS

24 visits

ETIOLOGY

- The pathophysiology of cervical myelopathy is based on the following three factors:
  - *Static mechanical factors* include the size of the spinal canal, which has shown to be correlated with cervical myelopathy when the sagittal diameter of the spinal cord was 12mm or less. This can be the result of degenerative processes, as well as congenital factors. Progressive cervical spondylitic changes have also been shown to be a key feature of this disorder. Intervertebral changes, including disc herniations, facet and ligamentous hypertrophy, and osteophyte formation, can all contribute in circumferential narrowing of the spinal canal.
  - *Dynamic mechanical factors* relate to the extent of mechanical compression the spinal cord is exposed to in positions such as cervical spine flexion and extension. In cervical spine flexion, the spinal cord has a higher vulnerability to prolonged axial tension, as well as ischemia. Anterior

osteophytes can also cause a tethering effect, which can contribute to overall excursion of the spinal cord and can act as a site of compression. In cervical spine extension, the spinal cord increases in cross-sectional area and the canal area reaches its maximum reduction in cross-sectional area, thus placing the spinal cord at significant risk. The ligamentum flavum may also contribute to this reduced cross-sectional area of the spinal canal in the posterior region.
  - *Ischemia* results when the blood vessels that supply the spinal cord are compressed by cervical spine structures that have undergone degenerative changes. Pathological manifestations of this may include gray matter changes, as well as spinal cord necrosis.

EPIDEMIOLOGY AND DEMOGRAPHICS

- Individuals over the age of 55
- A quarter of individuals that present with tetraparesis or paraparesis
- The overall prevalence is currently unknown

MECHANISM OF INJURY

Cervical myelopathy is a progressive disorder caused by degenerative changes within the cervical spine, with an insidious onset and not a result of a specific mechanism of injury or related traumatic episode.

COMMON SIGNS AND SYMPTOMS

- General symptoms can include any of the following:
  - Cervical, intrascapular, or shoulder area pain
  - Generalized nonspecific upper and/or lower extremity weakness and/or stiffness
  - Numbness or paresthesias in the upper or lower extremities
  - Clumsiness with hand function, which may be unilateral or bilateral
  - Gait ataxia
  - Sensory changes in the lower and/or upper extremities
  - Gait dysfunction
- Grade 1 (mild): Upper motor neuron signs with a normal gait
- Grade 2-5 (moderate to severe): Worsening gait disturbances and with a less favorable prognosis
- Upper motor neuron signs such as spasticity, clonus, a positive Babinski sign, a positive Hoffmann's sign, hyperreflexia, and bowel and/or bladder dysfunction
- Lower motor neuron signs such as hyporeflexia of the upper extremity, as well as weakness in a myotomal distribution

- Cervical myelopathy will commonly present with lower motor neuron signs at the level of spinal pathology and upper motor neuron signs below the level of spinal pathology

AGGRAVATING ACTIVITIES

No specific aggravating factors associated with this condition have been found in the literature, although the patient's functional limitations will be based on their current symptoms.

EASING ACTIVITIES

No specific easing factors associated with this condition have been found in the literature.

24-HOUR SYMPTOM PATTERN

There is no specific 24-hour pain or symptom pattern for this condition. The patient's performance when undertaking functional limitations may better guide clinically in regards to a potential symptom pattern.

PAST HISTORY FOR THE REGION

- There have been no studies that have looked at the statistical values (sensitivity, specificity, and likelihood ratios) regarding the patient's history in terms of assisting in the diagnosis of cervical myelopathy.
- Because of the progressive nature of this disorder, patients may or may not have had symptoms for some time before seeking care for their condition.
- There may or may not be reports of previous or ongoing neck pain.
- There may be no complaints of paresthesia. If there are reports of paresthesia, often these sensory changes appear after motor changes have already taken place.
- Sudden gait disturbances are the most common presentation, and the patient interview and history review should include any gait abnormalities.
- 55% of patients over the age of 65 were found to have numbness, decreased vibratory sense, and decreased fine motor control in the hands.
- As cervical myelopathy progresses, patients may start to report increasing gait difficulties, with varying degrees of proximal weakness.
- The following factors are as crucial when attempting to diagnosis cervical myelopathy:
  - It can cause a vast array of signs and symptoms.
  - There are no pathognomonic findings.
  - The onset of the pathology is insidious, with long periods of stable and fixed disability with episodic worsening.

PHYSICAL EXAMINATION

- Gait abnormalities and ataxia
- Reflex changes (hyperreflexia and/or hyporeflexia)

- Clonus
- Positive pathological reflexes (Babinski sign and Hoffmann's sign)
- Weakness/motor dysfunction in the lower or upper extremities
- Sensation changes in a nondermatomal pattern
- Spasticity
- Hand weakness, clumsiness, and possible visible muscle atrophy
- Decreased vibratory sense
- Bowel and bladder changes
- Paraparesis and/or tetraparesis

IMPORTANT OBJECTIVE TESTS

- Many of the clinical tests for cervical myelopathy have been shown to have relative poor sensitivity, therefore it is recommended that the clinician use a cluster of tests in assisting with shifting the probability of the pathology's presence or absence
- Finger escape sign
- Grip and release test
- Clonus
- Inverted supinator reflex
- Babinski sign
- Hoffmann sign
- Lhermitte sign
- Comprehensive neurological examination
- Gait assessment

DIFFERENTIAL DIAGNOSIS

- Cervical radiculopathy
- Diabetes
- Stroke
- Peripheral neuropathies
- Amyotrophic lateral sclerosis (ALS)
- Multiple sclerosis (MS)

CONTRIBUTING FACTORS

- Age >50 years
- Previous history of cervical spondylosis

TREATMENT

SURGICAL OPTIONS AND OUTCOMES

- The surgical treatment of choice to address cervical radiculopathy is the anterior cervical disc fusion (ACDF). Outcome for ACDF is good to excellent for the patient with a single level of impairment. Multiple disc segment involvement yielded less favorable responses: only 60% of patients had good-to-excellent results.
- Outcomes for patients with cervical myelopathy are mixed.
- Some report poor outcomes. In 1992, a thorough review of the literature pertaining to surgery for cervical myelopathy found that the chances for improvement after surgery were approximately 50%.

A separate 3-year prospective randomized trial found no significant difference between patients who were treated surgically and those who were treated conservatively in patients with mid to mild amounts of severity.

- Others report clinical improvement in 80% to 90% of patients after ACDF surgery.

REHABILITATION

- If the rehabilitation clinician suspects the presence of cervical myelopathy, the referring physician should be made aware of this suspicion. Further testing by the physician may be needed to rule out the presence of spinal cord involvement.
- If cleared by the physician, current best evidence for treating neck pain without any significant medical and/or psychosocial variables has focused on the use of a treatment-based classification schema in providing care.
- This classification system focuses on individuals with cervical spine ROM limitations, headaches of cervical nature, and/or radiating symptoms down the extremity.
- A recent article by Childs et al (2008) summarized the current best evidence for individuals presenting with neck pain.
- Strengthening exercises in the cervical spine, as well as the scapulohumeral area, have shown strong evidence for treating mechanical neck pain
- Exercises based on stretching and flexibility have shown weaker evidence, although exercises are valuable in treating anterior chest musculature (pectoralis major and minor) and local cervical spine musculature such as the scalenes, upper trapezius, and the levator scapulae.
- Neurodynamic mobilization procedures have shown moderate evidence in patients with neck and arm pain.
- Cervical immobilization is a common treatment to prevent spinal cord damage in the cervical spine. Its use has neither been validated nor refuted by research.

PROGNOSIS

A study of 27 patients treated conservatively for mild cervical myelopathy revealed that 10 would eventually need surgery and 17 responded favorably to conservative care when the myelopathy was due to cervical disc herniation.

SIGNS AND SYMPTOMS INDICATING REFERRAL TO PHYSICIAN

Spinal Fractures
- Major trauma (e.g. MVA, fall, or blow to the head) without proper imaging or the necessity for the Canadian C-Spine Rules
  - Severe limitations during neck active ROM in all directions

Cervical Myelopathy
- Sensory disturbances of the hands
  - Muscle wasting of the hand's intrinsic musculature
  - Unsteady gait
  - Positive Hoffmann's reflex
  - Hyperreflexia
  - Bowel and bladder disturbances
  - Multiple disc segmental weakness, sensory changes, or both

Neoplastic Conditions
- Age >50 years with a previous history of cancer
  - Unexplained weight loss
  - Constant pain with no relief with bed rest
  - Night pain

Upper Cervical Ligamentous Instability
- Occipital headache and numbness
- Severe limitation during neck active ROM in all directions
- Signs of cervical myelopathy

Vertebral Artery Insufficiency
- Drop attacks
- Dizziness or lightheadedness related to neck movement
- Dysphasia
- Dysarthria
- Diplopia
- Positive cranial nerve signs

Inflammatory or Systemic Disease
- Temperature >100° F
- Blood pressure >165/95 mm Hg
- Resting pulse >100 bpm
- Resting respiration >25 bpm
- Fatigue

SUGGESTED READINGS

Childs J, Cleland J, Elliott J, et al. Neck pain: clinical practice guidelines linked to the internal classification of functioning, disability, and health from the orthopaedic section of the american phyiscal therapy association. *J Orthop Sports Phys Ther.* 2008;38(9):A1-A34.

Childs J, Fritz J, Piva S, Whitman J. Proposal of a classification system for patients with neck pain. *J Orthop Sports Phys Ther.* 2004;34:686-696.

Clarke E, Robinson PK. Cervical myelopathy: a complication of cervical spondylosis. *Brain.* 1956;79(3):483-510.

Cleland J, Childs J, Fritz J, Whitman J, Eberhart S. Development of a clinical prediction rule for guiding treatment of a subgroup of patients with neck pain: use of thoracic spine manipulation, exercise and patient eduction. *Phys Ther.* 2007;87:9-23.

Cleland J, Fritz JM, Whitman JM, Heath R. Predictors of short-term outcome in people with a clinical diagnosis of cervical radiculopathy. *Phys Ther.* 2007;87(12):1619-1632.

Fehlings MG, Skaf G. A review of the pathophysiology of cervical spondylotic myelopathy with insights for potential novel mechanisms drawn from traumatic spinal cord injury. *Spine.* 1998;23(24):2730-2737.

Fritz JM, Brennan GP. Preliminary examination of a proposed treatment-based classification system for patients receiving physical therapy interventions for neck pain. *Phys Ther.* 2007;87(5):513-524.

Matsumoto M, Chiba K, Ishikawa M, et al. Relationships between outcomes of conservative treatment and magnetic resonance imaging findings in patients with mild cervical myelopathy caused by soft disc herniations. *Spine.* 2001;26(14):1592-1598.

McCormick WE, Steinmetz MP, Benzel EC. Cervical spondylotic myelopathy: make the difficult diagnosis, then refer for surgery. *Cleve Clin J Med.* 2003;70(10):899-904.

Moore AP, Blumhardt LD. A prospective survey of the causes of non-traumatic spastic paraparesis and tetraparesis in 585 patients. *Spinal Cord.* 1997;35(6):361-367.

Sampath P, Bendebba M, Davis J, Ducker T. Outcome of patients treated for cervical myelopathy: a prospective, multicenter study with independent clinical review. *Spine.* 2000;25(6):670-676.

Wainner RS, Fritz JM, Boninger M, Irrgang JJ, Delitto T, Allison SC. Reliability and diagnostic accuracy of the clinical examination and patient self-report measures for cervical radiculopathy. *Spine.* 2003;28(1):52-62.

Wainner RS, Gill HM. Diagnosis and non-operative management of cervical radiculopathy. *J Orthop Sports Phys Ther.* 2000;30:728-744.

AUTHOR: MICHAEL LEAL

Section III

ORTHOPEDIC PATHOLOGY

BASIC INFORMATION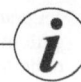

DEFINITION

Cervical radiculopathy is characterized by spinal nerve root dysfunction. Most commonly this is due to degenerative changes found within the spine that can either create a foraminal impingement on an associated cervical nerve root or create an inflammatory condition around the nerve itself. Pathologies, such as a cervical disc herniation or spondylosis, are common sources of this disorder.

SYNONYM

Cervical radiculitis

> **ICD-9CM CODES**
> 353.9 Unspecified nerve root and
>   plexus disorder
> 723.1 Cervicalgia
> 723.4 Cervical radiculitis

OPTIMAL NUMBER OF VISITS

8 visits

MAXIMAL NUMBER OF VISITS

12 visits

ETIOLOGY

- In the population younger than 40 years of age, cervical radiculopathy is hypothesized to occur via disc herniation or acute injury. These two pathologies will affect the foraminal circumference and create impingement on the exiting cervical nerve root.
- In the older population, it is speculated that degenerative changes, such as spondylosis, play a larger role on the cause of the nerve root impingement.
- The pathology is specific to nerve root dysfunction that can be caused from either a disc herniation, degenerative changes within the cervical spine creating foraminal narrowing, an inflammatory component of the nerve root itself or from surrounding structures, or a combination of all of the above.

EPIDEMIOLOGY AND DEMOGRAPHICS

According to a study by Wainner et al (2003), prevalence was reported as 23% in a sample of patients who underwent a standardized electrophysiological examination.

MECHANISM OF INJURY

- Injury or trauma related may involve extension of the cervical spine or any form of axial compression or loading.
- Insidious onset with a gradual buildup of symptoms involving the neck and arm over a certain time frame.

COMMON SIGNS AND SYMPTOMS

- Numbness and/or tingling in the arm or hand
- Weakness of hand musculature
- Pain in the cervical, scapular, intrascapular areas, as well as arm and/or hand
- Pain with limited cervical spine ROM
- Sensation changes along the dermatomal pattern of the suspected radiculopathy as follows:
  - A common pattern seen for this pathology may or may not include pain located in the neck, intrascapular, or arm area with radiation of symptoms extending into the shoulder, elbow, or distal component of the dorsal or volar aspect of the hand.
  - Numbness and/or tingling may be reported in a dermatomal pattern on the upper extremity, although current evidence is showing less support for a "specific" dermatomal pattern for lower cervical nerve root problems, so these results need to be analyzed with caution.

AGGRAVATING ACTIVITIES

Cervical spine ROM will often have a pattern of limitation highlighting extension, lateral bending, and rotation, either away from or toward the side of discomfort. With limitations toward the side of discomfort or pain, the cause may be more likely foraminal impingement, whereas limitations away from the side of discomfort or pain may be related to a disc or decreased mobility of the peripheral nerve trunk and/or brachial plexus.

EASING ACTIVITIES

- Cervical spine ROM or positions that would either "open" or decrease the mechanical load on the cervical spine nerve root.
- It has been reported that placing the arm on top of the head acts as a unloaded position for the nervous system and can be indicative of lower cervical nerve root dysfunction.

24-HOUR SYMPTOM PATTERN

The 24-hour symptom pattern may be mechanical or inflammatory, depending on the cause of the cervical nerve root dysfunction (e.g., inflammation around the nerve root versus an osteophyte or anatomical structure creating impingement in the foramen).

PAST HISTORY FOR THE REGION

- The past history may include progressive neck pain followed by sensation changes in the distal components of the arm or hand. This is usually of an insidious onset with no direct trauma or event.

- There may be associated trauma or a specific injury in certain instances involving head and/or neck trauma with associated neurological complaints (motor weakness and/or sensation changes).

PHYSICAL EXAMINATION

- Observation may include a cervical posture that is sidebent away from the area of pain, if the problem is due to compression or narrowing of the foramen. The cervical posture may also be sidebent toward the painful area to unload the nervous system, if nerve mobility is an issue or if the problem is a disc herniation. Commonly, there will also be posture abnormalities in the thoracic spine and the scapulothoracic area.
- Cervical ROM is usually limited in a pattern or direction that would either compress the nerve or position or mechanically challenge the nervous system in terms of mobility.
- The neurological examination may show lower motor neuron signs corresponding to the hypothesized level of the nerve root dysfunction such as hyporeflexia, decreased sensation to light touch, and motor weakness.
- Other associated findings may include pain with palpation over the local neck musculature, shortened anterior chest wall musculature, and decreased scapulothoracic muscle strength (lower trapezius, middle trapezius, and serratus anterior). Decreased motor control in the deep neck flexors may also be present and combined with overactive superficial muscle control.

IMPORTANT OBJECTIVE TESTS

- Many singular diagnostic special tests have questionable reliability and validity in diagnosing cervical radiculopathy.
- Test-item cluster for cervical radiculopathy
  - Test procedure: A test-item cluster (TIC) was developed by Wainner et al (2003) that looked at a combination of tests in determining the presence of cervical radiculopathy. The four variables that were found to increase the likelihood of cervical spine radiculopathy were the following:
    - The upper limb median nerve neurodynamic test (ULNT 1A)
    - Ipsilateral cervical rotation <60 degrees
    - A positive cervical distraction test
    - A positive Spurling's test
  - Positive tests:
    - 2/4 tests (sensitivity 0.39; specificity 0.56; positive likelihood ratio 0.88)
    - 3/4 tests (sensitivity 0.39; specificity 0.94; positive likelihood ratio 6.1)
    - 4/4 tests (sensitivity 0.24; specificity 0.99; positive likelihood ratio 30.3)

DIFFERENTIAL DIAGNOSIS

- Cervical strain or sprain
- Cervical spondylosis
- Cervical stenosis (central or foraminal stenosis)
- Cervical spondylolisthesis
- Cervical myelopathy
- Carpal tunnel syndrome
- First rib dysfunction
- Pancoast tumor
- Thoracic outlet syndrome
- T4 syndrome
- Brachial plexopathy
- Peripheral neuropathy

CONTRIBUTING FACTORS

- Posture
- Occupation (sitting, lifting, manual labor)
- Age

TREATMENT Rx

SURGICAL OPTIONS

Surgical options for cervical radiculopathy vary greatly, depending on the source of the nerve entrapment. See individual pathologies for surgical options and outcomes.

REHABILITATION

- Cleland et al (2005) showed that a multimodal treatment approach to patients with cervical spine radiculopathy was beneficial in terms of decreasing self-perceived disability. This multimodal approach included cervical spine mobilizations (lateral glides with the upper extremity in a neurodynamic position), thoracic spine manipulation, cervical traction, and scapulothoracic strengthening exercises.
- Preliminary data regarding patients who specifically benefit from a mechanical traction approach are also emerging. The preliminary clinical prediction rule is for those with cervical spine pain who would likely benefit from traction. The five variables that were determined from the analysis were as follows:
  - The patient reported peripheralization of symptoms with cervical spine mobility testing
  - Positive shoulder abduction sign

- Age >55 years
- Positive ULNT (median nerve)
- Relief of symptoms with manual distraction test
- Results: 3/5 variables present resulted in a positive likelihood ratio of 4.81 and 4/5 variables resulted in a positive likelihood ratio of 11.7; thus improving the posttest probability of success to 90.2%.

PROGNOSIS

- A study by Cleland et al (2007) looked at variables in the patient interview, as well as physical examination for those who were classified as having cervical radiculopathy and would demonstrate short-term favorable outcomes. The following variables were noted to be significant:
  - Age <54 years of age
  - Dominant arm is not affected
  - Looking down does not worsen symptoms
  - >30 degrees of cervical spine flexion
  - Mechanical traction
  - Thrust manipulation of the thoracic spine
  - No soft tissue mobilization
  - Multimodal treatment, including manual therapy, deep neck flexor training, cervical traction, and strengthening for at least 50% of their visits
- The following combination of these predictor variables resulted in the following probability of success:
  - 4 or more resulted in a 90.4% probability of success
  - 3 or more resulted in a 85.4% probability of success
  - 2 or more resulted in a 62.9% probability of success
  - 1 or more resulted in a 55.4% probability of success

SIGNS AND SYMPTOMS INDICATING REFERRAL TO PHYSICIAN

Spinal Fractures
- Major trauma (e.g. MVA, fall, blow to the head) without proper imaging or the necessity for the Canadian C-Spine rules
  - Severe limitations during neck active ROM in all directions

Cervical Myelopathy
- Sensory disturbances of the hands
  - Muscle wasting of the hand's intrinsic musculature

  - Unsteady gait
  - Positive Hoffmann's reflex
  - Hyperreflexia
  - Bowel and bladder disturbances
  - Multiple disc segmental weakness, sensory changes, or both

Neoplastic Conditions
- Age >50 years if age with a previous history of cancer
  - Unexplained weight loss
  - Constant pain with no relief with bed rest
  - Night pain

Upper Cervical Ligamentous Instability
- Occipital headache and numbness
- Severe limitation during neck active ROM in all directions
- Signs of cervical myelopathy

Vertebral Artery Insufficiency
- Drop attacks
- Dizziness or lightheadedness related to neck movement
- Dysphasia
- Dysarthria
- Diplopia
- Positive cranial nerve signs

Inflammatory or Systemic Disease
- Temperature >100° F
- Blood pressure >165/95 mm Hg
- Resting pulse >100 bpm
- Resting respiration >25 bpm
- Fatigue

SUGGESTED READINGS

Cleland JA, Whitman JM, Fritz JM, Palmer JA. Manual physical therapy, cervical traction, and strengthening exercises in patients with cervical radiculopathy: a case series. *J Orthop Sports Phys Ther.* 2005;35(12):802-811.

Cleland J, Fritz JM, Whitman JM, Heath R. Predictors of short-term outcome in people with a clinical diagnosis of cervical radiculopathy. *Phys Ther.* 2007;87(12):1619-1632.

Fritz JM, Brennan GP. Preliminary examination of a proposed treatment-based classification system for patients receiving physical therapy interventions for neck pain. *Phys Ther.* 2007;87(5):513-524.

Wainner RS, Fritz JM, Boninger M, Irrgang JJ, Delitto T, Allison SC. Reliability and diagnostic accuracy of the clinical examination and patient self-report measures for cervical radiculopathy. *Spine.* 2003;28(1):52-62.

Wainner RS, Gill HM. Diagnosis and non-operative management of cervical radiculopathy. *J Orthop Sports Phys Ther.* 2000;30:728-744.

AUTHOR: MICHAEL LEAL

BASIC INFORMATION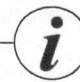

DEFINITION

Degenerative joint disease (DJD) can be defined as a breakdown of the cervical spine facet articular surfaces with a resultant loss of cartilage. This can occur in concert with degenerative disc disease (DDD) in which there is a loss of disc height. The breakdown of articular cartilage leads to a resultant inflammatory cascade that can result in bone spurs or osteophyte formation.

SYNONYMS

- Cervical spine osteoarthritis
- Cervical spine spondylosis

ICD-9CM CODES
721.0 Cervical spondylosis without myelopathy
721.1 Cervical spondylosis with myelopathy

OPTIMAL NUMBER OF VISITS

3 to 8 visits

MAXIMAL NUMBER OF VISITS

20 to 36 visits

ETIOLOGY

- Cervical DJD is generally the result of daily wear and tear in combination with various injuries sustained throughout life that cause the breakdown of healthy tissue.
- Physiologically, the wearing down of the hyaline cartilage leads to an inflammatory response. There is thickening and sclerosis of the subchondral bone and development of osteophytes or bone spurs. This leads to a narrowing of the joint space, loss of shock absorption, and pain.

EPIDEMIOLOGY AND DEMOGRAPHICS

- Nearly 10% of persons >30 years old show signs of cervical spine joint degeneration on x-ray.
- Seniors (osteoarthritis increases in prevalence 2% each year after 40 years of age) are more prone to cervical DJD.
- Men tend to have a higher prevalence than women.

MECHANISM OF INJURY

- Symptoms related to degenerative changes to the joint rarely occur as a result of direct trauma. Usually, it is a gradual process of physiological changes that eventually result in pain and dysfunction. Activities that can be associated with the degenerative changes include the following:
  - Daily use of the cervical spine
  - Excessive use/strain of the cervical spine secondary to work, obesity, or recreational activities
  - Injuries such as car accidents, slips and falls, and strains/sprains that cause inflammation in the cervical spine

COMMON SIGNS AND SYMPTOMS

- Unilateral pain in the neck
- Stiffness in the neck
- Cracking or crunching in the neck
- Loss of normal spinal curvature
- Facet joint pain tends to be localized over the area and surrounding paraspinal musculature and upper trapezius region, as follows:
  - Upper cervical facets (C2/3) will refer into the posterior aspect of the occiput and may result in headaches.
  - Midcervical facets (C3/4 and C4/5) will refer into the neck.
  - Lower cervical facets (C5/6 and C6/7) will refer into upper trapezius and rhomboid regions.
- If inflammation and/or stenosis occur (from the osteophytes) and narrow the nerve root foramen, there could be typical nerve root referral into the upper extremities
- Occasionally, temporomandibular joint (TMJ) dysfunction/pain may occur secondary to upper cervical facet dysfunction and its close proximity to the trigeminal nucleus

AGGRAVATING ACTIVITIES

- Inactivity leads to stiffness.
- Activity can irritate the joint surfaces.
- Inactivity allows the inflammation to "pool," which increases pressure leading to discomfort and loss of available movement.
- Typically, movements that "close down" the facet joints (extension, ipsilateral side flexion, and ipsilateral rotation) and cause more joint compression are more painful and limited.
- Joint movement increases "wear and tear" and inflammation/irritation to the articular surfaces. The more compression involved with the movement, the more "wear and tear" will occur.

EASING ACTIVITIES

- Gentle stretching and exercise, use of heat, massage, and antiinflammatory medications
- Generally, these activities lead to relaxation and loss of stiffness associated with this condition. It is hypothesized that these activities can promote circulation and increase synovial lubrication of the joint.

24-HOUR SYMPTOM PATTERN

- Stiffness may be present for the first 10 to 15 minutes in the morning
- Better after a warm shower and taking medication
- Can worsen with excessive movement
- Stiffens again in the evening

PAST HISTORY FOR THE REGION

- Jobs or recreational activities that require excessive use/strain of the cervical spine (looking upward, "craning" the neck, compression to the cervical spine through axial pressure, etc).
- Abnormal amount of damage due to injuries or accidents.
- The longer one lives the more likely degeneration will occur.

PHYSICAL EXAMINATION

- Loss of normal spinal curvature (most common is forward head with an loss of cervical lordosis)
- Loss of cervical ROM (especially extension, ipsilateral side flexion, and ipsilateral rotation)
- Localized pain, loss of passive physiological intervertebral movement, and loss of passive accessory joint movement
- Crepitus with movement
- Cervical musculature restrictions, unilateral guarding, muscle spasms, and tenderness

IMPORTANT OBJECTIVE TESTS

Common clinical assessment tools include the following:
- Active ROM (AROM) and passive ROM (PROM) will both be limited into extension, ipsilateral sidebending, and ipsilateral rotation.
- PROM tends to be greater than AROM as a result of muscle guarding.
- Unilateral posterior to anterior pressure on the pathological joint will be tender and lack mobility. Segmental rotation will be limited at the target segment.
- In the case of radiculopathies associated with cervical dysfunction, Wainner et al reported that the following clinical examination findings could be predictive of a cervical origin to radicular pain:
  - Positive Spurling's test
  - Positive neck distraction test
  - Positive upper limb tension test (ULTT) of the median nerve)
  - <60 degrees active cervical rotation to involved side
- If 3 out of 4 findings were positive, there was a 94% specificity that the symptoms were of cervical origin.
- If 4 out of 4 findings were positive, there was a 99% specificity that the symptoms were of cervical origin.

DIFFERENTIAL DIAGNOSIS

- DDD
- Cervical disc herniation

- Cervical sprain/strain, whiplash
- Nerve entrapment, "burners and stingers"
- TMJ dysfunction
- Meningitis
- Cardiac dysfunction
- Respiratory dysfunction
- Thyroid dysfunction
- Cancer

CONTRIBUTING FACTORS

- Age
- Gender: Men have a higher prevalence than women
- Past history of trauma to the region
- Repetitive activities that require neck motion
- Poor health (smoking, long-term use of steroids)
- Poor posture
- Poor thoracic mobility

TREATMENT

SURGICAL OPTIONS

- Cervical fusion (arthrodesis)
- Cervical laminectomy or laminoplasty
- Facet rhizotomy
- Cervical foraminotomy

REHABILITATION

- The focus of rehabilitation should be on the following:
  - Education regarding the correct use of ice/heat at home
  - Implementation of a home exercise program
  - Teach good body mechanics and encourage good posture
  - Teach good positioning for sleeping and good body mechanics for working or doing ADLs
  - Manual therapy (soft tissue mobilization, traction, or joint mobilization)
  - Modalities: ice/heat, ultrasound, electrical stimulation, or traction
- Initial exercises can include the following:
  - Stretches: upper trapezius, levator scapulae, pectoralis major and minor
  - Isometrics: cervical extension, cervical flexion, cervical side flexion, cervical rotation
  - Thoracic extension and shoulder extension/retraction exercises: Exercise ball, foam roller, Thera-Band rows
- Joint mobilization and manipulation may be used to unload the facet joints, lubricate the facet joint, and improve articular movement (localized and segments above and below).
- Soft tissue massage may be used to decrease pain by relaxing muscular tension and increase endorphin release.
- Exercise should focus on the following:
  - Decreasing muscular and joint stiffness
  - Improving joint alignment by increasing muscular support
  - Improving posture: Progressive thoracic extension and shoulder extension/retraction
  - Creating a sense of control over the symptoms and the condition
  - Generalized conditioning

PROGNOSIS

Long-term prognosis depends on the extent of wear and tear and ability to reduce the joint strain (posture, activity, etc). The condition is progressive, and the patient is likely to experience a pattern of symptom reduction followed by periods of symptom aggravation.

SIGNS AND SYMPTOMS INDICATING REFERRAL TO PHYSICIAN

- Unrelenting pain or unusual responses to therapy
- Possibility of cancer or meningitis
- Spinal cord symptoms
- Worsening nerve symptoms

SUGGESTED READINGS

Dugan SA. Exercise for health and wellness at midlife and beyond: balancing benefits and risks. *Phys Med Rehabil Clin N Am.* 2007;18(3):555-575.

Hoving JL. Manual therapy, physical therapy, or continued care by the general practitioner for patients with neck pain: long-term results from a pragmatic randomized clinical trial. *Clin J Pain.* 2006;22(4):370-377.

Manchikanti L, et al. Age-related prevalence of facet-joint involvement in chronic neck and low back pain. *Pain Physician.* 2008;11(1):67-75.

Rao RD, et al. Degenerative cervical spondylosis: Clinical syndromes, pathogenesis, and management. *J Bone Joint Surg Am.* 2007;89(6):1360-1378.

Wainner RS, Fritz JM, Boninger M, Irrgang JJ, Delitto T, Allison SC. Reliability and diagnostic accuracy of the clinical examination and patient self-report measures for cervical radiculopathy. *Spine.* 2003;28(1):52-62.

AUTHOR: SARA GRANNIS

BASIC INFORMATION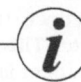

DEFINITION

- Rheumatoid arthritis (RA) is a systemic inflammatory condition that usually involves polyarthritis, which affects the smaller joints of the body such as the hands and feet. This progressive destruction of the joints leads to erosion and deformity, which then affects the patient's ROM and functional activities.
- Bouchaud-Chabot and Lioté reported that over half of RA patients will have some form of cervical spine involvement; the most common finding is atlantoaxial dislocation followed by atlantooccipital arthritis.

SYNONYMS

None known

ICD-9CM CODE
714.0 Rheumatoid arthritis

OPTIMAL NUMBER OF VISITS

6 visits

MAXIMAL NUMBER OF VISITS

36 visits

ETIOLOGY

A progressive buildup of articular inflammation, especially in the hands and feet, as a result of the immune system attacking the joints. RA is an autoimmune inflammatory disease and has been found to have no clear etiology or mechanism at this time.

EPIDEMIOLOGY AND DEMOGRAPHICS

- Approximately 1% of the population is affected, and women are affected 3 times more often than men.
- RA can occur at any age but tends to be found in older individuals because it is a progressive disorder with a peak incidence of individuals between the ages of 40 and 60 years.

MECHANISM OF INJURY

Insidious with a progressive onset of symptoms

COMMON SIGNS AND SYMPTOMS

- Symptoms of cervical myelopathy (neurological deficits)
- Subjective reports of instability
- Neck pain
- Stiffness in the cervical spine region as well as the distal extremities
- Pain with ROM
- Limited ROM in the neck and/or distal extremities

- Tenderness to palpation over local cervical spine musculature, as well as distal joints
- Swelling in the distal joints
- Deformities within the distal joints
- Visible rheumatoid nodules

AGGRAVATING ACTIVITIES

There are no specific aggravating factors found within the literature for this disorder, but based on the patient's current functional deficits, aggravating factors may be established. These may be based on the patient's current subjective complaints as well (stiffness, tenderness, and subjective reports of instability).

EASING ACTIVITIES

Like aggravating activities, there are no specific easing activities found within the literature for this disorder, but based on the patient's current functional deficits, easing factors may be established.

24-HOUR SYMPTOM PATTERN

There is no specific research to indicate a specific 24-hour pattern for this condition. Clinically, the patient's symptoms will wax and wane. Since inflammation is one of the hallmark signs of the pathology, stiffness may be present in the morning and with prolonged static positions. Muscle fatigue and soreness may be present as the day progresses; this is caused by joint laxity, which is another classic sign of RA.

PAST HISTORY FOR THE REGION

As RA may affect any age at any time in an individual's lifespan, symptoms may or may not have been present before seeking care. Patients may or may not have hand or foot symptoms and/or deformities, which are symptoms of the progressive polyarthritis that is a common sign of RA.

PHYSICAL EXAMINATION

- Neck pain and/or stiffness
- Stiffness in the hands or feet
- Tenderness of certain muscle groups
- Loss of joint ROM
- Cervical spine instability
- Decreased local and global neck and/or scapulothoracic musculature
- Limited anterior chest wall flexibility
- Visible deformities in the hands or feet
- Rheumatoid nodules

IMPORTANT OBJECTIVE TESTS

- The major concern with cervical RA is upper cervical instability. The Sharp-Purser test was developed to test for transverse ligament integrity in patients with RA. Sensitivity: 0.69; specificity: 0.96.
- Other tests commonly used to test for upper cervical ligament integrity include the alar ligament test, which tests the

integrity of the alar ligament and the tectorial membrane test, which tests the tectorial membrane. The validity and reliability of these tests have not been verified.

- Suspicions of upper cervical instability should be confirmed with radiographic studies. An atlantoaxial displacement of >3 mm on flexion-extension films is considered abnormal. Reported risk factors for cord compression based on radiographic examination measurement include:
  ○ Atlantoaxial subluxation of >9 mm
  ○ Space available for the cord of 14 mm or less
  ○ Presence of basilar invagination
- Cervical spine radiography should include lateral view radiographs taken in flexion and extension.

DIFFERENTIAL DIAGNOSIS

- Muscle strain
- Ligament sprain
- Radiculopathy
- Instability
- Myelopathy
- Spondylolysis
- Spondylolisthesis

CONTRIBUTING FACTORS

Contributing factors will be based on the patient interview, as well as the physical examination. Duration of symptoms, current job duties and workplace environment, and preexisting co-morbidities and musculoskeletal impairments can all potentially contribute to the outcome.

TREATMENT

SURGICAL INDICATORS

- Instability
- Intractable pain
- Neural involvement
- Combination of the three

SURGICAL OPTIONS

- Spinal fusion of the unstable or symptomatic segments is the most common surgical intervention for RA, as follows:
  ○ Gallie fusion of the first and second cervical vertebrae for atlantoaxial subluxation when there is failure of the transverse membrane or failure of the odontoid process
  ○ Fusion of the occiput and second cervical vertebra for superior migration of the odontoid process
  ○ Posterior fusion for subaxial subluxation

SURGICAL OUTCOMES

- In a study by Ranawat et al, 25 patients had posterior fusion; in 17 the condition was improved, in 5 there was no improvement, and in 3 the condition was worse. Of 19 patients with neural involvement, the condition was improved in 8, it was unchanged in 7, and it was made worse in 2. There were 3 postoperative deaths.

- In a separate study by Ronkainen et al, during the study period, 86 RA patients with atlantoaxial subluxation (AAS) underwent cervical spine surgery. The mean follow-up time was 7.5 years (range 5.0 to 9.8). During the follow-up, 32 patients (37%) died. The mean survival time after surgery was 7.2 years (95% CI 6.7-8.0). Seven patients experienced postoperative complications. Age, AAS other than horizontal, and occurrence of complications were independent predictors of mortality. In two-thirds of the patients, there was relief or decrease of pain and the functional capacity improved. Neurological deficits subsided in 53% of cases. The authors concluded that surgical treatments may not decrease the mortality of patients with RA, but it may result in more symptom-free life-years.
- van Asselt et al found that surgical treatment in the patients with symptoms of occipital neuralgia was successful in 62% of the patients studied.

REHABILITATION

- A thorough evaluation should be performed examining the upper cervical spine ligamentous structures before any form of intervention is applied.
- Rehabilitation should be based on the patient's current impairments linked to their functional limitations.
- Using current best evidence for the utilization of restoring tissue health should be implemented. Therapeutic exercises and muscle flexibility interventions addressing weakness in the local and global musculature.
- Manipulation, mobilization, and traction may all be contraindicated for the patient. The determining factor will be whether upper cervical instability is present. Careful screening should be conducted before any such treatments are implemented.

- Caution is always a wise approach with patients with cervical RA. Until you have a firm grasp of the patient's response to treatment, conservative management should be implemented because triggering a relapse is possible if treatment is too aggressive.
- Given the appropriate patient scenario, the patient should be progressed in terms of exercise and stretching similar to any other patient with cervical pain. Strengthening the local stabilizing muscles is appropriate because mild instabilities are present in many patients with cervical RA.

PROGNOSIS

- Recovery for patients with cervical RA is extremely variable. Some patient with mild involvement will live their daily lives with little to no functional limitations. Other with severe cases will be very limited in functional capacities as overuse can easily flair up a patient or trigger a relapse of symptoms.
- Surgical intervention for cervical RA should be undertaken with caution because the mortality rate is relatively high.

SIGNS AND SYMPTOMS INDICATING REFERRAL TO PHYSICIAN

Spinal Fractures
- Major trauma (e.g. MVA, fall, or blow to the head) without proper imaging or the necessity for the Canadian C-Spine Rules
  - Severe limitations during neck active ROM in all directions
Cervical Myelopathy
- Sensory disturbances of the hands
  - Muscle wasting of the hand's intrinsic musculature
  - Unsteady gait
  - Positive Hoffmann's reflex
  - Hyperreflexia
  - Bowel and bladder disturbances
  - Multiple disc segmental weakness, sensory changes, or both
Neoplastic Conditions
- Age >50 years with a previous history of cancer

  - Unexplained weight loss
  - Constant pain with no relief with bed rest
  - Night pain
Upper Cervical Ligamentous Instability
- Occipital headache and numbness
- Severe limitation during neck active ROM in all directions
- Signs of cervical myelopathy
Vertebral Artery Insufficiency
- Drop attacks
- Dizziness or lightheadedness related to neck movement
- Dysphasia
- Dysarthria
- Diplopia
- Positive cranial nerve signs
Inflammatory or Systemic Disease
- Temperature >100° F
- Blood pressure >165/95 mm Hg
- Resting pulse >100 bpm
- Resting respiration >25 bpm
- Fatigue

SUGGESTED READINGS

Bouchaud-Chabot A, Lioté F. Cervical spine involvement in rheumatoid arthritis. A review. *Joint Bone Spine.* 2002;69(2):141-154.

Cleland JA, Markowski AM, Childs JD. *The Cervical Spine: Physical Therapy Patient Management Utilizing Current Best Evidence.* American Physical Therapy Association, Orthopaedic Section; 2006.

Nguyen HV, Ludwig SC, Silber J, et al. Rheumatoid arthritis of the cervical spine. *Spine J.* 2004;4(3):329-334.

Ranawat CS, O'Leary P, Pellicci P, Tsairis P, Marchisello P, Dorr L. Cervical spine fusion in rheumatoid arthritis. *J Bone Joint Surg.* 1979;61(7):1003-1010.

Ronkainen A, Niskanen M, Auvinen A, Aalto J, Luosujärvi R. Cervical spine surgery in patients with rheumatoid arthritis: longterm mortality and its determinants. *J Rheumatol.* 2006;33(3):517-522.

Shen F, Samartzis D, Jenis L, An H. Rheumatoid arthritis: evaluation and surgical management of the cervical spine. *Spine J.* 2004;4(6):689-700.

van Asselt KM, Lems W, Bongartz E, et al. Outcome of cervical spine surgery in patients with rheumatoid arthritis. *Ann Rheum Dis.* 2001;60(5):448-452.

AUTHOR: MICHAEL LEAL

BASIC INFORMATION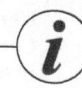

DEFINITION

- Torticollis is a rotational dysfunction of the upper neck musculature and is considered to be a form of cervical dystonia.
- Cervical dystonia is a syndrome in which an involuntary muscle contraction occurs that then causes abnormal posturing through frequent repetitive movements.

SYNONYMS

- Cervical dystonia
- Spasmatic torticollis

ICD-9CM CODES
723.5 Torticollis unspecified
333.83 Spasmodic torticollis
847.0 Torticollis traumatic, current

OPTIMAL NUMBER OF VISITS

6 visits

MAXIMAL NUMBER OF VISITS

24 visits

ETIOLOGY

- Torticollis is not a pathology but rather a physical manifestation of an underlying pathology. It is usually considered a protective mechanism imposed by the body to guard or protect the underlying pathology. The positioning of the head has usually been attributed to contraction of the sternocleidomastoid muscles, which results in a head posture of ipsilateral lateral cervical flexion and contralateral head rotation. Torticollis has been attributed to approximately 50 underlying pathologies. The following list includes those pathologies most commonly seen in orthopedic settings*:
- Congenital
  - Muscular torticollis
  - Positional deformation
  - Hemivertebra (cervical spine)
  - Unilateral atlantooccipital fusion
  - Klippel-Feil syndrome
  - Unilateral absence of sternocleidomastoid
- Trauma
  - Muscular injury (cervical muscles)
  - Atlantooccipital subluxation
  - Atlantoaxial subluxation
  - C2/3 subluxation
  - Rotary subluxation
  - Chiari malformation
  - Fractures

*Adapted from Spiegel DA, Hosalkar HS, Dormans JP, Drommond DS. The neck. In: Kliegman RM, Behrman RE, Jenson HB, Stanton BF: *Nelson Textbook of Pediatrics, 18th* ed. Philadelphia, PA: Saunders 2007.

- Inflammation
  - Cervical vertebral osteomyelitis
  - RA
  - Upper lobe pneumonia
- Neurological
  - Visual disturbances (nystagmus, superior oblique paresis)
  - Dystonic drug reactions (phenothiazines, haloperidol, or metoclopramide)
  - Cervical cord tumor
  - Posterior fossa brain tumor
  - Syringomyelia
- Other
  - Acute cervical disc calcification
  - Sandifer syndrome (gastroesophageal reflux, hiatal hernia)
  - Benign paroxysmal torticollis
  - Bone tumors (eosinophilic granuloma)
  - Soft tissue tumor
  - Hysteria

EPIDEMIOLOGY AND DEMOGRAPHICS

- The prevalence of torticollis is 8.9 per 100,000 people.
- A slight female predominance has been reported in the literature with an occurrence rate of men to women of 1:1.4.
- Familial basis for torticollis and hereditary muscle aplasia have been reported.

MECHANISM OF INJURY

- The mechanism of injury depends on the nature of the underlying pathology.
- In the case of congenital torticollis, the abnormal head positioning may be due to abnormal fetal positioning in utero. Muscle biopsies and MRI scans suggest that it may be caused by an intramuscular compartment syndrome. An injury while in the uterus may cause a localized inflammatory reaction, the result of which is fibrosis and muscular contraction.
- Like congenital torticollis, other pathology will either result in direct trauma to the sternocleidomastoid or a protective response by the muscle. The mechanism of injury for these pathologies can either be traumatic, repetitive, or have an insidious onset.

COMMON SIGNS AND SYMPTOMS

Patient is usually asymptomatic, but in the case of trauma, the patient's symptoms will take on the characteristics of the underling damaged tissue.

AGGRAVATING ACTIVITIES

- In many cases, the head position is asymptomatic, but in cases of symptom production, activities that require stretching of the affected sternocleidomastoid muscle will be symptomatic.
- Contraction of the sternocleidomastoid muscle, as well as ipsilateral lateral cervical flexion, cervical flexion, and contralateral cervical rotation, may also be symptomatic.

EASING ACTIVITIES

The posture of the torticollis itself is generally the easing position.

24-HOUR SYMPTOM PATTERN

Since the condition is generally asymptomatic, there is no 24-hour symptom pattern. In conditions where the posture is symptomatic, the patient's 24-hour pattern will take on the characteristics of the underlying pathology.

PAST HISTORY FOR THE REGION

- Stretch trauma in the birth canal or in utero
- Stretch trauma to the sternocleidomastoid such as whiplash
- History of congenital birth abnormalities
- History of head trauma

PHYSICAL EXAMINATION

- Since torticollis is a physical manifestation of some underlying disease process, other objective examinations will vary, based on the suspected causal pathology. Most patients will present with the following physical findings:
  - Head positioned in ipsilateral lateral cervical flexion and contralateral head rotation.
  - Decreased ROM into contralateral cervical lateral flexion or ipsilateral cervical rotation.
- In approximately 50% of the infants with congenital torticollis, a mass can be palpated with in the muscle belly of the sternocleidomastoid muscle. The mass disappears during infancy and is replaced by a fibrous band.
- Often, in the case of congenital torticollis, the patient will present with craniofacial asymmetries.
- The cervical region should be examined for signs of inflammation and infection.
- A complete neurological examination should be performed, including strength testing, sensory deficits, reflex testing, cranial nerve assessment, and gait.

IMPORTANT OBJECTIVE TESTS

- Crowner et al listed a series of key tests and measures to be performed while undertaking an examination of patient's with torticollis. They include a thorough postural examination in an attempt to distinguish which muscles have been overactive.
- Plain cervical radiographs, computed tomography (CT) scans, or MRI of the cervical spine should be ordered if fractures or C1/2 subluxation is suspected. MRI may also be used to rule out tumors or other soft tissue lesions.

DIFFERENTIAL DIAGNOSIS

There are approximately 50 potential sources of torticollis and the most common pathologies seen in orthopedics are listed under "Etiology."

CONTRIBUTING FACTORS

Approximately 5% to 8% of patients also have dysplasia of the hip.

TREATMENT

SURGICAL OPTIONS

- Surgery is usually not warranted to correct torticollis. Some of the underlying pathology, such as upper cervical subluxation, may require surgical interventions to correct the unstable segments. For a more detailed listing of surgeries, refer to the individual pathologies.
- BOTOX (botulinum toxin type A) injections may be considered in extreme cases of torticollis.

REHABILITATION

- Nonsurgical management involves identifying the underlying pathology and taking steps to correct the source pathology.
- Once the source pathology has been addressed, the torticollis will resolve.
- In cases of long-term torticollis in which fibrosis of the muscle is involved or congenital torticollis is involved, stretching of the involved sternocleidomastoid muscle is required (sidebend away and rotation toward the involved side).
- The patient or infant should be encouraged to look toward the involved side frequently. In infants, this may require changing the position of the crib so that the infant is forced to look toward the involved side.
- Carrying the child on the involved side (i.e., if torticollis is on the left side,

carry the child on the left side) will result in a stretch as the infant engages the head-righting mechanisms. Adding a stretch where the infant's head is then directed toward the floor will result in stretching of the sternocleidomastoid muscle.

PROGNOSIS

- The prognosis will depend on the underlying pathology.
- Most trauma-induced torticollis will resolve in 6 to 8 weeks.
- Congenital torticollis prognosis will vary, but most will resolve as the child develops.

SIGNS AND SYMPTOMS INDICATING REFERRAL TO PHYSICIAN

Spinal Fractures
- Major trauma (e.g. MVA, fall, or blow to the head) without proper imaging or the necessity for the Canadian C-Spine Rules
  - Severe limitations during neck active ROM in all directions

Cervical Myelopathy
- Sensory disturbances of the hands
  - Muscle wasting of the hand's intrinsic musculature
  - Unsteady gait
  - Positive Hoffmann's reflex
  - Hyperreflexia
  - Bowel and bladder disturbances
  - Multiple disc segmental weakness, sensory changes, or both

Neoplastic Conditions
- Age >50 years of age with a previous history of cancer
  - Unexplained weight loss
  - Constant pain with no relief with bed rest
  - Night pain

Upper Cervical Ligamentous Instability
- Occipital headache and numbness
- Severe limitation during neck active ROM in all directions
- Signs of cervical myelopathy

Vertebral Artery Insufficiency
- Drop attacks
- Dizziness or lightheadedness related to neck movement
- Dysphasia
- Dysarthria
- Diplopia
- Positive cranial nerve signs

Inflammatory or Systemic Disease
- Temperature >100° F
- Blood pressure >165/95 mm Hg
- Resting pulse >100 bpm
- Resting respiration >25 bpm
- Fatigue

SUGGESTED READINGS

Claypool DW, Duane DD, Ilstrup DM, et al. Epidemiology and outcome of cervical dystonia (spasmodic torticollis) in Rochester, Minnesota. *Mov Disord.* 1995;10(5):608–614.

Crowner BE. Cervical dystonia: disease profile and clinical management. *Phys Ther.* 2007;87:1511.

Duane DD. Spasmodic torticollis. *Adv Neurol.* 1988;49:135–150.

Ferreira JJ, Costa J, Coelho M, et al. The management of cervical dystonia. *Expert Opin Pharmacother.* 2007;8(2):129.

Gauthier S. Idiopathic spasmodic torticollis: pathophysiology and treatment. *Can J Neurol Sci.* 1986;13(2):88–90.

Sa DS, Mailis-Gagnon A, Nicholson K, et al. Posttraumatic painful torticollis. *Mov Disord.* 2003;18(12):1482–1491.

Singer C, Velickovic M. Cervical dystonia: etiology and pathophysiology. *Neurol Clin.* 2008;26:9–22.

Tonomura Y, Kataoka H, Sugie K, et al. Atlantoaxial rotatory subluxation associated with cervical dystonia. *Spine.* 2007;32(19):E561–E564.

van Herwaarden GM, Anten HW, Hoogduin CA, et al. Idiopathic spasmodic torticollis: a survey of the clinical syndromes and patients' experiences. *Clin Neurol Neurosurg.* 1994;96(3):222–225.

Velickovic M, Benabou R, Brin M. Cervical dystonia pathophysiology and treatment options. *Drugs.* 2001;61(13):1921–1943.

AUTHORS: MICHAEL LEAL and DERRICK SUEKI

Section III

ORTHOPEDIC PATHOLOGY

BASIC INFORMATION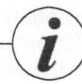

DEFINITION

Damage to the vertebral artery of the neck results in the loss of the arteries ability to supply blood to the brain and brainstem. Because the primary distribution of the basilar artery is the posterior aspect of the brain, loss of blood supply will affect the pons, medulla, thalamus, cerebellum, midbrain, and occipital region of the cortex.

SYNONYMS

- Vertebrobasilar ischemia
- Vertebral artery insufficiency
- Vertebrobasilar circulatory disorders

ICD-9CM CODES
433.2 Occlusion and stenosis of vertebral artery
435.1 Vertebral artery syndrome
435.3 Vertebrobasilar artery syndrome
443.24 Dissection of vertebral artery

OPTIMAL NUMBER OF VISITS

Patients are generally not treated for vertebrobasilar insufficiency (VBI).

MAXIMAL NUMBER OF VISITS

Patients are generally not treated for VBI.

ETIOLOGY

- The vertebral artery is a branch of the subclavian artery; the basilar artery and vertebral artery form the vertebrobasilar system. The vertebrobasilar system directly supplies the posterior aspect of the circle of Willis, while the carotid arteries supply blood to the anterior aspect of the circle of Willis. The left vertebral artery is usually larger and carries more blood.
- Anatomically, one vertebral artery is located on each side of the body. These arteries arise from the subclavian artery and then travel cortically to the C6 vertebrae where they enter the transverse foramen and travel the remainder of the cervical region in the transverse foramen of C2-C6. At the C2 level, the vertebral arteries travel posterior to the arch of the atlas before entering the foramen magnum. Inside the skull, the two vertebral arteries join to form the basilar artery at the base of the medulla oblongata. The basilar artery is the main blood supply to the brainstem. It then forms the circle of Willis with the carotid arteries. At each cervical level, the vertebral artery sends branches to the surrounding musculature via anterior spinal arteries.

- The vertebral artery can be divided by anatomical location into the following four parts:
  - Part 1 is located between the longus colli and the scalenus anterior.
  - Part 2 is the section that runs upward through the foramina in the transverse processes of the upper six cervical vertebrae.
  - Part 3 starts from the C2 transverse foramen, behind the superior articular process of the atlas, and then lies in the groove on the upper surface of the posterior arch of the atlas.
  - Part 4 pierces the dura mater of the foramen magnum and inclines up in front of the medulla oblongata. At the lower border of the pons, it unites with the vessel of the opposite side to form the basilar artery.
- Circulation through the vertebral or basilar arteries can be disrupted by several different conditions. The most common are atherosclerosis and artery dissection. In the case of atherosclerosis, fat deposits accumulate along the inner walls of the vertebral or basilar artery. These fat deposits trigger an inflammatory response in the area of the fat deposit, resulting in plaques that can either decrease the size of the lumen or clot to further decrease the size of the lumen. In either case, blood flow is impaired. A dissection is a tearing of the vertebral or basilar artery wall. The result of the tear is bleeding and formation of clots that can block the flow of blood cortically. Whereas atherosclerosis is generally the result of an ongoing physiological process, dissections may be caused by diseases or trauma to the neck. Other less common causes of vertebrobasilar vascular disorders include connective tissue diseases and vasculitis.
- There are three areas in which the vertebral artery is vulnerable to external compression, as follows:
  - At the level of the vertebral foramen of C6 by a contraction of the longus colli and the anterior scalene muscles
  - Within the transverse foramen between C2 and C6
  - At the level of C1/2
- Head and neck positions have been proposed to alter vertebral artery vascular flow. It has been speculated that end-range rotational activities could alter this vascular flow. The current research regarding cervical motion and circulation to the brain is mixed. Cadaveric studies have implicated rotation as the single movement most likely to alter blood flow. With rotation, the contralateral artery was compromised more often; however, when extension was coupled with rotation, the ipsilateral vertebral artery was involved as fre-

quently as the contralateral vessel. In 1998, Licht et al (2002) conducted several studies in which they found that there was no significant decrease in contralateral blood flow volume despite decreases in blood flow velocity. In 1999, Yi-Kai found vertebral artery flow to decrease with extension and rotation in both contralateral and ipsilateral vertebral arteries, with the most significant decrease in the contralateral artery.
- After an extensive review of studies on vertebral artery blood flow, Terrett reached the following conclusions: Rotation with and without extension applies the greatest stress to the vertebral arteries, and the greatest stress to the vertebral artery is between the atlas and axis transverse foramina. They determined that lateral flexion to the neck has little effect on vertebral artery blood flow.
- The Joint Study of Extracranial Arterial Occlusion as a Cause of Stroke reported that the frequency of atherosclerotic plaques was highest at the carotid bifurcation and the vertebral artery origin in a ratio of 2:1. The most common sites for atherosclerosis in the vertebrobasilar tree are at the origin of the vertebral artery and within the intradural segment.

EPIDEMIOLOGY AND DEMOGRAPHICS

- In the United States, 25% of the strokes are in a vertebrobasilar distribution.
- The incidence of VBI increases with age; the highest incidence is between 60 and 70 years of age.
- Men are more prone to VBI than women.
- African Americans have a greater prevalence than Caucasians.
- Risk factors include hypertension, diabetes, and smoking.

MECHANISM OF INJURY

- Occlusion of the vertebral or basilar arteries can potentially occur as a result of cervical rotation or rotation coupled with extension. Therefore activities, such as painting, yoga, backing out a car, and getting the hair washed, can all lead to symptoms of VBI.
- Dissections can be the result of MVAs, whiplash, and cervical manipulations.

COMMON SIGNS AND SYMPTOMS

- Primary signs of VBI include dizziness and gait disturbances. The joint and soft tissue structures in the cervical spine are abundantly supplied with proprioceptors. Altered afferent input from these proprioceptors and along their pathway to the higher centers caused by pathology can give rise to the symptoms of dizziness and cervical vertigo. Maigne has postulated that symptoms similar to VBI can be the products of stimulation of the vertebral nerve and the accompanying sympathetic plexus. This in turn can lead to spasm of the vertebrobasilar arteries and a cascade of symptoms, including vertigo, nausea, and headaches.

- Husni listed the frequency of symptoms in people who were known to have VBI, as follows:
  - Dizziness: 100%
  - Vertigo: 40%
  - Headache: 30%
  - Loss of consciousness: 25%
  - Visual disturbances: 15%
  - Gait disturbances: 15%
  - Upper extremity paresthesias: 10%
  - Nausea: 10%
- Occlusions at the vertebral artery origin tend to be asymptomatic, whereas intracranial vertebral artery lesions are more likely to be symptomatic (often in the form of a brain infarct).
- Secondary symptoms include the following:
  - Slurred speech
  - Nystagmus
  - Gait disturbances
  - Diplopia
  - Drop attacks
  - Dysarthria
  - Dysphasia
  - Tinnitus
  - Nausea
  - Occipital headaches
  - Facial paresthesia
  - Tingling in the upper limbs
  - Pallor
  - Blurred vision
  - Lightheadedness
  - Fainting and blackouts

AGGRAVATING ACTIVITIES

- Activities involving end-range rotation and/or extension
- Getting up too quickly from lying down
- Exercising the lower extremities vigorously

EASING ACTIVITIES

- Rest
- Avoiding aggravating positions

24-HOUR SYMPTOM PATTERN

Symptoms may occur several times throughout the course of the day but do not appear to be directly impacted by time of day. They are influenced to a greater extent by posture and head position.

PAST HISTORY FOR THE REGION

The patient may have a history of head trauma, whiplash, MVAs, or other trauma to the region.

PHYSICAL EXAMINATION

The diagnosis of VBI is a diagnosis of exclusion. To make a diagnosis, the clinician rules out other possible pathologies. In older patients, a cardiovascular risk-factor evaluation is important. This often includes a cholesterol level, lipid profile, electrocardiogram (ECG), and echocardiogram. Younger patients should have a work-up that includes hypercoagulable states such as lupus anticoagulant, anticardiolipin antibodies, protein C, protein S, and antithrombin III deficiencies.

IMPORTANT OBJECTIVE TESTS

- MRI or CT scans may be ordered by the physician to rule out other pathologies such as brain tumor.
- Angiogram or magnetic resonance angiography (MRA) can rule out blockage in the vertebral or basilar arteries.
- Doppler ultrasonography is not sensitive to VBI because of surrounding bone and because the most frequent site for occlusive disease is at the vessel origin, which is too deep for accurate imaging.
- Clinical vertebral artery testing is used to predict artery blood flow and is currently under question. Previously, the testing had been used frequently to diagnose the presence of vertebral occlusion. Recent studies have questioned the validity of the test, but it is still used as a first-line assessment and indicator of whether manipulation or end-range rotational mobilization techniques should be performed.
- Vertebral artery testing is performed with the patient sitting or supine and then sequentially taken into the following positions for 10 seconds while the patient is assessed for nystagmus or other VBI symptoms. Rotation to the right is thought to occlude the left vertebral artery. Symptom production would therefore suggest that the ipsilateral or right vertebral artery and the carotid arteries may not be providing adequate blood flow. The positions are as follows:
  - Cervical rotation to the right
  - Cervical rotation to the left
  - Cervical extension
  - Cervical extension and rotation to the right
  - Cervical extension and rotation to the left
  - Premanipulation position

DIFFERENTIAL DIAGNOSIS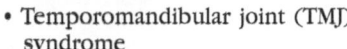

- Temporomandibular joint (TMJ) syndrome
- Bell's palsy

- MS
- Stroke
- Glossopharyngeal neuralgia
- Concussion
- Cervical strain or sprain
- Upper cervical instability
- Brain tumor
- Encephalitis
- Meningitis
- Cerebral aneurysms
- High blood pressure
- Medications
- Cervical spondylosis
- Cervical stenosis (central or foraminal stenosis)

CONTRIBUTING FACTORS

- Age
- Smoking
- Gender
- Diet
- Posture
- Daily activities
- Diabetes
- High blood pressure or very low blood pressure
- High cholesterol
- Heart irregularities or heart disease
- Circulation problems

TREATMENT

SURGICAL OPTIONS

- Surgical options are generally not warranted as a first-line treatment, but if conservative care fails, surgery can be performed to improve the artery's ability to transport blood. Surgical options include the following:
  - Intracranial angioplasty
  - Bypass grafting
  - Direct arterial anastomosis or transposition
  - Endarterectomy to remove plaque from the affected artery

SURGICAL OUTCOMES

Because of the small size of the vertebral artery, its convoluted route, and the challenges of surgical access to this region, combined morbidity and mortality rates are high.

MEDICAL OPTIONS

- Medically, the following treatments are common for VBI:
  - Initial treatment usually involves medications, such as antiplatelet agents (aspirin, clopidogrel, or aspirin/dipyridamole) or sometimes an anticoagulant (warfarin), once hemorrhage has been excluded by imaging. Research suggests that use of anticoagulant medication provides superior stroke reduction when compared to the use of aspirin in patients with intracranial lesions.

REHABILITATION

- If a patient is suspected of having VBI, the clinician should make sure that the patient's primary physician is aware of the problem. If the patient's physician is not aware of the issue, the patient should be referred back to the physician for assessment and testing.
- A patient is generally not sent to rehabilitation for VBI, but for the symptoms the patient is experiencing. Older patients will commonly complaint of leg weakness, loss of balance, and dizziness. Younger patients will complain of neck pain, headaches, and dizziness after trauma such as a car accident or fall.
- Rehabilitation usually involves lifestyle modifications. For example, if VBI is attributed mainly to postural changes, patients are advised to slowly rise to standing position after sitting for a long period of time. An appropriate exercise regimen for each patient can also be designed avoid excessive pooling of blood in the legs. Dehydrated patients are often advised to increase their water intake, especially in hot, dry climates. Finally, patients are often advised to stop smoking and to control their hypertension, diabetes, and cholesterol level.
- In the event that a patient suffers a "drop attack," patients should be advised to sit down at the first sign of dizziness rather than falling down if the symptoms are allowed to progress.
- Rehabilitation should also focus on lowering or eliminating risk factors, such as high blood pressure, high cholesterol, and smoking, and promoting a healthy diet and exercise.
- Manipulation and end-range rotational mobilization techniques should be avoided in this patient population.

PROGNOSIS

Symptoms and recurrence of symptoms will generally relapse and then remit. It is generally a recurrent problem.

SIGNS AND SYMPTOMS INDICATING REFERRAL TO PHYSICIAN

- Fainting
- Headaches that increase in intensity or frequency
- Loss of limb function
- Sensory disturbances of the hands
- Muscle wasting of the hand's intrinsic musculature
- Unsteady gait
- Bowel and bladder disturbances
- Severe limitation during neck active ROM in all directions
- Dysphasia
- Dysarthria
- Diplopia
- Temperature >100° F
- Blood pressure >165/95 mm Hg
- Resting pulse >100 bpm
- Resting respiration >25 bpm

SUGGESTED READINGS

Childs JD, Flynn TW, Fritz JM, et al. Screening for vertebrobasilar insufficiency in patients with neck pain: manual therapy decision-making in the presence of uncertainty. *J Orthop Sports Phys Ther.* 2005;35(5):300-306.

Davis JM, Zimmerman RA. Injury of the carotid and vertebral arteries. *Neuroradiology.* 1983;25:55-69.

Fields WS, North RR, Hass WK, et al. Joint study of extracranial arterial occlusion as a cause of stroke. I. Organization of study and survey of patient population. *JAMA.* 1968;203(11):955-960.

Husni EA, Storer J. The syndrome of mechanical occlusion of the vertebral artery; further observations. *Angiology.* 1967;18:106-116.

Kuether TA, Nesbit GM, Clark WM, Barnwell SL. Rotational vertebral artery occlusion: a mechanism of vertebrobasilar insufficiency. *Neurosurgery.* 1997;41:427-434.

Licht PB, Christensen HW, Høilund-Carlsen PF. Carotid artery blood flow during premanipulative testing. *J Manipulative Physiol Ther.* 2002;25(9):568-572.

Licht PB, Christensen HW, Høilund-Carlsen PF. Is there a role for premanipulative testing before cervical manipulation? *J Manipulative Physiol Ther.* 2000;23:175-179.

Mitchell JA. Changes in vertebral artery blood flow following normal rotation of the cervical spine. *J Manipulative Physiol Ther.* 2003;26:347-351.

Savitz SI, Caplan LR. Vertebrobasilar disease. *N Engl J Med.* 2005;352(25):2618-2622.

Terrett A. Missue of the literature by medical authors in discussing spinal manipulative therapy injury. *J Manipulative Physiol Ther.* 1995;18:203-210.

Yi-Kai L, Yun-Kun Z, Cai-Mo L, Shi-Zhen Z. Changes and implications of blood flow of the vertebral artery during rotation an extension of the head. *J Manipulative Physiol Ther.* 1999;22(2):91-95.

AUTHOR: DERRICK SUEKI

BASIC INFORMATION

DEFINITION

Whiplash technically cannot be considered a pathology but a mechanism of injury. It describes the process by which the head is forcefully displaced in one or multiple directions resulting in tissue damage. The group of pathologies that results from whiplash is often called *whiplash-associated disorders*.

SYNONYMS

- Whiplash-associated disorders
- Acceleration flexion-extension neck injury
- Soft tissue cervical hyperextension injury
- Cervical sprain
- Cervical strain
- Hyperextension injury

ICD-9CM CODE
847.0 Neck sprain

OPTIMAL NUMBER OF VISITS
6 visits

MAXIMAL NUMBER OF VISITS
24 visits

ETIOLOGY

- Whiplash injury continues to be a prominent medical issue in countries where automobile travel is prevalent. The use of seatbelts has decreased the number of fatalities, but with the increased usage of seatbelts has come an increase in more severe forms of whiplash injuries.
- The amount of available research on whiplash injury is overwhelming; some of the more significant findings regarding the etiology of whiplash injuries is included here.
- Many patients have pain and other symptoms long after normal healing time frames. Additionally, patients will experience severe pain and limitations after seemingly minor collisions. These factors have made the medical establishment question whether tissue damage actually occurs in MVAs or whether the majority of symptoms are psychological.
- Current research suggests that in most whiplash injuries, there is an objective pathological basis for the pain associated with whiplash. With the forced extension commonly experienced with whiplash, the cervical region is vulnerable to anterior muscle strains, anterior disc tears, and posterior compressive injuries to the synovial folds and articular surfaces of facet joints. It has also been suggested that hypersensitivity

in the central and peripheral nervous systems is responsible for some of the symptoms experienced with chronic pain after whiplash.
- Although tissue damage does occur after a whiplash injury, the exact biomechanics of whiplash have not been concretely established. This is due in part to the numerous factors involved in any whiplash injury. Directions of injury, forces involved, prior physical history, and type of restraint all play roles in the type and extent of tissue injury. With this in mind, several theories have been proposed to account for the tissue damage. Macnab suggested that hyperextension of the cervical spine causes the injuries. Based on the hyperextension theory as the injury mechanism in whiplash, the head restraint was designed to prevent neck injuries in rear-end collisions by blocking the hyperextension of the neck. With the introduction of head restraints, whiplash injuries decreased in number, but the restraint did not eliminate the injuries. In Sweden, the introduction of head restraints only decreased whiplash injuries by 20%. This suggests that other mechanisms besides pure hyperextension of the cervical spine are also responsible for the injuries. Panjabi suggested that the mechanism of injury is to the result of a biphasic response in the cervical spine. At initial rear impact, the cervical spine forms an "S" curve in which the lower cervical spine is forced into hyperextension and the upper cervical region is forced into extreme hyperflexion. The initial phase is followed by a phase in which the upper cervical and lower cervical regions extend. This extension never reaches end-ranges of motion. After the next extension, the cervical region will experience a period of maximal head flexion. Based on these findings, it has been suggested that tissue damage is due to the hyperextension of the lower cervical spine or hyperflexion of the upper cervical spine during initial impact.
- Kaneoka et al found that during a rear impact MVA, C6 starts to extend before the rest of the spine. This results in the S-shaped configuration of the spine described by Panjabi. As C6 extends, the rest of the spine initially flexes. After this initial response, the cervical spine extends, this results in an extreme rotational torque at the C5/6 level. At this point, there is a tensile force along the anterior longitudinal ligament and impaction of the C5/6 spinal segment as it is forced into a compacted position. It has been hypothesized that this may result in impingement and inflammation of the folds of synovial tissue between the zygapophyseal joints.

- Types of tissue damage seen with whiplash injuries are as follows:
  - Ligaments: Animal studies point to a strain on the capsular ligament around the facet joint. With rear impact injuries, most of the strain occurred in the *superior* and *anterior* portions of the capsule. The capsule most affected was ipsilaterally on the same side of the neck toward which the face was turned. The strain on the capsule with the head turned was twice what it was with the head facing forward at the point of impact.
  - Muscles: With an unexpected low-velocity frontal impact while the head was turned 45 degrees, it was found that the contralateral trapezius (right anterolateral impact and left trapezius) fired most vigorously (80% maximal voluntary contraction), while the splenius capitis and sternocleidomastoid muscles were not required to fire as much (50% maximal voluntary contraction). Subjects exhibited lower levels of their maximal voluntary contraction when the impact was expected and muscle responses were greater with higher levels of acceleration. Expecting or being aware of imminent impact plays a role in reducing muscle responses in low-velocity anterolateral impacts and with front off-center impacts, the contralateral muscle is at greatest risk of injury.
  - Muscles: Studies addressing the timing of muscle activation during a rear impact MVA discovered that none of the muscles of the neck became activated until about 100 milliseconds (msec). This was about 25 msec after the point at which the majority of the ligament injuries occurred. The anterior cervical muscles reach their maximum stretch at around 150 msec but are not fully recruited until later. The forces experienced by the anterior muscles were not as severe as the posterior muscles. The posterior cervical musculature became active at about 100 msec, so that they became fully contracted just when they reach their maximum stretch at 250 to 300 msec. The stresses and potential damage were higher in the posterior muscles than the anterior. The authors hypothesized that this would result in more potential muscle damage to the posterior muscles then the anterior.
  - Facets: Cervical zygapophyseal joint pain is common among patients with chronic neck pain after whiplash. In patients with pain after whiplash, research revealed that the prevalence of C2/3 zygapophyseal joint pain was 50%. Among those without C2/3 zygapophyseal joint pain, placebo-controlled blocks revealed that the

prevalence of lower cervical zygapophyseal joint pain was 49%. Overall, the prevalence of cervical zygapophyseal joint pain (C2/3 or below) was 60%.

EPIDEMIOLOGY AND DEMOGRAPHICS

- Around 20% of rear-end MVAs result in a whiplash injury.
- The incidence of neck injury to front-seat passengers is higher (16%) than for rear-seat passengers (10%) in rear-end collisions.
- Front-seat passengers have a higher prevalence for neck sprains (19%) than drivers (15%).

MECHANISM OF INJURY

- Motor vehicle accidents
  - Rear-end crashes are more likely to cause whiplash-associated pain than frontal impacts, although compression extension sprain can result from a blow to the front or the crown of the head.
  - Rear-end or side-impact MVAs are the number one cause of whiplash with injury.
- Falls
- Head trauma
- Child abuse
- Quick, sudden motions of the neck

COMMON SIGNS AND SYMPTOMS

- The following is a list of the ten most-reported symptoms, with their estimated prevalence:
  - Neck pain (97%)
  - Headache (97%)
  - Shoulder pain (65%)
  - Anxiety (55%)
  - Back pain (42%)
  - Depression (41%)
  - Visual symptoms (35%)
  - Thoracic outlet syndrome (33%)
  - Dizziness (23%)
- Symptoms can begin immediately after the injury, but most commonly patients will begin to experience pain several days after the injury. Common complaints include the following:
  - Headaches
  - Neck pain
  - Arm paresthesias
  - Nausea
  - Difficulty breathing
  - Difficulty swallowing
  - Inability to concentrate
  - Vision problems
  - Balance disorders
  - Tinnitus
  - Pallor
  - Blurred vision
  - Lightheadedness
  - Fainting and blackouts
  - Fatigue

AGGRAVATING ACTIVITIES

- Head motions
- Head will feel heavy and symptoms will increases as the day progresses
- Getting up too quickly from lying down

EASING ACTIVITIES

- Rest
- Avoiding aggravating positions
- Antiinflammatory medications
- Ice or heat
- Muscle relaxants
- Cervical soft collar

24-HOUR SYMPTOM PATTERN

- Patient will awaken in the morning with stiffness, which may take time to resolve.
- Symptoms will dissipate throughout the morning but will increase as the afternoon and evening approaches. Increases will be based on usage.
- At night the patient may have difficulty sleeping and once asleep may awaken because of increases in symptoms.

PAST HISTORY FOR THE REGION

May have history of head trauma, whiplash, MVAs, or other trauma to the region.

PHYSICAL EXAMINATION

- The clinician should first test the integrity of the upper cervical ligaments to rule out the presence of upper cervical ligament or odontoid injury.
- Generally, ROM is limited initially in all directions.
- Cranial nerve testing can help determine whether the brainstem was involved during the collision.
- Upper extremity neurological examinations are warranted if the patient is experiencing arm or hand symptoms.
- The clavicle, sternum, and thoracic spine should be examined; with impact, often the seatbelt shoulder strap will cause trauma to these structures.
- Clearing the lumbar spine is also an important aspect of the examination because both neck and low back pain often exist.
- Palpation will reveal guarding and tenderness in the trapezius posteriorly and the scalenes and sternocleidomastoid anteriorly.
- Tenderness will often be present in the upper cervical musculature because of the initial hyperflexion of the spine during impact.
- C5/6 and C2/3 will often be tender and guarded after a MVA because of the biphasic nature of whiplash during rear-end collisions.

IMPORTANT OBJECTIVE TESTS

- The first images generally ordered by the physician are plain radiographs. The patient should receive an open mouth x-ray to check the integrity of the odontoid process.
- MRI or CT scans may be ordered by the physician to rule out other pathologies such as soft tissue injuries or brain damage.
- Anterior widening of the atlantodens interval of more than 5 mm on the flexion view suggests that the transverse ligament is incompetent.
- Transverse ligament testing: Sensitivity: 0.69; specificity 0.96 for RA. No testing has been conducted validating its use on traumatic patients.
- Alar ligament testing: Reliability has not been established in literature.
- Angiogram or MRA is used to rule out blockage in the vertebral or basilar arteries.
- Clinical vertebral artery testing is used to predict artery blood flow and is currently under question. Previously, the testing had been used frequently to diagnose the presence of vertebral occlusion. Recent studies have questioned the validity of the test, but it is still used frequently as a first-line assessment and indicator of whether manipulation or end-range rotational mobilization techniques should be performed.
- Vertebral artery testing is performed with the patient sitting or supine and then sequentially taken into the following positions for 10 seconds while the patient is assessed for nystagmus or other VBI symptoms. Rotation to the right is thought to occlude the left vertebral artery. Symptom production would therefore suggest that the ipsilateral or right vertebral artery and the carotid arteries may not be providing adequate blood flow. The positions are as follows:
  - Cervical rotation to the right
  - Cervical rotation to the left
  - Cervical extension
  - Cervical extension and rotation to the right
  - Cervical extension and rotation to the left
  - Premanipulation position

DIFFERENTIAL DIAGNOSIS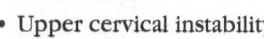

- Upper cervical instability
- Alar or transverse ligament damage
- Odontoid fractures
- Vertebral and basilar artery injury
- Concussion

CONTRIBUTING FACTORS

- Age
- Prior injury
- Force at impact
- Direction of impact
- Head position at impact

- Type of vehicle
- Seatbelt or airbag deployment
- Driver or passenger

TREATMENT

SURGICAL OPTIONS

Surgical options are generally not warranted as a first-line treatment, but if conservative care fails, surgery can be performed to address the underlying pathology. (See the underlying pathologies for specifics of surgical options and outcomes.)

MEDICAL OPTIONS

- Medically, the following treatments are common for whiplash associated disorders:
  - Antiinflammatories and muscle relaxants are prescribed initially.
  - Soft collars may be issued to unload the damaged tissue and to allow healing of the region without excessive motion.

REHABILITATION

- Initially, regardless of the tissue damaged, most whiplash injuries are treated similarly. The clinician should first assess for red flag pathology. Patient should be screened for upper cervical instability and VBI. If these tests are positive, the patient should be referred back to the physician for follow-up and additional testing to rule out these pathologies. See odontoid fracture, alar and transverse ligament damage, and VBI.
- If these tests prove negative, regardless of the tissue damage, the goal of the clinician is to decrease inflammation

and promote healing. Use of a soft collar for 1 to 2 weeks is often advisable. Cold packs and relative rest should be encouraged. Avoidance of strenuous activities should also be advised.
- As the inflammation and symptoms decrease, active rest can be initiated in which the patient is encouraged to return to most normal daily activities but with caution. Patients should rest if symptoms start to increase, but use and normal activity should be encouraged.
- After the inflammatory phase, the first 2 to 3 weeks, management of the patient will entail assessing and treating the specific tissue or tissues that were injured. The clinician is directed to the specific underlying tissue pathology or injury for further discussion and information regarding specific tissue pathology.

PROGNOSIS

About 20% of patients will develop some degree of chronic pain or stiffness, with about 5% having severe pain symptoms 3 to 6 months after the injury.

SIGNS AND SYMPTOMS INDICATING REFERRAL TO PHYSICIAN

- Fainting
- Headaches that increase in intensity or frequency
- Loss of limb function
- Sensory disturbances of the hands
- Muscle wasting of the hand's intrinsic musculature
- Unsteady gait
- Bowel and bladder disturbances
- Severe limitation during neck active ROM in all directions
- Dysphasia
- Dysarthria
- Diplopia
- Temperature >100° F
- Blood pressure >165/95 mm Hg
- Resting pulse >100 bpm
- Resting respiration >25 bpm

SUGGESTED READINGS

Kaneoka K, Ono K, Inami S, Hayashi K. Motion analysis of cervical vertebrae during whiplash loading. *Spine.* 1999;24(8):763-769.

Kumar S, Ferrari R, Narayan Y. Cervical muscle response to whiplash-type right anterolateral impacts. *Eur Spine J.* 2004;13(5):398-407.

Lord SM, Barnsley L, Wallis BJ, Bogduk N. Chronic cervical zygapophysial joint pain after whiplash: a placebo-controlled prevalence study. *Spine.* 1996;21(15):1737-1744.

Macnab I. The "whiplash syndrome". *Orthop Clin North Am.* 1971;2(2):389-403.

Panjabi MM. *New Findings About the Mechanism of Whiplash Injury.* Presented at the Twenty-First Annual Meeting of the American Society of Biomechanics, Clemson University, South Carolina. September 24-27, 1997.

Scholten-Peeters GG, Bekkering GE, Verhagen AP, et al. Clinical practice guidelines for the physiotherapy of patients with whiplash-associated disorders. *Spine.* 2002;27(4):412-422.

Siegmund GP, et al. Head-turned postures increase the risk of cervical facet capsule injury during whiplash. *Spine.* 2008;33(15):1643-1649.

Taylor J, Twomey L. Whiplash injury and neck sprain: a review of their prevalence, mechanisms, risk factors, and pathology. *Critica Reviews in Physical and Rehabilitation Medicine.* 2005;17(4):285-300.

Vasavada AN, Brault JR, Siegmund GP. Musculotendon and fascicle strains in anterior and posterior neck muscles during whiplash injury. *Spine.* 2007;32(7):756-765.

AUTHOR: DERRICK SUEKI

Section III

ORTHOPEDIC PATHOLOGY

BASIC INFORMATION

DEFINITION

Currently, there is no clear definition for costochondritis. It is considered a benign cause of chest pain resulting from an inflammatory process of the costochondral or costosternal joints. The diagnosis is made through exclusion rather than any specific testing methodology.

SYNONYMS

- Fibrositis
- Tietze's syndrome
- Idiopathic costochondritis

ICD-9CM CODE
733.6 Tietze's disease (costochondritis)

OPTIMAL NUMBER OF VISITS

6 to 20 visits

MAXIMAL NUMBER OF VISITS

20 visits

ETIOLOGY

It has been hypothesized that costochondritis is an inflammatory process involving the costosternal and costochondral joints. The pathology occurs from an acute or chronic inflammation response of the costosternal and costochondral joints. Any of the 7 costochondral junctions can be affected, although junctions 2-5 are generally the most frequently involved.

EPIDEMIOLOGY AND DEMOGRAPHICS

- Exact prevalence is unknown at this time.
- Chest pain of musculoskeletal origin occurs in 10% patients.
- In a study of an emergency room department, 30% of the patients seen for chest pain were diagnosed with costochondritis.
- Age prevalence is unknown.
- Disla et al reported that 69% of women were diagnosed with costochondritis versus 31% in the control group.

MECHANISM OF INJURY

- Often insidious
- Repetitive minor trauma

- Unaccustomed activity
- Bacterial or fungal infection in intravenous (IV) drug users
- Postthoracic surgery

COMMON SIGNS AND SYMPTOMS

- Localized chest pain/tenderness (costosternal and costochondral joints).
- Can be sharp, nagging, aching, or pressure-like.
- Can be severe in presentation.
- Can radiate extensively.

AGGRAVATING ACTIVITIES

- Symptoms can be exacerbated by the following:
  ○ Trunk movement
  ○ Deep inspiration and/or exertion

EASING ACTIVITIES

- Decreased movement
- Quiet breathing
- Change of position

24-HOUR SYMPTOM PATTERN

Typically a mechanical condition; activity affects symptomology.

PAST HISTORY FOR THE REGION

- Often insidious
- Repetitive minor trauma
- Unaccustomed activity
- Bacterial or fungal infection (in IV drug users)
- Postthoracic surgery

PHYSICAL EXAMINATION

Pain with palpation of costochondral joints (typically more common at the 2-5 costochondral junctions).

IMPORTANT OBJECTIVE TESTS

- Tenderness over the costochondral joints
- Tenderness associated with swelling, heat, and erythema may be a result of Tietze's syndrome

DIFFERENTIAL DIAGNOSIS

- Chest pain
- Angina
- Myocardial infarct
- Blunt abdominal trauma
- Acromioclavicular injury
- Sternoclavicular joint injury
- Anxiety
- Gout/pseudogout
- Herpes zoster

- Neoplasms (lung)
- Pericarditis
- Pleurodynia
- Polychondritis
- Fibromyalgia

TREATMENT

SURGICAL OPTIONS

Surgery is usually not warranted.

REHABILITATION

- Spinal manipulation (directed at posterior spinal and rib articulations)
- Posterior to anterior mobilization and manipulation
- Sustained natural apophyseal glide (SNAG) mobilizations (directed at rib angle)
- Motor control exercises for the scapular region

PROGNOSIS

- After 1 year, about half of patients may still have discomfort.
- One-third may still report tenderness with palpation.

SIGNS AND SYMPTOMS INDICATING REFERRAL TO PHYSICIAN

Any hypotheses in the differential diagnosis section, especially those of a severe nature.

SUGGESTED READINGS

Aspegren D, Hyde T, Miller M. Conservative treatment of a female collegiate volleyball player with costochondritis. *J Manipulative Physiol Ther.* 2007;30(4):321-325.

Disla E, Rhim HR, Reddy A, Karten I, Taranta A. Costochondritis. A prospective analysis in an emergency department setting. *Arch Intern Med.* 1994;154(21):2466-2469.

Mendelson G, Mendelson H, Horowitz SF, et al. Can (99m)-technetium methylene diphosphonate bone scan objectively document costochondritis? *Chest.* 1997;111(6):1600-1602.

Rabey I. Costochondritis: are the symptoms and signs due to neurogenic inflammation. Two cases that responded to manual therapy directed towards posterior spinal structures. *Man Ther.* 2008;13(1):82-86.

Wadhwa SS, Phan T, Terei O. Anterior chest wall pain in postpartum costochondritis. *Clin Nucl Med.* 1999;24(6):404-406.

AUTHOR: BRYAN DENNISON

BASIC INFORMATION

DEFINITION

Joint impairments of the first rib can be minor, such as lack of mobility, or can be a gross fracture of the rib itself. Often, these impairments will result in upper quadrant symptoms that can be local or radicular.

SYNONYMS

- Elevated first rib
- Hypomobile first rib
- Broken first rib

ICD-9CM CODES
739.2 Nonallopathic lesions – thoracic spine
848.9 Unspecified site of sprains and strains

OPTIMAL NUMBER OF VISITS

6 to 30 visits

MAXIMAL NUMBER OF VISITS

30 visits

ETIOLOGY

- Actual fractures to the first rib are rare. This may be a result of its limited size in comparison to other ribs and its protected position behind the clavicle. Despite its rarity, fractures of the first rib can cause subsequent trauma to the arteries, veins, and nerves of the upper extremity. Clinically, this would manifest itself as thoracic outlet syndrome or brachial plexus injury.
- Lindgren et al (1992) postulated that the first rib is "susceptible to subluxation because it lacks a superior supporting ligament."
- The subluxation of the first rib produces mechanical stress on adjacent local structures that produces symptoms. Specifically, Lindgren et al (1992) stated that "if the first rib is subluxed, the rib is situated somewhat cranially at the costotransverse joint. At this site, irritation of the nerve C8 and T1 and of the stellate ganglion situated nearby could explain the ulnar distribution of the radicular pain and symptoms resembling reflex sympathetic dystrophy (RSD) found in some patients."

EPIDEMIOLOGY AND DEMOGRAPHICS

- Exact numbers for first rib fracture were not found in literature, but clinically it rarely appears.
- First rib movement or mobility impairments may be more common, but once again, the actual prevalence is not known. Given the fact that females

are more prone to arterial and neural thoracic outlet syndrome, there is a potential that first rib dysfunction has a greater prevalence in females than males, but this is purely speculation.

MECHANISM OF INJURY

- First rib fracture may be from direct blows to the rib.
- Postulated "subluxation" of the first rib may be caused by the pull of the scalenes or may result from automobile accidents that may cause either compressive or tensile forces on the first rib.

COMMON SIGNS AND SYMPTOMS

- Neurological or vascular symptoms in the upper quarter region.
- Symptoms can be exacerbated with breathing.
- Radiating symptoms into the upper extremity, including numbness, tingling, decreased circulation resulting in skin pallor changes, and skin temperature changes.
- High stress environment can result increased forces on the first rib.
- Referral pattern for the pathology may include radiating symptoms into the upper extremity: unilateral or bilateral.

AGGRAVATING ACTIVITIES

- Abducting the arms
- Positioning the arms overhead
- Slouched posture
- Cervical motions away from the affected extremity

EASING ACTIVITIES

Avoiding arm abduction activities

24-HOUR SYMPTOM PATTERN

Symptoms are more mechanical in presentation and do not follow a 24-hour presentation.

PAST HISTORY FOR THE REGION

- Past history is unremarkable, although a history of motor vehicle accident (MVA) or trauma may predispose a patient to altered mechanics in region.
- Altered respiratory patterns and the inability to expand chest or engage the diaphragm may force the accessory muscles of respiration to overwork. Accessory muscles attach to the first rib and may be a source of altered first rib mechanics.

PHYSICAL EXAMINATION

- Subluxation of the first rib restricts cervical rotation and lateral flexion.
- Limited or "blocked" contralateral cervical spine flexion (the ear toward the chest [see Important Objective Tests]).

IMPORTANT OBJECTIVE TESTS

- Radiographs may be warranted to rule out fracture in cases of trauma.
- Cervical rotation lateral flexion (CRLF) test is used to assess first rib hypomobility.
  - Diagnostic accuracy (reliability): kappa = 1.0 (Flynn and Egan, 2006; Lindgren et al, 1992)
  - Description of test: With the patient sitting, passively maximally rotate the cervical spine to the side opposite being tested and then flex the cervical spine as far as possible moving the ear to the chest area
  - Positive test: When the lateral flexion movement is blocked
- First rib spring test is used to assess first rib hypomobility.
  - Diagnostic accuracy (reliability): kappa = 0.35
  - Description of test: The patient lays supine, the neck is positioned in slight flexion, and the cervical spine is rotated down to T1, fixating the cervical spine in this position with the opposite hand. With the free hand, press down on the first rib on the ipsilateral side in a ventral and caudal fashion. Assess the "springiness" of the rib and compare it to the contralateral side
  - Positive test: If the rib in question is more stiff than the contralateral side (Smedmark et al, 2000)

DIFFERENTIAL DIAGNOSIS

- Thoracic outlet syndrome
- Cervical radiculopathy
- Upper thoracic pain
- Cardiac and respiratory system pathology

CONTRIBUTING FACTORS

- Posture
- Trauma
- Accessory rib
- Osteoporosis
- Cardiac dysfunction or surgery
- Respiratory pathology
- Cervical rib

TREATMENT

SURGICAL INDICATORS

- Unremitting pain or symptoms
- Failed conservative management
- Fractures that threaten the underlying neurovascular structures

SURGICAL OPTIONS

Removal of the first rib

SURGICAL OUTCOME

Outcomes of surgery are unknown.

REHABILITATION

- Lindgren et al (1992) described the following management strategy; "Mobilization of the first ribs was initiated by isometric activation of the scalene muscles. This was performed by the patient, who pushed against the palm of his or her hand on the painful side. The patient pushed in each direction for one second and paused in between directions. This series of pushing movements was repeated ten times. The whole exercise was done ten times a day."
- Flynn and Egan described a seated high velocity, short amplitude thrust technique of the first rib in which a translatory mobilization is imparted to the first rib combined with exhalation.
- Initial exercises that can be utilized to promote healing are as follows:
  - Instruct the patient on first rib self-mobilization techniques (i.e., hold a towel over the first rib using one hand in front of the chest and a second hand behind the back).
  - Breathing activities with instruction on avoiding over utilization of accessory musculature.

PROGNOSIS

Generally, first rib dysfunction responds favorably to conservative management; surgery is very rarely required.

SIGNS AND SYMPTOMS INDICATING REFERRAL TO PHYSICIAN

- Signs suggesting progressively worsening neurological symptoms
- No response to conservative management

SUGGESTED READINGS

Brismee JM, Phelps V, Sizer P. Differential diagnosis and treatment of chronic neck and upper trapezius pain and upper extremity paresthesia: a case study involving the management of an elevated first rib and uncovertebral joint dysfunction. *J Manual & Manip Ther.* 2005;13(2):79-90.

Duane TM, O'Connor JV, Scalea TM. Thoracic outlet syndrome resulting from first rib fracture. *J Trauma.* 2007;62(1):231-233.

Egan WJ, Flynn TW. Thoracic Spine-Physical Therapy Patient Management Using Current Evidence. In: *The APTA-Orthopaedic Section's Home Study Course Series HHSC 16.2, Current Concepts of Orthopaedic Physical Therapy.* LaCrosse, WI; 2006.

Lindgren KA. Conservative treatment of thoracic outlet syndrome: a 2-year follow-up. *Arch Phys Med Rehabil.* 1997;78(4):373-378.

Lindgren KA, Leino E, Manninen H. Cervical rotation lateral flexion test in brachialgia. *Arch Phys Med Rehab.* 1992;73:735-737.

Lindgren KA, Leino E. Subluxation of the first rib: a possible thoracic outlet syndrome mechanism. *Arch Phys Med Rehabil.* 1988;69(9):692-695.

Smedmark V, Wallin M, Arvidsson I. Inter-examiner reliability in assessing passive intervertebral motion of the cervical spine. *Man Ther.* 2000;5(2):97-101.

AUTHOR: BRYAN DENNISON

BASIC INFORMATION

DEFINITION

- Osteoporosis is a disease process characterized by low bone mass and structural deterioration of bone tissue, which can lead to bone fragility and an increased susceptibility to fractures (National Osteoporosis Foundation).
  - Osteoporosis is defined as bone mineral density (BMD) 2.5 SDs below the mean of young adult women.
  - Osteopenia is defined as BMD 1.0 to 2.5 SDs below the mean of young adult women.
- Osteo- = bone; poros- = passage

SYNONYMS

- Osteopenia
- Brittle bone disease

ICD-9CM CODES
733.0   Osteoporosis
733.00 Osteoporosis unspecified
733.01 Senile osteoporosis
733.02 Idiopathic osteoporosis
733.03 Disuse osteoporosis
733.90 Osteopenia

OPTIMAL NUMBER OF VISITS

3 to 8 visits

MAXIMAL NUMBER OF VISITS

18 to 36 visits

ETIOLOGY

The rate of bone resorption from the osteoclasts outweighs the bone formation from the osteoblasts, and the bone loses overall density and mass.

EPIDEMIOLOGY AND DEMOGRAPHICS

- Osteoporosis affects over 10 million Americans.
- 27% of 80-year-olds are osteopenic and 70% are osteoporotic.
- The most common sites of osteoporosis are the hip, lumbar spine, and forearm.
- The bones most commonly fractured as a result of osteoporosis are the following:
  - Hip: 40% to 50%
  - Vertebral bodies (compression fractures): 19% to 41%
  - Wrist/distal forearm: 17% (usually secondary to a fall on an outstretched arm)
- The age group is most prone to osteoporosis is between 50 and 65 years of age.
- Females have a 40% to 50% risk of developing osteoporosis; males have a 13% to 22% risk of developing osteoporosis.
- Fractures typically happen 10 years later for men and their mortality after fracture is higher than for women.

- Asians and Caucasians have a higher risk of developing osteoporosis.
- $17.9 billion is spent annually for osteoporotic fractures; this amount is expected to increase to $50 billion by 2040.

MECHANISM OF INJURY

Osteoporosis itself is not painful, but the fractures that are a result of the condition are painful and debilitating. Some fractures (i.e., compression fractures) can occur insidiously with activities of daily living (ADLs) and some are a result of an injury like a fall.

COMMON SIGNS AND SYMPTOMS

- Loss in overall height
- Increased spinal curvatures (scoliosis, kyphosis, etc)
- Dowager's hump
- Back pain
- Fractures
- Depending on the area, pain can refer to the buttock, paraspinal muscles, and localized tissues

AGGRAVATING ACTIVITIES

- Poor posture
- Inactive lifestyle
- Unsafe movement choices (walking in the dark or unfamiliar locations)
- Eating poorly
- Smoking and drinking alcohol excessively
- The above activities aggravate osteoporosis because they cause the following:
  - Increase bony strain/stress
  - Decrease bone formation
  - Increase risk of trips and falls

EASING ACTIVITIES

- Gentle weight-bearing activities
- Maintaining good posture and positioning
- Eliminating unhealthy lifestyle choices (diet, smoking, alcohol consumption, etc)
- Fall prevention in home and work environments
- The above activities ease osteoporosis because they do the following:
  - Increase bone formation
  - Improve bone stress/strain distribution
  - Decrease risk of falls

24-HOUR SYMPTOM PATTERN

Pain pattern is more from the degenerative changes that typically occur with osteoporosis (fractures, arthritis, etc).

PAST HISTORY FOR THE REGION

- Family history of osteoporosis
- Endomorphic body type
- Poor diet
- Smoking and excessive alcohol consumption history
- Early menopause

- Long-term use of steroids (corticosteroids or otherwise)
- Kidney or liver failure

PHYSICAL EXAMINATION

- Increased spinal deformities (kyphosis, Dowager's hump, scoliosis)
- Low back pain
- Postoperative after a fall
- Hunched posture

IMPORTANT OBJECTIVE TESTS

Most diagnostic tests are done by a physician and include radiographs and dual energy x-ray absorptiometry (DEXA) scans.

DIFFERENTIAL DIAGNOSIS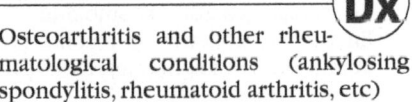

- Osteoarthritis and other rheumatological conditions (ankylosing spondylitis, rheumatoid arthritis, etc)
- Hip and wrist sprain/strain
- Lumbar sprain/strain
- Kidney dysfunction
- Osteogenesis imperfecta
- Bone cancer/tumors

CONTRIBUTING FACTORS

- Constitutional factors that make an individual at risk of developing osteoporosis include the following:
  - Gender: Females are more prone than males
  - Age: Older than 50 years of age
  - Race: Asians or Caucasians have a higher prevalence
  - Family history
  - Co-morbidity: Sex hormone deficiency (i.e., menopause), bone tumors, neuromuscular disorder (especially if on corticosteroids)
- Controllable risk factors include the following:
  - Weight: Underweight > overweight
  - Smoking
  - Excessive alcohol consumption
  - Prolonged immobilization
  - Diet: Low calcium and/or vitamin D

TREATMENT

SURGICAL OPTIONS

- Kyphoplasty (spine)
- Vertebroplasty (spine)
- Open reduction internal fixation (ORIF) and arthroplasties
- Kyphoplasty and vertebroplasty: 90% successful (vertebroplasty has a higher incidence of extravasation of cement)

REHABILITATION

- Benefits and risks of hormone replacement therapy (HRT) include the following:
  - Benefits: Reduces BMD loss, especially if menopause is early.

- ○ Risks: Cardiovascular disease, stroke, and invasive breast cancer risks are higher.
- Regular exercise has been shown to reduce the risk of fractures associated with osteoporosis.
- Regular resistance weight training can slow the rate of bone loss associated with osteoporosis.
- Research has demonstrated that women who walk a mile a day have 4 to 7 more years of bone in reserve than women who do not walk a mile a day.
- Rehabilitation programs should address the following:
  - ○ Encourage a balanced diet with adequate protein, calcium, and vitamin D
  - ○ Teach appropriate exercise and weight-bearing activities
  - ○ Encourage cessation of smoking
  - ○ Encourage reduction in alcohol consumption and maintenance of vision prescriptions
  - ○ Teach fall prevention and reduction of tripping hazards
  - ○ Encourage medication review with pharmacists/physician
- Initial exercises include the following:
  - ○ Walking and gentle weight-bearing activities (i.e., Tai Chi)
  - ○ Proprioception and balance training
  - ○ Weight lifting
  - ○ Core strengthening
- The role of exercise in osteoporosis rehabilitation includes the following:
  - ○ Supports bone formation
  - ○ Improves balance and decreases risk of falls
- Massage, joint mobilization, and manipulation can be used primarily for pain reduction; however, depending on the severity of the condition, joint mobilization/manipulation may not be indicated.

PROGNOSIS

Long-term prognosis for a patient with osteoporosis depends on the severity of the condition.

SIGNS AND SYMPTOMS INDICATING REFERRAL TO PHYSICIAN

- Suspicion of cancer or organ failure
- Alcoholism (for intervention)
- Suspicion of acute fracture
- Neurological involvement/spinal cord symptoms

SUGGESTED READINGS

Adler R. Osteoporosis in the male patient. *Clin Cornerstone*. 2006;8(suppl 3).

Bonnick S. Osteoporosis in men and women. *Clin Cornerstone*. 2006;8(1).

Delaney M. Strategies for the prevention and treatment of osteoporosis during early postmenopause. *Am J Obstet Gynecol*. 2006;194(suppl 2).

Dennison E, et al. Epidemiology of osteoporosis. *Rheum Dis Clin North Am*. 2006;32(4).

Gooren L. Osteoporosis and sex steroids. *The Journal of Men's Health & Gender*. 2007;4(2).

Lane N. Epidemiology, etiology, and diagnosis of osteoporosis. *Am J Obstet Gynecol*. 2006;194(suppl 2).

Lin J, Lane J. Rehabilitation of the older adult with an osteoporosis-related fracture. *Clin Geriatr Med*. 2006;22(2).

Lui P, et al. Tai chi chuan exercises in enhancing bone mineral density in active seniors. *Clin Sports Med*. 2008;27(1).

Pateder D, et al. Vertebroplasty and kyphoplasty for the management of osteoporotic vertebral compression fractures. *Orthop Clin North Am*. 2007;38(3).

Rizer M. Osteoporosis. *Primary Care: Clinics in Office Practice*. 2006;33(4).

Shedid D, et al. Kyphoplasty: vertebral augmentation for compression fractures. *Clin Geriatr Med*. 2006;22(3).

AUTHOR: SARA GRANNIS

BASIC INFORMATION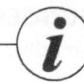

DEFINITION

A fractured rib refers to a loss of structural integrity of any one of the 24 rib bones. The integrity loss can vary in magnitude from a small hairline crack to a gross separation within the length of the rib.

SYNONYMS

- Broken rib bone
- Cracked ribs
- Flail chest

ICD-9CM CODES

807.00 Closed fracture of rib(s) unspecified
807.01 Closed fracture of one rib
807.02 Closed fracture of two ribs

OPTIMAL NUMBER OF VISITS

6 to 18 visits

MAXIMAL NUMBER OF VISITS

18 visits

ETIOLOGY

- Ribs are relatively flexible structures designed to protect the underlying visceral structures. As such, the ribs should be able to resist loading from multiple directions and of various forces. Fractures rarely occur in children because of the inherent pliability of the bony structures. Failure of the bone occurs when one of two circumstances exist: Forces exceed the capacity of the bony matrix or the bone becomes weakened or more brittle.
- The weakest portion of the rib is just anterior to the rib angle, but fractures can occur anywhere blunt trauma occurs. Although, in the case of axially loading onto the rib as in a fall onto lateral rib cage, the rib will fracture at its weakest point, which is just in front of the rib angle.
- Fractures of ribs are generally classified as fractures of ribs 1-4, ribs 5-9, or 10-12 and are grouped by the visceral structures they protect.
- Ribs 1-4 protect the arteries, veins, and nerves of the upper extremity. Therefore fractures of these ribs may be associated with neurovascular compromise of the brachial plexus or subclavian artery and vein.
- Ribs 5-9 protect the lungs and heart. Therefore fractures can result in damage to the lungs and subsequent pneumothorax if the ribs displace inward toward the lungs.
- Ribs 10-12 protect the kidneys, respiratory diaphragm, and spleen.

Therefore fractures can result in damage to the kidneys, spleen, and adrenal glands.

EPIDEMIOLOGY AND DEMOGRAPHICS

- 10% of blunt chest trauma patients have one or more rib fractures.
- Fourth through the ninth ribs are the most common fractured ribs. Other resources site the seventh and eighth ribs as the most commonly fractured.
- Rib fractures can happen at any age, although, because of the elasticity of their ribs, children are less likely to suffer a rib fracture.
- Gender and cultural prevalence are unknown.

MECHANISM OF INJURY

- Direct trauma results in a crush type fracture at the site of trauma
- Axial loading results in a torsional or bending fracture along the tensile side of the rib
- Tensile and torsional fracture is caused by forced twisting motions such as in baseball or golf
- Fracture from osteoporosis
- Coughing spells
- Recurrent arm movements can result in stress fractures
- Assault

COMMON SIGNS AND SYMPTOMS

- Severe pain on inspiration
- Tenderness to palpation
- Crepitus with movement and with breathing
- Ventilatory insufficiency (cyanosis, tachypnea, retractions, and use of accessory muscles)
- Pain referred along the entire length of the rib or just along portions of it

AGGRAVATING ACTIVITIES

- Inspiration
- Arm and/or trunk movement
- Twisting and rotational motions
- Coughing
- Direct pressure onto the fractures such as while sleeping

EASING ACTIVITIES

- Shallow breathing
- Accessory muscle breathing
- Splinting of the damaged area

24-HOUR SYMPTOM PATTERN

- Activity-dependent: Sleep will generally be disrupted because of pressure or twisting motions.
- Breathing will be hard and will increase symptoms during the course of the day.
- Stiffness may be present first thing in the morning.

PAST HISTORY FOR THE REGION

- A past history of osteoporosis or osteopenia may contribute to rib fractures.
- History of lung pathology will stiffen the region.
- History of cardiac, breast, or lung surgery may predispose a patient to fractures.
- Long-term use of steroids may also decrease the strength of bone.
- History of a hysterectomy may also lead to premature osteopenia.

PHYSICAL EXAMINATION

- Severe pain on inspiration
- Tenderness to palpation
- Crepitus with motion and with breathing
- Ventilatory insufficiency (cyanosis, tachypnea, retractions, and use of accessory muscles)

IMPORTANT OBJECTIVE TESTS

- X-rays are the primary diagnostic test of choice. A standard series of radiographs should be conducted to diagnose the presence of a rib fracture. Frontal, lateral, and off-lateral views should be taken. It has been reported that x-rays only detect 50% of the rib fractures.
- Computed tomography (CT) scan of the chest is an optional screening method for the presence of fracture.

DIFFERENTIAL DIAGNOSIS

- Abdominal trauma, blunt
- Back pain, mechanical
- Costochondritis
- Aortic dissection
- Domestic violence
- Elder abuse
- Esophagitis
- Clavicle fracture
- Sternal fracture
- Tension/traumatic pneumothorax
- Pulmonary embolism
- Upper genitourinary trauma

CONTRIBUTING FACTORS

- Osteoporosis or osteopenia
- Hysterectomy
- Long-term steroid use
- Balance disorders
- Lung pathology
- Prior cardiac surgery

TREATMENT

SURGICAL INDICATORS

Surgery is generally not indicated for these patients.

REHABILITATION

- Initial treatment should be geared toward pain prevention and promotion of healing, and these often go hand in hand. Taping of the damaged ribs, cryotherapy, and splinting or protecting the damaged ribs are all advisable first steps.

- Trunk and upper extremity movement should be encouraged as pain allows.
- Initial exercises utilized to promoted healing and proper rib function should include breathing and respiratory exercises.
- General range of motion (ROM) activities are advisable, but similar to other areas, restoring proper segmental mobility and proper activation of thoracic stabilizing muscles are important aspects of regaining proper mechanics through the region.

PROGNOSIS

- Full recovery is generally expected. In young patients, healing make take 6 weeks, with older patients longer time frames may be anticipated.

- Full functional recovery will depend on restoring normal biomechanics in the region. Proper thoracic mechanics are important aspects of cervical and upper extremity function and may predispose these regions to future pathology.
- A deformity may be observed on x-ray long after the fracture is healed.

SIGNS AND SYMPTOMS INDICATING REFERRAL TO PHYSICIAN

- Bleeding with respiration
- Pneumothorax
- Abdominal blunt trauma
- Aortic dissection
- Domestic violence
- Elder abuse
- Tension/traumatic pneumothorax
- Pulmonary embolism
- Upper genitourinary trauma

SUGGESTED READINGS

Bansidhar BJ, Lagares-Garcia JA, Miller SL. Clinical rib fractures: are follow-up chest X-rays a waste of resources? *Am Surg.* 2002;68(5):449-453.

Easter A. Management of patients with multiple rib fractures. *Am J Crit Care.* 2001;10(5):320-327; quiz 328-329.

Lee D. *The Thorax: An Integrated Approach.* 2nd ed. Minneapolis, MN: Orthopedic Physical Therapy Products (OPTP).

Wanek S, Mayberry JC. Blunt thoracic trauma: flail chest, pulmonary contusion, and blast injury. *Crit Care Clin.* 2004;20(1):71-81.

Ziegler DW, Agarwal NN. The morbidity and mortality of rib fractures. *J Trauma.* 1994;37(6):975-979.

AUTHOR: BRYAN DENNISON

BASIC INFORMATION

DEFINITION

Described by Holger Scheuermann as "a rigid kyphosis of the thoracic or thoracolumbar spine occurring in adolescents," Scheuermann's disease can be classified as an osteochondrosis of the spine.

SYNONYM

Juvenile "round back"

ICD-9CM CODE
732.0 Juvenile osteochondrosis of spine

OPTIMAL NUMBER OF VISITS

6 to 20 visits

MAXIMAL NUMBER OF VISITS

20 visits

ETIOLOGY

- Scheuermann's disease is an ossification of the ring apophysis (thoracic or thoracolumbar region). Currently, it is unclear whether the changes are as follows:
  - Primary structural changes caused by abnormal mechanical loading
  - A combination of genetic and environmental (loading) factors that result in disorganized endochondral ossification, reduction in collagen, and mucopolysaccharides

EPIDEMIOLOGY AND DEMOGRAPHICS

- There appears to be a genetic link
- 1% to 8% of the general population
- Overall incidence 0.4% to 10%
- Most common cause of kyphotic deformity in adolescents
- Second most common deformity issue in spine deformity clinics (idiopathic scoliosis: most common)
- Appears before puberty
- Diagnosed between ages 13 and 17 years, typically from late juvenile to 16 years of age, and commonly between 12 and 15 years
- No specific gender prevalence

MECHANISM OF INJURY

Ossification of the ring apophysis (thoracic or thoracolumbar region)

COMMON SIGNS AND SYMPTOMS

Two different curve patterns as follows:
- Thoracic pattern (most common form): Nonstructural hyperlordosis of the lumbar and cervical spine:
  - Type I spinal curve with the apex of the curve between T7 and T9
  - Bilateral hamstring tension

- Thoracolumbar pattern (most uncommon form): Expert opinion postulates that this form progresses in adulthood:
  - Type II spinal curve with the apex of the curve between T10 and T12
- Referral pattern for the pathology includes thoracic and/or thoracolumbar pain.

AGGRAVATING ACTIVITIES

- Many patients will be asymptomatic. The issue that brings them into their physician is poor posture or a referral from their school to screen for scoliosis.
- Sporting activities can aggravate symptoms.

EASING ACTIVITIES

Specific activities unknown (see Rehabilitation section)

24-HOUR SYMPTOM PATTERN

Can be activity related and not dependent on a specific time of day.

PAST HISTORY FOR THE REGION

Like other osteochondroses, patient may have a family history of the pathology or similar types of pathology.

PHYSICAL EXAMINATION

- Skin pigmentation over most prominent spinous processes (caused by friction of the back on supportive surfaces)
- Forward head
- Rounded shoulders (sometimes flexion contractures of shoulder joints)
- Hip joint flexion contractures
- Tight hamstrings
- Thoracolumbar form (type I; typically, these patients report the following:
  - Greater pain
  - Localized vertebral tenderness
  - Greater restriction with ADLs and physical exercise
- Lumbar form (type II); typically, these patients report persistent low back pain.

IMPORTANT OBJECTIVE TESTS

- Pediatric population
- Radiographs are required to visualize the following:
  - Vertebral body wedging
  - Vertebral endplate irregularity
  - Diminished anterior vertebral growth
  - Premature disc degeneration

DIFFERENTIAL DIAGNOSIS

- Postural kyphosis: Radiographically differentiated from Scheuermann's disease
- Postural kyphosis: Uniformly rounded kyphosis (nonstructural); absence of wedging of vertebral bodies; absence of disc degeneration

- Idiopathic kyphosis
- Spondylitis
- Osteochondral dystrophies
- Spondyloepiphyseal dysplasia
- Congenital kyphosis

CONTRIBUTING FACTORS

- Genetic predisposition
- Environmental triggers

TREATMENT

SURGICAL INDICATORS

- Recommended surgical criteria as follows:
  - Kyphoses >70 degrees
  - Progression of kyphosis despite bracing
  - Substantial kyphotic deformities in skeletally mature patients
  - Severity of localized and chronic pain refractory to conservative treatment
  - Neurological complications
  - A deformity that results in a cosmetic appearance affecting self-esteem/self-consciousness

SURGICAL OPTIONS

- Surgery is rarely needed. When surgery is needed (determined by preoperative evaluation of the patient), the following approaches are considered:
  - Posterior operative technique (Harrington rod most common): When indicated, performed for curves <70 degrees and if able to preoperatively correct a "flexible" kyphosis to approximately 50 degrees. Disadvantages include observed loss of correction, increased curve stiffness in adult patients; and a high degree of pseudoarthrosis if the curve is >70 degrees.
  - Combined anterior release with posterior instrumentation (release of anterior longitudinal ligament, complete diskectomy, excision of osteophytes, complete bridge of vertebral interspace, and bone graft): When indicated, increase rigidity in curves >75 degrees, skeletally immature >65 degrees, rigid kyphosis that is unable to be corrected to <60 degrees on hyperextension.

SURGICAL OUTCOME

- Surgeries are able to help improve deformities.
- Surgical improvements have been observed to revert.

REHABILITATION

- Bracing has been suggested (Milwaukee brace is the most common).
- The Milwaukee brace is used for the following:
  - Skeletally immature individuals
  - Flexible curve <65 degrees

- NOTE: Bracing is used to treat the postural dysfunction—not to resolve pain.
- The brace is used on a full-time basis (22 to 24 hours per day) for an average of 12 to 18 months.
- Weiss et al demonstrated favorable results to bracing in patients 17 to 21 year of age (n = 351) with painful Scheuermann kyphosis.
- Extension sports such as the following are encouraged:
  - Gymnastics
  - Aerobics
  - Swimming
  - Basketball
  - Cycling
  - Hyperextension exercises
- Jumping sports involving higher stress are discouraged.

PROGNOSIS

- The degree of kyphosis (severe) can cause neurological complications.

- A long-term study (32 year follow-up) by Murray, Weinstein, and Spratt found the following negative prognostic factors:
  - Mean kyphosis = 71 degrees.
  - Subjects worked in lighter jobs.
  - There was more severe back pain in individuals with Scheuermann's disease.
  - Subjects were more concerned with appearance but did not seem disabled.
  - Pain interfered with ADLs to a larger degree when compared to controls.

SIGNS AND SYMPTOMS INDICATING REFERRAL TO PHYSICIAN

- Not applicable unless red flags are detected.
- Development of neurological compromise.

SUGGESTED READINGS

Lowe TG, Line BG. Evidence based medicine: analysis of Scheuermann kyphosis. *Spine.* 2007;32(suppl 19):S115-S119.

Lowe TG. Scheuermann disease. *J Bone Joint Surg Am.* 1990;72(6):940-945.

Murray PM, Weinstein SL, Spratt KF. The natural history and long-term follow-up of Scheuermann kyphosis. *J Bone Joint Surg Am* 1993;75(2):236-248.

Scheuermann HW. Kyphosis dorsalis juvenilis. Ugeskrift for Læger. *Copenhagen.* 1920;82:385-393.

Scoles PV, Latimer BM, DiGiovanni BF, et al. Vertebral alterations in Scheuermann's kyphosis. *Spine.* 1991;16(5):509-515.

Weiss HR, Weiss G, Schaar HJ. Conservative management in patients with scoliosis–does it reduce the incidence of surgery? *Stud Health Technol Inform.* 2002;91:342-347.

AUTHOR: BRYAN DENNISON

BASIC INFORMATION

DEFINITION

- Scoliosis is a lateral curvature of the spine >10 degrees as measured using the Cobb method on a standing radiograph
- Idiopathic scoliosis is a structural curve with no clear underlying cause

SYNONYM

Curved spine

ICD-9CM CODES

737.10 Kyphosis (acquired) (postural)
737.11 Kyphosis due to radiation
737.12 Kyphosis postlaminectomy
737.19 Other kyphosis acquired

OPTIMAL NUMBER OF VISITS

6 to 20 visits

MAXIMAL NUMBER OF VISITS

20 visits

ETIOLOGY

- In most cases, the cause of scoliosis is idiopathic. Childhood classification of scoliosis is often based largely on when the spinal curvatures begin to appear. If the onset is before 3 years of age, the scoliosis is classified as infantile idiopathic scoliosis. If the onset is between 3 and 10 years of age, it is classified as juvenile and if the onset is after 10 years of age, it is classified as adolescent.
- As a whole, scoliosis can also be classified as functional, neuromuscular, or degenerative.
- Functional scoliosis is the result of abnormalities in the body that secondarily impact the spine. In the absence of the abnormalities, the spine would be normal. Leg length discrepancies or protective scoliosis secondary to a lumbar disc herniation are examples of functional scoliosis.
- Neuromuscular scoliosis develops secondary to problems during the development of the spine. Often, the bones of the spine will not form completely or they will fail to separate from each other and this results in the scoliosis. Scoliosis is caused by actual alterations in the structure of the spine and occurs in patients with Marfan syndrome, muscular dystrophy, or cerebral palsy.
- Degenerative scoliosis occurs as the body ages. Disc herniation, fractures, osteophytes, and other spinal changes create alterations in the normal spinal alignment. Unlike functional scoliosis, the spinal curves are a result of actual changes in the spinal vertebrae or discs.

EPIDEMIOLOGY AND DEMOGRAPHICS

- Prevalence of scoliosis
  - Infantile scoliosis: <1% of all cases.
  - Juvenile scoliosis: Between 12% and 21% of all patients with idiopathic scoliosis.
  - Adolescent idiopathic scoliosis: The majority of cases.
- Age group of scoliosis
  - Present in 2% to 4% of children between 10 and 16 years of age.
  - Prevalence of curves >30 degrees is 0.2%.
  - Prevalence of curves >40 degrees is 0.1%.
- Gender and culture prevalence of scoliosis are as follows:
  - Ratio of girls to boys is equal with curves of 10 degrees.
  - The ratio increases to 10:1 girls to boys in curves >30 degrees.
  - Females have a 10 times higher risk of curve progression.

MECHANISM OF INJURY

There is generally no specific mechanism of injury related to the development of scoliosis. The only exception is within the functional classification category in which disc herniations or injury to the lower extremity can create the curvatures seen in the spine.

COMMON SIGNS AND SYMPTOMS

- Pain, if present, may be referred anywhere along the spinal column and adjacent regions.
- Pain is not generally caused by the spinal curves, instead it is usually the curvature of the spine that places abnormal forces onto other tissues of the body. These abnormal forces cause failure of the tissue and resultant pain.

AGGRAVATING ACTIVITIES

Aggravating activities will be based on the tissue injured as a result of the scoliosis.

24-HOUR SYMPTOM PATTERN

24-hour pain pattern will take on the attributes of the specific tissue injured by the scoliosis.

PAST HISTORY FOR THE REGION

- Patient may have a family history of scoliosis.
- Patient may have history of lower extremity trauma or leg length discrepancies.

PHYSICAL EXAMINATION

- Cobb angle >10 degrees
- "Rib hump" in forward lumbar spine flexion (a hallmark sign of scoliotic curves >10 degrees)

- 90% of the curves are to the right
- Screen for leg length discrepancies

Risk of Curve Progression

Curve (Degree)	Growth Potential (Risser grade)	Risk*
10 to 19	Limited (2 to 4)	Low
10 to 19	High (0 to 1)	Moderate
20 to 29	Limited (2 to 4)	Low/ moderate
20 to 29	High (0 to 1)	High
>29	Limited (2 to 4)	High
>29	High (0 to 1)	Very high

*Low risk = 5% to 15%; moderate risk = 15% to 40%; high risk = 40% to 70%; very high risk = 70% to 90%.
Data from Reamy BV, Slakey JB: Adolescent idiopathic scoliosis: Review and current concepts, *Am Fam Physician.* 2001;64(1):111-116.

IMPORTANT OBJECTIVE TESTS

Radiographs are the most effective means of determining the nature and extent of spinal scoliosis.

DIFFERENTIAL DIAGNOSIS Dx

The clinician should screen for any of the pathology listed in the section on Contributing Factors.

CONTRIBUTING FACTORS

Secondary causes of scoliosis include the following:
- Inherited disorders of connective tissue
  - Ehlers-Danlos syndrome
  - Marfan syndrome
  - Homocystinuria
- Neurologic disorders
  - Syringomyelia
  - Tethered cord syndrome
  - Spinal tumor
  - Neurofibromatosis
  - Muscular dystrophy
  - Cerebral palsy
  - Poliomyelitis
  - Friedreich's ataxia
  - Familial dysautonomia (Riley-Day syndrome)
  - Werdnig-Hoffmann disease
- Musculoskeletal:
  - Leg length discrepancy
  - Developmental dysplasia of the hip
  - Osteogenesis imperfecta
  - Klippel-Feil syndrome

TREATMENT

SURGICAL OPTIONS

- Posterior instrumentation and spinal fusion

- Anterior instrumentation and arthrodesis
- Anterior spinal release
- Thoracoplasty

SURGICAL OPTIONS

If a spinal curve >45 degrees or if the curve is getting worse, surgery may be considered

SURGICAL OUTCOMES

- Patients have good long-term health-related quality of life after surgery for idiopathic scoliosis and spondylolisthesis in adolescence.
- Patients who have surgery for idiopathic scoliosis are likely to have better long-term outcomes than patients who have surgery for spondylolisthesis.
- In terms of types of surgeries, Cotrel-Dubousset instrumentation yielded better long-term functional and radiographic outcomes in patients with adolescent idiopathic scoliosis than did Harrington instrumentation. However, complications were more common in the Cotrel-Dubousset instrumentation group.

REHABILITATION

- Rehabilitation of scoliosis is based on the magnitude of the spinal curve and whether the curve is increasing. The type of scoliosis also plays a role in the choice of treatment methodology. Treatment choices generally will include observation, bracing, or surgery, depending on the age, type. and magnitude of the scoliosis.
- Observation is utilized for functional scoliosis, mild idiopathic scoliosis, and degenerative scoliosis. All of these will be monitored, and if there is no progression in symptoms, then no action need be taken. Functional scoliosis is addressed by treating the factors that contribute to the scoliosis. Shoe lifts, musculature strengthening, etc, can be utilized to address these factors. Once these changes are made, often the scoliosis

will self-correct because there are no spinal abnormalities present. Mild neuromuscular scoliosis will not correct itself, but as long as it is not worsening, no action need be taken. Degenerative scoliosis is only addressed if symptoms are present in structures adjacent to the scoliosis. Treatments will often be focused on the injury in adjacent tissue.
- Neuromuscular scoliosis has the greatest chance for poor outcomes. Observation and bracing do not normally work well for patients with this type of scoliosis. The majority of these patients will eventually need surgery to stop the curve from getting worse.
- Infantile scoliosis will generally get better without any intervention. Many children will grow out of the scoliosis as the child develops and grows. Bracing and surgery are not normally warranted.
- Juvenile idiopathic scoliosis has the highest risk for poor outcomes of all of the idiopathic types of scoliosis. Bracing is usually the first course of action. There are various types of bracing available that allow various types of freedom to the patient. Many bracing programs require 24-hour bracing, with the brace being removed only when the patient is bathing. These programs are difficult to comply with, considering the age of the patient and the social stigma that accompany the braces when they are worn. Electrical stimulation programs have been suggested to address this issue, but at this time their use has been limited to research. Bracing is generally tried early if the curve is not very severe. The goal is to prevent the curve from getting worse until the person stops growing. In a majority of patients with moderate to severe spinal curves, surgery is eventually needed.
- Adolescent idiopathic scoliosis is the most common form of scoliosis. Small curves require no bracing or intervention. If the curve is <25 degrees, no treatment is required. Bracing is utilized

for curves between 25 and 40 degrees. Curves >40 degrees usually require surgery.

PROGNOSIS

- The maximum progression of scoliosis will occur when a child exhibits Tanner stage 2 or 3 characteristics.
- Those who exhibit a greater growth potential and larger curve are prone to curve progression.
- If the curve are <40 degrees when the person stops growing, there curves will usually stabilize and not worsen. If the curve is greater than 40 degrees, the curve will likely get worse by 1 to 2 degrees annually for the remainder of their lives. This could potentially lead to future problems with degeneration in the spine and pathology in the viscera with digestion, heart, and lung function.

SIGNS AND SYMPTOMS INDICATING REFERRAL TO PHYSICIAN

- Worsening spinal curves
- Impaired lung or heart function
- Fevers or infection

SUGGESTED READINGS

Dubousset J. Scoliosis and its pathophysiology: do we understand it? *Spine.* 2001;26(9):1001.

Helenius I, Remes V, Lamberg T, Schlenzka D, Poussa M. Long-term health-related quality of life after surgery for adolescent idiopathic scoliosis and spondylolisthesis. *J Bone Joint Surg Am.* 2008;90(6):1231–1239.

Newton PO, Upasani VV, Lhamby J, Ugrinow VL, Pawelek JB, Bastrom TP. Surgical treatment of main thoracic scoliosis with thoracoscopic anterior instrumentation. A five-year follow-up study. *J Bone Joint Surg Am.* 2008;90(10):2077–2089.

Reamy BV, Slakey JB. Adolescent idiopathic scoliosis: review and current concepts. *Am Fam Physician.* 2001;64(1):111–116.

AUTHOR: BRYAN DENNISON

BASIC INFORMATION

DEFINITION

- Maitland described T4 syndrome in 1986 as "a clinical pattern that involves upper extremity paraesthesia and pain with or without symptoms into the neck and/or head."
- Evans further defined the condition as "a term used by clinicians for patients whose varied problems seem to be derived from the upper thoracic spine."

SYNONYMS

T4 syndrome is different than thoracic outlet syndrome, although the diagnosis may be made interchanging the two conditions.

ICD-9CM CODES
353.0 Nerve root and plexus disorders
353.3 Thoracic root lesions
353.8 Other nerve root and plexus disorders
353.9 Unspecified nerve root and plexus disorders

OPTIMAL NUMBER OF VISITS

6 to 20 visits

MAXIMAL NUMBER OF VISITS

20 visits

ETIOLOGY

- Evans notes that "entrapment of the segmental spinal nerves which are carrying afferent fibres from the sympathetic nerves; entrapment or ischemia of the sympathetic nerves (e.g. over the rib neck or osteophytes); referred pain from the heart, oesophagus, etc; referred pain from the thoracic spinal structure, and in the neck and dorsal spinal structure; referred pain from any structure in the forequarter."
- The pathology is hypothesized to be the result of arteriolar ischemia.
- Hypothesized scenarios, such as sustained or extreme postures, tax the arteriolar system of the sympathetic nervous system, causing microtrauma. Evans suggested that this repetitive process results in "scar formation, recurrent damage, attempted repair and patchy proliferating inflammatory tissue" that, by the repetitive process of injury and repair, results in arteriolar ischemia.

EPIDEMIOLOGY AND DEMOGRAPHICS

- The prevalence of the pathology is unknown.
- The age group most prone to the pathology is >35 years of age.
- Gender and culture prevalence is unknown.

MECHANISM OF INJURY

- Insidious
- After the start of a new job
- Change of work practice
- Taking up a new hobby
- Jobs that involve forward stooping and bending or sedentary positions

COMMON SIGNS AND SYMPTOMS

- Paraesthesia in all five fingers, in the whole hand, or in the forearm and hand (glove type long/short), in one hand or both.
- Hand feels hot or cold, and arm may feel heavy.
- Hands feel swollen, and they may actually be swollen.
- Aches and pains, nondermatomal, in arm and/or forearm.
- Pains may be crushing, bursting, or like a tight band.
- Combination of neck, upper thoracic, and cranial pain, without abnormal neurological signs.
- Headaches that present in a "cap" type presentation on the top of the head. Paraesthesia may involve the extremities and hands but not necessarily in a dermatomal pattern.

AGGRAVATING ACTIVITIES

Actual aggravating activities are unknown, although poor posture is suspected to play a role.

EASING ACTIVITIES

- Massage
- Hot showers
- Medication

24-HOUR SYMPTOM PATTERN

- Symptoms can come on in the morning and continue with aggravating activities (see Aggravating Activities section).
- After the symptoms start, positional changes do not seem to be effective in alleviating the symptoms.
- Symptoms may be worse at night and may even interrupt sleep.

PAST HISTORY FOR THE REGION

Symptoms can be insidious in their onset.

PHYSICAL EXAMINATION

- Posterior to anterior accessory mobilization at the T4 segment reproduces the patient's symptoms.
- Palpation of rib angles may elicit symptoms.
- Observation of trophic changes (i.e.. color: red/purple and temperature: hot/cold).
- Positive neurodynamic tests of the upper limb.

IMPORTANT OBJECTIVE TESTS

Radiographs and electromyographic studies are generally negative.

DIFFERENTIAL DIAGNOSIS

- Cardiac pain
- Thoracic outlet
- Gut problems
- Cervical spine dysfunction
- Neurological disease
- Spinal tumor
- Kidney disease
- Lumbar disc disease
- Diabetes
- Peripheral neuropathies

CONTRIBUTING FACTORS

- Sedentary lifestyle
- Posture

TREATMENT

SURGICAL INDICATORS

Unknown. Not reported in the literature.

SURGICAL OPTIONS

Unknown. Not reported in the literature.

SURGICAL OUTCOME

Unknown. Not reported in the literature.

REHABILITATION

- Manual therapy directed to the thoracic spine (thrust and nonthrust) pending determination of irritability clinically has proven effective in reducing the symptoms of T4 syndrome
- Postural education
- Movement reeducation after successful manual therapy interventions
- Postural retraining

PROGNOSIS

Long-term prognosis for a patient with a T4 syndrome is generally excellent if managed appropriately and no complicating factors arise.

SIGNS AND SYMPTOMS INDICATING REFERRAL TO PHYSICIAN

- Any signs or symptoms indicating the following:
  ○ Cardiac dysfunction
  ○ Neurological disease
  ○ Spinal tumor/metastases

- ○ Kidney disease
- ○ Gut problems

SUGGESTED READINGS

Conroy J, Schneiders A. The T4 syndrome. *Man Ther.* 2005;10(4):292–296.

DeFranca GG, Levine LJ. The T4 Syndrome. *J Manipulative Physiol Ther.* 1995; 18:34–37.

Evans P. The T4 syndrome: some basic science aspects. *Physiotherapy.* 1997;83:186–189.

Maitland GD. *Vertebral manipulation.* 5th ed. Boston, MA: Butterworth; 1986.

McGuckin N. The T4 syndrome. In: Grieve GP, ed. *Modern manual therapy of the vertebral column.* Edinburgh: Churchill Livingstone; 1994:370–376.

AUTHOR: BRYAN DENNISON

BASIC INFORMATION

DEFINITION

Loss of structural integrity in the vertebral body of one of the 12 thoracic vertebrae.

SYNONYMS

- Broken bone
- Broken back
- Wedge fracture
- Chance fracture
- Burst fracture

ICD-9CM CODE
805.2 Closed fracture of dorsal (thoracic) vertebra without spinal cord injury

OPTIMAL NUMBER OF VISITS

6 to 18 visits

MAXIMAL NUMBER OF VISITS

18 visits

ETIOLOGY

- Thoracic compression fractures occur most commonly in the lower thoracic spine (T10-T12). This is primarily a result of the increased load this region must carry. The amount of body weight the lower thoracic spine must support is much greater than the amount of weight the upper thoracic spine must carry.
- Anatomically, the majority of compression fractures occur in the anterior aspect of the vertebral body. The anterior aspect of the vertebral body is an area of relative weakness because of trabecular orientation. The trabeculae of the vertebral body are oriented in an angular pattern in both directions. The is a point in the anterior aspect of the vertebrae in which the trabeculae do not overlap. This is a point of relative weakness and the point most compression fractures occur.
- Biomechanically, the thoracic pain is kyphotic. As such, more load is placed on the anterior aspect of the vertebral body than the posterior aspect.
- In 1983, Denis proposed the 3-column model of the spine (anterior, middle, and posterior). Denis defines the anterior column as containing the anterior longitudinal ligament, the anterior half of the vertebral body, and the related portion of the intervertebral disc and its annulus fibrosus. The middle column contains the posterior longitudinal ligament, the posterior half of the vertebral body, and the intervertebral disc and its annulus. The posterior column contains the bony elements of the posterior neural arch and the ligamental elements, which include the ligamentum flavum, the interspinous ligaments, and the supraspinous ligaments. The joint capsule of the intervertebral articulations is also part of the posterior column. According to Denis, disruption of two or more columns results in an unstable configuration.
- Compression fractures can be divided into four major classifications based on mechanism of injury and divided into a column system (anterior, middle, and posterior columns):
  o Flexion and compression fractures are a result of the excessive forces applied with flexion and compression; there is failure in the anterior aspect of the vertebral body. This is the classic type of compression fracture. Because of the collapse that occurs in the anterior region and failure in the anterior column while the middle and posterior columns stay intact, the vertebra takes on a wedge appearance. This type of fracture may also be known as a wedge fracture.
  o Axial compression fractures are a result of compression loading on the spine, such as occurs in a fall, and there is failure at the anterior and middle column of the vertebra. This failure results in loss of overall vertebral body height and can also be called a burst fracture. Failure can occur at both superior and inferior endplates but most commonly occurs at the superior endplate.
  o Flexion and distraction fractures, unlike the other classifications, require failure of the posterior spinal column. If the force is applied into flexion and the force is in front of the anterior longitudinal ligament, a horizontal fracture occurs through the anterior and middle columns. The supraspinous ligament is also damaged. This type of fracture is called a chance fracture or seatbelt fracture. These fractures are usually stable because most of the posterior elements are still intact. If the direction of force is behind the anterior longitudinal ligament, damage to the posterior elements, such as the pars interarticularis, may occur. This leads to an unstable fracture because all three columns are generally affected.
  o Rotational fracture and dislocation fractures involve rotation and lateral flexion. Flexion and extension may or may not be involved. Because the mechanism is primarily rotation, the upper spinal vertebra rotates and takes the superior portion of the involved vertebral along with it. Failure occurs at the posterior and middle columns. The anterior column may or may not be involved. This mechanism of injury creates a slice type of appearance on radiographs. Because the pars interarticularis is involved, instability and neurological deficits are common findings.

EPIDEMIOLOGY AND DEMOGRAPHICS

- In the United States (US), it is estimated that 25% of white postmenopausal women are affected by fractures of the vertebrae.
- In persons 65 years of age or older, vertebral fractures account for 150,000 hospital admissions in the US annually.
- Spinal compression fractures occur in over 750,000 people per year in the US.
- About two-thirds of spinal compression fractures are never diagnosed because many patients and families think the back pain is merely a sign of aging and arthritis.
- Compression fractures are more prevalent in two patient populations: The elderly because of osteoporosis and increased fall risk and the young adult because of trauma such as MVAs or falls from a great height.

MECHANISM OF INJURY

- Falls onto tailbone or head
- Lifting heavy objects
- MVAs
- Coughing or sneezing

COMMON SIGNS AND SYMPTOMS

- Pain in the thoracic region over the affected vertebra may be severe, sharp, and exacerbated with motion
- Pain with lifting and carrying objects
- Pain with breathing
- May or may not have signs of cord compression, depending on magnitude of injury

AGGRAVATING ACTIVITIES

- Thoracic motion
- Pressure onto midback
- Inspiration and expiration
- Coughing
- Difficulty with lifting activities
- Pain with bending forward

EASING ACTIVITIES

- Rest
- Lying down
- Movement instability involved
- Abdominal bracing

24-HOUR SYMPTOM PATTERN

- Stiffness and pain in the morning lasting for 30 minutes or more
- Increased pain with prolonged activity and symptoms increase during the day
- Pain with lifting
- Sleeping may or may not be problematic

PAST HISTORY FOR THE REGION

- History of trauma: MVA, fall, etc
- History of osteoporosis or osteopenia

PHYSICAL EXAMINATION

- Pain with palpation of the involved segments
- Pain with active and passive range of motion (ROM) is present. Pain is usually worse with flexion but depends on type of fracture.

IMPORTANT OBJECTIVE TESTS

- Radiographs are the primary means of diagnosis. Plain radiographs are usually taken initially and can pick up major fractures, but often hairline or nondisplaced fractures can be overlooked.
- A CT myelogram can be used to determine the degree of impingement of the bony fragments on the thecal scan.
- MRI testing is the most sensitive tool for identifying the magnitude of the fracture and any soft tissue injuries that may be involved.

DIFFERENTIAL DIAGNOSIS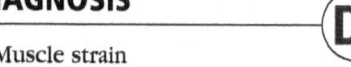

- Muscle strain
- Thoracic disc herniation
- Metastatic malignancy
- Spinal tumors
- Spinal infection
- Referred pain from other regions of the body
- Lung or heart pathology

CONTRIBUTING FACTORS

- Metastatic cancer especially lung and/or breast
- Osteoporosis
- Increased thoracic kyphosis
- Trauma

TREATMENT

SURGICAL OPTIONS

- Surgical approaches:
  - Posterior: Not used often because of limited exposure to the vertebral body.
  - Posterior lateral: Used only when anterior approach is not possible.
  - Anterior: Most common surgical approach because it allows for maximal access to the vertebral body.
- Surgical stabilization procedures:
  - Posterior lumbar interspinous fusion
  - Posterior rods
  - Cage
  - Z-plate anterior thoracolumbar plating system
- Each has different advantages and disadvantages based on the magnitude of the injury and the portions of the spine that have been involved.

REHABILITATION

- Many minor compression fractures will be treated conservatively. Patient is instructed to avoid heavy lifting and excessive forward flexion activities for 6 to 8 weeks. No bracing or surgery is required.
- In more moderate fractures or unstable fractures, the conservative treatment approach would be to have the patient wear a spinal brace for 6 to 8 weeks. Wearing a spinal brace is somewhat difficult, and outcomes are mixed. The braces allow for minimal amount of motion and do not stabilize the lower thoracic vertebrae well. Spinal body casting is better at stabilizing the spine but is uncomfortable and not well tolerated by patients.
- Early ambulation and walking programs are encouraged with all patients after compression fractures.
- Patients should be educated to avoid lifting and carrying objects. Forward-bending activities should be kept to a minimum.
- As patients progress, they may begin a program geared to increase trunk stability and promote thoracic extension.
- Lifting and carrying may be implemented once a good sign of bone healing is present.
- Full recovery may take up to a year.

PROGNOSIS

- There is a 23% mortality rate in those who develop compression fractures. This is in part a result of the prevalence of the pathology to the elderly or younger people with spinal trauma.
- In the general population the prognosis is good for return to all normal daily activities. Most thoracic compression fractures will heal but may produce permanent deformity.

SIGNS AND SYMPTOMS INDICATING REFERRAL TO PHYSICIAN

- Constant unremitting pain
- Neurological signs
- Worsening or progressing symptoms
- Bowel and bladder problems
- Spinal cord injury or cauda equina signs

SUGGESTED READINGS

Cooper C, Atkinson EJ, O'Fallon WM, Melton III LJ. Incidence of clinically diagnosed vertebral fractures: a population-based study in Rochester, Minnesota, 1985-1989. *J Bone Miner Res.* 1992;7:221-227.

Denis F. The three column spine and its significance in the classification of acute thoracolumbar spinal injuries. *Spine.* 1983; 8(8):817-831.

Evans AJ, Jensen ME, Kip KE, et al. Vertebral compression fractures: pain reduction and improvement in functional mobility after percutaneous polymethylmethacrylate vertebroplasty—retrospective report of 245 cases. *Radiology.* 2003;226:366-372.

Haczynski J, Jakimiuk A. Vertebral fractures: a hidden problem of osteoporosis. *Med Sci Monit.* 2001;7(5):1108-1117.

Lyles KW, Gold DT, Shipp KM, Pieper CF, Martinez S, Mulhausen PL. Association of osteoporotic vertebral compression fractures with impaired functional status. *Am J Med.* 1993;94:595-601.

Melton III LJ, Kan SH, Frye MA, Wahner HW, O'Fallon WM, Riggs BL. Epidemiology of vertebral fractures in women. *Am J Epidemiol.* 1989;129:1000-1011.

Ross PD, Davis JW, Epstein RS, Wasnich RD. Pain and disability associated with new vertebral fractures and other spinal conditions. *Am J Epidemiol.* 1994;47:231-239.

AUTHOR: DERRICK SUEKI

BASIC INFORMATION

The failure of either the nucleus pulposus or the annulus fibrosis of any of the discs in the thoracic region.

SYNONYMS

- Herniated thoracic disc
- Thoracic bulging disc
- Thoracic degenerative disc disease

ICD-9CM CODE
722.51 Degeneration of thoracic or thoracolumbar intervertebral disc

OPTIMAL NUMBER OF VISITS

8 to 24 visits

MAXIMAL NUMBER OF VISITS

24 visits

ETIOLOGY

- Disc herniation or disc bulges are synonymous terms utilized to describe a condition in which disc material extends beyond the perimeter of the normal disc space.
- The four common classes of disc herniations are as follows:
  - Disc *protrusion* occurs when the nucleus pulposus bulges outward into the annulus fibrosis but no damage is done to the annulus.
  - Disc *prolapse* occurs when the nucleus pulposus bulges outward into the annulus, and the annular lamina are damaged.
  - Disc *extrusion* occurs when the nucleus pulposus breaks past the outer lamina of the annulus fibrosis and into the space beyond.
  - Disc *sequestration* occurs when nucleus pulposus breaks free of annulus.
- The etiology is primarily degenerative. Disc pathology rarely occurs as a result of acute trauma alone. Disc injury in most cases result from a degenerative process. When the disc is loaded beyond its physiological capacity, the disc is likely to fail at the cartilaginous end plates. Injury to the endplates allow the contents of the vertebral body to enter into the nucleus of the disc. Chemically, the contents of the vertebral body will react with the contents of the nucleus to degrade the annulus from the inner lamina of the annulus outward. As the disc degrades, fewer annular lamina are available to resist loading and more stress is placed on each collagen fiber of the annulus. Further insults to the disc will increase the likelihood of additional degradation and eventually lead to the failure of the annulus and the development of a disc bulge.

EPIDEMIOLOGY AND DEMOGRAPHICS

- Reported as the least likely of the spinal regions for herniation, the thoracic spine region has been reported to account for 0.25% to 5.0% of all intervertebral disc herniations.
- One in a million patients will experience symptoms of a thoracic disc herniation every year.
- 2% of thoracic disc herniations occur at the lower thoracic spine (T11/12) with 70% of cases herniating in a posterolateral position.
- Age range has been reported to be between 11 and 82 years, with 40 to 50 years of age identified as the "peak age" for thoracic disc herniations.
- The condition appears to occur more commonly in men.
- Arce and Dohrmann reported that 60% of thoracic disc herniations occur in men and 40% of disc herniations occur in women.
- No apparent relationship exists between gender and the presence of disc herniation.

MECHANISM OF INJURY

- Degenerative changes resulting from repetitive flexion-based activities coupled with compressive loading such as bending and lifting objects
- Traumatic incident such as fall onto the buttock
- History of sudden strain such as coughing or sneezing

COMMON SIGNS AND SYMPTOMS

- Disc herniations in the thoracic spine may be asymptomatic.
- When pain is present, the distribution of the pain will be as follows:
  - Nonspecific pain (57%)
  - Involve sensory changes (24%)
  - Involve motor changes (17%)
  - Combination of motor and sensory disturbance (61%)
  - Bladder (sphincter) involvement (30%)
- Cyriax has described the clinical presentation of thoracic disc lesions as follows:
  - Intermittent backache
  - Acute thoracic lumbago
  - Thoracic root pain and paresthesia
  - Spinal cord compression symptoms

AGGRAVATING ACTIVITIES

- Sitting
- Coughing
- Bearing down

EASING ACTIVITIES

- Standing
- Lying supine

24-HOUR SYMPTOM PATTERN

- The patient with a disc injury will complain of stiffness and pain in the morning that lasts for more than 20 minutes.
- Symptoms will increase during the day if sitting too long.
- Sleeping may or may not be problematic.

PAST HISTORY FOR THE REGION

- There can be a history of trauma to the vertebral body.
- There may be history of a fall or MVA.

PHYSICAL EXAMINATION

- Restricted neck and back ROM in a noncapsular pattern (e.g., neck and back flexion usually more restricted than any other movement)
- Positive neural tension tests may be present (e.g., straight leg raise, slump test, femoral nerve stretch, or scapular retraction)
- Neurological signs may be present (e.g., nerve root palsy, decreased dermatomic sensation, altered deep tendon reflexes, or upper motor neuron signs)

IMPORTANT OBJECTIVE TESTS

- Radiographs may show spurring and failure at the vertebral endplates, but MRI scans are still the gold standard for diagnosing the presence of any disc pathology. The accuracy of this method specifically for the thoracic spine has not been determined by research.
- Straight leg raise testing has been utilized in the lumbar spine with good success to help rule in the presence of a lumbar disc; its use for disc pathology located in the thoracic spine is unknown.

DIFFERENTIAL DIAGNOSIS

- Thoracic disc pathology with chest wall pain
- Tietze's syndrome
- Costochondritis
- Rib trauma
- Painful rib swelling
- Slipping rib syndrome
- Costovertebral arthritis
- Painful xiphoid syndrome
- Traumatic muscle pain
- Ankylosing spondylitis
- Shingles
- Vertebral fracture

- Chest wall pain referral from the cervical spine, shoulders, thoracic outlet, or differential diagnosis for chest pain: Angina, lung or breast tumor, pleuritis, or intercostal neuritis (Bohlman, 1988)
- Patients with thoracic spine disc herniations are frequently misdiagnosed with the following:
  - Cardiac disorders
  - Pulmonary disorders
  - Gastrointestinal disorders
  - Renal disorders
  - Psychiatric disorders
  - Intercostal neuralgia
  - Neuritis
  - Cardiac neurosis
  - Pleurodynia
  - Esophagitis
  - Nephritis
  - Gastrointestinal ulcers
- Cholecystitis
- Shoulder impingement

CONTRIBUTING FACTORS

- Unknown because the frequency of positive MRI findings is relatively the same between asymptomatic and symptomatic individuals
- Increased thoracic kyphosis
- Activities requiring repetitive flexion combined with axial loading

TREATMENT

SURGICAL OPTIONS

- Costotransversectomy
- Laminectomy

SURGICAL OUTCOME

Costotransversectomy (80% success rate)

REHABILITATION

- Very little research has been conducted regarding rehabilitation of thoracic disc pathology. It seems a logical progression to utilize the principles learned from lumbar research to begin to build a rehabilitation program geared toward the thoracic spine.
- Initially, rehabilitation should focus on decreasing symptoms and promoting healing. This may be accomplished through a program of active rest. Care should be taken to offload the tissue through lying supine, but complete bed rest is not advisable because motion is need to help encourage healing and circulation. Therefore, the patient should be encouraged to walk frequently throughout the day. Lifting and carrying should be avoided.
- As symptoms decrease and healing progresses, patients can begin to normalize their mobility and movement patterns. Thoracic extension while prone and thoracic stabilization exercises should be encouraged.
- When motion is pain-free, loading the spine with functional activities can begin. Care should be taken to maintain core stability with all activities.
- Breathing should be utilized throughout the exercise regime because a large aspect of thoracic spine function involves the lungs.
- As with other regions, any rehabilitation program should identify the factors that contribute to the pathology and correct them whenever possible.

PROGNOSIS

Long-term prognosis is unknown, but clinically most patient make full functional recovery in 6 to 8 weeks.

SIGNS AND SYMPTOMS INDICATING REFERRAL TO PHYSICIAN

- Any patient presenting with symptoms indicating upper motor neuron involvement should be referred. Wilke et al noted that by the time a patient is diagnosed with thoracic disc herniation, 90% of the patients have signs of cord compression.
- Prolonged time without a diagnosis has contributed to permanent spastic paraplegia as a result of spinal cord compression.

SUGGESTED READINGS

Arce CA, Dohrmann GJ. Herniated thoracic discs. *Neurosurg Clin.* 1985;3:392.

Bohlman HH, Zdeblick TA. Anterior excision of herniated thoracic discs. *J Bone Joint Surg Am.* 1988;70(7):1038-1047.

Levi N, Gjerris F, Dons K. Thoracic disc herniation. *J Neurosurg.* 1998;88:148-150.

Mellion LR, Ladeira CE. The herniated thoracic disc, a review of the literature. *Journal of Manual and Manipulative Therapy.* 2001;9(3):154-163.

Whitcomb DC, Martin SP, Schoen RE, Jho HD. Chronic abdominal pain caused by thoracic disk herniation. *Am J Gastroenterol.* 1995;90:835-837.

Wilke A, Wolf U, Lageard P, Griss P. Thoracic disc herniation: a diagnostic challenge. *Man Ther.* 2000;5(3):181-184.

AUTHOR: BRYAN DENNISON

BASIC INFORMATION

DEFINITION

- Narrowing of the spinal cord space as a result of a space-occupying lesion may lead to spinal cord compression. The lesion is commonly caused by osteophytes, disc herniation, ligamentous thickening or calcification, or tumor.
- Cervical myelopathy is a form of central stenosis. It is compression of the spinal cord at the cervical level usually secondary to arthritic changes and possible disc degeneration. Generally, cervical myelopathy is a progression of cervical spondylosis.

SYNONYMS

- Spinal stenosis
- Myelopathy

ICD-9CM CODES
723.0 Spinal stenosis in cervical region
724.0 Spinal stenosis other than cervical
724.00 Spinal stenosis of unspecified region
724.01 Spinal stenosis of thoracic region
724.02 Spinal stenosis of lumbar region

OPTIMAL NUMBER OF VISITS

3 to 8 visits

MAXIMAL NUMBER OF VISITS

20 to 36 visits

ETIOLOGY

- Central stenosis can occur secondary to any of the following:
  - Disc pathology
  - Degenerative joint disease with osteophyte formation
  - Calcification of the posterior longitudinal ligament
  - Spondylolisthesis
  - Anterior cord compression from protruding disc or posterior osteophytes
  - Anterolateral compression from joints of Luschka in the neck
  - Lateral compression from cervical facets
  - Posterior compression from ligamentum flavum
- These problems/diagnoses may compress the spinal cord and cause damage to the tissues.
- Physiologically, bone spurs or osteophytes typically occur because of wear and tear to the joints. Disc herniations can occur from daily use and/or sudden injuries.

- These lesions narrow the space in which the spinal cord glides during normal movements. If the space is small enough or ragged enough, the cord or meninges are damaged.

EPIDEMIOLOGY AND DEMOGRAPHICS

- Lumbar spinal stenosis is a leading cause of impaired mobility and spinal surgery in the geriatric population, affecting 5 per 1000 Americans over the age 50.
- The age group most prone to central stenosis is between 50 and 60 years of age.
- There does not appear to be a gender preference for central stenosis.
- Cervical myelopathy may be underreported in western countries, since in Japan, it affects 5.7 per 100,000 people (Kokubun).
- Men are twice as likely to suffer from cervical myelopathy as women.

MECHANISM OF INJURY

- Wear and tear from normal or extreme use
- Previous injures to the spine, ligaments, or discs that lead to thickening, inflammation, and irregularities that line and form the spinal column

COMMON SIGNS AND SYMPTOMS

- Numbness, tingling, and muscular dysfunction in the extremities (lower extremities are more common than the upper extremities)
- Gait abnormalities such as decreased stride length and increased base of support
- Increased deep tendon reflexes
- Bowel and bladder dysfunction
- Deep spinal pain
- The following may occur in the cervical region:
  - Tingling in the hands and feet.
  - Weakness and heaviness in the hands; bilateral or unilateral; numbness in the hands and diminished sensation, coordination, fine motor control, and proprioception can also be noticed.
  - Heaviness and numbness can also be noticed in the forearms and upper arms.
  - Spasticity and weakness can also be noted in one or both legs. Patient will complain of balance, coordination, and gait disturbances.
  - Trunk numbness is sometimes experienced.
  - Bowel and bladder symptoms can occur if severe compression is present.
- The following may occur in the lumbar region:
  - Tingling in the feet

  - Saddle paresthesias
  - Changes in bowel or bladder function
  - Loss of balance during gait

AGGRAVATING ACTIVITIES

- Extension activities such as standing up straight, leaning backward, going down a hill or stairs, looking upward, or being upright or in positions that increase axial compression.
- These activities cause a narrowing of the central spinal column.

EASING ACTIVITIES

- Flexion activities such as walking and pushing a cart or walker, bending forward, riding a bike, or going down a hill or stairs.
- These activities increase the space for the spinal cord in the central column.

24-HOUR SYMPTOM PATTERN

- Morning stiffness that lasts for several minutes.
- Typically, symptoms are worse during the day when spinal movement is required for activities of daily living (ADLs).
- Depends on the activity or position of the affected spinal segment.
- Sleep is generally not impaired.

PAST HISTORY FOR THE REGION

- Excessive use or strain to the region.
- Traumatic injuries to spinal tissues.
- Being overweight or obese.
- Greater prevalence in the elderly since arthritic changes and progression of spondylitic changes result in spinal cord compression.
- Often the symptoms begin insidiously but are aggravated by prolonged hyperextension activities such as painting the ceiling or going to the hairdresser.

PHYSICAL EXAMINATION

- Postural deviations: inability to straighten (hunched or leaning forward) or stooped posture.
- Range of motion (ROM) is limited to extension.
- Joint mobility is reduced and painful.
- Traction decreases symptoms.
- Positive straight leg raise at 30 to 40 degrees.

IMPORTANT OBJECTIVE TESTS

- To date, many of the tests commonly used to assess central stenosis have not been validated by research. Common clinical assessment tools include the following:
  - Deep tendon reflex testing that should be hyperreflexic in the case of central stenosis. The increased reflex is an indication of upper motor neuron lesions.

- Straight leg raise testing can be used to test for central stenosis, but generally it has been used as an indicator of peripheral nerve entrapment by a lumbar disc. Its use in diagnosing central stenosis has yet to be validated.
- Balance testing often reveals inability to stand on one leg without losing stability.
- Babinski test will often be positive with central stenosis.
- Passive motion test will often reveal spasticity with motion.
- Quick stretching of calf may cause multiple beats of clonus.
- Dermatomal and myotomal assessment will be positive, but this does not help the clinician differentiate between an upper and lower neuron lesion.
- Vascular and neurological claudication can present similarly. Testing the reproduction of symptoms with a stationary bicycle and a treadmill can give insight to the problem. Vascular claudication will be symptomatic with both bicycle and treadmill testing. Neurogenic claudication will be present with treadmill testing but not present with bicycle testing.

DIFFERENTIAL DIAGNOSIS — Dx

- Spinal cord injury/trauma
- Vascular claudication
- Lower extremity osteoarthritis
- Multiple sclerosis (MS)
- Meningitis
- Somatic source of pain (kidneys, bowel/bladder, etc)
- Hydrocephalus

CONTRIBUTING FACTORS

- Work strain
- Repetitive overuse
- Excessive weight and obesity
- Family history of central stenosis

TREATMENT — Rx

SURGICAL OPTIONS AND OUTCOMES

- Surgical options for central stenosis include the following:
  - Discectomy with or without fusion.
  - Laminectomy: 64% to 85% had good to excellent outcomes at 2 years.
  - Foraminectomy.

- Lumbar stenosis
  - Little is presently known regarding the long-term outcome of surgery for lumbar spinal stenosis or how these outcomes compare to nonsurgical treatment.
  - Results reported thus far appear to indicate that short-term results are generally good with a high percentage of patients expressing satisfaction with their results.
  - The satisfaction tends to deteriorate with time, with only about 60% to 70% of patients satisfied 4 to 7 years after surgery.

REHABILITATION

- 30% to 40% of cervical stenotic patients with cord compression become stable with conservative treatment.
- Treatment should encourage flexion-based stabilization with the avoidance of extension.
- Strength and stabilization of the spinal musculature.
- Postural reeducation.
- Avoid extension, sidebending, and rotation for sustained periods.
- Solid collar may be indicated in the cervical region and lumbar braces in the lower back.
- Balance reeducation.
- Upper and lower extremity strengthening can be initiated, but care must be given to avoid undue stress on the spine.
- No manipulation is indicated in these patients, although mobilization can be used to alleviate joint stiffness and to promote circulation.
- Rehabilitation should include the following:
  - Education in correct use of ice/heat and equipment (traction or transcutaneous electrical stimulation [TENS] units) at home
  - Implementation of a flexion-based home exercise program
  - Teach good body mechanics and encourage good posture
  - Teach good positioning for sleeping or doing ADLs
  - Manual therapy (soft tissue mobilization, traction, or joint mobilization)
  - Modalities: Ice/heat, ultrasound, TENS, or traction
- Initial exercises to promote healing and pain abatement include the following:
  - Self-traction
  - Postural exercises

- Flexion-based ROM exercises within pain-free range
- Core stabilization exercises
- Joint mobilization/manipulation can be used to improve mobility of segments above and below the area and to promote the release of endorphins for pain relief.
- Massage decreases the muscular tension to the surrounding and affected areas, increases circulation to the area, and promotes the release of endorphins.
- Long-term exercises should be used to promote healing and prevent future injury. They should include the following:
  - Progressive stabilization exercises
  - Generalized conditioning exercises

PROGNOSIS

Long-term prognosis for a patient with a central stenosis depends on the severity of the stenosis and pain tolerance of the patient. Short-term relief of symptoms can be achieved in many patients, but symptoms are generally a recurrent problem caused by the degenerative and progressive nature of the pathology.

SIGNS AND SYMPTOMS INDICATING REFERRAL TO PHYSICIAN

- Unrelenting pain or unusual responses to therapy
- Possibility of cancer or organic dysfunction
- Spinal cord symptoms
- Worsening nerve symptoms

SUGGESTED READINGS

Asgarzadie F, Khoo L. Minimally invasive operative management for lumbar spinal stenosis: overview of early and long-term outcomes. *Orthop Clin North Am.* 2007;38(3).

Chad D. Lumbar spinal stenosis. *Neurol Clin.* 2007;25(2).

Dugan SA. The role of exercise in the prevention and management of acute low back pain. *Clin Occup Environ Med.* 2006;5(3):615-632, vi-vii.

Kokubun S, Sato T, Ishii Y, Tanaka. Cervical myelopathy in the Japanese. *Clin Orthop.* 1996;(323):129-138.

Markman J, Gaud C. Lumbar spinal stenosis in older adults: current understanding and future directions. *Clin Geriatr Med.* 2008;24(2).

AUTHOR: SARA GRANNIS

BASIC INFORMATION

DEFINITION

Degenerative joint disease (DJD) can be defined as a breakdown of the lumbar spine facet articular surfaces with a resultant loss of cartilage. This can occur in concert with DDD in which there is a loss of disc height. The breakdown of articular cartilage leads to a resultant inflammatory cascade that can result in bone spurs or osteophyte formation.

SYNONYMS

- Lumbar spine osteoarthritis
- Lumbar spine spondylosis
- Lumbar zygapophyseal (facet) joint pain/arthropathy

ICD-9CM CODES
721.3   Lumbosacral spondylosis without myelopathy
721.4   Thoracic or lumbar spondylosis with myelopathy

OPTIMAL NUMBER OF VISITS

3 to 8 visits

MAXIMAL NUMBER OF VISITS

20 to 36 visits

ETIOLOGY

- Lumbar DJD is generally the result of daily wear and tear in combination with various injuries sustained throughout life that cause the breakdown of healthy tissue.
- Physiologically, the wearing down of the hyaline cartilage leads to an inflammatory response. There is thickening and sclerosis of the subchondral bone and development of osteophytes or bone spurs. This leads to a narrowing of the joint space, loss of shock absorption, and pain.

EPIDEMIOLOGY AND DEMOGRAPHICS

- 15% to 45% of adults >30 years of age have radiological evidence of lumbar degenerative changes (prevalence increases with age).
- 40% to 85% of patients complaining of low back pain (LBP) as confirmed by computed tomography (CT) scans
- Facet degenerative changes seen level by level as follows:
  L1/2: 53%
  L2/3: 66%
  L3/4: 72%
  L4/5: 79%
  L5-S1: 59%
- Facet degenerative changes seen by decade of life:
  20-29 years of age: 57%
  30-39 years of age: 82%

40-49 years of age: 93%
50-59 years of age: 97%
>60 years of age: 100%
- Symptomatic lumbar DJD is rarely found in people younger than 40 years of age; it is more commonly found in people older than 60 years of age.
- Men have a higher prevalence and degree of facet degeneration than women.

MECHANISM OF INJURY

- Symptoms related to degenerative changes to the joint rarely occur as a result of direct trauma. Usually, it is a gradual process of physiological change that eventually results in pain and dysfunction. Activities that can be associated with the degenerative changes include the following:
  ○ Daily use of the lumbar spine
  ○ Excessive use/strain of the lumbar spine (including excessive weight)
  ○ Injuries, such as car accidents, slips and falls, and strains/sprains, that cause inflammation in the lumbar spine

COMMON SIGNS AND SYMPTOMS

- Unilateral pain in the back and gluteal region.
- Stiffness in the lumbar spine.
- Loss of normal lumbar lordosis.
- Facet joint pain tends to be localized over the area and surrounding paraspinal musculature and gluteal region.
- According to Fukui et al, the referral patterns of the lumbar zygapophyseal joint are as follows:
  L1/2: Lumbar spine
  L2/3: Lumbar spine and greater trochanter
  L3/4: Greater trochanter, lateral thigh, posterior thigh, and groin
  L4/5: Lumbar spine, greater trochanter, lateral/posterior thigh, and groin
  L5/S1: Gluteal, greater trochanter, lateral/posterior thigh, and groin
- If inflammation and/or stenosis occurs (from the osteophytes) and narrows the nerve root foramen, there could be typical nerve root referral into the lower extremities.

AGGRAVATING ACTIVITIES

- Inactivity leads to stiffness. Inactivity allows the inflammation to "pool" and increase pressure leading to discomfort and loss of available movement.
- Activity (especially weight-bearing activities) can irritate the joint surfaces.
- Typically, movements that "close down" the facet joints (extension, ipsilateral side flexion, and ipsilateral rotation) and cause more joint compression are more painful and limited.
- Joint movement increases "wear and tear" and inflammation/irritation to the

articular surfaces. The more compression involved with the movement the more "wear and tear" will occur.
- Walking.
- Standing.
- Bending backward.
- Lifting and carrying objects.

EASING ACTIVITIES

- Flexion-based activities
- Sitting
- Lying down with knees flexed
- Rest

24-HOUR SYMPTOM PATTERN

- Stiffness may be present for the first 10 to 15 minutes in the morning.
- Better after a warm shower and taking medication.
- Can worsen with excessive movement.
- Stiffens again in the evening.

PAST HISTORY FOR THE REGION

- Lengthy history of being overweight or obese.
- Heavy physical jobs or recreational activities that require excessive use/strain of the lumbar spine (lifting, bending, twisting, repetitive impact, or hypermobility).
- The longer one lives, the more likely degeneration will occur.

PHYSICAL EXAMINATION

- Loss of normal spinal curvature (most common is forward head with an loss of lumbar lordosis)
- Loss of trunk mobility or lumbar spine ROM (especially extension, ipsilateral side bend, and contralateral rotation)
- Localized pain, loss of passive physiological intervertebral movement, and loss of passive accessory joint movement
- Crepitus with movement
- Lumbar muscular restrictions and tenderness

IMPORTANT OBJECTIVE TESTS

- To date, many of the tests commonly used to assess lumbar DJD have not been validated by research. Common clinical assessment tools include the following:
  ○ AROM and PROM will both be limited into extension, ipsilateral sidebend, and contralateral rotation.
  ○ PROM tends to be greater than AROM because of muscle guarding.
  ○ Unilateral posterior to anterior pressure on the pathological joint will be tender and lack mobility. Segmental rotation will be limited at the target segment.
  ○ Lumbar quadrant testing similar to the cervical Spurling's test has been used as a provocative test to determine whether radicular pain into the

leg is of lumbar origin. Its reliability has yet to be established.

- o Neurological testing can be used to determine which nerve is affected by lumbar spine degeneration.

DIFFERENTIAL DIAGNOSIS

- DDD
- Lumbar disc herniation
- Lumbar sprain/strain
- Sacroiliac joint dysfunction
- Ankylosing spondylitis
- Nerve root pathology
- Kidney dysfunction
- Urogenital dysfunction
- Gastrointestinal dysfunction
- Cancer

CONTRIBUTING FACTORS

- Physical strain from job or recreational activities
- Repetitive injures to the lumbar spine
- Traumatic injuries to the lumbar spine
- Family history
- Obesity
- Poor posture
- Poor health (smoking, poor diet, or long-term use of steroids)

TREATMENT

SURGICAL OPTIONS

- Lumbar fusion
- Lumbar laminectomy or laminoplasty
- Foraminotomy
- Facet rhizotomy

SURGICAL OUTCOMES

- Fusion: Up to 90% success (especially if the patient had a positive response to facet nerve blocks)
- Laminectomy: 70% to 80% success

REHABILITATION

- The focus of rehabilitation should be on the following:

- o Education regarding the correct use of ice/heat at home.
- o Implementation of a home exercise program.
- o Teach good body mechanics and encourage good posture.
- o Teach good positioning for sleeping and good body mechanics for working or doing ADLs.
- o Manual therapy (soft tissue mobilization, traction, and joint mobilization).
- o Modalities: ice/heat, ultrasound, electrical stimulation, or traction.
- Initial exercises can include the following:
  - o Stretches: Double knee to chest, single knee to chest, hamstring, and piriformis
  - o Abdominal isometrics
  - o Core strengthening: Exercise ball, Pilates-based exercises, and mat exercises
  - o Aquatic exercises
- Joint mobilization and manipulation may be used to unload the facet joints, lubricate the facet joint, improve articular movement (localized and segments above and below).
- Soft tissue massage may be used to decrease pain by relaxing muscular tension and increase endorphin release.
- Exercise should focus on the following:
  - o Decreasing muscular and joint stiffness
  - o Improving joint alignment by increasing muscular support
  - o Improving posture: Progressive thoracic extension and shoulder extension/retraction
  - o Creating a sense of control over the symptoms and the condition
  - o Decrease pain by relaxing muscular tension and increase endorphin release
  - o Generalized conditioning
  - o Increasing metabolism and promoting weight loss/management

PROGNOSIS

Long-term prognosis for a patient with a lumbar DJD depends on the extent of

wear and tear and ability to reduce the joint strain (weight, posture, activity, etc). The condition is progressive and the patient is likely to experience a pattern of symptom reduction followed by periods of symptom aggravation.

SIGNS AND SYMPTOMS INDICATING REFERRAL TO PHYSICIAN

- Unrelenting pain, unusual response to therapy
- Possibility of cancer or meningitis
- Spinal cord symptoms
- Worsening nerve symptoms

SUGGESTED READINGS

Cohen SP, Srinivasa R. Pathogenesis, diagnosis, and treatment of lumbar zygapophysial (facet) joint pain. *Anesthesiology.* 2007;106(3).

Dugan SA. Exercise for health and wellness at midlife and beyond: balancing benefits and risks. *Phys Med Rehabil Clin N Am.* 2007;18(3):555-575.

Dugan SA. The role of exercise in the prevention and management of acute low back pain. *Clin Occup Environ Med.* 2006;5(3):615-632, vi-vii.

Eubanks JD, et al. Prevalence of lumbar facet arthrosis and its relationship to age, sex, and race: and anatomic study of cadaveric specimens. *Spine.* 2007;32(19):2058-2062.

Fukui S, Ohseto K, Shiotani M, Ohno K, Karasawa H, Naganuma Y. Distribution of referred pain from the lumbar zygapophyseal joints and dorsal rami. *Clin J Pain.* 1997;13(4):303-307.

Manchikanti L, et al. Age-related prevalence of facet-joint involvement in chronic neck and low back pain. *Pain Physician.* 2008;11(1):67-75.

AUTHOR: SARA GRANNIS

BASIC INFORMATION

DEFINITION

Interforaminal stenosis can be described as the loss of interforaminal area. This narrowing can result in impingement of the nerve root. The most common sources of lesions that decrease interforaminal space are loss of intervertebral disc height, inflammation, osteophytes, disc herniation, ligamentous thickening, calcification, and tumor.

SYNONYM

Spinal stenosis with radiculitis

ICD-9CM CODES
723.0 Spinal stenosis in cervical region
724.0 Spinal stenosis other than cervical
724.00 Spinal stenosis of unspecified region
724.01 Spinal stenosis of thoracic region
724.02 Spinal stenosis of lumbar region

OPTIMAL NUMBER OF VISITS

3 to 8 visits

MAXIMAL NUMBER OF VISITS

20 to 36 visits

ETIOLOGY

- Bone spurs or osteophytes typically occur because of wear and tear to the joints (facets and/or vertebral bodies). Disc herniations can occur from daily use and/or sudden injuries. Physiologically, these lesions narrow the space for the nerve to rest and glide during normal movements.
- Because of wear and tear or injury, the space that the nerve occupies shrinks and eventually the nerve becomes impinged. If the space is small enough or ragged enough, the nerve is damaged.
- The pathology depends on the source or sources of the stenosis. DJD, DDD, and disc herniations can occur because of wear and tear or injury. In any case, inflammation is the normal response of the body, but this, too, can decrease the space available for the nerve.

EPIDEMIOLOGY AND DEMOGRAPHICS

- Individuals >50 to 60 years of age are most prone to interforaminal stenosis.
- Both males and females are equally likely to suffer from interforaminal stenosis.

MECHANISM OF INJURY

- Interforaminal stenosis is rarely the result of direct or acute trauma. The narrowing of the space is generally a gradual, progressive disorder. Wear and tear from normal or extreme use can lead to physiological responses to the stressors.
- Over time, the body's response to the stressors can encroach into the interforaminal space.
- Injuries to the joint, ligaments, discs, or nerves lead to thickenings, inflammation, and irregularities that line and form the foramen.

COMMON SIGNS AND SYMPTOMS

- Limited movement and/or positions, especially those that close down the intervertebral foramen.
- Postural deformities that open up the foramen (leaning the head or body away from the affected foramen) are seen in highly irritable patients.
- In the spine, the nerve that is entrapped within the intervertebral foramen will vary. In the cervical spine, the spinal nerve root impacted will correspond with the lower vertebrae of the spinal unit (e.g., C5 nerve root will be entrapped within the C4/5 intervertebral foramen). In the lumbar and thoracic spine, the spinal nerve root impacted corresponds with the upper vertebrae of the spinal unit (e.g., the L5 nerve root will be entrapped within the L5/S1 spinal segment).
- Numbness and tingling along dermatomes occur if the nerve is involved.
- Pain is described as shooting, burning, stinging, electrical zapping, etc.
- Weakness and dysfunction of muscles within the affected myotomes.
- Radicular symptoms will follow the affected nerve root's dermatome, myotome, or sclerotome (cervical refers into the arm and hand, thoracic refers around the trunk, and lumbar refers into the leg and foot).

AGGRAVATING ACTIVITIES

- Movement that "closes down" the foraminal opening (extension, ipsilateral side flexion, and ipsilateral rotation). These movements physically narrow the foramen, creating less room for the nerve.
  - Lumbar and thoracic spine: Walking, standing, bending backward
  - Cervical spine: Driving, looking upward, washing hair
- Axial compression (external physical source or gravitational pull) such as lifting and carrying

EASING ACTIVITIES

- Movement that "opens up" the foraminal opening (flexion, contralateral side flexion, and contralateral rotation). These movements physically open up the foramen creating more room for the nerve.
  - Lumbar and thoracic spine: Sitting, bending forward
  - Cervical spine: Rotating toward or looking down
- Axial decompression (traction)

24-HOUR SYMPTOM PATTERN

- Stiffness may be present for the first 10 to 15 minutes in the morning.
- Typically worse during the day when spinal movement is required for ADLs.
- Depends on the activity or position of the affected spinal segment.
- Sleep can be affected in highly irritable patients.

PAST HISTORY FOR THE REGION

- Patient will commonly complain that symptoms began insidiously.
- Several years of history of back or neck pain that has been increasing in intensity and frequency with each new bout of pain.
- Daily activities that require excessive use of the region is common.
- Traumatic injuries to spinal tissues may be present.

PHYSICAL EXAMINATION

- Postural deviations: Head or trunk leans away from the side of pain.
- ROM is limited, and symptoms are increased with extension, ipsilateral side flexion, and ipsilateral rotation.
- Joint mobility is reduced at the affected segments.
- Axial compression increases symptoms; axial decompression decreases symptoms.

IMPORTANT OBJECTIVE TESTS

Common clinical assessment tools include the following:
- AROM and PROM will both be limited into extension, ipsilateral sidebending, and ipsilateral rotation.
- PROM tends to be greater than AROM because of muscle guarding.
- Unilateral posterior to anterior pressure on the pathological joint will be tender and lack mobility. Segmental rotation will be limited at the target segment.
- In the case of radiculopathies associated with cervical dysfunction, Wainner et al reported that the following clinical examination findings could be predictive of a cervical origin to radicular pain:
  - Positive Spurling's test
  - Positive neck distraction test
  - Positive ULTT of the median nerve
  - <60 degrees active cervical rotation to involved side

- If 3 out of 4 findings were positive, there was a 94% specificity that the symptoms were of cervical origin.
- If 4 out of 4 findings were positive, there was a 99% specificity that the symptoms were of cervical origin.
- Lumbar quadrant testing has been used as a provocative test to determine whether radicular pain into the leg is of lumbar origin. To date, its reliability has yet to be established.

DIFFERENTIAL DIAGNOSIS

- Spinal cord injury/trauma
- Vascular claudication
- Lower extremity osteoarthritis
- MS
- Neuropathy
- Localized peripheral nerve damage (i.e., "burners or stingers")
- Discogenic referred pain
- Somatic source of pain (lung, heart, gall bladder, spleen, etc.)

CONTRIBUTING FACTORS

- Work or repetitive activity strain
- Postural abnormality
- Genetic predisposition
- Past history of trauma
- Repetitive overuse
- Excessive weight
- Family history

TREATMENT

SURGICAL OPTIONS

- Laminectomy
- Foraminotomy
- Discectomy (microdiscectomy, discectomy with/without fusion, etc)

SURGICAL OUTCOMES

- Laminectomy: 64% to 85% had good to excellent outcomes at 2 years.

- Discectomy with fusion (cervical spine): 95% satisfied patients.

REHABILITATION

- Rehabilitation should include the following:
  - Education in the correct use of ice/heat and equipment (traction or TENS units) at home
  - Implementation of a flexion-based home exercise program
  - Teach good body mechanics and encourage good posture
  - Teach good positioning for sleeping or doing ADLs
  - Manual therapy (soft tissue mobilization, traction, and joint mobilization)
  - Modalities: Ice/heat, ultrasound, electrical stimulation, traction
- Self-traction, postural exercises, ROM exercises within pain-free range and core stabilization exercises can be used initially to promote healing.
- Joint mobilization and manipulation can be used to open up the foramen and allow decompression of the nerve. It can also allow for the injured section of the nerve to reposition and decrease the localized inflammation that may exist around the nerve.
- Massage can be used to decrease the muscular tension to the surrounding and affected areas and to increase circulation to the area. Massage may also result in the release endorphins in the body.
- Exercise is used to improve joint health and mobility, increase spinal support and improve posture, decrease muscular stiffness and spasms, and create a sense of control over the symptoms.
- Flexion-based exercises should be encouraged to open the intervertebral foramen and allow healing and circulation in the region. Extension-based exercises generally aggravate the patient's symptoms but can be used in adjacent

regions to decrease the stress placed on the affected spinal segments.
- Adjacent regions should be assessed and interventions implemented to address abnormalities that may contribute to the stenosis at the affected segment.

PROGNOSIS

Interforaminal stenosis is considered a progressive degenerative disorder. The clinician can alleviate the patient's current symptoms and focus treatment on preventing further episodes, but studies to date show a poor prognosis for long-term alleviation of symptoms.

SIGNS AND SYMPTOMS INDICATING REFERRAL TO PHYSICIAN

- Unrelenting pain or unusual responses to therapy
- Possibility of cancer or organic dysfunction
- Spinal cord symptoms
- Worsening nerve symptoms

SUGGESTED READINGS

Chad D. Lumbar spinal stenosis. *Neurol Clin.* 2007;25(2).

Dugan SA. The role of exercise in the prevention and management of acute low back pain. *Clin Occup Environ Med.* 2006;5(3):615-32, vi-vii.

Erickson M. Outpatient anterior cervical discectomy and fusion. *Am J Orthop.* 2007; 36(8):429-432.

Wainner RS, Fritz JM, Boninger M, Irrgang JJ, Delitto T, Allison SC. Reliability and diagnostic accuracy of the clinical examination and patient self-report measures for cervical radiculopathy. *Spine.* 2003;28(1):52-62.

AUTHOR: SARA GRANNIS

BASIC INFORMATION

DEFINITION

- Disc herniation or disc bulges are synonymous terms used to describe a condition in which disc material extends beyond the perimeter of the normal disc space.
- The four common classes of disc herniations are as follows:
  - Disc *protrusion* occurs when the nucleus pulposus bulges outward into the annulus fibrosis but no damage is done to the annulus.
  - Disc *prolapse* occurs when the nucleus pulposus bulges outward into the annulus and annular lamina are damaged.
  - Disc *extrusion* occurs when the nucleus pulposus breaks past the outer lamina of the annulus fibrosis and into the space beyond.
  - Disc *sequestration* occurs when nucleus pulposus breaks free of the annulus.

SYNONYMS

- Disc bulge
- Herniated disc

ICD-9CM CODES
722.10 Displacement of lumbar intervertebral disc without myelopathy
722.52 Degeneration of lumbar or lumbosacral intervertebral disc

OPTIMAL NUMBER OF VISITS

8 visits or less

MAXIMAL NUMBER OF VISITS

20 visits

ETIOLOGY

- In the lumbar region, disc herniations occur at L4/5 and L5/S1 90% of the time. L3/4 is the next most common disc to be injured.
- The disc can be injured anywhere along its periphery. Most disc bulges will occur in the posterior lateral aspect of the disc. The reason for this occurrence is the result of anatomical differences that occur in this region. There are fewer laminar layers of the annulus fibrosis, as well as a greater number of incomplete laminar layers. Additionally, blood supply enters the disc in the posterior lateral region. The penetration of the blood supply weakens the area.
- Disc pathology rarely occurs as a result of acute trauma alone. Disc injury in most cases results from a degenerative

process. When the disc is loaded beyond it physiological capacity, the disc is likely to fail at the cartilaginous endplates. Injury to the endplates allows the contents of the vertebral body to enter into the nucleus of the disc. Chemically, the contents of the vertebral body will react with the contents of the nucleus to degrade the annulus from the inner lamina of the annulus outward. As the disc degrades, fewer annular lamina are available to resist loading and more stress is placed on each collagen fiber of the annulus. Further insults to the disc will increase the likelihood of additional degradation and eventually lead to the failure of the annulus and the development of a disc bulge.
- As the disc bulges outward against the ligament and the dura of the lumbar spine, a dull, deep, poorly localized pain in the back is experienced.
- If the disc bulges posterolaterally against the nerve root, the result is a sharp nerve root pain.
- When the disc herniates and the thick gelatinous fluid of the nucleus pulposus flows around the dura and the nerve roots, an agonizing and persistent back pain will result.

EPIDEMIOLOGY AND DEMOGRAPHICS

- The most common age grouping for people to injure spinal discs is between 30 and 40 years of age. At this age, the disc is still gelatinous in nature. As a person ages, the water content within the disc diminishes.
- Most disc herniations do not hurt. In asymptomatic patients, magnetic resonance imaging studies have demonstrated that 39% to 50% of people had lumbar disc herniations, yet they were asymptomatic.

MECHANISM OF INJURY

- Bending forward with or without rotation
- Falling onto buttock with spine flexed
- Coughing and sneezing
- Bearing down for a bowel movement

COMMON SIGNS AND SYMPTOMS

- The disc will commonly refer pain locally into the low back, but in addition to this, the symptoms will commonly extend down posteriorly into the gluteal region. Pain that extends beyond the gluteal region and into the leg is most likely a result of nerve irritation. Symptoms can include referral to the lower thoracic or upper lumbar region, abdomen, flanks, groin, genitals, thighs, knees, calves, ankles, feet, and toes.

- With an L4/5 posterior lateral disc herniation, the L5 nerve root will be compressed.
- With an L4/5 central disc herniation, the L4 nerve root will be compressed.

AGGRAVATING ACTIVITIES

- Bending forward.
- Prolonged sitting.
- Driving.
- Lying for a prolonged period of time.
- Lifting activities.
- Coughing, sneezing, or bearing down to have a bowel movement.
- If disc pressure during upright standing is used as normal disc pressure, sitting increases the pressure on the disc 40%, bending forward will increase the disc pressure 50%, and seated flexion will increase the disc pressure 80%.
- Coughing, sneezing, and bearing down to have a bowel movement will also increase the patient's symptoms because of the increase in abdominal pressure, which in turn places a compressive load on the disc.

EASING ACTIVITIES

- Lying supine with the knee and hips flexed.
- Physicians will often prescribe anti-inflammatory medications, as well as muscle relaxants and pain medications to address the patient's symptoms.
- Walking.
- Repetitive lumbar extension motion.
- If disc pressure during upright standing is used as normal disc pressure, sidelying decreases the pressure on the disc 25% and lying supine will decrease the disc pressure 75%.
- Walking motion helps to promote circulation in the region of the disc.

24-HOUR SYMPTOM PATTERN

- The patient with a disc injury will complain of stiffness and pain in the morning that will last for more than 20 minutes.
- Symptoms will increase during the day and if sitting for too long.
- Sleeping may or may not be problematic.

PAST HISTORY FOR THE REGION

- Because of the degenerative and progressive nature of disc degradation, the patient will often complain of several bouts of LBP over the course of several years.
- The pain and discomfort will be present for several days to several weeks but will eventually resolve on its own.
- Each subsequent episode of LBP is generally worse than the prior episode.
- Exacerbating event is usually an activity that requires bending forward or flexion.

PHYSICAL EXAMINATION

- Patients with an injury to the disc will often present with a lateral shift.
- In the case of a disc injury, the curvature occurs away from the side of injury. Therefore a disc injury on the right side will result in a spinal curve to the left.
- The reason for this curve is that the injury will result in increased tissue sensitivity in the region of pathology. In response to this tissue sensitivity, the body will try to offload the region. This is accomplished through the lateral shift.
- It is important to note that this does not occur in all disc pathology, but when it does occur, disc pathology should move higher the list of possible pathology.
- Global muscles, such as the quadratus lumborum, iliopsoas, and gluteal muscles, are often tender to palpation.

IMPORTANT OBJECTIVE TESTS

- Lumbar ROM test
  - Flexion will be limited and will reproduce the patient's low back symptoms. Extension may be restricted, but the limitation will be stiffness instead of the patient's lumbar symptoms. Sidebend may be limited ipsilaterally.
- Straight leg raise test
  - Devillé et al compiled 15 studies that used straight leg raise tests to detect lumbar disc herniations.
  - Positive: Paresthesias in lower extremity that are changed with sensitizing maneuvers.
  - Sensitivity: 0.91; specificity: 0.26.
- Contralateral straight leg test
  - Devillé et al compiled eight studies that used cross straight leg raise tests to detect lumbar disc herniations.
  - Positive: Raising contralateral leg produces patient's symptoms in the involved extremity.
  - Sensitivity: 0.29; specificity: 0.88.
- When these tests results are positive, there is a 97% probability that a disc bulge is present in the lumbar spine.

DIFFERENTIAL DIAGNOSIS

- Muscle strain
- Ligament strain
- Stenosis
- DDD
- Spondylosis
- Spondylolysis
- Interforaminal stenosis
- Radiculopathy
- Instability

TREATMENT

SURGICAL OPTIONS

- Discectomy/microdiscectomy
- Percutaneous discectomy
- Laminectomy/laminotomy
- Anterior or posterior fusion
- Disc replacement
- Intradiscal electrothermal therapy
- Flexible posterior stabilizer
- Disc regeneration

SURGICAL OUTCOMES

- A review of literature indicated that both surgery and physical therapy produced good reduction in symptoms in 70% of patients.
- In a separate cross-sectional survey, the results of patients status postlumbar disc herniation surgery was reviewed. At 2 months postoperative, there was an 87% reduced leg pain and an 81% reduced back pain. Moderate-to-severe pain was still present in 25% in the leg and 20% in the back.

REHABILITATION

- The goal of rehabilitation is twofold: First, the focus should be on decreasing the patient's symptoms. Once the symptoms have diminished, then the focus of the rehabilitative process will turn to prevention of further episodes.
- As a result of injury, the body will attempt to protect the region. This is accomplished by contracting the large global muscles of the region, which is in response to the inflammation that will shut down the local muscle fibers. The body must protect and minimize stress to this area, and it does so by contracting the large muscle fibers. The lack of motion to the region impedes circulation to the region. Therefore chemical irritants that have been brought into the region in response to the injury do not leave the region.
- To decrease inflammation, the clinician should consider the following:
  - Myofascial release techniques to relax the large muscle groups
  - Joint mobilization
  - Lumbar traction
  - Walking
  - Exercises that promote movement of the region in a pain-free range
  - Cold or hot pack
  - Ultrasound
  - Electrical stimulation
- Once the inflammatory process has decreased, the focus of rehabilitation should be as follows:
  - Identifying the factors that contribute to the disc pathology. Although the disc has only a limited capacity

to repair itself, if the clinician can remove the factors that stress the region, then further insult to the injured disc can be prevented.

- Initially, exercises that minimize the stress to the disc should be used. If disc pressure during upright standing is used as normal disc pressure, lying in a hooklying position decreases intradiscal pressure by 65%. Exercises that take this into consideration will help to decrease the stress placed on the disc. Pain-free ROM exercises should also be implemented. Extension-based exercises are preferable to flexion exercises.
- Based on current evidence, intermittent or continuous traction as a single treatment for LBP cannot be recommended for mixed groups of patients with LBP with and without sciatica.
- Recent studies suggest that joint mobilization/manipulation is beneficial in a subset of patients with acute low back symptoms, but its efficacy in the treatment of chronic LBP is still in question.
  - In a mix of acute and chronic LBP patients, manipulation/mobilization provides either similar or better pain outcomes in the short- and long-term when compared with placebo and with other treatments, such as McKenzie therapy, medical care, management by physical therapists, soft tissue treatment, and back education programs.
- Massage has been shown to improve lymph drainage and increase superficial tissue temperature.
- In putting together the European guidelines for the management of chronic LBP, 40 different therapies were scrutinized for evidence of effectiveness and only the following 6 were ultimately recommended:
  - Weak opioids, supervised exercise, brief education on LBP, cognitive behavioral treatment, multidisciplinary biopsychosocial rehabilitation, and nonsteroidal antiinflammatory drugs (NSAIDs)
- Based on the works of McKenzie, it has been hypothesized that repetitive lumbar extension can reduce lower extremity paresthesias in patients with lumbar disc involvement. Clinically, repetitive extension has been observed to reduce leg paresthesias. This phenomenon has been termed *centralization*. McKenzie has hypothesized that the mechanism of centralization is the anterior migration of the nucleus with repetitive extension of the lumbar region. Studies suggest that when the annulus is intact the contents of the disc will move anteriorly with repetitive lumbar extension. When the annulus is not intact, lumbar

extension does not produce anterior translation of the disc.

- Initially, home exercises that minimize the stress to the disc should be used with progressive levels of stress being added as the disc heals. Exercises that stress the disc do so in the following manner:
  - Supine with lower extremity flexed to 45 degrees and knees extended increases pressure 50%, prone extension with upper and lower extremity extension increases pressure 80%, and supine curl up increases pressure 110%

CONTRIBUTING FACTORS

- Poor posture
- An occupation that requires repetitive bending or sitting
- Hypomobility in adjacent regions, especially the sacral iliac joint
- Leg length discrepancy
- Poor activation of local lumbar muscle groups such as the multifidus and the transverse abdominus muscles
- Tight muscle groups especially the hip flexors and hamstrings

PROGNOSIS

Most patients will fully recover from initial episodes of LBP that are the result of disc pathology. With severe symptoms, the patient and clinician can expect slow progress, depending on magnitude of herniation. On average, this process generally takes 6 weeks.

SIGNS AND SYMPTOMS INDICATING REFERRAL TO PHYSICIAN

- Constant unrelenting LBP: Infection or tumor
- Pain that does not change with position: Infection or tumor
- Significant and unexplained weight loss: Tumor
- Nocturnal Pain: Tumor
- Blood in urine or stool: Urinary pathology
- Saddle anesthesia: Cauda equina syndrome
- Major trauma: Fracture
- Fevers and chills: Infection or tumor
- Sudden onset of bowel and/or bladder dysfunction: Cauda equina syndrome
- Progressive bilateral lower extremity paresthesias that are nondermatomal: Cauda equina syndrome

SUGGESTED READINGS

Atlas SJ, et al. Long-term outcomes of surgical and nonsurgical management of sciatica secondary to a lumbar disc herniation: 10 year results from the Maine lumbar spine study. *Spine.* 2005;30:927-935.

Balague F, Mannion AF, Pellise F, Cedraschi C. Clinical update: low back pain. *Lancet.* 2007;369(9563):726-728.

Bronfort G, Haas M, Evans R, Bouter L. Efficacy of spinal manipulation and mobilization for low back pain and neck pain: a systematic review and best evidence synthesis. *The Spine Journal.* 2004;4(3):335-356.

Clarke JA, van Tulder M, Blomberg S, de Vet H, van der Heijden G, Bronfort G. Traction for low back pain with or without sciatica: an updated systematic review within the framework of the cochrane collaboration. *Spine.* 2006;31(14):1591-1599.

Deville WL, van der Windt DA, Dzaferagi A, Bezemer PD, Bouter LM. The test of Lasègue: systematic review of the accuracy in diagnosing herniated discs. *Spine.* 2000;25(9):1140-1147.

Flynn T, Fritz J, Whitman J, et al. A clinical prediction rule for classifying patients with low back pain who demonstrate short-term improvement with spinal manipulation. *Spine.* 2002;27:2835-2843.

Hakkinen A, et al. Pain, trunk muscle strength, spinal mobility, and disability following lumbar disc surgery. *J Rehabil Med.* 2003;35:236-240.

McKenzie RA, May S. *The Lumbar Spine. Mechanical Diagnosis and Therapy.* 2nd ed. Vols 1 and 2. Waikanae, New Zealand: Spinal Publications; 2003.

Wainner RS, Fritz JM, Irrgang JJ, Boninger ML, Delitto A, Allison S. Reliability and diagnostic accuracy of the clinical examination and patient self-report measures for cervical radiculopathy. *Spine.* 2003;28(1):52-62.

AUTHOR: DERRICK SUEKI

BASIC INFORMATION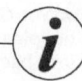

DEFINITION

Lumbar instability refers to excess motion in the lumbar spine segments in which a normal external force or load causes hypermobility and pain. Excessive motion is defined as an excessive rotational segmental angle or segmental translation >3 mm.

ICD-9CM CODE
724.6 Disorders of sacrum

OPTIMAL NUMBER OF VISITS

8 visits

MAXIMAL NUMBER OF VISITS

18 visits

ETIOLOGY

- Lumbar segmental instability can be caused by several factors.
- The excessive intervertebral motion may be due to degenerative changes in the intervertebral discs (DDD), spondylolisthesis, fracture, trauma, or a previous surgical procedure.
- The excessive motion can put pressure on the spinal cord, cauda equina, or nerve roots.
- Excessive intersegmental motion can also stress the joint capsule or ligaments.

EPIDEMIOLOGY AND DEMOGRAPHICS

- The primary age group to experience lumbar instability is 20 to 30 years of age.
- In the cases of instability caused by degenerative changes, the age group is >60 years of age.

MECHANISM OF INJURY

- Lumbar instability may be caused by a severe sprain, fracture, spondylolisthesis, or previous lumbar surgery.
- Degenerative mechanisms include DJD, DDD, and spondylosis.

COMMON SIGNS AND SYMPTOMS

- Patients with lumbar instability will usually report a history of recurrent/episodic locking, catching, or giving way of the low back during active motion.
- They may use terms like "clicking," "clunking," or "slipping" or may report a feeling of instability.
- Patients may report a sharp pain with motion or a painful arc of motion.
- They may report aching in the lumbar spine for several days after an episode of instability.

- They will usually report increased back pain after prolonged positioning and/or pain at the end-range of lumbar motion or on the return to neutral.
- The intensity of pain may seem excessive relative to the provoking force or activity. The symptom onset occurs after what seems to be a simple activity with minimal provocation, and the symptoms often resolve rapidly.
- There is no constant pattern of dysfunction or symptom onset.
- The pain is located in the lumbar region and may radiate into one or both buttocks or posterior thighs if the adjacent nerve root is irritated.
- Patients often report no relief or only temporary relief from previous intervention.

AGGRAVATING ACTIVITIES

- End-range positions.
- Sustained postures.
- Rapid movements.
- Patients often report no consistent findings for aggravating activities, positions, or motions.

EASING ACTIVITIES

- Moving slowly in midrange usually alleviates symptoms.
- Avoiding sustained activities or postures.

24-HOUR SYMPTOM PATTERN

- There is often no 24-hour pattern of symptoms.
- Sometimes symptoms are increased at the end of the day.
- They may report increased pain and stiffness first thing in the morning on arising if sustained sleeping postures are provocative.

PAST HISTORY FOR THE REGION

- Patients may report a history of back injury or trauma.
- There may be a history of trauma in which the passive ligamentous structures and joint capsule did not fully heal. The resultant scar tissue and collagen is not as strong or as regularly aligned to restrain outside forces.
- They often report a lack of response to intervention or only temporary symptom relief with intervention.
- They often report a long-term history of episodic back pain that is increasing in frequency and intensity.

PHYSICAL EXAMINATION

- Posterior skin creases in the trunk.
- Limited trunk ROM in a specific direction, possibly a painful arc of movement.
- They may demonstrate excessive ROM.
- Abnormal quality of movement, with hinging or catching.

- In the later stages, patients may be cautious or guarded with motion since they know which motions may provoke the symptoms.
- May need to use hands to walk up the thighs on the return from a forward-bent position (Gower's sign).
- Abnormal accessory movement testing indicating loss of stiffness or increased neutral zone at one segment.
- Local tenderness to palpation, "boggy" end-feel with accessory movement testing at the affected level. There may be palpable bands of local muscle hypertonicity.
- Excessive physiological movements on segmental testing, positive spring test, and positive anterior or posterior shear test.
- Positive H and I test for combined motion movement patterns.

Physical Examination Finding	Reliability
Painful arc in flexion	0.69
Painful arc on return to neutral from flexion	0.61
Instability catch: Sudden acceleration or deceleration of trunk motion outside the primary plane of motion	0.25
Reversal of lumbopelvic rhythm: On return from forward bend, shifts the pelvis anteriorly and flexes the knees	0.60
Posterior shear test	0.35
Prone instability test: symptom reproduction with prone over table edge posterior-anterior (PA) provocation, improved with PA while patient is actively extending legs off the floor	0.87

Lumbar Instability Finding	Sensitivity	Specificity
<37 years of age	0.57	0.81
Lumbar flexion range over 53 degrees	0.68	0.86
Total extension range over 26 degrees	0.50	0.76
Lack of hypomobility during intervertebral testing	0.43	0.95
Hypermobility during intervertebral motion testing	0.46	0.81
Passive lumbar extension test	0.84	0.90

- The presence of at least 53 degrees of lumbar flexion or a lack of hypomobility with intervertebral motion testing resulted in a positive likelihood ratio of 4.3 (95% CI: 1.8, 10.6), for predicting radiographic instability.

- The positive likelihood ratio of the passive lumbar extension test was 8.84 (95% confidence interval = 4.51-17.33).

IMPORTANT OBJECTIVE TESTS

- Positive radiographic findings for excessive translation with flexion or extension films.
- For instability to be diagnosed in the lumbar spine, there must be >3 mm of translation of the superior segment on the inferior segment with flexion/extension radiographs.
- Additional radiographic signs of instability include traction spurs, retrolisthesis or anterolisthesis, and/or degenerative scoliosis, and excessive angular or translational motion on flexion-extension radiographs.

DIFFERENTIAL DIAGNOSIS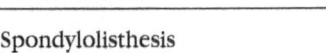

- Spondylolisthesis
- Fracture
- Strain/sprain
- DJD
- DDD
- Facet syndrome

CONTRIBUTING FACTORS

- A positive Beighton index
- Generalized ligamentous laxity
- History of trauma to the passive spinal restraints
- Degenerative changes
- Poor proprioception and muscular control/stability.

TREATMENT

SURGICAL OPTIONS

- Surgery may be indicated for progressive neurological deficit, lack of response to conservative intervention, and unrelenting symptoms.

- Fusion of the unstable segments is generally the surgical option of choice.

REHABILITATION

- Proprioceptive training.
- Specific exercises to facilitate recruitment of the stabilizing muscles, including deep fibers of the lumbar multifidi, transverse abdominus, and pelvic floor.
- Trunk stabilization and abdominal strengthening exercises.
- Strengthening exercises for the hip extensors and abductors.
- Manual therapy to restore lost motion in the joints and soft tissue structures.
- Patients should be educated to avoid sustained end-range positioning and to modify activity.
- Education should also include body mechanics training.

PROGNOSIS

- Prognosis is good with proper rehabilitation and activity modification.
- The prognosis is improved with decreased frequency of flare-ups and decreased intensity of the symptoms in those flare ups.
- If the patient is unable to control symptoms and symptoms progress, surgical fusion may be indicated.

SIGNS AND SYMPTOMS INDICATING REFERRAL TO PHYSICIAN

- Progressive neurological deficits
- Bowel/bladder dysfunction
- Unexplained weight loss
- Night pain
- Saddle anesthesia
- Gastrointestinal dysfunction
- Fever/chills/malaise

SUGGESTED READINGS

Abbott JH, McCane B, Herbison P, Moginie G, Chapple C, Hogarty T. Lumbar segmental instability: a criterion-related validity study of manual therapy assessment. *BMC Musculoskelet Disord*. 2005;7(6):56.

Cleland J. *Orthopaedic Clinical Examination: An Evidence-Based Approach for Physical Therapists*. Carlstadt, NJ: Icon Learning Systems; 2005.

Fritz JM, Piva SR, Childs JD. Accuracy of the clinical examination to predict radiographic instability of the lumbar spine. *Eur Spine J*. Oct 2005;14(8):743-750 [Epub 2005 Jul 27].

Fritz JM, Whitman JM, Childs JD. Lumbar spine segmental mobility assessment: an examination of validity for determining intervention strategies in patients with low back pain. *Arch Phys Med Rehabil*. 2005;86(9):1745-1752.

Hicks GE, Fritz JM, Delitto A, McGill SM. Preliminary development of a clinical prediction rule for determining which patients with low back pain will respond to a stabilization exercise program. *Arch Phys Med Rehabil*. 2005;86(9):1753-1762.

Hicks GE, Fritz JM, Delitto A, Mishock J. Interrater reliability of clinical examination measures for identification of lumbar segmental instability. *Arch Phys Med Rehabil*. 2003;84(12):1858-1864.

Kasai Y, Morishita K, Kawakita E, Kondo T, Uchida A. A new evaluation method for lumbar spinal instability: passive lumbar extension test. *Phys Ther*. 2006;86(12):1661-1667.

Landel R, Kulig K, Fredericson M, Li B, Powers CM. Intertester reliability and validity of motion assessments during lumbar spine accessory motion testing. *Phys Ther*. 2008;88(1):43-49 [Epub 2007 Nov 20].

Meadows J. *Orthopedic Differential Diagnosis in Physical Therapy*. New York, NY: McGraw Hill; 1999.

AUTHOR: PAMELA J. KIKILLUS

BASIC INFORMATION

DEFINITION

Lumbar ligament sprain is a tearing of the fibers of a lumbar ligament. If complete, it could lead to a lumbar segmental instability. A tear in a ligament can be complete or partial. A partial tear can be as small as a microtear in the substance of the ligament.

SYNONYMS

- Lumbar sprain and lumbar strains are often used interchangeably.
- A strain refers to injury to a musculotendinous structure while a sprain refers to injury to a ligamentous structure.

ICD-9CM CODES

846.0 Lumbosacral (joint) (ligament) sprain
847.2 Lumbar sprain
724.2 Lumbago
724.5 Backache unspecified

OPTIMAL NUMBER OF VISITS

6 visits

MAXIMAL NUMBER OF VISITS

18 visits

ETIOLOGY

- Ligament sprains occur when forces exceed the tissues' physiological capacities.
- Ligaments are designed to resist forces from multiple directs, unlike tendons that are designed to primarily to resist tensile forces.
- With excessive force, the ligament will fail at its weakest point:
  - In the elderly and the young, the weakest point is at the ligament-to-bone intersection.
  - In most adults, the weakest point is often at midsubstance. The weakest point will vary with each individual ligament. Some are more proximal in the ligament and others are more distal.
- Because ligaments are multipennated to resist forces from multiple directions, partial ligament ruptures or strains are common since the ligament may fail in one direction and continue to function in other directions.

EPIDEMIOLOGY AND DEMOGRAPHICS

Approximately 80% of people will experience LBP, and 80% of all back pain cases can be attributed to soft tissue injuries, grouped together as a sprain/strain.

MECHANISM OF INJURY

- A ligament sprain is usually caused by a trauma as opposed to an overuse syndrome.
- The trauma would include forced stretching of the ligament beyond its normal ROM, partially tearing the ligament. For example, a sprain of a posteriorly positioned ligament, such as the supraspinous ligament, would occur with a hyperflexion injury.
- A sprain of an anteriorly located ligament, such as the anterior longitudinal ligament, would occur with a hyperextension injury.
- Inflammation of the soft tissue after a strain causes localized pain.

COMMON SIGNS AND SYMPTOMS

- Signs and symptoms include localized LBP, generally without referral into the lower extremities.
- The pain is increased with stretching of the ligament.
- Pain is reported with sustained postures, with movement out of sustained postures, or at the end-range of motion.
- Signs and symptoms include pain and limited trunk ROM in a particular direction.
- Other directions may remain full and pain-free.

AGGRAVATING ACTIVITIES

- End-range positions or sustained postures aggravate the symptoms of the pathology.
- Sustained or end-range postures will fatigue or overstress the ligament.

EASING ACTIVITIES

- Rest
- Neutral postures
- Continual low-grade motion

24-HOUR SYMPTOM PATTERN

- Symptoms may be worse toward the end of the day or after activity.
- In some cases, symptoms are worse on arising in the morning after sustained sleep postures.

PHYSICAL EXAMINATION

- Patients usually present with painful, limited trunk motion in a given direction.
- Other motions may be full and pain-free.
- Active and resisted hip motions may elicit LBP.
- Active trunk motion may have a "hitch" or "catch" to the motion, and a Gower's sign may be present.
- In cases of a complete ligamentous tear, the ligament does not restrict segmental movement and excessive motion may be present.

- In cases of a partial ligamentous tear, stressing the ligament with stretch will cause pain.
- In some cases, findings are localized to a given spinal segment and in other cases, findings are multisegmental, depending on the span of the involved ligament.
- Similarly, some ligamentous tears will affect a single plane of motion, whereas other tears will affect motion in multiple planes.
- Any force (passive, active, or resisted) that stresses/stretches the involved ligament may elicit pain and/or excessive motion.
- If the ligamentous tear leads to segmental instability, the physical examination will include findings of instability (see section on Lumbar Instability).

DIFFERENTIAL DIAGNOSIS

- Lumbar strain
- Fracture
- Spondylolysis/spondylolisthesis

CONTRIBUTING FACTORS

- Obesity
- Smoking
- Deconditioning
- Poor body mechanics
- Limited hip flexibility/mobility
- Relatively poor trunk strength/dynamic stabilization

TREATMENT

SURGICAL OPTIONS

Surgery is not typically indicated for lumbar sprains; however, if a lumbar ligament sprain leads to an instability, spinal fusion surgery may be a consideration.

REHABILITATION

- In the early phases of rehabilitation, emphasis should be placed on pain-free motion. Early motion exercises can facilitate strong and aligned healing of the involved ligament. Motion and activity is also indicated to avoid the effects of immobility and deconditioning.
- As tolerated, strengthening exercises should include the abdominals, hip extensors, hip abductors, and spinal extensors.
- Later exercises include dynamic stabilization of the trunk.
- Rehabilitation should include patient education on body mechanics.
- General conditioning exercises should be included.

PROGNOSIS

- The prognosis is excellent, with over 90% of patients recovering within 1 to 2 months.

- In those cases in which a sprain leads to instability, the prognosis is not as favorable, and re-injury may occur more frequently or surgical intervention may be necessary.

SIGNS AND SYMPTOMS INDICATING REFERRAL TO PHYSICIAN

- Unrelenting pain
- Progressive neurological involvement

- Saddle anesthesia
- Bowel/bladder dysfunction
- Fever/malaise
- Gastrointestinal dysfunction
- History of cancer
- Unexplained weight loss

SUGGESTED READINGS

Dutton M. *Orthopedic Examination, Evaluation, and Intervention.* New York, NY: McGraw-Hill; 2004.

Hertling D, Kessler RM. *Management of Common Musculoskeletal Disorders: Physical Therapy Principles and Methods.* 4th ed. Philadelphia, PA: Lippincott Williams & Wilkins; 2006.

AUTHOR: PAMELA J. KIKILLUS

Section III

ORTHOPEDIC PATHOLOGY

BASIC INFORMATION

DEFINITION

A lumbar strain is a microtear of a lumbar muscle or tendon, most commonly at either the z-line or the musculotendinous junction. The most common lumbar muscle strained is the erector spinae muscle.

SYNONYMS

- Low back strain
- Muscle tear
- Pulled muscle

ICD-9CM CODES

846.0 Lumbosacral (joint) (ligament) sprain
847.2 Lumbar sprain

OPTIMAL NUMBER OF VISITS

6 visits

MAXIMAL NUMBER OF VISITS

16 visits

ETIOLOGY

- Muscle strains occur when forces exceed the muscle's physiological capacities.
- The contractile elements of the back can be considered as a muscle-tendon-bone complex.
- With excessive force, the muscle-tendon-bone complex will fail at its weakest point.
- In the elderly and the young, the weakest point is at the tendon-to-bone intersection.
- In most adults, the weakest point is at the myotendinous junction.

EPIDEMIOLOGY AND DEMOGRAPHICS

- The exact prevalence of lumbar strains is not known, but a lumbar strain is the most common injury to the low back.
- Lumbar strains can affect persons of any age group, but they occur most often in persons in their forties.

MECHANISM OF INJURY

- A lumbar muscle strain can occur from trauma or from overuse/misuse injuries.
- In the case of macrotrauma, the external forces on the lumbar muscles overcome the strength of the tendon and muscle. The mechanism for a traumatic strain is forced extension, usually from a position of trunk flexion or eccentric contractions of the lumbar extensors as they resist trunk flexion. The injury to the muscle or tendon can be caused by the stretching, tearing, or rupture.

- Overuse injuries generally result from repetitive use, misuse, or overuse of the lumbar muscles in a strenuous situation. The lumbar extensors act to extend the spine from a flexed position, either to neutral or past neutral to a position of extension. In addition, the misuse or overuse of the lumbar muscles in a person with a history of previous lumbar injury or deconditioned person can also lead to a lumbar strain.
- Activities, such as shoveling, gardening, and bending, can all cause a muscle strain. Pushing and pulling in sports, such as football and weightlifting, can cause a lumbar strain. Forceful twisting of the low back in sports, such as golf and baseball, can also cause this injury.

COMMON SIGNS AND SYMPTOMS

- The extensors act to extend the spine/trunk, usually from a flexed position, so the patient will report a resisted extension moment precipitating the pain.
- The pain is over a relatively broad area of the back.
- The pain does not usually radiate into the legs but may be felt into the buttocks.
- There may be tenderness with palpation or localized muscle spasm over the involved muscle. There may be localized swelling and inflammation. The pain is usually not located directly over the midline of the back but over the muscular regions along the side.
- Passive trunk extension is usually pain-free and unrestricted.

AGGRAVATING ACTIVITIES

- Lifting
- Twisting
- Forward bending
- Sitting
- Standing
- Walking
- There may be pain with sustained postures or positions

EASING ACTIVITIES

- Neutral postures
- Rest

24-HOUR SYMPTOM PATTERN

Symptoms are usually increased toward the end of the day and after activity.

PAST HISTORY FOR THE REGION

- The patient may have a history of previous low back injury.
- The patient is often deconditioned or not adequately conditioned enough to support performing the activity that preceded symptom onset.

PHYSICAL EXAMINATION

- Pain will be elicited with a resisted contraction of the involved lumbar muscle,

either with active contraction or with added resistance.
- There may be tenderness or muscle spasm locally on palpation.
- With a severe tear or strain, there may be a palpable divot in the muscle at the location of the injury.
- There may be pain with passive stretching of the lumbar extensors.
- The patient may have limited mobility at the hips, including the hamstrings and hip flexors.
- The patient may have relatively poor strength in the abdominals and poor trunk stability.

IMPORTANT OBJECTIVE TESTS

- A lumbar muscle strain will cause pain with active and resisted trunk extension:
  - If it is a minor strain, there will not be any associated weakness.
  - If it is a more extensive strain, there may be associated weakness of the involved muscle.

DIFFERENTIAL DIAGNOSIS

- Ligamentous sprain
- Fracture
- Spondylolysis

CONTRIBUTING FACTORS

- The major risk factor for LBP is a history of back pain.
- **Mismatched work load and patient strength.** A heavy workload or an activity with sustained or repeated lumbar motions in a person who has not properly conditioned for such an activity. Improper conditioning can include decreased endurance and weakened trunk muscles. Poor body mechanics and improper lifting can predispose an individual to a lumbar strain.
- Obesity.
- Smoking.
- Postural deformities do not necessarily increase a person's risk of lumbar muscle strain.

TREATMENT

SURGICAL OPTIONS

Surgery is not typically an intervention option for a lumbar muscle strain unless there is associated injury or co-morbidity that is treated surgically.

REHABILITATION

- A lumbar strain may take 4 to 12 weeks to heal.
- Initial intervention includes relative rest, ice, and pain-free exercise.

- Pain-free ROM exercises should be implemented as soon as possible, whether passive motion, active motion, or low-intensity resisted motion.
- In addition to spinal/trunk mobility, the hips and thoracic spine regions should also be included in mobility exercises.
- Early intervention should also include general conditioning exercises.
- As the patient progresses, exercises can target strengthening of the involved muscles, including both eccentric and concentric exercises at various speeds and at various muscle lengths.
- Core stabilization exercises target the abdominals and spinal extensors.
- Hip abductors and extensors should be included in a strengthening program.

PROGNOSIS

- The prognosis varies based on the severity of the strain and the intervention provided for the strain.
- Symptoms of a mild lumbar strain usually resolve within 2 to 3 weeks.

- Over 90% of people with a lumbar strain recover completely within 1 to 2 months.
- The risk of recurrence in the next few years is 60%.
- The prognosis is excellent for patients with a lumbar muscle strain, if they complete proper rehabilitation and modify their activity based on predisposing factors to the original injury. Modifications need to be made in lifting techniques, and improvements can be made in general strength and conditioning.
- After a severe strain, scar tissue formation may remain in the muscle after healing. Scar tissue has less flexibility than healthy muscle and tendon and may be the site of future injury.

SIGNS AND SYMPTOMS INDICATING REFERRAL TO PHYSICIAN

- Unrelenting pain
- Progressive neurological involvement
- Saddle anesthesia

- Bowel/bladder dysfunction
- Fever/malaise
- Gastrointestinal dysfunction
- History of cancer
- Unexplained weight loss

SUGGESTED READINGS

Dutton M. *Orthopedic Examination, Evaluation, and Intervention.* New York, NY: McGraw-Hill; 2004.

Hertling D, Kessler RM. *Management of Common Musculoskeletal Disorders: Physical Therapy Principles and Methods.* 4th ed. Philadelphia, PA: Lippincott Williams & Wilkins; 2006.

Van Dillen LR, Sahrmann SA, Wagner JM. Classification, intervention, and outcomes for a person with lumbar rotation with flexion syndrome. *Phys Ther.* 2005;85(4):336–351.

AUTHOR: PAMELA J. KIKILLUS

Section III

ORTHOPEDIC PATHOLOGY

BASIC INFORMATION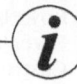

DEFINITION

Lumbar radiculopathy itself is not a cause of LBP, but a result of other lumbar pathology on the lumbar nerve root(s). If a lumbar nerve root is impinged or inflamed and causes neurological symptoms, the result is a lumbar radiculopathy. Lumbar radiculopathy causes pain, numbness, tingling, and weakness in the lower extremities. These neurological symptoms occur in the areas that are supplied by the involved nerve root (dermatome and myotome).

SYNONYMS

- Sciatica
- Pinched nerve

ICD-9CM CODES
724.3 Sciatica
724.4 Thoracic or lumbosacral radiculitis unspecified

NUMBER OF VISITS

The number of visits varies depending on the cause of the lumbar radiculopathy.

ETIOLOGY

- Lumbar radiculopathy is the result of other lumbar pathologies. Impingement or irritation of a lumbar nerve root causes neurological signs and symptoms in the corresponding dermatome/myotome/sclerotome.
- Lumbar nerve root irritation or impingement may be caused by a herniated disc, DDD, stenosis, spondylolisthesis, instability, or DJD. Any of these pathologies can compromise the size of the intervertebral foramen and impinge the lumbar nerve root.
- Sciatica is a type of lumbar radiculopathy with inflammation of the sciatic nerve in particular.

EPIDEMIOLOGY AND DEMOGRAPHICS

- 30% of those with back pain have a radiculopathy.
- The incidence ranges from 1% to 10%, affecting men and women equally.
- Symptoms occur most commonly in men in their forties and women in their fifties.

MECHANISM OF INJURY

- Lumbar radiculopathy can result from many lumbar pathologies, injuries, or degenerative processes that may compromise the nerve root.
- In the case of a herniated lumbar disc, the disc usually herniates in a posterior-lateral direction, potentially impinging the lumbar nerve root.

- DDD will decrease the disc height, decreasing the size of the intervertebral foramen.
- DJD with facet and ligament hypertrophy and lumbar stenosis can decrease the relative size of the intervertebral foramen.
- A forward slip of the superior vertebra in the case of a spondylolisthesis can also impinge the lumbar nerve root.

COMMON SIGNS AND SYMPTOMS

- Radiculopathy can cause pain, numbness, tingling, and weakness in a nerve root distribution pattern.
- The pain is described as sharp, shooting, or burning.
- The pain may begin in the low back or may start in the buttocks or thigh.
- Leg pain is often worse than back pain in those patients with radiculopathy.
- The onset of pain is often sudden.
- Most radiculopathies involve the lower lumbar nerve roots (L4-S1), sending symptoms below the level of the knee.
- The pain shoots from the buttocks to the posterior or posterior-lateral lower leg.
- Upper lumbar radiculopathies are not as common and cause pain in the anterior thigh but generally not below the knee.
- The referral pattern varies depending on the specific nerve root involved.
- Radicular pain, numbness, and tingling in the lower extremities are in a dermatomal pattern. A dermatome is a specific area in the lower extremity innervated by a specific lumbar nerve. It is more common to have sensory symptoms with radiculopathy, but muscle weakness may be present, especially in more severe instances.
- Muscle weakness and reflex changes will also occur in a specific myotomal pattern. A myotome is a motor function associated with a specific nerve root.

AGGRAVATING ACTIVITIES

- Coughing, sneezing, or bearing down may exacerbate the pain.
- Symptoms could worsen with prolonged sitting or moving from sitting to standing.
- Aggravating activities will vary depending on the cause of the radiculopathy.

- If a herniated disc is the cause, symptoms will worsen with lifting, bending, lumbar flexion, and sitting.
- If stenosis, DDD, or DJD is the cause, symptoms could worsen with standing, backward bending, and trunk extension.

EASING ACTIVITIES

- Depending on the cause of the radiculopathy, positions or activities that either open the intervertebral foramen, making more room for the nerve root, or that decrease the mechanical impingement on the nerve root will alleviate the symptoms of radiculopathy.
- Symptom centralization is an indicator of decreased pressure on the nerve root.

24-HOUR SYMPTOM PATTERN

Discogenic and arthritic/degenerative radiculopathy may be worse in the morning on arising

PAST HISTORY FOR THE REGION

- Patients may report a history of LBP or injury.
- Some patients report that when the radicular leg pain begins, the back pain goes away.

PHYSICAL EXAMINATION

- Patients may stand with the trunk side-bent away from the involved side, causing that side of the lumbar spine to have a convexity, opening the intervertebral foramen and decreasing the compression on the lumbar nerve root.
- Trunk motion may be limited in a pattern consistent with the structural cause of the radiculopathy. For example, if lateral stenosis is causing the radiculopathy, lumbar motion will likely be limited into extension or an extension quadrant.
- Straight leg raising test or slump test may be positive.
- Repeated lumbar movement may centralize symptoms, suggestive of a discogenic radiculopathy.
- The following table describes typical neurological involvement with lumbar radiculopathy. There is some overlap between adjacent dermatomes and myotomes.

Nerve Root	Sensory Disturbance	Motor Weakness	Diminished Reflex
L2	Proximal anterior thigh	Hip flexion, hip adduction	
L3	Anterior thigh to patella	Knee extension, hip adduction	
L4	Medial lower leg to medial malleolus	Ankle inversion, dorsiflexion	Patellar
L5	Dorsal foot and great toe	Great toe extension, hip abduction, ankle inversion, knee flexion	Medial hamstring
S1	Posterior calf, lateral foot, fifth toe	Ankle plantar flexion, eversion, knee flexion, hip extension	Achilles

IMPORTANT OBJECTIVE TESTS

- Electromyographic (EMG) studies
- Nerve conduction velocity (NCV) tests
- MRI
- Discogram
- Myelogram
- CT scan

DIFFERENTIAL DIAGNOSIS

- Degenerative disc disease
- Herniated disc
- Degenerative joint disease
- Spondylolisthesis
- Tumor
- Spinal stenosis
- Cauda equina syndrome
- Hip degenerative joint disease
- Piriformis syndrome
- Lateral femoral cutaneous nerve entrapment (meralgia paresthetica)
- Other peripheral nerve entrapment
- Diabetic neuropathy

CONTRIBUTING FACTORS

- A leg length discrepancy may contribute to radiculopathy. The longer leg side may have a relative ipsilateral concavity in the lumbar spine, decreasing the size of the intervertebral lumbar foramen.
- People who perform manual labor jobs that require heavy lifting and prolonged driving are at increased risk for developing radiculopathy. People between the ages of 30 and 40 are at increased risk for developing a herniated lumbar disc, one of the causes of lumbar radiculopathy. People with sedentary lifestyles are more likely than active people to develop lumbar radiculopathy.

TREATMENT

SURGICAL OPTIONS

- Decompression
- Discectomy
- Foraminotomy
- Laminectomy
- Fusion
- Indicators for surgery for patients with lumbar radiculopathy include the following:
  - Progressive neurological deficit
  - Cauda equine syndrome
  - Bowel/bladder dysfunction
  - Severe unrelenting pain

REHABILITATION

- Rehabilitation should be aimed at the involved anatomical structure causing the radicular symptoms.
- Rehabilitation for a radiculopathy caused by stenosis is different from that caused by a herniated disc.
- In general, rehabilitation is aimed at relieving the nerve root irritation and includes exercises for symptom centralization.
- In some cases, repeated lumbar extension centralizes the radicular symptoms from a herniated disc.
- Strengthening exercises for the abdominals and spinal extensors and trunk stabilization exercises are an important component of rehabilitation.
- Care should be taken to tailor the exercise program for the specific cause of the radiculopathy.
- For example, people with stenotic radiculopathy should not complete exercise that places the lumbar spine at end-range or sustained lumbar extension.
- Patient with a herniated disc should not sit for prolonged periods of time. Any exercises that peripheralize symptoms should not be included in a rehabilitation program.
- Antiinflammatory modalities may help to decrease local nerve root irritation.
- Lumbar traction may relieve symptoms, but it requires relatively high forces to distract the vertebrae.
- Manual therapy techniques may be incorporated to increase motion in hypomobile regions.
- These techniques may also be used during the recovery phase, with a lifelong home exercise program forming part of the maintenance phase.
- Rehabilitation should also include patient education on posture and body mechanics. The importance of a regular exercise program should also be emphasized.

PROGNOSIS

- Most cases of lumbar radiculopathy resolve in 1 to 2 months.
- 10% to 25% of patients will have symptoms that last longer than 6 weeks.
- It is important for patients who have had a lumbar radiculopathy to modify their activity and lifestyle to avoid recurrence.
- They should maintain flexibility, strength, stability, and endurance and should use proper body mechanics to minimize their risk of recurrence.

SIGNS AND SYMPTOMS INDICATING REFERRAL TO PHYSICIAN

- Unexplained weight loss
- Progressive neurological dysfunction
- Bowel/bladder dysfunction
- Gastrointestinal dysfunction
- Saddle anesthesia
- History of cancer
- Fever/chills/malaise
- Night pain

SUGGESTED READINGS

Barr KP, Griggs M, Cadby T. Lumbar stabilization: a review of core concepts and current literature, part 2. *Am J Phys Med Rehabil.* 2007;86(1):72-80.

Hahne AJ, Ford JJ. Functional restoration for a chronic lumbar disk extrusion with associated radiculopathy. *Phys Ther.* 2006;86(12):1668-1680.

Hyun JK, Lee JY, Lee SJ, Jeon JY. Asymmetric atrophy of multifidus muscle in patients with unilateral lumbosacral radiculopathy. *Spine.* 2007;32(21):E598-E602.

Lipetz JS. Pathophysiology of inflammatory, degenerative, and compressive radiculopathies. *Phys Med Rehabil Clin N Am.* 2002;13(3):439-449.

Tsao B. The electrodiagnosis of cervical and lumbosacral radiculopathy. *Neurol Clin.* 2007;25(2):473-494.

van Rijn JC, Klemetso N, Reitsma JB, et al. Symptomatic and asymptomatic abnormalities in patients with lumbosacral radicular syndrome: Clinical examination compared with MRI. *Clin Neurol Neurosurg.* 2006;108(6):553-557.

Weinstein JN, Tosteson TD, Lurie JD, et al. Surgical vs nonoperative treatment for lumbar disk herniation: the Spine Patient Outcomes Research Trial (SPORT): a randomized trial. *JAMA.* 2006;296(20):2441-2450.

AUTHOR: PAMELA J. KIKILLUS

BASIC INFORMATION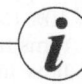

DEFINITION

Lumbar spondylolysis is a defect in the pars interarticularis. If the fracture defect widens and allows the superior segment to slip on the inferior segment, the result is a spondylolisthesis. *Spondylo* means spine, and *listhesis* means slippage. Therefore spondylolisthesis refers to a slippage of one spinal segment in relationship to its adjacent segment.

SYNONYMS

- Lumbar spondylolysis
- Lumbar spondylolisthesis

ICD-9CM CODES
738.4 Acquired spondylolisthesis
756.11 Congenital spondylolysis
　　　　lumbosacral region
756.12 Spondylolisthesis congenital

OPTIMAL NUMBER OF VISITS

6 visits

MAXIMAL NUMBER OF VISITS

18 visits

ETIOLOGY

- Spondylolysis is a fracture at the region of the pars interarticularis. It usually occurs at the fifth lumbar vertebra and next most frequently at the fourth lumbar vertebra.
- Spondylolisthesis results when the superior vertebra slips forward on the inferior vertebra. The most common spondylolisthetic level is L5/S1, followed by L4/5 and then L3/4.
- The four grades of spondylolisthesis are as follows:
  ○ A slippage of 0% to 25% is given a grade 1.
  ○ 25% to 50% a grade 2
  ○ 50% to 75% a grade 3
  ○ Over 75% a grade 4
- Spondylolisthesis is categorized into 5 different types, as follows:
  ○ *Dysplastic* is a true congenital spondylolisthesis. It is rare and usually has rapidly progressing neurological deficits. It is difficult to treat surgically because the posterior elements are not well formed for surgical fusion.
  ○ *Isthmic* refers to a pars defect that may be from a stress fracture. The defect in isthmic spondylolisthesis from repetitive hyperextension which causes shear of the posterior elements. Isthmic spondylolisthesis is most common at L5/S1. A lumbar spondylolysis is another term for isthmic spondylolisthesis.
  ○ *Degenerative* spondylolisthesis refers to a slippage of the superior vertebral segment because of facet arthritis. The facets have a more sagittal plane orientation, allowing the forward slip to occur.
  ○ *Traumatic* spondylolisthesis is caused by an acute fracture of the facet or pars interarticularis.
  ○ *Pathological* is caused by damage to the posterior elements from tumor, metastases, or metabolic bone disease.

EPIDEMIOLOGY AND DEMOGRAPHICS

- Dysplastic, traumatic, and pathological spondylolisthesis are very rare.
- Most spondylolistheses are isthmic or degenerative.
- Isthmic is the most common form and has a prevalence of 5% to 7% in the United States.
- The defect is usually acquired between the ages of 6 and 16.
- The majority do not become symptomatic; 90% of isthmic slips are low grade (<50%).
- Degenerative spondylolisthesis is found in older adults as the result of facet arthritis. There is a 30% incidence in Caucasian women over 65 years of age and 60% incidence in African-American women over age 65.
- 58% of adults have a bilateral defect in the pars interarticularis (spondylolysis), and the incidence of spondylolisthesis is 5% in the general population, but again, not all are symptomatic.
- Most isthmic slips occur during adolescence, but many are asymptomatic. Symptoms may not develop until adulthood, between the ages of 40 and 50.
- An increased incidence has been reported in football linemen, divers, dancers, gymnasts, weightlifters, and wrestlers.
- Spondylolisthesis is more common among 10 to 20 year olds.
- The incidence increases up to age 20 and then remains constant.
- 5% to 6% of males and 2% to 3% of females have a spondylolisthesis. The incidence in Eskimos is 50% and in African Americans is <3%.

MECHANISM OF INJURY

- Spondylolysis is a fracture at the region of the pars interarticularis, usually caused by forced extension of the lumbar spine. It occurs most frequently at L5, followed by L4, and more rarely at L3 or above. Less than half of the people with a spondylolysis will develop a spondylolisthesis.
- Spondylolisthesis can be the result of trauma, degenerative processes, or be congenital.

COMMON SIGNS AND SYMPTOMS

- Many people with a spondylolisthesis have no symptoms.
- In general, people with spondylolisthesis will report mild-to-moderate back and/or leg pain that is increased with extension positions. The pain may radiate into the buttocks, posterior thighs, or the lower legs.
- Degenerative spondylolisthesis will present with more of a stenotic history. The pain is made worse by extension activities, and symptoms of radiculopathy or neurogenic claudication, with or without LBP, may be present.
- Because of instability, patients may complain of catching or shifting in the back with motion.

AGGRAVATING ACTIVITIES

- Extension postures or activities
- A posterior to anterior shear force and compression through the shoulders in standing (which may increase the extension forces)
- Static postures will result in pain as lumbar muscles fatigue and slippage occurs

EASING ACTIVITIES

- Flexion postures or activities
- Relative rest

PHYSICAL EXAMINATION

- Increased lumbar lordosis
- Painful and limited trunk extension
- Tight hamstrings
- Weakness/pain in one or both lower extremities
- Posterior-anterior provocation will cause local pain
- Neurological signs may be present depending on the severity and chronicity of the condition
- If the spondylolysis has progressed to a spondylolisthesis, there may be a palpable "step-off" deformity when palpating the spinous processes

IMPORTANT OBJECTIVE TESTS

- Plain film radiographs in the oblique plane will show a fracture in the region of the pars interarticularis, known as a Scotty dog collar fracture.
- Tests for segmental instability, such as the sidelying segmental shear test, may reveal segmental laxity.
- The prone instability test has been suggested as a test for lumbar instability. The patient lies prone. A posterior-to-anterior directed force is applied to the unstable segment. If pain is produced, the patient is instructed to slightly extend their legs. The posterior-to-anterior force is applied once again. If symptoms are reduced, then instability may be present.

DIFFERENTIAL DIAGNOSIS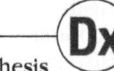

- Spondylolysis/spondylolisthesis
- Compression fracture
- Muscle strain
- Stenosis
- Degenerative joint disease

TREATMENT

SURGICAL OPTIONS AND OUTCOMES

- Surgery is indicated with progressive neurological deficits, severe restriction of activity, or pain that is not responding to conservative care.
- Surgery is also indicated for people with a high-grade spondylolisthesis (>50% slippage) versus a low-grade spondylolisthesis (<50% slippage).
- Surgical treatment is considered only after at least 6 weeks of conservative intervention that has not worked.
- Surgical options include the following:
  - Laminectomy
  - Decompression
  - Fusion
- Long-term outcomes for surgery include the following:
  - 57% were asymptomatic and 36% had mild symptoms as compared to nonsurgical intervention with 36% asymptomatic and 55% with mild symptoms.
  - Other studies show the outcome differences between surgical and nonsurgical intervention narrows with time.

REHABILITATION

- Initial intervention for spondylolysis/spondylolisthesis is nonsurgical.

  - The aggravating activities should be avoided until the symptoms go away.
  - Antiinflammatory medication (NSAIDs or steroids) may be prescribed to alleviate symptoms. Epidural steroid injections may be given to treat radicular pain.
  - Bracing with a (Thoraco-Lumbo-Sacral Orthosis (TLSO) or Lumbo-Sacral Orthosis (LSO) may be included.
  - Physical agents and modalities to relieve muscle spasm should be used only in conjunction with therapeutic exercise.
- Therapeutic exercises include the following:
  - Muscle strengthening for the abdominals and trunk stabilization.
  - A bias is given for flexion-based exercises.
  - Mobility into hip extension and hamstring flexibility exercise are included.

PROGNOSIS

- A unilateral pars defect has a better prognosis than a bilateral defect.
- Most patients benefit from nonsurgical intervention, including stabilization exercises and neuromuscular reeducation exercises.
- In a study of symptomatic adolescents with a spondylolysis, 95% had excellent results and 5% had good results with conservative care; none went on to surgery.

SIGNS AND SYMPTOMS INDICATING REFERRAL TO PHYSICIAN

- Unexplained weight loss/gain
- Saddle anesthesia/paresthesia
- Bowel/bladder dysfunction

- Night pain
- History of cancer
- Fever/chills/malaise
- Progressive neurological dysfunction

SUGGESTED READINGS

Harris IE, Weinstein SL. Long-term follow up of patients with grade III and IV spondylolisthesis. Treatment with and without posterior lateral fusion. *J Bone Joint Surg Am.* 1987;69(7):960-969.

Hosoe H, Ohmori K. Degenerative lumbosacral spondylolisthesis: possible factors which predispose the fifth lumbar vertebra to slip. *J Bone Joint Surg Br.* 2008;90(3):356-359.

Kalichman L, Hunter DJ. Diagnosis and conservative management of degenerative lumbar spondylolisthesis. *Eur Spine J.* 2008;17(3):327-335.

Kurd MF, Patel D, Norton R, Picetti G, Friel B, Vaccarro AR. Nonoperative treatment of symptomatic spondylolysis. *J Spinal Disord Tech.* 2007;20(8):560-564.

McNeely ML, Torrance G, Magee DJ. A systematic review of physiotherapy for spondylolysis and spondylolisthesis. *Man Ther.* 2003;2(8):80-91.

O'Sullivan PB, Phyty GD, Twomey LT, Allison GT. Evaluation of specific stabilizing exercise in the treatment of chronic low back pain with radiologic diagnosis of spondylolysis or spondylolisthesis. *Spine.* 1997;24(22):2959-2967.

Standaert CJ, Herring SA, Halpern B, King O. Spondylolysis. *Phys Med Rehabil Clin N Am.* 2000;11(4):785-803.

Vibert BT, Sliva CD, Herkowitz HN. Treatment of instability and spondylolisthesis: surgical versus nonsurgical treatment. *Clin Orthop Relat Res.* 2006;443:222-227.

AUTHOR: PAMELA J. KIKILLUS

BASIC INFORMATION

DEFINITION

Lumbar spondylosis is a term for lumbar DJD or osteoarthritis in which the thickness of the articular cartilage is decreased. In the advanced stages, subchondral bone is exposed, thus causing pain and symptoms. Bone spurs or osteophytes may form. Lumbar spondylosis is fusing of one or more lumbar vertebrae and may affect the facets and intervertebral discs and may impinge on the spinal nerves. Frequently, more than one segmental level is involved.

SYNONYMS

• Degenerative joint disease (DJD)
• Osteoarthritis

ICD-9CM CODES
721.3 Lumbosacral spondylosis
   without myelopathy
721.42 Spondylosis with myelopathy
   lumbar region
722.52 Degeneration of lumbar or
   lumbosacral intervertebral
   disc
724.2 Lumbago
724.5 Backache unspecified

OPTIMAL NUMBER OF VISITS

10 visits

MAXIMAL NUMBER OF VISITS

16 visits

ETIOLOGY

• Lumbar spondylosis is a degenerative process, associated with aging. It may be aggravated or accelerated by a low back injury.
• The degeneration of the facets can result in foraminal or central stenosis.
• The disc space decreases with disc degeneration, causing the discs to lose height.
• Lumbar ligaments hypertrophy and may calcify and impinge the adjacent lumbar nerve roots, causing radiculopathy.
• Additional degenerative changes include cartilage fibrillation and osteophyte formation.
• Spondylosis inhibits the normal spinal segmental motion. It can produce spinal instability and spinal deformity.

EPIDEMIOLOGY AND DEMOGRAPHICS

• Degenerative changes are very common in the older population and may not be symptomatic.
• Lumbar spondylosis is most common in those 45 years of age and older.

MECHANISM OF INJURY

Lumbar spondylosis may be the result of a traumatic spinal injury, aging and degeneration, or some type of rheumatoid disease process.

COMMON SIGNS AND SYMPTOMS

• Patients with lumbar spondylosis report increasing LBP.
• Morning stiffness.
• Difficulty moving early in the morning or after prolonged positioning.
• Symptoms may be most noticeable with repetitive movements such as bending backward or lifting.
• Patients may report pain, numbness, tingling, or weakness in the lower extremities if the lumbar nerve roots are affected.

AGGRAVATING ACTIVITIES

• Too much activity or strenuous activity can increase the symptoms, especially those requiring lumbar extension.
• Pain is increased after prolonged positioning if instability is involved.

EASING ACTIVITIES

Rest and moderation of activity/movement ease the symptoms.

24-HOUR SYMPTOM PATTERN

• Stiffness and pain is worse first thing in the morning on arising.
• Pain may increase again at the end of the day.

PAST HISTORY FOR THE REGION

• Patients may have a history of previous low back injury or trauma.
• They may have a personal or family history of osteoarthritis.

PHYSICAL EXAMINATION

• Limited trunk ROM into extension, with complaints of pain and stiffness.
• Segmental posterior-anterior provocation and spring testing is painful and stiff.

IMPORTANT OBJECTIVE TESTS

Plain film radiographs, MRI, or CT scan can demonstrate findings consistent with lumbar spondylosis.

DIFFERENTIAL DIAGNOSIS

• Central or lateral stenosis and DDD
• Diffuse idiopathic skeletal hyperostosis (DISH)
• Ankylosing spondylitis
• Rheumatoid arthritis

CONTRIBUTING FACTORS

• History of repetitive strenuous lifting or bending
• History or trauma or injury

TREATMENT

SURGICAL OPTIONS

• Decompression may be done to relieve nerve root impingement.
• In advanced cases where the degenerative process has led to instability or neural compromise, spinal fusion surgery may be performed.
• Most patients with lumbar spondylosis respond favorably to conservative intervention and do not require surgical intervention.
• Surgical indicators include the lack of response to conservative intervention, unrelenting pain, interference with ADLs, and progressive neurological compromise.

REHABILITATION

• Active pain-free movement exercises, including not only the lumbar spine, but adjacent regions of the hips and thoracic spine.
• Abdominal and trunk strengthening and stabilization exercises for core control.
• A warm water aquatic exercise program may be a good choice for individuals who cannot tolerate a land-based program because of high levels of pain.
• General conditioning exercises for weight loss and fitness can be beneficial.

PROGNOSIS

The degenerative process cannot be reversed, but patients may be able to increase their overall functional level and decrease their pain levels over time.

SIGNS AND SYMPTOMS INDICATING REFERRAL TO PHYSICIAN

• Progressive neurological deficits
• Bowel/bladder dysfunction
• Unexplained weight loss
• Night pain
• Saddle anesthesia
• Gastrointestinal dysfunction
• History of cancer
• Fever/chills/malaise

SUGGESTED READINGS

Bambakidis NC, Feiz-Erfan I, Klopfenstein JD, Sonntag VK. Indications for surgical fusion of the cervical and lumbar motion segment. *Spine*. 2005;30(suppl 16):S2–S6.

Gibson JN, Waddell G. Surgery for degenerative lumbar spondylosis. *Cochrane Database Syst Rev.* 2005;(2):CD001352.

Mata S, Fortin PR, Fitzcharles MA, et al. A controlled study of diffuse idiopathic skeletal hyperostosis. Clinical features and functional status. *Medicine (Baltimore).* 1997;76(2):104-117.

Roh JS, Teng AL, Yoo JU, Davis J, Furey C, Bohlman HH. Degenerative disorders of the lumbar and cervical spine. *Orthop Clin North Am.* 2005;36(3):255-262.

AUTHOR: PAMELA J. KIKILLUS

BASIC INFORMATION

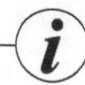

DEFINITION

Lumbar stenosis may be either central stenosis or lateral stenosis. Central stenosis is a narrowing of the central vertebral canal, and lateral stenosis is a narrowing of the intervertebral foramen. Central stenosis may compromise the spinal cord or cauda equina (dural sac), while lateral stenosis may compromise the nerve root or dorsal root ganglia.

SYNONYMS

- Degenerative disc disease
- Stenosis
- Foraminal stenosis
- Central stenosis
- Degenerative joint disease
- Neurogenic claudication

ICD-9CM CODES

724.02 Spinal stenosis of lumbar region
722.52 Degeneration of lumbar or lumbosacral intervertebral disc
724.4 Thoracic or lumbosacral neuritis or radiculitis unspecified

OPTIMAL NUMBER OF VISITS

8 visits or less

MAXIMAL NUMBER OF VISITS

20 visits

ETIOLOGY

- Lumbar stenosis is generally a degenerative process, with hypertrophy of the lamina, degenerative hypertrophy of the facets, or buckling or hypertrophy of the ligamentum flavum.
- The intervertebral disc may undergo degenerative changes. This degeneration causes disc collapse and facet arthritis, thus narrowing the intervertebral foramen.

EPIDEMIOLOGY AND DEMOGRAPHICS

- Lumbar stenosis is more common in people over 65 years of age.
- The onset of symptoms occurs in the fifth or sixth decade of life, and stenosis is evenly distributed in men and women.
- It is the most common cause of neurological leg pain in older adults.

MECHANISM OF INJURY

- Stenosis is a degenerative process without a specific history of macrotrauma.

- It is more often a cumulative trauma with stenosis being more common in people who have a long history of manual heavy labor jobs and repeat movement of bending and lifting.

COMMON SIGNS AND SYMPTOMS

- People with stenosis usually report the insidious onset of LBP and stiffness.
- Central stenosis can impinge the lumbar spinal cord or the cauda equina. Impingement of the spinal cord can cause upper motor neuron signs, including hyperreflexia, hypertonia, and decreased strength and sensation below the level of the pathology.
- Impingement of the cauda equina can cause lower motor neuron signs, including hyporeflexia, hypotonia, and decreased strength and sensation.
- Patients with either central or lateral stenosis have a low tolerance for trunk extension postures or activities.
- Patients with lateral stenosis may report pain or sensory changes in one or both lower extremities. Pain may be located below the buttocks or below the knees.

Sign/Symptom	Sensitivity	Specificity
Pain in legs with walking that is relieved with sitting	0.80	0.16
Walking is better when holding on to a shopping cart	0.63	0.67
Age over 65	0.77	0.69
Pain below knees	0.56	0.63
Pain below buttocks	0.88	0.34
No pain when seated	0.46	0.93
Severe lower extremity pain	0.65	0.67
Symptoms improve while seated	0.52	0.83

- L1/2 lateral stenosis will impinge the L1 nerve root.
- L2/3 lateral stenosis will impinge the L2 nerve root.
- L3/4 lateral stenosis will impinge the L3 nerve root.
- L4/5 lateral stenosis will impinge the L4 nerve root.
- L5/S1 lateral stenosis will impinge the L5 nerve root.

AGGRAVATING ACTIVITIES

- Lumbar extension postures and activities, such as standing and walking, will reproduce the back pain and neurological signs and symptoms.
- Symptoms are aggravated by overactivity.

EASING ACTIVITIES

- Lumbar flexion will alleviate the neurological signs and symptoms discussed above.
- Symptoms are eased with rest, sitting, and forward bending with the hands resting on the thighs to support the weight of the trunk.

PHYSICAL EXAMINATION

- Physical examination findings included decreased lumbar extension ROM with pain reproduction.
- Lower extremity pain is reproduced with trunk extension or active hip extension.
- A positive two staged treadmill test with increased time needed to develop symptoms when walking uphill and less recovery time needed as compared to level walking.
- Neurological findings may include an abnormal Romberg test, sensory vibration deficit (128 Hz tuning fork), lower extremity weakness, decreased peripheral deep tendon reflexes (in the corresponding dermatomes/myotomes).

IMPORTANT OBJECTIVE TESTS

- The two staged treadmill test is useful in diagnosing stenosis. Walking on a level treadmill compared to walking at a 15% inclined treadmill for 10 minutes with increased time needed to cause symptoms or longer walking time with uphill walking, and a longer recovery time needed after level walking.
- A treadmill versus bike test can differentiate lumbar stenosis from vascular claudication, as symptoms of stenosis will not be reproduced with a seated bicycle test but will be reproduced with treadmill ambulation.
- Plain film radiographs can confirm the diagnosis of stenosis.
- The following findings from Fritz, Katz, and Cleland are reported for specificity and sensitivity for clinical findings of people with stenosis:

Clinical Finding	Sensitivity	Specificity
Abnormal Romberg (10 seconds)	0.39	0.91
Vibration deficit to 128 Hz tuning fork at first metatarsal head	0.53	0.81
Decreased pin-prick sensation (dorsal foot, lateral calf)	0.47	0.81
Weakness in knee flexion, extension, great toe extension	0.47	0.78
Thigh pain during or after active hip extension	0.51	0.69
Absent Achilles reflex	0.46	0.78
Positive 2-staged treadmill test	0.68	0.85

DIFFERENTIAL DIAGNOSIS

- Any space-occupying lesion that could also compromise the size of the central canal or intervertebral foramen needs to be ruled out as a differential diagnosis
- Peripheral neuropathy
- Vascular claudication
- Tumor
- Cauda equina syndrome

CONTRIBUTING FACTORS

- Hypomobility in the areas adjacent to the lumbar spine including the sacroiliac region and the hips can contribute to stenosis.
- Repetitive forward bending and forceful extension/rotation can also contribute to degenerative process of stenosis.

TREATMENT

SURGICAL OPTIONS

Surgical options include:
- Laminectomy
- Laminotomy
- Fusion
- Surgery may be indicated for people with progressive neurological deficit and failure to respond favorable to conservative intervention

REHABILITATION

- Rehabilitation is focused on keeping the intervertebral foramen relatively open by biasing the lumbar spine into a flexion posture.
- Mobility exercises to maximize hip and thoracic extension ROM.
- Abdominal strengthening and trunk stabilization exercise are incorporated.
- Lumbar extension to symptom onset should be avoided.
- Manual therapy can restore motion at regions of hypomobility, including the hips and thoracic spine.
- Progressive ambulation on a treadmill or progressive body weight supported treadmill ambulation to symptom onset has been effective in increasing the functional tolerance of people with stenosis.

PROGNOSIS

- Lumbar stenosis is a degenerative process and cannot be reversed.
- The patient's overall function can be increased, although the stenosis will still be present on plain film radiographs.
- Symptoms may progress into advancing neurological compromise with ongoing nerve root compression.

SIGNS AND SYMPTOMS INDICATING REFERRAL TO PHYSICIAN

- Unexplained weight loss/gain
- Saddle anesthesia/paresthesia
- Bowel/bladder dysfunction
- Night pain
- History of cancer
- Fever/chills/malaise
- Gastrointestinal dysfunction

SUGGESTED READINGS

Atlas SJ, Keller RB, Wu YA, Deyo RA, Singer DE. Long term outcomes of surgical and non surgical management of lumbar spinal stenosis- 8-10 year results from the Maine lumbar spine study. *Spine.* 2005;30(8):936–943.

Chad DA. Lumbar spinal stenosis. *Neurol Clin.* 2007;25(2):407–418.

Cleland J. *Orthopaedic Clinical Examination: An Evidence-Based Approach for Physical Therapists.* Carlstadt, NJ: Icon Learning Systems; 2005.

Fritz JM, Delitto A, Welch WC, Erhard RE. Lumbar spinal stenosis: a review of current concepts in evaluation, management and outcome measurements. *Arch Phys Med Rehabil.* 1998;79(6):700–708.

Katz JN, Harris MB. Clinical practice lumbar spinal stenosis. *N Engl J Med.* 2008; 358(8):815–825.

Rittenberg JD, Ross AE. Functional rehabilitation for degenerative lumbar spinal stenosis. *Phys Med Rehabil Clin N Am.* 2003;14(1):111–120.

Weinstein JN, Tosteson TD, Lurie JD, et al. Surgical versus nonsurgical therapy for lumbar spinal stenosis. *N Engl J Med.* 2008;358(8):794–810.

Whitman JM, Flynn TW, Childs JD, et al. A comparison between two physical therapy treatment programs for patients with lumbar spinal stenosis: a randomized clinical trial. *Spine.* 2006;31(22):2541–2549.

AUTHOR: PAMELA J. KIKILLUS

Section III

ORTHOPEDIC PATHOLOGY

BASIC INFORMATION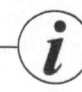

DEFINITION

- An abdominal muscle strain is a tearing injury to the abdominal muscles or tendons.
- An abdominal tendinopathy refers to a painful overuse chronic tendon.
- The term *tendonitis* also refers to a painful overuse tendon condition, but it implies an inflammation.
- Many chronic tendon conditions are not characterized by the presence of inflammatory cells when examined under a microscope.
- The term *tendinosis* refers to degenerative changes in the tendon, without inflammatory cells present.
- The term *tendinopathy* refers to a painful overuse tendon condition, without knowing whether or not inflammatory cells are present.
- A strain occurs when the fibers of the muscle or tendon are stretched too far and tear.
- Most tears are partial, caused by microscopic tear but tears can be complete ruptures.
- Strains usually occur at the musculotendinous junction or along the z-lines.
- Most abdominal strains occur to the rectus abdominus muscle but can affect the other abdominal muscles or tendons.
- Tendinopathy of the rectus abdominus usually affects the inferior aspect of the musculotendinous structure.

SYNONYMS

- Abdominal tendinopathy
- Abdominal hernia
- Abdominal tendinitis
- Stomach strain
- Pulled abdominal muscle

ICD-9CM CODES
726.9 Unspecified enthesopathy
789 Other symptoms involving abdomen and pelvis

OPTIMAL NUMBER OF VISITS

6 visits

MAXIMAL NUMBER OF VISITS

18 visits
- NOTE: Conditions of inflammation should respond quickly to intervention and require less time, whereas tendon degeneration conditions require longer time periods for tissue repair to occur. Tendinitis with inflammation should resolve in 3 to 14 days. Healing time for an uncomplicated tendinosis is 6 to 8 weeks and healing for a chronic complicated tendinosis is 3 to 6 months.

ETIOLOGY

- Abdominal tendinopathy is usually an overuse condition in which the tendon is partially torn and degeneration is likely evident at the cellular level.
- Excessive mechanical loading in activity or exercise is the main cause producing tendinopathy.
- Like other strains and tendinopathies, the muscle and tendon can be considered a functional unit. In normal adults, the weakest point of this unit is at the myotendinous junction. Therefore, most failures occur here. With children and with the elderly, the weakest point occurs at the tendon to bone interface. With this population, failure results in the tendon avulsing from the bone.

EPIDEMIOLOGY AND DEMOGRAPHICS

- Abdominal musculotendinous injuries occur in athletes whose sports require trunk rotation and forceful flexion/extension, such as gymnasts, throwers, tennis players, wrestlers, and pole vaulters.
- Repetitive motion in sport or occupation can damage the abdominal musculotendinous structures.
- Returning to sport or activity before the tendon has fully healed may predispose an individual to developing a tendinopathy.

MECHANISM OF INJURY

- Tendon injuries and pathologies can affect anyone and can be caused by sports injury, overuse, or aging.
- The muscle/tendon is excessively stretched and the tissue is torn.
- The abdominal muscles may be strained from or during abdominal exercises.
- Eccentric overload can cause tendinopathy or strain.
- Gradual wear and tear can damage the tissues.
- The onset can be gradual over time or sudden.
- A history of overuse or injury increases the likelihood of a sudden injury.

COMMON SIGNS AND SYMPTOMS

- Abdominal tendinopathy and abdominal strains cause localized pain in the area of injury.
- Tendinopathy caused stiffness, weakness of the affected structures.
- A low-grade (grade 1) strain may not have immediate pain, but the symptoms may arise after the aggravating activity.
- A more severe strain (grade 2 or 3) has immediate symptom onset during the activity.
- The pain may radiate over a diffuse abdominal area.

AGGRAVATING ACTIVITIES

Pain will increase with stretching or contraction of the involved structure.

EASING ACTIVITIES

Symptoms are eased with rest and avoiding contracting or stretching the abdominals.

24-HOUR SYMPTOM PATTERN

- Tendinopathy symptoms may be worse first thing in the morning and at night.
- Symptoms from a strain may increase later in the day after sustained activity.

PAST HISTORY FOR THE REGION

- Patients with abdominal tendinopathy may have a history of a previous abdominal injury, excessive training or increase in exercise regimen.
- A lack of complete healing from previous injury or preexisting tendon degeneration may increase the likelihood of injury, including tendon rupture.

PHYSICAL EXAMINATION

- Localized tenderness to palpation.
- Muscle spasms may be present.
- The tissue may be red, warm, bruised, or swollen.
- There may be a localized tender trigger point.
- There may be a palpable defect in the muscle or tendon with a complete tear/rupture.
- The underlying tissue may bulge through the torn abdominal muscle, causing a hernia.
- Attempted contraction or use of the involved muscle elicits pain and weakness.
- With a complete tear, there may be weakness, without pain provocation.
- There may be crepitus with contraction of the involved muscle.

IMPORTANT OBJECTIVE TESTS

Magnetic resonance imaging (MRI)

DIFFERENTIAL DIAGNOSIS

- Hip flexor strain
- Hip flexor abscess
- Abdominal hernia
- Gastrointestinal system pathology (such as appendicitis)

CONTRIBUTING FACTORS

- A sudden increase in the intensity of abdominal exercises.
- Excessive eccentric loading without proper training.
- A history of previous abdominal muscle injury that did not properly heal.

TREATMENT

SURGICAL OPTIONS

- Conservative measures are preferred initial management.
- If the patient does not respond and the symptoms are severe, surgery may be considered.
- Surgical options include:
  ○ Tenotomy
  ○ Fasciaplasty

SURGICAL OUTCOMES

- Most patients having rectus abdominus tenotomy in combination with fasciaplasty did not lose strength or power as compared to patients who did not have the surgery.

REHABILITATION

- Muscle strains should be treated with relative rest for 2-4 weeks, with pain-free exercises to restore mobility and strength.
- Exercise and activity is gradually progressed based on symptoms and patient response.
- Strains may take up to 3 months of rehabilitation.
- If inflammation is not present, the patient will not respond to antiinflammatory intervention.

- Intervention for a degenerative tendinosis or tendinopathy should emphasize collagen synthesis and tendon strength.
- Initial intervention for these conditions is conservative.
- Pain-free mobility and strengthening exercises are gradually progressed.
- Strengthening exercises emphasize eccentric training and eventually plyometric training and sport-specific exercises.
- Patient education and modification of activity or exercise/sport need to be included to decrease the external stress placed on the tendon until full healing is complete.

PROGNOSIS

- Many patients with tendinopathy do not respond favorably to intervention. Tissue healing and rehabilitation time can be lengthy. Returning to sport or activity too soon (before healing is complete) can result in re-injury.
- Outcomes for tendinopathy are varied and unpredictable.
- Tissue that has had an injury or degeneration is not as strong as healthy tissue without a history and may not have the strength to match external loads or physical demands placed on it.

SIGNS AND SYMPTOMS INDICATING REFERRAL TO PHYSICIAN

- Fever/chills/malaise
- Gastrointestinal dysfunction
- Unexplained weight loss
- Rebound tenderness
- Night pain
- History of cancer
- Bowel/bladder dysfunction

SUGGESTED READINGS

Johnson R. Abdominal wall injuries: rectus abdominis strains, oblique strains, rectus sheath hematoma. *Curr Sports Med Rep.* 2006;5(2):99-103.

Maquirriain J, Ghisi JP, Kokalj AM. Rectus abdominis muscle strains in tennis players. *Br J Sports Med.* 2007;41(11):842-848.

Maquirriain J, Ghisi JP. Uncommon abdominal muscle injury in a tennis player: internal oblique strain. *Br J Sports Med.* 2006;40(5):462-463.

Martens MA, Hansen L, Mulier JC. Adductor tendinitis and musculus rectus abdominis tendopathy. *Am J Sports Med.* 1987;15(4):353-356.

Wang JH, Iosifidis MI, Fu FH. Biomechanical basis for tendinopathy. *Clin Orthop Relat Res.* 2006;443:320-332.

AUTHOR: PAMELA J. KIKILLUS

Section III

ORTHOPEDIC PATHOLOGY

BASIC INFORMATION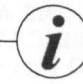

DEFINITION

Ankylosing spondylitis is a chronic inflammatory disease of unknown etiology and is classified as a spondyloarthropathy since it affects the joints of the spine. It typically affects fibrous tissue such as the entheses. Entheses are the insertions of ligaments, tendons, and capsules into bone.

SYNONYM

Spondyloarthropathy

ICD-9CM CODE
720.0 Ankylosing spondylitis

OPTIMAL NUMBER OF VISITS

6 visits or less

MAXIMAL NUMBER OF VISITS

24 visits

ETIOLOGY

- Ankylosing spondylitis is largely genetically determined. Those who have the antigen HLA-B27 are more likely to be diagnosed with ankylosing spondylitis than those without the antigen. The pathology may be triggered by an environmental stimulus; however, this stimulus may be ubiquitous.
- A familial history for ankylosing spondylitis is a strong risk factor.

EPIDEMIOLOGY AND DEMOGRAPHICS

- Males are two to three times more frequently diagnosed than females; however, females often have atypical presentations, thus they are not diagnosed as often with ankylosing spondylitis.
- The onset usually occurs in the teens, with peak onset at approximately age 28.
- Since the pathology has a strong association with HLA-B27, the prevalence of ankylosing spondylitis mirrors the frequency of this genetic expression in the different ethnic populations: white Americans 0.2%, white Germans 0.9%, and northern Norwegians 1.4%. African Americans are affected far less frequently than American whites.

MECHANISM OF INJURY

Insidious onset.

COMMON SIGNS AND SYMPTOMS

- The characteristics of inflammatory pain are reported, rather than a mechanically based pain syndrome. As ankylosing spondylitis progresses, ossification of the entheses and intervertebral discs typically occur, resulting in complaints of lumbopelvic tightness.
- The patient typically reports onset of gluteal pain of >3 months. It is often described as dull and is hard to localize. It may alternate from side to side and is typically unilateral and intermittent at onset. As the pathology progresses, the pain usually affects both gluteal regions and becomes constant. The pain is occasionally referred toward the iliac crest, greater trochanteric region, or down the posterior thigh. These symptoms are the manifestation of sacroiliitis.
- Lumbar pain and stiffness may occur with the initial onset of gluteal symptoms; however, it commonly follows the bilateral gluteal symptoms. This stiffness is worst during the morning.
- The patient may also describe chest pain and tenderness of the sternocostal region.
- Peripheral arthritis may be associated with this spondyloarthropathy, most commonly the hips, knees, and shoulders.
- Pain at the enthesis of the Achilles tendon and plantar fascia may be present as well.
- Redness of one eye at a time with pain and photophobia may be present.
- Cervical pain and stiffness is believed to be a late manifestation of ankylosing spondylitis.

AGGRAVATING ACTIVITIES

- Spinal rotation movements
- Coughing/sneezing, typically affecting the chest region
- After periods of prolonged rest

EASING ACTIVITIES

Patients commonly report decreased symptoms with exercise.

24-HOUR SYMPTOM PATTERN

The patient with ankylosing spondylitis will complain of stiffness and pain in the morning, lasting for more than 1 hour. As the day progresses and the patient is more active, his or her symptoms will typically lessen.

PAST HISTORY FOR THE REGION

Patients with ankylosing spondylitis typically have a history of intermittent gluteal and/or lumbar pain that began during the late adolescence or early adulthood, rarely after age 40. These symptoms typically become constant as the pathology progresses beyond this time frame.

PHYSICAL EXAMINATION

- Initially, there is a flattening of the normal lordotic spine. With continued progression of ankylosing spondylitis, there will be an increased thoracic kyphosis, forward head posture, and compensatory flexion of the hips and knees.
- The spine will erode at the adjacent corners of the vertebral body, leading to a "squaring" of the bodies. This results in the decrease of the lumbar lordosis. As the disease progresses, the spine will take on a "bamboo" appearance radiographically because of ossification of the annulus fibrosis, the anterior longitudinal ligament, and apophyseal joints, as well as the presence of bony bridges that form across the intervertebral spaces.
- Typically, there will be limited lumbar flexion range of motion (ROM) at the early onset of the disease. As the pathology progresses, the remaining cardinal planes of both the lumbar and thoracic regions will be limited. The amount of limitation usually parallels the progression of ankylosing spondylitis.
- Limited cervical extension is a later manifestation; however, it commonly precedes limitations in the remaining cervical cardinal planes.
- Viitanen et al (1995) found that the magnitude of the spinal ROM loss correlated with progressive radiological changes in both the lumbar and sacroiliac joints.
- Impaired myotomal strength, dermatomal sensation, and deep tendon reflexes are not common findings. As the pathology progresses, however, there may be co-morbidities that affect this portion of the examination.

IMPORTANT OBJECTIVE TESTS

- Spinal ROM testing
  - Schober test
  - Thoracolumbar rotation
  - Thoracolumbar flexion
  - Cervical rotation
- Chin:Chest distance
- Chest expansion
  - Viitanen found intraclass correlation coefficients of 0.53
- Occiput:Wall distance
  - Heuft-Dorenbosch found intraclass correlation of 0.94 to 0.96
- Tragus:Wall distance
  - Heuft-Dorenbosch found intraclass correlation of 0.93 to 0.95
- Provocation test
  - Robinson et al performed a study that included patients with the diagnosis of ankylosing spondylitis as part of the experimental group. They found the following provocation tests to be effective with diagnosing sacroiliac pain: sacroiliac compression (percent agreement ranged from 82% to 88% with kappa range of 0.48 to 0.67), sacroiliac distraction (82%, 0.63), posterior pelvic pain provocation test (also called the Gaenslen's test with 84% to 97% agreement and kappa

ranges of 0.74 to 0.76), Patrick-Fabere test (74% to 80%, 0.48 to 0.60), bilateral hip internal rotation passively (79%, 0.56), unilateral hip internal rotation passively (89% to 90%, 0.78 to 0.88), and the drop test (88% to 97%, 0.47 to 0.84). During the drop test, the patient performs a unilateral heel raise and then "drops down" onto the ipsilateral leg. Pain provocation is a positive finding.

- The absence of neurological findings in addition with inflammatory-based pain, objective evidence of spinal and chest wall tightness, and positive provocative testing tends to raise the suspicion of ankylosing spondylitis. A patient history that is significant for familial history of spondyloarthropathies, as well as the pain presentation discussed earlier, will further suggest the likelihood of ankylosing spondylitis.

DIFFERENTIAL DIAGNOSIS

- Lumbar disc pathology
- Lumbar facet arthropathy
- Gluteal strain
- Strain of lumbar musculature
- Ligament strain of the lumbopelvic spine
- Spondylosis
- Lumbopelvic instability
- Reiter's syndrome
- Diffuse idiopathic skeletal hyperostosis (DISH)
- Acquired immunodeficiency syndrome (AIDS)
- Psoriatic arthritis

TREATMENT

SURGICAL OPTIONS

- Total hip arthroplasty.
- Osteotomy of the spine may be performed to help correct severe spinal deformities.
- Spinal fusion may be an option in patients who have a single mobile segment that causes pain and limited function.
- These surgeries are not commonplace in patients with ankylosing spondylitis.

REHABILITATION

- Exercises that promote efficient posture and spinal mobility are advocated in this population. Breathing exercises are prescribed to increase thoracic, rib cage, and chest wall mobility. Cardiovascular exercise is helpful to maintain and progress overall fitness.
- Ince et al used a multimodal program including step exercises, stretching, and pulmonary exercises that lasted for

3 months and consisted of 3 sessions per week. They found improvements in chest expansion ($p = 0.04$), finger-to-floor distance ($p = 0.003$), chin-to-chest distance ($p = 0.03$), and occiput-to-wall distance ($p = 0.02$) compared to a control group. Significant improvements in inclinometric measurements were also detected with p values that ranged from 0.03 to 0.001. Physical work capacities improved in the exercise group ($p = 0.001$) and decreased in the control group ($p = 0.002$) at the end of 3 months. Vital capacity was maintained in the exercise group compared to a decrease in the control group ($p = 0.004$).

- Lubrano et al found that intensive, twice daily inpatient physical therapy treatment for 3 weeks produced a significant improvement in the assessment in ankylosing spondylitis (ASAS). The ASAS, which is a validated instrument for identifying treatment response, improved in 88.5% of the patients at the end of the structured visits. After this period, the patients were given a daily home exercise program. When they were reassessed 6 weeks later, the percentage of patients that remained to present with improvement decreased to 59.6%. After 12 weeks from the last visit, the percentage decreased further to 32.7%. This trend was statistically significant with p values of 0.001 for both subsequent follow-ups.

- Lim et al investigated the effectiveness of a home exercise program that was 30 minutes in duration, performed once daily, and lasted for 8 weeks. The program consisted of stretching, abdominal strengthening, hip extensor strengthening, and breathing exercises. When compared to a control group, there were improvements in joint mobility and spine flexibility ($p < 0.0001$) and depression ($p < 0.0001$). Functional capacity and pain also were reduced ($p < 0.0001$).

- Dagfinrud et al performed a review of the literature regarding physical therapy treatment and selected eleven trials for their conclusions. In summary, they found that an individual home-based or supervised exercise program is better than no intervention, that supervised group physical therapy is better than home exercises, and that combined inpatient therapy followed by group physical therapy is better than group physical therapy alone.

PROGNOSIS

- The prognosis of ankylosing spondylitis is good in the long term. Only 10% to 20% become significantly disabled over long periods (20 to 38 years after diagnosis); 85% to 90% are able to

maintain full-time jobs despite severe spinal restrictions that occur in approximately half of the patients.

- The earlier the onset of hip disease, the poorer the functional outcome generally is expected.
- Life expectancy is slightly reduced, but this may be due to related complications such as amyloidosis, spinal fractures, cardiovascular disease, gastrointestinal disease, and renal disease.

SIGNS AND SYMPTOMS INDICATING REFERRAL TO PHYSICIAN

- Acute fracture of the ankylosed spine, especially of the cervical spine after motor vehicle accidents (MVAs)
- Atlantoaxial subluxation
- Cauda equina syndrome
- Spinal stenosis
- Gastrointestinal symptoms caused by the typical prescription of nonsteroidal antiinflammatory drugs (NSAIDs) are found in this population
- Cardiac symptoms caused by aortic regurgitation and variable degrees of atrioventricular or bundle-branch block occur in approximately 5% of patients with ankylosing spondylitis

SUGGESTED READINGS

Alparslan L, et al. Imaging. In: Harris ED, et al., eds. *Kelley's Textbook of Rheumatology*. 7th ed. Philadelphia, PA: Elsevier Science; 2005 [Chapter 51].

Braun J, et al. Prevalence of spondyloarthropathies in HLA-B27 positive and negative blood donors. *Arthritis Rheum*. 1998;41:58-67.

Dagfinrud H, Kvien TK, Hagen KB. Physiotherapy interventions for ankylosing spondylitis. *Cochrane Database Syst Rev*. 2008;(1): CD002822.

Davis JC. Ankylosing spondylitis. In: Koopman W, Moreland LW, eds. *Arthritis and Allied Conditions: A Textbook of Rheumatology*. 15th ed. Philadelphia, PA: Lippincott Williams and Wilkins; 2005 [Chapter 63].

Fernandez-de-Las-Penas C, Alonso-Blanco C, Morales-Cabezas M, Miangolarra-Page JC. Two exercise interventions for the management of patients with ankylosing spondylitis: a randomized controlled trial. *Am J Phys Med Rehabil*. 2005;84(6):407-419.

Heikkila S, Viitanen JV, Kautiainen H, Kauppi M. Does improved spinal mobility correlate with functional changes in spondyloarthropathy after short term physical therapy? *J Rheumatol*. 2000;27(12):2942-2944.

Heikkila S, Viitanen JV, Kautiainen H, Kauppi M. Sensitivity to change of mobility tests; effect of short term intensive physiotherapy and exercise on spinal, hip, and shoulder measurements in spondyloarthropathy. *J Rheumatol*. 2000;27(5):1251-1256.

Heuft-Dorenbosch L, et al. Measurement of spinal mobility in ankylosing spondylitis: comparison of occiput-to-wall and tragus-to-wall distance. *J Rheumatol*. 2004;31(9):1779-1784.

Ince G, Sarpel T, Durgun B, Erdogan S. Effects of a multimodal exercise program for

Section III

ORTHOPEDIC PATHOLOGY

people with ankylosing spondylitis. *Phys Ther*. 2006;86(7):924-935.

Kraag G, Stokes B, Groh J, Helewa A, Goldsmith CH. The effects of comprehensive home physiotherapy and supervision on patients with ankylosing spondylitis-an 8-month follow up. *J Rheumatol*. 1994; 21(2):261-263.

Lawrence RC, et al. Estimates of the prevalence of arthritis and selected musculoskeletal disorders in the United States. *Arthritis Rheum*. 1998;41:778-799.

Lim HJ, Moon YI, Lee MS. Effects of home-based daily exercise therapy on joint mobility, daily activity, pain, and depression in patients with ankylosing spondylitis. *Rheumatol Int*. 2005;25(3):225-229.

Lubrano E, D'Angelo S, Parsons WJ, et al. Effectiveness of rehabilitation in active ankylosing spondylitis assessed by the ASAS response criteria. *Rheumatology*. Nov 2007;46(11):1672-1675.

Robinson HS, Brox JI, Robinson R, Bjelland E, Solem S, Telje T. The reliability of selected motion- and pain provocation tests for the sacroiliac joint. *Man Ther*. 2007;12(1):72-79.

Van Der Linden S, et al. Ankylosing spondylitis. In: Harris ED, et al., eds. *Kelley's Textbook of Rheumatology*. 7th ed. Philadelphia, PA: Elsevier Science; 2005 [Chapter 70].

Viitanen JV, et al. Correlation between mobility restrictions and radiologic changes in ankylosing spondylitis. *Spine*. 1995;20(4): 492-496.

AUTHOR: NEIL MCKENNA

BASIC INFORMATION

DEFINITION

An avulsion fracture of the ischial tuberosity is an injury in which the ischial apophysis dislocates from the innominate.

SYNONYMS

- Avulsion fracture of the ischial apophysis
- Grade IIIB strain of the hamstrings

ICD-9CM CODE
808.42 Closed fracture of ischium

OPTIMAL NUMBER OF VISITS

6 visits or less

MAXIMAL NUMBER OF VISITS

18 visits

ETIOLOGY

The ischial apophysis is a secondary ossification center that is first observed at 15 to 17 years of age and that fuses between ages of 19 to 25 years. It forms the ischial tuberosity. The developing apophysis is the weakest link in the chain of muscle, tendon, and bone. Chronic repetitive traction on the developing apophysis weakens this susceptible interface, allowing for the possibility of avulsion injuries. The strong sacrotuberous ligament helps to stabilize the rest of the ischium and generally prevents a large displacement of the avulsion.

EPIDEMIOLOGY AND DEMOGRAPHICS

- The prevalence of pelvic avulsion fractures is approximately 4%. Roughly 50% of pelvic avulsions are in the ischium.
- Adolescent cases are the most prevalent since the apophysis typically fuses after the age of 19 years.

MECHANISM OF INJURY

- The mechanism of injury is believed to be the result of a sudden forceful concentric or eccentric contraction of the hamstrings to accelerate or decelerate the body. The adductor magnus may be implicated in this injury as well, but it is less likely than the hamstrings.
- The avulsion may also occur as the result of a sudden lengthening of the hamstrings. These injuries typically occur during sport activity such as sprinting, long jumping, hurdling, and performing splits during gymnastics and dance.
- Often, there is no history of external trauma and the symptoms begin with a sudden, sharp pain associated with a "pop or snap."

COMMON SIGNS AND SYMPTOMS

- Pain at the ischial tuberosity
- Pain in the buttock
- Pain in the proximal posterior thigh
- Groin pain

AGGRAVATING FACTORS

- Pain with weight bearing through the affected limb, primarily if the patient is in the inflammatory phase of the fracture healing process
- Pain with sitting or moving on the involved tuberosity
- Activities, such as the following, that require contraction or stretch of the hamstrings and/or the adductor magnus:
  ○ Running/sprinting
  ○ Performing splits

EASING FACTORS

- If the time frame is during the stage of inflammation associated with the fracture, then the traditional rest, ice, compression, elevation (RICE) treatments help.
- Once the inflammatory phase ends, the only easing factor is usually one that decreases mechanical pressure on the ischial tuberosity.

24-HOUR SYMPTOM PATTERN

- During the inflammatory phase of bone healing, there may be more nocturnal pain with stiffness within 1 to 2 hours on rising.
- Beyond this phase, there will be no discernable diurnal pattern of pain.

PAST HISTORY FOR THE REGION

Because of the infrequency of this pathology, the diagnosis at onset of symptoms may be a hamstring tear. If this is the case, the patient may have already been treated with rest and physical therapy without return to pain-free activity. He or she will report pain with activities that require strong contractions and/or flexibility of the hamstring muscle group.

PHYSICAL EXAMINATION

- Swelling and tenderness at the ischial tuberosity
- Palpable "gap" at the origin of the hamstrings

IMPORTANT OBJECTIVE TESTS

- Pain reproduction with combined passive hip flexion and knee extension may indicate the possibility of an avulsion fracture. Further pain may be reported when the examiner adds hip abduction in this position.
- If the patient has progressed beyond the stages of bone healing, he or she may have weakness on manual muscle testing of the hamstrings.

DIFFERENTIAL DIAGNOSIS

- Hamstring strain (however, this may be a co-morbidity)
- Gluteal muscle strain
- Groin strain
- Piriformis syndrome
- Ischial, trochanteric bursitis
- Sacroiliac joint referral
- Lumbar facet referral
- Spondylolisthesis
- Lumbar disc referral
- Proximal femoral fracture
- Pelvic fracture, other than the ischial tuberosity

TREATMENT

SURGICAL OPTIONS

- Because this pathology is rare, there are limited studies regarding surgical outcomes. Case studies of surgical intervention typically demonstrate satisfactory results in which the patient is able to return to their prior level of sport activity.
- Open reduction internal fixation (ORIF) is typically recommended if the displacement is >2 cm.
- Excision of excessive callous formation may be performed if the symptoms are chronic and the patient did not require surgical fixation at the onset.

REHABILITATION

Nonsurgical Patients
- Metzmaker et al (1985) created a conservative program that utilizes phases of progression correlating to healing of the fracture zone. This included:
  ○ Rest and crutches: 7 days
  ○ Rest, crutches, ROM: 8-20 days
  ○ Mild resistance at midrange: 21-30 days
  ○ Full weight bearing, ROM, and resistance: 31-60 days
  ○ Sport training: 60 days, then return to normal activities

Internal Fixation of the Ischial Tuberosity
- Bed rest of 1 to 2 weeks is generally prescribed after surgery. Partial weight bearing is usually prescribed for 3-6 weeks after surgery.
- Allowed hip flexion ROM varied in the case studies from 1 to 6 weeks. Therefore the clinician should correspond with the surgeon regarding the time frame and allowance of hip flexion ROM.
- Union of the fracture area is typically complete by 3 to 4 months after fixation. By this point, the patient should have full ROM and strength to return to sport activities.

Stage	Days after Injury	Intervention	Radiographic Appearance
Rest	0-7 days	Ice and analgesics, with protected ambulation using crutches, bed rest 72 hours, and positioning in 25 degrees of knee flexion to reduce stress on the hamstring insertion.	Osseous separation
Increased excursion	7 to 14-20	Remains to use crutches and partial weight-bearing, moist heat, gentle passive ROM of the limb, and gentle active ROM in limited ROM.	Osseous separation
Progressive resistance	14-20 to 30	Use of mild resistance for midrange excursion once at least 75% of the hip flexion range is accomplished with the knee extended.	Early callus formation
Integration	30 to 60	Begins when 50% of strength is accomplished. Cycling, full weight bearing without assistive device, continued stretching and strengthening, and gentle sport patterns.	Maturing callus
Preparation to return to sport	60 to return to normal activities	Return to sport requires full strength, ROM, and integration of all activities without pain.	Maturing callus

PROGNOSIS

- The majority of those who sustained an avulsion fracture of the ischial apophysis generally do not require surgery. As long as the displacement was not significant (typically >2 cm), the patient typically returns to full activity without pain.
- The larger the fracture displacement without surgical intervention, the more likely the patient will report weakness of the hamstring, chronic pain, and limited ability to perform higher-level sport activities.

SIGNS AND SYMPTOMS INDICATING REFERRAL TO PHYSICIAN

- Sciatica is a complication of this injury because of the displaced apophysis and the development of callus formation around the fracture zone.
  - Therefore any dermatomal and/or myotomal disturbances should not be considered lightly.
- Progressive pain with ambulation and weakness of the hamstring may indicate further displacement of the apophysis.

- Intolerance to running >4 months after injury may indicate poor union of the fracture area.

SUGGESTED READINGS

Akova B, Okay E. Avulsion of the ischial tuberosity in a young soccer player: six years follow-up. *J Sports Sci Med.* 2002;1:27-30.

Buckwalter JA, et al. Basic science and injury of articular cartilage, menisci, and bone. In: DeLee JC, Drez D, eds. *DeLee and Drez's Orthopaedic Sports Medicine.* 2nd ed. Philadelphia, PA: Elsevier Science; 2003 [Chapter 2].

Dosani A, Giannoudis PV, Waseem M, et al. Unusual presentation of sciatica in a 14-year-old girl. *Injury.* 2004;35:1071-1072.

Gidwani S, Jagiello J, Bircher M. Avulsion fracture of the ischial tuberosity in adolescents: an easily missed diagnosis. *BMJ.* 2004;329:99-100.

Kujala UM, Orava S, Karpakka J, et al. Ischial tuberosity apophysis and avulsion among athletes. *Int J Sports Med.* 1997;18:149-155.

Mattick AP, Beattie TF, Macnicol MF. Just a pulled hamstring? *J Accid Emerg Med.* 1999;16(6):457-458.

Metzmaker JN, Pappas AM. Avulsion fractures of the pelvis. *Am J Sports Med.* 1985;13:349.

Miller A, Stedman GH, Beisaw NE, et al. Sciatica caused by an avulsion fracture of the ischial tuberosity. *J Bone Joint Surg.* 1987;69-A: 143-145.

Muscato M, Lim-Dunham J, Demos TC, et al. Avulsion fracture of the apophysis of the ischial tuberosity. *Orthopedics.* 2001; 24:1198-1200.

Nuccion SL, et al. Hip and pelvis. In: DeLee JC, Drez D, eds. *DeLee and Drez's Orthopaedic Sports Medicine.* 2nd ed. Philadelphia, PA: Elsevier Science; 2003 [Chapter 25].

Seo GS, Aoki J, Karakida O, Sone S, Ishii K. Ischiopubic insufficiency fractures: MRI appearances. *Skeletal Radiol.* 1997;26(12): 705-710.

Servant CT, Jones CB. Displaced avulsion of the ischial apophysis: a hamstring injury requiring internal fixation. *Br J Sports Med.* 1998;32(3):255-257.

Spinner RJ, Atkinson JL, Wenger DE, et al. Tardy sciatic nerve palsy following apophyseal avulsion fracture of the ischial tuberosity: case report. *J Neurosurg.* 1998;89:819-821.

Takami H, Takahashi S, Ando M. Late sciatic nerve palsy following avulsion of the biceps femoris muscle from the ischial tuberosity. *Arch Orthop Trauma Surg.* 2000;120(5-6):352-354.

Widmann RF. Fractures of the pelvis. In: Beaty JH, Kasser JR, eds. *Rockwood and Wilkins' Fractures in Children.* 6th ed. Philadelphia, PA: Lippincott Williams & Wilkins; 2006 [Chapter 20].

AUTHOR: NEIL MCKENNA

BASIC INFORMATION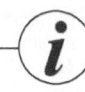

DEFINITION

Avulsion of the hamstring is an injury in which the origin of the semimembranosus, semitendinosus, and long head of the biceps femoris is displaced from the ischial tuberosity at the bone-tendon junction.

SYNONYM

Grade IIIA strain of the hamstrings

ICD-9CM CODE
848.9 Unspecified site of sprain and strain

OPTIMAL NUMBER OF VISITS

3 or less for those without surgical repair. In the case of surgery, 6 or less is the optimal number.

MAXIMAL NUMBER OF VISITS

36 for those without surgical repair. In the case of surgery, 70 may be the maximal number.

ETIOLOGY

- McMaster found that a healthy musculotendinous unit will not rupture through the tendon; however, it will rupture at the musculotendinous junction, the belly of the muscle, or at the bone-tendon junction.
- Garrett et al (1988) found injury and rupture at the musculotendinous junction whether the muscle was pulled from the origin or from the insertion at various rates of strain. They found that the muscles with a more pennate structure tended to elongate further under the strain before failure. The hamstrings are classified as a uni-pennate muscle, therefore they may be more susceptible to strain injuries.
- Garrett et al (1984) also classified the hamstrings to have a high proportion of type II fibers, which are important for rapid force production. This finding, as well as the susceptibility of these two-joint muscles to undergo large extrinsic factors, may predispose these muscles to injury.

EPIDEMIOLOGY AND DEMOGRAPHICS

- The prevalence of these injuries is very low.
- The injury is typically seen in adults since the ischial apophysis is typically fused by the age of 25. Therefore the younger population may be predisposed for avulsions of the ischial apophyses.
- Athletes are more likely to sustain this injury.

- Water skiers seem to have a higher risk for this injury as well.

MECHANISM OF INJURY

- The common mechanism for this injury is a rapid, forceful motion of hip flexion and knee extension, usually with contraction of the hamstring. Falling during water skiing is commonly reported as the mechanism since it involves these motions as the patient travels in a face-first dive into the water.
- Other common mechanisms are as follows:
  - Lifting heavy objects from the floor
  - Power lifting
  - Skating

COMMON SIGNS AND SYMPTOMS

Typically, the patient will report sharp, sudden, agonizing pain located at the posterior thigh. Sciatica symptoms may also be present after the initial onset of the injury.

AGGRAVATING ACTIVITIES

- At initial onset
  - Any activities requiring hip flexion and/or knee extension
  - Ambulation
  - Standing
  - Squatting
- Postinflammatory phase
  - Walking downhill
  - Running

EASING ACTIVITIES

- During the inflammatory phase, the patient will typically report pain relief with rest, use of ice and NSAIDs.
- Beyond the inflammatory phase, there are no significant easing factors.

24-HOUR SYMPTOM PATTERN

- During the inflammatory phase of soft tissue healing, there may be more nocturnal pain with stiffness within 1 to 2 hours on rising.
- Beyond this phase, there will be no discernable diurnal pattern of pain.

PAST HISTORY FOR THE REGION

Acute rupture of the hamstring tendons is rare and difficult to diagnose during the early phase of injury. Therefore the pathology may be conservatively managed for a prolonged period of time without full return to sport activities. The patient may report frequent hamstring "pulls" with higher level sport motions and may also complain of a chronically weak hamstring in comparison to the uninvolved side.

PHYSICAL EXAMINATION

- Large amounts of swelling and ecchymosis

- Presence of a posterior midthigh mass that retracts with contraction of the hamstrings
- Palpable gap at the origin of the hamstrings with pain generally on palpation

IMPORTANT OBJECTIVE TESTS

- Passive hip flexion combined with knee extension and manual muscle testing of the hamstring help to delineate the hamstring as the source of the patient's pain.
- If the clinician suspects an avulsion of the hamstrings, a referral to the physician may be warranted. The physician may then order a T2-weighted magnetic resonance imaging (MRI) or sonogram to help identify the severity of the injury.

DIFFERENTIAL DIAGNOSIS

- Sciatica
- Avulsion fracture of the ischial apophysis
- Proximal femoral fracture
- Gluteal muscle strain
- Piriformis syndrome
- Sacroiliac joint referral
- Lumbar facet referral
- Lumbar disc referral
- Ischial bursitis

CONTRIBUTING FACTORS

- Heiser et al, Jonhagen et al, and Orchard et al all reported that decreased hamstring torque production correlated with various levels of hamstring injuries.
- Jonhagen also found that sprinters who had a prior hamstring injury had significantly tighter hamstrings than uninjured sprinters.
- However, Orchard et al did not find a correlation of hamstring length and injury risk.

TREATMENT

SURGICAL OPTIONS

- Orava et al recommend early surgical treatment. They had better results when the surgery was performed within 2 months from the injury.
- Cross et al found an average hamstring strength grade of 60% when compared to the uninvolved side 2 years after the surgery. The average hamstring endurance was 57% of uninvolved side.
- Blasier et al found a 9% decrease in hamstring strength 7 years after surgery.

REHABILITATION

- Postsurgical patients
  - The postoperative protocols vary; therefore it would be best to contact

the referring surgeon regarding his or her protocol.

○ Physical therapy may not begin until 6 weeks after surgery. Typically, there is partial weight bearing after 2 weeks and full weight bearing after 4 weeks. ROM that produces strain on the hamstrings, such as combined hip flexion with knee extension, are best avoided for 1 month after surgery. ROM and strength should be maximized by 3 to 4 months after surgery in anticipation to return of full sport level.

• Nonsurgical patients

○ RICE should be instituted at the onset of the inflammatory process. Strength training should be progressed from isometrics to isotonics and then to isokinetics as the tissue progresses through the stages of healing. Along this continuum, integration of sport-specific training should be emphasized as well.

PROGNOSIS

• There are no case studies in the literature that discuss the prognosis of patients who do not have surgery. There are many cases in which the patient had persistent symptoms that limited them from their desired activities. These patients tended to seek the care of a surgeon.

• Generally, patients that receive surgery tend to return to their sport activity; however, weakness of the hamstring may remain.

SIGNS AND SYMPTOMS INDICATING REFERRAL TO PHYSICIAN

• Onset of neurological symptoms
• Inability to strengthen the hamstrings
• Continual pain extending beyond healing time frames

SUGGESTED READINGS

Blasier RB, et al. Complete rupture of the hamstring origin from a water skiing injury. *Am J Sports Med.* 1990;18(4):435-437.

Cross MJ, Vandersluis R, Wood D, Banff M. Surgical repair of chronic complete hamstring tendon rupture in the adult patient. *Am J Sports Med.* 1998;26:785-788.

Garrett WE, et al. Histochemical correlates of hamstring injuries. *Am J Sports Med.* 1984;12:98-103.

Garrett WE, Nikolaou PK, Ribbeck BM, et al. The effect of muscle architecture on the biomechanical failure properties of skeletal muscle under passive extension. *Am J Sports Med.* 1988;16:7-12.

Heiser TM, Weber J, Sullivan G, et al. Prophylaxis and management of hamstring muscle injuries in intercollegiate football players. *Am J Sports Med.* 1984;12:368-370.

Johnson AE, Granville RR, DeBerardino TM. Avulsion of the common hamstring tendon origin in an active duty airman. *Mil Med.* 2003;168(1):40-42.

Jonhagen S, Nemeth G, Ericsson E. Hamstring injuries in sprinters—The role of concentric and eccentric hamstring muscle strength and flexibility. *Am J Sports Med.* 1994;22:262-266.

Kujala UM, Orava S, Jarvinen M. Hamstring injuries; current trends in treatment and prevention. *Sports Med.* 1997;23:397-404.

McMaster PE. Tendon and muscle ruptures. Clinical and experimental studies on the causes and location of subcutaneous ruptures. *J Bone Joint Surg.* 1933;15:705-722.

Orava S, Kujala UM. Rupture of the ischial origin of the hamstring muscles. *Am J Sports Med.* 1995;23(6):702-705.

Orchard J, Marsden J, Lord S, Garlick D. Preseason hamstring muscle weakness associated with hamstring muscle injury in Australian footballers. *Am J Sports Med.* 1997;25:81-85.

AUTHOR: NEIL MCKENNA

BASIC INFORMATION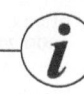

DEFINITION

The coccyx bone is composed of 3 to 5 separate or fused bony segments. Together they make up the lowest bone structures of the spinal column. Coccyx fracture refers to a break of this osseous structure.

SYNONYMS

- *Coccygodynia* and *coccydynia* are terms used to denote pain of the coccyx region
- Tailbone fracture

ICD-9CM CODE
805.6 Closed fracture of sacrum and coccyx without spinal cord injury

OPTIMAL NUMBER OF VISITS

6 visits or less

MAXIMAL NUMBER OF VISITS

18 visits

ETIOLOGY

The major complication associated with this fracture is resultant hypermobility of the coccyx, most likely from a sprain of the sacrococcygeal ligaments attributed to trauma. Hypermobility of the coccyx has been reported by Maigne et al (1996). He defined hypermobility when the coccyx flexed more than 25 degrees or displaced >25% compared to the sacrum. This movement was measured by the difference in coccyx angle from standing to sitting on lateral radiographs. Roughly 50% of patients with coccygodynia had hypermobility findings.

EPIDEMIOLOGY AND DEMOGRAPHICS

- It is relatively uncommon, and there are no published data on the prevalence of this pathology.
- There is no age group most at risk for this pathology. However, coccygodynia is more common in the 30- to 40-year-old bracket.
- Since the coccyx does not ossify until after birth, a coccyx fracture may also dislocate in the toddler age group. Raissaki et al found this situation in a 30-month-old child.
- There is no gender bias for coccyx fractures; however, women are 4 to 5 times more likely to develop coccygodynia.
- Ectomorphs, who are described as being long and thin, may be more susceptible to this fracture simply because they have less soft tissue mass of the gluteal region.

MECHANISM OF INJURY

- Axial impact on the most distal part of the spine is the most common mechanism for this fracture.
- Childbirth and obesity have been described in the literature as having roles in the development of coccygodynia.

COMMON SIGNS AND SYMPTOMS

Pain in the coccyx region

AGGRAVATING ACTIVITIES

- Sitting
- Sit-to-stand transfers
- Forward bending
- Bowel movements
- Pain with intercourse

EASING ACTIVITIES

- Sitting on the posterior thighs or just on one buttock
- Use of a sacral cushion

24-HOUR SYMPTOM PATTERN

There is no known diurnal pattern of symptoms for this patient population.

PAST HISTORY OF THE REGION

- These patients may develop a hypermobility syndrome of the coccyx that can lead to chronic coccygodynia. Maigne et al (2000) found hypermobility in 77% of patients who reported a traumatic event <1 month before their symptoms. Roughly 50% of patients with coccygodynia were classified as being hypermobile, whether they sustained a traumatic event or not.
- Patients who develop coccygodynia typically describe a trauma that was sustained years ago, even though their symptoms may have begun a few months ago.

PHYSICAL EXAMINATION

- Local swelling
- Tenderness of the superficial surface of the coccyx
- Pain with rectal examination of coccygeal motion

IMPORTANT OBJECTIVE TESTS

There are no specific objective tests designed to assess the integrity of the sacrococcygeal joint; however, joint assessment techniques may be employed to detect planes of restriction or excessive motion.

DIFFERENTIAL DIAGNOSIS

- Lumbar disc lesion
- Arachnoiditis of the lower sacral roots
- Tumors of the coccyx or sacrum
- Spasm of the pelvic floor musculature
- Anal, prostatic, or cervical infections

CONTRIBUTING FACTORS

Obesity and history of falls or childbirth have a relationship with the development of coccyx pain.

TREATMENT

SURGICAL INDICATORS

- Surgery is only performed initially if there are neurological complications such as bowel and bladder dysfunctions.
- Surgery is only recommended if the patient goes on to develop chronic coccygodynia.

SURGICAL OPTIONS

Total or partial coccygectomy may be performed, depending on the amount of hypermobility present.

SURGICAL OUTCOMES

The surgical outcomes reported in the data are typically 80% to 85% satisfactory.

REHABILITATION

- There are no specific rehabilitation interventions for someone who has sustained a coccyx fracture; however, there are several conservative treatment options for coccygodynia. They range from rectal mobilization of the coccyx, mobilization of the sacroiliac joint, and rectal soft tissue techniques/stretching of the levator anus.
- Maigne et al (2001) found satisfactory results for 25% of their cases using manual techniques.
- Wray et al used a rectal mobilization technique in addition to using injections of methylprednisolone and bupivacaine and reported an 85% cure rate with roughly 28% requiring repeat treatments.
- If the therapist is seeing a patient after a coccygectomy, it is very important to monitor healing of the surgical wound since infection of this site has been reported as a complication.

PROGNOSIS

The symptoms typically subside within weeks or months. Despite conservative treatment, approximately 20% remain to have pain. They may then be appropriate for a surgical intervention.

SIGNS AND SYMPTOMS INDICATING REFERRAL TO PHYSICIAN

- The presence of constitutional signs and symptoms should warrant referral to the physician.

- In the case that the patient received a coccygectomy, any indication of infection should indicate referral back to the surgeon.

SUGGESTED READINGS

Fogel GR, et al. Coccygodynia: evaluation and management. *J Am Acad Orthop Surg.* 2004;12:49-54.

Maigne JY, et al. Causes and mechanisms of common coccydynia: role of body mass index and coccygeal trauma. *Spine.* 2000;25(23):3072-3079.

Maigne JY, et al. Comparison of three manual coccydynia treatments: a pilot study. *Spine.* 2001;26(20):E479-483.

Maigne JY, et al. Standardized radiologic protocol for the study of common coccygodynia and characteristics of the lesions observed in the sitting position: Clinical elements differentiating luxation, hypermobility, and normal mobility. *Spine.* 1996;21(22):2588-2593.

Mouhsine E, et al. Posttraumatic coccygeal instability. *Spine J.* 2006;6(5):544-549.

Polkinghorn BS, et al. Chiropractic treatment of coccygodynia via instrumental adjusting procedures using activator methods chiropractic technique. *J Manipul Physiol Ther.* 1999;22:411-416.

Raissaki MT, et al. Fracture dislocation of the sacro-coccygeal joint: MRI evaluation. *Pediatr Radiol.* 1999;29(8):642-643.

Sehirlioglu A, et al. Coccygectomy in the surgical treatment of traumatic coccygodynia. *Injury.* 2007;38(2):182-187.

Wray CC, et al. Coccydynia: Aetiology and treatment. *J Bone Joint Surg Br.* 1991;73:335-338.

AUTHOR: NEIL MCKENNA

BASIC INFORMATION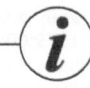

DEFINITION

- The description of the iliolumbar ligament differs among authors; however, they all agree that the attachment sites are the L5 transverse process and the ilium. Fujiwara et al (2000) found the ligament to consist of two separate bands. The anterior band originated from the anterior and lateral aspects of the L5 transverse process, inserted on the anterosuperior aspect of the ilium, and was connected to the anterior quadratus lumborum fascia. The posterior band originated from the posterior and inferior aspects of the L5 transverse process, inserted on the posteromedial ilium, and was connected to the posterior quadratus lumborum fascia. Sometimes this posterior band also attached to the dorsal sacroiliac ligament.
- The iliolumbar ligament functions to restrain motion at the L5-S1 segment, especially flexion and lateral bending.
- Pool-Goudzwaard et al found that severing the iliolumbar ligaments from cadavers led to increased sagittal plane motion of the sacroiliac joint. Therefore this ligament may have a role in stability of the sacroiliac joint as well.

ICD-9CM CODES
847.2 Lumbar sprain
846.0 Lumbosacral (joint) (ligament) sprain
848.5 Pelvic sprain

OPTIMAL NUMBER OF VISITS
8 visits or less

MAXIMAL NUMBER OF VISITS
24 visits

ETIOLOGY

- Snijders et al (2004) found that slouched sitting increased strain on the iliolumbar ligament. The mechanism of combined lumbar flexion with a posterior pelvic rotation produces a backward rotation of the sacrum (also called *counternutation*). This position produces strain at the iliolumbar ligament.
- The iliolumbar ligament is a highly innervated nociceptive tissue. Spinal ligaments generally have a high density of proprioceptive, mechanoreceptive, and nociceptive nerve fibers.
- The iliac periosteum on which the iliolumbar inserts also is highly innervated. Therefore any microtrauma at this junction could generate pain.
- Maigne et al postulated that edema and/or scarring of the iliolumbar ligament

may cause entrapment of the dorsal rami of the spinal nerves and therefore be a source of pain.

EPIDEMIOLOGY AND DEMOGRAPHICS

- Little attention has been paid to this ligament as a generator of symptoms in low back pain (LBP), therefore there is much to learn about its potential role. Binkley et al found that iliolumbar pathology could not be included as part of a classification scheme. This was due to a lack of specific diagnostic tests that indicate pathology of this structure, making it hard to delineate between closely related diagnoses.
- Therefore the prevalence of iliolumbar sprains is unknown.
- Fujiwara et al (2000) found the posterior band of the iliolumbar ligament in men to be shorter than the iliolumbar ligament in women. However, there has been no correlation of this finding with development of pain.
- Hanson et al found that the iliolumbar ligament in black people was one single, large band. White people had two smaller, distinct bands that originated from L5. There is a higher incidence of spondylolisthesis in both white men and women compared to black men and women. Hanson theorizes this may be due to the anatomical variations he isolated with his research.

MECHANISM OF INJURY

- Snijders et al (2004) found excessive strain at the iliolumbar ligament with dynamic slouching. They postulated that upper body weight and rectus abdominis activity would also increase strain at this ligament. Therefore microtrauma injury may occur if these activities were consistently repeated.
- The iliolumbar ligament has a role in controlling motion at the L5-S1 segments, especially with flexion and lateral flexion. Therefore an injury may be associated with these motions.

COMMON SIGNS AND SYMPTOMS

- Hirschberg et al described the "iliolumbar syndrome" as follows:
  ○ Spontaneous pain
  ○ Pain on the posterior aspect of the iliac crest
  ○ Pain that can vary from severe to a dull ache

AGGRAVATING ACTIVITIES

- Prolonged sitting or standing
- Transfers from bed

EASING ACTIVITY

Sitting with the use of a lumbar support

24-HOUR SYMPTOM PATTERN
There is typically no diurnal pattern.

PAST HISTORY OF THE REGION

- Past history is generally unremarkable.
- Fujiwara et al (1999) found that the morphology of the iliolumbar ligament can be a factor influencing the development of disc degeneration at L4/5 and L5-S1.
  ○ Therefore the patient may present with a pain history synonymous with hypermobility of the lower lumbar spine.

PHYSICAL EXAMINATION
The patient can usually place their finger on the exact site of pain.

IMPORTANT OBJECTIVE TESTS

- Pain can be reproduced with lateral flexion to the unaffected side.
- The neurological examination is typically negative.
- Repetitive lumbar motions should not refer pain below the knee.

DIFFERENTIAL DIAGNOSIS

- Lumbar disc pathology
- Spondylosis
- Spondylolisthesis (however, this may be a comorbidity)
- Sacroiliac pain referral
- Lumbar facet syndrome
- Myofascial pain of the gluteals, piriformis, iliopsoas, and quadratus lumborum

CONTRIBUTING FACTORS
Prolonged sitting and repetitive combined lumbar flexion with lateral flexion may affect the integrity of the iliolumbar ligament.

TREATMENT

SURGICAL OPTIONS

- There are no references indicating surgery for a direct iliolumbar ligament injury.
- However, Pool-Goudzwaard et al postulated that spinal surgery, which severs the iliolumbar ligament, may create sacroiliac hypermobility, thereby placing increased stress on the pelvic ligaments with possible pain provocation. This may partly explain failed back surgeries.

REHABILITATION
Programs developed to rehabilitate a patient with suspected iliolumbar ligament pathology should include the following:

- Prescribe the use of a lumbar support while sitting.

- Strengthen the patient's core muscles, with particular attention to the multifidus and the erector spinae.
  - Snijders et al (2007) found that activation of the multifidus and the erector spinae decreased stress at the iliolumbar ligament via its role in maintenance of the lumbar lordosis and pelvic position.
- Help to improve the patient's postural kinesthetic awareness.

PROGNOSIS

There are no specific data regarding the prognosis of iliolumbar ligament pathology, mainly because there is no currently accepted way to diagnose it.

SIGNS AND SYMPTOMS INDICATING REFERRAL TO PHYSICIAN

- As with all pathologies, the presence of constitutional signs and symptoms indicates referral to the physician.

- Since this pathology does not directly affect the peripheral nervous system, the presence of progressive neurological deficit warrants referral to a physician.

SUGGESTED READINGS

Binkley J, et al. Diagnostic classification of patients with low back pain: report on a survey of physical therapy experts. *Phys Ther*. 1993;73(3):138-150.

Fujiwara A, et al. Relationship between morphology of iliolumbar ligament and lower lumbar disc degeneration. *J Spinal Dis*. 1999;12(4):348-352.

Fujiwara A, et al. Anatomy of the iliolumbar ligament. *Clin Orthop Relat Res*. 2000; 380:167-172.

Hanson P, et al. Differences in the iliolumbar ligament and the transverse process of the L5 vertebra in young white and black people. *Acta Anat*. 1998;163:218-223.

Hirschberg GC, et al. Iliolumbar syndrome as a common cause of low back pain: diagnosis and prognosis. *Arch Phys Med Rehabil*. 1979;60:415-419.

Maigne JY, et al. Trigger point of the posterior iliac crest: painful iliolumbar ligament or cutaneous dorsal ramus pain? An anatomical study. *Arch Phys Med Rehabil*. 1991;72:734-737.

Pool-Goudzwaard A, et al. The iliolumbar ligament: its influence on stability of the sacroiliac joint. *Clin Biomechanics*. 2003;18: 99-105.

Sims JA, et al. The role of the iliolumbar ligament in low back pain. *Med Hypotheses*. 1996;46:511-515.

Snijders CJ, et al. The influence of slouching and lumbar support on iliolumbar ligaments, intervertebral discs and sacroiliac joints. *Clin Biomech (Bristol, Avon)*. May 2004;19(4):323-329.

Snijders CJ, et al. Effects of slouching and muscle contraction on the strain of the iliolumbar ligament. *Man Ther*. 2007;(in press).

AUTHOR: NEIL MCKENNA

BASIC INFORMATION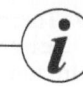

DEFINITION

- The obturator nerve arises from the ventral divisions of the second, third, and fourth lumbar nerves. It travels inferiorly along the psoas muscle, splits into anterior and posterior branches, and then enters the thigh through the obturator foramen.
- Brukner et al stated that its innervation includes the following:
  - Portions of the adductor magnus
  - Adductor longus
  - Adductor brevis
  - Gracilis
  - Obturator externus
  - Portions of the pectineus
- The obturator nerve innervates the medial distal two-thirds of the thigh, the hip joint, and the knee joint.

SYNONYM

Obturator nerve entrapment

ICD-9CM CODE
355.9 Mononeuritis of unspecified site

OPTIMAL NUMBER OF VISITS

12 visits or less

MAXIMUM NUMBER OF VISITS

56 visits

ETIOLOGY

- Bradshaw et al found that the most common site of entrapment for the obturator nerve was at the level of the obturator foramen and proximal thigh rather than in the obturator tunnel.
  - In this area, a fascial entrapment of the anterior branch of the obturator nerve is possible, particularly as the nerve passes over the adductor brevis muscle.
  - Less commonly, there may be pathology of the pelvis, such as fracture and inflammation, that could compress the nerve within the obturator tunnel.
- It is postulated that increased tension on the nerve is the likely culprit for symptom generation.
  - Bradshaw et al found an increased tendency for an obturator neuropathy in those with symptoms of an inguinal hernia. This could ultimately result in increased stretch of the obturator nerve.
- Another mechanism for obturator neuropathy is compression of the nerve at the fascial entrapment area near the adductor brevis.
- Topp et al discussed the effects of increased tension and compression on peripheral nerves. In summary, these

stressors can reduce intraneural blood flow, create demyelination, and disrupt axonal transport. These characteristically lead to symptom generation.

EPIDEMIOLOGY AND DEMOGRAPHICS

- The diagnosis of an obturator neuropathy is not very common.
- The likelihood of someone being diagnosed with an adductor strain is higher.
  - The prevalence rate of adductor strains amongst soccer players is between 10% and 18%.
- Men seem to be affected more than women.
  - Bradshaw et al stated that the anatomical difference of men having higher iliac bones, a smaller transverse diameter of the pelvic inlet, and a narrower subpubic angle may alter the angle in which the obturator nerve travels, thereby increasing the likelihood of excessive strain on the tissue.
- Athletes seem to be more at risk, as the reported cases tended to represent repetitive kicking, side-to-side movement, and twisting.

MECHANISM OF INJURY

- There is no specific mechanism of injury for this pathology. Rather, the symptoms are progressive with an insidious onset.
  - However, symptoms may occur after childbirth, pelvic fractures, and pelvic tumors.

COMMON SIGNS AND SYMPTOMS

- Symptoms near the adductor origin on the pubic bone.
- Pain in the ipsilateral anterosuperior iliac spine.
- The hallmark sign is symptom provocation during exercise. The symptoms usually become severe during this time.
  - This is typically when paresthesias are present; however, these are not commonplace and generally indicate more of a chronic situation.
- The pain is typically described as a deep ache.
- Complaints of weakness are common with this pathology.

AGGRAVATING FACTOR

- Generalized exercise involving the lower extremities
- Weakness with attempts of jumping during exercise

EASING FACTOR

Periods of rest

24-HOUR SYMPTOM PATTERN

There is no diurnal pattern of pain in the case of an obturator neuropathy.

PAST HISTORY FOR THE REGION

- The pain usually began insidiously. Commonly, the symptoms of inguinal hernia preceded the symptoms of an obturator neuropathy. These could be the following:
  - Lump or swelling of the groin
  - Abdominal pain
  - Groin pain
  - Sudden pain
- A history of inguinal hernia repair or adductor tenotomy may therefore be reported without resolution of the groin pain.
- Complaints of paresthesias along the medial thigh typically indicate a more chronic presentation.

PHYSICAL EXAMINATION

- Travell and Simons reported trigger points of the adductors longus, brevis, and magnus, as well as gracilis, that refer pain along the distribution of the obturator nerve.
  - Bradshaw et al found that the injection treatment provided by Travell and Simons was similar to the obturator block Bradshaw used.
  - Therefore palpation of these muscles may produce a referral indicative of an obturator neuropathy.
  - These patients may complain of a spasm in these areas.

IMPORTANT OBJECTIVE TESTS

- It is important to perform this portion of the examination after the patient has exercised and therefore is symptomatic.
- Manual muscle testing (MMT) of hip adduction will probably indicate weakness.
- Pain can be reproduced with resisted external rotation of the hip.
- Providing a pectineus stretch will provoke the symptoms.
  - While standing, the patient passively rotates the hip externally and abducts the affected lower extremity in a lunge-type position. The affected extremity will be the trailing limb in this position.
- Howship-Romberg sign: Medial knee pain as a result of forced hip abduction, extension, and internal rotation.
- Impaired sensation testing along the areas innervated by the obturator nerve.
- Diminished tendon reflex of the adductors with preservation of reflex testing all other muscles.

DIFFERENTIAL DIAGNOSIS

- Entrapments of the genitofemoral and ilioinguinal nerves

- Obturator and inguinal hernias
- Adductor muscle strain
- Stress fractures of the femur and pubic ramus
- Osteitis pubis
- Psoas bursitis or strain
- Osteomyelitis
- Referred pain from lumbar spine and sacroiliac joints
- Hip osteoarthritis or synovitis

CONTRIBUTING FACTORS

Sports activities that involve repetitive kicking, lateral motions, and twisting seem to predispose some for this pathology.

TREATMENT

SURGICAL OPTIONS

- Surgical decompression or release of the obturator nerve is the common practice.
  - This typically occurs at the thick fascia located between the pectineus and adductor longus.
- Candidates for this surgery include the following:
  - A patient who demonstrates positive electromyography (EMG) findings of denervation is likely to have surgery.
  - Patients typically will have the symptoms for at least 2 weeks before the EMG will be sensitive for demyelination. A repeat EMG may be provided 4 to 6 weeks later if the first one was inconclusive.

SURGICAL OUTCOMES

- Bradshaw et al reported success in all of their 32 cases.
- Siwinski et al "cured" 41 of 52 cases of chronic groin pain.
- Brukner et al found only one recurrence out of 150 patients.

REHABILITATION

- Whether the patient had decompressive surgery, Topp et al recommended that the clinician should focus on reducing inflammation, improving blood flow to the area, and enhancing the capacity of the nerve for strain and excursion along its full length.
  - Therefore mobilization techniques to affect the obturator nerve should be used.
- Butler described using the slump knee bend position to stress the obturator nerve.
  - In this case, the affected extremity will be on top with the patient in a sidelying position. The uninvolved extremity, which is closest to the table, will be flexed at both the knee and hip. The patient will maintain this posture using both hands on the knee.
  - The clinician then extends the involved hip slightly and abducts the leg. This is a sensitizing motion.
  - Another sensitizing motion involves cervical flexion and extension.
- A conservative program involving ultrasound, interferential treatment, soft tissue massage, adductor and pelvic strengthening exercises, oral antiinflammatory therapy, and groin stretching was advocated by Bradshaw.
- There is no other mention of specific physical therapy treatment in the literature for this pathology.
- Bradshaw et al stated that physical therapy might help to delay the progression to the more severe denervated state, which typically requires surgery.

PROGNOSIS

- There are no data regarding the prognosis from physical therapy treatment without surgery; however, it may delay or prevent the need for surgery.
- There is no information regarding the extent of symptom relief in this case.
- In addition to the excellent results of surgery, Brukner stated that patients typically were symptom-free with activity within 3 to 4 weeks from the surgical date.
  - They reported only 1 patient out of 150 that had a recurrence of their symptoms.

SIGNS AND SYMPTOMS INDICATING REFERRAL TO PHYSICIAN

- The presence of constitutional signs and symptoms
- Bowel or bladder dysfunction
- Progressive weakness of the adductors, or of muscles not innervated by the obturator nerve
- Pain when at rest, especially during the evening

SUGGESTED READINGS

Bradshaw C, et al. Obturator nerve entrapment: a cause of groin pain in athletes. *Am J Sports Med.* 1997;25(3):402-408.

Brukner P, et al. Obturator neuropathy: a cause of exercise-related groin pain. *The Physician and Sports Medicine.* 1999;27(5).

Butler DS. *The Sensitive Nervous System.* Adelaide: Noigroup Publications; 2000.

Morelli V, Weaver V. Groin injuries and groin pain in athletes: Part I. *Prim Care.* 2005;32:163-183.

Siwinski D. Neuropathy of the obturator nerve as a source of pain in soccer players. *Chir Narzadow Ruchu Ortop Pol.* 2005;70(3):201-204.

Topp KS, et al. Structure and biomechanics of peripheral nerves: nerve responses to physical stresses and implications for physical therapist practice. *Phys Ther.* 2006;86:92-109.

Travell J, Simons DG. *Myofascial Pain and Dysfunction: Volume 2. The Lower Extremities.* Baltimore, MD: Williams and Wilkins; 1992.

AUTHOR: NEIL MCKENNA

BASIC INFORMATION

DEFINITION

- The pudendal nerve is a mixed nerve that includes motor, sensory, and autonomic functions. It is derived from the S2-S4 roots and supplies the anal and urethral sphincters, as well as the pelvic floor musculature.
- The sensory distribution includes the following regions:
  ○ Perineal
  ○ Scrotal/vulval
  ○ Testicular/vaginal
  ○ Penile/clitoral

SYNONYM

Pudendal nerve entrapment (PNE)

ICD-9CM CODE
355.9 Mononeuritis of unspecified site

OPTIMAL NUMBER OF VISITS

12 visits or less

MAXIMUM NUMBER OF VISITS

56 visits

ETIOLOGY

- The pudendal nerve can become compressed at the following four areas:
  ○ At the level of the ischial spine: Antolak et al found anatomical variances in the ischial spine morphology of male patients who had pudendal entrapment:
  ○ At the sacrospinous and sacrotuberous ligaments.
  ○ By the obturator fascia in the pudendal canal (Alcock's canal).
  ○ By the piriformis muscle.
- Besides an entrapment, the pudendal nerve may be subject to mechanical tension leading to inflammation and possible fibrosis.
- Topp et al discussed the effects of increased tension and compression on peripheral nerves. In summary, these stressors can reduce intraneural blood flow, create demyelination, and disrupt axonal transport. These characteristically lead to symptom generation.

EPIDEMIOLOGY AND DEMOGRAPHICS

- Pudendal neuralgia is a very rare pathology with only a very few cases reported in the literature.
- Robert et al stated that roughly two-thirds of their cases were women. These tended to correlate with childbirth.
- Antolak et al found that men commonly had a history of playing sports, such as American football, and they wrestled or

lifted weights as teenagers. The researchers postulated that the increased use of the pelvic floor muscles led to hypertrophy. This could, in turn, have a role in the morphology of the developing ischial spine, increasing the susceptibility of the pudendal nerve in this region for compression.

MECHANISM OF INJURY

- Childbirth commonly precedes the symptoms of pudendal neuralgia
- After prolonged cycling
- Periods of pudendal traction during procedures such as hip surgeries
- Symptoms may occur after surgery of the following various regions:
  ○ Proctologic
  ○ Urologic
  ○ Gynecologic

COMMON SIGNS AND SYMPTOMS

- Pudendal neuralgia will present with pain in the urogenital or anorectal area
- Unilateral or bilateral symptoms
- Description of burning
- The pain can be sudden or develop over time
- Loss of sensation in the innervated regions
- Bowel, bladder, and sexual dysfunction may or may not be present
  ○ Urinary disturbances may not be prevalent
  ○ Generally, there may be difficulty with voiding
- Loss of libido because of the pain
- Depression

AGGRAVATING FACTORS

- Cycling
- Sitting

EASING FACTORS

- Sitting on toilet, since the painful region is free from contact
- Standing
- Lying supine

24-HOUR SYMPTOM PATTERN

Generally, the evenings and mornings are the best, with symptom progression through the day.

PAST HISTORY FOR THE REGION

- The symptoms commonly start as a relapsing course with symptom abatement. It can then mature to a chronic, progressive pain pattern.
  ○ Popeney et al stated that this chronic condition may be secondary to central sensitization because of the chronic nerve compression.

PHYSICAL EXAMINATION

Observable physical findings for this pathology are generally scarce.

IMPORTANT OBJECTIVE TESTS

- Popeney designed a protocol for diagnosis using techniques of nerve conduction velocity, EMG, and anesthetic nerve blocks.
- The patient would present with a normal lumbar myotomal and dermatomal examination.
- Palpation of the external entrapment sites with symptom reproduction should be helpful to the clinician, especially at the level of the ischial spine.

DIFFERENTIAL DIAGNOSIS

- Coccydynia
- Neuralgia of the ilioinguinal, iliohypogastric, or genitofemoral nerves
- Prostatitis
- Idiopathic vulvodynia
- Levator ani syndrome
- Urethral syndrome
- Endometriosis

CONTRIBUTING FACTORS

- Popeney et al found anatomical variations in the vast majority of their surgeries for entrapment of the pudendal nerve.
  ○ The nerve was typically compressed against or tethered to the lateral pelvic wall that led to impingement on pelvic floor muscle contractions.
- Antolak et al found a history in males suggesting increased pelvic floor development from athletic activity that may remodel the ischium and its associated ligaments.

TREATMENT

SURGICAL OPTIONS

- Decompression of one or both of the pudendal nerves. In this case, the nerve sheath is released with subsequent transposition from the area of compression.
  ○ Popeney et al found that 60% of the 58 patients responded favorably 1 year after the surgery.
  ○ Mauillon et al performed neurolysis-transpositions on 12 patients and had only 3 patients who were cured roughly 2 years later.

REHABILITATION

- Physical therapy treatment is referenced on a few occasions, but no specific interventions were included nor was it studied for efficacy.
- Treatment interventions that may provide relief for a patient with pudendal neuralgia include the following:
  ○ Whether the patient had decompressive surgery or not, Topp et al recommended that the clinician should

focus on reducing inflammation, improving blood flow to the area, and enhancing the capacity of the nerve for strain and excursion along its full length. Therefore mobilization techniques to affect the pudendal nerve should be used.

- ○ Soft tissue mobilization and possibly ultrasound in the vicinity of the ischial spine.
- ○ Sacroiliac treatment in response to the presence of a pelvic obliquity.
- ○ Stretching of the piriformis in an effort to reduce entrapment at this region.

PROGNOSIS

- Those who responded well to surgery typically responded well to injections before surgery.
- Conversely, those who were treated for depression had poorer surgical outcomes.

SIGNS AND SYMPTOMS INDICATING REFERRAL TO PHYSICIAN

- The presence of constitutional signs and symptoms.
- The presence of lumbar root signs and symptoms.
- Complaints of progressive bowel and bladder dysfunction.

SUGGESTED READINGS

Alevizon SJ, Finan MA. Sacrospinous colpopexy: management of postoperative pudendal nerve entrapment. *Obstet Gynecol.* 1996;88:713-715.

Amarenco G, et al. Electrophysiological analysis of pudendal neuropathy following traction. *Muscle Nerve.* 2001;24:116-119.

Antolak SJ, et al. Anatomical basis of chronic pelvic pain syndrome: the ischial spine and pudendal nerve entrapment. *Med Hypotheses.* 2002;59(3):349-353.

Mauillon J, et al. Results of pudendal nerve neurolysis-transposition in twelve patients suffering from pudendal neuralgia. *Dis Colon Rectum.* 1999;42:186-192.

Popeney C, et al. Pudendal entrapment as an etiology of chronic perineal pain: diagnosis and treatment. *Neurourol Urodyn.* 2007;26:820-827.

Ramsden CE, et al. Pudendal nerve entrapment as source of intractable perineal pain. *Am J Phys Med Rehabil.* 2003;82(6):479-484.

Robert R, Prat-Pradal D, Labat JJ, et al. Anatomic basis of chronic perineal pain: Role of the pudendal nerve. *Surg Radtol Anat.* 1998;20:93-98.

Topp KS, et al. Structure and biomechanics of peripheral nerves: nerve responses to physical stresses and implications for physical therapist practice. *Phys Ther.* 2006;86:92-109.

AUTHOR: NEIL MCKENNA

BASIC INFORMATION

DEFINITION

- Pelvic pain is a rather complex term with many joints and structures that can refer pain to its region. Sacroiliac joint pathology is typically a subclassification of this broader term.
- Sacroiliac joint pathology refers to dysfunction of the innominate articulations that exclusively create pelvic pain. The gold standard for verifying the sacroiliac articulation as the source of pain is the use of intraarticular anesthetic injections.

SYNONYM

Innominate obliquity/asymmetry

ICD-9CM CODES
724.6 Disorders of sacrum
846.9 Unspecified site of sacroiliac region sprain

OPTIMAL NUMBER OF VISITS

3 visits or less

MAXIMUM NUMBER OF VISITS

36 visits

ETIOLOGY

- The sacroiliac joint is an inherently stable structure designed for load transfer among the vertebral column, the lower extremities, and the ground.
- Goode et al performed a literature review and summarized the findings of motion along the X, Y, and Z axes. The X-axis corresponds with sacral rotation in the sagittal plane. The Y-axis corresponds with sacral rotation in the horizontal plane. Finally, the Z-axis corresponds with sacral rotation in the coronal plane.
  - Rotation in the X-axis ranged from −1.1 to 2.2 degrees with translation in this plane from −0.3 to 8 mm.
  - Rotation in the Y-axis ranged from −0.8 to 4 degrees with translation in this plane from −0.2 to 7 mm.
  - Rotation in the Z-axis ranged from −0.5 to 8 degrees with translation in this plane from −0.3 to 6 mm.
- Cibulka (2002) stated that the sacroiliac joint can move in only the following two directions:
  - Sagittal plane tilting of both innominates
  - One innominate tilting anteriorly and the other tilting posteriorly
- According to Cibulka (2002), the pubis should be considered as a fused articulation since it is fibrous joint.
  - Reports of pubic motion range from 0.5 to 2.5 mm, with more occurring

during pregnancy. However, Mens et al (1999) found significant differences in pubic bone alignment via x-ray in patients with pelvic girdle pain.
- Mens (1999), Hungerford (2004), and Snijders demonstrated aberrant motions of the sacroiliac joint, especially during closed-chain activities. The aberrant trend reported was anterior innominate rotation on the stance limb when the other limb was actively flexed at the hip (also known as the stork test, Gillet test, and one-leg standing test). Those without pelvic pain demonstrated posterior rotation on the stance limb.
- Hungerford (2003) and O'Sullivan (2007) postulated that improper motor control in the form of muscle sequencing allows for these abnormal motions to occur. This in turn could place increased strain on various pelvic structures, such as ligaments and muscles, resulting in pain.

EPIDEMIOLOGY AND DEMOGRAPHICS

- It is estimated that the incidence rate for sacroiliac joint pathology is 15%.
- Women seem to be more at risk. The female cases reported in the literature vastly outnumber the males.
- Men may be afflicted with this pathology less as their age progresses since bony fusion of the sacroiliac joints occurs more in men than women.
  - Dar et al showed that 23 out of 74 men in the 60- to 79-years-old group had fusion, compared to 1 out of 46 women in the same age group.
- Damen et al found via Doppler imaging that those with asymmetrical laxity of the sacroiliac joints correlated with moderate-to-severe levels of symptoms in subjects with pelvic pain. Generalized laxity bilaterally was not correlated with pelvic pain.

MECHANISM OF INJURY

- Dreyfuss et al stated that known causes of pain in this region are spondyloarthropathy, crystal and pyogenic arthropathy, fracture of the sacrum and pelvic, and diastasis resulting from pregnancy or childbirth.
- The most common correlation with development of pelvic pain is pregnancy.
- Other mechanisms of injury typically include activities that require opposing innominate motion in which one innominate is posteriorly rotated and the other is relatively anteriorly rotated.
  - The larger the difference in innominate rotation with the added comorbidity of asymmetrical sacroiliac joint laxity may lead to the development of pain with lunging, running, and twisting-based activities.

- Falling onto the buttocks and heavy lifting may be reported as well.

COMMON SIGNS AND SYMPTOMS

- Pain in the region of the sacral sulcus, just medial to the posterior superior iliac spine that may travel distally into the buttock and posterior thigh.
  - The symptoms typically do not extend to or beyond the knee.
- Pain of sacroiliac joint nature does not refer to the lumbar spine.

AGGRAVATING FACTORS

- Walking, running
- Cycling
- Sit to stand transfers
- Twisting activities, rolling over in bed
- Heavy lifting
- Prolonged sitting and standing

EASING FACTORS

- Crooklying and hooklying positions
- Use of antiinflammatory medication and ice

24-HOUR SYMPTOM PATTERN

Commonly, inflammatory type symptoms are reported. Therefore the patient may have increased pain and stiffness for the first 1 to 2 hours on waking.

PAST HISTORY FOR THE REGION

- Frequently, the initial onset occurs during or after pregnancy.
- There may been a traumatic fall onto one or both buttocks or stepping into a hole that preceded the onset of symptoms.

PHYSICAL EXAMINATION

- A patient with a sacroiliac joint dysfunction may present with an apparent leg-length difference, thereby influencing both lumbar and thoracic frontal plane curvature.
  - When observed dorsally, there may be presence of a scoliotic curve.

IMPORTANT OBJECTIVE TESTS

- The tests that identify sacroiliac joint pathology are classified into the following three categories:
  - Motion palpation tests to assess movement of the innominate
  - Pain provocation tests
  - Static palpation tests for symmetry; the common trend in the literature was that the most reliable tests were those of pain provocation; palpation is inherently unreliable
- When individual sacroiliac joint tests are performed, there is very low sensitivity and specificity for properly classifying this pathology:
  - Clusters of these tests have shown to increase the validity of objective testing for this region.

- Cibulka et al (1999) found 0.82 sensitivity and 0.88 specificity for sacroiliac joint pain when three out of four tests were positive. The tests were as follows:
  - Standing flexion test
  - Sitting posterior superior iliac spine (PSIS) palpation
  - Supine long-sitting test
  - Prone knee flexion test
- Laslett et al (2003) used a McKenzie evaluation followed with provocation testing and had a sensitivity of 91% with specificity being 83%. His likelihood ratio was 6.97.
  - The McKenzie method was used since Laslett has found patients with symptomatic lumbar discs to have false-positive responses to sacroiliac joint provocation testing.
  - Once he ruled out the possibility of a lumbar discal referral by the absence of centralization and peripheralization, the presence of pain with three or more of the following tests indicated that the patient was between 3 to 20 times more likely to have a had a positive diagnostic sacroiliac joint injection:
    - Distraction
    - Thigh thrust
    - Gaenslen's test
    - Compression
    - Sacral thrust
- Laslett et al (2005) found sensitivity of 94% and specificity of 78% in patients that had three or more of six positive sacroiliac joint tests. They used the same tests as described in the 2003 study, and Gaenslen's test was performed on each side.
  - When all six of the tests did not provoke symptoms, they were able to rule out the sacroiliac joint as a source of the pain.
- The use of the active straight leg test (ASLR) has been widely cited to be both specific and sensitive for sacroiliac joint pathology.
  - Mens et al (2002) found a high correlation of the severity of a positive ASLR test with the score on the Quebec Back Pain Disability Scale and isometric dynamometer strength readings of the hip adductors.
- Hungerford et al (2007) found the stork test, also called the Gillet test and one-leg standing test, to be reliable.
  - These tests evaluate the ability of a patient to stabilize their lumbosacral spine.
- Palpation of the sacral sulcus for symptom provocation is commonly employed in the literature; however, this alone does not constitute a sacroiliac joint pathology. Therefore the use of a cluster of examinations emphasizing sacroiliac joint provocative tests with the ASLR

test and the stork test is an effective means of evaluating this region, especially when repeated motions of the lumbopelvic spine have no influence on the symptoms.

DIFFERENTIAL DIAGNOSIS

- Lumbar disc pathology
- Lumbar spondylolysis
- Lumbar spondylolisthesis
- Lumbar radiculopathy
- Hip osteoarthritis
- Spondyloarthropathy such as ankylosing spondylitis
- Gluteal muscle strain
- Piriformis syndrome

CONTRIBUTING FACTORS

- Asymmetrical laxity of the sacroiliac joint was demonstrated by Damen et al.
- Pregnancy is another contributing factor.
- Ha et al found an incidence of sacroiliac joint degeneration in post-operative lumbar fusion patients of 75% compared to 38.2% of controls.
  - The degeneration incidence was higher in patients that underwent fusion including the S1 segment compared to those who had a fusion only to L5.

TREATMENT

SURGICAL OPTIONS

- Ferrante et al administered radiofrequency denervation of the sacroiliac joint and had a success rate of 36.4%.
  - They also found normalization of sacroiliac joint provocative tests with success of this technique.
- Ziran et al performed CT-guided stabilization of the sacroiliac joint with use of iliosacral screws into S1 and S2 in patients who had a reduction in pain from a preoperative injection.
  - They reported significant improvements in pain between the preintervention state with the postinjection and postsurgical states ($p < 0.0001$).
  - However, there was no significant change in the level of pain reported between the postinjection and postsurgical periods.

REHABILITATION

- Various methods of mobilization and manipulation of the sacroiliac joints are typically used during treatment of these patients; however, there is not much support in the literature for its use.
  - Tulberg found no change in the position of the sacroiliac joints after manipulation when assessed via roentgen stereophotogrammetric methods.

- Timgren and Soinila were able to produce symmetry of the pelvis in 87 of 106 patients using either a high-velocity, low-amplitude thrust technique through the ankle on the side of the dysfunctional sacroiliac joint or with a muscle energy technique. The weakness of this study was that they assessed the pelvic symmetry via palpation, which has been shown to be unreliable and has low sensitivity and specificity.
- Normalization of hip ROM may be helpful when treating patients with sacroiliac joint pathology (Warren).
- Motor training of the transverse abdominis, the transverse fibers of the internal oblique, and the pelvic floor muscles from supine positions to more functional, upright postures has been used by O'Sullivan et al (2007).
  - The abnormal kinematics of the diaphragm and pelvic floor during the ASLR improved as well as respiratory patterns.
  - The ability to consciously elevate the pelvic floor improved posttreatment as well.
  - Improvements in pain and disability were related with improvements in these variables.
- Strengthening of various core muscles is also advocated in the literature.
  - Hungerford et al (2003) found delayed activity of the internal oblique, multifidus, and gluteus maximus of the stance leg during the stork test in patients with sacroiliac joint pain.

PROGNOSIS

- The majority of the literature that demonstrates successful treatment of sacroiliac joint pathology conservatively includes aspects of specific motor control strategies.
  - The patient will need to practice these strategies frequently to have it become part of their motor program.
  - If the patient stops practicing these strategies before this happens, he or she will likely have recurrent symptoms.

SIGNS AND SYMPTOMS INDICATING REFERRAL TO PHYSICIAN

- The presence of constitutional signs and symptoms
- Bowel or bladder dysfunction
- Complaints of increasing morning stiffness of the lumbopelvic spine may be an early sign of ankylosing spondylitis

SUGGESTED READINGS

Cibulka MT, Koldehoff R. Clinical usefulness of a cluster of sacroiliac joint tests in patients with and without low back pain. *J Orthop Sports Phys Ther*. 1999;29(2):83-92.

Cibulka MT. Understanding sacroiliac joint movement as a guide to the management of a patient with unilateral low back pain. *Man Ther*. 2002;7(4):215-221.

Damen L, et al. Pelvic pain during pregnancy is associated with asymmetric laxity of the sacroiliac joints. *Acta Obstet Gynecol Scand*. 2001;80(11):1019-1024.

Dar G, et al. Sacroiliac joint fusion and the implications for manual therapy diagnosis and treatment. *Man Ther*. 2008;13:155-158.

Dreyfuss P, et al. The value of medical history and physical examination in diagnosing sacroiliac joint pain. *Spine*. 1996;21(22): 2594-2602.

Ferrante FM, et al. Radiofrequency sacroiliac joint denervation for sacroiliac syndrome. *Reg Anesth Pain Med*. 2001;26(2):137-142.

Goode A, et al. Three-dimensional movements of the sacroiliac joint: a systematic review of the literature and assessment of clinical utility. *Journal of Manual and Manipulative Therapy*. 2008;16(1):25-38.

Ha KY, et al. Degeneration of sacroiliac joint after instrumented lumbar or lumbosacral fusion: A prospective cohort study over five-year follow-up. *Spine*. 2008;33(11):1192-1198.

Hungerford B, et al. Evidence of altered lumbopelvic muscle recruitment in the presence of sacroiliac joint pain. *Spine*. 2003; 28(14):1593-1600.

Hungerford B, et al. Altered patterns of pelvic bone motion determined in subjects with posterior pelvic pain using skin markers. *Man Ther*. 2004;19:456-464.

Hungerford B, et al. Evaluation of the ability of physical therapists to palpate intrapelvic motion with the stork test on the support side. *Phys Ther*. 2007;87:879-887.

Laslett M, et al. Diagnosing painful sacroiliac joints: a validity study of a McKenzie evaluation and sacroiliac provocation tests. *Aust J Physiother*. 2003;49:89-97.

Laslett M, et al. Diagnosis of sacroiliac joint pain: validity of individual provocation tests and composites of tests. *Man Ther*. 2005;10:207-218.

Maigne JY, et al. Results of sacroiliac joint double block and value of sacroiliac pain provocation tests in 54 patients with low back pain. *Spine*. 1996;21(16):1889-1892.

Mens JM, et al. The active straight leg raising test and mobility of the pelvic joints. *Eur Spine J*. 1999;8:468-473.

Mens JM, et al. Responsiveness of outcome measurements in rehabilitation of patients with posterior pelvic pain since pregnancy. *Spine*. 2002;27(10):1110-1115.

O'Sullivan PB, Beales DJ. Diagnosis and classification of pelvic girdle pain disorders-Part I: a mechanism based approach within a biopsychological framework. *Man Ther*. 2007;12:86-97.

O'Sullivan PB, Beales DJ. Changes in pelvic floor and diaphragm kinematics and respiratory patterns in subjects with sacroiliac joint pain following a motor learning intervention: a case series. *Man Ther*. 2007;12:209-218.

Robinson HS, Brox JI, Robinson R, Bjelland E, Solem S, Telje T. The reliability of selected motion- and pain provocation tests for the sacroiliac joint. *Man Ther*. 2007;12(1):72-79.

Snijders CJ, Vleeming A, Stoeckart R. Transfer of lumbosacral load to iliac bones and legs I. Biomechanics of self-bracing of the sacroiliac joints and its significance for treatment and exercise. *Clin Biomech*. 1993;8:285-294.

Timgren T, Soinila S. Reversible pelvic asymmetry: an overlooked syndrome manifesting as scoliosis, apparent leg-length difference, and neurologic symptoms. *J Manipulative Physiol Ther*. 2006;29:561-565.

Tulberg T, et al. Manipulation does not alter the position of the sacroiliac joint: a roentgen stereophotogrammetric analysis. *Spine*. 1998;23(10):1124-1129.

Warren PH. Management of a patient with sacroiliac joint dysfunction: a correlation of hip range of motion asymmetry with sitting and standing postural habits. *The Journal of Manual and Manipulative Therapy*. 2003;11(3):153-159.

Ziran BH, et al. CT-guided stabilization for chronic sacroiliac pain: a preliminary report. *J Trauma*. 2007;63(1):90-96.

AUTHOR: NEIL MCKENNA

BASIC INFORMATION ⓘ

DEFINITION

Bell's palsy is defined as idiopathic cranial nerve VII paresis or paralysis.

SYNONYMS

- Peripheral facial palsy
- Idiopathic facial palsy
- Idiopathic facial nerve paralysis
- Acute peripheral facial palsy

ICD-9CM CODE
351.0 Bell's palsy

OPTIMAL NUMBER OF VISITS

Two-thirds of patients recover spontaneously without physical therapy treatment. Patients with slow (>3 months) or incomplete recovery might benefit from instruction in facial exercises, manual therapy for facial spasms, or treatment of pain. These services can be provided weekly, tapering down to monthly, and based on patient progress. Patient recovery is highly variable, so it is not possible to determine an optimal number of visits.

MAXIMAL NUMBER OF VISITS

Patient recovery is highly variable so it is not possible to determine a maximal number of visits.

ETIOLOGY

- Bell's palsy is a diagnosis of exclusion. However, the literature reports several possible causes of paralysis of cranial nerve VII. These include but are not limited to an adverse event of immunization, reactivation of herpes simplex virus type I, and upper respiratory tract infection.
- A virus-associated immune-mediated mechanism begins when a virus penetrates a cell of the geniculate ganglion in the host organism. After penetration, the virus parasitizes the host cell's replication proteins, producing a large number of progeny. The immune system mounts an inflammatory reaction as the host cells are destroyed by viral replication. Inflammation of the facial nerve alone can account for the symptoms of Bell's palsy. These symptoms can be further exacerbated if the swollen facial nerve becomes entrapped in the mental foramen and the labyrinthine segment of the temporal bone. In addition to immediate replication, a virus can enter a latent state so it is present but inactive in the host cell. The virus can be activated at a later date following trauma or other stressful events.

EPIDEMIOLOGY AND DEMOGRAPHICS

Peak incidence of Bell's palsy in the adult population occurs between the ages of 20 to 60 years. Estimated incidence is 13.1-20.2 per 100,000. It affects men and women equally. However, pregnancy increases the incidence of Bell's palsy to 45 per 100,000. In the pediatric population, Bell's palsy occurs in 2.7 per 100,000 children below the age of 10 and 10.1 per 100,000 children between the ages of 10 and 20.

MECHANISM OF INJURY

Injury might be instigated by viral infection inducing the inflammatory process, resulting in facial nerve demyelination/denervation. The reactivation of herpes simplex virus type I is thought to be the cause of most cases of Bell's palsy.

COMMON SIGNS AND SYMPTOMS

- Before onset of facial paralysis, patients often experience pain in or around the ear near the mastoid process, cervical pain, and facial numbness with no sensory loss.
- Within 24 hours of these symptoms, the following occur with varying extent, depending on the degree of facial nerve involvement and lesion location:
  - Progressive loss of motor control on one side of the face over 1 to 10 days
  - Loss of facial asymmetry at rest and with facial expressions
  - Nasal alar collapse, nasolabial flattening
  - Loss of taste on the anterior two-thirds of the tongue
  - Slowed or absent blink reflex
  - Hyperacusis
  - Excess or reduced salivation
  - Excess or reduced tearing
  - Facial muscle synkinesis
  - Facial spasms
- There can be referred pain around the ear and neck.

AGGRAVATING ACTIVITIES

None identified

EASING ACTIVITIES

None identified

PAST HISTORY FOR THE REGION

No common patient characteristics have been identified except possible exposure to herpes simplex virus type I.

PHYSICAL EXAMINATION

- Asymmetrical resting facial posture
- No or diminished voluntary facial movement with eyebrow raise, eye closure, smile, snarl, pucker, and frown
- Nasal, muffled speech
- Abnormal movement patterns (synkinesis)

IMPORTANT OBJECTIVE TESTS

- Because Bell's palsy is a diagnosis of exclusion, objective tests help determine the extent of the lesion but do not provide a definitive diagnosis.
- Electroneuronography to determine presence/absence of compound muscle action potentials (CMAP). CMAPs are the summed electrical activity of a population of muscle fibers. Absence of a CMAP, or a decrement relative to the unaffected side, are indicative of denervation.
- Surface or needle electromyography (EMG) to record facial muscle activity
- Nerve conduction velocity to determine excitability of facial nerve
- Magnetic resonance imaging (MRI) scan with gadolinium–DTPA contrast to assess inflammatory edema
- In addition to these electrodiagnostic and imaging techniques, clinicians may use the following to evaluate cranial nerve function and assess the extent of a patients impairments:
  - Cranial nerve assessment
  - Facial grading system
  - Facial disability index

DIFFERENTIAL DIAGNOSIS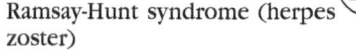

- Ramsay-Hunt syndrome (herpes zoster)
- Facial nerve trauma (temporal bone fractures, surgical incisions)
- Lyme disease (determined by presence of antibodies against *Borrelia burgdorferi* in the cerebral spinal fluid (CSF) or serum)
- Cerebellopontine angle lesions (acoustic neuromas, meningiomas) or parotid tumors (parotid gland subdivided into a superficial and deep part by emerging branches of the facial nerve)
- Facial nerve schwannomas
- Tumors of the external or internal acoustic meatus
- Nasopharyngeal carcinomas
- Diabetic cranial neuropathy
- Multiple sclerosis (MS)
- Paget disease
- Human immunodeficiency virus (HIV)
- Otitis media

CONTRIBUTING FACTORS

The true cause has not been agreed on, so factors contributing to the development of Bell's palsy have not been determined.

TREATMENT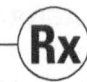

SURGICAL OPTIONS

- The use of steroids and antiviral agents has dramatically reduced the number of surgeries performed to alleviate the symptoms of Bell's palsy.
- Surgical decompression of cranial nerve VII might be indicated for patients who have >90% neural degeneration and no voluntary EMG potentials within 14 days of onset of weakness and do not respond to steroid/antiviral therapy. However, the literature supporting this is controversial because many studies do not support the use of this surgical technique.
- Lagophthalmos, or the inability to close the palpebral fissure when attempting to shut the eyelid, can result in exposure and injury of the cornea. At first, this can be treated by regular lubrication of the eye, manual blinking, and taping the eye shut at night. If the condition persists long enough that there is a danger of drying out the cornea, this can be treated by the surgical procedure known as *lid loading*. This procedure involves implantation of a gold weight on the upper eyelid to induce gravity-dependent lid closure. This is the most common surgical procedure in facial nerve palsy of any etiology. It provides good corneal protection with good cosmesis and maintenance of visual function.

REHABILITATION

Physical therapy interventions commonly used for the diagnosis of Bell's palsy include electrical stimulation, biofeedback, facial muscle exercises, massage, and pain relief. There is no evidence of benefit or harm for any of these treatments because studies performed have not been of sufficient strength or they have design flaws that do not allow conclusions to be drawn.

PROGNOSIS

- Complete recovery is experienced by 68% to 70% of patients; 13% to 27% of patients have nearly complete recovery, experiencing minimal weakness with volitional movement and slight asymmetry with eye closure and moving the corner of the mouth; and 5% to 16% of patients experience partial recovery with incomplete activation of the forehead muscles, difficulty closing eye with maximal effort, obvious asymmetry with movement of the corners of the mouth, synkinesis, contractures, and/or hemifacial spasm.
- Within 3 weeks, 70% of patients begin recovering volitional control of facial muscles; 85% of these patients have spontaneous complete recovery within 3 weeks; and the remaining 15% of patients experience complete recovery within 3 to 5 months. For patients that do not recover within 3 to 5 months, their symptoms can linger for >1 year and complete recovery is improbable.
- Age may influence extent of recovery: 90% of patients <14 years old recover completely, 84% of patients 15 to 19 years old recover completely, 75% of patients 30 to 44 years old recover completely, and 33% of patients >60 years old recover completely.
- Pregnancy appears to reduce the likelihood of complete recovery because 52% of pregnant patients experience complete recovery.
- A slow or absent blink reflex is associated with poor prognosis.

SIGNS AND SYMPTOMS INDICATING REFERRAL TO PHYSICIAN

- Sensory impairment with the exception of taste on the anterior two-thirds of the tongue
- Gradual onset of facial paralysis and facial pain
- Involvement of other cranial nerves
- Facial numbness
- Hearing loss or tinnitus
- Balance deficits
- Symptoms increasing over a period longer than 2 weeks are more suggestive of tumor or cholesteatoma

SUGGESTED READINGS

Alberts B, Bray D, Lewis J, Raff M, Roberts K, Watson JD. *Molecular Biology of the Cell*. 2nd ed. New York, NY: Garland Publishing Inc; 1989.

Brach JS, VanSwearingen JM, Lenert J, et al. Facial neuromuscular retraining for oral synkinesis. *Plast Reconstr Surg*. 1997;99:1922-1931.

Brach JS, VanSwearingen JM. Not all facial paralysis is Bell's palsy: a case report. *Arch Phys Med Rehabil*. 1999;80:857-859.

Evans AK, Licameli G, Brietzke S, Whittemore K, Kenna M. Pediatric facial nerve paralysis: Patients, management and outcomes. *Int J Pediatr Otorhinolaryngol*. 2005;69: 1521-1528.

Furuta Y, Fukuda S, Chida E, et al. Reactivation of herpes simplex virus type I in patients with Bell's palsy. *J Med Virol*. 1998;54:162-166.

Kiziltan ME, Akalin MA, Sahin R, Uluduz D. Peripheral neuropathy in patients with diabetes mellitus presenting as Bell's palsy. *Neurosci Lett*. 2007;427:138-141.

Kumar V, Cotran RS, Robbins SL. *Basic Pathology*. 7th ed. Philadelphia, PA: W.B. Saunders Company; 2003.

Ljostad U, Okstad S, Topstad T, Mygland A, Monstad P. Acute peripheral facial palsy in adults. *J Neurol*. 2005;252:672-682.

Ohtake PJ, Zafron ML, Potanki LG, Fish DR. Evidence in Practice. *Phys Ther*. 2006;86:1558-1564.

Peitersen E. Bell's palsy: the spontaneous course of 2,500 peripheral facial nerve palsies of different etiologies. *Acta Otolaryngol Suppl*. 2002;549:4-30.

Rath B, Linder T, Cornblath D, et al. All that palsies is not Bell's - The need to define Bell's palsy as an adverse event following immunization. *Vaccine*. 2007;26:1-14.

Rhaman I, Sadiq SA. Ophthalmic management of facial nerve palsy: a review. *Surv Ophthalmol*. 2007;52:121-143.

Yanagihara N, Honda N, Hato N, Murkami S. Edematous swelling of the facial nerve in Bell's palsy. *Acta Otolaryngol*. 2000;120:667-671.

AUTHOR: DEBORAH L. LOWE

Section III

ORTHOPEDIC PATHOLOGY

BASIC INFORMATION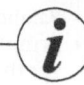

DEFINITION

Benign paroxysmal positional vertigo (BPPV) is the accumulation of calcium carbonate crystals (otoconia) in one of the three semicircular canals, resulting in episodic, positional vertigo.

SYNONYM

Benign paroxysmal positional nystagmus

ICD-9CM CODE
386.1 Other and unspecified peripheral vertigo

OPTIMAL NUMBER OF VISITS

The optimal number of visits varies according to the cause of BPPV—idiopathic versus traumatic. According to a study by Gordon et al, a single treatment rendered 33% of patients with traumatic BPPV asymptomatic, and 67% of patients with traumatic BPPV required multiple (2 to 4) treatments. In comparison, 86% of patients with idiopathic BPPV were asymptomatic after one treatment and only 14% required 2 to 4 treatments.

MAXIMAL NUMBER OF VISITS

Patients may require up to 4 visits for their symptoms to resolve; an occasional follow-up treatment may be needed if there is a recurrence.

ETIOLOGY

- Half (50%) of cases are idiopathic. Identifiable causes include head injury (i.e., whiplash or blunt head trauma), degenerative changes associated with aging leading to detachment of the otoconia from the otolith organs, viral infection, vascular lesion, migraine (can be associated with BPPV but may also be a separate diagnosis), and prolonged bed rest.
- Damage to the utricle results in displacement of the otoconia from the utricle to one or more of the semicircular canals. Two mechanisms have been postulated to explain the clinical presentation of BPPV. Otoconial debris can settle and become fixed in the cupula of the posterior semicircular canal (cupulolithiasis) or a free floating mass of otoconial debris migrates to the most dependent part of the canal when the head is moved so there is a discrepancy between a canal's plane and the pull (vector) of gravity (canalolithiasis). Canalolithiasis is thought to be the principal pathology for posterior canal involvement, whereas cupulolithiasis is thought to the principal pathology for horizontal canal involvement.
- Head injury can result in damage to the utricle and dislocation of otoconia normally attached to a membrane within the utriculus.

- Vasospasms associated with migraines can cause ischemic damage to the utricular maculae.

EPIDEMIOLOGY AND DEMOGRAPHICS

- BPPV is the most common peripheral vestibular disorder in adults and the most common cause of positional nystagmus. In specialized dizziness clinics, 20% to 30% of diagnoses are BPPV. According to the German National Telephone Health Interview Survey, 33% of the general population have a diagnosis of BPPV. The mean age of onset is 54 years with a range of 11 to 84 years.
- Nonidiopathic occurrence of BPPV occurs with the following frequency:
  ○ Vestibular neuronitis: 10% to 15%; head trauma: 17% to 20%.
  ○ BPPV rarely occurs in children, with a prevalence of 7.3%.
- The prevalence of BPPV increases with age: 18 to 39 years: 12%; 40 to 59 years: 40%; >60 years: 48%.
- BPPV is most common in the posterior semicircular canal (88%), the horizontal semicircular canal is affected in 10% of cases, and the anterior canal is affected in 2%.
- BPPV of idiopathic origin has 2.5% to 6.3% occurrence in both ears. BPPV of traumatic origin has 14.3% to 19% occurrence in both ears.

MECHANISM OF INJURY

- Trauma leading to dislocation of otoconia from utricle membrane.
- Degenerative changes associated with aging leading to detachment of the otoconia from the otolith organs.
- Ischemic episodes leading to damage to the utricle membrane and detachment of the otoconia.

COMMON SIGNS AND SYMPTOMS

- Vertigo is episodic (10 to 20 seconds).
- Vertigo is elicited by a particular rotational movement of the head as one changes position during tasks such as turning over in bed; lying down; standing up; or turning face up, down, or rapidly to one side.
- Dizziness.
- Lightheadedness.
- Disequilibrium.
- Initial onset of vertigo is often associated with nausea.
- Less common symptoms include the following:
  ○ Falling
  ○ Floating
  ○ Impulsion
  ○ Head heaviness or pressure
  ○ Burning or tingling inside the head with no clear spinning sensation
  ○ Neck pain and headache

AGGRAVATING ACTIVITIES

- Rotational movements of the head that occur when changing body position or direction of gaze.
- Changing positions (lying, sit-to-stand, etc).

EASING ACTIVITIES

Reducing speed of head and trunk movements may reduce the symptoms but they are inclined to exacerbate the pathology.

24-HOUR SYMPTOM PATTERN

- Symptom are episodic lasting only 10 to 20 seconds.
- Symptoms do not appear to increase in intensity or frequency as the day progresses.

PAST HISTORY FOR THE REGION

Patient may report history of trauma, such as motor vehicle accident (MVA), head trauma, or falls.

PHYSICAL EXAMINATION

- Physical findings will depend on which semicircular canal is involved. If the posterior canal is involved, the Dix-Hallpike maneuver will produce a stereotyped torsional and vertical nystagmus with the upper pole of the eye beating toward the dependent ear and the vertical nystagmus beating toward the forehead after a rapid position change from sitting to head-hanging in supine. The nystagmus typically begins after a 1-2 second latency, lasts for 10 to 20 seconds and is associated with a sensation of rotational vertigo. On returning the patient to the seated position, nystagmus is again observed, but the direction of nystagmus is reversed. Repetition of the Dix-Halpike maneuver results in a reduction in the intensity of vertigo and nystagmus.
- If the horizontal canal is involved, a vertigo and nystagmus beats in a direction opposite to the ground when the head is turned to either side of vertical when a patient is supine. The nystagmus exhibits no delay after the turning of the head and can last for several minutes.

IMPORTANT OBJECTIVE TESTS

- Dix-Hallpike maneuver.
- Roll test (rotation of the head in supine).
- Electronystagmography can distinguish peripheral from central signs.
- Bithermal caloric testing (caloric hypoexcitability in affected ear).

DIFFERENTIAL DIAGNOSIS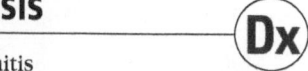

- Labyrinthitis
- Otitis media
- Intracranial tumors (vestibular schwannomas, meningiomas, gliomas, or lipomas)

- Vestibular hypofunction
- Ménière's disease
- Vertebrobasilar insufficiency (also associated with brainstem symptoms such as diplopia, dysarthria, and facial numbness)
- Panic attack
- Vestibular neuronitis (usually causes a single episode of vertigo lasting 1 to 2 days)
- Migraine-associated vertigo (highly variable in duration and usually proceeds or is accompanied by a headache; can also be accompanied by photophobia, phonophobia, and visual or other auras)
- Orthostatic dizziness.

CONTRIBUTING FACTORS

- Patients who present with BPPV have a higher incidence of the following comorbidities:
  - Hypertension: 52%
  - Elevated blood lipids: 55%
- The lifetime prevalence of BPPV is 50% higher in women than men.

TREATMENT

SURGICAL INDICATORS

- Chronic or recurrent symptoms that do not respond to conservative therapy and are debilitating.
- Surgery is rarely recommended for BPPV; only 3% to 5% of patients treated for BPPV require surgery.

SURGICAL OPTIONS

Posterior canal occlusion.

SURGICAL OUTCOMES

Posterior canal occlusion has a high cure rate with low incidence of hearing loss and other complications.

REHABILITATION

- Canalith repositioning maneuvers as follow:
  - Epley maneuver for posterior and anterior canal involvement.
  - Semont maneuver for posterior canal involvement.
  - Barbecue maneuver (lateral head turns in supine) for horizontal canal involvement.
- In a group of 592 patients with posterior, anterior, or horizontal canal involvement, 84% of patients had symptom remission after one canalith repositioning procedure; 13% required two treatments. For an average of 46 months of follow-up, 92% of patients reported no symptoms of vertigo.
- If BPPV occurs bilaterally, one ear should be treated at a time with 72 hours in between treatments. The response to a single canalith repositioning maneuver per ear is similar to unilateral cases.
- Patients that do not have symptom resolution after a single canalith repositioning

techniques often have a history of prior trauma or labyrinthitis.
- Patients with orthopedic restrictions can be successfully treated with vestibular habituation training.
- Traditionally, patients have been given the following posttreatment precautions:
  - Sleep semirecumbent for 2 nights, then sleep on a 30 degree wedge for 5 nights.
  - Avoid sleeping on the affected side.
  - Avoid vertigo-provoking head positions for 1 week.
  - Wear a cervical collar during the day between treatments.
- The necessity of these posttreatment precautions has recently been challenged. Patients treated with canalith repositioning maneuvers without posttreatment instructions are as successful as patients given posttreatment instructions.

CONTRIBUTING FACTORS

Enlarged vestibular aqueduct

PROGNOSIS

- Recurrence of vertiginous episodes is related to the cause of BPPV.
  - BPPV of traumatic origin has a 6- to 42-month recurrence rate of 57%.
  - BPPV of idiopathic origin has a 6- to 42-month recurrence rate of 19%.
  - Recurrence is not related to the number of treatments required to achieve a negative outcome for vertigo according to the Dix-Hallpike maneuver.

SIGNS AND SYMPTOMS INDICATING REFERRAL TO PHYSICIAN

- Failure to respond to the particle repositioning maneuver
- Tinnitus
- Hearing loss
- Duration of dizziness several minutes to days
- Cranial nerve signs
- Vertigo without positional dependence
- Cerebellar deficits

SUGGESTED READINGS

Balatsouras DG, Kaberos A, Assimakopoulou D, Katotomichelakis M, Economou NC, Korres SG. Etiology of vertigo in children. *Int J Pediatr Otorhinolaryngol.* 2007;71:487-494.

Baloh RW, Honrubia V, Jacobson K. Benign positional vertigo: cervical and oculographic features in 240 cases. *Neurology.* 1987;37:371.

Bertholen P, Tringali S, Faye MB, Antoine JC, Martin C. Prospective study of positional nystagmus in 100 consecutive patients. *Ann Otol Rhinol Laryngol.* 2006;115:587-594.

Brandt T, Steddin S. Current view of the mechanism of benign paroxysmal positioning vertigo: cupulolithiasis or canalolithiasis? *J Vestib Res.* 1993;3:373-382.

Del Rio M, Arriaga MA. Benign positional vertigo: Prognostic factors. *Otolaryngol Head Neck Surg.* 2004;130:426-429.

Dunniway HM, Welling DB. Intracranial tumors mimicking benign paroxysmal positional vertigo. *Otolaryngol Head Neck Surg.* 1998;118:429-436.

Epley JM. Positional vertigo related to semicircular canalithiasis. *Otolaryngol Head Neck Surg.* 1995;112:154-161.

Furman JM, Cass SP. Benign paroxysmal positional vertigo. *N Engl J Med.* 1999;341:1590-1597.

Gordon CR, Levite R, Joffe V, Gadoth N. Is post-traumatic benign paroxysmal positional vertigo different from the idiopathic form? *Arch Neurol.* 2004;61:1590-1593.

Horning E, Gorman SL. Case report: vestibular rehabilitation decreases fall risk and improves gaze stability for an older individual with unilateral vestibular hypofunction. *J Geriatr Phys Ther.* 2007;30:121-127.

House MG, Honrubia V. Theoretical models for the mechanisms of Benign Paroxysmal Positional Vertigo. *Audiol Neurootol.* 2003; 8:91-99.

Imai T, Takeda N, Ito M, et al. Benign paroxysmal positional vertigo due to a simultaneous involvement of both horizontal and posterior semicircular canals. *Audiol Neurootol.* 2006;11:198-205.

Katsarkas A, Kirkham TH. Paroxysmal positional vertigo – a study of 255 cases. *J Otolaryngol.* 1978;7:320-330.

Kovar M, Jepson T, Jones S. Diagnosing and treating benign paroxysmal positional vertigo. *J Gerontol Nurs.* 2006;12:22-27.

Manzari L. Enlarged vestibular aqueduct (EVA) related with recurrent benign paroxysmal positional vertigo (BPPV). *Med Hypotheses.* 2008;70:61-65.

Massoud EA, Ireland DJ. Post-treatment instructions in the nonsurgical management of benign paroxysmal positional vertigo. *J Otolaryngol.* 1996;25:121-125.

Neuhauser H, Lempert T. Vertigo and dizziness related to migraine: a diagnostic challenge. *Cephalagia.* 2004;24:83-91.

Nuti D, Nati C, Passali D. Treatment of benign paroxysmal positional vertigo: no need for postmaneuver restrictions. *Otolaryngol Head Neck Surg.* 2000;122:440-444.

Prokopakis EP, Chinona T, Tsagournisakis M, et al. Benign paroxysmal positional vertigo: 10-year experience in treating 592 patients with canalith repositioning procedure. *Laryngoscope.* 2005;115:1667-1671.

Sato S, Ohashi T, Koizuka I. Physical therapy for benign paroxysmal positional vertigo patients with movement disability. *Auris Nasus Larynx.* 2003;30:S53-S56.

Von Brevern M, Radtke A, Lezius F, et al. Epidemiology of benign paroxysmal positional vertigo: a population based study. *J Neurol Neurosurg Psychiatry.* 2007;78:710-715.

Wanamaker HH. Surgical treatment of benign paroxysmal positional vertigo. *Operative Techniques in Otolaryngology-Head and Neck Surgery.* 2001;12:124-128.

Welling DB, Barnes DE. Particle repositioning maneuver for benign paroxysmal positional vertigo. *Laryngoscope.* 1994;104:946-949.

Zappia JJ. Posterior semicircular canal occlusion for benign paroxysmal positional vertigo. *Am J Otol.* 1996;17:749-754.

AUTHOR: DEBORAH L. LOWE

BASIC INFORMATION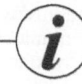

DEFINITION

Closed lock of the temporomandibular joint (TMJ) is the result of a nonreducing deformed disc acting as an obstacle to the sliding condylar head. The condition can be acute or chronic.

SYNONYMS

- Anterior disc displacement without reduction
- Anterior disc derangement

ICD-9CM CODE
524.6 Temporomandibular joint
    disorders

OPTIMAL NUMBER OF VISITS

12 to 24 visits, depending on the level of soft tissue structure involvement and documented functional gains

MAXIMAL NUMBER OF VISITS

24 visits

ETIOLOGY

- Closed lock of the TMJ results from mechanical stresses such as the following:
  - Traumatic events that result in stretching, tearing, or rupture of the disc, lateral ligament or capsule
  - Improper activity of the lateral pterygoid muscle resulting from hypertrophy, atrophy, or contracture
- The disc becomes anchored to the glenoid fossa; for the acute patient, it is possible to recapture the disc; for the chronic patient, it is not possible to recapture the disc.
- In response to mechanical stresses and resulting tissue damage, the inflammatory cascade is initiated. Proinflammatory markers, such as cytokines, interleukins, and tumor necrosis factor, have been detected in the synovial fluid of patients diagnosed with chronic-closed lock of the TMJ. This inflammatory cascade results in pathological soft tissue changes such as adhesions and cartilage degeneration.

EPIDEMIOLOGY AND DEMOGRAPHICS

- In the general population, 5% to 7 % will require treatment for temporomandibular dysfunction (TMD); chronic closed lock is a subset of TMD.
- TMD, including closed lock, are most common in the second through fourth decade.
- TMD of all etiologies is more common in women with a ratio of 4:1 to 6:1.

MECHANISM OF INJURY

The intraarticular disc may be injured whenever there is an alteration in the normal pathways of motion of the TMJ that involves the function of the articular disc. This may occur via acute or chronic trauma. If the trauma causes bleeding, there will be fibrotic intraarticular reactions leading to restricted mobility and pain. Less dramatic repetitive injury may lead to soft-tissue responses and permanent intraarticular changes.

COMMON SIGNS AND SYMPTOMS

- Restriction of translatory movements
- Absence or presence of clicking
- Deviation in opening the mouth toward the affected side
- Limitation in lateral movement toward the contralateral side
- Restriction in protrusive movements with the mandible shifting toward the affected side
- Pain present on palpation and during opening movements
- Symptoms develop in stages:
  - In the earliest stage a catching sensation may occur with mouth opening; noise and dysfunction are not evident.
  - In the next stage the articular disc has slipped forward, resulting in a clicking or popping sound with mouth opening and occasionally a reciprocal click with mouth closing. Joint pain, muscle pain, and headache may be present.
  - As the anterior displacement of the disc increases, the last stage occurs. The anteriorly displaced disc acts as an obstacle, and the joint appears locked. A patient will present with localized TMJ pain with mouth opening and chewing and joint tenderness on lateral palpation.
- Headache, facial muscle pain, toothache, and earache are all common symptoms associated with TMJ.

AGGRAVATING ACTIVITIES

- Activities that bring the mouth toward maximal opening such as yawning and singing
- Chewing hard objects such as nuts
- Repetitive chewing as with gum

EASING ACTIVITIES

The patient must reduce use of the jaw by not participating in activities that place prolonged stress on the TMJ such as the activities listed in the Aggravating Activities section.

24-HOUR SYMPTOM PATTERN

There is no common 24-hour pain pattern.

PAST HISTORY FOR THE REGION

Acute trauma or repetitive chronic strain on the soft tissue components of the TMJ that has altered biomechanical function

PHYSICAL EXAMINATION

- Maximal mouth opening <25 to 35 mm
- Maximal protrusion <5 mm
- Clicking and/or crepitation with mouth opening and closing, however, are not always present
- Tenderness with palpation of the lateral TMJ and/or muscles of mastication

IMPORTANT OBJECTIVE TESTS

There is no single definitive objective test for diagnosing closed lock of the TMJ. As with most conditions involving the TMJ, the clinician will use multiple resources to arrive at a diagnosis. Some of the objective tools are panoramic radiographs and MRI. Panoramic radiographs can be used to exclude dental, periodontal, and other problems of the oral region. MRI can be used to determine disc position in relation to TMJ position aiding in the differential diagnosis of TMDs.

DIFFERENTIAL DIAGNOSIS

- Toothache
- Pericoronitis
- Maxillary sinusitis
- Earache
- Salivary gland pathology
- Temporal arteritis
- Neuralgias
- Tension-type headache
- Degenerative conditions of the TMJ
- Myofascial pain and dysfunction

CONTRIBUTING FACTORS

- Personal habits that affect the use or position of the TMJ can contribute to the pathology. These include but are not limited to the following:
  - Gum chewing
  - Nail biting
  - Pipe smoking
  - Bruxism
  - Singing or yelling
  - Time spent in conversation
  - Dental health
  - Sleep position

TREATMENT

SURGICAL INDICATORS

Significant painful restricted vertical and horizontal mandibular movements, MRI findings of anterior nonreduced disc displacement, and failure of conservative therapy

SURGICAL OPTIONS

- Arthrocentesis (lavage of the upper joint compartment) with mandibular manipulation
- Arthroscopy procedure of lysis, lavage and capsular stretch and open-surgery high condylectomy with disc repositioning

SURGICAL OUTCOMES

- Arthrocentesis with mandibular manipulation has excellent-to-good results in 73% of patients with unilateral involvement.
- Visually guided TMJ irrigation has a 68% success rate.
- Open surgery high condylectomy with disc repositioning has a 90% success rate. The arthroscopy procedure of lysis, lavage, and capsular stretch has a 80% success rate. Success in both instances is defined as increased maximal mouth opening, decreased pain, and decreased joint dysfunction.

REHABILITATION

- Manual soft tissue therapy can be used to rehabilitate local myofascial and discoligamentous dysfunction and can occur via reduced local ischaemia, stimulation of proprioception, destruction of fibrous adhesions, stimulation of synovial fluid production, and reduction of pain. Commonly targeted muscles include but are not limited to muscles of mastication and the digastric, sternocleidomastoid, posterior cervical, scalene, and upper trapezius muscles.
- Physical therapy modalities may also be used to reduce symptoms of pain and deviations of jaw movement. Shortwave diathermy, megapulse, ultrasound, and soft laser have all been shown to provide statistically significant improvement when compared to placebo.
- Active and passive exercises can be used initially to promote appropriate TMJ motion; active and passive exercises can promote improved cervical and thoracic mobility; and isometric and isokinetic strengthening exercises can increase strength and recruitment of muscles of mastication and muscles of the cervical

and thoracic spine. Increased mobility and strength in these regions in addition to postural retraining will promote correction of forward head posture and other postural anomalies that can affect TMJ function. Head posture has been shown to be a significant contributor to TMD pathology, thus attention must be paid to retraining postural muscles. The mobility and strength of the upper quarter needs to be addressed for patients with myogenous involvement.

PROGNOSIS

- MRI findings, such as presence of joint effusion rupture of retrodiscal ligaments, or the thickness of the attachment of the external pterygoid muscle can be used as indirect signs of TMD such as closed-lock TMJ resulting from internal derangement.
- Cervical disorders can predispose one to TMJ dysfunction.
- 9% of reducing disc derangements progress to nonreducing disc derangements within 3 years.

SIGNS AND SYMPTOMS INDICATING REFERRAL TO PHYSICIAN

- Dental pain
- Psychosocial dysfunction
- Unremitting cervical pain or radiculopathies
- Migraine headaches

SUGGESTED READINGS

Al-Belasy FA. Arthrocentesis for the treatment of temporomandibular joint closed lock: a review article. *Int J Oral Maxillofac Surg.* 2007;36:773-782.

Cincaglini R, Colombo-Bolla G, Gherlone EF, et al. Orientation of craniofacial planes and temporomandibular disorder in young adults with normal occlusion. *J Oral Rehab.* 2003;30:878-886.

Gray RJM, Qualyle AA, Hall CA, Schofield MA. Temporomandibular pain dysfunction: Can electrotherapy help? *Physiotherapy.* 1995;81:47-51.

Hamada Y, Kondoh T, Holmlund AB, Sakota K, Nomura Y, Seto K. Cytokine and clinical predictors for treatment outcome of visually guided temporomandibular joint irrigation

in patients with chronic closed lock. *J Oral Maxillofac Surg.* 2008;66:29-34.

Ismail F, Demling A, Hessling K, Fink M, Stiesch-Scholz M. Short-term efficacy of physical therapy compared to splint therapy in treatment of arthrogenous TMD. *J Oral Rehabil.* 2007;34:807-813.

Kalamir A, Pollard H, Vitiello AL, Bonello R. Manual therapy for temporomandibular disorders: a review of the literature. *J Bodywork and Mvmt Therapies.* 2007;11:84-90.

Lundh H, Westesson PL, Kopp S. A three-year follow-up of patients with reciprocal temporomandibular joint clicking. *Oral Surg Oral Med Oral Pathol.* 1987;63:530-533.

McNeill C. History and evolution of TMD concepts. *Oral Surg Oral Med Oral Pathol Oral Radiol Endod.* 1997;83:51-60.

Molinari F, Manicone PF, Raffaelli L, Raffaelli R, Pirronti T, Bonomo L. Temporomandibular joint soft-tissue pathology, I: Disc Abnormalities. *Semin Ultrasound CT MR.* 2007;28:192-204.

Nicolakis P, Erdogmus B, Kopf A, Djaber-Ansari A, Piehslinger E, Fialka-Moser V. Exercise therapy for craniomandibular disorders. *Arch Phys Med Rehabil.* 2000;81:1137-1142.

Nitzan DW, Marmary Y. The "anchored disc phenomenon": a proposed etiology for sudden-onset, severe, and persistent closed lock of the temporomandibular joint. *J Oral Maxillofac Surg.* 1997;55:797-802.

Politi P, Sembronio S, Robiony M, et al. High condylectomy and disc repositioning compared to arthroscopic lysis, lavage, and capsular stretch for the treatment of chronic closed lock of the temporomandibular joint. *Oral Surg Oral Med Oral Pathol Oral Radiol Endod.* 200;103:27-33.

Sembronio S, Albiero AM, Toro C, Robiony M, Politi M. Is there a role for arthrocentesis in recapturing the displaced disc in patients with closed lock of the temporomandibular joint? *Oral Surg Oral Med Oral Pathol Oral Radiol Endod.* 2008;105:274-280.

Simons DG, Travell JG, Simons LS, et al. *Travell and Simons' Myofascial Pain and Dysfunction: The Trigger Point Manual, vol.* Baltimore, MD: Lippincott Williams and Wilkins; 1998:5-44, 103-164pp.

Tomas X, Pomes J, Berenguer J, Mercader JM, Pons F, Donoso L. Temporomandibular joint soft-tissue pathology, II: nondisc abnormalities. *Semin Ultrasound CT MR.* 2007;2:205-212.

AUTHOR: DEBORAH L. LOWE

BASIC INFORMATION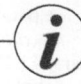

DEFINITION

Subluxation occurs when the hypermobile condyle moves horizontally beyond the anterior limit of the normal range of excursion. Subluxation is associated with wide mouth opening; the interincisal distance is 53 to 65 mm. It is a self-reducing, incomplete dislocation that can be unilateral or bilateral.

SYNONYMS

- Incomplete dislocation
- Self-reducing dislocation
- Hypermobility

ICD-9CM CODE
524.6 Temporomandibular joint
      disorders

OPTIMAL NUMBER OF VISITS

The optimal number of visits required for a subluxation of the temporomandibular joint will vary significantly. Non painful subluxations are common in the general public and often do not require medical attention. Painful subluxations will often follow normal tissue healing patterns with acute symptoms resolving within several weeks of the aggravating incident and complete tissue healing occurring within six weeks. Even with complete resolution of pain, subluxation may continue to occur. Optimally, the patient's acute symptoms can be managed within 4 – 6 visits. Long term resolution of the subluxation will be dependent upon patient compliance with home programs and whether anatomical or biomechanic issues factor into the subluxation.

MAXIMAL NUMBER OF VISITS

See Optimal Number of Visits.

ETIOLOGY

- The most likely explanations for unilateral subluxations are unilateral mastication on the contralateral side as a result of painful caries, unequal occlusal capacity, habit, or condylar fracture.
- Bilateral subluxation is frequently seen in patients who masticate with anterior teeth because of decreased molar occlusion, habit, overuse of the mandible as an instrument of expression, or protrusive manipulation of a bite piece during athletic competition.
- Causative factors include yawning to a point of subluxation, blows to the back of the head, falls, neck traction by means of head halters, whiplash injuries, muscle trismus, or loss of molar teeth.
- Repetitive subluxation of the condyle induces a thickening of the avascular connective tissue, the articular capsule and articular disc, which promotes the anterior position of the condyle.

EPIDEMIOLOGY AND DEMOGRAPHICS

- For patients with TMJ subluxation, anterior subluxation is the most common and lateral subluxation is rare.
- No research to date has demonstrated a correlation between age and TMJ subluxation.
- TMDs of all descriptions occur more frequently in women.

MECHANISM OF INJURY

- Forcible or lengthy opening of the mouth, such as occurs during the extraction of teeth; most commonly, downward pressure applied during the extraction of third molars
- Hypertonicity of the masticatory musculature from phenomena such as bruxism or other parafunctional masticatory habits that induce muscle fatigue

COMMON SIGNS AND SYMPTOMS

- Pain after a "pop" that may have been accompanied by an episode of acute dislocation; pain and limitation of excursion after initial subluxation
- Clicking in the other joint that may or may not be painful but may be hypermobile
- Interference with mandibular depression and deviation of the mandible toward the painful joint on opening; frequent clicking or jaw "sticks"
- Deviation of the mandible away from the subluxated side in unilateral subluxation
- Swelling in the area of the TMJ
- Pain on the side opposite the subluxated mandible from pressure of the condyle against the anterior wall of the auditory canal and the chorda tympanic nerve
- Pain, remote or local; clicking or grating noise in the TMJ region; visible presence of deformity from excursion of the condyles of the joints or from locking of the mouth in either the open or closed position or opening of the jaws beyond normal expectancy with sliding to one side
- Headaches in the region of distribution of the auricular tympanal nerve and along the distribution of the masseteric nerve involving all branches of the trigeminal nerve

AGGRAVATING ACTIVITIES

- Chewing gum
- Chewing tobacco or sticky substances such as taffy
- Excessive laughing or yawning

EASING ACTIVITIES

- Eating soft foods
- Reduce repetitive motion such as gum chewing
- Minimize mouth opening while talking, laughing, yawning, etc

24-HOUR SYMPTOM PATTERN

Pain on awakening, although no clear consistent pattern exists because symptoms and frequency of subluxation depend on patient's level of activity and the extent of degenerative joint changes.

PAST HISTORY FOR THE REGION

- Disc derangement
- Condylar fracture
- History of trauma

PHYSICAL EXAMINATION

- The anterior positioning of the condyle will spontaneously reverse
- Pain with palpation in the muscles of mastication
- Instability of the joint with active and passive movements
- Excessive mouth opening while the condyle is anterior to the articular eminence and excessive movement with anterior and or lateral glides
- Difficulty, instability, or pain with mastication
- Difficulty speaking because of joint instability
- Pain in the preauricular, facial, and cranial areas
- Joint noises during mandibular movement

IMPORTANT OBJECTIVE TESTS

- Radiographic analysis may demonstrate the following:
  - Displacement of the condyle anterior to the articular eminence
  - Flatness of the glenoid fossa with atrophy of the articular eminence

DIFFERENTIAL DIAGNOSIS

- Myofascial pain
- Acute closed lock of the TMJ meniscus
- Fracture/dislocations of the condylar neck
- Dislocation of TMJ (requires manual reduction)

CONTRIBUTING FACTORS

- Capsular laxity
- Trauma
- Abnormal chewing movements
- Internal derangement of the TMJ
- Occlusal disturbance
- Habitual rotational masticatory movements

TREATMENT

SURGICAL INDICATORS

Surgery is indicated for patients with significant, chronic pain, and/or recurrent subluxation with locking in the closed position.

SURGICAL OPTIONS

Extraarticular obstruction procedure

SURGICAL OUTCOMES

- 25 patients with subluxation associated with pain, clicking, audible cracking, and/or recurrent locking in the closed position who received the extraarticular obstruction procedure had the following results:
  - For the patients that reported preoperative pain: 52.9% were pain-free, 11.7% had reduced pain, and pain was unchanged for 35.2%.
  - For patients that reported painful clicking, audible cracking, or recurrent locking: 41.6% no longer experienced these symptoms, 29.1% were improved, and 25% reported no improvement.

REHABILITATION

- Similar courses of action are available for rehabilitating patients in whom surgery is not indicated and post-surgery.

- Eliminate the deforming forces such as soft diet in the short run, and encourage bilateral mastication if symptoms are unilateral.
- Treat pain resulting from acute joint strain or soft tissue injury with anti-inflammatories (topical or oral) and ice.
- Pain caused by muscle spasm may be addressed via myofascial release and other modalities, such as ultrasound and superficial heat, that reduce muscle spasm.
- Exercises need to address muscle imbalances that contributed to the initial condition.
- Isometric, active, and resisted exercises addressing strength of the masticatory muscles throughout their full range of motion (ROM).
- Positioning tongue on roof of mouth with active ROM (AROM) of mandible.
- Postural corrections for the craniomandibular region.

PROGNOSIS

Untreated TMJ subluxation often leads to TMJ dislocation.

SIGNS AND SYMPTOMS INDICATING REFERRAL TO PHYSICIAN

- Patient is unable to close mouth.
- Patient is unable to open mouth by more than 25 to 30 mm.

SUGGESTED READINGS

Caselli OJ. Treatment of the temporomandibular joint disturbances caused by chronic partial subluxation. *J Pros Den.* 1957;9:99-105.

Chausse JM, Richter M, Bettex A. Deliberate, fixed extra-articular obstruction. Treatment of choice for subluxation and true recurrent dislocation of the temporomandibular joint. *J Craniomaxillofac Surg.* 1987;15:137-140.

Gerry RG. Effects of trauma and hypermotility on the temporomandibular joint. *Proceedings of the New England Society of Oral Surgeons.* 1953;876-893.

Kummoona R. Surgical reconstruction of the temporomandibular joint for chronic subluxation and dislocation. *Int J Oral Maxillofac Surg.* 2001;30:344-348.

Luyk NH, Larsen PE. The diagnosis and treatment of the dislocated mandible. *Am J Emerg Med.* 1989;7:329-335.

Oh DW, Kim KS, Lee GW. The effect of physiotherapy on post-temporomandibular joint surgery patients. *J Oral Rehabil.* 2002;29:441-446.

Rosenbaum W. Sclerosing treatment for subluxation of the temporomandibular joint. *Am J Orthod Oral Surg.* 1946;32:551-571.

AUTHOR: DEBORAH L. LOWE

BASIC INFORMATION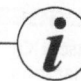

DEFINITION

- The acromioclavicular (AC) joint is the articulation between the acromion and the clavicle. An AC joint separation is a disruption in the ligamentous integrity of the AC joint.
- The ligaments providing stability to the AC joint include the following:
  - The superior and inferior AC ligaments
  - The coracoclavicular (CC) ligaments (conoid and trapezoid)

SYNONYMS

- AC joint separation
- Shoulder separation
- Separated shoulder
- NOTE: A shoulder separation is not the same as a shoulder dislocation. A shoulder separation injury occurs at the AC joint, whereas a shoulder dislocation occurs at the glenohumeral joint.

ICD-9CM CODES
718.91 Unspecified derangement of joint of shoulder region
719.91 Unspecified disorder of joint of shoulder region
831.04 Closed dislocation of acromioclavicular (joint)
831.14 Open dislocation of acromioclavicular (joint)
840.0 Acromioclavicular (joint) (ligament) sprain

OPTIMAL NUMBER OF VISITS

- 8 visits
- Optimal number of visits will vary by grade and severity of injury.

MAXIMAL NUMBER OF VISITS

36 visits

ETIOLOGY

- The AC joint is stabilized primarily by the ligaments and capsule that surround the joint. The AC joint is a diarthrodial articulation with a fibrocartilaginous meniscal disk that separates the acromial process and the distal clavicle.
- The joint capsule is reinforced by the AC ligaments. These include the superior, inferior, anterior, and posterior ligaments. The superior and inferior ligaments are stronger than the anterior and posterior ligaments.
- The AC ligaments are the principal restraint to anteroposterior translation, while the CC ligaments restrain vertical motions.
- The AC and CC ligaments are the passive stabilizers of the AC joint, and the deltoid and trapezius muscles are the dynamic stabilizers.

- The degree of clavicular displacement depends on the amount of damage the ligaments and the muscles that attach to the clavicle sustained.
- The first three types or grades of AC joint separations are as follows:
  - Grade I: Sprain of the AC ligaments without complete disruption; CC ligaments remain intact
  - Grade II: Complete disruption of the AC ligaments, with sprains of the CC ligaments
  - Grade III: Complete disruption of the AC and CC ligaments; CC interspace 25% to 100% greater than normal
- The next three types, grades IV through VI, may be classified as subtypes of grade III injuries, which include complete rupture of the AC and CC joints, as well as the following:
  - Grade IV: Avulsion of the CC ligament from the clavicle with superior and posterior displacement of the clavicle into or through the trapezius
  - Grade V: Exaggerated superior, vertical displacement of the clavicle from the scapular-CC interspace; 100% to 300% increase in CC interspace
  - Grade VI: Clavicle displaced inferior to coracoid (subcoracoid dislocation)

EPIDEMIOLOGY AND DEMOGRAPHICS

- AC joint separation injuries occur more frequently in men than in women, approximately 5:1.
- They account for approximately 12% of shoulder girdle injuries seen in clinical practice.
- Estimated as prevalent as 40% of all sports shoulder injuries, although this number may be greater since patients with minor sprains are less likely to seek medical attention.
- Most commonly occur in first 3 decades of life.
- Most common in young adults involved in contact sports such as football.
- Also common in soccer, rugby, hockey, and skiing.

MECHANISM OF INJURY

- Direct force
- Injury typically sustained secondary to a fall with direct impact onto the acromion
- Fall onto an adducted shoulder
- Indirect force
- Fall on an outstretched arm
- The force is transmitted through the humeral head on to the acromion, spraining the AC and/or CC ligaments
- Typical sports that may result in AC joint separations include the following:
  - Bicycle riding
  - Football
  - Rugby

  - Gymnastics
  - Martial arts

COMMON SIGNS AND SYMPTOMS

- Fairly localized pain
- Marked edema
- Abrasions
- Ecchymosis
- Local tenderness to palpation
- "Piano key" sign: hypermobile clavicle
- Step off deformity
- Pain aggravated with forced horizontal adduction

AGGRAVATING ACTIVITIES

Upper extremity movements, particularly flexion >90 degrees or adduction past midline

EASING ACTIVITIES

- Upper extremity supported by a sling or the other hand
- Glenohumeral joint at 0 degrees flexion, adducted at side, and internally rotated resting lower arm on abdomen

24-HOUR SYMPTOM PATTERN

- Symptoms are generally related to inflammation. Acutely seen, the patient will experience pain with most motions and have difficulty sleeping because of the pain.
- As the inflammation decreases, patient may experience some morning stiffness but this will resolve and will depend on use.
- The more the arm is used, the greater the stiffness and pain.
- Eventually, the symptoms will be only noted with motions above shoulder level and across midline.

PAST HISTORY FOR THE REGION

Generally, the injury is related to a traumatic injury. No prior history of pathology or injury need be associated with the separation.

PHYSICAL EXAMINATION

- Patient will present with arm in sling or supported by the other arm.
- Patient's movements will be guarded and protected.
- Patient will be unable to lift the arm overhead.
- Lifting and carrying objects with the arm will be painful.
- Patient will be unable to sleep on the affected shoulder.
- Step-off deformity will be noted at the AC joint.

IMPORTANT OBJECTIVE TESTS

- X-rays are taken as standard practice to diagnose AC joint disruption. They may also be necessary to rule out a fracture of the clavicle. In some cases, x-rays are taken while holding a weight in each hand to stress the joint.

- Magnetic resonance imaging (MRI) scans are not usually done.
- O'Brien test: Specificity: 92%; sensitivity: 100%.
- Cross-body adduction test: Specificity: 79%; sensitivity: 77%.
- AC-resisted extension test: Specificity: 85%; sensitivity: 72%.

DIFFERENTIAL DIAGNOSIS

- Shoulder dislocation
- Shoulder subluxation
- Clavicular fracture
- Humeral fracture
- Rotator cuff pathology
- Labral pathology
- Bone contusions

TREATMENT

SURGICAL OPTIONS

- AC joint injuries, grades I, II, or III, are typically managed conservatively, without surgical intervention.
- Grade III injuries managed conservatively compare favorably with those repaired surgically, with regard to outcome satisfaction, eliminating complications associated with surgery such as infection, the need for subsequent surgeries, and greater deformity.
- Grades IV, V, and VI require surgical intervention.
- Types of surgical intervention include the following:

  - Modified Weaver-Dunn procedure
  - Mumford procedure (distal clavicle excision)
  - Fixation with screws
  - Other procedures to stabilize region

REHABILITATION

- Topical cold packs can be used initially to reduce inflammation and pain.
- Rest is required during the acute phase of rehabilitation.
- Broad arm sling preferable while acute (typically first week of grade I, II, or III injury).
- AC, sternoclavicular, and glenohumeral joint mobilization may be indicated after the acute phase to restore normal joint kinematics.
- Passive range of motion (PROM) should be restored as pain allows.
- Active ROM (AROM) exercises should be incorporated to restore normal function.
- Movement reeducation is necessary to prevent scapular hiking and restore normal functional motions.
- Reacclimation to prior activities should be encouraged as pain allows. Functional training should be incorporated.
- Contact sports and heavy lifting (particularly bench press) should be avoided for 8 to 12 weeks after injury.

PROGNOSIS

- After rehabilitation, strength and endurance are similar to those of the uninvolved shoulder.
- Most patients return to prior levels of function, but because of altered AC joint function, the shoulder may be prone to subacromial pathologies later in life.

- Aching in the joint may be experienced for up to 6 months or longer; this is hypothesized to be secondary to degenerative changes in the joint.

SIGNS AND SYMPTOMS INDICATING REFERRAL TO PHYSICIAN

- Symptoms that do not improve within the first month should be referred to a physician for further evaluation.
- Signs of neurological or vascular involvement, such as distal weakness, paresthesias, or temperature change, should be referred to the physician to rule out neurovascular involvement.
- With the presence of a step-off sign, if the patient has not been seen initially by a physician, it is advisable for the patient to see a physician to rule out the possibility of fracture.

SUGGESTED READINGS

Fraser-Moodie JA, Shortt NL, Robinson CM. Injuries to the acromioclavicular joint. *J Bone Joint Surg Br*. 2009;90(6):697–707.

Larsen E, Bjerg-Nielsen A, Christensen P. Conservative or surgical treatment of acromioclavicular dislocation. A prospective, controlled, randomized study. *J Bone Joint Surg Am*. 1986;68(4):552–555.

Macdonald PB, Lapointe P. Acromioclavicular and sternoclavicular joint injuries. *Orthop Clin North Am*. 2008;39(4):535–545, viii.

Placzek JD, Boyce DA. *Orthopaedic Physical Therapy Secrets*. 2nd ed. St Louis, MO: Hanley & Belfus; 2006.

Powell JW, Huijbregts PA. Concurrent criterion-related validity of acromioclavicular joint physical examination tests: a systematic review. *J Man Manip Ther*. 2006;14(2):E19–E29.

AUTHOR: ROBERT S. BURNS

BASIC INFORMATION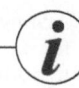

DEFINITION

- Adhesive capsulitis is a disorder in which the glenohumeral joint capsule becomes inflamed and stiff, developing adhesions. This process greatly restricts glenohumeral movement and is hallmarked by severe chronic pain and functional impairment.
- Adhesive capsulitis is a self limiting condition of uncertain etiology. It is characterized by clinically significant restriction of active and passive shoulder motion. This loss of motion occurs in the absence of a known intrinsic shoulder disorder.

SYNONYMS

- Frozen shoulder (FS)
- Frozen shoulder syndrome (FSS)
- Restrictive periarthritis
- Duplay's disease
- Scapulohumeral periarthritis

ICD-9CM CODE
726.0 Adhesive capsulitis of shoulder

OPTIMAL NUMBER OF VISITS

- 8 to 16 visits
- Literature is mixed regarding physical therapy's efficacy in treating patients with adhesive capsulitis. Some studies support high frequency of physical therapy visits, 4 to 5 per week for 2 weeks, optimally. Others suggest that patients will improve without physical therapy. Some studies suggest the patient should not expect to regain full glenohumeral range of motion (ROM) for 6 to 18 months.

MAXIMAL NUMBER OF VISITS

36 visits

ETIOLOGY

- Adhesive capsulitis may be broken down into the following two subcategories:
  - *Primary adhesive capsulitis* begins insidiously and without a clear mechanism of injury. While chronic inflammation, autoimmunity, and other systemic causes have been hypothesized as causes for primary adhesive capsulitis, objective data supporting these theories are lacking. Parallels have been drawn to Dupuytren's contracture, with regard to histological changes in the connective tissue.
  - *Secondary adhesive capsulitis* occurs in response to trauma or other precipitating event. These events often include rotator cuff impingement, bursitis, AC separation, or neuritis.

EPIDEMIOLOGY AND DEMOGRAPHICS

- Prevalence in the general population is 2%.
- It occurs more frequently between the fourth and sixth decades.
- 70% of cases occur in females and may affect women earlier than men.
- 12% to 16% of patients will experience symptoms in the contralateral shoulder.
- Contralateral adhesive capsulitis typically occurs within 5 years of initial onset of symptoms in the first shoulder.
- The frequency of bilateral involvement in patients with type 1 diabetes is elevated. Patients with type 2 diabetes have a 40% chance of developing adhesive capsulitis in their lifetimes.
- Hyperthyroidism and hypertriglyceridemia are also associated with elevated risk.

MECHANISM OF INJURY

- Mechanism may be related to an injury to the shoulder (secondary adhesive capsulitis) or may begin insidiously (primary adhesive capsulitis).
- The mechanism for secondary adhesive capsulitis may be a fall onto the hand or arm, surgery, or other trauma to the upper extremity.

COMMON SIGNS AND SYMPTOMS

- Painful, restricted glenohumeral AROM
- Pain in the deltoid region
- Pain both at rest and with activity
- Progressive stiffness
- Stage/phase I: The painful phase:
  - Insidious, predominantly nocturnal pain
  - Typically, no clear precipitating factor
  - Pain in deltoid region
  - Aggravated with movement to end-ranges
  - May have pain with rest
  - ROM is minimally restricted
  - Elastic glenohumeral joint end-feel
  - Stage/phase I lasts 2 to 9 months.
- Stage/phase II: The frozen or adhesive phase:
  - Pain associated with stage/phase I may persist but is normally diminished
  - Progressive ROM limitations in capsular pattern
  - Activities of daily living (ADLs) are severely affected
  - Pain in deltoid region and possibly into wrist
  - Pain with or without movement
  - Elastic or abrupt glenohumeral end-feel
- Stage/phase III: The thawing or regressive phase:
  - Pain progressively decreases
  - ROM progressively increases over 12 to 24 months
  - Pain into wrist

- Pain without movement
- Abrupt glenohumeral end feel
- Unable to lay sidelying

AGGRAVATING ACTIVITIES

- Combing hair
- Reaching for seatbelt
- Reaching into back pocket
- Fastening brassiere strap
- Reaching overhead

EASING ACTIVITIES

- Codman's (pendulum) exercises
- Corticosteroid injections
- Warm showers
- Many times, easing factors are not present and patient cannot identify an activity that decreases their symptoms

24-HOUR SYMPTOM PATTERN

- Nocturnal pain is a hallmark sign of adhesive capsulitis.
- The remainder of the day may or may not follow a distinctive pattern.
- Some patients will experience pain and stiffness on awakening and after prolonged periods of inactivity.

PAST HISTORY FOR THE REGION

- Patient may have a history of prior trauma to the region.
- Patient may have had a prior history of adhesive capsulitis to the affected or contralateral shoulder.

PHYSICAL EXAMINATION

- Patient will present with guarding or protected posturing of the shoulder.
- It may be positioned in slight flexion, abduction, and neutral rotation to place the glenohumeral joint in a more loose packed position.
- Very little arm swing on the affected limb is noted during gait.
- Patients presenting with stages I and II adhesive capsulitis will have pain on palpation of the anterior and posterior capsule and often will describe pain radiating to the deltoid insertion.
- Strength may or may not be symptomatic, depending on whether the rotator cuff muscles are involved with the pathology.
- Often, a reversal of normal scapular motion will be noticed. Decreased glenohumeral motion will be noted with a compensatory increase in scapulothoracic motion.

IMPORTANT OBJECTIVE TESTS

- Diagnosis of adhesive capsulitis is often a diagnosis of exclusion, thus other possible pathologies are ruled out. Therefore there are very few tests that are consistently witnessed across patients.
- Limited shoulder ROM is a consistent occurrence. Glenohumeral motion should be measured while stabilizing the scapula

to evaluate glenohumeral versus scapulothoracic ROM.

- The motions most limited by adhesive capsulitis will be external rotation, abduction, and internal rotation.
- X-rays are generally negative, although there may be evidence of osteopenia or osteoporosis.
- MRIs can be used to identify rotator cuff pathology in secondary adhesive capsulitis, but it is not routinely needed for diagnosis.

DIFFERENTIAL DIAGNOSIS

- Complex regional pain syndrome (CRPS) type I
- Brachial plexus injury
- Coronary or cardiac dysfunction
- Pancoast tumor
- Humeral fracture
- Rotator cuff pathology
- Heterotropic ossification
- Referral from the cervical and thoracic region

CONTRIBUTING FACTORS

- Endocrine system disorders
  ○ Diabetes
  ○ Thyroid disorders
  ○ Reproductive disorders
- There is some evidence of a genetic predisposition. Specific genetic abnormalities have been identified with this condition. There was an increase in trisomy 7 and trisomy 8 in the fibroblasts that were resected from the glenohumeral joint at time of surgery.

TREATMENT

SURGICAL OPTIONS

- Suprascapular nerve block and stellate block
- Intraarticular corticosteroid injection
- Closed manipulation under anesthesia (MUA) is performed in the following sequence:

  ○ Adducted shoulder and externally rotated
  ○ Abducted in the coronal plane
  ○ Externally rotated in abduction
  ○ Internally rotated in abduction
  ○ Forward flexed
  ○ Adducted and internally rotated
- Open or arthroscopic capsular release
- Hydroplasty

SURGICAL OUTCOMES

- Literature is mixed regarding the outcomes after manipulation.
- Some literature suggests that closed manipulation is an effective operative treatment for most patients with adhesive capsulitis; however, there is a high incidence of failure in patients with diabetes.
- Arthroscopy conducted after manipulation revealed that 79% of cases had a rupture of the capsule adjacent to the anterior inferior rim.
- Research from a long-term prospective study by Binder et al seems to indicate that subjects who are treated with vigorous shoulder manipulation fared worse than do those who are not treated at all.
- Literature also suggests that open and arthroscopic capsular releases are an effective treatment choice to immediately increase ROM, but long-term responses and functional changes have yet to be studied.

REHABILITATION

- The use and effectiveness of rehabilitation is controversial. Clinically, changes in function, motion and pain are seen, but these changes have not been backed up by research.
- Rehabilitation should initially focus on pain management and avoid painful overstretching, which may result in further loss of range.
- Data support the use of manual therapy to increase ROM. Gentle manual techniques recommended including grade I and II joint mobilization and myofascial release, as appropriate.
- Glenohumeral, AC, scapulothoracic, thoracic spine, and costotransverse joint

mobilization is advisable. Studies have demonstrated glenohumeral joint mobilization at end range to be more effective than midrange mobilization.
- Research is lacking regarding the effects of exercise on adhesive capsulitis. Therapeutic exercises include the following:
  ○ Active assist ROM (AAROM) stretching recommended, particularly performed in closed chain
  ○ Isometric glenohumeral joint AROM
  ○ Scapular exercises

PROGNOSIS

Adhesive capsulitis is considered a self-limiting disorder. Most patients will recover up to 90% of glenohumeral AROM in 2 years.

SIGNS AND SYMPTOMS INDICATING REFERRAL TO A PHYSICIAN

- Patients with increasing symptoms
- Patients with increasing neurological symptoms
- Patients with nocturnal pain coupled with dramatic unexplained weight loss
- Patients who are not responding to conservative interventions

SUGGESTED READINGS

Binder AI, Bulgen DY, Hazleman BL, et al. Frozen shoulder: a long-term prospective study. *Ann Rheum Dis.* 1984;43(3):361–364.

Callinan N, McPherson S, Cleaveland S, Voss DG, Rainville D, Tokar N. Effectiveness of hydroplasty and therapeutic exercise for treatment of frozen shoulder. *J Hand Ther.* 2003;16(3):219–224.

Mao CY, Jaw WC, Cheng HC. Frozen shoulder: correlation between the response to physical therapy and follow-up shoulder arthrography; *Arch Phys Med Rehabil.* 1997;78(8):857–859.

Sheridan MA. Upper extremity: emphasis on frozen shoulder. *Orthop Clin North Am.* 2006;37(4):531–539.

AUTHOR: ROBERT S. BURNS

Section III

ORTHOPEDIC PATHOLOGY

BASIC INFORMATION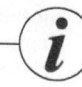

DEFINITION

A Bankart lesion is an avulsion of the anteroinferior glenoid labrum at its attachment to the inferior glenohumeral ligament (IGHL).

SYNONYMS

- Perthes lesion (a variant of the Bankart lesion)
- Labral tear

ICD-9CM CODE
840.7 Superior glenoid labrum lesion

OPTIMAL NUMBER OF VISITS

12 visits

MAXIMAL NUMBER OF VISITS

24 visits

ETIOLOGY

- The lesion is the result of anterior shoulder dislocation and is the primary lesion in recurrent anterior instability.
- Congenital anomalies of the labrum are often seen in the anterior and superior portions.
- When the humeral head is forced out anteriorly and inferiorly at the time of the initial injury, the anterior capsule and IGHLs are stretched. As a result of the traction, the fibrous labrum is pulled off from the inferior half of the anterior rim of the glenoid.
- The Bankart lesion results from the failure of healing of the anterior capsule and the labrum from the glenoid margin. This leaves a pouch in the front of the neck of the scapula, into which the head of the humerus easily re-dislocates.
- The oval-shaped glenoid is longest superiorly to inferiorly. The chondral surface of the glenoid is thickened by the labrum, which creates a greater concave surface to improve glenohumeral stability. The labrum is a fibrous structure that is firmly attached to the glenoid at its inferior rim and attached more loosely superiorly where it attaches to the long head of the biceps tendon. Howell and Galinat demonstrated that the labrum contributes approximately 50% of the total depth of the socket. Furthermore, they noted that detachment of the labrum anteriorly, as in a Bankart lesion, may reduce the depth of the socket in the anteroposterior direction from approximately 5 to 2.4 mm. Therefore loss of labral integrity greatly impacts glenohumeral joint stability.

EPIDEMIOLOGY AND DEMOGRAPHICS

- Bankart lesions occur more often in patients under 30 years of age.
- The lesions occur in >85% of traumatic anterior dislocations.

MECHANISM OF INJURY

- Trauma accounts for a vast majority of anteroinferior glenohumeral subluxations and dislocations. This can occur in the following ways:
  - Trauma, forced external rotation/abduction, with a posterior force at the glenohumeral joint
  - Traction onto the arm in an anterior direction
  - Fall onto outstretched hand (FOOSH) with arm abducted and externally rotated
  - Blunt trauma to the humerus in a posterior-to-anterior direction

COMMON SIGNS AND SYMPTOMS

- Moderate-to-severe pain and aching
- Feelings of instability
- Crepitus with motion of the arm
- Popping and locking with certain motions of the arm
- Recurrent dislocation

AGGRAVATING ACTIVITIES

- Actively moving the arm into scaption/flexion with external rotation, particularly with arm abducted to 90 degrees
- Lifting and carrying overhead
- Sleeping on the involved shoulder

EASING ACTIVITIES

- Placing the involved upper extremity in a resting sling
- Antiinflammatories
- Avoidance of aggravating activities

24-HOUR SYMPTOM PATTERN

- Initially, symptoms will be present with most motions.
- As the inflammation resolves, symptoms will be activity dependent.
- There will be no specific pattern related to time of day.

PAST HISTORY FOR THE REGION

- Recent anteroinferior humeral dislocation
- History of multiple joint laxity

PHYSICAL EXAMINATION

- Acutely, the patient presents in a "guarded" position; the arm is adducted and fully internally rotated.
- Pain is located in the anterior aspect of the shoulder.
- Patient will complain of instability and catching in the joint with motion.

IMPORTANT OBJECTIVE TESTS

- Active and passive motion testing

Labral (SLAP or Bankart) Tests		
Name of Test	Specificity of Tests (%)	Sensitivity of Tests (%)
Active compression	54-100	11-98.5
Anterior slide	8-78	84-91
Crank	35-91	56-93
Clunk	Not reported	Not reported
MRI	42-89	88-92

SLAP, Superior labrum from anterior to posterior.

- Sulcus sign: 1+ grade is equivalent to 1 cm inferior translation, 2+ is equal to 2 cm translation, etc.
- X-rays: Acute traumatic shoulder dislocations are evaluated with the standard anteroposterior, transscapular lateral, and axillary views. In more chronic instability, the West Point axillary view shows the anterior glenoid rim and may reveal bony Bankart lesions.
- MRI is usually the gold standard for picking up soft tissue injuries.

DIFFERENTIAL DIAGNOSIS

- Bankart lesions often occur with concomitant Hill-Sachs lesions.
- SLAP lesions
- Osseous contusion
- Biceps tendinopathy
- AC joint injury
- Cervical referral
- Rotator cuff tear
- Humeral fracture

CONTRIBUTING FACTORS

- Generalized ligament laxity: Congenital or disease related
- Age: Pathology will occur more often in the twenties and again later in the sixties
- Activities (involvement in sports that place the patient in compromised glenohumeral joint positions)
- Overhead throwers: Baseball, softball, volleyball, and swimming

TREATMENT

SURGICAL OPTIONS

- Arthroscopic labral repairs are often indicated
- Bankart operation
- Putti Platt procedure
- Bristow-Helfet procedure
- Saha procedure

REHABILITATION

- Phase I
  - Rest and immobilization
  - Pain control with nonsteroidal antiinflammatory drugs (NSAIDs) and cold packs
- Phase II
  - Isometric strengthening
  - Isotonic strengthening
  - Begin exercises with shoulder in adducted, forward-flexed position, progressing to abducted position (this position minimizes the stress placed on the glenohumeral joint)
  - Rotator cuff strengthening
  - Scapular stabilization
- Phase III
  - Endurance building with strengthening exercises
  - Progressive eccentric strengthening
  - Goal: Patient reaches 90% strength in the injured shoulder compared with the uninjured shoulder
- Phase IV
  - Increase activity to sport- or job-specific activities
  - Progressive, resisted internal rotation

PROGNOSIS

- The failure rates after open shoulder stabilization for recurrent anterior instability have been reported to be 3% to 9%.

- Bigliani et al reported only 67% of 63 throwing athletes were able to return to their pre-injury levels of competition after an open Bankart repair.
- Nearly all research demonstrates that arthroscopic stabilization resulted in a higher rate of recurrent instability when compared with traditional open techniques.
- Bottoni et al recently reported on a consecutive series of 64 patients who were prospectively randomized to either arthroscopic or open stabilization. They concluded that clinical outcomes were comparable; however, the mean loss of motion was greater in the open shoulders, although this difference was not statistically significant.

SIGNS AND SYMPTOMS INDICATING REFERRAL TO A PHYSICIAN

- Signs of unreduced shoulder dislocation
- Signs of neural or vascular involvement
- Sign of humeral or clavicular fracture

SUGGESTED READINGS

Bigliani LU, Kurzweil PR, Schwartzbach CC, et al. Inferior capsular shift procedure for anterior-inferior shoulder instability in athletes. Am J Sports Med. 1994;22:578-584.

Bottoni CR, Smith EL, Berkowitz MJ, et al. Arthroscopic versus open shoulder stabilization for recurrent anterior instability: a prospective randomized clinical trial. Am J Sports Med. 2006;34(11):1730-1737.

Dodson CC, Cordasco FA. Anterior glenohumeral joint dislocations. Orthop Clin North Am. 2008;39:507-518.

Fabbriciani C, Milano G, Demontis A, et al. Arthroscopic versus open treatment of Bankart lesion of the shoulder: a prospective randomized study. Arthroscopy. 2004;20:456-462.

Howell SM, Galinat BJ. The glenoid-labral socket. A constrained articular surface. Clin Orthop Relat Res. 1989;243:122-125.

Ide J, Maeda S, Yamaga M, Morisawa K, Takagi K. Shoulder strengthening exercise with an orthosis for multidirectional shoulder instability; quantitative evaluation of rotational shoulder strength before and after the exercise program; J Shoulder Elbow Surg. 2003;12(4):342-345.

AUTHOR: ROBERT S. BURNS

BASIC INFORMATION

DEFINITION

- Pathology involving the biceps tendon(s).
- Tendonitis is considered an acute inflammatory disorder. In response to trauma, the body produces inflammation that in turn irritates the biceps tendon.
- Tendinosis is considered a degenerative disorder. It involves an accumulation of microtrauma that can lead to degenerative changes in the tendon. These changes include fibrosis, adhesions, and microtears that cause pain and lead to more tendon damage as the disease progresses.
- Tendinitis is usually a precursor to tendinosis, although all tendonitis need not lead to tendinosis.
- Biceps tendinopathy refers to the injury of the biceps tendon as it runs in the intertubercular groove.
- Rupture of tendon involves loss of continuity of the biceps tendon and usually occurs at the long head of the biceps.

SYNONYMS

- Bicipital tendonitis
- Bicipital tendinosis
- Bicipital tenosynovitis
- Biceps tear
- Biceps tendon rupture

ICD-9CM CODES
726.1   Rotator cuff syndrome of shoulder and allied disorders
727.62 Nontraumatic rupture of tendons of biceps (long head)

OPTIMAL NUMBER OF VISITS

8 visits

MAXIMAL NUMBER OF VISITS

24 visits

ETIOLOGY

- Biceps musculotendinous junction is particularly susceptible to overuse injuries, especially in individuals performing lifting activities. Biceps tendinopathy is rarely seen in isolation. It is typically found with co-morbid rotator cuff pathology, subdeltoid bursitis, or glenohumeral instability.
- Bicipital tendinopathies are the result of excessive mechanical stress placed on the tendon(s), exceeding the tensile capacity of the tendon. These forces cause inflammatory response in the tendon with resultant pain and other symptoms. Stressors may be acute, resulting in tendonitis, or chronic, causing tendinosis.

- A flattened medial wall of the bicipital groove can predispose a patient subluxation of the tendon of the long head of the biceps, resulting in an increased risk for inflammation.
- A shallow bicipital groove can lead to tendon subluxation with lifting and carrying activities.
- Studies have found that up to 95% of patients with bicipital tendinitis have associated rotator cuff disease.
- A more recent study has noted biceps tendinopathy as a major source of anterior shoulder pain after a total shoulder arthroplasty.
- Three theories have been hypothesized to explain the tendon pathology:
  o Mechanical theory: Loading of the tendon exceeds its ability to repair itself
  o Vascular theory: Decreased vascularity in a region predisposes it to compromises in healing
  o Neural modulation theory: Tendinopathy results from neurally mediated mast cell degranulation and the release of substance P

EPIDEMIOLOGY AND DEMOGRAPHICS

- Bicipital tendinopathies occur frequently in concert with other shoulder pathologies.
- Typically, biceps pathology occurs in the younger, athletic populations, but a second peak of occurrence occurs in the elderly.
- Biceps tendon ruptures occur primarily in the elderly.
- The exact frequency of biceps tendinopathy has not been reported in the literature.
- Biceps tendon injury is less common than supraspinatus tendon injury.

MECHANISM OF INJURY

- Repetitive overhead activity.
- Resisted shoulder and/or elbow flexion involves a load greater than the physiological strength of the myotendinous complex.
- Injury to the biceps tendon can involve tendinosis from repetitive overhead use or repetitive activities, such as rowing or bench pressing, which cause the humeral head to translate anteriorly and superiorly, therefore impinging the biceps tendon.
- Common activities resulting in pathology are as follows:
  o Repetitive lifting overhead
  o Repetitive carry objects
  o Rowing
  o Bench pressing
  o Catching a heavy falling object
  o FOOSH

COMMON SIGNS AND SYMPTOMS

- Anterior glenohumeral pain at bicipital groove.
- Pain may radiate into elbow.
- Pain is usually exacerbated at initial onset of activities.
- Patient may experience weakness or fatigue in the shoulder.
- Nocturnal pain is not unusual.
- Biceps tendon ruptures are rare but easy to assess. They will present with loss of strength with overhead motions, poor strength with elbow flexion, and a bulge in the anterior aspect of the upper arm.
- Often patients will report feeling a "pop" in their arm with a lifting activity.

AGGRAVATING ACTIVITIES

- Pain aggravated by activities requiring shoulder flexion, elbow flexion, and/or supination
- Lifting overhead
- Repetitive lifting and carrying
- Reaching behind back

EASING ACTIVITIES

- Avoidance of aggravating activities
- Antiinflammatory and pain medications
- Heat
- Stretching

24-HOUR SYMPTOM PATTERN

- Nocturnal pain
- Pain early after prolonged rest
- Symptoms are activity dependent
- Symptoms increase with overuse

PAST HISTORY FOR THE REGION

- History of other past or concurrent shoulder pathology is not uncommon
- History of shoulder instability
- History of trauma involving the shoulder

PHYSICAL EXAMINATION

- Palpate for tenderness of bicipital tendons proximally near bicipital groove.
- Manual muscle tests (MMTs) are limited by pain.
- PROM and AROM are limited by pain (if limited at all).
- "Popeye" arm is seen in cases of tendon rupture. This finding is the result of the biceps brachii retracting toward the elbow in the absence of the counterforce generally provided by the long head of the biceps.
- Swelling and bruising may or may not be present in the case of a tendon tear.
- With tendon rupture, the myotendinous junction or distal tendon stump typically migrates distally and can be identified below the level of the pectoralis insertion on the humerus, which serves as a useful landmark.

IMPORTANT OBJECTIVE TESTS

- Selective tissue tension test (Cyriax) as follows:
  - Strong and painful resisted elbow flexion
  - Strong and painful resisted shoulder flexion
  - Strong and painful resisted supination

DIFFERENTIAL DIAGNOSIS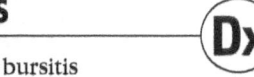

- Subacromial bursitis
- AC joint sprain
- Adhesive capsulitis
- Brachial neuritis
- Labral tear
- Rotator cuff pathology
- Referral from cervical or thoracic region
- Visceral referral

CONTRIBUTING FACTORS

- Impaired scapulothoracic rhythm
- Repetitive overhead/lifting activities

Biceps Tests

Name of Test	Specificity of Tests (%)	Sensitivity of Tests (%)
Yergason's	37	86
Speed's	70-83	33-38
O'Brien	50-55	47-68
Compression rotation	76	24
Biceps load 2	97	90

Dislocation/Instability Tests

Name of Test	Specificity of Tests (%)	Sensitivity of Tests (%)
Load-shift (under anesthesia)	83	100
Anterior drawer: Pain	71	28
Anterior drawer: Apprehension	85	53
Sulcus sign	Not reported	Not reported
Apprehension: Pain	56	50-53
Apprehension: Apprehension	96-99	53-72
Relocation: Pain	44-90	30-54
Relocation: Apprehension	90-99	67-81
Anterior release	92	89

Labral (SLAP or Bankart) Tests

Name of Test	Specificity of Tests (%)	Sensitivity of Tests (%)
Active compression	54-100	11-98.5
Anterior slide	8-78	84-91
Crank	35-91	56-93
Clunk	Not reported	Not reported
MRI	42-89	88-92

- Impingement syndrome/rotator cuff pathology
- Biceps tendon subluxation from bicipital groove
- Direct trauma
- Multidirectional shoulder instability
- Osteophyte formations
- Calcification of bicipital tendon
- Anatomical abnormalities

TREATMENT

SURGICAL OPTIONS

- Surgery reapproximation in cases of tendon rupture, but since it occurs most frequently in the elderly, surgery is not commonplace.
- Surgery is generally not indicated in cases of tendinosis or tendonitis.

REHABILITATION

Acute
- Rest
- Avoid aggravating activities
- Exercises that promote circulation such as pulleys or pendulum exercises

Subacute
- Manual therapy
  - Cross-friction massage to tendon
  - Release of muscles that prevent normal scapulothoracic and glenohumeral motions (i.e., posterior cuff, trapezius, and pectoralis muscles)
  - Joint mobilization may be used to stretch posterior and inferior cuff to allow normal glenohumeral joint mechanics
- Modalities
  - Electrical stimulation and heat may be beneficial to reduce muscle guarding and increase circulation.
- Exercise
  - First, focus on stabilizing the glenohumeral joint and preventing anterior translation of the humeral head; then, focus on normalizing scapulothoracic motion.
  - Progress to resistive exercises and functional activities as the patient improves the ability to stabilize glenohumeral joint and normalize the scapula.
  - Closed kinetic chain exercises are generally started first, with open kinetic chain exercises initiated later with sport-specific activities.
  - Address biomechanical factors that may be contributing to the biceps tendinopathy.

Long-Term
- Look for other causes or predisposing factors such as bony abnormalities, labral pathology, rotator cuff pathology, and radiculopathy.

PROGNOSIS

- Full recovery is anticipated in 6 to 8 weeks for tendonitis.
- Prognosis for tendinosis is variable and depends on the amount of degeneration that has occurred and whether the factors that contribute to the pathology can be changed.
- Tendon ruptures usually regain full mobility in 6 to 8 weeks. Strength overhead will be possible but will always be weaker because of loss of biceps contribution.

SIGNS AND SYMPTOMS INDICATING REFERRAL TO PHYSICIAN

Symptoms that may indicate further loss of tendon integrity include sudden increase in pain, erythema, or decrease in strength.

SUGGESTED READINGS

Beall DP, Williamson EE, Ly JQ, et al. Association of biceps tendon tears with rotator cuff

Section III

ORTHOPEDIC PATHOLOGY

abnormalities: degree of correlation with tears of the anterior and superior portions of the rotator cuff. *AJR Am J Roentgenol.* 2003;180:633-639.

Finlay K. Common tendon and muscle injuries: Upper extremities. *Ultrasound Clin.* 2007;2(4):577-594.

Harwood MI, Smith CT. Superior labrum, anterior-posterior lesions and biceps injuries: diagnostic and treatment considerations. *Prim Care.* 2004;31:831-855.

Middleton WD, Reinus WR, Totty WG, et al. Ultrasonographic evaluation of the rotator cuff and biceps tendon. *J Bone Joint Surg Am.* 1986;68:440-450.

Travis RD, Doane R, Burkhead WZ. Tendon ruptures about the shoulder. *Orthop Clin North Am.* 2000;31(2):313-330.

AUTHOR: ROBERT S. BURNS

BASIC INFORMATION

DEFINITION
Disruption of osseous integrity in the clavicle or collarbone.

SYNONYM
Broken collarbone

ICD-9CM CODES
810 Fracture of clavicle
767.2 Fracture of clavicle due to birth trauma

OPTIMAL NUMBER OF VISITS
8 visits

MAXIMAL NUMBER OF VISITS
24 visits

ETIOLOGY
- Result of trauma, typically nonaxial, directly onto clavicle
  - Class A: Middle-third fracture
  - Class B: Lateral-third fracture—the displacement is downward because of weight of arm
  - Class C: Medial-third fracture—the displacement is upward because of pull of sternocleidomastoid muscle
- The clavicle also elevates about 15 to 30 degrees and rotates posteriorly 30 to 50 degrees during shoulder elevation, therefore shoulder ROM may be limited or impaired after a clavicle fracture.
- During human development, the clavicle is the first bone to ossify; its ossification begins during the fifth week of gestation. It also the last bone to ossify. Late ossification occurs adjacent to the sternoclavicular joint. It does not fuse until after 20 years of age. The late fusion of the medial ossification center explains the physeal separation injuries commonly seen in young adults and children.
- Functionally, the clavicle acts as a long lever that connects the scapula to the thoracic spine. The length of this lever arm should be maintained to normalize normal mechanics and strength generation in the upper extremity.
- The clavicle also plays a protective role as it limits damage to the brachial plexus and vascular system beneath it. Injury to the clavicle could impact neural and vascular structures.

EPIDEMIOLOGY AND DEMOGRAPHICS
- 5% of all fractures seen in emergency department visits and up to 44% of all shoulder girdle fractures are clavicle fractures.
- They are the most common of all pediatric fractures.
- They constitute 4% to 10% of all adult fractures.
- There is a bimodal age distribution of incidence. The peaks of occurrence are under 40 years of age and over 70 years old.
- Middle-third clavicular fractures are the most common, accounting for 69% to 81% of all clavicular fractures because it is the thinnest section of the clavicle and devoid of muscle or ligament attachments.
- The lateral-third fracture accounts for 16% to 30% of all clavicular fractures.
- <3% of all clavicular fractures are medial-third fractures.

MECHANISM OF INJURY
- The young male will generally sustain a high energy mechanism such as direct trauma secondary to a motor vehicle accident (MVA) or a fall off a bicycle.
- The mechanism of injury in the elderly is due more often to a low energy load that is placed on insufficient bone such as in a fall onto the shoulder or an outstretched upper extremity (6% of cases).

COMMON SIGNS AND SYMPTOMS
- Pain
- Obvious deformity at region of fracture

AGGRAVATING ACTIVITIES
All shoulder motions, especially shoulder flexion or abduction

EASING ACTIVITIES
- Using a sling to support the arm and take weight off the shoulder
- Compression wrap
- Rest and ice
- Muscle relaxants, pain medications, and antiinflammatories

24-HOUR SYMPTOMS PATTERN
- Initially, pain is throughout the day because of inflammation.
- As inflammation diminishes, pain will be noted primarily with motion.
- Sleeping may be painful when patient rolls onto the affected shoulder.

PAST HISTORY FOR THE REGION
- Recent trauma
- No other pathology need be present in the region, although when fractures occur in the elderly, osteopenia or osteoporosis may be a factor

PHYSICAL EXAMINATION
- Deformity and osseous callous at fracture site
- Local edema
- Local tenderness to palpation at site of fracture
- Limited active and passive ranges of motion
- Because of its subcutaneous position, the clavicle may be fractured relatively easily and may occur in concert with concomitant injuries. Assess for the following injuries:
  - Costal fractures
  - Dislocations or subluxations of the shoulder
  - Sternal injury
  - AC separation
  - Sternoclavicular (SC) injury
  - Closed head injury
  - Pulmonary contusion
  - Pneumothorax or hemothorax

IMPORTANT OBJECTIVE TESTS
- Fracture is typically confirmed immediately on clinical examination via observation, postural, and palpatory assessments.
- A large hematoma may be present that may indicate damage to the subclavian vessels.
- X-rays are necessary to confirm the diagnosis. Computed tomography (CT) scans are generally not warranted unless to rule out soft tissue or vascular involvement.
- Assess distal upper extremity pulses (brachial, radial, and ulnar) and neurological systems.

DIFFERENTIAL DIAGNOSIS

- SC dislocations/subluxations
- AC joint separation/pathology
- Rib fracture
- Pneumothorax
- Rotator cuff pathology
- Thoracic outlet syndrome
- Brachial plexus injury
- Pathological fracture

CONTRIBUTING FACTORS
- Disorders compromising bone integrity, thus increasing susceptibility to fracture: osteopenia, osteoporosis
- Medications that reduce bone density such as corticosteroids
- Balance issues especially in the elderly

TREATMENT

SURGICAL OPTIONS
- Open clavicular fractures require urgent surgical consultation.
- Surgical fixation of the clavicle has generally been reserved for open fractures, associated neurovascular injuries, post-neurovascular repairs, scapulothoracic dissociations, and fractures with polytrauma.
- 90% of clavicular fractures are successfully healed without need for surgery.

- Surgery over time may be necessary if there is inadequate healing.
- Surgery often calls for implementation of a plate affixed by interosseous screws.

REHABILITATION

- Rehabilitation after clavicle fracture is started almost immediately.
- If there are no other injuries, the patient is allowed to continue working out all unaffected regions such as lower body, abdominals, or contralateral arm.
- Aerobic conditioning on an exercise bike or other low impact apparatus is advisable at first.
- The patient is allowed to immediately perform wrist and elbow ROM exercise, as well as grip strength maintenance exercises to maintain circulation and prevent clot formation.
- As the patient's symptoms improve, they can begin PROM exercises and isometric strengthening of the rotator cuff, deltoid, biceps, and triceps.
- Patient should be encouraged to resume normal daily activities and use the involved arm as much as pain allows.
- If surgery has been performed, the patient is generally limited to AROM below shoulder level for 6 to 8 weeks.

- In the absence of surgery, the patient can begin AROM as pain allows. Full ROM is attained within 4 to 6 weeks after injury.
- When the patient has full and pain-free AROM and there is good evidence of callus formation at the fracture site, the patient may begin resistive exercises.
- When the patient is pain-free and has functional ROM and normal return of strength, they can begin sports or functional retraining.
- Early symptoms may be managed through the following:
  - Modalities such as electrical stimulation and cryotherapy
  - Soft tissue techniques to the muscles of the shoulder girdle
  - Use of a sling is encouraged initially
- SC and AC joint mobilization may be required to restore normal clavicle mobility.
- Pectoralis major/minor and sternocleidomastoid stretching may be indicated.
- Cervical and thoracic screening should be completed and if warranted stretching of associated cervical and upper thoracic soft tissues may be beneficial.

PROGNOSIS

- Prognosis is excellent with proper follow-up care and treatment of complications.
- Most clavicle fractures should follow normal bone healing time frames; good callus formation and resolution of most symptoms should occur within 6 to 8 weeks.
- The majority of these patients will fully return to pre-injury functional status.

SIGNS AND SYMPTOMS INDICATING REFERRAL TO PHYSICIAN

- Sensory or motor impairment in the involved upper extremity
- Brachial plexus compression resulting from hypertrophic callus formation
- Signs of vascular interruption (1+ pulses)
- Cases of clavicular fracture with resultant subclavian artery transection, resulting in death, have been reported

SUGGESTED READINGS

Kim W, McKee MD. Management of acute clavicle fractures. *Orthop Clin North Am.* 2008;39:491-505.

AUTHOR: ROBERT S. BURNS

BASIC INFORMATION

DEFINITION

The Hill-Sachs lesion is an osteochondral lesion of the posterolateral humeral head caused by an acute anterior dislocation.

ICD-9CM CODES
715.31 Osteoarthrosis localized not specified whether primary or secondary involving the shoulder region
718.01 Articular cartilage disorder involving shoulder region
811.3   Open fracture of glenoid cavity and neck of scapula

OPTIMAL NUMBER OF VISITS

8 visits

MAXIMAL NUMBER OF VISITS

20 visits

ETIOLOGY

- A lesion occurs when the dislocated humeral head strikes the inferior margin of the glenoid, producing a "hatchet" compression fracture defect of the humeral head.
- This most commonly is the result of an anterior shoulder dislocation. The injury occurs when the head of the humerus retracts posteriorly toward the glenoid. The impaction results in the lesion.

EPIDEMIOLOGY AND DEMOGRAPHICS

- Injury occurs most frequently in males under 30 years of age and peaks again when people are in their fifties.
- 95% of first-time dislocations occur as a result of trauma.
- 98% of traumatic glenohumeral dislocations occur anteriorly.
- The prevalence of the Hill-Sachs lesion has been estimated to occur in 88% of all anterior shoulder dislocations and between 35% and 76% of all shoulder dislocations.

MECHANISM OF INJURY

- The mechanism of injury is similar to that seen in anterior dislocations. Dislocations are the result of any of the following:
  - Trauma, forced external rotation/abduction, with a posterior force at the glenohumeral joint
  - Traction onto the arm in an anterior direction
  - FOOSH, with arm abducted and externally rotated
  - Blunt trauma to the shoulder in a posterior-to-anterior direction

COMMON SIGNS AND SYMPTOMS

- Sulcus sign
- Deep ache and pain in the posterior aspect of the shoulder
- Pain with overhead motions of the arm
- Shoulder hiking with arm motions over shoulder level
- Weakness of the shoulder caused by muscle guarding and edema

AGGRAVATING ACTIVITIES

- Resisted AAROM in external rotation
- Overhead activities
- Activities that load the glenohumeral joint (e.g., isometric flexion)
- Closed-chain activities, such as push ups or pushing to get out of a chair, may or may not cause pain

EASING ACTIVITIES

- Rest
- Ice
- Avoidance of aggravating activities
- Antiinflammatories and muscle relaxants

24-HOUR SYMPTOM PATTERN

- Deep ache will be noted at night, and stiffness will be present first thing in the morning.
- Pain is activity dependent. When aggravating activities are involved, pain will increase.

PAST HISTORY FOR THE REGION

- Recent anterior dislocation
- Trauma
- History of repetitive shoulder dislocations

PHYSICAL EXAMINATION

- Posterior humeral head tender to palpation.
- Shoulder held in guarded posture.
- Humeral head may be positioned anteriorly.
- Poor scapulothoracic rhythm will be noted.
- Weakness and pain may be present with resisted shoulder abduction or external rotation.

IMPORTANT OBJECTIVE TESTS

- Apprehension test
  - Pain: Sensitivity: 0.50–0.53%; specificity: 0.56%
  - Apprehension: Sensitivity: 0.53–0.72%, specificity: 0.96–0.99%
- Relocation test
  - Pain: Sensitivity: 0.30–0.54%; specificity: 0.44–0.90%
  - Apprehension: Sensitivity: 0.67–0.81%; specificity: 0.90–0.99%
- Load-shift test
  - Load–shift (under anesthesia): Sensitivity: 100%; specificity: 83%

DIFFERENTIAL DIAGNOSIS

- Rotator cuff tear
- Fracture of greater tubercle
- Fracture of the scapula or glenoid rim
- Axillary nerve or brachioplexus injury
- Bankart lesion or other labral lesions
- Vascular injury/compression

CONTRIBUTING FACTORS

- Generalized joint laxity
- Systemic diseases that have ligament laxity: Ehlers-Danlos syndrome, rheumatoid arthritis, lupus
- Repetitive microtrauma to the shoulder in sports or daily activities:
  - Gymnasts, swimmers, and baseball players
- Weakness leads to stretching of capsule and associated ligaments

TREATMENT

SURGICAL OPTIONS

Most surgeries do not directly address the Hill-Sachs lesion directly. The surgeries are directed toward concomitant injuries such as anterior dislocations, rotator cuff tears, or labral tears. See these specific pathologies for recommended surgical interventions.

REHABILITATION

- It is important to note that undetected Hill-Sachs lesions will masquerade as rotator cuff injuries but will not improve on typical rotator cuff timelines. As a result, patient complaints will not be in typical rotator cuff patterns.
- Modalities and gentle soft tissue techniques for symptoms management can be used initially.
- As acute symptoms decrease, attention should turn toward increasing stability around the glenohumeral joint and normalizing scapulothoracic rhythm. Strengthening of rotator cuff, deltoid, pectoralis, latissimus dorsi, and scapular stabilizers should begin with this goal in mind.
- Since the majority of dislocations occur anteriorly, focus should be on strengthening the subscapularis muscle and performing exercises that will work on motor control of this muscle.
- Joint mobilization is appropriate but should be geared toward improving posterior joint mobility and allowing the humeral head to descend inferiorly.

PROGNOSIS

- May require up to 6 weeks after injury for marked subjective improvement.

Section III   ORTHOPEDIC PATHOLOGY

- Strength gains will progress slower than ROM changes.

SIGNS AND SYMPTOMS INDICATING REFERRAL TO PHYSICIAN

- Persistent complaints of pain while not progressing with conservative care
- Vascular or neural changes in the extremity

SUGGESTED READINGS

Burkhead WZ Jr, Rockwood CA Jr. Treatment of instability of the shoulder with an exercise program. *J Bone Joint Surg Am.* 1992;74:890-896.

Cicak N, Bilic R, Delimar D. Hill-Sachs lesion in recurrent shoulder dislocation: sonographic detection. *J Ultrasound Med.* 1998;17: 557-560.

Cordasco FA. Understanding multidirectional instability of the shoulder. *J Athl Train.* 2000;35(3):278-285.

Hayes K, Callanan M, Walton J, Paxinos A, Murrell GA. Shoulder instability: management and rehabilitation. *J Orthop Sports Phys Ther.* 2002;32:497-509.

Hegedus EJ, Goode A, Campbell S, et al. Physical examination tests of the shoulder: a systematic review with meta-analysis of individual tests. *Br J Sports Med.* 2008;42:80-92.

Lippitt S, Matsen F. Mechanisms of glenohumeral joint stability. *Clin Orthop Relat Res.* 1993;20-28.

AUTHOR: ROBERT S. BURNS

BASIC INFORMATION

DEFINITION

- Loss of structural osseous integrity of the humerus bone.
- Humeral fractures may occur along humeral diaphysis (shaft), surgical neck, anatomical neck, and greater or lesser tubercles.

ICD-9CM CODES
812   Fracture of humerus
812.41 Supracondylar fracture of
       humerus closed

OPTIMAL NUMBER OF VISITS

8 visits

MAXIMAL NUMBER OF VISITS

24 visits

ETIOLOGY

- Typically, humeral fractures occur as the result of direct trauma such as the following:
  - Tissue loading that exceeds the osseous tissues physiologically capacity results in tissue failure.
  - Pathological or occult fracture can occur secondary to systemic disease.
  - Infrequently, avulsion fractures may occur as a result of tractional forces.
- Fractures of the greater tuberosity can result in posterior and superior displacement as a result of the pull of the supraspinatus, infraspinatus, and teres minor. Similarly, fractures of the lesser tuberosity will displace the fragments anteriorly and medially because of the attachment of the subscapularis muscle.
- The axillary nerve is the most frequently injured portion of the brachial plexus associated with humeral fractures. Evidence of nerve injury is present on up to 45% of humeral neck fractures and dislocations. The suprascapular, radial, and musculocutaneous nerves are the next most commonly injured nerves.
- Neer has developed a four segment classification system based on the concept of four fragments. The central theory driving the classification system is the integrity of the blood supply to the humeral head. When any of the four major fragments is displaced >1 cm or angulated >45 degrees, the fracture is considered displaced.
- The Neer classification system includes four segments: I, II, III, and IV and also rates displacement and vascular isolation. The four segments are as follows:
  - Greater tuberosity
  - Lesser tuberosity
  - Humeral head
  - Shaft

EPIDEMIOLOGY AND DEMOGRAPHICS

- Proximal humeral fractures reportedly account for 4% to 5% of all fractures.
- Kannus et al reported an incidence of 40 proximal humerus fractures per 100,000 patients older than 60 years of age.
- Fractures are more likely to occur in older, osteoporotic patients with fragile bones or in the early adolescent patient who has open physes.
- Trauma accounts for most of the fractures in younger adults.
- Females are two times more likely to suffer a proximal humerus fracture, and these fractures are believed to be the result of osteoporosis.

MECHANISM OF INJURY

- FOOSH is the most common mechanism of injury.
- Falls onto the lateral shoulder, which will result in greater tuberosity fractures, are less common.
- Humeral head fractures may occur as result of dislocation (see Bankart Lesion).

COMMON SIGNS AND SYMPTOMS

- Persistent deep ache/pain in glenohumeral joint
- Pain or inability to actively move the involved arm immediately after the injury
- Guarding and protecting affected arm
- Strong and painful selective tissue tension tests for glenohumeral abduction, internal rotation, and external rotation

AGGRAVATING ACTIVITIES

- AROM as a result of muscular attachment site proximity to fracture site
- Pain with weight bearing onto the affected arm
- Pain when sleeping on affected arm
- Lifting or carry objects

EASING ACTIVITIES

- Cold packs
- Antiinflammatories, pain medications, or muscle relaxants
- Rest

24-HOUR SYMPTOM PATTERN

- Persistent ache that is present throughout the day
- Pain may increase during the night

PAST HISTORY FOR THE REGION

- Recent trauma to the shoulder
- May have a history of osteopenia or osteoporosis in the region

PHYSICAL EXAMINATION

- Swelling and tenderness will be palpable around the shoulder.
- Deformity can be seen in the presence of displaced fractures.
- Crepitus may be present if displaced fractures are present.
- Bruising is common, and discoloration will often extend past the elbow and into the lateral chest.
- AROM impairments will be present.
- Pain with muscle contraction caused by muscle guarding and swelling is present.
- Patient will guard the extremity in an adducted position.
- Patient will demonstrate positive impingement signs and will commonly be diagnosed as a rotator cuff strain.
- Pain with contraction of muscles that attach directly to the affected region is present.

IMPORTANT OBJECTIVE TESTS

- Radial and brachial pulses should be taken to rule out vascular involvement.
- Sensation testing is necessary to rule out neurological involvement, as follows:
  - The axillary nerve is the most commonly affected, therefore testing of sensation along the lateral upper arm is important.
  - Deltoid muscle strength can be tested to check motor involvement.
- Radiographic studies are needed to confirm diagnosis of humeral fracture.
- MRI or CT scan are generally not warranted but may be used to rule out concomitant soft tissue or neurovascular structures.

DIFFERENTIAL DIAGNOSIS **Dx**

- Proximal nondisplaced humeral fractures may present similarly to rotator cuff syndromes initially, but humeral fractures do not improve on typical rotator cuff timelines
- Bursitis
- Occult fracture
- Cervical radiculopathy
- Visceral referral
- Clavicular fractures
- AC separation
- Sternoclavicular separation
- Brachial plexus injury
- Axillary nerve injury

CONTRIBUTING FACTORS

- Disorders compromising osseous integrity
- Osteoporosis
- Osteopenia
- Long-term steroid use
- Cancer
- Occult fracture

TREATMENT

SURGICAL OPTIONS

- A review of the literature reveals that there is no good evidential support delineating whether surgery is superior to nonoperative treatment in the treatment of humeral fractures. There appears to be no consistent standards regarding which procedure is most effective for a specific fracture pattern.
- Most proximal humerus fractures are minimally displaced and can be treated nonoperatively.
- Open reduction and internal fixation (ORIF) are the most commonly used surgical techniques:
  - ○ Percutaneous reduction and pinning
  - ○ Plate fixation
  - ○ Kirschner wire and tension band
  - ○ Intramedullary fixation—ender nails
  - ○ Intramedullary nailing
- Humeral head replacements are utilized in severe cases.
- Closed reduction is used in most non-displaced fractures.

REHABILITATION

- Koval et al reported outcomes at an average of 41 months in 104 patients treated for one-part fractures. Results were excellent in 77% of patients, fair in 13%, and poor in 10%. The authors reported that patient age over 70 years and a delay of PROM exercises more than 14 days had detrimental effects on ROM outcome.
- A four-phase approach to rehabilitation, such as the following, should be used:
  - ○ First phase: PROM only until evidence of fracture healing is present. Most proximal humerus fractures are non-displaced or minimally displaced and can be treated with sling and early PROM exercises.
  - ○ Second phase: AROM and more aggressive stretching exercises are instituted. Early resistance exercises, both isometric and isotonic, can begin.
  - ○ Third phase: Increased focus on stretching, isotonic/isokinetic strengthening, restoring upper extremity motion quality and quantity, restoring shoulder strength, and restoring proprioception.
  - ○ Fourth phase: Return to sport and functional retraining.

PROGNOSIS

- Fracture healing in 4 to 6 weeks in absence of concomitant systemic pathology.
- Most patients with nerve injury after fracture will completely recover in 4 months.

SIGNS AND SYMPTOMS INDICATING REFERRAL TO PHYSICIAN

- Slow progress.
- Worsening pain complaints.
- Evidence of neurological or vascular compromise. The anterior humeral circumflex artery provides the main blood supply to the humeral head. Injury to this main blood supply of the humeral head with significant displacement of fracture fragments may result in avascular necrosis of the humeral head.
- Fractures involving the anatomical neck can disrupt the blood supply to the humeral head and can lead to avascular necrosis.
- Nonunions are most frequently encountered at the surgical neck and up to 23% may go on to nonunion.
- Nonunions are more frequent after ORIF.
- The most important factors in the development of avascular necrosis are fracture type, degree of displacement, and the treatment method selected. In four-part fractures, the reported incidence varies between 13% and 34%, whereas the incidence in three-part fractures is reported to range from 3% to 14%.
- Conditions that contribute to malunion or nonunion include osteoporotic bone, premature or aggressive rehabilitation, high-energy multitrauma, long head of biceps tendon interposition, and inadequate stability of operative stabilization.
- Myositis ossificans and heterotopic ossification can occur after fracture of the proximal humerus.

SUGGESTED READINGS

Dan G., Choi C-H, Cuomo F. In: DeLee JC, Drez D Jr, eds. *DeLee & Drez's Orthopaedic Sports Medicine: Principles and Practice.* 2nd ed. Philadelphia, PA: Saunders; 2003.

Drosdowech DS, Faber KJ, Athwal GS. Open reduction and internal fixation of proximal humerus fractures. *Orthop Clin North Am.* 2008;39:429-439.

Handoll HH, Gibson JN, Madhok R. Interventions for treating proximal humeral fractures in adults. *Cochrane Database Syst Rev.* 2003;(1):CD000434.

Kannus P, Palvanen M, Niemi S, et al. Osteoporotic fractures of the proximal humerus in elderly Finnish persons: sharp increase in 1970-1998 and alarming projections for the new millennium. *Acta Orthop Scand.* 2000;71(5):465-470.

Koval KJ, Blair B, Takei R, Kummer FJ, Zuckerman JD. Surgical neck fractures of the proximal humerus: a laboratory evaluation of ten fixation techniques. *J Trauma.* 1996;40(5):778-783.

Lanting B, MacDermid J, Drosdowech DS, et al. Proximal humeral fractures: a systematic review of treatment modalities. *J Shoulder Elbow Surg.* 2008;17(1):42-54.

AUTHOR: ROBERT S. BURNS

BASIC INFORMATION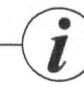

DEFINITION

Shoulder impingement syndrome is a generalized term used to describe the compression and resultant damage to soft tissue structures within the shoulder region.

SYNONYMS

- Subacromial impingement
- Subacromial compression
- Impingement syndrome

ICD-9CM CODES
840 Sprains and strains of shoulder and upper arm
840.4 Rotator cuff (capsule) sprain
840.6 Supraspinatus (muscle) (tendon) sprain
840.9 Sprain of unspecified site of shoulder and upper arm

OPTIMAL NUMBER OF VISITS

10 visits

MAXIMAL NUMBER OF VISITS

30 visits

ETIOLOGY

- Shoulder impingement can refer to several sites of entrapment. The most common site of impingement is the subacromial space. This was termed *impingement syndrome* by Neer.
- Dines et al described an impingement in the shoulder region involving the lesser tuberosity and the coracoid process. They called this occurrence *coracoid impingement syndrome*. These structures are impinged with a combined forward flexion, internal rotation, and adduction of the shoulder. Surgical examination of patients with coracoid impingement revealed fractures of the lesser tuberosity and calcification of the subscapularis tendon.
- Subacromial impingement occurs at the space between the inferior acromion and the superior humeral head, and this space is referred to as the *impingement interval*.
  - This space is narrowed during glenohumeral abduction.
- Impingement results from extrinsic compression superiorly from abnormalities of the acromion or inferiorly as the humeral head moves superiorly to entrap the tendons of the rotator cuff. The tendons most commonly entrapped are the supraspinatus and infraspinatus. The long head of the biceps can also be entrapped between the humeral head and the acromion.

- The compression to the tissue is applied perpendicular to the alignment of the fibers, thus, the tissue is not properly equipped to sustain the compressive load.
- Compressive forces cause erythremia, restrict blood flow to the tendon, and ultimately result in tissue failure.

EPIDEMIOLOGY AND DEMOGRAPHICS

- Neer stage I: Less than 25 years of age
- Neer stage II: 25 to 40 years of age
- Neer stage III: Older than 50 years of age

MECHANISM OF INJURY

- The mechanism of injury for subacromial impingement varies based on age bracket and aggravating usage. While the damage to the tissue is similar, regardless of the mechanism, the biomechanical factors that contribute to the injury are different.
- Neer has defined three stages of impingement that describe the differences in how the tendons can be injured:
- Neer stage I impingement:
  - Associated with overuse.
  - Typically occurs in patients younger than 25 years.
  - Reversing of the pathology is possible.
- Neer stage II impingement:
  - Found in patients 25 to 40 years of age.
  - Secondary to predisposing factors such as impaired scapulothoracic motion and stability.
  - Tendon changes are irreversible.
- Neer stage III impingement:
  - Generally occurs in patients over 50.
  - Frequently involves tendon rupture or tear.
  - Usually involves a process of attrition, culmination of chronic fibrosis, and tendinosis.
- Impingement syndromes can also be classified as external or internal.
- Primary external impingement:
  - Abnormalities of the superior structures result in impingement.
  - Diminished subacromial space.
  - Causes include congenital (os acromiale), osteophytes, and thickening of subacromial arch.
  - Generally occurs in patients older than 35 years of age.
- Secondary external impingement:
  - Excessive downward angulation of the acromion secondary to inadequate muscle stabilization of the scapula.
  - Anterior and inferior movement of the acromion encroaches into the subacromial space.
  - Patients are usually young, under 35 years.

  - Secondary external impingement is more prevalent in younger athletes with inadequate muscle control.
- Internal impingement:
  - Increased joint instability results in posterior impingement of the rotator cuff against the posterior and superior aspect of the glenoid labrum and the posterior humeral head.
  - The underside of the cuff rubs against the labrum, causing friction.
  - Internal impingement is commonly seen in overhead athletes such as baseball pitchers or tennis players.

COMMON SIGNS AND SYMPTOMS

- Pain
  - Anterior and lateral for external impingement.
  - Posterior for internal impingement.
- Weakness
  - Rotator cuff muscles that have been injured by the impingement.
  - Scapular control muscles, such as serratus anterior or levator scapulae, can be weak or exhibit more motor control.
- ROM impairment
  - External impingement: Pain in flexion and/or abduction.
  - Internal impingement: Increased external rotation and decreased internal rotation when range is tested at 90 degrees of abduction.
  - Coracoid impingement: Pain will be present with horizontal adduction.

AGGRAVATING ACTIVITIES

- Overhead activity
- Pain lying on either involved or uninvolved upper extremity

EASING ACTIVITIES

- Rest
- Cold packs
- Antiinflammatory medications
- Corticosteroid injections
- Avoidance of aggravating activities

24-HOUR SYMPTOM PATTERN

- Some stiffness may be present on awakening, depending of how the patient slept.
- Disturbed sleep pattern may be noted as patient rolls into aggravating positions.
- Generally, symptoms are related to usage and not to time of day.

PHYSICAL EXAMINATION

- Altered scapulohumeral rhythm
- Palpable tenderness at the involved tendons
- Weakness in the rotator cuff muscles if acute swelling or tissue damage is present

Section III

ORTHOPEDIC PATHOLOGY

- Weakness of serratus anterior
- Global muscle tightness caused by muscles that are recruited to compensate for weakened local stabilizers (i.e., upper trapezius tightness to compensate for supraspinatus injury)
- Poor scapular position may be noted
- Increased thoracic kyphosis may be present

IMPORTANT OBJECTIVE TESTS

Common Impingement Tests

Name of Test	Specificity of Tests (%)	Sensitivity of Tests (%)
Neer impingement	49-69	68-89
Hawkins-Kennedy	45-66	72-87
Cross-over	82	28
Painful arc sign	33	81
Supine impingement	9	97

- Modified Scapular Assist Test
  - Positive: Pain is reduced when scapula is assisted.
  - Good tester reliability.
  - Helps differentiate poor scapular mechanics as a contributor to the pathology.
- Park et al found that a combination of the Hawkins-Kennedy test, a painful arc sign, and the infraspinatus test or lag sign yielded the best post-test probability (95%) for any degree of impingement syndrome. Radiographic findings include the following:
  - MRI results may show degrees of inflammation and possible tearing of the tendons.
  - X-ray results may show arthritic changes in the subacromial space, along with acromial morphology.
  - Primary external: Positive.
  - Secondary external: Negative.
  - Internal: Negative.

DIFFERENTIAL DIAGNOSIS Dx

- Humeral head/neck fracture
- Subacromial spurring
- Type II and III acromions
- Thoracic outlet syndrome
- Cervical radiculopathy
- Cervical disk referral
- Visceral referral
- Lymphatic dysfunction
- Thoracic vertebral dysfunction
- Costotransverse dysfunction
- Costovertebral dysfunction

CONTRIBUTING FACTORS

- Impaired scapular stability causing secondary impingement

- Thicken subacromial bursa
- Forward shoulder posture
- Excessive anterior thoracic musculature shortness/tightness
- Structural anomalies (type II, III acromion)
- Calcific coracoacromial ligament
- AC arthritis
- Os acromiale, an unfused acromial apophysis

TREATMENT   Rx

SURGICAL OPTIONS

- Subacromial decompression is the most common technique used to address primary external impingement. The surgery involves resecting the inferior portion of the acromion to normalize its shape and increase subacromial space, which can be done open or arthroscopically. Arthroscopic decompression is the more common procedure.
- In severe cases of impingement, a Mumford procedure, which involves resection or removal of the end of the clavicle using arthroscopic techniques, may be warranted.
- Subacromial débridement may be warranted to clean out the debris within the subacromial space.

REHABILITATION

- Impingement is generally managed conservatively. If caught early enough, the subsequent sequelae of tendinopathy and tendon tears can be avoided.
- Begin by managing inflammation and pain with modalities and gentle manual techniques.
- Therapeutic exercise:
  - Begin with development of scapular stabilizers.
  - Progress from isometric, to concentric, to eccentric rotator cuff exercises.
  - Use sport-specific training.
  - Isotonic (fixed weight) exercises are preferable; free-weight resistance is recommended over band resistance.
  - Create scaled-down activities that require scapular stability and rotator cuff strength for functional rehabilitation.
- Joint mobilization:
  - Glenohumeral, AC, sternoclavicular, thoracic spine, and costotransverse joint mobilizations are appropriate.
- Range of motion:
  - Quality and quantity of shoulder ROM are equally important.
  - Attention should be on normalizing scapular motion and rhythm.

PROGNOSIS

- Stage I impingement usually respond favorably to conservative interventions.

- Stage II impingement may need surgery if predisposing factors cannot be rectified. Generally, these factors can be addressed through rehabilitation.
- Stage III impingement will respond to rehabilitation if caught early enough. If significant degeneration or significant changes in the acromion are present, surgery may be the only solution to resolve the patient's pain and restore shoulder function.

SIGNS AND SYMPTOMS INDICATING REFERRAL TO PHYSICIAN

- Nocturnal pain may indicate the presence of infection or tumor.
- Progressive weakness accompanied by arm paresthesias may indicate nerve involvement.
- Visceral structures can masquerade as impingement syndrome, so care must be taken to rule out cardiac, liver, lung, thyroid, and gall bladder pathology.

SUGGESTED READINGS

Dines DM, Warren RF, Inglis AE, Pavlov H. The coracoid impingement syndrome. *J Bone Joint Surg Br*. 1990;72(2):314-316.

Hawkins RJ, Kennedy JC. Impingement syndrome in athletes. *Am J Sports Med*. 1980;8:151-158.

Hawkins RJ, Mohtadi N. Rotator cuff problems in athletes. In: DeLee JC, Drez Jr D, eds. *Orthopaedic Sports Medicine: Principles and Practice*. Philadelphia, PA: WB Saunders; 1994.

Magee DJ. *Orthopedic Physical Assessment*. 2nd ed. Philadelphia, PA: WB Saunders; 1992.

Neer II CS. Anterior acromioplasty for the chronic impingement syndrome in the shoulder: a preliminary report. *J Bone Joint Surg Am*. 1972;54:41-50.

Park HB, Yokota A, Gill HS, El Rassi GE, McFarland EG. Diagnostic accuracy of clinical tests for the different degrees of subacromial impingement syndrome. *J Bone Joint Surg Am*. 2005;87(7):1446-1455.

Poppen NK, Walker PS. Normal and abnormal motion of the shoulder. *J Bone Joint Surg Am*. 1976;58:195-201.

Selkowitz DM, Chaney C, Stuckey SJ, Vlad G. The effects of scapular taping on the surface electromyographic signal amplitude of shoulder girdle muscles during upper extremity elevation in individuals with suspected shoulder impingement syndrome. *J Orthop Sports Phys Ther*. 2007;37(11):694-702.

AUTHOR: ROBERT S. BURNS

BASIC INFORMATION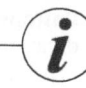

DEFINITION

A tear or disruption to the labrum of the shoulder

SYNONYMS

- Shoulder sprain/strain
- SLAP lesion
- Bankart lesion

ICD-9CM CODES
726.1 Rotator cuff syndrome of shoulder and allied disorders
726.19 Other specified disorders of bursae and tendons in shoulder region

OPTIMAL NUMBER OF VISITS

8 to 12 visits preoperative

MAXIMAL NUMBER OF VISITS

24 visits or less postoperative

ETIOLOGY

- The labrum is a fibrocartilage ring that sits on the glenoid fossa. It has the following functions:
  - Increases fit of the humeral head
  - Provides stability of the humeral head
- The long head of the biceps tendon has an attachment to the supraglenoid fossa, and in most cases, a significant portion of the tendon originates from the labrum, with a small attachment to the fossa.
- The biceps tendon also acts as a dynamic stabilizer for anterior stability of the glenohumeral joint.
- The inferior labrum is a rounded, fibrous structure, continuous with the articular cartilage. It blends in with the anterior IGHL. It provides inferior stability to the humeral head.
- Labral tears are classified as follows:
  - Superior labrum anterior to posterior (SLAP) lesions
  - Bankart lesions
  - Posterior labral lesions
- Snyder classified the SLAP lesions as follows:
  - Type I lesion: A degenerative process, common in ages 40 and older, marked by fraying of the superior labrum.
  - Type II lesion: Fraying of the superior labrum with a detached biceps anchor; majority of the lesions are type II.
  - Type III lesion: Bucket-handle tear of the superior labrum with a normal biceps tendon attachment.
  - Type IV lesion: Bucket-handle tear of the superior labrum with a tear of the biceps tendon.

- Injuries could be a combination of these lesions and can extend anteriorly, posteriorly, or inferiorly.
- Bankart lesions are tears of the anterior or inferior portion of the labrum, usually from 2 to 6 o'clock on the shoulder.
  - They are associated with anterior shoulder dislocations or subluxations.
  - They can be associated with Hill-Sachs lesions, which are bone divots in the humeral head caused by blunt trauma from the dislocation of the humeral head on the glenoid fossa.
- Posterior labral tears are associated with internal impingement of the shoulder, as described by Jobe.
  - In hypermobile shoulders, at end-range external rotation (i.e. cocking phase of throwing), the supraspinatus folds on itself and impinges between the greater tubercle and posterior superior labrum and can cause a labral tear.

EPIDEMIOLOGY AND DEMOGRAPHICS

- Younger groups are prone with repetitive overhead motions such as swimming, tennis, or throwing.
- Older groups are more prone to degenerative lesions, often associated with poor vascular supply.

MECHANISM OF INJURY

- FOOSH.
- Overhead repetitive activities such as throwing, swimming.
- Traction injuries (i.e., waterskiing, breaking fall from height, or pulling).
- Direct blow to the humerus.
- Dislocation/subluxations of the shoulder.
- Internal impingement.
- Degenerative processes.
- If the labrum is disrupted enough to get in the way of humeral head movement, this will cause pain with arm movement. Bucket-handle tear, fraying, detachment from the glenoid rim, and loose bodies from the labrum can all be sources of the shoulder symptoms.

COMMON SIGNS AND SYMPTOMS

- Aching of the shoulder region.
- Feeling of instability.
- Clicking or popping with motion.
- Catching of the shoulder with movement.
- Diffuse upper trapezius pain.
- Diffuse thoracic pain.
- If the shoulder is irritable, it may cause peripheral numbness or tingling caused by impingement of nerves through the shoulder complex. Symptoms will have a peripheral distribution, which is usually correlated with shoulder irritability.

AGGRAVATING ACTIVITIES

- Overhead activity
- Lifting objects
- Hand behind back
- Computer/desk work

EASING ACTIVITIES

- Out of aggravating position
- Activities and movements that facilitate scapular retraction
- Rest, ice, compression, and elevation (RICE)
- NSAIDs
- Shoulder adducted/internal rotated (loose packed position)

24-HOUR SYMPTOM PATTERN

- Morning pain: The shoulder may feel increased stiffness and pain, which may loosen up as the day goes on.
- Afternoon/evening pain: Pain in the injured region will typically increase as shoulder activity increases throughout the day.
- Sleeping may or may not be problematic.

PAST HISTORY FOR THE REGION

- History of secondary or internal impingement.
- History of overhead activity such as throwing.
- History of instability that includes dislocations, subluxations, and multidirectional instability.
- History of joint degeneration. Because of the degenerative and progressive nature of rotator cuff degradation, the patient will often complain of several bouts of shoulder pain over the course of several years.
- Each subsequent episode of shoulder pain is generally worse than the prior episode.
- Patient will often report latest episode as unresolved, with increasing loss of ROM.

PHYSICAL EXAMINATION

- Postural abnormalities
  - Forward shoulder
  - Protracted scapula
  - Scapular winging
  - Poor scapulohumeral rhythm with AROM
  - Sulcus sign
  - Excessive thoracic kyphosis
  - Internally rotated humerus
  - Overly developed anterior musculature with decreased tone in posterior musculature
- Palpation findings
  - Deep aching pain, general diffuse pain to palpation
  - Increased tone at upper trap
  - Increased tone/tightness at anterior shoulder
  - Increased tightness at posterior scapular muscles

- ○ Crepitus, clicking, popping with AROM/PROM
- Capsular findings
  - ○ Tight posterior capsule
  - ○ Hypermobile anterior capsule
  - ○ Multidirectional instability
  - ○ Positive sulcus
- Muscle strength findings
  - ○ Weak and/or painful with resistance of involved tendons
  - ○ Weak scapular stabilizers (lower trap, rhomboid, and serratus anterior)

IMPORTANT OBJECTIVE TESTS

- Most of the research with diagnostic orthopedic tests is inconclusive and contradictory. These tests should not be used as stand-alone findings to diagnose a labral tear, but rather, the combination of findings, a detailed history, and corroborating objective findings should be used to determine the most likely diagnosis.
- MRI results may show disruption of the labrum, but the severity and degree of tear will not be known without arthroscopic examination:
  - ○ False negatives of MRI are not uncommon.
  - ○ X-ray may reveal osteoarthritis, humeral head displacements, and Hill-Sachs lesions.

- O'Brien active compression test for superior labral integrity:
  - ○ Positive: Pain or clicking with forearm in pronation, alleviated with supination
  - ○ Reported sensitivity: 0.47 to 0.68
  - ○ Reported specificity: 0.50 to 0.55
- Compression-rotation test:
  - ○ Positive: Pain, clicking dunk
  - ○ Reported sensitivity: 0.24
  - ○ Reported specificity: 0.76
- Biceps load 2 test:
  - ○ Positive: Increased pain with elbow flexion
  - ○ Reported sensitivity: 0.90
  - ○ Reported specificity: 0.97
  - ○ A positive test would indicate a SLAP lesion
- Speed's test for biceps impingement and SLAP lesions:
  - ○ Positive: Bicipital groove pain
  - ○ Reported sensitivity: 0.18 to 0.38
  - ○ Reported specificity: 0.70 to 0.87

DIFFERENTIAL DIAGNOSIS **Dx**

- Biceps strain/rupture
- Shoulder dislocation/subluxation
- AC joint sprain
- Rotator cuff tear
- Cervical radiculopathy
- Fracture/Hill-Sachs lesion

TREATMENT

SURGICAL OPTIONS

- Surgical options for a SLAP lesion:
  - ○ Debridement of the labrum
  - ○ Anchoring of the labrum and/or the biceps attachment
- Surgical options for a Bankart lesion:
  - ○ Debridement of the labrum
  - ○ Anchoring of the labrum and/or IGHL/joint capsule
  - ○ Capsular shift

SURGERY OUTCOMES

80% to 95% of patients who received a SLAP lesion repair achieve a satisfactory result.

REHABILITATION

- Rehabilitation can be classified in two categories: preoperative/conservative treatment and postoperative treatment
- Preoperative:
  - ○ The main objective of the preoperative patient is to increase available ROM, prevent adhesive capsulitis, and strengthen surrounding muscles to prepare for possible postoperative rehabilitation. Also, the goal is to decrease irritability as much as possible.
  - ○ Once the inflammation process has decreased the focus of rehabilitation should be on increasing ROM and strength.
  - ○ Care should be taken for biceps irritation with a SLAP lesion.
  - ○ 90/90 shoulder position and inferior traction should be minimized with Bankart lesions.
- Postoperative:
  - ○ Most protocols after a SLAP lesion repair will call for no PROM into external rotation and no biceps AROM resisted for 4 weeks. The patient will be placed in a sling. The patient will receive pendulum exercises as postoperative instruction.
  - ○ Outpatient rehabilitation will start anywhere from 1 to 4 weeks postoperative, depending on the surgeon.
  - ○ Therapy will consist of PROM, AAROM, and AROM as tolerated.
  - ○ Strengthening exercises begins with isometrics and progresses as appropriate, usually after 2 to 4 weeks.
  - ○ Scapular mobilization can begin relatively early, depending on irritability. Benefits of scapular mobilization include improving scapulohumeral rhythm and decreasing upper trapezius tone and allow for proper muscle balance.

- Postoperative precautions or contraindications are as follows:
  - ○ A SLAP repair will call for no external rotation past 30 degrees and no resisted biceps for 4 weeks.
  - ○ A Bankart repair will call for no external rotation past 30 degrees for 4 weeks.
- Manual therapy:
  - ○ Using joint mobilization to manipulate humeral head posteriorly, so it is centered in the glenoid fossa will improve shoulder arthrokinematics and facilitate movement and decrease irritability.
  - ○ Care should be taken not to grind the humeral head against the glenoid fossa, irritating the labral repair.
  - ○ Using massage on the anterior soft tissue/musculature will help decrease forces into forward shoulder.
  - ○ Using massage on the upper trapezius will help alleviate pain caused by guarding and stress and the upper trap and facilitate proper shoulder arthrokinematics.
- Other factors to be considered with shoulder rehabilitation are as follows:
  - ○ Work and behavioral issues need to be addressed. The patient needs to be educated on the significance of forward shoulder and possible aggravating factors with daily activities.
  - ○ Core stability.
  - ○ Incorporate core stability exercises with elevation of shoulder, repetitive concerns, and functional tasks.

PROGNOSIS

- A shoulder with a labral tear will vary in terms of the length of rehabilitation. If the shoulder pain does not resolve in 4 weeks, the prognosis decreases significantly and surgery becomes more likely.
- 80% to 95% of patients who received a SLAP lesion repair achieve a satisfactory result.
- 82% to 98% of patients who received a Bankart repair achieve a satisfactory result.
- Outcomes will be limited by the following:
  - ○ An overly arthritic joint would limit the prognosis.
  - ○ Excessive labral damage.
  - ○ Rotator cuff lesions.
- Time frame of labral repair rehabilitation:
  - ○ 3 to 6 months: Fully functional for ADLs.
  - ○ 5 to 9 months: Fully functional for sports and overhead activities.

SIGNS AND SYMPTOMS INDICATING REFERRAL TO PHYSICIAN

- Constant unrelenting shoulder pain and pain that does not change with position can be associated with infection or tumor.

- Left chest or arm pain can be associated with cardiac pathology.
- Major trauma can be associated with a fracture.
- Shoulder not improving with conservative management may indicate the need for surgery.

SUGGESTED READINGS

Bankart ASB. The pathology and treatment of recurrent dislocation of the shoulder-joint. *Br J Surg*. 1938;26:23-29.

Hayes K, Callanan M, Walton J, Paxinos A, Murrell GAC. Shoulder instability: management and rehabilitation. *J Orthop Sports Phys Ther*. 2002;32(10):497-509.

Hegedus EJ, Goode A, Campbell S, et al. Physical examination tests of the shoulder: a systematic review with meta-analysis of individual tests. *Br J Sports Med*. 2008;42:80-92.

Itoi E, Kuechle DK, Newman SR, et al. Stabilising function of the biceps in stable and unstable shoulders. *J Bone Joint Surg Br*. 1993;75:546-550.

Jobe CM. Superior glenoid impingement. *Orthop Clin North Am*. 1997;28:137-143.

Kim SH, Ha KI, Kim SH, et al. Results of arthroscopic treatment of superior labral lesions. *J Bone Joint Surg Am*. 2002;84A:981-985.

Kim SH, Ha KL, Ahn JH, et al. Biceps load test II: a clinical test for SLAP lesions of the shoulder. *Arthroscopy*. 2001;17:160-164.

Pagnani MJ, Speer KP, Altchek DW, et al. Arthroscopic fixation of superior labral lesions using a biodegradable implant: a preliminary report. *Arthroscopy*. 1995;11:194-198.

Pal GP, Bhatt RH, Patel VS. Relationship between the tendon of the long head of biceps brachii and the glenoidal labrum in humans. *Anat Rec*. 1991;229:278-280.

Rathbun JB, Macnab I. The microvascular pattern of the rotator cuff. *J Bone Joint Surg Br*. 1970;52:540-553.

Resch H, Golser K, Thoeni H, et al. Arthroscopic repair of superior glenoid labral detachment (the SLAP lesion). *J Shoulder Elbow Surg*. 1993;2:147-155.

Samani JE, Marston SB, Buss DD. Arthroscopic stabilization of type II SLAP lesions using an absorbable tack. *Arthroscopy*. 2001;17:19-24.

Snyder SJ, Karzel RP, Del Pizzo W, et al. SLAP lesions of the shoulder. *Arthroscopy*. 1990;6:274-279.

Stetson WB, Snyder SJ, Karzel RP, et al. Long-term clinical follow-up of isolated SLAP lesions of the shoulder. Presented at the 65th annual meeting of the American Academy of Orthopaedic Surgeons, March 1998.

Yoneda M, Hirooka A, Saito S, et al. Arthroscopic stapling for detached superior glenoid labrum. *J Bone Joint Surg Br*. 1991;73:746-750.

AUTHOR: MICHAEL KO

BASIC INFORMATION

DEFINITION

- Osteoarthritis is a pathology associated with inflammation in the joints of the body. In the case of shoulder osteoarthritis, the arthritis and inflammation most commonly associated with a loss of glenoid and/or humeral head cartilage leading to shoulder pain.
- Osteoarthritis is a term derived from the Greek word "*osteo*" meaning "of the bone," "*arthro*" meaning "joint," and "*itis*" meaning "inflammation," even though the amount of inflammation present in the joint can range from excessive to little or no inflammation.

SYNONYMS

- Shoulder arthritis
- Shoulder degenerative joint disease

ICD-9CM CODES

715.11 Primary localized osteoarthrosis involving shoulder region
715.21 Osteoarthrosis localized secondary involving shoulder region

OPTIMAL NUMBER OF VISITS

3 to 6 visits

MAXIMAL NUMBER OF VISITS

20 to 36 visits

ETIOLOGY

- The wearing down of the hyaline cartilage leads to an inflammatory response. There is thickening and sclerosis of the subchondral bone and development of osteophytes or bone spurs. This leads to a narrowing of the joint space and ultimately pain.
- Daily wear and tear in combination with various injuries sustained throughout life is the most common cause of the breakdown of healthy tissue.
- Degeneration of the cartilage and the resultant arthritis can also be the result of other factors such as trauma or joint injury.
- At a cellular level, as a person ages, the number of proteoglycans in the articular cartilage decreases. Proteoglycans are hydrophilic and work within cartilage to bind water. With the reduction of proteoglycans comes a decrease in water content within the cartilage and a corresponding loss of cartilage resilience. With the decreases in cartilage resilience, collagen fibers of the cartilage become susceptible to degradation and injury. The breakdown of collagen and other cartilage tissue are released into the surrounding joint space.

Inflammation results as the body attempts to respond to the influx of byproducts from cartilage injury.
- As the cartilage degrades, the joint space narrows and ligaments become more lax. In response to the laxity, new bone outgrowths, called *spurs* or *osteophytes*, can form on the margins of the joints in an attempt to improve the congruence and passive stability of the articular cartilage surfaces.
- Primary osteoarthritis refers to joint degradation resulting from aging and tissue degeneration.
- Secondary osteoarthritis refers to joint degradation and tissue degeneration that result from factors other than aging such as obesity, trauma, and congenital disorders. Shoulder osteoarthritis can sometimes develop following lesions of the rotator cuff. It can also develop after vascular osteonecrosis.

EPIDEMIOLOGY AND DEMOGRAPHICS

- Arthritis and chronic joint symptoms affect one out of three adults, making it the most widespread disease in the United States.
- The prevalence of arthritis for all joints is higher in whites and men older than 45 years of age.
- Women older than 55 years of age, overweight and inactive persons, and persons with fewer than 8 years of education are also more likely to suffer from osteoarthritis.
- Osteoarthritis is less common in the shoulder than in weight-bearing joints.

MECHANISM OF INJURY

- Osteoarthritis is a pathology of overuse. The mechanism of injury is therefore the result of repetitive motions that stress the shoulder joint. The more cycles of an activity that the shoulder sees, the more likely the result will be anatomical damage.
- Daily use of the shoulder.
- Misalignment of the glenohumeral joint.
- Excessive use/strain of the shoulder.
- Injuries, such as fracture and strains/sprains, that cause inflammation and scar tissue in the shoulder.

COMMON SIGNS AND SYMPTOMS

- Forward humeral head, protracted scapula
- Deep, dull pain in the shoulder
- Limited ROM in the shoulder
- Cracking, deep crunching, or grinding in the shoulder
- The referral pattern for shoulder osteoarthritis is pain in the following:
  - Lateral upper arm
  - Upper trapezius region
  - Interscapular region

AGGRAVATING ACTIVITIES

- Inactivity allows the inflammation to "pool" and increase pressure, leading to discomfort and loss of available movement. Inactivity leads to stiffness.
- Reaching overhead.
- Throwing.
- Lifting.
- Reaching behind.
- Weight-bearing activities (like crawling or making a bed).

EASING ACTIVITIES

- Rest.
- Gentle motions of the shoulder joint.
- Gentle stretching and exercise.
- Use of heat.
- Massage.
- Taking antiinflammatory medication.
- Generally speaking, these activities lead to decreased wear and tear, increased joint lubrication, and loss of stiffness and inflammation associated with this condition.

24-HOUR SYMPTOM PATTERN

- Stiffness in the morning (10 to 15 minutes).
- Better after a warm shower and taking medication.
- Can worsen with excessive movement.
- Stiffens again in the evening.
- Stiffness after prolonged inactivity.

PAST HISTORY FOR THE REGION

- Jobs or recreational activities that require excessive use/strain of the shoulder (blue collar job, intense sport play, etc)
- Abnormal amount of damage due to injuries
- Poor posture or body mechanics

PHYSICAL EXAMINATION

- Forward head and shoulders (humeral head translated forward).
- Loss of shoulder ROM: All shoulder motions are generally limited to some extent, but flexion, abduction, and internal rotation are the most limited.
- Strength is generally limited by pain.
- Crepitus with movement.

IMPORTANT OBJECTIVE TESTS

- There are many special tests used in the shoulder region to aid in the differentiation process. However, none of the clinically based special tests have proven specific or reliable in diagnosing shoulder osteoarthritis.
- Radiographic testing, such as x-rays and MRIs, remains the gold standard for diagnosing shoulder osteoarthritis. The axillary view provides the best image to look for joint-space narrowing. Anteroposterior radiography, with the arm held at 45 degrees of abduction, may also show early joint-space narrowing.

DIFFERENTIAL DIAGNOSIS

- Shoulder sprain/strain
- Cervical spine radiculitis
- Thoracic outlet
- Tendonitis/impingement (biceps, rotator cuff)
- Frozen shoulder
- Cardiac pathology
- Respiratory pathology
- Liver pathology
- Fracture
- Bursitis

CONTRIBUTING FACTORS

- The shoulder is designed to handle normal daily use. When factors change the body's ability to respond to normal forces, damage occurs.
- Therefore the clinician should thoroughly interview the patient to determine which factors may contribute to the patient's symptoms.
- Factors that contribute or predispose an individual to shoulder osteoarthritis are as follows:
  - Physical strain from job or recreational activities
  - Overuse
  - Repetitive injuries to the shoulder
  - Traumatic injuries to the shoulder
  - Poor health (smoking, poor diet, and long-term use of steroids)

TREATMENT

Rx

SURGICAL OPTIONS

- Arthroscopic débridement.
- Hemiarthroplasty.
- Total shoulder replacement (arthroplasty):
  - Cemented
  - Biological fixation
- Arthroscopic débridement delays the need for a hemiarthroplasty or total shoulder replacement for younger and more active patients.
- Uncemented arthroplasty provides good pain relief and has good outcomes particularly for the younger and more active populations.

REHABILITATION

- Rehabilitation should focus on the following:
  - Education in correct use of ice/heat at home for pain abatement and edema control.
  - Implementation of a home exercise program.
  - Manual therapy (soft tissue mobilization, joint mobilization) can improve joint mobility and joint arthrokinematics and decrease pain.
  - Massage can decrease pain by relaxing muscular tension, improve circulation, and increase endorphin release.
  - Decreases muscular and joint stiffness.
  - Improves posture and joint mechanics.
  - Improves muscular support of the joint.
  - Improves functional mobility.
  - Creates a sense of control over the symptoms and the condition.
- Pathological changes to cartilage cannot be repaired by the body at this time. Even surgical advances have yet to solve the problems associated with cartilage damage. With this in mind, the focus of rehabilitation should focus on decreasing the stress placed on the damaged cartilage and correcting biomechanical and anatomical abnormalities that may predispose an individual to increased stress at the shoulder joint.
- The shoulder joint is a synovial joint. Therefore the cartilage heals and is affected by joint motion. It is aggravated by activities that excessively load the joint, but motion in a non-weight-bearing environment to a limited weight-bearing environment can greatly decrease the patient's symptoms.
- Initial exercises that promote healing include the following:
  - Stretches: Pectoralis major/minor and upper trapezius
  - Strengthening exercises (rotator cuff, middle and lower trapezius muscles, and rhomboids)
  - Postural exercises

PROGNOSIS

- Long-term prognosis for a patient with shoulder osteoarthritis depends on the extent of wear and tear and ability to reduce the joint strain placed on the joint (posture, activity, etc).
- For the most part, shoulder osteoarthritis is a degenerative condition. At earlier stages of the pathology, rehabilitation aimed at reducing the load placed on the joint can potentially slow or halt the progression of degeneration.
- For patients who are further along in the degenerative process, outcomes will be less favorable because cartilage has only a limited ability to repair itself.

SIGNS AND SYMPTOMS INDICATING REFERRAL TO PHYSICIAN

- Unrelenting pain may indicate the presence of infection or tumor.
- Unusual responses to therapy.
- Neurological signs.
- Red flag symptoms, such as excessive redness and swelling and generalized malaise and fatigue, may be signs of infection.

SUGGESTED READINGS

Dugan SA. Exercise for health and wellness at midlife and beyond: balancing benefits and risks. *Phys Med Rehabil Clin N Am*. 2007;18(3):555-575.

Krishnan SG, et al. Humeral hemarthroplasty with biologic resurfacing of the glenoid for glenohumeral arthritis. Surgical technique. *J Bone Joint Surg Am*. 2008;90(suppl 2):9-19.

Merolla G, Paladini P, Campi F, Porcellini G. Efficacy of anatomical prostheses in primary glenohumeral osteoarthritis. *Chir Organi Mov*. 2008;91(2):109-115.

National Center for Chronic Disease Prevention and Health Promotion: Division of Adult and Community Health. Arthritis: http://www.cdc.gov/arthritis/ (accessed August 2008).

Richards DP, Burkhart SS. Arthroscopic debridement and capsular release for glenohumeral osteoarthritis. *Arthroscopy*. 2007;23(9):1019-1022.

AUTHOR: SARA GRANNIS

Section III   ORTHOPEDIC PATHOLOGY

BASIC INFORMATION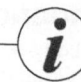

DEFINITION

- Disruption to the pectoralis major muscle fibers, usually by a sudden overload to the muscle
- The three grades of muscle strain are as follows:
  - Grade I: Local pain; mild swelling, ecchymosis, and tenderness; mild tightness or spasm locally; minimal loss of ROM and strength
  - Grade II: Similar to grade I; symptoms more pronounced
  - Grade III: Severe loss of ROM and strength, significant swelling and ecchymosis; may have a visible or palpable defect in the muscle

SYNONYMS

- Muscle pull
- Muscle tear
- Grade III: Muscle rupture

ICD-9CM CODE
840.9 Sprain of unspecified site of shoulder and upper arm

OPTIMAL NUMBER OF VISITS

- Grade I or II: 6 visits or less
- Grade III: 12 visits or less

MAXIMAL NUMBER OF VISITS

12 visits

ETIOLOGY

- The pectoralis major has two parts: the clavicular portion and the sternal portion.
- The clavicular portion has its origin at the sternal half of the clavicle; the sternal portion originates from the anterior surface of the sternum and ribs 1 to 7.
- They share a common insertion at the lesser tubercle of the humerus along the medial border of the bicipital groove.
- The clavicular portion is on greatest tension with horizontal abduction lower than 90° abduction; the sternal portion is on greatest tension with horizontal abduction greater than 90° abduction.

EPIDEMIOLOGY AND DEMOGRAPHICS

- The mechanism is usually a traumatic injury from unexpected resistance. As such, anyone who engages in activities that would put resistance on the shoulder is at risk for a pectoralis major strain.
- The most common site of muscle disruption occurs at the myotendinous junction in adults and at the tendon-to-bone attachment in the elderly and children.

MECHANISM OF INJURY

- A horizontal adduction motion with resistance; usually the resistance is sudden or heavier than expected. The following are activities that often cause pectoralis strains:
  - Pulling with one arm from an outstretched position to horizontal adduction
  - Pushing object away from chest
  - Stabilizing object that requires pectoralis recruitment (e.g., handlebars on motorcycle or steering wheel)

COMMON SIGNS AND SYMPTOMS

- Pain with horizontal adduction of the arm
- Pain with pushing things away from the chest
- Loss of strength with horizontal adduction or with push-ups
- Bruising in the chest region after initial aggravating event
- Swelling in the pectoral region

AGGRAVATING ACTIVITIES

- Overhead motion.
- Lifting (elbow curls or shoulder flexion).
- Scapular retraction.
- Prolonged side lying on affected side.
- Gripping activities.
- Deep exhalation/chest expansion.
- Any motion that requires pectoral recruitment will illicit pain. Any horizontal adduction activity will recruit pectorals (e.g., pressing off chest, pulling from arm abducted position across chest).
- Any motion that stretches the pectoralis muscle will illicit pain. Scapular retraction, chest expansion, or rib excursion can cause the pectorals to stretch. Sidelying on the affected side will cause tightness of the pectoral because of forward shoulder, and after prolonged sidelying, moving the shoulder out of forward shoulder will be painful.
- Any motion that requires stabilization of the shoulder complex will illicit pain. The pectorals are strong stabilizers of humeral movement. Gripping requires proximal stabilization. Holding a moving object in place requires proximal stabilization. The stronger the resistance, the harder the pectorals work to stabilize the entire upper extremity.

EASING ACTIVITIES

- RICE
- Physicians will often prescribe antiinflammatory medications, as well as muscle relaxants and pain medications to address the patient's symptoms
- Shoulder adducted/internal rotated (loose packed position)
- Soft tissue mobilization

24-HOUR SYMPTOM PATTERN

- Morning pain: The shoulder will feel increased stiffness and pain from inactivity of the muscle and associated inflammation causing general muscle stiffness. Also, the shoulder will likely have been in a prolonged shortened position, which would cause increased stiffness. The stiffness/pain should decrease as the shoulder warms up.
- Afternoon/evening pain: Pain in the injured region will typically increase as pectoral activity increases throughout the day.
- Sleeping may or may not be problematic.

PAST HISTORY FOR THE REGION

- The injury is usually acute, and the patient will usually not have any past history.
- There may be a history of similar injury to the same area, which would indicate a fibrotic change in the tissue.

PHYSICAL EXAMINATION

- Postural examination:
  - Patients will usually present with an internally rotated/adducted arm.
- Palpation: Point tender pain with possible palpable defect or swelling:
  - Defect is usually at the myotendinous junction for adults and at the insertion to the humerus for children or the elderly.
- ROM:
  - Pain and/or limitation with elevation and horizontal adduction.
  - Patient may also have pain with scapular retraction.
- Muscle testing: Depending on irritability and extent of injury, pain and/or loss of strength may occur with the following:
  - Horizontal adduction
  - Flexion
  - Internal rotation
  - Scapular protraction

IMPORTANT OBJECTIVE TESTS

- Shoulder ROM testing:
  - Shoulder elevation will be limited and will reproduce the patient's symptoms. Any movement that lengthens the pectoralis major may also illicit pain. The more acute the injury is, the more likely stiffness in forward shoulder will result in discomfort with lengthening. Horizontal abduction, external rotation, extension, and scapular retraction may be stiff and painful.
- Thoracic mobility:
  - A consideration that needs to be assessed later in rehabilitation is the thoracic and rib cage mobility. Since the pectoral has an attachment in close proximity to the ribs, addressing rib hypomobility may be an area to relieve pectoral tension.

DIFFERENTIAL DIAGNOSIS

- Shoulder joint sprain
- Intercostal muscle strain
- Sternocostal sprain
- Sternoclavicular joint sprain
- Rib fracture
- Subscapularis tendon strain
- Latissimus dorsi strain
- Bicipital tendonitis/tendinosis
- Left side angina

TREATMENT

SURGICAL OPTIONS

Surgery is not an option.

REHABILITATION

- The goal of rehabilitation of the patient is twofold. First, the focus should be on decreasing the patient's symptoms. Once the symptoms have diminished, the focus of the rehabilitative process will turn to increasing strength of the pectoral and shoulder girdle to return the patient to their prior level of function.
- Once the inflammation process has decreased, the focus of rehabilitation should be as follows:
  - Identifying the factors that contribute to forward shoulder. Scapular proprioceptive exercises may be indicated to minimize stiffness in the muscle.
  - Glenohumeral joint mobility, especially into the anterior posterior direction, should be assessed to minimize forward shoulder.
  - Cervical spine to scapular muscles can contribute to scapular stiffness (sternocleidomastoid, levator scapulae, or upper trapezius).
  - Rib cage mobility should be assessed. Rib cage breathing and mobilizations may help to decrease strain on the muscle.
  - Initially, exercises that promote scapular mobility and address forward shoulder should be used. Shoulder shrugs and pinches, upper trapezius and levator scapulae stretching, light pectoral stretching, and shoulder ROM can be done to tolerance.
  - Recent studies suggest that forward shoulder position puts strain on the shoulder girdle and negatively affects shoulder ROM. Joint mobilization would be used to counter this phenomenon.

CONTRIBUTING FACTORS

- Poor pectoral flexibility
- Forward shoulder/protracted scapula
- Decreased pectoral strength
- Poor rib cage excursion
- Increased thoracic kyphosis
- Weak scapular stabilizers
- General upper extremity weakness
- Poor body mechanics

PROGNOSIS

- Most patients will recover fully from a pectoral strain.
- Most patients will recover fully from a grade III pectoral strain, up to 6 to 8 weeks in time. However, depending on the severity of the injury, there may be residual stiffness and pain for an indeterminate amount of time.

SIGNS AND SYMPTOMS INDICATING REFERRAL TO PHYSICIAN

- Constant unrelenting shoulder pain can be associated with infection or tumor.
- Local pain with inhalations may indicate the presence of a rib fracture.
- History of cardiac disease.
- Angina-related pain may indicate myocardial infarction.
- Coughing up blood or inability to breathe may be associated with pneumothorax.

SUGGESTED READINGS

Bullock MP, Foster NE, Wright CC. Shoulder impingement: the effect of sitting posture on shoulder pain and range of motion. *Man Ther*. 2005;10(1):28-37.

AUTHOR: MICHAEL KO

Section III

ORTHOPEDIC PATHOLOGY

BASIC INFORMATION

DEFINITION

- A loss of muscle integrity to one of the four rotator cuff muscles.
- The most common muscle affected is the supraspinatus muscle.
- The three grades of impingement lesions and symptoms, according to Neer, are as follows:
  - Grade I: Subacromial bursitis/tendonitis: Local pain; mild swelling, ecchymosis, and tenderness; mild tightness or spasm locally; minimal loss of ROM and strength
  - Grade II: Partial rotator cuff tear: Symptoms similar to grade I; symptoms more pronounced
  - Grade III: Full thickness tear of rotator cuff: Severe loss of ROM and strength, significant swelling and ecchymosis
- Grade III tears are the focus of this section.

SYNONYM

Rotator cuff rupture

ICD-9CM CODES

726.1 Rotator cuff syndrome of shoulder and allied disorders
840.9 Sprain of unspecified site of shoulder and upper arm

OPTIMAL NUMBER OF VISITS

8 visits or less preoperative

MAXIMAL NUMBER OF VISITS

24 visits or less postoperative

ETIOLOGY

- A rotator cuff tear can be acute and traumatic or chronic and degenerative.
- Supraspinatus is the most prominent muscle and tendon in the subacromial space and therefore the most commonly injured.
- Any motion that puts strain on the rotator cuff can result in a tear. Lifting objects that are unexpectedly heavy, overhead throwing with increased velocity, or a FOOSH injury can all lead to a rotator cuff tear.
- Chronic and repetitive subacromial impingement can also lead to a rotator cuff tear. As the shoulder joint degenerates, bone spurs may develop in the subacromial area that may lead to increased impingement. Other factors, such as forward shoulder, increased thoracic spine kyphosis, weakness in the rotator cuff, and past shoulder history can all contribute to a degenerative tear in the rotator cuff.
- The primary function of the rotator cuff is to act as dynamic stabilizers. They hold the humeral head in place and counter forces caused by deltoid activation with elevation. This prevents subacromial impingement.
- The rotator cuff is comprised of the following four muscles:
  - Supraspinatus, which functions primarily as an arm abductor
  - Infraspinatus, which functions primarily as an arm external rotator
  - Teres minor, which functions primarily as an arm external rotator
  - Subscapularis, which functions primarily as an arm internal rotator
- Subscapularis has its distal attachment at the lesser tubercle; the other three muscles attach at the greater tubercle.

EPIDEMIOLOGY AND DEMOGRAPHICS

- The incidence of rotator cuff tears increases with age: 13% from ages 50 to 59 up to 51% incidence in ages greater than 80.
- The intrinsic and extrinsic factors that cause rotator cuff tears are as follows:
  - An example of an intrinsic factor is tendon blood supply. The blood supply to the rotator cuff diminishes with age and transiently with certain motions and activities. The diminished blood supply may contribute to tendon degeneration and complete tearing.
  - Extrinsic factors include acromion morphology, postural considerations, and behavioral considerations (such as repetitive stress).
- Acromial morphology
  - Grade I: Flat acromion, minimal impingement
  - Grade II: Curved acromion, moderate impingement
  - Grade III: Beaked acromion, maximal impingement
- Any age group is potentially at risk for acute, traumatic injury to the rotator cuff muscles. The risk of injury depends on activity level and baseline strength.
- Individuals 50 years of age and older are prone to degeneration of the rotator cuff.

MECHANISM OF INJURY

- The two separate mechanisms of injury are acute and degenerative.
  - An acute injury is any undue stress or strain on the tendon such as occurs with overhead throwing, FOOSH, or lifting heavy objects.
  - May be associated with other pathologies such as fractures, dislocations, and subluxations
- A degenerative injury is chronic and persistent subacromial impingement such as occurs with repetitive overhead motions (e.g., painting ceilings, construction, or overhead throwing).
  - Chronic and repetitive subacromial impingement can lead to a rotator cuff tear. As the shoulder joint degenerates, bone spurs may develop in the subacromial area that may lead to increased impingement. Other factors, such as forward shoulder, increased thoracic spine kyphosis, weakness in the rotator cuff, and past shoulder history, can all contribute to a degenerative tear in the rotator cuff.

COMMON SIGNS AND SYMPTOMS

- Lateral deltoid/arm pain.
- Point tender pain at greater tubercle.
- Diffuse upper trapezius pain.
- Diffuse thoracic/interscapular pain.
- If the shoulder is irritable, it may cause peripheral numbness or tingling from impingement of nerves through the shoulder complex. Symptoms will have a peripheral distribution and are usually correlated with shoulder irritability.

AGGRAVATING ACTIVITIES

- The supraspinatus is responsible for stabilizing the humeral head inferiorly during elevation, thus preventing subacromial impingement. Any elevation of the humerus with a compromised supraspinatus will cause impingement and pain.
- Active recruitment of a torn supraspinatus will illicit pain.
- Prolonged activities that promote forward shoulder will facilitate early subacromial impingement and cause pain when moving into elevation.
- Examples of these activities include the following:
  - Overhead activity
  - Lifting objects
  - Hand behind back
  - Computer/desk work
  - Lifting activities

EASING ACTIVITIES

- Out of aggravating position
- Activities and movements that facilitate scapular retraction
- RICE
- NSAIDs
- Shoulder adducted/internal rotated (loose packed position)

24-HOUR SYMPTOM PATTERN

- Morning pain: The shoulder may feel increased stiffness and pain, which may loosen up as the day goes on.
- Afternoon/evening pain: Pain in the injured region will typically increase as shoulder activity increases throughout the day.
- Sleeping may or may not be problematic.

PAST HISTORY FOR THE REGION

- Acute
  - Sudden onset of shoulder pain after specific activity.

○ Severe pain for first 24 to 72 hours with loss of sleep from throbbing.
○ Severe loss of ROM for first 1 to 2 weeks, improving as initial inflammation eases.
- Degenerative
  ○ Because of the degenerative and progressive nature of rotator cuff degradation, the patient will often complain of several bouts of shoulder pain over the course of several years.
  ○ Each subsequent episode of shoulder pain is generally worse than the prior episode.
  ○ Patient will often report latest episode not resolving, with increasing loss of ROM.

PHYSICAL EXAMINATION

- Patient will present with the arm close to body and internally rotated / adducted.
- Postural abnormalities may include the following:
  ○ Forward shoulder
  ○ Protracted scapula
  ○ Excessive thoracic kyphosis
  ○ Internally rotated humerus
- ROM testing:
  ○ Shoulder flexion and abduction will be significantly limited and will reproduce the patient's symptoms.
  ○ Excessive upper trapezius recruitment and scapular elevation to assist elevation may be present.
- Palpation findings:
  ○ Point tender pain at greater tubercle, acromion, and AC joint
  ○ Increased tone at upper trapezius muscle
  ○ Increased tone/tightness at anterior shoulder musculature (anterior deltoid, pectoralis major/minor)
  ○ Increased tightness at posterior scapular muscles

IMPORTANT OBJECTIVE TESTS

- Most of the research with the diagnostic orthopedic tests is inconclusive and contradictory. These tests should not be used as stand-alone finding to diagnose a rotator cuff tear, but rather, the combination of findings, a detailed history, and corroborating objective findings should be used to determine the most likely diagnosis.
- MRI is typically used to identify the tear and will determine the surgeon's desired plan of action.
- X-ray results will show arthritic changes in the subacromial space, as well as acromial morphology, but cannot be used to determine the extent of muscle damage.
- Park et al found that a combination of the drop arm test, a painful arc sign, and an infraspinatus test or lag sign yielded the best post-test probability (91%) for full thickness rotator cuff tears.

- Empty can test for supraspinatus integrity:
  ○ Positive: Pain, weakness
  ○ Reported sensitivity: 0.41 to 0.86
  ○ Reported specificity: 0.50 to 0.82
- Lift-off test for subscapularis integrity:
  ○ Positive: Inability to move hand off back and indicates subscapularis disruption
  ○ Reported sensitivity: 0.17 to 0.18
  ○ Reported specificity: 0.60 to 0.92
- Drop-arm test:
  ○ Positive: Patient unable to hold arm or lower eccentrically without pain
  ○ Sensitivity: 0.35; specificity: 0.88
  ○ A positive test would indicate a high probability of supraspinatus disruption
- Supine impingement test:
  ○ Positive: Pain
  ○ Sensitivity: 0.97; specificity: 0.09
  ○ A negative test would probably rule out a rotate cuff tear

DIFFERENTIAL DIAGNOSIS

- Biceps strain/rupture
- AC joint sprain
- Impingement syndrome
- Cervical radiculopathy
- Labral lesion
- Fracture

TREATMENT

REHABILITATION

- Conservative treatment: Approximately 50% of patients have decreased pain and improved motion and are satisfied with the outcome of nonsurgical treatment. Surgeons may recommend nonsurgical treatment for patients who are most bothered by pain, rather than weakness, because strength does not tend to improve without surgery.
- Predictors of poor outcome for nonsurgical treatment are as follows:
  ○ Long duration of symptoms (more than 6 to 12 months)
  ○ Large tears (more than 3 cm)
- Advantages of nonsurgical treatment include the following:
  ○ Patient avoids surgery and its inherent risks
  ○ Infection
  ○ Permanent stiffness
  ○ Anesthesia complications
  ○ Patient has no "down time"
- Disadvantages of nonsurgical treatment include the following:
  ○ Strength may not improve.
  ○ Tears may increase in size over time.
  ○ Patient may need to decrease or modify activity level to prevent further injury. If the patient does not improve satisfactorily with conservative treatment, a repair would be indicated.

SURGICAL OPTIONS

- Open rotator cuff repair
  ○ Full open procedure, with a 5 to 8 cm incision. Part of the deltoid is detached and the subacromial decompression and shoulder débridement are all done open.
- Mini open rotator cuff repair
  ○ The subacromial decompression and débridement are done arthroscopically; then a 3 to 5 cm incision is made and the deltoid is separated but not detached. This is a less invasive technique, which allows for minimal healing.
- Arthroscopic
  ○ The entire procedure is done arthroscopically. Currently, this is a high skill level procedure that requires a surgeon comfortable with working arthroscopically in the shoulder.
- Subacromial decompression: Shaving of the acromion in the subacromial space to allow increased space for the graft.

SURGICAL OUTCOMES

- 80% to 95% of patients achieve a satisfactory result.
- The following factors decrease the likelihood of a satisfactory result:
  ○ Poor tissue quality
  ○ Large or massive tears
  ○ Poor compliance with postoperative rehabilitation and restrictions
  ○ Patient age (older than 65 years)
  ○ Workers' compensation claims

REHABILITATION

- Rehabilitation can be classified in two categories: preoperative/conservative treatment and postoperative treatment.
- The main objective of the preoperative patient is to increase available ROM, prevent adhesive capsulitis, and strengthen surrounding muscles to prepare for possible postoperative rehabilitation. Also, the goal is to decrease irritability as much as possible.
- Once the inflammation process has decreased, the focus of rehabilitation should be increasing ROM and strength:
  ○ AAROM exercises
  ○ Scapular retraction
  ○ Joint mobilization/myofascial release
  ○ Progressive muscle strengthening
  ○ All strengthening should be pain-free
- Most postoperative protocols after a rotator cuff repair will call for no AROM for 4 weeks. The patient will be put in an immobilizer:
  ○ Rehabilitation will start anywhere from 1–4 weeks postoperative, depending on the surgeon
  ○ Therapy will consist of PROM, especially into flexion and external rotation
  ○ AAROM will be initiated from 1 to 4 weeks, depending on irritability

○ Once the patient has been removed from AROM restrictions, progressive strengthening begins with isometrics and progresses as appropriate

- Scapular mobilization can begin relatively early, depending on irritability; the benefits of scapular mobilization are as follows:
  ○ Improves scapulohumeral rhythm.
  ○ Decreases upper trapezius tone and allows for muscle balance.
- Rotator cuff repairs typically are immobilized for 4 to 6 weeks after surgery, and no AROM is allowed. The therapist must take care to not allow AROM or resisted motions into elevation to decrease the risk of a re-tear. The patient must be educated on the risks of a re-tear and how to prevent a re-tear from happening:
  ○ Because of this, the danger of adhesive capsulitis is great, and early PROM is encouraged.
  ○ The early PROM should focus on elevation and external rotation. Extension/internal rotation/hand behind the back tends to put the most strain on the graft and should be avoided in the early stages of PROM.
  ○ Joint mobilization may be used to position the humeral head posteriorly so it is centered in the glenoid fossa. This will improve shoulder arthrokinematics and facilitate movement and decrease irritability.
  ○ Using massage on the anterior soft tissue/musculature will help decrease forces into forward shoulder.
  ○ Using massage on the upper trapezius will help alleviate pain from guarding and stress and facilitate proper shoulder arthrokinematics.

PROGNOSIS

- Postsurgical prognosis
  ○ 4 to 6 weeks: Patient begins to decrease use of the shoulder immobilizer.
  ○ 10 to 16 weeks: Full functional ROM and strength for ADLs
  ○ 6 to 9 months: Fully functional with ADLs and no overhead activity
  ○ 9 to 12 months: Return to athletic activity involving arm/overhead sports

SIGNS AND SYMPTOMS INDICATING REFERRAL TO PHYSICIAN

- Postoperative
  ○ Possible re-tear of repair
  ○ Poor healing of incision
  ○ Unexpected and sudden loss of arm ROM

SUGGESTED READINGS

Bartolozzi A, Andreychik D, Ahmad S. Determinants of outcome in rotator cuff disease. *Clin Orthop Relat Res.* 1994;308:90-99.

Bigliani LU, Morrison DS, April EW. The morphology of the acromion and its relationship to rotator cuff tears. *Orthop Trans.* 1986;10:228.

Bokor DJ, Hawkins RJ, Huckell GH, Angelo RL, Schickendantz MS. Results of nonoperative management of full-thickness tears of the rotator cuff. *Clin Orthop Relat Res.* 1993;294:103-110.

Fukuda H, Hamada K, Yamanaka K. Pathology and pathogenesis of bursal-side rotator cuff tears viewed from an en bloc histologic sections. *Clin Orthop Relat Res.* 1990;254:75-80.

Hawkins RH, Dunlop R. Nonoperative treatment of rotator cuff tears. *Clin Orthop Relat Res.* 1995;321:178-188.

Hegedus EJ, Goode A, Campbell S, et al. Physical examination tests of the shoulder: a systematic review with meta-analysis of individual tests. *Br J Sports Med.* 2008;42:80-92.

Ianotti JP, Naranja J, Gartsman G. Surgical treatment of the intact cuff and repairable cuff defect: arthroscopic and open techniques, In: Norris TR, ed. *Orthopaedic Knowledge Update: Shoulder and Elbow.* Rosemont, IL: American Academy of Orthopaedic Surgeons; 1997:151-155.

Itoi E, Tabata S. Conservative treatment of rotator cuff tears. *Clin Orthop Relat Res.* 1992;275:165-173.

Neer CS. Impingement lesions. *Clin Orthop Relat Res.* 1983;173:70-77.

Rathbun JB, Macnab I. The microvascular pattern of the rotator cuff. *J Bone Joint Surg Br.* 1970;52:540-553.

Sigholm G, Styf J, Korner L, Herberts P. Pressure recordings in the subacromial bursa. *J Orthop Res.* 1988;6:123-128.

Tempelhof S, Rupp S, Seil R. Age-related prevalence of rotator cuff tears in asymptomatic shoulders. *J Shoulder Elbow Surg.* 1999;8:296-299.

AUTHOR: MICHAEL KO

BASIC INFORMATION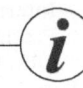

DEFINITION

- Shoulder tendonitis is an inflammation to one of the tendons in the shoulder region.
- Tendinosis is an accumulation of microtraumas that can lead to degenerative changes in the tendon. These changes include fibrosis, adhesions, and microtears that cause pain and lead to more tendon damage as the disease progresses.
- Tendinitis is usually a precursor to tendinosis, although all tendonitis need not lead to tendinosis.

SYNONYM

Shoulder sprain/strain

ICD-9CM CODES

726.1 Rotator cuff syndrome of shoulder and allied disorders
840.9 Sprain of unspecified site of shoulder and upper arm

OPTIMAL NUMBER OF VISITS

8 to 12 visits preoperative

MAXIMAL NUMBER OF VISITS

24 visits or less postoperative

ETIOLOGY

- The three grades of impingement lesions that can lead to a tendonitis or tendinosis, according to Neer, are as follows:
  - Grade I: Subacromial bursitis/tendonitis: local pain; mild swelling, ecchymosis, and tenderness; mild tightness or spasm locally; minimal loss of ROM and strength
  - Grade II: Partial rotator cuff tear; symptoms similar to grade I; symptoms more pronounced
  - Grade III: Full thickness tear of rotator cuff; severe loss of ROM and strength; significant swelling and ecchymosis
- Neer also identified the following three stages of impingement syndrome:
  - Stage 1: Benign, self-limiting overuse condition
  - Stage 2: Thickening and fibrosis of the tendon followed by repeated episodes of the first stage
  - Stage 3: Arthritic and bony changes in the subacromial space and humeral head, leading to more severe rotator cuff lesions
- Any conditions that would change the content of the tendon and make it fibrotic can potentially lead to tendinosis. A combination of overuse/repetitive injury and with decreased tendon blood supply would facilitate tendinosis.

- The blood supply to the rotator cuff diminishes with age and transiently with certain motions and activities. The diminished blood supply may contribute to tendon degeneration and complete tearing.

EPIDEMIOLOGY AND DEMOGRAPHICS

- Younger groups are prone to tendon pathology as a result of repetitive overhead motions.
  - Sports such as swimming, tennis, or baseball (throwing) can lead to tendon pathology.
- Older groups are more prone to tendon pathology because of degenerative lesions.
  - These lesions are often associated with poor vascular supply.

MECHANISM OF INJURY

- Impingement of the subacromial structures commonly leads to tendon pathology. The different types of impingement syndrome are as follows:
  - Primary impingement is described by Neer as impingement due to structural changes in the subacromial space.
  - Secondary impingement is impingement with similar presentation to the primary type but caused by instability of the shoulder. This is associated with high speed, aggressive overuse situations such as pitching a baseball. This injury usually occurs during the late cocking or early acceleration phase of throwing.
  - Internal impingement is due to contact between the posterior superior glenoid labrum and the insertion of the supra/infraspinatus at the greater tubercle and is also called *posterior superior glenoid impingement* (PGSI). PGSI is associated with extremes in abduction and external rotation. Pain is generally posterior, and the injury usually occurs during the late cocking phase of throwing. It is also associated with humeral retroversion, which is an adaptation of the shoulder into external rotation, thus decreasing relative internal rotation.
- Coracoid impingement: Anterior shoulder pain with flexion and internal rotation is related to decreased distance between the coracoid and anterior humeral structures.

COMMON SIGNS AND SYMPTOMS

- Lateral deltoid/arm pain.
- Point tender at greater tubercle pain.
- Diffuse upper trapezius pain.
- Diffuse thoracic/interscapular pain.
- Supraspinatus pain will be point tender at the greater tubercle and down the lateral deltoid.

- Biceps pain will be point tender at the bicipital groove anteriorly.
- If the shoulder is irritable, it may cause peripheral numbness or tingling from the impingement of nerves through the shoulder complex. Symptoms will have a peripheral distribution and are usually correlated with shoulder irritability.

AGGRAVATING ACTIVITIES

- The supraspinatus is responsible for stabilizing the humeral head inferiorly during elevation, thus preventing subacromial impingement. Any elevation of the humerus with a compromised supraspinatus will cause impingement and pain.
- Any activity that causes irritation of the involved tendon will illicit pain. This includes impingement and other stresses at the tendons.
- Prolonged activities that promote forward shoulder will facilitate early subacromial impingement, and cause pain when moving into elevation.
- With this in mind, the following activities may aggravate the symptoms:
  - Overhead activity
  - Lifting objects
  - Hand behind back
  - Computer/desk work

EASING ACTIVITIES

- Avoiding activities that aggravate the symptoms
- Activities and movements that facilitate scapular retraction
- RICE
- NSAIDs
- Shoulder adducted/internal rotated (loose packed position)

24-HOUR SYMPTOM PATTERN

- Morning pain: The shoulder may feel increased stiffness and pain, which may loosen up as the day goes on.
- Afternoon/evening pain: Pain in the injured region will typically increase as shoulder activity increases throughout the day.
- Sleeping may or may not be problematic.

PAST HISTORY FOR THE REGION

- Secondary or internal impingement
  - History of overhead activity such as throwing.
- Degenerative
  - Because of the degenerative and progressive nature of the subacromial space, that patient will often complain of several bouts of shoulder pain over the course of several years. Each subsequent episode of shoulder pain is generally worse than the prior episode.
  - Patient will often report latest episode not resolving, with increasing loss of ROM.

PHYSICAL EXAMINATION

- Postural findings:
  - Forward shoulder
  - Protracted scapula
  - Scapular winging
  - Poor scapulohumeral rhythm with AROM
  - Excessive thoracic kyphosis
  - Internally rotated humerus
  - Overly developed anterior musculature with decreased tone in posterior musculature
- Palpation findings:
  - Point tender pain at greater tubercle, acromion, or AC joint for supraspinatus tendon pathology
  - Tenderness at the bicipital groove anteriorly for biceps tendon pathology
  - Increased tone at upper trapezius
  - Increased tone/tightness at anterior shoulder musculature (anterior deltoid, pectoralis major/minor)
  - Increased tightness at posterior scapular muscles
  - Crepitus, clicking, popping with AROM
- Capsular findings:
  - Tight posterior capsule
  - Hypermobile anterior capsule
  - Multidirectional instability
  - Positive sulcus
- MMT findings:
  - Weak and/or painful with resistance of involved tendons
  - Weak scapular stabilizers (lower trapezius, rhomboid, or serratus anterior)

IMPORTANT OBJECTIVE TESTS

- Most of the research with the diagnostic orthopedic tests is inconclusive and contradictory. These tests should not be used as stand-alone findings to diagnose an impingement, but rather, the combination of findings, a detailed history, and corroborating objective findings should be used to determine the most likely diagnosis.
- Park et al found that a combination of the Hawkins-Kennedy test, a painful arc sign, and infraspinatus test or lag sign yielded the best post-test probability (95%) for any degree of impingement syndrome.
- Radiological findings include the following:
  - MRI results may show degrees of inflammation and possible tearing of the tendons.
  - X-ray results may show arthritic changes in the subacromial space, along with acromial morphology.

- Empty can test for supraspinatus integrity:
  - Positive: Pain, weakness
  - Reported sensitivity: 0.41 to 0.86
  - Reported specificity: 0.50 to 0.82
  - A positive test would confirm impingement
- Lift-off test for subscapularis integrity:
  - Positive: Inability to move hand off back; indicates infraspinatus disruption
  - A positive test would indicate a high probability of subscapularis disruption; a negative test would not rule it out
- Neer impingement sign:
  - Positive: Pain at subacromial space or anterior edge of acromion
  - Reported sensitivity: 0.68-0.89
  - Reported specificity: 0.49-0.69
  - This may be useful as a screen for impingement
- Hawkins-Kennedy test for impingement:
  - Positive: Pain at subacromial space
  - Reported sensitivity: 0.72-0.87
  - Reported specificity: 0.45-0.66
  - This may be useful as a screen for impingement
- Speed's test for deeps impingement and SLAP lesions:
  - Positive: Bicipital groove pain
  - Reported sensitivity: 0.33-0.38
  - Reported specificity: 0.70-0.83
- Drop arm test:
  - Positive: Patient unable to hold arm or lower eccentrically without pain
  - Sensitivity: 0.35; specificity: 0.88
  - A positive test would indicate a high probability of supraspinatas disruption
- Supine impingement test:
  - Positive: Pain
  - Sensitivity: 0.97; specificity: 0.09
  - A negative test would probably rule out a rotator cuff tear
- Modified scapular assist test:
  - Positive: Pain reduction when scapula is assisted
  - Good tester reliability
  - Helps differentiate poor scapular mechanics as a contributor to the pathology

DIFFERENTIAL DIAGNOSIS

- Biceps strain/rupture
- AC joint sprain
- Rotator cuff tear
- Cervical radiculopathy
- Labral lesion
- Fracture

CONTRIBUTING FACTORS

- Forward shoulder and increased thoracic kyphosis is a common physical finding. Forward shoulder is a descriptive term for a postural phenomenon that could include the following:
  - Anterior translation of the humeral head

- Internal rotation of the humerus
  - Protracted scapula
  - Elevated scapula
- Forward shoulder contributes to subacromial impingement for the following reasons:
  - If the humeral head is not seated in the glenoid fossa during shoulder elevation, the humeral head rides forward into the coracoid process and the subacromial arch, causing impingement and limiting maximal elevation.
  - If the humerus is internally rotated, the greater tubercle is positioned to ride into the subacromial arch, causing impingement and limiting maximal elevation.
  - If the scapula is protracted, the scapula cannot upwardly rotate soon enough or great enough to allow room for the humeral head to ride under the subacromial arch, thus disrupting normal scapulohumeral rhythm and causing impingement and limiting maximal elevation.
  - If the scapula is elevated, the scapula will tend to tip forward, causing the coracoid process to effectively ride into the humeral head, causing impingement with shoulder elevation and limiting maximal elevation.
  - Also, if the scapula is elevated, the scapula cannot depress early enough or adequately enough to facilitate normal scapulohumeral rhythm, which causes impingement and limits maximal elevation.

TREATMENT

SURGICAL OPTIONS

- Subacromial decompression
- Shaving of the acromion in the subacromial space to allow increased space for the graft
  - 80% to 95% of patients achieve a satisfactory result. Factors that decrease the likelihood of a satisfactory result are as follows:
    - Poor tissue quality
    - Large or massive tears
    - Poor compliance with postoperative rehabilitation and restrictions
    - Patient age (older than 65 years)
    - Workers' compensation claims

REHABILITATION

- Rehabilitation should be focused on decreasing subacromial impingement. This will include reducing the factors that facilitate forward shoulder, increasing stability of the humeral head, and facilitating proper scapulohumeral rhythm. The first priority should be to decrease irritability/inflammation.

- Exercises or tissue changes to help decrease forward shoulder include the following:
  - Increase anterior shoulder mobility
  - Pectoralis minor and major myofascial release
  - Posterior capsule mobility
  - Anterior-posterior glenohumeral joint mobilization
  - Pectoral stretch
  - Scapular retraction
  - Lower trapezius, rhomboid
  - Thoracic spine extension exercises
- Exercises or tissue changes to help increase humeral head stability include the following:
  - Pectoralis minor release: A tight pectoralis minor will cause the humeral head to stay anterior
  - Scapular release: A tight scapula on the thorax will increase mobility demands at the humeral head
  - Rotator cuff strengthening
  - Scapular stabilizing
  - Proprioceptive neuromuscular facilitation (PNF): Scapulothoracic and glenohumeral
- All of the above exercises can be used alone or in combination to improve scapulohumeral rhythm.
- Work and behavioral issues need to be addressed. The patient needs to be educated on the significance of forward shoulder and possible aggravating factors with daily activities.
- Incorporate core stability exercises with elevation of shoulder, repetitive concerns, and functional tasks.

PROGNOSIS

- Expected prognosis of a postoperative subacromial decompression:
  - 6 to 10 weeks: Should be fully functional.
  - An overly arthritic joint would limit the prognosis.
- Expected prognosis of a conservative nonsurgical shoulder rehabilitation:
  - A shoulder with good rehabilitation potential should resolve in 3 to 8 weeks, although depends on the amount of tissue changes needed to restore movement.
  - A more arthritic shoulder, or one with a partial rotator cuff tear, may not have full rehabilitation potential. A shoulder that does not reach full function at 8 weeks may have a poor rehabilitation potential.

SIGNS AND SYMPTOMS INDICATING REFERRAL TO PHYSICIAN

- Constant unrelenting shoulder pain and pain that does not change with position can be associated with infection or tumor
- Left chest or arm pain can be associated with cardiac pathology
- Major trauma can be associated with a fracture
- Nocturnal pain may be associated with a tumor
- Fevers and chills may indicate the presence of infection or tumor

SUGGESTED READINGS

Bigliani LU, Morrison DS, April EW. The morphology of the acromion and its relationship to rotator cuff tears. *Orthop Trans*, 1986;10:228.

Davidson PA, Elattrache NS, Jobe CM, Jobe FW. Rotator cuff and posterior-superior glenoid labrum injury associated with increased glenohumeral motion: a new site of impingement. *J Shoulder Elbow Surg*. 1995;4:384-390.

Fukuda H, Hamada K, Yamanaka K. Pathology and pathogenesis of bursal-side rotator cuff tears viewed from an en bloc histologic sections. *Clin Orthop Relat Res*. 1990;254:75-80.

Glousman R, Jobe F, Tibone J, Moynes D, Antonelli D, Perry J. Dynamic electromyographic analysis of the throwing shoulder with glenohumeral instability. *J Bone Joint Surg Am*. 1988;70:220-226.

Hawkins RH, Dunlop R. Non-operative treatment of rotator cuff tears. *Clin Orthop Relat Res*. 1995;321:178-188.

Hegedus EJ, Goode A, Campbell S, et al. Physical examination tests of the shoulder: a systematic review with meta-analysis of individual tests. *Br J Sports Med*. 2008;42:80-92.

Ianotti JP, Naranja J, Gartsman G. Surgical treatment of the intact cuff and repairable cuff defect: arthroscopic and open techniques. In: Norris TR, ed. *Orthopaedic Knowledge Update: Shoulder and Elbow*. Rosemont, IL: American Academy of Orthopaedic Surgeons; 1997:151-155.

Jobe CM, Coen MJ, Screnar P. Evaluation of impingement syndromes in the overhead-throwing athlete. *J Athl Train*. 2000;35(3):293-299.

Jobe CM. Superior glenoid impingement. *Orthop Clin North Am*. 1997;28:137-143.

Neer CS. Impingement lesions. *Clin Orthop Relat Res*. 1983;173;70-77.

Rabin A, Irrgang JJ, Fitzgerald GK, Eubanks A. The intertester reliability of the scapular assistance test. *J Orthop Sports Phys Ther*. 2006;36(9):653-660.

Rathbun JB, Macnab I. The microvascular pattern of the rotator cuff. *J Bone Joint Surg Br*. 1970;52:540-553.

Sigholm G, Styf J, Korner L, Herberts P. Pressure recordings in the subacromial bursa. *J Orthop Res*. 1988;6:123-128.

AUTHOR: MICHAEL KO

BASIC INFORMATION

DEFINITION

- A dislocation is a disarticulation of the humeral head out of the glenoid fossa that does not reduce spontaneously.
- A subluxation is a partial dislocation or a dislocation that immediately reduces spontaneously.

SYNONYM

Shoulder sprain/strain

ICD-9CM CODES

831.00 Closed dislocation of shoulder unspecified site
840.9 Sprain of unspecified site of shoulder and upper arm

OPTIMAL NUMBER OF VISITS

8 to 12 visits preoperative

MAXIMAL NUMBER OF VISITS

24 visits or less postoperative

ETIOLOGY

- The anterior glenohumeral ligament (AGHL) is the primary anterior stabilizer and prevents anterior movement of the humeral head.
- The AGHL is a thickening of the joint capsule that is composed of the following three parts:
  - The superior glenohumeral ligament primarily limits anterior and inferior translation with the humerus adducted.
  - The middle glenohumeral ligament limits anterior and inferior translation below 90 degrees of abduction.
  - The inferior glenohumeral ligament limits anterior, posterior, and inferior translation with the humerus abducted greater than 45 degrees.
- The labrum also contributes to stabilization of the shoulder.
  - The labrum can prevent translation of the glenohumeral joint by 20%.
- The primary function of the rotator cuff, along with the biceps tendon, is to act as dynamic stabilizers of the humeral head.
- The scapular stabilizers work to provide scapular control in upward rotation in sync with humeral elevation.
- Proper glenohumeral articulation is important to allow the dynamic and static stabilizers maximal stabilizing ability.

EPIDEMIOLOGY AND DEMOGRAPHICS

- 95% first-time dislocations occur from trauma.
- 98% of traumatic glenohumeral dislocations occur anteriorly.
- Most dislocations occur in those ages 11 to 30 years and those over 50 years.
- FOOSH is the major source of dislocations and subluxations in patients over the age of 60.
- It is hypothesized that the adolescent group tends to have poor techniques and adequate strength with sports.
- There is also speculation that the collagen makeup in adolescents makes them more susceptible to recurrent dislocations.
- 70% of redislocations occur within 2 years of the initial injury.
- Patients younger than 20 years of age have a recurrence rate of 90%.

MECHANISM OF INJURY

- Anterior dislocations and subluxations:
  - Trauma, forced external rotation/abduction, with a posterior force at the glenohumeral joint.
  - Traction onto the arm in an anterior direction.
  - FOOSH with arm abducted and externally rotated.
  - Blunt trauma to the shoulder in a posterior-to-anterior direction.
- Posterior dislocations and subluxations:
  - FOOSH with arm flexed, adducted, and internally rotated.
  - Blunt trauma to the shoulder in an anterior-to-posterior direction.
- Complicating factors commonly associated with a dislocation/subluxation:
  - Hill-Sachs lesion compression fractures and bony defects to the posterior humeral head caused by the humeral head impacting into the glenoid during anterior dislocations.
  - Fractures of the anterior glenoid rim can also occur with anterior shoulder dislocations.
  - Bankart lesions are lesions of the IGHL, inferior glenoid, and inferior labrum and can occur with shoulder dislocations.
  - Any of the peripheral nerves arising from the brachial plexus can be compromised. Damage can range from minor numbness or tingling to complete palsy of the nerve. The axillary nerve is especially susceptible.
  - Vascular damage can be caused by a shoulder dislocation. The brachial artery may be injured as it runs through the shoulder complex. Loss of vascular supply threatens the limb and must be identified immediately. Absence of the distal pulses will indicate a vascular compromise.

COMMON SIGNS AND SYMPTOMS

- With shoulder subluxations, a patient will commonly complain of generalized shoulder pain after traumatic injury to the shoulder or arm.
- With shoulder dislocations, a patient will complain of intense shoulder pain that is debilitating. Patient will not be able to move the arm and will have difficulty functioning because of the pain in the shoulder.
- Neural injury is not uncommon after a dislocation or subluxation. There can be sensory loss, numbness or tingling, weakness, or complete palsy, with a peripheral nerve distribution.

AGGRAVATING ACTIVITIES

- Acute dislocation:
  - Any movement
- Reduced dislocation or subluxation:
  - Shoulder abducted and externally rotated for anterior dislocations or flexed, adducted, and internally rotated with posterior dislocations
  - Overhead activity
  - Lifting objects
  - Hand behind back

EASING ACTIVITIES

- Out of aggravating position
- RICE
- Physicians will often prescribe antiinflammatory medications, muscle relaxants, and pain medications to address the patient's symptoms

24-HOUR SYMPTOM PATTERN

- Morning pain: The shoulder may feel increased stiffness and pain, which may loosen up as the day goes on.
- Afternoon/evening pain: Pain in the injured region will typically increase as shoulder activity increases throughout the day.
- Sleeping may or may not be problematic.

PAST HISTORY FOR THE REGION

- Acute dislocation/subluxation:
  - History of trauma with a fall, sports injury, or sudden jerk of the shoulder
- Chronic dislocation/subluxation.
- History of two or more episodes of dislocation/subluxation. Each subsequent episode of dislocation/subluxation is generally easier to provoke than the prior episode.
- Persistent popping, clicking, or clunking with or without pain.
- Subjective feelings of instability, dislocations, and apprehension.

PHYSICAL EXAMINATION

- Radiological findings:
  - MRI results could show labral tears and rotator cuff tears.
  - X-rays can show acute fractures and Hill-Sachs lesions.
  - X-ray results may show arthritic changes in the subacromial space and if there is chronic instability.

- Postural or observational findings:
  - For an acute dislocation, the patient will not be able to move the arm; it will feel locked, and any movement will be extremely painful.
  - The arm may be slightly abducted (anterior) or adducted (posterior), depending on the direction of the dislocation.
  - There might be an indentation in the deltoid patch, indicating humeral head deformity.
  - There may also be protrusions anteriorly or posteriorly, depending on direction of dislocation.
- For a dislocation that has been reduced, or a subluxation:
  - Generalized hypermobility.
  - Patients will present with arm held in internal rotation and adduction.
  - Anterior shoulder will lose its rounded appearance.
  - Loss of ROM and strength.
  - Patient will not be able to externally rotate their arm.
  - Poor scapular stability and dyskinesia with AROM.
  - Poor tone scapular stabilizers.
- Palpation findings:
  - Anterior shoulder pain
  - Increased tone at upper trapezius muscle
  - Increased tone/tightness at anterior shoulder musculature (anterior deltoid, pectoralis major/minor)
  - Increased tightness at posterior scapular muscles
  - Crepitus, clicking, popping with AROM
- Capsular findings:
  - Hypermobile joint capsule
  - Multidirectional instability
  - Positive sulcus
- Muscle strength findings:
  - Weak and/or painful with resistance of the shoulder muscles
  - Weak scapular stabilizers (lower trapezius, rhomboid, or serratus anterior)

IMPORTANT OBJECTIVE TESTS

- Most of the research with the diagnostic orthopedic tests is inconclusive and contradictory. The research points toward using the tests to check for apprehension and are less specific when testing for pain. These tests should not be used as stand-alone findings to diagnose a dislocation/subluxation, but rather, the combination of findings, a detailed history, and corroborating objective findings should be used to determine the most likely diagnosis.
- Anterior Drawer Test for anterior capsule laxity:
  - Pain: Sensitivity: 0.28; specificity: 0.71
  - Apprehension: Sensitivity: 0.53; specificity: 0.85
  - This is a good tool for a skilled practitioner to use for diagnosing anterior capsule laxity for apprehension.

- Apprehension/relocation test for anterior instability:
  - Positive: Increased external rotation with humeral head stabilized to pain and apprehension
  - Apprehension test: Pain: Sensitivity: 0.50 to 0.53; specificity: 0.56; and apprehension: Sensitivity: 0.53 to 0.72; specificity: 0.96 to 0.99
  - Relocation test: Pain: Sensitivity: 0.30 to 0.54; specificity: 0.44 to 0.90; and apprehension: Sensitivity: 0.67 to 0.81; specificity: 0.90 to 0.99
  - This is a good tool for diagnosing anterior capsule laxity for apprehension.

DIFFERENTIAL DIAGNOSIS

- Biceps strain/rupture
- AC joint sprain
- Rotator cuff tear
- Cervical radiculopathy
- Labral lesion
- Fracture/Hill-Sachs lesion

TREATMENT

SURGICAL OPTIONS

Bankart Repair
- Reattachment of the inferior labrum, along with an capsular tightening
- Redislocation rates after repair are as follows: Open: 11%; arthroscopic: 2% to 18%

Anterior Capsular Shift
- Open procedure involves overlaying the anterior capsule on itself, decreasing the amount of redundant capsule, and thus increasing stability of the shoulder.
- Over 75% of patients that receive a form of capsular shift have reported a satisfactory result, which would include the following:
  - No recurrence of dislocation
  - Decreased pain
  - Increased ROM

Thermal Capsulorrhaphy
- Arthroscopic procedure that involves thermally shrinking the anterior capsule.
- Long-term studies have yet to be performed and analyzed, but the initial reports are satisfactory.

REHABILITATION

- The ultimate goal of rehabilitation is to reduce the chance of redislocation or subluxation.
  - 70% of glenohumeral dislocation recur within 2 years of the initial injury.
- Rehabilitation should primarily focus on restoring ROM while taking care to not stress the joint capsule. Because of the capsular injury, manual techniques

and exercise should try to minimize capsular stretching.
- Efforts should also be focused on strengthening the shoulder muscles around the capsule, as well as the scapular stabilizers, allowing proper scapulohumeral rhythm to occur. This will minimize undue stresses at the glenohumeral joint with elevation.
- Tissue changes to help decrease humeral head displacement such as the following:
  - Pectoralis minor release: A tight pectoralis minor will cause the humeral head to stay anterior.
  - Scapular release: A tight scapula on the thorax will increase mobility demands at the humeral head.
- Exercises:
  - Rotator cuff strengthening exercises
  - Scapular stabilizer strengthening exercises
  - Proprioceptive neuromuscular facilitation: Scapulothoracic and glenohumeral
  - Closed-chain exercises to facilitate scapular stabilization
  - High level agility exercises that are specific to function and/or sport
- Other factors to be considered with shoulder rehabilitation are as follows:
  - Postural education/body mechanics: Work and behavioral issues need to be addressed; patient needs to be educated on the significance of forward shoulder and possible aggravating factors with daily activities.
  - Incorporate core stability exercises with elevation of shoulder, repetitive concerns, and functional tasks.

PROGNOSIS

- Expected time frame of a labral repair rehabilitation:
  - 3 to 6 months: Fully functional for ADLs
  - 5 to 9 months: Fully functional for sports or overhead activities
- 82% to 98% of patients who received a Bankart repair achieve a satisfactory result, which would include the following:
  - No recurrence of dislocation
  - Decreased pain
  - Increased ROM
- Factors limiting postsurgical recovery include the following:
  - An overly arthritic joint would limit the prognosis
  - Excessive labral damage
  - Rotator cuff lesions

Conservative Nonsurgical Shoulder Rehabilitation
- 4–6 weeks: functional ROM and strength
- The likelihood of a re-dislocation depends on the number of episodes, patient compliance with exercises, and patient compliance with risky activities.

SIGNS AND SYMPTOMS INDICATING REFERRAL TO PHYSICIAN

- Constant unrelenting shoulder pain and pain that does not change with position can be associated with infection or tumor.
- Left chest or arm pain can be associated with cardiac pathology.
- Major trauma can be associated with a fracture.

SUGGESTED READINGS

Bowen MK, Warren RF. Ligamentous control of shoulder stability based on selective cutting and static translation experiments. *Clin Sports Med.* 1991;10:757-782.

Burkhead WZ Jr, Rockwood CA Jr. Treatment of instability of the shoulder with an exercise program. *J Bone Joint Surg Am.* 1992;74: 890-896.

Cordasco FA. Understanding multidirectional instability of the shoulder. *J Athl Train.* 2000;35(3):278-285.

Goss TP. Anterior glenohumeral instability. *Orthopedics.* 1988;11:87-94.

Hawkins RJ, Bell RH, Hawkins RH, Koppert GJ. Anterior dislocation of the shoulder in the older patient. *Clin Orthop Relat Res.* 1986; 206:192-195.

Hayes K, Callanan M, Walton J, Paxinos A, Murrell GA. Shoulder instability: management and rehabilitation. *J Orthop Sports Phys Ther.* 2002;32:497-509.

Hegedus EJ, Goode A, Campbell S, et al. Physical examination tests of the shoulder: a systematic review with meta-analysis of individual tests. *Br J Sports Med.* 2008;42:80-92.

Hovelius L, Eriksson K, Fredin H, et al. Recurrences after initial dislocation of the shoulder. Results of a prospective study of treatment. *J Bone Joint Surg Am.* 1983;65: 343-349.

Lippitt S, Matsen F. Mechanisms of glenohumeral joint stability. *Clin Orthop Relat Res.* 1993;291:20-28.

Rowe CR. Prognosis in dislocations of the shoulder. *J Bone Joint Surg Am.* 1956;38A:957-977.

Walton J, Paxinos A, Tzannes A, Callanan M, Hayes K, Murrell GA. The unstable shoulder in the adolescent athlete. *Am J Sports Med.* 2002;30:758-767.

AUTHOR: MICHAEL KO

BASIC INFORMATION

DEFINITION

- Laxity of the shoulder joint capsule results in the humeral head having difficulty maintaining its articulation within the glenoid.
- A shoulder can be unstable in one direction (unidirectional instability) or in multiple directions (multidirectional instability).

SYNONYM

Shoulder sprain/strain

ICD-9CM CODES
831.00 Closed dislocation of shoulder unspecified site
840.9 Sprain of unspecified site of shoulder and upper arm

OPTIMAL NUMBER OF VISITS

8 to 12 visits preoperative

MAXIMAL NUMBER OF VISITS

24 visits or less postoperative

ETIOLOGY

- The anterior glenohumeral ligament (AGHL) is the primary anterior stabilizer of the glenohumeral joint.
- The AGHL is a thickening of the joint capsule and is composed of 3 parts:
  - The superior glenohumeral ligament primarily limits anterior and inferior translation with the humerus adducted.
  - The middle glenohumeral ligament limits anterior and inferior translation below 90 degrees abduction.
  - The inferior glenohumeral ligament limits anterior, posterior, and inferior translation with the humerus abducted greater than 45 degrees.
- The labrum also contributes to stabilization of the shoulder.
  - The labrum can prevent translation of the glenohumeral joint by 20%.
- The primary function of the rotator cuff and the biceps tendon is to act as dynamic stabilizers. They hold the humeral head in place and provide a counter forces to deltoid activation when the arm is elevated.
- Proper glenohumeral articulation is important to allow the dynamic and static stabilizers maximal stabilizing ability.

EPIDEMIOLOGY AND DEMOGRAPHICS

- Overhead sport athletes (i.e., swimmers and volleyball or baseball players) and patients with a history of dislocations/subluxations are the patient populations most likely to present with shoulder instability.
- Most dislocations occur ages 11-30 and over 50.
- The younger adolescent group is more likely to have shoulder instability because they are more active and tend to have poor technique and adequate strength with sports.
- There is also speculation that the collagen makeup in adolescents make them more susceptible to recurrent dislocations.
- The older group (over 60 years of age) is more likely to have shoulder instability because they are at higher risk for falls.

MECHANISM OF INJURY

- Shoulder instability can develop as the result of trauma. Usually, trauma will result in unidirectional instability. Laxity in most cases is felt in the anterior aspect of the joint. The typical unidirectionally unstable shoulder usually occurs after a shoulder dislocation or shoulder subluxation.
- Shoulder instability that is multidirectional may be the result of a genetic predisposition toward joint laxity. Generally, laxity is experienced in both shoulders, as well as other joints in the body.
- Co-morbidities associated with shoulder instability include the following:
  - Labral tears
  - Glenohumeral osteoarthritis
  - Subacromial bone spurs
  - Tendonitis/tendinosis
  - Shoulder impingement syndrome
  - Neurovascular compromise

COMMON SIGNS AND SYMPTOMS

- Generalized shoulder pain that can radiate down into the deltoid region of the shoulder.
- Patient will commonly complain of weakness in the shoulder and may complain of clicking or grinding with shoulder motion.
- Neural irritation is not uncommon in conjunction with shoulder instability. There can be sensory loss, numbness or tingling, weakness, or complete palsy, within a peripheral nerve distribution.

AGGRAVATING ACTIVITIES

- Apprehension position (arm abduction/extension rotation: 90/90):
  - The 90/90 position puts the glenohumeral joint and the anterior joint capsule on tension, giving the patient the feeling that the joint will disarticulate. This is more specific for an anterior dislocation/subluxation.
- Overhead activity
- Lifting objects
- Hand behind back
- Sidelying for a prolonged period of time

EASING ACTIVITIES

- Avoidance of aggravating positions
- RICE
- Physicians will often prescribe antiinflammatory medications, muscle relaxants, and pain medications to address the patient's symptoms

24-HOUR SYMPTOM PATTERN

- Morning pain: The shoulder may feel increased stiffness and pain, which may loosen up as the day goes on.
- Afternoon/evening pain: Pain in the injured region will typically increase as shoulder activity increases throughout the day.
- Sleeping may or may not be problematic.

PAST HISTORY FOR THE REGION

- History of two or more episodes of dislocation/subluxation
- Each subsequent episode of dislocation/subluxation is generally easier to provoke than the prior episode
- Persistent popping, clicking, or clunking with or without pain
- Subjective feelings of instability, dislocations, and apprehension

PHYSICAL EXAMINATION

- Postural or observational signs:
  - Generalized hypermobility
  - Loss of ROM and strength
  - Poor scapular stability and dyskinesia with AROM
  - Poor tone in scapular stabilizers
  - Forward shoulder, protracted scapulae
  - Winged scapula
  - Decreased thoracic spine mobility
- Palpation findings:
  - Increased tone at upper trapezius
  - Increased tone/tightness at anterior shoulder musculature (anterior deltoid, pectoralis major/minor)
  - Increased tightness at posterior scapular muscles
  - Crepitus, clicking, or popping with AROM
- Capsular findings:
  - Hypermobile joint capsule
  - Multidirectional instability
  - Positive sulcus
- Strength testing:
  - Weak and/or painful with resistance of the shoulder muscles
  - Weak scapular stabilizers (lower trapezius, rhomboid, and serratus anterior)

IMPORTANT OBJECTIVE TESTS

- Most of the research with the diagnostic orthopedic tests is inconclusive and contradictory. The research points toward using the tests to check for apprehension and are less specific when testing for pain. These tests should not be used as stand-alone findings to diagnose an unstable shoulder, but rather, the

combination of findings, a detailed history, and corroborating objective findings should be used to determine the most likely diagnosis.
- Radiological findings associated with unstable shoulders are as follows:
  ○ MRI results could show labral tears and rotator cuff tears. These pathologies are often associated with shoulder instability.
  ○ X-ray results may show arthritic changes in the subacromial space, as well as displacement of the humeral head.

- Anterior drawer test for anterior capsule laxity:
  ○ Pain: Sensitivity: 0.28; specificity: 0.71
  ○ Apprehension: Sensitivity: 0.53; specificity: 0.85
  ○ This is a good tool for a skilled practitioner to use for diagnosing anterior capsule laxity for apprehension.
- Apprehension/relocation test for anterior instability:
  ○ Positive: Increased external rotation with humeral head stablized to pain and apprehension
- Apprehension test:
  ○ Pain: Sensitivity: 0.50 to 0.53; specificity: 0.56
  ○ Apprehension: Sensitivity: 0.53 to 72; specificity: 0.96 to 0.99
- Relocation test:
  ○ Pain: Sensitivity: 0.30 to 0.54; specificity: 0.44 to 0.90
  ○ Apprehension: Sensitivity: 0.67 to 0.81; specificity: 0.90 to 0.99
  ○ This is a good tool for diagnosing anterior capsule laxity for apprehension.

DIFFERENTIAL DIAGNOSIS

- Biceps strain/rupture
- AC joint sprain
- Rotator cuff tear
- Cervical radiculopathy
- Labral lesion
- Hill-Sachs lesion/fracture

TREATMENT

SURGICAL OPTIONS

- Bankart repair
  ○ Reattachment of the inferior labrum and a capsular tightening
  ○ Redislocation rates: Open: 11%; arthroscopic: 2% to 18%
- Anterior capsular shift
  ○ Open procedure involves overlaying the anterior capsule on itself, decreasing the amount of redundant capsule, and thus increasing the stability of the shoulder.
  ○ Over 75% of patients that receive a form of capsular shift have reported

satisfactory results, which would include no recurrence of dislocation, decreased pain, and increased ROM.
- Thermal capsulorrhaphy
  ○ Arthroscopic procedure that involves thermally shrinking the anterior capsule.
  ○ Long-term studies have yet to be performed and analyzed, but the initial reports are satisfactory.

REHABILITATION

- The ultimate goal of rehabilitation is to reduce the chance of redislocation or subluxation.
- 75% to 93% of patients have been shown to have a satisfactory outcome (no redislocation) after conservative treatment.
- 70% of glenohumeral dislocations recur within 2 years of the initial injury.
- Rehabilitation should primarily be focused on restoring ROM while taking care to not stress the joint capsule. Manual techniques and exercise should minimize capsular stretching into the mechanism of injury.
- Efforts should also be focused on strengthening the dynamic, as well as scapular, stabilizers to allow proper scapulohumeral rhythm to occur. This will minimize undue stresses at the glenohumeral joint with elevation.
- Tissue changes that help decrease humeral head displacement include the following:
  ○ Pectoralis minor release: A tight pectoralis minor will cause the humeral head to stay anterior.
  ○ Scapular release: A tight scapula on the thorax will increase mobility demands at the humeral head.
- Exercises:
  ○ Rotator cuff strengthening
  ○ Closed-chain exercises to facilitate scapular stabilization and allow the humerus to stay in the glenoid
- Exercises to help facilitate scapulohumeral rhythm include the following:
  ○ Scapular stabilizer strengthening
  ○ PNF focusing on scapulothoracic rhythm
- Other factors that should be considered with shoulder rehabilitation are as follows:
  ○ Postural education/body mechanics
  ○ Core stability

PROGNOSIS

- Expected time frame of conservative treatment:
  ○ 3 to 6 weeks: Pain-free ROM
  ○ 4 to 8 weeks: Fully functional for ADLs
  ○ 6 to 10 weeks: Fully functional for sports, with modification to minimize chance of dislocation
- The likelihood of a redislocation depends on the following:
  ○ The number of episodes

- Patient compliance with exercises
- Patient compliance with risky activities
- Expected time frame of a stabilization surgery is as follows:
  ○ 4 to 6 weeks: Limited external rotation, abduction, and flexion to 90 degrees
  ○ 8 to 12 weeks: Fully functional ROM
  ○ 4 to 6 months: Return to athletic activity
- Factors that negatively impact the prognosis are as follows:
  ○ An overly arthritic joint would limit the prognosis
  ○ Excessive labral damage
  ○ Rotator cuff lesions

SIGNS AND SYMPTOMS INDICATING REFERRAL TO PHYSICIAN

- Left chest or arm pain can be associated with cardiac pathology.
- Major trauma can be associated with a fracture.
- Fevers and chills can be associated with infection or tumor.
- Shoulder not improving may indicate the need for surgery.
- Redislocation may indicate the need for surgery.

SUGGESTED READINGS

Bowen MK, Warren RF. Ligamentous control of shoulder stability based on selective cutting and static translation experiments. *Clin Sports Med.* 1991;10:757–782.

Burkhead WZ Jr, Rockwood CA Jr. Treatment of instability of the shoulder with an exercise program. *J Bone Joint Surg Am.* 1992;74:890–896.

Cordasco FA. Understanding multidirectional instability of the shoulder. *J Athl Train.* 2000;35(3):278–285.

Goss TP. Anterior glenohumeral instability. *Orthopedics.* 1988;11:87–94.

Hawkins RJ, Bell RH, Hawkins RH, Koppert GJ. Anterior dislocation of the shoulder in the older patient. *Clin Orthop Relat Res.* 1986;206:192–195.

Hayes K, Callanan M, Walton J, Paxinos A, Murrell GA. Shoulder instability: management and rehabilitation. *J Orthop Sports Phys Ther.* 2002;32:497–509.

Hegedus EJ, Goode A, Campbell S, et al. Physical examination tests of the shoulder: a systematic review with meta-analysis of individual tests. *Br J Sports Med.* 2008;42:80–92.

Hovelius L, Eriksson K, Fredin H, et al. Recurrences after initial dislocation of the shoulder. Results of a prospective study of treatment. *J Bone Joint Surg Am.* 1983;65:343–349.

Lippitt S, Matsen F. Mechanisms of glenohumeral joint stability. *Clin Orthop Relat Res.* 1993;291:20–28.

Rowe CR. Prognosis in dislocations of the shoulder. *J Bone Joint Surg Am.* 1956;38A:957–977.

Walton J, Paxinos A, Tzannes A, Callanan M, Hayes K, Murrell GA. The unstable shoulder in the adolescent athlete. *Am J Sports Med.* 2002;30:758–767.

AUTHOR: MICHAEL KO

BASIC INFORMATION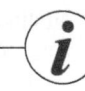

DEFINITION

Bursitis is an inflammation of the bursa sac. Subacromial bursitis refers to inflammation of the bursa that is situated in the subacromial space.

SYNONYM

Shoulder sprain/strain

ICD-9CM CODES
726.1 Rotator cuff syndrome of shoulder and allied disorders
727.3 Other bursitis disorders
840.9 Sprain of unspecified site of shoulder and upper arm

OPTIMAL NUMBER OF VISITS

6 to 8 visits

MAXIMAL NUMBER OF VISITS

12 to 16 visits

ETIOLOGY

- The following three grades of impingement lesions can lead to a bursitis, according to Neer:
  - Grade I: Subacromial bursitis/tendonitis: local pain; mild swelling, ecchymosis, and tenderness; mild tightness or spasm locally; minimal loss of ROM and strength
  - Grade II: Partial rotator cuff tear: symptoms similar to grade I; symptoms more pronounced
  - Grade III: Full thickness tear of rotator cuff: severe loss of ROM and strength; significant swelling and ecchymosis
- The subacromial bursa is the bursa involved with shoulder impingement. The bursa sits on the supraspinatus tendon and distal muscle belly beneath the acromion and deltoid. It can also extend anteriorly beneath the coracoid process.
- The primary function of the subacromial bursa is to facilitate humeral head movement under the subacromial arch.

EPIDEMIOLOGY AND DEMOGRAPHICS

- Younger groups are prone to tendon pathology as a result of repetitive overhead motions.
  - Sports, such as swimming or tennis, or throwing can lead to tendon pathology.
- Older groups are more prone to tendon pathology because of degenerative lesions that are often associated with poor vascular supply.

MECHANISM OF INJURY

- Impingement of the subacromial structures commonly leads to bursitis. The different types of impingement syndrome are as follows:
  - Primary impingement is described by Neer as impingement caused by structural changes in the subacromial space.
  - Secondary impingement is impingement with similar presentation to the primary type but caused by instability of the shoulder. This is associated with high speed, aggressive, overuse situations such as pitching a baseball. This injury usually occurs during the late cocking or early acceleration phase of throwing.
  - Internal impingement is due to contact between the posterior superior glenoid labrum and the insertion of the supra/infraspinatus at the greater tubercle and is also called *posterior superior glenoid impingement* (PGSI). PGSI is associated with extremes in abduction and external rotation. Pain is generally posterior, and the injury usually occurs during the late cocking phase of throwing. It is also associated with humeral retroversion, which is an adaptation of the shoulder into external rotation, thus decreasing relative internal rotation.
- Coracoid impingement: Anterior shoulder pain with flexion and internal rotation is related to decreased distance between the coracoid and anterior humeral structures.

COMMON SIGNS AND SYMPTOMS

- Lateral deltoid/arm pain.
- Point tender at greater tubercle pain.
- Diffuse upper trapezius pain.
- Diffuse thoracic/interscapular pain.
- Anteromedial pain
- If the shoulder is irritable, it may cause peripheral numbness or tingling caused by impingement of nerves through the shoulder complex. Spasm of the pectoralis minor may occur as irritability increases. Symptoms may occur in the fingers, hand, or forearm and may be intermittent and correlated with shoulder irritability.

AGGRAVATING ACTIVITIES

- The subacromial bursa is responsible for facilitating humeral head movement underneath the subacromial arch. If overhead activity is causing subacromial impingement, an inflamed bursa would illicit pain from the impingement. Activities include the following:
  - Overhead activity
  - Lifting objects
  - Hand behind back
  - Computer/desk work

- Prolonged activities that promote forward shoulder will facilitate early subacromial impingement and cause pain when moving into elevation.

EASING ACTIVITIES

- Avoidance of aggravating positions
- Activities and movements that facilitate scapular retraction
- RICE
- NSAIDs
- Shoulder adducted/internal rotated (loose packed position)
- Soft tissue mobilization

24-HOUR SYMPTOM PATTERN

- Morning pain: The shoulder may feel increased stiffness and pain, which may loosen up as the day goes on.
- Afternoon/evening pain: Pain in the injured region will typically increase as shoulder activity increases throughout the day.
- Sleeping may or may not be problematic.

PAST HISTORY FOR THE REGION

- Secondary or internal impingement:
  - History of overhead activity such as throwing.
- Degenerative:
  - Because of the degenerative and progressive nature of the subacromial space, that patient will often complain of several bouts of shoulder pain over the course of several years. Each subsequent episode of shoulder pain is generally worse than the prior episode.
  - Patient will often report latest episode not resolving, with increasing loss of ROM.

PHYSICAL EXAMINATION

- Postural findings:
  - Forward shoulder, protracted scapula, scapular winging, excessive thoracic kyphosis, and internally rotated humerus
  - Poor scapulohumeral rhythm with AROM
  - Overly developed anterior musculature with decreased tone in posterior musculature
- Palpation findings:
  - Point tender pain at greater tubercle, acromion, AC joint
  - Increased tone at upper trapezius and anterior shoulder musculature (anterior deltoid, pectoralis major/minor)
  - Increased tightness at posterior scapular muscles
  - Crepitus, clicking, or popping with AROM
- Capsular findings:
  - Tight posterior capsule and hypermobile anterior capsule
  - Multidirectional instability
  - Positive sulcus

- MMT findings:
  - Weak and/or painful with resistance of involved tendons
  - Weak scapular stabilizers (lower trapezius, rhomboid, and serratus anterior)

IMPORTANT OBJECTIVE TESTS

- MRI results may show degrees of inflammation and possible tearing of the tendons.
- X-ray results will show arthritic changes in the subacromial space, with acromial morphology.
- Most of the research regarding the diagnostic orthopedic tests is inconclusive and contradictory. These tests should not be used as stand-alone findings to diagnose a bursitis, but rather, the combination of findings, a detailed history, and corroborating objective findings should be used to determine the most likely diagnosis.
- In an isolated bursitis, resisted tests will be negative, while PROM tests will be positive.

- Empty can test for supraspinatus integrity:
  - Positive: Pain, weakness
  - Reported sensitivity: 0.41 to 0.86
  - Reported specificity: 0.50 to 0.82
  - A positive test would serve to confirm impingement.
- Neer impingement sign:
  - Positive: Pain at subacromial space or anterior edge of acromion
  - Reported sensitivity: 0.68 to 0.89
  - Reported specificity: 0.49 to 0.69
  - This may be useful as a screen, but has poor diagnostic value after meta-analysis was performed.
- Hawkins-Kennedy test for impingement:
  - Positive: Pain at subacromial space
  - Reported sensitivity: 0.72 to 0.87
  - Reported specificity: 0.45 to 0.66
  - This may be useful as a screen but has poor diagnostic value after meta-analysis was performed.
- Speed's test for biceps impingement and SLAP lesions:
  - Positive: bicipital groove pain
  - Reported sensitivity: 0.33 to 0.38
  - Reported specificity: 0.70 to 0.83
  - This is a poor diagnostic tool for biceps impingement or SLAP lesions.
- Supine impingement test:
  - Positive: Pain
  - Sensitivity: 0.97
  - Specificity: 0.09
  - A negative test would probably rule out a rotator cuff tear.

DIFFERENTIAL DIAGNOSIS

- Biceps strain/rupture
- AC joint sprain
- Rotator cuff tear
- Cervical radiculopathy
- Labral lesion
- Fracture

CONTRIBUTING FACTORS

- Forward shoulder is not necessarily slouching. It is possible to see a forward humeral head with decreased thoracic spine kyphosis or a flat spine. However, forward shoulder and increased thoracic kyphosis is a common physical finding.
- If the humeral head is not seated in the glenoid fossa, as seen in forward shoulder, during shoulder elevation, the humeral head rides forward into the coracoid process and the subacromial arch, causing impingement and limiting maximal elevation.
- If the humerus is internally rotated, the greater tubercle is positioned to ride into the subacromial arch, causing impingement and limiting maximal elevation.
- If the scapula is protracted, the scapula cannot upwardly rotate soon enough or great enough to allow room for the humeral head to ride under the subacromial arch, thus disrupting normal scapulohumeral rhythm and causing impingement and limiting maximal elevation.
- If the scapula is elevated, the scapula will tend to tip forward, causing the coracoid process to effectively ride into the humeral head, causing impingement with shoulder elevation and limiting maximal elevation.
- Also, if the scapula is elevated, the scapula cannot depress early enough or adequately enough to facilitate normal scapulohumeral rhythm, which causes impingement and limits maximal elevation.

TREATMENT

SURGICAL OPTIONS

- Subacromial decompression
- 80% to 95% of patients achieve a satisfactory result, which would include the following:
  - Decreased pain
  - Increased ROM
  - Increased ADLs/work
  - Return to recreational activity
- Factors that decrease the likelihood of satisfactory postsurgical results are as follows:
  - Poor tissue quality
  - Large or massive tears
  - Poor compliance with postoperative rehabilitation and restrictions
  - Patient age (older than 65 years)
  - Workers' compensation claims

REHABILITATION

- Rehabilitation should be focused on decreasing subacromial impingement and will include reducing the factors that facilitate forward shoulder, increasing stability of the humeral head, and

facilitating proper scapulohumeral rhythm. The first priority should be to decrease irritability/inflammation.
- Exercises or tissue changes to help decrease forward shoulder include the following:
  - Increase anterior shoulder mobility
  - Pectoralis minor and major myofascial release
  - Posterior capsule mobility
  - Anterior-posterior glenohumeral joint mobilization
  - Pectoral stretch
  - Scapular retraction
  - Lower trapezius, rhomboid
  - Thoracic spine extension exercises
- Exercises or tissue changes to help increase humeral head stability include the following:
  - Pectoralis minor release: A tight pectoralis minor will cause the humeral head to stay anterior
  - Scapular release: A tight scapula on the thorax will increase mobility demands at the humeral head
  - Rotator cuff strengthening
  - Scapular stabilizing
  - PNF: Scapulothoracic and glenohumeral
- All of these exercises can be used alone or in combination to improve scapulohumeral rhythm.
- Work and behavioral issues need to be addressed. The patient needs to be educated on the significance of forward shoulder and possible aggravating factors with daily activities.
- Incorporate core stability exercises with elevation of shoulder, repetitive concerns, and functional tasks.

PROGNOSIS

- Postoperative subacromial decompression surgery
  - 6 to 10 weeks: Fully functional.
  - An overly arthritic joint would limit the prognosis.
- Conservative nonsurgical shoulder rehabilitation
  - A shoulder with good rehabilitation potential should resolve in 3 to 8 weeks, depending on the amount of tissue changes needed to restore movement.
  - A more arthritic shoulder, or one with a partial rotator cuff tear, may not have full rehabilitation potential. A shoulder that does not reach full function at 8 weeks may have a poor rehabilitation potential (if goal is full function, ROM, and strength).

SIGNS AND SYMPTOMS INDICATING REFERRAL TO PHYSICIAN

- Constant unrelenting shoulder pain and pain that does not change with position can be associated with infection or tumor.

- Left chest or arm pain can be associated with cardiac pathology.
- Major trauma can be associated with a fracture.

SUGGESTED READINGS

Bigliani LU, Morrison DS, April EW. The morphology of the acromion and its relationship to rotator cuff tears. *Orthop Trans*. 1986;10:228.

Davidson PA, Elattrache NS, Jobe CM, Jobe FW. Rotator cuff and posterior-superior glenoid labrum injury associated with increased glenohumeral motion: a new site of impingement. *J Shoulder Elbow Surg*. 1995; 4:384-390.

Fukuda H, Hamada K, Yamanaka K. Pathology and pathogenesis of bursal-side rotator cuff tears viewed from an en bloc histologic sections. *Clin Orthop Relat Res*. 1990;254:75-80.

Glousman R, Jobe F, Tibone J, Moynes D, Antonelli D, Perry J. Dynamic electromyographic analysis of the throwing shoulder with glenohumeral instability. *J Bone Joint Surg Am*. 1988;70:220-226.

Hawkins RH, Dunlop R. Non-operative treatment of rotator cuff tears. *Clin Orthop Relat Res*. 1995;321:178-188.

Hegedus EJ, Goode A, Campbell S, et al. Physical examination tests of the shoulder: a systematic review with meta-analysis of individual tests. *Br J Sports Med*. 2008;42:80-92.

Ianotti JP, Naranja J, Gartsman G. Surgical treatment of the intact cuff and repairable cuff defect: arthroscopic and open techniques, In: Norris TR, ed. *Orthopaedic Knowledge Update: Shoulder and Elbow*. Rosemont, IL: American Academy of Orthopaedic Surgeons; 1997:151-155.

Jobe CM, Coen MJ, Screnar P. Evaluation of impingement syndromes in the overhead-throwing athlete. *J Athl Train*. 2000; 35(3):293-299.

Jobe CM. Superior glenoid impingement. *Orthop Clin North Am*. 1997;28:137-143.

Neer CS. Impingement lesions. *Clin Orthop Relat Res*. 1983;173:70-77.

Rathbun JB, Macnab I. The microvascular pattern of the rotator cuff. *J Bone Joint Surg Br*. 1970;52:540-553.

Sigholm G, Styf J, Korner L, Herberts P. Pressure recordings in the subacromial bursa. *J Orthop Res*. 1988;6:123-128.

Stallenberg B, Destate N, Feipel V, Gevenois PA. Involvement of the anterior portion of the subacromial-subdeltoid bursa in the painful shoulder. *AJR Am J Roentgenol*. 2006;187:894-900.

AUTHOR: MICHAEL KO

Section III

ORTHOPEDIC PATHOLOGY

BASIC INFORMATION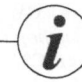

DEFINITION

Cubital tunnel syndrome is a form of mononeuropathy caused by entrapment, compression, stretch, ischemia, infection, or inflammation of the ulnar nerve in the cubital tunnel or surrounding tissues.

SYNONYMS

- Tardy ulnar palsy
- Ulnar neuritis
- Compression of ulnar nerve
- Ulnar neuropathy

ICD-9CM CODE
354.2 Lesion of ulnar nerve

OPTIMAL NUMBER OF VISITS

6 visits

MAXIMAL NUMBER OF VISITS

12 visits

ETIOLOGY

- The ulnar nerve injury in the cubital tunnel can occur with direct traumatic injury, repetitive stretching and stress to the nerve, or prolonged or repetitive compression.
- The injury that the nerve and the surrounding tissues sustain results in the progression of an inflammatory process. The result of the inflammatory process is tissue and neural ischemia with pain, paresthesia, and possibly strength and sensation changes and deficits. This ischemia and edema provide an ideal environment for increased fibroblast proliferation and fibrosis.
- Fibrosis to the nerve and/or its sheath decreases its extensibility and elasticity compromising the nerves overall mobility.
- Injury to a nerve is classified into three stages (I to III) based on the severity of the injury and the possibility of recovery.
  - Stage I: Neuropraxia is a distortion to the myelin sheath of the nerve producing a loss in conductivity.
  - Stage II: Axonotmesis is an interruption of the axon that initiates wallerian degeneration and repair.
  - Stage III: Neurotmesis is a complete disruption of the neuron and its supporting structures.
- As the damage to the nerve in each stage progresses, the length of time for recovery progresses and the possibility of recovery decreases.

EPIDEMIOLOGY AND DEMOGRAPHICS

- Cubital tunnel syndrome is the second most common nerve compression injury in the upper extremity, second only to carpal tunnel syndrome.
- Historically, the incidence of cubital tunnel syndrome is more commonly seen in men than women between the ages of 13 and 20 years.
- This is secondary to the males increased participation in repetitive and high velocity throwing activities. These activities have a high reported incidence compared to other sports-related activity.
- However, an increased incidence of ulnar neuritis in the workplace is on the rise in occupations of repetitive and prolonged compressive forces to the elbow. This type of neuritis is not age determined but is correlated to activity and time.

MECHANISM OF INJURY

- Several different mechanisms of injury have been identified for cubital tunnel syndrome. It can be caused by trauma, prolonged compressive or stretching forces, secondary trauma, or joint disfigurement or dysfunction.
- Joint disfigurement is secondary to osteophyte formation or changes in bony composition from previous fracture or trauma.
- Prolonged compressive or stretching forces are seen in patients with a history of sleeping in a position of prolonged flexion of the elbow, occupational positions with prolonged flexion of the elbow, or students/workers who spend a prolonged time working at a computer or desk leaning on the elbows or the proximal forearm.

COMMON SIGNS AND SYMPTOMS

- Initially the patient complains of pain, point tenderness, and swelling to the medial aspect of the elbow.
- This progresses to the patient describing a numb, tingling, and cold feeling to the medial distal third of the forearm and the little and ring fingers.
- This numbness progresses, and the individual with habitual inclination of sleeping with full flexion of the elbows will often complain of waking up at night with numbness and tingling to this area or an increase in symptoms during work or aggravating activity.
- As the patient's symptoms worsen, the signs and symptoms can progress to atrophy throughout the ulnar nerve distribution. More significantly, the patient will have difficulty gripping and will experience clumsiness, with complaints of frequently dropping of objects secondary to hand weakness.

AGGRAVATING ACTIVITIES

- The patient will complain of increased symptoms during activities that compress, stretch, or overload the cubital tunnel area.
- These activities can be sport specific, such as high-velocity pitching situation, or they can be positional.
- Positional activities that increase symptoms include resting elbows on a table or a surface for eating, reading, or resting.
- Sleeping can also be an aggravating activity in which the patient will report sleeping with elbows in a fully flexed position.

EASING ACTIVITIES

Patients will often report easing of symptoms with changing of position or cessation of aggravating activity, such as sleeping in a position with an arm in an outstretched position, or discontinuation of resting elbows on a table.

24-HOUR SYMPTOM PATTERN

- The 24-hour pattern varies according to the aggravating factors for the symptoms.
- For those patients with nighttime-aggravated cubital tunnel syndrome, initially the patient will be symptom-free during the daylight hours with increased numbness/tingling at night and difficulty sleeping.
- For patients with compressive issues, the patient will have symptoms associated with the compression activity with lingering of symptoms after stopping the activity.
- The amount of time the symptoms linger is directly proportional to the time duration and the intensity of the compressive force.
- Osteophytic compression will cause patients to have intermittent symptoms throughout the day depending on activity and position of the elbow.
- Patients with activity-related cubital tunnel symptoms will have increased symptoms while performing the activity and decreased symptoms once the activity is completed or stopped.
- Patients with long-term onset and progressive worsening of untreated cubital tunnel syndrome will generally complain of continuous symptoms of paresthesias and intermittent episodes of clumsiness and dropping objects.

PAST HISTORY FOR THE REGION

- Patients with cubital tunnel syndrome commonly have a past history of trauma or a space-occupying lesion that compresses on the ulnar nerve. However, the trauma can also be the result of prolonged positions or repetitive overuse from occupational and recreational hazards.
- It is common to find a history of recent fracture, dislocation, or traumatic

incident with injury to the nerve in the cubital tunnel space.

- Other considerations include systemic diseases and space-occupying lesions such as rheumatoid arthritis (RA), gout, ganglions, lipomas, osteophytes, hematoma, and anomalous muscles.

PHYSICAL EXAMINATION

- Observation
  - ○ The patient's forearm and hand of the affected limb should be compared to the forearm and hand of the unaffected limb.
  - ○ The therapist will note atrophic changes to the forearm and the hypothenar eminence, as well as hair growth, skin coloration, signs of deformity, or skin changes, such as dryness. Patients with significant progression of cubital tunnel syndrome will have significant changes to the upper extremity with atrophy of the hypothenar eminence, clumsiness, and hand weakness.
  - ○ The normal carrying angle at the elbow is 11 degrees for men and 13 degrees for women. This angle is measured by drawing a line through the length of the humerus and a line through the length of the forearm. It is not uncommon to see an increased angle, or valgus deformity, in throwing athletes secondary to adaptive changes or secondary to genetic abnormality. However, this increase in valgus deformity may lengthen the course of the ulnar nerve increasing its susceptibility to traction and injury.
  - ○ Wartenberg's sign: The patient will have an inability to hold the fifth digit into adduction against the fourth digit.
- Palpation
  - ○ Direct palpation and increases in numbness and tingling should be documented.
  - ○ Tenderness to the area of the nerve should be documented.
  - ○ Palpate during active flexion and extension of the elbow and for possible subluxation out of the cubital tunnel.
  - ○ Palpate for masses or deformities in the cubital tunnel and proximal and distal to the tunnel.
- Sensory testing
  - ○ Note the distribution and extent of the injury. Special attention should be given to the dorsal cutaneous branch of the ulnar nerve. This nerve branches proximal to the Guyon canal in the wrist and therefore is indicative of a forearm lesion when its distribution has decreased sensation.
- Range of motion (ROM) and manual muscle testing (MMT)
  - ○ Measurements to the elbow and wrist for ROM and strength should be documented.
  - ○ Quantifying grip strength is a useful tool as an objective measurement of documentation.
  - ○ The strength of the dorsal interossei and the abductor digit minimi muscles can indicate nerve damage. The dorsal interossei muscles are tested with the patient first spreading the fingers of both hands. Then the patient is asked to push the index fingers together, side to side with resistance. The examiner will note weakness that exists in the first dorsal interossei when one index finger overpowers the other.
  - ○ The abductor digiti minimi is tested in a similar fashion. The examiner has the patient turn the hands over and apply the same pressure through the little fingers side to side while wide spread. Weakness in which one finger overpowers the other indicates a positive test.
  - ○ Froment's sign: The examiner has the patient hold a piece of paper in a pincher grip between the thumb and index finger. The patient attempts to hold onto the paper as the examiner pulls away. A positive sign is a posture to the thumb with metacarpophalangeal (MCP) extension and distal interphalangeal (DIP) flexion to attempt to hold onto the paper.

IMPORTANT OBJECTIVE TESTS

- Elbow flexion test
  - ○ The patient is sitting, and the examiner directs the patient to fully flex the elbow and extend the wrist. The upper extremity is held in this position for up to 3 minutes. A positive test is indicated with the return of patient's symptoms. Buehler and Thayer found this test to have high reliability and validity for reproducing symptoms of cubital tunnel syndrome.
- Tinel's test
  - ○ Tinel's test is performed with the patient in sitting, the upper extremity at 90 degrees of elbow flexion, external rotation, and slight abduction of the shoulder. The examiner applies a percussive tap with his or her middle finger. A positive test is a reproduction of symptoms at the ulnar nerve distribution.
- Neural provocation testing
  - ○ The patient is taken into a series of movements to stretch the ulnar nerve so changes can be detected in neural mobility and the elasticity of a nerve. This testing is performed with the patient supine and taken into a progressive stretch to the nerve. The progression is shoulder depression, wrist extension, forearm pronation, elbow flexion, shoulder external rotation, and finally shoulder abduction. Symptom assessment is compared to the contralateral extremity to determine positive findings.

- Diagnostic testing ordered by the physician includes nerve conduction testing, x-rays for bony deformities, computed tomography (CT), magnetic resonance imaging (MRI), and ultrasonography for soft tissue encroachment or swelling.

DIFFERENTIAL DIAGNOSIS

- Cervical spine dysfunction
- Medial epicondylitis
- Brachial plexus injury
- Thoracic outlet syndrome
- Tumors
- Fractures
- Diabetic neuropathy
- RA
- Muscular dystrophy

CONTRIBUTING FACTORS

- The overall lifestyle of the patient contributes to this injury.
- A patient's occupation with prolonged flexion and repetitive motion in flexion can predispose the patient to changes in the cubital tunnel or surrounding tissue that increase the compression on the nerve.
- A patient's participation in sports activities can aggravate the ulnar aspect of the upper extremity.
  - ○ A pitcher with prolonged repetitive high intensity throwing has increased stress to the ulnar aspect of the elbow. This type of activity can damage, stretch, or compress the ulnar nerve or change the composition of the tissues surrounding the nerve, predisposing it to injury.
- Other contributing lifestyle factors can include sleeping patterns with the arms fully flexed and current position in life such as being a student with prolonged hours studying and compression through elbows using the computer.

TREATMENT

SURGICAL OPTIONS

- Epicondylectomy and transposition of the ulnar nerve are the surgical options for cubital tunnel syndrome, and the patient and physician should discuss these options.
- Transposition of the ulnar nerve is achieved through one of three methods: submuscular, subcutaneous, and intramuscular.
- Secondary to the scarring associated with the surgeries, the recommended

surgical approach is the epicondylec- tomy, which has excellent results.

- However, if transposition is desired, the approach with the greatest results and fewest complications from scarring is the subcutaneous method.
- The placement of the nerve during the intramuscular transpositions tends to have increased scar tissue formation and therefore is the less desirable of the three methods.

REHABILITATION

- Conservative rehabilitation for cubital tunnel syndrome is directed at symptoms.
- Initial rehabilitation should focus on decompression of the site of the ulnar nerve.
- Patients should change their lifestyles to decrease compression on the ulnar nerve such as the discontinuation of sleeping with elbows flexed or leaning onto elbows while studying or working on the computer.
- Initially, rest and protection to the area is the most important treatment. Night splints or rolled-up towels at the elbow may be used to ensure the patient does not flex the elbow(s) at night during sleep.
- Educating the patient about his or her symptoms and diagnosis, providing reassurance to the patient, and encour- aging compliance to physical therapy are important in the initial stages.
- During the initial time of rest, passive ROM (PROM), active assistive ROM (AAROM), and active ROM (AROM), neural flossing, and manual treatment is important to progress patients gently.
- Modalities can be used to decrease pain and swelling. Ice can be used for edema; however, care must be taken not to damage the ulnar nerve with increased ischemia and distal paresthesias during its use.
- Strengthening can be initiated as symp- toms subside; however, the therapist must pay special attention to symptom aggravation and onset of paresthesias during the patient's exercise regime. Return of paresthesias and feeling of weakness and clumsiness indicate nerve irritation and activity should be immedi- ately discontinued.
- The program should be advanced as tolerated with modification based on symptoms.
- For throwing athletes, complete ces- sation of symptoms before initiating a throwing program must be achieved. If symptoms return after initiation of the throwing program, the program must be regressed until the patient is again ready to return to the throwing program.
- Postsurgical rehabilitation programs vary according to the surgery performed.

Submuscular Transposition
- Weeks 1 to 2
  - Modalities to reduce pain and swell- ing and protection of the joint and the flexor pronator origin can begin.
- Week 2
  - ROM techniques can begin with AAROM, PROM, and progress as toler- ated to AROM.
- Weeks 2 to 8
  - AROM and against gravity strengthening.
  - Isometric strengthening.
  - Light lifting.
- Weeks 8 to 10
  - Aggressive strengthening can occur in this stage secondary to tendon-to- tendon healing.
- For throwing athletes, a throwing pro- gram cannot be initiated until the strength to the flexor-pronator group has returned and pain is resolved.
- Return to sport is approximately 6 months.

Subcutaneous Transposition
- Recovery and rehabilitation can be more aggressive.
- Days 7 to 10
  - ROM activities begin.
- Weeks 3 to 4
  - Strengthening to the upper extremity and particularly the flexor-pronator group can begin and progressed as tolerated.
- Week 8
  - An interval throwing program can be initiated.
- Weeks 12 to 16
  - Return to competition can occur.

Intramuscular Transposition
- With the intramuscular approach, the patient is immobilized and splinted for 3 weeks in a flexed and fully pronated position.
- After the 3-week immobilization
  - ROM can begin, and the patient pro- gressed through AROM and progres- sive strengthening.
  - Medial epicondylectomy seems to be the preferred approach with respect to early mobilization and decreased surgical complications.
  - No postoperative immobilization is required for this technique.
  - The patient has a soft dressing and is placed in a sling and allowed to per- form early active motion.
- Initial treatment started at weeks 1 to 2 with PROM, AAROM, and AROM, and the patient is progressed to resistive exercises as tolerated with respect to surgical area and pain/edema levels.

PROGNOSIS

- Early detection and treatment is import- ant for recovery and to decrease the chances of surgical intervention.

- Patients who seek help at the first sign of paresthesia to the ulnar distribution generally have the greatest response to conservative treatment outcome.
- Patients with symptoms of atrophy, weakness, clumsiness, and inability to hold their grip do not respond to conservative treatment and generally require surgical intervention. However, even with surgical intervention, these patients generally trend toward a poor outcome.
- Patients with normal motor strength and with paresthesias that undergo sur- gical intervention have a 90% recovery rate.
- Of the patients that have surgery to correct the problem, those that have subcutaneous transposition or medial epicondylectomy respond with excel- lent results.

SIGNS AND SYMPTOMS INDICATING REFERRAL TO PHYSICIAN

Patients who fail to respond to ther- apy with three to four visits or whose symptoms worsen require referral to a physician.

SUGGESTED READINGS

Buehler MJ, Thayer DT. The elbow flexion test. A clinical test for the cubital tun- nel syndrome. *Clin Orthop Relat Res.* 1988;233:213-216.

Coppieters MW, Bartholomeeusen KE, Stappaerts KH. Incorporating nerve-gliding techniques in the conservative treatment of cubital tunnel syndrome. *J Manipulative Physiol Ther.* 2004;27(9):560-568.

Deu RS, Carek PJ. Common sports injuries: upper extremity injuries. *Clinics in Family Practice.* 2005 June;7(2):259-260.

Elhassan B, Steinmann SP. Entrapment neuro- pathy of the ulnar nerve. *J Acad Orthop Surg.* 2007;15(11):672-681.

McFarland EG, Gill HS, Laporte DM, Streiff M. Miscellaneous conditions about the elbow in athletes. *Clin Sports Med.* 2004;23(4):743-763.

McPherson SA, Meals RA. Cubital tunnel syndrome. *Orthop Clin North Am.* 1992; 23(1):111-122.

Mowlavi A, et al. The management of cubital tunnel syndrome: a meta-analysis of clinical studies. *Plast Reconstr Surg.* 2000;106(2):327-334.

Novak CB, Lee GW, Mackinnon SE, Lay L. Provo- cative testing for cubital tunnel syndrome. *J Hand Surg Am.* 1994;19(5):817-820.

Rosati M, Martignoni R, Spagnolli G, Nesti C, Lisanti M. Clinical validity of the elbow flex- ion test for the diagnosis of ulnar nerve com- pression at the cubital tunnel. *Acta Orthop Belg.* 1998;64(4):366-370.

AUTHOR: LOU ANN MOORE

BASIC INFORMATION

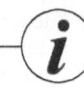

DEFINITION

Olecranon bursitis is the inflammation of the bursa, which is located superficially to the olecranon process of the ulna, secondary to traumatic injury or disease process. This bursa allows the gliding of tissue over the olecranon with decreased friction during flexion/extension of the elbow and provides protection to the bone from the external environment.

SYNONYMS

- Elbow bursitis
- Student's elbow
- Lunger elbow
- These terms indicate a typical mechanism of injury that may be discovered at evaluation such as a student leaning on the table studying for exams or a patient with chronic obstructive pulmonary disorder (COPD) leaning forward on his elbows to splint his thoracic cage for breathing purposes

ICD-9CM CODES
726.33   Olecranon bursitis
719.42   Pain in joint involving upper arm
727.3   Other bursitis disorders

OPTIMAL NUMBER OF VISITS

8 visits

MAXIMAL NUMBER OF VISITS

8 visits

ETIOLOGY

- Direct trauma to the tip of the olecranon process is the most common mechanism of injury for olecranon bursitis.
- However, other disorders can inflame the olecranon bursa in the absence of a traumatic event.
- Nontraumatic disorders include rheumatological disease, gout, systemic lupus erythematosus (SLE), chronic friction, infection, and repetitive overuse syndromes.
- Bursitis disorders can be classified acute, chronic, and septic.
  - Acute bursitis is secondary to direct trauma, which is seen in high impact sports such as football, wrestling, and volleyball, and direct trauma in the elderly typically from a fall.
  - Chronic bursitis is typically found in repetitive overuse activities and occupations in which there is repetitive rubbing and friction of the bursa.
  - Inflamed and possibly infected bursitis is secondary to an infectious process brought on by disease such as gout, rheumatological conditions, and SLE.

- When the cells in the bursa are irritated through acute or chronic conditions, they multiply and collagen production increases. This inflammation leads to production of fluid and increased capillary permeability allows fluid and proteinaceous exudates to flow into the bursa. This fluid can continue to accumulate even if treated properly. Generally, the fluid must decrease over time, secondary to the structure and blood supply of the bursa itself. Therefore it is important for early treatment to bring symptoms to resolution.

EPIDEMIOLOGY AND DEMOGRAPHICS

- Bursitis is not typically found in a specific age range or ethnic group.
- Young males do seem to be more commonly affected by acute olecranon bursitis secondary to their participation in high-impact sports.
- The chronic and infected bursitis does not have age or ethnic parameters and can occur in any age range and without specific mechanism of injury.

MECHANISM OF INJURY

- Olecranon bursitis can be caused by trauma, repetitive friction or compression, infection, systemic diseases, or deposition of crystals secondary to disease process.
- Bursitis is typically thought of as being caused by a direct blow to the tip of the olecranon that induces inflammation of the bursa.
- In traumatic bursitis, swelling ensues throughout the day after the incident.
- Inflammation in repetitive friction or compressive bursitis is secondary to frictional activity commonly seen with carpet layers and wrestlers or compressive activities as seen with students and patients with COPD. In the case of lunger elbow, for example, the patient with COPD attempts to improve his breathing and anterior/posterior chest diameter by leaning onto a table or counter with compression through the olecranon processes, inducing an inflammatory process in the elbows. Infectious olecranon bursitis can occur as traumatic and nontraumatic, as follows:
  - The bursa can become infected in a traumatic incident in which the bursa sustains a small laceration and infection develops in the area of the bursa.
  - In nontraumatic cases, the patient usually presents with an underlying primary disease process. Nontraumatic bursitis is probable in the presence of systemic or crystalline disease. A detailed history of an underlying disease process may reveal crystalline

deposition from gout, psoriasis, or RA or systemic disease prevalence such as diabetes mellitus, SLE, or uremia.

COMMON SIGNS AND SYMPTOMS

- Patients presenting with olecranon bursitis can have a combination of symptoms.
- Common signs and symptoms are localized swelling, warmth or heat to the posterior elbow, and palpable tenderness.
- Chronic bursitis frequently exhibits these symptoms with the exception of pain and tenderness.
- Other symptoms include increased heat or fever, erythema, cellulitis, and crystalline deposition, such as in the case of gout, and may lead to the diagnosis of infected and possible septic bursitis.
- Generally, the diagnosis of olecranon bursitis is localized to the posterior elbow; however, in cases of infection with joint involvement the elbow may become inflamed just proximally and distally to the joint line.

AGGRAVATING ACTIVITIES

The patient will report increased pain with full and forceful extension of the elbow, use of triceps tendon in area of the olecranon bursa, repetitive elbow extension movements, wearing a long-sleeved shirt, and prolonged compression to the olecranon process.

EASING ACTIVITIES

Patients will report decreased pain with rest to the area and guarding of elbow into slight flexion to decrease tension of triceps on the bursa and decrease compression through the elbow joint.

24-HOUR SYMPTOM PATTERN

- Generally, the patient will wake with stiffness in the morning secondary to inflammation and joint effusion.
- Pain decreases in the morning to early afternoon with mild-to-moderate activity and AROM to the joint.
- Patients will experience pain and inflammation that progressively worsens throughout the day into the evening with increased repetitive activity or prolonged compressive forces to the elbow.

PAST HISTORY FOR THE REGION

- Past history for this injury can include prior bursitis injury, occupational hazards, and athletic participation that may place the patient at risk in a repetitive motion, prolonged compression, or high velocity trauma situation.
- Illnesses and lifestyle can predispose a patient to bursitis and must be considered if an infected bursitis is

suspected. Patients may have a history of rheumatological disorders (RA and SLE), diabetes mellitus, gout, psoriasis, alcohol dependence, immunocompromised status, and inflammatory disease such as CREST (*c*alcinosis, *R*aynaud's phenomenon, *e*sophageal hypomobility, *s*clerodactyly, and *t*elangiectasia), and infection is sometimes present.

PHYSICAL EXAMINATION

- Swelling to the area of the posterior elbow at the olecranon process can range up to 6 cm in diameter and may have the appearance of a golf ball on the end of the elbow if fairly enlarged.
- Other observations to note are the appearance of erythema and possible crystalline deposits such as in the case of gout.
- During palpation, the examiner will notice an increase in warmth, tissue swelling, and local tenderness.

IMPORTANT OBJECTIVE TESTS

- Olecranon bursitis is easily identified and diagnosed secondary to the superficial location of the bursa to the elbow. A detailed history regarding the mechanism of injury, a review of the signs and symptoms, palpation, and observation of the tissue is all that is necessary to make the diagnosis.
- In some cases, the physician may order further diagnostic tools to identify the bursitis.
- Common diagnostic tools are ultrasonography, MRI, radiography, and bursal injection.
- The literature is undecided in support of the bursal injection, stating that this procedure may open the uncompromised bursa to the increased risk of infection.
- In cases of possible infected bursitis, the physician will generally aspirate the fluid to test for the infectious agent.

DIFFERENTIAL DIAGNOSIS

Dx

- The primary differentiation is to readily identify and report the possibility of an infectious bursitis. There is an increased danger of becoming septic with this diagnosis.
- Other disorders that may present as a bursitis include rare tumors, such as pigmented villonodular synovitis and xanthomas, and swelling to the olecranon bursa caused by rheumatoid nodules that can cause deposition of crystals.
- Other possible injuries to consider in regards to bursitis include the possibility of an underlying fracture with traumatic bursitis and tendinopathy/tendinitis or arthritis in the case of overuse or repetitive injury.

CONTRIBUTING FACTORS

- RA
- Gout
- Psoriasis
- Diabetes mellitus
- Arthritis
- Immunocompromise
- Alcohol dependency
- Current participation in sports can predispose patients to traumatic injury

TREATMENT

 Rx

SURGICAL OPTIONS

- Surgical excision of the bursa, bursectomy, is indicated in the patient with a bursa that is infected and unresponsive to treatment, not responding to repetitive draining, or the inflamed bursa is interfering with joint function and ROM.
- The two approaches to performing a bursectomy are the arthroscopic and open techniques.

REHABILITATION

- Initially, bursitis is treated conservatively with therapy, unless infection is suspected. Conservative treatment of olecranon bursitis consists of the acute, subacute, and progressive stages.
- Acute stage (weeks 1 to 2)
  ○ Therapy focuses on protection of the bursa and joint, initiating strengthening and ROM, and decreasing the inflammatory process.
  ○ This is accomplished with the application of ice, rest, and protection such as an elbow pad; antiinflammatory medications; and modalities to decrease pain and swelling.
  ○ The initiation of submaximal isometrics to the muscles surrounding the elbow joint and progressive resistive exercises (PREs) to those muscles of the joints distal and proximal to the elbow can be helpful in the initial stages of healing to promote blood flow and muscular reeducation. PREs are initiated with AROM against gravity and progressed to weighted resistance exercises as the patient tolerates.
  ○ Manual techniques can be employed to initiate ROM and to alleviate symptoms of tightness and spasm to the neck and thoracic spine secondary to muscular guarding. Gentle PROM to the elbow can be used at this time.
  ○ Modalities in this stage can include phonophoresis, iontophoresis, pulsed ultrasound, high-voltage pulsed galvanic stimulation (HVPGS), or interferential current. Each with its own benefit for decreasing inflammation. The literature does not specify a particular modality of preference.

- Subacute stage (weeks 3 to 4)
  ○ Progress patient to PREs of the elbow to increase strength and ROM exercises to improve motion. Start patient with AROM against gravity and let pain be a guide for progression into weight.
  ○ Manual therapy techniques should be progressed at this time as the patient tolerates progressive mobility and function.
  ○ Modalities should be continued in this stage to alleviate pain and inflammation that may be increased through the progression of resistance exercises.
- Progressive stage (weeks 4 and beyond)
  ○ The goal is to continue progression of strength and return to the previous level of function or sport. In the case of the throwing athlete, progressive strengthening to the elbow and rotator cuff is essential for the return to sport-specific activities. At this time, a progressive throwing program can be initiated if strength to the affected arm is 4+ or greater.
- Typically, initial therapy for the postoperative arthroscopic technique to bursectomy consists of a regime to protect the surgical area and progress the patient to function slowly. The site is protected, and modalities for the first 2 weeks are used to control pain and swelling. At 2 weeks, the patient can be progressed to isometrics of the joint and then further progressed to PREs as pain and edema allow.
- With the postoperative open technique, initial rehabilitation is slightly modified secondary to tissue disruption. Generally, the patient is placed in a compressive dressing for approximately 3 weeks to prevent re-infiltration and persistent edema to the area. Therapy is initiated at 3 weeks and can progress the same as for the arthroscopic technique.

PROGNOSIS

- There is a greater chance of recurrence of bursitis in those individuals with contributing factors such as disease processes, continuation of aggravating activity, or continuation of high-intensity sport subjecting the elbow to trauma.
- Patients with infectious bursitis generally respond well to aspiration of bursa and antibiotic treatment. The individual will continue to have an increased size of tissue surrounding the bursa area but will remain asymptomatic.
- Patients undergoing bursectomy generally do very well with full recovery of ROM and strength.

SIGNS AND SYMPTOMS INDICATING REFERRAL TO PHYSICIAN

- Patients who present to therapy with bursitis with significant erythema, heat, or fever to the area and increased tenderness to palpation require immediate referral to a physician because of the possibility of infectious bursitis.
- If a patient does not respond to conservative treatment of rest, protection, nonsteroidal antiinflammatories (NSAIDs), and modalities during a 2-week treatment regime, referral to a physician for possible drainage is mandatory.

SUGGESTED READINGS

Kerr DR. Prepatellar and olecranon arthroscopic bursectomy. *Clin Sports Med*. 1993; 12(1):137-142.

Liang KP, Matteson EL. Differentiation from problems in surrounding structures is difficult—Bursitis: common condition, uncommon challenge. *Journal of Musculoskeletal Medicine*. 2006;23(7):513-522.

McFarland EG, Gill HS, Laporte DM, Streiff M. Miscellaneous conditions about the elbow in athletes. *Clin Sports Med*. 2004;23(4):743-763.

McFarland EG, Mamanee P, Queale WS, Cosgarea AJ. Olecranon and prepatellar bursitis, treating acute, chronic, and inflamed. *The Physician and Sports Medicine*. 2000; 28(3):40-52.

AUTHOR: LOU ANN MOORE

BASIC INFORMATION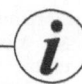

DEFINITION

The definition of elbow dislocation implies a complete discontinuity of the ulnohumeral articulation with associated radiocapitellar disruption. This can occur with or without proximal radioulnar disruption, associated neurovascular injury, and/or residual elbow instability.

SYNONYMS

- Elbow separation
- Subluxation

ICD-9CM CODES
718.22 Pathological dislocation of upper arm joint
718.32 Recurrent dislocation of upper arm joint
832.00 to 832.19 Range of various codes that can be used to describe clinically an elbow dislocation. There are specific codes that indicate type and directionality of the dislocation.

OPTIMAL NUMBER OF VISITS

16 visits

MAXIMAL NUMBER OF VISITS

16 visits

ETIOLOGY

- The most common type of elbow dislocation is posterior displacement of the olecranon in relation to the humerus. Two less common dislocations include anterior and divergent displacements.
- Dislocations occur in a three-stage process, called the circle of Horii, with progressive disruption of the congruency of the joint:
  - Stage I: A partial or complete disruption of the lateral collateral ligament (LCL)complex, including complete disruption of the lateral ulnar collateral ligament. The result is posterolateral rotator subluxation of the elbow that can spontaneously reduce.
  - Stage II: Further disruption to the joint anteriorly and posteriorly involving the joint capsule results in an incomplete dislocation posteromedially. The coronoid process of the ulna becomes perched on the humeral trochlea. This type of dislocation can reduce by self-manipulation and usually requires little force to correct.
  - Stage III: This stage is further divided into subcategories, as follows:
    - Stage IIIA: Disruption of all the soft tissues around and including the posterior part of the medial collat-

eral ligament except of the anterior bundle. This anterior bundle forms the pivot around which the elbow dislocates posteriorly by way of a posterolateral rotator mechanism.
    - Stage IIIB: Complete disruption of the medial collateral ligamentous complex of the elbow with severe instability.
    - Stage IIIC: Most severe, implies significant instability of the elbow complex so that the joint can dislocate even when immobilized in a cast at 90 degrees of flexion.

EPIDEMIOLOGY AND DEMOGRAPHICS

- The elbow is the second most commonly dislocated joint in the adult and the most common of all dislocations in the child.
- In the child, dislocation of the elbow is uncommon, therefore examination of the elbow for fracture must be considered.
- Over a lifetime, 6 of every 100,000 people will dislocate their elbow.
- Dislocations account for 10% to 25% of all injuries sustained to the elbow.
- The mean age for sustaining dislocations to the elbow is 30 years of age.
- 40% of all elbow dislocations occur during a sport activity; the most common sports are gymnastics, wrestling, basketball, and football.
- Dislocations in males occur 2 to 2.5 times more than in females.
- Lateral instability occurs 75% of the time after elbow dislocation.

MECHANISM OF INJURY

- A posterior elbow dislocation is caused by a fall on an outstretched arm with the elbow forced into hyperextension.
- Mechanically, the hand is supinated as the body rotates in a pronated direction in relation to the elbow, which causes a valgus force to the elbow.
- As the body continues in a forward motion, the elbow hyperextends and a posterior dislocation of the ulna in relation to the humerus occurs.

COMMON SIGNS AND SYMPTOMS

- Signs and symptoms of the acute elbow dislocation are as follows:
  - Very painful and increased swelling to the joint.
  - Elbow is held in 90 degrees of flexion, and the patient guards the upper extremity.
  - Forearm appears shorter when compared with the upper extremity or contralateral side.
  - All movement to elbow is painful.
  - Referral of paresthesias and cyanotic changes distal to injury with neurovascular compromise.

- Signs and symptoms of the subacute elbow dislocation are as follows:
  - Vague pain and soreness with activity to elbow.
  - Intermittent episodes of snapping, popping, or clicking to the joint with activity.
  - Episodes of apprehension or feeling of slipping to the lateral structures with activities.
  - Episodes of giving way or joint locking.
  - Difficulty lifting with forearm supinated, pushing, pulling, and pushing self out of chair.

AGGRAVATING ACTIVITIES

- For the throwing athlete who has sustained a dislocation injury of the elbow and possible postinjury instability, pain can be experienced during throwing.
- Pushing on armrests while rising from a chair.
- Pushing open a heavy door.
- Activities of daily living (ADLs) such as dressing, grooming, bathing, etc.

EASING ACTIVITIES

- For acute dislocation, symptoms will be eased with elbow held at 90 degrees and guarded close to the trunk.
- Easing activities for patients with chronic instability secondary to the dislocation include holding the elbow in a guarded position with forearm pronated. This position provides reassurance to the patient with the feeling of stability of the lateral structures.

24-HOUR SYMPTOM PATTERN

- Increased stiffness in the morning
- Pain with flexion and lifting activities
- Increased progression of soreness and fatigue with daily, functional, and recreational activities

PAST HISTORY FOR THE REGION

- The patient will have a recent history of dislocation to the elbow with possible history of recurrent elbow subluxation.
- The patient will report an injurious event of falling on an outstretched arm with body and arm rotation in opposite directions.

PHYSICAL EXAMINATION

- Observation
  - Carrying angle of the affected arm
  - Ecchymosis, edema, and wounds present
  - Patient's position and guarding the affected arm
  - Postural and proximal and distal joint asymmetries
- Palpation
  - Feel for warmth at or surrounding the joint and soft tissue structures.
  - Palpate for tenderness at the joint line and surrounding tissue structures

noting the intensity of tenderness in relation to aggressiveness of palpation.

- ○ Identify the muscular tone throughout the forearm and upper extremity.
- MMT and ROM testing
  - ○ Assess muscular strength and joint ROM throughout upper extremity.
  - ○ Take care with patients that feel sensation of instability to stabilize joint before testing.
  - ○ Assess pain inhibition of musculature and apprehensiveness of patient to hold contraction.

IMPORTANT OBJECTIVE TESTS

- The pivot shift test has been shown to be very effective at identifying instability at the elbow.
  - ○ In this test, the patient is supine and the affected arm is in full shoulder flexion.
  - ○ The examiner compresses through the shaft of the ulna, applies a valgus force at the elbow, and supinates the forearm while the shoulder is moved into extension, flexing at the elbow.
  - ○ A positive test is elicited if the patient is apprehensive or has pain or a palpable/observable divot is seen at the radial head.
- The milking maneuver can be effective in throwing athletes with a medial instability of the elbow.
  - ○ This test is performed with the patient sitting and the affected arm in shoulder abduction, external rotation, and elbow flexion.
  - ○ The examiner grabs the patient's thumb and pulls it into external rotation and extension.
  - ○ In a positive test, the examiner would recreate symptoms and see positive gapping at the radial head.
- Chair rise test
  - ○ This test is performed by having the patient actively push on the arm rests of a chair from a seated position with the elbows flexed at 90 degrees and the forearms in a supinated position.
  - ○ A positive test occurs when a patient either has a dislocation or apprehension of the movement.
- Floor push-up test
  - ○ This test is also positive if apprehension or dislocation occurs in extension.
  - ○ This test is performed with the patient doing an active floor push-up.
  - ○ The upper extremities are set initially at 90 degrees of elbow flexion and forearms supinated as the patient presses up into full elbow extension.

DIFFERENTIAL DIAGNOSIS

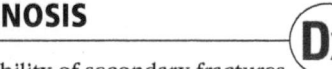

- Possibility of secondary fractures
- Valgus instability

- Radial tunnel syndrome
- Proximal radioulnar joint instability with dislocation
- Lateral or medial epicondylitis
- Ulnar neuritis

CONTRIBUTING FACTORS

- Contributing factors for this injury are generally specific to lifestyle.
- Individuals who participate in sporting activities that may predispose him or her to a falling incident are at risk of elbow dislocation.
- Other individuals that may be at risk of dislocation injury during a fall are those with natural joint laxity and flexibility.

TREATMENT

SURGICAL OPTIONS

- Generally, dislocations of the elbow alone do not require surgical intervention.
- In cases where there is an elbow fracture in association with the dislocation, surgical intervention may be necessary to stabilize the joint secondary to multiple traumas.
- Individuals who participate in an active lifestyle and have symptomatic recurring instability in the absence of a fracture may benefit from surgical intervention.
- Surgical intervention for this instability involves reconstruction through allograft or autograft tendon.

REHABILITATION

Postdislocation

- Initially the patient will be placed in a hinged elbow brace in full forearm pronation for 4 to 6 weeks. This position allows healing to take place within the ligamentous and soft tissue structures, preventing instability. Other than immobilization dislocation and postsurgical restrictions, rehabilitation can be relatively the same.

Postsurgical

- Initially, the patient is immobilized at 90 degrees flexion with the forearm in full pronation for 4 weeks. At week 4, mobilizations can begin in a hinged splint with the arm in pronation.
- Week 1
  - ○ Patient continues to wear brace.
  - ○ ROM exercises to wrist to decrease immobilization to multiple joints and promote blood flow and healing.
  - ○ Exercises to hand and wrist such as gripping, shoulder isometrics (no external rotation), and biceps isometrics.
  - ○ Cold pack application to control pain and swelling.

- Week 2
  - ○ Continue brace (both nonsurgical and surgical).
  - ○ Initiate wrist isometrics.
  - ○ Initiate elbow flexion/extension isometrics with forearm in brace and pronated.
- Weeks 3 to 4
  - ○ Continue with exercises and progress as tolerated with intensity of isometrics as tolerated.
  - ○ At week 4, begin mobilization of the upper extremity in the hinged brace and with forearm remaining in pronation.
- Weeks 5 to 6
  - ○ Patient continues wearing hinged brace.
  - ○ Continue with PROM techniques.
  - ○ Begin AROM and AAROM techniques.
  - ○ Begin light resistance exercises with the upper extremity, including wrist flexion/extension and elbow extension/flexion in forearm pronated position.
  - ○ Progress shoulder strengthening, continuing to avoid shoulder external rotation.
- Weeks 6 and beyond
  - ○ Brace is generally removed at this time.
  - ○ Progress AROM, AAROM, and PROM to promote improved motion to the elbow.
  - ○ Continue with strengthening and progress as tolerated.
  - ○ Initiate shoulder external rotation at this time and progress shoulder program as tolerated.
- For complex situations that involve multiple traumas to the elbow such as a fracture dislocation, refer to the surgeon for protocols and specific progression of the patient.

PROGNOSIS

- After reconstructive surgery, a mild flexion contracture of approximately 10 degrees is expected and acceptable.
- However, overall prognosis after surgery is reported, with good-to-excellent results at 85%.

SIGNS AND SYMPTOMS INDICATING REFERRAL TO PHYSICIAN

- Acute dislocations should have immediate orthopedic referral for relocation and examination to ensure minimal tissue and neurovascular damage.
- Patients who are not responding to therapy and continue to have instability issues resulting in a decrease in active lifestyle and neurovascular compromise with persistent paresthesias, cyanotic changes, and increased pain should be referred directly to a physician.

SUGGESTED READINGS

Burra G, Andrews JR. Acute shoulder and elbow dislocations in the athlete. *Orthop Clin North Am.* 2002;33(3):479-495.

Cheung EV. Chronic lateral elbow instability. *Orthop Clin North Am.* 2008;39:221-228.

Durig M, Mulller W, Reudi TP, et al. The operative treatment of elbow dislocation in the adult. *J Bone Joint Surg Am.* 1979;61:239-244.

Josefson PO, Gentz C, Johnell O, et al. Dislocations of elbow and intraarticular fractures. *Clin Orthop Relat Res.* 1998;246:126-130.

Josefson PO, Gentz C, Johnell O, et al. Surgical versus nonsurgical treatment of ligamentous injuries following dislocation of the elbow joint: A prospective randomized study. *J Bone Joint Surg Am.* 1987;69A:605-608.

Josefson PO, Johnell O, Gentz CF. Long term sequelae of simple dislocation of the elbow. *J Bone Joint Surg Am.* 1984;66:927-930.

Kuhn MA, Ross G. Acute elbow dislocations. *Orthop Clin North Am.* 2008;39(2):155-161.

Mehlhoff TL, Noble PC, Bennett JB, et al. Simple dislocation of the elbow in the adult. *J Bone Joint Surg Am.* 1988;70A:244-249.

Mehta JA, Bain GI. Elbow dislocations in adults and children. *Clin Sports Med.* 2004;23:609-627.

Morrey BF, An KN. Articular ligamentous contributions to the stability of the elbow joint. *Am J Sports Med.* 1983;11:315-319.

Morrey BF. Complex instability of the elbow. *J Bone Joint Surg.* 1997;79A:460.

Morrey BF. *Fractures and dislocations of the elbow.* Chicago: Year Book Publishers; 1993.

O'Driscoll SW, Bell DF, Morrey BF. Posterolateral rotatory instability of the elbow. *J Bone Joint Surg Am.* 1991;73A:440-446.

O'Driscoll SW, Morrey BF, Korinek S, et al. Elbow subluxation and dislocation: a spectrum of instability. *Clin Orthop Relat Res.* 1992;280:186-197.

Overly F, Steele DW. Common pediatric fractures and dislocations. *Clinical Pediatric Emergency Medicine.* 2002;3(2):106-117.

Plancher KD, Lucas TS. Fracture dislocations of the elbow in athletes. *Clin Sports Med.* 2001;20(1):59-75.

Protzman RR. Dislocation of the elbow joint. *J Bone Joint Surg Am.* 1978;60:539-541.

Smith JP 3rd, Savoie FH 3rd, Field LD. Posterolateral rotatory instability of the elbow. *Clin Sports Med.* 2001;20(1):47-57.

AUTHOR: LOU ANN MOORE

BASIC INFORMATION

DEFINITION

A fracture is defined as a defect or disruption and discontinuity in the surface and body of a bone that results in a crack or a complex break in the bone.

SYNONYMS

- Break
- Split
- Fissure
- Rupture
- Crack

ICD-9CM CODES

812.40	Fracture of unspecified part of lower end of humerus closed
812.41	Supracondylar fracture of humerus closed
812.42	Fracture of lateral condyle of humerus closed
812.43	Fracture of medial condyle of humerus closed
812.44	Fracture of unspecified condyle(s) of humerus closed
812.49	Other closed fractures of lower end of humerus
813.05	Fracture of head of radius closed
813.06	Fracture of neck of radius closed
813.15	Fracture of head of radius open
813.16	Fracture of neck of radius open
813.17	Other and unspecified open fractures of proximal end of radius (alone)
813.91	Fracture of unspecified part of radius (alone) open
813.01	Fracture of olecranon process of ulna closed
813.11	Fracture of olecranon process of ulna open

OPTIMAL NUMBER OF VISITS

24 visits

MAXIMAL NUMBER OF VISITS

36 visits

ETIOLOGY

- Types of fractures at the elbow include supracondylar, medial epicondyle, lateral epicondyle, radial neck or radial head fracture, olecranon fracture, coronoid fracture, and pediatric growth plate fracture. These fractures can exist as a union, nonunion, or compound fracture. The classification system varies for each type of fracture sustained and is beyond the scope of this chapter.

The reader is referred to the Suggested Readings section for this information.

- Fracture healing, as with most tissue injuries, occurs immediately after disruption of the bone. The process by which these fractures heal occurs in five stages. These stages remain the same for all fractures, whether union, nonunion, or comminuted; the difference is possible surgical intervention that may be required to approximate the fragments for healing to occur. The five stages of fracture are as follows:
  - Hematoma formation: During the initial 48 to 72 hours postinjury, a hematoma forms. This hematoma creates a fibrin meshwork that is the framework the fibroblasts and capillary buds use to surround the bony ends of the fracture.
  - Cellular proliferation: Osteogenic cells then begin to proliferate into the area and begin the process and progression of forming a fibrocartilage collar around the fracture site.
  - Callus formation: With the continuation of proliferation of the fibrocartilage collar, eventually the ends of the fragments of bone unite, creating a callus over the site of the fracture.
  - Ossification: As the osteoblasts continue to move into the site, the cartilage is slowly replaced by bone which causes a callus and ossification of the site.
  - Consolidation and remodeling: This stage completes the process as the callus is slowly reabsorbed and the bone remodels itself based on the mechanical stress placed on it. This phase can take up to a year to complete.
- The appropriate time of healing differs based on age. Children heal in approximately 4 to 6 weeks, adolescents in 6 to 8 weeks, and adults 10 to 18 weeks.
- Pediatric fractures must receive special mention secondary to the addition of the epiphyseal plate and their susceptibility to and response to injury. Fractures to the epiphyseal plate or in the bony tissue adjacent to it can disrupt the overall growth process to the limb and cause severe deformity if not addressed appropriately by the physician.
- These fractures are classified by physeal injury type. The most common and most widely used classification system is the Salter-Harris classification system as follows:
  - Type I fracture occurs through the hypertrophic cartilage that causes a widening to the epiphyseal plate. This is secondary to shearing, torsion, and avulsion movement producing a separation between the growth plate.
  - Type II fracture is the most common physeal plate fracture and rarely causes a functional deformity. This fracture extends through the physis and metaphysis.

- Type III fracture may cause chronic symptoms secondary to disruption of the articular surface of the bone. However, a type II fracture rarely causes deformity and has a good prognosis. This fracture extends through the physis and epiphysis, causing a disruption to the reproductive layer of the epiphysis.
- Type IV fracture is intraarticular and may result in chronic disability. It can disrupt the proliferative zone causing a gross deformity secondary to early fusion of the epiphysis. This fracture extends through the epiphysis, metaphysis, and physis.
- Type V fracture is a crush injury to the bone and generally results in premature closure of the growth plate and cessation of bone growth. On radiograph, this fracture is very difficult to diagnose, typically showing as a joint effusion.

EPIDEMIOLOGY AND DEMOGRAPHICS

- In adults, elbow fractures account for 7% of all fractures sustained.
- Of these fractures, approximately 30% involve the distal humerus, 33% are reported as radial head fractures, and 10% are reported as olecranon fractures.
- Distal humerus fractures are seen in two separate age groups, as follows:
  - Males between the ages of 12 to 19 years; fractures in this age group may be the result of high energy injuries sustained in motor vehicle accidents (MVAs) or falls from a height and sports.
  - Females older than 80 years of age; in this population, the occurrence of distal humerus fractures is >60% and occur from low-energy injuries such as falling from a standing position.
- Physeal type injuries account for 25% of all pediatric fractures with up to 30% showing growth disturbances and 2% showing observable growth deformity. The prevalence of Salter-Harris fractures at the elbow is as follows:
  - Type I fracture is commonly seen in infants and toddlers.
  - Type II fracture occurs most often in children older than 8 years of age.
  - Type III fracture is rarely seen at the elbow for any age of child.
  - Type IV fracture is not age-specific and occurs generally at the distal end of the humerus with the fracture passing through both the metaphyseal and epiphyseal plates.
- Supracondylar fractures account for 50% to 60% of all fractures to the upper extremities in children and type IV is the most common physeal fracture seen. Supracondylar fractures are more

common in children between the ages of 3 to 10 years and more prevalent in males. Lateral condyle fractures are seen primarily in the ages of 6 to 10 years, and medial fractures are seen in children 7 to 15 years of age. Avulsion fractures in which the tendon pulls a small piece of bone away when it ruptures are more commonly seen in adolescents.

MECHANISM OF INJURY

- Fractures to the upper extremity generally occur with a fall on an outstretched arm or through direct trauma onto the elbow. Some elbow fractures have specific mechanisms that predisposes their susceptibility to certain types of fractures.
- Amis and Miller found that coronoid and radial fractures occur with impact to a forearm at 80 degrees of flexion and distal humerus fractures with impact during flexion greater than 110 degrees, whereas olecranon fractures generally follow direct blows at 90 degrees of flexion.
- Olecranon fractures are secondary to a fall on an outstretched arm or through direct trauma onto olecranon with flexed elbow.
- Radial head fractures occur with a fall to an outstretched and supinated arm.
- Lateral condyle fractures occur with direct compression through a fall on an outstretched arm resulting in a shear force to the lateral condyle or through a varus-directed force to the elbow, causing an avulsion of the lateral condyle.
- Medial epicondyle fractures result from a valgus force with a combined contraction of the flexor muscles.
- Coronoid fractures are secondary to a hyperextension forces and will sometimes result in a dislocation and instability at the elbow. Coronoid fractures >50% cause significant instability and recurring dislocation that requires surgical stabilization.

COMMON SIGNS AND SYMPTOMS

- Signs and symptoms of a fracture at the elbow include pain, point tenderness, edema, ecchymosis, restricted motion, deformity, and weakness.
- For the medial and lateral epicondyle, swelling, point tenderness, and ecchymosis is localized to the respective area of injury.
- In acute supracondylar fractures, the first responder or emergency department physician will generally see a specific deformity pattern according to the direction of injury.
- In flexion fractures, the distal aspect of the fracture will shift anteriorly and the patient will hold the forearm at 90 degrees with increased guarding to the upper extremity.

- In extension fractures, the distal aspect of the fracture will shift posteriorly with a visible S-shaped deformity when the patient holds the arm at his side and an increased prominence of the olecranon process.
- Postsurgical symptoms include pain and soreness, decreased function with ADLs and functional activities, such as opening a jar or a door; tenderness to surgical area; difficulty applying pressure to elbow, such as resting on an armrest of a chair; difficulty extending arm when standing or walking; decreased strength throughout upper extremity including grip strength, ecchymosis, and swelling.

AGGRAVATING ACTIVITIES

- At the time of fracture the patient becomes guarded and movement is minimal.
- Aggravating activities include movement to the upper extremity that affects the elbow and palpation to the elbow.
- Postsurgical patients will generally complain of increased soreness and pain on movement of the elbow, wrist, and hand.
- All functional activities, such as eating, dressing, and bathing, will be difficult secondary to loss of motion and strength and therefore painful during the activity with latent soreness after cessation of the activity.

EASING ACTIVITIES

- Easing activities include guarding of the joint, splinting of the joint, pain medication, rest, elevation, and ice.
- The postsurgical patient will find increased easing of symptoms with use of medications: pain, muscle relaxer, or antiinflammatory. They will also report ease of symptoms with rest, use of sling, guarding to side of trunk, application of ice or heat modalities, and sleeping with arm propped on a pillow.

24-HOUR SYMPTOM PATTERN

- There is no specific 24-hour pattern for initial injury.
- The pain is constant and difficult to relieve.
- A 24-hour pattern for fractures that have been stabilized will generally continue with pain on activity and increase throughout the day; however, pain and stiffness will be present in the morning secondary to a persistent inflammatory process.
- The patient also complains of difficulty sleeping secondary to ROM issues with inability to get comfortable when sleeping or secondary to changing position in bed.

PAST HISTORY FOR THE REGION

- History of participation in high-impact sports.
- Past history of high-energy injury such as MVA or fall from a height.
- History of balance, weakness, and ataxia issues in the elderly.
- Postsurgical patients have recent history of decreased independence with ADLs requiring help with dressing, bathing, eating, etc. Recent history of decrease in functional activities such as opening a jar, turning a doorknob, pushing or pulling a door or car door, difficulty driving, and difficulty sleeping.

PHYSICAL EXAMINATION

- Typically, the clinician will receive a client status postsurgical intervention or after cast removal with healed or callused fracture to the elbow. The examination should include the following:
- Observation:
  - Signs of atrophy to elbow and muscles of proximal and distal joints
  - Signs of increased guarding of affected upper extremity
  - Malalignment post immobilization or surgery
- Inspection:
  - Incision site for closure of wound, drainage, or signs of infection
  - Ecchymosis or erythema to the area
  - Secondary wounds and changes in skin
- Girth measurements:
  - Elbow at epicondyles, proximal to joint line, and forearm to indicate edema and/or atrophy surrounding the injury
- Palpation:
  - Gentle-to-progressive palpation to joint and surrounding tissues in which therapist can identify atrophy, muscular tone, and edema in the tissues
  - Determine tenderness throughout and cold/warmth of tissue compared to contralateral side
  - Distal pulses for vascular compromise
  - Palpate for sensory deficits and paresthesias with light touch
- ROM testing:
  - Should be performed throughout upper extremity, proximal and distal joints, and secondary to overall immobility and decreased function to the limb.
  - Rule out cervical spine and thoracic spine deficits secondary to immobilization and wearing of sling or splint.
- MMT:
  - This testing may be deferred at initial examination based on tissue healing and appropriateness.
  - Test joint musculature proximal and distal to elbow if possible.

IMPORTANT OBJECTIVE TESTS

The identification of a fracture to the elbow is generally diagnosed through observation, palpation, mechanism of injury, and diagnostic testing. If fracture to the elbow is suspected by the physical therapist, manual manipulation to test the joint should be deferred until x-rays have been reviewed. See section on Elbow Dislocations regarding special testing for combination fracture dislocation and associated instability at the elbow.

DIFFERENTIAL DIAGNOSIS   Dx

- Postsurgical complicating factors as follows:
  - Neurovascular compromise and deficiency
  - Ligament instability and dislocation of the radial head or ulna
  - Forearm compartment syndrome
  - Volkmann's ischemic contracture
- Other diagnoses that may be secondary to a fracture postinjury and stabilization through the rehabilitation process as follows:
  - Medial or lateral epicondylitis
  - Elbow bursitis
  - Postinjury nerve entrapment secondary to osteophytes to radial, medial, or ulnar nerve

CONTRIBUTING FACTORS

- Participation in high-impact sports and intensity of sport.
- Home environment compounded with illness and weakness, such as in the elderly, in which lower extremity weakness, prior strokes, and disease processes contribute to balance issues that can predispose an elderly person to a fall.

TREATMENT   Rx

SURGICAL OPTIONS

- Surgical options are based on the site and type of fracture. Typically, surgical options involve an open reduction and internal fixation (ORIF).
- Supracondylar and medial/lateral epicondyle fractures:
  - These fractures generally require open fixation to promote early mobilization and improve prognosis for the patient. Types of procedures include transolecranon osteotomy, triceps sparring, triceps splitting, Bryan-Morrey approach, triceps reflecting anconeus pedicle approach, and arthroplasty just to name a few. An in-depth explanation of these and others can be found in the literature of each surgical approach.

- Olecranon fractures
  - Olecranon fractures considered nondisplaced and stable are treated nonoperatively. These are considered to be fractures with displacement less that 2 mm and no instability with flexion to 90 degrees and extension against gravity. Surgical techniques used to reduce a fracture to the olecranon process are the tension-band wire technique and limited contact dynamic compression plate fixation. Occasionally, nonunion fractures occur that require arthroplasty of the joint.
- Radial head fractures
  - Type II and above radial head fractures require intervention for the stability of the elbow complex. In fractures type II and above, the fracture segment is greater than 2 mm or comminuted, requiring surgical intervention to provide stability to the joint. Surgery can range from fixation of the fragment to radial head replacement. The type of surgery depends on the damage to the radial head. If the fragment is one-third of the radial head, the approach is replacement.
- Coronoid fractures
  - Type I coronoid fractures generally do not require internal fixation. However, type II and III fractures require ORIF secondary to instability of the joint and the importance that the coronoid process plays preventing posterior translation and dislocation of the ulna.
- Pediatric fractures
  - For children and type IV Salter-Harris fractures, ORIF must be done unless the fracture is nondisplaced.
  - For fractures at the ulnohumeral articulation in which the olecranon is fractured, an internal fixation is required if the fracture is >50%. This is secondary to the compromise to the stability of the joint.

REHABILITATION

- In any postoperative rehabilitation plan, it is important that the clinician refer to the physician's current protocols or contact the physician directly regarding ROM, healing stage, and activity modification.

Olecranon Fracture
- Posterior elbow splint is applied for 5 to 7 days after surgery.
- Weeks 1 to 8:
  - A removable splint is then applied and gentle AAROM and PROM initiated.
  - Instruct patient on use of opposite hand to assist in flexion-extension of the elbow gradually increasing the ROM.

- Instruct patient to remove splint several times a day to complete home program and allow gravity to assist in extension of the elbow.
- In weeks 1 to 2, begin strengthening and ROM techniques to the shoulder and wrist with use of isometrics, PROM, and manual techniques to ensure overall function of the upper extremity and progress of the elbow when strengthening to the elbow is allowed.
- Gentle isometrics can be initiated at 3 to 5 days postsurgically to unaffected joints. No active movement or resistance is allowed before week 8 secondary to the importance of callous formation at the olecranon.
- Weeks 8 to 10:
  - Active motion with progress into active resistance and PREs allowed at this time. Progress patient from isometrics, to AROM against gravity, and into resistance with light-heavy weights as tolerated.

Radial Head and Supracondylar Fracture
- Type I radial head fractures can be treated with a sling for 1 week with early AROM. Type II and above and supracondylar fractures can be treated aggressively if the joint is stabilized. This includes early mobilization with gentle PROM and AAROM progressing to AROM.
- Phase I: Day 3 (simple) or day 5 (complex) to 4 weeks postoperative
  - Gentle AROM and AAROM as tolerated.
  - Isometrics to uninvolved joints at 3 to 5 days postoperative.
  - At 4 weeks, initiate isometrics to elbow and flexor attachment.
- Phase II: Complex fractures 4-6 weeks
  - Complex fractures to begin gentle PROM in stable range. No aggressive PROM until 6 to 8 weeks.
  - Begin gentle prolonged low-load end-range stretching in pain-free range.
  - Grade I and II mobilizations employed for pain relief only.
  - Isometrics to elbow and flexor attachment musculature in stable range at 4 weeks. Start with submaximal and progress patient as tolerated.
- Phase II: Simple fractures
  - At 6 weeks, initiate light PREs per physician's protocol.
- Phase III: Complex fractures 6 to 8 weeks
  - Increase PROM per physician's protocol.
  - Aggressive PROM can begin 6 to 8 weeks postoperative.
  - Begin elbow and flexor attachment PREs per physician's direction. Initiate with AROM against gravity and slowly progress as tissue and patient tolerates.

- Phase IV: At 12 to 16 weeks for both simple and complex fractures
  - Work/leisure conditioning as tolerated.

Coronoid Fractures

- Coronoid fractures that are stabilized can withstand an accelerated rehabilitation program. At 2 days postsurgery, ROM is initiated. Patients may be in a continuous passive motion (CPM) apparatus to promote the return of pre-injury range.
  - Initiate day 2 with full AAROM into flexion with use of contralateral side.
  - Gravity-assisted extension.
  - Use nighttime extension splint for up to 16 weeks.
  - No strengthening until all fractures are confirmed healed.

PROGNOSIS

- 78% of patients with reduction of supracondylar fractures respond with good-to-excellent results secondary to early mobilization.
- Painful hardware irritation typically requiring removal
- Loss of motion at 10 to 15 degrees of extension even with early mobilization.
- With olecranon fixation, general outcomes are good to excellent with restoration of function in approximately 95% of patients.
- Approximately half (49%), of type III fractures, such as a supracondylar fracture, result in neurovascular compromise or forearm compartment syndrome.

- Fractures requiring >3 weeks immobilization have been associated with poor outcomes.
- Typical loss of 15% of strength to affected elbow.

SIGNS AND SYMPTOMS INDICATING REFERRAL TO A PHYSICIAN

- If the therapist is the first responder for the elbow fracture in the adult or the child, the treatment is initial splinting and immediate referral to physician so x-rays can be done to rule out fracture.
- Patients who are not responding to therapy with symptom increase; increase in neurovascular symptoms with paresthesias, temperature, and color changes; or patients who have not had surgery and have signs and symptoms of secondary injury, such as a dislocation or secondary fracture, should be referred to a physician for follow-up and further diagnostic studies.

SUGGESTED READINGS

Amis AA, Miller JH. The mechanisms of elbow fractures: an investigation using impact tests in vitro. *Injury*. 1995;26(3):163–168.

Anderson SJ. Sports Injuries. *Disease-A-Month*. 2005;51(8):438–542.

Carson S, Woolridge DP, Coletti J, Kilgore K. Pediatric upper extremity injuries. *Pediatr Clin North Am*. 2006;53(1):41–67.

Edwards GE, Rostrup O. Radial head prosthesis in the management of radial head fractures. *Can J Surg*. 1960;3:153–155.

Geel CW, Palmer AK, Ruedi T, et al. Internal fixation of radial head fractures. *J Orthop Trauma*. 1990;4:270–274.

Josefsson PO, Gentz C, Johnell O, et al. Dislocations of elbow and intra articular fractures. *Clin Orthop Relat Res*. 1998;246:126–130.

Morrey BF. Current concepts in the treatment of fractures of the radial head, the olecranon and the coronoid. *Instr Course Lect*. 1995;44:175–185.

Morrey BF. *Fractures and dislocations of the elbow*. Chicago: Year Book Publishers; 1993.

Newton EJ. Acute Complications of extremity trauma. *Emerg Med Clin North Am*. 2007;25(3);751–761.

Overly F, Steele DW. Common pediatric fractures and dislocations. *Clin Pediatr Emerg Med*. 2002;3(2):106–117.

Perron AD, Brady WJ. Evaluation and management of the high risk orthopedic emergency. *Emerg Med Clin North Am*. 2003;21(1):159–204.

Pollock JW, Faber KJ, Athwal GS. Distal humerus fractures. *Orthop Clin North Am*. 2008;39:187–200.

Swanson AB, Jaeger SH, LaRochelle D. Comminuted fracture of the radial head. The role of silicone-implant replacement arthroplasty. *J Bone Joint Surg Am*. 1981;63A:1039.

Szabo RM, Hotchkiss RN, Slater RR Jr. The use of frozen-allograft radial head replacement for the treatment of established symptomatic proximal translation of the radius: preliminary experience in five cases. *J Hand Surg Am*. 1997;22:269–278.

Turner RG, Faber KJ, Athwal GS. Complications of distal radius fractures. *Orthop Clin North Am*. 2007;38(2):217–228.

Veillette CJ, Steinmann SP. Olecranon fractures. *Orthop Clin North Am*. 2008;39:229–236.

AUTHOR: LOU ANN MOORE

BASIC INFORMATION

DEFINITION

Compartment syndrome is defined as a condition in which increased pressure in a limited space compromises the circulation and function of the tissue in the space. The forearm is separated into compartments by a very dense and strong fascia. When edema, hemorrhage, or external pressure is present, the pressure within these compartments can rapidly increase, causing compression that can compromise circulation and function of the forearm tissues.

SYNONYMS

No synonyms to describe this condition.

ICD-9CM CODES
729.71 Nontraumatic compartment syndrome of upper extremity
958.91 Traumatic compartment syndrome of upper extremity

OPTIMAL NUMBER OF VISITS

6 visits

MAXIMAL NUMBER OF VISITS

12 visits

ETIOLOGY

- The pathology for this syndrome is an increased pressure within one of the compartments of the forearm that compresses on the neural and vascular tissues and compromises their function. The three types of compartment syndrome are acute, chronic or exertional, and crush. There are three classifications of etiology for this diagnosis, as follows:
  - Decreased compartmental size
    - This can be caused by restrictive dressings, casts, and splints but also through excessive traction to the upper extremity or premature closure of fascia.
  - Increased compartment content
    - This may be caused by a fracture or vascular injury with increased bleeding into the compartment. This type of compartment syndrome can also be caused by overuse of muscles, burns, response to a chemical response such as a snake bite, or an infiltrated intravenous (IV) infusion
  - Externally applied pressure
    - A constrictive dressing or from prolonged compressive force, such as prolonged position of laying on the limb, can cause this syndrome, which is described as an edema-ischemia cycle. The damage to the compartment of the forearm through injury causes a rapid response by

the surrounding tissues. This rapid response brings an increased perfusion to the area that progresses to an ischemia at the capillary beds. This ischemia prevents venous emptying of the area. The capillaries dilate to increase the mean capillary pressure; however, this pressure continues to restrict the venous system from emptying the area. The body's response to this is increased histamine production and increased blood flow to the area with further continuation of increase in capillary dilation and permeability to the capillary walls. As this cycle persists, the interstitial pressure continues to rise and blood flow is cut off from the area. This ischemia then causes lactic acid release and damage to the surrounding tissues.

EPIDEMIOLOGY AND DEMOGRAPHICS

- Statistics on this specific condition are not well documented.
- Every year approximately 200,000 people are diagnosed with compartment syndrome. This number is a combination of forearm and lower extremity diagnoses.
- The prevalence of this syndrome is higher in males under the age of 35 years secondary to young males participating in and susceptibility to high-energy impact activities.
- Statistics show that fracture to the forearm and elbow tend to be the leading causative injury for compartment syndrome of the forearm.
- The elderly have a decreased incidence of compartment syndrome secondary to the elasticity of the tissue, decreased compartment size and volume, and generally a higher blood pressure that enhances perfusion and provides tolerance to higher tissue pressures.

MECHANISM OF INJURY

- Compartment syndrome is generally caused by acute trauma to the area or secondary to an injury such as a fracture or tight dressing/cast.
- Patients with chronic exertional forearm compartment syndrome are rare but have increased symptoms and pressure secondary to repetitive activities with the upper extremity and hands such as the repetitive and intense use of the forearms in motorcyclists.

COMMON SIGNS AND SYMPTOMS

- The common signs and symptoms for this condition are referred to as the 5 Ps: pallor, paresthesias, pulse deficit, paralysis, and pain on passive extension of the compartment.

- Pain is described as constant, deep, poorly localized, and dull ache to the arm not relieved with medication and typically out of proportion to the injury.
- In the later stages of this injury, paralysis and loss of distal pulses will be found.
- Chronic compartment syndrome will have increased pain with activity that is reduced quickly with rest from the activity.
- Other signs are numbness and tingling to the foot and distal leg and a feeling of tightness or fullness to the leg.

AGGRAVATING ACTIVITIES

- For the patient with chronic compartment syndrome, the activity precludes onset of symptoms.
- Chronic compartment syndrome is rare but can occur with high intensity and repetitive activity of the forearms and hands.
- The patient will complain of an increase in their intractable pain during passive stretching of the musculature within the affected forearm compartment.

EASING ACTIVITIES

- Patient's pain generally is not relieved in the later stages of this injury secondary to the progressive compression of the compartment.
- In the early stages of injury, the only easing activity is rest.
- The application is generally not relieving but aggravating, secondary to the ischemic nature of the application of ice.

24-HOUR SYMPTOM PATTERN

- Compartment syndrome is devoid of a 24-hour symptom pattern.
- Acute compartment syndrome is continuously painful and does not respond to pain medication.
- Chronic compartment syndrome is activity dependent.
- Onset of symptoms occurs during the pain-provoking activity and generally subsides when activity is ceased.

PAST HISTORY FOR THE REGION

Report of a recent traumatic event, such as fracture, dislocation, or direct compressive trauma, is common. The fracture can be the ensuing factor for this condition, or it can be a compressive dressing or cast that has been applied too tightly.

PHYSICAL EXAMINATION

- Observation
  - Increased edema to forearm comparative to contralateral side.
  - Appearance of tissue: Blanched, erythemic, cyanotic, or weeping.

- ○ Can patient find position of comfort while at rest?
- ○ Fracture blisters: Appearance of blisters on the skin may indicate pressure trying to be relieved.
- Palpation
  - ○ Tissue density and tightness.
  - ○ Response of the patient to light touch and pressure.
- MMT and ROM
  - ○ Generally unable to test without significant provocation of pain.
  - ○ Passive stretch to extremity causes significant pain.

IMPORTANT OBJECTIVE TESTS

- Currently, testing for compartment syndrome in the forearm or the leg can only be confirmed through the use of intramuscular needle pressure results.
- These signs and symptoms and passive stretch with production of increased noxious pain should convince the therapist to contact the physician for immediate follow-up.

DIFFERENTIAL DIAGNOSIS

- Stress fractures
- Volkmann's contracture

CONTRIBUTING FACTORS

- Traumatic injury to the forearm
- Recent fracture to the forearm
- Inappropriate application of casting to the upper extremity

TREATMENT

SURGICAL OPTIONS

- Compartment syndrome is a medical emergency and must be decompressed immediately once diagnosed.

- The only surgical option for this diagnosis is open fasciotomy in which the surgeon opens and releases the pressure in the compartment.

REHABILITATION

- If suspected, conservative management of this diagnosis before surgical fasciotomy consists of rest and antiinflammatory medications.
  - ○ Dressings and ice packs are contraindicated in this diagnosis secondary to the compressive and ischemic nature of these modalities.
  - ○ Elevation of the extremity is prohibited secondary to the poor perfusion and precipitation of further increased pressure in the compartment.

Postsurgical

- After fasciotomy, the patient will be relatively symptom-free and referral to physical therapy for postoperative diagnosis may be minimal.
- Week 1
  - ○ Initiate program with gentle PROM, AROM, and AAROM techniques throughout upper extremities.
  - ○ Address secondary joint issues such as neck, shoulder, upper back, and hand with ROM and manual techniques.
  - ○ Use of modalities to decrease any residual pain or swelling throughout limb such as interferential current. Continue with precaution regarding the application of ice packs secondary to the ischemic nature of forearm compartment syndrome. In patients with continued paresthesias, ice may be contraindicated secondary to decreased sensation.
- Week 2
  - ○ Initiate strength with AROM and progressing to PREs as tolerated and without symptom provocation.
  - ○ Progress aggressiveness of ROM exercises and techniques.

- ○ Initiate tissue mobilization to decrease scar tissue development.
- Weeks 3 to 4
  - ○ Continue progressive resistive exercises to return function.
  - ○ Modalities for reeducation of musculature such as neuromuscular electrical stimulation (NMES) and trigger point stimulation.

PROGNOSIS

- The prognosis for recovery and decreased residual effects of compartment syndrome are based on the early detection and diagnosis.
- Early surgical intervention, if indicated, is important to decrease the necrosis of tissue and possible loss of limb.

SIGNS AND SYMPTOMS INDICATING REFERRAL TO PHYSICIAN

Immediate referral to a physician is required if the physical examination and common signs and symptoms indicate possible forearm compartment syndrome.

SUGGESTED READINGS

Deu RS, Carek PJ. Common sports injuries: upper extremity injuries. *Clinics in Family Practice*. 2005;7(2):259-260.

Goubier JN, Saillant G. Chronic compartment syndrome of the forearm in competitive motor cyclists: a report of two cases. *Br J Sports Med*. 2003;37:452-454.

Harvey CV. Compartment syndrome: when it is least expected. *Orthop Nurs*. 2001;20(3):15-26.

McFarland EG, Gill HS, Laporte DM, Streiff M. Miscellaneous conditions about the elbow in athletes. *Clin Sports Med*. 2004;23(4):743-763.

McQueen MM, Gaston P, Court-Brown CM. Acute compartment syndrome. who is at risk? *J Bone Joint Surg Br*. 2000;82(2):200-203.

AUTHOR: LOU ANN MOORE

BASIC INFORMATION

DEFINITION

Tendinosis of the tendons, sheath, and muscular junction of the extensor carpi radialis brevis (ECRB) muscle and other extensor tendons on the lateral epicondyle of the humerus.

SYNONYMS

- Extensor tendinopathy
- Tennis elbow
- Epicondylalgia
- Tendinosis
- Lateral tendinopathy

ICD-9CM CODE
726.32 Lateral epicondylitis

OPTIMAL NUMBER OF VISITS

8 to 12 visits

MAXIMAL NUMBER OF VISITS

18 to 36 visits

ETIOLOGY

- The pathology occurs secondary to insidious, repetitive, eccentric contractions of the ECRB that cause microtrauma in the tendons at the lateral epicondyle.
- The primary muscles involved in tendon pathology are the ECRB and the extensor carpi radialis longus (ECRL). Secondary muscles of involvement are the anconeus and the extensor digitorum communis (EDC).
- Epicondylitis suggests an inflammatory process; however, acute inflammation only occurs in the early stages of the disease. Scientists and doctors have accepted the fact that tendonitis refers to the clinical syndrome and not the actual histopathology of the disorder, which is tendinopathy. Collagen becomes disorganized, with a loss of parallel orientation, asymmetrical crimping and loosening, and microtears. Because of hypovascularity of tendons, there is a propensity of the collagen fibers to breakdown during attempts to repair after excessive load and trauma.

EPIDEMIOLOGY AND DEMOGRAPHICS

- 5% to 10% of diagnosed patients are tennis players.
- 10% to 50% of tennis players are affected.
- 1% to 2% of the overall population is affected.
- Incidence is 5 to 9 times more common than medial epicondylitis.
- 7 to 10 times more prevalent than medial epicondylitis.

- Occurs in the dominant arm 75% of the time.
- Average age is 42 years.
- Age group is 35 to 50 years with median age 41 years.
- Young athletes suffer acute onset.
- Older patients suffer chronic symptoms.
- Incidence is 2 to 3.5 times higher in the over 40 age group.
- The incidence is higher for athletes who play >2 hours of tennis a day.
- The male-to-female ratio is equal.
- In tennis players, men are more affected than women.
- Prevalence worldwide depends on individual sports cultures, habits, and jobs.

MECHANISM OF INJURY

- The mechanism of injury is generally insidious; repetitive microtrauma caused by eccentric and concentric overloading of the ECRB will result in epicondylosis.
- Acute trauma to the lateral epicondyle can cause epicondylitis.

COMMON SIGNS AND SYMPTOMS

- Local tenderness directly over the lateral epicondyle with occasional forearm referral symptoms.
- Pain aggravated by strong gripping or decreased grip strength.
- Pain with passive stretching of the forearm muscles.
- Radiography reveals tendon calcification in 20% of patients.

AGGRAVATING ACTIVITIES

- Repetitive wrist turning or hand gripping, tool use, shaking hands, or twisting movements
- Baseball, fencing, swimming, and track and field throwing

EASING ACTIVITIES

Restful activities ease the pain of lateral epicondylitis/epicondylosis, as well as activity modification.

24-HOUR SYMPTOM PATTERN

- Nirschl classifies seven stages of pain caused by four stages of pathology.
  - In the early phase, pain is present at the lateral epicondyle during the offending activity, which lasts less than 24 hours.
  - As the pathology worsens, pain is present after exercise.
  - Symptoms progress into the later stages with pain affecting the performance of the activity and then affecting all ADLs.
  - Pain may also then progress to pain even while resting, affecting sleep.
  - Local swelling is rare but may be present because of early injury and inflammation.

- As the tendinopathy progresses, it is described as sharp, stabbing, long lasting, and present even at rest.
- At this point in the later phase, pain is described as a dull ache after activity.

PAST HISTORY FOR THE REGION

- Insidious, gradual worsening of pain that sometimes radiates down the forearm.
- Subjective history includes reports of engagement in activities that require repetitive wrist extension.
- Novice athletes are prone to microtrauma of the tendon because of the imperfection of form and technique.
- Patients also report progressive loss of grip strength.

PHYSICAL EXAMINATION

- Palpation
  - Tenderness to palpation over the anterior distal aspect of the lateral epicondyle over the extensor tendon insertion
- Resistive testing
  - Pain with resisted wrist extension, radial deviation, and forearm supination
  - Pain with resistive wrist extension while the elbow is in extension or when the forearm is in pronation
- Normal elbow ROM but may be slightly limited into wrist flexion with elbow extended
- Grip strength reduced and painful

IMPORTANT OBJECTIVE TESTS

- Pain with resisted wrist extension with elbow in full extension
- Pain with wrist extension with maximal wrist flexion and elbow in full extension
- Pain with resisted finger extension

DIFFERENTIAL DIAGNOSIS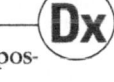

- Radial tunnel syndrome and posterior interosseus syndrome
- Intraarticular abnormalities: synovitis, plica, chondromalacia, and adolescent osteochondral defect
- Lateral collateral elbow instability
- Shoulder or neck pathology referred to as a deep ache:
  - C6/7 nerve root compression: Involvement along the dermatome and myotome
  - Ulnar nerve entrapment: Causes motor and sensory findings in the fourth and fifth fingers
  - Posterior tennis elbow: Extraarticular olecranon exostosis and bursitis
  - Rotator cuff tendonitis: A deep ache regardless of elbow AROM

CONTRIBUTING FACTORS

- High level of work-related, recreational, or sports activities requiring repetitive wrist extension

Section III   ORTHOPEDIC PATHOLOGY

- Activity level of three times a week or more at minimum of 30 minutes at a time
- Poor technique and a deconditioned musculoskeletal system
- Mesenchymal syndrome, or the tendency to develop tendinopathies in other tendons

TREATMENT

SURGICAL OPTIONS

- Open surgical treatments
  - Resection of part of the epicondyle
  - Partial resection of the annular ligament
  - Denervation
  - Nerve decompression
  - Lengthening of the involved tendons
- Arthroscopic lateral release
- Percutaneous release
- Regardless of technique, resolution of symptoms is successful and long lasting, as follows:
  - 91% patients report improvement at 4 years with tendon lengthening
  - 97.7% success at 2 years
  - 91% report success at 5 years
- Surgery is indicated if there is a persistence of pain and symptoms after 6 months of conservative management. Signs and symptoms should be severe enough to inhibit daily activities.

REHABILITATION

- Four phases foster healing. The goal is to reduce the stress at the tendons and enhance strength, flexibility, and endurance. As the pain decreases and function begins to improve, patients are able to progress from one phase to the next. Treatment will also include NSAIDs, topical analgesics, and corticosteroid injection.

Phase 1 (1 to 2 weeks)
- Minimize immobilization: May cause contractures and atrophy.
- Activity modification: Lift with forearm supinated, not pronated.
- Gentle stretching: Achieve and maintain full AROM/PROM.
- Modalities, such as the following, decrease pain/inflammation but no specific affect on collagen healing:
  - Corticosteroids: Effective for short-term relief, 2 to 6 weeks, and not long-term relief.
  - Ultrasound: Apply at the musculotendinous insertion at the medial epicondyle.
  - Deep tissue massage with trigger point pressure: Decreases the tension and spasm that occurs with the condition.
  - Cryotherapy: Effective for acute pain relief of tendinopathies.
  - Shock-wave therapy: Treatment through radio waves; efficacy is conflicting.

- HVPGS: Decreases synovitis and treats pain.
  - Iontophoresis with dexamethasone: Effectively reduces pain.
- Taping/bracing: Unloads the extensor bundle tension.
  - Splinting: Splint the wrist in 30 to 45 degrees of wrist extension.
  - Counterforce brace: Decreases the tendinous load during offending activities.
- Isometric exercises: Promote healing and prevent atrophy.

Phase 2 (2 to 4 weeks)
- Prepare the elbow for advanced activity, full ROM, and strengthen without pain.
- Progressive stretching: Move to the next stretch, only when no pain is felt.
  - Elbow bent at 90 degrees, elbow tucked by side, fingers open, forearm neutral, opposite hand stretches wrist flexion
  - Elbow bent at 90 degrees, elbow tucked by side, fingers fisted, forearm neutral, opposite hand stretches wrist flexion
  - Elbow straight, shoulder 90 degrees flexion, forearm pronated, finger loose, stretch wrist flexion
  - Elbow straight, shoulder 90 degrees flexion, forearm pronated, finger fisted, stretch wrist flexion
- Concentric exercises: Improves strength to a level greater than pre-injury.
- Neuromuscular reeducation: Enhances control during increased tendon load.
- Improve performance technique.
- Control intensity and duration.

Phase 3 (4 to 6 weeks)
- Patient must be 70% stronger compared to the contralateral side. Preparation to return to the offending activity.
- Eccentric strengthening promotes a higher return to premorbid activity, elimination of focal thickening of the tendon, and improved collagen fiber organization.
  - Progress at a slow pace with appropriate load to prevent regression
- Mild symptoms to the tendon are appropriate as long as functional limitations, pain, or edema do not persist or return.
- Avoid abrupt changes in training volume and speed.
- Aggressive strengthening, plyometrics, and power and endurance training.
- Improve biomechanics.
- Equipment:
  - Tennis and golf: Assess proper grip fit; proper club or racket weight, length, and structure
- Improper technique:
  - Tennis: Prevent hitting the ball late, with the head of the racket, and off the center point of the ball
  - Golf: Prevent breaking the swing at the top and using wrist flexion and pronation to hit the ball

- Occupations: Utilize ergonomically correct tools to reduce stress at the lateral elbow
- Occupational mechanics: Modify body mechanics
  - Address strength, stability, and endurance of the elbow and shoulder
- General body conditioning to improve neuromuscular education, minimize weight gain, and prevent loss of strength at surrounding structure.
- Wean off modalities and use mostly ice as needed.

Phase 4 (6 to 12 weeks)
- Progressive return to the offending activity, whether sports, occupation, or other ADLs.
- Use a structured return to an activity program such as the interval throwing program or programs for the golfer and tennis player.
- Satisfactory isokinetic testing to resume sports.

PROGNOSIS

- Short-term prognosis as follows:
  - 90% to 95% improvement of symptoms
  - 1 to 2 treatments give pain relief with deep tissue massage
  - 92% of patients reported improvement at 4 weeks
  - Increased grip strength at 6 weeks
  - Slow progression with greatest improvement at 12 weeks and lasting into week 52
- Long-term prognosis includes the following:
  - 91% success at 52 weeks
  - Approximately 10% recurrence of symptoms
  - Rehabilitation may take longer to reduce pain, but results are long term

SIGNS AND SYMPTOMS INDICATING REFERRAL TO PHYSICIAN

Pain is persistent after 6 to 12 months of conservative treatment and affects independent ADLs. In this case, surgery may be an option.

SUGGESTED READINGS

Anderson BC, Anderson RJ. Evaluation of the patient with elbow pain. Up To Date. http://www.uptodate.com/patients/content/topic.do?topicKey=~PAPPyTXhxRl9I

Anderson SJ. Sports injuries. *Curr Probl Pediatr Adolesc Health Care*. 2005;35:110–164.

Brosseau L, Casimiro L, Milne S, Robinson V, Shea B, et al. Deep transverse friction massage for treating tendonitis. *Cochrane Syst Rev*. 2002;4:CD003528 (from NIH/NLM MEDLINE).

Ciccotti MC, Schwartz MA, Ciccotti MG. Diagnosis and treatment of medial epicondylitis of the elbow. *Clin Sports Med*. 2004;23:693–705.

Chumbley EM, O'Connor FG, Nirschl RP. Evaluation of overuse elbow injuries. *Am Fam Physician*. 2000;61:691-700.

Davenport TE, Kulig K, Matharu Y, Blanco CE. The EdUReP model for non-surgical management of tendinopathy. *Phys Ther*. 2005;85(10):1093-1103.

Deu RS, Carek PJ. Common sports injuries: upper extremity injuries. *Clinics in Family Practice*. 2005;85(10):1093-1103.

Hart L. Short- and long-term improvement in lateral epicondylitis. *Clin J Sports Med*. 2007;17:513-514.

Maffulli N, Wong J, Almekinders LC. Types and epidemiology of tendinopathy. *Clin Sports Med*. 2003;22:675-692.

Nirschl RP, Ashman ES. Elbow tendinopathy: tennis elbow. *Clin Sports Med*. 2003; 22:813-836.

Pimentel L. Orthopedic trauma: office management of major joint injury. *Med Clin North Am*. 2006;90:355-382.

Sellards R, Kuebrich C. The elbow: diagnosis and treatment of common injuries. *Prim Care*. 2005;32:1-16.

Stracciolini A, Meehan WP, d'Hemecourt PA. Sports rehabilitation of the injured athlete. *Clin Pediatric Emerg Med*. 2007;8:43-53.

Whaley AL, Baker CL. Lateral epicondylitis. *Clin Sports Med*. 2004;23:677-691.

Wilk KE, Reinold MM, Andrews JR. Rehabilitation of the thrower's elbow. *Clin Sports Med*. 2004;23:765-801.

Wilson JJ, Best TM. Common overuse tendon problems: a review and recommendations for treatment. *Am Fam Physician*. 2005;72:811-818.

Woodley BL, Newsham-West RJ, Baxter GD. Chronic tendinopathy: effectiveness of eccentric exercise. *Br J Sports Med*. 2007;41:188-199.

AUTHOR: THERESA SCULLY

Section III

ORTHOPEDIC PATHOLOGY

BASIC INFORMATION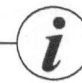

DEFINITION

Tendinosis of the tendons, sheath, and muscular junction of the flexor carpi radialis brevis (FCRB), the pronator teres, and other wrist flexor muscles that insert on the medial epicondyle of the humerus at the elbow.

SYNONYMS

- Golfer's elbow
- Reverse tennis elbow
- Thrower's elbow

ICD-9CM CODE
726.31 Medial epicondylitis

OPTIMAL NUMBER OF VISITS

12 to 18 visits

MAXIMAL NUMBER OF VISITS

18 to 36 visits

ETIOLOGY

- Repetitive concentric and eccentric stress placed on the flexor carpi radialis brevis (FCRB) and pronator teres muscles causes degeneration of the tendons at the medial epicondyle. Occasionally, the palmaris longus, flexor digitorum superficialis (FDS), and flexor carpi ulnaris (FCU) muscles are affected. The degeneration translates as pain, weakness, and reduced function of the wrist and elbow during activities that require wrist flexion with pronation.
- Epicondylitis suggests an inflammatory process; however, acute inflammation only occurs in the early stages of the disease. Scientists and doctors have accepted the fact that tendonitis refers to the clinical syndrome and not the actual histopathology of the disorder, which is tendinopathy. Collagen becomes disorganized, with a loss of parallel orientation, asymmetrical crimping and loosening, and microtears. Because of hypovascularity of tendons, there is a propensity of the collagen fibers to breakdown during attempts to repair after excessive load and trauma.

EPIDEMIOLOGY AND DEMOGRAPHICS

- Pimentel cites that 10% to 20% of all cases of epicondyltis involve the medial epicondyle.
- 64% are work-related activities requiring heavy load and repetitive hand functions.
- Occurrence is from 12 to 80 years old.
- More common in the 40 to 50 year olds.

- Baseball players ages 10 to 14 years old are at risk.
- Prevalent findings peak at 20-49 years.
- 75% present with symptoms in the dominant arm.
- Woodley reports a male-to-female ratio of 2:1.
- Others report an equal female-to-male ratio.
- Prevalence worldwide depends on individual sports cultures, habits, and jobs.

MECHANISM OF INJURY

- Onset is insidious and often due to repetitive motions and overuse.
- Less frequently, direct trauma to the medial epicondyle may lead to symptoms.
- Sudden eccentric contraction of the wrist and finger flexors may also lead to tendinopathy.

COMMON SIGNS AND SYMPTOMS

- Weak grasp/grip strength, pain with repetitive wrist flexion and pronation.
- Elbow flexion contracture seldom occurs but is noted in the throwing athlete.
- Pain is also described as a dull ache immediately after activity and at rest.
- Pain complaints are sharp or achy and radiate down medial forearm.

AGGRAVATING ACTIVITIES

- Golf, tennis, bowling, racquetball, football, archery, weightlifting, and javelin
- Carpentry, plumbing, and meat cutting
- Throwing in the late cocking and acceleration because of increased valgus stress

EASING ACTIVITIES

Restful activities ease the pain of medial epicondylitis, as well as activity modification.

24-HOUR SYMPTOM PATTERN

In the early phase, pain is present at the medial epicondyle with stiffness or achiness after the offending activity. After warming-up, the pain resolves. Symptoms progress into the later stages with pain during all activities, including competitive throwing, warm-ups. and during common ADLs. Local swelling is rare but may be present because of early injury and inflammation. As the tendinopathy progresses, it is described as sharp, stabbing, long lasting, and present even at rest. At this point in the later phase, pain is described as a dull ache after activity.

PAST HISTORY FOR THE REGION

- History of previous injury to shoulder, wrist, or forearm may be indicating

factors related to improper wrist mechanics.
- The history of the development of pain in relation to level of play and time of season also offers indicators as to the nature and structure of the injury.

PHYSICAL EXAMINATION

- Pain complaints: Sharp and achy during offending activity.
- Palpation: Tenderness that is 5 mm to 10 mm distal and anterior to the middle point of the medial epicondyle at the flexor insertion of the tendons.
  - Tenderness to palpation is positive over the flexor-pronator tendinous band and FCRB muscle.
  - Muscle atrophy may indicate the duration and chronicity of the tendinosis.
  - Localized increased temperature and swelling may not always be present.
- ROM: Generally normal, however, chronicity and severe pain may cause elbow flexion contractures.
- End-feel: Solid, firm, soft, or capsular may indicate other pathologies.
- Strength: Weakness of forearm pronation, wrist flexion, and grip strength.
- Important objective test: Resistive wrist flexion with pronation in a testing position of elbow extension.

DIFFERENTIAL DIAGNOSIS **Dx**

- Cervical radiculopathy: Rule out cervical nerve root impingement.
- Ulnar collateral ligament injury.
- Thoracic outlet syndrome.
- Ulnar neuritis: paresthesias in fourth and fifth finger.
- Snapping medial head of the triceps: Impingement of the ulnar nerve.
- Triceps tendonitis.
- Loose bodies or chondral involvement may cause crepitus.
- Multiple symptomatic tendons may indicate further evaluation for rheumatic disease.
- Avulsion of the apophysis in young athletes.

CONTRIBUTING FACTORS

- Age: Immaturity of the apophysis at the medial epicondyle.
- Premorbid ipsilateral injuries: Affects the ability to tolerate repetitive activity.
- Poor training: Poor technique, improper warm-up, improper training, and improper cool-down.
- Deconditioning: Individuals cannot tolerate repetitive demands of manual labor.
- Beginning a new activity or abruptly increasing the frequency or intensity of the offending activity may place increased load on the tendon.

- A history of frequent and forceful throwing in young boys contributes to medial tendinopathy.
- Improper biomechanics places repetitive load on the medial ligamentous and musculotendinous complex of the medial elbow.

TREATMENT

SURGICAL OPTIONS

- There are several classifications of surgery. Ciccotti categorizes surgery to five types, as follows:
  - Excision of the offending portion of the tendon
  - Increase local vascularity to stimulate the healing process
  - Reattachment of any prominent tendinous fibers to the origin
  - Repair of tendon defect
  - Management of coexisting ulnar nerve or ulnar collateral ligament pathology

SURGICAL OUTCOMES

- 8% to 17% failure rate with surgeries.
- At 6 years, 88% of clients report success.
- 19 out of 20 athletes returned to their previous level of sports.
- 14% noted a loss of endurance or strength.
- At 7-year follow-up, 87% reported success.
- 96% success rate with no ulnar nerve involvement.
- Surgery is indicated if there is no resolution of signs and symptoms at 3 to 6 months of conservative treatment. Elite athletes may receive surgery sooner, if objective physical examination and imaging reveal tendon disruption. Ligamentous instability is indicated for surgery as well.

REHABILITATION

- Length of conservative treatment is anywhere from 3 to 6 months. Treatment will include 3 to 4 phases of outpatient physical therapy, NSAIDs, topical analgesics, and corticosteroid injection.
- Phase 1 (Weeks 1 to 2)
  - Activity modification prevents increased damage to the tendon, reduces pain, and may assist with healing of the tendon. Activities that do not exacerbate the medial elbow pain may be continued.
  - Cryotherapy treats the inflammation of synovitis; increases tissue stiffness, so use after sports.
  - Splinting: Avoid full immobilization because of muscle atrophy and deconditioning.

- Counterforce brace decreases the tension created at the musculotendinous junction and assists in function during ADLs.
- Ultrasound at the musculotendinous insertion and into muscle belly of the wrist flexors.
- Shock wave therapy can be utilized to decrease inflammation and promote healing.
- HVPGS may decrease synovitis and treat pain.
- Corticosteroids treats synovitis instead of the actual tendinopathy.
- Phonophoresis and iontophoresis with dexamethasone treats synovitis.
- Deep transverse friction massage is commonly used, but efficacy is inconclusive.
- Isometric strengthening is performed first in elbow flexion to decrease strain at the medial epicondyle and then advance to elbow extension as long as response is pain-free.
- Pain-free stretching.
- Phase 2 (Weeks 2 to 4)
  - Full AROM for wrist and elbow without pain and 4/5 MMTs.
  - Progress strengthening from isometrics to concentrics as long as exercises are pain-free.
  - Eccentric exercises assist in remodeling the collagen fibers in the tendon.
  - Concentric exercises strengthen wrist flexors to greater than pre-injury strength.
  - Neuromuscular control exercises: Proprioceptive neuromuscular facilitation (PNF) activities to improve elbow stability
  - Address shoulder strength and begin strengthening as needed using thrower's ten exercise.
  - Sprint repetitions or plyometrics.
  - Activity simulation may begin once repetitive sprint repetitions may be performed to fatigue without symptoms.
  - Gradual return to sports or occupation ensures that symptoms do not return, maintaining strength and flexibility to tolerate repetitive stress.
  - Modalities as needed.
- Phase 3 (Weeks 4 to 6)
  - Improve biomechanics.
  - Review patient's sport equipment.
  - Tennis and golf: Assess proper grip fit; proper weight, length, and structure.
  - Play on softer surfaces to minimize stress when hitting the ball.
  - Review patient's technique.
  - Tennis: Prevent hitting the ball late, with the head of the racket, and off the center point of the ball.
  - Golf: Prevent breaking the swing at the top and using wrist flexion and pronation to hit the ball.

- Address strength, stability, and endurance of the elbow and shoulder.
- Wean off modalities and use mostly ice as needed.
- Phase 4 (Weeks 6 to 12)
  - Initiate and progress interval throwing program or swing programs for the tennis player and golfer.

PROGNOSIS

- Success rates are 85% to 90%.
- 5% to 15% have recurrent pain caused by incomplete rehabilitation.
- 26% of patients had a recurrence of symptoms.
- 40% had prolonged mild symptoms.
- At 6 months, 80% of patients reported full recovery.

SIGNS AND SYMPTOMS INDICATING REFERRAL TO PHYSICIAN

Refer to a physician if signs and symptoms do not subside with conservative treatment for 6 months and if differential diagnosis reveals another pathology for medial epicondyle pain.

SUGGESTED READINGS

Anderson SJ. Sports Injuries. *Curr Probl Pediatr Adolesc Health Care*. 2005;35:110-164.

Brosseau L, Casimiro L, Milne S, Robinson V, Shea B, et al. Deep transverse friction massage for treating tendonitis. *Cochrane Database Syst Rev*. 2002;(4):CD003528.

Cain EL Jr, Dugas JR. History and examination of the thrower's elbow. *Clin Sports Med*. 2004;23:553-566.

Cardone DA, Tallia AF. Diagnostic and therapeutic injection of the elbow region. *Am Fam Physician*. 2002;66:2097-2100.

Ciccotti MC, Schwartz MA, Ciccotti MG. Diagnosis and treatment of medial epicondylitis of the elbow. *Clin Sports Med*. 2004;23:693-705.

Khan K, Cook J. The painful nonruptured tendon: clinical aspects. *Clin Sports Med*. 2003;22:711-725.

Maffulli N, Wong J, Almekinders LC. Types and epidemiology of tendinopathy. *Clin Sports Med*. 2003;22:675-692.

Nourbakhsh MR, Fearon FJ. The effect of oscillating-energy manual therapy on lateral epicondylitis: a randomized placebo-control, double-blinded study. *J Hand Ther*. 2008;21:4-14.

Oken O, et al. The short-term efficacy of laser, brace, and ultrasound treatment in lateral epicondylitis: a prospective, randomized, controlled trial. *J Hand Ther*. 2008;21:63-68.

Pimentel L. Orthopedic trauma: office management of major joint injury. *Med Clin North Am*. 2006;90:355-382.

Reinold MM, Wilk KE, Reed J, et al. Interval sport programs: guidelines for baseball, tennis, and golf. *J Orthop Sports Phys Ther*. 2002;32:293-298.

Sellards R, Kuebrich C. The elbow: Diagnosis and treatment of common injuries. *Prim Care*. 2005;32:1-16.

Stracciolini A, Meehan WP, d'Hemecourt PA. Sports rehabilitation of the injured athlete. *Clin Pediatric Emerg med.* 2007;(8):43-53.

Whaley AL, Baker CL. Lateral epicondylitis. *Clin Sports Med.* 2004;23:677-691.

Wilk KE, Reinold MM, Andrews JR. Rehabilitation of the thrower's elbow. *Clin Sports Med.* 2004;23:765-801.

Wilson JJ, Best TM. Common overuse tendon problems: a review and recommendations for treatment. *Am Fam Physician.* 2005; 72:811-818.

Woodley BL, Newsham-West RJ, Baxter GD. Chronic tendinopathy: effectiveness of eccentric exercise. *Br J Sports Med.* 2007;41:188-199.

AUTHOR: THERESA SCULLY

BASIC INFORMATION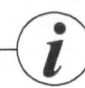

DEFINITION

Subluxation of the radial head from the annular ligament at the elbow.

SYNONYMS

- Toddler's elbow
- Pulled elbow
- Slipped elbow
- Annular ligament displacement

ICD-9CM CODES

832.09   Closed dislocation of other site of elbow
832.04   Closed lateral dislocation of elbow

OPTIMAL NUMBER OF VISITS

Not applicable.

ETIOLOGY

The head of the humerus is oval, and during forearm pronation, the more rounded shape articulates in the annular ligament and is prone to sublux through the ligament and cause impingement of the ligament. The common belief that nursemaid's elbow is due to children having a radial head smaller than the radial neck is incorrect. As children age, the ligament strengthens, making the condition less common.

EPIDEMIOLOGY AND DEMOGRAPHICS

- Mostly children 1 to 4 years of age, as young as 4 months, and as old as 15 years
- Left arm affected more than the right
- Occurs more commonly in females than males

MECHANISM OF INJURY

- A traction force at the elbow joint on an outstretched arm with forearm pronated.
- A fall is the second most common mechanism of injury.
- Infants may sublux when rolling independently or with assistance.
- 49% of cases in a study revealed a nontraction event.

COMMON SIGNS AND SYMPTOMS

- Immediate crying indicating pain
- Elbow postured in slight flexion and forearm pronation
- An aversion to using the arm
- Anterolateral tenderness over the radial head

AGGRAVATING ACTIVITIES

- Unable to use injured arm at onset
- Prone to re-injury after first onset

EASING ACTIVITIES

Not applicable for this pathology. Pain and symptoms are acute and not relieved until positional fault is reduced.

24-HOUR SYMPTOM PATTERN

Child presents with immediate pain and crying at onset and refusal to use arm. Arm is usually held in an adducted, elbow flexed, and forearm pronated position. Often, onset may be nontraumatic with insidious inability to use the arm. In this case, the pathology may not be noticed until several hours after onset.

PAST HISTORY FOR THE REGION

- A history of axial traction by a pull on the hand or wrist may be elicited by a caregiver as the child is resisting and not volunteering the arm.
- The history may also include, as common for other elbow fractures and dislocations, a fall on an outstretched arm. The injury may be insidious and not attributed to a traumatic fall or event.
- The child may abruptly fail to use the arm and be seen splinting the arm close to the body.
- A previous history of radial head subluxation may cause a recurrence as reported in 26.7% to 39% of injuries.

PHYSICAL EXAMINATION

- The child may appear anxious and protective of the affected arm. Usually the child is not in much pain, they are simply anxious.
- The patient will not be able to supinate or pronate the forearm, and they will also not be able to flex or extend the elbow.
- The child is generally afraid to move the hand and fingers.
- Visual inspection of the presence of deformity, ecchymosis, and asymmetry reveals no swelling or deformity.
- Tenderness at the anterolateral portion of the radial head.
- ROM assessment of the elbow and shoulder reveal that the arm is splinted against the side. Often, the weight of the affected arm is being held by the other hand in a supportive fashion.
- The forearm is positioned in a loose pack position for the radius, which is usually flexed 15 to 20 degrees at the elbow with the forearm partially pronated.
- Circulation and sensation testing should be normal. Neurovascular evaluation may reveal a competent nerve, artery, and vein.
- Muscle testing will be weak from muscle guarding.

IMPORTANT OBJECTIVE TESTS

- Diagnosis is made mostly on history of injury and physical examination.
- Radiographic studies may be completed to rule out the presence of a fracture.

DIFFERENTIAL DIAGNOSIS

- Elbow fracture
- Wrist fracture
- Soft tissue hand injury
- Radial head dislocation

CONTRIBUTING FACTORS

- No specific factors contribute to the pathology; research available on this information is lacking.
- The immaturity of the annular ligament and the tendency of stress to occur at the elbow because the caregiver handled the child incorrectly contribute to nursemaid's elbow.

TREATMENT

NONSURGICAL OPTIONS

- Two types of reductions are present: Hyperpronation and supination/flexion.
- In hyperpronation, the elbow is held in one hand, palpating the radial head, and the forearm is pronated.
- The second technique is supination/flexion, which is performed by taking the elbow and supinating the forearm and flexing the elbow. Often, a click is heard.
- One study mentioned that left arm injuries should be reduced with the hyperpronation technique since it may decrease the need for further treatment.
- One study reported that pronation/flexion for reduction may be less painful, especially for first reductions. The same study mentions that an audible click may indicate faster use of arm after reduction.

SURGICAL OPTIONS

Surgery is not necessary. Elbow is easily reduced.

REHABILITATION

- No physical therapy indicated. Usually, pain relief is immediate and there is no loss of AROM and strength after a reduction.
- Physical therapy may only be indicated as with any orthopedic pathology to treat loss of strength and function of the affected arm.
- The literature does not cite information on physical rehabilitation.

- Residual weakness caused by recurrent episodes or other complicating factors may need physical therapy to treat secondary effects.
- The approach is general strengthening, stretching, ROM, and functional rehabilitation of deficits assessed at evaluation.

PROGNOSIS

- Almost immediate use of elbow after reduction.
- Success rates are good with reports of 80.4% to 97.5% improvement with reduction.
- Recurrence rate is 26.7% to 30%.
- Return of use of arm occurs in 10 to 30 minutes
- A slow return to use of elbow is related to the child being younger than 2 years of age and not the time elapsed before reduction.
- 80.4% to 92% of elbows reduced through the supination/flexion technique are successful.
- 97.5% are successful with the hyperpronation method after the supination/flexion method.

SIGNS AND SYMPTOMS INDICATING REFERRAL TO PHYSICIAN

- Concern arises if the child does not use the arm after 15 minutes.
- X-rays will be acquired to assess for fracture. If there is no fracture, then the physician may place a posterior splint on the elbow and follow up in 24 hours.
- Referral to the physician is emergent in the presence of bony deformities, ecchymosis, swelling, and neurovascular findings such as radiculopathy and numbness.

SUGGESTED READINGS

Benjamin HJ, Hang BT. Common acute upper extremity injuries in sports. *Clin Pediatr Emerg Med.* 2007;8:15-30.

Carson S, Woolridge DP, Colletti J, Kilgore K. Pediatric upper extremity injuries. *Pediatr Clin North Am.* 2006;53:41-67.

Choung W, Heinrich S. Acute anular ligament interposition into the radiocapitellar joint in children (nursemaid's elbow). *J Pediatr Orthop.* 1995;15(4):454-456.

Kaplan RE, Lillis KA. Recurrent nursemaid's elbow (annular ligament displacement) treatment via telephone. *Pediatrics.* 2002;(110):171-174.

McDonald J, Whitelaw C, Goldsmith LJ. Radial head subluxation: comparing two methods of reduction. *Acad Emerg Med.* 1999;6(7):715-718.

Moses S. *Nursemaid's elbow. Family Practice Notebook.* http://www.fpnotebook.com/Ortho/Elbow/NrsmdsElbw.htm; 2008.

Moses S. *Radial head dislocation. Family practice notebook.* http://www.fpnotebook.com/Ortho/Elbow/RdlHdDslctn.htm; 2008.

Rooks YL, Corwell B. Common urgent musculoskeletal injuries in primary care. *Prim Care.* 2006;33:751-777.

Schunk JE. Radial head subluxation: epidemiology and treatment of 87 episodes. *Ann Emerg Med.* 1990;19:1019-1023.

Waander NA, Hellerstein E, Ballock RT. Nursemaid's elbow: pulling out the diagnosis. *Contemp Pediatr.* 2000;17(6):87.

Wolfram W. Pediatrics, Nursemaid elbow. Emedicine. http://www.emedicine.com/emerg/topic392.htm

AUTHOR: THERESA SCULLY

BASIC INFORMATION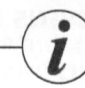

DEFINITION

Abnormal abutment of bone and soft tissue in the posterior compartment of the elbow.

SYNONYMS

- Posterior olecranon impingement
- Boxer's elbow
- Valgus extension overload syndrome

ICD-9CM CODES

715.12 Osteoarthrosis localized primary involving upper arm
718.12 Loose body in upper arm joint
719.42 Pain in joint involving upper arm
719.62 Other symptoms referable to upper arm joint

OPTIMAL NUMBER OF VISITS

8 to 12 visits

MAXIMAL NUMBER OF VISITS

18 to 36 visits

ETIOLOGY

- The pathology will occur secondary to a valgus force at the elbow that can bring into contact the medial tip of the olecranon process and the posteromedial tip of the olecranon fossa.
- There are two categories of posterior impingement. The first identifies impingement in elbows that present with functional stability of the medial and lateral ligaments and contribute the pathology to increased hyperextension forces. The other category identifies instability caused by functionally lengthened collateral ligaments, which then causes bony abutment of the olecranon in the humerus.
- Varus and posterolateral instability may cause impingement in the posterior compartment caused by the surface of the lateral edge of the olecranon compressing against the medial edge of the lateral wall of the olecranon fossa.
- Valgus instability causes impingement of the medial side of the olecranon on the lateral surface of the medial wall of the olecranon fossa.
- Because of this abutment, the elbow joint is prone to developing intraarticular loose bodies, osteophytes, and overall joint arthrosis relating not only to the humeral olecranon joint but also to the radiocapitellar joint.

EPIDEMIOLOGY AND DEMOGRAPHICS

- This pathology is mostly seen in overhead throwing athletes, such as in baseball, and in athletes involved in contact sports who experience hyperextension and valgus forces at the elbow such as football linemen and boxers.
- There is no specific gender or age group mentioned in the current literature.
- Athletes prone to posterior impingement are as follows:
  - Football linemen
  - Gymnasts
  - Rodeo participants
  - Weightlifters
  - Fast ball pitchers
  - Boxers

MECHANISM OF INJURY

Two mechanisms of injury are present: a valgus extension overload syndrome or a single traumatic hyperextension event such as a single hit in boxing.

COMMON SIGNS AND SYMPTOMS

- Pain in the posteromedial aspect of the elbow
- Joint swelling
- Onset insidious with loss of performance during throwing
- Elbow locking and crepitus
- Stiffness
- Coexisting valgus instability

AGGRAVATING ACTIVITY

Full extension of the elbow joint

EASING ACTIVITIES

Rest and immobilization

24-HOUR SYMPTOM PATTERN

- Patient presents with insidious onset of posterior elbow pain with extension during throwing.
- Progressive worsening of pain and function affects ability to perform the offending activity.
- Elbow locking and crepitus may also result with posterior medial impingement of the olecranon and in the olecranon fossa.

PAST HISTORY FOR THE REGION

- Ulnar collateral ligament instability
- Repetitive hyperextension a the elbow
- History of premorbid ipsilateral upper extremity pathology and muscle imbalance

PHYSICAL EXAMINATION

- ROM: Normal or below normal terminal elbow extension compared ipsilaterally.
- Positive crepitus or locking with full ROM:
  - Olecranon and coronoid bony contact
  - Decreased joint space of olecranon fossa
  - Loose osteophytes implanted in scar tissue

- Palpation of the posteromedial olecranon tip may reproduce pain.
- Mild anterior compartment contracture.
- Articular effusion (present on radiography).

IMPORTANT OBJECTIVE TESTS

- Passive elbow extension beyond AROM limits will elicit posterior elbow pain.
- Valgus stress with elbow extension and forearm pronated to prevent subluxation of the radius and ulna if positive for lateral collateral ligament disruption.
- Palpation to medial olecranon tip may illicit pain.
- Possible loss of terminal extension of elbow with reproducible pain on PROM into extension.
- Crepitus and/or locking with extension.

DIFFERENTIAL DIAGNOSIS

- Olecranon stress fracture
- Ulnar collateral ligament instability
- Triceps tendonitis

CONTRIBUTING FACTORS

- Ulnar collateral ligament instability
- Anterior compartment loose bodies
- Degeneration of the radiocapitellar joint

SURGICAL OPTIONS

- The arthroscopic procedure is usually chosen over open procedures. The goal of surgery is the debridement of loose bodies, osteophytes on the tip of the olecranon, and soft tissue lesions such as plica and synovitis and to deepen the olecranon. In surgery, the integrity of the ulnar collateral ligament will also be assessed and repaired as warranted.
- Arthroscopic treatment is particularly valuable because of increased intraarticular visualization of the anterior and posterior compartments and diminished soft tissue trauma.
- At an average follow-up of 40 months, a satisfactory subjective result of success was reported in 97% of patients. In the same study, satisfactory objective results of 91% have also been reported. Most athletes are able to return to the same level of their sport after arthroscopic surgery for posterior impingement of the elbow. At 1 year and 2 years, boxers and football linemen, respectively, reported good results.
- 74% of baseball players rated good to excellent results postoperative. In certain athletes, however, depending on the position played, re-operation rates are high, and return rates to the same level of competition can be less than in other athletes.

- Moskal notes that a retrospective review of re-operations in posterior elbow impingement arthroscopies reported that 25% needed ulnar collateral ligament reconstruction. Therefore physicians should fully assess concomitant elbow instability of candidates for posterior impingement arthroscopy.
- If conservative measures are not successful and there is a presence of osteophytes on the olecranon process or intraarticular loose bodies, surgery should be considered. Complicating pathology, such as valgus instability, also indicates surgery to treat the possible contributing factor to posterior impingement.

REHABILITATION

Phase 1 (Weeks 1 to 2)
- Rest and NSAIDs
- Modalities: Decrease pain and inflammation
  - Electrical stimulation: HVPGS and interferential current
  - Cryotherapy
  - Ultrasound: Decreases scar tissue and soft tissue adhesions
  - Iontophoresis with dexamethasone
  - Corticosteroids: Short-term relief

Phase 2 (Weeks 2 to 4)
- Address muscle imbalances
  - ECRB and longus muscles may be overused because of medial collateral ligament instability
  - FCRB and pronator teres muscles are hypertrophied
  - Shoulder rotator cuff strengthening
- Strengthening
  - Concentric elbow and wrist flexors and pronators
  - Isometrics of gripping, wrist flexion, and forearm pronation
  - Eccentrics of elbow flexors and wrist flexors and pronators
- Gentle stretching: Achieve and maintain full AROM/PROM and flexibility of wrist flexors and extensors

Phase 3 (Weeks 4 to 6)
- Progressive strengthening
  - Isokinetics
  - Plyometrics
  - Neuromuscular and proprioceptive training
- Sports-specific strengthening
  - Interval throwing program
  - Endurance training
- Improve biomechanics and address improper form

Phase 4 (Weeks 6 to 12)
- Progressive return to athletics
- Weight training with emphasis on high repetition and low weight
- Aerobic training
- Lower extremity and trunk conditioning

PROGNOSIS

Success rate for conservative treatment is usually around 80%.

SIGNS AND SYMPTOMS INDICATING REFERRAL TO PHYSICIAN

- After conservative treatment for more than 6 months and in some cases 18 months, operative management may be investigated.
- Any presence of intraarticular loose bodies, osteophytes at the tip of the olecranon, and ulnar collateral ligament instability may warrant elbow arthroscopy for debridement or ligament repair.

SUGGESTED READINGS

Hepler MD. Elbow arthroscopy in the treatment of posterior olecranon impingement. Presented at the American Academy of Orthopaedic Surgeons 65th Annual Meeting. http://www.medscape.com/viewarticle/427524

Moskal MJ. Arthroscopic treatment of posterior impingement of the elbow in athletes. *Clin Sports Med.* 2001;20(1):11-24.

Sellards R, Kuebrich C. The elbow: diagnosis and treatment of common injuries. *Prim Care.* 2005;32:1-16.

Stracciolini A, Meehan WP, d'Hemecourt PA. Sports rehabilitation of the injured athlete. *Clin Pediatric Emerg Med.* 2007;(8):43-53.

Valkering KP, van der Hoeven H, Pijnenburg BC. Posterolateral elbow impingement in professional boxers. *Am J Sports Med.* 2008;36(2):328-335.

AUTHOR: THERESA SCULLY

BASIC INFORMATION

DEFINITION

- A Barton's fracture is a fracture of the distal end of the radius bone in the forearm that is often accompanied by a fracture of the styloid of the ulna.
- Unlike Smith's and Colles' fractures, which are extraarticular, Barton's fractures involve the intraarticular joint of the radius and its adjoining carpal bones.
- Displacement or dislocation of the carpal bones distinguishes this type of fracture from Smith's or Colles' fractures.
- There are two types of Barton's fractures: dorsal and palmar. The latter is more common.

SYNONYMS

- Distal radius fracture
- Colles' fracture
- Smith's fracture

ICD-9CM CODE
813.41 Colles' fracture closed

OPTIMAL/MAXIMAL NUMBER OF VISITS

Highly variable, depending on specifics of fracture; length and type of immobilization; surgery; complications, including related injuries (ulnar styloid fracture, ligament injuries); and presence or absence of complex regional pain syndrome.

ETIOLOGY

- The fracture typically occurs from a fall on an outstretched hand.
- Falls from higher levels produce worse fractures. Specifics of the fall may account for associated injuries such as fracture of the ulnar styloid, ligament injuries, or carpal fracture or dislocation.
- The Barton's fracture is caused by a fall on an extended and pronated wrist. This increases carpal compression force onto the dorsal rim.
- Fractures that extend into the radiocarpal joint technically are considered Barton's fractures but commonly are categorized as Colles' fractures.

EPIDEMIOLOGY AND DEMOGRAPHICS

- The two peaks of incidence of distal radius fractures are ages 6 to 10 and 60 to 69 years.
  - In older adults, there is a 4:1 ratio of fractures in women. In adolescents, there is a 3:1 predominance of males.
  - In younger children, the higher incidence can be attributed to bone immaturity and increased likelihood of falls.
- Wrist fractures are more common in women over 65 years of age. There is an increase in incidence in white women between 45 and 60 years of age. The trend then stabilizes.
- Only 15% of wrist fractures occur in men; this incidence does not appear to increase as men age.
- In Europe, the annual incidence of distal forearm fractures in males and females was estimated at 1.7 and 7.3 per 1000 person-years, respectively.
- Distal forearm fractures can be used as an early and sensitive marker of male skeletal fragility.

MECHANISM OF INJURY

Fall on an outstretched hand, with the arm internally rotated at the shoulder, extended at the elbow, pronated at the forearm, and flexed (or extended) at the wrist, is the most common mechanism of injury.

COMMON SIGNS AND SYMPTOMS

After injury, the patient will report pain in the wrist, which may refer proximally into the forearm or distally into the hand. Movement may be limited by pain or physical block. Deformity in the wrist may be noted. Nerve symptoms, especially numbness or weakness in the median nerve distribution, may indicate serious complications.

AGGRAVATING FACTORS

- When seen acutely, wrist fractures will be limited in all motions. Forearm pronation and supination, gripping activities, lifting activities, and functional activities such as writing and typing will be limited and painful.
- When seen following immobilization or surgery, the patient will generally be limited in pronation and supination, therefore activities, such as turning doorknobs or typing, will be limited and aggravating.
- Activities, such as gripping, will be aggravating because wrist extension is needed to achieve a full grip.

EASING FACTORS

- Placing the wrist in a cast or splint is generally required to ease wrist symptoms and promote healing.
- Supporting the wrist with the other hand or a sling allows the hand and wrist to be in a rested position and a position of relative elevation.
- Elevation of the hand will help decrease the amount of dependent edema that can accumulate in the hand after an injury to the wrist.
- Ice is an appropriate modality to slow the production of inflammation and to modulate pain.
- Compression, like elevation, is used to limit the amount of edema that accumulates in the hand and wrist.
- Minimizing wrist and hand use.

24-HOUR SYMPTOM PATTERN

- As with most fractures, initially pain will be experienced most of the day and night. Patients will complain of a deep achiness in the wrist, and this pain will increase during the first 72 hours as the inflammatory phase peaks. Nocturnal achiness is common with fractures.
- As the fracture heals, achiness at night and with weather changes is still common. Morning stiffness that lasts over 30 minutes is not uncommon.
- Increased swelling and edema is normal at the end of the day and depends on use. As edema increases, it is not uncommon for patients to complain of achiness or tightness in the wrist.

PAST HISTORY FOR THE REGION

- In older individuals, history of osteopenia or osteoporosis is common.
- May have history of long-term use of steroids or other bone-weakening medications.

PHYSICAL EXAMINATION

- Pain in the wrist; generally pain and tenderness is located in the distal 2 inches of the radius or ulna. Pain and tenderness will progress distally into the radiocarpal joint. Pain will correlate with the location of the fracture, although the longer the time since injury, the more secondary and remote sites will be hypersensitized by the production of inflammation.
- Inability to move the wrist is experienced partly because of muscle guarding and partly because bony obstructions may prevent normal joint mechanics.
- Dinner-fork wrist deformity, or an anterior displaced wrist deformity, is a common deformity because of the displacement of the wrist and hand in relation to the remainder of the proximal forearm.
- Normal joint mechanics will be altered due to carpal displacement.
- Edema will be prevalent, especially in the acute phase. Muscle atrophy in the forearm will be noticed after casting. Edema may be present in the wrist even after several weeks of casting, but this edema is present secondary to disuse rather than from tissue injury.
- Bruising will be present acutely after a wrist fracture. Bone structures are highly vascularized, and injury to the tissue will result in damage to vascular structures. The damage to vascularized tissue will result in bruising.

IMPORTANT OBJECTIVE TESTS

Distal radius fracture is usually diagnosed with radiographs. Nondisplaced fractures may sometimes require computed tomography (CT).

DIFFERENTIAL DIAGNOSIS

- Although radiographs generally make differential diagnosis straightforward, other diagnoses to consider would include the following:
  - ○ Scaphoid fracture
  - ○ Ligament injury around the carpals
  - ○ Fracture of the distal ulna (uncommon in isolation)
  - ○ Triangular fibrocartilage complex tear
  - ○ Distal radioulnar joint dislocation
- These pathologies may also occur in conjunction with a distal radius fracture.

TREATMENT

SURGICAL OPTIONS

- Simple, stable fractures that can be reduced manually may require only casting.
- Unstable fractures may require percutaneous pinning or open reduction and hardware fixation.
- The success of surgery depends on the severity of the fracture (displacement, angulation, degree of bone compression, and whether the fracture is intraarticular or extraarticular) and the absence or presence of associated injuries.
- Surgery may be indicated if there is loss of bone length, unacceptable malalignment, or fracture into the joint, or if the fracture cannot be stabilized with a cast after closed reduction.

REHABILITATION

- The rehabilitation plan will be guided by the examination findings. Pain can be addressed with modalities, gentle manual techniques, and splinting for rest. When hypersensitivity is present, a desensitization program is indicated. Stiffness may benefit from joint and soft tissue mobilization and therapeutic exercise. Weakness will also respond to therapeutic exercise.
- The exercise program should start with gentle active and passive motion of the wrist, forearm, and fingers. Active and passive flexion of the finger metacarpophalangeal (MCP) joints in the maximum-tolerated range, including while the patient is casted, is important; this can prevent or decrease contractures that will be very difficult to correct once established.

PROGNOSIS

- In younger persons, the primary predisposing factors are lifestyle choices (e.g., participation in sports such as rollerblading or snowboarding). In older persons, impaired balance and osteopenia create increased risk of wrist fracture.
- Although the severity of the fracture must be considered, most patients will recover most or all of lost function and have little or no pain within 1 year after injury.
- Barton's fractures involve the radiocarpal joint. Because the fracture involves the joint space and the joint cartilage, prognosis for recovery is worse then for a distal radius fracture that does not involve the joint space or cartilage.
- Cartilaginous structures generally heal slowly, if at all.
- Restoration of normal radiocarpal joint alignment is difficult to achieve. As a result, it is difficult to restore normal joint biomechanics.

SIGNS AND SYMPTOMS INDICATING REFERRAL TO PHYSICIAN

Any indications of a distal radius fracture require immediate referral to a physician. If the injury is seen acutely, the patient should be encouraged to remove any rings from the fingers; otherwise, swelling may later necessitate that the rings be cut off.

SUGGESTED READINGS

Haentjens P, Johnell O, Kanis JA, et al. Evidence from data searches and life-table analyses for gender-related differences in absolute risk of hip fracture after Colles' or spine fracture: Colles' fracture as an early and sensitive marker of skeletal fragility in white men. *J Bone Miner Res.* 2004;19:1933-1944.

Hanel DP, Jones MD, Trumble TE. Wrist fractures. *Orthop Clin North Am.* 2002;33(1):35-57, vii.

Ismail AA, Pye SR, Cockerill WC, Lunt M, Silman AJ, et al. Incidence of limb fracture across Europe: results from the European Prospective Osteoporosis Study (EPOS). *Osteoporos Int.* 2002;13:565-571.

Owen RA, Melton LJ 3rd, Johnson KA, Ilstrup DM, Riggs BL. Incidence of Colles' fracture in a North American community. *Am J Public Health.* 1982;72:605-607.

AUTHORS: ROBIN BURKS and DERRICK SUEKI

BASIC INFORMATION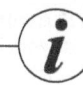

DEFINITION

A boutonnière deformity (BD) consists of proximal interphalangeal (PIP) joint flexion and distal interphalangeal (DIP) joint and MCP joint hyperextension of the finger.

SYNONYM

Buttonhole deformity

ICD-9CM CODE
736.21   Boutonnière deformity

OPTIMAL NUMBER OF VISITS

6 visits

MAXIMUM NUMBER OF VISITS

20 visits

ETIOLOGY

- BD begins with flexion of the PIP joint that is caused by a disruption of the common extensor tendon (central slip) that inserts on the base of the middle phalanx. This disruption results in the lateral bands migrating volarly to the PIP joint axis as the head of the proximal phalanx moves dorsally through the "hole" created by the central slip rupture.
- BD can occur as the result of mechanical trauma, rheumatoid arthritis (RA), burns, and infections. Trauma to the PIP joint may result in a laceration involving the central slip. Axial loading or forced flexion with the PIP in extension can cause closed disruption of the central slip. Volar dislocation of the PIP can cause avulsion of the central slip, as well.
- Chronic synovitis of a PIP joint with RA results in a slow, forced flexion. This causes the elongating of the central slip and ultimately leads to rupture. Subsequent volar displacement of the lateral bands below the axis of the PIP rotation creates increased tension on the DIP extensor mechanism, leading to hyperextension and limited flexion of the DIP.
- The difference between a fixed and a flexible boutonnière deformity is that a flexible BD is one in which the PIP joint can be passively extended. This is normally observed in acute or subacute cases. Rigid BDs are those in which the PIP joint cannot be extended with PROM as a result of oblique retinacular ligament (ORL) tightness. This occurs in more chronic and untreated cases.

EPIDEMIOLOGY AND DEMOGRAPHICS

Up to 50% of patients with RA are estimated to develop a BD in at least one digit.

MECHANISM OF INJURY

- Jamming the finger on the ground or another player in contact sports
- Burns
- Lacerations

COMMON SIGNS AND SYMPTOMS

Swelling and dorsal PIP joint tenderness to palpation

AGGRAVATING ACTIVITY

Continued flexion with gripping activities

EASING ACTIVITIES

- Rest will prevent aggravation of symptoms.
- Avoidance of flexion activities may slow progression of deformity.
- Early treatment and diagnosis will limit the discomfort.

24-HOUR SYMPTOM PATTERN

BDs are usually are not recognized in the early stages. As a result, many go untreated and become painful, chronic injuries. If a BD is suspected, treat it as such to limit the increased pain and deformity.

PAST HISTORY FOR THE REGION

- Recent trauma to the involved finger
- RA
- Osteoarthritis of the involved finger
- Recent burn or infection of the involved finger

PHYSICAL EXAMINATION

- PIP joint positioned in flexion, unable to actively extend
- DIP joint positioned in hyperextension, difficult to flex

IMPORTANT OBJECTIVE TESTS

- Test for extensor hood rupture: Finger is flexed to 90 degrees over edge of table. Patient is asked to extend the involved finger against resistance. The absence of extension force at the PIP joint and fixed extension of the DIP joint are signs of rupture of the central slip. Specificity and sensitivity unknown.
- Oblique retinacular ligament tightness test: PIP joint flexed is position of relaxation for the ORL, therefore the DIP joint should have more flexion than the PIP joint in extension. Specificity and sensitivity unknown.

DIFFERENTIAL DIAGNOSIS

- Phalanx fracture.
- Pseudoboutonnière deformity is a condition marked by PIP joint flexion contracture and restricted flexion of the DIP joint. This is commonly found in patients with RA. The characteristic hyperextension of the DIP joint in boutonnière deformity is not present. It often is the result of a hyperextension injury causing inflammation and contracture of the checkrein ligaments, the oblique retinacular ligaments, and possibly the first cruciate pulley. Pseudoboutonnière deformity must be distinguished from boutonnière deformity because pathophysiology and treatment are different.

CONTRIBUTING FACTORS

- Participation in contact sports.
- RA significantly increases the chances of having a boutonnière deformity.

TREATMENT

SURGICAL INDICATORS

Surgery may be indicated after conservative splinting treatments have failed or the injury is more than 8 weeks old. The patient and hand surgeon must carefully weigh and measure the risks and benefits before embarking on surgical planning.

SURGICAL OPTIONS

- When the central slip is avulsed with a bone fragment, the fragment should be either fixed or excised and the tendon reattached. The PIP joint then is held in extension with a Kirschner wire (K-wire) for a minimum of 10 days, followed by splinting.
- In closed volar dislocations warranting surgery or in open injuries, open reduction and repair of all soft tissue structures should occur, followed by stabilization of the PIP joint with a K-wire for at least 3 weeks. The PIP joint then is splinted for at least another 3 weeks while DIP joint motion is encouraged.
- Many surgical techniques have been described to repair a BD. The method for repair is determined by the condition of the central tendon and lateral bands. A sample of the many described techniques is as follows:
  - Using the superficial flexor tendon to reconstruct the central slip.
  - Using the lateral band on one side to reconstruct the central slip, while on the other side it is elongated to make use of a single lateral band.
  - Repositioning the lateral bands dorsally.
  - Separating the extrinsic and interosseous tendon from the lumbrical and oblique retinacular ligaments and centralize the lateral bands.

SURGICAL OUTCOMES

Deformities that can be passively corrected before surgery have better outcomes than those that remain rigid. Rigid deformities require extensive surgical release to correct, therefore putting the patient at risk for new postsurgical deformities.

REHABILITATION

- For deformities that the examiner is able to passively extend the PIP to 0 degrees, rehabilitation is as follows:
  - Edema control as needed, static splinting for PIP extension up to 6 weeks with full time wear. The splint should not interfere with MCP or DIP joint ROM. Initiate isolated DIP flexion exercises. Following the 6 weeks of total extension, flexion of the PIP joint is carefully initiated. Two to 4 weeks of extension should be continued following the initiation of flexion activities. Splinting is recommended only at night when full active extension is achieved and is maintained for subsequent visits.

- For patients with rigid PIP flexion contractures, rehabilitation is as follows:
  - Static PIP extension splinting for up to 8 weeks to regain full extension. The clinician may need to use serial casts that are changed weekly, depending on ROM progression. Continue isolated DIP flexion exercises. Resistant BDs may require treatment 6 to 9 months after injury, with full ROM requiring a full year of rehabilitation.

PROGNOSIS

- Prognosis is generally good for acute injuries and RA. Rarely will contracture and pain result in the need to amputate the digit.
- Participation in contact sports significantly increases your chances of having a BD.

SIGNS AND SYMPTOMS INDICATING REFERRAL TO PHYSICIAN

- If the patient reports trauma to the joint and a fracture is suspected, the patient should be referred to a hand surgeon for imaging studies.

- Patients with injuries not responding to conservative treatment of splinting and serial casting after 8 weeks should be referred to a hand surgeon.

SUGGESTED READINGS

Coons MS, Green SM. Boutonnière deformity. *Hand Clin.* 1995;11(3):387-402.

Harrison BP, Hilliard MW. Emergency department evaluation and treatment of hand injuries. *Emerg Med Clin North Am.* 1999;17(4):793-822.

Massengill JB. The boutonnière deformity. *Hand Clin.* 1992;8(4):787-801.

Towfigh H, Gruber P. Surgical treatment of the boutonnière deformity. *Oper Ortho Traumatol.* 2005;17(1):66-78.

AUTHOR: AUDRA PONCI BADO

BASIC INFORMATION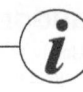

DEFINITION

A boxer's fracture occurs at the neck of the fifth metacarpal (MC) bone.

SYNONYM

Brawler's fracture

ICD-9CM CODE
815.04 Closed fracture of neck of metacarpal bones

OPTIMAL NUMBER OF VISITS

4 visits

MAXIMAL NUMBER OF VISITS

20 visits

ETIOLOGY

- A boxer's fracture most often occurs with all of the fingers flexed in a fist position with a force stronger than the bone directed at the MC head of the small finger.
- The fracture occurs at the MC neck, therefore the joint is not involved in the injury.
- The fracture could be unstable or displaced (rotated), causing possible complications for healing.
- Rotation of the fracture is exaggerated with all fingers flexed, at times causing the small finger to deviate underneath the ring finger.

EPIDEMIOLOGY AND DEMOGRAPHICS

- Boxer's fractures account for approximately 20% of all hand fractures.
- Boxer's fractures occur most often between the ages of 10 to 29 years.
- Males are more likely to have a boxer's fracture than females.

MECHANISM OF INJURY

- Motor vehicle accidents (MVAs)
- Bicycle accidents
- Fist fights
- Human or animal bites

COMMON SIGNS AND SYMPTOMS

- Loss of prominence of the small finger knuckle
- Loss of grip strength
- Pain, swelling, or bruising at the base of the small finger

AGGRAVATING ACTIVITIES

- Gripping
- Movement of the fingers

EASING ACTIVITIES

Immobilization of the fracture will provide support for the fragment and decrease the pain associated with the injury.

24-HOUR SYMPTOM PATTERN

An untreated fracture with become progressively swollen and stiff. Inflammation depends on use of finger as the day progresses.

PAST HISTORY FOR THE REGION

Physical trauma to the small finger

PHYSICAL EXAMINATION

- Wounds over the MC head as a result of a human bite or cut from the teeth require medical intervention to prevent infection.
- Tenderness to palpation over fracture site.
- Increased small finger rotation toward the thumb.
- Edema and bruising of the hand.
- Decreased ability to move the wrist, hand, or fingers.

IMPORTANT OBJECTIVE TESTS

- Radiographs should be performed from three different views: oblique, anteroposterior (AP), and true lateral.
- Radiographs should be performed 7 to 10 days after initial diagnosis to ensure proper healing alignment.

DIFFERENTIAL DIAGNOSIS

- Collateral ligament sprain
- Finger dislocation

CONTRIBUTING FACTORS

- Participation in high-contact or high-velocity sporting events
- Osteoporosis or osteopenia
- Taking medications or drugs that may decrease bone density

TREATMENT

SURGICAL INDICATORS

Research has great variability in the indicators for surgery. Some recommend surgical intervention if the fracture has more than 30 degrees of angulation. Others suggest nonsurgical intervention of active range of motion (AROM) for fractures with up to 70 degrees of angulation. The choice for surgery should be determined on an individual basis with a hand surgeon.

SURGICAL OPTIONS

The type of surgical intervention used is determined by the severity of the fracture. Treatments may include stabilization with percutaneous K-wires or internal fixation with plates and screws.

SURGICAL OUTCOMES

Surgical outcomes are unknown.

REHABILITATION

- Pain management is an important aspect of the rehabilitation process. Icing the fracture for 5 to 8 minute increments is a good way to control pain and edema. Antiinflammatory medications are excellent to use in combination with the ice treatment. Elevation of the hand is also important to reduce swelling.
- It is extremely important to know the stability of the fracture to determine treatment progression. When and how range of motion (ROM) exercises are initiated is determined on the fracture stability. Unstable closed reductions do not allow for ROM within the first 3 weeks. Stable semirigid fixations will allow protected AROM within the first few days. Communication with the hand surgeon will be essential to the patient's recovery.
- The boxer's fracture does not involve the PIP or the DIP joints of the hand. ROM of these joints should begin immediately, since this will not interfere with fracture healing. Movement will facilitate tendon gliding, as well as digital edema control.
- In general, it takes 6 weeks for a hand fracture to heal and a further 6 weeks to reach near normal strength. Very heavy lifting and contact sport should be avoided for approximately 8 to 12 weeks until the fracture healing has been confirmed.
- The types of splints used to promote boxer's fractures healing are as follows:
  - Depending on the severity of the fracture and the age and activity level of the patient, different types of splints may be used. The most protective splint is an ulnar gutter that includes the entire small and ring fingers up the forearm to include the wrist. The hand in a protected position with the MCP joints in 90 degrees of flexion and the interphalangeal (IP) joints fully extend.
  - A smaller splint that offers protection to a boxer's fracture is a hand-based ulnar gutter that allows full motion of the IP joints and wrist but protects the MCP joints of the small and ring fingers in 90 degrees of flexion.
  - Buddy taping the small finger to the ring finger has been shown to be effective for some boxer's fractures. This type of soft splinting is usually initiated 4 weeks postsurgical intervention. The tape can be manipulated to correct small amounts of digital rotation in nonsurgical cases.
- Possible complications with the rehabilitation of a boxer's fracture are as follows:

○ The extensor mechanism is vulnerable to adhesions during the period of immobilization. It is important to instruct the patient in protected ROM exercises as soon as indicated by the hand surgeon. IP joints usually have no movement restrictions and therefore can maintain extensor tendon motion.

○ Extensor lag is an additional concern of the extensor mechanism. Lag can occur if the MCP joint loses more than 3 mm of length because of fracture. The resultant slack does not allow the mechanism to fully extend the small finger. Early imaging and proper stabilization via splint or surgical intervention are necessary to avoid this complication.

○ Edema is a common complication during the rehabilitation process. It is important to resolve this issue to increase ROM and decrease pain for the patient. Retrograde massage and Coban wrap can be used to eliminate this problem.

○ A fracture callus is a bony lump that may appear at the fracture site as the bone heals. This is a normal part of the healing process and usually gets smaller over 6 to 12 months.

PROGNOSIS

Perfect alignment of the bone on x-ray is not always necessary to maintain full hand function. There are 25 to 40 degrees of compensatory movement at the small finger carpal MC (CMC) joint to make up for deformity at the fracture site.

SIGNS AND SYMPTOMS INDICATING REFERRAL TO PHYSICIAN

If the clinician suspects a boxer's fracture, the patient should be referred to a hand surgeon for proper imaging to confirm the diagnosis and initiate treatment to facilitate an excellent recovery.

SUGGESTED READINGS

Hardy MA. Principles of metacarpal and phalangeal fracture management: a review of rehabilitation concepts. *J Orthop Sports Phys Ther*. 2004;34:781-799.

Poolman RW, Goslings JC, Lee JB, Statius Muller M, Stelle EP, Struijs PA. Conservative treatment for closed fifth (small finger) metacarpal neck fractures. *Cochrane Database Syst Rev*. 2005;20(3):CD003210.

AUTHOR: AUDRA PONCI BADO

BASIC INFORMATION

DEFINITION

Carpal tunnel syndrome is compression of the median nerve in the wrist as it passes within the carpal tunnel, which is a structure bordered by the carpal bones and roofed by the transverse carpal ligament.

SYNONYMS

None in common usage. Carpal tunnel syndrome is a diagnosis often incorrectly used by clinicians for a variety of other hand conditions involving pain.

ICD-9CM CODE
354.0 Carpal tunnel syndrome

OPTIMAL NUMBER OF VISITS

6 visits

MAXIMAL NUMBER OF VISITS

20 visits

ETIOLOGY

Carpal tunnel syndrome occurs when either the volume of the carpal tunnel decreases or the volume of the contents increases, resulting in increased pressure within the tunnel. The increased pressure leads to ischemia or axonal compression of the median nerve, experienced by the patient as pain, paresthesias, and/or numbness in the volar aspect of the radial three digits. Advanced cases may include weakness and atrophy in the thenar muscles and lumbrical muscles to the index and middle fingers, or hypohidrosis (decreased sweating) as a result of involvement of the sympathetic nerves.

EPIDEMIOLOGY AND DEMOGRAPHICS

- The prevalence of carpal tunnel syndrome is approximately 50 cases per 1000 population in the United States (US).
- Peak age of onset is 45 to 60 years.
- Prevalence is 3 to 10 times as high in women as in men; prevalence is higher in whites than nonwhites.

MECHANISM OF INJURY

- Compression of the median nerve often results from sleeping with the wrists positioned in full flexion.
- Activities involving prolonged repetitive activity of the hands (e.g., keyboarding), vibration (e.g., riveting), or physical pressure over the volar wrist can cause or worsen nerve compression.

COMMON SIGNS AND SYMPTOMS

- The symptom pattern for carpal tunnel syndrome is specific and characteristic. Pain and paresthesias/numbness are felt in the volar aspect of the index and middle fingers and in the radial aspect of the ring fingers and the thumb, as well as the dorsum of these digits distal to the DIP joint.
- The palm is not involved.
- If there is weakness, it will be noted as decreased strength for thumb opposition.
- In addition to these symptoms, patients may complain of pain in the volar forearm, anterior upper arm, and even shoulder.
- Sympathetic nerve involvement may manifest as decreased sweating in the involved area.
- Patients may report difficulty manipulating small objects such as earrings or buttons.

AGGRAVATING ACTIVITIES

- Carpal tunnel syndrome is aggravated by prolonged positioning in wrist flexion or extension or with the weight of the hand producing pressure on the volar wrist or by sustained activities involving repetitive motion such as keyboarding.
- Prolonged exposure to vibration, such as while using power tools, can also provoke symptoms.

EASING ACTIVITIES

Avoiding aggravating factors relieves symptoms; splinting to prevent end-range wrist positions and frequent rest breaks during sustained activities are the primary methods.

24-HOUR SYMPTOM PATTERN

Carpal tunnel syndrome symptoms can occur at any time; however, it is common for the initial symptoms to appear at night, often waking the patient.

PAST HISTORY FOR THE REGION

There is no consistent prior local history; however, injuries to the wrist area, such as a distal radius fracture, may be noted.

PHYSICAL EXAMINATION

- Initial complaints are of pain and decreased sensation.
- Little objective evidence will be found in most patients; in more advanced cases, thenar weakness or atrophy or hypohidrosis in the involved area may be noted.

IMPORTANT OBJECTIVE TESTS

- Clinical tests
  - Carpal tunnel compression test

  - Phalen's test
  - Tinel's test at the wrist
- Nerve conduction studies are the gold standard for carpal tunnel syndrome. They are highly specific but not very sensitive when the condition is mild (complaints primarily of intermittent pain). Concurrent compression of proximal nervous structures (double or multicrush syndrome) may be overlooked.

DIFFERENTIAL DIAGNOSIS

- The primary pathology to rule out is nerve compression proximal to the carpal tunnel; cervical nerve roots, brachial plexus, and areas around the elbow should all be considered and examined.
- One helpful finding is the presence or absence of sensory changes and hypohidrosis in the palm.
- Since this area is supplied by a branch of the median nerve that does not pass through the carpal tunnel, symptoms in the palm suggest more proximal compression.

CONTRIBUTING FACTORS

- Factors that may decrease the volume of the tunnel include the following:
  - Arthritic spurs in the radiocarpal or intercarpal joints
  - Synovitis caused by RA
  - Tumor formation such as a ganglion cyst
  - Chronic positioning in mid- to end-ranges of wrist flexion or extension
- Factors that may increase the volume of the contents include the following:
  - Systemic conditions that increase fluid retention such as hypothyroidism and pregnancy
  - Irritation of the tendon sheath because of overuse
  - Congenital anomalies such as unusually proximal lumbrical origin on the flexor digitorum profundus tendon
- Other risk factors include diabetes, smoking, obesity, and alcoholism.

TREATMENT   Rx

SURGICAL OPTIONS

- Surgery involves release of the transverse carpal ligament. There are two primary types of surgery: open and endoscopic. There is little difference in long-term outcomes for the two groups other than a 5% recurrence problem with endoscopic surgery caused by incomplete release.
- Estimates of effectiveness of carpal tunnel release vary from 46% to 87%.
- Surgery is indicated in the presence of constant measurable sensory loss or weakness/atrophy of the thenar mus-

cles. Surgery may also be indicated for patients with intermittent pain or sensory changes who fail to improve with conservative treatment.

REHABILITATION

- Patients with carpal tunnel syndrome should be fitted with a prefabricated or custom splint designed to hold the wrist in neutral position. The splint should be worn when sleeping and whenever the patient performs activities that provoke symptoms.
- Patients should be instructed in activity modification to decrease the effects of the aggravating factors.
- Pulsed ultrasound, nerves gliding exercises, carpal bone mobilization, magnetic therapy, and yoga have also been shown to be helpful with some patients.
- A home program of nerve gliding exercises may be useful.

PROGNOSIS

- The long-term outlook for patients with mild carpal tunnel syndrome treated conservatively is good for symptom control, although long-term splint wear and/or activity modification may be necessary.
- If the patient returns to the same activities without modification and discontinues splint wear, the symptoms may return.
- Long-term outcomes after surgery are generally good, but weakness/atrophy may not be reversible and advanced sensory loss may not recover fully.
- Some patients experience pain ("pillar pain") in the thenar and hypothenar areas after surgery that generally resolves in about 3 months. A small number of patients do not fully regain ROM.

SIGNS AND SYMPTOMS INDICATING REFERRAL TO PHYSICIAN

Worsening sensory symptoms or the development of atrophy/weakness in the thenar muscles may indicate the need for surgery.

SUGGESTED READINGS

Ashworth NL. *Carpal Tunnel Syndrome.* Retrieved November 23, 2007, from http://www.emedicine.com/pmr/topic21.htm; 2006.

Muller M, Tsui D, Schnurr R, Biddulph-Deisroth L, Hard J, MacDermid JC. Effectiveness of hand therapy interventions in primary management of carpal tunnel syndrome: a systematic review. *J Hand Ther.* 2004;17(2):210–228.

AUTHOR: ROBIN BURKS

BASIC INFORMATION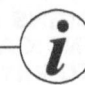

DEFINITION

A chauffeur's fracture is an avulsion fracture of the distal end of the radial styloid process.

SYNONYMS

- Distal radius fracture
- Radial styloid fracture

ICD-9CM CODE
813.41 Colles' fracture closed

OPTIMAL/MAXIMAL NUMBER OF VISITS

Highly variable, depending on specifics of fracture; length and type of immobilization; surgery; complications, including related injuries (ulnar styloid fracture, ligament injuries); and presence or absence of complex regional pain syndrome.

ETIOLOGY

- The fracture typically occurs from a fall on an outstretched hand.
- Falls from higher levels produce worse fractures. Specifics of the fall may account for associated injuries such as fracture of the ulnar styloid, ligament injuries, or carpal fracture or dislocation.
- A strong radiocarpal ligament, particularly the radioscaphocapitate ligament, results in failure at the bone rather than disruption of the ligaments. The relative weakness of the bone results in avulsion of the radial styloid from the metaphysis of the radius.

EPIDEMIOLOGY AND DEMOGRAPHICS

- The two peaks of incidence of distal radius fractures are ages 6 to 10 and 60 to 69 years.
  - In older adults, there is a 4:1 ratio of fractures in women. In adolescents, there is a 3:1 predominance of males.
  - In younger children, the higher incidence can be attributed to bone immaturity and increased likelihood of falls.
- Wrist fractures are more common in women over 65 years of age. There is an increase in incidence in white women between 45 and 60 years of age. The trend then stabilizes.
- Only 15% of wrist fractures occur in men; this incidence does not appear to increase as men age.
- In Europe, the annual incidence of distal forearm fractures in males and females was estimated at 1.7 and 7.3 per 1000 person-years, respectively.

- Distal forearm fractures can be used as an early and sensitive marker of male skeletal fragility.

MECHANISM OF INJURY

- Fall on an outstretched hand with the wrist ulnar deviated and supinated.
- Radial styloid fractures most commonly occur from tension forces sustained during the ulnar deviation and supination of the wrist.

COMMON SIGNS AND SYMPTOMS

- After injury, the patient will report pain in the wrist that may refer proximally into the forearm or distally into the hand.
- Movement may be limited by pain or physical block.
- Deformity in the wrist may be noted.
- Nerve symptoms, especially numbness or weakness in the median nerve distribution, may indicate serious complications.

AGGRAVATING FACTORS

- When seen acutely, wrist fractures will be limited in all motions. Forearm pronation and supination, gripping activities, lifting activities, and functional activities, such as writing and typing, will be limited and painful.
- When seen following immobilization or surgery, the patient will generally be limited in pronation and supination, therefore activities, such as turning doorknobs or typing, will be limited and aggravating.
- Activities, such as gripping, will be aggravating because wrist extension is needed to achieve a full grip.

EASING FACTORS

- Placing the wrist in a cast or splint is generally required to ease wrist symptoms and promote healing.
- Supporting the wrist with the other hand or a sling allows the hand and wrist to be in a resting position and a position of relative elevation.
- Elevation of the hand will help to decrease the amount of dependent edema that can accumulate in the hand after an injury to the wrist.
- Ice is an appropriate modality to slow the production of inflammation and to modulate pain.
- Compression, like elevation, is used to limit the amount of edema that accumulates in the hand and wrist.
- Minimizing wrist and hand use.

24-HOUR SYMPTOM PATTERN

- As with most fractures, initially pain will be experienced most of the day and night. Patients will complain of a deep achiness in the wrist, and this pain will

increase during the first 72 hours as the inflammatory phase peaks. Nocturnal achiness is common with fractures.
- As the fracture heals, achiness at night and with weather changes is still common. Morning stiffness that lasts over 30 minutes is not uncommon.
- Increased swelling and edema is normal at the end of the day and depends on use. As edema increases, it is not uncommon for patients to complain of achiness or tightness in the wrist.

PAST HISTORY FOR THE REGION

- In older individuals, history of osteopenia or osteoporosis is common.
- May have history of long-term use of steroids or other bone-weakening medications.

PHYSICAL EXAMINATION

- Pain in the wrist; generally pain and tenderness is located at the radial styloid process. Pain will correlate with the location of the fracture, although the longer the time since injury, the more secondary and remote sites will be hypersensitized by the production of inflammation.
- Inability to move the wrist is experienced partly because of muscle guarding and partly because bony obstructions may prevent normal joint mechanics. Limitations will be especially be noted into ulnar deviation and pronation.
- Edema will be prevalent, especially in the acute phase. Muscle atrophy in the forearm will be noticed after casting. Edema may be present in the wrist even after several weeks of casting, but this edema is present secondary to disuse rather than from tissue injury.
- Bruising will be present acutely after a wrist fracture. Bone structures are highly vascularized, and injury to the tissue will result in damage to vascular structures. The damage to vascularized tissue will result in bruising.
- Numerous ligamentous attachments generally maintain the alignment of the radial styloid in relationship to the carpus, but the styloid may be markedly displaced from the rest of radius.
- The brachioradialis, extrinsic wrist/finger flexors, and wrist/finger extensors will exert a powerful displacing force on the carpus/radial styloid complex.
- Fractures of the styloid process are frequently accompanied by dislocations of lunate.

IMPORTANT OBJECTIVE TESTS

- Distal radius fracture is usually diagnosed with radiographs. Nondisplaced fractures may sometimes require CT scan.
- The styloid is best visualized radiographically in a partially pronated view.

- Identification of scapholunate diastasis requires supinated view.

DIFFERENTIAL DIAGNOSIS

- Although radiographs generally make differential diagnosis straightforward, other diagnoses to consider would include the following:
  - Scaphoid fracture
  - Lunate dislocation or fracture
  - Ligament injury around the carpals
  - Triangular fibrocartilage complex tear
  - Distal radioulnar joint dislocation
- These pathologies may also occur in conjunction with a distal radius fracture.

TREATMENT Rx

SURGICAL OPTIONS

- Simple, stable fractures that can be reduced manually may require only casting.
- Unstable fractures may require percutaneous pinning or open reduction and hardware fixation.
- The success of surgery depends on the severity of the fracture (displacement, angulation, degree of bone compression, and whether the fracture is intraarticular or extraarticular) and the absence or presence of associated injuries.
- Surgery may be indicated if there is loss of bone length, unacceptable malalignment, or fracture into the joint, or if the fracture cannot be stabilized with a cast after closed reduction.

REHABILITATION

- The rehabilitation plan will be guided by the examination findings. Pain can be addressed with modalities, gentle manual techniques, and splinting for rest. When hypersensitivity is present, a desensitization program is indicated. Stiffness may benefit from joint and soft tissue mobilization and therapeutic exercise. Weakness will also respond to therapeutic exercise.
- The exercise program should start with gentle active and passive motion of the wrist, forearm, and fingers. Active and passive flexion of the finger MCP joints in the maximum-tolerated range, including while the patient is casted, is important; this can prevent or decrease contractures that will be very difficult to correct once established.

PROGNOSIS

- In younger persons, the primary predisposing factors are lifestyle choices (e.g., participation in sports such as rollerblading or snowboarding). In older persons, impaired balance and osteopenia create increased risk of wrist fracture.
- Although the severity of the fracture must be considered, most patients will recover most or all of lost function and have little or no pain within 1 year after injury.

SIGNS AND SYMPTOMS INDICATING REFERRAL TO PHYSICIAN

Any indications of a distal radius fracture requires immediate referral to a physician. If the injury is seen acutely, the patient should be encouraged to remove any rings from the fingers; otherwise, swelling may later necessitate that the rings be cut off.

SUGGESTED READINGS

Haentjens P, Johnell O, Kanis JA, et al. Evidence from data searches and life-table analyses for gender-related differences in absolute risk of hip fracture after Colles' or spine fracture: Colles' fracture as an early and sensitive marker of skeletal fragility in white men. *J Bone Miner Res*. 2004;19:1933-1944.

Hanel DP, Jones MD, Trumble TE. Wrist fractures. *Orthop Clin North Am*. 2002;33(1):35-57, vii.

Ismail AA, Pye SR, Cockerill WC, Lunt M, Silman AJ, et al. Incidence of limb fracture across Europe: results from the European Prospective Osteoporosis Study (EPOS). *Osteoporos Int*. 2002;13:565-571.

Owen RA, Melton LJ 3rd, Johnson KA, Ilstrup DM, Riggs BL. Incidence of Colles' fracture in a North American community. *Am J Public Health*. 1982;72:605-607.

AUTHORS: ROBIN BURKS and DERRICK SUEKI

BASIC INFORMATION

DEFINITION

- A Colles' fracture is a fracture of the distal end of the radius bone in the forearm, often accompanied by fracture of the styloid of the ulna.
- The fracture usually occurs about an inch or two proximal to the radiocarpal joint.
- The distal portion of the wrist and hand are displaced posterior and laterally, resulting in the characteristic dinner-fork deformity.

SYNONYM

Distal radius fracture

ICD-9CM CODE
813.41 Colles' fracture closed

OPTIMAL/MAXIMAL NUMBER OF VISITS

Highly variable, depending on specifics of fracture; length and type of immobilization; surgery; complications including related injuries (ulnar styloid fracture, ligament injuries); and presence or absence of complex regional pain syndrome.

ETIOLOGY

- The fracture typically occurs from a fall on an outstretched hand.
- Falls from higher levels produce worse fractures. Specifics of the fall may account for associated injuries such as fracture of the ulnar styloid, ligament injuries, or carpal fracture or dislocation.
- The posterior and lateral displacement of the hand and wrist are usually the result of a fall in which the arm is internally rotated at the shoulder, extended at the elbow, pronated at the forearm, and extended at the wrist.
- Fractures that extend into the radiocarpal joint technically are considered Barton's fractures but commonly are categorized as Colles' fractures.

EPIDEMIOLOGY AND DEMOGRAPHICS

- The two peaks of incidence of distal radius fractures are ages 6 to 10 and 60 to 69 years.
  - In older adults, there is a 4:1 ratio of fractures in women. In adolescents, there is a 3:1 predominance of males.
  - In younger children, the higher incidence can be attributed to bone immaturity and increased likelihood of falls.
- Wrist fractures are more common in women over 65 years of age. There is an increase in incidence in white women between 45 and 60 years of age. The trend then stabilizes.
- Only 15% of wrist fractures occur in men; this incidence does not appear to increase as men age.
- In Europe, the annual incidence of distal forearm fractures in males and females was estimated at 1.7 and 7.3 per 1000 person-years, respectively.
- Distal forearm fractures can be used as an early and sensitive marker of male skeletal fragility.

MECHANISM OF INJURY

Fall on an outstretched hand, with the arm internally rotated at the shoulder, extended at the elbow, pronated at the forearm, and extended at the wrist, is the most common mechanism of injury.

COMMON SIGNS AND SYMPTOMS

- After injury, the patient will report pain in the wrist that may refer proximally into the forearm or distally into the hand.
- Movement may be limited by pain or physical block.
- Deformity in the wrist may be noted.
- Nerve symptoms, especially numbness or weakness in the median nerve distribution, may indicate serious complications.

AGGRAVATING FACTORS

- When seen acutely, wrist fractures will be limited in all motions. Forearm pronation and supination, gripping activities, lifting activities, and functional activities, such as writing and typing, will be limited and painful.
- When seen following immobilization or surgery, the patient will generally be limited in pronation and supination, therefore activities, such as turning doorknobs or typing, will be limited and aggravating.
- Activities, such as gripping, will be aggravating because wrist extension is needed to achieve a full grip.

EASING FACTORS

- Placing the wrist in a cast or splint is generally required to ease wrist symptoms and promote healing.
- Supporting the wrist with the other hand or a sling allows the hand and wrist to be in a resting position and a position of relative elevation.
- Elevation of the hand will help to decrease the amount of dependent edema that can accumulate in the hand after an injury to the wrist.
- Ice is an appropriate modality to slow the production of inflammation and to modulate pain.
- Compression, like elevation, is used to limit the amount of edema that accumulates in the hand and wrist.
- Minimizing wrist and hand use.

24-HOUR SYMPTOM PATTERN

- As with most fractures, initially pain will be experienced most of the day and night. Patients will complain of a deep achiness in the wrist, and this pain will increase during the first 72 hours as the inflammatory phase peaks. Nocturnal achiness is common with fractures.
- As the fracture heals, achiness at night and with weather changes is still common. Morning stiffness that lasts over 30 minutes is not uncommon.
- Increased swelling and edema is normal at the end of the day and depends on use. As edema increases, it is not uncommon for patients to complain of achiness or tightness in the wrist.

PAST HISTORY FOR THE REGION

- In older individuals, history of osteopenia or osteoporosis is common.
- May have history of long-term use of steroids or other bone-weakening medications.

PHYSICAL EXAMINATION

- Pain in the wrist; generally pain and tenderness is located in the distal 2 inches of the radius or ulna. Pain will correlate with the location of the fracture, although the longer the time since injury, the more secondary and remote sites will be hypersensitized by the production of inflammation.
- Inability to move wrist is experienced partly because of muscle guarding and partly because bony obstructions may prevent normal joint mechanics.
- Dinner-fork wrist deformity is common because of the posterior displacement of the wrist and hand in relationship to the remainder of the proximal forearm.
- Edema will be prevalent, especially in the acute phase. Muscle atrophy in the forearm will be noticed after casting. Edema may be present in the wrist even after several weeks of casting, but this edema is present secondary to disuse rather than from tissue injury.
- Bruising will be present acutely after a wrist fracture. Bone structures are highly vascularized, and injury to the tissue will result in damage to vascular structures. The damage to vascularized tissue will result in bruising.

IMPORTANT OBJECTIVE TESTS

Distal radius fracture is usually diagnosed with radiographs. Nondisplaced fractures may sometimes require CT scans.

DIFFERENTIAL DIAGNOSIS

- Although radiographs generally make differential diagnosis straightforward, other diagnoses to consider would include the following:
  - Scaphoid fracture
  - Ligament injury around the carpals
  - Fracture of the distal ulna (uncommon in isolation)
  - Triangular fibrocartilage complex tear
  - Distal radioulnar joint dislocation
- These pathologies may also occur in conjunction with distal radius fracture.

TREATMENT

SURGICAL OPTIONS

- Simple, stable fractures that can be reduced manually may require only casting.
- Unstable fractures may require percutaneous pinning or open reduction and hardware fixation.
- The success of surgery depends on the severity of the fracture (displacement, angulation, degree of bone compression, and whether the fracture is intraarticular or extraarticular) and the absence or presence of associated injuries.
- Surgery may be indicated if there is loss of bone length, unacceptable malalignment, or fracture into the joint, or if the fracture cannot be stabilized with a cast after closed reduction.

REHABILITATION

- The rehabilitation plan will be guided by the examination findings. Pain can be addressed with modalities, gentle manual techniques, and splinting for rest. When hypersensitivity is present, a desensitization program is indicated. Stiffness may benefit from joint and soft tissue mobilization and therapeutic exercise. Weakness will also respond to therapeutic exercise.
- The exercise program should start with gentle active and passive motion of the wrist, forearm, and fingers. Active and passive flexion of the finger MCP joints in the maximum-tolerated range, including while the patient is casted, is important; this can prevent or decrease contractures that will be very difficult to correct once established.

PROGNOSIS

- In younger persons, the primary predisposing factors are lifestyle choices (e.g., participation in sports such as rollerblading or snowboarding). In older persons, impaired balance and osteopenia create increased risk of wrist fracture.
- Although the severity of the fracture must be considered, most patients will recover most or all of lost function and have little or no pain within one year following injury.

SIGNS AND SYMPTOMS INDICATING REFERRAL TO PHYSICIAN

Any indications of a distal radius fracture require immediate referral to a physician. If the injury is seen acutely, the patient should be encouraged to remove any rings from the fingers; otherwise, swelling may later necessitate that the rings be cut off.

SUGGESTED READINGS

Haentjens P, Johnell O, Kanis JA, et al. Evidence from data searches and life-table analyses for gender-related differences in absolute risk of hip fracture after Colles' or spine fracture: Colles' fracture as an early and sensitive marker of skeletal fragility in white men. *J Bone Miner Res.* 2004;19:1933-1944.

Hanel DP, Jones MD, Trumble TE. Wrist fractures. *Orthop Clin North Am.* 2002;33(1):35-57.

Ismail AA, Pye SR, Cockerill WC, Lunt M, Silman AJ, et al. Incidence of limb fracture across Europe: results from the European Prospective Osteoporosis Study (EPOS). *Osteoporos Int.* 2002;13:565-571.

Owen RA, Melton LJ 3rd, Jonson KA, Ilstrup DM, Riggs BL. Incidence of Colles' fracture in a North American community. *Am J Public Health.* 1982;72:605-607.

AUTHORS: ROBIN BURKS and DERRICK SUEKI

BASIC INFORMATION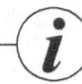

DEFINITION

Irritation of the extensor pollicis brevis (EPB) and abductor pollicis longus (APL) tendons on the radiodorsal aspect of the wrist

SYNONYMS

- Stenosing tenosynovitis of the first dorsal compartment
- Radial styloid tenosynovitis

ICD-9CM CODE
727.04 Radial styloid tenosynovitis

OPTIMAL NUMBER OF VISITS

8 visits

MAXIMAL NUMBER OF VISITS

18 visits

ETIOLOGY

- Pathologically, de Quervain's tenosynovitis refers to chronic irritation of the EPB and APL tendons as they pass deep to the extensor retinaculum in the first dorsal compartment.
- The pathology occurs secondary to overuse or misuse, often the result of a change in customary use patterns for the wrist and thumb, and leads to inflammation. The condition may be precipitated by discrete trauma, such as a blow to the wrist, but onset is usually gradual.
- Initially, physical irritation results in acute inflammation of the tendon sheath. Over time, chronic degenerative changes develop as a result of this inflammation, leading to tendinosis.

EPIDEMIOLOGY AND DEMOGRAPHICS

This relatively common problem is equally frequent in people of all races but is somewhat more common in women than men.

MECHANISM OF INJURY

Repeated wrist radial deviation and/or thumb palmar or radial abduction, especially under load.

COMMON SIGNS AND SYMPTOMS

Pain in the radial aspect of the wrist, especially over the involved tendons, refers into the thumb and up the radial side of the forearm.

AGGRAVATING ACTIVITIES

Activities involving wide grip and resistance to ulnar deviation such as pouring from a bottle of milk, using a hammer, or lifting an infant.

EASING ACTIVITIES

- Rest
- Ice
- Splinting (thumb spica)
- Possibly heat, if chronic
- Avoiding aggravating activities

24-HOUR SYMPTOM PATTERN

Symptoms are generally worse with activity and may seem worse at night when distractions are absent.

PAST HISTORY FOR THE REGION

- Recurrent episodes are common.
- Work requiring aggravating activities is often cited.
- Onset in women after the birth of a child is probably caused by altered hand use in lifting the infant and positioning for breast feeding.

PHYSICAL EXAMINATION

- Tenderness over the involved tendons may be severe.
- Resisted use of the involved tendons will be painful.
- There may be visible or palpable edema in the radial side of the wrist.

IMPORTANT OBJECTIVE TESTS

Finkelstein's test, which involves active flexion of the thumb into the palm, closing a fist over it, and then ulnarly deviating the wrist, is the gold standard for testing de Quervain's tenosynovitis.

DIFFERENTIAL DIAGNOSIS

- Scaphoid fracture
- Scapholunate dissociation
- Thumb CMP joint arthritis
- Intersection syndrome
- Local radial sensory nerve irritation
- Radial nerve impingement in the arm
- C6 radiculopathy

CONTRIBUTING FACTORS

Wearing constrictive watches or bracelets may increase irritation on the tendons.

TREATMENT

SURGICAL OPTIONS

- The usual surgery is a release of the first dorsal compartment.
- Surgery is often successful but technically challenging.
- Problems include failure to release all slips of the tendon, injury to the superficial radial nerve, and tendon adhesions in the scar bed.
- Surgery should be considered if 6 to 8 conservative treatments do not relieve symptoms at least 75%.

REHABILITATION

- Without surgery, the most important single aspect of treatment is protecting the tendons from stress through activity modification and splinting (thumb spica splint). Modalities, including heat, ice, ultrasound, and iontophoresis with dexamethasone, play a secondary role in recovery.
- After surgery, the patient may need a splint to protect the area while healing. Activity modification remains important to prevent recurrence. Scar mobilization and joint mobilization may assist in restoration of motion, as may therapeutic exercises. Gentle strengthening of EPB and APL will minimize scarring around the tendons.
- Initially, exercise may worsen the condition until the inflammation has been controlled.
- Later in recovery or when tendinosis is suspected, careful progression of eccentric palmar abduction exercises for the thumb may be helpful.

PROGNOSIS

- De Quervain's tenosynovitis may resolve if treated promptly and if biomechanical aggravating factors are well controlled.
- Recurrences are common, probably a result of the patient returning to prior provocative activities.

SIGNS AND SYMPTOMS INDICATING REFERRAL TO PHYSICIAN

The patient should be referred to a physician if the symptoms started after a fall (scaphoid injury should be ruled out) or if conservative treatment is not producing marked improvement in a few weeks.

SUGGESTED READINGS

Foye PM, Stitik TP. DeQuervain tenosynovitis. Retrieved April 21, 2008 http://www.emedicine.com/pmr/TOPIC36.HTM; 2006.

AUTHOR: ROBIN BURKS

Section III   ORTHOPEDIC PATHOLOGY

BASIC INFORMATION

DEFINITION

Dupuytren's contracture is a benign, slowly progressive fibroproliferative disease of the palmar fascia that has no clear etiology or pathogenesis.

SYNONYMS

- Dupuytren's disease
- Palmar fasciitis
- Palmar fibromatosis
- Viking disease

ICD-9CM CODE
728.6 Contracture of the palmar fascia

OPTIMAL NUMBER OF VISITS

5 visits

MAXIMAL NUMBER OF VISITS

15 visits

ETIOLOGY

- Dupuytren's contracture is an autosomal dominant disease, characterized by fibroblast proliferation and collagen deposition. It is not known why the uncontrolled proliferation of palmar fascia begins and why it continues to the point of debilitating flexion contractures.
- The pathognomonic feature of Dupuytren's contracture is a firm nodule in the palm, often found near the distal palmar crease. Multiple nodules are common and may or may not be tender to palpation.
- Nodules are a result of fibroblast and myofibroblast proliferation. The palmar skin becomes pitted and thick with the progressive contracture of the underlying subcutaneous tissue.
- With disease progression, cords begin to develop proximal to the nodules.
- Advanced disease is characterized by the regression of nodules and progression of MCP and PIP joint contractures. The fibrosis of the palmar fascia creates tendon-like cords adhering to underlying structures such as tendon sheaths.

EPIDEMIOLOGY AND DEMOGRAPHICS

- Males are more likely to be affected than females. The male disease also tends to be more severe.
- Dupuytren's disease is very common in northern Europe, the United Kingdom, and in countries inhabited by immigrants from these areas such as Australia, Canada, and the US.
- Approximately 5% to 15% of males older than 50 years of age are affected

in the US, reflecting immigration from Northern Europe.
- In Norway, approximately 5.6% of individuals older than 60 years are affected.
- In Australia, 26% of males and 20% of females older than 60 years are affected.
- Incidence of Dupuytren's disease is less than 3% in blacks and Asians.
- Among Indians, Native Americans, and individuals of Hispanic descent, the incidence of Dupuytren's disease is less than 1%.
- Increased severity of disease is associated with an earlier age of initial presentation.
- Dupuytren's contracture most often affects the ring and small fingers.

MECHANISM OF INJURY

There is no common physical reason to develop Dupuytren's disease, since it has a genetic predisposition. However, it can be triggered by a fall onto the hand.

COMMON SIGNS AND SYMPTOMS

- Nodules in the hand are normally not painful.
- Flexion contracture of the MCP or PIP joints.

AGGRAVATING ACTIVITIES

- Patient with MCP contractures of 30 degrees or more complain of the following:
  ○ Difficultly shaking hands
  ○ Difficulty getting their finger in and out of pockets

EASING ACTIVITIES

Attempts to stop the progression of this contracture via splinting have failed.

PAST HISTORY FOR THE REGION

Some research has shown trauma to the hand may trigger development of a contracture.

PHYSICAL EXAMINATION

- Firm nodules that may be tender to palpation
- Painless, tendon-like cords proximal to the nodules
- Skin blanching on active finger extension
- Atrophic grooves or pits in the skin, denoting adherence to the underlying fascia
- Presence of MCP or PIP joint contractures

IMPORTANT OBJECTIVE TESTS

- Tabletop test
  ○ Place the palm on a table. If the hand can flatten onto the table, then no surgical intervention should be needed.

If the palm cannot reach the table, MCP or PIP joint contractures are demonstrated, indicating that surgical intervention should be considered.

DIFFERENTIAL DIAGNOSIS

Palmar tendinitis

CONTRIBUTING FACTORS

Risk factors may include prior hand trauma, alcoholism, smoking, diabetes mellitus, and thyroid conditions.

TREATMENT

SURGICAL INDICATORS

- MCP joint contracture of 30 degrees or more. When the MCP joint is involved, surgical intervention is not urgent because even long-standing and severe contractures of the MCP joint are usually corrected readily after surgery and usually do not recur.
- PIP joint contractures do not carry the same prognosis because more than one fascial band causes this contracture. Removing the involved fascia may not correct the joint contracture, particularly those of long duration. Patients should be informed that surgery can improve but may not completely correct the contracture.
- Functional disability is a subjective symptom that may be an indication for surgery. It is essential the patient clearly understands the potential morbidity and that the process is occasionally exacerbated by the operation.

SURGICAL OPTIONS

- The goal of surgical intervention is to excise the diseased fascia to make the hand functional for the patient. This treatment does not cure the disease but is meant to prevent progression to severe debilitating joint contractures.
- Fasciotomy is a surgery performed with local anesthesia. A stab wound is made, which blindly cuts the contracted fascia. This procedure can be more thorough when an incision over the diseased cord is made to visualize and dissect the diseased fascia.
- Regional fasciotomy involves removing the involved fascia and may provide short-term relief but is also associated with a very high recurrence rate. This procedure may correct an MCP joint contracture but almost certainly will not correct a PIP joint deformity. This procedure should be reserved for elderly or debilitated patients who are unable to tolerate a more lengthy procedure.

- Extensive fasciectomy involves removing as much fascia as possible, including the grossly normal. Today, this procedure is not commonly performed because of the increased associated morbidity, including hematoma risk and prolonged postoperative edema and stiffness. Some authors prefer to leave the skin wound open to heal by secondary intention as a means of decreasing hematoma risk.
- Dermofasciectomy removes the diseased fascia and the overlying skin. Resurface the wound with a full-thickness skin graft. Recurrence rates are quite low with this approach. Because of the radical nature of this procedure, it is usually reserved for patients with recurrent or severe disease.

SURGICAL OUTCOMES

- Long-term overall recurrence is approximately 50% and can be in the same area of the hand or in a new area.
- MCP joint contractures are readily corrected with surgery and usually do not recur.
- PIP joint contractures are usually not completely corrected and are occasionally exacerbated by surgery.

REHABILITATION

- Postsurgical
  - Preoperative hand therapy management of Dupuytren's contracture with modalities or splinting is not supported by scientific evidence.
  - Postoperative rehabilitation is a gradual process of increasing activity and decreased splinting to achieve optimal restoration of movement. Frequent visits to a hand therapist help restore preoperative flexion and maintain extension gained at the time of surgery is vital to the recovery process. Edema control, wound care, and scar management are also essential.
  - A hand-based dorsal or volar splint is used to keep the fingers and hand open while the wound heals. This should be removed three times per day for AROM and PROM of the fingers.
  - Postoperative splinting can also be used to statically progress remaining flexion contractures at the PIP joint.
  - After surgery the splint must be worn 24 hours a day. It should only be removed for wound care and ROM. After 3 weeks, weaning from the splint may begin at the discretion of the hand therapist and surgeon. Be sure that the patient is provided with adequate oral analgesics to promote comfort and therapy compliance.
  - Final results are realized in approximately 6 weeks. After this period, patients should wear the splint only at night for an additional 3 to 6 months, at the discretion of the hand therapist and surgeon. This is important to maintain extension and prevent scar contracture. Silicone gel sheets and scar massage are useful adjuncts to promote scar softening and maturation.

PROGNOSIS

Experiments are being performed with enzyme injections that may be able to break down the tough bands and improve motion without surgery. Early results are promising, but these injections are not available for general use at this time.

SIGNS AND SYMPTOMS INDICATING REFERRAL TO PHYSICIAN

- If a painful lump is present, an injection from a physician may help diminish the pain.
- If contractures have developed that cause the patient to lose functional use of the hand, the patient should be referred to a physician.

SUGGESTED READINGS

Shaw RB Jr, Chong AK, Zhang A, Hentz VR, Chang J. Dupuytren's disease: history, diagnosis, and treatment. *Plast Reconstr Surg.* 2007;120(3):44e-54e.

Trojian TH, Chu SM. Dupuytren's disease: diagnosis and treatment. *Am Fam Physician.* 2007;76(1):86-89.

AUTHOR: AUDRA PONCI BADO

BASIC INFORMATION

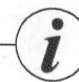

DEFINITION

Finger dislocation occurs when the two articular joint surfaces loose complete contact because of a traumatic force.

SYNONYMS

- Coach's finger
- Baseball finger
- "Jammed" finger

ICD-9CM CODE
834 Dislocation of finger

OPTIMAL NUMBER OF VISITS

3 visits

MAXIMAL NUMBER OF VISITS

15 visits

ETIOLOGY

- Finger dislocations occur from high-speed forces of hyperflexion, hyperextension, radial or ulnar stress, axial compression, or direct pressure.
- A dislocation may or may not involve a fracture.
- DIP joint dislocations are rare because of the stability of the collateral ligaments and the terminal attachments of the flexor and extensor tendons.
  - If the DIP joint does dislocate, it is most often dorsal and associated with an avulsion fracture.
- Dorsal PIP dislocations most commonly occur because of axial stress and hyperextension, causing failure of one or more of the collateral ligaments and the volar plate.
- An avulsion fracture of the middle phalanx is commonly a result of volar plate rupture from its insertion. This injury is frequently reduced on the athletic field before proper medical evaluation. It is essential that the dislocation is identified as dorsal, volar, or lateral to implement the correct splinting method for recovery.
- Volar PIP dislocations are rare and are usually associated with rupture of the central slip, collateral ligament, and volar plate. This may require surgical reduction and repair of the damaged soft tissue.
- MCP joint dislocations are more rare than PIP dislocations because of the increased mobility of the MCP joint and position at the base of the finger. The condyloid shape of the joint allows lateral mobility to dissipate disruptive forces. The collateral ligaments are taut only in flexion. This allows a more extended digit increased mobility.
  - When MCP dislocations occur, they are most common in the dorsal direction as a result of a hyperextension force. The volar plate and at least one of the collateral ligaments are usually ruptured.
  - The dislocation is often associated with a fracture of the MCP head.

EPIDEMIOLOGY AND DEMOGRAPHICS

Dorsal dislocations of the PIP joint of the second through fifth digits are the most common dislocations within the hand.

MECHANISM OF INJURY

- The finger is hit with a ball or another player during a sporting event.
- The finger is stepped on during a football game.

COMMON SIGNS AND SYMPTOMS

- Finger deformity
- Swelling
- Decreased ROM
- Pain over the affected joint

AGGRAVATING ACTIVITIES

- Movement of the dislocated digit
- Gripping
- Pinching
- Carrying objects

EASING ACTIVITIES

Reduction of the dislocated joint.

24-HOUR SYMPTOM PATTERN

If left untreated, the dislocated finger may demonstrate neurovascular changes, increased edema, and progressive stiffness.

PHYSICAL EXAMINATION

- Limited ROM of the finger
- Laxity or rupture of one or both collateral ligaments and/or volar plate
- Tenderness over the affected joint
- Deformity of the finger

IMPORTANT SUBJECTIVE INFORMATION

- Time of injury
- Exact position of the hand during the injury
- Direction of the traumatic force
- Interventions that were attempted such as number of relocation attempts
- Previous traumas to the finger
- Joint laxity from previous dislocations may predispose the joint to future dislocations

IMPORTANT OBJECTIVE TESTS

Radiographs

DIFFERENTIAL DIAGNOSIS

- Avulsion fracture
- Volar plate rupture
- Fracture
- Tendon rupture
- Central slip rupture (BD)

CONTRIBUTING FACTORS

- Participation in high-velocity and/or contact sporting events
- Systemic pathology, such as RA, Down syndrome, or SLE, may predispose a patient to dislocation because of joint laxity

TREATMENT

SURGICAL INDICATORS

- Indicators for surgery include the following:
  - PIP dorsal dislocations requiring more than 25 degrees of flexion to maintain reduction
  - Volar PIP dislocations with ruptures of the central slip
  - Joints not successfully reduced with closed reduction attempts
  - Fractures involving more than 30% of the articular surface
  - Delay in seeking proper treatment

SURGICAL OPTIONS

- PIP dorsal dislocation options may include dynamic skeletal traction, extension block pinning, force couple splinting, and volar plate arthroplasty.
- MCP dorsal dislocations may need surgical reduction to displace the volar plate lodged inside the MCP joint. This is normally done via a longitudinal incision through the volar plate.

REHABILITATION

- Goals of rehabilitation after a finger dislocation are as follows:
  - Maintain reduction of the joint
  - Maintain soft tissue gliding
  - Prevent swelling and edema
  - Maintain ROM with protected splinting
- DIP joint dislocation:
  - Closed reduction can usually be obtained with the DIP joint. Dorsal dislocations require immobilization in neutral or slight flexion for 1 to 2 weeks to maintain reduction. The joint should be protected for 4 to 6 weeks after the injury.
  - Volar dislocations of the DIP joint are treated as an avulsion fracture or mallet injury. Treatment requires extension immobilization for 4 to 6 weeks.

- PIP joint dislocation:
  - Dorsal closed reductions of the PIP joint can begin AROM using a dorsal extension block (DEB) splint. The MCP should be positioned in 30 degrees of flexion, and the IP joints blocked in full extension. This position will limit extension to 30 degrees to maintain the joint congruity.
  - The figure-of-eight splint is an example of a DEB that allows functional mobility of the hand while protecting the damaged joint.
  - Resultant flexion contractures after PIP joint dorsal dislocation are often misdiagnosed as a BD. With the extensor tendon intact, the DIP joint will remain flexible. This positioning is termed a pseudoboutonnière deformity.
  - Volar PIP joint dislocations usually involve rupture of the central slip and lateral bands. The PIP joint should be treated with immobilization splinting in full extension. Rehabilitation requires up to 6 weeks of PIP joint immobilization splinting or surgical repair of the tendon.
  - Central slip extensor tendon ruptures that go undiagnosed with PIP joint volar dislocations become BDs.

- MCP joint dislocation:
  - Dorsal MCP joint dislocations should be immobilized with a DEB splint in more than 50 degrees of flexion at the MCP joint. This position maintains the reduction and lengthens the collateral ligaments.
  - Full ROM of the IP joints and flexion of the MCP joint should be maintained during the immobilization. The joint should also be included in the DEB splint.
  - The buddy tape technique can be used to protect a dislocation for up to 3 months after initial injury.

- Potential complications after a finger dislocation:
  - If the dislocation is not reduced properly or reduction is delayed, the joint may have future instability, stiffness, or deformity.
  - Fractures are a common complication after overly aggressive attempts to reduce a finger dislocation.
  - Recurrent dislocations are common if the finger was not properly immobilized after the initial reduction.
  - Muscle contractures will result with a prolonged immobilization.
  - Infections may result from an open fracture not treated with antibiotics and tetanus prophylaxis.

PROGNOSIS

The more quickly the finger dislocation is properly assessed and treatment implemented, the less likely long-term complications will exist.

SIGNS AND SYMPTOMS INDICATING REFERRAL TO PHYSICIAN

An assessment from a hand surgeon is important for appropriate imaging studies and to rule out secondary injuries associated with the dislocation.

SUGGESTED READINGS

Leggit JC, Meko CJ. Acute finger injuries: Part I. Tendons and ligaments. *Am Fam Physician*. 2006;73(5):810–816.

Leggit JC, Meko CJ. Acute finger injuries: Part II. Fractures, dislocations, and thumb injuries. *Am Fam Physician*. 2006;73(5):827–834.

Zemel NP. Metacarpophalangeal joint injuries in fingers. *Hand Clin*. 1992;8(4):745–754.

AUTHOR: AUDRA PONCI BADO

Section III

ORTHOPEDIC PATHOLOGY

BASIC INFORMATION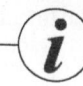

DEFINITION

A fracture is a complete or incomplete break in a bone because of a failure of the material.

SYNONYMS

- Phalanx fracture
- P1, P2, P3 fracture
- Phalangeal fractures
- Mallet fracture (see section on Mallet Finger)
- Boxer fracture (see section on Boxer's Fracture)

ICD-9CM CODES

816   Fracture of one or more phalanges of hand
815   Fracture of metacarpal bone(s)

OPTIMAL NUMBER OF VISITS

6 visits

MAXIMAL NUMBER OF VISITS

24 visits

ETIOLOGY

- Phalanx fractures are produced through axial compression or spiral or transverse forces on semiflexed or hyperextended digits. Fractures of the proximal phalanx are potentially the most disabling fractures in the hand; direct blows tend to cause transverse or comminuted fractures, whereas twisting injury may cause an oblique or spiral fracture.
- Proximal fragments are usually flexed by intrinsic muscles, whereas distal fragments are extended because of extrinsic compressive forces.
- A frequent complication of both proximal and middle phalanx fractures is the adhesion of the extensor mechanism causing loss of motion in the finger. These fractures can also damage the gliding surface of the flexor tendon sheath as a result of to periosteal injury.
- The periosteum of the bone forms the dorsal wall of the fibroosseous tunnel in which the tendon glides. Adhesion of the tunnel would result in loss of motion of the digit and potentially the entire hand.
- Tendons can also cause increased fracture instability from their opposite directions of pull. For example, a mallet fracture is due to the terminal tendon in avulsion from the DIP joint. A portion of the distal phalanx will move dorsal with the extensor tendon and a portion will move volar with the flexor tendon.

EPIDEMIOLOGY AND DEMOGRAPHICS

- Many different groups of people are prone to finger fractures. Children commonly have proximal phalanx base fractures from getting their fingers stuck in doors or drawers. The elderly sustain fractures from falls, 10- to 29-year-olds suffer fractures from sport-related injuries, and 40- to 69-year-olds fracture their fingers most frequently in machinery accidents.
- Middle phalanx fractures account for 8% to 12% of hand fractures.
- Distal phalanx fractures are reported as the most frequent of all hand fractures in adults at a rate of 40% to 50%.
- The proximal phalanx was the most frequently fractured bone among the phalanges in children.
- Salter-Harris fractures are unique to children as they are through the growth plate. The classification system is based on the site and extent of the injury and therefore can determine possible long-term complications.
- Salter-Harris type II is the most common injury. This describes a fracture where a piece of the metaphysis breaks off the epiphysis. The bone may have minimal shortening but will usually not result in functional limitations.

MECHANISM OF INJURY

A finger fracture usually occurs from hitting a hard object with the finger, being hit by a ball, getting the hand slammed in a door, or falling onto the hand. These injuries are common in ball-handling sports.

COMMON SIGNS AND SYMPTOMS

- Pain, decreased ROM
- Swelling
- Ecchymosis
- Finger deformity

AGGRAVATING ACTIVITIES

- Any movement that stresses the unstable bone will cause pain
- Gripping
- Pinching
- Lifting objects
- Carrying objects

EASING ACTIVITIES

Ice, elevation, and compression can help limit the edema associated with the fracture.

24-HOUR SYMPTOM PATTERN

If the fracture goes untreated, the pain and swelling will increase while the ROM begins to decrease.

PAST HISTORY FOR THE REGION

- The patient will report a trauma to the hand. It is extremely important to know exactly how the fracture occurred to determine the mechanism of fracture to realize the stability of the fragment.
- Patient may or may not report prior injury to the region.

PHYSICAL EXAMINATION

- Tenderness or pain over the site of fracture
- Ecchymosis
- Loss of ROM
- Rotational deformity is indicated if the fingers do not point toward the proximal portion of the scaphoid with the hand in a fist position

IMPORTANT OBJECTIVE TESTS

Stress radiography: It is important to have stress put through the fracture to determine the true stability of the bone. The periosteum can give the appearance of a stable fracture in a nonstressed image.

DIFFERENTIAL DIAGNOSIS

Pathological nontraumatic fracture (enchondroma)

CONTRIBUTING FACTORS

- High-velocity sports
- Osteoporosis or osteopenia
- Long-term use of the following:
  - Prednisone
  - Methotrexate
  - Corticosteroids

TREATMENT

SURGICAL INDICATORS

- Volarly angulated or condylar fracture
- Spiral oblique fractures are inherently unstable and require internal fixation
- Phalanx fractures involving more than 30% of the joint surface

SURGICAL OPTIONS

- Open reduction and internal fixation (ORIF) with screws and/or plates
- Intramedullary nailing
- Pin fixation
- External fixation

SURGICAL OUTCOMES

- Surgery can be extremely effective in terms of stabilizing the fracture.
- Research has reported complications such as plate fixation interfering with the extensor apparatus, faulty technique, and malunion.

REHABILITATION

- It is essential for the clinician to know the location, pattern, and stability of the fracture. Postoperatively the clinician should know the surgical intervention performed and the stability of the fragment.

- Generally speaking, stable, nonoperative fractures can begin protected AROM 1 to 3 weeks after injury. PROM for closed reductions can usually be initiated at 5 weeks once the surgeon believes that the fracture is sufficiently healed. Operative fixations allow for early movement at approximately 3 to 10 days after surgery, if the surgeon believes sufficient stabilization was achieved. After surgery, PROM should not normally begin for 6 to 8 weeks.

- A proximal phalanx fracture may require a hand-based splint with MCP flexed to 90 degrees and IP joints in full extension with a dorsal extension block. Full-fist ROM is allowed. Middle and at times proximal phalanx fractures will be sufficiently stabilized with a finger-based splint. This splint should remain on at all times, with the exception to remove for therapeutic exercise. Splinting can usually be discontinued by 4 to 6 weeks, unless the patient is participating in contact sports. Use of splinting and/or buddy taping may help maintain stabilization of the injury site with return to activity.

- Buddy taping is used for stable, nonangulated phalanx fractures. This technique encourages the patient to move the finger but keeps it protected while it heals.

- Taping technique can also be used to correct varus and valgus deformities of the finger.

- Fingers can be casted or splinted with the finger flexed or straight. When the finger is immobilized in an extended position, there must be at least 60 degrees of MCP joint flexion. This position can be used for stable fractures that require a reduction. Unstable, transverse fractures are immobilized in a flexed position.

REHABILITATIVE COMPLICATIONS OF FINGER FRACTURES

- Flexion contractures of the PIP joint are a serious complication after a proximal phalanx fracture. It is important to splint the PIP in extension to avoid this deformity. Contractures occur at this joint because of the large flexion force and relatively weak extensor forces.

- Another complication is tendon adherence, which is evident when the patient has limited AROM and full PROM extension of the finger. An important exercise is to limit MCP hyperextension to focus the extensor force at the PIP joint.

PROGNOSIS

Most simple finger fractures heal without any problem. If the fracture goes into a joint, the finger may continue to feel stiff and may lose some mobility.

SIGNS AND SYMPTOMS INDICATING REFERRAL TO PHYSICIAN

Because of the critical nature of early intervention with finger fractures, it is essential that the patient see a hand surgeon for accurate imaging and diagnosis.

SUGGESTED READINGS

Davis TR, Stothard J. Why all finger fractures should be referred to a hand surgery service: a prospective study of primary management. *J Hand Surg Br.* 1990;15:299-302.

Hardy MA. Principles of metacarpal and phalangeal fracture management: a review of rehabilitation concepts. *J Orthop Sports Phys Ther.* 2004;34:781-799.

AUTHOR: AUDRA PONCI BADO

Section III

ORTHOPEDIC PATHOLOGY

BASIC INFORMATION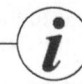

DEFINITION

Tendinopathy refers to pathology of the tendon. It can include tendinitis, tendinosis, or rupture of the flexor carpi ulnaris (FCU) tendon.

SYNONYMS

- FCU tendinitis
- FCU tendinosis
- FCU strain
- Calcific FCU

ICD-9CM CODE
726.9 Unspecified enthesopathy

OPTIMAL NUMBER OF VISITS

6 visits

MAXIMAL NUMBER OF VISITS

12 visits

ETIOLOGY

- Microscopic damage to the tendon causes an inflammatory response and degeneration to the tendon or tendon-muscle attachment.
- Tendons possess the highest tensile strength of any tissue in the body. This is in part a result of its high concentration of collagen and partly because of the parallel orientation of tendon fibers. As a result of this, tendons are designed to resist tensile loading, therefore other factors should be considered when assessing the root cause of tendon pathology.
- Tendonitis refers to the acute inflammatory response witnessed in tissue initially after injury to a tendon. Tendinosis refers to the degenerative process that occurs at a tendon as a result of repetitive injury, but unlike tendonitis, very little inflammation is seen with tendinosis.
- In a rehabilitation setting, the prevalence of tendinosis far outweighs the presence of tendonitis.
- The FCU is the only tendon at the wrist without a synovial sheath, and it is partially attached to the volar surface of the flexor retinaculum.
- The FCU inserts into the pisiform bone and then via ligaments into the hamate bone and fifth MC bone, acting to flex and adduct the wrist joint.
- Calcific tendinopathy is commonly seen just proximal to the tendon's insertion onto the pisiform bone.

EPIDEMIOLOGY AND DEMOGRAPHICS

- Racquet sports or other sports requiring ulnar deviation (e.g., baseball).

- Occupations that require repetitive ulnar deviation of the wrist (e.g., carpenters).
- Age: Immature tendons are generally weaker then mature tendons, and there is no significant difference in strength between mature tendons and old tendons. Therefore age does not appear to play a role in the occurrence of tendon pathology from a tissue perspective. Tendons are designed to maintain their strength through the lifespan. There is an increased likelihood of tendon pathology in youth because the tendons have yet to reach the strength they will gain at maturity.

MECHANISM OF INJURY

- Because tendons are designed to maintain their strength over time, the mechanism of injury is generally related to factors that may weaken or impact the performance of the tendon. The following should be considered:
- Extrinsic causes:
  - Overuse and repetitive strain
  - Compression loading
  - Prolonged exercise
  - Intense exercise
  - Immobilization
  - NSAIDs
- Intrinsic causes:
  - Endocrine (i.e., increased catecholamine and glucocorticoids)
  - Nutritional (i.e., iron or calcium deficiency)
  - Vascularity (i.e., decreased from diabetes)

COMMON SIGNS AND SYMPTOMS

Aching pain and swelling proximal to the pisiform and along the FCU tendon

AGGRAVATING ACTIVITIES

- Wrist flexion
- Ulnar deviation
- Exercise, increased activity, or movement with the involved extremity
- Gripping or lifting objects

EASING ACTIVITIES

- Activity avoidance
- Ice
- Antiinflammatory or pain medications
- Splinting of the wrist

24-HOUR SYMPTOM PATTERN

- Symptoms are related to movement.
- Generally, no stiffness or pain is noted at a specific time of day.
- Symptoms will increase with use of the involved tendon.

PAST HISTORY FOR THE REGION

- Repetitive movement or trauma to the involved upper extremity

- Past history of fracture of the wrist such as a Colles' type fracture.
- Fracture of the scaphoid or instability of the carpals may lead to increased force and demand at the ulnar aspect of the wrist.
- History of diabetes or RA.

PHYSICAL EXAMINATION

- Painful to palpation around the FCU tendon, pisiform, or distal insertion.
- Wrist flexion and ulnar deviation against resistance will be painful.
- Very little swelling will generally be present.

IMPORTANT OBJECTIVE TESTS

- Difficult to objectively confirm tendonitis.
- X-ray may reveal calcific deposits or spurring in the structure adjacent to the tendon.

DIFFERENTIAL DIAGNOSIS

- De Quervain's disease
- Tendonitis of other wrist flexors and extensors
- Pisotriquetral arthritis
- Ulnar neuritis
- Tendinosis, tenosynovitis

CONTRIBUTING FACTORS

- Training error.
- Lack of strength or flexibility.
- Malalignment.
- Tendon healing is affected by age. Vascular supply diminishes as one gets older.

TREATMENT

SURGICAL OPTIONS

- Surgery is generally not required, and most patient recover when treated conservatively. In cases where surgery is required, the following surgeries may be employed:
  - Removal of adhesions or degenerative tissue.
  - Repair of torn tissue.
  - In severe cases of tendon degeneration, fusion of the wrist may be considered a measure of last resort.

SURGICAL INDICATORS

Failed conservative management

REHABILITATION

- Tendinosis is a chronic condition. Some management of inflammation and pain is needed, but they are not generally the primary consideration. Focus should be on increasing strength, eliminating factors that may be causing compression and looking to other regions of the body that may be helping to perpetuate the problem.

- Relative rest is advisable early on. Patients may require splinting initially to decrease the load placed on the tendon. Especially when completing work or activities requiring use of the wrist and hand.
- Posture and positioning should be assessed to eliminate weakness that may contribute to excessive forces at the wrist.
- Although not specifically addressed or studied in literature, eccentric training of chronic tendon pathology has proved beneficial and should be considered as tissue irritability allows.

- ○ Gradually progressive strength and endurance program should be implemented.
- ○ Strengthening should progress from isometric to isotonic and then eccentric exercises.
- ○ High repetition exercises are not recommended.
- Gradual return to sport or activity as symptoms allow.

PROGNOSIS

Time to recovery depends on the ability of the patient to comply with conservative methods for decreasing stress to the area and stopping the inflammatory cascade. Once healing begins, it will take about 6 weeks for the body to go through the stages of healing.

SIGNS AND SYMPTOMS INDICATING REFERRAL TO PHYSICIAN

Any indication of tendon rupture such as the inability to flex or ulnarly deviate the wrist.

SUGGESTED READINGS

Finlay K, Friedman L. Common tendon and muscle injuries: Upper extremities. *Ultrasound Clinics*. 2007;2(4):577-594.

Uhl TL, Madaleno JA. Rehabilitation concepts and supportive devices for overuse injuries of the upper extremities. *Clin Sports Med*. 2001;20:621-639.

AUTHOR: AKEMI RICO

Section III

ORTHOPEDIC PATHOLOGY

BASIC INFORMATION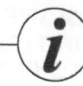

DEFINITION

- Disruption of any of the nine flexor tendons
- Classification into five zones is based on location of injury:
  - Zone 1: From insertion of the FDS in the middle phalanx to the insertion of the FDP in the base of distal phalanx.
  - Zone 2: From the fibrosseous tunnel at the A1 pulley to the FDS insertion; both FDS and FDP tendons travel together in this area.
  - Zone 3: From the distal border of the carpal tunnel to the proximal border of the A1 pulley; marked externally by the distal palmar crease, including both FDS and FDP tendons, lumbrical muscles, and common digital nerves and vessels.
  - Zone 4: Includes the carpal tunnel and all nine digital flexors and median nerve.
  - Zone 5: Includes the forearm from the musculotendinous junction of the extrinsic flexors to the proximal border of the transverse carpal ligament.

SYNONYM

Rupture of the FDP is also known as Jersey finger.

ICD-9CM CODES
883.2 Open wound of fingers with tendon involvement
882.2 Open wound of hand except fingers alone with tendon involvement
881.22 Open wound of wrist with tendon involvement

OPTIMAL NUMBER OF VISITS

6 visits

MAXIMAL NUMBER OF VISITS

24 visits

ETIOLOGY

- Tendon laceration is associated with an open injury and is often caused by puncture wounds or lacerations.
- Tendon ruptures are often associated with a closed injury and can be traumatic or the result of chronic friction. Disease processes or medications that weaken the tendons play major roles in the pathology. Neurovascular deficits can also work to weaken the tendon.
- The hand has a complex interplay of multiple tendons, pulleys, and joints. When injury occurs to one of the elements, the remainder of the systems in the region are usually impacted. As the pulley and sheath system loses its

structural integrity, centers of rotation for joints and lever arms of pull change. The result is often bowstringing of the tendons away from the bone.

EPIDEMIOLOGY AND DEMOGRAPHICS

- Flexor tendon lacerations and ruptures are common, although no resource was found that listed prevalence rates.
- Single tendon ruptures are more common than multiple tendon involvement.

MECHANISM OF INJURY

- Accidental laceration with broken glass, kitchen knives, or table saws; MVA; crush injury; or suicide attempt.
- Resisted digital flexion against a strong extensor force such as getting a finger caught in a jersey.
- Nontraumatic rupture: Chronic friction, which might occur with prolonged inflammatory tenosynovitis, rheumatoid pathology, Kienböck disease, scaphoid nonunion, hamate fracture, or Colles' fracture.

COMMON SIGNS AND SYMPTOMS

- Inability to flex one or more fingers
- Weakened grip strength
- Stiffness of adjoining joints
- Pain with digital ROM
- Open injury to the flexor side of the fingers, palm, wrist, or forearm
- Swelling and tenderness to palpation

AGGRAVATING ACTIVITY

Movement

EASING ACTIVITIES

- Rest
- Ice
- Immobilization via casting, taping, or splinting

24-HOUR SYMPTOM PATTERN

- Symptoms are related to movement of the injured hand.
- Some morning stiffness may be present but as inflammation resolves, stiffness will also resolve.

PAST HISTORY FOR THE REGION

- Working with sharp objects, mishandling of glass
- History of endocrine diseases
- History of steroid use

PHYSICAL EXAMINATION

- Suspected
  - Lack of digital flexion while squeezing the flexor muscles of the forearm
  - Absence of a tenodesis effect with flexion and extension of the wrist
  - Abnormal resting position of the digits
- Postoperative
  - Inspection of incision site and sutures

- Assess wound drainage, erythema, edema, odor, skin temperature, and vascularity.
- Palpation of forearm, wrist, hand, and fingers.
- Assess AROM and PROM of joints not restricted by postsurgical precautions.
- Strength assessment is contraindicated until after postoperative week 8.
- Assess tendon gliding and presence of adhesions.
- Assess sensory changes along dermatomes. Evaluation with Semmes-Weinstein monofilaments is indicated with history of nerve injury or trophic changes.
- Assess edema with circumferential measurement.

IMPORTANT OBJECTIVE TESTS

- X-ray to rule out fracture.
- Ultrasound or magnetic resonance imaging (MRI) to visualize the damage.
- Passively moving the wrist through flexion and extension results in extension and flexion of the digits, respectively. When intact, the normal tenodesis in the wrist will produce the movement of the fingers. If disrupted, the finger motion will not occur.
- Compression or squeezing of the forearm flexion muscles can be used to test the integrity of the flexor tendons in the hand. When the forearm is squeezed, the digits are drawn into flexion. This will not occur if the tendons are no longer intact.

DIFFERENTIAL DIAGNOSIS

- Digital fractures
- Muscle weakness caused by nerve pathology
- RA
- Osteoarthritis

CONTRIBUTING FACTORS

- Dangerous working conditions
- RA
- Endocrine diseases
- Steroid use

TREATMENT

SURGICAL INDICATORS

Based on functional loss or if greater than 60% of the tendon is lacerated, surgery is indicated for most flexor tendon laceration injuries.

SURGICAL OPTIONS

- The retracted ends of the tendons are retrieved and sutured.
- Method of suturing will vary, depending on the surgeon.

SURGICAL OUTCOMES

A delay between injury and surgical repair allows for the development of scar tissue and adhesions, reducing the likelihood of regaining full function. Ideally, the repair should be performed within 2 weeks of injury.

REHABILITATION

- Treatment and hand rehabilitation should be guided by tendon physiology and healing principles. Healing of the flexor tendon system has the following four stages:
  - Hemostasis involves clot formation, vasoconstriction, and platelet deposition. Healing is impacted by the fibrosis and adhesions that can occur as a result of clot formation.
  - Inflammation: Scar tissue and adhesions continue to be deposited. Inflammatory factors result in swelling, stiffness, and pain.
  - Proliferation is characterized by a marked rise in fibroblast proliferation occurring within 1 cm of the repair site. The proliferation phase lasts 2 to 28 days. Collagen deposition rises markedly and rapidly as the fibroblasts proliferate. Adhesions continue to form and mature.
  - Remodeling: Collagen fibers reorganize and strengthen in a pattern parallel to the uninjured tendon fibers. Begins at approximately 6 weeks after injury.
- The repaired tendons are weakest between 6 and 12 days postoperatively and continue to mature with time. With this in mind, care should be taken in rehabilitating all flexor tendon lacerations and ruptures. The primary goals of

the process are protection of the tendon and prevention of tendon adhesions. Strengthening is not a primary consideration initially. Strength will occur as function improves.

- Tendon gliding exercises and splinting are mainstays of early tendon repair rehabilitation.
- Zone 1: See Jersey Finger
- Zones 2 to 5:
  - Splinting may be used for weeks 1 to 4 maintaining the wrist in 20% to 30% flexion and 60% to 70% MCP flexion with IP joints in extension. A dorsal splint may be used until week 5 or 6.
  - Home exercise program should include a progression of tendon gliding at all joints.
  - AROM of the involved digits may be contraindicated until after week 4 unless specifically cleared for early active motion.
  - Resisted ROM can begin at 8 to 12 weeks.

REHABILITATIVE COMPLICATIONS OF FLEXOR TENDON LACERATION

- Restriction of AROM for at least 72 hours postsurgical repair is presumed to be beneficial in regards to reduction of edema and inflammation at the repair site.
- Adhesions, trigger finger, tendon rupture, and bowstringing are all possible complications.
- Modification to treatment may be necessary, depending on what additional structures are damaged, including the following:
  - Vincula, which provide nutritional support to flexor tendons in zones 1 and 2
  - Fracture, pulley, nerve, or vessel repair

  - Patient cognition necessary to comply with a home exercise program
  - Infection

PROGNOSIS

- Outcomes depend on type and severity of injury, timing of surgical repair, age and underlying health of the patient, and the ability of the patient to understand and comply with precautions and the home exercise program.
- Injuries with involvement of tendon, bone, nerve, and/or vessels have a poorer prognosis than simple laceration.
- Average expected recovery is the following:
  - 75% of grip strength
  - 77% of finger pressure
  - 75% of pinch strength
  - 76% of PIP motion
  - 75% of DIP motion

SIGNS AND SYMPTOMS INDICATING REFERRAL TO PHYSICIAN

Undiagnosed suspected laceration must be referred immediately to avoid development of adhesions and scarring.

SUGGESTED READINGS

Dovelle S, Heeter PK. The Washington regimen: rehabilitation of the hand following flexor tendon injuries. *Phys Ther*. 1989;69:1034–1040.

Groth GN. Current practice patterns of flexor tendon rehabilitation. *J Hand Ther*. 2005;18:169–174.

AUTHOR: AKEMI RICO

Section III

ORTHOPEDIC PATHOLOGY

BASIC INFORMATION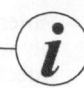

DEFINITION

A ganglion cyst is a fluid-filled lump that grows out of a joint or tendon sheath similar to a balloon on a stalk.

SYNONYM

Bible bump

> **ICD-9CM CODE**
> 727.4 Ganglion and cyst of synovium tendon and bursa

OPTIMAL NUMBER OF VISITS

2 visits

MAXIMAL NUMBER OF VISITS

8 visits

ETIOLOGY

- Ganglion cysts are usually attached to a nearby joint or tendon sheath. This condition is due to a defect in the synovium or joint capsule, but the exact cause of a ganglion is unknown.
- Dorsal wrist ganglions are more common than volar.
- Ganglions often change in size with increased activity and may even spontaneously disappear.
- Ganglion cysts are not malignant.
- The cyst contains a thick, clear, mucus-like fluid similar to the fluid found in the joint.

EPIDEMIOLOGY AND DEMOGRAPHICS

- Ganglion cysts occur most often in the 20 to 60 age group.
- Women are three times more likely than men to develop a ganglion cyst.

MECHANISM OF INJURY

There are no known causes for ganglion cysts; however, they may result from increased repetitive use of wrist or finger flexion activity.

COMMON SIGNS AND SYMPTOMS

- Nail deformities may occur as the result of a ganglion from the DIP joint.
- Blister-like bump gets large with activity and shrinks with rest.
- A ganglion cyst can be quite painful if it presses on nerves, even if the cyst is quite small. In contrast, a large cyst without nerve involvement may be completely painless.

AGGRAVATING ACTIVITIES

- Waiting tables.
- Gymnastics.
- Weight lifting.

- Playing musical instruments.
- Irritation of a ganglion depends on where it develops. A cyst on the dorsal wrist could be irritated with wrist extension, whereas a cyst that develops from the flexor tendon sheath could be irritated with finger flexion activity.

EASING ACTIVITIES

- Resting the involved ganglion joint may decrease pain and may reduce the size of the cyst.
- Immobilization of the wrist or fingers with splinting is an effective way to allow the joint to rest.

24-HOUR SYMPTOM PATTERN

Ganglions may be smaller and less painful in the morning. The afternoon and evening hours may bring more pain as a result of increased activity of the affected joint.

PAST HISTORY FOR THE REGION

There is no common past history for the development of a ganglion.

PHYSICAL EXAMINATION

- Blister-like bumps may or may not be painful.
- Ganglion cysts occur 60% to 70% of the time on the dorsal side of the wrist. They can also be found on the volar wrist, proximal volar side of the finger, or on the base of the fingernail just below the cuticle.
- The ganglia that arise from small joints, such as the DIP, are the result of osteoarthritis.
- Volar retinacular ganglia arise from the flexor sheath of fingers or the thumb. These ganglia can be closely associated with digital nerves and can make treatment more difficult.

IMPORTANT OBJECTIVE TESTS

Usually the diagnosis can be easily made from the appearance and location of the cyst. A hand surgeon may wish to obtain radiographs to look for associated joint abnormalities.

DIFFERENTIAL DIAGNOSIS

- Arthritis
- Bone tumor
- MC boss

CONTRIBUTING FACTORS

- Possible genetic predisposition
- Gender
- Osteoarthritis
- Repetitive use

TREATMENT

SURGICAL INDICATORS

A ganglion cyst that has failed multiple aspirations, remains painful, limits activity, or that has an appearance unacceptable to the patient may warrant surgical removal.

SURGICAL OPTIONS

- The ganglion cyst can be removed in outpatient surgery. This procedure includes removing the outer shell and cauterizing the stalk of the ganglion so that it may never reform and reappear.
- Aspiration is an office procedure conducted by the hand surgeon. The area around the cyst is numbed, and a needle is used to puncture the ganglion and drain the fluid. Recurrence is common after one aspiration; however, research has shown three or more aspirations have an 85% cure rate.

SURGICAL OUTCOMES

- Surgical removal of a ganglion cyst has a lower recurrence rate than aspiration; however, this does not guarantee the cyst will not return in the future.
- Research suggests that surgical removal of the cyst can cause additional problems for the patient such as joint instability and persistent symptoms.

REHABILITATION

- Typically, rehabilitation for a ganglion cyst is unnecessary. The majority of patients only require explanation that the cyst is benign. Nearly half of all ganglions can disappear without any treatment at all. It is important to continue observation of the cyst to make sure that no unusual changes occur.
- Initial exercises
  - Immobilization is a safe and effective way to reduce pain and appearance of the ganglion cyst. Activity often causes the ganglion to increase in size. This increase in size is due to increased pressure on nerves, causing pain. A wrist brace or splint may relieve symptoms by allowing the ganglion to decrease in size.
- Postsurgical
  - A bulky compressive dressing will be applied after surgery. Gentle AROM exercise can be initiated to avoid stiffness of the joint. A custom splint may be fabricated to provide rest for the joint once the surgical dressing is removed. Usual recovery time for ganglion cysts ranges from 2 to 3 weeks for small ganglions of the finger and 6 to 8 weeks for ganglions involving the wrist.

PROGNOSIS

The exact cause for ganglions in unknown; however, vocations or hobbies that force the wrist and hand into extreme positions may increase a person's chance of a cyst. Many cysts will resolve spontaneous and others will be present long term. Even if cysts are aspirated, many cysts will reappear spontaneously.

SIGNS AND SYMPTOMS INDICATING REFERRAL TO PHYSICIAN

If any unusual changes are observed in the cyst, referral to a hand surgeon is rec-ommended. It may also be beneficial to the patient to see a hand surgeon to provide imaging to rule out abnormal anatomy under the skin causing the cyst to become painful.

SUGGESTED READINGS

Mehdian H, McKee MD. Scapholunate instability following dorsal wrist ganglion excision: a case report. *Iowa Orthop J.* 2005;25:203-206.

Stephen AB, Lyons AR, Davis TR. A prospective study of two conservative treatments for ganglia of the wrist. *J Hand Surg Br.* 1999;24(1):104-105.

Zubowicz VN, Ishii CH. Management of ganglion cysts of the hand by simple aspiration. *J Hand Surg Am.* 1987;12(4):618-620.

AUTHOR: AUDRA PONCI BADO

BASIC INFORMATION

DEFINITION

Intersection syndrome is a tenosynovitis that primarily affects the radial wrist extensors. The condition is so-named because symptoms present near the "intersection" of the extensor carpi radialis brevis (ECRB) and extensor carpi radialis longus (ECRL) muscles and the overlying muscle bellies of the extensor pollicis brevis (EPB) and APL.

SYNONYMS

- Tenosynovitis of the radial wrist extensors
- Peritendinitis crepitans
- Subcutaneous perimyositis
- Crossover syndrome
- Oarsman syndrome
- Bugaboo forearm
- Squeaker's wrist

ICD-9CM CODE
727.05 Other tenosynovitis of hand and wrist

OPTIMAL NUMBER OF VISITS
4 visits

MAXIMAL NUMBER OF VISITS
12 visits

ETIOLOGY

- The EPB and APL muscles lie dorsal to the tendons of the ECRB and ECRL approximately 4 cm proximal to the carpal joint line
- This point lies just superior to Lister's tubercle and is where the wrist and thumb tendons and muscles "intersect" or "crossover" each other
- Because of the close proximity, repetitive use of the wrist extensors can cause friction trauma to their synovial sheaths and concurrent irritation of the overlying EPB and EPL

EPIDEMIOLOGY AND DEMOGRAPHICS

- Intersection syndrome is found about equally in males and females.
- Canoeists, skiers, and weightlifters have the highest incidence of the disorder.

MECHANISM OF INJURY

- Repetitive extension of the wrist as occurs in weightlifting, shoveling, rowing, and raking.
- Intersection syndrome is also found in tennis players and downhill skiers who are inclined to "plant" or drag their ski poles in deep snow, thereby increasing resistance to wrist extension.

COMMON SIGNS AND SYMPTOMS

- Pain with thumb extension and abduction
- Pain with wrist extension
- Crepitus with wrist movements
- Redness and edema
- "Squeaky" feeling during wrist movements

AGGRAVATING ACTIVITIES

- Repeated wrist extension
- Repeated ulnar/radial deviation, pronation, supination
- Pressure over the distal portion of the dorsal wrist and forearm
- Activities such as rowing, raking, shoveling, skiing, and weightlifting

EASING ACTIVITIES

- Rest and modified activities that decrease wrist extension and other wrist movements
- Ice and elevation

24-HOUR SYMPTOM PATTERN

- Although there is no typical 24-hour variation in symptoms, the associated pain and swelling may increase throughout the day as a result of cumulative use.
- Early morning pain and swelling may result from immobility.

PAST HISTORY FOR THE REGION

- Recent increase in activities that involve resisted wrist movements
- Involvement in rowing, racket sports, or skiing

PHYSICAL EXAMINATION

- Palpation along the dorsal aspect of the wrist will reveal tenderness and swelling approximately 4 cm distal to Lister's tubercle.
- The pain of de Quervain's syndrome will be localized more radially toward the base of the thumb.
- Guarding and pain may limit active and to a lesser extent passive movements of the wrist in all directions, especially in the sagittal plane.

IMPORTANT OBJECTIVE TESTS

- First CMC grind test to rule out involvement of CMC
- Finkelstein's test to rule out de Quervain's syndrome
- Tinel's test of the radial nerve to rule out Wartenberg syndrome
- Watson's test (scaphoid shift)

DIFFERENTIAL DIAGNOSIS

- De Quervain's tenosynovitis
- Arthritis of the first CMC
- Fracture of radial styloid

- Fracture of the scaphoid or scapholunate separation
- Wartenberg syndrome

CONTRIBUTING FACTORS

- Prior tendinopathies
- Preexisting circulatory problems
- Inflammatory disorders
- Advanced age

SURGICAL OPTIONS

- Surgery is not necessary except in rare instances.
- The most common surgical option is a tenosynovectomy of the ECRL and ECRB.
- After tenosynovectomy, the thumb is placed in a volar spica splint for 1 to 2 weeks, and physical or occupational therapy is initiated.
- Surgery is usually an effective option when conservative treatments are not.

TREATMENT

REHABILITATION

- Use of modalities, heat, ice, and electrical stimulation to control swelling and pain.
- Splinting to facilitate healing and prevent exacerbation during the acute stages of healing (most commonly a spica splint with a bias toward 20 to 30 degrees of extension).
- 2 to 4 weeks of splinting will allow adequate healing in uncomplicated cases; however, healing depends on age and abstention from overuse of the wrist musculature.
- Focus of treatment should be regaining and maintaining ROM through passive and active movement of the thumb and wrist.
- As pain and symptoms subside, strengthening of the wrist and thumb should commence with isometrics, followed by gentle contractions against gravity with progression to very light resistance.

PROGNOSIS

- Typically, a 3-week course of splinting will lead to symptom resolution in 60% of patients.
- The majority of patients will find relief within a few months.

SIGNS AND SYMPTOMS INDICATING REFERRAL TO PHYSICIAN

- Lack of progress with conservative care
- Complications due to splint use
- Suspicion of an undiagnosed fracture

SUGGESTED READINGS

Dobyns JH, Sim FH, Linscheid RL. Sports stress syndromes of the hand and wrist. *Am J Sports Med.* 1978;6:236-254.

Hanlon DP, Luellen JR. Intersection syndrome: a case report and review of the literature. *J Emerg Med*. 1999;17(6):969-971.

de Lima J, Kim HJ, Albertotti F, Resnick D. Intersection syndrome: MR imaging with anatomic comparison of the distal forearm. *Skeletal Radiol*. 2004;33(11):627-631.

Pantukosit S, Petchkrua W, Stiens SA. Intersection syndrome in Buriram Hospital: a 4-yr prospective study. *Am J Phys Med Rehabil*. 2001;80(9):656-661.

Parellada AJ, Gopez AG, Morrison WB, et al. Distal intersection tenosynovitis of the wrist: a lesser-known extensor tendinopathy with characteristic MR imaging features. *Skeletal Radiol*. 2007;36(3):203-208. Epub 2006 Dec 20.

Verdon ME. Overuse syndromes of the hand and wrist. *Prim Care*. 1996;23(2):305-319.

AUTHOR: SON TRINH

BASIC INFORMATION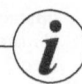

DEFINITION

- Rupture or avulsion of the flexor digitorum profundus (FDP).
- Classification is based on how far the tendon retracts, which in turn will affect the success of surgical repair.
  - A type I injury retracts all the way to the palm. The vincula brevis and longus are ruptured and blood supply is interrupted. Extensive scarring can develop within the tendinous sheath, therefore surgical repair is indicated within 7 to 10 days.
  - Type II retracts to the PIP joint. The long vinculum may still be intact, and a small chip of bone may be avulsed with the tendon. The avulsed end may become entrapped at the flexor digitorum superficialis (FDS) chiasma, causing a flexion contracture.
  - Type III occurs when a bony fragment is avulsed and remains attached to the tendon, which is then unable to retract through the A4 pulley. The tendon remains in the synovial sheath.

SYNONYMS

- FDP avulsion
- Rugby finger

ICD-9CM CODES
727.6 Rupture of tendon nontraumatic
883.2 Open wound of fingers with tendon involvement

OPTIMAL NUMBER OF VISITS

6 visits

MAXIMAL NUMBER OF VISITS

24 visits

ETIOLOGY

- Rupture or avulsion of the FDP tendon can occur during activities that require sustained digital flexion against forceful or unexpected resistance, resulting in hyperextension of the DIP joint and rupture of the FDP tendon.
- Rupture of the FDP tendon commonly occurs when an athlete's finger catches on another player's clothing in sports such as football.

EPIDEMIOLOGY AND DEMOGRAPHICS

Ring finger (fourth digit) is the most common involvement. It is the weakest and accounts for 75% of all cases.

MECHANISM OF INJURY

- Forceful passive extension of the digit while the FDP is in maximal contraction.

- The injury causes forced extension of the DIP joint during active flexion and can occur if the force is concentrated at the middle phalanx or at the distal phalanx.
- Sports such as the following:
  - Football
  - Rugby

COMMON SIGNS AND SYMPTOMS

- Pain
- Swelling
- Inability to flex the PIP joint

AGGRAVATING ACTIVITIES

- Movement of the affected finger
- Gripping
- Lifting activities
- Shaking hands

EASING ACTIVITIES

- Rest
- Splinting
- Ice

24-HOUR SYMPTOM PATTERN

- Pain consistent with movement (e.g., lifting or weight bearing with the affected hand).
- If left untreated, inflammation can lead to fibrosis of the FDP tendon and quadriga.

PAST HISTORY FOR THE REGION

- There may be a history of repetitive movements requiring flexion against resistance.
- Trauma caused by a sudden unexpected force that occurs while trying to maintain a grip on a rope, such as might occur while restraining a dog on a leash, or holding onto a jersey during a football game.
- Tendon may have been weakened by steroid use or disease processes that weaken tendon integrity.

PHYSICAL EXAMINATION

- A patient with jersey finger may present with pain and swelling at the palmar aspect of the DIP joint.
- The finger may be extended with the hand at rest because of lack of flexor counterforce.
- There may be a tender fullness or lump if the tendon has been retracted.
- Palpation to the involved palm will be painful and may reveal the retracted distal end of the ruptured tendon.

IMPORTANT OBJECTIVE TESTS

- The integrity of the FDP tendon can be tested by stabilizing the MCP and PIP joints in extension while having the patient attempt to flex the DIP. If the patient is unable to flex the DIP, the tendon is ruptured.

- The FDS tendon can be evaluated and differentiated from the profundus by holding the unaffected fingers in extension and asking the patient to flex the injured finger. An injured FDS tendon will produce no movement.
- Ultrasound of the flexor sheath to visualize the location and status of the avulsed end of the tendon can be used.
- X-rays will generally not reveal pathology, MRI scans can be used, but the results should be backed up by other clinical findings.
- Strength will reveal weakness of the FDP and ROM testing may reveal hypermobility into DIP extension. In the case of long-term pathology, extension may be limited by scar tissue and adhesions.

DIFFERENTIAL DIAGNOSIS

- Anterior interosseous nerve paralysis
- Trigger finger
- Swan-neck deformity
- Jammed finger

CONTRIBUTING FACTORS

- Any activity requiring repetitive resisted flexion such as participation in contact sports, walking the dog, or starting a lawnmower.
- Long-term steroid use.
- Endocrine system pathology.

TREATMENT

SURGICAL INDICATORS

- Type I injuries: Surgical repair is indicated within 7 to 10 days because of the risk of inflammation and scarring at the end of the ruptured tendon, making it impossible to thread the tendon back through the tendinous sheath.
- Type II injuries: Surgical repair is indicated within up to 4 weeks from the date of injury.
- Type III injury: Surgical repair can be successful after 4 weeks because the distal end of the tendon has not retracted all the way through the synovial sheath.

SURGICAL OPTIONS

- Type I injuries: The distal end of the tendon must be trimmed because of the lack of blood supply. Likelihood of success decreases with time: Surgery is indicated within 7 to 10 days of injury because of the inflammatory response. Surgical options beyond this time frame include tendon excision and DIP fusion.
- Type II injury: The flexor tendon must be reattached and can be rethreaded with a silicone flexible tendon.

- Type III injury: The flexor tendon must be reattached.

SURGICAL OUTCOMES

- Injury to the A4 pulley may impair DIP flexion.
- Tethering or fibrosis of the FDP tendon (quadriga) caused by scarring may result in loss of ROM and decreased grasp strength in the remaining digits.
- Type I injury: Repair can be difficult if the tendon has retracted all the way into the palm because of inflammation, avulsed vinculum, and inability to re-thread the tendon. This may result in compromised PIP ROM.
- Type II injury: Blood supply and vinculum remain intact. Fibrosis at the FDS chiasm may impair tendon gliding.
- In the case of a chronic rupture, or a type II or III injury more than 4 weeks since the injury, consideration should be given to whether there is enough of a functional impairment to warrant intervention. Tenodesis, arthrodesis, or free tendon grafting may also be considered.

REHABILITATION

- Postsurgical repair
  - Forearm-based dorsal block splint for 4 to 5 weeks with wrist and MCPs at 30 degrees of flexion and IPs in full extension. The involved finger should be held at 45 degrees of DIP flexion, positioning the FDP tendon proximal to the skin incision.
  - In general, active finger and wrist flexion and passive finger extension are contraindicated for the first 3 to 4 weeks.
  - Passive wrist and finger flexion and passive wrist extension are allowed. Functional movement of the hand is allowed after 4 weeks, and splint may be discontinued at 5 weeks.
  - Resistance should be avoided for 7 to 8 weeks.
- Nonsurgical repair
  - Resection of the retracted tendon and/or DIP joint fusion.
  - If there are minimal functional impairments, further intervention is not required.

REHABILITATIVE COMPLICATIONS OF JERSEY FINGER

- If the tendon is not repaired surgically, there is an increased risk of continued pain in the palm and finger and possible development of carpal tunnel syndrome caused by inflammation.
- Quadriga may occur because of adhesions or scarring of the involved digit restricting flexion of the other digits.

Pain may persist in the palm or involved digit.

PROGNOSIS

- Average recovery expected is as follows:
  - 75% of grip strength
  - 77% of finger pressure
  - 75% of pinch strength
  - 76% of PIP motion
  - 75% of DIP motion

SIGNS AND SYMPTOMS INDICATING REFERRAL TO PHYSICIAN

Because of the critical nature of the timing of surgical repair, a suspected FDP rupture must be referred immediately to a physician for assessment.

SUGGESTED READINGS

Bois AJ, Johnston G, Classen D. Spontaneous flexor tendon ruptures of the hand: Case series and review of the literature. *J Hand Surg Am.* 2007;32:1061-1071.

Hankin FM, Peel SM. Sport-related fractures and dislocations in the hand. *Hand Clin.* 1990;6:429-453.

Hofmeister EP, Craven CE. Zone I rupture of the flexor digitorum profundus tendon caused by blunt trauma: A case report. *J Hand Surg Am.* 2008;33:247-249.

AUTHOR: AKEMI RICO

Section III

ORTHOPEDIC PATHOLOGY

BASIC INFORMATION

DEFINITION

Mallet finger is a zone I injury to the extensor tendon mechanism at or near the DIP joint. Mallet finger is the result of excessive stretching or tearing of the extensor tendon, or in some cases, an avulsion fracture at the distal phalanx.

SYNONYMS

- Baseball finger
- Dropped finger
- Hammer finger

ICD-9CM CODE
736.1 Mallet finger

OPTIMAL NUMBER OF VISITS

12 visits

MAXIMAL NUMBER OF VISITS

24 visits

ETIOLOGY

- The digital extensor tendon terminates as a flattening of the lateral bands, which are the terminal offshoots of the more proximal extensor hood. This hood runs along the dorsal aspect of the phalanges, tapering and inserting into the distal phalanx.
- The extensor tendon may rupture or tear when a tensile load is placed on it.
- When stressed at a slow rate, the tendon may undergo microdamage that causes some fraying or stretching.
- With more rapid loading, the less elastic tendon bone interface can avulse.
- Since the extensor tendon undergoes very little excursion during normal movement, a large flexor moment, applied rapidly, causes a fulcrum at the DIP joint. Given sufficient force and velocity, hyperflexion at the DIP results in failure of the tendon or its attachment to the distal phalanx. The latter may result in avulsion fractures.
- Subtypes are as follows:
  - Type I: Avulsion of the extensor tendon
  - Type II: Lacerated tendon
  - Type III: Avulsion involving both skin and tendon
  - Type IV: Injury of the tendon with associated fracture

EPIDEMIOLOGY AND DEMOGRAPHICS

Commonly affects athletes, such as baseball and softball players, although it is also associated with basketball, football, and soccer.

MECHANISM OF INJURY

- Forceful impact to the finger causing high-velocity DIP flexion.
- Laceration of the extensor tendon(s).
- Trauma (MVA, crush injuries).
- The most common mechanism of injuries include two baseball-related injuries: being struck by a ball at the distal phalanx and hyperflexion of the distal phalanx against a base pad while executing a "slide" maneuver.

COMMON SIGNS AND SYMPTOMS

- Weak or loss of active extension at the DIP joint (passive extension may be intact)
- Resting DIP flexion ("dropped finger") from unopposed activity of the FDP
- Redness and edema
- Ecchymosis
- Pain (although the injury may present as painless especially in the absence of a concomitant fracture)
- Swan-neck deformity (caused by compensatory hyperextension at the PIP joint during function)

AGGRAVATING ACTIVITIES

- Continued activity with the affected hand
- Pressure or impact to the affected finger
- Attempts to actively extend DIP joint

EASING ACTIVITIES

- Rest
- Immobilization
- Icing
- Elevation

24-HOUR SYMPTOM PATTERN

- Increased swelling in the morning or with long periods of immobility
- Pain and swelling may increase later in the day with increased activity

PAST HISTORY FOR THE REGION

- Past injury
- Circulatory compromise
- Lack of DIP flexion ROM
- Involvement in high-risk activities such as baseball or basketball

PHYSICAL EXAMINATION

- Palpate for tenderness along the dorsal aspect of the affected digit, particularly along the distal phalanx.
- Observe and feel for signs of inflammation (erythema, edema, etc).
- Test distal phalangeal extension by isolating at the DIP joint: Test should reveal loss of active extension with partial or complete preservation of PROM.
- Compare affected digit with its counterpart on the opposite hand to check for increased DIP flexion, especially if the extensor tendon has avulsed.

IMPORTANT OBJECTIVE TESTS

- X-ray and MRI may help to determine the presence of fracture and underlying damage to the tendon, as well as to nearby muscles and ligaments.
- Radiographs may also help to differentiate fracture types (middle phalangeal, shaft or Tuft fracture, etc).

DIFFERENTIAL DIAGNOSIS

- Tuft fracture deformity
- Phalangeal fracture
- Swan-neck deformity

CONTRIBUTING FACTORS

- Intrinsic weakness of the tendon (caused by disease or steroid use)
- Advanced age
- Decreased blood supply to the hand and/or digits
- Tendency to hold digits in a rigid position

TREATMENT

SURGICAL OPTIONS

- Indications for and benefits of surgery remain controversial.
- Fixation is often advocated for fractures associated with volar displacement of the distal digit.
- Surgery will usually involve reduction, realignment, and placement of a K-wire to fixate the fractured fragments and allow balance between flexor and extensor tone.
- Surgical outcomes are typically very good.

REHABILITATION

- Ice and antiinflammatories as needed.
- Interventions vary as a function of injury type.
- For type I injuries, recommended course is splinting into extension for 4 to 6 weeks (more if continued extensor lag is noted) followed by a weaning period of approximately 2 weeks and a night splinting period of 2 to 6 weeks.
- For athletes, additional splinting during activity for as much as 8 weeks.
- Type II injuries may require surgery followed by splinting (see type I).
- Type III protocol is similar to that of type I but may also include surgery to repair the tendon and restore the integrity of the overlying skin.
- Type IV injuries respond best to fracture reduction followed by a splinting protocol (see type I).
- PROM should begin as soon as possible to maintain DIP flexion and extension along with motion throughout the affected digit.
- AROM can commence after 6 weeks.

PROGNOSIS

- With uninterrupted splinting, outcomes are excellent for pain reduction, ROM recovery, and cosmesis.

- Minor extension lag of a few degrees may persist along with residual swelling that normally remits within a few months.
- Prognosis will depend largely on compliance with splinting schedules.

SIGNS AND SYMPTOMS INDICATING REFERRAL TO PHYSICIAN

- Deep lacerations
- Signs and symptoms of infection
- Suspected fracture not previously diagnosed
- Development of necrosis or ulcerations secondary to splint use

SUGGESTED READINGS

Peterson JJ, Bancroft LW. Injuries of the fingers and thumb in the athlete. *Clin Sports Med*. 2006;25(3):527-542.

Rocchi L, Genitiempo M, Fanfani F. Percutaneous fixation of mallet fractures by the "umbrella handle" technique. *J Hand Surg Br*. 2006;31(4):407-412.

Simpson D, McQueen MM, Kumar P. Mallet deformity in sport. *J Hand Surg Br*. 2001;26(1):32-33.

Teoh LC, Lee JY. Mallet fractures: a novel approach to internal fixation using a hook plate. *J Hand Surg Eur Vol*. 2007; 32(1):24-30.

Tuttle HG, Olvey SP, Stern PJ. Tendon avulsion injuries of the distal phalanx. *Clin Orthop Relat Res*. 2006;445:157-168.

AUTHOR: SON TRINH

BASIC INFORMATION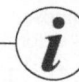

DEFINITION

- Osteoarthritis is a pathology associated with inflammation in the joints of the body. In the case of hand osteoarthritis, the arthritis and inflammation most commonly associated with a loss of carpal, MC, or phalanges glenoid cartilage leading to hand pain.
- Osteoarthritis is a term derived from the Greek word "*osteo*" meaning "of the bone," "*arthro*" meaning "joint," and "*itis*" meaning inflammation even though the amount of inflammation present in the joint can range from excessive to little or no inflammation.

SYNONYMS

- Hand arthritis
- Hand degenerative joint disease

ICD-9CM CODES
715.14 Osteoarthrosis localized
             primary involving hand
715.24 Osteoarthrosis localized
             secondary involving hand

OPTIMAL NUMBER OF VISITS

3 to 6 visits

MAXIMAL NUMBER OF VISITS

20 to 36 visits

ETIOLOGY

- The wearing down of the hyaline cartilage leads to an inflammatory response. There is thickening and sclerosis of the subchondral bone and development of osteophytes or bone spurs. This leads to a narrowing of the joint space, loss of shock absorption, and ultimately pain.
- Daily wear and tear in combination with various injuries sustained throughout life is the most common cause of the breakdown of healthy tissue.
- Degeneration of the cartilage and resultant arthritis can also be the result of other factors such as trauma or joint injury.
- At a cellular level, as a person ages, the number of proteoglycans in the articular cartilage decreases. Proteoglycans are hydrophilic and work within cartilage to bind water. With the reduction of proteoglycans comes a decrease in water content within the cartilage and a corresponding loss of cartilage resilience. With the decreases in cartilage resilience, collagen fibers of the cartilage become susceptible to degradation and injury. The breakdown of collagen and other cartilage tissue is released into the surround joint space. Inflammation results as the body attempts to respond to the influx of byproducts from cartilage injury.
- As the cartilage degrades, the joint space narrows and ligaments become more lax. In response to the laxity, new bone outgrowths, called *spurs* or *osteophytes,* can form on the margins of the joints in an attempt to improve the congruence and passive stability of the articular cartilage surfaces.
- Primary osteoarthritis refers to joint degradation resulting from aging and tissue degeneration.
- Secondary osteoarthritis refers to joint degradation and tissue degeneration that results from factors other than aging such as obesity, trauma, and congenital disorders.

EPIDEMIOLOGY AND DEMOGRAPHICS

- Adults in the US over 60 years of age:
  - 58% had Heberden's nodes.
  - 29.9% had Bouchard's nodes.
  - 18.2% had first CMC deformities.
- Symptomatic hand osteoarthritis occurs in 8% to 15% of the elderly.
- Symptomatic osteoarthritis occurs in the following:
  - 5.4% to 35% at the DIP joints (especially the second)
  - 4.7% to 18% at the PIP joints (especially the third)
  - 1.9% to 21% at the first CMC joints (adults 40 years of age and older)
- 30% of all joints affected by osteoarthritis are joints in the hand, as follows:
  - 21% in the first CMC joint
  - 35% in the second DIP joint
  - 18% in the third PIP joint
- Individuals over 55 years old are the most prone to hand osteoarthritis.
- Women (24% of those over 60 years of age) have a higher prevalence than men (10.3% of 60-year-olds).
- Usually the osteoarthritis is found more in the dominant hand.

MECHANISM OF INJURY

- Osteoarthritis is a pathology of overuse. The mechanism of injury is therefore the result of repetitive motions that stress the hand and finger joints. The more cycles of an activity that the hand sees, the more likely the result will be anatomical damage.
- Daily use of the hand/fingers
- Excessive use/strain of the hand/fingers
- Injuries, such as fracture and strains/sprains, that cause inflammation and scar tissue in the hand or fingers

COMMON SIGNS AND SYMPTOMS

- Deformities (Heberden's nodes, Bouchard's nodes)
- Pain in the hand or fingers
- Stiffness in the hand or fingers
- Cracking or deep crunching in the hand or finger joints
- Inflammation and thickening of the hand or finger joints
- The American College of Rheumatology's criteria for hand osteoarthritis includes pain, ache, and stiffness, plus at least three of the following:
  - Bony thickening at the third DIP joint
  - Bone thickening at the second and third PIP joints
  - Bone thickening at the first CMC joint
  - Bony thickening of at least two DIP joints
  - Swelling of at least three MCP joints
  - Deformity of at least 1 of the 10 aforementioned joints

AGGRAVATING ACTIVITIES

- Inactivity allows the inflammation to "pool" and increase pressure leading to discomfort and loss of available movement. Inactivity leads to stiffness.
- Reaching overhead.
- Throwing, lifting, reaching behind.
- Weight-bearing activities such as crawling or making a bed.

EASING ACTIVITIES

- Rest
- Gentle motions of the hand and finger joints
- Gentle stretching and exercise, heat, massage, antiinflammatory medications, non-weight–bearing activities, and leg elevation
- Generally speaking, these activities lead to decreased wear and tear, increased joint lubrication, and loss of stiffness and inflammation associated with this condition

24-HOUR SYMPTOM PATTERN

- Stiffness in the morning (first 10 to 15 minutes)
- Better after a warm shower and taking medication
- Can worsen with excessive movement
- Stiffens again in the evening

PAST HISTORY FOR THE REGION

- Jobs or recreational activities that require excessive use/strain of the hand (dancing, walking, running, jumping, etc)
- Abnormal amount of damage from injuries

PHYSICAL EXAMINATION

- Joint thickening (bony changes and inflammation)
- Loss of hand/finger ROM
- Localized pain and loss of joint mobility
- Crepitus with movement

IMPORTANT OBJECTIVE TESTS

- The standard test for differentiating hand or finger osteoarthritis is x-ray. MRIs may be warranted if soft tissue damage is suspected.
- No one specific clinical test has proved reliable in differentiating hand or finger osteoarthritis. Common clinical assessments are as follows:
  - Palpation: Composite compression test (through the MCP joints) and specific joint compression
  - Alignment assessment
  - AROM and PROM
  - Joint mobility
  - Strength tests (grip and pinch dynamometers)

DIFFERENTIAL DIAGNOSIS

- Hand/finger sprain/strain
- Tendonitis (de Quervain's syndrome)
- RA
- Trigger finger
- Reflex sympathetic dystrophy
- Complex regional pain syndrome
- Cervical radiculopathy

CONTRIBUTING FACTORS

- Uncontrolled risk factors that contribute or predispose an individual to hand osteoarthritis pathology are as follows:
  - Gender (females more than males)
  - Age (increase 2% per year after age 40 years)
  - Genetics
- Modifiable risk factors that contribute or predispose an individual to continue or to progress to hand osteoarthritis are as follows:
  - Weight
  - Work or recreational activities
  - Repetitive or significant traumatic injuries to the hip
  - Poor health (smoking, long-term use of steroids)

TREATMENT

SURGICAL OPTION

Fusion (arthrodesis)

REHABILITATION

- Rehabilitation regimes should address the following:
  - Education regarding correct use of ice/heat at home
  - Give home exercise program/ADL training
  - Body mechanics and joint protection (use of assistive devices) training with ADLs
  - Manual therapy (soft tissue mobilization, joint mobilization)
  - Modalities: Heat, paraffin, ultrasound, electrical stimulation, tape/splints
- Initial exercises used to promote healing are as follows:
  - Therapeutic exercises: ROM, isometrics (for painful joints), and progressive resistive exercises (for minimal to nonpainful joints)
  - Agility exercises
- Manual therapy (soft tissue mobilization, joint mobilization) can improve joint mobility and joint arthrokinematics and decrease pain.
- Massage can decrease pain by relaxing muscular tension, improving circulation, and increasing endorphin release.
- Exercise should be used to do the following:
  - Decrease muscular and joint stiffness
  - Improve joint alignment by increasing muscular support
  - Improve functional mobility
  - Create a sense of control over the symptoms and the condition

PROGNOSIS

- Long-term prognosis for a patient with hand osteoarthritis depends on the extent of wear and tear and the ability to reduce the joint strain placed on the joint (posture, activity, etc).

- For the most part, hand osteoarthritis is a degenerative condition. At earlier stages of the pathology, rehabilitation aimed at reducing the load placed on the joint can potentially slow or halt the progression of degeneration.
- For patients who are further along in the degenerative process, outcomes will be less favorable because cartilage has only a limited ability to repair itself.

SIGNS AND SYMPTOMS INDICATING REFERRAL TO PHYSICIAN

- Unrelenting pain
- Unusual responses to therapy
- Neurological symptoms
- Signs of infection, reflex sympathetic dystrophy, or complex regional pain syndrome

SUGGESTED READINGS

Dillon CF, Hirsch R, Rasch EK, Gu Q. Symptomatic hand osteoarthritis in the United States: prevalence and functional impairment estimates from the third U.S. National Health and Nutrition Examination Survey, 1991-1994. *Am J Phys Med Rehabil.* 2007;86(1):12-21.

Dugan SA. Exercise for health and wellness at midlife and beyond: balancing benefits and risks. *Phys Med Rehabil Clin N Am.* 2007;18(3):555-575.

Glass GG. Osteoarthritis. *Dis Mon.* 2006;52(9):343-362.

Rogers MW. The effects of strength training among persons with hand osteoarthritis: a two-year follow-up study. *J Hand Ther.* 2007;20(3):244-249. quiz 250.

Wilder FV. Joint-specific prevalence of osteoarthritis of the hand. *Osteoarthritis Cartilage.* 2006;14(9):953-957.

AUTHOR: SARA GRANNIS

BASIC INFORMATION

DEFINITION

Rheumatoid arthritis (RA) is a systemic inflammatory disease that results in cartilage and bone destruction. RA is characterized by a typical pattern and distribution of synovial joint involvement. Disorganization of the joint leads to deformities and loss of function.

SYNONYMS

- Rheumatic disease
- Rheumatism

ICD-9CM CODE
714.0 Rheumatoid arthritis

OPTIMAL NUMBER OF VISITS

3 visits

MAXIMAL NUMBER OF VISITS

20 visits

ETIOLOGY

- Currently, the cause of RA is unknown, although there are several theories. Evidence points to a combination of environmental and genetic factors.
- RA progresses in four stages. Joints most commonly affected are those with the highest ratio of synovium to articular cartilage.
  - The first stage is the swelling of the synovial lining, causing pain, warmth, stiffness, redness, and swelling around the joint. This stage is the most painful and usually causes patients to seek medical care.
  - The second stage is characterized by the rapid division and growth of cells, or pannus, which causes the synovium to thicken. In this stage the pannus extends beyond the cartilage to adjacent ligaments and tendons. Pain decreases during this stage, and the joints do not yet exhibit deformities.
  - The third stage is known as the chronic active phase. The inflamed cells release enzymes that may digest bone and cartilage, often causing the involved joint to lose its shape, alignment, and ROM. Joint deformities become significant and irreversible in the phase.
  - The fourth stage is the chronic inactive phase. Skeletal collapse occurs with the presence of dislocation and spontaneous fusions.
- About 10% to 20% of RA patients have a sudden onset of the disease, followed by many years with no symptoms. This is considered a prolonged remission.
- Some RA patients experience periods of few or no symptoms between flare ups

that can last for months. This is referred to as intermittent symptoms of RA.
- The majority of RA patients have the chronic, progressive type of RA that requires long-term medical management.

EPIDEMIOLOGY AND DEMOGRAPHICS

- Approximately 1.3 million people in the US have RA.
- All races and ethnicities are affected by RA.
- Onset usually occurs between 30 and 50 years of age. Earlier onset is associated with a more severe disease process.
- Women are two to three times more likely to be diagnosed with RA than men; however, men are more severely affected.

MECHANISM OF INJURY

RA commonly begins in the smaller joints of the fingers, hands, and wrists.

COMMON SIGNS AND SYMPTOMS

- Sausage-shaped (fusiform) swelling of the finger
- A soft lump over the back of the hand that moves with the extensor tendons
- Crepitus with movement
- Shifting of the fingers as they drift away from the thumb (ulnar drift)
- Swelling and inflammation of the flexor tendons resulting in clicking or triggering of the fingers
- Tendon ruptures eliminating the ability to flex or extend the fingers or the thumb
- Unstable joints in the wrist, fingers, and thumb
- Boutonnière and swan-neck deformities

AGGRAVATING ACTIVITIES

- Gripping activities
- Brushing hair
- Opening a door

EASING ACTIVITIES

- Rest
- Supportive splinting
- Medications

24-HOUR SYMPTOM PATTERN

- The patient may experience stiffness in the morning lasting more than 1 hour.
- Patient may require frequent breaks to complete tasks caused by fatigue and weakness.

PAST HISTORY FOR THE REGION

- Symmetrical, multijoint pain
- Stiffness in the morning lasting more than 45 minutes
- Pain in your hands, wrists, and/or feet
- Feelings of weakness or fatigue

PHYSICAL EXAMINATION

- The most common deformity is ulnar deviation of the MP joint. To examine the true amount of deviation the hand should be unsupported.
- Other common deformities include the following:
  - Thumb deformities
  - Distal ulna dorsal subluxation
  - Volar subluxation of the carpal bones on radius
  - Ulnar displacement of the proximal carpal row causing radial deviation of the wrist
- Skin changes present warm and red in the acute stage, but chronically the skin thins and easily bruises as a result of steroid use.
- Nodules with or without pain occur at joints or along tendons and most often the largest is at the elbow.
- Synovitis around the joint capsule. Chronicity thickens the synovitis and leads to instability, misalignments, restricted ROM, and eventual deformities.
- Loss of ROM is caused by tendon rupture; tendons weaken from inflamed synovium and rupture from gliding over rough bony areas.
- Boutonnière and swan-neck deformities in the fingers and thumbs.

IMPORTANT OBJECTIVE TESTS

- Diagnosing RA is a process. There no one specific test that will positively diagnosis RA. A physician relies on a number of tools to determine the best treatment for the symptoms of the patient.
- Possible laboratory tests include the following:
  - Complete blood count (CBC)
  - Erythrocyte sedimentation rate (ESR, or sed rate)
  - C-reactive protein (CRP)
  - Rheumatoid factor
  - Antinuclear antibodies (ANA)
  - Imaging studies, such as radiographs and MRI, may also be indicated

DIFFERENTIAL DIAGNOSIS **Dx**

- Connective tissue diseases such as scleroderma and systemic lupus erythematosus (SLE)
- Fibromyalgia
- Hemochromatosis
- Infectious endocarditis
- Polyarticular gout
- Polymyalgia rheumatica
- Sarcoidosis
- Thyroid disease
- Viral arthritis

CONTRIBUTING FACTORS

- Female gender
- Family history

- Older age
- Silicate exposure
- Smoking

TREATMENT

SURGICAL INDICATORS

Debilitating pain and loss of functional use of the hand

SURGICAL OPTIONS

- Synovectomy reduces the amount of inflammatory tissue by removing the diseased synovium or lining of the joint. It may result in less swelling and pain. This surgery may also slow or prevent further joint damage.
- Arthroscopic surgery can be used as a treatment or diagnostic tool. Tissue samples can be obtained, loose cartilage removed, tears in the soft tissue repaired, joint surfaces smoothed, and diseased synovial tissue removed.
- Osteotomy cuts the bone to increase stability by redistributing the weight on the joint. Osteotomy is not often used with rheumatoid patients because there are many other options available.
- Joint replacement surgery or arthroplasty involves the removal of the joint, resurfacing and relining of the ends of bones, and replacement with a man-made component. This procedure is usually recommended for people over 50 years of age or those who have severe disease progression. Typically, a new joint will last between 20 and 30 years.
- Arthrodesis or fusion fuses two bones together. Although it limits movement, it also decreases pain and increases stability of the joints.
- Tendon ruptures occur frequently in the rheumatoid hand, and multiple surgical procedures are used to restore finger flexion, extension, and thumb ROM. Choice of procedure depends on how many tendons have ruptured and current status of the remaining tendons available for transfer.

SURGICAL OUTCOMES

Unfortunately, there is no cure for RA. However, surgical procedures can often help correct deformities, relieve pain, and improve function.

REHABILITATION

- Treatment must be tailored to the individual, taking into account the severity of the arthritis, individual lifestyle, and co-morbidities.
- Current treatment methods focus on relieving pain, reducing inflammation, stopping or slowing joint damage, and improving overall function and sense of well-being.
- Joint deformities should be palpated to determine if they are rigid or flexible. The clinician should not attempt to correct a rigid deformity; instead, the joint should be protected from further deformity progression.
- Because of the chronic nature of RA, the patient should be educated on healthy lifestyle choices that may decrease the severity and progression of the disease. These changes include the following:
  - Staying healthy and fit with regular exercise
  - Activity and rest
  - Managing stress, depression, and fatigue
  - Avoiding joint pain and injury
  - Using preventive medications
- Equipment: Today, many devices are available to help decrease pain and increase functional use of the hand. Electric knives, scissors, and jar openers are simple devices that can reduce hand damage. Ergonomic door handles and writing devices are examples of utensils that can preserve the joints of the hand.
- Splinting: Custom splints allow painful joints to rest while a person is sleeping.
  - Splints are worn during the day to increase function and limit pain.
  - Splints should only be used to support the hand and prevent further pain and deformity. Research has demonstrated that corrective splinting is unsuccessful.
  - During stage one, resting splints should be used to reduce pain. These can be worn selectively during the day or night.
  - During stage two, night splints should be used to prevent future deformity and reduce pain.
  - During stage three, the patient will need splints during the day to increase functional use of the hand. Night splinting may also prevent further deformity.
  - During stage four, splinting increases joint stability and function during the day. Night splinting provides comfort.
- Therapeutic exercise should avoid all painful ROMs and overstretching the already unstable joints. Gentle wrist and finger flexion and extension and thumb opposition AROM can be used to maintain function.
  - Strengthening should be used with extreme caution because it may increase deformities of the hand. Strengthening activities should not be painful.

PROGNOSIS

- There is no known cure for RA.
- Factors influencing the prognosis for RA include the following:
  - Lower education level and socioeconomic status
  - Early involvement of multiple joints
  - Markers for inflammation are elevated on laboratory tests (elevated CRP and ESR)
  - Significant joint damage already evident on radiographs at diagnosis
  - Testing positive for rheumatoid factor or anti-cyclic citrullinated peptide antibody (anti-CCP)

SIGNS AND SYMPTOMS INDICATING REFERRAL TO PHYSICIAN

Joint destruction begins within a few weeks of symptom onset. Early treatment decreases the rate of disease progression. If RA is suspected, refer the patient to a rheumatologist.

SUGGESTED READINGS

Biese J. Therapist's evaluation and conservative management of rheumatoid arthritis in the hand and wrist. In: Mackin EJ, Callahan AD, Osterman AL, Skirven TM, Schneider LH, and Hunter JM. *Hunter, Mackin & Callahan's Rehabilitation of the Hand and Upper Extremity*. 5th ed. vol. 2. St. Louis, Missouri: Mosby; 2002:1569–1582.

Rindfleisch JA, Muller D. Diagnosis and management of rheumatoid arthritis. *Am Fam Physician*. 2005;72:1037–1047.

AUTHOR: AUDRA PONCI BADO

BASIC INFORMATION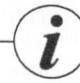

DEFINITION

The scaphoid is the most frequently fractured carpal. The fracture is classified by the region of the bone in which it occurs: proximal pole, middle (waist), or distal pole.

SYNONYM

Navicular fracture

ICD-9CM CODE
814.11 Open fracture of navicular (scaphoid) bone of wrist

OPTIMAL NUMBER OF VISITS

10 visits

MAXIMAL NUMBER OF VISITS

24 visits

ETIOLOGY

- A scaphoid fracture most commonly occurs as the result of a sudden impact to the palm with the wrist hyperextended. Less common mechanisms may involve forced flexion and axial loading of the wrist with the hand in a fist position.
- The waist of the scaphoid accounts for 70% of all fractures.
- The proximal pole fractures occur 20% of the time.
- Distal pole fractures occur only 10% of the time.
- The amount of blood supply determines how fast or how complete a scaphoid fracture will heal. The majority of blood supply to the carpal, 70% to 80%, enters distally. The proximal pole has no direct blood supply, so it must depend on vessels that primarily supply the waist. Diminished blood flow to the proximal pole is noted in about one-third of fractures at the waist level. This reduced blood supply may result in avascular necrosis of the proximal pole of the scaphoid. Almost 100% of proximal pole fractures result in aseptic necrosis. Displaced scaphoid fractures have a nonunion rate of 55% to 90%.
- Frequently, the diagnosis of a scaphoid fracture is delayed. Late diagnosis may alter the prognosis for fracture union and dramatically increase the long-term likelihood of arthritis.
- Proper immobilization, and surgery if needed will contribute to the rate of healing.

EPIDEMIOLOGY AND DEMOGRAPHICS

- Approximately 35,000 scaphoid fractures occur annually in the US, with occult fractures representing 12% to 16% of the total.
- Young males have a peak incidence between the ages of 15 to 35 years.

MECHANISM OF INJURY

Common mechanism of injury may involve using the hand to brace a fall or may result from an athlete running into another person or a wall during competition.

COMMON SIGNS AND SYMPTOMS

- Swelling in the wrist
- Tenderness or pain within the anatomical snuffbox

AGGRAVATING ACTIVITY

Heavy gripping activities such as holding a baseball bat or a tennis racket

EASING ACTIVITY

Rest of the involved hand should decrease discomfort

24-HOUR SYMPTOM PATTERN

Symptoms may or may not increase as the day progresses, depending on use of the hand.

PAST HISTORY FOR THE REGION

Patients will report persistent wrist pain and previous trauma to the hand.

PHYSICAL EXAMINATION

- Loss of wrist motion, especially radial deviation
- Snuffbox tenderness
- Pain with resisted forearm rotation

IMPORTANT OBJECTIVE TESTS

CT and radiographs

DIFFERENTIAL DIAGNOSIS **Dx**

- Radial sensory nerve neuritis
- de Quervain's tenosynovitis
- CMC joint arthritis

CONTRIBUTING FACTORS

- Participation in high-contact sports such as football or basketball
- Osteoporosis or osteopenia
- Long-term use of the following:
  - Prednisone
  - Methotrexate
  - Corticosteroids

TREATMENT **Rx**

Fractures to the waist or distal pole that are nondisplaced can heal with closed treatment and do not require surgery

SURGICAL INDICATORS

- Poor vascularity and instability of the bone fragment
- Associated fractures of the distal radius
- Nondisplaced fractures that do not show evidence of healing after 6 weeks of immobilization
- Displaced fractures

SURGICAL OPTIONS

- Displaced or unstable fractures require percutaneous pin fixation or compression screw fixation to prevent malunion.
- Internal fixation is accomplished with either smooth K-wires or a Herbert screw.
- Nonunion scaphoid fractures are the result of a patient failing to seek timely medical attention, a misdiagnosis of a wrist sprain, or failure to heal with cast immobilization. Bone grafting is necessary for healing of nonunion fractures.
  - Nonunions of the scaphoid can be treated with radial styloidectomy, excision of the proximal bone fragment, proximal row carpectomy, total or partial wrist arthrodesis, or traditional bone grafting.
  - Avascular necrosis develops in 30% to 40% of nonunion scaphoid fractures, most frequently in a fracture of the proximal third of the scaphoid bone.

SURGICAL OUTCOMES

Research has shown a return to sport occurs at an average of 7 weeks after Herbert screw fixation, compared to a 15 to 26 week return after closed treatment.

REHABILITATION

- Postsurgical
  - If rigid internal fixation is used, such as a Herbert screw, AROM can begin as early as 10 to 14 days when the cast is removed. A thumb spica should be fabricated for the patient to wear 24 hours a day with removal only for therapeutic ROM exercises. Edema control and ROM for the hand should begin immediately after surgery.
  - At 4 to 6 weeks, controlled loading of the wrist is initiated, as well as the introduction of strength training. Progression of wrist activities is determined by the healing of the fracture using radiograph. It is recommended that an athlete wear a Nirschl R-U wrist brace to limit extreme wrist extension on the initial return to sport.
- Nonsurgical Patient
  - Initially, nondisplaced fractures are treated with long-arm thumb spica cast with the wrist in neutral position for 6 weeks, followed by a short-arm

spica cast for an additional 6 weeks until roentgenographic union is evident.

○ Active ROM exercises to the forearm, wrist, and thumb should be performed 6 to 8 times daily after immobilization. A wrist and thumb static splint with wrist in neutral should be worn between exercise sessions and at night until ROM and strength gains have occurred.

○ Using this nonoperative casting technique, the expected rate of union is 95% within 10 weeks.

• Average rate of healing for a scaphoid fracture heal as follows:

○ Fractures of the middle third of the scaphoid heal on average in 6 to 12 weeks.

○ Distal third fractures of the scaphoid heal on the average in 4 to 8 weeks.

○ Proximal third fractures of the scaphoid heal on the average in 12 to 20 weeks.

PROGNOSIS

• Prognosis is less favorable if the fracture is displaced, diagnosis is delayed, or the fracture is in the proximal or middle third of the scaphoid bone.

• Chronic pain, decreased ROM, and decreased grip strength may result.

SIGNS AND SYMPTOMS INDICATING REFERRAL TO PHYSICIAN

Immediate referral to a hand surgeon is essential if a scaphoid fracture is suspected. Prompt diagnosis and treatment will significantly improve prognosis and recovery.

SUGGESTED READINGS

Gutow AP. Percutaneous fixation of scaphoid fractures. *J Am Acad Orthop Surg.* 2007;15(8):474-485.

Yin ZG, Zhang JB, Kan SL, Wang P. Treatment of acute scaphoid fractures: systematic review and meta-analysis. *Clin Orthop Relat Res.* 2007;460:142-151.

AUTHOR: AUDRA PONCI BADO

Section III

ORTHOPEDIC PATHOLOGY

BASIC INFORMATION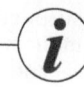

DEFINITION

- A Smith's fracture is a fracture of the distal end of the radius bone in the forearm, often accompanied by fracture of the styloid of the ulna.
- The fracture usually occurs about an inch or two proximal to the radiocarpal joint.
- The distal portion of the wrist and hand are displaced anteriorly in relationship to the proximal forearm.

SYNONYM

Distal radius fracture

ICD-9CM CODE
813.41 Colles' fracture closed

OPTIMAL/MAXIMAL NUMBER OF VISITS

Highly variable, depending on specifics of fracture; length and type of immobilization; surgery; complications, including related injuries (ulnar styloid fracture, ligament injuries); and presence or absence of complex regional pain syndrome.

ETIOLOGY

- The fracture typically occurs from a fall on an outstretched hand.
- Falls from higher levels produce worse fractures. Specifics of the fall may account for associated injuries such as fracture of the ulnar styloid, ligament injuries, or carpal fracture or dislocation.
- The anterior displacement of the hand and wrist is usually the result of a fall in which the arm is internally rotated at the shoulder, extended at the elbow, pronated at the forearm, and flexed at the wrist.
- Fracture can also occur if the shoulder is externally rotated, extended at the elbow, supinated at the forearm, and extended at the wrist during a fall.
- Fractures that extend into the radiocarpal joint technically are considered Barton's fractures but commonly are categorized as Colles' or Smith's fractures.

EPIDEMIOLOGY AND DEMOGRAPHICS

- The two peaks of incidence of distal radius fractures are ages 6 to 10 and 60 to 69 years.
  - In older adults, there is a 4:1 ratio of fractures in women. In adolescents, there is a 3:1 predominance of males.
  - In younger children, the higher incidence can be attributed to bone immaturity and increased likelihood of falls.
- Wrist fractures are more common in women over 65 years of age. There is an increase in incidence in white women between 45 and 60 years of age. The trend then stabilizes.
- Only 15% of wrist fractures occur in men; this incidence does not appear to increase as men age.
- In Europe, the annual incidence of distal forearm fractures in males and females was estimated at 1.7 and 7.3 per 1000 person-years, respectively.
- Distal forearm fractures can be used as an early and sensitive marker of male skeletal fragility.

MECHANISM OF INJURY

Fall on an outstretched hand, with the arm internally rotated at the shoulder, extended at the elbow, pronated at the forearm, and flexed at the wrist, is the most common mechanism of injury.

COMMON SIGNS AND SYMPTOMS

- After injury, the patient will report pain in the wrist that may refer proximally into the forearm or distally into the hand.
- Movement may be limited by pain or physical block.
- Deformity in the wrist may be noted.
- Nerve symptoms, especially numbness or weakness in the median nerve distribution, may indicate serious complications.

AGGRAVATING ACTIVITIES

- When seen acutely, wrist fractures will be limited in all motions. Forearm pronation and supination, gripping activities, lifting activities, and functional activities, such as writing and typing, will be limited and painful.
- When seen after immobilization or surgery, the patient will generally be limited in pronation and supination, therefore activities, such as turning doorknobs or typing, will be limited and aggravating.
- Activities, such as gripping, will be aggravating because wrist extension is needed to achieve a full grip.

EASING ACTIVITIES

- Placing the wrist in a cast or splint is generally required to ease wrist symptoms and promote healing.
- Supporting the wrist with the other hand or a sling allows the hand and wrist to be in a rested position and in a position of relative elevation.
- Elevation of the hand will help decrease the amount of dependent edema that can accumulate in the hand after an injury to the wrist.
- Ice is an appropriate modality to slow the production of inflammation and to modulate pain.
- Compression, like elevation, is used to limit the amount of edema that accumulates in the hand and wrist.
- Minimizing wrist and hand use.

24-HOUR SYMPTOM PATTERN

- As with most fractures, initially, pain will be experienced most of the day and night. Patients will complain of a deep achiness in the wrist, and this pain will increase during the first 72 hours as the inflammatory phase peaks. Nocturnal achiness is common with fractures.
- As the fracture heals, achiness at night and with weather changes is still common. Morning stiffness that lasts over 30 minutes is not uncommon.
- Increased swelling and edema is normal at the end of the day and depends on use. As edema increases, it is not uncommon for patients to complain of achiness or tightness in the wrist.

PAST HISTORY FOR THE REGION

- In older individuals, history of osteopenia or osteoporosis is common.
- May have history of long-term use of steroids or other bone weakening medications.

PHYSICAL EXAMINATION

- Pain in the wrist; generally pain and tenderness is located in the distal 2 inches of the radius or ulna. Pain will correlate with the location of the fracture, although the longer the time since injury, the more secondary and remote sites will be hypersensitized by the production of inflammation.
- Inability to move wrist is experienced partly because of muscle guarding and partly because bony obstructions may prevent normal joint mechanics.
- Wrist deformity is common because of the anterior displacement of the wrist and hand in relationship to the remainder of the proximal forearm.
- Edema will be prevalent, especially in the acute phase. Muscle atrophy in the forearm will be noticed after casting. Edema may be present in the wrist even after several weeks of casting, but this edema is present secondary to disuse rather than from tissue injury.
- Bruising will be present acutely after a wrist fracture. Bone structures are highly vascularized and injury to the tissue will result in damage to vascular structures. The damage to vascularized tissue will result in bruising.

IMPORTANT OBJECTIVE TESTS

Distal radius fracture is usually diagnosed with radiographs. Nondisplaced fractures may sometimes require CT.

DIFFERENTIAL DIAGNOSIS

- Although radiographs generally make differential diagnosis straightforward, other diagnoses to consider include the following:
  - ○ Scaphoid fracture
  - ○ Ligament injury around the carpals
  - ○ Fracture of the distal ulna (uncommon in isolation)
  - ○ Triangular fibrocartilage complex tear
  - ○ Distal radioulnar joint dislocation
- These pathologies may also occur in conjunction with distal radius fracture.

TREATMENT

SURGICAL OPTIONS

- Simple, stable fractures that can be reduced manually may require only casting. Unstable fractures may require percutaneous pinning or open reduction and hardware fixation.
- The success of surgery depends on the severity of the fracture (displacement, angulation, degree of bone compression, and whether the fracture is intraarticular or extraarticular) and the absence or presence of associated injuries.
- Surgery may be indicated if there is loss of bone length, unacceptable malalignment, or fracture into the joint, or if the fracture cannot be stabilized with a cast after closed reduction.

REHABILITATION

- The rehabilitation plan will be guided by the examination findings. Pain can be addressed with modalities, gentle manual techniques, and splinting for rest. When hypersensitivity is present, a desensitization program is indicated. Stiffness may benefit from joint and soft tissue mobilization and therapeutic exercise. Weakness will also respond to therapeutic exercise.
- The exercise program should start with gentle active and passive motion of the wrist, forearm, and fingers. Active and passive flexion of the finger MCP joints in the maximum-tolerated range, including while the patient is casted, is important; this can prevent or decrease contractures that will be very difficult to correct once established.

PROGNOSIS

- In younger persons, the primary predisposing factors are lifestyle choices (e.g., participation in sports such as rollerblading or snowboarding). In older persons, impaired balance and osteopenia create increased risk of wrist fracture.
- Although the severity of the fracture must be considered, most patients will recover most or all of lost function and have little or no pain within 1 year after injury.

SIGNS AND SYMPTOMS INDICATING REFERRAL TO PHYSICIAN

Any indications of a distal radius fracture require immediate referral to a physician. If the injury is seen acutely, the patient should be encouraged to remove any rings from the fingers; otherwise, swelling may later necessitate that the rings be cut off.

SUGGESTED READINGS

Haentjens P, Johnell O, Kanis JA, et al. Evidence from data searches and life-table analyses for gender-related differences in absolute risk of hip fracture after Colles' or spine fracture: Colles' fracture as an early and sensitive marker of skeletal fragility in white men. *J Bone Miner Res.* 2004;19:1933-1944.

Hanel DP, Jones MD, Trumble TE. Wrist fractures. *Orthop Clin North Am.* 2002;33(1):35-57, vii.

Ismail AA, Pye SR, Cockerill WC, Lunt M, Silman AJ, et al. Incidence of limb fracture across Europe: results from the European Prospective Osteoporosis Study (EPOS). *Osteoporos Int.* 2002;13:565-571.

Owen RA, Melton LJ 3rd, Johnson KA, Ilstrup DM, Riggs BL. Incidence of Colles' fracture in a North American community. *Am J Public Health.* 1982;72:605-607.

AUTHORS: ROBIN BURKS and DERRICK SUEKI

Section III

ORTHOPEDIC PATHOLOGY

BASIC INFORMATION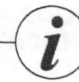

DEFINITION

A swan-neck deformity is defined as PIP joint hyperextension with concurrent DIP joint flexion.

SYNONYMS

None

> **ICD-9CM CODE**
> 814.1 Open fracture of carpal bones

OPTIMAL NUMBER OF VISITS

3 visits

MAXIMAL NUMBER OF VISITS

8 visits

ETIOLOGY

- Swan-neck deformities can be divided into three categories: congenital, traumatic, or secondary to RA.
- RA is the most common disease affecting the PIP joint. Chronic inflammation of the PIP joint puts a stretch on the volar plate. As the volar plate weakens, the PIP joint becomes loose and falls into hyperextension. The lateral bands slip dorsal to the joint axis, increasing the PIP hyperextension force. This change relaxes the tension on the terminal extensor tendon, allowing the DIP joint to fall into flexion. As the DIP joint flexes and the PIP joint hyperextends, the swan-neck deformity occurs.
- Congenital swan-neck deformity is the result of intrinsic muscle tightness. The muscular contracture can develop from hand trauma, cerebral palsy, Parkinson's disease, or stroke. The muscle imbalance tends to weaken the volar plate and pull the PIP joint into extension.
- Trauma to a finger that forces the PIP joint into hyperextension can also rupture or stretch the volar plate. This laxity may then lead to a swan-neck deformity.
- Trauma to the finger that forces the DIP into hyperflexion and rupturing the terminal tendon results in a mallet deformity. Hyperextension of the PIP occurs secondary to a swan-neck deformity.

EPIDEMIOLOGY AND DEMOGRAPHICS

Approximately 50% of patients with RA develop a swan-neck deformity.

MECHANISM OF INJURY

- The finger fractures from MVA or stepped on during a sporting competition can cause adhesions.
- Burns to the finger may cause an interruption in the vascular supply.

- Hyperextension force from a ball hitting the finger.
- Forced flexion of the DIP from a ball hitting the finger causing a tendon avulsion.

COMMON SIGNS AND SYMPTOMS

- Inability to close the hand because of the finger locking into extension at the PIP joint.
- PIP edema or tenderness.

AGGRAVATING ACTIVITIES

- Activities that place the hand in MCP flexion and IP extension exacerbate intrinsic tightness.
- Holding a newspaper or resting the chin on the dorsal fingers should be avoided.

EASING ACTIVITIES

Stretching the MCP into extension and the PIP into flexion at the same time elongates the intrinsic muscles of the hand and attempts to ease the deformity

24-HOUR SYMPTOM PATTERN

Swan-neck deformities are insidious, and there are no 24-hour symptom changes.

PAST HISTORY FOR THE REGION

- Trauma or neurological conditions such as cerebral palsy, stroke, Parkinson's disease, and traumatic brain injury
- Recent trauma to the involved digit
- RA

PHYSICAL EXAMINATION

- Terminal tendon rupture or attenuation with secondary hyperextension of PIP
- PIP hyperextension from laxity within the volar capsule secondary to synovitis
- FDS rupture
- Intrinsic tightness secondary to MCP pathology

IMPORTANT OBJECTIVE TESTS

- Intrinsic Tightness test: More MCP flexion with the PIP in flexion than the PIP in extension indicates intrinsic muscles tightness. Sensitivity and specificity unavailable.
- ORL test: Tightness exists if the DIP has greater flexion with the PIP flexed rather than extended. Sensitivity and specificity unavailable.
- Radiography to rule out fracture.

DIFFERENTIAL DIAGNOSIS

- Fracture
- Dislocation
- Tendon rupture

CONTRIBUTING FACTORS

- Rheumatic diseases, such as SLE and scleroderma, may increase changes of development of swan-neck deformities.
- Parkinson's disease and cerebral vascular accidents are examples of insults on the central nervous system that can predispose a patient to a swan-neck deformity.

TREATMENT

SURGICAL INDICATORS

Pain, loss of finger function caused by deformity, and failure of conservative treatment methods

SURGICAL OPTIONS

- PIP joint arthroplasty: Swan-neck deformity with a stiff PIP joint may require replacement of the PIP joint. The surgeon works from the dorsal surface of the finger to remove both surfaces of the PIP joint to make room for the new implant. With the new joint in place, the surgeon balances the soft tissues around the joint to ensure that the new joint can easily bend and straighten.
- Joint fusion: Fusing the two joint surfaces together eases pain, makes the joint stable, and helps prevent additional joint deformity. The PIP joint is usually fused in a bent position, between 25 and 45 degrees. If the PIP joint remains flexible, the DIP joint may be fused in full extension.
- Early swan-neck deformity can be corrected by intrinsic release, flexor synovectomy, the correction of PIP joint hyperextension with capsulodesis or tenodesis, or a combination of these.

SURGICAL OUTCOMES

- On average, there is less functional improvement in swan-neck deformities caused by RA than in those resulting from trauma.
- Patients have reported significant pain relief after PIP joint synovectomy.

REHABILITATION

- Successful nonsurgical treatment is based on restoring balance in the structures of the hand and fingers. The approach depends on whether the PIP joint is flexible or stiff.
- A flexible PIP joint deformity can benefit from a splint keeping the PIP joint in slight flexion to avoid locking into the hyperextend position. This form of splinting allows for full flexion of the finger to increase functional mobility of the hand. These splints are shaped like jewelry rings and are available in stainless steel, sterling silver, or gold.

This approach works best for mild cases of swan-neck deformity as a result of RA.

- Treatment of stiff PIP joint deformities is usually not successful despite a rigorous splinting therapy program. It is difficult to correct the muscle imbalance that is responsible for the swan-neck deformity. However, many hand surgeons will try 6 weeks with the splint and exercise to improve PIP joint mobility before performing surgery.
- Splinting that prevents complete extension of the PIP joint is needed to decrease the imbalance force of the lateral bands. It should also allow full motion of all joints, except to prevent total extension of the PIP joint.
  - Splinting will not permanently correct the deformity; however, it will hold the finger in a functional position. Preventing extreme hyperextension of the PIP joint will allow the patient functional use of the hand.
    - Thermoplastic figure-eight and Silver Ring splints are commonly used for this deformity.
- Exercises with PIP joint flexion and MPC extension are good because they promote an intrinsic muscle stretch. It is also important to educate patients to avoid activities or exercises that place the hand in prolonged MCP flexion and IP extension, or intrinsic plus position, since this position will only encourage deformity.

PROGNOSIS

The prognosis is determined by the primary cause of the deformity and the speed of intervention. The quicker the treatment is implemented the better the outcome. For this reason, determining the primary cause of the deformity is essential.

SIGNS AND SYMPTOMS INDICATING REFERRAL TO PHYSICIAN

If a swan-neck deformity is suspected, the patient should be evaluated by a hand surgeon to determine the best course of treatment.

SUGGESTED READINGS

Boyer MI, Gelberman RH. Operative correction of swan-neck and boutonnière deformities in the rheumatoid hand. *J Am Acad Orthop Surg*. 1999;7(2):92–100.

Nalebuff EA. The rheumatoid swan-neck deformity. *Hand Clin*. 1989;5(2):203–214.

AUTHOR: AUDRA PONCI BADO

BASIC INFORMATION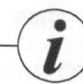

DEFINITION

Thumb CMC arthritis describes the deterioration of the articular cartilage and development of new bone formation between the trapezium and first MC bone in the hand.

SYNONYM

Basal joint arthritis

ICD-9CM CODE
715.04 Osteoarthrosis generalized
        involving hand

OPTIMAL NUMBER OF VISITS

2 visits

MAXIMAL NUMBER OF VISITS

20 visits

ETIOLOGY

- The exact cause of thumb arthritis, as with osteoarthritis in general, is not known. Researchers suspect that it is a combination of factors, including being overweight, the aging process, joint injury or stress, heredity, muscle weakness, and cumulative load.
- With thumb CMC arthritis, the cartilage that covers the ends of the bones deteriorates and its smooth surface becomes rough. The bones then rub against each other, resulting in friction and joint damage.
- The body attempts to repair the damage by making new bone. Unfortunately, this new bone manifests along the sides of the existing bone, resulting in spurs that may be palpable over the joint.
- The MC bone moves in a dorsal radial direction from the trapezium as a result of ligament failure. The MCP joint then becomes positioned in hyperextension.
- Most patients have osteoarthritis for years and do not have any pain. The initiating event for the inflammatory process can be genetic, metabolic, systemic, or traumatic.

EPIDEMIOLOGY AND DEMOGRAPHICS

- Thumb arthritis usually occurs after 40 years of age.
- Physiologically, thumb CMC arthritis is more common in women than in men. Recent evidence has shown that the female hormones estrogen and relaxin in the joint ligaments may play a part in thumb arthritis.

MECHANISM OF INJURY

- Generally, thumb symptoms will increase in frequency and intensity over the course of several months to years.
- Repetitive use of thumb for ADLs.
- Repeated pinching or gripping activities.

COMMON SIGNS AND SYMPTOMS

- Swelling, stiffness, and tenderness at the base of the thumb
- Decreased strength when pinching or grasping objects
- Decreased thumb ROM
- Enlarged, bony or out-of-joint appearance of the first CMC joint
- General discomfort or aching after continued use
- A sense of instability

AGGRAVATING ACTIVITIES

- Tip to tip pinch: Zipping up a zipper
- Heavy gripping: Holding heavy bags of groceries
- Lateral pinch with a twisting motion: Starting a car

EASING ACTIVITIES

- Since much of the pain is related to activity, relief is related to rest.
- Wrist splints that provide a thumb support (forearm thumb spica splint) allow the joint to rest with functional mobility of the fingers.

24-HOUR SYMPTOM PATTERN

The pain, stiffness, and decreased movement may be minimal or significant, depending on the severity of the condition and how patients use their hands in work and recreation.

PAST HISTORY FOR THE REGION

- Past injuries to the basal joint such as fractures and sprains
- Repetitive use of hands for work or leisure

PHYSICAL EXAMINATION

- Pain with palpation of the first CMC joint
- Bump at the base of the first CMC joint (shoulder sign)
- Muscle atrophy of thenar eminence
- Adducted web space

IMPORTANT OBJECTIVE TESTS

- Grind test
- X-rays
- CT scans
- MRI scans

DIFFERENTIAL DIAGNOSIS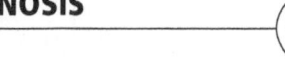

- Gout
- RA
- De Quervain's tenosynovitis
- Scaphotrapeziotrapezoid (STT) arthritis
- Radiocarpal or scaphoid instability
- Flexor pollicis longus (FPL) tenosynovitis
- Flexor carpi radialis insertional tendonitis
- Dorsal or volar ganglion

CONTRIBUTING FACTORS

- Age
- Gender
- Ligamentous laxity
- Autoimmune diseases such as RA
- Excessive use of the basal joint
- History of previous basal joint injury

TREATMENT

SURGICAL INDICATORS

- Failure of conservative treatment consisting of splinting, corticosteroid injections, and oral anti-inflammatory drugs
- Pain or deformity that interferes with daily function

SURGICAL OPTIONS

- Joint fusion (arthrodesis): Surgeons permanently fuse bones in a joint to increase stability and reduce pain. The fused joint can bear weight without pain but has no flexibility.
- Osteotomy: In this procedure, sometimes called bone cutting, surgeons reposition your bones to help correct deformities.
- Trapeziectomy: The surgeon removes the trapezium that sits adjacent to the joint. The trapezium may be partially or completely removed, depending on the surgical procedure.
- Joint replacement (arthroplasty): In this procedure, the surgeon removes part or all of the joint and replaces it with a graft from one of the patient's tendons. New plastic or metal devices, called prostheses, are also being developed to replace the joint.
- Hematoma and distraction arthroplasty: Excision of the entire trapezium and K-wire immobilization of the first MC bone in opposition and slight distraction.

SURGICAL OUTCOME

It is extremely difficult to measure the success of surgical procedures through research. No surgeon can agree as to which outcome measures are most important or how each should be measured. The majority of the studies seem to indicate ligamentous reconstruction and tendon interposition (LRTI) as the surgical method of choice.

REHABILITATION

- Initial treatment of thumb arthritis of any stage is activity modification, NSAIDs, and resting the joint with splinting.
- Treatment focuses on helping to reduce pain, maintain or improve joint movement, and minimize disability.

- Splints can be used to support the joint and limit the movement of thumb and wrist. Splints help decrease pain, encourage proper positioning, and give the joint time to rest. Depending on individual needs, the patient may wear a splint overnight or throughout the day.
- Splinting in conjunction with a corticosteroid injection may be the best solution for reducing acute inflammation.
- Several types of splints are available. Some are prefabricated and can be found in medical supply or drugstores. Others can be custom fabricated to fit the hand. Research is extensive regarding which type of custom splint is the best for the treatment of thumb CMC osteoarthritis.
- The type of splint used will depend on the source of the pain, the amount of stabilization needed, how positioning effects the other joints of the hand, and how the design and material ultimately affects total function.
- Often a patient will need more not less stability from a splint. A custom rigid plastic forearm splint with a thumb spica can be the most comfortable way to immobilize the wrist for a painful thumb.
- Modifying household equipment:
  - Consider purchasing adaptive equipment such as jar openers, key turners and large zipper pulls.
  - Enlarge the grasp on garden tools, kitchen utensils, and writing devices or buy items with large handles.
  - Replace traditional door handles, which you must grasp with your thumb, with levers.
  - Adaptive equipment is often available by catalog or internet.
- The patient should use other joints when possible. For instance, instead of grasping a doorknob to open a door, push it open with your shoulder.
- Education:
  - Teach the patient how to assess what causes their pain and how to avoid aggravation.
  - The more the patient knows about their condition, the better they will be at recognizing the motions that produce pain.
- Both heat and ice can be used in the treatment of CMC osteoarthritis. Heat can help ease pain, decrease joint stiffness, and relax tense muscles. Cold can also be helpful for reducing pain during flare-ups or after the patient has had too much physical activity.
- If oral medications and splinting are not effective in reducing pain in the thumb, a hand surgeon may recommend injecting a long-acting corticosteroid into the first CMC joint. Corticosteroid injections can offer some pain relief and reduce inflammation. Corticosteroid injections are only a temporary solution. Frequent use of corticosteroids can result in side effects such as nerve damage and decreased resistance to infection.

PROGNOSIS

Patients who are educated early on in the disease process have a good opportunity to limit the severity of disease. For those that will require surgery, procedures are continually researched and refined to give optimal results.

SIGNS AND SYMPTOMS INDICATING REFERRAL TO PHYSICIAN

Imaging of the joint to determine the stage and diagnosis of the disease is an important tool. A hand surgeon and a hand therapist can develop the most effective plan for the patient.

SUGGESTED READINGS

Croog AS, Rettig ME. Newest advances in the operative treatment of basal joint arthritis. *Bull NYU Hosp Jt Dis.* 2007;65(1):78–86.

Gray KV, Meals RA. Hematoma and distraction arthroplasty for thumb basal joint osteoarthritis: minimum 6.5 year follow-up evaluation. *J Hand Surg (Am).* 2007;32(1):23–29.

Martou G, Veltri K, Thoma A. Surgical treatment of osteoarthritis of the carpometacarpal joint of the thumb: a systematic review. *Plast Reconstr Surg.* 2004;114(2):421–432.

AUTHOR: AUDRA PONCI BADO

BASIC INFORMATION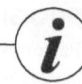

DEFINITION

The triangular fibrocartilage complex (TFCC) is a bi-concave structure that transmits 20% of force across the wrist from the hand through the distal radial ulnar (DRU) joint. The TFCC also provides a smooth, gliding surface for the ulna to indirectly articulate with the triquetrum and the lunate.

SYNONYM

Wrist sprain

ICD-9CM CODE
848.9 Unspecified site of sprain and strain

OPTIMAL NUMBER OF VISITS

5 visits

MAXIMAL NUMBER OF VISITS

20 visits

ETIOLOGY

- The components of the TFCC include the following:
  - Triangular fibrocartilage (TFC), also known as the articular disc, has a central avascular core with a hard outer vascularized layer
  - Dorsal and volar radioulnar ligaments
  - Ulnocarpal ligament (ulnolunate and ulnotriquetral)
  - Extensor carpi ulnaris (ECU) sheath
  - Lunotriquetral interosseous ligament
- TFCC injuries can be caused by any of the following:
  - DRU joint incongruity and distal radius fractures may cause an increase in axial load through the ulnar wrist. This change can result in damage to the TFCC.
  - Ulnar variance can significantly impact the load to the TFCC. The ulnar head moves distally with activities of pronation. An ulnar-positive (head is positioned above the articular surface of the radius) position will increase forces to the ulnar side of the wrist in a neutral position but will increase force with activities of pronation moving the head even more distally into the TFCC.
  - Falling onto pronated hyperextended wrist.
  - Distraction force applied to the volar forearm or wrist with twisting.
  - Disruption of ECU excursion causes damage to the TFCC because the sheath is part of the complex. The tendon is normally stabilized in the groove on the ulnar head. Subluxation may occur with forearm rotation as the tendon shifts from a strong ulnar

deviator with pronation to a primary extensor with supination.

EPIDEMIOLOGY AND DEMOGRAPHICS

- Degeneration of the TFCC begins in the third decade of life and progressively increases in frequency and severity in subsequent decades. After the fifth decade of life, studies have observed no normal appearing TFCCs.
- Gymnasts and males more than females suffer from TFCC injuries that result from using the wrist as a weight-bearing joint.

MECHANISM OF INJURY

- Falling onto the hand
- Having an opponent grab and forcefully twist the forearm in a wrestling match
- Repetitive use such as long-term use of crutches or walkers
- May be precipitated by a distal wrist fracture

COMMON SIGNS AND SYMPTOMS

- Catching or snapping in the ulnar aspect of the wrist
- Swelling that increases with activity and decreases with rest
- Complaints of weakness
- Pain with grip and twist motions.

AGGRAVATING ACTIVITIES

- Weight bearing through the wrist
- Activities that require ulnar deviation are as follows:
  - Opening a jar
  - Pouring from a gallon of milk
  - Scrubbing the surface of a table

EASING ACTIVITY

Rest in the form of splint immobilization.

24-HOUR SYMPTOM PATTERN

Intensity and frequency of pain may increase throughout the day, depending on the use of the hand for aggravating activities.

PAST HISTORY FOR THE REGION

- Reports may include a rotational injury or stress to the DRU joint
- Pain or swelling that improves with rest and worsens with activity
- Past injuries to the distal radius, proximal ulna, or radial head

PHYSICAL EXAM

- Decreased grip strength caused by pain
- Limited wrist ROM secondary to pain
- Ulnar variance (positive or negative)
- Pain with ulnar deviation of the wrist
- Tenderness at the base of the ulnar styloid
- Pain with compression of the DRU joint and forearm rotation

IMPORTANT OBJECTIVE TEST

- Arthrogram of the radiocarpal and distal radioulnar joints
- MRI, alone or enhanced with gadolinium or saline
- Ulnar grind test

DIFFERENTIAL DIAGNOSIS

- Metabolic diseases such as inflammatory arthritis or hyperlaxity
- Congenital abnormalities
- Degenerative problems
- Lunotriquetral joint instability
- Fracture of ulnar styloid
- ECU tendonitis or instability
- FCU tendonitis
- Ulnar nerve compression
- Midcarpal instability
- DRU joint instability

CONTRIBUTING FACTORS

- Diabetes
- Rheumatoid diseases

TREATMENT

SURGICAL INDICATORS

Surgery is only indicated after the lesion has failed to respond to conservative treatment.

SURGICAL OPTIONS

- Open or arthroscopic surgery with débridement or repair.
  - The central avascular area of the articular disc must be débrided since it has no healing potential. The periphery has good blood supply, therefore tears can be repaired in this region. Wrist arthroscopy is the criterion standard; it can be a diagnostic or therapeutic tool.
- Two types of ulnar shortening are as follows:
  - 2 to 3 mm osteotomy with rigid plate fixation is combined with a débridement for an articular disc tear.
  - 1 to 2 mm excision of the ulnar head.

SURGICAL OUTCOMES

Research has shown that independent of open or arthroscopic surgery, 75% to 90% of patients achieve at least 80% or greater of their original grip strength.

NONSURGICAL MANAGEMENT

- A combination of the following pain control management may help reduce symptoms: NSAIDs, cortisone injection, or iontophoresis with dexamethasone.
- Immobilization: The specific type of splint needed will depend on the findings from the objective tests. Initial

treatment of both symptomatic degenerative and traumatic tears lasts 8 to 2 weeks. Types of immobilization splints may include the following:

- Short-arm splint limits all wrist ROM, except forearm rotation.
- Long-arm splint, such as a Munster or Sugar Tong, limits wrist and forearm movement.
- Ulnar gutter splint limits all wrist motion, except forearm rotation.

POST SURGICAL MANAGEMENT

- All patients are immobilized immediately after surgery.
- If debridement alone is performed, patients are placed in a bulky dressing and started on motion exercises at days 5 to 7. Movement should be limited to a pain-free ROM. The patient may have a removable wrist splint for an additional 2 weeks before returning to all previous activities.
- All other surgical patients are placed in a long-arm splint.
- TFCC repairs need time for the tissues to heal before weight-bearing activities

can begin. This can require up to 8 weeks of immobilization in a long-arm cast followed by an additional 1 to 2 months in a removable splint to advance ROM exercises.

- Ulnar shortening with osteotomy and rigid plate fixation may require up to 6 weeks of immobilization with a long-arm cast. Once removed, an ulnar gutter splint may be used for protection for an addition 2 weeks.
- Strengthening should begin with the forearm in a supinated position for both surgical and nonsurgical patients. In supination, the ulna is in a shortened position unloading the TFCC. If no pain is felt in this position, the patient can be slowly progressed to exercises in neutral and finally pronation.

PROGNOSIS

Good prognosis can be expected; however, prognosis depends on the extent of the TFCC injury, how quickly the patient is diagnosed and treated and the compliance of the patient to the rehabilitation program.

SIGNS AND SYMPTOMS INDICATING REFERRAL TO PHYSICIAN

Failure of 4 to 6 weeks of conservative treatment involving immobilization and modalities for pain would warrant referral to a hand surgeon.

SUGGESTED READINGS

Cooney WP. Tears of the triangular fibrocartilage of the wrist. In: Cooney WP, Linscheid RL, Dobyns J, eds. *The wrist: diagnosis and operative treatment*. St. Louis, Missouri: Mosby; 1998:710-742.

Ekenstam F. Osseous anatomy and articular relationships about the distal ulna. *Hand Clin.* 1998;14(2):161-164.

LaStayo P, Weiss S. The GRIT: a quantitative measure of ulnar impaction syndrome. *J Hand Ther.* 2001:14;173-179.

AUTHOR: AUDRA PONCI BADO

BASIC INFORMATION

DEFINITION

Trigger finger is a tenosynovitis of the digital flexor tendons. It is often associated with repetitive, forceful gripping of the hands and with systemic diseases like gout, which cause pathological changes in tendons. The hallmark sign of the disorder is catching or "triggering" of the flexor tendons during active or passive flexion/extension of the digits.

SYNONYMS

- Stenosing tenosynovitis of the digits
- Digital tenovaginitis stenosans

ICD-9CM CODE
727.03 Trigger finger (acquired)

OPTIMAL NUMBER OF VISITS

6 visits

MAXIMAL NUMBER OF VISITS

14 visits

ETIOLOGY

- Repetitive use, inflammation, and fluid stasis within the fibroosseous tunnel surrounding the digital flexor tendons have all been implicated in trigger finger.
- Often, a fibrous nodule will form along the tendon of the FDS as it passes under the A1 pulley.
- In other cases, morphological changes in the pulley or FDS/FDP tendons can interfere with smooth passage of these tendons through the volar pulley system.
- Changes in the tendon and pulley can include nodular formation, peritendinous edema, and metaplasia of the chondrocytes.
- The bottom line in trigger finger is that the flexor tendon (usually FDS) is mismatched to the size of the retinacular tunnel through which it passes.
- In some cases the condition may be idiopathic, although there is often a history of diabetes or RA.

EPIDEMIOLOGY AND DEMOGRAPHICS

- More commonly found in females between the ages of 40 and 70 years
- Higher incidence in those with diabetes, rheumatoid conditions, and gout
- Found more often in manual laborers, farmers, musicians and others whose occupations involve prolonged and/or forceful gripping
- Trigger finger usually affects the dominant hand

MECHANISM OF INJURY

- In some cases, the condition may come on insidiously.
- In other cases, there is a history of repetitive hand use that leads to tendon hypertrophy and subsequent triggering caused by the pulley system being unable to accommodate the enlarged tendon or the nodule that sometimes forms.

COMMON SIGNS AND SYMPTOMS

- Pain and tenderness along the volar surface of the palm and digit
- Stiffness, catching, locking, cracking, or popping with flexion or extension
- Locking at any point in flexion/extension range and with passive or active movement
- Symptoms are most commonly found in the first, third, and fourth digits
- Symptoms may worsen after periods of inactivity and lessen with movement

AGGRAVATING ACTIVITIES

- Repeated gripping, flexion, and extension of the affected digits (especially at the MCP joint), and general hand movements
- After periods of inactivity, flexion and extension or gripping causes increased pain

EASING ACTIVITIES

- Decreased activity, rest, and immobilization
- Inactivity, however, may lead to increased stiffness
- Taking antiinflammatory medications

24-HOUR SYMPTOM PATTERN

- Catching, stiffness, and locking may be worse in the morning because of prolonged inactivity.
- Symptoms usually improve at the end of the day.

PAST HISTORY FOR THE REGION

- Frequent use of the fingers, especially gripping
- Involvement in work that requires repetitive use of the hands for gripping
- Repetitive flexion and extension of the fingers
- Underlying inflammatory condition such as diabetes or gout
- Possible history of carpal tunnel syndrome and/or de Quervain's syndrome

PHYSICAL EXAMINATION

- Sometimes a palpable nodule will be present on the volar surface of the digit near the MC head.
- Tenderness may be present at the site of the A1 pulley and near the junc-

tion of the MC head and proximal phalanx.
- Hypomobility may be noted with passive and active flexion/extension of the MCP joint; this may sometimes be accompanied by crepitus and locking.
- If "stuck," the joint may require overpressure to "break free."

IMPORTANT OBJECTIVE TESTS

No specific test has been objectified. Diagnosis is generally made via palpation of the A1 pulley and catching when finger is flexed and extended.

DIFFERENTIAL DIAGNOSIS

- Locking/subluxation of the MCP joint
- Injury/swelling of the FDP or FDS tendons
- Nodule formation on the FDP
- Tendinous tumor

CONTRIBUTING FACTORS

- RA
- Diabetes mellitus
- Hypothyroid conditions
- Gout
- Amyloidosis
- Advanced age

TREATMENT

SURGICAL OPTIONS

- Surgical excision of the A1 pulley through a "percutaneous release" procedure is advocated when conservative measures fail to resolve triggering.
- Success rates are usually high (up to 95%) compared to corticosteroids (90%) and splinting alone (60%).
- Rare risks include severance of digital nerves or of the A2 pulley.
- The latter may result in "bowstringing" of the flexor tendons and associated impairments in finger flexion.

REHABILITATION

- Iontophoresis may be helpful for delivery of antiinflammatory agents.
- Splinting for up to 6 weeks, depending on symptom resolution and activity level
- Painless ROM exercises should begin as early as possible (this should include flexion and extension at the MCP and interphalangeal joints).
- AROM should begin once pain and swelling decrease.
- Myofascial release.
- Joint mobilization (if indicated).

PROGNOSIS

Prognosis is good to excellent for recovery within an average of 6 weeks.

SIGNS AND SYMPTOMS INDICATING REFERRAL TO PHYSICIAN

Continued loss of range, weakness, and pain in spite of continued treatment, especially beyond 6 weeks' duration.

SUGGESTED READINGS

Freiberg A, Mulholland RS, Levine R. Nonoperative treatment of trigger fingers and thumbs. *J Hand Surg Am*. 1989; 14(3):553-558.

Griggs SM, Weiss AP, Lane LB, et al. Treatment of trigger finger in patients with diabetes mellitus. *J Hand Surg Am*. 1995; 20(5):787-789.

Moriya K, Uchiyama T, Kawaji Y. Comparison of the surgical outcomes for trigger finger and trigger thumb: preliminary results. *Hand Surg*. 2005;10(1):83-86.

Peters-Veluthamaningal C, Winters JC, Groenier KH, et al. Corticosteroid injections effective for trigger finger in adults in general practice: a double-blinded randomized placebo controlled trial. *Ann Rheum Dis*. 2008;67(9):1262-1266.

Sampson SP, Badalamente MA, Hurst LC, et al. Pathobiology of the human A1 pulley in trigger finger. *J Hand Surg Am*. 1991; 16(4):714-721.

Turowski GA, Zdankiewicz PD, Thomson JG. The results of surgical treatment of trigger finger. *J Hand Surg Am*. 1997;22(1): 145-149.

AUTHOR: SON TRINH

Section III

ORTHOPEDIC PATHOLOGY

BASIC INFORMATION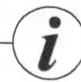

DEFINITION

The ulnar collateral ligament (UCL) of the thumb attaches the first MC bone to the proximal phalanx at the MCP joint. Forces onto the thumb in a lateral direction may tear fibers of the UCL. The strength of this ligament is so great that forces on the UCL may not tear it, but instead the ligament will detach from the insertion with a small piece of bone. This condition is called an avulsion fracture.

SYNONYMS

- Gamekeeper's thumb
- Skier's thumb
- Biker's thumb

ICD-9CM CODE
718.34 Recurrent dislocation of hand joint

OPTIMAL NUMBER OF VISITS

4 visits

MAXIMAL NUMBER OF VISITS

10 visits

ETIOLOGY

- Forced abduction of the first MCP joint. The UCL may be partially or completely torn with or without an avulsion fracture. This may result from chronic stress to the joint or from a sudden traumatic event.
- "Gamekeeper's thumb" was derived from the chronic injury to thumbs of British gamekeepers caused by the repeated twisting of the necks of rabbits.
- "Skier's thumb" is used to describe the common acute injury to thumbs of skier's falling on their hands while holding a ski pole.
- "Biker's thumb" describes the acute injury of mountain bike riders that fall over the tops of their handlebars injuring the thumb.

EPIDEMIOLOGY AND DEMOGRAPHICS

- UCL injuries occur nine times more than radial collateral ligament (RCL) injuries.
- Patients who are active in sports, such as skiing and mountain bike riding, are prone to this injury.
- There does not appear to be a gender prevalence.

MECHANISM OF INJURY

- A UCL tear most often occurs as the result of a sports injury when the thumb is forced into abduction.

- When the thumb is forced into the ground during a falling.
- When the thumb is jammed on a ball or another player.
- Fall over bicycle handlebars.
- Fall while holding ski poles.

COMMON SIGNS AND SYMPTOMS

- Patients with an acute tear of the UCL will complain of pain and swelling directly over the torn ligament at the base of the thumb. Pain may also be reported along the ulnar side of the MCP joint.
- Chronic UCL laxity or tears may present with complaints of weakness with grip or pinching activities.

AGGRAVATING ACTIVITIES

Pinching or gripping activities such as holding a tennis racket or throwing a baseball.

EASING ACTIVITIES

Stabilizing the MCP joint of the thumb with a spica splint will serve as a substitute for the lack of ligament stability and allow the joint to rest in a pain-free position.

24-HOUR SYMPTOM PATTERN

- Increased pain after prolonged activity of the thumb.
- Days without much thumb use will be less symptomatic.

PAST HISTORY FOR THE REGION

- Reports of an acute trauma to the thumb.
- Chronic cases of weakness or an inability to grasp or pinch using the thumb are common.

PHYSICAL EXAM

- Swelling at the MCP joint.
- Discoloration and tenderness to palpation along the ulnar volar aspect of the thumb.
- Significant swelling and ecchymosis are suggestive of severe UCL damage.
- Most UCL tears occur distally near the insertion of the ligament into the proximal phalanx.

IMPORTANT OBJECTIVE TESTS

- Valgus stress test of the thumb: A negative finding shows minimal or no instability. A negative test is classified as less than 30 degrees of laxity or less than 15 degrees more laxity than in the noninjured thumb. Although the preferred technique is to examine the thumb in full extension, a complete evaluation of the UCL should also include assessment of the thumb in full flexion when the ligament is maximally taut.

- Plain radiographs are used to assess for possible thumb fracture or subluxation. An avulsion fracture of the volar base of the proximal phalanx commonly accompanies UCL injuries.
- Stress radiographs are used to assess the severity of damage to the thumb and UCL. A joint opening that is >30 degrees while the MCP is fully flexed is consistent with complete rupture of the UCL; if the joint opening is <30 degrees, one can assume that part of the ligament remains intact. If questions arise regarding the degree of joint opening and the severity of damage, stress radiographs of the uninjured thumb can be obtained for comparison.
- MRI is useful for evaluating UCL injuries, but it is expensive and not always necessary.

DIFFERENTIAL DIAGNOSIS

- RCL sprain
- Fracture
- Dislocation of the MCP joint

CONTRIBUTING FACTORS

Hobbies or occupational hazards that cause a repetitive strain to the thumb and stretching of the UCL.

TREATMENT

SURGICAL INDICATORS

- Indications for surgery include the following:
  ○ Complete rupture of UCL.
  ○ Unstable and displaced avulsion fracture.
  ○ Stenner lesion is a condition in which the UCL is completely ruptured and the adductor pollicis muscle fragments interfere with ligament healing. If treated nonsurgically, this results in permanent instability at the first MCP joint.

SURGICAL OPTIONS

- Suture repair: If possible, the surgeon will repair the torn ends of the ligament back together. If the ligament is torn from the bone, the torn end will be sutured down to the bone itself. Surgery is usually most effective when performed within the first few weeks after injury.
  ○ If the injury to the ulnar collateral ligament is older, it is likely that a direct repair will not be possible. In this case, either another structure will be transferred to reconstruct the UCL or one of the muscles at the base of the thumb will be advanced to compensate for the torn ligament.

○ A pin is often placed across the MCP joint to prevent any stress on the repair site. It is usually removed 4 weeks after surgery.

- Fusion surgery is used for chronic instabilities to keep the MCP joint from moving. A fusion procedure is often the best choice when a patient's job involves heavy labor that would continue to put too much strain on the unstable thumb. When the joint is fused, a person's ability to complete daily tasks is not significantly changed because of the normally limited ROM at the first MCP joint. Fusion keeps the joint from moving, but it also protects it from eventually becoming arthritic and painful.

SURGICAL OUTCOMES

Surgical outcomes are unknown.

REHABILITATION

- Nonsurgical patients
  - ○ Incomplete UCL rupture can be treated conservatively with proper immobilization. The patient is placed in a cast or splint that includes the wrist with a thumb spica for 2 to 4 weeks. The MCP joint is positioned in 20 degrees of flexion with mild adduction to reduce stress on the ligament. The IP joint remains free to begin AROM to avoid tendon adhesions.
  - ○ After 2 to 4 weeks of immobilization for an incomplete UCL tear, reassess the thumb. If swelling and tenderness have diminished and the joint remains stable, the patient should continue to wear a thumb spica splint for an additional 2 to 4 weeks. The splint can be shortened to a hand-based spica splint to give the patient back wrist mobility. The patient should now be instructed to remove the splint several times daily for gentle AROM exercises.

  - ○ If the joint remains significantly unstable after 3 to 4 weeks of immobilization, operative repair should be considered.
  - ○ It is important to teach the patient that a stable thumb is much more important than obtaining end-ranges of motion. Increased movement can lead to instability and result in chronic pain.
- Strengthening for the nonsurgical UCL tear
  - ○ Lateral or key pinches can be initiated after 4 weeks of immobilization. The strength exercises should not illicit any pain at the UCL. Tip pinch should be avoided for approximately 8 weeks.
- Return to skiing after a UCL tear
  - ○ If there is a clinical decision to allow the patient to continue skiing after a recent injury to the UCL at the thumb, then protective splinting should be considered. Options include moldable fiberglass splints that can be adapted to the ski pole, athletic taping, either in wrist/thumb spica style, or the figure-eight approach. Before these interventions, the patient should have a clear understanding that there is a potential for their condition to worsen from further injury.
- Surgical patients
  - ○ After surgery, patients are placed in a cast or splint for 4 to 6 weeks to protect the repaired ligament. A radial-sided buttress can added on the spica to protect from any forces of radial deviation. IP joint ROM exercises are used to avoid adhesions of the extensor hood.
  - ○ After cast or splint removal, the patient will continue immobilization in a hand-based removable thumb spica splint for an additional 2 to

4 weeks. The splint is removed only for AROM exercise of the CMC and IP and gentle PROM of the MCP joint.
  - ○ Strengthening exercises can be used to help the return of full function. Tip pinch should be avoided until approximately 8 weeks after surgery.
  - ○ The patient should be weaned slowly from the splint over a 2 to 6 week period of time. Most patients are able to play sports 3 to 4 months after surgery.

PROGNOSIS

- With avulsions of the UCL, cartilage damage may occur that does not show up on radiographs. This occasionally results in long-term pain and eventual arthritis. Some patients may benefit from cortisone injections or eventual surgery.
- When properly treated, patients with a UCL injury have a good prognosis for returning to their prior level of function.

SIGNS AND SYMPTOMS INDICATING REFERRAL TO PHYSICIAN

Because avulsion fractures are common with UCL injuries, an evaluation from a hand surgeon with proper imaging is in the best interest of the patient.

SUGGESTED READINGS

Fricker R, Hintermann B. Skier's thumb. Treatment, prevention and recommendations. *Sports Med*. 1995;19(1):73-79.

Newland CC. Gamekeeper's thumb. *Orthop Clin North Am*. 1992;23(1):41-48.

Peterson JJ, Bancroft LW. Injuries of the fingers and thumb in the athlete. *Clin Sports Med*. 2006;25(3):527-542, vii-viii.

AUTHOR: AUDRA PONCI BADO

Section III

ORTHOPEDIC PATHOLOGY

BASIC INFORMATION

DEFINITION

Adductor tendinopathy most commonly refers to proximal adductor tendon pathology that acutely involves microtears and inflammation and chronically involves degeneration and cellular and collagen abnormalities.

SYNONYMS

Tendonitis and tendinosis, depending on the stage of pathology

> **ICD-9CM CODES**
> 726.5 Enthesopathy of hip region
> 726.9 Unspecified enthesopathy

OPTIMAL NUMBER OF VISITS

Approximately 12 visits; number depends on the stage of tissue pathology.

MAXIMAL NUMBER OF VISITS

25 visits

ETIOLOGY

- Adductor longus and gracilis tendons are the most commonly affected tendons and anatomically lie close to one another on the pubic bone.
- The enthesis or insertion of the tendon receives some of the highest stress concentration and therefore is the tendon most commonly injured.
- When the adductor tendons are constantly exposed to repetitive loading, which happens in certain sports activities that involve twisting and turning, traction is applied across the enthesis. Repeated activity can cause further tearing and inflammation. As blood supply to the tendon is relatively poor, the rate of healing is not enough to prevent further injury and pathology. As degeneration progresses, tissue maladaption advances, causing weakening of the tendon. Furthermore, as the tear spreads from the fibrocartilage to the pubic bone, fluid collects between the tendon and bone, which restricts healing.
- Initially the inflammatory reaction is the cause of acute adductor tendinitis pain. Under constant stress and strain, the tendon undergoes oxidative stress and apoptosis, causing a disorganized and immature matrix to be formed. Anoxia is theorized to stimulate nociceptors. With continued stress, more and more of the normal tendon matrix is replaced with a weaker and painful substitute. Chronic pain results from infiltration of vascular and neuronal tissue, which can be accompanied by adrenergic involvement.

EPIDEMIOLOGY AND DEMOGRAPHICS

- Tendinopathy can affect active individuals of any age. It is more commonly studied in younger populations but has been reported in studies to range from the second to the fifth decade of life. Older, active individuals are more susceptible to tendon pathology in which injury occurs with lower loads, and injuries can be more severe because there is less tendon integrity. There is also an increased incidence in men.
- In comparing symptomatic athletes to asymptomatic athletes, significant adductor enthesis changes on magnetic resonance imaging (MRI) are only found in the symptomatic groups, indicating that once a tear has progressed to a certain point, all individuals will have pain. However, in other areas of the body, degenerative changes have been found in asymptomatic tendons.

MECHANISM OF INJURY

- The adductor tendon is commonly injured with repetitive loading activities such as the following:
  - Twisting and direction changes
  - Kicking
  - Rapid lateral movements

COMMON SIGNS AND SYMPTOMS

- The pain pattern can be very similar to other hip and pelvic pathologies and includes unilateral groin, pubic, and medial thigh pain.
- Sensory and motor innervation is from the obturator nerve. The pectineus is innervated by the femoral nerve. Therefore symptoms will be affiliated with the respective nerve.

AGGRAVATING ACTIVITIES

- Running, especially with direction changes or uneven surfaces.
- Jumping, hopping.
- Kicking.
- Single-leg exercises.
- Side to side exercises/activities (cutting, lunges).
- Other activities with resisted hip adduction.
- These activities all require high contractility and power of the adductor muscles for stabilization and movement; for the pelvis and trunk to maintain a stable position the adductor muscles are very active. With a weakened adductor tendon, these activities can further aggravate tears and prevent adequate healing.

EASING ACTIVITIES

- Rest from aggravating activities.
- Physicians will often prescribe antiinflammatory medications, muscle relaxants, and pain medications to address the patient's symptoms.
- Depending on the phase of tendinopathy, ice and antiinflammatory approaches will have different success rates.
- The stress placed on the adductor tendon is less, inflammation (if present) can be decreased, and healing can occur.

24-HOUR SYMPTOM PATTERN

- The patient with tendinopathy will complain of stiffness and pain in the morning.
- Symptoms will increase with activity, usually activities involving higher levels of exertion than activities of daily living (ADLs).
- Sleeping may or may not be problematic.

PAST HISTORY FOR THE REGION

- Symptoms may occur after one direct injury or can occur insidiously over time. The symptoms will progress with continued activity until eventually the individual is unable to continue with the sport or exercise.
- Lower extremity tendinopathies can follow other injuries, such as low back pain, which is believed to alter trunk muscle activation, resulting in delayed stabilization of the pelvic ring. Injury to more distal parts of the kinetic chain can alter biomechanics and the load placed on the adductor muscles.

PHYSICAL EXAMINATION

- The causes of pain in the adductor region are hard to differentiate, and there are no specific clinical findings for adductor tendinopathy. Several studies have found subjects actually have multiple pathologies involved (in addition to adductor tendinopathy).
- All the adductor muscles can be symptomatic to palpation: Adductor brevis, adductor longus, adductor magnus, pectineus, and gracilis.

IMPORTANT OBJECTIVE TESTS

- Range of motion (ROM) tests for the hip
  - Hip passive abduction and external rotation may be limited by pain because of the stretch on the muscle and tendon.
- Resisted isometric hip adduction
  - Resisted hip adduction with the hip in neutral (no flexion or extension) will target adductor longus and brevis. Adding resisted knee flexion will help to target gracilis. Pectineus is easier to provoke with the hip in 90 degrees of flexion.
  - Positive: Pain and weakness in the adductor tendon.
  - Pain with isometric hip adduction is not a specific finding for adductor pathology.

- Palpation of the adductor tendon and surrounding structures
  - Palpation of the proximal bilateral adductor tendon, muscle, and pubic bone.
  - Positive: Pain is localized over adductor tendon (usually unilateral) but can radiate to pubic bone and into the muscle. Change in tissue compliance is also a positive finding.
  - Not a specific test for adductor tendinopathy.
- The tests will help localize the cause of the pain to the adductor region, but imaging is necessary to determine the exact pathology for certain diagnoses (osteitis pubis, adductor strain).

DIFFERENTIAL DIAGNOSIS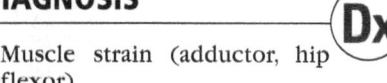

- Muscle strain (adductor, hip flexor)
- Osteitis pubis
- Other hip pathology
- Lumbar pathology
- Avulsion or heterotopic ossification
- Hernia (inguinal, femoral, or sports-related)
- Sacroiliac joint pathology
- Peripheral nerve entrapment
- Visceral pathology (urological, gynecological, or gastrointestinal)

TREATMENT

SURGICAL OPTIONS

- Tenotomy of the adductor tendon.
- Local anesthetic injection.
- Surgery is reserved for chronic, intractable adductor tendinopathy; usually, steroid injection has been attempted without long-standing success.
- Tenotomy has been found to be successful for nonspecific groin pain. Studies usually release the adductor longus tendon, but success has also been reported with the release of adductor brevis and gracilis.
  - Return to sport has been reported as early as 3 months after adductor longus tenotomy.

REHABILITATION

- The goals of rehabilitation of the tendon are to reverse pathological changes, return the individual to previous activity level, educate the patient in the management of activity level, and prevent recurrent injury to the muscle.
- Initially a rest period is enforced. Rehabilitation of adductor tendon injury is slower than rehabilitation of an adductor strain. Once pain and local tenderness have decreased, gentle stretching and strengthening are started. Gradual

reloading of the tendon followed by appropriate activity progression is necessary throughout rehabilitation and even during initial return to sport. Functional deficits and compensations must be identified and corrected before return to activity and sports.
- Initially, the primary focus of rehabilitation should be to decrease inflammation. Then the following can be used to reduce swelling:
  - Rest from aggravating activities
  - Correction of altered mechanics in other parts of the kinetic chain (strength, ROM of the lower extremity and trunk)
  - Soft tissue mobilization (STM) or myofascial release techniques to relax the adductors
  - Exercises that promote movement of the region in a pain-free range
  - Cold or hot pack
  - Ultrasound
  - Electrical stimulation
- Once the inflammation process has decreased, the focus of rehabilitation should be to restore normal biomechanics and decrease compensations, which are the factors that may contribute to the pathology. This is important not only while unloading the tendon but for proper reloading.
- Abdominal and trunk muscles are important during rehabilitation from groin pain. In a study by Cowan et al, a delay in transversus abdominis activation was found during straight leg raise in subjects with chronic groin pain. Trunk and pelvic strength and stability are important for healing, as well as injury prevention. Exercises to promote adequate hip ROM and strength, without increasing adductor pain, are necessary to restore correct motor control and performance.
- Current evidence has only explored the use of eccentric exercises for tendinopathy in other regions of the body (Achilles and patellar tendons). However, histological changes in tendinopathy are similar in different areas of the body, and eccentric exercises have been found to have beneficial effects if progressed slowly while monitoring for changes in function.
- STM of the adductor tendinopathy is limited by anatomical limitations. Friction and tendon mobilization techniques are generally used to decrease pain and increase mobility and flexibility.
- The role of exercise specifically for adductor tendinopathy has not been thoroughly researched, but its effectiveness for other tendinopathies is well known. Symptom resolution has been reported to be as high as 100% for an eccentric strengthening program for Achilles tendinopathy.

- In a study on adductor-related groin pain (at least 2 months duration), the group undergoing active strengthening and coordination exercises had significantly better outcomes than the group receiving only stretching, laser, transverse friction, and transcutaneous electrical nerve stimulation (TENS). Successful outcomes were based on return to sports activity, absence of pain with palpation, and isometric adduction (Holmich). The specific cause of groin pain was not identified, and radiological signs of osteitis pubis were present in more than half of the groups.
- Correct training intensity is important not only during healing phases but also for prevention of overuse injuries. During exercise, attention needs to be focused on signs and symptoms of continuing or new overuse pathology with unloading of the tissue as necessary. Even when symptoms are not present, adequate strengthening, conditioning, and recovery times need to be followed.

CONTRIBUTING FACTORS

- Abrupt changes in training intensity
- Technique errors
- Lower extremity impairments
- Poor activation of trunk muscle groups such as the multifidus and the transverse abdominis muscles
- Inadequate strength and ROM of the hip

PROGNOSIS

Most patients will recover fully or have minimal pain with high adductor-loading activities only.

SIGNS AND SYMPTOMS INDICATING REFERRAL TO PHYSICIAN

- Pain that does not change with position: Infection or tumor
- Nocturnal pain and significant and unexplained weight loss: Tumor
- Saddle anesthesia: Cauda equina syndrome
- Major trauma: Fracture
- Fevers and chills: Infection or tumor

SUGGESTED READINGS

Cook JL, Purdam CR. Rehabilitation of lower limb tendinopathies. *Clin Sports Med.* 2003;22:777-789.

Cowan SM, Schache AG, Brukner P, et al. Delayed onset of transversus abdominis in longstanding groin pain. *Med Sci Sports Exerc.* 2004;36(12):2040-2045.

Cunningham PM, Brennan D, O'Connell M, MacMahon P, O'Neil P, Eustace S. Patterns of bone and soft-tissue injury at the symphysis pubis in soccer players: observations at MRI. *AJR Am J Roentgenol.* 2007;188:W291-W296.

Davenport TE, Kulig K, Matharu Y, Blanco CE. The EdUReP model for nonsurgical management of tendinopathy. *Phys Ther.* 2005;85(10):1093-1103.

Holmich P, Uhrskou P, Ulnits L, et al. Effectiveness of active physical training as treatment for long-standing adductor-related groin pain in athletes: randomised trial. *Lancet*. 1999;353:439-443.

Robinson P, Barron DA, Parsons W, Grainger AJ, Schilders EM, O'Connor PJ. Adductor-related groin pain in athletes: correlation of MR imaging with clinical findings. *Skeletal Radiol*. 2004;33:451-457.

Xu Y, Murrell GA. The basic science of tendinopathy. *Clin Orthop Relat Res*. 2008;466:1528-1538.

AUTHOR: ALISON R. SCHEID

BASIC INFORMATION

DEFINITION

Avascular necrosis of the hip is the destruction and death of bone in the hip region as a result of ischemia.

SYNONYM

Osteonecrosis of the femoral head

ICD-9CM CODES
733.42 Aseptic necrosis of head and neck of femur

OPTIMAL NUMBER OF VISITS

Depends on surgical intervention

MAXIMAL NUMBER OF VISITS

Depends on surgical intervention

ETIOLOGY

- Numerous factors may be associated with blood loss to the hip such as femoral neck fractures, posterior hip dislocation, hip surgeries, corticosteroid use, alcoholism, smoking, renal and cardiac transplants, systemic lupus erythematosus (SLE), gout, diabetes, sickle cell and other anemias, septic conditions of the hip, Gaucher's disease, slipped capital femoral epiphysis, decompression sickness (Caisson's disease), pregnancy, radiation therapy, tumors, chronic pancreatitis, or chronic liver diseases or an idiopathic cause.
- The pathophysiology of osteonecrosis is attributed to several theories such as an alteration in intravascular blood flow, direct cellular toxicity, and impaired mesenchymal cellular differentiation. A change in the cells' balance of bone and adipose formation has been theorized to not only change bone composition but possibly alter blood flow to the femoral head. Without proper blood supply, the bone does not receive oxygen and cell death occurs causing small fractures and eventually bone collapse.
- The initial injury occurs in the subchondral bone of the femoral head. Medullary infarcts may also occur but are more stable and clinically silent.
- The articular cartilage initially spared because the cartilage is able to receive nutrients from the synovial fluid of the joint.
- Many patients will experience pain before the head of the humeral head collapses, which is theorized to be caused by the focal osteonecrosis process, as well as marrow edema of the femur.
- Once the femoral head has collapsed, the joint space narrows and cartilage damage occurs.

EPIDEMIOLOGY AND DEMOGRAPHICS

- The most common age group affected is 30 to 50 years of age.
- Many people with only a small area of necrosis or the absence of marrow edema are asymptomatic. However, once the area of involvement is increased and edema is present, most people will develop hip or groin pain.

MECHANISM OF INJURY

- Most causes of avascular necrosis do not have a mechanism of injury.
- Hip fractures of the femoral neck can predispose individuals to avascular necrosis.
- Nondisplaced stress fractures, such as insufficiency and fatigue fractures, are theorized to result from repetitive cyclical activities such as running, marching, jumping, and strenuous cycling.
- Since the amount of vascular injury in undisplaced fractures is less, it is less common to see osteonecrosis result from these fractures. However, cases of femoral neck tension fatigue fractures can lead to displaced fractures.
- Traumatic hip fractures leading to displaced hip fractures can result from the following:
  - Motor vehicle accidents (MVAs)
  - Falling
  - Other high-energy trauma

COMMON SIGNS AND SYMPTOMS

- Groin and thigh pain are the major symptoms of hip pathology. The hip joint receives innervation from the obturator, femoral, superior gluteal, and sciatic nerves.
- Some people may also experience buttock pain from the multiple innervation. Symptoms can go as far distally as the medial knee because of the innervation by the obturator nerve.
- ROM and joint stiffness is present, as well as muscle spasms in response to pain.

AGGRAVATING ACTIVITIES

- Standing
- Walking
- Running, jumping
- Climbing or descending stairs
- Lifting activities
- Other weight-bearing activities

EASING ACTIVITIES

- Lying supine, prone, and on the contralateral side
- Physicians will often prescribe antiinflammatory medications, muscle relaxants, and pain medications to address the patient's symptoms
- Sitting

24-HOUR SYMPTOM PATTERN

- The pain is slowly progressing, usually over weeks to months with symptoms related more to activity rather than time of day.
- Sleeping may or may not be problematic, depending on the severity of the necrosis.
- Initially, pain is only present with weight-bearing activities and resolves with rest.
- As the disease progresses, pain becomes more constant until it is present at rest.

PAST HISTORY FOR THE REGION

- Patient may or may not have a history of trauma to the area.
- Childhood history of hip pathology, torsions, or dysplasia may be present.

PHYSICAL EXAMINATION

- Patients with an injury to the hip will often present with a lateral trunk lean away from the affected side. Weight bearing can be shifted primarily to the contralateral leg in an attempt to remove weight from the painful hip.
- Often large muscles, such as the iliopsoas, rectus femoris, and sartorius, will spasm to create a splint for the painful hip.
- Posterior hip muscles, such as the gluteals and piriformis, can be very tender to palpation.
- As pain and postural changes progress, patients may also eventually develop pain and spasm in the muscles of the back.

IMPORTANT OBJECTIVE TESTS

- Hip ROM testing
  - In early stages, ROM is normal. As the joint destruction progresses, limitations in extension, internal rotation, and abduction can be seen, with pain possibly accompanying the movement.
- Diagnosis is usually based on imaging findings (MRI, x-ray, and computed tomography [CT] scans).

DIFFERENTIAL DIAGNOSIS

- Muscle strain
- Ligament strain
- Fracture (stress, traumatic)
- Tendinopathies
- Meralgia paresthetica
- Sacroiliac joint pathology
- Symphysis pubis pathology
- Lumbar spine pathology
- Hernia
- Ankylosing spondylitis
- Visceral pathology (urological, gynecological, or gastrointestinal)

TREATMENT

SURGICAL OPTIONS

- Once the hip becomes symptomatic and/or the stage of collapse is advanced, surgery is generally recommended. If the lesion has not caused the femoral head to collapse or the collapsed area is small enough, the femoral head is preserved and surgical options, such as core decompression and osteotomy, are performed.
- Surgeries
  - Total hip replacement
  - Resurfacing hemiarthroplasty
  - Resurfacing total hip replacement
  - Standard hemiarthroplasty
  - Vascularized bone grafting
  - Nonvascularized bone graft
  - Osteotomy
  - Core decompression with bone graft or graft substitute
  - Core decompression without graft or substitution

SURGICAL OUTCOMES

- Core compression has demonstrated effectiveness in managing small- to moderate-sized lesions.
- Osteotomy is also effective in reducing pain, but just like hip resurfacing, bone grafting, and core decompression, pain may develop years later and require a total hip arthroplasty (THA).
- THA has been shown to effectively decrease pain within 1 year of surgery.

REHABILITATION

- Initial rehabilitation focuses on patient education for given precautions and timeline for progression of activity, which vary based on the type of surgery.
  - Cemented THA allows for full weight bearing after surgery although certain hip ROM precautions apply.
  - Noncemented THA may have more weight-bearing precautions as well as ROM restrictions.
  - Osteotomy and decompression are usually limited to partial weight bearing for up to 3 to 6 months after surgery but allow active ROM (AROM) as tolerated.
  - Pain management and regaining functional mobility of the joint are important to resuming daily tasks and transitions.
- Inflammation can be decreased, using the following:
  - STM
  - Safe joint mobilization
  - Exercises that promote movement of the region in a pain free range
  - Cold or hot pack
  - Ultrasound
  - Electrical stimulation

- Initially, exercises should address the following:
  - Strength of the areas above and below the hip joint is essential for support of the hip. As pain and disability may have occurred for a prolonged time period before the surgery, core, knee, and foot/ankle strength may be significantly decreased, in addition to muscles around the hip.
  - Depending on the surgical approach, different muscles of the hip may have been split and reflected and may require healing time. If the gluteals and deep rotators of the hip can be strengthened, modified weight-bearing exercises for the hip can be initiated.
  - The type, frequency, and number of exercises are important to monitor and progress according to patient tolerance during healing phases. The major healing phase for bone, muscle, and the joint capsule is from 1 to 3 months after surgery, and even after this period, muscles are usually easily fatigued. Total healing time is estimated to take up to 1 year for joint replacements.
- STM can improve lymph drainage, decrease muscle spasm and pain, decrease scar adhesion and increase tissue extensibility as tissue temperature increases.
- Exercises to continue to increase muscle strength at the hip are important after any of the surgical alternatives. If only one muscle decreases its function across the joint, the compressive force on the cartilage can exceed the person's body weight by four times, which is an important consideration for the remaining joint surfaces and/or the preservation of the joint arthroplasty.
- For joint arthroplasty and resurfacing, wear on the components is a concern for the joint lifespan of the younger patient. Stress to the joint can be minimized by avoiding excessive joint loading during jogging and jumping.

CONTRIBUTING FACTORS

- Loosening of the joint component
- Dislocation of the hip
- According to some references, steroid-induced avascular necroses have a higher rate of revision after THA and may have less success after resurfacing
- Leg length discrepancy or joint malalignment in the knee or foot
- Hip abductor weakness
- Poor activation of local lumbar muscle groups such as the multifidus and the transversus abdominis muscles
- Nerve injury
- Muscle contracture (iliopsoas, rectus femoris, tensor fascia latae, or adductors)

PROGNOSIS

- With the exception of very small lesions without collapse, nonoperative treatment is generally unsuccessful.
- Core decompression generally has higher rates of success in patients without steroid and alcohol use risks.
- Hip resurfacing procedures have shown a good survival rate at an average of 6 years and have been found to be the most successful in males with excellent bone stock. Since most of the bone is preserved with joint resurfacing, it allows for possible secondary procedures in younger patients.
- Osteotomy has a high conversion rate to total hip replacement; however, survival rates may be higher with vascularized transplants.
- THA for more advanced lesions and collapse have been found to have a high survival rate after 10 to 20 years. Conversion to THA after other procedures is not uncommon.

SIGNS AND SYMPTOMS INDICATING REFERRAL TO PHYSICIAN

- Increased calf swelling, localized tenderness, erythema, and possible pain with ankle dorsiflexion: Deep vein thrombosis (DVT) or infection (if located more proximally)
- Constant unrelenting pain or pain that does not change with position (nonmechanical): Infection or tumor
- Major trauma and severe pain with movement: Fracture (traumatic or periprosthetic)
- If the patient is unable to fully weight bear on the affected lower extremity: Fracture
- If pain continues, becomes significant at rest, awakens the patient from sleep, or is associated with significant swelling or redness, tests should be performed to rule out other causes such as tumor or osteomyelitis

SUGGESTED READINGS

Lavernia CJ, Sierra RJ, Grieco FR. Osteonecrosis of the femoral head. *J Am Acad Orthop Surg.* 1999;7:250-261.

Petrigliano FA, Lieberman JR. Osteonecrosis of the hip: novel approaches to evaluation and treatment. *Clin Orthop Relat Res.* 2007; 465:53-62.

Pihlajamaki HK, Ruohola J, Kiuru MJ, Visuri TI. Displaced femoral neck fatigue fractures in military recruits. *J Bone Joint Surg Am.* 2006;88(9):1989-1997.

Zacher J, Gursche A. Regional musculoskeletal conditions: 'hip' pain. *Best Pract Res Clin Rheumatol.* 2003;17(1):71-85.

AUTHOR: ALISON R. SCHEID

BASIC INFORMATION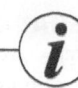

DEFINITION

A stress fracture is defined as the alteration of bone resulting from the inability to withstand nonviolent stress that is applied in a rhythmic, repeated, and subthreshold manner. Stress fractures of the femur are most commonly found at the femoral neck, medial aspect of the proximal shaft, and distal shaft.

SYNONYMS

- Femoral fatigue fracture
- Femoral insufficiency fracture

ICD-9CM CODES
733.95   Stress fracture of other bone
820   Fracture of neck of femur
821.0   Fracture of shaft or unspecified part of femur closed
821.2   Fracture of lower end of femur closed

OPTIMAL NUMBER OF VISITS

8 visits

MAXIMAL NUMBER OF VISITS

18 visits

ETIOLOGY

Physiological Mechanisms of Stress Fractures
- Stress fractures develop when the accumulation of microfractures at a uniform location cannot be accommodated by the normal physiological bone remodeling process.
  - Tension fractures result from cyclic loads causing osteon debonding and microfractures, thereby forming gross fatigue fractures. This further leads to higher stresses and rapid failure of the bone, and displacement may occur.
  - Compressive fractures occur with cyclic loads of shear microfractures disrupting the osseous microcirculation. Bone necrosis results, and osteoclastic bone remodeling occurs.
- Femoral neck stress fractures
  - In normal single-leg stance: Compressive strain occurs at the inferior aspect of the femoral neck with minimal forces applied to the superior aspect of the femoral neck. The downward-bending tension stress at the superior aspect of the femoral neck is counteracted by contraction of the abductors. This further produces a compensatory compressive strain on the superior aspect of the femoral neck.
  - The three categories of femoral neck stress fractures are *compressive stress fractures* that occur on the inferomedial

aspect of the femoral neck with little risk for displacement; *tension stress fractures* that occur on the superolateral aspect of the femoral neck and are at risk for fracture displacement; and *displaced stress fractures* caused by the complete disruption of the femoral neck that is the result of continued weight bearing of a tension stress fracture.
- Proximal shaft stress fracture
  - During normal running, compressive forces are placed on the medial aspect, while tensile forces are placed on the lateral side of the femur.
  - Additionally, the adductors and vastus medialis muscles apply a compressive load to the medial aspect.
- Distal shaft stress fracture
  - During normal running, the distal femur has the largest shear, compression, and torsional forces.

Types of Stress Fractures
- Fatigue fracture occurs in normal bone from repetitive mechanical stress as repetitive loading results in a decrease in the bone's failure strength.
- Insufficiency fracture occurs in bone with lowered bone fatigue strength such as osteomalacia, osteoporosis, or other disease states. Fracture may occur with lower loads or fewer loading cycles.

Location of Femoral Stress Fractures
- The three different types of femoral neck stress fractures are as follows:
  - Type I: Those with only an endosteal callus, periosteal callus, or both, without an overt fracture line
  - Type II: Those with a fracture line in the calcar region or across the neck but without displacement
  - Type III: Those in which displacement occurs
- Proximal shaft stress fractures: Have a greater occurrence on the medial aspect.
- Distal shaft stress fractures: occur between the distal one-third and femoral condyles.

EPIDEMIOLOGY AND DEMOGRAPHICS

- Prevalence is not well documented for the general population. It is estimated that 10% of all stress fractures occur at the femur and 5% of all stress fracture occur at the femoral neck.
- In runners, femoral stress fractures account for 4% to 14% of all stress fractures.
- In military recruits, femoral stress fractures account for 10% to 33% of all stress fractures.
- 3.5% to 20% of femoral stress fractures are at the femoral shaft.
- It is estimated 50% of femoral stress fractures occur at the femoral neck and 3.5% to 20% occur at the proximal shaft.

- Insufficiency fractures typically occur in the elderly.
- Fatigue fractures typically occur in younger populations.
- Runners, ballet dancers, athletes, and military trainees have an increased risk for fatigue stress fractures because of the initiation of new activity or the increase in frequency or intensity of a current activity.
- Postmenopausal women have an increased risk for insufficiency fractures.

MECHANISM OF INJURY

- Femoral stress fractures result from repetitive activity in weight bearing. The change in activity level or training, such as increasing the duration, frequency, and/or intensity of activity or training without allowing for proper bone and supporting muscle adaptation, can result in microscopic damage to the bone, which cannot be healed quickly.
- Athletic activities include but are not limited to the following:
  - Running
  - Military training
  - Ballet dancing

COMMON SIGNS AND SYMPTOMS

- Deep ache or stabbing pain at the hip or groin
- Hip, thigh, and/or knee pain that may not correlate with the region of the stress fracture
- Tenderness to palpation over the anterior aspect of the hip in the case of femoral neck stress fractures
- Painful weight bearing and difficulty with ambulation
- Painful activity that worsens with physical exertion
- Complaints of pain for several days, weeks, or months without traumatic incident
- Pain from femoral stress fractures can radiate into the hip, thigh, and knee

AGGRAVATING ACTIVITIES

- Weight-bearing activities: Walking, climbing or descending stairs, squatting, patient-specific sport or activity.
- Resistive exercises of the hip or knee musculature may cause pain, depending on site of the fracture.

EASING ACTIVITIES

- Rest from activity
- Non-weight–bearing activities
- Compression may help with pain relief

24-HOUR SYMPTOM PATTERN

- Morning soreness
- Aching in the hip on the first few steps in the morning or after prolonged rest
- Pain gradually increasing throughout the day with prolonged weight bearing
- Nighttime pain may be present

PAST HISTORY FOR THE REGION

Recurrence of femoral stress fractures is possible if rehabilitation was not completed properly.

PHYSICAL EXAMINATION

- Femoral neck stress fracture
  - Pain at end-range of motion, flexion, external rotation and internal rotation
  - Antalgic gait
  - Painful single-leg stance
  - Painful percussion at greater trochanter, tenderness to palpation at anterior aspect of the hip
- Femoral shaft stress fracture
  - No limitation in hip ROM
  - Antalgic gait
  - Painful single-leg stance

IMPORTANT OBJECTIVE TESTS

- There no objective tests in physical therapy that completely rule in or rule out a femoral stress fracture. A strong subjective and cluster of findings may best indicate a stress fracture. Radiographs, bone scintigraphy, and MRI are useful to visualize the fracture site.
- Femoral shaft stress fracture: Fulcrum test or "Hang" test—no specificity, sensitivity, or predictive value is currently reported.
  - Positive test includes an exacerbation of sharp thigh pain and apprehension and is shown to have a high clinical correlation for femoral shaft stress injuries.
- Ausculatory patella-pubic percussion test: Sensitivity: 0.96; specificity: 0.76; positive predictive value: 0.98
  - Positive test includes diminished or muffled sound quality and is indicative of bony disruption along the conduction path (femur). This is then followed up with MRI or a bone scan.
- Cyriax's seven "signs of the buttock"
  - Positive test is indicative of possible serious pathology.

DIFFERENTIAL DIAGNOSIS

- Hip synovitis
- Acute fracture
- Pubic ramus stress fracture
- Adductor strain
- Trochanteric bursitis
- Tendonitis: Iliopsoas or rectus femoris
- Snapping hip syndrome
- Sacroiliac joint dysfunction
- Degenerative arthritis
- Lumbar spine referred pain

CONTRIBUTING FACTORS

- Increase in gravitational force causes increased tensile stress in the femoral neck.

- Abductor muscle fatigue/weakness: Unable to counteract the tensile stress causing increased tensile stress at the femoral neck.
- Muscle fatigue limits shock-absorbing capabilities, thus increasing stresses on the femur. Additionally, gait is altered by muscle fatigue placing additional stress on bone.
- Metabolic and biochemical disorders: Rheumatoid arthritis (RA), hyperparathyroidism, hypogonadism, nutritional insufficiency (anorexia nervosa), menstrual disturbances, and long-term steroid use affecting the bone remodeling process.
- Osteopenia and reduced bone density.
- Structural and biomechanical influences include leg length discrepancy, femoral anteversion, coxa vara, or excessive pronation.
- Lack of physical training or conditioning.
- History of previous stress fractures.

TREATMENT

SURGICAL OPTIONS

- Tension and displaced stress fractures typically require surgical stabilization with screws and/or pins. Open reduction internal fixation (ORIF) or a THA is required for displaced fractures, depending on age and activity level.
- Compression type stress fractures do not typically require surgery except in instances where healing may not occur.

SURGICAL OUTCOMES

- Fixation failure rate within 3 months of surgery occurs in 12% to 24% of displaced femoral neck fractures treated by internal fixation. This is usually to the result of complications from fracture displacement or delayed diagnosis.
- In tension type stress fractures of the femoral neck, nonoperative management has been used in distinct cases. High patient compliance and careful supervision is required. Additionally, early detection of the stress fracture is necessary.
- Surgical indicators are as follows:
  - Displaced stress fractures require surgical intervention.
  - Typically, stress fractures at risk for displacement require surgery. The physician may monitor the fracture for a week or two to see if the pain lessens and the fracture begins to heal. If pain does not resolve or if evidence of fracture line expansion is noted, surgery is indicated.
  - If other forms of immobilization fail or cannot be used.

REHABILITATION

- The goals of physical therapy are to promote healing, prevent complications, and return to premorbid level of function.
- Initially, patients are educated to rest to minimize stress on the fracture site.
  - Non-weight–bearing with use of crutches or appropriate assistive device
  - Non-weight–bearing exercises painfree: Hip, knee, and ankle ROM, stretching and strengthening exercises for hip and knee musculature in open chain
  - Non-weight–bearing aerobic exercise: Swimming, low-resistance stationary bike exercise, upper body ergometry
- As symptoms resolve, weight-bearing status is gradually progressed.
  - Toe-touch weight bearing to partial weight bearing to weight bearing as tolerated based on pain.
  - No pain should be present for weight bearing to be progressed.
  - Physiological time frames usually indicate roughly 4 to 6 weeks for full weight bearing.
- As weight bearing is progressed, it is important to identify and address biomechanical faults and contributing factors to the stress fracture.
- Initiation of light weight-bearing strengthening exercises follows full weight bearing without pain.
  - Radiographic evidence of proper healing of bone is a good indicator to progress to light weight-bearing strength activities.
  - Low-impact aerobic exercise may also begin at this time.
- A prescribed walk-to-run program may be initiated after light weight-bearing strengthening exercises and prolonged ambulation are pain-free.
  - No ROM or strength limitations should be present to initiate this part of rehabilitation.
- After the walk-to-run program has been completed, gradual progression of distance, pace, surface and frequency are allowed.
  - Generally, pace or distance is not increased by more than 10% per week.
  - Sport-specific drills and higher intensity activities should be gradually introduced and progressed.
  - Activities are to remain pain-free. If pain recurs, then activity should be stopped.
- Education from physical therapy should include prevention of recurrence of stress fractures; contributing factors to the stress fractures, including biomechanical, nutritional, and endocrine factors; maintenance of proper flexibility, strength, and fitness; and cross-training or preconditioning for participation in sports.

PROGNOSIS

- At the femoral neck, prognosis depends on the nature of the fracture and any complications that arise.
- Compression type stress fractures usually have an excellent prognosis with proper rehabilitation.
- In nondisplaced femoral neck stress fractures, early diagnosis and proper treatment may prevent displacement of the fracture, thus improving the prognosis.
- Up to 25% of patients may have residual pain and discomfort of gait difficulties.
- Displaced fractures typically have the worst prognosis.
- Complications are usually associated with fracture displacement or delay in diagnosis. Most common complications include delayed union, nonunion, refracture, osteonecrosis, and avascular necrosis.

SIGNS AND SYMPTOMS INDICATING REFERRAL TO PHYSICIAN

- Suspicion of a fracture or any other serious pathology warrants referral to a physician

- Constant, unrelenting hip pain: Infection or tumor
- Pain that does not change with position or with non-weight-bearing: Tumor or infection
- Fevers and chills: Infection or tumor
- Significant and unexplained weight loss: Tumor
- Inability to bear weight on affected limb: Fracture, slipped capital femoral epiphysis, Legg-Calvé-Perthes disease, or avascular necrosis

SUGGESTED READINGS

Aro H, Dahlstrom S. Conservative management of distraction-type stress fractures of the femoral neck. *J Bone Joint Surg Br.* 1986;68(1):65-67.

Blickenstaff LD, Morris JM. Fatigue fractures of the femoral neck. *J Bone Joint Surg Am.* 1966;48:1031-1047.

Devas MB. Stress fractures of the femoral neck. *J Bone Joint Surg Br.* 1965;47(4):728-738.

Edwards WB, Gillette JC, Thomas JM, Derrick TR. Internal femoral forces and moments during running: implications for stress fracture development. *Clin Biomech (Bristol, Avon).* 2008;23(10):1269-1278.

Egol KA, Koval KJ, Kummer F, Frankel VH. Stress fractures of the femoral neck. *Clin Ortho Relat Res.* 1998;348:72-75.

Gurney B, Boissonnault WG, Andrews R. Differential diagnosis of a femoral neck/head stress fracture. *J Orthop Sports Phys Ther.* 2006;36(2):80-88.

McBryde AM. Stress fractures in athletes. *J Sports Med.* 1975;3:212-217.

Tountas AA. Insufficiency fractures of the femoral neck in elderly women. *Clin Orthop Rel Res.* 1993;292:202-209.

Weishaar MD, McMillian D, Moore JH. Identification and management of 2 femoral shaft stress injuries. *J Orthop Sports Phys Ther.* 2005;35(10):665-673.

AUTHOR: STEPHANIE S. SAITO

Section III

ORTHOPEDIC PATHOLOGY

BASIC INFORMATION

DEFINITION

- Greater trochanteric pain syndrome is a clinical syndrome based on the presence of symptoms over the greater trochanter of the hip, including bursitis, gluteal tendinopathy, and iliotibial band (ITB) pathology.
- The three common greater trochanter bursa are as follows:
  - The gluteus minimus bursa lies above and slightly anterior to the proximal and superior part of the greater trochanter.
  - The subgluteus medius bursa lies beneath the gluteus medius muscle, posterior and superior to the proximal greater trochanter.
  - The subgluteus maximus bursa is lateral to the greater trochanter, lying between the gluteus medius and the converging fibers of the gluteus maximus and the tensor fasciae latae as they form the ITB. It also separates the fibers of the gluteus maximus and the vastus lateralis origin.

SYNONYM

Greater trochanteric bursitis

ICD-9CM CODE
726.5 Enthesopathy of hip region

OPTIMAL NUMBER OF VISITS

8 to 12 visits

MAXIMAL NUMBER OF VISITS

25 visits

ETIOLOGY

- Originally, the most commonly assumed cause of pain for the lateral hip region was the subgluteus maximus bursa. Now other pathologies have been found to be just as prevalent including gluteal tendinopathy and atrophy and tensor fasciae latae tendinopathy.
- The gluteus medius tendon is more commonly found to be the pathological structure; however, in many cases of greater trochanteric pain, gluteus medius pathology is in conjunction with other pathologies. In terms of atrophy, one study found the gluteus minimus muscle is more commonly involved (Woodley et al).
- The causes of trochanteric pain are based on theories that suggest the ITB or iliotibial tract is rubbing over the gluteus medius tendon over time or that injury to the lateral hip structures follows direct trauma and strain. Most commonly, it is believed to be from repetitive microtrauma to the muscles

that insert on the greater trochanter while they try to stabilize the hip during periods of altered lower extremity biomechanics.
- Initially, the inflammatory reaction is the cause of bursitis or tendinitis pain. Under continued stress and strain, the tendon undergoes oxidative stress and apoptosis, causing a disorganized and immature matrix to be formed. Anoxia is theorized to stimulate nociceptors. With continued stress, more and more of the normal tendon matrix is replaced with a weaker and painful substitute. Chronic pain results from infiltration of vascular and neuronal tissue, which can be accompanied by adrenergic involvement.

EPIDEMIOLOGY AND DEMOGRAPHICS

- The most common age groups for trochanteric pain is middle-aged women (fourth decade of life) and the elderly (sixth decade of life).
- In a study by Woodley et al, almost half of the cases with bursitis diagnosed on MRI were in asymptomatic hips; however, osteoarthritis and tendon pathology were more commonly reported in symptomatic hips. There are also cases where no pathology was found on MRI, but the individuals still experienced lateral hip pain that was believed to be independent from lumbar referral.

MECHANISM OF INJURY

- In the case of trauma, the mechanism of injury for greater trochanteric pain syndrome:
  - Hyperadduction of the hip
  - Direct blow or fall onto the lateral hip
- As mentioned, the more common mechanism for injury is overuse of the hip structures for stabilization that causes repetitive microtrauma.

COMMON SIGNS AND SYMPTOMS

- Pain will be over the posterior lateral hip and buttock and can extend down the lateral thigh. Rarely, pain extends beyond the knee and into the posterior thigh and is usually chronic and intermittent. Individuals can report numbness in the upper thigh and a snapping sensation near the greater trochanter.
- The L2-L4 nerve roots can refer pain to the greater trochanter region and parts of the thigh. The L5 dermatome is slightly more posterior but can still refer to the lateral thigh region.
- The superior and inferior gluteal nerves innervate the gluteal and tensor fasciae latae muscles while the deep external rotators of the hip receive direct innervation from the sacral plexus. The lateral femoral cutaneous nerve gathers

sensory input from the lateral hip and thigh. The lateral cutaneous branch of the iliohypogastric nerve provides sensory innervation of the lateral and superior gluteal/hip region.

AGGRAVATING ACTIVITIES

- Ipsilateral side lying.
- Prolonged standing.
- Crossing the legs.
- Rising from a chair.
- Climbing and descending stairs or walking uphill.
- Hip external rotation and abduction movements.
- Running and jumping.
- Climbing activities.
- All of these activities create increased stress or pressure on the hip joint, requiring more stabilization from muscle-tendon units and their surrounding structures. Running, jumping, and climbing all require a high level of gluteal muscle contraction with both concentric and eccentric control.

EASING ACTIVITIES

- Rest from aggravating activities.
- Physicians will often prescribe antiinflammatory medications to address the patient's symptoms.
- Lying supine.
- Contralateral side lying with pillow between knees.
- These positions will decrease the demand on the surrounding structures, as well as decreasing the pressure directly on the lateral hip.
- Antiinflammatory medications may have more of an effect early during the presence of inflammation, and its effectiveness will decrease as the symptoms become chronic.

24-HOUR SYMPTOM PATTERN

- The severity of morning and sleeping symptoms depend on sleep position (see section Aggravating Activities). Symptoms may include stiffness and pain on waking.
- Symptoms will increase during the day if standing for too long or if sitting with crossed legs or with the aggravating activities as listed.

PAST HISTORY FOR THE REGION

- Symptoms may occur after one direct injury or can occur insidiously over time.
- Although a causal relationship has not necessarily been shown, greater trochanteric pain syndrome has been associated with lower extremity pathology and low back pain. Previous pain of the lower extremities and back can alter lower extremity biomechanics, leading to a gradual onset of lateral hip pain.

- With overuse the onset is very gradual, with pain increasing over time. Snapping may be present early or later on.

PHYSICAL EXAMINATION

- Patients with an injury to the lateral hip structures will often have altered gait mechanics. As the muscles attaching to the greater trochanter are responsible for pelvic and trunk stability during stance phases of gait, a contralateral pelvic drop can occur during stance on the painful limb (Trendelenburg's sign).
  - A leg length discrepancy may also be found.
  - For runners, crossover past midline may be observed and excessive lateral wearing of their shoes.
- More global muscles, such as the quadratus lumborum, and iliopsoas muscles are often tender to palpation. Any of the muscles attaching to or close to the greater trochanter may be tender to palpation (gluteals, tensor fasciae latae, and ITB).

IMPORTANT OBJECTIVE TESTS

- Hip ROM testing: Flexion, adduction, and/or internal rotation will be limited and painful because of the stretch on the gluteals and tensor fasciae latae.
- Palpation around the greater trochanter should be performed with the patient in sidelying, with the response compared to palpation of the opposite hip.
  - Positive: Pain reproduction
  - Many studies use tenderness to palpation as part of their diagnostic criteria for greater trochanteric pain syndrome. Woodley et al found all symptomatic hips with bursitis and/or tendon pathology to be positive to pain provocation with palpation in their study.
- Resisted hip abduction can be assessed with the patient either in supine with the hip abducted 45 degrees (Bird et al) or in sidelying with the hip abducted with slight extension and external rotation for gluteus medius and pure abduction for gluteus medius (Woodley et al).
  - Positive: Pain reproduction and/or weakness.
  - Bird et al reported a sensitivity of 73% and an even lower specificity of 46% with this test when based on the presence of pain as a positive response.
  - Woodley et al reported a sensitivity of 47% and a specificity of 86% when based on the presence of pain as a positive response and 80% sensitivity and 57% to 71% specificity when the presence of weakness was used as a positive response.
- Trendelenburg's sign/test can be assessed during single-leg stance and during walking.
  - Positive: Excessive contralateral pelvic drop. For Woodley et al, a positive test was the inability to hold a level pelvic position for 30 seconds.
  - Bird et al found Trendelenburg's sign to have 73% sensitivity and 77% specificity, whereas Woodley et al reported 23% sensitivity and 94% specificity.
- Resisted internal and external rotation of the hip can be performed in sitting and supine with the hip externally rotated for the internal rotation resistance and with the hip internally rotated for the external rotation resistance.
  - Positive: Pain and weakness.
  - Specificity and sensitivity have not been reported as very high, if reported at all.
- These tests represent only a few of the many tests of the hip in attempt to identify pathologic structures. However, their ability to predict greater trochanter pain syndrome requires further research and consensus on how to perform the tests.
- After ruling out other regions of pathology, these tests can be useful to assist in isolating the greater trochanter structures as the cause of symptoms while making other diagnoses less likely.

DIFFERENTIAL DIAGNOSIS (Dx)

- Other hip pathology (osteoarthritis, labral pathology)
- Lumbar spine pathology (including radiculopathy)
- Sacroiliac joint pathology
- Meralgia paresthetica
- Femoral nerve irritation
- Fibromyalgia
- Other muscle or ligament injury

TREATMENT (Rx)

SURGICAL OPTIONS

- Corticosteroid injections
- Bursal sac and calcification excision
- ITB release or lengthening
- Tendon anchor repair
- Trochanteric reduction osteotomy

SURGICAL OUTCOMES

- Local injections have results ranging from 50% to 100% success rates for pain alleviation, but symptoms have been found to return during long-term follow-up in some subjects.
- These surgeries have reported good outcomes over long-term follow-up but most of the studies have small subject numbers. Outcomes of conservative treatment in comparison to surgical options have not been well investigated.

REHABILITATION

- The goal of rehabilitation is to decrease further injury to the structures surrounding the greater trochanter, decrease inflammation if present, and regain ROM and strength. In the case of a traumatic injury, a rest period must be enforced while inflammation is being managed.
- The clinician may employ the following to address the initial pain and inflammation:
  - Rest from aggravating activities, including use of pillow between the knees with contralateral sidelying (avoiding ipsilateral sidelying)
  - Correction of altered mechanics in other parts of the kinetic chain (strength, ROM of the lower extremity and trunk)
  - Shoe lift if leg length discrepancy present
  - STM or myofascial release techniques
  - Joint mobilization
  - Exercises that promote movement of the region in a pain-free range
  - Cold or hot pack
  - Ultrasound
  - Electrical stimulation
- Once the inflammation process has decreased, the focus of rehabilitation should be on identifying the factors that contribute to the greater trochanteric pain syndrome such as abnormal biomechanics, poor use of trunk muscles, and decreased flexibility and ROM.
- Trunk and pelvic strength and stability are important for healing as well as injury prevention. Exercises to promote adequate hip ROM and strength, without increasing lateral hip pain are necessary to restore correct motor control and performance.
- STM is an important tool in improving ITB mobility without having to place much stress over the greater trochanter. As stretching this large and thick structure is difficult based on structure, as well as the tendency to place increased stress on the greater trochanter, STM can be an early intervention to decrease pain and prevent further stress to pathological structures. STM is also useful in improving flexibility in other hip muscles.
- Physical therapy interventions for greater trochanteric pain syndrome have not been well researched or compared to other treatment options.
  - Eccentric gluteal exercises may help in tendon healing and strengthening, as well as contribute to dynamic pelvic stability.
  - As the correlation of greater trochanter pain with low back pain has been reported, the importance of trunk muscle strength and stability may play a very important role in rehabilitation.

- Maintaining adequate hip and trunk muscle strength, as well as avoiding aggravating activities, if other lower extremity injuries occur (causing alteration of normal biomechanics). Modification of running to avoid crossing midline, as well as running only on level surfaces, will help prevent injury. Athletic footwear must provide adequate stability and shock absorption and need to be replaced regularly. Correction of leg length discrepancy must be maintained to prevent recurrence.

CONTRIBUTING FACTORS

- Poor walking or running mechanics
- An occupation that requires prolonged sitting or standing
- Lumbar or sacroiliac pathology
- Leg length discrepancy
- Poor activation of local lumbar muscle groups such as the multifidus and the transversus abdominis muscles
- Tight muscle groups especially the hip flexors, adductors, and hamstrings

PROGNOSIS

Most patients will recover fully from conservative management of the symptoms, and recurrence is not commonly reported in the literature.

SIGNS AND SYMPTOMS INDICATING REFERRAL TO PHYSICIAN

- Constant unrelenting low back or hip pain: Infection or tumor
- Pain that does not change with position: Infection or tumor
- Significant and unexplained weight loss: Tumor
- Major trauma: Fracture
- Fevers and chills: Infection or tumor

SUGGESTED READINGS

Bird PA, Oakley SP, Shnier R, Kirkham BW. Prospective evaluation of magnetic resonance imaging and physical examination findings in patients with greater trochanteric pain syndrome. *Arthritis Rheum.* 2001;44(9):2138-2145.

Braun P, Jensen S. Hip Pain: a focus on the sporting population. *Aust Fam Physician.* 2007;36(6):406-413.

Segal NA, Felson DT, Torner JC, et al. Greater trochanteric pain syndrome: epidemiology and associated factors. *Arch Phys Med Rehabil.* 2007;88:988-992.

Shbeeb MI, Matteson EL. Trochanteric bursitis (greater trochanteric pain syndrome). *Mayo Clin Proc.* 1996;71:565-569.

Tortolani PJ, Carbone JJ, Quartararo LG. Greater trochanteric pain syndrome in patients referred to orthopedic spine specialists. *Spine J.* 2002;2:251-254.

Woodley SJ, Nicholson HD, Livingstone V, et al. Lateral hip pain: findings from magnetic resonance imaging and clinical examination. *J Orthop Sports Phys Ther.* 2008;38(6):313-328.

AUTHOR: ALISON R. SCHEID

BASIC INFORMATION

DEFINITION

- Hamstring tendinopathy refers to tendon pathology that acutely involves microtears and inflammation and chronically involves degeneration and cellular and collagen abnormalities.
- Hamstring strain is a tissue deformation in response to stress of the biceps femoris (short or long head), semimembranosus, and/or semitendinosus, occurring at the musculotendinous junction or muscle belly.
- The three grades of muscle strain are as follows:
  - Grade I is defined by pain with minimal or no strength and ROM loss. Very minimal tissue disruption has occurred.
  - Grade II is defined by tissue damage that results in decreased muscle strength and function. Muscle fiber disruption has occurred.
  - Grade III is defined by complete muscle disruption resulting in complete strength and functional losses.

SYNONYM

Pulled hamstring

ICD-9CM CODES
843.8   Sprain of other specified sites of hip and thigh
726.5   Enthesopathy of hip region
726.9   Unspecified enthesopathy

OPTIMAL NUMBER OF VISITS

8 visits

MAXIMAL NUMBER OF VISITS

20 visits

ETIOLOGY

- The biceps femoris is the most commonly strained muscle. The hamstrings as a group are the most commonly strained muscles, partially as a result of its biarticular anatomy.
- Strains most commonly occur at the musculotendinous junction, which is present along the entire length of the hamstring muscles. Most tendon injuries occur in the proximal hamstring tendons, close to their insertion on the ischial tuberosity.
- Hamstring strain is the result of an indirect injury or trauma. A strong eccentric load placed across these muscles, usually during sport activities, exceeds the tissue's deformation capacity, causing inflammation, possible tearing, and bleeding of the muscle.
- Hamstring tendon injury occurs when exposed to repetitive loading as in certain sports activities involving running and sprinting where traction is applied across the enthesis. Repeated activity can cause further tearing and inflammation. As blood supply to the tendon is relatively poor, the rate of healing is not enough to prevent further injury and pathology. As degeneration advances, tissue maladaption progresses, causing weakening and thickening of the tendon. Furthermore, as the tear spreads from the fibrocartilage to the ischial tuberosity, fluid collects between the tendon and bone, which restricts healing. Bone cortical defects can be present near the insertion site.
- Damage to the muscle triggers an inflammatory response that causes edema, warmth, redness, and pain. Damage can also occur to small blood vessels, causing bleeding and pain.
- Tendons originally undergo inflammation, but because of their relatively poor blood supply in comparison to the muscle belly and continued stress placed on them, poor healing occurs leading to chronic tendinopathy or tendinosis. A disorganized and immature matrix is formed, and anoxia is theorized to stimulate nociceptors. With continued stress, more and more of the normal tendon matrix is replaced with a weaker and painful substitute. Chronic pain results from infiltration of vascular and neuronal tissue, which can be accompanied by adrenergic involvement.

EPIDEMIOLOGY AND DEMOGRAPHICS

- Older age ranges are usually associated with increased hamstring injury caused by nonmodifiable changes with aging. In a study of competitive soccer players, a lower risk of sustaining a hamstring injury was found in the 17- to 22-year-old age group (Woods et al).
- Most clinical definitions of a muscle strain rely on the presence of pain, and all grades of muscle strain involve pain. Cases of muscle tissue deformation in the absence of pain are not commonly reported or investigated.
- Degenerative changes may be found in the tendon before symptoms of tendinopathy are present.
- Studies have reported up to 45% of reported hamstring injuries had no signs of muscle damage on MRI, suggesting other areas, such as the lumbar spine, may be involved in the presence of hamstring pain.

MECHANISM OF INJURY

- The hamstrings are commonly injured with noncontact eccentric activities such as the following:
  - Rapid acceleration of running speed (sprints)
  - Repetitive hip stretching exercises that require larger ROMs
  - Fall during a sporting event
  - Jumping
  - Kicking, lunging

COMMON SIGNS AND SYMPTOMS

- Hamstring tendinopathy will present as gluteal pain usually with point tenderness but can occasionally lead to pain within the muscle. Hamstring strain can cause pain anywhere within the muscle.
- The sciatic nerve travels deep to the hamstrings in close proximity to the proximal hamstring tendons. The sciatic nerve separates to form the tibial and the common peroneal (fibular) nerves. The tibial nerve innervates all of the hamstring muscles except the short head of the biceps femoris, which receives its innervation from the common peroneal nerve.

AGGRAVATING ACTIVITIES

- Running, sprinting.
- Jumping.
- Kicking.
- Dance, yoga, and martial arts activities involving hamstring lengthening.
- Lunging.
- Hiking.
- These activities require the hamstrings to work to decelerate knee extension (eccentric action), which causes tension while lengthening the muscle. Repetitive activities like running and sprinting require the hamstrings to rapidly change from the eccentric extension at the knee to concentric extension at the hip.
- Dance, yoga, and martial arts require a lot of hip motion and hamstring flexibility that can also injure the hamstring muscles with repetitive excessive lengthening activities.

EASING ACTIVITIES

- Slow walking on level surfaces.
- Physicians will often prescribe antiinflammatory medications, muscle relaxants, and pain medications to address the patient's symptoms.
- Rest from aggravating activities.
- Positions of hip neutral and knee flexion, which can be accompanied by posterior pelvic tilt and lumbar spine flexion.
- Slow, level walking decreases the stress and stretch placed on the muscles and decreases the rapid change from eccentric to concentric contraction.
- Antiinflammatory medications will be more effective during acute injury phases.
- Positioning the hip and knee to avoid excessive stretch on the muscles generally provides relief. Anterior tilt positions stretch the hamstrings from their proximal attachment site.

Section III   ORTHOPEDIC PATHOLOGY

24-HOUR SYMPTOM PATTERN

- The patient with a muscle strain or tendinopathy will complain of stiffness and pain in the morning.
- At the beginning of exercise or sport activity, the muscles feel stiff and painful.
- Symptoms will increase with higher level activities, and soreness can continue afterward.
- Sleeping is usually not a problem.

PAST HISTORY FOR THE REGION

- Symptoms may occur after one direct injury or can occur insidiously over time. The symptoms will progress with continued activity until eventually the individual is unable to continue with the sport or exercise.
- Lower extremity tendinopathies can follow other injuries such as low back pain, which is believed to alter trunk muscle activation resulting in delayed stabilization of the pelvic ring. Early activation of the biceps femoris has been found following sacroiliac joint pain, potentially predisposing the hamstring to injury during a stabilization task (Hungerford et al). Hamstrings have also been found to be prematurely active with walking in subjects with chronic low back pain (Vogt et al).
- Injury to more distal parts of the kinetic chain can alter biomechanics and the demand on the hamstring muscles.

PHYSICAL EXAMINATION

- Although not specific for type of hamstring injury, signs of inflammation can be observed, including ecchymosis, and swelling can be present with initial injury. Atrophy may be present in chronic injuries.
- Attention should be paid to pelvis and lumbar spine posture as the physical findings will direct treatment approaches. Anterior pelvic tilt and increased lumbar lordosis may add stress to the hamstrings, while a posterior tilt may be the result of trying to unload the injured muscle.
- Possible gait changes with hamstring injury will include decreased ipsilateral step length to decrease the demand and time in swing phases.
- All the hamstring muscles can be symptomatic to palpation: Biceps femoris (short or long head), semimembranosus, and/or semitendinosus. Other muscles surrounding the knee can also be symptomatic: gastrocnemius, tensor fasciae latae, and the ITB. The global trunk muscles may also be symptomatic.

IMPORTANT OBJECTIVE TESTS

- Hip and lumbar ROM testing
  - Flexion of the hip and spine/pelvis will be limited and will reproduce the patient's hamstring symptoms, especially with knee extension. Knee extension with the hip in flexion will be limited and painful.
- Manual muscle tests (MMTs)
  - The hamstrings are given isometric resistance with the patient in prone with the tibia internally then externally rotated to differentiate between the semimembranosus/semitendinosus and biceps femoris respectively.
  - Positive: Pain and weakness in the hamstrings.
- Slump test
  - With the patient sitting, the spine is flexed or slumped forward, including the cervical spine. The knee is slowly passively extended with the ankle held in dorsiflexion until pain is reported. Symptom change with cervical spine extension is recorded, as well as knee extension angle. Test is performed bilaterally.
  - Positive: Pain in the posterior thigh that is the same with cervical spine extension suggests hamstring injury. Relief of symptoms with cervical spine extension reflects positive neural tension. However, neural tension has been suggested to be responsible for recurrent hamstring injury.
  - Lew and Briggs measured the change in hamstring tension and electromyogram (EMG) activity to establish that hamstring length did not vary with cervical position supporting the finding that increased symptoms with cervical flexion are due to neural structures.
- Taking off the shoe test
  - With the patient standing, the hip is externally rotated approximately 90 degrees and about 20 to 25 degrees of knee flexion. The knee is then forcefully flexed as if to pull the ipsilateral shoe off from the heel by pressing it against the contralateral foot's longitudinal arch.
  - Positive: Sharp pain over the biceps femoris.
  - Zeren and Oztekin described this test in a group of 140 male soccer players. Within the first 2 weeks of hamstring injury the sensitivity and specificity of the test was 100% for biceps femoris strain when the contralateral leg was used as the control. They found this test to be more sensitive and specific than ROM tests.
- These tests will assist in isolating the hamstrings as the cause of symptoms while making other diagnoses, such as referred posterior thigh pain, less likely.

DIFFERENTIAL DIAGNOSIS

Dx

- Lumbar pathology
- Other hip pathology
- Peripheral nerve pathology (piriformis syndrome)
- Sacroiliac joint pathology
- Ischiogluteal bursitis or apophysitis
- Ischial tuberosity avulsion or muscle ossification
- Compartment syndrome of posterior thigh
- Other muscle strain (adductor magnus, tensor fascia latae/ITB)
- Posterior knee pathology (meniscus, Baker's cyst)

TREATMENT

SURGICAL OPTIONS

- Hematoma evacuation puncture
- Repair of tendon rupture (proximal or distal)
- Local anesthetic injection

SURGICAL OUTCOMES

Surgery is rarely used to treat muscle strain or hamstring tendinopathy. Good to excellent results for return to preinjury sports level for complete tendon tears have been reported, and similar success rates have been reported with partial tears in distal and proximal tendons. Most studies recommend early surgery, but results for delayed repairs are comparable.

REHABILITATION

- The goal of rehabilitation of a hamstring injury is to decrease further injury, hemorrhaging, and inflammation; regain ROM; prevent atrophy; and regain strength and endurance to return to exercise and sport activity. Once the individual has returned to sports and activities, the goal is to avoid re-injury.
- Interventions used initially to address inflammation and pain should include the following:
  - Rest from aggravating activities
  - Correction of altered mechanics in other parts of the kinetic chain (strength, ROM of the lower extremity and trunk)
  - STM or myofascial release techniques
  - Walking on level surfaces
  - Exercises that promote movement of the hip and knee in a pain free range
  - Cold or hot pack, compression, and elevation
  - Ultrasound
  - Electrical stimulation
- Once the inflammation process has decreased, the focus of rehabilitation should be on identifying the factors that contribute to the hamstring injury such as abnormal biomechanics, poor use of trunk muscles, and decreased flexibility and ROM.
- Isometric followed by concentric and eccentric; pain-free exercises can be

used to prevent atrophy as well as cardiovascular exercise initially. Stretching of the hamstrings, as well as improving the flexibility of other muscles, is important for normal biomechanics. In a study by Malliaropoulos et al, increased stretching frequency of daily static, pain-free stretches was found to accelerate rehabilitation.

- Joint mobilization can increase the ROM of the hip and other joints in attempts to normalize lower extremity and trunk biomechanics to decrease the stress put on the injured muscles.
- One of the most important rehabilitation goals with hamstring injuries is prevention of recurrence. Exercises to establish proper flexibility, strength ratios, and stability of the surrounding joints are required before return to activities.
- In a study comparing stretching, isolated hamstring progressive exercise, and icing to a second intervention group consisting of progressive agility and trunk stabilization exercises and icing, return to sport time was the same. However, in a 1-year follow-up, the rates of recurrence were significantly less in the agility and stabilization group, suggesting the importance of including such exercises in a rehabilitation program (Sherry and Best).
- Eccentric hamstring strengthening is important since most injuries occur with eccentric contractions.
- Maintaining adequate muscular strength and endurance, even during the off-season is important in injury prevention. Correct training intensity is important not only during healing phases but also for prevention of injuries. Adequate abdominal, lumbar, pelvic, and gluteal muscle strength is important for healing and injury prevention.
- A regular hamstring stretching regimen has been associated with decreased injury in soccer players (Witvrouw et al). Strength of the hamstrings has been used to predict injury and has also been found to significantly decrease the chances of injury after an eccentric loading program (Askling).

CONTRIBUTING FACTORS

- Poor warm-up
- Imbalance in strength between the quadriceps and hamstrings
- Hypomobility of the hip and in adjacent regions (lumbar spine and pelvis)
- Fatigue of the muscles
- Poor activation of local lumbar muscle groups such as the multifidus and the transversus abdominis muscles
- Tight muscle groups especially the hip flexors, erector spinae, and hamstrings
- Poor running technique and biomechanics
- Neural tension

PROGNOSIS

The highest risk for injury recurrence is within the first 2 weeks of return to sport. Estimates for sprinters have been as high as 50% in those who had suffered previous strains. Re-injury estimates reported range from 12% to 34%.

SIGNS AND SYMPTOMS INDICATING REFERRAL TO PHYSICIAN

- Pain that does not change with position: Infection or tumor
- Sciatic neuropathy, progressing pain, thigh fullness/swelling: Compartment syndrome
- Dark urine with muscle pain and weakness: Rhabdomyolysis
- Saddle anesthesia: Cauda equina syndrome
- Major trauma: Fracture
- History of cancer: Metastatic disease
- Fevers and chills: Infection or tumor
- Sudden onset of bowel and/or bladder dysfunction: Cauda equina syndrome
- Progressive bilateral lower extremity paresthesias that are nondermatomal: Cauda equina syndrome

SUGGESTED READINGS

Askling C, Karlsson J, Thorstensson A. Hamstring injury occurrences in elite soccer players after preseason strength training with eccentric overload. *Scand J Med Sci Sports.* 2003;13:244-250.

Bencardino JT, Mellado JM. Hamstring injuries of the hip. *Magn Reson Imaging Clin N Am.* 2005;13(4):677-690.

Hoskins W, Pollard H. The management of hamstring injury – part 1: issues in diagnosis. *Man Ther.* 2005;10:96-107.

Hoskins W, Pollard H. Hamstring injury management – part 2: treatment. *Man Ther.* 2005;10:180-190.

Hungerford B, Gilleard W, Hodges P. Evidence of altered lumbopelvic muscle recruitment in the presence of sacroiliac joint pain. *Spine.* 2003;28(14):1593-1600.

Lempainen L, Sarimo J, Heikkila J, Mattila K, Orava S. Surgical treatment of partial tears of the proximal origin of the hamstring muscles. *Br J Sports Med.* 2006;40:688-691.

Lempainen L, Sarimo J, Mattila K, Heikkila J, Orava S. Distal tears of the hamstring muscles: review of the literature and our results of surgical treatment. *Br J Sports Med.* 2007;41:80-83.

Lew PC, Briggs CA. Relationship between the cervical component of the slump test and change in hamstring muscle tension. *Man Ther.* 1997;2(2):98-105.

Malliaropoulos N, Papalexandris S, Papalada A, Papacostas E. The role of stretching in rehabilitation of hamstring injuries: 80 athletes follow-up. *Med Sci Sports Exerc.* 2004;36(5):756-759.

Petersen J, Holmich P. Evidence based prevention of hamstring injuries in sport. *Br J Sports Med.* 2005;39:319-323.

Sherry MA, Best TM. A comparison of 2 rehabilitation programs in the treatment of acute hamstring strains. *J Orthop Sports Phys Ther.* 2004;34:116-125.

Witvrouw E, Danneels L, Asselman P, D'Have T, Cambier D. Muscle flexibility as a risk factor for developing muscle injuries in male professional soccer players. A prospective study. *Am J Sports Med.* 2003;31(1):41-46.

Woods C, Hawkins RD, Maltby S, Hulse M, Thomas A, Hodson A. The Football Association Medical Research Programme: an audit of injuries in professional football – analysis of hamstring injuries. *Br J Sports Med.* 2004;38:36-41.

Vogt L, Pfeifer K, Banzer W. Neuromuscular control of walking with chronic low back pain. *Man Ther.* 2003;8(1):21-28.

Zeren B, Oztekin HH. A new self-diagnostic test for biceps femoris muscle strains. *Clin J Sports Med.* 2006;16(2):166-169.

AUTHOR: ALISON R. SCHEID

BASIC INFORMATION

DEFINITION

- A tear in the groin muscles allows the intestines to slide out of the abdomen.
- Several types of hernias occur in the hip and thigh regions.
  - Sports hernias involve a weakening of the posterior inguinal wall, made up of the transversalis fascia, which results in chronic pain with activity. A clinically obvious hernia is usually absent.
  - Inguinal hernias involve a weakening of the aponeurosis of the external oblique muscle, allowing the intestines or the greater omentum to be forced anteriorly into the deep inguinal ring and inguinal canal (superior to the inguinal ligament). This is the most common type of inguinal hernia and considered an indirect inguinal hernia. A direct inguinal hernia enters through the posterior inguinal wall not the inguinal ring. Both inguinal hernias can extend into the scrotum.
  - Femoral hernias involve a weakening inferior to the inguinal ligament, allowing the intestines to push inferiorly into the femoral triangle.

SYNONYMS

- Sportsman hernia, hockey hernia, or athletic pubalgia
- Incipient hernia
- Gilmore's groin
- Hockey groin syndrome
- Pre-hernia complex

ICD-9CM CODES

550.9 Inguinal hernia without mention of obstruction or gangrene
550.10 Unilateral or unspecified inguinal hernia with obstruction without gangrene
551.0 Femoral hernia with gangrene
552.0 Femoral hernia with obstruction
553.0 Femoral hernia without mention of obstruction or gangrene
553.8 Hernia of other specified sites without obstruction or gangrene

OPTIMAL NUMBER OF VISITS

Depends on surgical approach

MAXIMAL NUMBER OF VISITS

Depends on surgical approach

ETIOLOGY

- Inguinal hernias are the most common lower abdominal hernia and can affect different age groups. Since the diagnosis of a sport's hernia is difficult, many individuals may receive different diagnoses.
- The lower quarter of the abdomen has a very thin posterior wall because the internal oblique and transversus abdominis muscles will insert anterior to the rectus abdominis, leaving only the transversalis fascia to form the posterior wall. This is believed to create a vulnerable area for a direct hernia and is the most often injured for a sports hernia. For inguinal hernias, the deep inguinal ring is the most common area for herniation because it is a weak point of the lower abdominal wall (indirect inguinal hernia).
- High pressures from one area escape through weak abdominal and inguinal areas. For a sports hernia, this area is the posterior wall, and for some inguinal hernias, this area is the deep inguinal ring, as well as other surrounding structures (conjoined tendon, internal oblique muscle fibers, etc). A patent processus vaginalis from fetal development creates an opening or weak area of the abdomen for an indirect hernia. For a femoral hernia, the weak area is within the femoral canal, allowing abdominal contents to pass distally.
- A weak posterior wall is encouraged by muscle imbalances, theorized to occur when the adductors have a strong pull, while the abdominal muscles provide poor stabilization, leading to tearing of the transversalis fascia and other layers.
- The pressure and tearing of the abdominal and inguinal walls can cause pain, as well as resulting pressure on the abdominal contents that enter the inguinal canal in the case of inguinal hernias.
- For femoral and inguinal hernias, pain may not result from the initial displacement of the bowels but may develop from the ischemia and necrosis if the condition progresses and is left untreated (strangulation).

EPIDEMIOLOGY AND DEMOGRAPHICS

- Indirect inguinal hernias can occur at any age including infants, adolescents, and young adults. Direct inguinal hernias are more common from ages 40 to 50 years and older. Inguinal hernias are more common in men. Sports hernias are more common in athletes, and most of the cases studied include young male athletes. Femoral hernias are more common in females approximately 30 to 70 years of age; however, rare cases in young adults and children have been reported.
- The inguinal canal is larger in males than females, since only the round ligament passes through the canal in females and in males the spermatic cord must be able to pass through, creating a larger opening for abdominal contents to enter.

- Not all people with hernias experience pain. Early inguinal and femoral hernias may not cause pain as the displaced abdominal contents are able to retract and/or the area of involvement may be small. However, in the case of sports hernias, a true hernia is not present even though pain persists. Some studies have reported inconsistencies between the side of anatomical pathology and side of pain, but pathology is usually present when pain is present.
- All femoral hernias and irreducible inguinal hernias require further testing to prevent strangulation of the intestines.

MECHANISM OF INJURY

- The abdominal and inguinal wall are commonly injured with straining (Valsalva maneuver) and high-exertion activities such as the following:
  - Lifting a heavy object
  - Coughing and sneezing
  - Bearing down to have a bowel movement
  - Twisting or fast directional change with the hip forced into abduction, adduction, or extension
  - Repetitive slap-shots by hockey players

COMMON SIGNS AND SYMPTOMS

- All of these hernias, if symptomatic, will present with groin pain that is worse with exertion. The lower abdomen and inguinal region may also be painful, and pain can be unilateral or bilateral. Pain can radiate to the proximal and medial thigh, as well as the perineum.
- For inguinal hernias, pain and signs of an enlarged scrotum may be present with exertion or standing. If the bowel is actually obstructed, the person may not only have pain in the obstructed area but also nausea and vomiting, with no bowel movements or flatulence. For sports hernias, pain is usually dull and diffuse over the groin and pubic regions. Femoral hernias have very similar signs and symptoms as inguinal hernias, but a bulge will be present below the inguinal ligament instead of the scrotum.
- Several peripheral nerves can be affected and there are many anatomical variations from person to person. The femoral, ilioinguinal, iliohypogastric, genitofemoral, and lateral femoral cutaneous nerves are found in and around the inguinal canal.

AGGRAVATING ACTIVITIES

- Forward bending can be painful.
- Active hip adduction or sit-up.
- Endurance running.
- Lifting activities.
- Kicking.
- Sudden changes in direction.

- Coughing, sneezing, or bearing down to have a bowel movement (Valsalva maneuvers).
- Coughing, sneezing, and bearing down to have a bowel movement will also increase the patient's symptoms because of the increase in abdominal pressure, which in turn creates an externally driven force on the abdominal wall and can increase protrusion of abdominal contents.
- Lifting, kicking, running, direction changes, or hip adduction all require stabilization of the hip and trunk using the abdominal muscles, and potentially quick maximal exertion can create stress in the inguinal area.

EASING ACTIVITIES

- Rest
- Avoidance of aggravating activities

24-HOUR SYMPTOM PATTERN

- The patient with a hernia may complain of pain in the morning with getting out of bed because straining may occur.
- Symptoms will increase during the day if coughing or activities requiring increased abdominal pressure transpire.
- Rest and sleep are usually not a problem unless serious pathology exists and strangulation of the abdominal contents occurs (inguinal and femoral hernias).

PAST HISTORY FOR THE REGION

- A sports hernia may not have any specific signs or symptoms in the region leading up to the hernia, and athletes often report a specific incident when the pain began. If symptoms do precede the sports hernia, they can include groin pain, which may change the normal biomechanics of the lower extremities.
- Inguinal and femoral hernias may follow a chronic cough, chronic constipation, heavy physical labor and straining, and pregnancy.
- Hernias may be reported as a problem in the past, since the rates of recurrence are high and the abdominal wall has a demonstrated weakness.

PHYSICAL EXAMINATION

- Patients with a painful inguinal or femoral hernia will prefer to be supine or sitting reclined versus standing or bending forward because of the pressure on the abdominal contents in upright or forward positions. It is therefore recommended that all tests be performed in supine and standing.
- The abdominal muscles, the pubic crest and tubercle, the inguinal canal, and adductor muscle and tendon can all be painful with a hernia. Spasm of the adductor or hip flexor muscles can also be present, which can be misleading as to the cause of pain.

- An enlargement or dilation of the superficial inguinal ring can be found in both sports and inguinal hernias, and a bulge may be present.

IMPORTANT OBJECTIVE TESTS

- Active straight leg raise (ASLR) test or resisted hip flexion
  - Active hip flexion or resistance during hip flexion during varying degrees of hip flexion/extension
  - Positive: Pain and weakness
  - Not a specific test for hernias
- Bilateral resisted hip adduction
  - Bilateral isometric resisted hip adduction with legs flexed or extended on the table, pushing against the clinician's forearms
  - Positive: Pain and weakness
  - Not a specific test for hernias
- Active sit-up
  - Examine trunk flexion in the sagittal plane and into bilateral rotation with hips in flexion and extension. Can add resistance while palpating inguinal region.
  - Positive: Pain and weakness; possible bulge for inguinal and femoral hernias
- Cough test
  - Cough with palpation of inguinal region
  - Positive: Pain for all hernias with palpable bulge for inguinal and femoral hernias
- Palpation of superficial inguinal ring
  - Commonly performed by inverting the scrotum with the examiner's small finger with the patient standing. Assessment is made bilaterally.
  - Positive: Pain and widening of the ring.

DIFFERENTIAL DIAGNOSIS

- Muscle strain (adductor, hip flexor, rectus abdominis)
- Ligament strain
- Lumbar pathology
- Enlarged lymph node (lymphadenopathy) or lipoma
- Psoas abscess
- Osteitis pubis or chronic pubic pain
- Genitourinary pathology
- Gastrointestinal pathology
- Stress fracture (femur, pubic ramus)
- Hip pathology
- Peripheral nerve entrapment (ilioinguinal, obturator, or femoral)

TREATMENT

SURGICAL OPTIONS

- Herniorrhaphy (laparoscopic or open)
- Hernioplasty
- Adductor release

- Open rectus abdominis repair (pelvic floor repair)
- Neurotomy

SURGICAL OUTCOMES

- Most results for conservative management of symptomatic hernias are not successful.
- Success rates after surgery range from 70% to 100% (based on return to previous functional or sport activities). However, return to functional activities and sports does not necessarily indicate relief from symptoms, and some studies have reported as many as 30% of patients after inguinal herniorrhaphy still had pain 2 to 3 years later.

REHABILITATION

- The goal of rehabilitation is twofold. First, the focus should be on healing and decreasing the patient's symptoms. Once the symptoms have diminished and healing has progressed, the focus of the rehabilitative process will turn to strengthening to prevent further episodes and return to activities and sports.
- For the first 1 to 3 weeks after surgery, rest is encouraged, along with techniques to decrease inflammation, with rest time depending on type of surgery.
- Initial inflammation can be addressed using the following:
  - STM and/or myofascial release techniques to relax the large muscle groups
  - Graded joint mobilization
  - Walking on level surfaces
  - Cold or hot pack
  - Ultrasound
  - Electrical stimulation
- Once the inflammation process has decreased, the focus of rehabilitation should be on identifying the factors that contribute to altered lower extremity biomechanics or decreased core strength and stability, including the pelvic floor muscles. Proper strength and ROM will be important to prevent re-injury. Establishing correct body mechanics with lifting and bending will also be important for prevention, starting without any weight.
- Establishing correct body mechanics with lifting and bending will also be important for prevention, starting without any weight.
- Stretches within a pain-free range, as well as aerobic exercise, are important after the initial rest period. Diaphragmatic breathing exercises are very important for establishing normal rib movement, lymphatic flow, and normal breathing mechanics because the origin of the abdominal muscles involve the ribs and spine.

- STM has been shown to improve lymph drainage and can increase pain-free ROM and superficial tissue temperature.
- Adequate amounts of cardiovascular exercise are important for overall fitness, but in the case of femoral and inguinal hernias are necessary for maintaining a healthy body weight. Diet also plays a large part in maintaining a healthy body weight, including adequate amounts of fiber to avoid straining with bowel movements. Avoiding smoking is important not only for healing, but also because not smoking decreases chronic coughing.
- Maintaining adequate lower extremity ROM and strength (especially in the hip) is crucial for sports, as well as to avoid unnecessary strain in the abdominal area with lifting. Proper lifting mechanics and avoidance of large loads are essential for healing and prevention of reoccurrence after surgery, particularly for inguinal and femoral hernias.
- Sports-specific training and strengthening are important for prevention of recurrence with return to high-level activity.

CONTRIBUTING FACTORS

- Chronic cough (smoking, chronic bronchitis)
- An occupation that requires repetitive bending, lifting, and standing (inguinal and femoral)
- Excessive body weight
- Pregnancy
- Poor activation of local lumbar, abdominal, and pelvic muscle groups during activity, as well as poor hip muscle strength
- Tight muscle groups, especially around the hip
- History of previous hernias
- Family history of hernias (more common for inguinal)

PROGNOSIS

- In studies done on soccer players with sports hernias who had open repairs, running is resumed at about 4 to 5 weeks and return to play by 6 to 8 weeks. Laparoscopic repairs have similar success rates for sports hernias, and this less invasive surgery may allow for early return to activities. Rates of re-injury or recurrence of sports hernia are not well documented, but the rates that are reported are usually low; however, cases of continued pain after surgery hand limitations in sports can occur in up to 20% or more.
- Some researchers recommend examination and exploration of the contralateral groin for possible prevention of future hernias.
- After inguinal herniorrhaphy, symptoms are expected to resolve by 3 months. Severe preoperative groin pain and postoperative complications (infection, hematoma) have been found to independently predict postoperative inguinal pain. One study reported approximately 30% of patients have continued pain and discomfort 2 to 3 years after the surgery with a reoccurrence rate reported at 4.5%.

SIGNS AND SYMPTOMS INDICATING REFERRAL TO PHYSICIAN

- Pain that does not change with position: Infection or tumor
- Significant and unexplained weight loss: Tumor
- Blood in urine or stool: Urinary pathology
- Saddle anesthesia: Cauda equina syndrome
- Fevers and chills: Infection or tumor
- Sudden onset of bowel and/or bladder dysfunction: Cauda equina syndrome
- Progressive bilateral lower extremity paresthesias that are nondermatomal: Cauda equina syndrome

SUGGESTED READINGS

Alimoglu O, Kaya B, Okan I, et al. Femoral hernia: a review of 83 cases. *Hernia.* 2006;10:70-73.

Braun P, Jensen S. Hip pain: a focus on the sporting population. *Aust Fam Physician.* 2007;36(6):406-413.

Ferzli GS, Edwards E, Al-Khoury G, Hardin R. Postherniorrhaphy groin pain and how to avoid it. *Surg Clin North Am.* 2008;88:203-216.

Jenkins JT, O'Dwyer PJ. Inguinal hernias. *BMJ.* 2008;336:269-272.

Lynch SA, Renstrom PA. Groin injuries in sport: treatment strategies. *Sports Med.* 1999; 28(2):137-144.

Swan KG, Wolcott M. The athletic hernia: a systematic review. *Clin Orthop Relat Res.* 2007;455:78-87.

AUTHOR: ALISON R. SCHEID

BASIC INFORMATION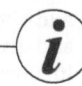

DEFINITION

- Muscle strains of the hip flexor and adductor muscles are tissue deformations in response to stress of the iliopsoas; rectus femoris; sartorius; adductors longus, brevis, and magnus; gracilis; and pectineus muscles occurring at the musculotendinous junction or muscle belly.
- The three grades of muscle strain are as follows:
  - Grade I is defined by pain with minimal or no strength and ROM loss. Very minimal tissue disruption has occurred.
  - Grade II is defined by tissue damage that results in decreased muscle strength and function. Muscle fiber disruption has occurred.
  - Grade III is defined by complete muscle disruption resulting in complete strength and functional losses.

SYNONYMS

- Groin strain
- Rider's strain

ICD-9CM CODE
843.8 Sprain of other specified site of hip and thigh

OPTIMAL NUMBER OF VISITS

8 to 10 visits

MAXIMAL NUMBER OF VISITS

20 visits

ETIOLOGY

- Adductor longus is the most frequently strained adductor muscle, and the rectus femoris and iliopsoas are the most commonly strained hip flexors. Adductor strains are more common than hip flexor strains.
- The musculotendinous junction is the most commonly reported injury site, located near the groin area.
- A strong eccentric load placed across these muscles, usually during sport activities, exceeds the tissue's deformation capacity causing inflammation, possible tearing, and bleeding of the muscle.
- Damage to the muscle triggers an inflammatory response that causes edema, warmth, redness, and pain. Damage can also occur to small blood vessels, causing bleeding and pain.

EPIDEMIOLOGY AND DEMOGRAPHICS

- Muscle strains can occur at any age, and hip flexor and adductor muscle strains are more commonly reported in relation to sports activity instead of age. However, musculotendinous changes with age can increase risk for injury.
- As most clinical definitions of a muscle strain rely on the presence of pain, all grades of muscle strain involve pain. Cases of muscle tissue deformation in the absence of pain are not commonly reported or investigated.

MECHANISM OF INJURY

- The hip flexor muscles are commonly injured with flexion activities such as the following:
  - Kicking a ball
  - Running uphill
  - Hurdles
  - Jumping
  - Ballet and martial arts positions
- The adductor muscles are commonly injured with quick lateral loading movements such as the following:
  - Twisting and direction changes
  - Kicking
  - Rapid lateral movements (jumps, sprints)

COMMON SIGNS AND SYMPTOMS

- Hip flexor muscle strains can refer pain from the groin area to the anterior and medial thigh, depending on what muscles are involved. The rectus femoris muscle will result in more anterior thigh pain because of its two-joint coverage and anatomy.
- The adductor muscles will refer pain from the groin and into the medial thigh.
- The femoral nerve supplies all of the hip flexors, except the psoas major, which receives direct innervations from the lumbar plexus. The adductors are innervated by the obturator nerve, and the pectineus is innervated by the femoral nerve.

AGGRAVATING ACTIVITIES

- Running, especially with direction changes or uneven surfaces.
- Jumping, hopping.
- Kicking.
- Single-leg exercises.
- Side-to-side exercises/activities (cutting, lunges, and twisting).
- Other activities with resisted hip flexion or adduction.
- Dance moves requiring increased hip flexor use (grande battement, développé, and rond de jambe en l'air).
- These activities all require high contractility and power of the hip flexor and adductor muscles for stabilization and movement. For the pelvis and trunk to maintain a stable position, the adductor muscles must be very active. These activities also require maximal ROMs for the hip muscles that can stress and stretch injured muscle tissue.

EASING ACTIVITIES

- Rest from aggravating activities.
- Physicians will often prescribe antiinflammatory medications, muscle relaxants, and pain medications to address the patient's symptoms.
- Walking on level surface, normal velocity.
- These activities prevent excessive stress and stretching from being placed on the muscle and allow for tissue healing to occur. Walking can place minimal stress on the hip flexor and adductor muscles if performed without extreme hip ROMs.

24-HOUR SYMPTOM PATTERN

- The patient with a muscle strain will complain of stiffness and pain in the morning.
- At the beginning of exercise or sport activity, the muscles feel stiff and painful. Symptoms will increase with higher level activities, and soreness can continue after.
- Sleeping is usually not a problem.

PAST HISTORY FOR THE REGION

- Symptoms usually follow one distinct injury. The symptoms will progress with continued activity until eventually the individual is unable to continue with the sport or exercise.
- Injury to more distal parts of the kinetic chain can alter biomechanics and the load placed on the adductor muscles. Poor trunk stabilization with activities can place increased strain on both the hip flexor and adductor muscles.

PHYSICAL EXAMINATION

- Many of the physical findings used to diagnose a hip flexor and adductor muscle strain are also used to diagnose other causes of groin pain. Signs of inflammation can be observed, including ecchymosis and swelling, which can be present with initial injury.
- In severe cases of hip flexor strain, gait will be affected, causing a decreased step length bilaterally (compensation to decrease the stretch of the muscle and weakness in hip active flexion). Other gait deviations with hip flexor pain and weakness may be increased hip external rotation to assist with limb clearance.
- In severe cases of adductor muscle strains, step length and time spent in swing phases may be decreased to minimize the stabilizing and dynamic role of these muscles.
- It is not uncommon to have multiple muscle pathologies (adductor, hip flexor, and abdominal), and they can cause various gait deviations.
- The affected adductor and hip flexor muscles will be tender to palpation. Global muscles, such as the abdominals and large lumbar extensors, may also be tender as they try to control pelvic stability.

IMPORTANT OBJECTIVE TESTS

- ROM tests for the hip
  - Hip passive abduction and external rotation may be limited by pain because of the stretch on the adductor muscles.
  - The Thomas test for hip extension will be positive for pain reproduction in different positions, depending on muscle involvement. Positions of hip extension with knee flexion and extension, as well as hip extension with abduction, should be assessed.
- Resisted isometric hip adduction
  - Resisted hip adduction with the hip in neutral (no flexion or extension) will target the adductor longus and brevis muscles. Adding resisted knee flexion will help to target the gracilis muscle. The pectineus muscle is easier to provoke with the hip in 90 degrees of flexion, but if other hip flexor muscles are injured, this test will be positive.
  - Positive: Pain and weakness in the adductor muscle.
  - Pain with isometric hip adduction is not a specific finding for adductor pathology.
- Resisted hip flexion
  - Performed isometrically or moving into hip flexion. The hip and knee position and resistance can be varied to target different muscles (knee flexion/extension, hip adduction/abduction, or internal/external rotation).
  - Positive: Pain, weakness, or painful snapping.
  - Not a specific test to target hip muscle strain and rule out other local pathology.
- Palpation of the muscles and surrounding structures
  - Palpation of bilateral hip flexors and adductor muscle.
  - Positive: Pain localized over involved muscles (usually unilateral). Change in tissue consistency indicating a muscle defect is also a positive finding.
  - Very commonly performed in addition to isometric tests to diagnose muscle strain, but other pathologies will present with a positive test.
- These tests will help localize the cause of the pain to the groin region, but further tests are necessary to rule out other pathologies such as osteitis pubis or hernia.

DIFFERENTIAL DIAGNOSIS   **Dx**

- Osteitis pubis
- Other hip pathology
- Iliopsoas abscess, bursitis
- Lumbar pathology
- Avulsion or heterotopic ossification
- Hernia (inguinal, femoral, sports)

- Sacroiliac joint pathology
- Peripheral nerve entrapment
- Visceral pathology (urological, gynecological, or gastrointestinal)
- Rhabdomyolysis

TREATMENT   **Rx**

SURGICAL OPTIONS

- Tenotomy of the adductor tendon
- Local anesthetic injection

SURGICAL OUTCOMES

- Surgery is rarely used to treat muscle strain. Local injections are tried first; in chronic cases, surgery becomes an option after attempts with conservative management and physical therapy fail. All other causes for groin pain should be thoroughly ruled out as a muscle strain will usually resolve without the need for surgery.
- Tenotomy has been found to be successful for nonspecific groin pain. Studies usually release the adductor longus tendon, but success has also been reported with the release of the adductor brevis and gracilis muscles.

REHABILITATION

- The goal of rehabilitation of the hip muscle strain is to decrease further injury and inflammation, regain ROM, prevent atrophy, and regain strength and endurance to return to exercise and sport activity.
- In the presence of hematoma, especially in the quadriceps, rehabilitation will be much slower than for other muscle strain caused by the risk of calcification or myositis ossificans. Stretching and vigorous STM can do more harm in the presence of muscle hematoma and calcification.
- To decrease inflammation, the clinician can utilizes the following:
  - Rest from aggravating activities
  - Short-term use of protected weight bearing
  - Correction of altered mechanics in other parts of the kinetic chain (strength, ROM of the lower extremity and trunk)
  - STM or myofascial release techniques to relax the adductors
  - Exercises that promote movement of the region in a pain-free range
  - Cold or hot pack
  - Ultrasound
  - Electrical stimulation
- Once the inflammation process has decreased the focus of rehabilitation should be on identifying the factors that contribute to the muscle strain such as hip ROM limitations and other lower extremity abnormal biomechanics. Pain-free strengthening can begin

and should include the gluteal muscles and trunk muscles, in addition to the involved muscles.
- Trunk and pelvic strength and stability are important for healing, as well as injury prevention. Exercises to promote adequate hip ROM and strength, without increasing hip flexor or adductor pain are necessary to restore correct motor control and performance.
- Joint mobilization can increase the ROM of the hip and other joints in an attempt to normalize lower extremity and trunk biomechanics to decrease the stress put on the injured muscles.
- STM can be useful to decrease pain and muscle spasm and increase muscle flexibility by increasing superficial tissue temperature and lymphatic drainage in an area with lots of superficial lymph nodes.
- The role of exercise in comparison to surgery for hip flexor and adductor muscle strains has not been thoroughly researched; this may be partly due to the fact that conservative treatments are successful and surgical treatments are rarely required.
- In a study on conservatively managed adductor-related groin pain (at least 2 months duration), the group undergoing active strengthening and coordination exercises had significantly better outcomes than the group receiving only stretching, laser, transverse friction, and TENS. Successful outcomes were based on return to sports activity, absence of pain with palpation, and isometric adduction (Hölmich et al). The specific cause of groin pain was not identified and radiological signs of osteitis pubis were present in more than half of the groups.
- Maintaining strength and ROM, even during off-season is important in injury prevention. Correct training intensity is important not only during healing phases but also for prevention of injuries. Adequate abdominal, lumbar, pelvic, and gluteal muscle strength is important for healing and injury prevention.
- In a preseason exercise study done by Tyler et al on professional ice hockey players, a six-week adductor-strengthening program was given to athletes with an abductor to adductor strength ratio less than 80%. A significant reduction in adductor injury risk was achieved during the season.

CONTRIBUTING FACTORS

- Multiple sites of pathology with diffuse symptoms
- Early return to sport activity resulting in inadequate healing time
- Previous hip muscle strain or other preexisting injury

- Leg length discrepancy or other lower extremity malalignment
- Poor activation of local lumbar muscle groups such as the multifidus and the transversus abdominis muscles
- Tight muscle groups, especially the hip flexors and hamstrings
- Decreased hip ROM and strength

PROGNOSIS

Recurrence rate for high-level athletes has been reported to be high for adductor strains, up to 44%. Most athletes are able to return to the same level of sporting activity with minimal or no pain.

SIGNS AND SYMPTOMS INDICATING REFERRAL TO PHYSICIAN

- Blood in urine or stool: Urinary pathology
- Dark urine with muscle pain and weakness: Rhabdomyolysis
- Saddle anesthesia: Cauda equina syndrome
- Major trauma: Fracture
- Sudden onset of bowel and/or bladder dysfunction: Cauda equina syndrome
- Progressive bilateral lower extremity paresthesias that are nondermatomal: Cauda equina syndrome

SUGGESTED READINGS

Fricker PA. Management of groin pain in athletes. *Br J Sports Med.* 1997;31:97-101.

Hölmich P. Long-standing groin pain in sportspeople falls into three primary patterns, a "clinical entity" approach: a prospective study of 207 patients. *Br J Sports Med.* 2007;41:247-252.

Hölmich P, Uhrskou P, Ulnits L, et al. Effectiveness of active physical training as treatment for long-standing adductor-related groin pain in athletes: randomised trial. *Lancet.* 1999;353:439-443.

Ibrahim A, Murrell GA, Knapman P. Adductor strain and hip range of movement in male professional soccer players. *J Orthop Surg (Hong Kong).* 2007;15(1):46-49.

Lynch SA, Renstrom PA. Groin injuries in sport: treatment strategies. *Sports Med.* 1999;28(2):137-144.

Morelli V, Smith V. Groin injuries in athletes. *Am Fam Physician.* 2001;64:1405-1414.

Nicholas SJ, Tyler TF. Adductor muscle strains in sport. *Sports Med.* 2002;32(5):339-344.

Tyler TF, Nicholas SJ, Campbell RJ, Donellan S, McHugh MP. The effectiveness of a preseason exercise program to prevent adductor muscle strains in professional ice hockey players. *Am J Sports Med.* 2002;30(5):680-683.

AUTHOR: ALISON R. SCHEID

BASIC INFORMATION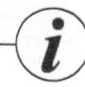

DEFINITION

ITB friction syndrome (ITBFS) is an injury caused by repetitive friction of the ITB at the lateral femoral epicondyle. Pain may also occur at the distal insertion (Gerdy's tubercle), along the ITB or at the greater trochanter.

SYNONYM

ITB syndrome

> **ICD-9CM CODE**
> 728.89   Other disorders of muscle ligament and fascia

OPTIMAL NUMBER OF VISITS

8 visits or less

MAXIMAL NUMBER OF VISITS

16 visits

ETIOLOGY

- Overuse, positional faults, weakness, and/or tightness cause abnormal stress on the ITB.
- As a result, pain occurs in response to the inflammatory process from prolonged or excessive friction caused by the impingement.
- At the lateral femoral condyle to lateral tibial plateau, the synovium, also known as the lateral synovial recess, becomes irritated and inflamed with the repetitive stress placed on it. Hyperplasia of the synovium occurs in response to the stress.
- Impingement of the ITB at the lateral epicondyle of the femur when the knee flexes between 20 to 30 degrees.
- During knee flexion past 20 to 30 degrees, the ITB to moves posteriorly along the lateral femoral epicondyle. In extension the ITB is anterior to the femoral epicondyle.
- Repetitive friction of the ITB at the greater trochanter during the hip flexion and extension, abduction and adduction, and internal and external rotation.
- Trigger point pain along the ITB may be present along with myofascial restrictions along the ITB.
- Overuse injuries may result from errors in training such as changes in surface, distance, speed, shoes, and frequency.

EPIDEMIOLOGY AND DEMOGRAPHICS

- Reported incidence as high as 22.2% of all lower extremity injuries.
- Age group most prone to the pathology include the following:
  - Children with cerebral palsy or muscular dystrophy with altered muscle tone, abnormal weight bearing, and muscle imbalances
  - Adolescents who have had recent growth spurts in which soft tissues have not adapted to bone growth
  - Active, exercising adults
- Populations that have a higher prevalence of the pathology include the following:
  - Runners: This population has an incidence as high as 12% of all running-related injuries, and long distance runners are affected more than sprinters
  - Cyclists
  - Persons in a new regime of activity or training (e.g., military training)
  - Vigorous exercisers
  - Females may be more affected than males because of anatomical differences in femoral pelvic angles

MECHANISM OF INJURY

- Running: Typical knee flexion angle during initial contact while running is roughly 21 degrees. Since friction of the ITB at the lateral femoral epicondyle occurs between 20 to 30 degrees of knee flexion, each step causes repetitive friction during long distance running.
- Cycling: Seat height too high or lower extremity in excessive internal or external rotation with cleats causes friction at the ITB during flexion to extension moments during cycling.
- Excessive training.

COMMON SIGNS AND SYMPTOMS

- Lateral knee pain or ache
- Lateral hip pain
- Tenderness to palpation
- Limitation in duration of activity run or cycling; pain comes on about same time or distance
- Longer runs, downhill running, or altered courses are painful
- Pain with climbing or descending stairs
- Pain with walking in prolonged cases
- Pain at lateral hip that may or may not radiate along ITB to knee
- Pain at lateral knee, local to Gerdy's tubercle or lateral femoral epicondyle

AGGRAVATING ACTIVITIES

- Walking may be painful the longer the pathology exists
- Downhill running: Knee flexion angle during initial contact is less, therefore has more repetitive friction
- Cycling
- Stairs: Climbing or descending
- Repetitive knee and hip flexion extension activities

EASING ACTIVITIES

- Rest and ice
- Light stretching
- The physician may prescribe antiinflammatories to assist with pain control

24-HOUR SYMPTOM PATTERN

- Generally little difference throughout the day and night.
- Usually has pain after repetitive activity, which subsides with rest. May have a feeling of tightness or ache afterward.
- In chronic cases, person may have pain with walking and climbing or descending stairs.

PAST HISTORY FOR THE REGION

- May have had similar symptoms in the past.
- Recent changes in training variables such as shoes, bicycle, distance, surface, intensity, or frequency.
- Other recent injury, such as foot, ankle, or knee injury, affecting the entire lower extremity chain.

PHYSICAL EXAMINATION

- Weak hip abductors, gluteus medius
- Weak knee flexion
- Weak knee extension
- Tenderness along ITB, myofascial restrictions
- Tightness of hip flexors, gluteus maximus
- Limitation of hip adduction ROM
- Positive Trendelenburg's sign
- Limited patella glides medially

IMPORTANT OBJECTIVE TESTS

- Ober's test assesses the soft tissue mobility or length of the ITB.
- Thomas test evaluates hip flexor length.

DIFFERENTIAL DIAGNOSIS

- Symptoms at the hip region are as follows:
  - Lumbar spine radiculopathy
  - Snapping hip syndrome
  - Stress fracture
  - Sacroiliac joint dysfunction
  - Gluteus medius muscle strain
  - Tensor fascia lata muscle strain
  - Trochanteric bursitis
- Symptoms at lateral knee region are as follows:
  - Tendonitis: Biceps femoris, vastus lateralis, popliteus
  - Lateral meniscus tear
  - Lateral collateral ligament sprain
  - Degenerative joint disease
  - Gastrocnemius muscle strain
  - Lumbar spine radiculopathy
  - Stress fracture

CONTRIBUTING FACTORS

- Positional faults, such as leg length discrepancy, excessive foot pronation, lateral pelvic tilt, or improper alignment on equipment, may place abnormal stresses along the ITB.
- Weakness of supporting hip musculature, such as the hip abductors or

tightness of hip musculature caused by myofascial restrictions, may place undue stress along the ITB.
- See section on Etiology for additional factors contributing to ITBFS.

TREATMENT

SURGICAL OPTIONS
- ITB release: Z-lengthening
  - Resection of triangular portion of posterior ITB over lateral femoral epicondyle with knee flexed to 30 degrees
  - Resection of synovial tissue at lateral condyle

SURGICAL OUTCOMES
- Return to activity in 3 to 7 weeks on average with ITB release.
- Positive results for the resection of posterior ITB.
- May have complications of synovial tissue resection such as chronic effusion and hematoma formation.
- Surgical indicator would be lack of relief from conservative care 3 to 6 months in duration.
- Conservative care includes rest, physical therapy, and local steroid injections.

REHABILITATION
- Acute stage: Primary focus is to decrease pain and inflammation.
  - Activity modification and patient education
  - Local modalities for inflammation: Ice, phonophoresis, or iontophoresis
- Subacute stage: Treatment of impairments
  - Biomechanical evaluation: Correction of external biomechanical faults such as seat height, pedal position, and proper shoe wear/support.
  - STM: Trigger point release, scar tissue mobilization, and mobilization of restrictions along the ITB. Cross-friction is not indicated as friction is the pathology that occurs.
  - Stretching: Hip flexors, hip extensors, hip abductors, and hip adductors to restore optimal flexibility.
  - Manual therapy: Treatment of joint restrictions contributing to biomechanical flaws.
- Recovery stage: Restore muscle function
  - Strengthening: typically hip abductors require strengthening.
- Open- and closed-chain exercises
- Concentric and eccentric muscle function
  - Neuromuscular reeducation: Proper position and alignment during activity
- Return to activity: Running, cycling
  - Return to activity once open- and closed-chain exercises are performed in proper form and pain-free.
  - Gradual incorporation of distance and frequency is required to return to full activity.

PROGNOSIS
- Conservative management is usually successful in mild-to-moderate cases.
- Runners may typically return to running by approximately 6 weeks.

SIGNS AND SYMPTOMS INDICATING REFERRAL TO PHYSICIAN
- Constant of unrelenting hip pain: Infection or tumor
- Pain that does not change with position or with non-weight–bearing: Tumor or infection
- Fevers and chills: infection or tumor
- Significant and unexplained weight loss-tumor
- Inability to bear weight on affected limb: Fracture, slipped capital femoral epiphysis, Legg-Calvé-Perthes disease, avascular necrosis
- Trauma: Fracture
- Inability to weight bear: Fracture, stress fracture

SUGGESTED READINGS
Fredericson M, Cookingham CL, Chaudhari AM, Dowdell BC, Oesteicher CL, Sahrmann SA. Hip abductor weakness in distance runners with iliotibial band syndrome. *Clin J Sports Med.* 2000;10:169–175.

Fredericson M, Weir A. Practical management of iliotibial band fraction syndrome in runners. *Clin J Sports Med.* 2006;16(3):261–268.

Gose JC, Schweizer P. Iliotibial Band Tightness. *J Orthop Sports Phy Ther.* 1989;10(10): 399–407.

Hertling D, Kessler RM. *Management of Common Musculoskeletal Disorders: Physical Therapy Principles and Methods.* Philadelphia, PA: Lippincott Williams & Wilkins; 2006;240–243, 535–536.

AUTHOR: STEPHANIE S. SAITO

Section III

ORTHOPEDIC PATHOLOGY

BASIC INFORMATION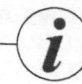

DEFINITION

Ischiogluteal bursitis is the inflammation of the bursa that lines the ischial tuberosity and hamstrings tendon covered by the gluteus maximus.

SYNONYMS

- Weaver's Bottom
- Taylor's Bottom

ICD-9CM CODE
726.5 Enthesopathy of hip region

OPTIMAL NUMBER OF VISITS

6 visits or less

MAXIMAL NUMBER OF VISITS

12 visits

ETIOLOGY

- Ischiogluteal bursitis usually occurs with local trauma to the bursa, repetitive use of the hamstrings and gluteus maximus, crystal deposits from system inflammatory disease or infection: Septic arthritis.
- The ischiogluteal bursa is a synovial fluid lubricating sac that reduces friction between the ischial tuberosity, hamstrings tendon, and gluteus maximus. When the bursa becomes irritated, swelling and pain occur. The condition can be acute, recurrent, or chronic.
- With irritation to the bursa, the synovial lining becomes thickened, which further produces excessive synovial fluid and inflammatory chemicals, resulting in localized swelling and pain.

EPIDEMIOLOGY AND DEMOGRAPHICS

- In general, bursitis is a common diagnosis within the 150 plus bursa located throughout the body. Specific to ischiogluteal bursitis, it less prevalent than trochanteric bursitis.
- May be more common in sedentary elderly persons.
- May also be common in middle age.
- In general, septic arthritis occurs more frequently in men.
- The bursitis diagnosis is also common in runners.

MECHANISM OF INJURY

- Occupations with prolonged sitting
- Prolonged sitting sustaining vibration such as using a sewing machine "weaver," tractor, or road equipment machines
- Prolonged sitting activity in sitting such as cycling

- Prolonged sitting with spinal cord injury
- Falling onto buttocks

COMMON SIGNS AND SYMPTOMS

- Local pain at gluteal region
- Pain radiating into lower extremity with "sciatica" feeling
- Impaired ambulation
- Impaired sitting
- Referral of pain into the posterior thigh
- If it has affected the sciatic nerve, then pain and symptoms follow sciatic nerve pattern

AGGRAVATING ACTIVITIES

- Direct pressure onto the bursa as in sitting
- Walking
- Climbing uphill
- Climbing or descending stairs
- Flexed hip activities

EASING ACTIVITIES

Patient may have pain at rest and with activity.

24-HOUR SYMPTOM PATTERN

- Limited ability to sit or walk throughout the day
- Limited ability to find comfortable sleeping position ("toss and turn")

PAST HISTORY FOR THE REGION

- Patient may have had ischiogluteal bursitis previously
- History of hamstring tendonitis
- See section on Contributing Factors

PHYSICAL EXAMINATION

- Local tenderness at ischiogluteal bursa
- Pain with passive hip flexion
- Pain with resisted hip extension
- May have limited hip ROM caused by pain
- In the case of chronic bursitis, hamstrings and gluteals may present with weakness

IMPORTANT OBJECTIVE TESTS

- Palpatory tenderness of the ischiogluteal bursa is an indicator of local pathology. However, other structures are local to that area. No specificity, sensitivity, or positive likelihood ratio is available.
- In cases where other pathology is suspected, MRI may be used to differentiate masses at the ischiogluteal region.

DIFFERENTIAL DIAGNOSIS

- Hamstrings tendonitis
- Lumbar spine herniated disc
- Lumbar spine radiculopathy

- Pudendal neuralgia
- Piriformis syndrome
- Lumbar facet dysfunction

CONTRIBUTING FACTORS

- Medical conditions increasing risk of infection, autoimmune diseases, RA, arthritis, and/or gout
- Spinal cord injury
- Sedentary job requiring prolonged sitting.
- Sporting activities requiring prolonged sitting

TREATMENT

SURGICAL OPTIONS

- Typically, medical procedures used are aspiration or drainage of the bursa.
- Bursectomy of the chronically inflamed bursa may be an option.
- Surgery is not usually required. Conservative care typically assists in nonseptic bursitis.
- Surgical indicators include lack of relief from conservative care and after corticosteroid injections.

REHABILITATION

- Initial focus of rehabilitation is to decrease inflammation at the bursa.
  - Patient education: Rest, decrease resting pressure on ischiogluteal bursa, modify seat with a cushion, address the underlying cause of bursitis.
  - Modalities: Ice, phonophoresis, or iontophoresis to assist with inflammation and pain.
- As the inflammatory process becomes controlled, rehabilitation should focus on the contributing factors to the bursitis.
  - STM: The role of soft tissue is limited for ischiogluteal bursitis. It will affect hamstrings tendonitis; however, will not affect ischiogluteal bursitis and may actually irritate it.
  - Exercises: Initiation of gentle and pain-free stretching of the hip, stretching of tight of hip musculature, and strengthening of weak hip musculature.
- Additionally, rehabilitation should address outside factors such as prolonged sitting, poor seating posture, adjustment of equipment for activities. (e.g., bicycle seat, saddle, wheel chair, etc).

PROGNOSIS

- Generally, bursitis resolves with conservative treatment.
- Bursitis may return in the presence of preexisting medical conditions or without change in activity that led to bursitis.

SIGNS AND SYMPTOMS INDICATING REFERRAL TO PHYSICIAN

- Constant unrelenting pain: Tumor or infection
- Fevers and chills: Infection or tumor
- Local skin infection or open sore at buttock region: Infection
- Warmth and redness: Infection
- Loss of bowel or bladder function: Urogenital
- Unresponsive to conservative care

SUGGESTED READINGS

Cho K, Lee SM, Lee YH, et al. Noninfectious ischiogluteal bursitis: MRI findings. *Korean J Radiol.* 2004;5:280-286.

Malone TR, McPoil T, Nitz A. *Orthopedic and Sports Physical Therapy.* St. Louis, MO: Mosby; 1997;498-499.

AUTHOR: STEPHANIE S. SAITO

BASIC INFORMATION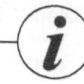

DEFINITION

A labral tear is a tear of the cartilage lining the acetabulum of the hip joint.

SYNONYMS

- Hip labral tear
- Acetabular labral tear
- Acetabular rim syndrome

ICD-9CM CODES
718.05 Articular cartilage disorder involving pelvic region and thigh
715.15 Osteoarthrosis localized primary involving pelvic region and thigh

---

OPTIMAL NUMBER OF VISITS

8 visits or less

MAXIMAL NUMBER OF VISITS

20 visits

ETIOLOGY

- Degenerative tears are related to the degree of degenerative changes present in the joint.
- The tear or fraying of the cartilage that lines and cushions the acetabulum decreases the ability of the joint to maintain a good contour, changing the kinematics and compromising the stability. Mechanical symptoms occur as a result of the tear.
- A tear may cause fluid to leak, increasing friction of the femoral head on acetabulum.
- Tears associated with hip dysplasia, capsular laxity, or femoroacetabular impingement (FAI) typically occur because of an impingement of the labrum between the acetabulum and femoral head.
- Traumatic tears occur from the direction of force and extent of trauma to the labrum.
- The four types of tears that have been identified are as follows:
  - Radial flap tear: Most common type, disruption of the free margin of the labrum
  - Radial fibrillation tear: Fraying of the free margin, associated with degenerative joint disease
  - Abnormally mobile tears: Detached labrum, similar to a Bankart lesion of the shoulder
  - Longitudinal peripheral tear: Least common type, tear in longitudinal direction in the peripheral aspect of the labrum
- Labral tears are most common (92%) in an anterior and anterosuperior location of the inner aspect of the labrum.

EPIDEMIOLOGY AND DEMOGRAPHICS

- There is a higher prevalence of hip labral tears in athletes who have groin pain: Approximately 25%.
- Greater chance of pathology among persons with hip structure abnormalities or previous hip pathologies: Hip dysplasia, slipped capital femoral epiphysis, femoral head anteversion, coxa vara, extreme coxa valga, Legg-Calvé-Perthes disease, capsular laxity, or FAI.
- Repetitive motion tears: Microtrauma tends to occur in persons participating in sports and repetitive work/job activities.
- Highly active individuals in the 20 to 40 years age group have a higher prevalence.
- Labral tears and fraying in patients older than 60 years of age occur as a result of degenerative changes.
- Females have a higher prevalence than males.

MECHANISM OF INJURY

- In a traumatic event, such as dislocation, subluxation, or fracture, disruption of the cartilage occurs. Activities with sudden twisting, pivoting, hyperflexion, or squatting may cause a sudden tear.
- Repetitive microtrauma applies a general wear and tear on the joint surfaces.
- No specific mechanism may occur, especially in individuals with degenerative changes or predisposing factors such as FAI, capsular laxity, or hip dysplasia.

COMMON SIGNS AND SYMPTOMS

- Locking, clicking, or catching sensation in the hip joint
- Pain in the groin or deep hip region
- Stiffness of hip joint
- Instability or giving way
- Limited painful hip ROM
- Intraarticular hip pathologies can refer pain to the anterior groin, buttock, greater trochanter, thigh, and/or medial knee
- Labral tears commonly refer pain to the anterior groin region

AGGRAVATING ACTIVITIES

- Pivoting or twisting
- Deep squatting
- Crossing legs (e.g., to tie shoes)
- Walking
- Climbing or descending stairs
- Sitting

EASING ACTIVITIES

- Rest in open pack position
- Hip distraction
- Antiinflammatories or muscle relaxants may be prescribed by the physician

24-HOUR SYMPTOM PATTERN

- In the morning, the patient may have stiffness at the hip joint
- As the day progresses, increased pain with weight bearing and irritation to the labral tear
- Soreness, ache at the end of the day
- Sleep: Difficulty finding a comfortable position

PAST HISTORY FOR THE REGION

- Osteoarthritis or articular cartilage degeneration
- Previous hip pathology: Slipped capital femoral epiphysis, Legg-Calvé-Perthes disease
- Capsular laxity
- Femoroacetabular impingement
- Hip dysplasia
- Previous injuries in hyperextension

PHYSICAL EXAMINATION

- Resting position in hip flexion, abduction or external rotation if joint effusion is present.
- Trendelenburg's gait may be present with decreased loading on the affected side, increased knee flexion in stance to absorb shock, and decreased stride length.
- A majority of tests for labral pathology provide more general information regarding the possibility for lumbosacral spine, intraarticular, and/or extraarticular hip pathology.
- Intraarticular lesion tests
  - FABER test: is positive and the patient may have limited ROM.
  - Scour test: Positive test produces pain and/or clicking as compressive forces are applied to acetabulum.
  - Resisted straight leg raise: Positive test produces pain as the resistance loads the joint anterosuperiorly and reproduces pain to the anterior groin when a lesion is present.
  - FAI test: Positive test produces pain as the movement engages the femoral head-neck junction into the superior labrum and acetabular rim.
- Capsular laxity tests
  - Log-roll test: Positive test reproduces a click, which is suggestive of a labral tear; increased external rotation ROM indicates iliofemoral laxity.
  - Long-axis distraction: Positive result for capsular laxity may have increased motion and a feeling of apprehension with this maneuver. With capsular hypomobility, there will be decreased motion and relief of pain.
- Articular cartilage degeneration (osteoarthritis) ROM
  - Pain and/or limited hip ROM into internal rotation is the most predictive of mild-to-moderate hip osteoarthritis
  - Limited hip flexion ROM

IMPORTANT OBJECTIVE TESTS

- FABER test: Hip pain was 0.88 sensitive for intraarticular hip pathology. No correlation was found between a positive FABER test and specific hip pathology.
- Hip ROM: Single hip motion limited into flexion; external or internal rotation had 0.86 sensitivity, 0.54 specificity, 1.9 positive likelihood ratio for identifying mild-to-moderate radiographic evidence of osteoarthritis (Martin et al). Additionally, individuals with <15 degrees of internal rotation and hip flexion ≤115 degrees were classified as having osteoarthritis with a sensitivity of 0.86 and specificity of 0.75.
- Diagnostics
  - MRA: Sensitivity: 66%-95%; specificity: 71% to 88% in diagnosing labral tears.

DIFFERENTIAL DIAGNOSIS

- FAI
- Capsular laxity
- Articular cartilage degeneration
- Snapping hip syndrome
- Contusion
- Strains
- Osteitis pubis
- Piriformis syndrome
- Bursitis (trochanteric, ischiogluteal, or iliopsoas)
- Lumbar spine referred pain
- Sacroiliac joint referred pain

CONTRIBUTING FACTORS

- Conditions that commonly affect the joint typically include FAI, capsular laxity, or hip dysplasia.
- FAI: Decreased joint clearance between the femur and acetabulum causing labral tears and contributing to a progressive degenerative process leading to osteoarthritis.
- Capsular laxity: Lack of joint stability causes inability to absorb stress and subjects the labrum to abnormal stress and pathology. Additionally, a tear in the labrum decreases the ability to stabilize the joint, which puts greater force on the iliofemoral ligament and creates anterior capsular laxity.
- Dysplasia: A shallow acetabular socket decreases the normal bony stability of the hip, placing additional stress on the capsule and labrum. Over time, stress on these structures leads to labral tears.
- Articular cartilage degeneration or inflammatory arthropathies.

TREATMENT

SURGICAL OPTIONS

- Arthroscopic debridement
- Open labral surgery

SURGICAL OUTCOMES

- Arthroscopy for the hip is the gold standard in both the diagnosis and treatment of labral tears. Débridement has a 91% success rate in the relief of symptoms.
- 2 years after arthroscopic surgery (McCarthy et al):
  - For minor lesions, 91% had good-to-excellent results.
  - With marked degenerative changes: 78% were associated with a poor result, 43% went on to total joint arthroplasty with 2 years of arthroscopy.
- Surgical indicator is progression of symptoms with determination of structural abnormality.

REHABILITATION

- Primary focus of rehabilitation is to decrease pain and the inflammatory process at the hip joint.
  - Joint mobilization/distraction.
  - Modalities: Cold packs and hot packs, electrical stimulation.
  - Assistive device may be issued to support the lower extremity to decreased gait abnormalities.
- Identification of impairments and contributing factors to the labral pathology.
- Joint mobilizations: Hip distraction and glides to improve ROM and joint mechanics.
- Exercises to include improving flexibility of hip musculature.
  - Stretching of hip flexors, external rotators, and adductors.
  - Addressing strength deficits of the hip to improve hip stabilization, core stabilization, and proprioception.
  - Cross-training in pain-free activities to decrease strain on the hip.
- Movement reeducation: Correction and reeducation of abnormal movement patterns.

PROGNOSIS

No research studies were found comparing the prognosis of patients undergoing physical therapy versus surgical intervention because arthroscopic surgery is the gold standard for diagnosis and treatment of symptomatic labral tears.

SIGNS AND SYMPTOMS INDICATING REFERRAL TO PHYSICIAN

- Acute hip pain in combination with the following could indicate possible infection or tumor, septic arthritis, osteomyelitis, or other inflammatory condition:
  - Fever and chills
  - Night sweats
  - Drastic weight loss
  - Night pain
  - Intravenous drug abuse
  - History of cancer
  - Compromised immune system
- Significant trauma, pain with any and all movements, or inability to walk or weight bear through affected extremity and/or in the presence of a shortened externally rotated lower extremity: Fracture
- History of corticosteroid exposure or alcohol abuse: Avascular necrosis
- Pain exacerbated by coughing, sneezing, or resisted sit-up: Hernia
- Pain with inability to weight bear: Slipped capital femoral epiphysis, Legg-Calvé-Perthes disease
- Lack of improvement with conservative care and physical therapy

SUGGESTED READINGS

Burnett RS, Della Rocca GJ, Prather H, Curry M, Maloney WJ, Clohisy JC. Clinical presentation of patients with tears of the acetabular labrum. *J Bone Joint Surg Am.* 2006;88:1448-1457.

Fitzgerald RH. Acetabular labrum tears: diagnosis and treatment. *Clin Orthop Relat Res.* 1995;311:60-68.

Martin RL, Enseki KR, Draovitch P, Trapuzzano T, Philippon MJ. Acetabular labral tears of the hip: examination and diagnostic challenges. *J Orthop Sports Phys Ther.* 2006;36(7):503-515.

Martin RL, Sekiya JK. The interrater reliability of 4 clinical tests used to assess individual with musculoskeletal hip pain. *J Orthop Sports Phys Ther.* 2008;38(2):71-77.

McCarthy J, Noble P, Aluisio FV, Schuck M, Wright J, Lee J. Anatomy, pathologic features, and treatment of acetabular labral tears. *Clin Orthop Relat Res.* 2003;406:38-47.

Mitchell B, McCrory P, Brukner P, O'Donnell J, Colson E, Howells R. Hip joint pathology: clinical presentation and correlation between magnetic resonance arthrography, ultrasound, and arthroscopic findings in 25 consecutive cases. *Clin J Sports Med.* 2003;13(3):152-156.

Schmerl M, Pollard H, Hoskins W. Labral injuries of the hip: a review of diagnosis and management. *J Manipulative Physiol Ther.* 2005;28:632.

AUTHOR: STEPHANIE S. SAITO

BASIC INFORMATION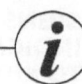

DEFINITION

Multiple definitions for osteitis pubis exist, and there is much disagreement in the use of the term *osteitis pubis*. Most commonly, it is defined as the chronic inflammation of the symphysis pubis caused by injury or infection. More recently, radiology-based definitions of osteitis pubis have been developed that use the presence of bone marrow edema at the pubic symphysis.

SYNONYMS

- Pubic bone stress injury
- Pubic instability

ICD-9CM CODES
848.5 Pelvic sprain
665.6 Obstetrical damage to pelvic
      joints and ligaments

OPTIMAL NUMBER OF VISITS

14 visits

MAXIMAL NUMBER OF VISITS

25 visits

ETIOLOGY

- Limited hip ROM, weakness of hip adduction or abduction, a rapid increase in a training program (intensity, frequency, and duration), and skeletal immaturity. Speculation on abnormal biomechanics as a predisposing factor exist; excessive mobility at the symphysis and hypomobility of the hip and sacroiliac joints have been proposed but little evidence exists.
- Injury can result from athletic activities, such as soccer, fencing, football, and hockey, as well as after operations of the bladder and prostate.
- It is suggested that microtears of the adductors muscles occurs first, causing muscular instability, laxity, and impaction at the symphysis. A physiological cleft develops in the area of the tendon insertion to the symphysis and is believed to restrict healing. Continued activity causes the tear to progress, causing continued pain and inflammation of the symphysis pubis and leading to osteitis pubis. Cortical bone changes, including erosions, cysts, osteophytic spurs and areas of heterotopic calcification, demonstrate degenerative changes at the symphysis. Bone marrow edema develops, indicating stress injury to the trabecular bone.
- Adductor muscle spasms can cause pain and aggravate the symphysis pubis area.

EPIDEMIOLOGY AND DEMOGRAPHICS

- Average age varies significantly, but a majority of studies on osteitis pubis focus on young athletic populations where average age is around 30 years, with a higher proportion of males to females.
- Many patients with bone marrow edema suggesting stress injury are asymptomatic. Articular surface irregularities at the pubic symphysis, as well as herniation of the fibrocartilage disc, is found in both symptomatic and asymptomatic hips. The diagnosis of osteitis pubis is based on the presence of pain in the area. Linear parasymphysial T2 hyperintensity on MRI has been used to help to diagnose osteitis pubis.

MECHANISM OF INJURY

- The pubic symphysis is commonly injured with repetitive trauma and stress to the abdominals and adductor muscles that may occur during the following:
  - Pregnancy or postpartum periods (laxity and increased joint stress)
  - Contact sports and weightlifting (primary trauma)

COMMON SIGNS AND SYMPTOMS

- Injury to the symphysis results in pain in the groin, medial thigh, perineum, and lower abdominal area. Pain can be sharp or aching and is usually gradual in onset unless after direct trauma.
- Acute illness (possibly with fever) or chronic pain in the region as described (most commonly occurs after urological or gynecological procedures).

AGGRAVATING ACTIVITIES

- Twisting and turning.
- Walking.
- Running, hopping.
- Kicking.
- Sit to stand transition.
- Lifting activities.
- Single-leg stance.
- Other activities with resisted hip adduction.
- High intensity exercises, direction changes, and single-leg activities place shearing forces, as well as traction from pelvic muscles. Running and jumping place repetitive cyclical stresses across the pelvis.

EASING ACTIVITIES

- Lying down or hooklying may be more comfortable than sidelying.
- Occasionally, sitting can provide relief.
- Physicians will often prescribe antiinflammatory medications or injections to address the patient's symptoms.
- Pelvic muscles can relax and weight-bearing stresses are no longer placed through the joint.

24-HOUR SYMPTOM PATTERN

The patient with osteitis pubis will have pain that is responsive to exercise and activity. After high intensity or aggravating activities, pain may be worse in the evening.

PAST HISTORY FOR THE REGION

Because of the overuse nature of osteitis pubis, the patient will often complain of gradual onset of symptoms that progressed with continued activity or exercise over the period of weeks to months.

PHYSICAL EXAMINATION

- Just as the subjective findings are not very specific for osteitis pubis, physical findings are also helpful in ruling out other areas of pathology (lumbar spine, hip), but specifically reaching a differential diagnosis for the local sources of pain (i.e., adductor tendinopathy, hernia) is very difficult.
- The hip adductor muscles with their origin near the symphysis tend to be very tender to palpation. Lower abdominal muscles may also be tender to palpation.

IMPORTANT OBJECTIVE TESTS

- Palpation of the symphysis pubis
  - Local tenderness over the symphysis or pubic bone is generally present but not necessarily specific for osteitis pubis.
- Hip ROM test
  - Limited hip ROM, especially internal and external rotation
- Squeeze test
  - Maximal adduction of the hips around the clinician's fist with the hips flexed to 45 degrees, knees flexed to 90 degrees (Verall et al, 2005b); can also be performed with varying degrees of hip flexion
  - Positive: Weakness and pain
  - Not a specific test for osteitis pubis
- Bilateral hip adduction test
  - Bilateral isometric-resisted hip adduction with legs extended on the table, pushing against the clinician's forearms (Hölmich et al). The test has also been described with the subject actively maintaining 30 degrees of hip flexion with slight hip abduction and internal rotation while the examiner resists hip adduction (Verrall et al, 2005b).
  - Positive: Pain and weakness.
  - Not a specific test for osteitis pubis.
- Single adductor test
  - The last of the three tests described by Verrall et al, (2005b) has the subject positioned with one hip flexed 30 degrees and hip adduction resisted, the other lower extremity rests on the table. Both legs are tested.
  - Positive: Pain and weakness on the tested leg or pain of the contralateral leg.
  - Not a specific test for osteitis pubis.

- ASLR test
  - Used to identify pelvic ring instability in addition to pubic pathology.
  - The patient performs an ASLR test about 20 cm off the mat, and the performance is graded by the clinician on a 5-point scale.
  - Difficulty in raising the leg is associated with poor stabilization of the pelvic ring (abdominals, pelvic floor).
- Research on the usefulness of these tests is very limited. Many other objective tests are used clinically but lack sufficient research and description of performance.
  - The ASLR, though not specific for diagnosing osteitis pubis, is a valid test to assess for mobility of the pelvic joints. An impairment of the ASLR correlates strongly with a unilateral increase in pubic symphysis movement on radiographs in peripartum women. In an athletic male population with chronic groin pain, ASLR impairment correlates with a delayed onset in the transversus abdominis muscle.
  - Verrall et al (2005b) compared and gave descriptions for three of these tests (single adductor, squeeze, and bilateral adductor) and found a high positive predictive value for all three positive tests, with the signs and symptoms of chronic groin pain (pain to palpation of the pubic symphysis or ramus and groin pain) correlating with pubic bone marrow edema.
  - In another study by Verrall et al (2005a), a reduction in hip internal and external rotation ROM was found in athletes with chronic groin injury diagnosed as pubic bone stress injury, which is believed to cause traumatic osteitis pubis.

DIFFERENTIAL DIAGNOSIS

- Adductor muscle strain
- Ligament strain
- Adductor tendinopathy
- Labral tear of the hip
- Sacroiliitis and other sacroiliac joint pathology
- Hernia (inguinal, femoral, sports)
- Other hip pathology
- Lumbar spine pathology
- Nerve entrapments (obturator, femoral)
- Myositis ossificans
- Visceral pathology (urological, gynecological, or gastrointestinal)

TREATMENT

SURGICAL OPTIONS

- Tenotomy of the adductor tendon
- Correction of other pathology (hernia, muscle tear)

- Local anesthetic injection
- Wedge resection of the symphysis
- Complete resection of the symphysis
- Symphysiodesis

SURGICAL OUTCOMES

- Surgery is rarely required, and conservative management of symptoms is usually successful. However, a larger portion of patients with infectious osteitis pubis have to undergo surgery.
- Complete resection of the joint has been found to cause pelvic instability and continued pain. Wedge resection theoretically maintains more pelvic stability, but there are very few studies with small sample sizes to demonstrate this and some studies report posterior pelvic instability over time. Persistent pain after surgery is not uncommon after symphysiodesis and resection.

REHABILITATION

- Rest from aggravating activities and sports to alleviate pain is the first step. Once the symptoms have diminished, the focus of the rehabilitative process will turn to prevention of further episodes.
- Osteitis pubis is believed to be a self-limiting condition, but multiple treatment approaches that focus on rest, appropriate stretching, and strengthening programs to restore normal movement patterns may improve recovery and recovery time.
- Initial treatments should include the following:
  - STM
  - Graded joint mobilization
  - Exercises that promote movement of the region in a pain-free range
  - Cold or hot pack
  - Ultrasound
  - Electrical stimulation
  - A physician may prescribe use of nonsteroidal antiinflammatory drugs (NSAIDs) and/or corticosteroid injection
- Physical therapy focusing on core stability has been shown to reduce symptom recurrence.
- Adductor and abductor strengthening, balance exercise, and lumbar extensor strengthening
- Pelvic floor muscle strengthening will promote further pelvic stability and should be addressed either in isolation or in combination with other core exercises.
- Early muscular reeducation is necessary to gain pelvic stability and control as a foundation for further stretching and strengthening exercises.
- A graduated return to sport and activities is necessary to prevent further injury and promote continued healing.

- In an uncontrolled study using conservative treatment for 12 weeks to treat pubic stress injury in athletes, the results were comparable to surgery and injections for return to sport time (Verrall et al, 2007).
- Improvement in muscle balance (strength, flexibility) and movement patterns can promote healing, as well as prevent further injury. Such exercises should address core, pelvis, hip muscles and joints, and any other lower extremity joint dysfunction. Balance and proprioceptive exercises should also be used long term. Proper footwear for the given sport and/or activity level should be maintained for shock absorption and traction.

CONTRIBUTING FACTORS

- Deconditioning
- Repetitive exposure to high-load activities
- Hypomobility in adjacent regions, especially the hip joint
- Other injuries to local or adjacent areas
- Poor or delayed activation of pelvic and core muscle groups such as the transversus abdominis muscles
- Muscle imbalances (flexibility, strength, and endurance)

PROGNOSIS

Most patients will have symptom resolution 6 to 9 months after conservative treatment. Return to sports has been reported as ranging from 3 to 6 months or more. If conservative treatment fails, surgery is considered. Recurrence rates have been reported to be around 25% in males.

SIGNS AND SYMPTOMS INDICATING REFERRAL TO PHYSICIAN

- Constant unrelenting pain: Infection or tumor
- Blood in urine or stool: Urinary or gastrointestinal pathology
- Major trauma or severe pain with movement: Fracture
- Fevers and chills: Infection or tumor
- Sudden onset of bowel and/or bladder dysfunction: Cauda equina syndrome
- Progressive bilateral lower extremity paresthesias that are nondermatomal: Cauda equina syndrome

SUGGESTED READINGS

Braun P, Jensen S. Hip pain: a focus on the sporting population. *Aust Fam Physician.* 2007;36(6):406–413.

Cowan SM, Schache AG, Brukner P, et al. Delayed onset of transversus abdominus in long-standing groin pain. *Med Sci Sports Exerc.* 2004;36:2040–2045.

Cunningham PM, Brennan D, O'Connell M, MacMahon P, O'Neil P, Eustace S. Patterns of bone and soft-tissue injury at the symphysis pubis in soccer players: observations at MRI. *AJR Am J Roentgenol.* 2007;188:W291-W296.

Lynch SA, Renstrom PA. Groin injuries in sport: treatment strategies. *Sports Med.* 1999;28(2):137-144.

McCarthy A, Vicenzino B. Treatment of osteitis pubis via the pelvic muscles. *Man Ther.* 2003;8(4):257-260.

Mens JM, Vleeming A, Snijders CJ, Stam HJ, Ginai AZ. The active straight leg raising test and mobility of the pelvic joints. *Eur Spine J.* 1999;8:468-473.

Verrall GM, Hamilton IA, Oakeshott RD, Spriggins AJ, Barnes PG, Fon GT. Hip joint range of motion reduction in sports-related chronic groin injury diagnosed as pubic bone stress injury. *J Sci Med Sport.* 2005a;8(1):77-84.

Verrall GM, Slavotinek JP, Barnes PG, Fon GT. Description of pain provocation tests used for the diagnosis of sport-related chronic groin pain: relationship of tests to defined clinical (pain and tenderness) and MRI (pubic bone marrow oedema) criteria. *Scand J Med Sci Sports.* 2005b;15:36-42.

Verrall GM, Slavotinek JP, Fon GT, Barnes PG. Outcome of conservative management of athletic chronic groin injury diagnosed as pubic bone stress injury. *Am J Sports Med.* 2007;35(3):467-474.

AUTHOR: STEPHANIE S. SAITO

BASIC INFORMATION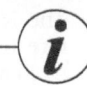

DEFINITION

- Osteoarthritis is a pathology associated with inflammation in the joints of the body. In the case of hip osteoarthritis, the arthritis and inflammation most commonly associated with a loss of acetabular and/or femoral head cartilage, leading to hip, groin, and buttock pain.
- Osteoarthritis is a term derived from the Greek word "*osteo*", meaning "of the bone," "*arthro*," meaning "joint," and "*itis*," meaning inflammation, even though the amount of inflammation present in the joint can range from excessive to little or no inflammation.

SYNONYMS

- Hip arthritis
- Hip degenerative joint disease

ICD-9CM CODES

715.15 Osteoarthrosis localized primary involving pelvic region and thigh
715.25 Osteoarthrosis localized secondary involving pelvic region and thigh

OPTIMAL NUMBER OF VISITS

3 to 6 visits (12 visits if status post arthroplasty)

MAXIMAL NUMBER OF VISITS

20 to 36 visits (60 visits if status post arthroplasty)

ETIOLOGY

- The wearing down of the hyaline cartilage leads to an inflammatory response in which there is thickening and sclerosis of the subchondral bone and development of osteophytes or bone spurs. This leads to a narrowing of the joint space, loss of shock absorption, and ultimately pain.
- Daily wear and tear in combination with various injuries sustained throughout life is the most common cause of the breakdown of healthy tissue.
- Degeneration of the cartilage and resultant arthritis can also be the result of other factors such as trauma or joint injury.
- At a cellular level, as a person ages, the number of proteoglycans in the articular cartilage decreases. Proteoglycans are hydrophilic and work within cartilage to bind water. With the reduction of proteoglycans comes a decrease in water content within the cartilage and a corresponding loss of cartilage resilience. With the decreases in cartilage resilience, collagen fibers of the cartilage become susceptible to degradation and

injury. The breakdown of collagen and other cartilage tissue are released into the surround joint space. Inflammation results as the body attempts to respond to the influx of byproducts from cartilage injury.
- As the cartilage degrades, the joint space narrows and ligaments become more lax. In response to the laxity, new bone outgrowths, called *spurs* or *osteophytes*, can form on the margins of the joints in an attempt to improve the congruence and passive stability of the articular cartilage surfaces.
- Primary osteoarthritis refers to joint degradation resulting from aging and tissue degeneration.
- Secondary osteoarthritis refers to joint degradation and tissue degeneration that results from factors other than aging such as obesity, trauma, and congenital disorders.
- The stages of hip osteoarthritis are as follows:
  - Stage I: Slight cartilage wearing, slight joint space narrowing, and small osteophytes
  - Stage II: Moderate cartilage wearing, moderate joint space narrowing, and cyst formation on the femoral head; increased number and size of osteophytes
  - Stage III: Complete cartilage deterioration, very narrow or absent joint space, significant bony sclerosis, and large osteophytes and bony cysts

EPIDEMIOLOGY AND DEMOGRAPHICS

- Symptomatic hip osteoarthritis occurs in 3% of the adults 55 years of age and older
  - Osteoarthritis is the number one cause of disability.
  - 70% of all individuals older than 70 years of age have x-ray evidence of hip osteoarthritis. Only one-third to one-half are symptomatic.
- Individuals older than 60 years of age are most prone to hip osteoarthritis.
- There is a higher prevalence of hip arthritis in women than men, and there is a higher prevalence of hip osteoarthritis in white Americans than Chinese and Chinese Americans.
- 150,000 hip replacements are performed each year.
- $54 billion per year is spent annually in medical costs and lost wages related to osteoarthritis.

MECHANISM OF INJURY

- Osteoarthritis is a pathology of overuse. The mechanism of injury is therefore the result of repetitive motions that stress the hip joint. The more cycles of an activity that the hip performs, the more likely the result will be anatomical damage.

- Daily use of the hip in weight-bearing positions
- Misalignment of the femur (anteversion abnormalities)
- Excessive use/strain of the hip secondary to work, obesity, or recreational activities
- Injuries, such as fracture and strains/sprains, that cause inflammation and scar tissue in the hip

COMMON SIGNS AND SYMPTOMS

- Pain in the groin, inner thigh, and/or buttock
- Stiffness in the hip
- Cracking or deep crunching in the hip
- Difficulty crossing legs
- Limping (ipsilateral lurch during weight bearing)
- Anterior hip pain with walking or standing
- Anterior hip pain or inability to tie shoes

AGGRAVATING ACTIVITIES

- Weight-bearing activities (walking, running, dancing, jumping, etc)
- Long-term standing, especially on harder surfaces like concrete
- Walking
- Squatting or kneeling
- Tying shoes or putting on socks
- Crossing legs
- Standing after prolonged sitting or lying down; inactivity leads to stiffness
- Inactivity allows the inflammation to "pool" and increase pressure, leading to discomfort and loss of available movement

EASING ACTIVITIES

- Rest
- Gentle motions of the hip joint
- Gentle stretching and exercise, heat, massage, antiinflammatory medication, non–weight-bearing activities, and leg elevation
- Generally speaking, these activities lead to decreased wear and tear, increased joint lubrication, and loss of stiffness and inflammation associated with this condition

24-HOUR SYMPTOM PATTERN

- Stiffness in the morning (10 to 15 minutes)
- Better after a warm shower and taking medication
- Can worsen with excessive movement
- Stiffens again in the evening
- Stiffness after prolonged inactivity

PAST HISTORY FOR THE REGION

- Jobs or recreational activities that require excessive use/strain of the hip (walking, running, jumping, dancing, gymnastics, etc)

- Abnormal amount of damage because of injuries
- Obesity
- Past history of injury to the hip or any part of the lower extremity
- Past history of injury to the contralateral lower extremity can create increased loading onto the now symptomatic hip joint
- Childhood history of hip joint pathology or lower extremity torsions

PHYSICAL EXAMINATION

- Loss of hip ROM, especially hip flexion and hip internal rotation
- Hip adduction, flexion, and internal rotation combined will cause anterior hip pain
- Crepitus with movement
- Decreased weight bearing in stance phase of gait
- Increased hip external rotation with all phases of gait
- Possible Trendelenburg's weakness on the affected limb
- Pain with resisted hip flexion and resisted hip adduction

IMPORTANT OBJECTIVE TESTS

- Possible leg length discrepancies
- FABER test

DIFFERENTIAL DIAGNOSIS **Dx**

- Hernia
- Hip sprain/strain
- Sacroiliac joint dysfunction
- Lumbar spine dysfunction
- Tendonitis (hip flexor, ITB)
- Bursitis (trochanteric)
- Dislocation
- Avascular necrosis of the femoral head
- Osteochondritis desiccans
- Pelvic dysfunction such as endometriosis, ovarian cysts, or prostate enlargement
- Sigmoid colon pathology
- Appendicitis

CONTRIBUTING FACTORS

- The hip is designed to handle normal daily use. When factors change the body's ability to respond to normal forces, damage occurs.
- Therefore the clinician should thoroughly interview the patient to determine which factors may contribute to the patient's symptoms.
- Uncontrolled risk factors that contribute or predispose an individual to hip osteoarthritis pathology:
  ○ Gender (females more than males)
  ○ Age (increase 2% per year after age 40 years)
  ○ Genetics
  ○ Prior history of injury to either lower extremity

  ○ Prior history of childhood hip pathology
  ○ Leg length discrepancies
- Modifiable risk factors that contribute or predispose an individual to continue or progress to hip osteoarthritis:
  ○ Weight
  ○ Work or recreational activities
  ○ Repetitive or significant traumatic injuries to the hip
  ○ Poor health (smoking, long-term use of steroids)

TREATMENT

SURGICAL OPTIONS

- Total hip replacement (arthroplasty): Cemented or biological fixation; anterior or posterior approach
- Osteotomy
- Factors affecting choice of hip surgery:
  ○ Cemented: Younger, high level of activity, overweight/obese
  ○ Uncemented: Older, inactive, frail
  ○ Osteotomy: Very young (<50 years of age); postpones arthroplasty
- Lifespan of total hip replacements is 15 to 20 years of age

REHABILITATION

- Rehabilitation should focus on the following:
  ○ Education in correct use of ice/heat at home for pain abatement and edema control.
  ○ Implementation of a home exercise program.
  ○ Teach proper footwear with or without orthotics. Correction of foot alignment and reduction of loading on the joint are important factors related to hip osteoarthritis.
  ○ Manual therapy (STM, joint mobilization) can be used to improve joint mobility and arthrokinematics and to decrease pain.
  ○ Massage can be used to decrease pain by relaxing muscular tension, improving circulation, and increasing endorphin release.
- Pathological changes to cartilage cannot be repaired by the body at this time. Even surgical advances have yet to solve the problems associated with cartilage damage. With this in mind, rehabilitation should focus on decreasing the stress placed on the damaged cartilage and correcting biomechanical and anatomical abnormalities that may predispose an individual to increased stress at the hip joint.
- The clinician should also evaluate the patient for leg length discrepancies that would cause abnormal stresses to placed onto the hip joint. Shoe lifts can be recommended to equalize the length of the legs during function.

- The hip joint is a synovial joint. Therefore the cartilage heals and is affected by joint motion. It is aggravated by activities that excessively load the joint, but motion in a non–weight-bearing to a limited weight-bearing environment can greatly decrease the patient's symptoms.
- Exercises include the following:
  ○ Stretches: Hip flexors, piriformis, quadriceps, ITB, hamstrings to decrease the stresses placed across the joint
  ○ Strengthening exercises: Quadriceps, hamstrings, hip abductors, hip adductors, hip extensors, hip internal/external rotators
  ○ Proprioceptive exercises to improve balance and function
  ○ Cardiovascular exercises, such as bicycle, progressing to treadmill, promote circulation and healing
- Exercises creates a sense of control over the symptoms and the condition.
- Modalities: Ice/heat, ultrasound, electrical stimulation, and tape/braces can be used as adjuncts to improve the healing environment.
- Factors that contribute to abnormal joint mechanics and loading should be determined and addressed.

PROGNOSIS

- Long-term prognosis for a patient with hip osteoarthritis depends on the extent of wear and tear and ability to reduce the joint strain placed on the joint (posture, activity, etc).
- For the most part, hip osteoarthritis is a degenerative condition. At earlier stages of the pathology, rehabilitation aimed at reducing the load placed on the joint can potentially slow or halt the progression of degeneration.
- For patients who are further along in the degenerative process, outcomes will be less favorable because cartilage has only a limited ability to repair itself.

SIGNS AND SYMPTOMS INDICATING REFERRAL TO PHYSICIAN

- Unrelenting pain
- Unusual responses to therapy
- Neurological signs
- Red flag symptoms such as excessive redness and swelling and generalized malaise and fatigue: Infection

SUGGESTED READINGS

Dugan SA. Exercise for health and wellness at midlife and beyond: balancing benefits and risks. *Phys Med Rehabil Clin N Am.* 2007;18(3):555-575.

Glass GG. Osteoarthritis. *Dis Mon.* 2006;52(9):343-362.

Jensen LK. Hip osteoarthritis: influence of work with heavy lifting, climbing stairs or ladders, or combining kneeling/squatting with heavy lifting. *Occup Environ Med.* 2008;65(1):6-19.

Jones CA, et al. Total joint arthroplasties: Current concepts of patient outcomes after surgery. *Rheum Dis Clin North Am.* 2007;33(1):71-86.

MacDonald CW, Whitman JM, Cleland JA, Smith M, Hoeksma HL. Clinical outcomes following manual physical therapy and exercise for hip osteoarthritis: A case series. *J Orthop Sports Phys Ther.* 2006;36(8):588-99.

O'Connor M. Osteoarthritis of the hip and knee: Sex and gender differences. *Orthop Clin North Am.* 2006;37(4):559-568.

St. Clair S, et al. Hip and knee arthroplasty in the geriatric population. *Clin Geriatr Med.* 2006;22(3):515-533.

AUTHOR: SARA GRANNIS

Section III

ORTHOPEDIC PATHOLOGY

BASIC INFORMATION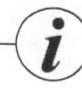

DEFINITION

Piriformis syndrome is a condition of the piriformis muscle causing local pain in the buttocks with or without referred symptoms into the lower extremity caused by compression of the sciatic nerve.

SYNONYMS

- Piriformis impingement
- Sciatica
- Pelvic outlet syndrome

ICD-9CM CODES
724.3 Sciatica
355.0 Lesion of sciatic nerve

OPTIMAL NUMBER OF VISITS

6 visits or less

MAXIMAL NUMBER OF VISITS

16 visits

ETIOLOGY

- Myofascial pain occurs from local trauma that causes hematoma formation followed by adhesion formation, which irritates the piriformis muscle.
- Compression or irritation of the sciatic nerve from trauma may occur; this is due to the inflammation that causes chemical irritation of the sciatic nerve.
- Muscle strains and myofascial pain occur from muscle strains. As a result of the strain, scar tissue may occur that would restrict muscle mobility. If atrophy occurs, then shortening of the piriformis muscle by loss of sarcomeres of the myofibrils occurs.
- Nerve entrapment/impingement occurs in cases in which the sciatic nerve pierces through the piriformis muscle, creating neural irritation and inflammation of the sciatic nerve when the piriformis muscle is compressed.
- Classification of piriformis syndrome is as follows:
  - Primary piriformis syndrome: All pathology intrinsic to the piriformis muscle secondary to an inciting event such as trauma is included.
  - Secondary piriformis syndrome: All other causes in which the symptoms of posterior buttock pain with or without radiation down the leg depend on the location of the pathology in relation to the structures adjacent to the sciatic notch, provided that spinal pathology is excluded.

EPIDEMIOLOGY AND DEMOGRAPHICS

- 15% to 20% of the population has the sciatic nerve passing through the piriformis muscle.
- 6% of sciatica diagnoses are due to piriformis syndrome.
- Generally found in patients 30 to 40 years old.
- Female versus male at a ratio of 3:1 for myofascial pain and a ratio of 6:1 for entrapment/impingement pain.

MECHANISM OF INJURY

- Trauma such as a fall on the buttock
- Prolonged sitting
- Excessive physical strain of the muscle
- Pregnancy
- Insidious onset

COMMON SIGNS AND SYMPTOMS

- Cardinal features of piriformis syndrome are as follows:
  - History of local trauma
  - Pain in the buttocks/gluteal region, deep with difficulty walking
  - Acute pain brought on by stooping or lifting
  - Palpable spindle or sausage-shaped mass, tender to palpation at piriformis region
  - Positive Lasègue's sign
  - Gluteal atrophy in chronic cases
- Intolerance for sitting
- Pain with bowel movements
- Dyspareunia
- Radicular-type symptoms into the lower extremity posterior thigh and calf following the sciatic nerve pattern in cases with nerve irritation: "Wallet sign"

AGGRAVATING ACTIVITIES

- Sitting
- Putting shoes on
- Crossing legs while sitting
- Squatting
- Lunging
- Ascending steps
- Motions of hip adduction and internal rotation

EASING ACTIVITIES

- Out of stretch position of the piriformis, supine with lower extremity externally rotated
- Standing with lower extremity externally rotated
- Standing from seated position
- Traction

24-HOUR SYMPTOM PATTERN

- If inflammation is the source of symptoms, patient may experience stiffness in the morning.
- If muscle strain or injury is the source, the soreness may increase throughout the day, but this will depend on how often aggravating activities are completed.

PAST HISTORY FOR THE REGION

- History of low back pain: Radiculopathy or disc herniation
- History of hip pathology or surgery

PHYSICAL EXAMINATION

- Tenderness at piriformis muscle belly with palpable difference in muscle tone
- Limited ROM: Internal rotation limited below 60 degrees of hip flexion; external rotation limited at 90 degrees of hip flexion
- Pain with resisted abduction and external rotation
- Trendelenburg's sign
- Cluster of signs to assist with diagnosis of piriformis syndrome are as follows:
  - Lasègue sign: Pain is present in the vicinity of the greater sciatic notch during extension of the knee with the hip flexed to 90 degrees, tenderness to palpation of the greater sciatic notch is noted.
  - Pace sign: Pain and weakness are present on resisted abduction-external rotation of the thigh.
  - Freiberg sign: Pain occurs with passive internal rotation of the extended thigh when the patient is supine.
  - Pain with flexion adduction and internal rotation position (FADIR, or FAIR, test)
  - Straight leg raise with hip adduction; altered with foot dorsiflexion and plantarflexion

IMPORTANT OBJECTIVE TESTS

- FADIR (or FAIR) test: Sensitivity: 0.88; specificity: 0.83; positive likelihood ratio: 5.2, negative likelihood ratio: 0.14.
- Palpation: Local tenderness or palpable spindle with reproductions of pain.
- EMG: Testing for Hoffman reflex (H reflex) in FADIR delays H reflexes; expected delays in hamstring and gluteus maximus
- CT and MRI for lumbar pathology

DIFFERENTIAL DIAGNOSIS

- Lumbar spine pathology: Herniated disc, facet dysfunction, stenosis, L5-S1 radiculopathy
- Bursitis/tendonitis gluteus or hamstring
- Sacroiliac joint dysfunction
- Pelvic or genitourinary pathology

CONTRIBUTING FACTORS

- Weak gluteal muscles
- Weak core stabilizers
- Increased lumbar spine lordosis
- Fibrosis caused by trauma at piriformis/gluteal region
- Partial or total nerve anatomical abnormalities
- Occupations requiring prolonged sitting or driving

TREATMENT Rx

SURGICAL OPTIONS

Surgical release of the piriformis muscle with or without surgical neurolysis.

SURGICAL OUTCOMES

- Surgical intervention is invasive, with varying results, and the last resort to assisting with the pain.
- Excellent in 11 of 15 patients, good in 4 of 15 patients (Benson and Schutzer).
- A surgical indicator would be the inability of conservative treatments, such as physical therapy, massage therapy, medication, and injections, to be effective for pain.

REHABILITATION

- The focus of physical therapy is to address the impairments leading to the piriformis syndrome and restore function.
- Initially, treatment assists in reducing pain to the area.
  - The patient should be educated on the reduction of irritation to the piriformis region. This may include things like standing frequently if his or her occupation requires prolonged sitting. Placing the muscle in a slacked position may also help relieve pain.
- Exercises: Gentle hip ROM and stretching of the piriformis can be used.
- Use of modalities, such as ultrasound, vasocoolant spray, and massage, to assist with muscle flexibility and pain management. Additionally, local ice may help with pain and any inflammation.
- After the initial acute pain has subsided, the focus is to restore flexibility and address contributing factors.

- Exercises: Gentle stretching should be gradually progressed. Strengthening for gluteal muscles and core stabilizers can be used.
  - STM can be used to assist in releasing the piriformis muscle for greater flexibility.
  - Joint mobilizations include sacroiliac joint and hip joint mobility.
  - Modalities are used as needed.
- In later stages of rehabilitation, the return to previous level of function is the goal.
  - Neural mobilization improves mobility of the sciatic nerve to prevent further entrapment.
  - Correction and reeducation of abnormal movement patterns and functional exercises are goals.
  - Pain-free activities without neurological symptoms are required before fully returning to prior level of function activities.

PROGNOSIS

- Conservative treatment is usually sufficient in most cases.
- Success rate is approximately 85% after conservative treatment with manual therapy and local injections.
- After surgery, return to activity is 2 to 3 months.

SIGNS AND SYMPTOMS INDICATING REFERRAL TO PHYSICIAN

- Constant unrelenting hip pain: Infection or tumor

- Constant pain that is severe and worse with movement: Fracture
- Pain that does not change with position change: Infection or tumor
- Fevers and chills: Infection
- Inability to weight bear on lower extremity: Fracture, stress fracture, Legg-Calvé-Perthes disease, slipped capital femoral epiphysis, or avascular necrosis.

SUGGESTED READINGS

Benson ER, Schutzer SF. Posttraumatic piriformis syndrome: diagnosis and results of operative treatment. *J Bone Joint Surg Am.* 1999;81(7):941-949.

Cleland J. *Orthopaedic Clinical Examination: An Evidence Based Approach for Physical Therapists.* Carlstadt, NJ: Icon learning systems; 2006:269.

Fishman LM, Dombi GW, Michaelsen, C, et al. Piriformis syndrome: diagnosis, treatment, and outcome- a 10 - year study. *Arch Phys Med Rehabil.* 2002;83:295-301.

Hertling D, Kessler RM. *Management of Common Musculoskeletal Disorders: Physical Therapy Principles and Methods.* Philadelphia, PA: Lippincott Williams & Wilkins; 2006:243-245.

Papadopoulos EC, Khan SN. Piriformis syndrome and low back pain: a new classification and review of the literature. *Orthop Clin North Am.* 2004;35:65-71.

AUTHOR: STEPHANIE S. SAITO

Section III

ORTHOPEDIC PATHOLOGY

BASIC INFORMATION

DEFINITION

Posterior compartment syndrome is defined as an elevation of the interstitial pressure of the posterior compartment of the thigh, which is comprised of the hamstrings and sciatic nerve, resulting in microvascular compromise and possible tissue damage.

SYNONYMS

- Compartment syndrome
- Recurrent compartment syndrome
- Exertional compartment syndrome

ICD-9CM CODES

729.72 Nontraumatic compartment
        syndrome of lower extremity
958.8   Other early complications of
        trauma
958.92 Traumatic compartment
        syndrome of lower extremity

OPTIMAL NUMBER OF VISITS

6 visits

MAXIMAL NUMBER OF VISITS

24 visits

ETIOLOGY

- Acute compartment syndrome (ACS)
  - Usually occurs in response to a decrease in compartment volume, an increase in compartmental contents, or externally applied pressure.
  - Increase in interstitial pressure occurs in response to a decrease in compartment volume, an increase in compartment contents, or externally applied pressure.
  - As the duration and magnitude of interstitial pressure increases, arterioles collapse with elevated pressure above diastolic blood pressure, myoneural function is impaired, ischemia occurs, and soft tissue necrosis eventually occurs.
  - Partial ischemia and intracompartmental compression is followed by necrosis of muscle tissue.
  - Finally, regeneration of fibrous tissue causes a contracture.
- Chronic compartment syndrome (CCS)
  - Also known as recurrent compartment syndrome or exertional compartment syndrome, CCS occurs with repetitive activity and microtrauma.
  - Since muscle bulk increases approximately 20% during exercise, there is an increase in intracompartmental pressure.
  - Repetitive muscle contractions increase intramuscular pressure to cause transient ischemia, therefore causing high pressure between successive contractions, impeding blood flow.
  - Intracompartmental pressure increases to levels causing transient ischemia. Tissue necrosis does not occur because symptoms typically resolve when the activity is stopped and the patient rests.
  - As pressure rises, arterial flow decreases during relaxation, resulting in muscle cramping.

EPIDEMIOLOGY AND DEMOGRAPHICS

- The thigh has the potential space to allow for swelling and an increase in the interstitial pressure before circulation is compromised.
- ACS is usually prevalent in younger populations who engage in athletic or military activities.
- CCS typically occurs in endurance athletes or military personnel.

MECHANISM OF INJURY

- Compartment syndrome, in general, may be secondary to the following:
  - Proximal extracompartmental occlusion of the main artery supplying the compartment
  - Intracompartmental injury to either the bone, soft tissue, or both, resulting in hemorrhage
- In ACS, decrease in compartment volume from the following:
  - Reduction of femoral fracture through traction
  - Stretch of hamstrings with knee flexion contracture
  - Closure of fascia defect, scarring and contraction of skin and/or fascia (e.g., with burns)
- In ACS, an increase in compartment contents from the following:
  - Intracompartmental bleeding, swelling and edema from hamstring avulsion, hamstring tear, contusions and hemorrhages after blunt trauma, surgical fixation, or total hip arthroplasty
- In ACS, externally applied pressure from the following:
  - Compression garments, casts, tight dressings, lower extremity resting (pressure caused by body weight)
  - Sciatic nerve palsy or stretch injury
- The mechanism of injury for CCS is repetitive activities such as long distance running, basketball, skiing, and soccer

COMMON SIGNS AND SYMPTOMS

- Aching muscular pain that is out of proportion to the injury
- 5 Ps: Pain, pallor, paresthesias, paralysis, and pulselessness
- Coolness of the skin
- Tension or tightness in the limb
- Posterior thigh pain, with sciatic nerve compression: Radiation into sciatic nerve distribution

AGGRAVATING ACTIVITIES

- ACS is aggravated over the course of time. Additionally, use of hamstrings, compressing the posterior compartment, and passive stretching will aggravate.
- CCS is aggravated by overuse of hamstrings and passive stretching.

EASING ACTIVITIES

- ACS: Rest limb at heart level; relieve possible causes of the syndrome.
- CCS: Rest and decreasing level of activity and symptoms typically subside.

24-HOUR SYMPTOM PATTERN

- ACS: Over the course of time pressure continues to build in the compartment.
- CCS: Ache worsens after activity then improves with rest. There may be no difference in day or night unless person continues to exert posterior compartment contents throughout the day.

PAST HISTORY FOR THE REGION

- Severe thigh contusion
- Severe injury to hamstrings
- Multiple traumas to the area
- Recent casting or bandaging

PHYSICAL EXAMINATION

- 5 Ps: Pain, pallor, paresthesias, paralysis, and pulselessness
- Tightness of the posterior compartment
- Pain with passive stretch of hamstrings
- Pressure changes of the compartment

IMPORTANT OBJECTIVE TESTS

- Compartment pressure testing is the gold standard.
- ACS
  - Measured pressure of the compartment: 30 mm Hg for a normotensive person or 10 to 30 mm Hg below diastolic blood pressure for hypotensive person
- CCS
  - A resting compartment pressure ≥15 mm Hg
  - A 1-minute postexercise compartment pressure ≥30 mm Hg
  - A 5-minute postexercise compartment pressure ≥20 mm Hg (Pedowitz)

DIFFERENTIAL DIAGNOSIS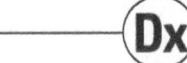

- Muscle strains
- Stress fractures
- Sciatica
- Intermittent neural or vascular claudication

CONTRIBUTING FACTORS

- Chronic anticoagulation therapy
- Systemic hypotension

TREATMENT

SURGICAL OPTIONS

- Decompressive fasciotomy also known as compartment release
  - Single or double incision
  - Debridement of necrotic tissue

SURGICAL OUTCOMES

- Surgery in ACS is generally successful to relieve pressure in the leg. However, persistent deficits in sensory or motor function may occur, depending on the delay to diagnosis and treatment.
- In CCS, open fasciotomy has low risk and good results.
- Early return to running reported as early as 1 week after surgery, generally at 6 weeks.
- Surgical indicators are as follows:
  - ACS is limb threatening. Surgery is indicated with high pressures without relief in 30 to 60 minutes of conservative care.
  - CCS: Lack of resolution with conservative care for 3 to 6 months.

REHABILITATION

- ACS requires operative management
  - Postoperative care depends on primary pathology that lead to the compartment syndrome.
  - Initially, postoperative ambulation with physical therapy to assist with limited weight bearing using assistive devices can be done.
  - As tissue heals, gradual increases in weight bearing provided there is no contraindication to weight bearing.
  - Gentle ROM and flexibility exercises: Ankle, knee, and hip without excessive strain on posterior compartment or contents.

- Once healing has occurred, then gradual progressive resistance exercises are allowed.
- CCS without surgery
  - Initial goals of physical therapy are to reduce symptoms into the lower extremity.
  - Instruction to rest lower extremities and prevent further increase in compartment pressure.
  - No compression should be applied to the thigh.
  - As symptoms resolve, emphasis should be placed on gradual incorporation of exercise and activity without increasing compartment pressure.
  - Exercises may include gentle stretching of lower extremities. Aerobic exercise may gradually be incorporated with emphasis on cross-training to limit repetitive stress and muscle contraction of the posterior compartment.
  - STM may help with facial release and facilitate lymph drainage.
  - Addressing biomechanical issues, including strength, flexibility, proper equipment (i.e., shoes, orthotics) and gradual incorporation of exercise and activity.
- CCS with surgery
  - Ambulation immediately postoperative: Weight bearing as tolerated with crutches.
  - ROM exercises as tolerated.
  - After surgery, early return to activity allows fascia to heal in an expanded state.
  - Gradually add progressive resistance exercises and sport-specific exercises.
  - Cross-training with bike or swimming for ROM and water jogging will help regain strength and flexibility without loading the compartment.

PROGNOSIS

- ACS: If a fasciotomy is performed within a good time frame (tissue necrosis occurs after 4 to 6 hours with ischemia) and

without complications, then prognosis is good. With tissue necrosis and further complications, prognosis is poor. Sensory or motor deficits may persist at 1-year follow-up in patients despite early treatment.
- CCS has had good prognosis in case studies of long distance runners receiving a fasciotomy after failure of conservative care.

SIGNS AND SYMPTOMS INDICATING REFERRAL TO PHYSICIAN

- Increasing lower extremity pressure and pain: ACS, DVT, peripheral vascular injury
- Major trauma: Fractures, ACS
- Fever and chills: Infection, necrotizing fasciitis, cellulitis
- Unrelenting pain in lower extremity: Infection or tumor

SUGGESTED READINGS

Clancey GJ. Acute posterior compartment syndrome in the thigh. A case report. *J Bone Joint Surg Am.* 1985;67:1278-1280.

Pedowitz RA, Hargens AR, Mubarak SJ, Gershuni DH. Modified criteria for the objective diagnosis of chronic compartment syndrome of the leg. *Am J Sports Med.* 1990;18:35-40.

Raether PM, Lutter LD. Recurrent compartment syndrome in the posterior thigh: report of a case. *Am J Sports Med.* 1982;10:40-43.

Salter RB. *Textbook of Disorders and Injuries of the Musculoskeletal System.* Baltimore, MD: Lippincott Williams & Williams.

Schwartz JT Jr, Brumback RJ, Lakatos R, Poka A, Bathon GH, Burgess AR. Acute compartment syndrome of the thigh. A spectrum of injury. *J Bone Joint Surg.* 1989;71(3):392-400.

AUTHOR: STEPHANIE S. SAITO

Section III

ORTHOPEDIC PATHOLOGY

BASIC INFORMATION

DEFINITION

A stress fracture is defined as the alteration of bone caused by the inability to withstand nonviolent stress that is applied in a rhythmic, repeated, and subthreshold manner. Stress fractures of the pubic ramus typically occur at the inferior pubic ramus more than at the superior pubic ramus.

SYNONYMS

- Pelvic stress fracture
- Pelvic insufficiency fracture
- Pelvic ring stress fracture
- March fractures

ICD-9CM CODES
733.95 Stress fracture of other bone
808.2 Closed fracture of pubis

OPTIMAL NUMBER OF VISITS

8 visits

MAXIMAL NUMBER OF VISITS

18 visits

ETIOLOGY

- Fatigue fracture occurs in normal bone because of repetitive mechanical stress. Repetitive loading results in a decrease in the bone's failure strength.
- Insufficiency fracture occurs in bone with lowered bone fatigue strength such as occurs in osteomalacia, osteoporosis, or other disease states. This fracture may occur with lower loads or fewer loading cycles.
- The inferior pubic ramus has opposing tensile-based stresses placed on it during stance and swing phases of the gait cycle.
- The adductor and external rotator muscles are attached to the pubic arch in two groups on either side of the ischiopubic line. As the hip is extended, tensile forces on the medial portion of the pubic ramus are produced by strong muscle pulls on the lateral part of the pubic ramus and ischium.
- During stance, the hip adductors resist the force of the abductors to stabilize the femur as the limb progresses into hip extension.
- During the swing phase of ambulation, external rotators contract to compensate for the rotation of the pelvis toward the opposite limb.
- The continuous and repetitive muscular pulling on the bony insertion during activity causes local bony absorption and osteoporosis, leading to microfractures.
- Stress fractures develop when the accumulation of microfractures at a uniform location cannot be accommodated by the normal physiological bone remodeling process.
- Tension fractures result from cyclic loads causing osteon debonding and microfractures, thereby forming gross fatigue fractures. This further leads to higher stresses and rapid failure of the bone; displacement may occur.

EPIDEMIOLOGY AND DEMOGRAPHICS

- Stress fractures of the pubic ramus are infrequent.
- Insufficiency fractures typically occur in the elderly.
- Fatigue fractures typically occur in younger populations.
- Pubic stress fractures occur in females more often than males; the pelvis is typically more slender, the pubic symphysis is more shallow, margins of the ischiopubic rami are less everted, and the obturator foramen is more triangular, altering forces placed. Additionally, it is hypothesized that females rely on greater hip-extension forces during running, causing more tensile stresses in the medial portion of the pubic ramus.
- Caucasian.
- 12% in female Caucasian-American recruits.
- Long distance or marathon runners.
- Military recruits: Mixed training of males and females.
- Younger athletes.

MECHANISM OF INJURY

- Jogging, running
- Military training (marching)
- Fencing
- Jumping

COMMON SIGNS AND SYMPTOMS

- Pain in the groin, buttock, or thigh.
- Painful weight bearing.
- Pain may be noted suddenly after running or during a training session. Typically, there is a gradual increase in discomfort after long distance running or a marathon, which has been shown from 0 to 5 weeks afterward.
- Tenderness to palpation at pubic ramus.
- Pain may refer from the groin or buttock into the thigh.

AGGRAVATING ACTIVITIES

- Weight-bearing activities: Jogging, running, or jumping

EASING ACTIVITIES

- Resting from activity
- Decreased weight bearing and muscle activation

24-HOUR SYMPTOM PATTERN

- Morning soreness

- Aching in the hip on the first few steps in the morning or after prolonged rest
- Pain gradually increasing throughout the day with prolonged weight bearing
- Night-time pain may be present

PAST HISTORY FOR THE REGION

- Previous operations of the hip
- Past history of hip pathology

PHYSICAL EXAMINATION

- Tenderness locally at pubic ramus.
- Tenderness at adductor origin.
- ROM typically not limited and may have pain with abduction.
- Pain may occur with resisted adduction and external rotation of the hip.
- Antalgic gait pattern.

IMPORTANT OBJECTIVE TESTS

There no objective tests in physical therapy that rule in or rule out a pelvic ramus stress fracture. A strong subjective and cluster of findings may best indicate a stress fracture. Radiographs, bone scintigraphy, and MRI are useful to visualize the fracture site.

DIFFERENTIAL DIAGNOSIS

- Groin strain
- Adductor tendinopathy
- Adductor avulsions
- Osteitis pubis
- Sacroiliac joint dysfunction
- Labral tear or intraarticular pathology

CONTRIBUTING FACTORS

- Change in activity level or training: Increasing the duration, frequency, and/or intensity of activity or training without allowing for proper bone and supporting muscle adaptation, resulting in microscopic damage to the bone, which cannot be healed quickly.
- Lack of physical training or conditioning.
- Osteopenia and reduced bone density.
- Metabolic and biochemical disorders: RA, hyperparathyroidism, hypogonadism, nutritional insufficiency (anorexia nervosa), menstrual disturbances, and long-term steroid use affecting the bone remodeling process.
- Structural and biomechanical influences: Leg length discrepancy, excessive pronation.
- Obesity or increase in gravitational force causes increased tensile stress.
- Instability at the sacroiliac joint may place undue stress on the pelvic ring.

TREATMENT

SURGICAL OPTIONS

- ORIF
- Retrograde medullary screw

SURGICAL OUTCOMES

- Stress fractures at the pubic ramus do not usually require surgical intervention. Therefore success rates for pubic ramus stabilization are usually following trauma with high instability.
- Surgical indicators are as follows:
  - Prolonged nonunion stress fractures or widely displaced fractures
  - Failure of conservative management

REHABILITATION

- The goals of physical therapy are to promote healing, prevent complications, and return to premorbid level of function.
- Initially, patients are educated to rest to minimize stress on the fracture site.
  - No pain should be present with weight bearing, otherwise, non-weight-bearing activity should be followed with crutches or appropriate assistive device.
  - Initial exercises should be pain-free: Hip, knee, and ankle ROM, stretching and strengthening exercises for hip and knee musculature in open chain.
  - Aerobic exercise: Swimming, low resistance stationary bike exercise for patients unable to tolerate weight-bearing activity and low-impact aerobic exercise for patients able to tolerate weight bearing.
- As weight-bearing activity is progressed, it is important to identify and address biomechanical faults and those factors that contributed to the stress fracture.
  - A prescribed walk-to-run program may be initiated after light weight-bearing strengthening exercises and prolonged ambulation are pain-free.
  - No ROM or strength limitations should be present when this part of rehabilitation is initiated.
  - The walk-to-run training program should provide a cyclical exposure to stress with rest days, rather than a progressive and continuous increase.
- Sport-specific drills and higher intensity activities should be gradually introduced and advanced.
  - Activities are to remain pain-free. If pain recurs, the activity should be stopped.
  - Education from physical therapy should include prevention of recurrence of stress fractures, understanding those factors that contributed to the stress fractures, including biomechanical, nutritional, and endocrine factors; maintenance of proper flexibility, strength, and fitness; and cross-training or preconditioning for participation in sports.

PROGNOSIS

After proper medical management and successful rehabilitation, patients are able to return to previous level of activities.

SIGNS AND SYMPTOMS INDICATING REFERRAL TO PHYSICIAN

- If a fracture or any other serious pathology is suspected, referral to a physician is warranted
- Constant of unrelenting hip/pelvic pain: Infection or tumor
- Pain that does not change with position or non–weight-bearing: Tumor or infection
- Fevers and chills: Infection or tumor
- Significant and unexplained weight loss: Tumor
- Inability to bear weight on affected limb: Fracture
- Rapidly progressing stress fracture: Malignancy

SUGGESTED READINGS

Hill PF, Chatterji S, Chambers D, Keeling JD. Stress fractures of the pubic ramus in female recruits. *J Bone Joint Surg Br.* 1996;78:383–386.

Lee SW, Lee CH. Fatigue stress fractures of the pubic ramus in the army: imaging features with radiographic, scintigraphic and MR imaging findings. *Korean J Radiol.* 2005;6:47–51.

Pavlov H, Nelson TL, Warren RF, Torg JS, Burstein AH. Stress fractures of the pubic ramus. A report of twelve cases. *J Bone Joint Surg Am.* 1982;64:1020–1025.

Thienpont E, Bellemans J, Samson I, Fabry G. Stress fracture of the inferior and superior pubic ramus in a man with anorexia nervosa and hypogonadism. *Acta Orthop Belg.* 2000;66(3):297–301.

AUTHOR: STEPHANIE S. SAITO

Section III

ORTHOPEDIC PATHOLOGY

BASIC INFORMATION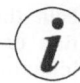

DEFINITION

Quadriceps contusion is an area of local muscle damage and bleeding that is usually caused by a direct trauma, specifically at the quadriceps.

SYNONYMS

- Charley horse
- Cork thigh
- Quad bruise

ICD-9CM CODES
924.00 Contusion of thigh
924.01 Contusion of hip

OPTIMAL NUMBER OF VISITS

6 visits or less

MAXIMAL NUMBER OF VISITS

10 visits

ETIOLOGY

- The pathology is generally the result of direct trauma or a blow to the quadriceps, usually the anterior portion.
- Bruises are caused by blood that pools from damaged capillaries into interstitial tissues.
- Bleeding causes increased tissue pressure by also stimulating the inflammatory reaction. Although the inflammatory process is important for muscle regeneration, it further causes increased tissue pressure as a result of the macrophage action, phagocytosis, and stimulation of capillary production. Increased tissue pressure caused by edema leads to anoxia and cell death.
- The more severe contusions have a higher risk for traumatic myositis ossificans complications.
- Severity of the hematoma is based on the degree of passive knee flexion after 24 hours.
  - Mild: 90 degrees plus flexion
  - Moderate: 45 to 90 degrees flexion
  - Severe: <45 degrees flexion
- The pathology usually occurs in a single quadriceps muscle.

EPIDEMIOLOGY AND DEMOGRAPHICS

- Contusions are common in contact sports where direct blow or trauma may occur.
- Also common in sports with a ball or object travelling at high speeds.
- Typically occurs in younger populations because of activities in which they participate.
- Contact sports such as football, basketball, hockey, and martial arts.
- Sports with high velocity objects.

MECHANISM OF INJURY

- Direct blow or trauma to the muscle belly.
- Helmet contact is common in football.
- Knee to thigh is common in basketball or soccer.
- Kicks to the thigh with martial arts.
- Objects, such as hockey pucks, impacting area.

COMMON SIGNS AND SYMPTOMS

- Patient may not recall a specific incident in less severe cases; more severe cases will usually recall incident.
- May continue with activity with soreness after cooling down or after period of rest in mild-to-moderate cases. In severe cases, may not be able to continue with activity.
- Local formation of a bruise.
- Onset of soreness can be immediate or soon after activity.
- Usually pain is local to injury; blood from the contusion may track down to the knee region causing irritation.

AGGRAVATING ACTIVITIES

- Depending on the severity of the contusion, activities involving isometric contractions and concentric and eccentric contractions may be aggravating
- Walking, running
- Climbing or descending stairs or steps
- Squatting
- Sitting to standing
- Passive knee flexion: Stretching of the contusion
- Active knee extension: Concentric
- Controlled knee flexion: Eccentric
- Excessive activity using quadriceps muscle

EASING ACTIVITIES

- Resting
- Gentle activity may help with pain

24-HOUR SYMPTOM PATTERN

- Generally sore and stiff in the morning
- Improves with gentle activity but resumes stiffness after inactivity

PAST HISTORY FOR THE REGION

- Previous history of contusions
- A series of minor contusions during a game have a cumulative effect

PHYSICAL EXAMINATION

- Local tenderness to palpation
- Swelling
- Bruising
- Increased circumference
- Limited ROM into flexion
- Loss of strength

- Gait deviations: Difficulty weight bearing, walks with knee locked in extension (quadriceps avoidance pattern)

IMPORTANT OBJECTIVE TESTS

- Combination of findings such as palpation, ROM, and observation.
- MRI will show the extent of edema in the involved muscle and have the greatest specificity and sensitivity for quadriceps disorder.

DIFFERENTIAL DIAGNOSIS

- Quadriceps sprain/strain/tear
- Stress fracture
- Compartment syndrome
- Myositis ossificans
- Delayed onset muscle soreness, muscle cramps, or muscle spasms

CONTRIBUTING FACTORS

- Lack of adequate padding to the quadriceps region in contact sports
- Previous history of quadriceps contusions

TREATMENT

SURGICAL OPTIONS

Unless a compartment syndrome occurs, there usually is no surgical intervention.

REHABILITATION

- Initial goals of physical therapy are to address the inflammatory process and control the hemorrhage.
  - To control the hemorrhage the knee is initially wrapped with a compression wrap in 120 degrees of flexion.
  - Modalities: Ice, electrical stimulation for pain.
  - STM is contraindicated at this time.
  - Exercise: Gentle ROM.
- After the inflammatory process is controlled, the goal is to restore ROM and increase strength while monitoring swelling.
  - Exercises should focus on restoring ROM and improving tolerance for weight bearing and light quadriceps muscle activation.
  - STM is used to improve lymph drainage.
  - Modalities can be used as necessary.
- Finally, rehabilitation should focus on returning to functional and recreational activities and sport.
  - Care is taken to ensure proper rehabilitation without re-injury. Emphasis is on proper padding to avoid a delay in recovery or increasing the severity of the damage from the original contusion.
  - Exercises for concentric and eccentric strength, functional activities, multidirectional activities, and sport-specific activities.

PROGNOSIS

- The degree of severity determines the prognosis: Lesser severity usually requires several days to resolve versus weeks to resolve.
- More severe cases may have other symptoms such as knee joint irritation.
- In cases in which other complications occur, such as myositis ossificans, the recovery usually takes longer.

SIGNS AND SYMPTOMS INDICATING REFERRAL TO PHYSICIAN

- Physical symptoms similar to a contusion without corresponding history: Fracture, tumor, or metabolic process
- Area of calcification with pain: Myositis ossificans
- Increase in pain, not in proportion to the injury: Compartment syndrome
- Trauma: Fracture
- Unrelenting pain: Tumor
- Fever and chills: Infection or tumor

SUGGESTED READINGS

Brukner P, Khan K. *Clinical Sports Medicine*. Australia: McGraw-Hill.

Diaz JA, Fischer DA, Rettig AC, Davis TJ, Shelbourne KD. Severe quadriceps muscle contusions in athletes; a report of three cases. *Am J Sports Med.* 2003;31:289–293.

Hertling D, Kessler RM. *Management of Common Musculoskeletal Disorders: Physical Therapy Principles and Methods*. Philadelphia, PA: Lippincott Williams & Wilkins; 2006:532–533.

Jackson DW, Feagin JA. Quadriceps contusions in young athletes. Relation of severity to injury to treatment and prognosis. *J Bone Joint Surg Am.* 1973;55:95–105.

AUTHOR: STEPHANIE S. SAITO

BASIC INFORMATION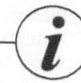

DEFINITION

Quadriceps strain is damage or tear of the quadriceps (vastus medialis, vastus lateralis, vastus intermedius, and rectus femoris) muscle group or musculotendinous junction, ranging from grade I to III.

SYNONYMS

- Quadriceps pull
- Quadriceps tear

ICD-9CM CODES

843.8 Sprain of other specified sites of hip and thigh

843.9 Sprain of unspecified site of hip and thigh

844.8 Sprain of other specified sites of knee and leg

844.9 Sprain of unspecified site of knee and leg

OPTIMAL NUMBER OF VISITS

6 visits

MAXIMAL NUMBER OF VISITS

36 visits

ETIOLOGY

- A quadriceps strain occurs as a result of a rapid concentric or eccentric load placed on the muscle. Additionally, it can occur from extensive overuse of the muscle group.
- Strains are graded by the severity of damage, as follows:
  - First degree: Mild —damage to a minimal number of muscle fibers
  - Second degree: Moderate—damage to more extensive number of muscle fibers
  - Third degree: Severe—complete rupture of the muscle that results in loss of function of the muscle, tendon, or attachment
- The strain can be at the musculotendinous junction or in the muscle belly itself.
- The rectus femoris is the most commonly strained quadriceps muscle because of the actions of hip flexion and knee extension and the potential to be forced through large length changes.
- The most site of rupture is at the distal musculotendinous junction.
- The second most common location is proximal within the muscle belly.
- The strain occurs at the weakest part of the muscle-tendon unit. Muscles fibers fail to hold against the demands placed on them, causing tearing in the muscle, the musculotendinous junction, or damage to the tendon to bony attachment.

EPIDEMIOLOGY AND DEMOGRAPHICS

- In general, lower extremity muscle strains are common, especially in the two joint muscles.
- It is common among all age groups and has a high frequency in middle-aged athletes.
- It is generally found in athletes involved in sports in which sprinting, jumping, or kicking is required.

MECHANISM OF INJURY

- Rapid acceleration or deceleration of the quadriceps
- Sprinting
- Jumping
- Kicking
- General functional overload of the quadriceps muscle

COMMON SIGNS AND SYMPTOMS

- May have felt tearing or popping during the injury
- Tenderness at site of tear
- Pain with activity or muscle contraction of quadriceps
- Local swelling/inflammation
- Local bruising
- Pain: After cool down in less severe cases
- Antalgic gait
- The referral of the muscle generally follows the line of the quadriceps muscle group

AGGRAVATING ACTIVITIES

- Depending on the severity of the muscle strain, a variety of activities can be aggravating. These activities involve isometric contractions and concentric and eccentric contractions
  - Walking, running
  - Climbing or descending stairs
  - Squatting
  - Sitting to standing
  - Passive knee flexion: Stretching

EASING ACTIVITIES

- Rest, ice, and compression
- Lower extremity positioned with slack on quadriceps muscle

24-HOUR SYMPTOM PATTERN

- Soreness/stiffness in the morning, better after warms up
- Worse throughout the day with activity using the muscle
- Fatigue with muscle use

PAST HISTORY FOR THE REGION

- Recent hamstring strain or quadriceps strain
- Recurring strain

PHYSICAL EXAMINATION

- Limited knee ROM

- Limited quadriceps strength: Extensor lag may indicate partial and complete tears; no extension may indicate complete tear
- Limited quadriceps flexibility
- Gait deviations: Walks with knee locked in full extension to avoid use of quadriceps

IMPORTANT OBJECTIVE TESTS

- Clusters of finding help diagnose the muscle strain:
  - Thomas test: Pain with stretch of the rectus femoris
  - ASLR: Pain with activation of the rectus femoris
  - Palpation of deficit in the quadriceps muscle, musculotendinous junction
  - Limitation of strength at quads
- Other diagnostic tests from the physician can be used for diagnosis. MRIs have the greatest specificity and sensitivity for quadriceps disorders. Ultrasound may help diagnose severe tears.

DIFFERENTIAL DIAGNOSIS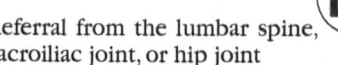

- Referral from the lumbar spine, sacroiliac joint, or hip joint
- Femoral neuropathy
- Quadriceps contusion
- Femoral stress fracture
- Sartorius muscle strain
- Anterior compartment syndrome

CONTRIBUTING FACTORS

- Muscle inflexibility
- Overstretching
- Imbalance in strength
- Leg length discrepancy
- Improper warm up

SURGICAL OPTIONS

Surgical repair of the muscle belly or musculotendinous junction of nonhealing strains or complete ruptures

SURGICAL OUTCOMES

- In cases of complete rupture, surgery is effective. Good outcomes are shown for return to functional activities. Return to previous level of activity and sport varies.
- Conservative management has been shown to be the standard of care or just as effective for first- and second-degree injuries.
- Surgery was indicated for patients with the following:
  - Nonhealing severe strain/rupture
  - Inability to actively extend knee
  - Bunching of quadriceps muscle, as in a rupture of the quadriceps tendon

REHABILITATION

- Goals of physical therapy are to restore pain-free ROM of the hip, knees, ankle and foot; normalize gait pattern, and ultimately return to previous functional status for ADLs and vocational, recreational, and sport activities. The extent of rehabilitation depends on the severity of the strain.

- Initially, the inflammatory process is addressed.
  - Modalities for pain and swelling such as electrical stimulation, iontophoresis, phonophoresis, compression, or ice
  - For severe strains, crutches may be indicated to limit gait deviations caused by pain
  - Gentle ROM: Pain-free stretching and passive ROM (PROM)
  - Gentle STM to promote lymph drainage
  - Gentle isometric exercises
- After addressing the acute inflammatory phase, the focus of rehabilitation is to return to functional activities, then progress to recreational activities and sport.
  - STM can be used to limit adhesions and improve lymph drainage.
  - Strengthening and stretching exercises: Pain-free exercises initially to promote proper scar tissue formation. Emphasis is on flexibility exercises of quadriceps, retraining of quadriceps, and addressing muscular imbalances.
  - Long-term exercises: Emphasis is on proper warm-up and cool-down exercises, stretching, and cross-training to prevent overuse injuries.

PROGNOSIS

Recurrences of the quadriceps strains is common. Proper rehabilitation minimizes recurrence of strains.

SIGNS AND SYMPTOMS INDICATING REFERRAL TO PHYSICIAN

- Lack of healing or complications at the site of injury: Other pathology such as a femoral stress fracture
- Trauma: Fractures at the hip or femur
- Increase in swelling, pain, and thigh pressure: Compartment syndrome
- Constant unrelenting pain: Bone tumor or infection
- Nocturnal pain: Tumor

SUGGESTED READINGS

Brukner P, Khan K. *Clinical Sports Medicine*. Australia: McGraw-Hill.

Cross T, Gibbs N, Houang M, Cameron M. Acute quadriceps muscle strains: magnetic resonance imaging features and prognosis. *Am J Sports Med.* 2004;32(3):710–719.

Hertling D, Kessler RM. *Management of Common Musculoskeletal Disorders: Physical Therapy Principles and Methods.* Philadelphia: Lippincott Williams & Wilkins; 2006.

McMaster P. Tendon and muscle ruptures: clinical and experimental studies on the causes and location of subcutaneous ruptures. *J Bone Joint Surg Am.* 1933;15:705–722.

Orchard J. Biomechanics of muscle strain injury. The Dr Matt Marshall Lecture. *NZJ Sport Med.* 2002;92–98.

Temple H, Kuklo T, Sweet D, Gibbons CL, Murphey M. Rectus femoris muscle tear appearing as a pseudotumor. *Am J Sports Med.* 1998;26:544–548.

AUTHOR: STEPHANIE S. SAITO

BASIC INFORMATION

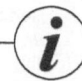

DEFINITION

Snapping hip syndrome is a condition of the hip characterized by an audible and/or palpable snap or click that may be painful or painless.

SYNONYMS

- Coxa saltans
- Iliopsoas syndrome
- Trochanteric syndrome

ICD-9CM CODES
719.65 Other symptoms referable to joint of pelvic region and thigh
843.8 Sprain of other specified sites of hip and thigh
843.9 Sprain of unspecified sites of hip and thigh
843.0 Iliofemoral (ligament) sprain
843.1 Ischiocapsular (ligament) sprain

OPTIMAL NUMBER OF VISITS

6 visits or less

MAXIMAL NUMBER OF VISITS

16 visits

ETIOLOGY

- External snapping hip syndrome
  - External snapping hip syndrome refers to the "snapping" sound and/or feeling that occurs at the lateral hip, which is caused by the tensor fascia lata, ITB, anterior fibers of the gluteus maximus, or a combination sliding over the greater trochanter.
  - The ITB translates posterior over the greater trochanter when the hip extends from a flexed position. Likewise, the ITB translates anterior over the greater trochanter when the hip is flexed from an extended position.
  - The gluteus maximus and tensor fascia lata influence the ITB because of the insertions and actions of the muscle fibers.
  - External snapping hip is the most common cause of the snapping hip syndrome.
  - Increased friction at the greater trochanter results in irritation and inflammation of those tissues, typically the ITB, tensor fascia lata, gluteus maximus or a combination of the three. Degenerative changes, such as hypertrophy or thickening, may rise, causing the tissues to snap over the greater trochanter.
  - The physiological process is the same as tendonitis, tendinosis, or trochanteric bursitis.

- Internal snapping hip syndrome
  - Internal snapping hip syndrome refers to the "snapping" sound and/or feeling that occurs at the hip, which is caused by the iliopsoas tendons flipping over the iliopectineal eminence or femoral head, iliopsoas tendon snapping over the anterior inferior iliac spine or bony ridge of the lesser trochanter, or iliofemoral ligaments moving over the femoral head or anterior capsule of the hip.
  - The most common cause of internal snapping hip syndrome is the iliopsoas tendon sliding over the iliopectineal eminence. This typically occurs as the hip moves into extension from a flexed and externally rotated position.
  - Physiologically, irritation, inflammation, or degenerative changes to the capsule, iliopsoas, or bursa causes as the normal iliopsoas motion across the femoral head and iliopectineal eminence change to painful snapping and locking.
  - The physiological process is the same as iliopsoas tendonitis, iliopsoas tendinosis, or iliopsoas bursitis.
- Intraarticular snapping hip syndrome refers to the "clicking" or "catching" that occurs at the hip, which is caused by labral tears, loose bodies, displaced osteochondral fracture fragments, synovial chondromatosis or ligamentum teres disruptions.
  - Physiologically, lesions of the hip alter the hip's motion as a result of mechanical incongruence producing a "click" or "snap."

EPIDEMIOLOGY AND DEMOGRAPHICS

- Most commonly noted in ages 15 to 40 years.
- Ballet dancers, gymnasts, track and field athletes, cyclists, runners, soccer players, and martial artists are affected by repetitive hip flexion and extension with internal and external rotation.
- Typically, females are affected more than males. The difference is thought to be a result of anatomical differences in pelvic/hip and hip/knee angles.

MECHANISM OF INJURY

- Insidious onset
- Sudden or repetitive loading of the hip joint into a flexed position, such as occurs when landing a jump
- Repetitive overuse or over training with hip flexion and extension activities with or without internal and external rotation

COMMON SIGNS AND SYMPTOMS

- May or may not have pain and discomfort. Pain will be of a dull pain or deep ache, with location of "snapping" at lateral or anterior and deep hip.
- During repetitive flexion and extension activities, person will be able to hear and/or feel click or snap. Hip internal or external rotation may be associated with hip flexion.
- Intermittent symptoms may occur at first, then followed by a known movement pattern that reproduces the symptoms. Over time, the symptoms may be caused by passive motion.
- Generally local symptoms, but in certain instances, pain may radiate laterally along ITB and/or into lumbar spine.

AGGRAVATING ACTIVITIES

- Repetitive hip flexion and extension activities with or without internal and external rotation
- High hip flexion activities: Hip hyperflexion

EASING ACTIVITIES

- Rest
- Limitation of activities causing snapping
- Physician may prescribe antiinflammatories or muscle relaxers or give a local injection

24-HOUR SYMPTOM PATTERN

- Better in the morning after rest.
- Worse after aggravating activities with dull pain or deep ache.
- Sleep is generally not affected in cases of internal snapping hip syndrome. In cases of external snapping hip syndrome, lateral weight-bearing on the affected hip may be painful.

PAST HISTORY FOR THE REGION

- History of hip injury altering biomechanics with secondary hip bursitis or tendonitis
- History of surgical procedures at the hip, altering biomechanics such as hip arthroplasty
- Altered biomechanics of the hip from other lower extremity injuries or surgeries

PHYSICAL EXAMINATION

- Palpation: Tenderness at lateral ITB and gluteus maximus with external snapping hip syndrome; may have tenderness at femoral triangle with internal snapping hip syndrome.
- Gait abnormalities.
- Reproduction of external snapping hip syndrome during hip internal and external rotation in hip flexion.
- Reproduction of internal snapping hip symptoms during flexion, abduction, and external rotation to extension, adduction, and internal rotation.
- Common impairments found with snapping hip syndromes include tightness of hip flexors, soft tissue restrictions of the

hip flexors and ITB, hip joint hypomobility, weakness of hip abductors, external rotators and core stabilizers, and postural and biomechanical faults.

IMPORTANT OBJECTIVE TESTS

- Ober's test assesses the soft tissue mobility or length of the ITB.
- Thomas test evaluates hip flexor length.

DIFFERENTIAL DIAGNOSIS

- ITBFS
- Acetabular labral tear
- Bursitis
- Muscle strain
- Intraarticular loose body or lesion
- Stress fracture
- Lumbar spine referral
- Sacroiliac dysfunction

CONTRIBUTING FACTORS

- Leg length discrepancy
- Variations of ITB width
- Coxa vara
- Poor posture
- Weak core stabilizers, anterior pelvic tilt, and excessive lumbar spine lordosis
- Changes in training or exercise
- Recent adolescent growth spurt

TREATMENT

SURGICAL OPTIONS

- External snapping hip syndrome
  - Z-plasty: Lengthening of the ITB
  - Anchoring of the iliotibial tract to the trochanter
  - Resection of the posterior half of the tract at the gluteus maximus insertion with excision of the trochanteric bursa
  - Elliptical resection of part of the ITB at the greater trochanter with removal of the trochanteric bursa
- Internal snapping hip syndrome
  - Lengthening of the iliopsoas tendon
  - Resection of the bony prominence of the lesser trochanter
  - Complete release of iliopsoas tendon

SURGICAL OUTCOMES

- Surgical intervention is rarely necessary for external and internal snapping hip syndromes.
- Surgical intervention for external snapping hip syndrome is generally good for resolution of the snapping symptom and pain.

- Results for return to activity are unclear. Studies reported patients returning to activities, such as running, cycling, and hiking, after Z-plasty surgery and were involved in sports after elliptical resection surgery.
- The results for patient requiring surgery for snapping hip surgery vary from no change in symptoms to improvement in symptoms and function.
- Complications occurred in one-third of patients of a separate study. These included hip flexor weakness, persistent hip pain, and sensory deficits.
- Return to function was reported, with 73% of patients returning to previous athletic activities and 45% returning to their previous level of athletic activity after surgery.
- Surgical indicator: Lack of symptom relief from conservative care for 6 to 12 months for internal snapping hip syndrome.

REHABILITATION

- Initially address pain and the inflammatory process with the following:
  - Local modalities such as hot or cold packs, ultrasound or phonophoresis for external snapping hip, iontophoresis: External snapping hip, electrical stimulation.
  - Hip joint mobilization: Distraction for pain relief.
  - Exercise: Pain-free ROM of the hip.
  - Activity modification for pain relief and avoidance of the snapping symptom. Emphasis is on resting, especially from repetitive overuse activities.
- Address impairments, abnormal movement patterns, and biomechanical faults that contribute to the snapping hip syndrome.
  - STM: Breaks up adhesions and fibrosis within the tissue to reduce tissue tension and stiffness.
  - Exercises: Stretching of hip musculature, initiation of strengthening exercises for hip stability.
  - Joint mobilization/distraction: Improves joint mechanics and restores deficits in hip ROM.
  - Integration of necessary structural and biomechanical components such as orthotics.
- Integration of high level exercise and activities
  - Progress to gradual return to functional activities, recreational activities, and sport with emphasis on proper training.

PROGNOSIS

- Conservative treatment usually fares well.
- Stretching, physical therapy, activity modification, antiinflammatories, and/or injections are the typical conservative treatments.
- Surgical intervention is rarely necessary.

SIGNS AND SYMPTOMS INDICATING REFERRAL TO PHYSICIAN

- Constant unrelenting pain or pain that does not change with position: Infection or tumor
- Night sweats, night pain: Tumor
- Fevers and chills: Infection or tumor
- Inability to weight bear: Fracture, avascular necrosis, slipped capital femoral epiphysis, Legg-Calvé-Perthes disease
- Major trauma: Fracture
- Painful and limited PROM: Intraarticular lesion
- Urogenital discomfort or changes

SUGGESTED READINGS

Brignall CG, Brown RM, Stainsby GD. Fibrosis of the gluteus maximus as a cause of snapping hip. A case report. *J Bone Joint Surg Am.* 1993;75:909-910.

Brignall CG, Stainsby GD. The snapping hip: treatment by Z-Plasty. *J Bone Joint Surg Br.* 1991;73:253-254.

Gose JC, Schweizer P. Iliotibial band tightness. *J Orthop Sports Phys Ther.* 1989;10(10):399-407.

Hertling D, Kessler RM. *Management of Common Musculoskeletal Disorders: Physical Therapy Principles and Methods.* Philadelphia, PA: Lippincott Williams & Wilkins; 2006.

Provencher MT, Hofmeister EP, Muldoon MP. The surgical treatment of external coxa saltans (the snapping hip) by Z-pasty of the iliotibial band. *Am J Sport Med.* 2004; 32(2):470-476.

Schaberg J, Harper M, Allen W. The snapping hip syndrome. *Am J Sport Med.* 1984;12(5): 361-365.

Wahl CJ, Warren RF, Adler RS, Hannafin JA, Hansen B. Internal coxa saltans (snapping hip) as a result of overtraining: a report of 3 cases in professional athletes with a review of causes that the role of ultrasound in early diagnosis and management. *Am J Sport Med.* 2004;32(5):1302-1309.

White RA, Hughes MS, Burd T, Hamann J, Allen WC. A new operative approach in the correction of external coxa saltans: the snapping hip. *Am J Sport Med.* 2004;32(6): 1504-1508.

AUTHOR: STEPHANIE S. SAITO

BASIC INFORMATION

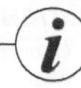

DEFINITION

- A sudden or violent twist or wrench of the tibiofemoral joint results in the stretching or tearing of the anterior cruciate ligament (ACL).
- The ACL is a tough band of fibrous tissue that connects the bones of the upper and lower leg at the knee joint.
- Like other types of sprains, knee sprains are classified according to the following grading system:
  - Grade I (mild): This injury stretches the ligament, which causes microscopic tears in the ligament. These tiny tears do not significantly affect the overall ability of the knee joint to support the body's weight.
  - Grade II (moderate): The ligament is partially torn, and there is some mild-to-moderate instability (or periodic giving out) of the knee while standing or walking.
  - Grade III (severe): The ligament is torn completely or separated at its end from the bone, and the knee is more unstable.

SYNONYMS

- ACL tear
- ACL sprain

ICD-9CM CODES
848.9 Unspecified site of sprain and strain
717.83 Old disruption of anterior cruciate ligament
844.2 Sprain of cruciate ligament of knee

OPTIMAL NUMBER OF VISITS

8 or fewer

MAXIMAL NUMBER OF VISITS

12

ETIOLOGY

- The ACL, like all other ligaments, is composed of type I collagen. The ultrastructure of a ligament is close to that of tendons, but the fibers in a ligament are more variable and have a higher elastin content.
- Ligaments receive their blood supply from their insertion sites. The vascularity within a ligament is uniform, and each ligament contains mechanoreceptors and free nerve endings that are hypothesized to aid in stabilizing the joint.
- Avulsion of ligaments generally occurs between the unmineralized and mineralized fibrocartilage layers. The more common ACL tear, however, is a midsubstance tear. This type of tear occurs primarily as the ligament is transected by the pivoting lateral femoral condyle.
- No one single cause accounts for this injury. ACL injuries can be related to extrinsic and intrinsic factors. Numerous studies document the fact that poor levels of conditioning correlate directly with increased levels of injury. Research also has demonstrated that improved conditioning results in reduced numbers of injuries.
- Body movement and positioning play a big role in ACL injuries. Noyes et al demonstrated that most ACL injuries (78%) occur without contact, and most of these injuries occur on landing after a jump. The Noyes study involved only female basketball players, but the capacity of the knee to plant and turn or absorb the shock of a jump is relevant to both male and female athletes in all sports.
- Muscle strength is the last of the extrinsic factors that affects the ACL. The hamstring is an ACL agonist working in concert with the ACL to prevent anterior tibial translation. Conversely, the quadriceps acts as an antagonist to the ACL, generating force that promotes anterior tibial translation. Ideally, a balance exists between these opposing forces to protect the knee; however, the quadriceps averages 50% to 100% greater muscle strength than the hamstring. Strength coaches often emphasize quadriceps strengthening and ignore hamstring strengthening, further exacerbating the inequality.
- Several intrinsic factors can contribute to ACL injuries, as follows:
  - Joint laxity is one of these factors. Significant controversy surrounds this topic, since published studies are contradictory about whether increased laxity contributes to ACL injuries. Acasuso-Diaz et al and Kibler et al concurred that a strong relationship exists; however, Godshall and Jackson et al maintain that ACL laxity does not predispose to ACL injury.
  - The Q angle is the acute angle between the line connecting the anterior superior iliac spine, the midpoint of the patella, and the line connecting the tibial tubercle with the same reference point on the patella. Theoretically, larger Q angles signal increases in the lateral pull of the quadriceps muscle on the patella and put medial stress on the knee. Shambaugh et al studied 45 athletes and found that the average Q angles of athletes sustaining knee injuries were significantly larger than the average Q angles for players who were not injured. Because lower extremity alignment cannot be altered, no recommendation can help minimize the athlete's risk of ACL rupture; however, the dynamic position of the tibia can be improved with internal rotation exercises for the tibia (e.g., medial hamstrings).
  - A narrow intercondylar notch may be a predictive factor for ACL rupture. According to various reports, athletes who sustain ACL injuries often have narrow notch widths compared to fellow athletes with uninjured knees. The notch width index (NWI), defined by Souryal et al, is "the ratio of the width of the intercondylar notch to the width of the distal femur at the level of the popliteal groove on a tunnel view radiograph." Another study by Souryal et al established that NWI measurements fall along a gaussian curve, indicating that measurement is reproducible. Results showed that athletes sustaining ACL injuries had the lowest NWI. The critical NWIs were calculated as 1 standard deviation (SD) below the gender-dependent mean. Athletes falling into this critical range, according to data reported, are 26 times more susceptible to ACL injuries than other athletes.
  - Repetitive friction has been found to occur at the posterior edge of the band, which is felt to be tighter against the lateral femoral condyle than the anterior fibers. The friction causes a gradual development of a reddish-brown bursal thickening at the lateral femoral condyle.

EPIDEMIOLOGY AND DEMOGRAPHICS

- ACL injuries occur most commonly in individuals aged 14 to 29 years. These years correspond to a high degree of athletic activity.
- Epidemiological studies estimate that approximately 1 in 3000 individuals sustain an ACL injury each year in the United States. This figure corresponds to an overall injury rate approaching 200,000 injuries annually.
- Female athletes are 2.4 to 9.5 times more likely to sustain an ACL injury than male athletes. There have been studies correlating menstruation with ACL tears in women.
- Estrogen and progesterone receptor sites have been reported in human ACL cells. It has been reported that levels of these hormones may have deleterious effects on the tensile strength of the ACL.
- Female athletes are more susceptible to ACL injuries. Studies have shown a twofold increase in female collegiate soccer players and a fourfold increase in female basketball players compared with their male counterparts.

- Differences may be due to experience, differences in training, different strength-to-weight ratios, limb alignment, joint laxity, muscle recruitment patterns, and NWI, but further studies to document a definitive cause are ongoing. A recent study has determined that ACL laxity does not vary with the menstrual cycle, thus dismissing this possible etiology.
- Unlike ACL injuries, which occur at a higher rate in females, lateral collateral ligament (LCL) and medial collateral ligament (MCL) injuries occur at an equal rate in males and females.

MECHANISM OF INJURY

- The ACL and the posterior cruciate ligament (PCL) bridge the inside of the knee joint, forming an "X" pattern that stabilizes the knee against front-to-back and back-to-front forces.
- The ACL typically sprains during one of the following knee movements: A sudden stop; a twist, pivot, or change in direction at the joint; extreme over-straightening (hyperextension); or a direct impact to the outside of the knee or lower leg.
- These injuries are seen among athletes in football, basketball, soccer, rugby, wrestling, gymnastics, and skiing.
- The ACL provides 85% of the total restraining force to anterior translation of the tibia. This injury usually occurs during a sudden cut or deceleration, as it typically is a noncontact injury. The patient states, "I planted, twisted, and then heard a pop."
- Often, the mechanism of injury results in injuries to multiple structures. The most common structures to be injured in association with the ACL are the MCL and the medial meniscus.

COMMON SIGNS AND SYMPTOMS

- Pain
- Feeling or hearing an audible pop
- Feeling the knee give out
- Inability to continue playing sport
- Swelling or large hemarthrosis
- Instability and giving away
- Loss of knee motion

AGGRAVATING ACTIVITIES

- Ambulation
- Going up and down stairs in a reciprocal pattern
- Returning to normal activities or sport
- Change of direction
- Cutting
- Pivoting
- Jumping

EASING ACTIVITIES

- Elevation

- Prescription antiinflammatory medications, muscle relaxants, and pain medications.
- Ice
- Rest

24-HOUR SYMPTOM PATTERN

Within 1 to 2 hours, a large hemarthrosis may develop.

PAST HISTORY FOR THE REGION

- Patient may report prior history of knee injury that has affected the mechanics of the knee.
- Prior injuries to the ankle or hip may also predispose the patient to increased stresses at the knee.

PHYSICAL EXAMINATION

- Joint examination: Observe any gross effusion or bony abnormality
- Immediate effusion indicates significant intraarticular trauma. Effusion that takes many hours to accumulate usually indicates an extraarticular trauma or meniscal involvement
- The presence of bruising is also a good indicator of tissue injury. Extraarticular injured tissue, such as an MCL, results in visible bruising. Intraarticular injured tissue, such as the ACL, does not result in visible bruising.
- In the absence of bony trauma, an immediate effusion is believed to have a 72% correlation with an ACL injury of some degree.
- Ligamentous laxity

IMPORTANT OBJECTIVE TESTS

- Lachman's test is the most sensitive test for acute ACL rupture.
  - Sensitivity: 0.82; specificity: 0.97 (Katz et al)
- Pivot shift test
  - Sensitivity: 0.82; specificity: 0.98 (Katz et al)
- Anterior drawer test
  - Sensitivity: 0.41; specificity: 0.95 (Katz et al)

DIFFERENTIAL DIAGNOSIS

- Muscle strain
- Myofascial pain
- Patellofemoral stress syndrome
- Early degenerative joint disease
- Popliteal or biceps femoris tendinitis
- Common peroneal nerve injury
- Tendinitis
- Referred pain from the lumbar spine or hip
- Femoral stress fracture
- Infection
- Neoplasm
- Tibial spine fracture
- Tibial plateau fractures

- Osteochondral fracture
- Knee dislocation
- Meniscal tear
- Multiligamentous injury
- Posterolateral instability
- Osteochondral fracture
- Extensor mechanism rupture
- Osteonecrosis of the femoral epicondyle
- Osteonecrosis of the tibial condyle
- Inflammatory conditions (systemic disease)

CONTRIBUTING FACTORS

- Football, baseball, soccer, skiing, and basketball account for up to 78% of sports-related injuries.
- 100-fold increase in the incidence of ACL injury in college football players when compared to the general population.
- Female athletes are more susceptible to ACL injuries
- Femoral notch stenosis (the ratio of the femoral notch width to the width of the femoral condyles). NWI <0.2 is defined as notch stenosis.

TREATMENT

SURGICAL OPTIONS

- Intraarticular reconstruction of the ACL
  - Bone-patella-bone autografts
  - Hamstring tendon grafts
  - Allografts
- Surgical reconstruction
  - Autograft
  - Patellar tendon
  - Quadriceps tendon
  - Hamstring tendons
  - Medial head of gastrocnemius
- Allograft
  - Achilles tendon
  - Patellar tendon
  - Quadriceps tendon
  - Hamstring tendons
- Mid-patellar tendon graft had been the treatment of choice, but the recent trend has been to use arthroscopic techniques and reconstruct the ligament with an allograft. Rationales for this change are varied, but in general it is believed that use of the allograft minimizes the trauma to the knee extensor mechanism. Patellar tendon problems were common after the midpatellar tendon autograft technique.
- Allograft use
  - Pros: Less invasive to patient, with a quicker return to function
  - Cons: Disease and infection (sterilized via gamma radiation and ethylene oxide) and weaker than autografts (radiation decreases strength by 26% and stiffness by 12%)
  - Can result in rejection

- Autograft strength: Normalized to the patellar tendon
  - Normal ACL: 100%
  - Bone–patellar tendon–bone: 175%
  - Semitendinosus: 75%
  - Gracilis: 49%
  - Iliotibial tract: 38%
  - Tensor fascia lata (TFL): 36%
- Surgical indicators, as follows:
  - Desire to return to high-demand sports
  - Associated injuries (e.g., MCL or meniscal involvement)
  - Abnormal laxity

REHABILITATION

- Rehabilitation of the ACL depends on whether surgery was performed. In patients who underwent surgery, several factors need to be taken into consideration. They include the following:
  - Graft maturation and ligamentation process
  - Autographs are strong at implantation.
  - Autografts undergo "ligamentation," which is a gradual biological transformation of tissue.
  - Collagen forms, remodels, and matures for 1 to 2 years after surgery.
  - The transplanted graft never obtains all of the cellular features of normal ACL tissue.
- Stages of ligamentation
  1. Necrosis (1 to 3 weeks): Cells of graft die because blood supply is interrupted. Collagen matrix remains intact.
  2. Revascularization (6 to 8 weeks): New blood vessels grow into graft. Process occurs from peripheral to central.
  3. Cellular proliferation (8 weeks +): New cells can proliferate into graft as early as the first week. The cells are thought to arise from extrinsic sources (synovial fluid and bone marrow) and intrinsic sources (surviving original cells)
  4. Collagen formation, remodeling, and maturation (8 weeks +): Cell proliferation takes place as a continuing process throughout the maturation process. New cells proliferate into graft from the new blood sources, as well as from synovium, ostium, and fat pads.

GENERAL ACL REHABILITATION GUIDELINES

Phase I: Acute Inflammatory Phase (Days 0 to 14 after injury)
- When to progress to phase: Initial injury to the ligament
- Goals of phase
  - Maintain range of motion (ROM).
  - Decrease inflammation and irritation and promote healing.
- Interventions
  - Medications: Antiinflammatories and/or muscle relaxants

- Modalities: Electrical stimulation for quadriceps contraction, ultrasound, ice after activity
- Myofascial release to global muscles as needed
- Lower extremity flexibility: Hamstrings, iliotibial band (ITB), and hip flexors
- Home exercise program: ROM exercises; lower extremity flexibility; hip strengthening; and rest, ice, compression, and elevation (RICE)

Phase 2: Reparative Phase (Days 15 to 21 after injury)
- When to progress to phase: Progress as pain allows
- Goals of phase
  - Restore normal ROM.
  - Achieve full extension ROM.
  - Minimize swelling.
- Interventions
  - Medications as needed
  - Modalities as needed
  - Myofascial release to global muscles; progress as needed.
  - Lower extremity flexibility: Hamstrings and hip flexors
  - Home exercise program: Walking program, lower extremity flexibility, and strengthening

Phase 3: Remodeling Phase (Days 22 to 60 after injury)
- When to progress to phase
  - Pain-free ROM
  - No functional limitations
- Goals of phase
  - Increase agility
  - Progress to return to sports
  - Address contributing factors
- Interventions
  - Medications and myofascial release as needed
  - Home exercise program: Progress lower extremity flexibility and strengthening program.
  - Other: Address contributing factors

Phase 4: Remodeling Phase (Days 60 to 360 after injury)
- When to progress to phase: No functional limitations
- Goals of phase
  - Correction of contributing factors that result in ligament injury
  - Retraining muscle activity to account for functional activities
- Interventions
  - Medications and myofascial release as needed
  - Home exercise program: Progress lower extremity flexibility and strengthening program.
  - Other: Address contributing factors, functional rehabilitation, and retraining.

PROGNOSIS

- Patients treated with surgical reconstruction of the ACL have long-term success rates of 82% to 95%.

- Recurrent instability and graft failure is seen in approximately 8% of patients.
- Patients with ACL ruptures, even after successful reconstruction, are at risk for osteoarthrosis.
- The goal of surgery is to stabilize the knee, decrease the chance of future meniscal injury, and delay the arthritic process.

SIGNS AND SYMPTOMS INDICATING REFERRAL TO PHYSICIAN

- Constant unrelenting leg pain or pain that does not change with position may indicate infection or tumor.
- Significant and unexplained weight loss or nocturnal pain may indicate the presence of a tumor.
- Major trauma may necessitate radiographs to rule out the presence of a fracture.
- A history of cancer may indicate the need to rule out metastatic disease if all other musculoskeletal factors have been eliminated.

SUGGESTED READINGS

Acasuso Diaz M, Collantes Estevez E, Sanchez Guijo P. Joint hyperlaxity and musculoligamentous lesions: study of a population of homogeneous age, sex and physical exertion. *Br J Rheumatol*. 1993;32(2):120-122.

Beynnon BD, Johnson RJ, Abate JA, Fleming BC, Nichols CE. Treatment of anterior cruciate ligament injuries, part I. *Am J Sports Med*. 2005;33(10):1579-1602.

Browner BD. *Skeletal Trauma: Fractures, Dislocations, Ligamentous Injuries*. Philadelphia: WB Saunders; 1998.

Dugan SA. Sports-related knee injuries in female athletes: what gives?. *Arch Phys Med Rehabil*. 2005;84(2):122-130.

Dutton M. *Orthopaedic Examination, Evaluation, & Intervention*. New York: McGraw-Hill; 2004.

Godshall RW. The predictability of athletic injuries: an eight-year study. *J Sports Med*. 1975;3(1):50-54.

Hastings DE. The non-operative management of collateral ligament injuries of the knee joint. *Clin Orthop*. 1980;(147):22-28.

Jackson DW, Jarrett H, Bailey D, et al. Injury prediction in the young athlete: a preliminary report. *Am J Sports Med*. 1978;6(1):6-14.

Kibler WB, Chandler TJ, Uhl T, et al. A musculoskeletal approach to the preparticipation physical examination. Preventing injury and improving performance. *Am J Sports Med*. 1989;17(4):525-531.

Maday MG, Harner CD, Fu FH. Evaluation and treatment. In: Feagin JA, ed. *The Crucial Ligaments: Diagnosis, Treatment of Ligamentous Injuries About the Knee*. 2nd ed. New York: Churchill Livingstone; 1994:711-723.

Noyes FR, Mooar PA, Matthews DS, et al. The symptomatic anterior cruciate-deficient knee. Part I: the long-term functional disability in athletically active individuals. *J Bone Joint Surg [Am]*. 1983;65(2):154-162.

Quarles JD, Hosey RG. Medial and lateral collateral injuries: prognosis and treatment. *Prim Care*. 2004;31(4):957-975, ix.

Shambaugh JP, Klein A, Herbert JH. Structural measures as predictors of injury basketball players. *Med Sci Sports Exerc*. 1991;23(5):522-527.

Souryal TO, Freeman TR. Intercondylar notch size and anterior cruciate ligament injuries in athletes. A prospective study [published erratum appears in Am J Sports Med 1993;21(5):723]. *Am J Sports Med*. 1993;21(4):535-539.

Souryal TO, Moore HA, Evans JP. Bilaterality in anterior cruciate ligament injuries: associated intercondylar notch stenosis. *Am J Sports Med*. 1988;16(5):449-454.

Strayer RJ, Lang ES. Evidence-based emergency medicine/systematic review abstract. Does this patient have a torn meniscus or ligament of the knee? *Ann Emerg Med*. 2006;47(5):499-501.

Wiener SL. *Differential diagnosis of acute pain by body region*. New York: McGraw-Hill; 1993.

AUTHOR: BERNARD LI

BASIC INFORMATION

DEFINITION

- Articular cartilage damage occurs either by acute trauma or by degenerative changes.
- Osteoarthritis occurs when progressive erosion and loss of the articular cartilage lining the ends of the femur and the tibia occur.
- Trauma can include damage to the cartilage or underlying bone.

SYNONYMS

- Osteochondral lesion
- Osteochondral fracture
- Osteochondritis dissecans (OCD)
- Osteoarthritis
- Degenerative joint disease

ICD-9CM CODES

715.16 Osteoarthrosis localized
       primary involving lower leg
718.0 Articular cartilage disorder

OPTIMAL NUMBER OF VISITS

8

MAXIMAL NUMBER OF VISITS

30

ETIOLOGY

Degenerative
- Cartilage destruction results from a combination of excess or abnormal biomechanical and biochemical forces on weight-bearing surfaces.
- Erosion and loss of cartilage is progressive over time and more commonly occurs in the medial compartment of the knee.
- Once osteoarthritis begins, the rate of tibial cartilage loss per year markedly increases in comparison to healthy knees.
- Osteoarthritis occurs when catabolism exceeds cartilage synthesis. Cytokines (proteolytic digestion of cartilage), growth factors (cartilage repair/synthesis), and collagenolytic enzymes (cartilage breakdown) play a role in the pathophysiology of the pathology.
- Structural changes include joint space narrowing, osteophytes, and subchondral bone cysts and sclerosis.

Traumatic
- Osteochondral fractures usually occur on weight-bearing surfaces. Surfaces commonly injured include the lateral talus, patella, femur, or tibia. These fractures commonly involve both the articular cartilage and its underlying bone. Generally, only one fracture occurs at a time.

- OCD most commonly occurs secondary to a compressive type of trauma. The pathophysiology of OCD involves the following three stages:
  - Stage 1: Thickening and swelling of the intraarticular and periarticular structures. Thinning of the adjacent metaphysis.
  - Stage 2: Thinning and disruption of the subcortical zone of rarefaction. Fragmentation of the epiphysis and disruption of blood flow to the epiphysis.
  - Stage 3: Repair in which granulation tissue replaces necrotic tissue.
- In the knee joint, the medial femoral condyle is the most commonly involved site, occurring 75% of the time. OCD rarely occurs on the medial tibial plateau.

EPIDEMIOLOGY AND DEMOGRAPHICS

- Osteoarthritis is the most common joint disorder in the world.
- Approximately 11% of individuals older than 64 years have symptomatic osteoarthritis of the knee.
- Risk factors associated with aggressive progression are high body mass index (BMI), meniscal lesion, and subchondral bone marrow edema.
- Other risk factors associated with the development of osteoarthritis are female gender, previous joint injury, and age.
- In femoral condyles, OCD has been estimated to occur in 6 per 10,000 men and in 3 per 10,000 women younger than 50 years.
- OCD of the ankle occurs in 2 per 100, [2 per 100,000], regardless of age and sex
- OCD average age of occurrence is in the mid-20s.

MECHANISM OF INJURY

- Degenerative
  - Primarily nontraumatic, insidious onset, and progressive with age
  - Patients with a previous history of knee trauma or surgery are at greater risk of developing osteoarthritis at an earlier age.
- Traumatic
  - In the knee, osteochondral fractures typically result when you twist your knee badly.
  - Direct trauma (sudden, forceful injury) to the inner or outer part of the femur at the knee can lead to these lesions.
  - In the ankle, these fractures occur by a force directed from the joint surface of the tibia (shin bone), across the joint, and into the talus.
  - Most osteochondral fractures to the outer side of the talus result from

trauma. Injuries to the inner side of the talus may result from a recurring ankle injury such as a sprain.
  - OCD commonly occurs as a result of compressive loading of the joint and cartilage.

COMMON SIGNS AND SYMPTOMS

- Knee joint pain and effusion
- Crepitus
- Grinding
- Clicking
- Decreased ROM
- Pain with weight-bearing activities
- Morning stiffness lasting 30 minutes or less
- Joint instability or buckling
- There is generally no referral pattern for osteoarthritis of the knee.

AGGRAVATING ACTIVITIES

- Prolonged walking or standing
- Stairs
- Squatting
- Sit to stand

EASING ACTIVITIES

- Non–weight-bearing activities
- Rest
- Heat or ice, depending on stage of healing

24-HOUR SYMPTOM PATTERN

Morning stiffness that lasts <30 minutes

PAST HISTORY FOR THE REGION

- Meniscal damage
- Knee surgery or trauma

PHYSICAL EXAMINATION

- Decreased ROM
- Joint enlargement or deformity
- Tenderness to palpation at the medial or lateral joint line
- Palpable joint effusion
- Degenerative
  - Radiographic features: loss of joint space, sclerosis, and osteophytes
- Traumatic
  - Evidence of lesions or fractures

IMPORTANT OBJECTIVE TESTS

- Degenerative
  - Radiographic features: Loss of joint space, sclerosis, and osteophytes
  - Positive McMurray's test: Osteoarthritis is often associated with meniscal derangement.
- Traumatic
  - X-rays often show no sign of OCD; therefore, computed tomography (CT) scans, magnetic resonance imaging (MRI), and ultrasound are often recommended to rule out the presence of OCD.

DIFFERENTIAL DIAGNOSIS

- Meniscal derangement
- Patellofemoral pain syndrome
- Referred pain from hip joint pathology

TREATMENT

SURGICAL OPTIONS

- Total knee arthroplasty (TKA)
- Unicompartmental knee arthroplasty (partial knee replacement)
- Arthroscopic debridement and chondroplasty
- Microfracture
- Osteotomy

INDICATIONS FOR SURGERY

- TKA is indicated in cases of severe arthritis with total loss of cartilage and significant functional limitation.
- Unicompartmental knee replacement is recommended when arthritis is localized to only one side of the knee, the patient is not obese, and ligaments are intact.
- Osteotomy: Joint damage is localized to only one side, leading to either a genu varum or genu valgum deformity in the knee. The patient is typically active and younger, and the purpose of this procedure is to delay progression of arthritis and the need for a total knee replacement.
- Arthroscopy is generally performed on mild cases of osteoarthritis or OCD to remove loose bodies and debris and to trim damaged cartilage.
- Surgery may be required to remove the intraarticular loose body and/or correct the resulting degenerative changes

SURGICAL OUTCOME

- Total and partial knee arthroplasties typically result in good long-term outcomes.
- Partial knee replacements have a faster recovery rate because of the less-invasive nature of the procedure.

- In total knee replacements, >90% of patients have successful outcomes and are able to return to low-impact activities.
- Arthroscopic debridement and chondroplasty: Review of literature reveals that this may not be effective in treating knee osteoarthritis.
- Osteotomy: Candidates for surgery must be very carefully selected to ensure a successful outcome. If the surgery is successful, the results of the surgery can last from 8 to 10 years.

REHABILITATION

- Treatment for OCD and degenerative changes to cartilage are both similar.
- Goals: Restore ROM and strength, decrease pain and swelling, and reduce stress to the knee joint to delay progression and promote healing for return to normal function.
- Initial exercises used to promote healing are as follows:
  o ROM and strengthening exercises within limited weight-bearing conditions (open kinetic chain) promote joint lubrication and decrease stress on the menisci and articular cartilage.
  o Avoid exercises involving heavy loads with rotation to the knee joint if meniscal damage is present.
  o Stationary bicycle
  o Aquatic therapy
  o Low-load knee flexion/extension exercises in supine: Heel slides, quad sets, straight leg raises, bridging, leg press in supine
  o Hamstring and quadriceps stretching
- Recommendations to the patient to delay the progression of osteoarthritis and achieve optimal outcomes after surgery.
  o Weight loss
  o Proper footwear to maximize shock absorption during gait; avoid high heels
  o Assess the need for custom or over-the-counter foot orthotics to decrease medial or lateral knee joint stress.
  o Participate in low-impact activities and avoid high-impact, repetitive activities such as running and jumping.

PROGNOSIS

- For partial and total knee replacements, prosthetic survival rates typically range from 10 to 15 years.
- OCD and osteochondral fractures have excellent prognosis for full recovery.

SIGNS AND SYMPTOMS INDICATING REFERRAL TO PHYSICIAN

- Postoperative indicators
  o Signs of infection: Excessive pain, swelling, redness, fever, malaise
  o Signs of deep vein thrombosis (DVT): Calf pain/tenderness, redness, and swelling
- Failure to respond to conservative treatment

SUGGESTED READINGS

Felson DT, Zhang Y. An update on the epidemiology of knee and hip osteoarthritis with a view to prevention. *Arthritis Rheum.* 1998;41:1343-1355.

Kocher MS, Tucker R, Ganley TJ, Flynn JM. Management of osteochondritis dissecans of the knee: current concepts review. *Am J Sports Med.* 2006;34(7):1181-1191.

Laupattarakasem W, Laopaiboon M, Laupattarakasem P, Sumananont C. Arthroscopic debridement for knee osteoarthritis. *Cochrane Database Syst Rev.* 2008;Issue 1. Art. No.: CD005118. DOI: 10.1002/14651858.CD005118.pub2.

Vad V, Hong HM, Zazzali M, Agi N, Basrai D. Exercise recommendations in athletes with early osteoarthritis of the knee. *Sports Med.* 2002;32(11):729-739.

Weigl M, Angst F, Aeschlimann A, Lehmann S, Stucki G. Predictors for response to rehabilitation in patients with hip or knee osteoarthritis: a comparison of logistic regression models with three different definitions of responder. *Osteoarthritis and Cartilage.* 2006;14(7):641-651.

Wluka A, Forbes A, Wang Y, Hanna F, Jones, G, Cicuttini FM. Knee cartilage loss in symptomatic knee osteoarthritis over 4.5 years. *Arthritis Res Ther.* 2006;8(4):1-9.

AUTHOR: DELLA LEE

BASIC INFORMATION

DEFINITION

- A Baker's cyst is a fluid-filled mass located in the popliteal fossa and most commonly observed as a distention of a bursa located posterior to the medial femoral condyle, between the tendons of the medial head of the gastrocnemius and semimembranosus muscles.
- The bursa communicates with the knee joint via a valvular opening at the posteromedial aspect of the knee capsule just superior to the joint line

SYNONYMS

- Popliteal cyst
- Synovial cyst

ICD-9CM CODES
727.51 Synovial cyst of popliteal space

OPTIMAL NUMBER OF VISITS
6

MAXIMAL NUMBER OF VISITS
12

ETIOLOGY

- A Baker's cyst results from intraarticular pathologies, such as meniscal tears, primary osteoarthritis, and rheumatoid arthritis (RA) that may lead to joint effusion.
- The bursa serves as a protective mechanism for the knee joint, allowing effusion to be displaced into the cyst to reduce potentially abnormal, destructive pressure in the joint space.
- Because of the bursa's valve-like communication with the knee, fluid does not flow in the reverse direction, thus trapping the effusion and causing abnormal distention of the bursa.
- There are two types of Baker's cysts, classified anatomically and clinically as follows:
  - Primary cyst: Occurs when the distention of the bursa arises independently with no direct communication to the joint and in the absence of intraarticular pathology.
  - Secondary cyst: Results from an intraarticular pathology and there is direct communication of the bursa to the joint. This is the most common type of cyst.

EPIDEMIOLOGY AND DEMOGRAPHICS

- Adults: 5% to 20% will experience a Baker's cyst.
  - 70% of cysts are associated with medial meniscus tears

- 85% associated with chondral lesions
- Secondary cysts are most commonly observed in adults.
- In adults, they are most often found in patients with meniscal lesions, osteoarthritis, chondromalacia, loose bodies, and RA.
- Children: 6.3% will experience a Baker's cyst.
  - In children and adolescents, the majority of the cysts are the primary type, typically developing before the age of 15 years.

MECHANISM OF INJURY

- Baker's cysts are not directly caused by trauma.
- Primary cysts occur as the result of excessive joint effusion secondary to an intraarticular pathology (traumatic or inflammatory disease process).

COMMON SIGNS AND SYMPTOMS

- Posterior knee pain
- Complaints of knee ache and fullness
- Stiffness
- Effusion
- In children, it is typically asymptomatic.

AGGRAVATING ACTIVITIES
No specific aggravating activities

EASING ACTIVITIES
No specific easing activities

24-HOUR SYMPTOM PATTERN
No specific pattern. Stiffness may be noted with prolonged inactivity or first thing in the morning.

PAST HISTORY FOR THE REGION
History of trauma causing mechanical intraarticular derangement, osteoarthritis, or an inflammatory disease process

PHYSICAL EXAMINATION
Posterior knee joint swelling or a palpable mass located posterior to the medial femoral condyle between the tendons of the medial head of the gastrocnemius and semimembranosus muscles

IMPORTANT OBJECTIVE TESTS

- Confirmed via MRI or ultrasonography
- Diagnostic arthroscopy

DIFFERENTIAL DIAGNOSIS **Dx**

- DVT
- Popliteal artery aneurysm
- Soft tissue tumor (benign or malignant)
- Ganglion cyst
- Pseudothrombophlebitis

TREATMENT **Rx**

SURGICAL OPTIONS
Surgery is uncommon for this pathology; however, surgical excision may be indicated in cases unresponsive to conservative treatment.

CONTRIBUTING FACTORS

- Osteoarthritis
- Internal derangement of the knee (meniscal tears, ACL tears, or osteochondral fractures)
- RA
- Gout
- Hemophilia
- Juvenile RA
- Psoriasis
- Terythematosus (SLE)

REHABILITATION
Baker's cysts are typically treated conservatively, with the goal of reducing the swelling via modalities and antiinflammatory agents and treating the underlying cause of the cyst, which is typically osteoarthritis or an internal derangement.

PROGNOSIS
Baker's cysts typically do not cause any long-term functional limitations or disability. They resolve over time once the underlying cause of the cyst is corrected.

SIGNS AND SYMPTOMS INDICATING REFERRAL TO PHYSICIAN

- Leakage of cyst
- Rupture or dissection of cyst
- Hemorrhage
- DVT
- Infection
- Posterior compartment syndrome

SUGGESTED READINGS

De Maeseneer M, Debaere C, Desprechins B, Osteaux M. Popliteal cysts in children: prevalence, appearance and associated findings at MR imaging. *Pediatr Radiol.* 1999;29(8):605-609.

Fritschy D, Fasel J, Imbert J, Bianchi S, Verdonk, R, Wirth CJ. The popliteal cyst. *Knee Surg Sports Traumatol Arthrosc.* 2006;14:623-628.

Miller TT, Staron RB, Koenigsberg T, Levin TL, Feldman F. MR imaging of Baker cysts: association with internal, effusion and degenerative arthropathy. *Radiology.* 1996;210(1):247-250.

Rupp S, Seil R, Jochum P, Kohn D. Popliteal cysts in adults. Prevalence, associated intraarticular lesions, and results after arthroscopic treatment. *Am J Sports Med.* 2002;30(1):112-115.

Sansone V, De Ponti A. Arthroscopic treatment of popliteal cyst and associated intra-articular knee disorders in adults. *Arthroscopy.* 1999;15(4):368-372.

AUTHOR: DELLA LEE

BASIC INFORMATION

DEFINITION

Iliotibial band friction syndrome (ITBFS) is a repetitive stress injury resulting from friction of the ITB as it slides over the prominent lateral femoral condyle at approximately 30 degrees of knee flexion. Friction tends to occur at the posterior edge of the band because fibers in this region are tighter against the lateral femoral condyle than the anterior fibers. The friction gradually causes bursa thickening at the lateral femoral condyle.

SYNONYMS

- Iliotibial band syndrome (ITBS)
- Iliotibial band friction syndrome (ITBFS)

ICD-9CM CODES
722.10 Displacement of lumbar intervertebral disc without myelopathy

---

OPTIMAL NUMBER OF VISITS

8 or fewer

MAXIMAL NUMBER OF VISITS

12

ETIOLOGY

- This pathology is a repetitive stress injury resulting from friction of the ITB as it slides over the prominent lateral femoral condyle at approximately 30 degrees of knee flexion.
- A small recess forms between the lateral femoral epicondyle and the ITB as it travels along the lateral thigh to the tibial plateau. This space was believed to have a separate bursa lying deep to the band, but studies have revealed it to be synovium that is a lateral extension and invagination of the actual knee joint capsule (lateral synovial recess).
- Histological analysis demonstrates inflammation and hyperplasia in the synovium, whereas MRI studies show diffuse signal abnormality below the band and in the synovium but not the ITB. This finding suggests that ITBS is not a tendinopathy. Variance is observed in the congenital thickness of the band, so patients with thicker bands may be predisposed to ITBFS.

EPIDEMIOLOGY AND DEMOGRAPHICS

- ITBFS is the most common overuse syndrome of the knee and is particularly common in long distance runners who run 20 to 40 miles per week. In addition, long distance runners who train on

hilly terrain, graded slopes, or road cambers are also at risk, especially if their runs include downhill running, which positions the knee in significantly less flexion than normal at initial contact. Finally, running on canted surfaces can result in a leg-length inequality and a change in Q angle, which can increase the stress on the ITB.
- Although most cases of ITBFS have been reported in distance runners, anyone engaging in activity that requires repetitive knee flexion and extension, such as downhill skiing, circuit training, weight lifting, cycling, and jumping sports, is prone to developing this pathology.
- ITBFS is common in cyclists. This is thought to be due to the pedaling stroke, which causes the ITB to be pulled anteriorly on the downstroke and posteriorly on the upstroke. Extrinsic factors include excessive bike seat height or cleat position on the pedal. If the cleats are excessively internally rotated on the pedal, the tibia also internally rotates, resulting in a valgus force on the knee and increased tension of the ITB.
- More common in repetitive stress activities

MECHANISM OF INJURY

Repetitive friction has been found to occur at the posterior edge of the band, which is felt to be tighter against the lateral femoral condyle than the anterior fibers. The friction causes a gradual development of a reddish-brown bursal thickening at the lateral femoral condyle.

COMMON SIGNS AND SYMPTOMS

- Subjectively, the patient reports pain with the repetitive motions of the knee.
- Lateral hip, thigh, or knee pain and snapping as the ITB passes over the greater trochanter
- Swelling or thickening of the tissue at the point where the band moves over the femur
- Pain may not occur immediately during activity but may intensify over time, especially as the foot strikes the ground.

AGGRAVATING ACTIVITIES

- Climbing or descending stairs
- Downhill skiing
- Long distance running
- Circuit training
- Weight lifting
- Jumping sports
- Cycling

EASING ACTIVITIES

- Lying supine with the knee and hips flexed

- Prescription antiinflammatory medications, muscle relaxants, and pain medications to address the patient's symptoms
- Walking
- Ice
- Rest

24-HOUR SYMPTOM PATTERN

Symptoms are generally activity related; however, individuals may experience pain with walking as the syndrome progresses.

PAST HISTORY FOR THE REGION

- Patients commonly report a change in activity level immediately preceding the onset of pain.
- Past injury to ipsilateral or contralateral lower extremity is not uncommon.

PHYSICAL EXAMINATION

- Localized tenderness to palpation at the lateral femoral condyle or Gerdy's tubercle on the anterolateral portion of the proximal tibia.
- Pain is localized along the lateral knee; it also can include the hip. Pain may radiate from the knee proximally or distally.
- Tenderness is over the lateral knee, with a tender point at the lateral femoral condyle, approximately 1 to 2 cm proximal to the lateral joint line. Pain can be elicited with active flexion-extension of the knee within the first 30 degrees as the thumb presses over the epicondyle and ITB.
- Crepitation may be felt.
- Restriction in hip adduction indicates tightness in the ITB and TFL.
- Observe restrictions in iliopsoas, rectus femoris, gastrocnemius, and soleus muscle function.
- Examination usually reveals restriction of hip adduction and weakness of the hip abductors, specifically the gluteus medius.

IMPORTANT OBJECTIVE TESTS

- Resisted tests are likely to be negative for pain.
- Positive Ober's test
- Positive Noble compression test
- Positive creak test
- Thomas test

DIFFERENTIAL DIAGNOSIS

- Muscle strain
- Myofascial pain
- Patellofemoral stress syndrome
- Early degenerative joint disease
- Lateral meniscal pathology
- Superior tibiofibular joint sprain
- Popliteal or biceps femoris tendinitis

- Common peroneal nerve injury
- Tendinitis
- Referred pain from the lumbar spine.
- Femoral stress fracture
- Infection
- Neoplasm

CONTRIBUTING FACTORS

- ITBS usually is caused by overuse, mostly caused by errors in training. Sudden changes in surface (i.e., soft to hard, flat to uneven, or decline), speed, distance, shoes, and frequency can break down the body faster than it can heal, causing injury.
- Leg length difference (with the syndrome developing on the shorter side)
- Genu varum
- Overpronation cavus foot (calcaneal varus) structure
- Hip adductor weakness
- Myofascial restriction
- Muscle fatigue
- Internal tibial torsion (increases lateral retinaculum tension)
- Anatomically prominent lateral femoral epicondyle
- Long distance runners with ITBS have weaker hip abduction strength in the involved leg compared with the uninvolved leg.
- Excessive frontal plane movement occurs during stance phase. The gluteus medius and TFL must exert a continuous hip abductor movement. Fatigued runners or those with weak gluteus medius muscles are prone to increased thigh adduction and internal rotation at midstance. This in turn leads to an increased valgus vector at the knee and increased tension on the ITB, making it more prone to impingement.

TREATMENT

INDICATIONS FOR SURGERY

- Surgical intervention is not indicated for ITBS except in rare cases in which prolonged conservative treatment has failed to either alleviate the patient's symptoms or resolve the ITBS.
- Surgical intervention, consisting of resection of the posterior half of the ITB at the level that passes over the lateral femoral condyle, is reserved for the more recalcitrant cases.

SURGICAL OPTIONS

- A portion of the ITB where it comes into contact with the lateral femoral epicondyle is removed.
- Z-lengthening of the ITB at the level of the lateral epicondyle has also been proposed.

REHABILITATION

- The goal of following conservative interventions consists of activity modification to reduce the irritating stress (decreasing mileage, changing the bike seat position, and changing the training surfaces and new running shoes):
  - Heat or ice application
  - Strengthening the hip abductors
  - Stretching the ITB
  - Nonsteroidal antiinflammatory drugs (NSAIDS)

Phase I: Acute Inflammatory Phase (Days 0 to 14 after injury)
- When to progress to phase: Initial injury to the ITB region
- Goals of phase
  - Rest by decreasing the amount of exercise or training
  - Decrease inflammation and irritation and promote healing.
- Interventions
  - Medications: Antiinflammatories/muscle relaxants
  - Modalities: Heat, ultrasound, and stretching before exercise; phonophoresis or iontophoresis; ice after activity
  - Myofascial release to TFL, hip flexors, and ITB as needed.
  - Lower extremity flexibility: Hamstrings, ITB, and hip flexors
  - Home exercise program: Walking program, lower extremity flexibility, hip strengthening

Phase 2: Reparative Phase (Days 15 to 21 after injury)
- When to progress to phase: Progress as pain allows
- Goals of phase
  - Improve lower extremity flexibility in hips and ITB.
  - Strengthening hips, knee, back, and core
- Interventions
  - Medications as needed
  - Modalities as needed
  - Myofascial release to global muscles. Progress as needed.
  - Lower extremity flexibility: Hamstrings and hip flexors
  - Home exercise program: Improve strength in hips, knees, abdominals, and back.

Phase 3: Remodeling Phase (Days 22 to 60 after injury)
- When to progress to phase
  - Pain-free ROM
  - No functional limitations
- Goals of phase
  - Identify factors that contribute to ITB.
  - Address contributing factors.
- Interventions
  - Medications and myofascial release as needed
  - Home exercise program: Progress lower extremity flexibility and strengthening program.
  - Other: Address contributing factors.

Phase 4: Remodeling Phase (Days 60 to 360 after injury)
- When to progress to phase: No functional limitations
- Goals of phase:
  - Correction of contributing factors
  - Retraining muscle activity to account for functional activities
- Interventions
  - Medications and myofascial release as needed
  - Home exercise program: Progress lower extremity flexibility and strengthening program.
  - Other: Address contributing factors, functional rehabilitation, and retraining.

PROGNOSIS

The prognosis for ITBS is excellent if the athlete maintains ITB flexibility and corrects the intrinsic factors that lead to this injury. The athlete must also avoid the extrinsic factors that provoke ITBS.

SIGNS AND SYMPTOMS INDICATING REFERRAL TO PHYSICIAN

- Constant unrelenting low back pain: Infection or tumor
- Pain that does not change with position: Infection or tumor
- Significant and unexplained weight loss: Tumor
- Nocturnal pain: Tumor
- Major trauma: Fracture
- History of cancer: Metastatic disease
- Fevers and chills: Infection or tumor

SUGGESTED READINGS

Adams WB. Treatment options in overuse injuries of the knee: patellofemoral syndrome, iliotibial band syndrome, and degenerative meniscal tears. *Curr Sports Med Rep.* 2004;3(5):256–260.

Dutton M. *Orthopaedic Examination, Evaluation, & Intervention.* New York: McGraw-Hill; 2004.

Fredericson M, Cookingham CL, Chaudhari AM. Hip abductor weakness in distance runners with iliotibial band syndrome. *Clin J Sport Med.* 2000;10(3):169–175.

Fredericson M, Weir A. Practical management of iliotibial band friction syndrome in runners. *Clin J Sport Med.* 2006;16(3):261–268.

Fredericson M, Wolf C. Iliotibial band syndrome in runners: innovations in treatment. *Sports Med.* 2005;35(5):451–459.

Khaund R, Flynn SH. Iliotibial band syndrome: a common source of knee pain. *Am Fam Physician.* 2005;71(8):1545–1550.

Wiener SL. *Differential Diagnosis of Acute Pain By Body Region.* New York: McGraw-Hill; 1993.

AUTHOR: BERNARD LI

BASIC INFORMATION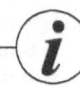

DEFINITION

- A sudden or violent twist or wrench of the tibiofemoral or tibiofibular joint results in the stretching or tearing of the lateral collateral ligament (LCL).
- The LCL is a tough band of fibrous tissue that connect the bones of the upper and lower leg at the knee joint. The LCL supports the outer side of the knee.
- Like other types of sprains, knee sprains are classified according to the following grading system:
  ○ Grade I (mild): This injury stretches the ligament, which causes microscopic tears in the ligament. These tiny tears do not significantly affect the overall ability of the knee joint to support the body's weight.
  ○ Grade II (moderate): The ligament is partially torn, and there is some mild-to-moderate instability (or periodic giving out) of the knee while standing or walking.
  ○ Grade III (severe): The ligament is torn completely or separated at its end from the bone, and the knee is more unstable.

SYNONYMS

- LCL tear
- LCL sprain

ICD-9CM CODES
848.9 Unspecified site of sprain and
      strain
844.0 Sprain of lateral collateral knee

OPTIMAL NUMBER OF VISITS

8 or fewer

MAXIMAL NUMBER OF VISITS

12

ETIOLOGY

- LCL, like all other ligaments, is composed of type I collagen. The ultrastructure of a ligament is close to that of tendons, but the fibers in a ligament are more variable and have a higher elastin content.
- Ligaments receive their blood supply from their insertion sites. The vascularity within a ligament is uniform, and each ligament contains mechanoreceptors and free nerve endings that are hypothesized to aid in stabilizing the joint.
- Avulsion of ligaments generally occurs between the unmineralized and mineralized fibrocartilage layers. The LCL injury occurs most commonly at the fibular attachment (75% of the time).

- Overstressing of the ligament occurs with a varus force placed at the knee. This excessive loading results in ligament failure.
- No one single cause accounts for this injury. LCL injuries can be related to extrinsic and intrinsic factors. Numerous studies document the fact that poor levels of conditioning correlate directly with increased levels of injury. Research also has demonstrated that improved conditioning results in reduced numbers of injuries.

EPIDEMIOLOGY AND DEMOGRAPHICS

- The LCL sprain is the least common of all knee ligament injuries.
- Injuries to the LCL are rare, accounting for only 2% of all knee injuries.
- It is the least likely knee ligament to be sprained because most LCL injuries are caused by a blow to the inside of the knee and that area usually is shielded by the opposite leg.

MECHANISM OF INJURY

- The LCL controls varus loading and external rotation of the tibia.
- Contact injuries involve a direct varus load to the knee. This is the usual mechanism in a complete tear. The most common method of injury is a direct varus force with the foot plantar flexed and the knee in extension.
- Related injuries include injuries to the peroneal nerve, posterolateral capsule damage, or PCL damage.
- The mechanism of knee adduction, flexion, and external rotation of the femur on the tibia is much less common. With excessive force, the LCL is usually disrupted initially, followed by the capsular ligaments, the arcuate ligament complex, the popliteus, the ITB, the biceps femoris, and the common peroneal nerve; one or both cruciate ligaments may be disrupted

COMMON SIGNS AND SYMPTOMS

- Mild-to-moderate knee pain
- Patient reports feeling a pop in the knee
- Bruising in the lateral knee is often present since the LCL is an extraarticular structure.
- Swelling builds up slowly over several days.
- Instability and giving away may be noted.
- Loss of knee motion and moderate stiffness
- Lateral joint line pain may be reported.

AGGRAVATING ACTIVITIES

- Starting a run
- Walking longer distances

- Uneven ground may lead to a sensation of instability.
- Cutting or change of direction actions, especially turning ipsilaterally

EASING ACTIVITIES

- Elevation
- Prescription antiinflammatory medications, muscle relaxants, and pain medications to address the patient's symptoms
- Ice
- Rest

24-HOUR SYMPTOM PATTERN

- Redness, swelling, and bruising may appear within the first 72 hours after injury.
- Stiffness in the knee joint is present after prolonged activity or prolonged inactivity.
- Sleeping may be painful if sleeping sidelying with no support under the knee.

PAST HISTORY FOR THE REGION

- Patient may report prior history of knee injury that has affected the mechanics of the knee.
- Prior injuries to the ankle or hip may also predispose the patient to increased stresses at the knee.

PHYSICAL EXAMINATION

- Joint examination: Observe for any gross effusion or bony abnormality.
- Partially full or functional ROM
- Point tenderness is present over the LCL, especially at its fibular attachment.
- Immediate effusion indicates significant intraarticular trauma. Effusion that takes many hours to accumulate usually indicates an extraarticular trauma or meniscal involvement.
- The presence of bruising is also a good indicator of tissue injury. Extraarticular injured tissue, such as an LCL or MCL, will result in visible bruising. Intraarticular injured tissue does not result in visible bruising.
- Ligamentous laxity

IMPORTANT OBJECTIVE TESTS

LCL or varus stress test

DIFFERENTIAL DIAGNOSIS

- Muscle strain
- Myofascial pain
- Early degenerative joint disease
- Popliteal or biceps femoris tendinitis
- Tendinitis
- Referred pain from the lumbar spine or hip
- Femoral stress fracture
- Infection
- Neoplasm

Section III

ORTHOPEDIC PATHOLOGY

- Osteochondral fracture
- Knee dislocation
- Peroneal nerve injury
- Meniscal tear
- Multiligamentous injury
- Extensor mechanism rupture
- Osteonecrosis of the femoral epicondyle
- Osteonecrosis of the tibial condyle
- Inflammatory conditions (systemic disease)

CONTRIBUTING FACTORS

- Football, baseball, soccer, skiing, and basketball account for up to 78% of sports-related injuries.
- Long-term use of corticosteroids can weaken knee ligaments.
- Systemic diseases, such as RA or lupus, can predispose a patient to joint laxity.

TREATMENT

SURGICAL OPTIONS

- Lesser injuries can be treated nonsurgically based on the symptoms present, although a completely torn ligament will likely require surgery. LCL surgery reconstructs the ligament by direct repair of the torn ligament or reconstruction, depending on the severity and chronicity of the injury. In extreme cases in which the ligament is irreparable, reinforcement with a tendon graft is considered. Several different methods have been developed for LCL reconstruction. They include the following:
  - Ligament repair: If the ligament has been detached from the bone, it is reattached using either large sutures or suture anchors. Tears in the midsubstance of the ligament are usually repaired by suturing the ends together.
  - Ligament reconstruction: Chronic swelling or instability caused by a collateral ligament injury may require a surgical reconstruction. A reconstruction operation entails either tightening up the loose ligament or replacing the loose ligament with a tendon graft.
  - Ligament tightening: Ligament tightening involves detaching one end of the ligament from its bony attachment. The ligament is then reattached to the bone and tightened in the new place with sutures or metal staples.
  - Autograft method: Autografts are generally the treatment of choice if ligament replacement is required. The semitendinosus is the most commonly used autograft. Studies have shown that this tendon can be removed without affecting the strength of the leg because other uninvolved hamstring

muscles can take over the function of the tendon that is removed.
  - Allograft method: Allografts can be used similar to other knee ligament repairs. (See section on ACL Sprain for guidelines.)

REHABILITATION

- Patients are strongly advised to follow the recommendations about how much weight to place on the leg while standing or walking. After a ligament repair, patients are instructed to put little or no weight on their foot when standing or walking for up to 6 weeks. Weight bearing may be restricted for up to 12 weeks after a ligament reconstruction. The MCL is well vascularized, and as a result, surgery is rarely required. Instead, the knee is braced for the first 72 hours to prevent valgus stresses to the knee. After this initial period, the knee should be protected to avoid excessive valgus loading for 6 weeks. During this time, it is hoped that scar tissue will form to reinforce the damaged ligament.
- In rare cases, surgery is performed. Arthroscopic surgery is not indicated since the structure is extraarticular. Instead, a small incision is made adjacent to the injured ligament and the ligament is sutured together or to the bone.
- Rehabilitation of the LCL depends on whether surgery was performed or not.
- Caution should be used immediately after surgery. Some surgeons use a continuous passive motion (CPM) machine initially. Regardless, the knee is braced into full extension for 3 to 4 weeks, and the patient may come out of the brace to use the CPM machine. At 5 to 6 weeks, the patient will progress to a knee brace with a hinge to protect the knee during ambulation. Complete recovery generally takes between 6 months and a year.

GENERAL LCL REHABILITATION GUIDELINES

Phase I: Acute Inflammatory Phase (Days 0 to 14 after injury)
- When to progress to phase: Initial injury to the ligament
- Goals of phase:
  - Maintain ROM.
  - Protect the joint and ligament.
  - Decrease inflammation and irritation and promote healing.
- Interventions
  - Medications: Antiinflammatories/muscle relaxants
  - Modalities: Electrical stimulation for quadriceps contraction, ultrasound, ice after activity
  - Myofascial release to global muscles as needed

  - Lower extremity flexibility: Hamstrings, ITB, and hip flexors
  - Home exercise program: ROM exercises, lower extremity flexibility, hip strengthening, RICE

Phase 2: Reparative Phase (Days 15 to 21 after injury)
- When to progress to phase: Progress as pain allows
- Goals of phase
  - Restore normal ROM.
  - Minimize swelling.
- Interventions
  - Medications as needed
  - Modalities as needed
  - Myofascial release to global muscles; progress as needed.
  - Lower extremity flexibility: Hamstrings and hip flexors
  - Home exercise program: Walking program, lower extremity flexibility and strengthening

Phase 3: Remodeling Phase (Days 22 to 60 after injury)
- When to progress to phase:
  - Pain-free ROM
  - No functional limitations
- Goals of phase
  - Increase agility.
  - Progress to return to sports.
  - Address contributing factors.
- Interventions
  - Medications and myofascial release as needed
  - Home exercise program: Progress lower extremity flexibility and strengthening program.
  - Other: Address contributing factors.

Phase 4: Remodeling Phase (Days 60-360 after injury)
- When to progress to phase: No functional limitations
- Goals of phase
  - Correction of contributing factors that result in ligament injury
  - Retraining muscle activity to account for functional activities
- Interventions
  - Medications and myofascial release as needed
  - Home exercise program: Progress lower extremity flexibility and strengthening program.
  - Other: Address contributing factors, functional rehabilitation, and retraining.

PROGNOSIS

- Most patients have excellent outcomes.
- The goal of surgery is to stabilize the knee, decrease the chance of future meniscal injury, and delay the arthritic process.
- Early diagnosis allows 85% of patients requiring surgery to be able to return to their preinjury activity level. Only 65% of patients who have surgical treatment for a chronic complete tear of their LCL will return to full activity.

- The ability of a torn ligament to heal depends on a variety of factors, including anatomical location and the presence of associated injuries.
- Typically, grade I sprains of the LCL should get better within 4 to 6 weeks. Grade II tears should rehabilitate within 2 months. Grade III tears require up to 3 months. If patients are still having problems after 3 months, they will likely need surgery. Severe tears or ruptures of the LCL are the trickiest because they tend to leave the knee joint the most unstable, and patients with this condition typically do not do well with non-surgical care.

SIGNS AND SYMPTOMS INDICATING REFERRAL TO PHYSICIAN

- Constant unrelenting leg pain or pain that does not change with position may indicate infection or tumor.
- Significant and unexplained weight loss or nocturnal pain may indicate the presence of a tumor.
- Major trauma may necessitate radiographs to rule out fracture.
- A history of cancer may indicate the need to rule out metastatic disease if all other musculoskeletal factors have been eliminated.

SUGGESTED READINGS

Browner BD. *Skeletal Trauma: Fractures, Dislocations, Ligamentous Injuries.* Philadelphia: WB Saunders; 1998.

Dugan SA. Sports-Related knee injuries in female athletes: What gives?. *Arch Phys Med Rehabil.* 2005;84(2):122-130.

Dutton M. *Orthopaedic Examination, Evaluation, & Intervention.* New York: McGraw-Hill; 2004.

Hastings DE. The non-operative management of collateral ligament injuries of the knee joint. *Clin Orthop.* 1980;(147):22-28.

Quarles JD, Hosey RG. Medial and lateral collateral injuries: prognosis and treatment. *Prim Care.* 2004;31(4):957-975, ix.

Strayer RJ, Lang ES. Evidence-based emergency medicine/systematic review abstract. Does this patient have a torn meniscus or ligament of the knee? *Ann Emerg Med.* 2006;47(5):499-501.

Wiener SL. *Differential Diagnosis of Acute Pain By Body Region.* McGraw-Hill Inc. Health Professions Division; 1993.

AUTHOR: BERNARD LI

BASIC INFORMATION

DEFINITION

- A sudden or violent twist or wrench of the tibiofemoral joint results in the stretching or tearing of the medial collateral ligament (MCL).
- The MCL is a tough band of fibrous tissue that connects the bones of the upper and lower leg at the knee joint.
- Like other types of sprains, knee sprains are classified according to the following grading system:
  - Grade I (mild): This injury stretches the ligament, which causes microscopic tears in the ligament. These tiny tears do not significantly affect the overall ability of the knee joint to support the body's weight.
  - Grade II (moderate): The ligament is partially torn, and there is some mild-to-moderate instability (or periodic giving out) of the knee while standing or walking.
  - Grade III (severe):The ligament is torn completely or separated at its end from the bone, and the knee is more unstable.

SYNONYMS

- MCL tear
- Medial collateral ligament sprain

ICD-9CM CODES
848.9 Unspecified site of sprain and
      strain
844.1 Sprain of medial collateral knee

OPTIMAL NUMBER OF VISITS

8 or fewer

MAXIMAL NUMBER OF VISITS

12

ETIOLOGY

- The MCL, like all other ligaments, is composed of type I collagen. The ultrastructure of a ligament is close to that of tendons, but the fibers in a ligament are more variable and have a higher elastin content.
- Ligaments receive their blood supply from their insertion sites. The vascularity within a ligament is uniform, and each ligament contains mechanoreceptors and free nerve endings that are hypothesized to aid in stabilizing the joint.
- The MCL restrains valgus stress and external rotation of the tibia. A blow to the outside of the knee, therefore, is the most common cause of injury.
- Anatomically, it is composed of two layers: the superficial and the deep.

- Avulsion of ligaments generally occurs between the unmineralized and mineralized fibrocartilage layers. The MCL injury occurs most commonly at the femoral attachment (65% of the time).
- No one single cause accounts for this injury. MCL injuries can be related to extrinsic and intrinsic factors. Numerous studies document the fact that poor levels of conditioning correlate directly with increased levels of injury. Research also has demonstrated that improved conditioning results in reduced numbers of injuries.

EPIDEMIOLOGY AND DEMOGRAPHICS

- MCL sprain is the most common of all ligament injuries.
- The MCL is often injured in conjunction with other structures such as the ACL or medial meniscus.

MECHANISM OF INJURY

- Contact injuries involve a direct valgus load to the knee. This is the usual mechanism in a complete tear.
- Noncontact, or indirect, injuries are observed with deceleration, cutting, and pivoting motions. These mechanisms tend to cause partial tears.
- Overuse injuries of the MCL have been described in swimmers. The whip-kick technique of the breaststroke has been implicated. This technique involves repetitive valgus loads across the knee.
- The MCL supports the knee along the inner side of the leg. Like the ACL, the MCL can be torn by a direct sideways blow to the outside of the knee or lower leg, which is the kind of blow that can happen in football, soccer, hockey, and rugby. The MCL can be injured by a severe knee twist during skiing or wrestling, particularly when a fall twists the lower leg outward, away from the upper leg.

COMMON SIGNS AND SYMPTOMS

- Mild-to-moderate knee pain
- Patient reports feeling a tearing in the knee, not a pop
- Bruising in the medial knee is often present since the MCL is an extraarticular structure.
- Swelling builds up slowly over several days.
- The patient walks with a limp and has pain with knee extension since it stretches the ligament.
- Instability and giving away may be noted.
- Loss of knee motion and moderate stiffness
- Medial joint line pain may be reported.

AGGRAVATING ACTIVITIES

- Extension of the knee
- Initial contact position of gait
- Ascending or descending stairs or an incline
- Walking downhill
- Starting a run
- Walking longer distances
- Uneven ground may lead to a sensation of instability.
- Cutting or change of direction actions, especially turning contralaterally

EASING ACTIVITIES

- Elevation
- Prescription antiinflammatory medications, muscle relaxants, and pain medications to address the patient's symptoms
- Ice
- Rest

24-HOUR SYMPTOM PATTERN

- Redness, swelling, and bruising may appear within the first 72 hours after injury.
- Stiffness in the knee joint is present after prolonged activity or prolonged inactivity.
- Sleeping may be painful if sleeping side-lying with no support under the knee.

PAST HISTORY FOR THE REGION

- Patient may report prior history of knee injury that has affected the mechanics of the knee.
- Prior injuries to the ankle or hip may also predispose the patient to increased stresses at the knee.

PHYSICAL EXAMINATION

- Joint examination: Observe any gross effusion or bony abnormality
- Partially full or functional ROM
- Point tenderness over the MCL, especially at its femoral attachment
- Immediate effusion indicates significant intraarticular trauma. Effusion that takes many hours to accumulate usually indicates an extraarticular trauma or meniscal involvement.
- The presence of bruising is also a good indicator of tissue injury. Extraarticular injured tissue, such as an MCL sprain, will result in visible bruising. Intraarticular injured tissue does not result in visible bruising.
- Ligamentous laxity

IMPORTANT OBJECTIVE TESTS

MCL or valgus stress test

DIFFERENTIAL DIAGNOSIS

- Muscle strain
- Myofascial pain

- Patellofemoral stress syndrome
- Early degenerative joint disease
- Popliteal or biceps femoris tendinitis
- Tendinitis
- Referred pain from the lumbar spine or hip
- Femoral stress fracture
- Infection
- Neoplasm
- Osteochondral fracture
- Knee dislocation
- Meniscal tear
- Multiligamentous injury
- Extensor mechanism rupture
- Osteonecrosis of the femoral epicondyle
- Osteonecrosis of the tibial condyle
- Inflammatory conditions (systemic disease)

CONTRIBUTING FACTORS

- Football, baseball, soccer, skiing, and basketball account for up to 78% of sports-related injuries.
- Long-term use of corticosteroids can weaken the knee ligaments.
- Systemic diseases, such as RA or lupus, can predispose a patient to joint laxity.

TREATMENT

SURGICAL OPTIONS

- Several different methods have been developed for MCL reconstruction. They include the following:
  - Distal advancement involves pulling the ligament distally to suture or reattach the ligament.
  - Proximal advancement involves pulling the ligament proximally to suture or reattach the ligament.
  - Direct repair involves directly suturing the ligament together.
  - Augmentation involves using the semitendinosus tendon for augmentation of medial collateral repair. Because it loses some of its initial strength in the revascularizing and remodeling process, it is not strong enough to replace the ligament but is useful in augmenting or protecting of repaired MCL.

REHABILITATION

- The MCL is well vascularized. As a result, surgery is rarely required. Instead, the knee is braced for the first 72 hours to prevent valgus stresses to the knee. After this initial period, the knee should be protected to avoid excessive valgus loading for 6 weeks. During this time, it is hoped that scar tissue will form to reinforce the damaged ligament.

- The ability of a torn ligament to heal depends on a variety of factors, including anatomical location and the presence of associated injuries. Typically, a grade I or grade II MCL injury will heal within 11 to 20 days. Grade III injuries may take 6 months to a year to heal.
- In rare cases, surgery will be performed. Arthroscopic surgery is not indicated since the structure is extraarticular. Instead, a small incision is made adjacent to the injured ligament and the ligament is sutured together or to the bone.
- Rehabilitation of the MCL depends on whether surgery was performed or not.
- In the case of surgery, patients are fitted with braces close to full extension for the first 3 to 4 weeks. The brace may be removed frequently for specific active ROM (AROM) and active-assisted ROM (AAROM) exercises. The splint should be used to protect the graft. At 5 to 6 weeks, a long leg splint or knee immobilizer may be replaced with a hinged device, or a previously locked hinge can be unlocked. This brace is kept on until 6 weeks after surgery. The hinged brace is also removed for specific ROM exercises and then is reapplied. It is also worn at night. Complete rehabilitation takes 6 months.

GENERAL MCL REHABILITATION GUIDELINES

Phase I: Acute Inflammatory Phase (Days 0 to 14 after injury)
- When to progress to phase: Initial injury to the ligament
- Goals of phase
  - Maintain ROM.
  - Protect the joint and ligament.
  - Decrease inflammation and irritation and promote healing.
- Interventions:
  - Medications: Antiinflammatories/muscle relaxants
  - Modalities: Electrical stimulation for quadriceps contraction, ultrasound, ice after activity
  - Myofascial release to global muscles as needed
  - Lower extremity flexibility: Hamstrings, ITB, and hip flexors
  - Home exercise program: ROM exercises, lower extremity flexibility, hip strengthening, RICE
Phase 2: Reparative Phase (Days 15 to 21 after injury)
- When to progress to phase: Progress as pain allows
- Goals of phase
  - Restore normal ROM.
  - Protect full extension ROM as it stretches the MCL.
  - Minimize swelling.

- Interventions
  - Medications as needed
  - Modalities as needed
  - Myofascial release to global muscles. Progress as needed.
  - Lower extremity flexibility: Hamstrings and hip flexors
  - Home exercise program: Walking program, lower extremity flexibility and strengthening
Phase 3: Remodeling Phase (Days 22 to 60 after injury)
- When to progress to phase:
  - Pain-free ROM
  - No functional limitations
- Goals of phase
  - Increase agility.
  - Progress to return to sports.
  - Address contributing factors.
- Interventions
  - Medications and myofascial release as needed
  - Home exercise program: Progress lower extremity flexibility and strengthening program.
  - Other: Address contributing factors
Phase 4: Remodeling Phase (Days 60 to 360 after injury)
- When to progress to phase: No functional limitations
- Goals of phase
  - Correction of contributing factors that result in ligament injury
  - Retraining muscle activity to account for functional activities
- Interventions
  - Medications and myofascial release as needed
  - Home exercise program: Progress lower extremity flexibility and strengthening program.
  - Other: Address contributing factors, functional rehabilitation, and retraining.

PROGNOSIS

- Most patients have excellent outcomes.
- The goal of surgery is to stabilize the knee, decrease the chance of future meniscal injury, and delay the arthritic process.

SIGNS AND SYMPTOMS INDICATING REFERRAL TO PHYSICIAN

- Constant unrelenting leg pain or pain that does not change with position may indicate infection or tumor.
- Significant and unexplained weight loss or nocturnal pain may indicate the presence of a tumor.
- Major trauma may necessitate radiographs to rule out the presence of a fracture.
- A history of cancer may indicate the need to rule out metastatic disease if all other musculoskeletal factors have been eliminated.

SUGGESTED READINGS

Browner BD. *Skeletal Trauma: Fractures, Dislocations, Ligamentous Injuries.* Philadelphia: WB Saunders; 1998.

Dugan SA. Sports-related knee injuries in female athletes: What gives? *Arch Phys Med Rehabil.* 2005;84(2):122-130.

Dutton M. *Orthopaedic Examination, Evaluation, & Intervention.* New York: McGraw-Hill; 2004.

Hastings DE. The non-operative management of collateral ligament injuries of the knee joint. *Clin Orthop.* 1980;(147):22-28.

Quarles JD, Hosey RG. Medial and lateral collateral injuries: prognosis and treatment. *Prim Care.* 2004;31(4):957-975, ix.

Strayer RJ, Lang ES. Evidence-based emergency medicine/systematic review abstract. Does this patient have a torn meniscus or ligament of the knee? *Ann Emerg Med.* 2006;47(5):499-501.

Wiener SL. *Differential Diagnosis of Acute Pain By Body Region.* New York: McGraw-Hill; 1993.

AUTHOR: BERNARD LI

BASIC INFORMATION

DEFINITION

A tear or degeneration of the semilunar, fibrous piece of cartilage located in the knee joint is diagnosed arthroscopically (gold standard) or by MRI. Pathology can be found in either the medial or lateral meniscus or both.

SYNONYMS

- Meniscus tear
- Meniscal derangement
- Internal derangement
- Cartilage tear

ICD-9CM CODES
717 Internal derangement of knee
717.3 Other and unspecified derangement of medial meniscus
717.4 Derangement of lateral meniscus

OPTIMAL NUMBER OF VISITS
12

MAXIMAL NUMBER OF VISITS
30

ETIOLOGY

- Meniscal tears can result from major or minor trauma to the knee or from degeneration of the meniscus.
- Acute tears most commonly result from a sudden twisting motion or rapid change in direction.
- Degenerative tears are age related or may result from repetitive activities over time such as squatting and kneeling.
- The medial meniscus is more commonly injured because of its attachment to the joint capsule, making it less mobile than the lateral meniscus.
- Meniscal tears are often associated with anterior collateral ligament (ACL) tears.
- The several types of tears based on the location of the tear are as follows:
  - Bucket-handle tear is a vertical tear with displacement of the inner margin, most often associated with an ACL tear and more commonly observed in the medial meniscus.
  - Radial tear is most often found in the medial aspect of the lateral meniscus and may be associated with an ACL tear; it commonly results from trauma and is often observed in young, active individuals.
  - Horizontal tears are degenerative and often found in older patients with osteoarthritis.
  - Longitudinal tear usually involves the posterior portion of the meniscus, the most common type of tear, and is typically associated with an ACL tear.
  - Flap tear is a displaced flap that is a secondary result from a radial, bucket-handle, or horizontal tear.
  - Oblique tear is a full-thickness tear that runs obliquely from the inner edge of the meniscus out into the body of the meniscus.
- Menisci play a major role in joint lubrication and support, and they act to cushion compressive loads to the knee to protect the tibiofemoral joint, thus making it susceptible to injury.
- Degenerative tears occur as a natural part of the aging process when the collagen fibers within the meniscus begin to break down and give less support to the structure of the meniscus.

EPIDEMIOLOGY AND DEMOGRAPHICS

- Degenerative tears: Age is a risk factor, since 60% of individuals older than 65 years have degenerative tears.
- Young, active, or athletic individuals are more susceptible to acute, traumatic meniscal tears.

MECHANISM OF INJURY

- Traumatic tears
  - Compressive force coupled with a rotation while the knee is in a flexed position.
  - Most tears occur from a noncontact event such as landing from a jump, pivoting, decelerating, or cutting.
- Degenerative tears
  - Most commonly observed in individuals older than 65 years and are often nontraumatic, common resulting from repetitive activities over time or from a previous history of trauma to the knee such as an ACL tear or previous history of knee surgery.

COMMON SIGNS AND SYMPTOMS

- Clicking, popping, locking, giving way, catching
- Pain with weight bearing
- Joint line tenderness/pain
- Swelling, decreased or painful knee ROM
- Meniscal injury does not have a referral pattern.

AGGRAVATING ACTIVITIES

- Walking
- Running
- Squatting
- Climbing stairs
- Pivoting
- Cutting
- Prolonged weight bearing

EASING ACTIVITIES

Any position of non–weight-bearing

24-HOUR SYMPTOM PATTERN

Pain may increase with increased activity throughout the day.

PAST HISTORY FOR THE REGION

- Knee joint osteoarthritis
- Previous history of knee trauma or surgery
- ACL tear or other ligament damage

PHYSICAL EXAMINATION

- Medial or lateral joint line tenderness
- Decreased knee ROM or pain with AROM
- Pain at end-range knee flexion with overpressure
- Knee joint swelling

IMPORTANT OBJECTIVE TESTS

- No single special test when used alone can accurately diagnose a meniscus tear; however, combined results of McMurray's test, Apley's test, joint line tenderness, and the subjective history improves diagnostic accuracy.
  - McMurray's test: Sensitivity: 70.5%; specificity: 71.1%
  - Joint line tenderness: Sensitivity: 63.3%; specificity: 77.4%
  - Apley's test: Sensitivity: 60.7; specificity: 70.2%
  - Thessaly test (at 20 degrees of knee flexion): Sensitivity: 92%; specificity: 96% (for lateral meniscus tear), 94% (for medial meniscus tears)
  - Ege's test: Specificity: 81% (for medial meniscus tears), 90% (for lateral meniscus tears)

DIFFERENTIAL DIAGNOSIS

- Osteoarthritis
- Patellofemoral pain syndrome
- ACL or PCL tear
- Medial or LCL tear
- ITBFS
- Pes anserine bursitis/tendinitis
- Knee OCD

CONTRIBUTING FACTORS

- Age (degenerative tears)
- Weight
- Previous surgical history
- Previous knee trauma

TREATMENT

INDICATIONS FOR SURGERY

- Repair is recommended for active individuals younger than 50 years or older individuals who remain athletically active.
- Partial meniscectomy is recommended for tears that occur in the avascular

region of the meniscus or for complex tears that can not be repaired.

- Meniscal repairs are recommended for tears that occur in the outer edges (vascular region) of the meniscus. Tears should be longer than 1 cm, and the depth should be greater than 50% of the thickness of the meniscus.
- Meniscal transplantation is recommended for patients with a previous total meniscectomy, who are younger than 50 years, and who have evidence of articular cartilage damage or symptoms involving the tibiofemoral joint, and 2 mm or more of tibiofemoral joint space on 45-degree weight-bearing anteroposterior radiographs.
- Normal limb alignment and knee stability is also required to minimize transplant failure.

SURGICAL OPTIONS

- Arthroscopy: partial meniscectomy or meniscal repair
- Meniscal transplantation

SURGICAL OUTCOME

- Tears located in the peripheral one-third vascularized region have high success rates with repairs.
- Meniscal transplantation is generally successful if performed before the advanced onset of tibiofemoral joint osteoarthritis.

REHABILITATION

- Goals are to restore ROM and lower extremity strength while protecting the meniscus as it heals.

- Limit high compressive and shear forces that could disrupt the healing process of a repair or meniscal transplant by controlling excessive weight bearing.
- Initial interventions can minimize stress to the meniscus and thus decrease pain and promote healing (acute, postoperative phase).
- Lower extremity strengthening and ROM exercises with limited weight-bearing (open kinetic chain exercises): Heel slides, quadriceps sets, straight leg raises, stationary bicycle, hip abduction exercises
- Patellar mobilization
- Stretching/soft tissue mobilization (STM) techniques for hamstrings, quadriceps, gastrocnemius to improve knee ROM
- Gait training with assistive device
- Decrease pain and inflammation via modalities.

PROGNOSIS

- Results are variable, since they depend on the extent and location of the tear and the presence of comorbidities, but the majority of patients have a favorable outcome and are able to return to daily activities and sports.
- Patients with a meniscal lesion are at greater risk for developing osteoarthritis in the long term.

SIGNS AND SYMPTOMS INDICATING REFERRAL TO PHYSICIAN

- Failure to respond to conservative treatment

- Signs of infection: Fever, malaise, redness, swelling, unrelenting pain

SUGGESTED READINGS

Fritz JM, Irrgang JJ, Harner CD. Rehabilitation following allograft meniscal transplantation: A review of the literature and case study. *J Orthop Sports Phys Ther.* 2006;24(2):98-107.

Heckmann TP, Barber-Westin SD, Noyes FR. Meniscal repair and transplantation: Indications, techniques, rehabilitation, and clinical outcome. *J Ortho Sports Phys Ther.* 2006;36(10):795-815.

Hegedus EJ, Cook C, Hasselblad V, Goode A, McCrory DC. Physical examination tests for assessing a torn meniscus in the: A systematic review with meta-analysis. *J Orthop Sports Phys Ther.* 2007;37(9):541-550.

Karachalios T, Hantes M, Zibis AH, Zachos V, Karantanas AH, Malizos KN. Diagnostic accuracy of a new clinical test (the Thessaly test) for early detection of meniscal tears. *J Bone Joint Surg Am.* 2005;87(5):955-962.

Mackenzie R, Dixon AK, Keene GS, Hollingworth W, Lomas DJ, Villar RN. Magnetic resonance imaging of the knee: assessment of effectiveness. *Clin Radiol.* 1996;51(4):245-250.

AUTHOR: DELLA LEE

BASIC INFORMATION

DEFINITION

- Osteoarthritis is a pathology associated with inflammation in the joints of the body. In the case of ankle osteoarthritis, the arthritis and inflammation most commonly affects the tibiofemoral or patellofemoral joints, leading to knee pain.
- Osteoarthritis is a term derived from the Greek word *osteo,* meaning "of the bone," *arthro,* meaning "joint," and *itis,* meaning inflammation, even though the amount of inflammation present in the joint can range from excessive to little or no inflammation.

SYNONYMS

- Knee arthritis
- Knee degenerative joint disease

ICD-9 CODES
715.16 Osteoarthrosis localized primary involving lower leg
715.26 Osteoarthrosis localized secondary involving lower leg

OPTIMAL NUMBER OF VISITS

3 to 6 (12 if status post arthroplasty)

MAXIMAL NUMBER OF VISITS

20 to 36 (60 if status post arthroplasty)

ETIOLOGY

- The wearing down of the hyaline cartilage leads to an inflammatory response. There is thickening and sclerosis of the subchondral bone and development of osteophytes or bone spurs. This leads to a narrowing of the joint space, loss of shock absorption, and ultimately pain.
- Daily wear and tear in combination with various injuries sustained throughout life is the most common cause of the breakdown of healthy tissue.
- Degeneration of the cartilage and resultant arthritis can also be the result of other factors such as trauma or joint injury.
- At a cellular level, as a person ages, the number of proteoglycans in the articular cartilage decreases. Proteoglycans are hydrophilic and work within cartilage to bind water. With the reduction of proteoglycans comes a decrease in water content within the cartilage and a corresponding loss of cartilage resilience. With the decreases in cartilage resilience, collagen fibers of the cartilage become susceptible to degradation and injury. The breakdown of collagen and other cartilage tissue are released into

the surround joint space. Inflammation results as the body attempts to respond to the influx of byproducts from cartilage injury.
- As the cartilage degrades, the joint space narrows and ligaments become more lax. In response to the laxity, new bone outgrowths, called *spurs* or *osteophytes,* can form on the margins of the joints in an attempt to improve the congruence and passive stability of the articular cartilage surfaces.
- Primary osteoarthritis refers to joint degradation resulting from aging and tissue degeneration
- Secondary osteoarthritis refers to joint degradation and tissue degeneration that results from factors other than aging such as obesity, trauma, and congenital disorders.
- Stages of knee osteoarthritis:
  - Stage I (mild): Mild joint space narrowing, cartilage fissuring
  - Stage II (moderate): Cartilage erosion, osteophytes, sclerosis, and moderate joint space narrowing
  - Stage III (moderate severe): Significant joint space narrowing, larger and more numerous osteophytes, sclerosis, and significant cartilage erosion
  - Stage IV (severe): Obliteration of joint space, large osteophytes, significant sclerosis, complete erosion of cartilage, and large osteophytes

EPIDEMIOLOGY AND DEMOGRAPHICS

- The Framingham study has revealed that radiographic knee osteoarthritis occurs in at least 33% of persons aged 60 years and older.
- Approximately 6% of 30-year-old adults have knee pain from osteoarthritis on most days; 10% to 15% of 60-year-old adults have this same pain.
- As the American population gets older and more overweight, the prevalence will grow.
- 70% of all individuals older than 70 years of age have x-ray evidence. Only one-third to one-half has symptoms.
- Changes can usually be seen in persons older than 30 years, with significant impairments noted in persons older than 50 years.
- In general, there is a higher prevalence of osteoarthritis in women than in men after the age of 50 years. For persons with diagnosed osteoarthritis before the age of 50 years, there are more men than women.
- Whites and African Americans have similar prevalence, but African Americans may be more disabled from their pathology. Chinese Americans have a higher prevalence of knee osteoarthritis than Whites. Few data are found

about Hispanic Americans, but it is theorized that the prevalence is high.
- 200,000 knee replacements are performed each year.

MECHANISM OF INJURY

- Osteoarthritis is a pathology of overuse. The mechanism of injury is therefore the result of repetitive motions that stress the hip joint. The more cycles of an activity that the ankle performs, the more likely the result will be anatomical damage.
- Daily use/misuse of the knee
- Misalignment of the tibiofemoral joint or patellofemoral joint
- Excessive use/strain of the knee secondary to work, obesity, or recreational activities
- Injuries, such as fracture and strains/sprains, that cause inflammation and scar tissue in the knee
- Poor foot or hip mechanics

COMMON SIGNS AND SYMPTOMS

- Deep pain in the knee
- Difficulty localizing the exact location of the pain
- Stiffness in the knee with inactivity
- Cracking or deep crunching in the knee
- Inflammation and thickening of the knee
- Knee flexion contracture
- Joint deformity (valgus or varus)
- Pain tends to be localized to the affected joints (usually anterior knee or on either joint line) and surrounding tissues
- Studies have shown subjectively that inactivity stiffness, pain on using stairs, and night pain have high reliability (0.80 to 0.90 kappa value) are predictors of knee osteoarthritis.

AGGRAVATING ACTIVITIES

- Inactivity leads to stiffness
- Weight-bearing activities (walking, running, dancing, jumping, etc.)
- Long-term standing, especially on harder surfaces like concrete
- Poor footwear (i.e., high heels)
- Inactivity allows the inflammation to "pool" and increase pressure, leading to discomfort and loss of available movement.
- Joint movement increases "wear and tear" and inflammation/irritation of the articular surfaces. The more compression involved with the movement, the more "wear and tear" and irritation will occur.

EASING ACTIVITIES

- Rest
- Pain-free motion of the ankle joint
- Gentle stretching and exercise, use of heat/ice, massage, taking antiinflammatory

medication, non–weight-bearing positions, and ankle elevation

- Generally speaking, these activities lead to decreased wear and tear, increased joint lubrication, and loss of stiffness and inflammation associated with this condition.

24-HOUR SYMPTOM PATTERN

- Stiffness in the morning
- Better after a warm shower and taking medication
- Can worsen with excessive movement.
- Stiffens again in the evening
- Deep achiness in the knee at night described as throbbing

PAST HISTORY FOR THE REGION

- Jobs or recreational activities that require excessive use/strain of the knee (walking, running, jumping, dancing, baseball catcher, etc.)
- Prior history to injury in either the foot or hip
- Prior history of injury to the knee
- Obesity
- Prior history of knee surgery

PHYSICAL EXAMINATION

- Genu valgum or genu varum
- Decreased weight bearing noted during stance phase of gait
- Decreased knee flexion during swing phase of motion
- Joint thickening (bony changes and inflammation)
- Loss of knee ROM: End-range flexion and extension may be limited.
- Localized pain when palpating the medial and lateral margins of the patella and when palpating the tibiofemoral joint line
- Loss of joint mobility when testing tibiofemoral or patellofemoral accessory motions
- Crepitus with movement with patellofemoral osteoarthritis

IMPORTANT OBJECTIVE TESTS

- Alignment assessment
- AROM and passive ROM (PROM)
- Joint mobility
- Special tests: Ligament stability, meniscal integrity, and patellar grind
- Strength tests
- In studies focusing on knee osteoarthritis, the following tests have the highest reliability factor in predicting pathology:
  - Medial instability test at full knee extension (0.66 kappa value)
  - Lateral instability test at full knee extension (0.88 kappa value)
  - Values are less for instability tests when knee is flexed slightly.
  - Posterior drawer test (0.82 kappa value)

DIFFERENTIAL DIAGNOSIS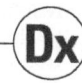

- Knee sprain
- Tendinitis (patellar, iliotibial, or pes anserine)
- Bursitis (patellar, pes anserine)
- RA
- Septic arthritis
- Meniscal injury
- Ligament injury
- Fracture
- Referral from the lumbar region

CONTRIBUTING FACTORS

- The knee is designed to handle normal daily use. When factors change the body's ability to respond to normal forces, damage occurs.
- Uncontrolled risk factors that contribute or predispose an individual to knee osteoarthritis pathology:
  - Gender (females > males)
  - Age (increase 2%/year after age 40 years)
  - Genetics
  - Prior history of injury to either lower extremity
  - Prior history of childhood hip pathology
  - Leg length discrepancies
- Modifiable risk factors that contribute or predispose an individual to continue or progress ankle osteoarthritis include the following:
  - Weight
  - Work or recreational activities
  - Repetitive or significant traumatic injuries to the hip
  - Poor health (smoking, long-term use of steroids)
  - Muscle or tissue restrictions such as tight ITB, calf, or hip flexors

TREATMENT

SURGICAL OPTIONS

- Arthroscopic debridement for mild-to-moderate symptoms
- Total knee replacement (TKA)
  - Noncemented for younger (40 to 50 years of age) patients
  - Cemented for older or overweight patients
  - Replacement tends to last 15 to 20 years.
- Osteotomy (for deformity) for young patients to postpone the need for arthroplasty
- Osteochondral drilling

REHABILITATION

- Rehabilitation should focus on the following:
  - Education in correct use of ice/heat at home for pain abatement and edema control

- Implementation of a home exercise program
- Teach proper footwear with or without orthotics. Correction of foot alignment and reduction of loading on the joint are important factors related to hip osteoarthritis.
- Manual therapy (STM, joint mobilization) can improve joint mobility and arthrokinematics and decrease pain.
- Massage can decrease pain by relaxing muscular tension, improving circulation, and increasing endorphin release.
- Pathological changes to cartilage cannot be repaired by the body at this time. Even surgical advances have yet to solve the problems associated with cartilage damage. With this in mind, rehabilitation should focus on decreasing the stress placed on the damaged cartilage and correcting biomechanical and anatomical abnormalities that may predispose an individual to increased stress at the knee joint.
- The clinician should also evaluate the patient for leg length discrepancies that would cause abnormal stresses to placed on the hip joint. Shoe lifts can be recommended to equalize the length of the legs during function.
- The knee joint is a synovial joint. Therefore the cartilage has the potential to heal. Joint motion can influence the healing process. It is aggravated by activities that excessively load the joint, but motion in a non–weight-bearing to a limited weight-bearing environment can greatly decrease the patient's symptoms.
- Exercises include the following:
  - Stretches: Calf (gastrocnemius and soleus), quadriceps, ITB, hamstrings
  - Strengthening exercises: Quadriceps (VMO), hamstrings, hip abductors, hip adductors, hip extensors
  - Proprioceptive exercises
  - Cardiovascular exercises: Bicycle progressing to treadmill to promote circulation and healing.
- Exercise creates a sense of control over the symptoms and the condition.
- Modalities: Ice/heat, ultrasound, electrical stimulation, and tape/braces can be used as adjuncts to improve the healing environment.
- Factors that contribute to abnormal joint mechanics and loading should be determined and addressed.

PROGNOSIS

- Long-term prognosis for a patient with knee osteoarthritis depends on the extent of wear and tear and ability to reduce the joint strain placed on the joint (posture, activity, etc).
- For the most part, knee osteoarthritis is a degenerative condition. At earlier

stages of the pathology, rehabilitation aimed at reducing the load placed on the joint can potentially slow or halt the progression of degeneration.

- For patients who are further along in the degenerative process, outcomes will be less favorable because cartilage has only a limited ability to repair itself.

SIGNS AND SYMPTOMS INDICATING REFERRAL TO PHYSICIAN

- Unrelenting pain
- Unusual responses to therapy
- Neurological signs

- Red flag symptoms such as excessive redness and swelling and generalized malaise and fatigue: Infection

SUGGESTED READINGS

Amin S. Cigarette smoking and the risk for cartilage loss and knee pain in men with knee osteoarthritis. *Ann Rheum Dis.* 2007;66(1):18-22.

St Clair SF, Higuera C, Krebs V, Tadross NA, Dumpe J, Barsoum WK. Hip and knee arthroplasty in the geriatric population. *Clin Geriatr Med.* 2006;22(3):515-533.

Dugan SA. Exercise for health and wellness at midlife and beyond: balancing benefits and risks. *Phys Med Rehabil Clin N Am.* 2007;18(3):555-575.

Glass GG. Osteoarthritis. *Dis Mon.* 2006;52(9).

Hinman RS. Patellofemoral joint osteoarthritis: an important subgroup of knee osteoarthritis. *Rheumatology (Oxford)* 2007;46(7):1057-1062.

Jones CA, et al. Total joint arthroplasties: current concepts of patient outcomes after surgery. *Rheum Dis Clin North Am* 2007;33(1).

O'Connor M. Osteoarthritis of the hip and knee: sex and gender differences. *Orthop Clin North Am.* 2006;37(4).

AUTHOR: SARA GRANNIS

BASIC INFORMATION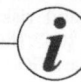

DEFINITION

- Patellar dislocation occurs when there is no contact between the patella and the trochlear groove.
- Patellar subluxation is a temporary, partial dislocation of the patella from the trochlear groove.

SYNONYMS

Patellar instability

ICD-9CM CODES
836.3 Dislocation of patella closed

OPTIMAL NUMBER OF VISITS

8

MAXIMAL NUMBER OF VISITS

20

ETIOLOGY

- Acute dislocations can occur with direct trauma such as a fall or a direct blow to the knee; however, most occur from a noncontact mechanism, typically frequent exposure to the primary mechanism of injury.
- Most dislocations/subluxations occur laterally, resulting in severe disruption of the extensor mechanism as a result of the patella sliding over the lateral portion of the trochlear groove.

EPIDEMIOLOGY AND DEMOGRAPHICS

- Acute patellar dislocations account for 2% to 3% of all knee injuries.
- First-time dislocations with a history of prior subluxation are most observed in girls 10 to 17 years of age, but subluxations/dislocations are most often observed in young, athletic individuals.
- Younger children and preadolescents have higher rates of recurrence and greater underlying mechanical risk factors.
- In those treated nonoperatively after a one-time dislocation, up to 44% will dislocate again and >50% will report symptoms associated with recurrent instability.

MECHANISM OF INJURY

Dislocation/subluxation most often results from a noncontact, lower extremity internal rotation and knee valgus stress on a fixed distal extremity.

COMMON SIGNS AND SYMPTOMS

- Patients present with a vague anterior knee pain and swelling, with complaints of giving way with specific activities such as jumping, running, or making quick stops and quick changes in direction.
- In recurrent instability, symptoms are typically episodic and long term.

AGGRAVATING ACTIVITIES

- Jumping
- Running
- Quick stops
- Quick changes in direction

EASING ACTIVITIES

Inactivity and rest

24-HOUR SYMPTOM PATTERN

No specific pattern

PAST HISTORY FOR THE REGION

History of one-time dislocation or recurrent subluxations leading to patellar instability.

PHYSICAL EXAMINATION

- Dislocated patella: Patella is positioned laterally over the femoral trochlear groove.
- Decreased knee ROM
- Palpable tenderness and swelling over the lateral condyle and medial soft tissue structures
- Injury to the medial patellofemoral ligament (MPFL) may be inferred if it is painful with palpation at its origin at the adductor tubercle.
- Weak hip abductors/external rotators, weak quadriceps
- Excessive foot pronation/pes planus; midfoot hypermobility
- Genu valgum
- Patellar hypermobility

IMPORTANT OBJECTIVE TESTS

- Positive patellar apprehension test
- Laterally subluxated patella on plain Mercer-Merchant view (sunrise view) radiographs
- MRI findings of a large disruption of the MPFL–vastus medialis oblique (VMO)–adductor mechanism

DIFFERENTIAL DIAGNOSIS

- Patellofemoral pain syndrome
- ITBFS
- Meniscal derangement
- ACL tear
- Patellar tendinopathy
- Chondromalacia
- OCD
- Patellar fracture

CONTRIBUTING FACTORS

- Age: Young, active
- Gender: Female
- Increased Q angle
- Genu valgum
- Patella alta
- Increased femoral anteversion
- Coxa valga
- Family history of dislocation
- Trochlear dysplasia
- Abnormal foot mechanics: Excessive foot pronation that leads to genu valgum
- Weak hip abductors and external rotators may lead to genu valgum.
- Gross ligamentous laxity
- Excessive foot pronation

TREATMENT

SURGICAL OPTIONS

- Open and arthroscopic techniques are available, if the pathology is associated with fractures, to repair/remove loose bodies and repair soft tissue structures.
- Medial repair (open): Repair of the MPFL, plication of the medial patellar retinaculum, VMO plasty (VMO removed and reinserted 10 to 15 mm distally from its insertion on the patella).

SURGICAL OUTCOME

- VMO-plasty at 5-year follow-up has a re-dislocation rate of 7%.
- Repair or reconstruction of the MPFL is key to preventing lateral patellar dislocations/subluxations.

INDICATIONS FOR SURGERY

- Surgery is not often performed and is typically reserved for complicated dislocations with associated osteochondral fractures or patients who fail to respond to physical therapy. In general, if patients have no anatomical abnormalities and no evidence of intraarticular damage, conservative treatment is the optimal intervention.
- Surgery is recommended for patients with recurrent subluxations/dislocations with normal anatomy or for patients who have an anatomical abnormality and who experience an acute episode of dislocation or a later episode of subluxation/dislocation.
- Presence of palpable disruption of the MPFL-VMO-adductor mechanism and MRI evidence of a large complete rupture of the MPFL
- Open repairs are recommended if the osteochondral fracture is greater than 10% of the patella articular surface or part of the weight-bearing portion of the lateral femoral condyle, as long as the fragment is amenable to fixation.

REHABILITATION

- Acute injury
  - Bracing to immobilize the patella for 2 to 3 weeks, reduce pain and swelling via modalities, cease activities that

cause increased stress on the patell-ofemoral joint.

○ Therapeutic goals for successful rehabilitation of patellar instability

○ Restore normal patellar tracking and activity modification to reduce patellofemoral joint stress.

• Interventions to promote healing

○ Quadriceps strengthening exercises in ranges that place the least amount of stress on the patellofemoral joint.

○ Proper footwear and assess the need for orthotics if excessive pronation or pes planus is present, contributing to genu valgum posture.

○ Hip abduction and external rotation strengthening exercises to minimize femoral adduction and internal rotation, which may contribute to increased genu valgum posture in squat positions.

○ Patellar taping to assist in normal patellar tracking during exercise.

○ Improve ITB flexibility to decrease lateral pull on patella.

○ Medial patellar glides to stretch lateral patellar retinacular soft structures.

PROGNOSIS

• Based on the literature, prognosis is variable for first-time dislocations. However, it has been reported that for patients who undergo nonoperative interventions, there is a 44% re-dislocation rate and >50% chance of having symptoms associated with recurrent instability.

• Prognosis is also variable for patients who undergo surgery.

• With conservative or nonconservative interventions, the prognosis for return to normal function and return to athletic activity is favorable overall, but the risk of re-dislocation/subluxation or recurrent instability is high.

SIGNS AND SYMPTOMS INDICATING REFERRAL TO PHYSICIAN

• Signs associated with postoperative infection indicate referral to a physician.

SUGGESTED READINGS

Fithian DC, Paxton EW, Stone ML, et al. Epidemiology and natural history of acute patellar dislocation. *Am J Sports Med.* 2004;32(5):1114–1121.

Hinton RY, Sharma KM. Acute and recurrent patellar instability in the young athlete. *Orthop Clin N Am.* 2003;34(3):385–396.

Krause F, Kolling C, Brantschen R, Sieber HP. Medium-term results after m. vastus medialis obliquus-plasty for lateral patellar dislocation. *Orthopade.* 2006;35(1):94–101.

Stefancin JJ, Parker RD. First-time traumatic patellar dislocation. A systematic review. *Clin Orthop Relat Res.* 2007;455(2):93–101.

AUTHOR: DELLA LEE

BASIC INFORMATION

DEFINITION

A patellar fracture is the cracking or breaking of the patella bone in the knee.

SYNONYMS

Broken knee cap

ICD-9CM CODES
822.0 Closed fracture of patella
822.1 Open fracture of patella

OPTIMAL NUMBER OF VISITS

6

MAXIMAL NUMBER OF VISITS

18

ETIOLOGY

- A compressive force (direct blow) to the patella or a forceful contraction of the quadriceps while the knee is extended (eccentric contraction) results in excessive tensile force on the patella.
- May occur as a result of postoperative complication or diseases such as the following:
  - ACL reconstruction with patellar tendon autograft
  - TKA
  - Pathological fracture secondary to an infection, primary or metastatic tumors (benign or malignant), metabolic disease
- Types of patellar fractures
  - Transverse fracture is the most common. It results from a direct blow and has only one fracture line that is typically in the central aspect or distal one third of the patella.
  - Stellate fracture occurs with a direct blow to the patella, resulting in a comminuted fracture pattern.
  - Vertical fracture is rare, with a fracture line that runs in the sagittal plane, from the superior to inferior aspect of the patella.
  - Marginal fracture occurs at the edge of the patella and does not extend across the bone.
  - Osteochondral fracture results from a direct or indirect blow or from an acute patellar dislocation injury; it often occurs in children and adolescents secondary to patellar hypermobility. The bone and articular cartilage covering the fragment has been fractured and may separate and become a loose body within the knee joint.
  - Sleeve fracture is an uncommon type of osteochondral fracture that involves an avulsion of a large portion of the articular cartilage. When the inferior pole is involved, it is typically the result of high-impact jumping activities (forceful eccentric quadriceps contraction).

EPIDEMIOLOGY AND DEMOGRAPHICS

- 68% in patients after a TKA
- Accounts for approximately 1% of all musculoskeletal injuries in adults and children.
- Osteochondral and sleeve fractures most commonly affect children and adolescents.
- Fractures resulting from postoperative complications are most often observed in osteoporotic and elderly patients.

MECHANISM OF INJURY

- Direct fall onto the knee
- Motor vehicle accidents (MVAs) in which the knee is forced into the dashboard
- Acute patellar dislocations
- High-impact jumping activities

COMMON SIGNS AND SYMPTOMS

- Persistent patellar tenderness and swelling
- History of a direct blow or trauma to the knee
- Pain with weight bearing
- Difficulty with active knee flexion and extension
- Decreased knee ROM
- Patellar fracture has no referral pattern.

AGGRAVATING ACTIVITIES

- Knee flexion and extension
- Weight-bearing activities
- Prolonged sitting

EASING ACTIVITIES

- Rest
- Non–weight-bearing positions

24-HOUR SYMPTOM PATTERN

No specific pain pattern

PAST HISTORY FOR THE REGION

- Trauma
- Knee surgery
- Osteoporosis
- Patellar instability
- Benign or malignant tumor

PHYSICAL EXAMINATION

- Decreased or painful knee ROM
- Point tenderness over the patella
- Knee joint effusion

IMPORTANT OBJECTIVE TESTS

- X-rays
- CT scan

DIFFERENTIAL DIAGNOSIS

- Patellofemoral pain syndrome
- Bipartite patella
- Quadriceps/patellar tendinopathy
- Patellar tendon rupture
- Quadriceps tendon rupture

CONTRIBUTING FACTORS

- Infection
- Benign, malignant, or metastatic tumors
- Degenerative/metabolic disease
- TKA
- Obesity
- Osteoporosis
- Excessive knee flexion
- High activity level
- RA
- Resurfaced patella

TREATMENT

SURGICAL OPTIONS

- Fixation of the fragment using screws and wires.
- Partial or complete patellectomies are performed in rare cases with severe comminution of the patella, in which fixation is not possible.

INDICATIONS FOR SURGERY

- Patients with a minimally displaced or nondisplaced fracture who are able to perform a straight leg raise may not require surgical intervention.
- Displaced patellar fragments amenable to fixation may require surgery.

REHABILITATION

- Initial rehabilitation is started once the patient is cleared from all precautions.
  - Early focus should be on achieving normal knee ROM as soon as possible.
  - Progressive weight-bearing exercises to promote return to normal gait without the use of assistive devices if possible.
  - Progressive, resistive lower extremity strength program
- Initial exercises to promote healing are as follows:
  - Heel slides
  - Quad sets, straight leg raises, knee extension exercises
  - Soft tissue stretching exercise
  - Stationary bicycle
  - Calf and hip strengthening exercises
  - Bridging
  - Walking

PROGNOSIS

- Prognosis is variable, depending on whether the normal anatomy of the patellofemoral joint was restored during the surgery.

- Intraarticular damage or incongruities place the patient at greater risk for developing early-onset osteoarthritis.
- The patient is also at risk for developing arthrofibrosis if prolonged immobilization occurs postoperatively.

SIGNS AND SYMPTOMS INDICATING REFERRAL TO PHYSICIAN

- Signs of infection
- Decreased knee ROM caused by arthrofibrosis: Patient may require manipulation under anesthesia.
- Lack of improvement with rehabilitation or continued severe pain

- Nonunion
- Loss of fixation or reduction because of inadequate fixation or aggressive physical therapy.
- Hardware prominence: Some patients require hardware removal once the fracture is healed.

SUGGESTED READINGS

Ortiguera CJ, Berry DJ. Patellar fracture after total knee arthroplasty. *J Bone Joint Surg Am*. 2002;84:532–540.

Papageorgiou CD, Kostopoulos VK, Moebius UF, Petropoulou KA, Georgoulis AD, Soucacos PN. Patellar fractures associated with medial-third bone-patellar tendon-bone autograft ACL reconstruction. *Knee Surg Sports Traumatol Arthrosc*. 2001;9(3):151–154.

Parvizi J, Kim K, Oliashirazi A, Ong A, Sharkey PF. Periprosthetic patellar fractures. *Clin Orthop*. 2006;446(5):161–166.

Shabat S, Mann G, Kish B, Stern A, Sagiv P, Nyska M. Functional results after patellar fractures in elderly patients. *Arch Gerontol Geriatr*. 2003;37(1):93–98.

AUTHOR: DELLA LEE

Section III

ORTHOPEDIC PATHOLOGY

BASIC INFORMATION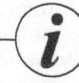

DEFINITION

- Patellar tendinitis is acute inflammation of the patellar tendon.
- Patellar tendinosis is a chronic pathology involving degeneration of the patellar tendon.

SYNONYMS

Jumper's knee

ICD-9CM CODES

726.90 Enthesopathy of unspecified site

OPTIMAL NUMBER OF VISITS

6

MAXIMAL NUMBER OF VISITS

24

ETIOLOGY

- Results from overuse activity, primarily involving patients that participate in sports such as basketball, volleyball, soccer, skiing, tennis, and track and field.
- Tendon overload occurs when 3% to 8% strain is applied to the tendon, which results in microlesions to the collagen fibers.
- Extrinsic and intrinsic factors may play a role in patellar tendinopathy: Decreased muscle flexibility, strength deficits or imbalances, patellar alignment, age, inappropriate footwear, excessive training intensity or duration.
- An acute inflammatory (tendinitis) or chronic, noninflammatory condition (tendinosis) involving the midsubstance of the patellar tendon or its proximal insertion at the inferior pole of the patella or its distal insertion at the tibial tubercle.
- Tendinosis describes histopathological changes to the tendon that occur over time in chronic conditions, ultimately resulting in a failed tissue healing response.
- Repetitive strain of the tendon eventually exceeds the capacity of the tendon to repair itself from the microlesions, ultimately resulting in microtrauma to the tendon.
- Tendons have a low metabolic rate, thus the demand for collagen and matrix production exceeds its reparative capacity.
- In tendinosis, collagen fibers repair and regenerate into a disorganized and discontinuous pattern, often marked by variable fibrosis and neovascularization.

EPIDEMIOLOGY AND DEMOGRAPHICS

- Approximately 15% of all soft tissue injuries are patellar tendinopathies.
- Significantly more common in aging athletes, with the peak incidence between 30 and 50 years of age.

MECHANISM OF INJURY

- Repetitive jumping and running
- Repetitive eccentric loading of the tendon

COMMON SIGNS AND SYMPTOMS

- Localized pain and possible swelling in the region of the patellar tendon, most often located at the proximal insertion at the inferior pole of the patella.
- Pain during or after activities
- Insidious onset of symptoms
- There is no referral pattern for patellar tendinopathy.

AGGRAVATING ACTIVITIES

- Running
- Jumping activities
- Going up and down stairs
- Squatting

EASING ACTIVITIES

- Rest
- Patellar tendon bracing
- Symptoms may improve during activity only to worsen after cessation of activity.

24-HOUR SYMPTOM PATTERN

- May be stiff initially after prolonged sitting or inactivity.
- Symptoms may be worse after completing aggravating activity.

PAST HISTORY FOR THE REGION

- No previous history of trauma
- Recent onset of a new activity/sport or recent increased activity

PHYSICAL EXAMINATION

- Palpable tenderness and swelling over the patellar tendon (swelling is absent in tendinosis)
- Point tenderness at the origin or insertion of the patellar tendon
- Pain with passive knee flexion and active, resisted knee extension
- Normal, but pain with knee ROM
- Hamstring and quadriceps tightness
- Quadriceps weakness
- Abnormal patellar alignment

IMPORTANT OBJECTIVE TESTS

- Diagnosis of patellar tendinopathy is largely based on the subjective history and physical examination findings.
- Diagnostic testing is rarely necessary; however, MRI and ultrasonography are highly sensitive for detecting tendon abnormalities.

DIFFERENTIAL DIAGNOSIS

- Patellofemoral pain syndrome
- Prepatellar bursitis
- Osgood-Schlatter disease
- Pes anserine bursitis
- Meniscal lesions

CONTRIBUTING FACTORS

- Excessive training intensity or duration
- Increased Q angle
- Genu valgum/varum
- Decreased muscle flexibility
- Abnormal patellar alignment
- Improper footwear
- Muscle weakness

TREATMENT

SURGICAL OPTIONS

- Open tenotomy with excision of macroscopic necrotic area
- Arthroscopic patellar tenotomy
- Drilling/resection of the inferior pole of the patella
- Resection of the tibial attachment with realignment and quadriceps bone-tendon graft
- Longitudinal or percutaneous longitudinal tenotomy

INDICATIONS FOR SURGERY

Surgery is indicated if the patient fails to respond to physical therapy and symptoms continue beyond 6 months after the start of treatment.

SURGICAL OUTCOME

For chronic proximal tendon pathologies, success rates generally are greater than 80%.

REHABILITATION

- Correction of the intrinsic and extrinsic risk factors
- Activity modification
- Improve quadriceps and hamstring flexibility
- Correct any biomechanical abnormalities, such as excessive foot pronation/pes planus or abnormal patellar tracking
- Emphasize the importance of rest and stopping all aggravating activities
- Cryotherapy
- Literature currently supports the use of eccentric exercise training for chronic tendinopathy. Results from studies are variable; however, the consensus is in favor of eccentric training.
- Eccentric training exercise: Patient stands on a 25-degree decline board (maximizes the load on the patellar tendon) on the affected limb only and slowly lowers into a single-limb squat

to 90 degrees of knee flexion. Patient then uses both legs to return to the start position. Double-limb eccentric squats may be performed if patient is unable to perform a single-limb squat.

PROGNOSIS

- Prognosis is favorable for the majority of patients to return to normal function or sport after physical therapy.
- 50% to 70% chance of recovering from chronic patellar tendinopathy with eccentric training program

SIGNS AND SYMPTOMS INDICATING REFERRAL TO PHYSICIAN

- Signs associated with infection (postoperative)
- Evidence of complete patellar tendon rupture

SUGGESTED READINGS

Almekinders LC, Temple JD. Etiology, diagnosis, and treatment of tendonitis: an analysis of the literature. *Med Sci Sports Exerc.* 1998;30(8):1183–1190.

Frohm A, Halvorson K, Thorstensson. Patellar tendon load in different types of eccentric squats. *Clin Biomech.* 2007;22(6):704–711.

Frohm A, Saartok T, Halvorsen K, Renstrom P. Eccentric treatment for patellar tendinopathy: a prospective randomized short-term pilot study of two rehabilitation protocols. *Br J Sports Med.* 2007;41(7):e7.

Leadbetter WB. Cell-matrix response in tendon injury. *Clin Sports Med.* 1992;11:533–578.

Linenger JM, West LA. Epidemiology of soft-tissue/musculoskeletal injury among U.S. Marine recruits undergoing basic training. *Mil Med.* 1992;157:491–493.

Mafi N, Lorentzon R, Alfredson H. Superior short-term results with eccentric calf muscle training compared to concentric training in a randomized prospective multicenter study on patients with chronic Achilles tendinosis. *Knee Surg Sports Traumatol Arthrosc.* 2001;9:42–47.

Peers KHE, Lysens RJJ. Patellar tendinopathy in athletes. Current diagnostic and therapeutic recommendations. *Sports Med.* 2005;35(1):71–87.

Visnes H, Bahr R. The evolution of eccentric training as treatment for patellar tendinopathy (jumper's knee): a critical review of exercise programmes. *Br J Sports Med.* 2007;41(4):217–223.

AUTHOR: DELLA LEE

BASIC INFORMATION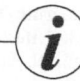

DEFINITION
Rupture of the tendon that runs over the patella to the tibial tubercle.

SYNONYMS
Patellar ligament rupture

ICD-9CM CODES
844.8 Sprain of other specified sites of knee and leg
727.66 Nontraumatic rupture of patellar tendon

OPTIMAL NUMBER OF VISITS
12

MAXIMAL NUMBER OF VISITS
36

ETIOLOGY
- Typically occurs unilaterally as a result of a traumatic athletic activity involving a severe overloading of the extensor mechanism.
- May also occur after chronic tendon degeneration caused by repetitive microtrauma, systemic disease, or history of prior steroid injections.
- With unilateral, traumatic ruptures, when the knee is in a flexed knee position, the patellar tendon sustains greater stress than the quadriceps tendon and the tensile load is much higher at the insertion sites than in the midsubstance of the tendon, resulting in ruptures most often observed at the inferior pole of the patella.
- Histological studies of ruptured tendons primarily demonstrate grossly attenuated tendons, with chronic degenerative and reparative changes.

EPIDEMIOLOGY AND DEMOGRAPHICS
- Patellar tendon ruptures are rare; however, they are the third most common cause of disruption of the knee extensor mechanism.
- Ruptures most commonly occur in individuals younger than 40 years, with peak incidence between ages 30 to 40 years, who participate in athletic activities that overload the extensor mechanism.
- Patients with systemic disorders, such as SLE, diabetes mellitus, rheumatological disease, chronic renal insufficiency, and hyperparathyroidism, are at a higher risk for a rupture.
- Patients who have received a local injection of corticosteroids are at higher risk for a rupture. A history of receiving

2 to 3 steroid injections to the tendon before the rupture was found in 60% of patients with a patellar tendon rupture.
- May occur as a surgical complication in patients who have undergone a TKA or ACL reconstruction using a patellar tendon autograft.

MECHANISM OF INJURY
- An activity that results in a very strong quadriceps contraction that coincides with sudden knee flexion such as landing from a jump.
- A force 17.5 times the body weight is necessary to rupture a healthy patellar tendon in a young individual.
- In patients with systemic disease, the patellar tendon tends to tear midsubstance.

COMMON SIGNS AND SYMPTOMS
- Inability to extend the knee and inability to walk
- Patient reports immediate severe pain, popping, or tearing sensation and inability to stand up or walk immediately after the injury
- Immediate swelling after the injury
- Complaints of instability or giving way

AGGRAVATING ACTIVITIES
- Walking
- Knee extension
- Squatting
- Going up and down stairs

EASING ACTIVITIES
Inactivity

24-HOUR SYMPTOM PATTERN
None

PAST HISTORY FOR THE REGION
History of patellar tendinopathy or a surgical complication after TKA or ACL reconstruction with a patellar tendon autograft

PHYSICAL EXAMINATION
- Pain, diffuse swelling, ecchymosis, hemarthrosis
- Palpable defect distal to the patella
- Palpable or observable patella alta
- Quadriceps manual muscle testing grade 1/5
- Inability to extend the knee
- Quadriceps atrophy

IMPORTANT OBJECTIVE TESTS
- Patella is superiorly displaced and observed as patella alta on radiographs.
- MRI
- Ultrasonography

DIFFERENTIAL DIAGNOSIS
- Quadriceps tendon rupture
- Patellar fracture
- Patellar dislocation

CONTRIBUTING FACTORS
- Systemic disease: RA, diabetes mellitus, chronic renal failure
- History of ACL repair with patellar tendon autograft
- History of multiple corticosteroid injections to the patellar tendon

TREATMENT

SURGICAL OPTIONS
- Repair typically involves suturing the patellar tendon back onto the tibial tubercle and repair of any retinacular tears that typically accompany a patellar tendon rupture.
- In chronic ruptures, extensive release of scar tissue and the use of a tendon allograft or autograft may be required.

INDICATIONS FOR SURGERY
Any patellar tendon rupture should be surgically repaired for optimal outcomes.

SURGICAL OUTCOME
- Outcomes depend largely on time between rupture and repair.
- Patients who are able to have surgery immediately after the injury have a good chance of achieving full knee ROM with full return of strength and function.

REHABILITATION
- Days 3 to 13
  - Non–weight-bearing, immobilized
  - Control of inflammation and pain via modalities and medication
  - Gentle hamstring and quadriceps isometric exercises (no straight leg raises)
  - Gentle patellar mobilizations
  - Passive knee extension to 0 degrees; gentle active knee flexion up to 45 degrees
- Weeks 2 to 4
  - Gait training with toe touch weight bearing with hinged knee brace locked in extension
  - Inflammation and pain control
  - Maintain passive knee extension to 0 degrees and gentle active knee flexion up to 90 degrees
  - Maintain patellar mobility
  - Continue with isometric hamstring and quadriceps exercises (no straight leg raises)

- Weeks 4 to 6
  - Weight-bearing gait training as tolerated with assistive device or if possible discontinue use of crutches with hinged knee brace locked in extension
  - Active and passive knee flexion exercises as tolerated
  - Continue with isometric hamstring and quadriceps exercises (no straight leg raises)
- Weeks 6 to 12
  - Gait training without assistive device with hinged knee brace locked in extension until normal gait and good quadriceps control are achieved.
  - Begin straight leg raises (no resistance).
  - Stationary bicycle at 8 weeks
- Weeks 12 to 16
  - Full weight-bearing gait training without brace
  - Balance/proprioception training
  - Continue to progress with hamstring and quadriceps strengthening exercise
- Weeks 16 to 24
  - Begin running and work-specific or sport-specific training.
- At 6 months
  - Begin jumping and contact sports-specific training
- Basic postoperative goals after repair of a patellar tendon
  - 2 weeks: Full passive knee extension, between 45 and 60 degrees of active knee flexion ROM
  - 4 to 6 weeks: Up to 90 degrees of active knee flexion ROM
  - 6 to 8 weeks: Full knee flexion ROM
  - 4 months: Negative extensor lag with a straight leg raise
  - 6 months: Jumping and sports-related activities
- Complications may occur during rehabilitation such as the following:
  - Patellar tendinitis
  - Patellofemoral pain syndrome
  - Chondromalacia of the patella

PROGNOSIS

- Prompt diagnosis and repair is very important to a favorable prognosis.
- Patients with chronic ruptures have less-favorable outcomes because of development of scar tissue and the proximal retraction of the tendon, complicating the repair.
- Rehabilitation time increases in chronic cases because of severe muscle atrophy and pronounced long-term functional limitations.

SIGNS AND SYMPTOMS INDICATING REFERRAL TO PHYSICIAN

- DVT
- Signs associated with infection

SUGGESTED READINGS

Enad JG, Loomis LL. Patellar tendon repair: Postoperative treatment. *Arch Phys Med Rehabil.* 2000;81(6):786-788.

Kannus P, Jozsa L. Histopathological changes preceding spontaneous rupture of a tendon. A controlled study of 891 patients. *J Bone Joint Surg Am.* 1991;73:1507-1525.

Kasten P, Schewe B, Maurer F, Gosling T, Krettek C, Weise K. Rupture of the patellar tendon: a review of 68 cases and a retrospective study of 29 ruptures comparing two methods of augmentation. *Arch Orthop Trauma Surg.* 2000;121:578-582.

Kellersman R, Blattert, TR, Weckbach A. Bilateral patellar tendon rupture without predisposing systemic disease or steroid use: a case report and review of the literature. *Arch Orthop Trauma Surg.* 2005;125:127-133.

Kelly DW, Carter VS, Jobe FW, Kerlan RK. Patellar and quadriceps tendon ruptures—jumper's knee. *Am J Sports Med.* 1984;12(5):375-380.

Rose PS, Frassica FJ. Atraumatic bilateral patellar tendon rupture. *J Bone Joint Surg Am.* 2001;83(9):1382-1386.

Zernicke RF, Garhammer J, Jobe JF. Human patellar-tendon rupture. *J Bone Joint Surg Am.* 1977;59:179-183.

AUTHOR: DELLA LEE

BASIC INFORMATION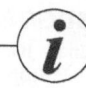

DEFINITION

Pain located behind or around the patella.

SYNONYMS

- Runner's knee
- Chondromalacia patella
- Retropatellar pain syndrome
- Anterior Knee Pain Syndrome

ICD-9CM CODES

719.46 Pain in joint involving lower leg

OPTIMAL NUMBER OF VISITS

6

MAXIMAL NUMBER OF VISITS

24

ETIOLOGY

- Repetitive, overuse activities cause increased force at the patellofemoral joint, resulting in pain during flexion and extension activities.
- Factors that may lead to abnormal patellofemoral joint compression forces include the following:
  - Decreased knee extensor or gluteal muscle strength
  - Pes planus or pes cavus
  - Excessive foot pronation
  - Wide Q angle
  - Increased tibial torsion or femoral anteversion
  - Decreased flexibility of quadriceps, hamstrings, or ITB
  - Genu recurvatum, genu valgus, or genu varus
  - Lateral retinaculum tightness
  - Patella alta or patella baja
  - Patellar instability
- Patellofemoral joint pain occurs when increased or abnormal amounts of stress are placed on the undersurface of the patella as it tracks up and down in the trochlear groove during knee flexion and extension.
- Excessive joint loading secondary to abnormal patellofemoral joint mechanics during flexion-extension activities results in pain and inflammation.
- As the knee moves from extension to flexion, the quadriceps must increase force to counter the flexion moment. This leads to increased compressive loads at the patellofemoral joint as the knee moves into greater degrees of flexion. Therefore, to minimize patellofemoral joint stress, the greatest amount of patellar contact surface area should ideally be when compressive loads on the joint are at their highest.
- Abnormal patellar tracking may increase stress to the patellofemoral joint if the articulating surface area of the patella changes or decreases as it glides up against the patellar articulating surface of the femur as the knee moves into flexion.

EPIDEMIOLOGY AND DEMOGRAPHICS

- Patellofemoral pain syndrome is the most common problem involving the knee, accounting for 25% of knee injuries.
- Most cases commonly occur in adolescents and young adults, especially active individuals.
- More commonly affects females than males.

MECHANISM OF INJURY

No specific mechanism of injury. Typically results from one or a combination of multiple factors, resulting in abnormal patellofemoral joint mechanics.

COMMON SIGNS AND SYMPTOMS

- Generalized knee pain, pain behind the patella, or peripatellar pain
- Swelling
- Crepitus
- Pain typically increases with prolonged or repeated activity
- There is no referral pattern for patellofemoral pain syndrome.

AGGRAVATING ACTIVITIES

- Prolonged sitting ("movie-goers' knee" or "theater sign")
- Running
- Walking
- Ascending or descending stairs
- Squatting
- Bicycling

EASING ACTIVITIES

Avoidance of knee-flexion activities or prolonged flexed postures

24-HOUR SYMPTOM PATTERN

Increased pain with increasing activity throughout the day

PAST HISTORY FOR THE REGION

- Patellar subluxation or dislocation
- ACL reconstruction with patellar tendon graft
- Trauma
- History of chronic knee pain
- Recent change in activity (increase)

PHYSICAL EXAMINATION

- Pain with patellar compression into the trochlear groove (patellar grind test)
- Laterally tilted patella
- Hypomobile medial patellar glide
- Midfoot hypermobility
- Pes planus or pes cavus
- Knee extensor weakness
- Hip extensor or abductor weakness
- Decreased hip external rotation ROM
- Decreased hamstring, quadriceps, or ITB flexibility
- Q angle greater than 17 degrees
- Generalized ligamentous laxity
- Femoral anteversion

IMPORTANT OBJECTIVE TESTS

Laboratory examinations are typically not necessary to diagnose this pathology; however, plain radiographs may be helpful to see the position of the patella.

DIFFERENTIAL DIAGNOSIS

- Tibial-femoral joint osteoarthritis
- Meniscal lesion
- ACL or PCL tear
- Patellar tendinopathy
- Osgood-Schlatter disease
- OCD
- Chondromalacia patella
- ITBFS

CONTRIBUTING FACTORS

Hip or ankle pathology or altered biomechanics in these regions are major factors that contribute to patellar femoral pain.

TREATMENT

SURGICAL OPTIONS

Surgery is rarely performed; however, an arthroscopic lateral retinacular release may be performed in chronic cases.

INDICATIONS FOR SURGERY

Surgery indicators include failure to respond to physical therapy and a stable patella that is excessively laterally tilted because of tight retinacular tissue, preventing normal tracking of the patella in the trochlear groove.

SURGICAL OUTCOMES

Lateral retinacular releases are generally unsuccessful if performed on patients with patellar instability, but they have been shown to have good success rates if performed on a stable patella.

REHABILITATION

- Chief goal is to identify the impairments that are the primary contributing factors leading to abnormal patellar tracking such as abnormal foot alignment or mechanics, decreased flexibility of lateral hip and knee soft tissue structures, or weak hip abductors or external rotators.

- Avoid the following activities and exercises that increase patellofemoral joint stress:
  - Deep squatting activities
  - Stairs and step ups
  - Avoiding the last 30 degrees of knee extension with long arc quad exercises
  - ROMs that increase stress at the patellofemoral joint
  - Open kinetic chain exercises: Between 0 and 30 degrees of knee flexion
  - Closed kinetic chain exercises: Limit knee flexion range up to 60 to 90 degrees.
- Specific interventions may be beneficial in treating patellofemoral pain syndrome
  - Medial patellar glides and tilts improve patellar mobility medially and stretch the lateral retinaculum.
  - STM and stretching of the proximal lateral hip musculature and ITB may help to decrease the lateral pull of the patella.
  - Patellar taping promotes normal patellar tracking.

- Use of orthotics to correct foot malalignment (typically pes planus or excessive foot pronation)
- Quadriceps strengthening within the ranges that minimize patellofemoral joint stress
- Knee extension, avoiding the terminal knee extension range
- Seated and supine leg press, avoiding knee flexion range greater than 60 degrees

PROGNOSIS

The majority of patients have good success with conservative treatment.

SIGNS AND SYMPTOMS INDICATING REFERRAL TO PHYSICIAN

Failure to respond to conservative treatment

SUGGESTED READINGS

Boling MC, Bolgla LA, Mattacola CG, Uhl TL, Hosey RG. Outcomes of a weight-bearing rehabilitation program for patients diagnosed with patellofemoral pain syndrome. *Arch Phys Med Rehabil*. 2006;87(11):1428-1435.

Brushoj C, Holmich P, Nielsen MB, Albrecht-Beste E. Acute patellofemoral pain: aggravating activities, clinical examination, MRI and ultrasound findings. *Br J Sports Med*. 2008;42(1):64-67.

Fredericson M, Yoon K. Physical examination and patellofemoral pain syndrome. *Am J Phys Med Rehabil*. 2006;85(3):234-243.

MacIntyre NJ, Hill NA, Fellows RA, Ellis RE, Wilson DR. Patellofemoral joint kinematics in individuals with and without patellofemoral pain syndrome. *J Bone Joint Surg Am*. 2006;88-A(12):2596-2605.

Steinkamp LA, Dillingham MF, Markel MD, Hill JA, Kaufman KR. Biomechanical considerations in patellofemoral joint rehabilitation. *Am J Sports Med*. 1993;21(3):339-444.

Willson JD, Davis IS. Lower extremity mechanics of females with and without patellofemoral pain across activities with progressively greater task demands. *Clin Biomech*. 2008;23(2):203-211.

AUTHOR: DELLA LEE

BASIC INFORMATION

DEFINITION

- The Pellegrini-Stieda sign, a finding seen on x-rays of the knee, is a calcium deposit on the medial side of the knee, where the tibial collateral ligament (TCL) attaches to the femur. A Pellegrini-Stieda sign is often seen in people who have had a TCL injury.
- Pellegrini-Stieda syndrome occurs when there is pain over this calcium deposit.

SYNONYMS

- TCL sprain
- Medial collateral ligament sprain
- Köhler-Pellegrini shadow
- Köhler-Stieda-Pellegrini syndrome
- Pellegrini's disease
- Pellegrini's syndrome
- Stieda's fracture
- Stieda's lesion
- Stieda-Pellegrini disease

ICD-9CM CODES
726.62 Tibial collateral ligament bursitis

OPTIMAL NUMBER OF VISITS

8 or less

MAXIMAL NUMBER OF VISITS

12

ETIOLOGY

- Pellegrini-Stieda syndrome is a result of ossification of the superior portion of the TCL of the knee, usually caused by trauma with subsequent hemorrhage.
- Subsequently, there is formation of bone in soft tissue that is neither needed nor desired.
- Physiologically, there is direct trauma to the area, which produces abnormal bone formation.

EPIDEMIOLOGY AND DEMOGRAPHICS

- Pellegrini-Stieda syndrome can occur at any age.
- Both genders appear to be equally affected.

MECHANISM OF INJURY

- The pathology appears after valgus force is applied to the knee.
- Direct trauma to the medial aspect of the knee can also result in Pellegrini-Stieda syndrome.

COMMON SIGNS AND SYMPTOMS

- Swelling
- Decreased ROM

- Tenderness on palpation and pressure over the internal condyle of the femur
- Possibly a palpable mass over the TCL
- Pain is generally localized to regions directly adjacent to the TCL. There is typically no referral of symptoms.

AGGRAVATING ACTIVITIES

- Walking
- Changing direction
- Cutting
- Running
- Standing
- Climbing stairs

EASING ACTIVITIES

- Elevation
- Prescription antiinflammatory medications, muscle relaxants, and pain medications to address the patient's symptoms
- Ice
- Rest

24-HOUR SYMPTOM PATTERN

- Initially, symptoms follow normal inflammatory patterns. The knee is stiff and painful for 30 minutes in the morning and with overuse.
- As the inflammatory phase diminishes, the morning stiffness abates, but pain with overuse continues.

PAST HISTORY FOR THE REGION

The pathology is typically a result of trauma. No other prior history of pathology needs to be present.

PHYSICAL EXAMINATION

- Tenderness along the course of the TCL, especially at its femoral attachment
- Swelling is often present in the medial aspect of the knee.

IMPORTANT OBJECTIVE TESTS

- Valgus stress test positive is initially and may or may not be positive as time progresses and the TCL heals.
- X-ray reveals calcification of the TCL.

DIFFERENTIAL DIAGNOSIS

- Muscle strain
- Myofascial pain
- Patellofemoral stress syndrome
- Early degenerative joint disease
- Lateral meniscal pathology
- Superior tibiofibular joint sprain
- Popliteal or biceps femoris tendinitis
- Common peroneal nerve injury
- Tendinitis
- Referred pain from the lumbar spine or hip.
- Femoral stress fracture

- Infection
- Neoplasm
- Tibial spine fracture
- Tibial plateau fractures
- Osteochondral fracture
- Knee dislocation
- Patella dislocation
- Meniscal tear
- Multiligamentous injury
- Knee dislocation
- Posterolateral instability
- Osteochondral fracture
- Tibial plateau fracture
- Extensor mechanism rupture
- Osteonecrosis of the femoral epicondyle
- Osteonecrosis of the tibial condyle
- Inflammatory conditions (systemic disease)

CONTRIBUTING FACTORS

Direct and indirect trauma

TREATMENT

INDICATIONS FOR SURGERY

- Conservative treatment fails
- Significant decrease in knee ROM
- Knee contracture
- Limitation in function

SURGICAL OPTIONS

- Arthroscopic surgery
  - Arthroscopic release
  - Partial removal of ossification

REHABILITATION

- Rehabilitation mirrors a traditional TCL rehabilitation program. The focus is on the following:
  - Encourage ROM
  - Strengthen the lower extremities: quadriceps, hamstrings, hips
  - Proprioceptive training

Phase I: Acute Inflammatory Phase (Days 0 to 14 after injury)
- When to progress to phase: Initial injury to the ligaments
- Goals of phase
  - Decrease inflammation and promote healing.
  - Maintain ROM.
- Interventions
  - Medications: Antiinflammatories and/or muscle relaxants
  - Modalities: Ice
  - Myofascial release to global muscles
  - Lower extremity flexibility: Hamstrings and hip flexors
  - Home exercise program: RICE, lower extremity flexibility, and ROM

Phase 2: Reparative Phase (Days 15 to 21 after injury)
- When to progress to phase: Progress as pain allows
- Goals of phase

○ Restore normal ROM.
○ Achieve full-extension ROM.
○ Strengthening
○ Minimize swelling.
• Interventions
○ Medications as needed
○ Modalities as needed
○ Myofascial release to global muscles; progress as needed.
○ Lower extremity flexibility: Hamstrings and hip flexors
○ Home exercise program: Walking program, lower extremity flexibility and strengthening.

Phase 3: Remodeling Phase (Days 22 to 60 after injury)
• When to progress to phase
○ Pain-free ROM
○ No functional limitations
• Goals of phase
○ Increase agility.
○ Progress to return to sports.
○ Address contributing factors.
• Interventions
○ Medications and myofascial release as needed
○ Home exercise program: Progress lower extremity flexibility and strengthening program.
○ Other: Address contributing factors.

Phase 4: Remodeling Phase (Days 60 to 360 after injury)
• When to progress to phase: No functional limitations
• Goals of phase
○ Correction of contributing factors
○ Retraining muscle activity to account for functional activities
• Interventions
○ Medications and myofascial release as needed
○ Home exercise program: Progress lower extremity flexibility and strengthening program.
○ Other: Address contributing factors, functional rehabilitation, and retraining.

PROGNOSIS

Most patients have excellent outcomes.

SIGNS AND SYMPTOMS INDICATING REFERRAL TO PHYSICIAN

• Constant unrelenting leg pain: Infection or tumor
• Pain that does not change with position: Infection or tumor
• Major trauma: Fracture
• History of cancer: Metastatic disease
• Fevers and chills: Infection or tumor

SUGGESTED READINGS

Dutton M. *Orthopaedic Examination, Evaluation, & Intervention*. McGraw-Hill Inc; 2004.

Hastings DE. The non-operative management of collateral ligament injuries of the knee joint. *Clin Orthop*. 1980;(147):22-28.

Mendes LF, Pretterklieber ML, Cho JH, Garcia GM, Resnick DL, Chung CB. Pellegrini-Stieda disease: a heterogeneous disorder not synonymous with ossification/calcification of the tibial collateral ligament-anatomic and imaging investigation. *Skeletal Radiol*. 2006;35(12):916-922.

Niitsu M, Ikeda K, Iijima T, Ochiai N, Noguchi M, Itai Y. MR Imaging of Pellegrini-Stieda disease. *Radiat Med*. 1999;17(6):405-409.

Quarles JD, Hosey RG. Medial and lateral collateral injuries: prognosis and treatment. *Prim Care*. 2004;31(4):957-975, ix.

Wang JC, Shapiro MS. Pellegrini-Stieda syndrome. *Am J Orthop*. 1995; 24(60):493-497.

Wiener SL. *Differential Diagnosis of Acute Pain By Body Region*. New York: McGraw-Hill; 1993.

AUTHOR: BERNARD LI

Section III

ORTHOPEDIC PATHOLOGY

BASIC INFORMATION

DEFINITION

- Pes anserinus means "goose's foot," and this is a literal description of the webbed foot-like structure. The conjoined tendon lies superficial to the tibial insertion of the MCL of the knee.
- The tendon inserts into the anteromedial proximal tibia. From anterior to posterior, the three tendons inserting from the sartorius, gracilis, and semitendinosus along the medial tibial plateau are collectively called the pes anserinus
- This condition can involve any of the bursae lying between the various tendons of the superficial pes anserinus or a bursa between the MCL and the superficial pes anserinus.
- Inflammation of the bursae is common in novice swimmers and long-distance runners.

SYNONYMS

Breaststroker's knee

ICD-9CM CODES
726.61 Pes anserinus tendinitis or
        bursitis

OPTIMAL NUMBER OF VISITS

6 or fewer

MAXIMAL NUMBER OF VISITS

12

ETIOLOGY

- Acute trauma to the medial knee
- Athletic overuse
- Chronic mechanical and degenerative processes
- Obesity is associated with pes anserine bursitis, particularly in middle-aged women.
- Pes planus (i.e., flat foot) may predispose patients to this bursitis and other problems in the medial knee.
- Sporting activities that require side-to-side movement or cutting have been associated with pes anserine bursitis.
- Local trauma, exostosis, and tendon tightness may predispose the patient to inflammation.
- Pes anserine bursitis is most common in young individuals involved in sporting activities and in obese middle-aged women.
- This condition also is common in patients aged 50 to 80 years who have osteoarthritis of the knees.
- The sartorius, gracilis, and semitendinosus muscles are primary flexors of the knee. These muscles also influence internal rotation of the tibia and protect the knee against rotary and valgus stress.

Theoretically, bursitis results from stress to this area.
- A number of bursae are situated in the soft tissues around the knee joint. The bursae reduce friction and cushion the movement of one body part over another. The bursae become inflamed.

EPIDEMIOLOGY AND DEMOGRAPHICS

- Obese middle-aged women
- Older individuals with arthritis
- A slight preponderance of females over males.
- Incidence of bursitis in runners may be as high as 10%.

MECHANISM OF INJURY

- The sartorius, gracilis, and semitendinosus muscles influence internal rotation of the tibia and protect the knee against rotary and valgus stress.
- Excessive stress to the bursae

COMMON SIGNS AND SYMPTOMS

The hallmark physical finding is pain over the proximal medial tibia at the insertion of the conjoined tendons of the pes anserinus, approximately 2 to 5 cm below the anteromedial joint margin of the knee.

AGGRAVATING ACTIVITIES

- Ascending stairs
- Descending stairs
- Arising from a seated position
- Sport that requires side-to-side movement or cutting
- Swimming, occasionally called breaststroker's knee

EASING ACTIVITIES

- Rest
- Ice
- Prescription antiinflammatory medications, muscle relaxants, and pain medications to address the patient's symptoms

24-HOUR SYMPTOM PATTERN

- Weight-bearing activity.
- Symptoms increase during the day and if sitting too long.
- Sleeping may or may not be problematic.

PAST HISTORY FOR THE REGION

- Repetitive injury or trauma to the area
- The pain and discomfort are present for several days to several weeks but eventually resolve on their own.

PHYSICAL EXAMINATION

- The bursa usually is not palpable unless effusion and thickening are present.

- Valgus stress may reproduce the symptoms in athletic individuals, making it hard to distinguish from MCL injuries. Typically, painful tenderness in association with MCL injuries is superior and posterior to the pes anserine bursa.
- If swelling can be traced more proximally along the pes anserinus tendons, a formal tendinitis may be present, and a snapping of the pes anserinus tendons can occur.
- An exostosis of the tibia has been described in athletes and may contribute to chronic symptoms.
- Distal insertion of the sartorius, gracilis, and semitendinous tendons along the medial tibial plateau

IMPORTANT OBJECTIVE TESTS

The hallmark physical finding is pain over the proximal medial tibia at the insertion of the conjoined tendons of the pes anserinus, approximately 2 to 5 cm below the anteromedial joint margin of the knee.

DIFFERENTIAL DIAGNOSIS

- Fibromyalgia
- Hamstring strain
- MCL and LCL injuries
- Myofascial pain
- Osteoarthritis
- Patellofemoral syndrome
- Prepatellar bursitis
- Stress fracture

TREATMENT

SURGICAL OPTIONS

In cases of disability, such as those causing 6 to 8 weeks of limitation among athletes, some surgeons advocate resection, especially if mature exostosis is present and causing irritation. The operation includes excision of the bursa and any bony exostosis.

REHABILITATION

- The goal of rehabilitation is twofold. First, the focus should be on decreasing the patient's symptoms. Once the symptoms have diminished, the focus of the rehabilitative process turns to preventing further episodes.
- Rest and nonsteroidal antiinflammatory drugs (NSAIDs) are first-line treatment.
- Ice in foam cups can be applied and rubbed directly on the patient's skin (ice massage) for up to 10 minutes at a time. Other forms of cryotherapy (e.g., cold packs) also may be used.
- Ultrasound has been reported to be effective in reducing inflammation associated with pes anserine bursitis.

- Electrical stimulation has been used in other forms of bursitis, although its use has not been documented specifically in pes anserine bursitis.
- Rehabilitation exercise for athletes with significant medial knee stress follows general physiatric principles for knee disorders (stretching and strengthening of the adductor and quadriceps groups [especially the last 30 degrees of knee extension using the vastus medialis muscle] and stretching of the hamstrings). For cases caused by restricted flexibility of muscles and/or tendons, stretching may promote significant reduction of tension over the bursa.
- Advise older patients and those with chronic pain to avoid muscle atrophy from disuse. Address obesity in cases where it is a contributing factor.
- Exercises that promote movement of the region in a pain-free range
- Intrabursal injection with local anesthetics and/or corticosteroids
- Initially, exercises that minimize the stress to the pes anserine area should be used. Lower extremity flexibility should be used to increase ROM.

Phase I: Acute Inflammatory Phase (Days 0 to 14 after injury)
- When to progress to phase: Initial injury to the pes anserinus region
- Goals of phase
  - Decrease inflammation and irritation and promote healing.
- Interventions
  - Medications: Antiinflammatories and/or muscle relaxants
  - Modalities: Ultrasound and ice massage to break pain cycle
  - Myofascial release to global muscles (sartorius, gracilis, and semitendinosus)
  - Lower extremity flexibility: Hamstrings and hip flexors
  - Home exercise program: Walking program, lower extremity flexibility

Phase 2: Reparative Phase (Days 15–21 after injury)
- When to progress to phase
  - Progress as pain allows

- Goals of phase:
  - Restore normal ROM
  - Return patient to prior functional status
- Interventions:
  - Medications as needed
  - Modalities as needed.
  - Myofascial release to global muscles; progress as needed.
  - Lower extremity flexibility: Hamstrings and hip flexors
  - Home exercise program: Walking program, lower extremity flexibility and strengthening.

Phase 3: Remodeling Phase (Days 22 to 60 after injury)
- When to progress to phase
  - Pain-free ROM
  - No functional limitations
- Goals of phase
  - Identify factors that contribute to pes anserinus syndrome
  - Address contributing factors.
- Interventions
  - Medications and myofascial release as needed
  - Home exercise program: Progress lower extremity flexibility and strengthening program.
  - Other: Address contributing factors.

Phase 4: Remodeling Phase (Days 60 to 360 after injury)
- When to progress to phase: No functional limitations
- Goals of phase
  - Correction of contributing factors
  - Retraining muscle activity to account for functional activities
- Interventions
  - Medications and myofascial release as needed
  - Home exercise program: Progress lower extremity flexibility and strengthening program.
  - Other: Address contributing factors, functional rehabilitation, and retraining

CONTRIBUTING FACTORS

- Acute trauma to the medial knee
- Athletic overuse
- Chronic mechanical and degenerative processes

- Obesity is associated with pes anserine bursitis, particularly in middle-aged women.
- Pes planus (i.e., flat foot) may predispose patients to this bursitis and other problems in the medial knee.
- Sporting activities that require side-to-side movement or cutting have been associated.
- Tight muscle groups, especially the hip flexors and hamstrings
- Local trauma, exostosis, and tendon tightness may predispose the patient to inflammation.

PROGNOSIS

- Patients with pes anserine bursitis generally are treated successfully with conservative measures and are recommended for outpatient physical therapy.
- Surgical intervention is required only rarely. Rest, administration of NSAIDs, or injection brings about resolution in most cases. Chronic arthritic diseases that often accompany bursitis obviously persist, but identification and treatment of pes anserine bursitis can reduce pain significantly. Most athletes return to play sports.

SIGNS AND SYMPTOMS INDICATING REFERRAL TO PHYSICIAN

- Tenderness in the distal or middle third of the bone: Stress fracture of the tibia
- Recurrent episodes of deep, distal calf pain: Compartment syndrome
- Tenderness over the adjacent muscle at the tibial margin: Medial tibial stress syndrome
- Major trauma: Fracture
- History of cancer: Metastatic disease
- Fevers and chills: Infection or tumor

SUGGESTED READINGS

Dutton M. *Orthopaedic Examination, Evaluation, & Intervention.* New York: McGraw-Hill; 2004.

Wiener SL. *Differential Diagnosis of Acute Pain by Body Region.* New York: McGraw-Hill; 1993.

AUTHOR: BERNARD LI

Section III

ORTHOPEDIC PATHOLOGY

BASIC INFORMATION

DEFINITION

- A sudden or violent twist or wrench of the tibiofemoral joint that results in stretching or tearing of the posterior cruciate ligament (PCL).
- The PCL is a tough band of fibrous tissue that connects the bones of the upper and lower leg at the knee joint.
- Like other types of sprains, knee sprains are classified according to the following grading system:
  - ○ Grade I (mild): This injury stretches the ligament, which causes microscopic tears in the ligament. These tiny tears don't significantly affect the overall ability of the knee joint to support your weight.
  - ○ Grade II (moderate): The ligament is partially torn, and there is some mild to moderate instability (or periodic giving out) of the knee while standing or walking.
  - ○ Grade III (severe): The ligament is torn completely or separated at its end from the bone, and the knee is more unstable.

SYNONYMS

- PCL tear
- PCL sprain

ICD-9CM CODES
848.9 Unspecified site of sprain and strain
717.84 Old disruption of posterior cruciate ligament
844.2 Sprain of cruciate ligament of knee

OPTIMAL NUMBER OF VISITS

8 or fewer

MAXIMAL NUMBER OF VISITS

12

ETIOLOGY

- The PCL, like all other ligaments, is composed of type I collagen. The ultrastructure of a ligament is close to that of tendons, but the fibers in a ligament are more variable and have a higher elastin content.
- Ligaments receive their blood supply from their insertion sites. The vascularity within a ligament is uniform, and each ligament contains mechanoreceptors and free nerve endings that are hypothesized to aid in stabilizing the joint.
- The PCL functions to control posterior tibia translation, knee hyperextension, and tibial internal rotation.
- Anatomically, it is composed of two bundles, the anterolateral bundle, which is

taut in flexion, and the posteromedial, which is taut in extension.
- Avulsion of ligaments generally occurs between the unmineralized and mineralized fibrocartilage layers. The PCL injury occurs most commonly at the tibial attachment (70% of the time).
- No one single cause accounts for this injury. PCL injuries can be related to extrinsic and intrinsic factors. Numerous studies document the fact that poor levels of conditioning correlate directly with increased levels of injury. Research also has demonstrated that improved conditioning results in reduced numbers of injuries.

EPIDEMIOLOGY AND DEMOGRAPHICS

PCL is the strongest of all ligaments and less commonly injured (3% to 20% of all knee injuries)

MECHANISM OF INJURY

- The patient with an ACL tear reports an active mechanism of injury. Conversely, most PCL injuries are the result of passive external forces being applied to the knee.
- A posteriorly directed force on a flexed knee, such as the anterior aspect of the flexed knee striking a dashboard, may cause PCL injury.
- A fall onto a flexed knee with the foot in plantar flexion and the tibial tubercle striking the ground first, directing a posterior force to the proximal tibia, may result in injury to the PCL.
- Hyperextension alone may lead to an avulsion injury of the PCL from the origin. This kind of injury may be amenable to repair.
- An anterior force to the anterior tibia in a hyperextended knee with the foot planted results in combined injury to the knee ligaments along with knee dislocation.

COMMON SIGNS AND SYMPTOMS

- Mild knee pain
- Unlike the patient with an ACL injury, these patients rarely report feeling or hearing an audible pop.
- Moderate swelling or hemarthrosis
- Instability and giving away
- Loss of knee motion and moderate stiffness
- Medial joint line pain may be reported.
- Retropatellar pain symptoms
- Swelling and stiffness may be reported in cases of chondral damage.

AGGRAVATING ACTIVITIES

- Semiflexed position
- Ascending or descending stairs or an incline
- Starting a run

- Lifting a load
- Walking longer distances
- Uneven ground may lead to a sensation of instability.

EASING ACTIVITIES

- Elevation
- Prescription antiinflammatory medications, muscle relaxants, and pain medications to address the patient's symptoms.
- Ice
- Rest

24-HOUR SYMPTOM PATTERN

Minimal pain and minimal hemarthrosis noted.

PAST HISTORY FOR THE REGION

- Patient may report prior history of knee injury that has affected the mechanics of the knee.
- Prior injuries to the ankle or hip may also predispose the patient to increased stresses at the knee.

PHYSICAL EXAMINATION

- Joint examination: Observe any gross effusion or bony abnormality.
- Minimal to no pain may be noted by the patient.
- Minimal hemarthrosis is usually noted by the patient.
- Partially full or functional ROM
- Contusion may be present over the anterior tibia.
- Immediate effusion indicates significant intraarticular trauma. Effusion that takes many hours to accumulate usually indicates an extraarticular trauma or involvement of the meniscus.
- The presence of bruising is also a good indicator of tissue injury. Extraarticular injured tissue, such as an MCL or LCL, results in visible bruising. Injuries to intraarticular tissue, such as the ACL and PCL, do not result in visible bruising.
- Ligamentous laxity

IMPORTANT OBJECTIVE TESTS

- Posterior tibial sag sign
- Posterior sag sign during extension
- Positive quadriceps active test
- Posterior drawer test
- MRI is the standard radiographic study if PCL injury is suspected. MRI has been shown to be 96% to 100% sensitive in picking up PCL tears.

DIFFERENTIAL DIAGNOSIS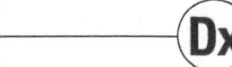

- Muscle strain
- Myofascial pain
- Patellofemoral stress syndrome
- Early degenerative joint disease
- Popliteal or biceps femoris tendinitis

- Tendinitis
- Referred pain from the lumbar spine or hip
- Femoral stress fracture
- Infection
- Neoplasm
- Tibial spine fracture
- Tibial plateau fractures
- Osteochondral fracture
- Knee dislocation
- Meniscal tear
- Multiligamentous injury
- Posterolateral instability
- Osteochondral fracture
- Extensor mechanism rupture
- Osteonecrosis of the femoral epicondyle
- Osteonecrosis of the tibial condyle
- Inflammatory conditions (systemic disease)

CONTRIBUTING FACTORS

- Football, baseball, soccer, skiing, and basketball account for up to 78% of sports-related injuries.
- Long-term use of steroids can weaken knee ligaments.
- Systemic diseases, such as RA or lupus, can predispose a patient to joint laxity.

TREATMENT

SURGICAL OPTIONS

Several different methods have been developed for PCL reconstruction. Unfortunately, no current technique has met with reproducibly excellent results. With this in mind, numerous variables exist involving graft placement, graft choice, type of fixation, and postoperative rehabilitation. Generally, arthroscopic surgery is the treatment of choice.

SURGICAL RECONSTRUCTION

- Autograft
  - Patellar tendon
  - Quadriceps tendon
  - Hamstring tendons
  - Medial head of gastrocnemius
- Autograft strength: Normalized to the patellar tendon
  - Normal ACL: 100%
  - Bone-patellar tendon-bone: 175%
  - Semitendinosus: 75%
  - Gracilis: 49%
  - Iliotibial tract: 38%
  - TFL: 36%
- Allograft
  - Achilles tendon
  - Patellar tendon
  - Quadriceps tendon
  - Hamstring tendons
- Allografts can be rejected.
- Pros:
  - Less invasive to patient
  - Quicker return to function

- Cons:
  - Disease and infection (sterilized via gamma radiation and ethylene oxide)
  - Weaker than autografts (radiation decreases strength by 26% and stiffness by 12%)

SURGICAL INDICATORS

- Desire to return to high-demand sports
- Associated injuries (involvement of MCL or meniscus)
- Abnormal laxity

REHABILITATION

- Whether to have surgery or not is controversial. Many sources suggest nonoperative treatment of PCL injuries. Dandy and Pusey treated 20 patients with persistent knee symptoms caused by unrecognized, isolated PCL injury. At 7.2 years of follow-up, 18 of the 20 had a good functional result. Tietjens recommended that patients with isolated PCL injuries be treated nonoperatively after reporting 80% good or excellent functional results in 50 patients. The remaining 20%, however, had either disabling instability or meniscal tears.
- Rehabilitation of the PCL depends on whether surgery was performed. In patients who underwent surgery, several factor need to be taken into consideration. They include the following:
  - Graft maturation and ligamentation process
  - Autographs are strong at implantation.
  - Autografts undergo "ligamentation," which is a gradual biological transformation of tissue.
  - Collagen forms, remodels, and matures for 1 to 2 years after surgery.
  - The transplanted graft never obtains all of the cellular features of normal PCL tissue.
- Stages of ligamentation
  1. Necrosis (1 to 3 weeks): Cells of graft die because blood supply is interrupted. Collagen matrix remains intact.
  2. Revascularization (6 to 8 weeks): New blood vessels grow into graft. Process takes place peripheral to central.
  3. Cellular proliferation (8 weeks +): New cells can proliferate into graft as early as the first week. The cells are thought to arise from extrinsic sources (synovial fluid and bone marrow) and intrinsic sources (surviving original cells).
  4. Collagen formation, remodeling, and maturation (8 weeks +): Cell proliferation takes place as a continuing process throughout the maturation process. New cells proliferate into graft from the new blood sources, as well as from synovium, ostium, and fat pads.

GENERAL PCL REHABILITATION GUIDELINES

Phase I: Acute Inflammatory Phase (Days 0 to 14 after injury)
- When to progress to phase: Initial injury to the ligament
- Goals of phase
  - Maintain ROM.
  - Decrease inflammation and irritation and promote healing.
- Interventions
  - Medications: Antiinflammatories and/or muscle relaxants
  - Modalities: Electrical stimulation for quadriceps contraction, ultrasound, ice after activity
  - Myofascial release to global muscles as needed
  - Lower extremity flexibility: Hamstrings, ITB, and hip flexors
  - Home exercise program: ROM exercises, lower extremity flexibility, hip strengthening, RICE

Phase 2: Reparative Phase (Days 15 to 21 after injury)
- When to progress to phase: Progress as pain allows
- Goals of phase
  - Restore normal ROM.
  - Achieve full-extension ROM.
  - Minimize swelling.
- Interventions
  - Medications as needed
  - Modalities as needed
  - Myofascial release to global muscles; progress as needed.
  - Lower extremity flexibility: Hamstrings and hip flexors
  - Home exercise program: Walking program, lower extremity flexibility and strengthening

Phase 3: Remodeling Phase (Days 22 to 60 after injury)
- When to progress to phase
  - Pain-free ROM
  - No functional limitations
- Goals of phase
  - Increase agility
  - Progress to return to sports
  - Address contributing factors
- Interventions
  - Medications and myofascial release as needed
  - Home exercise program: Progress lower extremity flexibility and strengthening program.
  - Other: Address contributing factors.

Phase 4: Remodeling Phase (Days 60 to 360 after injury)
- When to progress to phase: No functional limitations
- Goals of phase
  - Correction of contributing factors that result in ligament injury
  - Retraining muscle activity to account for functional activities

- Interventions
  ○ Medications and myofascial release as needed
  ○ Home exercise program: Progress lower extremity flexibility and strengthening program.
  ○ Other: Address contributing factors, functional rehabilitation, and retraining

PROGNOSIS

- Most patients have excellent outcomes.
- The goal of surgery is to stabilize the knee, decrease the chance of future meniscal injury, and delay the arthritic process.

SIGNS AND SYMPTOMS INDICATING REFERRAL TO PHYSICIAN

- Constant unrelenting leg pain or pain that does not change with position: Infection or tumor
- Significant and unexplained weight loss or nocturnal pain: Tumor
- Major trauma: Fracture
- History of cancer: Metastatic disease if all other musculoskeletal factors have been eliminated.

SUGGESTED READINGS

Beynnon BD, Johnson RJ, Abate JA, Fleming BC, Nichols CE. Treatment of anterior cruciate ligament injuries, part I. *Am J Sports Med.* 2005;33(10):1579-602.

Browner BD. *Skeletal Trauma: Fractures, Dislocations, Ligamentous Injuries.* Philadelphia: WB Saunders; 1998.

Dandy DJ, Pusey RJ. The long-term results of unrepaired tears of the posterior cruciate ligament. *J Bone Joint Surg Br.* 1982;64:92-94.

Dugan SA. Sports-related knee injuries in female athletes: What gives? *Arch Phys Med Rehabil.* 2005;84(2):122-130.

Dutton M. *Orthopaedic Examination, Evaluation, & Intervention.* New York: McGraw-Hill; 2004.

Hastings DE. The non-operative management of collateral ligament injuries of the knee joint. *Clin Orthop.* 1980;(147):22-28.

Maday MG, Harner CD, Fu FH. Evaluation and treatment. In: Feagin J.A., ed. *The Crucial Ligaments: Diagnosis, Treatment of Ligamentous Injuries About the Knee.* 2nd ed. New York: Churchill Livingstone; 1994:711-723.

Strayer RJ, Lang ES. Evidence-based emergency medicine/systematic review abstract. Does this patient have a torn meniscus or ligament of the knee? *Ann Emerg Med.* 2006;47(5):499-501.

Tietjens BR. Posterior cruciate ligament injuries. *J Bone Joint Surg Br* 1985;67:674.

Wiener SL. Differential diagnosis of acute pain by body region. New York: McGraw-Hill; 1993.

AUTHOR: BERNARD LI

BASIC INFORMATION

DEFINITION

- Prepatellar bursitis is inflammation of the bursa that lies superficial to the patella.
- The prepatellar bursa is a thin synovial lining located between the skin and the anterior aspect of the patella.
- The pathology is commonly seen in patients who experience recurrent minor trauma of the anterior knee. Those whose occupations require long periods of kneeling are particularly at risk.

SYNONYMS

- Housemaid's knee
- Carpenter's knee
- Gardener's knee

ICD-9CM CODES
726.65 Prepatellar bursitis

OPTIMAL NUMBER OF VISITS
4 or fewer

MAXIMAL NUMBER OF VISITS
12

ETIOLOGY

The prepatellar bursa is a flat, round synovium-lined structure; its main function is to separate the patella from the patellar tendon and skin. This bursa is superficial, suggesting that it is undeveloped at birth. Within the first few months to years of life, the bursa arises from direct pressure and friction. The function of the bursa is to reduce friction and allow maximal ROM. Injury occurs when the prepatellar bursa is subjected to blunt trauma or repetitive microtrauma over the anterior knee.

EPIDEMIOLOGY AND DEMOGRAPHICS

- Prepatellar bursitis affects all age groups; however, in the pediatric age group, it is likely to be septic and to develop in an immunocompromised host.
- Incidence of prepatellar bursitis is greater in males than females.

MECHANISM OF INJURY

- Prepatellar bursitis can occur as a result of the following:
  - Direct trauma (e.g., a fall on the patella or direct blow to the knee)
  - Recurrent minor injuries associated with overuse (e.g., repeated kneeling)
  - Septic or pyogenic process
  - Infection is commonly from *Staphylococcus aureus* (usually from a break in the skin)
  - Can be mistaken for pyogenic arthritis

- Crystal deposition (e.g., gout, pseudogout)
- History of inflammatory disease
- Occupation (carpet layer, coal miner, roofer, plumber, or homemaker)
- Injury occurs when the prepatellar bursa is subjected to blunt trauma or repetitive microtrauma over the anterior knee. Either type of loading can result in swelling of the bursa.

COMMON SIGNS AND SYMPTOMS

- Tenderness of the patella to palpation
- Anterior knee pain
- Localized swelling and erythema of the anterior region of the knee
- Difficulty with ambulation
- Inability to kneel on the affected side
- Relief of pain with rest
- History of repetitive motion
- History of occupation requiring excessive kneeling
- History of a fall on the knee or blunt trauma to the knee (with presentation of symptoms up to 10 days after the incident)
- Fluctuant edema over the lower pole of the patella
- Crepitation of the knee
- Decreased knee flexion secondary to pain

AGGRAVATING ACTIVITIES

- Repetitive motion
- Weight-bearing position
- Going up and down stairs in a reciprocal pattern
- Any increase in pressure to the prepatellar bursitis with an increase in pain

EASING ACTIVITIES

- Relief of pain with rest
- Ice
- Antiinflammatory medications
- Elevation of affected leg
- Braces
- Unloading the prepatellar bursa

24-HOUR SYMPTOM PATTERN

Symptoms are generally activity related. The more aggravating activities experienced during the day, the more pain experienced in the knee.

PAST HISTORY FOR THE REGION

- Patient will presents with a history of repetitive movement leading to microtrauma or blunt trauma.
- Patient may also have an activity or occupation that requires repetitive kneeling.

PHYSICAL EXAMINATION

- Common physical findings include the following:
  - Decreased knee flexion secondary to pain

- Tenderness of the patella to palpation
- Fluctuant edema over the lower pole of the patella
- Erythema of the knee
- Crepitation of the knee
- Decreased knee flexion secondary to pain

IMPORTANT OBJECTIVE TESTS

- Laboratory studies (to rule out other pathologies)
  - White blood cell (WBC) count: >5000 per µL
  - Elevated protein
  - Elevated lactate
  - Decreased glucose
  - Gram-negative results in septic bursitis
  - Monosodium urate crystals found in gout.
  - Calcium pyrophosphate crystals found in pseudogout.
  - Cholesterol crystals found in rheumatoid bursitis.
- Imaging studies
  - Plain radiographs may show soft tissue swelling; however, radiographs are necessary only if other conditions are suggested (e.g., fracture and/or dislocation).
  - CT scan and MRI are reserved for cases that have been difficult to manage (e.g., failure of initial treatment for septic prepatellar bursitis).

DIFFERENTIAL DIAGNOSIS

- Patellar fracture or bruising
- ACL injury
- MCL and LCL Injuries
- Osteoarthritis
- Pes anserinus bursitis
- PCL Injury
- RA
- Cellulitis
- Connective tissue disorders

CONTRIBUTING FACTORS

- Direct trauma
- Overuse
- History of inflammatory disease
- Repetitive kneeling

TREATMENT

MEDICAL/SURGICAL OPTIONS

- Aspiration of prepatellar bursa fluid may be indicated because sepsis is common.
- Consider injecting the prepatellar bursa with corticosteroids only when infection has been excluded.
- Select position of maximal fullness as the site for injection.

- Complications of injection include but are not limited to the following: Infection, bleeding, postinjection inflammation and erythema, postinjection pain, tendon rupture, and subcutaneous atrophy.
- Incision and drainage of the prepatellar bursa usually is performed when symptoms of septic bursitis have not improved significantly within 36 to 48 hours. Surgical removal of the bursa (i.e., bursectomy) may be necessary for chronic or recurrent prepatellar bursitis. Arthroscopic or endoscopic excision of the bursa has more recently been reported to have satisfactory results with less trauma than open excision.

REHABILITATION

- After the initial period of rest, the goal of physical therapy is to regain any loss of ROM, while increasing the flexibility of the quadriceps and hamstrings.
- Use of therapeutic modalities can be helpful to assist stretching in this period.
- As a result of injury, the body attempts to protect the region. This is accomplished by contracting the large global muscles of the region. This is in response to the fact that inflammation shuts down the local muscle fibers. The body must protect and minimize stress to this area. It does so by contracting the large muscle fibers. The lack of motion to the region impedes circulation to the region. Therefore chemical irritants that have been brought into the region in response to the injury do not leave the region.
- Myofascial release techniques can be used to relax the large muscle groups.
- Joint mobilization
- Walking
- Exercises that promote movement of the region in a pain-free range
- Cold or hot pack
- Ultrasound
- Electrical stimulation
- Initially, exercises should be chosen that minimize the stress to the prepatellar bursa such as lower extremity flexibility and knee ROM.

Phase I: Acute Inflammatory Phase (Days 0 to 14 after injury)
- When to progress to phase: Initial injury to the prepatellar region.
- Goals of phase:
  ○ Decrease inflammation and irritation and promote healing.
- Interventions
  ○ Medications: Antiinflammatories and/or muscle relaxants
  ○ Modalities: Ultrasound and ice massage to break pain cycle.
  ○ Myofascial release to global muscles (quadriceps and hamstrings)
  ○ Lower extremity flexibility: Hamstrings and hip flexors
  ○ Home exercise program: Walking program, lower extremity flexibility.

Phase 2: Reparative Phase (Days 15 to 21 after injury)
- When to progress to phase: Progress as pain allows.
- Goals of phase
  ○ Restore normal ROM.
  ○ Return patient to prior functional status.
- Interventions
  ○ Medications as needed
  ○ Modalities as needed.
  ○ Myofascial release to global muscles; progress as needed.
  ○ Lower extremity flexibility: Hamstrings and hip flexors
  ○ Home exercise program: Walking program, lower extremity flexibility and strengthening.

Phase 3: Remodeling Phase (Days 22 to 60 after injury)
- When to progress to phase
  ○ Pain-free ROM
  ○ No functional limitations
- Goals of phase
  ○ Identify factors that contribute to bursitis.
  ○ Address contributing factors.
- Interventions
  ○ Medications and myofascial release as needed
  ○ Home exercise program: Progress lower extremity flexibility and strengthening program.
  ○ Other: Address contributing factors.

Phase 4: Remodeling Phase (Days 60 to 360 after injury)
- When to progress to phase: No functional limitations

- Goals of phase
  ○ Correction of contributing factors that result in ligament sprain
  ○ Retraining muscle activity to account for functional activities
- Interventions
  ○ Medications and myofascial release as needed
  ○ Home exercise program: Progress lower extremity flexibility and strengthening program.
  ○ Other: Address contributing factors, functional rehabilitation, and retraining,

PROGNOSIS

Prognosis is excellent with correct treatment. Most patients make a full recovery to prior level of function.

SIGNS AND SYMPTOMS INDICATING REFERRAL TO PHYSICIAN

- High-velocity trauma: Patellar fracture
- Pain, edema, tenderness, deformity, ecchymosis in supracondylar region: Supracondylar fracture of the femur
- Acute monarthritis with aching or throbbing pain, swelling, redness, tenderness, and warmth, or fever, chills, weakness, diaphoresis, and malaise: Septic prepatellar bursitis (patient may require administration of intravenous [IV] antibiotics.)
- Pain that does not change with position: Infection or tumor
- Significant and unexplained weight loss: Tumor
- Nocturnal pain: Tumor
- History of cancer: Metastatic disease
- Fevers and chills: Infection or tumor

SUGGESTED READINGS

Dutton M. *Orthopaedic Examination, Evaluation, & Intervention.* New York: McGraw-Hill; 2004.

Wiener SL. *Differential Diagnosis of Acute Pain by Body Region.* New York: McGraw-Hill; 1993.

AUTHOR: BERNARD LI

BASIC INFORMATION

DEFINITION

Rheumatoid arthritis (RA) is a chronic, multisystem, progressive, systemic, and inflammatory disease of connective tissue characterized by spontaneous remissions and exacerbations (flare-ups). It is the second most common rheumatic disease after osteoarthritis, but it is the most destructive to synovial joints. Unlike osteoarthritis, RA involves primary tissue inflammation rather than joint degeneration. Although most individuals who develop RA do so in early-to-middle adulthood, some experience a late-onset RA (LORA) in their older years.

SYNONYMS

- RA
- LORA

ICD-9CM CODES
714.0 Rheumatoid arthritis
719.36 Palindromic rheumatism
         involving lower leg

OPTIMAL NUMBER OF VISITS

12 or fewer

MAXIMAL NUMBER OF VISITS

20

ETIOLOGY

- The exact etiology of RA is unclear; it is considered one of many autoimmune disorders. Abnormal immunoglobulin (Ig) G and IgM antibodies develop in response to IgG antigens to form circulating immune complexes. These complexes lodge in connective tissue, especially synovium, and create an inflammatory response. Inflammatory mediators, including cytokines (e.g., tumor necrosis factor), chemokines, and proteases, activate and attract neutrophils and other inflammatory cells. The synovium thickens, fluid accumulates in the joint space, and a pannus forms, eroding joint cartilage and bone. Bony ankylosis, calcifications, and loss of bone density follow.
- The role of genetic influences in the etiology of RA was established by the demonstration of an association with the class II major histocompatibility complex gene product, HLA-DR4.

EPIDEMIOLOGY AND DEMOGRAPHICS

- RA may begin at any age, but there is a peak in onset in women of childbearing years and a second peak in elderly men and women.
- The onset is most frequent during the fourth and fifth decade of life; with 80% of all patients developing the disease between the ages of 35 and 50 years.
- Most individuals who develop RA do so in their early-to-middle adulthood; some experience a LORA in their older years.
- Women are approximately three times as likely to develop RA than men are.
- RA affects approximately 1% of the population worldwide.
- RA is seen throughout the world and affects all races.
- Family studies indicate a genetic predisposition.

MECHANISM OF INJURY

- There is no specific mechanism of injury, but patients with RA generally manifest symptoms that include both joint involvement and systemic problems.
- Although the exact cause of RA is still unknown, it is thought to result from a combination of genetic susceptibility and exposure to a trigger.
- The trigger for onset of RA has yet to be identified. However, stressors to the body, either physical or emotional, result in an abnormal immune response.

COMMON SIGNS AND SYMPTOMS

- Rheumatoid disease typically begins in the joints of the arm or hand.
- The individual complains of joint stiffness lasting longer than 30 minutes on awakening.
- Unlike osteoarthritis, the distal interphalangeal joints of the fingers usually are not involved in RA.
- Characteristically a chronic polyarthritis
- Pain
- Swelling
- Heat (synovitis)
- Generalized weakness
- Vague musculoskeletal weakness
- Fatigue
- Anorexia
- Low-grade fever
- Mild weight loss
- Symmetrical arthritis of small joints of the hands, wrists, feet, and knees
- Rheumatoid nodules
- Over time, disease progression may include the following:
  - Systemic manifestations increase
  - Potentially life-threatening organ involvement begins
  - Cardiac problems such as pericarditis and myocarditis
  - Respiratory complications, such as pleurisy, pulmonary fibrosis, and pneumonitis, are common.
  - As the disease worsens, joints become deformed.
  - Secondary osteoporosis can result in fractures.
  - Hand and finger deformities are typical in the advanced stages of the disease.
  - Palpable subcutaneous nodules, often appearing on the ulnar surface of the arm, are associated with a severe, destructive disease pattern.
- Pathologies commonly associated with RA include the following:
  - Sjögren's syndrome is characterized by dryness of the eyes (keratoconjunctivitis), mouth (xerostomia), and other mucous membranes.
  - Felty's syndrome is characterized by leukopenia and hepatosplenomegaly, often leading to recurrent infections. It encompasses a diverse group of pathogenic mechanisms in RA, all of which result in decreased levels of circulating neutrophils.

AGGRAVATING ACTIVITIES

- Pain in affected joints is aggravated by excessive movement and overuse.
- Weight-bearing activities increase symptoms.

EASING ACTIVITIES

- Heat
- Rest
- Gentle pain-free motion
- Swimming

24-HOUR SYMPTOM PATTERN

- Generalized stiffness is common and is usually greatest after periods of inactivity.
- Stiffness in the morning is present.

PAST HISTORY FOR THE REGION

- Initially, the patient may have no prior indicators or symptoms.
- Stress, emotional or physical, may precede initial onset.
- Flu or illness may precede initial onset.
- There may be a family history of autoimmune disorders.

PHYSICAL EXAMINATION

- Typical picture of bilateral symmetrical inflammatory polyarthritis involving small and large joints in both the upper and lower extremities, with sparing of the axial skeleton except the cervical spine, suggesting the diagnosis.
- Morning stiffness
- Subcutaneous nodules
- Presence of rheumatoid factor and inflammatory synovial fluid with increased numbers of polymorphonuclear leukocytes
- Radiographic findings of juxtaarticular bone demineralization and erosion of the affected joints
- Guidelines for classification of RA: Four of the following seven criteria are

required to classify a patient as having RA:

- ○ Morning stiffness: Stiffness in and around the joints lasting 1 hour before maximal improvement
- ○ Arthritis of three or more joint areas: At least three joint areas, observed by a physician simultaneously, have soft tissue swelling or joint effusion, not just bony overgrowth. The 14 possible joint areas involved are right or left proximal interphalangeal, metacarpophalangeal, wrist, elbow, knee, ankle, and metatarsophalangeal joints.
- ○ Arthritis of hand joints: Arthritis of wrist, metacarpophalangeal joint, or proximal interphalangeal joint
- ○ Symmetrical arthritis: Simultaneous involvement of the same joint areas on both sides of the body
- ○ Rheumatoid nodules: Subcutaneous nodules over bony prominences, extensor surfaces, or juxtaarticular regions observed by the physician.
- ○ Serum rheumatoid factor (RF): Demonstration of abnormal amounts of serum RF by any method for which the result has been positive in less than 5% of normal control subjects.
- ○ Radiographic changes: Typical changes of RA on posteroanterior hand and wrist radiographs that must include erosions or unequivocal bony decalcification localized in or adjacent to the involved joints.
- Patients with two or more clinical diagnoses are not excluded.

IMPORTANT OBJECTIVE TESTS

No single test or group of laboratory tests can confirm a diagnosis of RA, but they can support the findings from the patient's history and the physical findings. A number of immunological tests, such as RF and antinuclear antibody (ANA) titer are available to aid diagnosis. Normal values differ, depending on the precise laboratory technique used.

DIFFERENTIAL DIAGNOSIS

- Gout and pseudogout
- Osteoarthritis
- SLE
- Psoriatic arthritis
- Lyme disease
- Reactive arthritis (Reiter's disease)
- Ankylosing spondylitis
- Sarcoidosis, amyloidosis, Whipple's disease
- Rheumatic fever
- Gonococcal

CONTRIBUTING FACTORS

- RA is a chronic, multisystem disease of unknown etiology.

- Family studies indicate a genetic predisposition.
- Illness or infection
- Stress: Emotional or physical

TREATMENT

SURGICAL OPTIONS

- Joint arthroplasties and total joint replacements
- Open or arthroscopic synovectomy

REHABILITATION

- The goals of physical therapy for RA patients are as follows:
  - ○ Relief of pain
  - ○ Reduction of inflammation
  - ○ Preservation of functional capacity
  - ○ Resolution of the pathologic process
  - ○ Facilitation of healing
- To decrease inflammation, rehabilitation may include the following:
  - ○ Patient education and rest ameliorates symptoms and can be an important component of the total therapeutic program.
  - ○ Myofascial release techniques to relax the large muscle groups
  - ○ Joint mobilization
  - ○ Exercises directed at maintaining muscle strength and joint mobility without exacerbating joint inflammation
  - ○ Cold or hot pack
  - ○ Ultrasound
  - ○ Electrical stimulation

Phase I: Acute Inflammatory Phase (Days 0 to 14 after injury)

- When to progress to phase: Initial onset of symptoms
- Goals of phase
  - ○ Decrease inflammation
  - ○ Provide pain relief
  - ○ Promote healing
- Interventions
  - ○ Medications: Antiinflammatories and/or muscle relaxants
  - ○ Modalities: Superficial or deep heat is an effective modality to relieve joint pain and stiffness and is administered by hot packs, electric mittens, a hot shower, spas, ultrasound, diathermy, or paraffin. Cold is preferable for treatment of an acutely inflamed joint.
  - ○ Myofascial release to global muscles to regain ROM
  - ○ Home exercise program: Aerobic conditioning and resistive exercises

Phase 2: Reparative Phase (Days 15 to 21 after injury)

- When to progress to phase: Progress as pain allows
- Goals of phase
  - ○ Increase ROM
  - ○ Increase strength and endurance
  - ○ Return patient to prior functional status

- Interventions
  - ○ Medications as needed
  - ○ Modalities as needed
  - ○ Myofascial release to global muscles; progress as needed.
  - ○ Lower extremity flexibility: Hamstrings and hip flexors
  - ○ Home exercise program: Walking program, lower extremity flexibility and strengthening

Phase 3: Remodeling Phase (Days 22 to 60 after injury)

- When to progress to phase
  - ○ Pain-free ROM
  - ○ No functional limitations
- Goals of phase
  - ○ Increase strength and endurance.
  - ○ Address contributing factors.
- Interventions
  - ○ Medications and myofascial release as needed
  - ○ Home exercise program: Progress lower extremity flexibility and strengthening program.
  - ○ Other: Address contributing factors.

Phase 4: Remodeling Phase (Days 60 to 360 after injury)

- When to progress to phase: No functional limitations
- Goals of phase
  - ○ Prevention and corrections of deformities
  - ○ Retraining muscle activity to account for functional activities
- Interventions
  - ○ Medications and myofascial release as needed
  - ○ Home exercise program: Progress lower extremity flexibility and strengthening program.
  - ○ Other: Address contributing factors, functional rehabilitation, and retraining.

PROGNOSIS

- The course of RA is quite variable and difficult to predict in an individual patient. Most patients experience persistent but fluctuating disease activity accompanied by a variable degree of joint deformity.
- After 10 to 12 years, less than 20% of patients have no evidence of disability or deformity.
- Features of patients that predict the development of disability include older age, female gender, more severe radiographic involvement, and the presence of rheumatoid nodules or elevated titers of RF.
- Approximately 15% of patients with RA have a short-lived inflammatory process that remits without major deformity.
- Remissions of disease activity are most likely to occur during the first year.
- Persons who present with higher titers of RF, C-reactive protein, and hapto-

globin also have a worse prognosis, as do individuals with subcutaneous nodules or radiographic evidence of erosions at the time of initial evaluation.

• The median life expectancy of persons with RA is shortened by 3 to 7 years.

SIGNS AND SYMPTOMS INDICATING REFERRAL TO PHYSICIAN

• Sudden, unexplained swelling and pain in any joints
• Joint pain associated with a fever or rash
• Pain that is so severe that the patient cannot use the joint
• Side effects that occur with large doses of NSAIDs or other medication used to treat the arthritis
• Mild-to-moderate joint pain that continues and has not improved for more than 6 weeks

SUGGESTED READINGS

Alamanos Y, Voulgari PV, Drosos AA. Incidence and prevalence of rheumatoid arthritis, based on the 1987 American College of Rheumatology criteria: a systematic review. *Semin Arthritis Rheum*. 2006;36(3):182-188.

de Jong Z, Munneke M, Zwinderman AH, Kroon HM, Jansen A, Ronday KH, van Schaardenburg D, Dijkmans BA, Van den Ende CH, Breedveld FC, Vliet Vlieland TP, Hazes JM. Is a long-term, high-intensity exercise program effective and safe in patients with rheumatoid arthritis? *Arthritis Rheum*. 2003;48(9):2415-2424.

Harris Jr ED. Clinical features of rheumatoid arthritis. In: Harris Jr ED et al., eds. *Kelley's Textbook of Rheumatology*. 7th ed. vol. 2. Philadelphia: Elsevier Saunders; 2005:1043-1078.

Kasper DL, Braunwald E, Hauser S, Longo D, Jameson JL, Fauce AS, eds. *Harrison's Principles of Internal Medicine*. 16th ed. New York: McGraw-Hill; 2004.

Majithia V, Geraci SA. Rheumatoid arthritis: diagnosis and management. *Am J Med*. 2007;120(11):936-939.

Murray MT, Pizzorno Jr JE. Rheumatoid arthritis. In: Pizzorno JE, Murray MT, eds. *Textbook of Natural Medicine*. 3rd ed. vol. 2. St. Louis: Churchill Livingstone Elsevier; 2006:2089-2108.

O'Dell J. Therapeutic strategies for rheumatoid arthritis. *N Engl J Med*. 2004;350(25):2591-2602.

O'Dell JR. Rheumatoid arthritis: The clinical picture. In: Koopman WJ, Moreland LW, eds. *Arthritis and Allied Conditions: A Textbook of Rheumatology*. 15th ed. vol. 1. Philadelphia: Lippincott Williams and Wilkins; 2005:1165-1194.

Turesson C, O'Fallon WM, Crowson CS, Gabriel SE, Matteson EL. Extra-articular disease manifestations in rheumatoid arthritis: incidence trends and risk factors over 46 years. *Ann Rheum Dis*. 2003;62(8):722-727.

AUTHOR: BERNARD LI

BASIC INFORMATION

DEFINITION

- The tibiofibular joint is a relatively immobile structure that joins the two shin bones: the fibula (outer) and the tibia (inner). It is separated into two parts: the proximal, or upper joint, just below the knee and the distal joint, which lies above the ankle joint.
- The joints function as follows:
  - Limit the movement between the two shin bones caused by twisting movements of the leg. It is composed of strong ligamentous bands that pass diagonally between the tibia and the fibula.
  - Accept one-sixth of the axial load of the leg.
  - Resist torsional stresses originating from the ankle.
  - Resist tensile forces created with weight bearing.
  - Resist lateral bending forces.
- Subluxation is common in preadolescent girls and resolves with skeletal maturity.

SYNONYMS

- Tibiofibular dislocation
- Proximal tibiofibular (PTF) subluxation

ICD-9CM CODES
836.50　Closed dislocation of knee unspecified part

OPTIMAL NUMBER OF VISITS

6 or fewer

MAXIMAL NUMBER OF VISITS

12

ETIOLOGY

- Injuries are typically seen in activities requiring aggressive twisting motions of the knee.
- The population most commonly affected by this injury is athletes. There does not appear to be an age or gender more prone to superior tibiofibular injury.
- Superior tibiofibular injuries occur secondary to impact or falls with the knee in a fully flexed position, with the foot pointing inward (inversion) and downward.

MECHANISM OF INJURY

- The isolated dislocations are typically seen in activities requiring aggressive twisting motions of the knee such as the following:
  - Soccer
  - Parachuting
  - Horseback riding

- In traumatic cases, the superior tibiofibular injury may occur with the following:
  - Posterior hip dislocation
  - Open tibiofibular fracture
  - Ankle fracture
  - Twisting injury or direct blow

COMMON SIGNS AND SYMPTOMS

- Lateral knee pain
- Pain at the head of the fibula or lateral shin
- Ankle motion may elicit pain.
- May have locking or popping.
- Aggravated by direct pressure over the fibular head.
- Patient may be unable to bear weight.

AGGRAVATING ACTIVITIES

- Full flexion of the knee
- Ankle inversion or motion exacerbates knee
- Weight bearing
- These activities cause increased pressure to the proximal tibiofibular joint.

EASING ACTIVITIES

- Rest
- Ice

24-HOUR SYMPTOM PATTERN

Weight-bearing activity

PAST HISTORY FOR THE REGION

- Repetitive injury or trauma to the area
- The pain and discomfort are present for several days to several weeks.

PHYSICAL EXAMINATION

- Irritability and tenderness noted at the fibular head.
- The following muscles or structures are symptomatic with palpation:
  - LCL (tibial collateral ligament)
  - Biceps femoris muscle
  - Peroneal muscles and nerve

IMPORTANT OBJECTIVE TESTS

- Palpation
- Radiolucent sign
  - Elicited in prone position
  - One hand stabilizes the thigh and the leg is internally rotated in an attempt to produce anterior fibular subluxation.
- Helfet sign
  - Patient bears full weight through the affected limb.
  - Patients PTF instability, they will hook the contralateral limb around the affected calf in an attempt to stabilize the PTF joint.
- Imaging
  - Plain radiographs in true anteroposterior (AP) and lateral planes (72% sensitive)

  - Comparison radiographs of the contralateral extremity (increases sensitivity to 82%)
  - Resnick's line follows the lateral tibial spine and should be found over the midpoint of the fibular head.
  - Computed tomography (CT) scan, if diagnosis is equivocal (86% sensitivity compared with 82% on plain films).

DIFFERENTIAL DIAGNOSIS

- Distal ITB syndrome
- Hamstring strain
- LCL injury
- Myofascial pain
- Osteoarthritis
- Patellofemoral syndrome
- Prepatellar bursitis
- Stress fracture

TREATMENT

SURGICAL OPTIONS

- Acute dislocation: 57% (N = 33) of patients with acute dislocations require surgery for recurrent symptoms.
- Closed reduction under general or local anesthesia
- Open reduction
  - For failed closed reductions
  - Posteromedial and superior dislocations
- Arthrodesis
- Resection of fibular head
- Reconstruction of the PTF joint

REHABILITATION

- The nonsurgical management is usually successful in treating superior tibiofibular injuries.
- Casting for 2 to 3 weeks can be used to immobilize the joint.
- Strap applied 1 cm below fibular head can be used to stabilize the joint.
- Avoid activities that place the knee in hyperflexion.
- Early ROM after casting is recommended to prevent joint contractures.

Phase I: Immobilize in Extension (Days 0 to 21 after injury)
- When to progress to phase: Initial injury to the superior tibiofibular joint
- Goals of phase
  - Decrease inflammation and irritation and promote healing
  - Early passive exercise to maintain mobility and strength without weight bearing
  - Maximize patient independence with an assistive device to maintain non-weight-bearing status
  - Strengthening program

- Interventions
  - Medications: Antiinflammatories and/or muscle relaxants
  - Modalities: Heat and stretching prior to exercise and ice after exercise
  - Myofascial release to global muscles of the knee, ankle, and hip
  - Lower extremity flexibility: Knee, hip, and ankle ROM
  - Home exercise program: Knee ROM, hip strengthening, and lower extremity flexibility

Phase 2: Progressive Weight Bearing (Days 28 to 42 after injury)

- When to progress to phase: Delay until fracture heals
- Goals of phase
  - Restore normal ROM.
  - Proprioceptive exercises
  - Increased attention to lateral and rotatory movements.
  - Focus on strengthening peroneal muscles, extensor hallucis longus, and extensor digitorum longus, all of which assist in superior tibiofibular stabilization.
  - Improve lower extremity flexibility in hips and knees.
  - Active exercises for mobility and strength
  - Strengthening hips, knees, back, and core
- Interventions
  - Medications as needed

- Modalities as needed
- Myofascial release to global muscles; progress as needed.
- Lower extremity flexibility: Stretching biceps femoris and soleus; strengthening of these muscles is not encouraged because these muscles produce posterior excursion of the superior tibiofibular joint.
- Home exercise program: Improve strength in hips, knees, and abdominals.

Phase 3: Full Weight Bearing (Days 42 to 84 after injury)

- When to progress to phase: Return to full weight bearing when tissue healing is evident.
- Goals of phase
  - Gain 5/5 lower extremity strength
  - Address contributing factors.
- Interventions
  - Medications and myofascial release as needed
  - Home exercise program: Progress lower extremity flexibility and strengthening program.
  - Other: Address contributing factors.

SIGNS AND SYMPTOMS INDICATING REFERRAL TO PHYSICIAN

- Tenderness in the distal or middle third of the bone: Stress fracture of the tibia

- Recurrent episodes of deep, distal calf pain: Compartment syndrome
- Tenderness over the adjacent muscle at the tibial margin: Medial tibial stress syndrome
- Major trauma: Fracture
- History of cancer: Metastatic disease
- Fevers and chills: Infection or tumor

SUGGESTED READINGS

Dutton M. *Orthopaedic Examination, Evaluation, & Intervention*. New York: McGraw-Hill; 2004.

Halbrecht JL, Jackson DW. Recurrent dislocation of the proximal tibiofibular joint. *Orthop Rev*. 1991;20:957-960.

Sekiya JK, Kuhn JE. Instability of the proximal tibiofibular joint. *J Am Acad Orthop Surg* 2003;11:120-128.

Semonian RH, Denlinger PM, Duggan RJ. Proximal tibiofibular subluxation relationship to lateral knee pain: a review of proximal tibiofibular joint pathologies. *J Orthop Sports Phys Ther*. 1995;21:248-257.

Wiener SL. *Differential Diagnosis of Acute Pain By Body Region*. New York: McGraw-Hill; 1993.

AUTHOR: BERNARD LI

Section III

ORTHOPEDIC PATHOLOGY

BASIC INFORMATION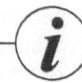

DEFINITION

- Plica is defined as an extension of the synovial capsule of the knee.
- Synovial plica syndrome occurs when the plica becomes irritated or inflamed.
- Once an inflammatory process is established, the normal plical tissue may hypertrophy into a truly pathological structure.

SYNONYMS

- Medial synovial shelf
- Meniscus of the patella
- Plica synovialis
- Superomedial plica
- Plica synovialis patellaris
- Infrapatellar septum

ICD-9CM CODES
727.83 Plica syndrome

OPTIMAL NUMBER OF VISITS

8 or fewer

MAXIMAL NUMBER OF VISITS

12

ETIOLOGY

- The etiology of symptomatic plica is unclear.
- Potential causes of inflammation include repetitive stress, a single blunt trauma, loose bodies, OCD, meniscal tears, or other aggravating knee pathology.
- A popular theory for the initiation of inflammation is that the plica is converted to a bowstring, which causes it to contact the medial femoral condyle. During flexion of the knee, the plica abrades the condyle, causing symptoms to occur.
- An inflammatory process then leads to edema and thickening and decreased elasticity of the plica. The plica may develop irregular edges and may snap over the femoral condyle, leading to a secondary synovitis and chondromalacia. Loose areolar fatty tissue appears to become gristle-like. When plicae are soft, wavy, and vascular with synovial covered edges, they are not pathological.

EPIDEMIOLOGY AND DEMOGRAPHICS

Plica syndrome is a common overuse syndrome of the knee that appears more commonly with repetitive stress activities.

MECHANISM OF INJURY

No specific mechanism of injury has been implicated, but potential mechanisms include repetitive stress, blunt trauma, or inflammation secondary to other knee pathology.

COMMON SIGNS AND SYMPTOMS

- A diverse and broad range of symptoms makes this pathology difficult to diagnose.
- Symptoms resemble or overlap with other pathology.
- Reported symptoms include anterior or anteromedial knee pain, intermittent or episodic pain, clicking, high-pitched snapping, occasional giving way, locking (pseudolocking), and catching.
- Meniscal tears, patellar tendinitis, Osgood-Schlatter disease, Sinding-Larsen-Johansson disease, and patellar instability are the most commonly found concomitant conditions.

AGGRAVATING ACTIVITIES

- Prolonged standing
- Squatting
- Sitting
- Stair climbing

EASING ACTIVITIES

- Ice
- Rest

24-HOUR SYMPTOM PATTERN

Symptoms are generally activity related; however, individuals may experience pain with walking and stair climbing as the syndrome progresses.

PAST HISTORY FOR THE REGION

Patient may or may not report history of knee pain or trauma.

PHYSICAL EXAMINATION

- Plica syndrome is difficult to differentiate from other pathology and remains a diagnosis of exclusion.
- Palpable tenderness along either or both the medial and inferior aspect of the patella.
- The inferomedial quadrant is generally the most consistently painful.

IMPORTANT OBJECTIVE TESTS

- Palpation: Tenderness one fingerbreadth medial to the medial border of the patella.
- A positive TARP sign:
  - *T*aut
  - *A*rticular
  - *R*eproduces
  - *P*ain

DIFFERENTIAL DIAGNOSIS

- Muscle strain
- Myofascial pain
- Patellofemoral stress syndrome
- Early degenerative joint disease
- Medial or lateral meniscal pathology
- Tendinitis
- Osgood-Schlatter disease
- Sinding-Larsen-Johansson disease
- Patellar instability

CONTRIBUTING FACTORS

- Athletic activity that requires repetitive stress to the knee, such as running and jumping
- Hip adductor weakness

TREATMENT

INDICATIONS FOR SURGERY

6 months of failed conservative nonoperative treatment

SURGICAL OPTIONS

- Arthroscopic surgery
- Plica resection
- Surgical results are very good for patients who are selected properly.

REHABILITATION

- A patient-centered flexibility and strengthening program often leads to some improvement.
- Optimize patient's knee strength and flexibility.
- Stretching the hip flexors
- Strengthening of the hip abductors

Phase I: Acute Inflammatory Phase (Days 0 to 14 after injury)
- When to progress to phase: Initial injury to the plica.
- Goals of phase
  - Decrease inflammation and irritation and promote healing.
- Interventions
  - Medications: Antiinflammatories and/or muscle relaxants
  - Modalities: Ultrasound and ice massage to break pain cycle
  - Myofascial release to global hips and hamstrings to gain ROM
  - Lower extremity flexibility: Hamstrings and hip flexors
  - Home exercise program: Walking program, lower extremity flexibility.

Phase 2: Reparative Phase (Days 15 to 21 after injury)
- When to progress to phase: Progress as pain allows.
- Goals of phase
  - Optimize patellofemoral mechanics.
  - Strengthening and flexibility
  - Return patient to prior functional status
- Interventions
  - Medications as needed
  - Modalities as needed
  - Myofascial release to global muscles; progress as needed.

○ Lower extremity flexibility: Hamstrings and hip flexors
○ Home exercise program: Walking program, lower extremity flexibility and strengthening

Phase 3: Remodeling Phase (Days 22 to 60 after injury)
• When to progress to phase
  ○ Pain-free ROM
  ○ No functional limitations
• Goals of phase
  ○ Address contributing factors.
• Interventions
  ○ Medications and myofascial release as needed
  ○ Home exercise program: Progress lower extremity flexibility and strengthening program.
  ○ Other: Address contributing factors.

Phase 4: Remodeling Phase (Days 60 to 360 after injury)
• When to progress to phase: No functional limitations
• Goals of phase

○ Correction of contributing factors
○ Retraining muscle activity to account for functional activities
• Interventions
  ○ Medications and myofascial release as needed
  ○ Home exercise program: Progress lower extremity flexibility and strengthening program.
  ○ Other: Address contributing factors, functional rehabilitation, and retraining.

PROGNOSIS

The prognosis for plica syndrome is very good.

SIGNS AND SYMPTOMS INDICATING REFERRAL TO PHYSICIAN

• Pain that does not change with position: Infection or tumor
• Major trauma: Fracture
• History of cancer: Metastatic disease
• Fever and chills: Infection or tumor

SUGGESTED READINGS

Broom MJ, Fulkerson JP. The plica syndrome: a new perspective. *Orthop Clin North Am.* 1986;17(2):279–281.

Dutton M. *Orthopaedic Examination, Evaluation, & Intervention.* New York: McGraw-Hill; 2004.

Dupont JY. Synovial plicae of the knee. Controversies and review. *Clin Sports Med.* 1997;16(1):87–122.

O'Dwyer KJ, Peace PK. The plica syndrome. *Injury.* 1988;19(5):350–352.

Tindel NL, Nisonson B. The plica syndrome. *Orthop Clin North Am.* 1992;23(4):613–618.

Wiener SL. *Differential Diagnosis of Acute Pain by Body Region.* New York: McGraw-Hill; 1993.

AUTHOR: BERNARD LI

BASIC INFORMATION

DEFINITION

A tibial plateau fracture occurs at the top of the shin bone and involves the cartilage surface of the knee joint.

SYNONYMS

- Fender fracture
- Bumper fracture
- ITBFS

ICD-9CM CODES
823.0 Fracture of upper end of tibia and fibula closed

OPTIMAL NUMBER OF VISITS

12 or fewer

MAXIMAL NUMBER OF VISITS

36

ETIOLOGY

- Tibial plateau fractures can occur as a result of high-energy trauma or low-energy trauma.
- The fracture is the act or process of breaking a bone or the state of being broken.
- Fractures occur when bone cannot withstand outside forces.
- The integrity of the bone has been lost, and the bone structure fails.
- The closed pack position of the tibiofemoral joint is extension. Therefore the most force will be placed onto the tibia when the knee is fully extended.

EPIDEMIOLOGY AND DEMOGRAPHICS

- Fractures of the tibial plateau in older persons are more common than in the general population.
- In younger patients, tibial plateau fractures typically affect men because of their greater involvement in high-energy contact sports such as wrestling and boxing.
- The frequency of tibial plateau fractures is higher in older women than in older men because of the greater incidence of osteoporosis in women.
- Tibial plateau fracture has no racial predilection.

MECHANISM OF INJURY

- Force is directed from the femoral condyles onto the medial and lateral portions of the tibial plateau.
- Axial loading from a fall
- Automobile bumper impact
- Lateral direct forces
- Falls
- Twisting injury

COMMON SIGNS AND SYMPTOMS

- Severe pain
- Weight-bearing limitations
- Knee effusion
- Joint stiffness
- Pain from a tibial plateau fracture refers into the tibial plateau and along the tibial shaft.

AGGRAVATING ACTIVITIES

- Weight bearing
- Walking
- Ascending or descending stairs
- Closed pack position of the knee

EASING ACTIVITIES

- Ice
- Rest
- Open pack position of the knee

24-HOUR SYMPTOM PATTERN

Symptoms are generally activity related; however, individuals may experience pain at night.

PAST HISTORY FOR THE REGION

Because of the traumatic nature of the pathology, there is often no past history within the knee.

PHYSICAL EXAMINATION

- Localized tenderness to palpation at the osseous structures of the knee joint that include the following:
  - Tibia
  - Fibula
  - Femur
  - Patella
- Localized tenderness to the following structures:
  - PCL
  - Popliteal artery
  - Lateral stabilization complex of the knee
  - Tibialis anterior

IMPORTANT OBJECTIVE TESTS

- X-rays, as follows:
  - AP
  - Cross-table lateral
  - Patellar (sunrise)
  - Oblique views
- CT scan: Characterize fractures of the tibial plateau and assess the depression of the tibia and the degree of diastasis (splitting) of the fractured parts to plan for surgical intervention.
- MRI: Assessment of soft tissue structures. Excellent for depicting ligamentous and meniscal injuries.
- Arteriography or MR angiography is used if popliteal artery injury is suspected.
- Schatzker system to classify tibial plateau fractures as follows:
  - Type I fractures are split fractures of the lateral tibial plateau, usually in

younger patients. No depression is seen at the articular surface.
  - Type II fractures are split fractures with depression of the lateral articular surface and typically are seen in older patients with osteoporosis.
  - Type III fractures are characterized by depression of the lateral tibial plateau, without splitting through the articular surface.
  - Type IV fractures involve the medial tibial plateau and may be split fractures with or without depression.
  - Type V fractures are characterized by split fractures through both the medial and lateral tibial plateaus.
  - Type VI fractures are the result of severe stress and result in dissociation of the tibial plateau region from the underlying diaphysis.

DIFFERENTIAL DIAGNOSIS

- Muscle strain
- Myofascial pain
- Patellofemoral stress syndrome
- Early degenerative joint disease
- Lateral meniscal pathology
- Superior tibiofibular joint sprain
- Popliteal or biceps femoris tendinitis
- Common peroneal nerve injury
- Tendinitis
- Referred pain from the lumbar spine or hip
- Femoral stress fracture
- Infection
- Neoplasm

CONTRIBUTING FACTORS

- Decrease in bone density caused by osteopenia or osteoporosis
- Long-term use of steroids or medications, such as prednisone, which diminishes bone density.

TREATMENT

INDICATIONS FOR SURGERY

Recommend open reduction and internal fixation (ORIF) for fractures that show greater than 5 mm of depression or 1 mm displacement.

SURGICAL OPTIONS

- Displaced fractures often require surgery to realign the bones and restore stability and alignment of the knee joint.
- Recommend ORIF for fractures that show greater than 5 mm of depression or 1 mm displacement.
- Several surgical options in the treatment of tibial plateau fractures; choosing the

type of procedure depends on the fracture pattern: Certain types of fractures may or may not be amenable to treatment with a particular type of surgery.
• ORIF

SURGICAL OUTCOMES

ORIF with the restoration of the articular surfaces promotes the best outcomes, with satisfactory results 75% of the time.

REHABILITATION

• Early ROM of the knee and the maintenance of non–weight-bearing status on the affected leg are generally considered critical. Prolonged immobilization in a cast has been found to increase stiffness that is not amenable to physical therapy.
• The goal should be to gain 90 degrees of flexion ROM by 4 weeks.
• After 12 weeks, patients can do full weight bearing if there is radiographic evidence of healing. Progression to partial and full weight-bearing status per the surgeon.
• Nondisplaced fractures generally require 3 months of partial to non-weight-bearing status. Some nondisplaced fractures are at risk for displacing immediately after the injury. These injuries must be followed closely by an orthopedic surgeon. If displacement occurs, surgery may be required to stabilize and realign the knee.

• Displaced fractures often require surgery to realign the bones and restore stability and alignment of the knee joint. Each surgeon has specific requirements, but generally weight bearing is limited for the first 2 months, with x-ray evidence of bone formation before allowing full weight-bearing status.
• Recovery from a tibial plateau fracture can take several months to a full year. Times are determined by several factors, including age, gender, magnitude of fracture, whether the cartilage was involved, and the expected demands of daily life.
• If the cartilage surface of the joint is involved, the knee must be protected from weight bearing until the fracture has healed. Most commonly, patients are allowed to actively and passively move the knee, but non–weight-bearing status must be maintained until evidence of sufficient bone formation is present in x-rays.
• Initial exercises should include the following:
  ○ Knee extension exercises for ROM. (e.g., prone knee hang)
  ○ Knee flexion exercises. (e.g., heel slides)

PROGNOSIS

Long-term prognosis depends on the type of fracture, age of patient, bone quality, and concomitant injury, as discussed in the beginning of this standard of care.

Time frame can be from several months to more a year.

SIGNS AND SYMPTOMS INDICATING REFERRAL TO PHYSICIAN

• Calf tenderness: DVT
• Significant redness and swelling: Infection
• Blood in urine or stool: Urinary pathology
• Fevers and chills: Infection or tumor

SUGGESTED READINGS

Anglen JO, Healy WL. Tibial plateau fractures. *Orthopedics*. 1988;11(11):1527–1534.

Barrow BA, Fajman WA, Parker LM, et al. Tibial plateau fractures: evaluation with MR imaging. *Radiographics*. 1994;14(3):553–559.

Bennett WF, Browner B. Tibial plateau fractures: A study of associated soft tissue injuries. *J Orthop Trauma*. 1994;8:183–188.

Dutton M. *Orthopaedic Examination, Evaluation, & Intervention*. New York: McGraw-Hill; 2004.

Lachiewicz PF, Funcik T. Factors influencing the results of open reduction and internal fixation of tibial plateau fractures. *Clin Orthop*. 1990;(259):210–215.

Watson J, Schatzker J. *Skeletal Trauma*. 2nd ed. Philadelphia: WB Saunders; 1998.

Wiener SL. *Differential Diagnosis of Acute Pain by Body Region*. New York: McGraw-Hill; 1993.

AUTHOR: BERNARD LI

Section III

ORTHOPEDIC PATHOLOGY

BASIC INFORMATION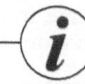

DEFINITION

- Achilles tendinopathy can be defined as a painful overuse tendon condition and can be classified as tendinitis or tendinosis.
  - Tendinitis is defined as a painful overuse tendon injury with the presence of inflammatory cells.
  - Tendinosis is defined as to the degeneration of the tendon in the absence of inflammatory cells.

SYNONYMS

- Achilles tendinitis
- Achilles tendinosis
- Achilles tendinopathy
- Partial rupture
- Tenosynovitis
- Peritendinitis
- Achillodynia

ICD-9CM CODES
726.71 Achilles bursitis or tendinitis
845.09 Other ankle sprain
727.82 Calcium deposits in tendon and bursa

OPTIMAL NUMBER OF VISITS

3 or 4 with proper patient education

MAXIMAL NUMBER OF VISITS

12, if additional rehabilitation is needed.

ETIOLOGY

- The actual physiological cause of Achilles tendinopathy remains largely misunderstood and has not been clarified. However, the common presumption is that the tendon has failed to heal normally. Achilles tendon studies have shown that there is increased neurovascularization of the tendon at the site of pain. In addition, it has been found that increased glutamate and substance P, which are powerful neurotransmitters, are present in the region of the tendon. Scientists believe that the combination of increased neurovascularization and presence of increased neurotransmitters may be responsible for pain that is present with tendinopathy.
- The primary site of tendon injuries is just proximal (2 to 6 cm) to the tendon's insertion.
- This part of the tendon is noted to be a region of hypovascularity and has an increased susceptibility to injury.
- Achilles tendinopathy typically results from some form of excessive overuse, and the causes are usually multifactorial. Acute tendinopathy is usually caused by trauma, muscle fatigue, or excessive use.

EPIDEMIOLOGY AND DEMOGRAPHICS

- Achilles tendinopathy is most common in older male athletes (teenagers) who participate in running activities.
- Achilles tendinopathy occurs most often in people who participate in running activities or jumping sports.
- Incidence of Achilles tendinopathy has been reported as 11% in runners, 9% in dancers, and 5% in gymnasts.

MECHANISM OF INJURY

Achilles tendon injuries are typically the result of excessive eccentric loading that results from training errors, changes in training, increased distance, and changes in terrain.

COMMON SIGNS AND SYMPTOMS

- Patients typically report pain at the insertion site and/or just above (2 to 6 cm) the insertion site.
- Patients typically present with swelling and thickening of the tendon at the site of injury.

AGGRAVATING ACTIVITIES

- Walking
- Running
- Jumping activities

EASING ACTIVITIES

- Pain relief is usually noted with rest.
- Nonsteroidal antiinflammatory drugs (NSAIDs) may be prescribed by physicians and may be beneficial in acute cases but have been found to be largely ineffective with chronic Achilles tendinopathies.
- Heel lifts and walking-cast boots may be useful in controlling pain with weight-bearing activities during acute phases.

24-HOUR SYMPTOM PATTERN

- Patients commonly complain of morning stiffness. Pain is otherwise noted with walking and sports-specific activities.
- Pain is more commonly present during daily activities in more severe cases.

PAST HISTORY FOR THE REGION

Patients may or may not report prior history of injury or pain in this area. Patients typically report participation in some sort of sporting activity, usually running activities; however, this is not always the case.

PHYSICAL EXAMINATION

- Swelling and thickening of the Achilles tendon
- Pain with contraction of calf muscle
- Increased pronation through stance
- Avoidance of terminal stance phase in gait

IMPORTANT OBJECTIVE TESTS

- Currently, there are no validated tests for diagnosing Achilles tendinopathies. Diagnosis is largely based on subjective information and physical findings.
- Ultrasonography is commonly used to verify a diagnosis of Achilles tendinopathy.
- Magnetic resonance imaging (MRI) may also be used for clarification of diagnosis but is not commonly performed because of the cost.

DIFFERENTIAL DIAGNOSIS

- Calf strain
- Partial rupture of the calf
- Lumbar radiculopathy
- Os trigonum
- Retrocalcaneal bursitis
- Sever's disease or calcaneal apophysitis (pediatric patients)
- Sural nerve entrapment
- Systemic inflammatory disorders

CONTRIBUTING FACTORS

- Increased pronation
- Pes planus
- Increased rearfoot mobility
- Calf weakness
- Poor footwear
- Changes in training program
- Diabetes
- Obesity
- Steroid exposure
- Hypertension
- Quinolone antibiotics

TREATMENT

SURGICAL OPTIONS

- Surgery for Achilles tendinopathy is usually performed when conservative treatment has failed.
- There are several surgical options for Achilles tendinopathy such as the following:
  - Tendon debridement
  - Para tendon debridement
  - Debridement with lesion removal
  - Achilles tendon reconstruction
- Results suggest that of the patients who undergo surgical repair, 75% have favorable outcomes and return to premorbid function. Poorer outcomes are reported to be associated with advanced age, intertendon lesions, and partial tendon ruptures.

REHABILITATION

- The treatment approach for these patients depends on the stage in which they present. For acute cases, the primary goal of therapy is to decrease the inflammatory process.

- Acute Achilles tendinitis
  - Compression
  - Cryotherapy
  - Rest
  - Heel wedge
  - Walking boot
  - Soft tissue mobilization (STM)
  - Activity modification
- Chronic Achilles tendinopathies
  - Stretching
  - Night splints
  - Strengthening
  - Orthotic therapy
  - Biomechanical correction
  - Sclerotic therapy
  - Extracorporeal shockwave therapy (ESWT)
- Stretching is one of the most common treatments prescribed for Achilles tendinopathies despite a lack of strong evidence to support its effectiveness. Current scientific theory states that stretching facilitates decreased muscle and tendon stiffness and increases muscle length, therefore reducing the force transmitted through the musculotendinous unit. There is no evidence available that stretching alone is an effective treatment for Achilles tendinopathy
- Night splints have shown some effectiveness in relieving pain at a 12-month follow-up when used alone or in conjunction with an eccentric exercise program.
- Strengthening
  - Heavy-load eccentric strengthening has been shown to be extremely effective in the treatment of Achilles tendinopathy. Alfredson and Cook reported 89% long-term improvement in patients who underwent a 12-week eccentric strengthening program for chronic Achilles tendinopathy. All patients from this study were surgical candidates and had failed to respond to conservative treatments that included rest, use of NSAIDs, footwear changes, orthoses, physical therapy, and other training programs.
- Eccentric training program
  - In a treatment created by Alfredson, patients were instructed to perform 3 sets of 15 repetitions of heel drops off the edge of the stairs with both the knee straight and the knee bent, for both the gastrocnemius and soleus muscles. Patients were instructed to lower themselves over a 6-second

period to the point when maximal stretch was felt. At this point the patients were to return to the starting position using the opposite leg. If the patient did not experience pain with each repetition, they were instructed to increase the load through the use of weights or a weight machine.
- Evidence does not support the use of concentric strengthening exercises alone for the treatment of Achilles tendinopathy.
- Excessive pronation, pes planus, and excessive rearfoot motion are considered factors that may predispose people to the development of Achilles tendinopathy. Correction of the abnormal foot mechanics may help to prevent the recurrence of injury.
- Biomechanical corrections
  - Altered lower extremity biomechanics have been reported as a possible contributing factor for abnormal loading of the Achilles tendon. Correction of the abnormal biomechanics may be beneficial for preventing the recurrence of Achilles tendinopathy. Therapists should consider including a lower extremity biomechanical evaluation in patients with Achilles tendinopathy.
- Sclerotic therapy
  - Recent research in the treatment of tendon pain has focused on the use of sclerosing agents. Small randomized controlled trials have shown sclerosing agents to be effective at 2-year follow-up in the treatment of pain in patients with chronic Achilles tendinopathy.
  - Abolishment of the neovascularization in and around the tendon is believed to be responsible for the reduction of pain after injections of sclerosing agents.
- ESWT
  - Increasing evidence is emerging advocating ESWT for chronic Achilles tendinopathy. Several small controlled trials have shown excellent-to-good results at 12-month follow-up in patients who were treated with ESWT.

PROGNOSIS

- The prognosis for patients with Achilles tendinopathy is highly variable. The prognosis depends on several factors, including interventions. Patients who

undergo heavy-load eccentric strengthening have been shown to have a excellent-to-good prognosis.
- Emerging research has shown an improved prognosis for patients who undergo sclerotic and shockwave therapy. However, additional research is needed to validate these treatment interventions.
- Patients with circulatory disorders, long-term steroid use, obesity, hypertension, and partial tendon ruptures have a poorer prognosis.

SIGNS AND SYMPTOMS INDICATING REFERRAL TO PHYSICIAN

Patients should be referred to a physician if they show signs of complete tendon rupture.

SUGGESTED READINGS

Alfredson H, Cook J. A treatment algorithm for managing Achilles tendinopathy: new treatment options. *Br J Sports Med.* 2007; 41(4):211–216.

Alfredson H. Conservative management of Achilles tendinopathy: new ideas. *Foot Ankle Clin.* 2005;10(2):321–329.

Furia JP. High-energy extracorporeal shock wave therapy as a treatment for chronic noninsertional Achilles tendinopathy. *Am J Sports Med.* 2008;36(3):502–508.

Holmes GB, Lin J. Etiologic factors associated with symptomatic Achilles tendinopathy. *Foot Ankle Int.* 2006;27(11):952–959.

Mahieu NN, McNair P, Cools A, D'Haen C, Vandermeulen K, Witvrouw E. Effect of eccentric training on the plantar flexor muscle-tendon tissue properties. *Med Sci Sports Exerc.* 2008;40(1):117–123.

Paavola M, Kannus P, Jarvinen TA, Khan K, Jozsa L, Jarvinen M. Achilles tendinopathy. *J Bone Joint Surg Am.* 2002;84-A(11):2062–2076.

Park DY, Chou L. Stretching for prevention of Achilles tendon injuries: a review of the literature. *Foot Ankle Int.* 2006;27(12): 1086–1095.

Reischl SF, Noceti-dewit LM. The Foot and Ankle: Physical Therapy Patient Management Utilizing Current Evidence. In: *Current Concepts of Orthopaedic Physical therapy.* 2nd ed. La Crosse, Wi: Orthopaedic Section; 2006.

Rompe JD, Nafe B, Furia JP, Maffulli N. Eccentric loading, shock-wave treatment, or a wait-and-see policy for tendinopathy of the main body of tendo Achillis: a randomized controlled trial. *Am J Sports Med.* 2007;35(3):374–383.

AUTHOR: JASON TONLEY

Section III

ORTHOPEDIC PATHOLOGY

BASIC INFORMATION

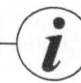

DEFINITION

Ankle dislocation is defined as a displacement of the talus out of the ankle mortise.

SYNONYMS

- Dislocated ankle
- Ankle fracture
- Ankle sprain
- Broken ankle
- Posterior ankle dislocation
- Anterior ankle dislocation
- Superior ankle dislocation
- Lateral ankle dislocation

ICD-9CM CODES
837.0 Closed dislocation of ankle
837.1 Open dislocation of ankle

OPTIMAL NUMBER OF VISITS

12 (Visits depend on whether surgical intervention is involved.)

MAXIMAL NUMBER OF VISITS

24 (Complicated dislocations require more time.)

ETIOLOGY

- Ankle dislocations are usually caused by a traumatic event and the result of a high-energy force being applied to the ankle joint while in maximal plantar flexion. The direction of the dislocation is a result of which direction from which the force is applied.
- The talus is trapezoidal, with the greater width anterior. As the joint moves into plantar flexion, the talus becomes narrower, resulting in a decrease in stability.
- Ankle dislocations most commonly occur in the posterior direction followed by medial and lateral dislocations.
- Isolated dislocations are unusual. Most dislocations to the tibiotalar joint are associated with a fracture of either the medial or lateral malleolus or the posterior edge of the tibia. Depending on the application of force, fracture of the talus may occur as well.
- Most ankle dislocations are open dislocations resulting in increased damage to the surrounding soft tissue and increased risk for infection.
- A primary concern with any dislocation is damage to neurovascular structures and avascular necrosis of the talus.

EPIDEMIOLOGY AND DEMOGRAPHICS

- Isolated dislocation without fracture is very rare.

- Ankle dislocations are more likely to occur in younger male patients because of the generally higher association they have with traumatic events.
- The literature states that most ankle dislocations result from falls of >3 meters (>9 feet), motorcycle accidents, motor vehicle accidents (MVAs), and sports (basketball, volleyball, and soccer).

MECHANISM OF INJURY

- Posterior dislocations
  - The talus moves in a posterior direction in relation to the distal tibia as force drives the foot backward. The wider anterior talus wedges back, resulting in forced widening of the joint. This must be accompanied by either a disruption of the tibiofibular syndesmosis or a fracture of the lateral malleolus. This occurs most commonly when the ankle is plantar flexed.
- Anterior dislocations
  - The talus moves anteriorly in relation to the tibia. These injuries typically occur with the foot fixed, and a posterior force is applied to the tibia or with forced dorsiflexion.
- Lateral dislocations
  - The talus is displaced laterally in relation to the tibia. These dislocations usually result from forced eversion while in planter flexion.
  - Lateral dislocations are associated with fractures of either or both the malleoli or the distal fibula.
- Medial dislocations
  - The talus is displaced medially with relation to the distal tibia.
  - These dislocations usually result from forced inversion with the ankle in plantar flexion.
  - Medial dislocations are associated with fractures of the medial and/or lateral malleoli, as well as damage to the lateral capsule and ligament structures.
- Superior dislocations
  - Diastasis occurs when a force drives the talus upward into the mortise. These dislocations usually are the result of a fall from a height. In such cases, the patient should be evaluated carefully for concomitant spine injury and fracture of the calcaneus.

COMMON SIGNS AND SYMPTOMS

- Ankle dislocations are a medical emergency and are generally not seen acutely in a rehabilitation setting.
- Patients, at initial injury, typically present with severe pain, deformity, inability to bear weight, open laceration of the skin, tenting of the skin, and tenderness to palpation of the joint and associated ligament structures.

AGGRAVATING ACTIVITIES

- Standing
- Walking
- Ankle ROM
- Resisted activities

EASING ACTIVITIES

- Rest
- Ice
- NSAIDs
- Immobilization
- Non–weight-bearing positions

24-HOUR SYMPTOM PATTERN

- Patients typically report stiffness and mild-to-moderate pain in the morning that should improve or resolve within 30 to 60 minutes on rising.
- Pain may increase during the day, depending on how much weight-bearing activity is performed.

PAST HISTORY FOR THE REGION

- Because of the traumatic nature of ankle dislocations, patients do not typically present with a prior history of injury.
- In cases of recurrent or nontraumatic dislocations, a prior history of ankle instability may be reported.
- Treatment prior to physical therapy:
  - This depends on the severity of the initial injury. If the patient suffered a closed dislocation without fracture, the dislocation is reduced and the ankle is placed in a short leg cast. Weight bearing is typically restricted for 4 to 6 weeks. Once the cast is removed, progressive weight bearing is normally allowed.
  - If the patient suffered an open dislocation or other injures, such as fracture, osteochondral lesions, or a grade III syndesmotic sprain that required operative treatment, weight-bearing restrictions are longer and depend on the surgical intervention or healing of fracture.

PHYSICAL EXAMINATION

- Depending on the severity of the dislocation, patients present to physical therapy as early as 2 to 3 weeks or as late as 12 weeks.
- Common physical findings for patients with ankle dislocations at initial evaluation of physical therapy are as follows:
  - Pain
  - Swelling
  - Restricted or limited weight bearing
  - Impaired ankle range of motion (ROM)
  - Impaired proprioception
  - Ambulation with an assistive device
  - Decreased strength
  - Impaired sensation may or may not be present.

IMPORTANT OBJECTIVE TESTS

- At initial injury, the patient should undergo examination for neurovascular injury. A sensation examination and assessment of pedal and tibial pulses should be performed.
- X-ray is the most common diagnostic test performed. X-rays assist in the assessment of a dislocation if it has not been reduced already, as well as determining if fractures are present.
- In the case of closed dislocations, an MRI may be performed to determine the extent of soft tissue damage present to capsular, ligament, and other soft tissue structures.
- No routine diagnostic testing has been consistently reported in the literature to determine if impaired blood flow to the talus is present for determining risk of avascular necrosis.

DIFFERENTIAL DIAGNOSIS

- Fracture: Malleoli, tibia, talus, calcaneus, or navicular
- Ligament disruption: Lateral and medial collateral
- Syndesmotic injures
- Neurovascular injuries
- Tendon injuries
- Subtalar dislocations
- Talonavicular dislocations
- Os trigonum

CONTRIBUTING FACTORS

- Internal malleolus hypoplasia
- Ligamentous laxity
- Peroneal muscle weakness
- Previous ankle sprains
- Participation in sports

TREATMENT

SURGICAL OPTIONS

- Open reduction and internal fixation (ORIF)
- External fixation
- Capsular or ligament reconstruction
- Arthrodesis
- Talectomy
- Tibiocalcaneal arthrodesis
- Amputation
- Predictors of negative or positive surgical outcome are as follows:
  - Postsurgical infection
  - Avascular necrosis

REHABILITATION

- Rehabilitation of ankle dislocations should focus on an impairment-based treatment approach. Initial treatment should be directed at management of

pain and edema, protection of surgical repair (if necessary), and initiation of weight-bearing tolerance. As pain decreases and weight-bearing tolerance improves, progression of the program to increased ROM, strengthening of local and proximal muscles, proprioceptive training, and return to function should be emphasized.
- In the case of an open dislocation or a dislocation that requires a surgical intervention, the therapist must pay attention to signs of infection or avascular necrosis during the initial portion of the rehabilitation process.
- Treatment to decrease inflammation is as follows:
  - Myofascial release techniques to reduce edema
  - Joint mobilization: Grade I or II
  - Pain-free ROM as tolerated
  - Cold or hot pack
  - Ultrasound
  - Electrical stimulation
  - Compression garments
  - Partial weight bearing
- Weight-bearing status is highly variable and depends on the procedures performed at the time of initial injury. In closed dislocations, patients typically initiate weight bearing at weeks 4 to 6 and should be full weight bearing within a 4- to 6-week period. For patients undergoing some form of fixation, fracture reduction, or ligament reconstruction, weight bearing as tolerated or partial weight bearing may begin as early as week 5 or 6, with precautions being extended for up to 8 to 12 weeks.
- During early phases of rehabilitation, patients should be in a general body cardiovascular program to improve cardiovascular health.
- Based on available research, patients with ankle injuries are noted to have changes in proximal hip neuromotor control and strength. Therefore early implementation of proximal hip strengthening should be a part of the patient's initial rehabilitation program.
- Rehabilitation should focus on progressing to full weight bearing and restoration of normal ankle motion, normal gait mechanics without the use of an assistive device, and strengthening. Treatment should include the following:
  - Joint mobilizations
  - ROM exercises
  - Strengthening
  - Proprioceptive training
  - Gait training
  - Functional exercise/activity training

PROGNOSIS

- Patients who suffer closed dislocations tend to have a good recovery. The available

research states that patients with isolated closed dislocations tend to have full recovery and return to sporting activities.
- Patients who suffer open dislocations, fractures, or ligament disruption or who require surgical fixations should not expect to make a full recovery but should expect to return to daily activities with minimal-to-no restriction.
- Patient who require removal of the talus or fusion can expect to have a poor prognosis to return to full function but should be able to return normal daily activities with minimal restriction.

SIGNS AND SYMPTOMS INDICATING REFERRAL TO PHYSICIAN

- Signs of postsurgical infection include the following:
  - Fever
  - Increased redness around the incision
  - Increased swelling around the incision
  - Drainage from the wound for more than 5 days after surgery
  - Drainage from the wound that is cloudy, yellow, or foul smelling
  - Pain that is increasing and becoming constant
- Signs of avascular necrosis include the following:
  - Pain that is progressively worsening
  - Pain that is not relieved by rest
  - Decreased tolerance to weight bearing
  - Progressively increasing joint pain

SUGGESTED READINGS

Colville MR, Colville JM, Manoli II A. Posteromedial dislocation of the ankle without fracture. *J Bone Joint Surg Am* 1987;69(5):706-711.

Fernandes TJ. The mechanism of talo-tibial dislocation without fracture. *J Bone Joint Surg Br.* 1976;58(3):364-365.

Moehring HD, Tan RT, Marder RA, et al. Ankle dislocation. *J Orthop Trauma.* 1994;8(2):167-172.

Toohey JS, Worsing Jr RA. The long-term follow-up study of tibiotalar dislocations without associated fractures. *Clin Orthop.* 1989;239:207-210.

Wehner J, Lorenz M. Lateral Ankle Fracture without Trauma, *J Orthop Trauma.* 1990;4(3):362-365.

Wilson J, Michele A, Jacobsen E. Ankle Dislocations without Fracture. *J Bone Joint Surg Am.* 1939;21:198-204.

Wroble RR, Nepola JV, Malvitz TA. Ankle dislocation without fracture. *Foot Ankle.* 1988;9(2):64-74.

AUTHOR: JASON TONLEY

BASIC INFORMATION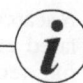

DEFINITION

- Osteoarthritis is a pathology associated with inflammation in the joints. In the case of ankle osteoarthritis, the arthritis and inflammation most commonly affects the talocrural joint.
- Osteoarthritis is a term derived from the Greek word *osteo*, meaning "of the bone, *arthro*, meaning "joint," and *itis*, meaning "inflammation," even though the amount of inflammation present in the joint can range from excessive to little or no inflammation.

SYNONYMS

- Ankle arthritis
- Ankle degenerative joint disease

ICD-9 CODES
715.17 Osteoarthrosis localized primary involving ankle and foot
715.27 Osteoarthrosis localized secondary involving ankle and foot

OPTIMAL NUMBER OF VISITS

3 to 6

MAXIMAL NUMBER OF VISITS

20 to 36

ETIOLOGY

- The wearing down of the hyaline cartilage leads to an inflammatory response. There is thickening and sclerosis of the subchondral bone and development of osteophytes or bone spurs. This leads to a narrowing of the joint space, loss of shock absorption, and ultimately pain.
- Daily wear and tear in combination with various injuries sustained throughout life is the most common cause of the breakdown of healthy tissue.
- Degeneration of the cartilage and resultant arthritis can also be the result of other factors such as trauma or joint injury.
- At a cellular level, as a person ages, the number of proteoglycans in the articular cartilage decreases. Proteoglycans are hydrophilic and work within cartilage to bind water. With the reduction of proteoglycans comes a decrease in water content within the cartilage and a corresponding loss of cartilage resilience. With the decreases in cartilage resilience, collagen fibers of the cartilage become susceptible to degradation and injury. The breakdown of collagen and other cartilage tissue are released into the surrounding joint space. Inflammation results as the body attempts to respond to the influx of byproducts from cartilage injury.

- As the cartilage degrades, the joint space narrows and ligaments become more lax. In response to the laxity, new bone outgrowths, called *spurs* or *osteophytes*, can form on the margins of the joints in an attempt to improve the congruence and passive stability of the articular cartilage surfaces.
- Primary osteoarthritis refers to joint degradation resulting from aging and tissue degeneration.
- Secondary osteoarthritis refers to joint degradation and tissue degeneration that results from factors besides aging such as obesity, trauma, and congenital disorders.

EPIDEMIOLOGY AND DEMOGRAPHICS

- About 50% of people in their sixties and seventies have ankle or foot osteoarthritis as seen on x-ray.
- Symptomatic ankle osteoarthritis is not very common in the general population; there is an increased prevalence in persons with a history of significant ankle trauma or extreme sports or activities (i.e., dance).
- Osteoarthritis is the number one cause of disability.
- Seniors, especially those with a history of long-term abnormal use (poor footwear, excessive injuries, career or recreational overuse, or obesity) are more prone to ankle osteoarthritis.
- Women have more ankle osteoarthritis than men.
- $54 billion per year in medical costs and lost wages

MECHANISM OF INJURY

- Osteoarthritis is a pathology of overuse. The mechanism of injury is therefore the result of repetitive motions that stress the hip joint. The more cycles of an activity that the ankle sees, the more likely the result will be anatomical damage.
- Daily abuse of the ankle (3-inch heels increase foot and ankle stress 7 times compared to 1-inch heels)
- Misalignment of the foot and or toes
- Excessive use or strain of the ankle
- Injuries, such as fracture and strains or sprains, that cause inflammation and scar tissue in the ankle

COMMON SIGNS AND SYMPTOMS

- Pain in the ankle
- Stiffness in the ankle
- Cracking or deep crunching in the ankle joint
- Inflammation and thickening of the ankle
- Gait abnormalities (increased foot pronation, out-toeing, or limp)
- Anterior ankle pain with descending stairs
- Deep achiness in the ankle region
- Achiness in the ankle at night

AGGRAVATING ACTIVITIES

- Inactivity leads to stiffness
- Weight-bearing activities such as walking, running, dancing, jumping, etc.
- Long-term standing, especially on harder surfaces like concrete
- Poor footwear (e.g., high heels)
- Inactivity allows the inflammation to "pool" and increase pressure, leading to discomfort and loss of available movement.
- Joint movement increases wear and tear and inflammation and irritation of the articular surfaces. The more compression involved with the movement, the more wear and tear and irritation will occur.

EASING ACTIVITIES

- Rest
- Pain-free motion of the ankle joint
- Gentle stretching and exercise, use of heat or ice, massage, taking antiinflammatory medication, non–weight-bearing positions, and ankle elevation
- Generally speaking, these activities lead to decreased wear and tear, increased joint lubrication, and loss of stiffness and inflammation associated with this condition.

24-HOUR SYMPTOM PATTERN

- Stiffness in the morning (10 to 15 minutes)
- Better after a warm shower and taking medication
- Can worsen with excessive movement
- Stiffens again in the evening

PAST HISTORY FOR THE REGION

- Jobs or recreational activities that require excessive use or strain of the ankle such as walking, running, jumping, etc.
- Abnormal amount of damage from injuries
- Obesity
- History of injury to either lower extremity

PHYSICAL EXAMINATION

- Ankle thickening (bony changes and inflammation)
- Loss of ankle ROM, especially dorsiflexion
- Localized pain and loss of joint mobility
- Crepitus with movement
- Decreased dorsiflexion noted with midstance to terminal-stance phase of gait
- Decrease talocrural joint accessory motion

IMPORTANT OBJECTIVE TESTS

- No specific clinical testing regimen has been developed to positively confirm the presence of ankle osteoarthritis.
- Diagnosis is made by a combination of radiographic evidence coupled with clinical and subjective examination.

DIFFERENTIAL DIAGNOSIS

- Ankle sprain
- Tendinitis
- Rheumatoid arthritis (RA)
- Talar dome cartilage damage
- Sesamoiditis (os trigonum)
- Osteochondritis desiccans
- Ankle fracture
- Referral from the lower lumbar region
- Pitting edema secondary to cardiac pathology

CONTRIBUTING FACTORS

- The ankle is designed to handle normal daily use. When factors change the body's ability to respond to normal forces, damage occurs.
- Uncontrollable risk factors that contribute or predispose an individual to ankle osteoarthritis pathology are as follows:
  - Gender (females > males)
  - Age (increase 2% per year after age 40 years)
  - Genetics
  - Prior history of injury to either lower extremity
  - Prior history of childhood hip pathology
  - Leg length discrepancies
- Modifiable risk factors that contribute or predispose an individual to continue or progress ankle osteoarthritis:
  - Weight
  - Work or recreational activities
  - Repetitive or significant traumatic injuries to the hip
  - Poor health (smoking, long-term use of steroids)

TREATMENT **Rx**

SURGICAL OPTIONS

- Ankle fusion
- Ankle arthroplasty (replacement)
- Arthroscopic debridement
- Postsurgical outcome as follows:
  - Fusion: Most commonly used, but controversies exist regarding significant loss of motion.
  - Arthrodesis: Need for revision is 5% after 1 year and 11% after 5 years; need for subtalar fusion at 5 years is higher than arthroplasty.
  - Arthroplasty: Need for revision is 9% after 1 year and 23% after 5 years.

REHABILITATION

- Pathological changes to cartilage cannot be repaired by the body at this time. Even surgical advances have yet to solve the problems associated with cartilage damage. With this in mind, the focus of rehabilitation should be on decreasing the stress placed on the damaged cartilage and correcting biomechanical and anatomical abnormalities that may predispose an individual to increased stress at the talocrural joint.

- Decreased ankle dorsiflexion is a common restriction in patients with ankle osteoarthritis. Improving ankle dorsiflexion is an important component of the ankle's ability to absorb shock. Anterior to posterior talocrural joint mobilization, ankle traction mobilization, and STM to the calf can help increase ankle dorsiflexion.
- Midfoot dysfunction can also affect talocrural joint function. Increased pronation is often associated with decreased ankle dorsiflexion. This motion should be controlled, but making the midfoot too rigid prevents it from dissipating shock. Instead, this shock is transferred to the arthritic talocrural joint. Orthotics or foot and ankle exercises can be used to control foot pronation.
- Hip external rotation weakness or femoral torsions can also affect ankle function and should be assessed and corrected.
- The clinician should also evaluate the patient for leg length discrepancies that would cause abnormal stresses to be placed onto the ankle joint.
- Rehabilitation should focus on the following:
  - Education in correct use of ice and heat at home for abatement of pain and control of edema
  - Implementation of a home exercise program
  - Teach proper footwear with or without orthotics. Correction of foot alignment and reduction of loading on the joint are important factors related to ankle osteoarthritis.
  - Manual therapy (STM, joint mobilization) can be used to improve joint mobility and arthrokinematics and to decrease pain.
  - Modalities: Ice or heat, ultrasound, electrical stimulation, and tape or braces can be used as adjuncts to improve the healing environment.
  - Factors that contribute to abnormal joint mechanics and loading should be determined and addressed.
- The ankle joint is a synovial joint. Therefore the cartilage heals and is affected by joint motion. It is aggravated by activities that excessively load the joint, but motion in a non-weight-bearing to a limited weight-bearing environment can greatly decrease the patient's symptoms.
- Exercises include the following:
  - Stretches to the calf (gastrocnemius and soleus) to decrease muscular and joint stiffness
  - "Arch forming" exercises to improve midfoot joint alignment by increasing muscular support
  - Proprioceptive exercises to improve balance and function
  - Cardiovascular exercises, bicycle progressing to treadmill, to promote circulation and healing

  - Hip weakness and restriction and foot abnormalities are contributing factors often associated with ankle osteoarthritis. These factors should be addressed in the patient's exercise regimen.
  - Exercises create a sense of control over the symptoms and the condition.
- Massage can decrease pain by relaxing muscular tension, improving circulation, and increasing endorphin release.

PROGNOSIS

- Long-term prognosis for a patient with ankle osteoarthritis depends on the extent of wear and tear and the ability to reduce the joint strain (posture, activity, etc).
- For the most part, ankle osteoarthritis is a degenerative condition. At earlier stages of the pathology, rehabilitation aimed at reducing the load placed on the joint can potentially slow or halt the progression of degeneration.
- For patients who are farther along in the degenerative process, outcomes will be less favorable because cartilage has only a limited ability to repair itself.

SIGNS AND SYMPTOMS INDICATING REFERRAL TO PHYSICIAN

- Unrelenting pain
- Unusual responses to therapy
- Red flag symptoms such as excessive redness and swelling and generalized malaise and fatigue: Infection

SUGGESTED READINGS

Abidi NA, Gruen GS, Conti SF, et al. Ankle arthrodesis: indications and techniques. *J Am Acad Ortho Surg*. 2000;8:200-209.

Dugan SA. Exercise for health and wellness at midlife and beyond: balancing benefits and risks. *Phys Med Rehabil Clin N Am*. 2007;18(3):555-575.

Easley ME, Vertullo CJ, Urban WC, Nunley JA, et al. Total ankle arthroplasty. *J Am Orthop Surg*. 2002;10:157-167.

Frey CZ. The Effects of obesity on orthopaedic foot and ankle pathology. *J Foot Ankle Int*. 2007;28(9):996-999.

Glass GG. Osteoarthritis. *Dis Mon*. 2006;52(9).

Huang YC. Effects of ankle-foot orthoses on ankle and foot kinematics in patient with ankle osteoarthritis. *Arch Phys Med Rehabil*. 2006;87(5):710-716.

Thomas R. Gait analysis and functional outcomes following ankle arthrodesis for isolated ankle arthritis. *J Bone Joint Surg Am*. 2006;88(3):526-535.

Valderrabano V, Nigg BM, von Tscharner V, Stefanyshyn DJ, Goepfert B, Hintermann B, et al. Gait analysis in ankle osteoarthritis and total ankle replacement. *Clinical Biomech (Bristol, Avon)* 2007;22(8):894-904.

Valderrabano V. Lower leg muscle atrophy in ankle osteoarthritis. *J Orthop Res*. 2006; 24(12):2159-2169.

AUTHOR: SARA GRANNIS

Section III

ORTHOPEDIC PATHOLOGY

BASIC INFORMATION

DEFINITION

- The term sprain indicates that the structural integrity of the ligament(s) at the ankle has been altered.
- The three classes of ankle sprains are:–
  - Lateral ankle sprains, which occur when the ligaments on the lateral portion of the ankle are injured. The most common ligaments injured are the anterior tibiofibular ligament and the calcaneal fibular ligament.
  - Syndesmotic sprains, which are synonymous with high ankle sprains and anterior tibiofibular ligaments sprains. These sprains occur when there is an injury to the ligaments between the two major bones of the lower leg (tibia and fibula) at the level of the ankle.
  - Medial ankle sprains, which are the rarest and occur when there is an injury to the deltoid ligament.
- Sprains are divided into the following three groups, depending on the severity of damage to the involved ligament:
  - Grade I sprain: The most common sprain requires the least amount of treatment and recovery. The ligaments connecting the ankle bones are often over stretched and damaged microscopically but not actually torn. The ligament damage has occurred without any significant instability developing.
  - Grade II (second-degree) sprain: A more severe sprain indicates that the ligament has been more significantly damaged, but there is no significant instability. The ligaments are often partially torn.
  - Grade III (third-degree) sprain: A grade III sprain is the most severe. This indicates that the ligament has been significantly damaged and that instability has resulted. A grade III injury means that the ligament has been torn.

SYNONYMS

- Ankle strain/sprain
- Ankle instability
- Twisted ankle
- High ankle sprain

ICD-9CM CODES
845.00 Unspecified site of ankle
     sprain
845.01 Deltoid ligament ankle
     sprain
845.02 Calcaneofibular (ligament)
     ankle sprain
845.03 Tibiofibular (ligament) sprain
     distal

OPTIMAL NUMBER OF VISITS
6

MAXIMAL NUMBER OF VISITS
20

ETIOLOGY

- The lateral ligaments and the anterior-lateral capsule are the most commonly injured structures. The most commonly damaged ligament is the anterior talofibular ligament followed by the calcaneal-fibular ligament.
- Ankle sprains usually occur as a result of trauma. As the ligament is loaded or stretched beyond its normal physiological capabilities, microtearing of the fibers occurs. If the loading continues, there will be gross tearing of the ligament, resulting in permanent deformation of the ligament and resultant joint instability.

EPIDEMIOLOGY AND DEMOGRAPHICS

- Approximately 1 to 10,000 people per day experience an ankle sprain daily or between 5000 to 27,000 sprains occur daily.
- Lateral ankle sprains account for 10% to 15% of all sports-related injuries.
- Injury to the anterior talofibular ligament occurs about 65% of the time.
- Syndesmotic sprains are responsible for approximately 10% of all ankle sprains.
- Medial ankle sprains are reported to be responsible for 5% to 10% of all ankle sprains.
- Ankle sprains most commonly occur in patients younger than 35 years, with the highest occurrence in the 15 to 19 years of age range.

MECHANISM OF INJURY

- Low ankle sprain: Lateral ankle ligament injuries are usually the result of a rapid inversion movement at the ankle. Patients commonly report they rolled their ankle or state they heard a pop during activities such as the following:
  - Planting the foot when running
  - Stepping up or down
  - Stepping or landing on an uneven surface
- High ankle sprain: Syndesmotic sprains are believed to occur when the ankle is planted in dorsiflexion with external rotation of the lower leg. Most syndesmotic ankle sprains are believed to occur because of direct contact.
- Medial ankle sprains occur with plantar flexion with eversion.

COMMON SIGNS AND SYMPTOMS

- Common signs and symptoms of ankle sprains include the following:
  - Ecchymosis
  - Bruising

- Redness
- Tenderness
- Instability
- Loss of ROM
- Inability to bear full weight
- Ankle ligament injuries commonly refer pain locally in the region of the ligament.
- Syndesmotic injuries may mimic pain similar to a lateral ankle sprain.

AGGRAVATING ACTIVITIES

Ankle sprains are usually aggravated with weight-bearing activities such as walking. Depending on the particular ligament that is injured, pain results with open-chain movements that increase stress on the injured ligament.

EASING ACTIVITIES

- Non–weight-bearing positions usually are the least painful. Patients are frequently advised to use ice, antiinflammatory medications, and pain medications during the acute stage of recovery.
- Some patients may be immobilized with a removable ankle brace or walking boot during the initial injury to help reduce pain during weight-bearing activities.

24-HOUR SYMPTOM PATTERN

During the acute stage, patients may feel pain throughout the day. As the healing process continues, patients may note stiffness in the morning for 30 to 60 minutes, followed by pain with progressive weight-bearing activities.

PAST HISTORY FOR THE REGION

- Patients frequently have recurrent ankle sprains of the same ankle, particularly if they did not participate in a rehabilitation program.
- Commonly, patients report that they have had an ankle injury in the past.

PHYSICAL EXAMINATION

- Patients usually present with limited weight bearing on the affected lower extremity.
- The patient may have limited ROM, depending on the grade of injury and which ligament is injured.
- Localized tenderness of the ligament
- Pain with ligament stress tests
- Hindfoot varus alignment
- Peroneal tendon insufficiency
- Congenital tarsal coalitions

IMPORTANT OBJECTIVE TESTS

- Lateral ligament sprains
  - Anterior drawer test is considered the hallmark test for lateral ankle instability, predominantly for the anterior tibiofibula ligament. Hertel et al reported sensitivity of 0.78 and specificity of 0.75.

- Syndesmotic sprains
  - Fibular translation test: Beumer et al. reported sensitivity of 0.82 and specificity of 0.88.
  - External rotation test: Although this is a common test performed for syndesmotic sprains, it has not been well researched. Beumer et al found high specificity of 0.95 but did not report on sensitivity.
- Medial ankle sprain
  - Valgus stress test: The reliability of this test has not been reported in the literature.

CONTRIBUTING/PREDISPOSING FACTORS

Strauss et al found that 64% of patients have some extraarticular pathology associated with lateral ankle sprains. The most common pathologies include peroneal tendon injuries (28%), os trigonum (13%), and os subfibulare and other lateral gutter ossicles (10%).

DIFFERENTIAL DIAGNOSIS

- Fibularis tendinitis
- Fracture
- Nerve injury
- Nerve entrapment
- Os trigonum
- Osteochondral defect
- Peripheral neuropathy
- Posterior tibial tendinitis
- Subluxing fibularis tendon
- Subluxed fibula
- Subtalar joint sprain
- Tarsal tunnel syndrome
- Vascular injury

TREATMENT

SURGICAL OPTIONS

- Surgery is not usually indicated for ankle sprains, especially grade I and II sprains. Patients may undergo surgery for grade III sprains.
- Patients with grade III syndesmotic sprains are usually treated with some form of internal fixation procedure. Surgical procedures vary, depending on the physician.
- Surgical reconstruction of the anterior tibiofibular ligament and/or calcaneal fibular ligament may be performed for chronic lateral ankle instability.
- Surgery has not been established as the treatment of choice for grade III sprains and usually is performed only after conservative care has failed.

SURGICAL OUTCOMES

Colville reported that 85% of all lateral ankle reconstructions were successful regardless of the surgical procedure used.

REHABILITATION

- Patients with ankle sprains should be taken through the following three-phase process, according to the stage of healing:
  - Phase one, or acute phase, should emphasize inflammation control, decreasing edema, and protection from further injury.
  - Phase two, or subacute stage, should emphasize decreasing pain, increasing pain free ROM, and limited loss of strength and proprioception.
  - Phase three should emphasize restoration of full ROM, strength, and proprioception with return to function.
- Several treatment options are available, including ankle braces, air cast, walking boot, or ankle taping.
- Several taping options are available. Tradition ankle taping for medial and lateral ankle stability has been regularly used during this phase. In addition, the Mulligan taping for lateral ankle sprain can be extremely effective.
- Crutches, walker, or other assistive devices may be used, depending on the severity of the sprain.
- Gentle joint mobilizations can be effective for pain and edema during the acute phase of injury. In addition, early mobilization has been found to assist in formation and orientation of collagen bundles during the healing process.
- For patients with lateral ankle sprains, a therapist should evaluate if pain is originating from the distal tibiofibular joint. This can be easily assessed by assessing pain and ROM with lantar flexion and inversion, then comparing this when assessing plantar flexion and inversion while applying a posterior/superior glide to the distal fibula. A decrease in pain and/or increased ROM indicates injury to the tibiofibular joint and not the anterior talofibular ligament.

PROGNOSIS

- Wester et al reported that 17% to 58% of people who experience ankle sprains are likely to experience recurrent sprains.
- Several factors are reported to contribute to recurrent ankle sprains that include joint laxity, muscular weakness, proprioceptive deficits, and delayed neuromuscular response.
- Recurrent ankle sprains are commonly reported in the literature. Both the use of ankle braces and taping have been found to be effective in reducing the risk of recurrence.
- The use of the posterior fibular glide taping has been reported by Moiler et al to be more effective than traditional ankle taping in preventing ankle sprains in competitive basketball players.
- The integration of proprioceptive retraining has also been found to be as effective as bracing in preventing recurrent lateral ankle sprains.

SIGNS AND SYMPTOMS INDICATING REFERRAL TO PHYSICIAN

- The modified Ottawa rules for the foot and ankle indicate the necessity of radiographs or referral to a physician.
- Radiographs are warranted if the patient is unable to bear weight immediately after injury or during examination.
- Radiographs are also warranted if bone tenderness is present at any one or more of the following:
  - Crest or midportion of the lateral or medial malleolus
  - Navicular
  - Base of the fifth metatarsal

SUGGESTED READINGS

Ankle sprains. *The Center for Orthopaedics & Sports Medicine*. www.arthroscopy.com/sp09005.htm; 2003.

Colville MR. Surgical treatment of the unstable ankle. *J Am Acad Orthop Surg.* 1998;6:368-377.

Colville MR, Grondel RJ. Anatomic reconstruction of the lateral ankle ligaments using a split peroneus brevis tendon graft. *Am J Sports Med.* 1995;23:210-213.

Moiler K, Hall T, Robinson K. The role of fibular tape in the prevention of ankle injury in basketball : A pilot study. *J Orthop Sports Med.* 2006;36(9):661-667.

Reischl SF, Noceti-Dewit LM. The foot and ankle: physical therapy patient management utilizing current evidence. In: *Current Concepts of Orthopaedic Physical therapy*. 2nd ed. La Crosse, Wi: Orthopaedic Section; 2006.

Seto JL, Brewster CE. Treatment approaches following foot and ankle injury. *Clin Sports Med.* 1994;13(4):695-719.

Strauss JE, Forsberg JA, Lippert 3rd FG. Chronic lateral ankle instability and associated conditions: a rationale for treatment. *Foot Ankle Int.* 2007;28(10):1041-1044.

Wester JU, Jespersen SM, Nielsen KD, Neumann L. Wobble board training after partial sprains of the lateral ligaments of the ankle: a prospective randomized study. *J Orthop Sports Phys Ther.* 1996;23(3):332-336.

Wolfe MW, Uhl ML, Mccluskey LC. Management of Ankle Sprains. *Am Fam Physician.* 2001;63:93-104.

Young CC. Ankle sprain. *EMedicine Journal.* 2002;3(1).

AUTHOR: JASON TONLEY

BASIC INFORMATION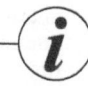

DEFINITION

- Compartment syndrome is defined as a condition in which increased pressure within a limited space compromises the circulation and function of the tissues within that space.
- There are two types of compartment syndrome: acute and chronic.
- There are separate compartment syndromes listed for different locations of involvement.

SYNONYMS

- Acute
  - Volkmann ischemia
  - Anterior shin splints
  - Calf hypertension
  - Traumatic tension in muscles
- Chronic
  - Chronic exertion compartment syndrome
  - Exercise-induced compartment syndrome
  - Anterior or medial tibial pain syndrome
  - Polyalgia

ICD-9CM CODES
728.9 Unspecified disorder of muscle ligament and fascia
958.8 Other early complications of trauma

OPTIMAL NUMBER OF VISITS
4

MAXIMAL NUMBER OF VISITS
16

ETIOLOGY

- Compartment syndrome (CS) is a condition in which there is substantial increased tissue pressure within a confined space. It can be an acute pathology if the mechanism of injury is sudden such as a blunt trauma, burn, or crush injury. It can be chronic if the tissue pressure is the result of an overuse or repetitive microtraumatic injury.
- It typically occurs from a traumatic injury or after an ischemic reperfusion injury. It may also be a result of a burn, prolonged limb compression after drug overdose, or poor positioning during surgery.
- Because the connective tissue that defines the compartment does not stretch, a small amount of bleeding into the compartment or swelling of the muscles within the compartment can cause immense pressure to rise.
- Chronic CS (CCS) is caused by repetitive heavy use of the muscles, as in a runner. Loss of circulation can cause

temporary or permanent damage to nearby nerves and muscle if the problem is not addressed.

- Physiologically, capillary blood flow is compromised with any pressure increases in the compartment. Edema of the soft tissue within the compartment further raises the intracompartment pressure, which compromises venous and lymphatic drainage of the injured area. Pressure, if further increased in a reinforcing vicious cycle, can compromise arteriole perfusion, leading to further tissue ischemia.
- Small vessels in the tissue become compressed when the pressure is ≥30 mm Hg. This leads to reduced nutrient blood flow, ischemia, and pain. If the diastolic blood pressure exceeds compartment pressure by < 30 mm Hg, it is considered an emergency.

EPIDEMIOLOGY AND DEMOGRAPHICS

- Approximately 40% of CS occurs with persons experiencing tibial shaft fractures; 17% of individuals experiencing a tibial fracture have a CS in which the anterior compartment may be affected. Soft tissue injuries without fractures account for another 23%. Incidence in complex pelvic surgeries is 1 in 500.
- Acute CS (ACS) is seen more commonly in the population younger than 35 years as a result of activity level. This can later lead to loss of function and affect long-term productivity.

MECHANISM OF INJURY

- Acute
  - Blunt trauma
  - Crush injuries
  - Fractures
  - Tight cast or brace
  - Muscle rupture
  - Vascular puncture
  - IV injections
  - Ischemic-reperfusion post injury
  - Burns
  - Prolonged limb compression (i.e., cast or antishock garment)
  - Prolonged surgery in lithotomy positions (i.e., pelvic and perineal surgery)
- Chronic
  - Overuse injuries (i.e., runners, cyclists, and athletes in other sports that demand running)
  - Previous fracture, extremity surgery, or casting

COMMON SIGNS AND SYMPTOMS

- The pain after a sudden mechanism of injury in ACS may be beyond the physical response of the injury. It usually does not improve with medications.

The swelling and tension of the soft tissue may appear minimal, but the pain and loss of voluntary movement may be severe. There may be possible motor and sensory deficits to certain areas following a nerve distribution.

- In CCS, symptoms occur gradually, depending on the demand or loading of the muscle(s) involved. This usually occurs in individuals participating in a repetitive athletic event such as running, cycling, and sometimes dancing. It may be concurrent with other overuse syndromes (e.g., tibial stress fractures). A gradual dull achy "tightness" may be experienced in a specific or multiple compartments. Muscles are tender to touch. It may progress to numbness and paresthesia, as with the acute onset, but the gradual onset depends on the intensity of the activity.
- Referral pattern
  - Anterior CS: Pain is local to the location of the injury, with pain radiating to its periphery. Numbness and paresthesia may be an issue because of the anterior tibial artery and the deep peroneal nerve, which supplies sensation to the first web space.
  - Posterior CS: Sensation to the lateral foot and distal calf may be affected if the sural nerve is compromised.
  - The plantar surface of the foot may experience sensation deficits and pain if the tibial nerve is affected.

AGGRAVATING ACTIVITIES

- Excessive walking
- Running (high intensity, duration, and uneven surface)
- Tight clothing

EASING ACTIVITIES

- Rest
- Lying supine with legs elevated
- Pain medications
- Antiinflammatory medications

24-HOUR SYMPTOM PATTERN

There is no literature to confirm any pattern regarding time of day. CCS depends on activity type and intensity.

PAST HISTORY FOR THE REGION

Individuals who have previously experienced a CS may have higher predisposition to a recurrent problem. Unfortunately, the literature does not confirm any specified number at this time. Previous fractures, extremity surgery, or casting is considered to have some relevance in recurrence of the problem.

PHYSICAL EXAMINATION

- ACS
  - 5 Ps: Pain, paralysis, paresthesia, pallor, and pulselessness

- o Decreased acuity to two-point discrimination
- o Impaired capillary refill of >3 seconds
- o Pulselessness may not be evident unless very severe.
- CCS
  - o Mild muscle tenderness
  - o Muscular herniation
  - o Capillary refill, skin color, skin temperature, ROM, and tendon reflexes are usually normal except in severe cases.
- Anterior CS
  - o Swelling and tautness in involved region (skin and muscle)
  - o Decreased function of ankle dorsiflexion (tibialis anterior muscle) with possible footdrop
  - o Decreased function of toes into extension (long toe extensors)
  - o Paresthesia in the web space between the first and second toes
  - o Possible palpable muscle herniation (approximately 40% of cases)
- Posterior CS
  - o Decreased function of the plantar flexor and invertors of the foot
  - o Decreased function of long toe flexors
  - o Paresthesia at the plantar surface of the foot
  - o Pain with stretch
  - o Pain with muscular activity (if able)

IMPORTANT OBJECTIVE TESTS

- There are no specific physical objective tests noted in any literature at this time.
- Since the 1970s, a number of devices were developed to facilitate early diagnosis by identifying the increased intracompartmental pressure in all cases.
  - o Examples of some of these systems are wick catheter, slit catheter, and solid-state transducer intracompartmental catheter.
  - o The transducer-tipped probe has been shown to be easy to use and highly accurate according to Willy et al.

DIFFERENTIAL DIAGNOSIS

- Anterior CS
  - o Shin splints
  - o Tibial stress fractures
  - o Fibular stress fractures
  - o Severe muscle trauma
  - o Neurapraxia of the deep or superficial peroneal nerve
  - o Arterial occlusion of the anterior tibial artery
- Posterior CS
  - o Arterial occlusion of the peroneal artery
  - o Deep vein thrombosis (DVT)
  - o Atherosclerosis with vascular claudication

- o Severe muscle trauma
- o Neurapraxia of the tibial and sural nerve
- o Cellulitis
- o Popliteal artery compression from aberrant insertion of the medial gastrocnemius
- o Muscle hyperdevelopment
- o Cystic adventitial disease

CONTRIBUTING FACTORS

- Length of procedure or surgery
- Amount of leg elevation
- Amount of perioperative blood loss
- Peripheral vascular disease
- Obesity
- Diabetes
- Poor running mechanics with excessive ankle pronation

TREATMENT

- ACS is a medical emergency requiring immediate surgical treatment (known as a fasciotomy) to allow the pressure to return to normal. This treatment may be a subcutaneous fasciotomy or open fasciectomy.
- Subacute CS, while not quite as much of an emergency, usually requires urgent surgical treatment similar to acute compartment syndrome.
- CCS in the lower leg can be treated conservatively or surgically. Conservative treatment includes rest, antiinflammatories, elevation of the limb, and manual decompression. Patients should be educated on the proper footwear with possible orthotics to improve foot mechanics for increased pronation. They should also be educated on the type of running surface, intensity of activity, and monitoring the extremity for physical changes.
- In cases where symptoms persist, the condition should be treated by a surgical procedure. Without treatment, CCS can develop into the acute syndrome. A possible complication of surgical intervention for CCS can be chronic venous insufficiency.

SURGICAL OPTIONS

- Subcutaneous fasciotomy
- Open fasciectomy
- Amputation

SURGICAL OUTCOMES

- Subjects with ACS after fasciotomy are expected to have more complications because of its sudden onset. Mortality rates are 10% to 15% with a profound morbidity. Diminished limb function is rated relatively high at 27%, and amputation rates are in the 10% to 20% range.
- In a study of individuals who have undergone a fasciotomy for CCS, 70% of patients had good-to-excellent outcomes. Another study reports an 80% to

90% success rate with decreased symptoms and return to sports. Recurrence rate of 3% to 20% was reported, with possible relationship to excessive scar tissue formation and inadequate fascial release.

REHABILITATION

- The goal of rehabilitation is individualized to each person's needs because of the lack of literature to support any specific protocol.
- Rehabilitation of CCS has not been fully explored.
- Nonsurgical rehabilitation should include the following:
  - o Rest
  - o Analysis of the lower extremity biomechanics
  - o Proper footwear and orthotics to address possible excessive foot pronation
  - o Correction of training errors: Intensity, duration, and type of progression
- Postsurgical rehabilitation should include the following:
  - o Proper skin care
  - o Correction of footdrop with possible ankle-foot orthosis
  - o Gait training with initial status of weight bearing as tolerated (WBAT)
  - o Gentle ROM exercises after day of surgery
  - o Gradual strengthening and return to activities in the following 1 to 2 weeks
  - o Return to prior functional status within 8 to 12 weeks

PROGNOSIS

- Some specialists report that conservative treatment has a 100% failure rate. For those who undergo surgery, there is an 80% to 90% success rate.
- Untreated CS-mediated ischemia of the muscles and nerves leads to eventual irreversible damage and death of the tissues within the compartment.

SIGNS AND SYMPTOMS INDICATING REFERRAL TO PHYSICIAN

- Contractures
- Paralysis
- Infection
- Gangrene
- Myoglobinuria
- Kidney failure
- Nerve damage

SUGGESTED READINGS

Elliott K, Johnstone A. Diagnosing acute compartment syndrome. *J Bone Joint Surg.* 2003;85-B:625–632.

Frontera WR, Silver JK, Rizzo TD, Rizzo Jr TD. Essentials of physical medicine and rehabilitation: musculoskeletal disorders, pain, rehabilitation. 2008;325–330.

Section III

ORTHOPEDIC PATHOLOGY

Heemskerk J, Kitslaar P. Acute compartment syndrome of the lower leg: retrospective study on prevalence, technique, and outcome of fasciotomies. *World J Surg.* 2003;27:744-747.

Leversedge FJ, Casey PJ, Seiler 3rd JG, et al. Endoscopically assisted fasciotomy: description of technique and in vitro assessment of lower-leg compartment decompression. *Am J Sports Med.* 2002;30(2):272-278.

Mubarak SJ, Owen CA, Garfin S, et al. Acute exertional superficial posterior compartment syndrome. *Am J Sports Med.* 1978;6(5): 287-290.

Schepsis AA, Gill SS, Foster TA. Fasciotomy for exertional anterior compartment syndrome: is lateral compartment release necessary? *Am J Sports Med.* 1999;27:430-435.

Swain R, Ross D. Lower extremity compartment syndrome: when to suspect acute or chronic pressure buildup. *Postgrad Med.* 1999;105:159-162,165,168.

Willy C, Gerngross H, Sterk J. Measurement of intracompartment pressure with the use of a new electronic transducer-tipped catheter system. *J Bone Joint Surg Am.* 1999;81-A:158-168.

AUTHOR: STEVEN M. YUN

BASIC INFORMATION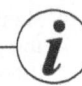

DEFINITION

Anterolateral impingement is the impingement of soft tissue structures: capsule ligament or synovium or bone in the anterolateral gutter of the ankle caused by trauma, infection or rheumatological or degenerative disease states.

SYNONYMS

- Ankle impingement
- Chronic ankle pain
- Synovitis
- Ankle strain or sprain
- Syndesmotic sprain

ICD-9CM CODES

No ICD-9 code exists for anterolateral ankle impingement; however, the following are possible codes to be used:
845.00 Unspecified site of ankle sprain
719.27 Villonodular synovitis involving ankle and foot
726.90 Enthesopathy of unspecified site
959.7 Other and unspecified injury to knee leg ankle and foot
729.5 Pain in limb
719.57 Stiffness of joint not elsewhere classified involving ankle and foot

OPTIMAL NUMBER OF VISITS

8 visits or fewer

MAXIMAL NUMBER OF VISITS

Up to 70 visits (if postsurgical)

ETIOLOGY

- Ankle impingement is most typically the result of a posttraumatic event at the ankle. Repetitive injury is also noted as a common cause leading to development of anterolateral ankle impingement.
- Impingement may be caused by bone or soft tissue. In the case of a traumatic injury, a loose body may develop in the joint space or gets lodged in the joint space with dorsiflexion. In the case of soft tissue impingement, after injury, thickening of the synovium or capsule or a thickened hyaline band of connective tissue, called a *meniscoid lesion*, forms in the joint space, causing impingement within the anterolateral joint space.
- Bone spurs are considered a primary cause of pain in anterolateral impingement syndrome.
- McMurray described the spurs as traction spurs that develop as a result of frequent impact in plantar flexion; when kicking a ball, spurs form at the connection of the capsule to the bone. A recent study by Tol et al found that the

joint capsule attaches 4.3 mm above the region where these bone spurs form and they are unlikely to be caused by repetitive traction stress. Currently, best evidence suggests that these spurs are caused by repetitive microtrauma or macrotrauma to the joint cartilage that extends 2 to 3 mm above the weight-bearing surface.
- Tibial spurs usually form on the anterolateral surface, and talar bone spurs are usually found medial to midline.
- Recent evidence suggests that syndesmotic sprains can cause a tear in the anteroinferior tibiofibular ligament (AITFL). A tear of the AITFL can create the a fascicle that can become lodged in the anterolateral ankle with dorsiflexion or may cause synovitis in the anterolateral joint space.

EPIDEMIOLOGY AND DEMOGRAPHICS

- It has been reported that 20% to 40% of people have chronic ankle pain after ankle sprains and that one third of those patients have pain related to some form of impingement syndrome.
- Anterolateral impingement syndrome most commonly occurs in a population younger than 40 years, with a mean age of 33 to 35 years old.
- Impingement most commonly occurs in the athletic population: Basketball, soccer, and volleyball players, as well as dancers.

MECHANISM OF INJURY

Anterolateral ankle impingement is usually the result of an injured ankle sprain or a repetitive microtrauma. In the case of dancers, mechanism of injury is reported to be caused by excessive talar dome compression secondary to excessive dorsiflexion with the demi-plié position.

COMMON SIGNS AND SYMPTOMS

- Patients report a history of vague or sharp anterolateral ankle pain located in the lateral gutter region.
- Patients may also report complaints of catching, locking, or giving way in the ankle.

AGGRAVATING ACTIVITIES

- Activities requiring dorsiflexion typically aggravate the ankle. During dorsiflexion the pathological structure is compressed between the tibia and the talar head. These activities include the following:
  ○ Walking
  ○ Squatting
  ○ Stairs
  ○ Cutting
  ○ Pivoting

EASING ACTIVITIES

- Rest
- Ice
- Unweighting activities
- Cessation of activity
- Bracing

24-HOUR SYMPTOM PATTERN

- Patients typically complain of pain with aggravating activities.
- Patients may present with signs of pain and stiffness after activity.
- Pain and/or stiffness are the result of an inflammatory process.

PAST HISTORY FOR THE REGION

Patients typically report a history of an ankle sprain, blunt trauma, or repetitive injury to the lateral ankle. Some patients, such as dancers, may report a history of activity that requires excessive dorsiflexion.

PHYSICAL EXAMINATION

- Swelling in the sinus tarsi region
- Palpable pain and tenderness in the lateral gutter region
- Pain with palpation of the AITFL
- Decreased proprioception
- Limited dorsiflexion: This may be by only a few degrees as compared to the other side.
- Positive Molloy impingement test/forced dorsiflexion test

IMPORTANT OBJECTIVE TESTS

- Molloy impingement test/forced dorsiflexion test
  ○ The patient is in a sitting position. This test consists of placing thumb pressure into the anterolateral portion of the talus while forcefully dorsiflexing the foot. A positive test reproduces pain in the anterolateral region of the ankle.
  ○ Sensitivity: 0.95; specificity: 0.88
- A clinical prediction rule has been developed by Lui et al for anterolateral impingement. The clinical prediction rule states that five of the six symptoms in the following list are positive for anterior ankle impingement:
  ○ Anterolateral joint tenderness
  ○ Anterolateral joint swelling
  ○ Pain with forced dorsiflexion
  ○ Pain with single-leg squat
  ○ Pain with activities
  ○ Absence of joint instability
  ○ Sensitivity: 0.94; specificity: 0.75
- X-rays are useful in identifying bone spurs that cause impingement.
- MRI findings are positive 30% of the time in patients with ankle impingement. The result is usually a low-density signal, indicating a meniscoid mass.
- MRI, computed tomography (CT) scan, and bone scan maybe more useful in ruling out other pathologies for differential diagnosis.

Section III

ORTHOPEDIC PATHOLOGY

- Haller et al reported that MRI did not accurately diagnose impingement but was more helpful in determining intraarticular versus extraarticular joint pathology. Additionally, no benefit was found from performing MR arthrography (MRA) as compared to MRI.

DIFFERENTIAL DIAGNOSIS

- Osteochondral lesions
- Calcific ossicles
- Peroneal subluxation
- Degenerative joint disease
- Peripheral nerve entrapment
- Fracture
- Subtalar joint dislocation

CONTRIBUTING FACTORS

- Previous ankle sprains
- Joint laxity
- Excessive calcaneal valgus
- Excessive pronation
- Peroneal weakness
- Participation in sports that involve cutting, pivoting, and jumping
- Poor footwear
- Poor lower extremity biomechanics

TREATMENT

SURGICAL OPTIONS

- The current literature indicates that patients are candidates for surgery if symptoms fail to improve or plateau after 3 months of conservative care that includes medical management, modalities, bracing, and rehabilitation.
- Surgical options include either arthroscopic debridement or open arthrotomy.
- The primary goal of surgery is to debride or remove the pathological tissue or bone spur causing the impingement.
- Arthroscopic versus open debridement:
  - Scanton and McDermott found that patients recovered more quickly with arthroscopic debridement.
  - Coull et al reported excellent results in 92% of patient at a 5- to 9-year follow-up provided they did not have preoperative joint space narrowing.

SURGICAL OUTCOMES

- Surgery is a very viable option for anterolateral impingement. Several authors report high satisfaction rates with full return to premorbid activity levels.
- Van Dijk et al reported an overall 73% excellent or good result 2 years postsurgery, 90% if no joint space narrowing was noted.
- Tol et al reported at a mean follow-up of 6.5 years, 77% of patients with no osteoarthritis or grade I osteoarthritis had excellent or good results, and 53% of patients with grade II osteoarthritis had excellent or good results.

REHABILITATION

- Since many of these patients usually present with a traumatic injury or are post-surgical, treatment should initially focus on control of inflammation and edema. Treatment can include the following:
  - STM for edema
  - Joint mobilization: Grades 1 and 2
  - Use of an assistive device for ambulation
  - Pain free ROM exercise
  - Proximal strengthening
  - Cold or hot pack
  - Ultrasound
  - Electrical stimulation
  - Bracing or taping
- Treatment should focus on normalizing impairments at the ankle and addressing contributing factors. Since many of these patients present with limited ROM, limited strength, and decreased strength, the following are considered treatment options:
  - Joint mobilization: Talocrural joint to promote dorsiflexion
  - Joint mobilization: Subtalar joint to promote inversion
  - Proprioceptive exercises
  - Strengthening
  - Stretching
  - Biomechanical corrections
  - Bracing or taping
  - Orthotics
- Compression of the anterolateral structures is considered a cause of impingement. The following are considered possible biomechanical faults that can cause increased compression of lateral structures:
  - Excessive midfoot pronation
  - Calcaneal valgus
  - Valgus moment at the knee
  - Femoral adduction or medial rotation
- Patients who are noted to have hypermobility of the midfoot or excessive calcaneal eversion should be considered for orthotics. Patients who are unable to correct or control these positions with strengthening and muscle reeducation should be considered candidates for surgery.

PROGNOSIS

- Long-term prognosis appears to be primarily affected by the amount of joint space narrowing prior to injury. Studies indicate that the greater amount of osteoarthritis present at the time of injury, the poorer the prognosis.
- Patients can usually return to sporting activities as tolerated at 4 to 6 weeks. Patients with syndesmotic injuries may require a longer period of time before returning to participating in sports.

SIGNS AND SYMPTOMS INDICATING REFERRAL TO PHYSICIAN

- Patients should be referred to the physician if they present with signs and symptoms such as the following:

  - Significant decrease in weight-bearing tolerance: Fracture
  - Increased unrelenting pain and fever: Infection
  - Pain that is progressively worsening or that is not relieved by rest, decreased tolerance to weight bearing, progressively increasing joint pain: Avascular necrosis

SUGGESTED READINGS

Bassett 3rd FH, Gates 3rd HS, Billys JB, Morris HB, Nikolaou PK. Talar impingement by the antero-inferior tibiofibular ligament. A cause of chronic pain in the ankle after inversion sprain. *J Bone Joint Surg Am.* 1990;72(1):55-59.

Coull R, Raffiq T, James LE, Stephens MM. Open treatment of anterior impingement of the ankle. *J Bone Joint Surg Br.* 2003; 85-B:550-553.

Haller J, Bernt R, Seeger T, Weissenback A, Tuchler H, Resnick D. MR-imaging of anterior tibiotalar impingement syndrome: agreement, sensitivity and specificity of MR-imaging and indirect MR-arthrography. *Eur J Radiol.* 2006;58(3):450-460.

Hauger O, Moinard M, Lasalarie JC, Chauveaux D, Diard F. Anterolateral compartment of the ankle in the lateral impingement syndrome: appearance on CT arthrography. *AJR Am J Roentgenol.* 1999;173(3):685-690.

Henderson I, La Valette D. Ankle impingement: combined anterior and posterior impingement syndrome of the ankle. *Foot Ankle Int.* 2004;25(9):632-638.

Liu SH, Nuccion SL, Finerman G. Diagnosis of anterolateral ankle impingement. Comparison between magnetic resonance imaging and clinical examination. *Am J Sports Med.* 1997;25(3):389-393.

McMurray TP. Footballer's ankle. *Lancet.* 1955;2:1219-1220.

Molis MA. Ankle impingement syndromes. *EMedicine Journal.* 2006.

Molloy S, Solan MC, Bendall SP. Synovial impingement in the ankle. A new physical sign. *J Bone Joint Surg Br.* 2003;85(3):330-333.

Nihal A, Rose DJ, Trepman E. Arthroscopic treatment of anterior ankle impingement syndrome in dancers. *Foot Ankle Int.* 2005;26(11):908-912.

Nikolopoulos CE, Tsirikos AI, Sourmelis S, Papachristou G. The accessory anteroinferior tibiofibular ligament as a cause of talar impingement: a cadaveric study. *Am J Sports Med.* 2004;32(2):389-395.

Scanton PE, McDermott JE. Anterior tibiotalar spurs: a comparison of open versus arthroscopic debridement. *Foot and Ankle.* 1992;13:125-129.

Tol JL, van Dijk CN. Etiology of the anterior ankle impingement syndrome: a descriptive anatomical study. *Foot Ankle Int.* 2004;25(6):382-386.

Urguden M, Soyuncu Y, Ozdemir H, Sekban H, Akyildiz FF, Aydin AT. Arthroscopic treatment of anterolateral soft tissue impingement of the ankle: evaluation of factors affecting outcome. *Arthroscopy.* 2005;21(3):317-322.

van Dijk CN, Tol JL, Verheyen CC. A prospective study of prognostic factors concerning the outcome of arthroscopic surgery for anterior ankle impingement. *Am J Sports Med.* 1997;25:737-745.

AUTHOR: JASON TONLEY

BASIC INFORMATION

DEFINITION

Deep vein thrombosis (DVT) or thrombophlebitis is a partial or complete occlusion of a vein by a thrombus with secondary inflammatory reaction in the wall of the deep small vein

SYNONYMS

- Deep venous thrombosis
- Thrombophlebitis
- Calf vein thrombosis
- Economy class syndrome

ICD-9CM CODES
453.40 Venous embolism and thrombosis of unspecified deep vessels of lower extremity

OPTIMAL NUMBER OF VISITS

Not applicable

MAXIMAL NUMBER OF VISITS

Not applicable

ETIOLOGY

- DVT is a formation of a blood clot in a deep vein. It commonly affects the veins in the lower extremity (femoral or popliteal vein) but occasionally affects the veins of the arm (Paget-Schrötter disease).
- According to Virchow's triad, venous thrombosis occurs via three mechanisms: Decreased flow rate of blood, damage to the blood vessel wall, and increased tendency of the blood to clot.
- Thrombus formation is usually attributed to venous stasis, hypercoagulability, or injury to the venous wall, although other risk factors are present. Commonly, at least two of the three conditions (see risk factors in section on Treatment) must be present for thrombi to form.
- Trauma to the endothelium of the vein wall exposes subendothelial tissues to platelets in the venous blood, initiating a blood clot or thrombosis. Platelets on the vein wall attract the deposition of fibrin, leukocytes, and erythrocytes, forming a thrombus. Secondary inflammatory changes develop as it forms scarring of the vein wall and destruction of the valves when the thrombus is invaded by fibroblasts.

EPIDEMIOLOGY AND DEMOGRAPHICS

- DVT is the third most common cardiovascular disease after acute coronary artery episodes and cerebrovascular accidents. Up to 2 million Americans are affected annually or about 1 per 1000 persons per year. Approximately 30% of people undergoing major surgical procedures develop DVT up to 2 weeks postoperatively. About 1% to 5% die from complications (e.g., pulmonary embolism).
- The prevalence is highest in people older than 40 years. Different sources vary the age from 40 to 60 years.
- Women are more susceptible to developing DVT because risk factors include pregnancy, childbirth, and hormone supplements or replacements. There are also genetic and lifestyle factors that influence its probability such as use of oral contraceptives and smoking.

MECHANISM OF INJURY

- Physical immobility
- Trauma
- Surgery

COMMON SIGNS AND SYMPTOMS

- 50% of individuals may have no signs or symptoms in the affected extremity in the early stages.
- Classics symptoms may include the following:
  - Swelling
  - Tightness
  - Ache
  - Pain with possible redness.
- Symptoms may occur bilaterally, although they are usually unilateral. The condition is more severe when symptoms involve the entire extremity.
- Signs are often absent. There may be slight swelling in the involved leg, slight fever, or tachycardia. These are unreliable and may occur without DVT.
- In phlegmasia alba dolens, the leg is pale and cool, with a diminished arterial pulse as a result of spasm. It usually results from acute occlusion of the iliac and femoral veins caused by DVT.
- In phlegmasia cerulea dolens, there is an acute and nearly total venous occlusion of the entire extremity outflow, including the iliac and femoral veins. The leg is usually painful, cyanosed, and edematous. Venous gangrene may supervene.

AGGRAVATING ACTIVITIES

- Walking
- Calf exercises: Resistive or passive stretch
- Exercise that increases cardiovascular activity
- Wearing tight-fitting clothes

EASING ACTIVITIES

- Lying supine with legs elevated above the heart
- Medications

24-HOUR SYMPTOM PATTERN

- Patient may have nocturnal cramping in severe cases.
- Symptoms may increase with increased activities.

PAST HISTORY FOR THE REGION

There is a 5% probability of DVT recurrence if treatment was insufficient or risk factors were not monitored properly.

PHYSICAL EXAMINATION

- Currently, duplex venous ultrasound is the most common test used to diagnose deep vein clots. It is reported to have high sensitivity, specificity, and reproducibility. It is used to evaluate the blood flow in the veins and can detect the presence and specific location of blood clots. During a venous ultrasound, the technologist applies pressure when scanning the arm or leg. If the vein does not compress with pressure, it may indicate a blood clot is present. This may or may not be used with impedance plethysmography or Doppler ultrasonography.
- Intravenous (IV) venography is less often used because it is invasive, but it still remains the gold standard in detecting DVT. It may be performed if the duplex ultrasound does not provide a clear diagnosis. During the procedure, a contrast material (dye) is injected into the veins to make the vein and the blood clot visible on x-ray.
- Other tests that may be performed to detect a blood clot include MRI, MR venography (MRV), and CT scan.
- D-dimer is a fibrin degradation product present in the blood after a blood clot is degraded by fibrinolysis. This test is used primarily to rule out the pathology rather than ruling it in. A negative test (low score) virtually rules out thrombosis at 1% to 5% probability that it may exist with 0.93 sensitivity. A positive test (high score) requires further testing according to its low specificity at 0.44.
- If the physician suspects that an inherited disorder could be causing the clots, he or she may conduct a series of blood tests such as the following:
  - Complete blood count (CBC)
  - Primary coagulation studies: prothrombin time (PT), activated partial thromboplastin time (APTT), fibrinogen, and liver enzymes
  - Renal function and electrolytes
- These tests may be important if the patient has the following:
  - Repeated blood clots that cannot be linked to any other cause
  - A blood clot in a vein at an unusual location such as in a vein from the intestines, liver, kidney, or brain
  - A strong family history of blood clots.

Section III

ORTHOPEDIC PATHOLOGY

IMPORTANT OBJECTIVE TESTS

- Scarvelis and Wells Clinical Prediction Rules
  ○ Sensitivity: 0.78; specificity: 0.98
- Wells score or criteria (possible score −2 to 9)
  ○ Active cancer (treatment within last 6 months or palliative): 1 point
  ○ Calf swelling >3 cm compared to other calf (measured 10 cm below tibial tuberosity): 1 point
  ○ Collateral superficial veins (nonvaricose): 1 point
  ○ Pitting edema (confined to symptomatic leg): 1 point
  ○ Swelling of entire leg: 1 point
  ○ Localized pain along distribution of deep venous system: 1 point
  ○ Paralysis, paresis, or recent cast immobilization of lower extremities: 1 point
  ○ Recently bedridden >3 days or major surgery requiring regional or general anesthetic in past 12 weeks: 1 point
  ○ Previously documented DVT: 1 point
  ○ Alternative diagnosis at least as likely: Subtract 2 points
- Interpretation
  ○ Score of 2 or higher: DVT is likely. Consider imaging the leg veins.
  ○ Score of less than 2: DVT is unlikely. Consider blood test such as D-dimer test to further rule out DVT.
- Homans' test: Dorsiflexion of foot elicits pain in posterior calf. However, it must be noted that it is of little diagnostic value and is theoretically dangerous because of the possibility of dislodging a of loose clot.
  ○ Sensitivity: 0.35 to 0.48; specificity: 0.41
- Pratt's sign: Squeezing posterior calf elicits pain.
  ○ Sensitivity: 0.82; specificity: 0.72

DIFFERENTIAL DIAGNOSIS **Dx**

- Superficial phlebitis or superficial venous thrombosis
- Achilles tendinitis
- Gastrocnemius and plantar muscle injury
- Baker's cyst

CONTRIBUTING FACTORS

- Immobility
  ○ Hospitalization or prolonged bed rest
  ○ Neurological disorder (spinal cord injury, stroke, etc)
  ○ Chronic disorder (cardiac disease)
  ○ Cancer and chemotherapy treatments
  ○ Long travel
- Trauma
  ○ Major surgery
  ○ Recent injury
  ○ Fracture or dislocation
  ○ Childbirth
  ○ Sclerosing agent
- Lifestyle
  ○ Smoking
  ○ Oral contraceptive use
  ○ Hormone replacement therapy or medication
  ○ Pregnancy
  ○ In vitro fertilization
- Hypercoagulation
  ○ Hereditary thrombotic disorders
  ○ Neoplasm
  ○ Increased levels of coagulation factors (VII, XI)
  ○ Increased levels of homocysteine
  ○ Prothrombin mutation
  ○ Activated protein C syndrome
- Others
  ○ Genetics
  ○ Age older than 40 years
  ○ Obesity
  ○ Diabetes mellitus

TREATMENT **Rx**

- Depending on the condition, the patient may be admitted to the hospital for DVT treatment or may receive outpatient treatment.
- According to a meta-analysis by the Cochrane Collaboration, hospitalization is considered if the patient has more than two of the following risk factors:
  ○ Bilateral DVT
  ○ Renal insufficiency
  ○ Body weight less than 70 kg
  ○ Recent immobility
  ○ Chronic heart failure
  ○ Cancer
- The main goals in treating DVT are the following:
  ○ Stop the clot from getting bigger
  ○ Prevent the clot from breaking off in the vein and moving to the lungs
  ○ Reduce the risk of another blood clot
  ○ Prevent long-term complications from the blood clot (chronic venous insufficiency or postthrombotic syndrome)

NONSURGICAL OPTIONS

- *Anticoagulants* (sometimes called blood thinners) decrease the blood's ability to clot but do not break up blood clots that have already formed.
  ○ First priority is prompt anticoagulation with heparin to prevent local extension, embolization, and recurrence of venous thromboembolic disease. This continues for 3 to 5 days until the patient is stable.
  ○ Two options for acute anticoagulant treatment are IV unfractionated heparin (UH) and subcutaneous low-molecular-weight heparin (LMWH). Physicians may choose enoxaparin sodium (Lovenox) or Fragmin sodium (dalteparin sodium). Fondaparinux sodium (Arixtra) may be used in conjunction with these for quicker results.
  ○ Weight-based IV heparin has been shown to achieve therapeutic anticoagulation more rapidly than traditional approaches. This protocol achieved therapeutic anticoagulation in 97% of patients within 24 hours in a randomized controlled trial. It was shown to be more effective, safer, and superior to the standard therapy. Patients treated with UH should remain hospitalized until they are therapeutically anticoagulated with oral warfarin.
  ○ LMWH has been used since 1998 for acute outpatient management of DVT after approval of enoxaparin. The advantage includes fixed dosing, subcutaneous route of administration, and more predictable anticoagulant response. Laboratory monitoring is unnecessary except in patients with renal insufficiency. In comparison with unfractionated heparin, LMWH significantly reduced the risk of death over 3 to 6 months. A subsequent meta-analysis of 13 randomized controlled trials with a total of 4447 patients with venous thromboembolism had statistically significant reduction in mortality with reduction in the risk of recurrent thromboembolism and major bleeding.
  ○ Second treatment uses oral warfarin (Coumadin) therapy in conjunction on the first day of treatment to establish the therapeutic international normalized ratio (INR) after heparin loading is complete. Pregnant women cannot take warfarin and are treated with heparin or LMWH only. Antithrombotic effect of warfarin is best established after 3 to 5 days, thus the reason for overlap with heparin. There has been improved success in achieving a stable and therapeutic INR by day 5 with less initial risk of hemorrhagic complication.
  ○ No randomized or cohort studies directly compare inferior vena caval interruption with standard anticoagulation therapy. A recent clinical trial in 400 anticoagulated patients revealed a significant decrease in pulmonary embolism assessed at day 12 of therapy but a significant increase in the rate of recurrent symptomatic DVT over the next 2 years by 9.2%. Available evidence does not support the use of vena caval filters in managing the patient with an initial and uncomplicated DVT.
- *Thrombolytics* are medications given to actually dissolve the blood clot that has already formed. It may be generally

reserved for extensive clot (e.g. an iliofemoral thrombosis). Drugs such as streptokinase, urokinase, and tissue plasminogen activator are infused into a vein in the arm or foot or in some cases directly at the clot using a catheter and x-ray control. Because they increase the risk of bleeding, they are only used in special situations determined by the physician. These situations may include massive swelling of an arm or leg or in situations where a blood clot in the lungs (pulmonary embolism) has left the patient very short of breath or with low blood pressure. Thrombolysis appears to offer advantages in terms of reducing postthrombotic syndrome and maintaining venous patency after DVT. Use of strict eligibility criteria has improved the safety and acceptability of this treatment. The optimum drug, dose, and route of administration have yet to be determined. Bleeding complications, stroke, or intracerebral hemorrhage are potential adverse events for both treatments.

• *Elastic compression stockings* should be routinely applied within 1 week of diagnosis and up to at least 1 year for best results. They can reduce the chronic swelling that can occur in the leg after a blood clot has developed. The swelling often occurs because the valves in the leg veins have become damaged or the vein remains blocked from the blood clot.

  ○ Most compression stockings are worn just below the knee. These stockings are tight at the ankle and become looser as they go up the leg. This causes gentle external compression (or pressure) on the leg.

MEDICAL (SURGICAL AND NONSURGICAL) OPTIONS

• *Catheter-directed thrombolytic therapy* is a nonsurgical treatment to dissolve blood clots. The patient receives a sedative with topical anesthesia to the area where the procedure is to be performed. A sheath (thin, plastic tube) is inserted into the vein along with a catheter. It is guided through the vein to the segment in which the blood clot is located. Thrombolytic medication is infused through the catheter into the clot. The medication takes effect in a matter of hours to a few days. The physician often uses a venogram or duplex ultrasound to evaluate the progress of the medication. At times, the narrowed area of the vein needs to be treated with angioplasty to prevent further clots from forming.

• *Angioplasty* is a nonsurgical treatment for DVT that is used to widen the vein after the blood clot has been dissolved. During angioplasty, a small balloon at the tip of the catheter is inflated to stretch the vein open and increase blood flow. A stent may be necessary at times and is placed during the angioplasty procedure to keep the vein open.

• *Vena cava filters* are used when the patient cannot take medications (heparin, LMWH, or fondaparinux) to thin the blood or if the patient is taking blood thinners and continues to develop clots. The filter can prevent blood clots from moving from the vein in the legs to the lung (pulmonary embolism). During a small surgical procedure, the filter is inserted through a catheter into a large vein in the groin or neck, then into the vena cava (the largest vein in the body). It can catch clots as they move through the body to the lungs. This treatment helps prevent a pulmonary embolism but does not prevent the development of more clots.

REHABILITATION

• Two goals of rehabilitation are to return patients to their prior level of activity and to prevent future risks of DVT.

• Once DVT occurs, getting around may become more difficult at first. Patients should gradually return to normal activities. In addition, patients should be advised to do the following:

  ○ Drink plenty of water. Avoid consuming alcohol or caffeine.

  ○ Get out of bed and move around as soon as you are able after surgery or illness.

  ○ Stand up and walk for a few minutes every hour while awake. Avoid prolonged stationary positions.

  ○ Exercise lower leg muscles when sitting: Raising and lowering heels while keeping toes on the floor and raising and lowering toes while keeping heels on the floor.

  ○ Avoid wearing tight-fitting clothes because they may decrease the circulation.

  ○ Wear compression stockings as prescribed if recommended by your doctor.

  ○ Lie on your back with the heels elevated 5 to 6 inches, if your legs feel heavy or swollen.

  ○ Avoid activities that may cause a serious injury or trauma.

  ○ Progress to regular cardiovascular exercises. Avoid smoking.

• If patients have had DVT, then they need to prevent further clots from developing by doing the following:

  ○ Take medications as prescribed to prevent or treat blood clots.

  ○ Schedule follow-up appointments with the physician to monitor response to medications and other treatments.

PROGNOSIS

• A return to normal health and activity can be expected within 1 to 3 weeks for a person with calf DVT. It may take up to 6 weeks for a person with thigh or pelvic DVT.

• Prognosis depends on the size of the vessel involved, the presence of collateral circulation, and the underlying cause of the thrombosis.

• Postphlebitic syndrome occurs in 15% of patients with DVT.

• There is a 5% chance for recurrence, depending on related risk factors or insufficient treatment.

• Treatment for DVT with anticoagulants usually lasts for 3 to 6 months. The following situations may change the length of treatment:

  ○ If the blood clot occurred after a short-term risk like surgery or trauma, treatment with anticoagulants may be shorter.

  ○ If the patient has had clots before, longer treatment may be needed.

  ○ If the patient is being treated for another illness (such as cancer), an anticoagulant may need to be taken as long as the risk factor is present.

SIGNS AND SYMPTOMS INDICATING REFERRAL TO PHYSICIAN

• The most common side effect of anticoagulants is bleeding. The physician should be called immediately if the patient is experiencing easy bruising or bleeding.

• Postphlebitic syndrome symptoms may include the following:

  ○ Leg edema and pain

  ○ Nocturnal cramping

  ○ Venous claudication

  ○ Skin pigmentation

  ○ Dermatitis and ulceration

• Pulmonary embolism symptoms may include the following:

  ○ Sudden shortness of breath

  ○ Sharp chest pain

  ○ Pain in back

  ○ Cough with or without bloody sputum

  ○ Excessive sweating

  ○ Rapid pulse or breathing

  ○ Lightheadedness or loss of consciousness

SUGGESTED READINGS

Bates SM, Kearon C, Crowther M, et al. A diagnostic strategy involving a quantitative latex D-dimer assay reliably excludes deep venous thrombosis. *Ann Intern Med.* 2003;138(10):787-794.

Geerts WH, Pineo GF, Heit JA, et al. Prevention of venous thromboembolism: the Seventh ACCP Conference on Antithrombotic and Thrombolytic Therapy. *Chest.* 2004;126: 338S-400S.

Neff MJ. ACEP releases clinical policy on evaluation and management of pulmonary embolism. *Am Fam Physician.* 2003; 68(4):759–?.

Othieno R, Abu Affan M, Okpo E. Home versus in-patient treatment for deep vein thrombosis. *Cochrane Database Syst Rev.* 2007;(3):CD003076.

Scarvelis D, Wells P. Diagnosis and treatment of deep-vein thrombosis. *CMAJ.* 2006;175(9): 1087–1092.

Snow V, Qaseem A, Barry P, et al. Management of venous thromboembolism: a clinical practice guideline from the American College of Physicians and the American Academy of Family Physicians. *Ann Intern Med.* 2007; 146(3):204–210.

Tsai A, Cushman M, Rosamond W, Heckbert S, Polak J, Folsom A. Cardiovascular risk factors and venous thromboembolism incidence: the longitudinal investigation of thromboembolism etiology. *Arch Intern Med.* 2002;162(10):1182–1189.

Virchow R. Ueber die Erweiterung kleinerer Gefäfse. *Arch Pathol Anat Physiol Klin Med.* 1851;3:427–462.

Watson L, Armon M. Thrombolysis for acute deep vein thrombosis. *Cochrane Database Syst Rev.* 2004:CD002783.

Wells PS, Anderson DR, Rodger M, et al. Evaluation of D-dimer in the diagnosis of suspected deep-vein thrombosis. *N Engl J Med.* 2003;349(13):1227–1235.

Wells PS, Owen C, Doucette S, Fergusson D, Tran H. Does this patient have deep vein thrombosis? *JAMA.* 2006;295(2):199–207.

AUTHOR: STEVEN M. YUN

BASIC INFORMATION

DEFINITION

Fracture caused by excessive bone loading that is a common cause of lateral leg pain in athletes in running, jumping, and high-impact sports.

SYNONYMS

- Fatigue fracture
- Insufficiency fracture

ICD-9CM CODES

733.93 Stress fracture of tibia or fibula

OPTIMAL NUMBER OF VISITS

4 or fewer

MAXIMAL NUMBER OF VISITS

12

ETIOLOGY

- Stress fractures generally occur as a result of repetitive loading of the bone that exceeds its ability to repair itself.
- Bone that is repetitively loaded develops microdamage. As a result of Wolff's law, bone increases development where stress is placed on it. During remodeling from microdamage, breakdown via osteoclastic activity often occurs faster than osteoblastic rebuilding, leading to a weakening of the bone if sufficient healing time is not granted. If continued microdamage occurs, a stress reaction can result. The patient may be symptomatic at this time, although there may be no change seen radiographically. If continued loading occurs, the stress reaction progresses to form a stress fracture.
- The fibula is injured most often in the distal one third, but injury can be in the proximal one third as well.

EPIDEMIOLOGY AND DEMOGRAPHICS

- Fibular stress fractures are uncommon, accounting for only 10% of all stress fractures.
- One study has shown an incidence of 1.9% of all athletes suffer from a stress fracture each year.
- Stress fractures tend to be more related to activity than age. However, they should not be overlooked in children, as well as adults, who may have decreased bone mineral density (BMD).
- Women are more likely than men to suffer a stress fracture. This is especially true in women with eating disorders. Women with stress fractures should be queried about amenorrhea and dietary habits.

- Risk factors for developing a fibular stress fracture include the following:
  - Participation in sports involving running and jumping
  - Rapid increase in a physical training program
  - Poor preparticipation physical condition
  - Female gender
  - Hormonal or menstrual disturbances
  - Low bone turnover rate
  - Decreased BMD
  - Decreased thickness of cortical bone
  - Nutritional deficiencies (including dieting)
  - Extremes of body size and composition
  - Running on irregular or angled surfaces
  - Inappropriate footwear
  - Inadequate muscle strength
  - Poor flexibility

MECHANISM OF INJURY

Patients often report a change in their training regimen, often increasing their mileage or intensity.

COMMON SIGNS AND SYMPTOMS

- Gradual onset. Early in the process, the patient may complain of pain toward the end of activity. Later in the process, pain may occur earlier in activity and not abate with rest.
- Pain is often localized and dull and tends to worsen during weight bearing.
- It is often tender to palpation over the injury site.
- Patients may complain of nocturnal symptoms.
- Stress fractures tend to have a very localized pain pattern.

AGGRAVATING ACTIVITIES

- Weight-bearing activities such as walking, running, and jumping
- Sporting activities that require repetitive loading

EASING ACTIVITIES

- Non–weight-bearing positions
- Physicians often prescribe antiinflammatories to address the patient's symptoms, but these drugs are unlikely to relieve the symptoms completely.
- Cryotherapy may relieve the symptoms.

24-HOUR SYMPTOM PATTERN

- Pain tends to be activity related rather than temporal.
- The patient may complain of dull pain at night because of the fracture.

PAST HISTORY FOR THE REGION

- 60% of people with a stress fracture have had a previous stress fracture.
- Patients may report other episodes of overuse injuries in their lower extremities.

PHYSICAL EXAMINATION

- On visual inspection, there may be redness or edema over the painful area.
- The patient often walks with an antalgic gait since weight bearing is painful.
- The site of injury is often painful with palpation. There may be a palpable bump in the area of pain from a periosteal reaction.
- Plain radiographs may not be positive for a few weeks after onset of symptoms.
- Bone scan is better for diagnosing early; sensitivity nears 100%, specificity is poor.
- MRI: High sensitivity. Specificity is greater than for bone scans.
- Therapeutic ultrasound
  - Boam et al compared 2.0 MHz ultrasound with bone scans and found poor sensitivity (0.43) and specificity (0.49).
  - Romani et al compared 1 MHz continuous ultrasound with MRI and found that none of the stress fractures found with MRI were identified with ultrasound.
- Tuning fork
  - Lesho compared a 128 Hz tuning fork to a bone scan for identifying stress fractures. The sensitivity and specificity of the tuning fork test were 75% and 67%, respectively.

DIFFERENTIAL DIAGNOSIS

- Fibularis tendinitis or muscle strain
- Shin splints
- Compartment syndrome
- Superficial fibular nerve entrapment

TREATMENT

SURGICAL OPTIONS

Surgery is rarely necessary for a fibular stress fracture. Most fibular stress fractures heal in 4 to 6 weeks with conservative treatment.

REHABILITATION

- The initial goal of rehabilitation of a fibular stress fracture is to remove the offending activity to allow the bone to heal.
- Modified rest should occur until the patient has been pain-free for 2 to 3 weeks.
- Aircast splinting is appropriate if the patient has severe symptoms.
- Non–weight-bearing cross-training exercises can be implemented early on in rehabilitation.
- NSAIDs and cryotherapy can be used to decrease inflammation.

- Low-intensity pulsed ultrasound (<0.1 W/cm²) has been shown in multiple studies to aid in the healing of delayed union, nonunion, and acute fractures.
- Once the inflammation process has diminished, the focus of rehabilitation should be on the following:
  - Identifying the factors that contribute to the formation of a stress fracture.
  - A program to address any biomechanical faults and strength, flexibility, or coordination deficits should be developed.
- One goal during rehabilitation from a stress fracture should be the maintenance of fitness. The patient may have restricted weight bearing initially, so this should be taken into consideration in the exercise program. Cross-training that avoids excessive loading of the affected bone, such as low-resistance cycling, swimming, or aqua jogging, can maintain fitness while allowing healing.
- It is recommended that the patient be pain-free with weight bearing for 2 to 3 weeks before returning to the sport or activity program.
- Footwear advice is an important consideration in the rehabilitation program.
  - Runners should replace their shoes every 300 miles

- People with high arched feet should use shoes that provide maximal cushioning.
- People with flexible feet should use shoes that provide support or motion control.
- To prevent fibular stress fractures, the following should be considered:
  - Preparticipation physicals should be completed to screen for risk factors.
  - Preseason conditioning and training
  - Appropriate training plan for gradual progression of distance and intensity (no more than 10% change in volume per week)

CONTRIBUTING FACTORS

- Prior foot or ankle injuries
- Training errors: Too much too soon
- Nutritional deficiencies, eating disorders
- Improper footwear
- Femoral or tibial torsion

PROGNOSIS

- 60% of people with a stress fracture have had a previous stress fracture
- In a study of healing in stress fractures, the majority of detected areas of bone stress reaction disappeared when follow-up imaging was taken at the conclusion of a 5-month training program.

SIGNS AND SYMPTOMS INDICATING REFERRAL TO PHYSICIAN

- Constant unrelenting pain: Infection or tumor
- Pain that does not change with position: Infection or tumor
- Significant and unexplained weight loss: Tumor
- Nocturnal pain: Tumor
- Major trauma: Fracture
- History of cancer: Metastatic disease

SUGGESTED READINGS

Boam WD, Miser WF, Yuill SC, Delaplain CB, Gayle EL, MacDonald DC. Comparison of ultrasound examination with bone scintiscan in the diagnosis of stress fractures. *J Am Board Fam Pract.* 1996;9(6):414–417.

Lesho EP. Can tuning forks replace bone scans for identification of tibial stress fractures? *Mil Med.* 1997;1162:802–803.

Romani WA, Perrin DH, Dussault RG, Ball DW, Kahler DM. Identification of tibial stress fractures using therapeutic continuous ultrasound. *J Orthop Sports Phys Ther.* 2000;30:444–452.

Sanderlin BW, Raspa RF. Common stress fractures. *Am Fam Physician.* 2003;68(8): 1529–1532.

AUTHOR: BENJAMIN CORNELL

BASIC INFORMATION

DEFINITION

- Tendinopathy can be defined as a painful overuse tendon condition without implying a microscopic finding. It can be further classified as tendinitis or tendinosis.
  - Tendinitis is defined as painful overuse tendon injury with the presence of inflammatory cells.
  - Tendinosis is defined as to the degeneration of the tendon in the absence of inflammatory cells.

SYNONYMS

- Tendon tear
- Subluxation
- Tendon dislocation
- Muscle strain
- Tendinitis
- Tenosynovitis

ICD-9CM CODES
719.47 Pain in joint involving ankle or foot
726.7   Enthesopathy of ankle and tarsus
726.79 Other enthesopathy of ankle and tarsus
727.06 Tenosynovitis of foot and ankle

OPTIMAL NUMBER OF VISITS
3

MAXIMAL NUMBER OF VISITS
36

ETIOLOGY

- Both fibularis brevis and longus tendons are susceptible to injury. Dombek et al reported the incidence of fibularis brevis tendon injuries was of 88% as compared to 13% for the fibularis longus tendon. Injury of both occurred 37% of the time.
- Isolated fibular tendon injuries rarely occur. Acute injuries typically have the following two mechanisms as the cause:
  - Inversion ankle injury is often seen with associated anterior talofibular ligament and/or calcaneofibular ligament disruption.
  - A powerful contraction of the fibularis muscles with a forcefully dorsiflexed foot. Chronic injuries are usually associated with ankle or subtalar joint arthritis and ankle instability.
- Common biomechanical factors that predispose someone to fibular tendinopathies include the following:
  - Gait abnormalities. Patients may present with excessive supination, placing constant strain on the fibularis tendon.
  - Pes cavus
  - Equinus or restricted ankle dorsiflexion
  - Anterolateral ankle impingement
  - Poor-fitting equipment such as ice skates or basketball high-top shoes

EPIDEMIOLOGY AND DEMOGRAPHICS

- The occurrence rate of injuries to the fibular tendons is not actually known. DiGiovanni et al found that 25% to 77% of patients with chronic lateral ankle instability had some type of injury to the fibular tendons. Fallat et al noted that out of 638 acute ankle sprains only 83 involved damage to the fibular tendons.
- In a retrospective study by Dombek et al, found the average age for patients with fibular tendon injuries to be 42 years.
- A recent study suggested that the distribution of blood vessels supplying the fibular tendons are not homogenous and three distinct avascular zones exist. The fibularis brevis tendon has one avascular zone in the region where the tendon turns around the lateral malleolus. The fibularis longus has two avascular zones. One region begins where the tendon turns around the lateral malleolus and extends to the fibular tubercle of the calcaneus. The second avascular zone occurs where the tendon turns around the cuboid. These zones correspond well with the most common locations of fibular tendinopathy.

MECHANISM OF INJURY

- Acute injury involves forceful dorsiflexion with contraction of the fibular muscles or an inversion injury with a high load. Most acute injuries have subacute and chronic tendinopathies.
- Chronic injury involves repeated inversion injuries, damage to the posterior talofibular and lateral malleolar retinaculum, and/or recurrent dislocation of the fibular tendons, leading to chronic tears and lateral ankle instability.

COMMON SIGNS AND SYMPTOMS

- Patients typically present with lateral ankle or foot pain, pain along the tendon, or pain at the insertion sites. Signs and symptoms of typical fibular tendon injuries are as follows:
- Fibular tendinitis
  - Symptoms of pain behind and distal to the lateral malleolus or lateral foot.
  - Swelling and tenderness may also be present.
- Fibular tendinosis
  - Swelling is not typically present, pain may or may not be present, but weakness is often noted.
- Fibular tendon subluxation
  - Snapping along the lateral ankle is present, with a sense of weakness or pain.
  - With acute injury, pain and swelling are noted over the posterolateral aspect of the ankle. Chronic ankle injuries can lead to subluxation, including recurrent inversion injuries, leading to lateral ankle instability and painful snapping across the ankle.
- Fibular tendon tears
  - With acute injury, pain and swelling are inferior and posterior to the lateral malleolus. The patient may have had pain before the injury, but now the pain is debilitating and strength is decreased.
  - Chronic injury results in the subtle, insidious onset of pain posterior to lateral malleolus that progressively worsens in terms of both function and the level of pain.

AGGRAVATING ACTIVITIES

- Fibular tendinopathies may be aggravated with resisted eversion and raising on the toes.
- The patient may complain of pain with terminal stance in gait.

EASING ACTIVITIES

Pain is usually eased with non–weight-bearing activities, especially rest and ice for those with acute tendinitis.

24-HOUR SYMPTOM PATTERN

- The 24 hour pattern for acute fibular tendinitis is similar to that of other types of tendinitis.
- Patients with fibular tendinopathies may report complaints of stiffness and/or weakness in the morning. The patient may or may not report pain with use during the day.

PAST HISTORY FOR THE REGION

- The patient with acute tendinitis reports repetitive or prolonged activities or a traumatic event.
- A patient with chronic tendinopathy likely reports past history of ankle sprain, instability, or foot injury. The patient may report a longer history of lateral foot pain that has not resolved with conventional treatment.

PHYSICAL EXAMINATION

- Acute tendinitis is characterized by the gradual onset of pain, swelling, and warmth in the posterolateral ankle. Pain is exacerbated by passive hindfoot inversion and ankle dorsiflexion and by active hindfoot eversion and ankle plantar flexion
- For tendinosis, patients may or may not have pain with resisted movements, but weakness is likely to be present. Patients likely do not have swelling or

inflammation in the posterior lateral malleolar region or foot.

- Cuboid syndrome may manifest with symptoms similar to a fibular tendinopathy and should be ruled out. Patients with cuboid syndrome present with a painful and hypomobile cuboid. Treatment of the cuboid mobility restriction usually results in the resolution of pain with contraction of the fibularis muscles.

IMPORTANT OBJECTIVE TESTS

- Fibularis manual muscle test
  - Patients with acute tendinitis present with pain and reproduction of symptoms with the manual muscle test.
  - Patients with fibular tendinosis may or may not present with pain with manual muscle testing, but weakness may or may not be present secondary to the compensatory actions of other foot evertors.
  - No other specific objective tests have been validated in the literature to aid in the diagnosis of fibular tendinopathies.
  - Patients should undergo an examination that includes evaluation of posture, gait, and lower functional examination. An evaluation of talocrural, subtalar, and first ray joint mobility should be included in the examination. Patients should also be evaluated for lateral ankle instability as part of their evaluation. (See the section on Ankle Sprains for details.)

DIFFERENTIAL DIAGNOSIS

- Cuboid fracture
- Cuboid syndrome
- Köhler's disease
- Lateral ankle sprain
- Lumbar radiculopathy
- Superficial nerve entrapment

CONTRIBUTING FACTORS

- Ankle sprains or instability
- Hindfoot varus
- Limited talocrural joint dorsiflexion, subtalar joint eversion, first ray mobility
- Pes cavus
- Lateral ankle impingement
- Hypertrophic fibular tubercle
- Bony spurring
- Poor footwear
- Training errors
- Poor trunk lower extremity mechanics

TREATMENT

SURGICAL OPTIONS

- Lateral retinacular repair
- Fibular tendon repair
- Fibular tendonotomy
- Calcaneal osteotomy
- Hunter rod and flexor hallucis tendon transfer
- Deepening of the fibular groove

SURGICAL OUTCOMES

- Patients who undergo surgery have typically failed conservative treatment or have recurrent tendon ruptures.
- Retinacular repairs and fibular groove deepening have been shown to be very successful in limiting recurrence of fibular tendon subluxation and further tendon damage. Kollias reported that all patients had no incidence of tendon instability and 82% of patients reported no complaints of pain.
- Patients undergoing tendon repairs typically have good-to-excellent outcomes.
- Patients' average return to full active function is reported between 3 and 4 months.

REHABILITATION

- There is little to no evidence reported in the literature specific to fibular tendonopathies. Therefore, treatment guidelines follow treatment of other lower extremity tendon disorders.
- Treatment of patients with acute fibular tendinitis is similar to treatment of other types of tendinitis. Initial treatment should emphasize rest, ice, and elevation. The use of a lateral wedge may assist in decreasing demand on the fibular tendons. In severe cases, a walking boot may be used to help control pain and inflammation.
- Initial exercise should be aimed at decreasing pain, swelling, and inflammation. The use of pain-free active ROM (AROM) would be best during the acute stage of fibular tendinitis.
- Once symptoms have subsided or when treating chronic tendinopathies, the use of STM, joint mobilization, strengthening, orthotic therapy, and bracing should be implemented.
- STM may be used to help normalize peripheral soft tissue structure to allow normal mobility. Cross-friction massage over the tendon may be used to break adhesions in the tendon and has been shown to be helpful for chronic tendon injuries
- Joint mobilization may be used to normalize talocrural and subtalar joint and first ray mobility.

- Strengthening has been shown to be effective in reducing pain and preventing recurrent episodes. In the case of tendinosis, eccentric strengthening versus concentric strengthening should be strongly considered, based on effectiveness in treating other tendinosis.
- Orthotic therapy or a lateral wedge can be used to correct of hindfoot varus or pes cavus foot.
- If tendon instability is present, external bracing or taping may be helpful in decreasing the strain or limiting recurrent subluxation of the fibular tendons.

PROGNOSIS

There is no current evidence that reports the long-term prognosis of patients with fibular tendinopathy. However, postsurgical prognosis appears good to excellent for full return to function.

SIGNS AND SYMPTOMS INDICATING REFERRAL TO PHYSICIAN

Patients who are unsuccessful with conservative therapy should be referred to a physician for further diagnostic testing to rule out tendon tears. If the physical therapist is the initial person seeing the patient for an acute traumatic injury and the patient is showing signs of fracture, the patient should be referred to a physician before treatment is implemented.

SUGGESTED READINGS

DiGiovanni BF, Fraja CJ, Cohen BE, Shereff MJ. Associated injuries found in chronic lateral ankle instability. *Foot Ankle.* 21:805-815.

Dombek MF, Lamm BM, Saltrick K, Mendicino RW, Catanzariti AR. Fibular tendon tears: a retrospective review. *J Foot Ankle Surg.* 2003;42(5):250-258.

Fallat L, et al. Sprained ankle syndrome: review and analysis of 639 acute injuries. *J Foot Ankle Surg.* 1998;37(4):280-285.

Kollias SL, Ferkel RD. Fibular grooving for recurrent fibular tendon subluxation. [see comment] *Am J Sports Med.* 1997;25(3):329-335. UI: 9167812.

Saxena A, Cassidy A. Fibular tendon injuries: an evaluation of 49 tears in 41 patients. *J Foot Ankle Surg.* 2003;42(4):215-220.

Selmani E, Gjata V, Gjika E. Current concepts review: Fibular tendon disorders. *Foot Ankle Int.* 2006;27(3):221-228.

Wapner KL, Taras JS, Lin SS, Chao W. Staged reconstruction for chronic rupture of both fibular tendons using Hunter rod and flexor hallucis longus tendon transfer: a long-term follow up study. *Foot Ankle Int.* 2006;27(8):591-597.

AUTHOR: JASON TONLEY

BASIC INFORMATION

DEFINITION

- A Maisonneuve fracture of the proximal fibula occurs after eversion and external rotation injury of the ankle.
- Injury can also occur to the following structures:
  - Deltoid ligament
  - AITFL
  - Interosseous membrane
  - Medial malleolar avulsion fracture
  - Proximal tibiofibular joint

SYNONYMS

Fibula fracture

ICD-9CM CODES
823.1   Fracture of upper end of tibia and fibula open
823.2   Fracture of shaft of tibia and fibula closed

OPTIMAL NUMBER OF VISITS

12 or fewer

MAXIMAL NUMBER OF VISITS

24

ETIOLOGY

- An external rotation force on the talus in the ankle mortise produces torque on the interosseous membrane and through the proximal third of the fibula
- The injury involves a spiral or oblique fracture of the superior fibula, with or without syndesmosis, deltoid ligament, or medial malleolus injuries.

EPIDEMIOLOGY AND DEMOGRAPHICS

- Approximately 5% of all fractures treated surgically are Maisonneuve fractures.
- More commonly they are seen in young adults because the injuries are often sports related.
- In senior adults, the recovery period tends to be significantly longer.

MECHANISM OF INJURY

- The most common mechanism of injury is a twisting injury of the ankle during sports activity.
- Severe external rotation of the foot causes a torque of the talus within the ankle mortise, leading to disruption of the interosseous membrane and fracture of the proximal fibula.

COMMON SIGNS AND SYMPTOMS

- Inability to bear weight because of pain
- Ankle pain and edema

- Pain over the proximal tibiofibular joint
- As a result of the extent of tissue damage, pain can be very diffuse in the lower extremity.

AGGRAVATING ACTIVITIES

- Weight bearing such as walking or standing
- Ankle and knee movement

EASING ACTIVITIES

- Maintaining non–weight-bearing positions
- Immobilization of the extremity
- Physicians may prescribe antiinflammatory and pain medications to address the patient's pain symptoms.

24-HOUR SYMPTOM PATTERN

- Patients may report increased stiffness in the morning caused by edema.
- Nocturnal pain is also common and manifests as a deep achiness.

PAST HISTORY FOR THE REGION

- The patient may have had one or more previous ankle injuries.
- Ankle sprains that have not been fully rehabilitated place the patient at greater risk for further ankle injuries.

PHYSICAL EXAMINATION

- Prominence of the proximal tibiofibular joint.
- Edema and discoloration of the ankle.
- Proximal tibiofibular joint, medial malleolus, syndesmosis, AITFL, deltoid ligament, and proximal tibiofibular joint are symptomatic with palpation.
- Most movements of the ankle are painful, but external rotation of the ankle is most painful because of the stress it places on the injured structures.

IMPORTANT OBJECTIVE TESTS

- Syndesmosis squeeze test
  - The lower leg is grasped at the midcalf with both hands, and the tibia and fibula are squeezed together.
  - Pain can indicate a fibular fracture or syndesmosis sprain.
  - Reliability of this test has been found to be good. Sensitivity and specificity have not been reported.
- Ottawa Ankle Rules: An x-ray should be performed if any of the following are present:
  - Pain and tenderness at the distal 6 cm of the medial or lateral malleolus
  - Pain and tenderness at the navicular bone
  - Pain and tenderness at the base of the fifth metatarsal
  - Inability to bear weight or ambulate on the foot
- Multiple studies have demonstrated a sensitivity of 100%.

DIFFERENTIAL DIAGNOSIS

- Syndesmosis sprain
- Deltoid ligament sprain
- Ankle (inversion) sprain
- Tibialis posterior tendinopathy
- Fracture of the sustentaculum tali

TREATMENT

SURGICAL OPTIONS

- Closed or open reduction of the proximal fibula fracture
- Reduction of the syndesmosis tear via screw fixation
- Closed or open reduction of any medial malleolar fracture

SURGICAL OUTCOMES

- Studies have shown that return to function is directly related to the amount of tissue damage.
- Return to sport with normal ROM and strength can be expected in a high percentage of patients who suffer Maisonneuve fractures.

REHABILITATION

- Management of the patient usually involves immobilization.
- The patient will be on non–weight-bearing status for 6 to 8 weeks in a short leg cast.
- While the patient is immobilized, fitness can be maintained via upper body ergometry. Strengthening exercises for the uninvolved muscles of the lower extremities should be performed to offset the losses caused by immobilization.
- After immobilization, the following objective tests should be performed:
  - ROM of the talocrural and subtalar joints
  - Joint mobility of the talocrural and subtalar joints
  - The gastrocnemius, soleus, tibialis anterior and posterior, and fibularis muscle groups should be tested with manual muscle tests.
- Once the patient is no longer immobilized, the focus of rehabilitation should be on the following:
  - ROM and strengthening of the foot and ankle and the entire lower extremity should be progressed to proprioceptive training and return to sport or leisure activities when appropriate.
  - AROM and passive ROM (PROM) in all planes should be performed to promote healing.
  - After prolonged immobilization, joint mobilization is necessary to decrease stiffness and increase ROM

of the talocrural, subtalar, and mid-tarsal joints.

○ Caution should be used early with anterior-to-posterior mobilization to avoid spreading the healing ankle mortise and interosseous membrane.

○ Mobilization with movement has been shown to be effective in increasing pain-free dorsiflexion.

○ STM may help increase tissue extensibility after immobilization.

○ Stretching should be used to assist with ROM.

○ Strengthening of muscles of the foot and ankle and the entire lower extremity is necessary to allow return to normal activity.

○ Proprioceptive training should not be overlooked because lack of proprioception can be one of the contributing factors to the injury.

CONTRIBUTING FACTORS

• Decreased BMD as seen in osteoporosis or long-term steroid use
• Prior history of ankle injury

PROGNOSIS

Most patients return to full activities after a Maisonneuve fracture, even with surgery. Older patients should expect a longer recovery. If significant tissue damage occurs in the initial injury, prognosis is less favorable. Possible sequelae include early talocrural arthrosis, widening of the syndesmosis, and subchondral sclerosis. Full recovery can take between 6 and 12 months.

SIGNS AND SYMPTOMS INDICATING REFERRAL TO PHYSICIAN

• Positive Ottawa Ankle Rules: Fracture
• Increased feeling of instability: Widening of mortise
• Abnormal redness, warmth, or edema: Postoperative infection

SUGGESTED READINGS

Alonso A, Khoury L, Adams R. Clinical tests for ankle syndesmosis injury: Reliability and prediction of return to function. *J Orthop Sports Phys Ther.* 1998;27(4):276-284.

Duchesneau S, Fallat LM. The Maisonneuve fracture. *J Foot Ankle Surg.* 1995;34(5):422-428.

Pankovich AM. Maisonneuve fracture of the fibula. *J Bone Joint Surg Am.* 1976;58:337-342.

Savoie FH, Wilkinson MM, Bryan A, Barrett GR, Shelton WR, Manning JO. Maisonneuve fracture dislocation of the ankle. *J Athl Train.* 1992;27(3):268-269.

Sproule JA, Khalid M, O'Sullivan M, McCabe JP. Outcome after surgery for Maisonneuve fracture of the fibula. *Injury Int J Care Injured* 2004;35:791-798.

AUTHOR: BENJAMIN CORNELL

BASIC INFORMATION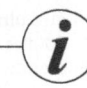

DEFINITION

- A periosteal contusion results from a direct blow from a hard object or compression between two hard surfaces.
- When trauma occurs, blood vessels are damaged or broken and blood seeps into adjoining tissue.

SYNONYMS

Bone bruise

ICD-9CM CODES
924.9 Contusion of unspecified site

OPTIMAL NUMBER OF VISITS

4 or fewer

MAXIMAL NUMBER OF VISITS

12

ETIOLOGY

- A periosteal contusion is bruising or damage that occurs to the outer covering of the bone.
- This outer covering of the bone is known as the periosteum. The periosteum is divided into an outer fibrous layer and an inner cambium layer.
- The fibrous layer contains fibroblasts, whereas the cambium layer contains progenitor cells that eventually become osteoblasts.
- Orthopedically, the periosteum contains nociceptive nerve endings that account for the pain experienced with a periosteal contusion.
- The periosteum is also rich in blood vessels; damage to these vessels can account for the delay in healing of the periosteum and underlying bone.

EPIDEMIOLOGY AND DEMOGRAPHICS

- Alanan et al found that 27% of those who suffered an inversion injury to the ankle had evidence of a bone bruise.
- Sijbrandij et al reported that 18% of patients undergoing MRIs for persistent pain after an ankle sprain had evidence of subchondral abnormalities.
- For sports-related injuries, periosteal contusions tend to be more common in teens and young adults.
- Periosteal contusions caused by trauma can occur at any age.
- There appears to be no gender or cultural prevalence with periosteal contusion.

MECHANISM OF INJURY

- Direct blow from a blunt object (such as a baseball, ski, dashboard) or falls

- Talar contusions often occur with inversion injuries of the ankle as the talus becomes lodged against the tibia.

SIGNS AND SYMPTOMS

- Pain with activities that place stress through the injured area
- Localized pain and possibly edema over the area of injury
- Pain with palpation over the injured area
- Deep achiness in region of injury

AGGRAVATING ACTIVITIES

- Direct pressure on the area of periosteal contusion
- If contusion occurs within the joint, weight bearing is painful.

EASING ACTIVITIES

- Antiinflammatory medication or modalities.
- Non–weight-bearing status if the contusion is located within a joint

24-HOUR SYMPTOM PATTERN

Early after injury, the patient may report morning pain and stiffness caused by inflammation.

PAST HISTORY FOR THE REGION

- No specific history would predispose the patient to a periosteal contusion.
- Symptoms increase with use.
- Nocturnal pain is common with periosteal contusion.

PHYSICAL EXAMINATION

- Contraction of muscles attaching to periosteum may produce pain.
- Local tenderness over the area of contusion
- Overlying muscles or soft tissue are also often injured. Therefore surface bruising may appear.
- Local areas of edema or hypertrophy may be palpated.

IMPORTANT OBJECTIVE TESTS

- There are no specific tests to rule in a periosteal contusion, although empirically it seems logical that clinical tests used to diagnose fractures may also produce symptoms with periosteal contusion.
- Therapeutic ultrasound
  ○ Boam et al. compared 2.0 MHz ultrasound with bone scans and found poor sensitivity (0.43) and specificity (0.49).
  ○ Romani et al compared 1 MHz continuous ultrasound with MRI and found that none of the stress fractures found with MRI were identified with ultrasound.
- Tuning fork
  ○ Lesho compared a 128 Hz tuning fork to a bone scan for identifying stress fractures. The sensitivity and specificity

of the tuning fork test were 75% and 67%, respectively.

DIFFERENTIAL DIAGNOSIS

- Heterotopic ossification
- Osteochondroma
- Myositis ossificans
- Stress fracture
- Shin splints
- Medial tibial stress syndrome
- Tendinopathy
- Compartment syndrome

TREATMENT

SURGICAL OPTIONS

Surgery is uncommon after a periosteal contusion.

REHABILITATION

- In most cases, periosteal contusions are self-limiting. Pain relieving and antiinflammatory modalities can be used early in the process.
- Initially, inflammation and pain can be decreased by using the following:
  ○ Exercises that promote movement of the region in a pain-free range
  ○ Cold pack
  ○ Ultrasound
  ○ Electrical stimulation
  ○ Ice massage has been clinically proved very effective in treating bone bruises.
- Once the inflammation process has decreased, there likely are few impairments that need to be addressed. The goals of rehabilitation are to return patients to their prior level of activity when pain permits.

CONTRIBUTING FACTORS

Playing a sport that can produce direct blows (baseball, soccer, hockey, or football)

PROGNOSIS

The majority of patients incurring a periosteal contusion injury return to their former activities. Pain complaints can continue for a number of months, and this injury may take longer to heal than an actual fracture.

SIGNS AND SYMPTOMS INDICATING REFERRAL TO PHYSICIAN

- Constant unrelenting pain: Infection or tumor
- Significant and unexplained weight loss: Tumor
- Nocturnal pain: Tumor
- Major trauma: Fracture
- History of cancer: Metastatic disease
- Fevers and chills: Infection or tumor

SUGGESTED READINGS

Alanen V, Taimela S, Kinnunen J, Koskinen SK, Karaharju E. Incidence and clinical significance of bone bruises after supination injury of the ankle. *J Bone Joint Surg Am.* 1998;80(3):513-515.

Boam WD, Miser WF, Yuill SC, Delaplain CB, Gayle EL, MacDonald DC. Comparison of ultrasound examination with bone scintiscan in the diagnosis of stress fractures. *J Am Board Fam Pract.* 1996;9(6):414-417.

Gaebler C, Kukla C, Breitenseher MJ, et al. Diagnosis of lateral ankle ligament injuries: Comparison between talar tilt, MRI and operative findings in 112 athletes. *Acta Orthop Scand.* 1997;68(3):286-290.

Lesho EP. Can tuning forks replace bone scans for identification of tibial stress fractures? *Mil Med.* 1997;1162:802-803.

Romani WA, Perrin DH, Dussault RG, Ball DW, Kahler DM. Identification of tibial stress fractures using therapeutic continuous ultrasound. *J Orthop Sports Phys Ther.* 2000;30:444-452.

Sijbrandij ES, van Gils APG, Louwerens JWK, de Lange EE. Posttraumatic subchondral bone contusions and fractures of the talotibial joint: Occurrence of "kissing" lesions. *AJR.* 2000:175.

AUTHOR: BENJAMIN CORNELL

BASIC INFORMATION

DEFINITION

Posterior impingement syndrome occurs when the posterior aspect of the talus impinges with the posterior tibia in end-range plantar flexion.

SYNONYMS

- Os trigonum syndrome
- Posterior tibiotalar impingement syndrome (PTTIS)

ICD-9CM CODES
726.71 Achilles bursitis or tendinitis

OPTIMAL NUMBER OF VISITS

8 or fewer

MAXIMAL NUMBER OF VISITS

16

ETIOLOGY

- Forced or repetitive plantar flexion causes the talus and nearby soft tissue to be compressed between the calcaneus and tibia.
- Posterior impingement can occur because of any of the following:
  - Impingement of the talus and posterior aspect of the tibia
  - The presence of a Stieda process or an os trigonum
  - Synovitis or posterior capsule thickening of either the tibiotalar or subtalar joints
  - After severe ankle sprains, scar tissue can impinge between the medial aspect of the talus and the posterior aspect of the medial malleolus.
- Os trigonum syndrome refers to an unfused area in the posterior process of the talus that is present in approximately 10% of the population.

EPIDEMIOLOGY AND DEMOGRAPHICS

- Posterior ankle impingement is an uncommon (5 to 100 per 100,000) disorder.
- Adolescents and young adults are more likely to suffer from posterior ankle impingement.
- Sports or activities that have a higher prevalence of posterior ankle impingement include those that require significant plantar flexion.
  - Ballet
  - Swimming
  - Kicking
  - Gymnastics
  - Downhill running

MECHANISM OF INJURY

- Repetitive or forceful plantar flexion

- Traumatic injury involving end-range plantar flexion and compression of the ankle

COMMON SIGNS AND SYMPTOMS

- Posterior ankle pain and edema at the posterior ankle
- Tenderness just behind the inferior portion of the fibula
- Pain is worse when the foot is plantar flexed.
- A painful clicking sensation may be reported.
- Catching may be felt in forced plantar flexion.

AGGRAVATING ACTIVITIES

Activities requiring end-range plantar flexion

EASING ACTIVITIES

- Avoidance of end-range plantar flexion
- Antiinflammatory medications or modalities

24-HOUR SYMPTOM PATTERN

The symptoms in posterior impingement are activity driven, rather than temporal in nature. Therefore, symptoms increase in direct relation to the amount of aggravating activity the patient engages in.

PAST HISTORY FOR THE REGION

Patients may report prior ankle sprains or instability.

PHYSICAL EXAMINATION

- Palpation should include the following structures:
  - Posterior inferior fibula
  - Posterior talus
  - Posterior talocrural joint line
- Ankle instability tests should be conducted to determine whether ankle instability is contributing to the impingement.

IMPORTANT OBJECTIVE TESTS

- Passive ankle plantar flexion
  - Pain reproduced with passive plantar flexion can indicate a posterior impingement problem.
- Anesthetic injection
  - Gold standard
  - Local anesthetic is injected around posterior talus. Passive ankle plantar flexion is repeated.
  - If pain is relieved, symptoms are due to impingement.
- Resisted plantar flexion should not reproduce pain if symptoms are due to posterior ankle impingement.
  - Pain would be more indicative of soft tissue injury.
- X-rays may be beneficial to rule out the presence of an os trigonum.

- Bone scans may show areas of inflammation localized to the posterior aspect of the talus or the posterior aspect of the tibia.

DIFFERENTIAL DIAGNOSIS

- Achilles tendinitis
- Achilles tendon rupture
- Retrocalcaneal bursitis
- Flexor hallucis longus tendinitis
- Ankle joint arthritis
- Ankle sprain
- Osteochondral lesion
- Haglund deformity
- Calcaneal fracture
- Sever disease
- Lumbar radiculopathy

TREATMENT

SURGICAL OPTIONS

- Removal of posterior talar process
- Removal of os trigonum

SURGICAL OUTCOMES

Studies have shown excellent and good postoperative results in approximately 84% at 2 to 5 years of follow-up

REHABILITATION

- The goals of rehabilitation are to decrease the patient's symptoms and inflammation, as well as to retrain and provide stability during activities requiring plantar flexion.
- To decrease inflammation, the clinician can use the following:
  - Bracing or taping to prevent excessive plantar flexion
  - Exercises that promote ankle movement in a pain-free range
  - Cold pack
  - Ultrasound
  - Electrical stimulation
  - The muscles of the ankle should be strengthened.
- Once inflammation has slowed, the focus of rehabilitation should turn to movement reeducation for painful activities and activities to promote stability of the unstable ankle.
- Joint mobilization and manipulation
  - Talocrural mobilization may improve mobility of the talus in the ankle mortise to make it better able to avoid posterior impingement.
- Other factors to consider include the following:
  - Prior history of ankle sprains or instability. Proprioceptive training can be used to improve stability.
  - Movement reeducation for proper foot and ankle positioning during activities requiring plantar flexion may reduce the impingement position.

CONTRIBUTING FACTORS

- Performance of activities that require forceful or repetitive plantar flexion
- Talar instability after ankle sprain

PROGNOSIS

- Patients with posterior ankle impingement resulting from instability have a higher likelihood of success with conservative measures.
- Patients with diagnosed structural changes likely require surgery to continue with activity.

- Most patients who have conservative or surgical treatment can return to their prior activities.

SIGNS AND SYMPTOMS INDICATING REFERRAL TO PHYSICIAN

- Constant unrelenting pain: Complex regional pain syndrome (CRPS)
- Major trauma: Fracture
- History of cancer: Metastatic disease
- Fevers and chills: Infection or tumor

SUGGESTED READINGS

Best A, Giza E, Linklater J, Sullivan M. Posterior impingement of the ankle caused by anomalous muscles. A report of four cases. *J Bone Joint Surg Am.* 2005;87(9):2075–2079.

Bureau NJ, Cardinal E, Hobden R, Aubin B. Posterior ankle impingement syndrome: MR imaging findings in seven patients. *Radiology.* 2000;215(2):497–503.

AUTHOR: BENJAMIN CORNELL

BASIC INFORMATION

DEFINITION

- Posterior tibial tendinopathy encompasses a range of conditions from tendinitis to rupture. It is a common cause of foot dysfunction and pain.
- The following are the four stages of posterior tibial tendon dysfunction:
  ○ Stage 1: Mild swelling, medial ankle pain
  ○ Stage 2: Progressive arch flattening, weakness of inversion of the foot. Rearfoot valgus and forefoot abduction appear but are flexible.
  ○ Stage 3: Deformity of hindfoot (rearfoot valgus) becomes fixed.
  ○ Stage 4: Talus in valgus tilt in talocrural joint resulting in tibiotalar degeneration
- The primary roles of the tibialis posterior include the following:
  ○ Prevention of the collapse of the medial longitudinal arch during weight bearing
  ○ Rearfoot inversion
  ○ Forefoot adduction

SYNONYMS

Posterior tibialis tendon dysfunction

ICD-9CM CODES
726.72 Tibialis tendinitis

OPTIMAL NUMBER OF VISITS

6 or fewer

MAXIMAL NUMBER OF VISITS

16

ETIOLOGY

- This pathology was previously thought to be an inflammatory process. Although this may be the case at the onset, surgical exploration has not confirmed the presence of inflammatory cells.
- Characteristics of the analyzed tissue include fibroblast hypercellularity, mucinous degeneration, and neovascularization.
- Ultrasound imaging demonstrates tendon thickening, irregular tendon structure, and synovial sheath effusion. These are characteristic of tendinosis rather than tendinitis.
- Physiologically, excessive loading causes the pathology. The proximal and distal components of the myotendinous junction are most susceptible to damage. If local damage occurs there, loads are shifted to the midsubstance of the tendon. Overuse in this area can produce microtears representing collagen fiber disruption or rupture. Continued overuse may prevent tenocytes from providing optimal healing of the tendon, thereby compromising the tendon structure.

EPIDEMIOLOGY AND DEMOGRAPHICS

- The most affected group with posterior tibial tendinopathy is overweight, white females, ages 45 to 65 years old. Ruptures are most common in this group as well.
- Posterior tibial tendinopathy is also a common overuse injury in weight-bearing sports.

MECHANISM OF INJURY

There are multiple causes of posterior tibial tendinopathy. These include overuse and age-related degeneration. Tendon ruptures can occur from trauma or atraumatically following prolonged degeneration.

COMMON SIGNS AND SYMPTOMS

- Medial ankle pain and possible swelling
- Pain in the medial plantar arch or radiating into the proximal calf
- Progressive collapse of the medial longitudinal arch
- Patients may report abnormal shoe wear in chronic conditions caused by walking with weight more medially.

AGGRAVATING ACTIVITIES

- Weight bearing
- Walking
- Standing on toes

EASING ACTIVITIES

- Non–weight-bearing activity
- Wearing full contact, supportive orthotics
- Supportive shoes
- Arch support

24-HOUR SYMPTOM PATTERN

- Symptoms can be worse with first steps in the morning if feet have been in a position of plantar flexion at night.
- If the patient works in a standing or walking occupation, pain tends to worsen throughout the day.

PAST HISTORY FOR THE REGION

Patients should be screened for previous overuse injuries of the lower extremity and prior injuries in the foot or ankle.

PHYSICAL EXAMINATION

- Patients present with a pronated foot, navicular drop, and abducted forefoot.
- Tibialis posterior and possibly the flexor hallucis longus are symptomatic with palpation.

IMPORTANT OBJECTIVE TESTS

- Manual Muscle Testing: Tibialis posterior is weak and painful.

- Single leg heel rise test
  ○ The patient performs weight-bearing plantar flexion on one foot. Weak or absent inversion of the calcaneus is evidence of posterior tibial tendon dysfunction. Dysfunction may also be evident if the patient is unable to rise on the toes. Patients may report pain at their medial ankle.
- First metatarsal rise sign
  ○ Test is performed with the patient standing on both feet. The examiner passively externally rotates the tibia of one leg. The first metatarsal head rises in the patient with posterior tibial tendon dysfunction and stays on the floor if posterior tibial tendon function is normal.
- Joint mobility
  ○ The following joints should be checked for accessory mobility: talocrural, subtalar, and midtarsal.
  ○ With long-standing pronation, the patient is likely to lose talocrural dorsiflexion as well as subtalar inversion.
- ROM
  ○ Dorsiflexion loss caused by Achilles tendon contracture often occurs after long-standing hindfoot valgus.
  ○ Calcaneal inversion and inversion, as well as rearfoot to forefoot angle, may be helpful in treatment, especially with orthotic intervention.

DIFFERENTIAL DIAGNOSIS

- Calcaneonavicular (spring) ligament sprain
- Arthritis of the ankle joint
- Arthritis of the talonavicular joint
- Neuropathy
- Lumbar radiculopathy
- Deltoid ligament sprain

TREATMENT

SURGICAL OPTIONS

- Synovectomy
- Debridement/excision

SURGICAL OUTCOMES

Teasdale found that 16 of 19 patients felt much better, and 74% had complete resolution of symptoms at 30-month follow-up

REHABILITATION

- Davenport et al developed the EdUReP model for the nonsurgical management of tendinopathy. It consists of the following components:
  ○ **Ed**ucation
  ○ **U**nloading
  ○ **Re**loading
  ○ **P**revention

- Patient education in the rehabilitation of posterior tibial dysfunction includes the following:
  - Patients should understand tendinopathy and behavioral risk factors.
  - Patients should be advised on avoidance of behavioral risk factors and educated in preventive and restorative strategies for their condition.
- Tissue unloading includes the following:
  - Mechanical unloading of an affected tendon can be provided in a number of ways, including orthoses, taping, bracing, and workplace ergonomic modifications.
  - McNair et al demonstrated that instructions to change lower extremity position during landing were effective in reducing ground reaction forces at the ankle, including tendon structures.
- The proper means to reload the injured tissue includes the following:
  - Body weight support initially such as a swimming pool
  - Weaning from supportive devices such as braces and orthotics
  - Gradual increase in weight bearing
  - Strengthening tendon both concentrically and eccentrically
  - Functional exercise progression for return to sport or activity
- Preventive measures should be as follows:
  - The topics addressed in the education portion of the model should be reemphasized at this time.
- Once the inflammation process has decreased, the focus of rehabilitation should be on manual and exercise interventions to address ROM, strength, and motor control impairments.

- The following interventions should be included in an exercise program for posterior tibial tendinopathy:
  - Stretching and ROM exercises to improve talocrural dorsiflexion ROM.
  - Closed-chain exercises to teach control of pronation through the stance phase of gait.
  - Strengthening of the tibialis posterior. It has been suggested that eccentric strengthening may be more effective in cases of tendinosis.
  - Balance and proprioceptive exercises to improve arch control during dynamic activities.
  - With prolonged dysfunction, patients exhibit decreased talocrural dorsiflexion and calcaneal inversion. Joint mobilization can assist in restoring these motions.
  - Mobilization with movement has been shown to be effective in increasing pain-free dorsiflexion.
  - In a study by Kulig et al (2005), wearing custom orthotics and shoes improved selective activation of the tibialis posterior.

CONTRIBUTING FACTORS

- An occupation that requires prolonged standing or walking
- Increased rearfoot eversion
- Increased medial longitudinal arch angle
- Increased forefoot abduction

PROGNOSIS

Prognosis is good if symptoms are caught before structural changes occur in the foot. If fixed structural changes, such as calcaneal varus, have occurred, external support will likely be needed.

SIGNS AND SYMPTOMS INDICATING REFERRAL TO PHYSICIAN

- Constant unrelenting pain: Infection or tumor
- Significant and unexplained weight loss: Tumor
- Nocturnal pain: Stress fracture
- Major trauma: Fracture
- History of cancer: Metastatic disease
- Fevers and chills: Infection or tumor

SUGGESTED READINGS

Davenport TE, Kulig K, Matharu Y, Blanco CE. The edurep model for nonsurgical management of tendinopathy. *Phys Ther.* 2005;85:1093-1103.

Geideman WM, Johnson JE. Posterior tibial tendon dysfunction. *J Orthop Sports Phys Ther.* 2000;30(2):68-77.

Kulig K, Burnfield JM, Requejo SM, Sperry M, Terk M. Selective activation of tibialis posterior: Evaluation by magnetic resonance imaging. *Med Sci Sports Exerc.* 2004;36(5):862-867.

Kulig K, Burnfield JM, Reischl S, Requejo SM, Blanco CE, Thordarson DB. Effect of foot orthoses on tibialis posterior activation in persons with pes planus. *Med Sci Sports Exerc.* 2005;37(1):24-29.

McNair PJ, Prapavessis H, Callender K. Decreasing landing forces: effect of instruction. *Br J Sports Med.* 2000;34:293-296.

Tome J, Nawoczenski DA, Flemister A, Houck. Comparison of foot kinematics between subjects with posterior tibialis tendon dysfunction and healthy controls. *J Orthop Sports Phys Ther.* 2006;36(9):635-644.

AUTHOR: BENJAMIN CORNELL

BASIC INFORMATION

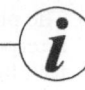

DEFINITION

- Pott's fracture involves one or both of the malleoli.
- The three common classifications of malleolar fractures are as follows:
  - First degree: Injury of the medial malleolus only
  - Second degree (bimalleolar): Fracture of both the medial and lateral malleoli, which often appears as an inversion deformity of the foot
  - Third degree (trimalleolar): Fracture of the medial and lateral malleoli, as well as a fracture of the posterior aspect of the tibia; often associated with a posterior dislocation of the talocrural joint

SYNONYMS

- Ankle fracture
- Malleolar fracture
- Bimalleolar fracture
- Trimalleolar fracture

ICD-9CM CODES
824.0 Fracture of medial malleolus closed
824.1 Fracture of medial malleolus open
824.2 Fracture of lateral malleolus closed
824.3 Fracture of lateral malleolus open
824.4 Bimalleolar fracture closed
824.5 Bimalleolar fracture open
824.6 Trimalleolar fracture closed
824.7 Trimalleolar fracture open

OPTIMAL NUMBER OF VISITS

8 or fewer

MAXIMAL NUMBER OF VISITS

20

ETIOLOGY

- Most often, an abduction and external rotation force at the ankle causes a fracture of one of the malleoli. In some cases, an adduction force causes the fracture.
- A combined abduction external rotation force of the ankle sprains the deltoid ligament. This force can also avulse the medial malleolus. As the talus continues to rotate and move laterally, it can fracture the lateral malleolus or cause sufficient external rotation of the fibula to cause a tear of the syndesmosis and a fracture of the proximal fibula.

EPIDEMIOLOGY AND DEMOGRAPHICS

- 15% of all patients evaluated for ankle injuries have a fracture.

- Pott's fracture is most common among young adults who play contact sports, may occur in older people because of tripping and falling, and is rare in children.
- Males are twice as likely to have a Pott's fracture compared to females in the general population. Women older than 40 years have the highest incidence of fracture dislocations.

MECHANISM OF INJURY

- Fracture of the medial malleolus
  - Abduction injury: Avulsion of the medial malleolus
  - Adduction injury: Fracture superior to joint line
- Fracture of the lateral malleolus
  - Abduction or external rotation injury
- Fracture of the lateral malleolus and deltoid ligament tear
  - Abduction or external rotation injury
- Bimalleolar fracture
  - Abduction or external rotation injury
- Trimalleolar fracture
  - External rotation with posterior displacement of the talus

COMMON SIGNS AND SYMPTOMS

- Inability to bear weight because of pain
- Ankle pain, edema, and bruising
- Pain over the malleoli

AGGRAVATING ACTIVITIES

- Weight-bearing activity
- Moving the ankle in any direction

EASING ACTIVITIES

- Maintaining non–weight-bearing activity
- Immobilization of the extremity
- Physicians may prescribe antiinflammatories and pain medications to address the patient's pain symptoms.

24-HOUR SYMPTOM PATTERN

- Patients may report increased stiffness in the morning because of edema.
- Nocturnal pain is very common.
- The first 72 hours after injury are typically the worst as swelling and inflammation peak. Symptoms should diminish as the fracture heals and inflammation decreases.

PAST HISTORY FOR THE REGION

The patient may have had one or more previous ankle injuries. Ankle sprains that have not been fully rehabilitated place the patient at greater risk for further ankle injuries.

PHYSICAL EXAMINATION

- Prominence of the proximal tibiofibular joint

- Edema and discoloration of the ankle
- Medial malleolus, lateral malleolus, syndesmosis, anterior inferior tibiofibular ligament, and deltoid ligament may be symptomatic to palpation.
- Most or all movements are painful, but external rotation of the ankle is most painful because of the stress it places on the injured structures
- Because of the mechanism of injury, neurovascular status should be checked, including pedal pulse

IMPORTANT OBJECTIVE TESTS

- Ottawa Ankle Rules: An x-ray should be performed if any of the following are present:
  - Pain and tenderness at the distal 6 cm of the medial or lateral malleolus
  - Pain and tenderness at the navicular bone
  - Pain and tenderness at the base of the fifth metatarsal
  - Inability to bear weight or ambulate on the foot
- Multiple studies have demonstrated a sensitivity of 100%.
- Tests for ligamentous laxity: Talar tilt and anterior drawer help rule out ligamentous injury.

DIFFERENTIAL DIAGNOSIS

- Ankle (deltoid, anterior talofibular, or calcaneofibular) sprain
- Syndesmosis sprain
- Tibialis posterior tendinopathy
- Peroneal (fibularis) tendinopathy
- Stress fracture
- Fracture of the sustentaculum tali

TREATMENT

SURGICAL OPTIONS

- ORIF
- Closed reduction

REHABILITATION

- The patient is non–weight-bearing for 4 to 6 weeks in a short leg cast. In some cases, weight bearing is allowed in a cam rocker boot.
- Fitness can be maintained via upper body ergometry. Strengthening exercises for the uninvolved muscles of the lower extremities should be performed to offset the losses resulting from immobilization.
- Initially, the clinician can use the following to decrease inflammation:
  - Compression
  - Elevation of the lower extremity
  - Exercises that promote movement of the region in a pain-free range
  - Cold pack
  - Ultrasound
  - Electrical stimulation

- The following objective tests should be checked after immobilization:
  - ROM of the talocrural and subtalar joints
  - Joint mobility of the talocrural and subtalar joints
  - Manual muscle tests of the gastrocnemius, soleus, tibialis anterior, and posterior and fibularis muscle groups should be tested.
- Once the patient is no longer immobilized, the focus of rehabilitation should be:
  - ROM and strengthening of the foot and ankle, as well as the entire lower extremity. These should be progressed to proprioceptive training and return to sport or leisure activities when appropriate.
- After prolonged immobilization, joint mobilization is necessary for decreaseing stiffness and increasing ROM of the talocrural, subtalar, and midtarsal joints.
- Mobilization with movement has been shown to be effective in increasing pain-free dorsiflexion.
- Caution should be used early with anterior-to-posterior mobilization to avoid spreading the healing ankle mortise and interosseous membrane if either was injured.
  - STM may help increase tissue extensibility after immobilization.
  - Stretching should be used to assist with ROM.
  - Strengthening of muscles of the foot and ankle, as well as the entire lower extremity, is necessary for return to normal activity.
  - Proprioceptive training should not be overlooked since impaired proprioception can be one of the factors contributing to the injury.

CONTRIBUTING FACTORS

- Age: Young adults and the elderly
- Past history of ankle sprains or other foot or ankle injuries
- Osteoporosis osteopenia
- Long-term use of steroids or other medications that decrease BMD

PROGNOSIS

- Posttraumatic arthritis is expected after both bimalleolar and trimalleolar fractures.

- The posterior tibial tendon can become interposed after disruption of the deltoid ligament or fracture of the medial malleolus.
- In one study, 73% reported good-to-excellent overall results after bimalleolar fractures and 63% reported good-to-excellent results after trimalleolar fractures.

SIGNS AND SYMPTOMS INDICATING REFERRAL TO PHYSICIAN

- Positive Ottawa Ankle Rules: Fracture
- Decreased pedal pulses: Consult a vascular surgeon

SUGGESTED READINGS

Bachmann LM, Kolb E, Koller MT, Steurer J, ter Riet G. Accuracy of Ottawa ankle rules to exclude fractures of the ankle and mid-foot: systematic review. *BMJ.* 2003;326:417.

AUTHOR: BENJAMIN CORNELL

BASIC INFORMATION

DEFINITION

- Shin splits is a general term for pain along the distal two thirds of the posterior medial tibia and can be a debilitating injury in runners.
- Medial tibial stress syndrome is a more specific label that excludes diagnoses of stress fracture or posterior compartment syndrome.

SYNONYMS

- Medial tibial stress syndrome
- Medial tibial syndrome
- Stress-related anterior lower leg pain
- Periostalgia

ICD-9CM CODES
844.9 Sprain of unspecified site of knee and leg

OPTIMAL NUMBER OF VISITS

8 or fewer

MAXIMAL NUMBER OF VISITS

12

ETIOLOGY

- James et al have classified the etiology of overuse injuries into the following three categories:
  - Anatomical and biomechanical factors
  - Training errors
  - Interaction between shoes and the running surface
- There are multiple causes of shin splints, including the following:
  - Periostitis at the posterior medial border of the distal tibia
  - The soleus has been reported in recent studies to be a likely contributor to medial shin pain.
  - The flexor digitorum longus and the deep crural fascia may also be sources of shin splints, since they attach to the tibia in a location similar to that of the symptoms in shin splints
- Microscopic findings include vasculitis, increased medial periosteal formation, and cortical hypertrophy along the distal one third of the posterior medial tibial border.

EPIDEMIOLOGY AND DEMOGRAPHICS

- Shin splints have been reported as one of the top two most commonly diagnosed injuries in recreational runners.
- Studies have shown that shin splints account for 13.1% of running injuries and 22% of aerobic dancing injuries.
- Shin splints are most common among teens to young adults who are involved in running or jumping activities; how-

ever, they may be seen in any population of active people.
- Clement et al reported that the incidence of shin splints is higher among female runners (16.8%) than male runners (10.7%).

MECHANISM OF INJURY

Overuse or unaccustomed use are the most common factors leading to shin splints.

COMMON SIGNS AND SYMPTOMS

- Pain to palpation over the middle to distal third of the posterior medial border of the tibia
- Pain described as dull ache but can be intense pain
- Increased by weight-bearing exercise
- Pain may last hours to days after exercise.

AGGRAVATING ACTIVITIES

- Walking, as well as ballistic weight-bearing exercise such as running or jumping
- Downhill walking or running can be especially painful because of the increased eccentric load placed on the pretibial muscles.

EASING ACTIVITIES

- Non–weight-bearing activities
- Rest

24-HOUR SYMPTOM PATTERN

Pain tends to be activity dependent. In the acute phase, pain may be more pronounced first thing in the morning because of edema.

PAST HISTORY FOR THE REGION

In one study, previously injured runners were twice as likely to incur shin splints; however, this was not statistically significant.

PHYSICAL EXAMINATION

- Foot overpronation is commonly seen in those suffering from shin splints.
- The following structures are symptomatic with palpation:
  - Posterior medial distal tibia
  - Tibialis posterior muscle

IMPORTANT OBJECTIVE TESTS

- Navicular drop test: The height of the navicular from the ground is measured in subtalar neutral and relaxed standing.
  - A drop greater than 10 mm is considered abnormal.
  - Interrater reliability is 0.73, and intrarater reliability is 0.78–0.98.
- The diagnosis of shin splints is often one of omitting other sources such as tibial stress fracture and posterior tibial tendinitis. Therefore tests for these

conditions should be performed to rule them out as a source of symptoms. (See sections on Posterior Tibial Tendinopathy and Tibial Stress Fracture for further details.)

DIFFERENTIAL DIAGNOSIS

- Stress fracture
- Myositis
- Periostitis
- Posterior tibial tendinitis
- Compartment syndrome
- Fasciitis
- Saphenous or superficial fibular nerve entrapment

TREATMENT

SURGICAL OPTIONS

Fasciotomy of the superficial posterior compartment of the leg is a common surgical option.

SURGICAL OUTCOMES

- Holen et al reported on 35 athletes undergoing fasciotomy of the superficial posterior compartment of the leg; of the 35, 23 improved, 7 had no change, and 2 reported poor results.
- In a study by Yates et al, after deep posterior fasciotomy, 72% had significant reductions in pain; however, only 41% of those undergoing surgery returned to their presymptom level of activity.

REHABILITATION

- The initial goal of rehabilitation of the patient with shin splints is activity modification to allow the tissue to heal.
- At this time, activities and exercise should be not be painful.
- Non–weight-bearing exercise, such as swimming or aqua jogging, can help the patient maintain fitness while the tissues are healing.
- Education regarding risk factor modification should be taught early in the rehabilitation process and reiterated at discharge.
- Strength, ROM, endurance, and proprioceptive impairments and contributing factors should be addressed during the rehabilitation process.
- External devices, such as taping or orthotics, may be necessary.
- To decrease inflammation, the clinician should use the following:
  - Exercises that promote movement of the region in a pain-free range
  - Cold or hot pack
  - Ultrasound
  - Electrical stimulation
- Once the inflammation process has decreased, the focus of rehabilitation should be on the following:

○ Addressing impairments that led to the pathology, including strength and ROM deficits

○ Stretching to improve dorsiflexion and decrease pronation.

○ Strengthening of the muscles that control pronation

○ Exercises to improve motor control of pronation during dynamic activities

○ Mobilization of a restricted talocrural joint to improve dorsiflexion may help decrease pronation at the midfoot and forefoot.

• In a study by Kulig et al, wearing custom orthotics and shoes improved selective activation of the tibialis posterior. This may assist in controlling pronation.

• Advice on footwear should include the following:

○ Runners should replace their shoes every 300 miles.

○ People with high arched feet should use shoes that provide maximal cushioning.

○ People with flexible feet should use shoes that provide support or motion control.

CONTRIBUTING FACTORS

• Bennett et al found that excessive navicular drop measurements correctly identified 64% of medial tibial stress syndrome cases in high school cross-country runners.

• Higher body mass index (BMI) in runners increased the likelihood of medial tibial stress syndrome.

• Multiple studies have shown a relationship with increased pronation and increased incidence of shin splints.

PROGNOSIS

• With proper rehabilitation and behavioral modification, most people with shin splints can return to their prior activities in 6 to 8 weeks.

• Patients who have suffered a lower extremity overuse injury have a much higher likelihood of future overuse injuries.

SIGNS AND SYMPTOMS INDICATING REFERRAL TO PHYSICIAN

• Constant unrelenting shin pain or pain that does not change with position: Infection or tumor

• Nocturnal pain: Tumor or fracture

• Major trauma: Fracture

• History of cancer: Metastatic disease

SUGGESTED READINGS

Bennett JE, Reinking MF, Pluemer B, Pentel A, Seaton M, Killian C. Factors contributing to the development of medial tibial stress syndrome in high school runners. *J Orthop Sports Phys Ther.* 2001;31(9):504-510.

Clement DB, Taunton JE, Smart GW, Mcnicol KL. A survey of overuse running injuries. *Phys Sportsmed.* 1981;9:47-58.

Holen KJ, Engebretsen L, Grøntvedt T, Rossvoll I, Hammer S, Stoltz V. Surgical treatment of medial tibial stress syndrome (shin splint) by fasciotomy of the superficial posterior compartment of the leg. *Scand J Med Sci Sports.* 1995;5(1):40-43.

James SL, Bates BT, Osternig LR. Injuries to runners. *Am J Sports Med.* 1978;2:40-50.

Kulig K, Pomrantz AB, et al. Non-operative management of posterior tibialis tendon dysfunction: design of a randomized clinical trial. *BMC Musculoskelet Disord.* 2006;7:49.

Mizel MS, Hecht PJ, Marymount JV, Temple HT. Evaluation and treatment of chronic ankle pain. *J Bone Joint Surg Am.* 2004;86(3):622-632.

Plisky MS, Rauh MJ, Heiderscheit B, Underwood FB, Tank RT. Medial tibial stress syndrome in high school cross-country runners: incidence and risk factors. *J Orthop Sports Phys Ther.* 2007;37(2):40-47.

Yates B, Allen MJ, Barnes MR. Outcome of surgical treatment of medial tibial stress syndrome. *J Bone Joint Surg Am.* 2003;85(10):1974-1980.

AUTHOR: BENJAMIN CORNELL

BASIC INFORMATION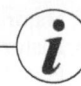

DEFINITION

- Tarsal tunnel syndrome is entrapment of the tibial nerve as it courses through the tarsal tunnel posterior to the medial malleolus. It normally manifests as burning or paresthesias in the sole of the foot.
- The flexor retinaculum, the superior aspect of the calcaneus, the medial side of the talus, and the distal-medial portion of the tibia make up the tarsal tunnel.
- The flexor hallucis longus tendon, flexor digitorum longus muscle, tibialis posterior muscle, tibial nerve, and posterior tibial artery and vein are located within the tarsal tunnel.

SYNONYMS

- Tarsal tunnel neuropathy
- Entrapment neuropathy of the tibial nerve
- Posterior tibial nerve neuralgia

ICD-9CM CODES
355.5 Tarsal tunnel syndrome

OPTIMAL NUMBER OF VISITS

8 or fewer

MAXIMAL NUMBER OF VISITS

16

ETIOLOGY

- The entrapment of the tibial nerve in the tarsal tunnel can be a result of trauma, foot deformities, space-occupying lesions, ganglia, tumors, or talocalcaneal coalition.
- 50% of cases are thought to be idiopathic.

EPIDEMIOLOGY AND DEMOGRAPHICS

- Tarsal tunnel syndrome is rare, affecting less than 0.05% of the population.
- Tarsal tunnel syndrome is more related to activity than age.
- Women and men seem to have an equal prevalence.

MECHANISM OF INJURY

- 50% of cases are thought to be idiopathic.
- Result from injury such as inversion injury to the ankle
- Repetitive stress associated with excessive pronation

COMMON SIGNS AND SYMPTOMS

- Sensory disturbances in the medial ankle and plantar portion of the foot can include burning, tingling, aching, or numbness. Patients may present with tenderness along the medial ankle.
- In more chronic cases, atrophy of the muscles innervated by the tibial nerve may be present. These muscles include the great toe flexors. Atrophy may be evident by hollowing of the arch of the foot or clawing of the toes.
- The tibial nerve root is compressed. This can cause problems along its branches, the medial and lateral plantar nerves.

AGGRAVATING ACTIVITIES

- Weight-bearing activities
- Walking
- The tarsal tunnel has been shown to decrease in diameter with any movement that takes the ankle out of a neutral position.

EASING ACTIVITIES

Non–weight-bearing activities with the ankle in a neutral position

24-HOUR SYMPTOM PATTERN

- The patient with tarsal tunnel syndrome often has pain that is worse at night.
- If the patient has an occupation that involves standing or walking, pain may intensify as the day progresses.

PAST HISTORY FOR THE REGION

Because of the double crush phenomenon, other nerve entrapments of the lower extremity should be ruled out.

PHYSICAL EXAMINATION

- It is common for a patient with tarsal tunnel syndrome to have increased foot pronation.
- The following structures are symptomatic with palpation:
  - A ganglion or cyst may be palpable along the medial ankle.
  - Tenderness over the tarsal tunnel is common.

IMPORTANT OBJECTIVE TESTS

- Dorsiflexion-eversion test
  - In this test the ankle is placed in maximal dorsiflexion and eversion with the metatarsophalangeal joint in extension and held for 5 to 10 seconds. A positive test reproduces the patient's symptoms.
- Straight leg raise (SLR) test
  - Tibial nerve bias (dorsiflexion and eversion) may be provocative.
- Tinel's sign at the tarsal tunnel
  - Test is performed by tapping over the tibial nerve in the tarsal tunnel.
  - Positive: Distal symptoms are reproduced.
  - To increase sensitivity of the test, it can be checked in the position of the dorsiflexion eversion test.
- Neurological examination: Neurological signs that indicate radiculopathy should be ruled out, including dermatomal, myotomal, and reflex changes.
- Nerve conduction studies are the gold standard for diagnosis
- Ultrasound and MRI can identify any space-occupying lesions.

DIFFERENTIAL DIAGNOSIS

- Lumbar radiculopathy
- Plantar fasciitis
- Posterior tibial tendinopathy
- Interdigital neuroma
- Peripheral neuropathy
- Peripheral vascular disease
- Medial calcaneal nerve entrapment

TREATMENT

SURGICAL OPTIONS

Tarsal tunnel release or tibial nerve decompression

SURGICAL OUTCOMES

- Takakura et al reported that an excellent result can be expected from surgical treatment in cases in which a definite lesion is identified as the cause of tarsal tunnel syndrome.
- Surgery is significantly more successful when performed soon after the onset of symptoms.

REHABILITATION

- The goals of rehabilitation should be to reduce inflammation, improve neural mobility, and correct impairment leading to the pathology.
- To decrease inflammation, the clinician should use the following:
  - Corticosteroid injection
  - Cold pack
  - Ultrasound
  - Electrical stimulation
- Once the inflammation process has decreased, the focus of rehabilitation should be on the following:
  - Identifying the factors that contribute to the tarsal tunnel pathology. These are likely to be impairments leading to increased foot pronation, such as lack of dorsiflexion ROM, decreased gastrocnemius and soleus extensibility, and weakness of the muscles that control pronation.
- Initially, exercises that minimize the stress to the tibial nerve should be used. It has been shown that Neutral

dorsiflexion has been shown to place the least pressure on the tarsal tunnel.
- If increased foot pronation is a cause of the patient's symptoms, mobilization of a restricted talocrural joint to improve dorsiflexion may help decrease pronation at the midfoot and forefoot.
- STM along the entrapment sites of the tibial nerve and its branches can help with neural mobility.
- Orthotics may decrease foot pronation, which can relieve the traction force on the tibial nerve.
- Arch taping can be an effective adjunct for control of foot pronation.
- In a case study by Meyer et al, a patient with subcalcaneal pain reproduced by SLR testing was treated with slump neural mobilization as part of his overall rehabilitation. By the end of treatment, the patient had an increased SLR test that did not reproduce the symptoms.
- An exercise regimen should address the following:
  - Stretching of the gastrocnemius and soleus to increase dorsiflexion
  - Strengthening of the muscles that control pronation
  - Exercises for motor control to decrease excessive pronation during dynamic activities

CONTRIBUTING FACTORS

- Increased foot pronation or flatfoot deformity
- An occupation that requires prolonged standing
- Existence of talocalcaneal coalition, accessory muscles, and bony fragments around the tarsal tunnel
- Studies have shown that many patients with tarsal tunnel syndrome have had previous trauma to the ankle or calcaneus.

PROGNOSIS

The majority of patients are able to return to their sport after treatment.

SIGNS AND SYMPTOMS INDICATING REFERRAL TO PHYSICIAN

- Constant unrelenting pain: Complex regional pain syndrome (CRPS)
- Major trauma: Fracture
- History of cancer: Metastatic disease
- Fevers and chills: Infection or tumor
- Symptoms in a dermatomal or myotomal pattern: Radiculopathy

SUGGESTED READINGS

Kinoshita M, Okuda R, Morikawa J, Jotoku T, Abe M. The dorsiflexion-eversion test for diagnosis of tarsal tunnel syndrome. *J Bone Joint Surg Am.* 2001;83(12):1835-1839.

Meyer J, Kulig K, Landel R. Differential diagnosis and treatment of subcalcaneal heel pain: A case report. *J Orthop Sports Phys Ther.* 2002;32:114-124.

Mizel MS, Hecht PJ, Marymount JV, Temple HT. Evaluation and treatment of chronic ankle pain. *J Bone Joint Surg Am.* 2004;86(3):622-632.

Takakura Y, Kitada C, Sugimoto K, Tanaka Y, Tamai S. Tarsal tunnel syndrome. Causes and results of operative treatment. *J Bone Joint Surg Br.* 1991;73(1):125-128.

AUTHOR: BENJAMIN CORNELL

BASIC INFORMATION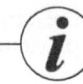

DEFINITION
Tibial stress fracture is the result of excessive bone loading that is a common cause of shin pain in athletes in running, jumping, and impact sports.

SYNONYMS
- Fatigue fracture
- Insufficiency fracture

ICD-9CM CODES
733.93 Stress fracture of tibia or fibula

OPTIMAL NUMBER OF VISITS
4 or fewer

MAXIMAL NUMBER OF VISITS
12

ETIOLOGY
- Repetitive loading of the bone exceeds its ability to repair itself and results in a stress fracture.
- Physiologically, bone that is repetitively loaded develops microdamage. As a result of Wolff's law, bone increases development where stress is placed on it. During remodeling as a result of microdamage, breakdown via osteoclastic activity occurs faster than osteoblastic rebuilding, leading to a weakening of the bone if sufficient healing time is not granted. If continued microdamage occurs, a stress reaction can occur. The patient may be symptomatic at this time, although there may be no change seen radiographically. If continued loading occurs, the stress reaction progresses to form a stress fracture.
- In adults, tibial stress fractures tend to occur in the middle to distal one third. In adolescents and children, these fractures tend to occur in the proximal one third.

EPIDEMIOLOGY AND DEMOGRAPHICS
- Tibial stress fractures are the most common type of stress fracture, accounting for nearly 50% of all stress fractures.
- One study has shown that 1.9% of all athletes suffer from a stress fracture each year.
- Stress fractures tend to be more related to activity than age. However, they should not be overlooked in children, as well as adults, who may have decreased BMD.
- Women are more likely than men to suffer a stress fracture. This is especially true in women with eating disorders. Women with stress fractures should be queried about amenorrhea and dietary habits.

- Risk factors for developing a tibial stress fracture include the following:
  - Participation in sports involving running and jumping
  - Rapid increase in a physical training program
  - Poor preparticipation physical condition
  - Female gender
  - Hormonal or menstrual disturbances
  - Low bone turnover rate
  - Decreased bone density
  - Decreased thickness of cortical bone
  - Nutritional deficiencies (including dieting)
  - Extremes of body size and composition
  - Running on irregular or angled surfaces
  - Inappropriate footwear
  - Inadequate muscle strength
  - Poor flexibility

MECHANISM OF INJURY
It is typical for the patient to report a change in his or her training regimen, often increasing mileage or intensity; 86% of athletes with stress fractures reported an increase in training before their stress fracture.

COMMON SIGNS AND SYMPTOMS
- Gradual onset: Early in its process, the patient may complain of pain toward the end of activity. Later in the process, pain may occur earlier in activity and not abate with rest.
- Pain is often localized and dull and tends to worsen during weight bearing.
- It is often tender to palpation over the injury site.
- The patient may complain of nocturnal symptoms.
- Stress fractures tend to have a very localized pain pattern.

AGGRAVATING ACTIVITIES
- Weight-bearing activities
- Sporting activities

EASING ACTIVITIES
- Non–weight-bearing positions
- Physicians often prescribe antiinflammatories to address the patient's symptoms, but medications are unlikely to relieve symptoms completely.
- Cryotherapy may relieve the symptoms.

24-HOUR SYMPTOM PATTERN
Pain tends to be activity related rather than temporal. The patient may, however, complain of pain at night.

PAST HISTORY FOR THE REGION
- 60% of people with a stress fracture have had a previous stress fracture.
- Patients may report other episodes of overuse injuries in their lower extremities.

PHYSICAL EXAMINATION
- There may be redness or edema present over the painful area.
- The patient often walks with an antalgic gait because weight bearing is painful. The site of injury is often painful. There may be a palpable bump in the area of pain from a periosteal reaction.

IMPORTANT OBJECTIVE TESTS
- Plain radiographs may not be positive for a few weeks after onset of symptoms.
- Bone scan is better for diagnosing early; sensitivity nears 100%, specificity is poor.
- MRI: High sensitivity; specificity is greater than for bone scans.
- Therapeutic ultrasound
  - Boam et al compared 2.0 MHz ultrasound with bone scans and found poor sensitivity (0.43) and specificity (0.49).
  - Romani et al compared 1 MHz continuous ultrasound with MRI and found that none of the stress fractures found with MRI were identified with ultrasound.
- Tuning fork
  - Lesho compared a 128 Hz tuning fork to a bone scan for identifying stress fractures. The sensitivity and specificity of the tuning fork test were 75% and 67%, respectively.

DIFFERENTIAL DIAGNOSIS
- Medial tibial stress syndrome (MTSS)
- Shin splints
- Compartment syndrome
- Posterior tibial tendinitis or muscle strain
- Anterior tibial tendinitis or muscle strain
- Periosteal contusion

TREATMENT

SURGICAL OPTIONS
Rarely, surgery must be performed. Surgical fixation may be necessary if the fracture progresses to a nonunion fracture.

REHABILITATION
- The initial goal of rehabilitation of the patient with a tibial stress fracture is to abandon the offending activity to allow the bone to heal.
- Modified rest should occur until the patient has been pain-free for 2 to 3 weeks.
- Aircast splinting is appropriate if the patient has severe symptoms.
- Non–weight-bearing cross-training exercises

- To decrease inflammation, the clinician can use the following:
  - NSAIDs
  - Cryotherapy
- Low-intensity pulsed ultrasound ($<0.1W/cm^2$) has been shown in multiple studies to aid in the healing of delayed union, nonunion, and acute fractures.
- Once the inflammation process has decreased, the focus of rehabilitation should be as follows:
  - Identifying the factors that contribute to the formation of a stress fracture. A program to address any biomechanical faults and strength, flexibility, or coordination deficits should be developed.
  - One goal during rehabilitation from a stress fracture should be the maintenance of fitness. The patient may have restricted weight-bearing activities initially, so this should be taken into consideration in the exercise program. Cross-training that avoids excessive loading of the affected bone, such as low-resistance cycling, swimming, or aqua jogging, can maintain fitness while allowing healing.
- It is recommended that patients are pain-free with weight bearing for 2 to 3 weeks before returning to a sport or activity program.

- Footwear advice should include the following:
  - Runners should replace their shoes every 300 miles.
  - People with high arched feet should use shoes that provide maximal cushioning.
  - People with flexible feet should use shoes that provide support or motion control.
- Programs to prevent stress fractures should include the following:
  - Preparticipation physicals should be completed to screen for risk factors.
  - Preseason conditioning and training should be implemented.
  - Appropriate training plan for gradual progression of distance and intensity (no more than 10% change in volume per week)

CONTRIBUTING FACTORS

- Training errors, too much too soon
- Nutritional deficiencies, eating disorders
- Improper footwear

PROGNOSIS

- 60% of people with a stress fracture have had a previous stress fracture.
- In a study of healing in stress fractures, the majority of detected areas of bone stress reaction disappeared when follow-up imaging was taken at the conclusion of a 5-month training program.

SIGNS AND SYMPTOMS INDICATING REFERRAL TO PHYSICIAN

- Constant unrelenting pain or pain that does not change with position: Infection or tumor
- Significant and unexplained weight loss: Tumor
- Major trauma: Fracture
- History of cancer: Metastatic disease

SUGGESTED READINGS

Boam WD, Miser WF, Yuill SC, Delaplain CB, Gayle EL, MacDonald DC. Comparison of ultrasound examination with bone scintiscan in the diagnosis of stress fractures. *J Am Board Fam Pract.* 1996;9(6):414-417.

Lesho EP. Can tuning forks replace bone scans for identification of tibial stress fractures? *Mil Med.* 1997;1162:802-803.

Romani WA, Perrin DH, Dussault RG, Ball DW, Kahler DM. Identification of tibial stress fractures using therapeutic continuous ultrasound. *J Orthop Sports Phys Ther.* 2000;30:444-452.

Sanderlin BW, Raspa RF. Common stress fractures. *Am Fam Physician.* 2003;68(8):1529-1532.

AUTHOR: BENJAMIN CORNELL

BASIC INFORMATION

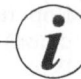

DEFINITION

Stress fractures are generally closed incomplete fractures through the cortex and into the trabecular bone matrix of the calcaneus. Stress fractures and stress reactions, both repetitive stress injuries (RSIs) of bone, are a reaction of bone to repetitive and abnormal forces.

SYNONYMS

• Fatigue fracture
• Insufficiency fractures
• Chronic repetitive stress injury of bone
• Stress reaction

ICD-9CM CODES
825.0 Fracture of calcaneus closed
733.95 Stress fracture of other bone

OPTIMAL NUMBER OF VISITS

Physical therapy for this condition depends on the intervention chosen by the physician. Generally, a boot is used for a period of time and a home exercise program can be initiated. Return to function may require 4 to 8 visits over a number of weeks.

MAXIMAL NUMBER OF VISITS
12

ETIOLOGY

• The initial injury involves the bone matrix, which may be the result of a biological or biochemical abnormality or failure at the cellular or bone multicellular unit (BMU) level.
• An excessive amount of stress or repetitive stress occurs, causing microdamage; the bone had inadequate rest to allow for adaptation to the stress. The stress that creates these injuries is too much, too soon for the bone.
• Over time with repeated stressors and overload to the bone, bone resorption takes place without significant bone production. The forces contributing to the injury include both direct impact to the bone and forces generated by the pull of ligaments and tendons on the bone.
• Normal stress to abnormally weakened bone (e.g., osteoporosis) can lead to insufficiency fractures.

RISK FACTORS

• Repetitive activity such as sports (e.g., distance running) or in military recruits
• Increases in intensity, frequency, and loading of training or activity

• Hyperthyroidism, hyperparathyroidism, and use of fluoride treatment for osteoporosis
• White women who smoke and are sedentary
• Systemic diseases that weaken bone such as (RA), lupus, osteoarthrosis, pyrophosphate arthropathy, renal disease, osteoporosis, joint replacement, or nutritional deficiency
• Low bone mineral density (BMD), especially after prolonged immobilization and not bearing weight.
• Prior history of nontraumatic fracture
• Low calcium and magnesium intake (<1000 mg per day)
• General joint laxity and possibly first ray dorsal hypermobility
• Pes planus foot type has been correlated with stress fractures.
• Running >20 miles per week. especially on hard surfaces
• Overtraining without adequate rest periods
• Delayed menarche
• Poor nutrition
• Amenorrhea

EPIDEMIOLOGY AND DEMOGRAPHICS

General Prevalence
• Generally, stress fractures constitute 10% of all athletic injuries.
  ○ Tibia: ≈50%; tarsals: 25%; and metatarsals: 9% of all lower extremity stress fractures
  ○ Bilateral in 16%
• Calcaneal stress fractures occur far less often (<10% of all stress fractures) than calcaneal fractures. Calcaneal stress fractures occur second most often, next to fractures of the metatarsals. There is a 2.6 per 10,000 incidence rate in military recruits.
• The posterior superior or posterior calcaneus is most often involved and has a vertical orientation.
• 5% to 10% of heel pain is nonmechanical and can stem from a systemic origin.
Gender or Cultural Prevalence
• Prior and continued athletic activity increases calcaneal stiffness in postmenopausal women, thereby reducing the chance of stress fracture.
• Relative risks:
  ○ Females > males (relative risk = 3.5)
  ○ White males > black males (relative risk = 4.7)
  ○ White females > black females (relative risk = 8.5)
• Females with low body mass index (BMI) and fractal analysis of calcaneal radiographic images are more prone to stress fracture.
• Track and field athletes and runners sustain this fracture most often.

• Females who overtrain and develop the athlete's triad have menstrual irregularities 50% of the time and thus have reduced bone density.
• Males can lower testosterone after 2 days of hard training by up to 25%, which increases osteoclast development and bone resorption.
Age Prevalence
• Calcaneal stress fractures can occur in any age group, especially active and athletic individuals.
• The prevalence is higher in adolescent girls and inactive elderly women, who show signs of osteopenia or osteoporosis. Children younger than 5 years who have gait abnormalities are also more susceptible.

MECHANISM OF INJURY

• Repetitive weight-bearing activities without sufficient recovery time
• Excessive muscle forces
• Muscle fatigue
• Biomechanical forces: Hyperpronators or supinators, hallux valgus, genu varum or genu valgum, leg length discrepancy, hip retroversion, or changes in footwear or training surface.
• Most calcaneal fractures are the result of a traumatic event—most commonly, falling from a height. A smaller number of calcaneal fractures are *stress* fractures, caused by overuse or repetitive stress on the heel bone. Bone is noted to fail more readily in tension than in compression. An intact plantar aponeurosis is necessary to affect the calcaneus in fracture loads.
• Repetitive downward force by the talus compressing vertically can affect beneath the outer two thirds of the posterior facet and create a superior portion stress fracture of the calcaneus.
• The trabecular system of the calcaneus is designed to resist all forces relative to a standing position so that the anteroposterior and anterior oblique trabeculae resist tension, while the dorsal-plantar oriented trabeculae resist compressive loads. The subsequent location and orientation of the stress fracture may provide a clue to the source of the dysfunction.
• Calcaneal stress reactions occurred in a group of military recruits; the majority (56%) of reactions were in the posterior third of the bone, and 79% occurred in the upper half of the calcaneus. The majority of stress injuries of the calcaneus occur in the posterior part of the bone, but a considerable proportion can generally be found in the middle and anterior part.
• Insufficiency fractures are typically present in patients with RA or neurological disorders.

CONTRIBUTING FACTORS

- Dramatic changes in training such as increased mileage, twice daily runs, speed work, a new pair of running shoes, poor shoe quality, or aging running shoes.
- Menstrual irregularity, oligomenorrhea (six times greater chance of problem in track athletes), osteoporosis, menopause, diabetic or idiopathic neuropathy, smoking and alcohol intake, hypothyroidism, lower contraceptive use, anorexia nervosa, Paget's disease, neurological disorders, and RA.
- Menopause and age-related decreases occur in the H-mean parameter of fractal analysis of calcaneal trabecular bone. This may demonstrate a greater chance of incurring a stress fracture in post-menopausal women.
- Heel pad atrophy increases stress to the calcaneus in loading.

COMMON SIGNS AND SYMPTOMS

- A good patient history that exposes a relatively sudden or subacute onset of injury, a changing pattern of exercise, and particularly one that notes the onset and character of the pain is very important when differentiating between plantar fasciitis and calcaneal stress fractures.
- Often, calcaneal stress fractures are misdiagnosed and continue unrecognized because of improvement through treatments that are aimed at plantar fasciitis.
- Tenderness and diffuse pain over the medial and lateral calcaneus
- Rule out systemic problems, such as RA, by determining if the patient has morning pain, swelling, forefoot problems, stiffness longer than 2 hours, involvement of the hands, skin lesions, hair loss, fatigue, back or hip pain, recent sexually transmitted diseases, penile discharge, or vision changes
- Diffuse heel pain
- Deep ache after rapid training change
- Pain progression: Pain after activity followed by pain with activity and finally pain at rest
- Pain with walking
- Night pain rarely occurs (consider another diagnosis)
- Fracture site: Intense localized pain
- Tenderness to palpation over the medial and lateral aspects of the calcaneus
- Tenderness on lateral compression of the body, rather than at the medial calcaneal tuberosity or tenderness that is only plantar to the calcaneus
- Positive percussion of bone distant from symptomatic site
- Vibrating tuning fork (128 Hz) at suspected site
- Local swelling over site

AGGRAVATING ACTIVITIES

- Gradual onset of pain related to activity, relieved with rest but may linger, pain may become constant if activities are not modified.
- Walking in hard-soled shoes
- Standing and walking on hard surfaces such as tile or concrete
- Running or walking downhill
- Jumping on hard surfaces
- Progressing return to activity and intensity too quickly

EASING ACTIVITIES

- Rest
- Immobilization
- Ice
- Certain modalities
- Rocker heel shoe use

24-HOUR SYMPTOM PATTERN

- Depending on the severity of the stress reaction, more chronically there is pain at rest after activity that eases in the morning.
- Night pain can occur if the fracture is more severe and chronic.

PAST HISTORY FOR THE REGION

- Osteopenia
- Osteoporosis
- Prolonged heel pain
- Specific high-intensity vertical-loading activities.

PHYSICAL EXAMINATION

- Tenderness to palpation, lateral compression of the body, rather than at the medial calcaneal tuberosity, or tenderness that is only plantar to the calcaneus
- Percussion of bone distant from symptomatic site elicits pain at the suspected site.
- Weaker dorsiflexors in muscle testing
- Calcaneal compression test may be positive.
- Vibrating tuning fork (128 Hz) at suspected site
- Lower limb tension tests
- Palpation over painful site
- Reduced talocrural joint dorsiflexion range of motion (ROM)
- Positive side-to-side glide of calcaneus (pain)
- Foot postural malalignment with forefoot pronation (in one third of patients with Sever's disease)
- Gait may be changing: Involved foot position with excessive varum or valgum during weight acceptance or omit direct heel contact altogether in stance.

IMPORTANT OBJECTIVE TESTS

- Cup heel and move side to side to elicit pain.

- Hop test (not validated for this condition)
- Percussion over the site of pain versus remotely
- Therapeutic ultrasound is unreliable over the actual site of fracture.
- Assess the lower extremities for muscle imbalances, including weakness, length, static strength, dynamic strength, function, and other painful areas.
- Radiographic findings are rarely abnormal in the early phases of the disorder and only 50% display significant changes in follow-up. There is no actual fracture line in most grades of this injury, especially early after onset. The lack of evidence is most pronounced when radiographs are obtained soon after the onset of symptoms, before the appearance of a fracture line or new bone formation, and when the patient has osteopenia. Detecting stress fracture radiographically offers a 26% sensitivity and 10% specificity.
- To obtain a diagnosis, magnetic resonance imaging (MRI) is warranted if plain radiography does not show abnormalities in a physically active patient with exercise-induced pain in the ankle or heel.
- MRI demonstrates characteristic findings that include the following:
  - Bandlike areas of very low signal intensity in the medullary space, which usually extend to the cortex
  - Surrounding alteration in signal intensity in the marrow space
  - Low signal intensity on T1-weighted images
  - High signal intensity in fat-suppressed T2-weighted images and increased short TI inversion recovery (STIR), which represents medullary edema and hemorrhage
  - As the injury progresses to a stage of increasing severity, a low signal fracture line and bone callus may be visible. This process of calcification typically takes about 4 to 6 weeks to see on plain x-ray; therefore, periodic follow-up x-rays may aid in diagnosing a stress fracture of the heel.
- Tests, such as bone scans, computed tomography (CT), or MRI, usually demonstrate the fracture. A three-phase technetium bone scan can help differentiate the location and degree of inflammation in the calcaneus (specificity: 100%; sensitivity: 76%). Bone scintigraphy is considered sensitive, and MRI is considered to be both sensitive and specific.
- CT scans are less sensitive.

Radiological Grading System for Stress Fractures

Grade	Radiograph	Bone Scan	MRI	Treatment
1	Normal	Mild uptake confined to one cortex	Positive STIR image	Rest for 3 weeks
2	Normal	Moderate activity; larger lesion confined to unicortical area	Positive STIR and T2-weighted images	Rest for 3-6 weeks
3	Discrete line (±), periosteal reaction (±)	Increased activity (>50% width of bone)	No definite cortical break; positive T1- and T2-weighted images	Rest for 12-16 weeks
4	Fracture or periosteal reaction	More intense bicortical uptake	Fracture line; positive T1- and T2-weighted images	Rest for 16+ weeks

Adapted with permission from Arendt EA, Griffiths HJ: The use of MR imaging in the assessment and clinical management of stress reactions of bone in high-performance athletes, *Clin Sports Med* 16:291-306, 1997.
MRI, Magnetic resonance imaging; *STIR*, short TI inversion recovery.

DIFFERENTIAL DIAGNOSIS   **Dx**

- A number of conditions may confound diagnosis and appear similar to stress fracture on certain imaging studies. In other cases, asymptomatic bone marrow edema may be visible on MRI.
- Primary benign bone neoplasm
- Rheumatological diseases (RA, seronegative spondyloarthropathies)
- Osteoid osteoma
- Ostcoblastoma
- Eosinophilic granuloma
- Infections: Chronic or subacute osteomyelitis
- Crohn's disease or ulcerative colitis, sarcoidosis, Behçet's syndrome (1% to 5% incidence).
- Chronic musculoskeletal soft tissue injury
  - Tendinopathy
  - Muscle strain
  - Chronic compartment syndrome
- Metastatic neoplasm
  - Prostate cancer
  - Breast cancer
  - Myeloma
- Primary malignant bone neoplasms
  - Osteosarcoma
- Nerve compression syndromes
  - Tarsal tunnel syndrome (Tinel's sign, electromyogram [EMG], weakness)
  - Carpal tunnel syndrome
  - Ulnar tunnel syndrome
  - Herniated intervertebral disc
- Osteoarthritis
- Ankylosing spondylitis (in 15- to 35-year-olds with heel pain)
- Gout

- Hypertrophic pulmonary osteoarthropathy
- Reiter's syndrome (laboratory tests, pedal involvement, periostitis at posterior calcaneus, keratoderma blennorrhagicum)

RELATED DIAGNOSES

- A stress fracture of the calcaneus is a condition that is often overlooked in the differential diagnosis of heel pain. Plantar fasciitis (also called heel spur syndrome) is so common that most health care providers default to plantar fasciitis as a primary diagnosis when evaluating heel pain.
- Radicular pain from lumbosacral origin (EMG, MRI, clinical)
- Lumbar stenosis (MRI)
- Tarsal tunnel syndrome and compartment syndromes (EMG, sensation, Tinel's sign, weakness, palpation, pressure measures)
- Achilles or retro calcaneal bursitis (resisted manual muscle testing [MMT], palpation, MRI)
- Local tendinopathy or ligament sprain (resisted MMT, palpation, MRI)
- Haglund's deformity (radiograph, MRI)
- Osteoid osteoma (pain at night relieved with analgesics, CT scan)
- Osteomyelitis (radiograph, laboratory tests)
- Osteosarcoma (radiograph)
- Ewing tumor (radiograph)
- Bone metastases (radiograph)
- Osteochondral fracture (bone scintigraphy, radiograph)
- Accessory navicular (painful)
- Inflammatory disorders (psoriatic arthritis)
- Medial tibial stress syndrome (radiograph)

TREATMENT   **Rx**

SURGICAL OPTIONS

- Surgical indicators
  - High-risk fractures for nonunion
  - Nonhealing fractures that last longer than 4 to 6 months
- Surgical options
  - Surgery is rarely required for a calcaneal stress fracture.
  - Placement of a calcaneal intermedullary screw or nail has been used successfully in severe cases.
  - Focal drilling or bone grafting has been used successfully.
- Surgical outcomes
  - Recurrence and concomitant problems often arise over time.
  - Calcaneal stress fracture has been reported after surgery for Achilles tendinosis.

REHABILITATION

- Initial exercises and procedures: Experimental and anecdotal
  - Electromagnetic field devices (expensive, lacks evidence).
  - Electrical stimulation may be used for patients who have delayed healing.
- Initial management
  - Rest for 4 to 7 weeks (may require up to 3 months) or until local tenderness subsides, which must be monitored weekly.
  - Non–weight-bearing to slowly progressive weight-bearing with assistive devices until assessed pain-free walking. The degree of pain should guide the progression. Severe pain involves non–weight-bearing or partial weight-bearing with assistive devices until the pain subsides (usually 7 to 10 days).
  - Immobilization: A cam walker, pneumatic walker, or low pneumatic walker for 4 to 6 weeks may alleviate pain faster and be clinically superior to a postoperative shoe for stress reactions of the metatarsal area and for other foot stress reactions. An added benefit of the pneumatic walker is that it can be removed for hygiene purposes and to allow limited exercise of the limb. This walker makes showers easier and allows the patient to do ROM exercises of the leg.
- Short leg casting indications include noncompliance and high risk for nonunion such as the following:
  - Navicular stress fracture
  - Metatarsal stress fracture
  - Reduce compression in weight bearing
- Prevention and education for the patients and coaches as follows:
  - Do not increase exercise intensity >10% per week.
  - Stretch and warm-up before exercise.

- ○ Choose level running surfaces.
- ○ Shoes should be lightweight and in good condition.
- ○ Consider orthoses to correct biomechanical factors.
- ○ Avoid barefoot walking.
- ○ Shock-absorbing insoles may be beneficial.
- ○ A slow and easy approach to increasing exercise is helpful.
- ○ Dietary calcium should reach recommended levels. Supplements may assist in this. Calcium has been found at lower levels in athletes who incur a stress reaction. Make certain to also meet daily requirements of vitamin D, which aids in both absorption of calcium and in the development of bone.

TREATMENT   **Rx**

- Conservative treatment works well for most stress fractures and stress reactions of bone.
- Assess and retrain adjacent and distal muscles.
- Restore joint ROM and muscle and connective tissue flexibility and extensibility. Notably restoring ankle dorsiflexion is vital from a non-weight-bearing to weight-bearing progression as tolerated.
- Progressive pain-free weight bearing
- Active rest (cross-training) goals
  - ○ Cardiovascular conditioning
  - ○ Flexibility
  - ○ Proprioception
  - ○ Strength
- Asymptomatic weight-bearing progression activities
  - ○ Maintenance of upper body strength
  - ○ Swimming
  - ○ Pool running with float vest
  - ○ Biking
  - ○ Elliptical trainer
  - ○ Progressive walking
  - ○ Stair climbing machines (later stages) to use the gastrocnemius/soleus group concentrically
  - ○ Running at 17 to 26 weeks after injury
- Return to function
  - ○ Eliminate the pain of weight bearing where forces should be sufficiently low for healing and remodeling to take place.
  - ○ Use a training log.
  - ○ Progressive pain-free strengthening and cardiovascular-based exercise
  - ○ Sport-specific training
  - ○ Previous radiographic changes are absent.

PROGNOSIS

- Long-term prognosis: Most lower extremity stress reactions take between 8 and 26 weeks for full recovery, although symptoms generally resolve in 6 to 8 weeks with proper rest and rehabilitation. The calcaneus has a rich blood supply, so it generally heals more readily than the adjacent tarsal bones.
- Slow progression of forces act on the stress fracture. Superior and posterior locations of a stress fracture would limit the action of the ankle plantar flexors.
- Regression of stress fractures:
  - ○ Stage I: Crack initiation: Areas of stress concentration
  - ○ Stage II: Crack propagation: No repair or more damage than repair
  - ○ Stage III: Final fracture: Cracks coalesce, enlarge, ultimate failure
- Symptoms and disability may continue for months along with adaptive movement patterns in compensation if progressed too rapidly.
- Lower than normal BMD has been seen 1 to 2 years after lower extremity surgery

SIGNS AND SYMPTOMS INDICATING REFERRAL TO PHYSICIAN

- Subjective history consistent with mechanism of injury
- >3 weeks with acute localized pain
- Lack of progression
- Other possible diagnoses, especially systemic red flags
- The necessity for imaging or other diagnostic tests

SUGGESTED READINGS

Akkus O, Rimnac CM. Cortical bone tissue resists fatigue fracture by deceleration and arrest of microcrack growth. *J Biomech.* 2001;34:757–764.

Aldridge T. Diagnosing heel pain in adults. *Am Fam Physician.* 2004;70(2):332–338.

Bennell KL, Malcolm SA, Thomas SA, Ebeling PR, McCrory PR, Wark JD, Brukner PD. Risk factors for stress fractures in female track-and-field athletes: a retrospective analysis. *Clin J Sport Med.* 1995;5(4):229–235.

Bradley WB, Slomiany WP. Shin pain treatments get active patiens back on track. *Biomechanics.* 2008;31–38.

Breithaupt J. Zur pathologie des menschlichen fussess. *Medizin Zeitung.* 1855;24:169–177.

Fredericson M, Bergman AG, et al. Tibial stress reaction in runners. Correlation of clinical symptoms and scintigraphy with a new magnetic resonance imaging grading system. *Am J Sports Med.* 1995;23(4):472–481.

Geffen A, Seliktar R. Comparison of trabecular architecture and the isostatic stress flow in the human calcaneus. *Med Eng Phys.* 2004;26(2):119–129.

Hastings MK, et al. Bone mineral density of the tarsals and metatarsals with reloading: case report. *Phys Ther.* 2008;88(6):766–779.

Jansen M. March foot. *J Bone Joint Surg.* 1926;8:262–272.

Jones BH, Thacker SB, Gilchrist J, Kimsey CD Jr, Sosin DM. Prevention of lower extremity stress fractures in athletes and soldiers: a systematic review. *Epidemiol Rev.* 2002; 24(2):228–247.

Kaczander BI, Shapiro J. Consider systemic causes of heel pain. *Biomechanics.* 2005:59–61.

Lebrun M. The female athlete triad: What's a doctor to do? *Curr Sports Med Rep.* 2007;6:397–404.

Leroux JL, et al. Fractures of the calcaneus during fluoride treatment for osteoporosis. *Sem Hop.* 1983;8,59(45):3140–3142.

Lespessailles E, Poupon S, Niamane R, Loiseau-Peres S, Derommelaere G, Harba R, Courteix D, Benhamou CL. Fractal analysis of trabecular bone texture on calcaneal radiographs. *Osteoporosis Int.* 2002;13(5):366–372.

Matheson GO, Clement DB, McKenzie DC, Taunton JE, Lloyd-Smith DR, MacIntyre JG. Stress fractures in athletes. A study of 320 cases. *Am J Sports Med.* 1987;15(1):46–58.

Meyer J, Kulig K, Landel R. Differential diagnosis and treatment of subcalcaneal heel pain: a case report. *JOSPT.* 2002;32(3):114–125.

Niva MH, Sormaala MJ, Kiuru MJ, Haataja R, Ahovuo JA, Pihlajamaki HK. Bone stress injuries of the ankle and foot: an 86-month magnetic resonance imaging-based study of physically active young adults. *Am J Sports Med.* 2007;35(4):643–649.

Prouteau S, Ducher G, Nanyan P, Lemineur G, Benhamou L, Courteix D. Fractal analysis of bone texture: a screening tool for stress fracture risk? *Eur J Clin Invest.* 2004;34(2):137–142.

Sormaala MJ, Niva MH, Kiuru MJ, Mattila VM, Pihlajamäki HK. Stress injuries of the calcaneus detected with magnetic resonance imaging in military recruits. *J Bone Joint Surg Am.* 2006;88:2237–2242.

Stafford SA, Rosenthal DI, Gebhardt MC, Brady TJ, Scott JA. MRI in stress fracture. *AJR Am J Roentgenol.* 1986;147:553–556.

Stechow. Fussödem und Röntgenstrahlen. *Deutsche Militärärztliche Zeitschrift.* 1897;26:465.

Swenson EJ Jr, DeHaven KE, Sebastianelli WJ, Hanks G, Kalenak A, Lynch JM. The effect of a pneumatic leg brace on return to play in athletes with tibial stress fractures. *Am J Sports Med.* 1997;25(June):322–328.

Verma RB, Sherman O. Athletic Stress fractures: Part1–3. *Am J Orthop.* 2001;30(11):798–806.

Weber JM, Vidt LG, Gehl RS, Montgomery T. Calcaneal stress fractures. *Clin Podiatr Med Surg.* 2005;22(1):45–54.

Zager E, et al. Conservative approach benefits Calcaneal fracture treatment. *Biomechanics.* 2005;35–47.

AUTHOR: STEPHEN PAULSETH

BASIC INFORMATION

DEFINITION

A disruption or subluxation of the cuboid affects the structural congruity of the calcaneocuboid portion of the midtarsal joint.

SYNONYMS

- Subluxed cuboid
- Locked cuboid
- Dropped cuboid
- Cuboid fault syndrome
- Peroneal cuboid syndrome

ICD-9CM CODES

726.70 Enthesopathy of ankle and tarsus unspecified

OPTIMAL NUMBER OF VISITS

6 or fewer

MAXIMAL NUMBER OF VISITS

16

ETIOLOGY

- The cuboid and the calcaneus articulate to form the calcaneocuboid joint. Structural integrity of this joint is important for the maintenance of lateral foot stability. The cuboid plays a unique role in that it is the only bone that articulates with the midtarsal and tarsometatarsal joints. It also is the only bone to link the lateral column to the transverse plantar arch. Proper alignment and mechanics of this bone are critical for the stability and mobility of the foot.
- A subluxation or misalignment of the cuboid can potentially irritate the surrounding joint capsule, ligaments, and fibularis longus tendon.
- The dorsal and plantar calcaneocuboid, dorsal and plantar cuboidconavicular, dorsal and plantar cuboideometatarsal, and the long plantar ligament all act to passively stabilize the cuboid in the lateral column of the foot. These ligaments are more taut dorsal medially than plantar laterally. Therefore the calcaneocuboid joint rotates around a medially positioned axis.
- The function and the stability of the cuboid is affected by the fibularis longus muscle. The muscle's tendon travels anteromedially through the cuboid's peroneal groove and inserts on the lateral base of first metatarsal and first cuneiform. The fibularis longus muscle's strength and function depends on proper position and stability of the cuboid as it uses the bone as a lever to generate force and stabilize the foot.
- Fibularis longus is most active during the stance phase of gait. It contracts midway

through the midstance phase and continues to contract through the terminal stance phase. As the foot supinates during the terminal phase of gait, the fibularis longus muscle acts as a dynamic stabilizer of the forefoot as it assists in plantar flexion of the first ray while using the cuboid as a pulley, increasing the mechanical advantage of the muscle.
- Cuboid syndrome involves the subluxation or displacement of the cuboid bone. The subluxation is often caused by plantar flexion inversion ankle sprains. As the foot and ankle are placed into plantar flexion and inversion, the fibularis longus tendon places a dorsal and lateral force on the forefoot, creating a close packed position and forcing the cuboid in an inferomedial direction and tearing the interosseous ligaments. The force on the cuboid is further increased by the stretch reflex. When the foot is rapidly plantar flexed and inverted, the fibularis longus muscle is quickly stretched and responds with a more forceful contraction.

EPIDEMIOLOGY AND DEMOGRAPHICS

- It has been hypothesized that 4% of athletic foot injuries involve the cuboid.
- 6.7% of patients with low ankle sprains have a displaced cuboid.
- In ballet dancers, 17% of foot injuries involve the cuboid. In male dancers, the mechanism appears to related to trauma, whereas in female dancers it appears to involve repetitive use.

MECHANISM OF INJURY

- Plantar flexion and inversion (low ankle) sprain
- Repetitive use on an unstable foot. If the patient lacks foot stability, the fibularis longus muscle is required to work harder to stabilize the foot. If joint laxity is present, the cuboid is pulled out of alignment by the continuous force of the fibularis longus.
- Ballet, due to the stress of jumping and landing with poor foot support

COMMON SIGNS AND SYMPTOMS

- Symptoms can begin rapidly as a result of injury or more gradually as a result of overuse.
- Tenderness is present locally at the plantar surface of the cuboid bone.
- Pain is also commonly experienced in the medial arch or along the fourth metatarsal bone.
- Pain is most often present with weight-bearing activities such as walking and standing.
- Symptoms are most commonly experienced at the terminal stance phase of gait.

- Patients also experience weakness when rising up onto their toes or with jumping.

AGGRAVATING ACTIVITIES

- Walking
- Walking barefoot
- Standing
- Jumping
- Coming up onto toes
- Ballet dancing

EASING ACTIVITIES

- Non–weight-bearing activities
- Rest
- Cold pack or compress

24-HOUR SYMPTOM PATTERN

- Symptoms may be better during the morning, especially after sleeping with the foot elevated.
- Symptoms may worsen during the day with increased weight-bearing activities.

PAST HISTORY FOR THE REGION

- Previous history of ankle injury
- History of trauma to the foot
- History of repetitive use coupled with poor foot stability

PHYSICAL EXAMINATION

- Pain at the terminal stance phase of gait. Decreased stride length noted as a compensatory mechanism.
- Weakness when testing the patient's ability to rise up onto the toes
- MMT of the fibularis longus muscle is weaker than the contralateral side because of the altered cuboid position.
- Inversion ROM testing may be limited or painful.
- Point tenderness at the plantar surface of the cuboid
- If the cuboid is severely displaced, there may be a sulcus present over the dorsal aspect of the cuboid.
- Altered midfoot mobility is noted (abnormal pronation or supination when compared with the contralateral side).
- Neural dynamic testing should be normal. Abnormal findings may indicate that the pain is not from the cuboid but from lateral plantar nerve.
- Poor ankle proprioception is often present.

IMPORTANT OBJECTIVE TESTS

- MRI, x-ray, and ultrasound have not been found to be beneficial in diagnosing cuboid syndrome. The alterations in structural alignment are too small to be picked up on imaging studies. Imaging may be appropriate to rule out other potential pathology and in identifying joint destruction or inflammatory processes.
- No one specific clinical test has been shown to definitively identify the

presence of cuboid syndrome, but the following three findings are often positive:
- ○ Decreased fibularis longus strength
- ○ Decreased ability to come up onto the toes
- ○ Pain on the plantar aspect of the cuboid

DIFFERENTIAL DIAGNOSIS

- Jones fracture
- Tumor
- Fracture of the anterior calcaneal process
- Tarsal coalition
- Peroneal and extensor digitorum brevis tendinitis
- Subluxing peroneal tendons
- Arthritis
- Gout
- Sinus tarsi syndrome
- Lateral plantar nerve entrapment
- Lisfranc injuries
- Stress fractures of the cuboid
- Lyme disease
- Metatarsal stress fractures

CONTRIBUTING FACTORS

- Overpronation
- Poorly constructed orthoses
- Running on uneven surfaces
- Poor shoe construction
- Inversion ankle injuries
- Chronic ankle sprain
- Balance disorder
- History of ankle instability
- Participation in high-level athletic sports or dance

TREATMENT

MEDICAL

- Surgery is not typically performed on patients with cuboid syndrome.
- Medically, the physician may prescribe antiinflammatory medications to reduce the irritation and swelling in the region.
- In severe cases, a walking boot or cast may be used to reduce the loading on the foot.

REHABILITATION

- Cuboid syndrome responds favorably and quickly to manipulative therapy.

The effectiveness of treatment has been attributed to the fact that most patients with cuboid syndrome have pain and dysfunction caused by a malalignment of the cuboid bone. When the cuboid is returned to its normal position, symptoms resolve and function improves.
- Two common techniques used in the clinic and described in research are the cuboid whip and the cuboid squeeze techniques.
  - ○ Cuboid whip: Jennings and Davies found that 7 of 104 patients with lateral ankle sprains had subluxed cuboids. A cuboid whip manipulation was performed on all seven subjects. Symptoms were assessed immediately after the manipulation. All of the patients reported substantial reductions in pain and symptoms. Two of the seven required one additional manipulation, and the authors attributed the need to be a result of the longer duration that the symptoms had been present. A 2- to 8-month follow-up with the patients revealed no return of symptoms in any of the 7, and all had returned to prior levels of function.
  - ○ Cuboid squeeze: Marshall and Hamilton described a cuboid squeeze technique performed on three subjects, all of whom had complete resolution of symptoms after one or two treatments. In a 5-year follow up, none of the three subjects had a return of symptoms.
- Low dye taping with or without cuboid pads is commonly used in clinic to support and stabilize the subluxed cuboid. Clinicians also use the taping to support a cuboid immediately after a manipulative technique.
- Once the patient's cuboid has been reduced, it is wise to have the patient refrain from sports for several days after the manipulation to ensure that the cuboid remains in its normal position. If the patient remains symptom-free, they can begin to return to sport.
- The patient can return to sport, but care must be taken to slowly progress the loading through the cuboid. Full return to sport can occur when all biomechanical contributing factors have been addressed, balance and proprioception are normal, and strength is at least 90% that of the contralateral side.

PROGNOSIS

- The prognosis for patients with cuboid syndrome is generally good.
- If the factors resulting in abnormal forces being placed on the cuboid can be eliminated, then the patient should heal.
- Symptoms usually abate rapidly once the cuboid is aligned correctly. The challenge for the clinician is preventing future subluxations.

SIGNS AND SYMPTOMS INDICATING REFERRAL TO PHYSICIAN

- Red flag signs in the foot are usually few. If the patient is not improving over the course of a month, the patient should be referred to a physician.
- If there is suspicion of tumors (unremitting or nonmechanical pain), referral to a physician is warranted.
- Suspicions of gout should also be referred back to the referring physician for medical workup. Unresolving inflammation may be an indication of gout or other systemic inflammatory disorders.

SUGGESTED READINGS

Caselli MA, Pantelaras N. How to treat cuboid syndrome in the athlete. *Podiatry Today*. 2004;117(10):76-80.

Jennings J, Davies GJ. Treatment of cuboid syndrome secondary to lateral ankle sprains: a case series. *J Orthop Sports Phys Ther.* 2005;335(7):409-415.

Leerar PJ. Differential diagnosis of tarsal coalition versus cuboid syndrome in and adolescent athlete. *J Orthop Sports Phys Ther.* 2001;331(12):702-707.

Marshall P, Hamilton WG. Cuboid subluxation in ballet dancers. *Am J Sports Med.* 1992;220(2):169-175.

Mooney M, Maffey-Ward L. Cuboid plantar and dorsal subluxations: assessment and treatment. *J Orthop Sports Phys Ther.* 1994;220(4):220-226.

Newell SG, Woodle A. Cuboid syndrome. *Physician Sports Med.* 1981;9:71-76.

Patterson S. Cuboid syndrome: a review of literature. *J Orthop Sports Phys Ther.* 2006;5:597-606.

Subotnick SI. Peroneal cuboid syndrome. *J Am Podiatr Med Assoc.* 1989;779(8):413-414.

AUTHOR: DERRICK SUEKI

BASIC INFORMATION

DEFINITION

Fat pad contusion is a condition in which force or trauma is applied to the fat pad of the heel; this force results in damage to the fat pad and the subsequent inflammatory response results in irritation of the fat pad. Contusion occurs when the force is great enough to bruise the underlying bone as well.

SYNONYMS

- Bruised heel
- Fat pad irritation
- Policeman's heel
- Fat pad syndrome

ICD-9CM CODES
924.2   Contusion of ankle and foot, excluding toe(s)

OPTIMAL NUMBER OF VISITS

6 or fewer

MAXIMAL NUMBER OF VISITS

16

ETIOLOGY

- Anatomically, the fat pad is a protective layer on the plantar surface of the calcaneus. Normally, it is about 1 inch thick and composed of fibrous tissue septa, which separates the closely packed fat cells. This structure allows the heel fat pad to act as a shock absorber.
- Contusion or bruising of the heel can occur when the septa holding the fat pad together are damaged. This allows the fat pad to move laterally along the surface of the calcaneus when force is placed on the heel. The slippage of the fat pad leaves the calcaneus with less cushion and as a result, more force is delivered to the heel itself. Ultimately, the increased force on the calcaneus bone results in damage and irritation of the bone.

EPIDEMIOLOGY AND DEMOGRAPHICS

The prevalence of fat pad contusion is unknown. Calcaneal fractures account for approximately 2% of all body fractures.

MECHANISM OF INJURY

- Repetitive use such as walking or running
- Poor footwear such as marching in hard boots
- Falls on the heel
- Walking barefoot on hard surfaces

COMMON SIGNS AND SYMPTOMS

- Pain is worse with weight bearing.
- Swelling and tenderness on the plantar surface of the heel. Usually, the pain is more posterior on the heel as opposed to heel spurs or plantar fasciitis, which is more anterior
- Pain increases with walking.

AGGRAVATING ACTIVITIES

- Walking
- Walking in hard-soled shoes
- Walking barefoot
- Standing
- Landing during jumping

EASING ACTIVITIES

- Non–weight-bearing activities
- Rest
- Cold pack or compress
- Wearing cushioned insoles in the shoes

24-HOUR SYMPTOM PATTERN

- Symptoms may be better during the morning, especially after sleeping with the foot elevated.
- Symptoms may worsen during the day with increased weight-bearing activities.

PAST HISTORY FOR THE REGION

- Previous history of chronic ankle sprain
- History of ankle instability may place abnormal forces onto the calcaneus.
- History of falls onto the foot
- History of repetitive use coupled with poor or no footwear

PHYSICAL EXAMINATION

- Local tenderness at the posterior aspect of the calcaneus
- Pain during heel strike or initial contact phase of gait
- Increased foot pronation or increased calcaneal eversion may be present, which would place more pressure onto the medial aspect of the calcaneus during gait. This could result in breakdown of the fat pad in the posteromedial aspect of the heel and damage to the underlying bone.
- Increased foot supination or increased calcaneal inversion results in a decreased ability of the foot to absorb shock and therefore greater force placed on the posterolateral aspect of the calcaneus.
- ROM testing may reveal decreased dorsiflexion of the ankle, which could contribute to the heel pain.
- Neural dynamic testing should be normal. Abnormal findings may indicate that the pain is not from the fat pad but from nerve entrapment. Entrapment of

the tibial nerve in the tarsal tunnel may manifest as heel pain.
- Muscle weakness (e.g., in the posterior tibialis muscle) may affect the biomechanics of the foot and result in abnormal loading on the calcaneus.

IMPORTANT OBJECTIVE TESTS

- Radiographic imaging
  - ○ A painful heel fat pad can be confused with nerve irritation or plantar fasciitis. MRI can also help distinguish between these conditions.
  - ○ Heel fat pad pathology can demonstrate changes in signal intensity; low-signal-intensity bands represent fibrosis and decreased height of the fat pad.
  - ○ Fat pad inflammation demonstrates edematous changes in the fat pad, with ill-defined areas of decreased signal intensity on T1-weighted images that increase in signal intensity on T2-weighted images.
  - ○ MRI is also useful in identifying space-occupying lesions within the fat pad from peripheral nerve sheath tumors or rheumatoid nodules.

DIFFERENTIAL DIAGNOSIS

- Plantar fasciitis
- Tibial nerve entrapment
- Retrocalcaneal bursitis
- Heel bone spurs
- Tarsal tunnel syndrome
- Talus fracture
- Calcaneus fracture

CONTRIBUTING FACTORS

- Osteoporosis or osteopenia
- Balance disorder
- Chronic ankle sprain
- History of ankle instability
- Participation in high-level athletic sports
- Footwear
- Overpronation or over supination
- Repetitive walking on hard surfaces

TREATMENT

MEDICAL

- Surgery is generally not warranted in patients with fat pad contusions. The physician may prescribe antiinflammatory medications to reduce the irritation and swelling in the region.
- In severe cases, a walking boot or cast may be used to reduce the loading on the heel.
- If conservative care fails, the physician may inject corticosteroids into the fat pad to reduce the inflammation and pain.

REHABILITATION

- The bone under the fat pad has the potential to heal, but the load on the bone must be reduced and then gradually reintroduced so that inflammation can be eliminated and then proper bone healing can occur.
- Rehabilitation involves decreasing the inflammatory response and addressing the factors that contribute to increased loading on the heel.
- To reduce inflammation, the clinician can use cryotherapy, ultrasound, or electrical stimulation. Ice massage is an effective way to deliver localized treatment to the calcaneus.
- Reducing the loading on the calcaneus is also an important aspect of rehabilitation. Cushioned heel pads can cushion the shoe during gait. Advising the patient to wear low heels may also reduce some of the load on the heel during gait.
- Improving the mechanics of the foot can also place the heel in a better position during gait. Orthotics may help improve foot position during gait, although it is questionable whether the orthotics benefit the patient during the heel-strike portion of gait.
- Improving the mobility of the subtalar joint and the calf can improve ankle dorsiflexion. This is often needed to help improve the biomechanics of the foot, but it is questionable what effect the increased dorsiflexion will have on foot mechanics during initial contact of gait.
- Taping of the heel, clinically, has proved effective at stabilizing the fat pad and not allowing it to slip or migrate. Patients often experience significant pain abatement with heel taping.

PROGNOSIS

- The prognosis for patients with fat pad contusions or irritation is generally good.
- If the factors resulting in abnormal calcaneal forces can be eliminated, then the patient should heal.
- Normal healing generally takes 6 to 8 weeks. Reducing the loading in a commonly used area in the body, such as the foot, is difficult. Healing may take a little longer as a result.

SIGNS AND SYMPTOMS INDICATING REFERRAL TO PHYSICIAN

- The red flag signs in the heel are usually few. If the patient is not improving over the course of a month, they should be referred back to their physician
- If there is suspicion of tumors (unremitting or nonmechanical pain), a referral to the physician is warranted.
- Infections from cuts or insect bites can also result in swelling and inflammation of the heel. If this is suspected, a referral to the physician should be made.

SUGGESTED READINGS

DiMarcangelo MT, Yu TC. Diagnostic imaging of heel pain and plantar fasciitis. *Clin Podiatr Med Surg.* 1997;14:281–301.

Karr SD. Subcalcaneal heel pain. *Orthop Clin North Am.* 1994;25:161–173.

Narvaez JA, Narvaez J, Ortega R, Aguilera C, Sanchez A, Andia E. Painful heel: MR imaging findings. *Radiographics.* 2000;20:333–352.

AUTHOR: DERRICK SUEKI

BASIC INFORMATION

DEFINITION

Injury to the tendon of the flexor hallucis longus (FHL) muscle can include an acute inflammatory response, in which case the tendon injury is labeled tenosynovitis. If the tendon injury is more chronic, the injury is considered a tenosynovitis. Complete disruption of the tendon is considered a tendon rupture.

SYNONYMS

- Dancer's tendinitis
- FHL tendinitis
- FHL tendinosis
- FHL rupture
- FHL tenosynovitis

ICD-9CM CODES
727.06 Tenosynovitis of foot and
        ankle

OPTIMAL NUMBER OF VISITS

6 or fewer

MAXIMAL NUMBER OF VISITS

16 or more

ETIOLOGY

- The FHL muscle attaches proximally at the posterior superior third of the fibula and distally attaches at the base of the distal phalanx of the hallux. It functions to flex all the joints of the big toe and also acts to plantar flex the ankle joint.
- Together with the flexor digitorum longus (FDL) tendon and the posterior tibialis tendon, the FHL tendon passes behind the medial malleolus and through the tarsal tunnel. Grooves on the talus and calcaneus contain the tendon of the muscle and are lined by a mucous sheath.
- A continuum of injuries can involve the FHL tendon and its associated sheath. In the past, the term *tendinitis* was used to explain all pathology that occurred within a tendon. As the knowledge base has expanded, the definitions of tendon pathology have also changed.
  - *Tendinitis* usually refers to an acute injury in which there is damage and inflammatory response to the tendon.
  - *Tendinosis* usually refers to a chronic condition in which there still may be an inflammatory response, but degeneration of the tendon and alteration in tissue has begun to occur. Inflammation is minimal.
  - *Paratenonitis* occurs when there is irritation of the outer layers of the paratenon and epitenon. Acute edema and hyperemia of the paratenon result.

The paratenon is the tissue between a tendon sheath and its tendon. The paratenon surrounds and nourishes the tendon.
  - *Tenosynovitis* is inflammation of the fluid-filled synovial sheath (called the *synovium*) that surrounds a tendon. Tenosynovitis refers to the chronic degenerative state of the tenosynovium.
  - Partial or complete tendon tears can occur centrally, in the intrasubstance, or at the external margins of the tendon. Tendon retraction may or may not occur in the case of complete tendon tears. Complete ruptures of the FHL are rare.
  - Tendon entrapment or checkrein deformity is tethering or entrapment of the FHL tendon that can occur under or just proximal to the flexor retinaculum.
  - Tendon subluxation or dislocation can occur as the tendon travels posterior to the medial malleolus.
- Injury to the FHL tendon can occur in the following regions:
  1. Within the tarsal tunnel
  2. At the knot of Henry, under the base of the first metatarsal. where the FDL tendon crosses the FHL tendon
  3. Where the FHL tendon passes between the great toe sesamoids beneath the metatarsal head

EPIDEMIOLOGY AND DEMOGRAPHICS

The prevalence of FHL tendon pathology is not documented in the literature. FHL injuries as a whole are more prominent in ballet dancers and in sports requiring repetitive plantar flexion of the foot.

MECHANISM OF INJURY

- FHL injuries generally result from repetitive plantar flexion combined with vertical loading. Common mechanisms include ballet, because dancers are required to repetitively come up onto their toes. It can also occur in runners who run long distances downhill. Running downhill requires more plantar flexion than running uphill.
- Synovitis and tenosynovitis may also occur as a result of inflammatory diseases such as RA. Synovitis and interosseous muscle atrophy of the interosseous muscles commonly seen in RA can result in misalignments of the foot and ankle joints.
- Other mechanisms of injury include the following:
  - Repetitive use during walking or standing
  - Poor footwear such as wearing shoes that are too tight
  - Walking in high heels
  - Repetitive jumping sports

COMMON SIGNS AND SYMPTOMS

- Insidious onset of posteromedial ankle pain.
- Localized swelling in the region of entrapment that is generally at the tarsal tunnel.
- If scar tissue or fibrosis has occurred, clicking or catching may be noted at the site of entrapment.
- Pain is noted with repetitive plantar flexion of the foot and ankle.

AGGRAVATING ACTIVITIES

- Walking or running down hill
- Rising up onto toes
- Walking in high heels
- Standing
- Jumping

EASING ACTIVITIES

- Non-weight-bearing activities
- Rest
- Cold pack or compress

24-HOUR SYMPTOM PATTERN

- Symptoms may be better during the morning, especially after sleeping with the foot elevated.
- Symptoms may worsen during the day with increased weight-bearing activities.

PAST HISTORY FOR THE REGION

- Previous history of ankle or foot injury
- History of trauma to the foot
- History of repetitive use coupled with poor or no footwear

PHYSICAL EXAMINATION

- Point tenderness at the site of entrapment is generally posterior to the medial malleolus but can also occur under the base of the first metatarsal where the FDL tendon crosses the FHL tendon or where the FHL tendon passes between the great toe sesamoids beneath the metatarsal head.
- Crepitus or catching of the tendon may be palpable at the site of entrapment.
- Increased foot pronation or increased calcaneal eversion may be present, which would place more pressure onto the medial aspect of the foot and during gait.
- ROM testing may reveal decreased dorsiflexion of the ankle, which could contribute to the foot dysfunction.
- Resisted muscle testing of the FHL may produce pain.
- Pain is also present when patients are asked to rise up onto their toes.
- Neural dynamic testing should be normal. Abnormal findings may indicate that the pain is from the tibial nerve.
- Balance and proprioception are often poor in these patients.
- Muscle weakness (e.g., in the posterior tibialis muscle) may affect the biomechanics

of the foot and result in abnormal loading on the metatarsal heads.

IMPORTANT OBJECTIVE TESTS

- MRI, x-ray, and ultrasound have been found to be beneficial in ruling out other potential pathology and in identifying joint destruction or other inflammatory processes.
- Fluid in the synovial sheath is common in 20% of patients because the FHL tendon sheath communicates with the ankle joint.
- No one specific clinical test has been shown to definitively identify the presence of flexor hallucis longus tendinopathy.

DIFFERENTIAL DIAGNOSIS

- Posterior impingement syndrome
- Achilles tendinopathy
- Tibial nerve irritations
- Lumbar spine nerve entrapment
- Os trigonum syndrome
- Tarsal tunnel syndrome
- Osteoarthritis
- RA
- Tibialis posterior tendinopathy
- Subtalar coalition
- Fractured Stieda process
- Calcaneal fractures with impingement

CONTRIBUTING FACTORS

- Entrapment of the FHL tendon may be due to an enlarged os trigonum, an associated calcaneal fracture, or fracture dislocation
- Overpronation
- Hallux limitus
- Balance disorders
- Chronic ankle sprain
- History of ankle instability
- Participation in high-level athletic sports that require repetitive plantar flexion
- Footwear
- Ballet and dance

TREATMENT

MEDICAL

- Surgery is generally only considered if all conservative options have been exhausted. The physician may prescribe antiinflammatory medications to reduce the irritation and swelling in the region. Steroid injections may be used to reduce inflammation locally around the region of irritation.
- In severe cases, a walking boot or cast may be used to reduce the loading on the forefoot.

- In cases where conservative treatment has failed to relieve symptoms, surgical intervention may be required. If a patient has a complete tear with marked tendon retraction, some surgeons administer a trial of conservative treatment. However, surgical repair with reapposition of the torn ends of the tendon is eventually performed.
- In patients with chronic dislocation or subluxation, surgery is performed. The surgery may involve resection of abnormal ossific structures, repositioning of hardware, or fixation of fractures in patients with previous ankle and foot fracture, depending on the structures that are causing tendon irritation.

SURGICAL OUTCOMES

Success and complications rates vary, depending on the nature and magnitude of the surgery, but general postsurgical outcomes are good.

REHABILITATION

- The body has a remarkable ability to heal. The synovium of the metatarsal joint is no different. The key to healing FHL tendinopathy is identification of the structural and biomechanical abnormalities that are leading to the stress placed on the tendon.
- Rehabilitation initially involves decreasing the inflammatory response. Medications, ice, and elevation are appropriate measures to address the inflammation that is present. To reduce the stress placed on the tendon, devices such as foot orthotics have proved effective in reducing the loading on the tendon and improving the mechanics of the foot so that the loads are subsequently reduced. Therapy must allow the inflammation to subside or resolve by relieving the repeated excessive stress and irritation.
- Improving the mobility of the talocrural joint and the calf can improve ankle dorsiflexion. This is often needed to help improve the biomechanics of the foot during the mid-to-late stance phases of gait.
- The patient can return to sport, but care must be taken to slowly progress the loading through the tendon so that appropriate tissue remodeling can occur. Full return to sport can occur when all biomechanical contributing factors have been addressed, balance and proprioception are normal, and strength is at least 90% that of the contralateral side.
- Eccentric training programs have shown good results in patients with chronic tendon pathology.

- Strengthening must increase gradually and should be relatively pain free.
- Programs focusing on training and strengthening of the posterior tibialis muscle are currently being studied and show good potential for improving the mechanics of the foot and ankle, therefore reducing the stress placed on the tendon.

PROGNOSIS

- The prognosis for patients with FHL tendinopathy is generally good.
- If the factors resulting in abnormal forces being placed on the metatarsal joint can be eliminated, then the patient should heal.
- Normal healing would generally take 6 to 8 weeks. Reducing the loading in a commonly used area in the body, such as the foot, is difficult. Healing may take a little longer as a result.
- The prognosis for patients with complete ruptures or dislocation or subluxation of the tendon is not as good as for tenosynovitis.

SIGNS AND SYMPTOMS INDICATING REFERRAL TO PHYSICIAN

- Red flag signs in the ankle and foot are less common. If the patient is not improving over the course of a month, they should be referred back to their physician.
- If there is suspicion of tumors (unremitting or nonmechanical pain), a referral to the physician is warranted.
- Suspicion of gout should also be referred back to the referring physician for medical workup. Nonresolving inflammation may be an indication of gout or other systemic inflammatory disorders.

SUGGESTED READINGS

Boruta PM, Beauperthuy GD. Partial tear of the flexor hallucis longus at the knot of Henry: presentation of three cases. *Foot Ankle Int.* 1997;18(4):243-246.

Bureau NJ, Cardinal E, Hobden R, Aubin B. Posterior ankle impingement syndrome: MR imaging findings in seven patients. *Radiology.* 2000;215(2):497-503.

Sammarco GJ, Cooper PS. Flexor hallucis longus tendon injury in dancers and nondancers. *Foot Ankle Int.* 1998;19(6):356-362.

Trevino S, Baumhauer JF. Tendon injuries of the foot and ankle. *Clin Sports Med.* 1992;11(4):727-739.

AUTHOR: DERRICK SUEKI

BASIC INFORMATION

DEFINITION

- Osteoarthritis is a pathology associated with inflammation in the joints of the body. In the case of foot osteoarthritis, the arthritis and inflammation most commonly affects the midfoot, hindfoot, or forefoot.
- Osteoarthritis is a term derived from the Greek word *osteo*, meaning "of the bone," *arthro*, meaning "joint," and *itis*, meaning inflammation, even though the amount of inflammation present in the joint can range from excessive to little or no inflammation.

SYNONYMS

- Foot arthritis
- Foot degenerative joint disease

ICD-9 CODES

715.17 Primary localized osteoarthritis, ankle and foot
715.27 Secondary localized osteoarthritis, ankle and foot

OPTIMAL NUMBER OF VISITS

3 to 6

MAXIMAL NUMBER OF VISITS

20 to 36

ETIOLOGY

- The wearing down of the hyaline cartilage leads to an inflammatory response. There is thickening and sclerosis of the subchondral bone and development of osteophytes or bone spurs. This leads to a narrowing of the joint space, loss of shock absorption, and ultimately pain.
- Daily wear and tear in combination with various injuries sustained throughout life is the most common cause of the breakdown of healthy tissue.
- Degeneration of the cartilage and resultant arthritis can also be the result of other factors such as trauma or joint injury.
- At a cellular level, as a person ages, the number of proteoglycans in the articular cartilage decreases. Proteoglycans are hydrophilic and work within cartilage to bind water. With the reduction of proteoglycans comes a decrease in water content within the cartilage and a corresponding loss of cartilage resilience. With the decreases in cartilage resilience, collagen fibers of the cartilage become susceptible to degradation and injury. The breakdown of collagen and other cartilage tissue is released into the surround joint space. Inflammation results as the body attempts to respond to the influx of byproducts from cartilage injury.

- As the cartilage degrades, the joint space narrows and ligaments become more lax. In response to the laxity, new bone outgrowths, called *spurs* or *osteophytes*, can form on the margins of the joints in an attempt to improve the congruence and passive stability of the articular cartilage surfaces.
- Primary osteoarthritis refers to joint degradation resulting from aging and tissue degeneration.
- Secondary osteoarthritis refers to joint degradation and tissue degeneration that result from factors besides aging such as obesity, trauma, and congenital disorders.

EPIDEMIOLOGY AND DEMOGRAPHICS

- About 50% of people in their sixties and seventies have ankle or foot osteoarthritis as seen on x-ray.
- Symptomatic foot osteoarthritis is not very common in the general population; there is an increased prevalence in persons with a history of significant foot trauma or extreme sports or activities (e.g., dance)
- Seniors, especially those with a history of long-term abnormal use (poor footwear, excessive injuries, career or recreational overuse, or obesity)
- Females have more ankle and foot osteoarthritis than males.

MECHANISM OF INJURY

- Osteoarthritis is a pathology of overuse. The mechanism of injury is therefore the result of repetitive motions that stress the foot. The more cycles of an activity that the foot sees, the more likely the result will be anatomical damage.
- Daily use or misuse of the foot (3-inch heels increase foot and ankle stress 7 times compared to 1-inch heels)
- Misalignment of the foot and/or toes
- Excessive use or strain of the foot
- Injuries, such as fracture and strains or sprains, that cause inflammation and scar tissue in the foot or toes

COMMON SIGNS AND SYMPTOMS

- Pain in the foot or toes
- Stiffness in the foot or toes
- Cracking or deep crunching in the foot or toe joints
- Inflammation and thickening of the foot or toe joints
- Misalignment of foot and toe bones
- Gait abnormalities (increased foot pronation, out-toeing, or limp)

AGGRAVATING ACTIVITIES

- Inactivity leads to stiffness
- Weight-bearing activities (like walking, running, dancing, jumping, etc)

- Long-term standing, especially on harder surfaces like concrete, and wearing tight and/or poorly supportive shoes
- Inactivity allows the inflammation to pool and increase pressure, leading to discomfort and loss of available movement.
- Joint movement and weight bearing increases wear and tear and inflammation/irritation to the articular surfaces.
- Poor footwear (i.e., high heels)

EASING ACTIVITIES

- Gentle stretching and exercise, use of heat/ice, massage, taking antiinflammatory medication, non–weight-bearing activities, and elevating the feet
- Generally speaking, these activities lead to decreased wear and tear and loss of the stiffness and inflammation associated with this condition.

24-HOUR SYMPTOM PATTERN

- Stiffness in the morning
- Better after a warm shower and taking medication
- Can worsen with excessive movement
- Stiffens again in the evening

PAST HISTORY FOR THE REGION

- Jobs or recreational activities that require excessive use or strain of the foot (dancing, walking, running, jumping, etc)
- Abnormal amount of damage from injuries
- Past history of poor footwear

PHYSICAL EXAMINATION

- Joint thickening (bony changes and inflammation)
- Loss of foot or toe ROM
- Localized pain and loss of joint mobility
- Crepitus with movement

IMPORTANT OBJECTIVE TESTS

- No specific clinical testing regimen has been developed to positively confirm the presence of foot osteoarthritis.
- Diagnosis is made by a combination of radiographic evidence coupled with clinical and subjective examination.

DIFFERENTIAL DIAGNOSIS

- Foot or toe sprain
- Tendinitis
- RA
- Sesamoiditis
- Bunions
- Fallen arches
- Plantar fasciitis
- Gout
- Referral from the lower lumbar region
- Pitting edema secondary to cardiac dysfunction

CONTRIBUTING FACTORS

- Uncontrollable risk factors that contribute or predispose an individual to ankle osteoarthritis pathology are as follows:
  - Gender (females > males)
  - Age (increase 2% per year after age 40 years)
  - Genetics
  - Prior history of injury to either lower extremity
- Modifiable risk factors that contribute or predispose an individual to continue or progress ankle osteoarthritis are as follows:
  - Weight
  - Work or recreational activities
  - Repetitive or significant traumatic injuries to the hip
  - Poor health (smoking, long-term use of steroids)
  - Poor footwear

TREATMENT

SURGICAL OPTIONS

- Fusion (arthrodesis)
- Bunionectomy

REHABILITATION

- Pathological changes to cartilage cannot be repaired by the body at this time. Even surgical advances have yet to solve the problems associated with cartilage damage. With this in mind, rehabilitation should focus on decreasing the stress placed on the damaged cartilage and correcting biomechanical and anatomical abnormalities that may predispose an individual to increased stress at the talocrural joint.
- Decreased ankle dorsiflexion is a common restriction in patients with foot osteoarthritis. Improving ankle dorsiflexion is an important component of the ankle's ability to absorb shock. Anterior-to-posterior talocrural joint mobilization, ankle traction mobilization, and soft tissue mobilization (STM) to the calf can help to increase ankle dorsiflexion.
- Midfoot dysfunction can also affect hindfoot and forefoot function. Increased pronation is often associated with decreased ankle dorsiflexion and a plantar flexed first ray. This motion should be controlled, but making the midfoot too rigid prevents it from dissipating shock. Instead, this shock is transferred to the talocrural joint and to the forefoot. Orthotics or foot and ankle exercises can be used to control foot pronation.
- Hip external rotation weakness or femoral torsions can also affect ankle and foot function and should be assessed and corrected.
- The clinician should also evaluate the patient for leg length discrepancies that cause abnormal stresses to be placed onto the ankle joint.
- Rehabilitation should focus on the following:
  - Education in correct use of ice and heat at home
  - Providing a home exercise program
  - Teaching proper footwear with or without orthotics
  - Manual therapy (STM, joint mobilization); may be able to teach patients self-mobilization techniques.
  - Modalities: Ice or heat, ultrasound, electrical stimulation, tape or braces
- Initial exercises to promote healing and pain abatement include the following:
  - Stretches: Calf (gastrocnemius and soleus), toe flexors, plantar fascia
  - Theraband exercises
  - Arch forming exercises
  - Toe strengthening exercises
  - Proprioceptive exercises
  - Pain-free foot motions such as foot alphabets
  - Joint mobilization and manipulation can be used to improve arthrokinematics, decrease pain, and increase ROM
  - Massage can decrease pain by relaxing muscular tension and increasing endorphin release.
- Exercise should be used to do the following:
  - Decrease muscular and joint stiffness.
  - Improve joint alignment by increasing muscular support.
  - Improve functional mobility: gait and recreational needs.
  - Improve proprioception and balance.
  - Create a sense of control over the symptoms and the condition.

PROGNOSIS

- Long-term prognosis for a patient with foot osteoarthritis depends on the extent of wear and tear and ability to reduce the joint strain (posture, activity, etc).
- For the most part, ankle osteoarthritis is a degenerative condition. At earlier stages of the pathology, rehabilitation aimed at reducing the load placed on the joint can potentially slow or halt the progression of degeneration.
- For patients who are farther along in the degenerative process, outcomes will be less favorable because cartilage has only a limited ability to repair itself.

SIGNS AND SYMPTOMS INDICATING REFERRAL TO PHYSICIAN

- Unrelenting pain
- Unusual responses to therapy
- Red flag symptoms, such as excessive redness and swelling and generalized malaise and fatigue may be signs of infection.
- Neurological symptoms

SUGGESTED READINGS

Dugan SA. Exercise for health and wellness at midlife and beyond: balancing benefits and risks. *Phys Med Rehabil Clin N Am.* 2007;18(3):555-575.

Frey C, Zamora J. The effects of obesity on orthopaedic foot and ankle pathology. *Foot Ankle Int.* 2007;28(9):996-999.

Glass GG. Osteoarthritis. *Dis Mon.* 2006;52(9).

Jung HG, Myerson MS, Schon LC. Spectrum of operative treatments and clinical outcomes for atraumatic osteoarthritis of the tarsometatarsal joints. *Foot Ankle Int.* 2007;28(4):482-489.

Mahiquez MY. Positive hindfoot valgus and osteoarthritis of the first metatarsophalangeal joint. *Foot Ankle Int.* 2006;27(12):1055-1059.

Valderrabano V, Nigg BM, von Tscharner V, Stefanyshyn DJ, Goepfert B, Hintermann B. Gait analysis in ankle osteoarthritis and total ankle replacement. *Clin Biomech (Bristol, Avon).* 2007;22(8):894-904.

AUTHOR: SARA GRANNIS

BASIC INFORMATION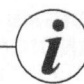

DEFINITION

- The term *Jones fracture* is controversial because it has been used indiscriminately to describe any fracture of the proximal portion of the fifth metatarsal.
- Jones fracture was described by Rosenberg as a fracture of the fifth metatarsal between the diaphysis and metaphysis. It is an intraarticular fracture involving the articulation between the fourth and fifth proximal metatarsals. It is an acute injury without precursory symptoms and is often confused with a tuberosity avulsion fracture.
- The location of the fracture is associated with a watershed area of the bone; thus the Jones fracture is notorious for poor healing and nonunion.

SYNONYMS

Fracture of the base of the fifth metatarsal

ICD-9CM CODES
825.25 Fracture of metatarsal bone(s) closed

OPTIMAL NUMBER OF VISITS

6 or fewer

MAXIMAL NUMBER OF VISITS

18

ETIOLOGY

- Jones fracture occurs when an acute external force is applied to the lateral foot while it is in plantar flexion, such as with a misstep to the lateral border of the foot, with cutting or pivoting with the foot planted and body weight on the metatarsal heads, in crossover maneuvers (soccer), or with repeated deceleration.
- The Jones fracture does not occur as a result of peroneus brevis or plantar aponeurosis avulsion of the tubercle. This is classified as an avulsion fracture.
- The pathology involves a fracture of the fifth metatarsal between the diaphysis and metaphysis that does not extend beyond the articulation of the fourth and fifth proximal metatarsals.
- Physiologically, a large external load into adduction is applied at the head of the fifth metatarsal, causing a bending moment that surpasses the bone's tensile strength laterally. This results in a fracture between the diaphysis and metaphysis at the proximal metatarsal.

EPIDEMIOLOGY AND DEMOGRAPHICS

- Jones fractures can occur at any age because they are the result of trauma.
- As a result of the rich innervation of the bone, periosteum and surrounding soft tissue pain is usually associated with the fracture.

MECHANISM OF INJURY

- Jones fracture commonly occurs with a large external load into adduction and with the foot plantar flexed during activities such as the following:
  - Misstep off a step or curb onto the lateral forefoot
  - Cutting or pivoting off the lateral forefoot with most of body weight on the foot
  - Sudden deceleration with the foot in plantar flexion and forefoot inversion.
  - Crossover maneuvers in sports such as soccer, basketball, and football

COMMON SIGNS AND SYMPTOMS

- Pain at the lateral aspect of the foot over the base of the fifth metatarsal
- Swelling and bruising at the base of the fifth metatarsal
- Difficulty walking or weight-bearing on the affected foot.

AGGRAVATING ACTIVITIES

- Walking
- Running
- Ascending and descending stairs
- Position of injury (plantar flexion and forefoot adduction)

EASING ACTIVITIES

- Elevation
- Ice
- Often, pain medication is prescribed; the use of antiinflammatories is controversial in patients with fracture because they have been associated with delayed bone healing.
- Non–weight-bearing activities
- Bracing to prevent position of injury

24-HOUR SYMPTOM PATTERN

- The patient with a Jones fracture may experience stiffness in the foot on waking.
- Symptoms increase during the day if the foot is in a gravity-dependent position for the majority of the day.
- Sleeping may or may not be problematic, depending on the foot's position.

PAST HISTORY FOR THE REGION

Because of the acute nature of this fracture, no previous history is required.

PHYSICAL EXAMINATION

- The patient may avoid symmetrical weight-bearing positions on the involved foot, especially along the lateral surface of the foot.
- Body weight may be biased on the heel of the involved foot to avoid pressure on the distal aspect of the fifth metatarsal (long lever arm).
- Tenderness from guarding the affected foot may be observed in the peroneals, long toe flexors, and gastrocnemius/soleus complex.

IMPORTANT OBJECTIVE TESTS

- Ottawa Rules: Set of two findings for the foot and ankle may implicate fracture.
- A foot radiographic series is recommended if the patient presents with pain in the midfoot and any one of the following findings:
  - Tenderness with palpation over the navicular or over the base of the fifth metatarsal
  - Inability to bear weight on the affected foot immediately after injury and in the office for four steps.
- An ankle radiographic series is recommended if the patient presents with pain in the malleolar region and any one of the following findings:
  - Bone tenderness with palpation in the distal 6 cm of the tibia to the medial malleolus or distal 6 cm of the fibula to the lateral malleolus
  - Inability to bear weight on the affected foot immediately after injury and for four steps in the office.
  - 100% sensitive

DIFFERENTIAL DIAGNOSIS

- Dancer's fracture
- March fracture
- Avulsion fracture
- Lisfranc dislocation
- S1 radiculopathy
- Sural nerve pathology

TREATMENT

SURGICAL OPTIONS

- Fixation with intermedullary screw
- Bone graft
- Indications for surgery
  - Nonunion of fracture after 6 to 8 weeks in non–weight-bearing cast immobilization

REHABILITATION

- After immobilization, the following should be done:
  - Control any residual inflammation
  - Restore normal weight bearing and gait
  - Perform active ROM (AROM) and passive ROM (PROM), especially at the talocrural, subtalar, and midfoot joints. Also, assessment and treatment of knee and hip mobility must also be considered as the patient has been on non–weight-bearing status for 6 to 8 weeks.

- ○ Address strengthening. Since the patient has been immobilized for 6 to 8 weeks, consider a certain amount of atrophy and weakness, not only in the involved calf but also of the proximal musculature of the involved side.
- ○ Perform balance and proprioceptive training, especially with progression into previous level of function, activity, and/or sport.
- Postsurgical: Manage edema and the wound and scar. Watch for signs of infection.
- Nuneley gives the following recommendation after surgery:
  - ○ Usually, the patient is toe-touch weight bearing for 2 weeks postsurgery
  - ○ After 2 weeks, the patient uses a walking boot to bear weight as tolerated. AROM is also encouraged.
  - ○ After the fourth week, the walking boot is discontinued and the patient is instructed to wear a tennis shoe with orthotic or insert to ensure stiffness of the sole to prevent stress at the fracture site.
- Before clearing the patient to bear weight as tolerated, rehabilitation can focus on proximal strengthening, edema management, early AROM in a pain-free ROM, and scar management.
  - ○ Weight-bearing, gait training, strengthening, and AROM and PROM as per non-surgical rehabilitation once cleared.
  - ○ Once cleared, weight bearing should be encouraged. A study by Vorlat et al reported that the greatest predictor for poor functional outcome is the amount of time spent in non–weight-bearing. In this study, 38 subjects with either Jones or tuberosity avulsion fractures were followed for 490 days, with function measured using the Olerud ankle score and pain and comfort measured using analog scales.
  - ○ Frangolias et al presented a case study in which an elite runner sustained a Jones fracture, opted for nonsurgical casting, and used deep water running to maintain aerobic capacity. He participated in deep water training from 4 weeks after fracture to week 15, combination water running and land run-walk from weeks 16 to 21, and land runs from weeks 25 to 31. X-rays at weeks 4, 8, and 11 showed normal healing and, at week 16, union of fracture. Maximal oxygen uptake (VO_2 max) testing at weeks 29 and 30 was 83% of his preinjury VO_2 max testing.

- To reduce inflammation, the clinician may consider the following:
  - ○ Lymphatic massage
  - ○ Joint mobilization: *Not* at involved site
  - ○ Elevated AROM within a pain-free ROM
  - ○ Exercises that promote movement of the region in a pain-free range
  - ○ Cold or hot pack
  - ○ Ultrasound: *Only* if there is union of the fracture and *no* surgical fixation.

CONTRIBUTING FACTORS

- No contributing factors are necessary.
- A study by Yu et al reported possible increased risk in fracture or injury to the fifth metatarsal with basketball players wearing over-the-counter medial arch supports. In this study of 14 males, plantar forces and pressures beneath the fifth ray were assesses during two basketball tasks: One foot landing after lay-up and shuttle run. They found that with use of the orthoses, there was an increase in the angle of maximal ankle inversion and increased pressure over the fifth metatarsal head and base with both landing on one foot and with the shuttle run.

PROGNOSIS

- Reported rates of nonunion in nonsurgical cases of non–weight-bearing in a cast for 6 to 8 weeks to be between 7% and 28%.
- Successful union of fracture in nonsurgical cases has been reported to take up to 21.2 weeks.
- After failure of conservative care, with surgical intervention of intermedullary screw or bone graft, time to union was reported as approximately 21 weeks.
- Vorlat et al reported the greatest predictor for poor functional outcome is the amount of time spent in non-weight-bearing activity. In this study, 38 subjects with either Jones or tuberosity avulsion fractures were followed for 490, days with function measured using the Olerud ankle score and pain and comfort measured using analog scales. However, limitations in his study include a small number of subjects with Jones fracture (6), and his population was generally a sedentary group.
- Nuneley reported that if union is confirmed, return to running after surgical fixation can occur approximately 5 to 6 weeks after surgery and return to sport by 8 weeks.

SIGNS AND SYMPTOMS INDICATING REFERRAL TO PHYSICIAN

- No change or worsening of symptoms: Nonunion of fracture
- Major trauma (if patient comes in without diagnosis): Fracture
- Purulent exudate from surgical site: Infection
- Significant edema, erythema, and tracking: Infection
- Fevers and chills: Infection or tumor
- Association with myotomal weakness, dermatomal pattern, and possible (not required lumbosacral symptoms) L5/S1 radiculopathy
- Hyperalgesia, allodynia, temperature changes, edema: Complex regional pain syndrome

SUGGESTED READINGS

Fetzer GB. Wright RW. Metatarsal shaft fractures and fractures of the proximal fifth metatarsal. *Clin Sports Med.* 2006;25:139-150.

Frangolias DD, Taunton JE, Rhodes EC, McConkey JP, Moon M. Maintenance of aerobic capacity during recovery from right foot Jones fracture: a case report. *Clin J Sports Med.* 1997;7:54-58.

Hawkins BJ. Fractures of the metatarsals and phalanges of the foot. In: Calhoun JH, Laughlin RT, eds. *Fractures of the Foot and Ankle: Diagnosis and Treatment of Injury and Disease.* Boca Raton, FL: Taylor and Francis Group; 2005.

Nuneley JA. Fractures of the base of the fifth metatarsal: the Jones fracture. *Orthop Clin North Am.* 2001;32(1).

Rosenberg GA, Sferra JJ. Treatment strategies for acute fractures and nonunions of the proximal fifth metatarsal. *J Am Acad Orthop Surg.* 2000;8:332-338.

Stiell IG, Greenberg GH, McKnight RD, et al. Decision rules for the use of radiography in acute ankle injuries: refinement and prospective validation. *JAMA.* 1993;269(1):127-132.

Stroud CC. Fractures of the midtarsals, metatarsals, and phalanges. In: Richardson EG, ed. *Orthopedic Knowledge Update: Foot and Ankle.* Rosemont, IL: American Academy of Orthopedic Surgeons; 2004.

Vorlat P, Achtergael W, Haentjens P. Predictors of outcome of non-displaced fractures of the base of the fifth metatarsal. *Int Orthop.* 2007;31:5-10.

Yu B, Preston JJ, Queen RM, et al. Effects of wearing foot orthosis with medial arch support on the fifth metatarsal loading and ankle inversion angle in selected basketball tasks. *J Orthop Sports Phys Ther.* 2007;37(4):186-191.

AUTHOR: MILDRED V. LIMCAY

BASIC INFORMATION

DEFINITION

- Ligament injuries of the phalanges include attenuation or rupture of the medial collateral ligament (MCL), lateral collateral ligament (LCL), dorsal ligament, and/or volar (plantar) plate of toes 2 to 5.
- Grading of ligament sprains is as follows:
  - Grade I: Partial tear of a ligament without mechanical instability
  - Grade II: Incomplete tear of a ligament with mild-to-moderate instability
  - Grade III: Complete tear and loss of integrity of a ligament; mechanical instability

SYNONYMS

Toe sprain

ICD-9CM CODES

845.13 Interphalangeal (joint) toe sprain
845.12 Metatarsophalangeal (joint) sprain

OPTIMAL NUMBER OF VISITS

3 or fewer

MAXIMAL NUMBER OF VISITS

36

ETIOLOGY

- The second toe is usually the most affected because is normally longer than toes 3 to 5.
- Usually the ligaments at the metatarsophalangeal (MTP) joints are most affected, possibly as result of the greater amount of motion at this joint versus the proximal and distal interphalangeal joints.
- Ligament injuries can result from a sudden trauma that exceeds the tensile strength of the ligament, causing attenuation and partial or complete rupture.
- Thornton and associates found ligaments to be more susceptible to injury with repeated loading versus static loading in less time when using the same load.
- In acute injuries, nociceptors within ligaments and joint capsules are stimulated with attenuation or tear. Inflammation resulting from ligamentous injury bathes the area in chemical mediators (substance P, bradykinin, etc) that can sensitize neurons, thus perpetuating pain.
- Edema within the joint can produce feelings of pressure and ache.

EPIDEMIOLOGY AND DEMOGRAPHICS

- The pathology is not specific to any age group.

- Early stage symptoms are inflammation and acute ligament damage. Once inflammation has cleared, instability can remain, which predisposes the joint to abnormal shear forces that may produce symptoms.

MECHANISM OF INJURY

- Hyperextension: Plantar plate disruption
  - Fall with landing axially on the lesser toes with toes dorsiflexed
  - Long-term wearing of high-heel shoes
  - Sudden planting and stopping with toes impacting shoe toebox
- Hyperflexion: Dorsal plate disruption
  - Fall with landing axially on the lesser toes with toes dorsiflexed
  - Sudden planting and stopping with toes impacting shoe toebox
- Varus stress loading: LCL disruption
- Valgus stress loading: MCL disruption
- Dislocation: Multiple ligaments
  - High-energy trauma, causing hyperflexion or extension of the toes such as a fall, motor vehicle accident (MVA), or toe(s) getting caught in moving bicycle spoke.
  - Preexisting condition causing ligamentous laxity such as RA

COMMON SIGNS AND SYMPTOMS

- Pain, discoloration, and edema over the affected toe
- Depending on severity of injury, patients may avoid normal weight-bearing positions through the forefoot during gait.

AGGRAVATING ACTIVITIES

- Depending on grade of injury:
  - Weight-bearing
  - Extension of the affected toe, passively or actively
  - Flexion of the affected toe, passively or actively
  - Compression of the forefoot, type of shoe worn (tight toebox)
  - Walking, especially barefoot or in flexible-soled shoes
  - Running
  - Rising up onto toes (heel raise)
- Activities and positions that require MTP dorsiflexion and/or toe extension places stress on the attenuated or torn plantar support structures. MTP plantar flexion and/or phalangeal flexion places stress on the attenuated or torn dorsal support structures. In the presence of interarticular edema, symptoms can be aggravated with either position.
- With walking, symptoms are exacerbated with weight bearing and progression of the body over the forefoot with the transition from midstance to terminal stance.

EASING ACTIVITIES

- Non–weight bearing or partial weight-bearing activities

- Wearing firm-soled or rocker-bottom shoes that prevent extension at the MTP during walking, thus not allowing attenuation of plantar support structures.
- Medication (antiinflammatories, pain relievers)
- Ice
- In presence of acute injury, ice and medication can address inflammation.

24-HOUR SYMPTOM PATTERN

- If swelling is present, the patient can have feelings of stiffness in the affected joint in the morning.
- The patient is usually more symptomatic by the end of the day with time spent on the feet and time spent with the foot in a gravity-dependent position.

PAST HISTORY FOR THE REGION

- With cases of traumatic onset, there does not have to be a history of injury to the foot and ankle predisposing to injury.
- Chronic cases do involve a previous history of one or a repeated injury to the affected joint's support structures, which has caused complete disruption of the capsuloligamentous structures.
- Chronic cases caused by systemic inflammatory disorders can involve other joints of the foot.

PHYSICAL EXAMINATION

- The patient may avoid weight-bearing positions on the affected side.
- With a chronic injury that has resulted in disruption of second MTP stabilizers, the second toe may be deviated or deformed. The most common presentation is attenuation or disruption of the LCL of the second MTP, causing angulation toward the great toe.

IMPORTANT OBJECTIVE TESTS

- AROM and PROM testing
  - In acute injury, both flexion and extension of the involved toe are limited, more so toward the direction of the mechanism of injury due to pain.
  - In subacute and especially chronic phases, hypermobility may be noted toward the direction of the injury caused by attenuation of the capsule and ligaments.
  - If the end-feel is hard or blocked, one should suspect a foreign body within the joint.
- Varus and valgus testing to assess for compromise of MCL and LCL of the involved joint.
- Accessory mobility (drawer testing)
  - Depending on severity of injury and capsuloligamentous damage, laxity or instability with arthrokinematic motion assessment is associated with direction of injury.

○ For example, with the hyperextension mechanism at the second MTP, there may be laxity in end-feel and hypermobility in dorsal glide of the proximal phalanx relative to the metatarsal.

DIFFERENTIAL DIAGNOSIS

- Freiberg's infraction
- Interdigital neuroma
- Phalanx fracture
- Dislocation at the interphalangeal or MTP joint
- Metatarsal fracture
- Osteoarthritis
- Rupture of flexor or extensor tendons of the lesser toes
- Gout
- Systemic inflammatory disorders (systemic lupus erythematosus [SLE], psoriatic arthritis, or Reiter's syndrome)

TREATMENT

SURGICAL OPTIONS

- Surgery is considered if instability is present and conservative treatment has failed.
- Type of intervention depends on severity of deformity and instability.
- Surgery for MTP disorders can be the following:
  ○ Plantar plate repair
  ○ Capsular reefing
  ○ Capsular reefing with tendon transfer
  ○ Weil osteotomy
- Surgery for disorders within the digit can be as follows:
  ○ Proximal interphalangeal (PIP) resection arthroplasty
  ○ PIP fusion
  ○ Tendon transfer
  ○ Amputation

SURGICAL OUTCOMES

- Coughlin reported good to excellent results in 93% of cases of surgical reduction and reconstruction for second MTP joint instability.
- Bouche and Heit evaluated outcomes 1 year after plantar plate repair with tendon transfer in 15 subjects:
  ○ All patients reported pain relief after surgery: 60% had full pain relief, 33% had occasional pain, and 7% had moderate pain.
  ○ Function: 67% reported no limitation, 26% reported mild limitation with some weight-bearing exercise, and 7% reported mild limitation with all weight-bearing exercises
- Surgical complications include the following:
  ○ Metatarsalgia
  ○ Loss of ROM
  ○ Recurrence of deformity

REHABILITATION

Nonoperative
- Acute stages: Address inflammation and pain
- Use taping and external support (orthoses) to decrease load and protect the injured digit
- Modify activity (use rigid-soled shoes)
- As pain reduces, restore of normal foot mechanics and weight bearing with walking, functional tasks, and sport
- Address limitation in mobility of the foot and ankle.

Postsurgical
- Acute stages: Rest, ice, compression, and elevation (RICE).
  ○ Use of modalities such as ultrasound and electrical stimulation are *contraindicated* with metal implantation.
- Later stages
  ○ Gait training, with or without assistive device
  ○ Restore ROM at the affected digit, foot, and ankle
  ○ Proprioceptive and balance training
  ○ Strength training
  ○ Progressive return to previous level of activity
  ○ Consider possibility of orthoses to protect area
- To decrease inflammation, the clinician should consider the following:
  ○ Lymphatic massage
  ○ ROM in a pain arc
  ○ Cold pack
  ○ Joint mobilization: Time frame and surgery specific
  ○ Ultrasound: Contraindicated in patients with metal fixation
  ○ Electrical stimulation: Contraindicated in patients with metal fixation
- Once the inflammation process has decreased, the focus of rehabilitation should be on the following:
  ○ Identify the factors that would further aggravate the injured digit
  ○ Gait training: Emphasis on normal weight bearing and progression over forefoot
  ○ Restore ROM at the affected digit, foot, and ankle, especially if the patient had a period of immobilization.
  ○ Proprioceptive and balance training
  ○ Strength training of the affected lower extremity to address weakness resulting from disuse due to surgery or immobilization.
  ○ Progressive return to previous level of activity
- Initial exercises that can be used to promoted healing include:
  ○ If nonoperative: AROM in a pain-free range to stimulate circulation and reduce edema
- Postoperative: Highly dependent on type of surgery and postsurgical precautions

○ Tendon transfers: Early active ROM is contraindicated.
○ Joint mobilization or manipulation: Appropriate at nonaffected joints (such as talocrural) that may contribute to excessive loading at the toes. At the affected joint, mobilization may be indicated postsurgically if immobilization rendered the joint hypomobile. Caution should be used in mobilization toward in the direction that would stress the injured ligament. Postsurgically, mobilization is a possibility after healing is confirmed, but caution should be used.

Massage
- Acute stages: Can help with lymph circulation to address edema
- Later stages: STM is appropriate in addressing soft tissue restriction in joint ROM.

Exercise: To regain strength lost in the affected lower extremity caused by immobilization.

CONTRIBUTING FACTORS

- Systemic inflammatory diseases and disorders (RA, SLE)
- Repetitive loading injury at the toes (e.g., jumpers, dancers, sprinters)
- Long-term steroid use
- Forefoot equinus
- Medial column instability
- Severe calcaneovalgus deformity

PROGNOSIS

Depending on severity and treatment of initial injury: A less severe sprain with immediate treatment has better long-term results.

SIGNS AND SYMPTOMS INDICATING REFERRAL TO PHYSICIAN

- Constant unrelenting foot pain: Infection or tumor
- Pain that does not change with position or weight bearing: Infection or tumor
- Allodynia, hyperesthesia, sympathetic changes: Reflex sympathetic dystrophy (RSD)
- Streaking along skin toward lymph nodes: Infection
- Purulent exudate from surgical site: Infection
- Significant and unexplained weight loss: Tumor
- Nocturnal pain: Tumor
- Worsening or no improvement of symptoms: Fracture, infection
- Major trauma: Fracture
- Fevers and chills: Infection or tumor

SUGGESTED READINGS

Bouche RT, Heit EJ. Combine plantar plate and hammertoe repair with flexor digitorum longus tendon transfer for chronic, severe sagittal plane in stability of the lesser metatarsophalangeal joints: preliminary observations. *J Foot Ankle Surg.* 2008;47(2):125–137.

Coughlin MJ. Common causes of pain in the forefoot in adults. *J Bone Joint Surg (Br).* 2000;28-B(6):781–790.

Coughlin MJ, Grimes JS, Schenck RC. Lesser toe deformities. In: Porter DA, Schon LC, eds. *Baxter's The Foot and Ankle in Sport.* Philadelphia: Mosby; 2008.

Leung WY, Wong SH, Lam JJ, Ip FK, Ko PS. Presentation of a missed injury of a metatarsophalangeal joint dislocation in the lesser toes. *J Trauma.* 2001;50:1150–1152.

Prisk VR, O'Loughlin PF, Kennedy JG. Forefoot injuries in dancers. *Clin Sports Med.* 2008;27:305–320.

Sferra JJ. Lesser toe deformities, Freiberg's infraction and bunionette deformity. In: Richardson EG, ed. *Orthopedic Knowledge Update: Foot and Ankle.* Rosemont, IL: American Academy of Orthopedic Surgeons; 2004.

Thornton GM, Schwab TD, Oxland TR. Fatigue is more damaging than creep in ligament revealed by modulus reduction and residual strength. *Ann Biomed Eng.* 2007;35(10):1713–1721.

AUTHOR: MILDRED V. LIMCAY

BASIC INFORMATION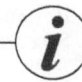

DEFINITION
Metatarsal stress fractures are closed incomplete fractures through the cortex and into the trabecular bone matrix in the shaft of a metatarsal bone. Stress fractures and stress reactions, both RSIs of bone, are a reaction of bone to repetitive and abnormal forces.

SYNONYMS
- Fatigue fracture
- Insufficiency fracture
- Chronic RSI of bone
- Stress reaction
- March fracture

ICD-9CM CODES
733.94 Stress fracture of the
        metatarsals

OPTIMAL NUMBER OF VISITS
Physical therapy for this condition depends on the intervention chosen by the physician. Generally, a boot is used for a period of time and a home exercise program can be initiated. Return to function may require 4 to 8 visits over a number of weeks.

MAXIMAL NUMBER OF VISITS
<13 (depends on union time of bone healing; should be <7 months)

ETIOLOGY
- This injury is caused by repetitive (usually submaximal) stress and overload to the forefoot and metatarsal bones. Over time with repeated stressors, bone resorption may take place without adequate bone production. The forces contributing to the injury include both direct impact and forces generated by the pull of ligaments and tendons on the bone. These forces are compressive, tensile, or complex.
- Normal stress to abnormal bone (e.g., osteoporosis) can lead to insufficiency fractures.
- The initial injury involves the bone matrix, which may be the result of a biological or biochemical abnormality or failure at the cellular or BMU level, and is difficult to clinically measure or detect.
- Each bone in the foot has a potentially different bone density, which varies with loading (weight-bearing patterns).
- The trabecular system of the metatarsals is designed to resist all forces relative to a standing position, so that the anteroposterior and anterior oblique resist tension and the dorsal plantar-oriented trabeculae resist compressive loads. The

subsequent location and orientation of the stress fracture may provide a clue to the source of the dysfunction.
- Insufficiency fractures typically are present in patients with RA or neurological disorders.
- Any of the metatarsals can incur a stress fracture, but fractures of the second and fifth are most common.
- Second metatarsal stress fracture usually occurs in the shaft and/or neck.
- Fractures to the fifth metatarsal are Jones, tuberosity avulsion (the most common), and diaphyseal stress fractures.
- Stress reactions can occur with periosteal changes and remodeling that does not disrupt the bone.
- The first metatarsal carries twice the load of each lesser metatarsal.
- The second to fourth metatarsals are weakest cross-sectionally.
- BMD decreases rapidly with prolonged non–weight-bearing status. Maximizing the BMD response to reloading activities is critical to minimizing fracture risk. BMD of the metatarsal is more vital than bone geometry for determining the strength of the bone.
- There is an imbalance between bone resorption and formation that occurs with muscle atrophy or osteopenia from prolonged rest. Advancing activities too rapidly and intensely can increase the chance of injury.
- During balanced standing, the maximum von Mises stresses were at the shaft and the bases of the metatarsals, and the maximum strains of bony regions are found around metatarsal cavities. Among plantar soft tissues, relatively high tensions are borne by plantar fascia, followed by the long plantar ligament. The minimum tensions occurred in plantar intrinsic muscles.
- Risk factors include the following:
  - Low BMD, especially after prolonged immobilization and non–weight-bearing position
  - Prior history of nontraumatic fracture
  - Low calcium and magnesium intake (<1000 mg per day).
  - General joint laxity and possibly first Ray dorsal hypermobility
  - Pes planus or overpronatory foot type has been correlated to stress fractures
  - Supinators and pes cavus foot type
  - Run ning more than 20 miles per week, especially on hard surfaces
  - Low volume of training is associated with proximal second metatarsal stress fractures.
  - Overtraining without adequate rest periods (muscle fatigue)
  - Delayed menarche
  - Poor nutrition
  - Amenorrhea
  - Repetitive activity such as sports (distance running) or that done by military recruits.

  - Increases in intensity, frequency, and loading of training or activity without adequate rest intervals.
  - Hyperthyroidism, hyperparathyroidism, and use of fluoride treatment for osteoporosis
  - White women who smoke and are sedentary
  - Systemic diseases that weaken bone such as RA, SLE, osteoarthrosis, pyrophosphate arthropathy, renal disease, sleep deprivation, collagen deficiencies, osteoporosis, joint replacement, or nutritional deficiency (dieting)

EPIDEMIOLOGY AND DEMOGRAPHICS
- Generally, stress fractures account for 0.7% to 20% of all sports clinic injuries, especially among military recruits and runners.
- Metatarsal stress fractures: 9% to 25% of stress fractures in the lower extremity
- Tibia: ≈50%; tarsals: 25%; and metatarsals: 9% of all lower extremity stress fractures
- Bilateral in16%
- Stress fractures to the metatarsals occur to the diaphysis of the second and third metatarsal 80% to 90% of the time.
- 95% of second metatarsal stress fractures occur at the distal end.
- Fifth metatarsal fractures occur most often, especially after an inversion ankle injury.
- Generally found in younger athletes but can occur in the active elderly.
- Ballet dancers have this condition at the base of the second metatarsals most often.
- Track and field runners are more prone to stress fractures of the metatarsal.
- Female athletes who overtrain and develop the athlete's triad have menstrual irregularities 50% of the time and thus have a reduced BMD.
- White women who smoke and are sedentary
- Males can lower testosterone after 2 days of hard training by up to 25%, which increases osteoclast development and bone resorption.
- Females have a higher predisposition than males: Relative risk = 3.5.
- White males have a higher predisposition than black males: Relative risk = 4.7.
- White females have a higher predisposition than black females: Relative risk = 8.5.

MECHANISM OF INJURY
- Recent evidence suggests that the loading pattern of the foot during walking or running may alter the magnitude of response of BMD in individual bones of the foot and is linked to several foot impairments.

- Tightness of the gastrocnemius/soleus complex increases forefoot pressure, which can induce stress increases.
- Excessive femoral anteversion can increase hyperpronation at the foot, which may lead to a lower extremity stress reaction.
- A short first metatarsal (i.e., 80% of the second metatarsal length) can increase stress to the second metatarsal, especially proximally.
- With muscle fatigue during running, there is an increased maximal force, peak pressure, and impulse under the second and third metatarsal head and under the medial arch. Contact area and time are only slightly affected. The mean EMG activity is significantly reduced in the medial gastrocnemius, lateral gastrocnemius, and soleus muscles in some runners. Thus there is an increased forefoot loading with fatigue that could lead to a metatarsal stress fracture over time.
- Imbalances in muscle forces since muscle strength increases faster than bone strength.

CONTRIBUTING FACTORS

- Foot type: Individuals with a low arch index are more susceptible to metatarsal stress fractures. Individuals with a high arch index typically incur a more proximal stress injury, although hindfoot valgus can also contribute.
- Biomechanical factors: First ray hypermobility, short first metatarsal (Morton's toe), hallux rigidus, hallux valgus, Achilles contracture, leg length differences, genu varum, and external hip rotation.
- Abnormal menses
- Different bones in the foot heal at different rates and have distinct bone densities.
- Cortical bone responds slower to loading and reloading than trabecular bone.
- Eating disorders
- Osteoporosis
- Female athlete's triad with associated eating disorders
- Rigid surfaces
- Changes in foot gear
- Proximal stress fractures are chronic and more common in those with tight Achilles tendons and metatarsal length differences and those with prior stress fractures, a low level of training, and a high BMI.

COMMON SIGNS AND SYMPTOMS

- Insidious onset of midfoot or forefoot pain for 2 to 3 weeks, although a sudden onset can occur after or during a run.
- The symptoms are stress pain and aching at rest after training.

- Deep ache after rapid training change
- Pain progression: Initially, the patient experiences pain after activity, which progresses to pain with activity. As the pathology progresses, the patient experiences pain with walking. Finally, the patient experiences pain at rest.
- Intense localized pain at the fracture site
- Tenderness to palpation and compression induces pain.
- Percussion of bone distant from a symptomatic site

AGGRAVATING ACTIVITIES

- Weight-bearing activity
- Change in training schedule, surface, intensity, or mileage

EASING ACTIVITIES

- Rest
- Ice

24-HOUR SYMPTOM PATTERN

- Night pain rarely occurs.
- Symptoms increase with activity as the day continues.

PAST HISTORY FOR THE REGION

- General health changes, medication, diet, and occupation
- Hormonal, nutritional, and medical abnormalities
- Those with a prior history have a higher chance of another stress fracture.
- Symptoms lasting >3 months suggests the possibility of a proximal metatarsal stress fracture.

PHYSICAL EXAMINATION

- Local palpation yields tenderness and periosteal thickening.
- Local swelling, ecchymosis, pain, and deformity
- Reduced mobility of adjacent rays in non-weight-bearing positions.
- A vibrating tuning fork (128 Hz) can be used at the suspected site.

- Biomechanical evaluation includes limb length differences, excessive hindfoot pronation, muscle length imbalances and strength imbalances.
- Gait: Reduced heel rise and push-off in terminal stance.

IMPORTANT OBJECTIVE TESTS

- There are very few physical tests for this condition, although a hop test or running may reproduce symptoms.
- Diagnostics (proceed in the following order)
  - Stress fracture x-ray
  - Stress fracture bone scan
  - Stress fracture CT
  - Stress fracture MRI
- Quantitative CT assesses 3-dimensional volume of bone density of specific bones of the foot.
- Radionuclide bone scanning has high sensitivity but lacks specificity since it is hard to visualize the fracture line. Bone scans lag behind clinical improvements so they should not be used to monitor healing and return to activity.
- Technetium bone scanning is highly sensitive but has low specificity.
- Bone scintigraphy is more sensitive than MRI (which has higher specificity) initially but can be overly sensitive with increased false positives. MRI is useful in monitoring healing progression and distinguishing soft tissue lesions from bone.
- Quantitative ultrasound (QUS) can be used to measure low BMD.
- Initial radiographs are often negative (≈50%) and have low sensitivity. The only x-ray findings seen are those that show up toward the end of the healing process, sometimes as long as several months after the injury. The fracture is not directly visualized; instead, calcification occurs in the late phases of the healing process.

Radiological Grading System for Stress Fractures

Grade	Radiograph	Bone Scan	MRI	Treatment
1	Normal	Mild uptake confined to one cortex	Positive STIR image	Rest for 3 weeks
2	Normal	Moderate activity; larger lesion confined to unicortical area	Positive STIR and T2-weighted images	Rest for 3-6 weeks
3	Discrete line (±), periosteal reaction (±)	Increased activity (>50% width of bone)	No definite cortical break; positive T1- and T2-weighted images	Rest for 12-16 weeks
4	Fracture or periosteal reaction	More intense bicortical uptake	Fracture line; positive T1- and T2-weighted images	Rest for 16+ weeks

MRI, magnetic resonance imaging; STIR, short T1 inversion recovery.
Adapted with permission from Arendt EA, Griffiths HJ: The use of MR imaging in the assessment and clinical management of stress reactions of bone in high-performance athletes, *Clin Sports Med* 16:291-306, 1997.

- Torg et al explained the healing potential of fifth metatarsal diaphyseal stress fractures. They divided diaphyseal stress fractures into acute injuries and those that develop into delayed unions or nonunions. An acute fracture is characterized by a fracture line with sharp margins, without widening or radiolucency, and with minimal cortical hypertrophy or evidence of periosteal reaction to chronic stress. A delayed union is characterized by a previous injury or fracture, a fracture line that involves both cortices and displays associated periosteal new bone, a widened fracture line with adjacent radiolucency due to bone resorption, and evidence of intramedullary sclerosis. The features of a nonunion are a history of repetitive trauma and recurrent symptoms, a wide fracture line with periosteal new bone and radiolucency, and complete obliteration of the medullary canal at the fracture site by sclerotic bone.

DIFFERENTIAL DIAGNOSIS **Dx**

- It has been reported that 22 patients with 23 Jones fractures had delayed union in 12 (67%) of 18 patients treated nonoperatively. However, in 9 of the 22 patients, the clinical and radiographic evidence was more characteristic of a stress fracture. Further, in 20 fractures of the proximal fifth metatarsal there was a 25% incidence of nonunion. Most of the injuries were diaphyseal stress fractures.
- Periostitis
- Infection
- Avulsion fractures
- Muscle strain
- Bursitis or tendinosis
- Neoplasm
- Exertional compartment syndromes
- Nerve entrapment
- Lisfranc fracture or dislocation.
- Primary benign bone neoplasm such as osteoid osteoma, osteoblastoma, and eosinophilic granuloma
- Infections: Chronic or subacute osteomyelitis
- Metastatic neoplasm: Breast cancer or prostate cancer
- Primary malignant bone neoplasms: Osteosarcoma
- Nerve compression syndromes such as tarsal tunnel syndrome or herniated intervertebral disc
- Osteoarthritis
- Hypertrophic pulmonary osteoarthropathy

TREATMENT

SURGICAL OPTIONS

- Nonacute fifth metatarsal stress fractures of the diaphysis do well with either closed axial intramedullary-screw fixation or autogenous corticocancellous grafting, especially with delayed union or nonunion. Torg type II and type III fractures usually require operative intervention consisting of closed axial intramedullary-screw fixation, tricortical inlay bone grafting, or a combination of the two techniques.
- General guidelines for surgery include the following:
  - If imaging is negative, progress to rehabilitation.
  - If imaging is positive and the patient is a high-demand athlete, progress to surgery.
  - If imaging is positive and the patient is a low-demand athlete, determine if the fracture is displaced or nondisplaced.
  - If the fracture is nondisplaced, progress to rehabilitation.
  - If the fracture is displaced, progress to surgery.
- At high risk for nonunion
  - Nonhealing fractures
  - Specific high-risk sites such as navicular or tibial stress fracture
  - Base of fifth metatarsal stress fracture

SURGICAL OUTCOMES

When indicated, surgery is very successful, especially in nonunions.

REHABILITATION

Prevention

- Identify and correct predisposing factors such as footwear problems. Shoes should be lightweight and in good condition.
- Accommodative (shock absorbent) shoe inserts or foot orthoses. The use of orthotic devices reduced stress fracture in the femur in patients with high arches and the incidence of metatarsal stress fracture in those with low arches.
- Reduce overtraining and use an adequate rest period.
- Increase calcium intake to 1000 mg per day
- Hormone replacement therapy with contraceptives or estrogen may hasten healing.
- Do not increase exercise intensity more than 10% per week
- Stretch and warm-up before exercise
- Choose level running surfaces.
- Shock-absorbing insoles may be beneficial.

Nonsurgical Treatment

- A cam walker, pneumatic walker, or low pneumatic walker may alleviate pain faster and be clinically superior to a postoperative shoe for stress reactions of the metatarsal area and for other foot stress reactions.
- Non–weight-bearing status in a short leg cast or boot for 1 to 8 weeks (may take 3 months) to see if symptoms reduce and the patient can walk pain-free.
- Immobilization
  - Short-leg casting indications include noncompliance and high risk for nonunion, especially metatarsal stress fracture.
  - Pneumatic brace (air cast): Support results in quicker recovery and less pain.
  - Active rest (cross training) to enhance cardiovascular conditioning, flexibility, proprioception, and strength. This can include swimming, pool running with a float, biking, or stair machines (later stages).
- If symptoms continue after 3 weeks of non–weight-bearing status for fifth metatarsal fracture, then possible surgical options need to be explored.

Postsurgical Rehabilitation

- A pneumatic brace or boot may be used.
- Electromagnetic field therapy: Pulsed electromagnetic fields were used to treat a series of nine fractures of the proximal fifth metatarsal that developed into delayed unions or nonunions, and all fractures healed in a mean time of 4 months.
- Have the patient keep an exercise log daily of no-load, low-load, and high-load activities.
- Initiate physical therapy ≈4 weeks postoperatively.
- Non–weight-bearing ROM exercises at 4 weeks and scar management.
- Progressive weight bearing and weaning from boot at 6 weeks
- Inversion and eversion motion at 8 to 10 weeks

PROGNOSIS

- Safe reloading can increase bone density within 26 weeks from 12% to 34%.
- Certain stress fractures do not respond to immobilization and may require surgery.
- It can take up to 2 years before BMD measures are equal in both feet after a stress fracture.
- Ballet dancers with base of second metatarsal stress fractures have returned successfully at 6 to 8 weeks after diagnosis.
- Proximal second metatarsal fractures heal much slower, and delayed union is common if the bone is completely fractured.
- After open reduction internal fixation (ORIF) of the fifth metatarsal fracture, full return to activities can occur in 8 to 10 weeks.

SIGNS AND SYMPTOMS INDICATING REFERRAL TO PHYSICIAN

- Delayed healing or nonprogression
- Proximal fractures usually require surgery and are slower to heal.
- Other red flags or complications in the patient.

SUGGESTED READINGS

Akkus O, Rimnac CM. Cortical bone tissue resists fatigue fracture by deceleration and arrest of microcrack growth. *J Biomech.* 2001;34:757-764.

Armagan OE, Shereff MJ. Injuries to the toes and metatarsals. *Orthop Clin North Am.* 32(1):1-10.

Bennell KL, Malcolm SA, Thomas SA, Ebeling PR, McCrory PR, Wark JD, Brukner PD. Risk factors for stress fractures in female track-and-field athletes: a retrospective analysis. *Clin J Sport Med.* 1995;5(4):229-235.

Boden BP, Osbahr DC. High-risk stress fractures: evaluation and treatment. *J Am Acad Orthop Surg.* 2000;8:344-353.

Bradley WB, Slomiany WP. Shin pain treatments get active patiens back on track. *Biomechanics.* 2008;31-38.

Breithaupt J. Zur pathologie des menschlichen fusses. *Medizin Zeitung.* 1855;24:169-177.

Buckwalter JA, Brandser EA. Stress and insufficiency fractures. *Am Fam Physician.* 1997;56(1):175.

Chuckpaiwong B, Cook C, Pietrobon R, Nunley JA. Second metatarsal stress fracture in sport: comparative risk factors between proximal and non-proximal locations. *Br J Sports Med.* 2007;41(8):510-514.

Fredericson M, Bergman AG, et al. Tibial stress reaction in runners. Correlation of clinical symptoms and scintigraphy with a new magnetic resonance imaging grading system. *Am J Sports Med.* 1995;23(4):472-481.

Glasoe WM, et al. Dorsal first ray in women athletes with a history of stress fracture of the 2/3 MT. *JOSPT.* 2002;32(11):565-567.

Hastings MK, et al. Bone mineral density of the Tarsals and Metatarsals with reloading: case report. *Phys Ther.* 2008;88(6):766-779.

Jansen M. March foot. *J Bone Joint Surg.* 1926;8:262-272.

Jones BH, et al. *Epidemiol Rev.* 2002;24: 228-247.

Lebrun M. The female athlete triad: what's a doctor to do? *Curr Sports Med Rep.* 2007;6:397-404.

Matheson GO, Clement DB, McKenzie DC, Taunton JE, Lloyd-Smith DR, MacIntyre JG. Stress fractures in athletes. A study of 320 cases. *Am J Sports Med.* 1987;15(1):46-58.

Niva MH, Sormaala MJ, Kiuru MJ, Haataja R, Ahovuo JA, Pihlajamaki HK. Bone stress injuries of the ankle and foot: an 86-month magnetic resonance imaging-based study of physically active young adults. *Am J Sports Med.* 2007;35(4):643-649.

O'Malley MJ, Hamilton WG, Munyak J, DeFranco MJ. Stress fracture at the base of the second MT in ballet dancers. *Foot Ankle Int.* 1996;17(2):89-94.

Orava S, Hulkko A, Koskinen S, Taimela S. Links [Stress fractures in athletes and military recruits. An overview][Article in German]. Orthopade. 1995;24(5):457-466.

Proteau S, Ducher G, Nanyan P, Lemineur G, Benhamou L, Courteix D. Fractal analysis of bone texture: a screening tool for stress fracture risk? *Eur J Clin Invest.* 2004;34(2):137-142.

Reeder MT, Dick BH, Atkins JK, Pribis AB, Martinez JM. Stress fractures: current concepts of diagnosis and treatment. *Sports Med.* 1996;22(3):198-212.

Rosenberg GA, Sferra JJ. Treatment strategies for acute fractures and nonunions of the proximal 5th metatarsal. *J Am Acad Orthop Surg.* 2000;8(5):332-338.

Sanderlin BW, Raspa RF. Common stress fractures. *Am Fam Physician.* 2003;68(8): 1527—1532.

Simmons. *AAFP Sports Med Review.* 1997.

Simkin A, Leichter I, Giladi M, Stein M, Milgrom C. Combined effect of foot arch structure and an orthotic device on stress fractures. *Foot Ankle.* 1989;10(1):25-29.

Stafford SA, Rosenthal DI, Gebhardt MC, Brady TJ, Scott JA. MRI in stress fracture. *Am J Roentgenol.* 1986;147:553-556.

Stechow. Fussödem und Röntgenstrahlen. *Deutsche Militärärztliche Zeitschrift.* 1897; 26:465.

Swenson EJ, DeHaven KE, Sebastianelli WJ, Hanks G, Kalenak A, Lynch JM. The effect of a pneumatic leg brace on return to play in athletes with tibial stress fractures. *Am J Sports Med.* 1997;322-328.

Torg JS, Balduini FC, Zelko RR, Pavlov H, Peff TC, Das M. Fractures of the base of the fifth metatarsal distal to the tuberosity: classification and guidelines for non-surgical and surgical management. *J Bone Joint Surg Am.* 1984;66:209-214.

Verma RB, Sherman O. Athletic stress fractures: Part 1-3. *Am J Orthop.* 2001;30(11):798-806.

Warren MP, Brooks-Gunn J, Fox RP, Lancelot C, Newman D, Hamilton WG. Lack of bone accretion and amenorrhea: evidence for a relative osteopenia in WB bones. *J Clin Endocrinol Metab.* 1991;72(4):847-853.

Weist R, Eils E, Rosenbaum D. The influence of muscle fatigue on electromyogram and plantar pressure patterns as an explanation for the incidence of metatarsal stress fractures. *Am J Sports Med.* 2004;32(8):1893-1898.

Wu L, Zhong S, Zheng R, Qu J, Ding Z, Tang M, Wang X, Hong J, Zheng X, Wang X. Clinical significance of musculoskeletal finite element model of the 2-5th MT cavities and sinus. *Surg Radiol Anat.* 2007;29(7):561-567.

AUTHOR: STEPHEN PAULSETH

Section III

ORTHOPEDIC PATHOLOGY

BASIC INFORMATION

DEFINITION

Metatarsal joint synovitis is inflammation of the synovium surrounding the metatarsophalangeal (MTP) joint. The actual pain experienced with this condition is often called metatarsalgia. Metatarsalgia can also be caused by other pathologies such as Morton's neuroma or avascular necrosis.

SYNONYMS

• Metatarsalgia
• MTP joint synovitis
• Enthesopathy of the metatarsal

ICD-9CM CODES
726.70   Enthesopathy of ankle and
         tarsus unspecified

OPTIMAL NUMBER OF VISITS
6 or fewer

MAXIMAL NUMBER OF VISITS
16

ETIOLOGY

• Metatarsal joint synovitis can occur at either of the joints at which the metatarsal bone articulates, either the tarsal-metatarsal joint or the metatarsalphalangeal joint. Pathology most commonly occurs at the latter.
• The MTP joint is enclosed by a capsule. The inside of the capsule is lined with synovial cells that produce joint fluid. If the covering of the capsule is inflamed, the problem is capsulitis. If the cells inside the capsule are inflamed, the problem is synovitis.
• The synovium and synovial cells of the metatarsal joint can be irritated by intrinsic and extrinsic factors. Intrinsically, pathologies, such as RA or gout, can result in joint destruction. This destruction ultimately leads to an inflammatory response and irritation of the synovium. Extrinsically, repetitive loading or traumatic loading of the MTP joint can result in injury to the bone, cartilage, or surrounding tissue. In response to the injury, inflammation results, that ultimately affects the synovium and synovial cells.

EPIDEMIOLOGY AND DEMOGRAPHICS

The prevalence of metatarsal joint synovitis is not documented in the literature. Metatarsalgia, as a whole, has the highest prevalence in relationship to other causes of foot pain. Pain in the forefoot region is eight times more common than in other regions of the foot.

MECHANISM OF INJURY

• MTP joint pain is often associated with biomechanical abnormalities. Misalignment of the joint surfaces can result in altered foot mechanics. The result of the altered mechanics can cause joint subluxations, capsular impingement, and joint cartilage damage. The byproducts of this process are joint and synovial inflammation. Directly, misaligned joints may cause synovial impingement and synovitis.
• MTP joint synovitis may also occur as a result of inflammatory diseases such as RA. Synovitis and interosseous muscle atrophy of the interosseous muscles commonly seen in RA can result in misalignments of the MTP joints, which can lead to hammer toe deformities. The metatarsal fat pad, which usually cushions the stress between the metatarsals and interdigital nerves during gait, moves distally under the toes. Calluses and bursitis may result from the loss of cushion. Digital nerves may also become entrapped by the misalignments.
• Other mechanisms of injury include the following:
  ○ Repetitive use during walking or standing
  ○ Poor footwear such as shoes that are too tight
  ○ Walking in high heels
  ○ Repetitive jumping sports
  ○ Ballet
  ○ Walking barefoot on hard surfaces

COMMON SIGNS AND SYMPTOMS

• Pain at one or more of the metatarsal heads
• Pain is most commonly located in the second, third, and fourth metatarsal heads.
• Poorly localized forefoot and midfoot pain are often present in athletes who participate in sports that require jumping.
• The pain is typically aggravated during the midstance and terminal phases of walking or running.
• A history of a gradual, chronic onset is more common than an acute presentation.
• Chronic symptoms may be of gradual onset over a 6-month period.

AGGRAVATING ACTIVITIES

• Walking
• Walking in high heels
• Walking barefoot
• Standing
• Jumping

EASING ACTIVITIES

• Non–weight-bearing activities
• Rest
• Cold pack or compress
• Wearing cushioned insoles in the shoes

24-HOUR SYMPTOM PATTERN

• Symptoms may be better during the morning, especially after sleeping with the foot elevated.
• Symptoms may worsen during the day with increased weight-bearing activities.

PAST HISTORY FOR THE REGION

• Previous history of ankle injury
• History of bunions or hammer toes
• History of trauma to the foot
• History of repetitive use coupled with poor or no footwear

PHYSICAL EXAMINATION

• Point tenderness at the distal end of the plantar metatarsal fat pad and at the plantar surface of the involved metatarsal head
• Calluses may be present at the plantar aspect of the MTP joint.
• Increased foot pronation or increased calcaneal eversion may be present, which places more pressure onto the medial aspect of the forefoot during gait. This could result in increased force placed on the first, second, and third MTP joints, resulting in damage to the underlying bone and joint.
• Increased foot supination and increased calcaneal inversion or pes cavus could result in a decreased ability for the foot to absorb shock and therefore greater force to be placed on the lateral aspect of the forefoot.
• ROM testing may reveal decreased dorsiflexion of the ankle that could contribute to the foot dysfunction.
• A shortened first metatarsal bone can result in abnormal subtalar joint pronation, which would shift the weight to the second metatarsal during gait.
• Neural dynamic testing should be normal. Abnormal findings may indicate that the pain is not from the metatarsal joint but from interdigital neuromas.
• Muscle weakness (e.g., in the posterior tibialis muscle) may affect the biomechanics of the foot and result in abnormal loading on the metatarsal heads.

IMPORTANT OBJECTIVE TESTS

• MRI, x-ray, and ultrasound have been found to be beneficial in ruling out other potential pathology and in identifying joint destruction or inflammatory processes.
• No one specific clinical test has been shown to definitively identify the presence of metatarsal joint synovitis.

DIFFERENTIAL DIAGNOSIS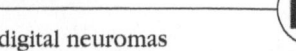

• Interdigital neuromas
• Tibial nerve and plantar nerve entrapment
• Tumor

- Arthritis
- Gout
- Lisfranc fracture
- Lyme disease
- Osteomyelitis
- Sesamoiditis
- Metatarsal stress fractures

CONTRIBUTING FACTORS

- Pes cavus
- Overpronation
- Hallux limitus
- Morton's foot: A shortened first metatarsal causing excess pressure to go through the second MTP joint.
- Tight extensor tendons of the toes.
- Osteoporosis or osteopenia
- Balance disorder
- Chronic ankle sprain
- History of ankle instability
- Participation in high-level athletic sports
- Footwear
- Repetitive walking on hard surfaces

TREATMENT

MEDICAL

- Surgery is generally only considered if all conservative options have been exhausted. Medically, the physician may prescribe antiinflammatory medications to reduce the irritation and swelling in the region.
- In severe cases, a walking boot or cast may be used to reduce the loading on the forefoot.
- In cases in which conservative treatment has failed to provide relief of symptoms, surgical intervention may be required, including operative synovectomy, arthroplasty, wedge osteotomies of the metatarsal bases, ligamentous release, and tendon transfer.

SURGICAL OUTCOMES

Success and complications rates vary. The osteotomy of the second and third metatarsals has been shown to be an effective and safe procedure for the treatment of metatarsalgia.

REHABILITATION

- The body has a remarkable ability to heal. The synovium of the metatarsal joint is no different. The key to healing most metatarsal joint issues is identifying the structural abnormalities that are leading to stress placed on the joint.
- Rehabilitation initially involves decreasing the inflammatory response. Medications, ice, and elevation are appropriate measures to address the inflammation that is present. To reduce the stress placed on the joint, devices such as foot orthoses or metatarsal pads have proved effective in reducing the loading on the metatarsal joint and improving the mechanics of the foot so that the loads are subsequently reduced. Therapy must allow the inflammation to subside or resolve by relieving the repeated excessive pressure.
- Improving the mobility of the talocrural joint and the calf can improve ankle dorsiflexion. This is often needed to help improve the biomechanics of the foot during the midstance to late stance phases of gait.
- The patient can return to sport, but care must be taken to slowly progress the loading through the metatarsal so that appropriate bone remodeling can occur. Full return to sport can occur when all biomechanical contributing factors have been addressed, balance and proprioception are normal, and strength is at least 90% of that of the contralateral side.
- Long-axis distraction and dorsal/plantar glides of the MTP joint are mobilization techniques that can be used to restore normal metatarsal joint mobility.

PROGNOSIS

- The prognosis for patients with metatarsal joint synovitis is generally good.
- If the factors resulting in abnormal forces being placed on the metatarsal joint can be eliminated, then the patient should heal.
- Normal healing would generally take between 6 to 8 weeks. Reducing the loading in a commonly used area in the body, such as the foot, is difficult. Healing may take a little longer as a result.

SIGNS AND SYMPTOMS INDICATING REFERRAL TO PHYSICIAN

- The red flag signs in the forefoot are usually few. If the patient is not improving over the course of a month, he or she should be referred back to the physician
- If tumors are suspected (unremitting or nonmechanical pain), a referral to the physician is warranted.
- Suspicions of gout should also be referred back to the referring physician for medical workup. Unresolving inflammation may be an indication of gout or other systemic inflammatory disorders.

SUGGESTED READINGS

Coughlin MJ. Common causes of pain in the forefoot in adults. *J Bone Joint Surg Br.* 2000;82(6):781-790.

Kang JH, Chen MD, Chen SC, Hsi WL. Correlations between subjective treatment responses and plantar pressure parameters of metatarsal pad treatment in metatarsalgia patients: a prospective study. *BMC Musculoskelot Disord.* 2006;7:95.

Kennedy JG, Deland JT. Resolution of metatarsalgia following oblique osteotomy. *Clin Orthop Relat Res.* 2006;453:309-313.

Miller SD. Technique tip: forefoot pain: diagnosing metatarsophalangeal joint synovitis from interdigital neuroma. *Foot Ankle Int.* 2001;22(11):914-915.

Mizel MS, Yodlowski. Disorders of the lesser metatarsophalangeal joints. *J Am Acad Orthop Surg.* 1995;3:166-173.

Tóth K, Huszanyik I, Kellermann P, Boda K, Ródc L. The effect of first ray shortening in the development of metatarsalgia in the second through fourth rays after metatarsal osteotomy. *Foot Ankle Int.* 2007;28(1):61-63.

Trepman E, Yeo SJ. Nonoperative treatment of metatarsophalangeal joint synovitis. *Foot Ankle Int.* 1995;16(12):771-777.

AUTHOR: DERRICK SUEKI

BASIC INFORMATION

DEFINITION

The midtarsal joint is composed of the calcaneocuboid and talonavicular joint. It is a synovial joint that runs through the medial and lateral arches of the foot. A sprain occurs when the ligament is stressed beyond its physical capabilities. If forces continue and the ligament fails, dislocation and fracture can occur.

SYNONYMS

- Chopart joint sprain
- Midfoot sprain
- Chopart joint fracture
- Midfoot fracture

ICD-9CM CODES
825.2 Fracture of other tarsal and metatarsal bones closed
825.3 Fracture of other tarsal and metatarsal bones open
838.2 Dislocation of the foot, mid tarsal joint
848.9 Unspecified site of sprain and strain

OPTIMAL NUMBER OF VISITS

Depends on nature of injury

MAXIMAL NUMBER OF VISITS

Depends on nature of injury

ETIOLOGY

- Midtarsal joint injuries are uncommon, partly a result of the strong ligamentous structures around the midtarsal joint. The strongest ligamentous structures of the midtarsal joint are on the plantar side, which is protected by the long and short plantar ligament, bifurcate ligament, and the plantar calcaneonavicular or spring ligament. All of these are important supports for the arch of the foot.
- A continuum of injuries may occur within the midtarsal joint. The nature and extent of the injury are influenced greatly by the magnitude and direction of the forces applied on the midtarsal joint during injury.
- Traumatic forces applied to one side of the midfoot are transmitted to the other side, so the clinician must look to both sides of the foot for damage. Midfoot fractures may result from forced eversion, inversion, plantar flexion or dorsiflexion, or crushing of the foot.
- Since there are two primary articulations composing the joint, injuries can involve one or both of the articulations, as follows:
  - *Medial-directed forces* can result in sprains of the lateral calcaneocuboid region or progression of the sprain to dislocations or fractures. In cases of dislocation, the forefoot is displaced medially in relationship to the hindfoot. Swivel-type dislocations can also occur as the talonavicular joint is dislocated and the calcaneocuboid joint remains intact.
  - *Longitudinal-directed forces:* When compressive forces are applied to a plantar flexed foot, forces are transmitted longitudinally through the forefoot to the midtarsal joint. The result of these forces is generally a fracture of the navicular or cuboid bone. If the foot is in less plantar flexion, fracture-dislocation may occur.
  - *Lateral-directed forces:* Excessive lateral forces result in sprains of the medial talonavicular joint. If the forces continue, the ligament will fail and the forefoot will displace laterally in relationship to the hindfoot. Swivel dislocations can also occur if the calcaneocuboid joint is dislocated as the talonavicular joint remains intact.
  - *Plantar-directed forces:* With excessive plantar flexion, the ligaments on the plantar surfaces of the midtarsal joint may be strained. In the event of ligament failure, dislocation may occur through the talonavicular joint, calcaneocuboid joint, or both. These are strong ligamentous structures; therefore dislocation is relatively rare.
  - *Crush forces:* Crush injuries usually result in fracture of the cuboid or navicular bones.

EPIDEMIOLOGY AND DEMOGRAPHICS

- The prevalence of navicular stress fractures has been estimated at 35% of all stress fractures and is generally the result of running or jumping.
- Chopart joint injuries (talonavicular and calcaneocuboid joints) are less common than Lisfranc joint injuries (tarsal metatarsal joint).
- The dislocation is typically medial or lateral (rarely anterior or posterior). Medial dislocation is more common, occurring in 80% of the midfoot dislocations.
- Midfoot dislocations are more common in young men because of the higher prevalence of MVAs and traumatic injuries in young men.
- In a study of 100 patients with Chopart joint dislocations, pure Chopart joint dislocations were observed 25% of the time, fracture dislocations occurred 55% of the time, and combined Chopart and Lisfranc joint fracture dislocations occurred 20% of the time.

MECHANISM OF INJURY

- In most cases, midtarsal joint injuries are the result of trauma.

- In a study reviewing Chopart dislocation injuries, the most common cause of injury was vehicular trauma. Other causes included falls and motorcycle accidents.
- Directional mechanisms of injury include the following:
  - Medial-directed forces: Inversion sprains of the ankle, falls onto an inverted foot
  - Longitudinal-directed forces: Falls onto a plantar flexed foot
  - Lateral-directed forces: Falls or missteps that force the foot into eversion or valgus positions
  - Plantar-directed forces: MVA or accidents in which the forefoot is pinned under an object while force is applied in a plantar-flexed direction
  - Crush forces: Objects landing or rolling over the top of the foot

COMMON SIGNS AND SYMPTOMS

- Signs and symptoms depend on which bodily tissue has been injured and the magnitude of tissue damage.
- Pain is generally localized around the area damaged.
- Dislocations manifest with visible alteration in structural alignment.
- Pain is noted during the stance phase of gait. The greater the magnitude of injury, the more severely gait will be altered. With minor sprains, the patient can ambulate with only minor pain and alteration in gait mechanics. With unreduced dislocations, the patient cannot ambulate.
- Palpable tenderness is present at the site of injury.
- Bruising and swelling is common in the foot after sprains, fractures, and dislocations.
- Nocturnal achiness is common if fractures are present.
- The pain is typically aggravated during the midstance and terminal phases of walking or running.

AGGRAVATING ACTIVITIES

- Foot motions
- Walking
- Running
- Marching
- Walking in heels
- Walking barefoot
- Standing
- Jumping

EASING ACTIVITIES

- Non-weight-bearing activities
- Rest
- Elevation of the foot
- Cold pack or compress

24-HOUR SYMPTOM PATTERN

- Symptoms may be better during the morning, especially after sleeping with the foot elevated.

- Symptoms may worsen during the day with increased weight-bearing activities.
- If irritated, the forefoot may ache at night.
- Fractures may also ache at night.

PAST HISTORY FOR THE REGION

Injury is usually the result of trauma. No prior history of injury need be present.

PHYSICAL EXAMINATION

- The physical examination depends on the tissues injured. In all dislocations or fractures, neurological and vascular screening of the foot should be completed. If compromise is suspected, the dislocation or displaced fracture should be reduced immediately. Radiographic images of the foot should be taken before reduction is performed.
- Lateral midtarsal sprain
  - Palpable tenderness at the ligament
  - Increased mobility noted between the calcaneus and cuboid bones
  - Bruising and swelling may be present around the sprained ligament.
  - Pain with midstance to terminal stance of gait
  - Altered pronation and supination of the foot is noted.
  - Pain with rising up onto the toes
- Midtarsal joint complete dislocation
  - Palpable tenderness at the midtarsal joint
  - Visible deformity of the forefoot is displaced either medially or laterally in comparison to the hindfoot.
  - Bruising and swelling may be present around the midtarsal region.
  - Patients cannot ambulate and may have difficulty moving the foot because of the pain.
- Midtarsal joint swivel dislocations
  - Palpable tenderness at displaced joint articulation; either calcaneocuboid or talonavicular joint
  - Decreased mobility noted between the calcaneus and cuboid bones or the talus and the navicular bone. The hypomobility is present at the dislocated or subluxed joint.
  - Bruising and swelling may be present around the dislocated region.
  - Altered pronation and supination of the foot are noted.
  - Pain with midstance to terminal stance of gait
  - Pain with raising up onto the toes
- Navicular fracture
  - Palpable tenderness at the navicular bone
  - Decreased mobility noted between the talus and navicular bones.
  - Bruising and swelling may be present around the navicular bone.
  - Altered pronation and supination of the foot are noted.

- Pain with midstance to terminal stance of gait
- Pain with raising up onto the toes.
- Cuboid fracture
  - Palpable tenderness at the cuboid
  - Decreased mobility noted between the calcaneus and cuboid bones.
  - Bruising and swelling may be present around the cuboid.
  - Altered pronation and supination of the foot are noted.
  - Pain with midstance to terminal stance of gait
  - Pain with rising up onto the toes.

IMPORTANT OBJECTIVE TESTS

- MRI, x-ray, and ultrasound have been found to be beneficial in diagnosing the presence of a fracture and dislocation.
- Plain radiographs may not be positive for a few weeks after onset of symptoms. Bone scan is a better choice for early diagnosis because it has high sensitivity but poor specificity. MRI also has a high sensitivity, and its specificity is greater than that of bone scans.
- Therapeutic ultrasound: Poor sensitivity (0.43) and specificity (0.49) at identifying stress fractures
- Tuning fork: Sensitivity and specificity of a 128-Hz tuning fork test were 75% and 67%, respectively.

DIFFERENTIAL DIAGNOSIS

- Lisfranc joint injury
- Plantar fasciitis
- Tibial nerve and plantar nerve entrapment
- Tumor
- Arthritis
- Gout
- Lyme disease
- Osteomyelitis
- Metatarsal joint synovitis

CONTRIBUTING FACTORS

Since the mechanism of injury is generally traumatic, no contributing factors have to be present. Risk factors may include the type of sport or occupation. High-impact sports or occupations that risk falls from heights may predispose a patient to midfoot injuries. Osteoporosis or osteopenia may also predispose a patient to fracture.

TREATMENT

MEDICAL AND SURGICAL

- For midfoot dislocations, the primary treatment is surgery. Surgery usually involves stabilizing the displaced segments with an ORIF. Whether surgery is

or is not performed, the ankle is generally placed in a cast for 6 to 8 weeks.
- Surgery is rarely performed for ligament sprains. Generally, they are only considered if all conservative options have been exhausted. Medically, the physician may prescribe antiinflammatory medications to reduce the irritation and swelling in the region.
- A walking boot or cast may be used to reduce the loading on the forefoot.

REHABILITATION

- Rehabilitation of midtarsal joints initially depends on the nature of the injury. Sprains require rest initially. Treatment should focus on decreasing inflammation and promoting healing. This can be accomplished through RICE. Severe sprains may require a walking boot to reduce the loads placed on the sprained ligament.
- Fractures and dislocations require casting initially to allow the bones and ligaments to heal.
- If using the walking boot, the patient can be allowed to remove it for bathing and for non–weight-bearing activity, but in all weight-bearing settings, boot use should be encouraged.
- Exercising while in the boot should be initiated. The patient can ride a recumbent bicycle while in the boot and should remove the boot several times during the day to complete ROM exercises.
- Once the bone or ligaments have healed, rehabilitation should focus on normalizing midtarsal joint mobility. Stiffness is common after the immobilization process. Mobilization should be completed on the talonavicular and calcaneocuboid joints. After ORIF surgery, the hardware may prevent the joint from moving. Also, if the joint has dislocated, mobilization may not be warranted because the patient needs stability in the joint, not mobility.
- Strengthening and proprioceptive training are important aspects of the rehabilitation process. Both are likely impaired by the injury and require retraining to normalize gait and weight-bearing function.
- The patient can return to sport, but care must be taken to slowly progress the loading through the metatarsal so that appropriate bone remodeling can occur. Full return to sport can occur when all biomechanical contributing factors have been addressed, balance and proprioception are normal, and strength is at least 90% that of the contralateral side.
- Improving the mobility of the talocrural joint and the calf can improve ankle dorsiflexion. This is often needed to help improve the biomechanics of the foot during the midstance to late-stance phases of gait.

PROGNOSIS

- Sprains and strains generally resolve without long-term functional impairments. Medial fracture-dislocations and swivel dislocations are successfully treated by prompt reduction and immobilization. Medial joint sprains have better recovery potential than lateral joint sprains.
- Longitudinal injuries may recover, but the results depend on the severity of the injury. Recovery potential is strongly influenced by the integrity of the medial longitudinal arch. If the stability of the arch is maintained, recovery potential is good.
- Fractures of the navicular and cuboid bones have good recovery potential if they occur in isolation. Both of these fractures rarely occur without secondary injuries. The greater the injury to other tissue, the worse the ultimate prognosis.

- In a study of patients with midfoot dislocations, 48% of patients with midfoot dislocations had a fair or poor result at follow-up 20 to 56 months after the injury. Functionally, these people had substantial limitations of daily activities. The authors found that the quality of the initial reduction was the major determinant for obtaining an excellent long-term result.

SIGNS AND SYMPTOMS INDICATING REFERRAL TO PHYSICIAN

- The red flag signs in the forefoot are usually few. If the patient is not improving over the course of a month, the patient should be referred back to the physician
- If tumors are suspected (unremitting or nonmechanical pain), a referral to the physician is warranted.

- Suspicions of gout should also be referred back to the physician for medical workup. Inflammation that does not resolve may be an indication of gout or other systemic inflammatory disorders.

SUGGESTED READINGS

Coughlin MJ. Common causes of pain in the forefoot in adults. *J Bone Joint Surg Br.* 2000;82(6):781-790.

Disraeli P. Managing foot fractures in urgent care. *JUCM.* 2008.

Jones M. Navicular stress fractures. *Clin Sports Med.* 2006;25(1):151-158.

Main BJ, Jowett RL. Injuries of the midtarsal joint. *J Bone Joint Surg Br.* 1975;57B(1):89-97.

Perron AD, Brady WJ, Keats TE. Orthopedic pitfalls in the ED: Lisfranc fracture-dislocation. *Am J Emerg Med.* 2001;19(1):71-75.

Wagner R, Blattert TR, Weckbach A. Talar dislocations. *Injury.* 2004;35(suppl 2):SB36-SB45.

AUTHOR: DERRICK SUEKI

BASIC INFORMATION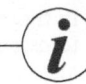

DEFINITION

- Morton's neuroma is irritation and swelling of the intermetatarsal plantar digital nerve as it passes beneath the intermetatarsal ligament.
- It is a chronic nerve compression and not a true neuroma.

SYNONYMS

- Interdigital neuroma
- Interdigital plantar nerve entrapment
- Interspace neuroma
- Morton's neuralgia

ICD-9CM CODES
355.6 Morton's metatarsalgia, neuralgia, neuroma

OPTIMAL NUMBER OF VISITS

6 or fewer

MAXIMAL NUMBER OF VISITS

24

ETIOLOGY

- 95% of cases occur in the third webspace, though it can also occur in the second web space between the second and third metatarsal heads. It is less likely in the first or fourth webspace.
- The area of the nerve most often injured is the interdigital nerve, proximal to bifurcation of the nerve into the toes, beneath and distal to the intermetatarsal ligament. Branches of the medial and lateral plantar nerve from the posterior tibial nerve (L4/S1) make up the interdigital nerve.
- Initial irritation can lead to inflammation of the nerve beneath the transverse intermetatarsal ligament, causing swelling, pain, and degeneration of the neural fibers. The nerve enlarges and continues to get impinged, and inflamed, leading to fibrotic scarring.
- Results from constant traction and impingement of the nerve against the transverse intermetatarsal ligament during the following:
  - Lateral deviation of the forefoot such as with hyperpronation, forefoot varus, or hallux valgus.
  - Mediolateral compression such as with footwear (narrow toe box)
  - Hyperextension of the MTP joint, which may occur with habitual use of high-heeled shoes or with direct trauma
- The patient experiences pain as a result of the following factors:
  - Compression of the enlarged nerve mediolaterally by the metatarsals, as well as dorsoventrally by the transverse intermetatarsal ligament.

- Localized pain commonly accompanied by pain, burning, or tingling into the toes and reports of clicking or popping between the toes as the neuroma slides beneath the transverse intermetatarsal ligament.

EPIDEMIOLOGY AND DEMOGRAPHICS

- The most common age group affected is between 40 and 60 years of age.
- It is 5 to 10 times more likely to occur in women than men with a correlation with footwear, especially high-heeled shoes.

MECHANISM OF INJURY

- Results from constant traction and impingement of the nerve against the transverse intermetatarsal ligament during the following:
  - Lateral deviation of the forefoot such as with hyperpronation, forefoot varus, or hallux valgus
  - Mediolateral compression such as with footwear (narrow toe box)
  - Hyperextension of the MTP joint, which may occur with habitual use of high-heeled shoes or with direct trauma

COMMON SIGNS AND SYMPTOMS

- Localized sharp pain on the plantar aspect between or immediately distal to the metatarsal heads
- Burning, pain, or tingling into the two adjacent toes
- Popping or clicking at the affected interspace
- The following nerves are affected:
  - The interdigital nerve at the affected interspace
  - The interdigital nerve arises from the medial and lateral plantar nerves from the posterior tibial nerve.

AGGRAVATING ACTIVITIES

- Walking
- Running
- Tight toe box of a shoe
- Wearing high-heeled shoes.
- Heel raise (caused by extension at the MTPs)
- Circumferential compression at the metatarsal heads elicits pressure on the neuroma.
- Extension at the MTP joint tightens the transverse intermetatarsal ligament and compresses the neuroma beneath it.

EASING ACTIVITIES

- Rest
- Avoid footwear with a tight toe box
- Avoid high-heeled shoes
- These activities prevent compression of the nerve, thus easing disc herniation.

24-HOUR SYMPTOM PATTERN

- Depends on activity and footwear

PAST HISTORY FOR THE REGION

- No previous history of neuroma needs to be present for occurrence.
- Inflammation of the intermetatarsal bursa or thickening of the transverse metatarsal ligament.
- History of direct trauma to the forefoot may also contribute to a Morton's neuroma.

PHYSICAL EXAMINATION

- May avoid bearing weight over the affected side.
- May avoid trailing limb posture in gait as a result of the MTP extension normally found in this phase of gait.
- No muscles are tender to palpation.
- Space between metatarsal heads, palpated plantar and dorsally, are painful.

IMPORTANT OBJECTIVE TESTS

- Morton's test
  - The metatarsal heads are grasped and squeezed together as the MTP joints are passively extended. Reproduction of symptoms indicates a positive test. This can reproduce a click or pop referred to as *Mulder's click*.
- Mulder's sign
  - The foot is squeezed at the level of the metatarsal heads in a medial-to-lateral direction. Palpation of the affected webspace occurs concurrently, which may result in a click or grinding. Reproduction of symptoms is considered a positive test. Clicking or grinding without symptoms is considered a normal finding.

DIFFERENTIAL DIAGNOSIS

- Metatarsalgia
- Freiberg's disease
- Synovial cyst
- Referred pain from tarsal tunnel syndrome
- Referred pain from S2 nerve root

TREATMENT

NONSURGICAL OPTIONS

- Local corticosteroid injection
- Modification of footwear or orthotics
- Physical therapy

SURGICAL OPTIONS

- Nerve resection with or without transposition into the intermuscular space
- Release of transverse intermetatarsal ligament (with or without neurolysis)
- Excision of the neuroma proximal to the metatarsal head

- Surgical indicators are failure of conservative treatment such as corticosteroid injections, physical therapy, and footwear modification.

SURGICAL OUTCOMES

- 5-year follow-up study of interdigital neuroma resection showed an overall satisfaction rate of good or excellent in 85% of patients.
- Most common postsurgical complication is symptomatic recurrent neuroma; 10% in primary resection, 40% in revision resections.

REHABILITATION

- Local irritation and inflammation should be addressed first, followed by modification of footwear and activity for prevention of recurrence.
- To address inflammation, the clinician may consider the following:
  - Use of a metatarsal bar or pad to offload the area.
  - Patient education regarding footwear
  - Ice or cold packs
  - Ultrasound
  - Light therapy
- Rehabilitation should focus on preventing of recurrence, including education regarding footwear and possible fabrication of orthoses. Use of metatarsal pads or bars decreases the irritation of the neuroma by spreading the metatarsal heads apart. Also, physical therapy should address impairments that lead to excessive stress at the forefoot, such as lack of talocrural mobility, especially in the context of the aggravating activity (e.g., running)
- Exercises may include the following:
  - Stretching of the talocrural joint, if a soft tissue limitation has been identified.
  - Modification of cardiovascular exercise to partial weight-bearing or non-weight-bearing exercise (e.g., biking or swimming versus running)
  - If postsurgical: AROM exercises can improve local circulation and aid in reducing edema.

CONTRIBUTING FACTORS

- Activity that involves repetitive impact in the forefoot
- Narrow or tight toe box in shoes
- High-heeled shoes with narrow toe boxes
- Intermetatarsal bursitis
- Thickening of the transverse metatarsal ligament

PROGNOSIS

- Approximately one third of patients respond to modification in footwear and use of devices such as a metatarsal pad to unload and spread the metatarsals.
- In those who receive surgical excision of a neuroma, the success rate is approximately 85%.
- In those who have recurrence of symptoms, success for re-excision is approximately 60% to 70%.

SIGNS AND SYMPTOMS INDICATING REFERRAL TO PHYSICIAN

- Unrelenting pain, worsening pain, or no response to interventions: Infection, fracture, or tumor
- Pain that does not change with position: Infection or tumor
- Purulent discharge from postsurgical incision (if applicable): Infection
- Major trauma: Fracture
- Fevers and chills: Infection

SUGGESTED READINGS

Beskin JL. Nerve entrapment syndromes of the foot and ankle. *J Am Acad Orthop Surg.* 1997;5:261–269.

Chao W. Interdigital neuroma and tarsal tunnel syndrome. In: Richardson EG, ed. *Orthopedic Knowledge Update: Foot and Ankle*. Rosemont, IL: American Academy of Orthopedic Surgeons; 2004.

Dellon AL. Nerve disorders and plantar heel pain. In: Porter DA, Schon LC, eds. *Baxter's the Foot and Ankle in Sport*. Philadelphia: Mosby; 2008.

Foot and Ankle Surgery. In: Skinner EB, ed. *Current Diagnosis and Treatment in Orthopedics*.

AUTHOR: MILDRED V. LIMCAY

BASIC INFORMATION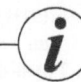

DEFINITION

- A navicular fracture is the osseous disruption of the navicular bone.
- Avulsion
  - Dorsal lip avulsion caused by deltoid ligament insertion
  - Plantar or medial lip avulsion caused by posterior tibialis tendon or spring ligament
  - Constitutes 50% of all navicular fractures
- Body: Half of fractures occur vertically through the midbody portion and are classified as the following:
  - Type I: Separates the navicular into dorsal and plantar sections (fracture through the transverse plane). No forefoot deformity, and the superior fragment is dorsally displaced.
  - Type II: Most common type of this fracture. Oblique fracture runs dorsolaterally to plantar medially, with the more medial fragment being displaced dorsomedially. The forefoot appears adducted, and the talonavicular joint is often subluxed or dislocated entirely.
  - Type III: Comminuted fracture of the navicular with or without displacement. Affects the midlateral portion of the navicular, also disrupting the naviculocuneiform joint. The forefoot appears to be in abduction and there a loss of height in the medial longitudinal arch.
- Tuberosity
  - Similar to the type II body injury, but the fragment is laterally displaced and smaller. Also, the amount of displacement is not as significant.
- Stress
  - Two major fracture patterns are avulsion and body fractures.
  - Isolated acute navicular fractures are rare.
  - The navicular bone is the keystone of the medial longitudinal arch of the foot.
  - Articulation of the navicular bone with the talus is responsible for 80% of rearfoot motion, and it is responsible for midfoot pronation and supination.

SYNONYMS

- Midfoot fracture
- Deltoid avulsion fracture

ICD-9CM CODES
733.95 Stress fracture of other bone
825.22 Fracture of navicular (scaphoid) bone of foot closed

OPTIMAL NUMBER OF VISITS
3 or fewer

MAXIMAL NUMBER OF VISITS
18

ETIOLOGY

- The most commonly fractured areas are as follows:
  - Dorsal aspect of the navicular tuberosity (avulsion fracture)
  - Vertically through midbody (body fracture)
  - Midbody: The most watershed area (stress fracture)
- Avulsion fractures occur because of the following:
  - Dorsal aspect avulsion of the navicular tuberosity: By the deltoid ligament in hyperplantarflexion of the midfoot or plantar flexion–eversion injury.
  - Medial and plantar aspect avulsion of the navicular tuberosity: By the posterior tibialis tendon or spring ligament during excessive eversion.
- Body fractures occur vertically through the midbody as a result of the following:
  - High-impact axial loading
  - Crush injuries
- Stress fracture: Midbody (the most watershed area)
- Pain is experienced because of the following:
  - Bone and periosteum are highly innervated. Fracture stimulates nociceptors and relay pain signals; this type of pain is often referred to as "bone pain." After fracture, inflammatory mediators bathe the area and stimulate nociceptors.
  - Local nerves (e.g., medial plantar nerve) in the immediate area are also irritated by inflammatory mediators.
  - Depending on the type of severity of navicular fracture, there may be attenuation or disruption of the interosseous ligaments of the tarsals.

EPIDEMIOLOGY AND DEMOGRAPHICS

- Body and tuberosity fractures can occur with any age because they are preceded by significant trauma.
- The elderly are more likely to have stress fractures due to the loss of vascularization, with aging, to the navicular, especially the central portion. This area of the navicular is considered the "watershed" area and is the most common site for stress and insufficiency fractures.
- Stress fractures also affect persons participating in certain types of sports. Khan and associates summarized populations over three studies consisting of 122 total subjects, as follows:
  - Track and field: 72 subjects (59%)

- Football, soccer, and rugby: 30 subjects (25%)
- Basketball: 14 subjects (11%)
- Racquet sports: 3 subjects (2.5%)
- Ballet, gymnastics: 3 subjects (2.5%)
- Most people with navicular fractures experience pain caused by the rich innervation present in bones and periosteum.

MECHANISM OF INJURY

- Avulsion fractures
  - Dorsal aspect avulsion of the navicular tuberosity: By the deltoid ligament in hyperplantarflexion of the midfoot or plantar flexion-eversion injury.
  - Medial and plantar aspect avulsion of the navicular tuberosity: By the posterior tibialis tendon or spring ligament during excessive eversion.
- Body fractures
  - High-velocity, high-force injury as occurs with traffic accidents and falls from a significant height
- By classification
  - Type I are caused by forces running along the central longitudinal axis of the foot.
  - Type II occur from axial compression, crush injuries, and dorsomedial forces on the forefoot.
  - Type III occur from laterally directed axial forces.
- Stress fractures:
  - Overuse with high loading activities
  - Training errors
- Pathological stress fractures caused by conditions, disorders, or medications facilitating fractures such as the following:
  - Tumors
  - Infections
  - Osteoporosis
  - Osteogenesis imperfecta
  - Long-term steroid use
  - Long-term alcohol use
  - Immunosuppressant use (e.g., methotrexate)

COMMON SIGNS AND SYMPTOMS

- Insidious onset of nagging, dull ache along the dorsomedial or plantar-medial midfoot
- Pain with ambulation

AGGRAVATING ACTIVITIES

- Walking
- Running
- Standing
- Ascending or descending stairs
- Rising up onto toes
- During gait, motion at the talonavicular joint is crucial for shock absorption (midfoot pronation during loading response) and for progression of body weight over a rigid foot (midfoot

supination during terminal stance to preswing).
- Similar mechanics are necessary for stair climbing, rising up onto toes, and standing.

EASING ACTIVITIES
- Non–weight-bearing positions: Sitting, lying down
  - Non–weight-bearing positions reduce load and shear on the navicular.
  - In cases of severe stress fracture and acute fracture, pain can occur at rest as well.
- Pain medications
  - Use of antiinflammatory medications with fracture has been controversial because of the inhibition of prostaglandins that are required for bone healing.
  - Pain medication modulates the body's pain perception via attenuating conduction or by stimulating the body's own pain-suppressing pathways.
- Ice reduces edema and neural conduction velocity, thereby slowing pain signals.
- Mild compression for edema

24-HOUR SYMPTOM PATTERN
- Inflammation can cause stiffness in the morning.
- May worsen throughout the day if the foot is left in a gravity-dependent position that would facilitate edema.

PAST HISTORY FOR THE REGION
- Acute fracture: No predisposing injury or condition required
- Stress fracture
  - No history of foot or ankle injury is necessary
  - Some hypothesize presence of a short first metatarsal; excessive pes cavus or pes planus predisposes to stress fracture.
  - Associated with onset of overtraining or overuse

PHYSICAL EXAMINATION
- Patients avoid weight bearing on the involved foot.
- Ankle is in loose pack position, approximately 30 degrees plantar flexion.
- Because of guarding after trauma, all global muscles around the foot and ankle tender, especially the posterior tibialis, gastrocnemius, and soleus.

IMPORTANT OBJECTIVE TESTS
Modified Ottawa Ankle Rules
- Tenderness or pain on palpation of the following:
  - Navicular
  - Base of the fifth metatarsal
  - Tip of each malleolus to 6 cm proximal
- Inability to weight bear immediately after injury or during evaluation for a total of four steps

- Considered positive if there exists tenderness with one site of palpation and inability to bear weight.
- Springer and associates showed physical therapists were just as skilled as orthopedic surgeons in detecting a positive sign.

Interobserver Agreement
- Kappa coefficient:
  - 0.82 for ankle injuries
  - 0.88 for foot injuries
  - Sensitivity 100%
  - Specificity for ankle injuries 46%
  - Specificity for foot injuries 79%
- MMT of the posterior tibialis may exacerbate symptoms if navicular fracture is suspected because of its attachment to the navicular tuberosity.
- PROM
  - Subtalar joint: Passive eversion at the subtalar joint stresses the deltoid ligament and could reproduce symptoms of an avulsion fracture.
  - Talonavicular joint: Limited by pain

DIFFERENTIAL DIAGNOSIS

- Accessory navicular fracture
- Posterior tibialis tendinopathy
- Anterior tibialis tendinopathy
- Navicular apophysitis (Köhler's disease)
- Deltoid ligament sprain
- Spring ligament sprain
- Medial plantar neuropathy
- Saphenous neuropathy
- Plantar fasciitis
- Charcot arthropathy
- Osteoarthritis
- Systemic inflammatory disorders (RA, Reiter's syndrome, ankylosing spondylitis)
- L4, L5 or S2 radiculopathy

TREATMENT

SURGICAL OPTIONS
- Avulsion fractures: Surgery is performed only with large avulsed fragments through percutaneous pinning or screw.
- Body fractures: Surgery is performed only when displacement is present.
  - ORIF
  - External fixation
  - Bone grafting
- Fractures that cannot be reconstructed.
  - Arthrodesis: Navicular to the first and second cuneiforms

SURGICAL OUTCOMES
- Outcome of surgery correlated with accuracy of reduction
  - <60% report accuracy related to poorer prognosis.
  - 83% report good outcome for primary line of treatment.

- 68% report good outcome for surgery as a second line of treatment.
- Possible postsurgical complications
  - Avascular necrosis
  - Nonunion: Usually occurs in fractures through the central portion of the navicular. Related to severity of the fracture and the patient's age caused by receding vascularity of this region with age.

REHABILITATION
- Nonoperative treatment
  - Common with stress fractures and nondisplaced, small avulsion fractures
  - Short leg cast with non–weight-bearing status for 6 to 8 weeks. After this period of time, transition to a walking boot is made with progressive weight bearing over 4 to 6 weeks. Time frame depends on fracture healing.
  - After removal of the cast, regaining foot and ankle mobility through active ROM and STM. With confirmed union, joint mobilization may be employed.
  - Gait training throughout course of rehabilitation to address weight-bearing ability
  - Proprioceptive and balance training
- In both nonoperative and operative treatments, immobilization with non-weight-bearing is part of the protocol, with immobilization lasting anywhere from 6 to 8 weeks. Exercise is significant in regaining strength to those muscles that have undergone disuse atrophy not only around the foot and ankle but also along the entire affected lower quarter.
- Postoperative
  - Weight-bearing status and progression of weight bearing depends on surgical intervention, severity of fracture, and fracture healing.
  - Active ROM: Degree depends on procedure and healing times
  - Gait training, with and without assistive devices
  - Proprioceptive and neuromuscular reeducation
  - Strengthening
  - Joint mobilization and STM to restore mobility
- To decrease inflammation, the clinician may consider the following:
  - Lymphedema massage
  - Myofascial release
  - Joint mobilization
  - AROM in a pain-free range
  - Cold pack
  - Modalities, such as electric stimulation and ultrasound, are *not* appropriate if metal fixation is present.
- Progression of treatment should include the following:
  - Restoration of mobility via STM and joint mobilization
  - Restoration of normal gait (within weight-bearing precautions)

○ Balance and proprioceptive training: Tropp and associates identified rehabilitation using balance discs to prevent occurrence and recurrence of inversion ankle injuries by addressing functional instability and impaired postural control after ankle injury.

• Strength training around the ankle and proximal hip musculature: Mediolateral sway is controlled primarily at the foot and ankle, secondarily by the hip.

• Initial exercises should include exercises in non–weight-bearing that actively go through pain-free ROM to promote circulation and reduce edema. Must take into consideration any precautions with ROM.

• Joint mobilization and manipulation are appropriate in the later phases of rehabilitation after confirmation of fracture healing to address joint-specific mobility restrictions after immobilization at the tarsal, subtalar, talocrural, and tibiofibular joints.

• Massage can be used in early rehabilitation (lymphatic massage or myofascial release) to reduce edema.
  ○ In later stages, STM is appropriate to address soft tissue restrictions in mobility

• Exercise has a significant role in the prevention or recurrence of inversion ankle injuries, specifically those that target proprioceptive and balance training.
  ○ In both nonoperative and operative treatments, immobilization with non–weight-bearing status is part of the protocol, with immobilization lasting anywhere from 4 to 6 weeks. Exercise is significant in regaining strength to those muscles that have undergone disuse atrophy, not only around the foot and ankle but also along the entire affected lower quarter.

• Long-term exercise
  ○ Proprioceptive and balance training can prevent inversion ankle injury, which is the most common cause of osteochondral lesions. Also, this helps prevent dynamic instability of the talocrural joint, which can also lead to other foot and ankle disorders.
  ○ Exercises targeting the proximal hip musculature would assist in prevention, according to Bullock-Saxton, who identified a delay in hip muscle function after severe ankle sprain.

CONTRIBUTING FACTORS

• Age
• Osteoporosis
• Smoking
• Diabetes
• Vascular disease
• Long-term steroid use
• Long-term alcohol use
• Immunosuppressant use (e.g., methotrexate)

PROGNOSIS

• Prognosis depends on type and severity of fracture and factors that would impair bone healing (see previous list).
• Stress fracture: Khan et al reported an 86% healing rate of the navicular after 6 to 8 weeks in a non–weight-bearing cast, with return to activity averaging 5.6 months.
• Acute traumatic fracture: More severe, comminuted fractures have a poor prognosis, especially if they could not be reconstructed or if the accuracy of reduction would be <60%.

SIGNS AND SYMPTOMS INDICATING REFERRAL TO PHYSICIAN

• Severe swelling, pain, erythema, signs of vascular compromise (slowing or loss of capillary refill, pulses): Compartment syndrome or deep vein thrombosis

• Constant unrelenting pain: Infection or tumor
• Pain that does not change with position: Infection or tumor
• Nocturnal pain: Tumor
• Streaking: Infection
• Purulent discharge: Infection
• Fevers, fatigue, and chills: Infection or tumor

SUGGESTED READINGS

Burne SG, Mahoney CM, Forster BB, Koehle MS, Taunton JE, Khan KM. Tarsal navicular stress injury: long-term outcome and clinicoradiological correlation using both computed tomography and magnetic resonance imaging. *Am J Sports Med.* 2005;33(12):1875–1881.

DiGiovanni CW. Fractures of the navicular. *Foot Ankle Clin North Am.* 2004;9:25–63.

Goulart M, O'Malley MJ, Hodgkins CW, Charlton TP. Foot and ankle fracture in dancers. *Clin Sports Med.* 2008;27:295–305.

Khan KM, Fuller PJ, Brukner PD, Kearney C, Burry HC. Outcome of conservative and surgical management of navicular stress fractures in athletes: 86 cases proven with computerized tomography. *Am J Sports Med.* 1992;20:657–666.

Luthje P, Nurmi I. Fracture-dislocation of the tarsal navicular in a soccer player. *Scand J Med Sci Sports.* 2000;12:236–240.

Ostlie DK, Simons SM. Tarsal navicular stress fracture in a young athlete: case report with clinical, radiologic and pathophysiologic correlations. *J Am Board Fam Pract.* 2001;14(5):381–385.

Stroud CC. Fractures of the midtarsals, metatarsals, and phalanges. In: Richardson EG, ed. *Orthopedic Knowledge Update: Foot and Ankle.* Rosemont, IL: American Academy of Orthopedic Surgeons; 2004.

AUTHOR: MILDRED V. LIMCAY

Section III

ORTHOPEDIC PATHOLOGY

BASIC INFORMATION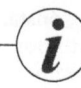

DEFINITION

- The two categories of phalanges fractures are as follows:
  - Hallucal fractures: Fracture of the proximal and/or distal phalanges
  - Fractures of the lesser toes: Fracture of any part of the distal and/or proximal phalanges of toes 2 to 5.
- Most common fractures of the forefoot.

SYNONYMS

- Broken toe
- Fracture of the base of the fifth proximal phalanx
  - Bedroom fracture
  - Nightwalker fracture
  - Nightstand fracture
- Phalanx fracture

ICD-9CM CODES
827.0 Fracture, phalanges of 1 foot

OPTIMAL NUMBER OF VISITS
6 or less

MAXIMAL NUMBER OF VISITS
18

ETIOLOGY

- The most commonly injured toe: Fractures of the lesser toes are most common versus that of the great toe; 76% to 83% of phalangeal fractures involve the lesser toes.
- Phalangeal fractures occur by direct trauma such as a "crush injury" or blunt force trauma.
- Phalangeal fractures also occur by indirect trauma such as the following:
  - Hyperextension injury at the MTP joint
  - Hyperflexion injury at the MTP joint
  - Abduction or adduction force
  - Stress fracture
- Patients experience pain because of the following:
  - The bone and periosteum itself is innervated and capable of sending nociceptive input after fracture.
  - Postfracture edema with inflammatory and pain mediators floods the area and irritate the surrounding nociceptive fibers.
  - Possible secondary damage to other innervated structures caused by mechanism of injury (ligaments, tendons, or if skin is broken during an open fracture)

EPIDEMIOLOGY AND DEMOGRAPHICS

- Incidence: 14 in 10,000
- Ratio of occurrence in males versus females is 1:6.

- Most with fractures of the first digit experience pain because of the weight-bearing load required in this region.
- Occasionally, those with lesser toe fractures, estimated at 10% to 25%, experience few to no symptoms, including pain.

MECHANISM OF INJURY

- Direct trauma
  - "Crush injury" or blunt force trauma
  - Dropping an object on the toe is the most common mechanism of distal phalanx fracture. Often associated with soft tissue and nail damage in addition to development of a subungual hematoma.
- Indirect trauma
  - Hyperextension injury at the MTP joint results from a fall onto toes and can lead to fracture and dorsal dislocation of proximal phalangeal condyles at the interphalangeal or MTP joint. Typically of the great toe, proximal phalanx with hyperextension and loading at the first MTP causing a transverse or oblique fracture. Fracture can extend through the joint surface at the first MTP joint.
  - Most common is a sudden abduction force of the fifth digit causing a transverse or oblique fracture of the proximal phalanx.
  - Stress fracture occurs mostly in athletes, especially in the presence of hallux valgus, at the medial base of the first proximal phalanx as a result of repetitive forced hyper extension of the first MTP joint. In the presence of a hallux valgus with repetitive forced hyperextension, tension through the MCL propagates microtrauma at its insertion at the base of the first proximal phalanx.

COMMON SIGNS AND SYMPTOMS

- Edema of the toe and possibly into the dorsum of the foot.
- Ecchymosis
- Subungual hematoma
- Toe deviation, angulation, or deformation
- Symptoms are typically local to region of injury, although edema could spread to the dorsum of the foot.

AGGRAVATING ACTIVITIES

- Weight-bearing activity
- Wearing shoes
- Walking
- Rising up onto toes

EASING ACTIVITIES

- Limited or non–weight-bearing activities
- Shoes with large toebox and rigid sole
- Elevation
- Ice

24-HOUR SYMPTOM PATTERN
Symptoms depend on activity; however, if the foot remains in a dependent position, edema and discomfort may be worse at the end of the day.

PAST HISTORY FOR THE REGION

- No previous injury is necessary for fractures caused by blunt trauma.
- For fracture as a result of indirect mechanisms, patients may have a history of previous hyperextension or hyperflexion injury to the affected toe resulting in ligamentous laxity.
- With stress fracture, patient may report history of pain with worsening over time at the site of fracture. Patient may also have hallux valgus.

PHYSICAL EXAMINATION

- The patient avoids weight bearing over the forefoot. In standing, the patient may bias body weight toward the heel on the affected side.
- Long and short toe flexors may be tender to palpation.

IMPORTANT OBJECTIVE TESTS

- Digit ROM testing
  - Flexion and extension are limited because of pain and/or swelling. Limitation in motion can occur at the interphalangeal or metacarpophalangeal (MCP) joint depending on location of the fracture and extent of edema.
- Vibratory testing with tuning fork or percussion
  - Anecdotal examination to identify stress fracture; has not been validated.
  - Use of 512 cycles per second tuning fork, applied to the affected site. Reproduction of symptoms is thought to implicate fracture.

DIFFERENTIAL DIAGNOSIS

- Sprain of the phalangeal ligaments
- Turf toe
- Interdigital neuroma
- Distal metatarsal fracture
- Sesamoiditis
- Fractured sesamoid
- Phalangeal dislocation
- Freiberg's infraction
- MTP instability
- Gout
- Distal tendon avulsion of toe flexors or extensors

CONTRIBUTING FACTORS

- Female athlete's triad
- Dancing over 5 hours per day
- Excessive training
- Osteoporosis

TREATMENT

SURGICAL OPTIONS

- For fractures of the lesser toes, surgery is not usually indicated unless an open fracture is present.
  - In closed fractures, buddy taping with a pad between the toes is used to stabilize the fracture for approximately 4 to 6 weeks.
- Fractures of the great toe indications for surgery:
  - Long oblique, spiral, or comminuted fractures are considered unstable and require fixation.
  - Failure to close or reduce a fracture
  - Intraarticular fractures
- Surgical interventions can do the following:
  - Remove small loose fragments
  - Use Kirschner wires to stabilize larger or intraarticular fragments.

REHABILITATION

- The goal of rehabilitation is to restore ROM, especially if the first MTP joint is involved. Dorsiflexion is needed for progression of the body over the forefoot during gait.
- The rest of the foot and ankle should be evaluated for loss of ROM and strength during the healing of the fracture.
- Restore strength, balance, and proprioceptive loss and tolerance to weight bearing over the affected digit.
- Progression to premorbid activity level.
- To address inflammation, the clinician should consider the following:
  - Lymphatic massage

  - Exercises that promote movement of the region in a pain-free range
  - Cold pack
- Initial exercises
  - Weight bearing as tolerated is usually allowed after surgery. At this point, physical therapy focuses on gait training in the prescribed protective device (surgical shoe or short leg cast) and assistive device.
  - AROM of the talocrural and subtalar joints within a pain-free ROM in an elevated position. Active contraction can assist in edema control and preserve motion at nonaffected joints.
  - Once cleared for AROM of the toes, flexion-extension exercises, such as towel curls, can begin.
  - Weight bearing over the affected region can begin with partial weight bearing in supine or sitting, eventually progressing from double-limb to single-limb stance.

PROGNOSIS

- Some residual angulation may be present. This usually occurs in fractures of the proximal phalanx in the second, third, or fourth toe.
- If malunion does occur, a plantar prominence can occur that may be removed by exostectomy.

SIGNS AND SYMPTOMS INDICATING REFERRAL TO PHYSICIAN

- Nonhealing wound or wound with purulent exudates: Infection
- Streaking: Infection
- Major trauma: Fracture

- Fevers and chills: Infection or tumor
- Allodynia, hyperalgesia, or swelling: Chronic regional pain syndrome

SUGGESTED READINGS

Armagan OE, Shereff MJ. Injuries to the toes and metatarsals. *Orthop Clin North Am.* 2001;32(1).

Goulart M, O'Malley MJ, Hodgkins CW, Charlton TP. Foot and ankle fracture in dancers. *Clin Sports Med.* 2008;27:295-305.

Hawkins BJ. Fractures of the metatarsals and phalanges of the foot. In: Calhoun JH, Laughlin RT, eds. *Fractures of the Foot and Ankle: Diagnosis and Treatment of Injury and Disease.* Boca Raton, FL: Taylor and Francis Group; 2005.

Sauer ST, Hanson TW, Marymont JV. Disorders of the subtalar joint, including subtalar sprains and tarsal coalitions. In: Porter DA, Schon LC, eds. *Baxter's The Foot and Ankle in Sport.* Philadelphia: Mosby, Inc; 2008.

Schnaue-Constantouris EM, Birrer RB, Grisafi PJ, Dellecorte MP. Digital foot trauma: emergency diagnosis and treatment. *J Emerg Med.* 2002;22(2):163-170.

Stroud CC. Fractures of the midtarsals, metatarsals, and phalanges. In: Richardson EG, ed. *Orthopedic Knowledge Update: Foot and Ankle.* Rosemont, IL: American Academy of Orthopedic Surgeons; 2004.

AUTHOR: MILDRED V. LIMCAY

BASIC INFORMATION

DEFINITION

- Plantar fasciitis is classically defined as inflammation of the plantar fascia, most common at its proximal insertion at the medial tubercle of the calcaneus. However, active inflammation is not necessary.
- Bone spurs at the attachment site of the plantar fascia are common co-findings; however, there is no evidence that this is the pain-generating structure in plantar fasciitis.
- It is a chronic, overuse disorder causing repetitive microtears and thus pain in the plantar aspect of the foot, anywhere along the course of the plantar fascia, but most commonly at the proximal medial edge.

SYNONYMS

- Painful heel syndrome
- Runner's or jogger's heel
- Heel spur syndrome
- Traction periostitis of the plantar fascia

ICD-9CM CODES
728.71 Plantar fasciitis

OPTIMAL NUMBER OF VISITS

6 or fewer

MAXIMAL NUMBER OF VISITS

24

ETIOLOGY

- The plantar aponeurosis is most often injured at the proximal attachment of the plantar fascia into the medial calcaneal tubercle.
- Typically, plantar fasciitis occurs as an overload injury caused by a combination of physiological or structural and external considerations. Examples of physiological and structural components include body weight, presence of pes cavus or pes planus deformities, and inadequate dorsiflexion at the talocrural joint. Examples of external considerations include footwear, change in exercise regimen, and the type of surface on which the patient trains or walks.
- Physiologically, there is no one accepted pathogenesis, though plantar fasciitis is widely accepted to be a result of a mechanical abnormality.
- General belief: Excessive tension through the plantar fascia causing chronic inflammation and microtears, especially at its proximal insertion.
- Presence of inflammation is controversial: Histological findings do not necessarily support presence of inflammatory cells.

- Presence of a low medial longitudinal arch is thought to increase the tensile force within the plantar fascia, thus causing microtearing.
- The patient experiences pain as explained in the following:
  ○ Wearing et al hypothesized the presence of free nerve endings in the plantar fascia, which would act as nociceptors when stimulated.
  ○ Chang et al reports association with medial plantar neuropathy with plantar fasciitis. In their 2006 study, they sampled 26 patients with clinically and ultrasonographically diagnosed plantar fasciitis and performed nerve conduction studies of the sural, posterior tibial, and lateral and medial calcaneal nerves. When results were compared with 20 age-matched controls, a significant difference was found in those with plantar fasciitis—specifically, latency in conduction and a decrease in sensory nerve action potential of the medial calcaneal nerve.

EPIDEMIOLOGY AND DEMOGRAPHICS

- Plantar fasciitis can occur at any age, and it most commonly occurs in those 40 to 60 years of age.
- There is a higher prevalence in females.
- Prevalence is not dependent on race or ethnicity.
- Obese individuals, male runners, and athletes have a higher prevalence.

MECHANISM OF INJURY

- Plantar fasciitis usually occurs as a result of overuse with faulty biomechanics.
- The function of the plantar fascia has been likened to a "Spanish windlass." It allows passive stability of the osseous structures of the foot when tensioned via rearfoot supination and toe dorsiflexion. This allows progression of body weight over a rigid and stable foot.
- An increase in tensile load to the plantar fascia as a result of obesity, excessive time spent on the feet, or pathomechanics have been identified as mechanisms of plantar fasciitis.
  ○ Specifically, excessive pronation at the midfoot, especially with walking, to excessively stress or tension the plantar fascia, causing microtears and degeneration.
  ○ The aforementioned pathomechanics has been hypothesized to be a compensatory strategy in individuals with inadequate talocrural dorsiflexion ROM. As a result of this lack of dorsiflexion in gait, the individual may progress through the midfoot via pronation.

COMMON SIGNS AND SYMPTOMS

- Insidious onset of progressively worsening medial heel pain
- Pain is worst in the morning or after periods of non–weight-bearing position followed by standing and walking
- Pes planus
- Limited gastrocnemius and soleus flexibility

AGGRAVATING ACTIVITIES

- First steps in the morning
- Direct pressure over the insertion of the plantar fascia into the calcaneus
- Ascending or descending stairs
- Squatting
- Walking barefoot
- Running
- Prolonged standing
- In extended periods of non–weight-bearing or partial weight-bearing positions, such as sleeping or sitting, the plantar fascia is not stressed because of the resting position of the foot and ankle (talocrural plantar flexion and toes in neutral) and does not tension the plantar fascia. Also, because the patient is not weight bearing, the mechanism for which the plantar fascia is engaged for the support of the medial longitudinal arch is not activated. On the first steps in the morning, sudden tensioning of the plantar fascia, especially with terminal stance, creates the pain and discomfort the patient feels.

EASING ACTIVITIES

- Sitting or lying down
- Wearing shoes with a small heel
- These are positions in which the plantar fascia is not tensioned

24-HOUR SYMPTOM PATTERN

- Symptoms are the worst in the morning with first steps.
- Improvement with subsequent steps to a certain extent; then worsens in correlation to the amount of time the patient spends on his or her feet.

PAST HISTORY FOR THE REGION

- Not necessary for the onset of plantar fasciitis
- Possible history of injury that would limit flexibility of the talocrural joint into dorsiflexion, which may lead to compensatory progression of body weight through the midfoot via pronation, thus stressing the plantar fascia.

PHYSICAL EXAMINATION

- The patient with plantar fasciitis often shifts the the body away from weight bearing on the affected side.
- Gastrocnemius, soleus, and the intrinsic muscles of the foot are often tender to palpation.

IMPORTANT OBJECTIVE TESTS

- Functional tests
  - Gait: May avoid terminal stance or preswing during gait, as this is the phase when the plantar fascia is most stressed. Can appreciate if the patient is progressing through the midfoot as opposed to the talocrural joint and first ray, which would contribute to pathology.
  - Squat (single- and double-limb): may be symptomatic, especially if there is a lack of talocrural dorsiflexion and the affected foot compensates via midfoot pronation, thus tensioning the plantar fascia.
- Straight leg raise (SLR) and/or slump testing
  - To determine or differentially diagnose symptoms of neural origin.
  - Tibial nerve bias of talocrural dorsiflexion and subtalar eversion may replicate patients' symptoms. If changed with sensitizing maneuvers, medial plantar nerve involvement can be suspected.

DIFFERENTIAL DIAGNOSIS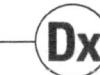

- S2 radiculopathy
- Plantar nerve entrapment
- Calcaneal stress fracture
- Sever's disease
- Bone bruise of the calcaneus
- Systemic arthritic condition such as RA, SLE, or spondyloarthropathies

TREATMENT

SURGICAL OPTIONS

- Partial fasciotomy
- Complete fasciotomy

SURGICAL OUTCOMES

- Only recommended after all conservative treatments have failed. Possible adverse effects include complete release that may lead to flattening of the medial longitudinal arch because of resection of the plantar fascia and neurovascular complications.
- Fishco et al, in a retrospective study 20.9 months after plantar fasciotomy, reported that out of 83 patients, 93.5% reported a successful outcome with 95.7% reporting they would recommend the procedure to others.
- Jerosch et al reported improvement of symptoms in 13 out of 17 patients, approximately 18 months after endoscopic partial release of the plantar fascia as measured by the Ogilvie-Harris score.

CONSERVATIVE MEDICAL MANAGEMENT

- Extracorporeal shockwave therapy (ESWT)
- Local injection of a corticosteroid
- Night dorsiflexion splint
- Foot orthoses

REHABILITATION

- Riddle et al established talocrural dorsiflexion as the most significant risk factor in plantar fasciitis. Rehabilitation should then focus on regaining mobility at the talocrural joint and neuromuscular retraining so that compensatory mechanisms that cause undue tension at the plantar fascia can be avoided.
- Improving talocrural dorsiflexion may be achieved via the following:
  - Joint mobilizations at the talocrural joint, as well as proximal and distal tibiofibular articulations, if warranted
  - STM of the gastrocnemius and soleus complex
  - Stretching of the gastrocnemius and soleus complex
  - Use of medial longitudinal arch (Holms et al) or calcaneal taping (Hyland et al) has been recommended to alleviate symptoms and decrease stress on the plantar fascia.
  - Identification of the need for foot orthoses
- Initial exercises should include the following:
  - Stretching of the gastrocnemius/soleus complex, as well as the plantar fascia
  - Strengthening of postural stabilizers at the ankle and hip
  - Strengthening of the intrinsic and extrinsic dynamic medial longitudinal arch stabilizers
  - Self-STM of the plantar fascia
  - Balance exercises with preservation of the medial longitudinal arch
- Joint mobilization
  - If the hypothesized contributing factor or risk factor for plantar fasciitis is lack of talocrural dorsiflexion and the result of joint restrictions, mobilizations of the talocrural and/or proximal and distal tibiofibular joints are appropriate.
- Massage
  - If the hypothesized contributing factor or risk factor for plantar fasciitis is lack of talocrural dorsiflexion and a result of muscular restriction, STMs of the gastrocnemius and soleus are appropriate.
  - STM directly to the plantar tissues of the foot may help to increase circulation and healing.
- Long-term exercises
  - Maintenance of talocrural dorsiflexion via stretching
  - Neuromuscular reeducation, including balance training to avoid excessive stresses at midfoot, specifically at the talonavicular joint to prevent further stress of the plantar fascia.

CONTRIBUTING FACTORS

- Irving et al suggested a pronated foot position and obesity to be risk factors. Riddle et al assessed risk factors in those with plantar fasciitis. Primary risk factors include the following:
- Inadequate talocrural dorsiflexion ROM (odds ratio at 95% confidence interval)
  - 6 to 10 degrees dorsiflexion, odds ratio 2.1
  - 1 to 5 degrees dorsiflexion, odds ratio 8.2
  - ≤0 degree dorsiflexion, odds ratio 23.3
- BMI >25 (odds ratio at 95% confidence interval)
  - 25 to 30, odds ratio 2.0
  - >30, odds ratio 5.6

PROGNOSIS

- A study done by Davis et al evaluated conservative treatment of nonspecific heel pain consisting of NSAIDs, relative rest, heel cushions, Achilles tendon stretching exercises, and injections (not with every subject). After 12 months of conservative treatment, 89.5% of patients improved to some extent.
- Batt et al studied the use of a dorsiflexion night splint, and out of 33 cases, 30 subjects improved as reported via pain scale (visual analog scale), plantar fascia tenderness, and ankle ROM.

SIGNS AND SYMPTOMS INDICATING REFERRAL TO PHYSICIAN

- Exquisite tenderness with presence of erythmosis and edema: Infection
- Pain that does not change with position: Infection
- Major trauma: Fracture
- Sudden onset of bowel and/or bladder dysfunction: Cauda equina syndrome
- Progressive bilateral lower extremity paresthesias: Cauda equine syndrome
- No improvement of symptoms after 4 months of conservative care: Possible need for surgical intervention

SUGGESTED READINGS

Batt ME, Tanji JL, Skattum N. Plantar fasciitis: a prospective randomized clinical trial of the tension night splint. *Clin J Sport Med.* 1996;6:158-162.

Chang CW, Wang YC, Hou WH, Lee XX, Chang KF. Medial calcaneal neuropathy is associated with plantar fasciitis. *Clin Neurophysiol.* 2007;118:119-123.

Cornwall MW, McPoil TG. Plantar fasciitis: etiology and treatment. *J Orthop Sports Phys Ther.* 1999;29(12):756-760.

Davis PF, Severud E, Baxter DE. Painful heel syndrome: results of nonoperative treatment. *Foot Ankle Int.* 1994;15:531-535.

Fishco WD, Goecker RM, Schwartz RI. The instep plantar fasciotomy for chronic plantar fasciitis. A retrospective review. *J Am Podiatr Med Assoc.* 2000;90(2):66-69.

Holmes CF, Wilcox D, Fletcher JP. Effect of a modified, low-dye medial longitudinal arch taping procedure on the subtalar joint neutral position before and after light exercise. *J Orthop Sports Phys Ther.* 2002;32:194-201.

Hyland MR, Webber-Gaffney A, Cohen L, Lichtman SW. Randomized controlled trial of calcaneal taping, sham taping and plantar fascia stretching for short term management of plantar heel pain. *J Orthope Sports Phys Ther.* 2006;36(6):365-371.

Irving DB, Cook JL, Young MA, Menz HB. Obesity and pronated foot type may increase the risk of chronic plantar heel pain: a matched case-control study. *BMC Musculoskelet Disord.* 2007;8(41):1-8.

Jerosch J, Schunck J, Liebsch D, Filler T. Indication, surgical technique and results of endoscopic fascial release in plantar fasciitis (EFRPF). *Knee Surg Sports Trauma Arthrosc.* 2004;12:471-477.

La Porta GA, La Fata PC. Pathologic conditions of the plantar fascia. *Clin Podiatr Med Surg.* 2005;22:1-9.

Riddle DL, Pulisic M, Pidcoe P, Johnson RE. Risk factors for plantar fasciitis: a matched case-control study. *J Bone Joint Surg Am.* 2003;85:872-877.

Wearing SC, Smeathers JE, Urry SR, Hennig EM, Hills AP. The pathomechanics of plantar fasciitis. *Sports Med.* 2006;36(7):585-611.

AUTHOR: MILDRED V. LIMCAY

BASIC INFORMATION

DEFINITION

- Posterior impingement causes pain by entrapping soft tissue or osseous structures at the posteromedial or posterolateral aspect of the talocrural joint in plantar flexion.
- Possible impingement occurs in one or more of the following structures:
  - Hypertrophic tissue (caused by previous injury) of the posterior tibiotalar band of the deltoid ligament
  - Transverse tibiotalar ligament
  - Posterior synovial inflammation, with or without hypertrophy caused by chronic stress
  - Loose body
  - Unstable os trigonum
  - Osteophytic formation
  - Trigonal process of the talus

SYNONYMS

Ankle impingement

ICD-9CM CODES
726.71 Achilles bursitis or tendinitis

OPTIMAL NUMBER OF VISITS
6 or fewer

MAXIMAL NUMBER OF VISITS
24

ETIOLOGY

- Posterior impingement can occur either posteromedially or posterolaterally at the talocrural joint.
- Can occur after trauma, as the result of soft tissue hypertrophy or the resultant instability of the talocrural joint.
  - Inversion sprain: Deep posterior fibers of the deltoid ligament or the posteromedial joint capsule could get pinched and damaged between the medial malleolus and calcaneus during inversion sprain. Scarring, hypertrophy, and possible calcification ensues and facilitates impingement between medial malleolus and calcaneus with plantar flexion at the talocrural joint.
  - Osseous structures: Presence of an os trigonum or hypertrophied posterior talar prominence in addition to event or repetitive activity that would facilitate soft tissue entrapment.
- Hypertrophied soft tissue (ligament, capsule) can produce a sharp pain when impinged between the talus and mortise with plantar flexion.
- Presence of os trigonum or prominent posterior talar prominence alone does not create a posterior impingement or pain.

EPIDEMIOLOGY AND DEMOGRAPHICS

- The following groups of people are most likely to present with posterior impingement:
  - Dancers, especially those on pointe or demi-pointe
  - Athletes or physically active individuals
  - Because posterior impingement can occur from either trauma or overuse, it can occur across the lifespan.

MECHANISM OF INJURY

- Posterior impingement from overuse is caused by repetitive plantar flexion, usually in ballet dancers and runners.
  - Forceful, repetitive plantar flexion associated with these activities increases plantar flexion ROM, thus allowing more approximation between the posterior aspect of talus and mortise and/or the calcaneus and mortise.
  - Greater approximation can entrap soft tissues between these osseous structures, leading to inflammation and tissue hypertrophy, which makes it easier to get impinged.
  - Calcification of soft tissue or joint capsule may also occur.
- Posttraumatic posterior impingement is a result of instability, as well as soft tissue damage, leading to hypertrophy and formation of scar tissue.

COMMON SIGNS AND SYMPTOMS

Localized sharp pain over the site of entrapment, either posteromedially or posterolaterally.

AGGRAVATING ACTIVITIES

- Rising up onto toes
- Running, especially down hill
- Dancing on pointe or demi-pointe
- Wearing heels
- Plantar flexion, active or passive
- Dorsiflexion in some
- Plantar flexion approximates the posterior talus and calcaneus to the posterior mortise, thus allowing compression of the soft tissues or bone fragments between these osseous structures.
- In some, dorsiflexion can also aggravate symptoms by stretching the affected posterior joint capsule and/or posterior talofibular ligament, which is attached to the posterior talar process.

EASING ACTIVITIES

- Avoidance of end-range plantar flexion
- Medications, such as pain relievers, may help; however, depending on duration of symptoms, antiinflammatories may not assist in easing symptoms.
- Allow greater space between the posterior ankle mortise, talus, and calcaneus.

24-HOUR SYMPTOM PATTERN

Symptoms depend more on position and activity, as opposed to depending on time or fatigue.

PAST HISTORY FOR THE REGION

- May have had ankle sprain(s) previously, which led to instability in the talocrural joint.
- May have history of activity that involved repetitive plantar flexion (e.g., ballet, running).

PHYSICAL EXAMINATION

- Depending on how severe the symptoms are, patients may avoid bearing weight on the affected side.
- Tenderness can be present in the muscles of the posterior and lateral compartments of the lower leg, especially if the ankle is unstable.

IMPORTANT OBJECTIVE TESTS

- Forced plantar flexion
  - Weight-bearing versus non–weight-bearing positions
  - If posterior impingement, both conditions should reproduce symptoms because soft tissue and/or osseous structure(s) are caught between the posterior talus and mortise.
- Resistive tests of the posterior tibialis and FHL differentiate between a tendinopathy and posterior impingement.
- SLR testing can differentiate between neurodynamic source of symptoms as opposed to posterior impingement
  - Positive: Symptom reproduction

DIFFERENTIAL DIAGNOSIS

- Posterior tibialis tendinopathy
- FHL tendinopathy
- Peroneal tendinopathy
- Achilles tendinopathy
- Retrocalcaneal bursitis
- Sever's disease
- Calcaneal fracture
- Osteochondral lesion of the talus
- Syndesmotic injury (high ankle sprain)
- Osteomyelitis
- Systemic inflammatory disease: Spondyloarthropathies, RA
- S1 or S2 radiculopathy

TREATMENT

SURGICAL OPTIONS

- Open or arthroscopic debridement of soft tissues and/or osseous structures
  - Removal of os trigonum
  - Removal of hypertrophic bone
  - Removal of hypertrophic soft tissues

SURGICAL OUTCOMES

- According to Willits et al, in a study of an open surgical technique of debridement for posterior impingement, 10% had neurological consequences. In a review of 16 patients with posterior arthroscopic approach, no neurological compromise occurred, 15 of 16 were able to return to sport, and patients were all moderately to very satisfied with results.
- A review by Niek van Dijk reported half the recovery time in patients undergoing arthroscopic as opposed to open debridement. Evaluation of 57 patients undergoing endoscopic surgery for posterior impingement, after a mean follow-up of 38 weeks, was as follows:
  - Overall return to work: 3 weeks
  - Overall return to sports activities: 9 weeks
  - Overall percentage of good or excellent results: 80%

REHABILITATION

- Conservative care
  - Niek van Dijk recommends the use of corticosteroid injections and heel lifts in the early phase.
  - Joint mobilization to address any limitation of the talocrural, proximal and distal tibiofibular, and subtalar joints that may facilitate posterior impingement
  - Balance and stability training: As the pathomechanics are related to functional and/or structural instability.
- Postoperative
  - Myofascial release to address soft tissue limitation of mobility
  - Joint mobilization
  - Exercises that promote movement of the region in a pain-free range
  - Proprioceptive training or neuromuscular reeducation
  - Gait training
  - Cold or hot pack
  - Ultrasound
- Once the inflammation process has decreased, rehabilitation should focus on the following:
  - Restoration of full AROM and PROM
  - Functional stability of the ankle to prevent recurrence, specific to previous tasks, activities, sport that aggravated symptoms.
- Initial exercises should include AROM through a pain-free ROM.
- Joint mobilization and manipulation
  - Presurgical and postsurgical mobilization would be appropriate to address joint-related restriction in ROM that would facilitate posterior impingement (e.g., lack of anterior glide of the talus during plantar flexion facilitates approximation of the posterior talus and/or calcaneus with the mortise).
- Massage, in preoperative and postoperative situations, would be helpful in restoring talocrural ROM lost by soft tissue restrictions.
  - Lymphatic massage may be used to reduce the amount of postoperative edema.
- Exercise: The main role of exercise would be to gain functional stability of the talocrural joint via strengthening and neuromuscular reeducation.
- Long-term exercises
  - Proprioceptive and balance training can prevent recurrent inversion ankle injury by addressing the dynamic instability of the talocrural and subtalar joints, which is associated with the pathomechanics of posterior impingement syndrome.
  - Exercises targeting the proximal hip musculature would assist in prevention, according to Bullock-Saxton, who identified a delay in hip muscle function after severe ankle sprain.
  - For those active in sport, external bracing should be considered.

CONTRIBUTING FACTORS

- Instability of the talocrural joint such as after an inversion or eversion ankle sprain
- Activities that require jumping and running such as sports and dance
- Hypertrophied posterior talar process
- Presence of an os trigonum

PROGNOSIS

- Willits et al studied the recovery of 23 patients after arthroscopic treatment of posterior impingement syndrome and determined prognosis after surgery was good, as follows:
  - Average time to return to work: 1 month
  - Average time to return to sport at pre-injury level: 5.8 months
  - ROM within 5 degrees of contralateral foot
  - No reports of neurological deficit

SIGNS AND SYMPTOMS INDICATING REFERRAL TO PHYSICIAN

- Pain that does not change with position: Infection or tumor
- Significant and unexplained weight loss: Tumor
- Nocturnal pain: Tumor
- Major trauma: Fracture
- Fevers and chills Infection or tumor
- Purulent discharge from incision site: Infection

SUGGESTED READINGS

Best A, Giza E, Linklater J, Sullivan M. Report of four cases: Posterior impingement of the ankle caused by anomalous muscles. *J Bone Joint Surg Am.* 2005;87(9):2075-2079.

Bullock-Saxton JE. Local sensation changes and altered hip muscle function following severe ankle sprain. *Phys Ther.* 1994;74:23-37.

Hamilton WG, Geppert MJ, Thompson FM. Pain in the posterior aspect of the ankle in dancers: differential diagnosis and operative treatment. *J Bone Joint Surg Am.* 1996;78:1491-1500.

Niek van Dijk C. Anterior and posterior ankle impingement. *Foot Ankle Clin North Am.* 2006;11:663-683

Paterson RS, Brown JN, Roberts SNJ. The posteromedial impingement lesion of the ankle: A series of six cases. *Am J Sports Med.* 2001;29(5):550-557.

Tropp H, Askling C, Gillquist J. Prevention of ankle sprains. *Am J Sports Med.* 1985;13:259-262.

Watson AD. Ankle instability and impingement. *Foot Ankle Clin North Am.* 2007;12:177-195.

Willits K, Sonneveld H, Amendola A, et al. Outcome of posterior ankle arthroscopy for hindfoot impingement. *Arthrosc: J Arthrosc elat Surg.* 2008;24(2):196-202.

AUTHOR: MILDRED V. LIMCAY

BASIC INFORMATION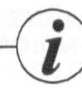

DEFINITION

- Retrocalcaneal bursitis is an inflammation of the retrocalcaneal bursa that can occur independently or with inflammation to the Achilles tendon or paratendon.
- The retrocalcaneal bursa is located just anterior to the Achilles tendon at its insertion to the calcaneus and functions to protect the tendon from shearing by the underlying bone with talocrural dorsiflexion.
- It can occur independently, but when concurrent with Achilles tendinitis superficial patellar bursitis, and a prominent bursal-calcaneal projection, this grouping of disorders is known as Haglund's disease.

SYNONYMS

- Pre-Achilles bursitis
- Bursitis of the heel

ICD-9CM CODES
726.70   Enthesopathy of ankle and tarsus unspecified
727.9   Unspecified disorder of synovium tendon and bursa
727.3   Other bursitis disorders

OPTIMAL NUMBER OF VISITS

6 or fewer

MAXIMAL NUMBER OF VISITS

24

ETIOLOGY

- The patient experiences pain because the bursa has nociceptive innervation. Chemical mediators associated with inflammation bathe not only the bursa but also surrounding tissues.
- Patients with a structural predisposition have a prominent posterior-superior aspect of the calcaneus, which can compress the retrocalcaneal bursa against the shoe counter.
- Repetitive compression and friction caused by ill-fitting footwear can create the pathology, specifically, shoes with a firm heel counter that hits at the level of the attachment of the Achilles or calcaneus.

EPIDEMIOLOGY AND DEMOGRAPHICS

- Individuals most likely to present with retrocalcaneal bursitis are as follows:
  - Those with systemic inflammatory diseases (RA, Reiter's syndrome)
  - Those with prominent posterosuperior calcanei
  - Runners (especially long-distance runners)
  - Older recreational athletes: "weekend warriors"
  - Poor shoe fit at the heel counter
- Because of the inflammatory nature of the disorder, which can trigger nociceptors both on the retrocalcaneal bursa and on surrounding tissues, most people with retrocalcaneal bursitis experience pain.

MECHANISM OF INJURY

- Presence of a bone prominence on the superior calcaneal tuberosity can compress and irritate the retrocalcaneal bursa, especially with dorsiflexion.
- Ill-fitting footwear with a firm or rigid heel counter facilitates repeated compression of the retrocalcaneal bursa with talocrural dorsiflexion.
- Repetitive compression between the Achilles and calcaneus with tasks requiring repetitive loaded dorsiflexion (such as uphill running)

COMMON SIGNS AND SYMPTOMS

Pain is located anterior to the attachment of the Achilles tendon on the calcaneus without radiation of symptoms.

AGGRAVATING ACTIVITIES

- Uphill walking or running
- Activities requiring talocrural dorsiflexion: Squatting, stair climbing
- Wearing certain types of shoes
- These types of activities facilitate compression of the bursa between the posterosuperior calcaneus and distal Achilles tendon, especially if the bursa is already enlarged and inflamed.

EASING ACTIVITIES

- Non–weight-bearing activities
- Assuming a plantar-flexed talocrural position
- Avoiding shoes with a firm heel counter
- Ice
- Antiinflammatory medications
- Reduction of compression of the bursa
- Reduction of inflammation reduces both noxious inflammatory mediators and size of bursa, which reduces compression between the calcaneus and Achilles tendon.

24-HOUR SYMPTOM PATTERN

- As with other inflammatory conditions, symptoms of stiffness occur first in the morning, with gradual improvement with continued walking.
- Worsening of symptoms with prolonged walking and/or footwear that aggravates symptoms

PAST HISTORY FOR THE REGION

No previous history necessary in the foot and ankle.

PHYSICAL EXAMINATION

- Patients may avoid equal weight-bearing activities onto involved side.
- Rearfoot varus
- Rigid plantar-flexed first ray
- There should not be tenderness with direct palpation over the distal attachment of the Achilles tendon, but if palpation is firm enough, symptoms may be reproduced because of compression of the underlying retrocalcaneal bursa.

IMPORTANT OBJECTIVE TESTS

- Passive dorsiflexion should be painful.
- Active-resisted plantar flexion, especially in a dorsiflexed talocrural position, may reproduce pain
- Pinch or two-finger squeeze test
  - Pinching on either side of the Achilles immediately anterior and proximal to its insertion onto the calcaneus should reproduce symptoms with palpable warmth and soft tissue engorgement.

DIFFERENTIAL DIAGNOSIS

- Insertional or midsubstance Achilles tendinitis
- Achilles tendinosis
- Achilles paratenonitis
- Haglund's deformity
- Tendo-Achilles bursitis
- Sever's disease (pediatric population)
- Calcaneal fracture
- Achilles tendon rupture
- Posterior tibialis tendinopathy
- FHL or FDL tendinopathy
- Haglund's syndrome (retrocalcaneal bursitis, Achilles tendinitis, and supracalcaneal bursitis)
- S1 or S2 radiculopathy
- Systemic inflammatory diseases (RA, ankylosing spondylitis, Reiter's syndrome)

TREATMENT

SURGICAL OPTIONS

- Resection of the retrocalcaneal bursa with or without debridement of the Achilles tendon
- Calcaneal resection

SURGICAL OUTCOMES

- In the 24 cases reported by Schepsis of retrocalcaneal debridement, 75% reported good-to-excellent results based on subjective report. No time frame was given.
- van Dijk reported on 21 procedures in 20 patients and evaluated results of endoscopic calcaneoplasty. Mean follow-up was 3.9 years.
  - Based on Ogilvie-Harris score: 15 excellent, 4 good, 1 fair result
  - Average recovery time: 7 weeks

- ○ Average time for return to work: 7 weeks
- ○ Average time for return to sport: 12 weeks

REHABILITATION

- Use of a heel wedge to decrease the angle of calcaneal pitch, thereby reducing compression of the retrocalcaneal bursa.
- Footwear modification: With athletic shoe, well-padded heel counter with notch to accommodate the Achilles tendon
- Activity modification
  - ○ Running regimen to avoid uphill running until symptoms subside, then slow reintroduction after addressing muscle length or biomechanical issues; change running surface (soft ground).
  - ○ Cross-training to avoid repetitive insult
- STM and stretching of the gastrocnemius and soleus complex
- To diminish inflammation, the following should be considered:
  - ○ Soft tissue techniques for tissue extensibility and edema reduction
  - ○ Joint mobilization
  - ○ Exercises that promote movement of the region in a pain-free range
  - ○ Cold or hot pack
  - ○ Ultrasound or phonophoresis
  - ○ Iontophoresis or electrical stimulation
- Once the inflammation process has decreased, the focus of rehabilitation should be on identifying the factors that caused pathology
  - ○ Biomechanical factors (via joint mobilization and/or STM, stretching, strengthening, orthoses, change in footwear)

- ○ Faulty mechanics with specific task or sport (neuromuscular re-education, proprioceptive training, orthoses)
- ○ If systemic inflammatory disorder, refer to physician.
- Initial exercises: AROM in a pain-free range
- Long-term exercises
  - ○ Stretching the gastroc nemius/soleus complex
  - ○ Specific to each aggravating task; address any restriction or compensation pattern up and down the kinetic chain that would lead to recurrence of symptoms

CONTRIBUTING FACTORS

- Rearfoot varus
- Rigid plantar-flexed first ray
- Restricted talocrural dorsiflexion (by joint or soft tissue changes)
- Sedentary lifestyle with sudden onset of activity
- Running terrain
- Use of shoes with firm heel counters that hit directly at Achilles insertion

PROGNOSIS

- In a study done by van Dijk, the following postsurgical results were reported:
  - ○ Average recovery time: 7 weeks
  - ○ Average time for return to work: 7 weeks
  - ○ Average time for return to sport: 12 weeks
- Nonsurgical prognosis is good, although retrocalcaneal bursitis can recur if the patient returns to previous habits.

SIGNS AND SYMPTOMS INDICATING REFERRAL TO PHYSICIAN

- Constant unrelenting pain: Infection or tumor
- Pain that does not change with position: Infection or tumor
- Major trauma: Fracture
- History of cancer: Metastatic disease
- Fevers and chills: Infection or tumor
- Purulent exudate: Infection
- Progressive bilateral lower extremity paresthesias that are nondermatomal: Cauda equina syndrome

SUGGESTED READINGS

Aronow MS. Posterior heel pain (retrocalcaneal bursitis, insertional and noninsertional Achilles tendinopathy). *Clin Podiatr Med Surg.* 2005;22:19–43.

Leitze Z, Sella EJ, Aversa JM. Endoscopic decompression of the retrocalcaneal space. *J Bone Joint Surg Am.* 2003;85-A:1488–1496.

Pavlov H, Ditchek J, Potter HG, Schneider R. Imaging of the hindfoot and ankle. In: Ranawat CS, Positano RG, eds. *Disorders of the Heel, Rearfoot, and Ankle*. Philadelphia: Churchill Livingstone; 1999.

Schepsis AA, Wagner C, Leach RE. Surgical management of Achilles tendon overuse injuries: a long-term follow-up study. *Am J Sports Med.* 1994;22:611–619.

Title CI, Schon LC. Achilles tendon disorders including tendinosis and tears. In: Porter DA, Schon LC, eds. *Baxter's the Foot and Ankle in Sport*. Philadelphia: Mosby; 2008.

van Dijk CN, van Dyk GE, Scholten PE, Kort NP. Endoscopic calcaneoplasty. *Am J Sports Med.* 2001;29:185–189.

AUTHOR: MILDRED V. LIMCAY

BASIC INFORMATION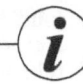

DEFINITION

- The sesamoid bones are located on the plantar surface of the head of the first metatarsal encapsulated by the flexor hallucis brevis tendon:
  - Normally transmits 50% of body weight and with push-off can transmit >300% of body weight.
  - Normal function is to provide shock absorption to the first MTP joint and provide increased mechanical leverage to the great toe flexors and to protect the FHL tendon.
- The following disorders may occur to the sesamoid bones:
  - Sesamoiditis is a general term for pain around the sesamoid region as a result of soft tissue (bursa, flexor tendon) pathology with normal radiographs and MRI; this is a diagnosis of exclusion.
  - Sesamoid fracture most often occurs to the tibial (most medial) sesamoid.
  - Sesamoid degeneration is associated with chondromalacia, osteophytes, and gout.
  - Avascular necrosis of the sesamoid: Traumatic or nontraumatic
  - Osteomyelitis of the sesamoid: Direct relation to plantar wound or ulcer or puncture wound

SYNONYMS

Sesamoiditis

ICD-9CM CODES
733.99 Other disorders of bone and cartilage

OPTIMAL NUMBER OF VISITS

6 or fewer

MAXIMAL NUMBER OF VISITS

18

ETIOLOGY

- The most commonly injured sesamoid bones are as follows:
  - The tibial sesamoid is fractured because of its larger size and weight-bearing responsibility.
  - The fibular sesamoid is more involved in avascular necrosis.
- Sesamoid bones are injured by overuse and repetitive soft tissue injury: Sesamoiditis.
- Sesamoid fracture
  - Acute: Trauma involving hyperdorsiflexion of the first MTP joint
  - Stress fracture: Related to activities involving repetitive loading through a dorsiflexed first MTP joint, as with dancers and runners

- Avascular necrosis of the sesamoids: Each sesamoid bone receives its blood supply mainly from one sesamoid artery off the medial and/or lateral plantar artery. With trauma, blood flow can be disrupted, leading to avascular necrosis.
- The patient experiences pain as a result of the following:
  - Sesamoiditis: Inflammation of soft tissue structures leads to pain and edema
  - Fractures: Nociceptors within the bone stimulated with fracture of either type, especially when weight bearing
  - Avascular necrosis: Pain caused by bone deterioration and collapse

EPIDEMIOLOGY AND DEMOGRAPHICS

- Sesamoid injury accounts for 9% of foot and ankle injuries and 1.2% of all running injuries.
- Sesamoid injury can occur within any age group, especially traumatic sesamoid injuries.
- Insufficiency fractures of the sesamoids occur more in the middle-aged to elderly population.
- The people most likely to develop an overuse or repetitive sesamoid injury are those who often load through a dorsiflexed first ray (e.g., runners, dancers, and those who wear high-heeled shoes).
- Infection of the sesamoids is most likely to occur in those who are immunosuppressed (via medication or disease), those who have lost sensation in the feet resulting in plantar ulcers (diabetes, peripheral neuropathies), those with poor circulation leading to plantar ulcers (those with atherosclerosis or peripheral vascular disease), or those who have had a puncture wound to the foot.
- Not all sesamoid abnormalities manifest with pain, such as a congenital bipartite sesamoid is present in 7.8% to 35% of the population. This can often be mistaken for a fractured sesamoid.

MECHANISM OF INJURY

- Sesamoiditis: Overuse, repetitive pressure soft tissue injury
  - Possibility of congenital predisposition if there exists asymmetry in size of the sesamoid, rotation of the sesamoid, or condylar malformation of the first metatarsal.
- Acute sesamoid fracture
  - Trauma involving hyperdorsiflexion of the first MTP joint
  - Direct axial load to a dorsiflexed first ray such as with a fall
  - Can also occur with dislocation of the first MTP joint.
- Stress fracture is related to activities involving repetitive loading through a dorsiflexed first MTP joint, as with dancers and runners.

- Avascular necrosis of the sesamoids can occur with trauma, after a crush injury, or with stress fracture. As a result of poor vascularization, the patient is susceptible to nontraumatic avascular necrosis caused by the following:
  - Emboli
  - Blood disorders such as sickle cell anemia
  - Long-term steroid use
  - Long-term alcohol use
  - Decompression disease
- Infections
  - Plantar ulcers associated with insensitivity or poor circulation
  - Puncture wounds
  - Use of medications that lower resistance to infections (e.g., antirheumatics such as methotrexate)

COMMON SIGNS AND SYMPTOMS

- Localized pain and tenderness on the plantar surface of the first MTP joint with or without swelling
- May complain of a grinding sensation.

AGGRAVATING ACTIVITIES

- Rising up onto toes
- Running
- Walking (especially terminal stance)
- Stair climbing
- Standing
- Wearing high-heeled shoes
- These activities produce direct pressure onto the sesamoids and mimic mechanism of injury in traumatic cases.
- These activities compress the sesamoids against the first MTP joint.

EASING ACTIVITIES

- Non-weight-bearing status, although in more severe and progressive cases of avascular necrosis, patients may have pain while not bearing weight as well
- Ice
- Antiinflammatory medications
- Avoid first MTP dorsiflexion: Use taping or a splint.
- Use over-the-counter turf toe pads
- Wearing firm-soled or rocker-bottomed shoes
- Ice and antiinflammatories address the inflammation and edema component of pain, if present.
- Turf toe pad, non-weight-bearing positions, and avoiding first MTP dorsiflexion ease symptoms because they do not allow direct pressure onto the sesamoid bones.

24-HOUR SYMPTOM PATTERN

- If inflammation is present, the patient can present with stiffness in the morning with gradual improvement.
- In most sesamoid disorders, symptoms are most apparent with weight-bearing activities.

- In later stages of avascular necrosis and with infections, there is constant pain throughout the day.

PAST HISTORY FOR THE REGION

- For acute fracture: Traumatic event without previous incident or injury to the foot or ankle.
- For stress fracture and avascular necrosis: May have previous history of pain over the plantar surface of the first MTP.
- Osteomyelitis: History of plantar pressure ulcer (and neurological deficit) or puncture wound that would account for the introduction of infection.

PHYSICAL EXAMINATION

- Avoidance of weight-bearing or asymmetrical weight-bearing activities that favor the involved foot.
- During gait, patients may reveal lack of trailing limb posture and a shortened stance phase on the affected side
- Flexor hallucis brevis and longus may be tender to palpation or may even elicit pain at the sesamoids because of the close anatomical relationship of their distal tendons and the sesamoids.

IMPORTANT OBJECTIVE TESTS

- No specific physical tests for sesamoids: Because of the close and intricate relationship between the sesamoids, the first MTP joint, and the flexor tendons, it is difficult to isolate a sesamoid pathology, which is why radiographs are often recommended to rule out fracture, osteoarthritis, and avascular necrosis.
- First ray ROM
  - Symptoms may be reproduced with passive dorsiflexion of the first ray.
- First MTP joint mobility or stability
  - Differentiates between first MTP instability or rigidus versus sesamoid injury
- Compression of the sesamoids to provoke symptoms
  - Reproduction of grinding may indicate osteoarthritis
- Palpation of region for edema and warmth

DIFFERENTIAL DIAGNOSIS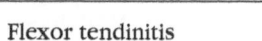

- Flexor tendinitis
- Turf toe
- Interdigital neuroma
- Gout
- RA
- Intractable plantar keratosis
- Osteoarthritis of the first MTP joint
- Osteonecrosis of the sesamoid
- Absent sesamoid
- Bipartite sesamoid

TREATMENT

SURGICAL OPTIONS

- Sesamoidectomy
- Curettage and grafting
- Bone graft for midwaist fractures
- Internal fixation

SURGICAL OUTCOME

- Sesamoidectomy
- Literature reports between 42% and 50% complete pain relief after sesamoidectomy.
- Although sesamoidectomy may relieve symptoms, the literature reports several complications postsurgically, as follows:
  - Intrinsic minus or cock-up deformity of the great toe
  - Hallux varus deformity
  - Exacerbation of a hallux valgus deformity
  - Hallux rigidus
  - Overload to the first MTP leading to osteoarthritis
- Curettage and grafting has been reported to be 89% successful without report of these complications.

REHABILITATION

- First course of action is nonsurgical treatment for at least 3 months for most sesamoid injuries. Usually this involves a period of casting or splinting and limited weight-bearing activities, depending on severity and type of disorder.
- Acute disorders should be treated using activity modification and RICE to relieve symptoms.
- Focus is on offloading the sesamoids with activity via orthoses, metatarsal pads, or devices to limit hallux dorsiflexion.
- Strengthening and proprioceptive or balance training address loss caused by immobilization and disuse.
- To decrease inflammation, the clinician may consider the following:
  - Pain-free AROM
  - Cold pack
  - Ultrasound: If no fracture or tumor is present
  - Electrical stimulation
- Once the inflammation process has decreased, the focus of rehabilitation should be on the following:
  - Eliminating the source of repetitive stress
  - External considerations such as taping, pads to offload sesamoids (placed proximal to sesamoids), and/or orthoses
- Early exercises in non–weight-bearing positions that actively go through pain-free ROM to promote circulation and reduce edema.

- Joint mobilization and manipulation are appropriate in the later phases of rehabilitation to address limitations in first MTP motion, specifically hallux dorsiflexion.
- Massage can be used in early rehabilitation (lymphatic massage or myofascial release) to reduce edema.
- In later stages, STM is appropriate for addressing soft tissue restrictions in mobility.
- Exercise plays a significant role in regaining strength and proprioceptive loss caused by disuse and immobilization.

CONTRIBUTING FACTORS

- Failure to incorporate modifications to footwear and activity
- Factors that contribute to nontraumatic sesamoid disorders are as follows:
  - Blood disorders that facilitate ischemia such as sickle cell anemia
  - Long-term steroid use
  - Long-term alcohol use
  - Systemic inflammatory disorders
  - Diabetes (neuropathic pressure ulcers)
  - Those who are immunosuppressed

PROGNOSIS

- Prognosis depends on type and severity of disorder such as the following:
  - Sesamoiditis and disorders responding to conservative care should continue to be asymptomatic with continued modification of activity and footwear.
  - Avascular necrosis or infection will likely require sesamoidectomy, which can resolve pain; however, iatrogenic complications are likely to cause other symptoms in patients.

SIGNS AND SYMPTOMS INDICATING REFERRAL TO PHYSICIAN

- Constant unrelenting pain: Infection or tumor
- Pain that does not change with position: Infection or tumor
- Major trauma: Fracture
- Fevers, fatigue, and chills: Infection or tumor
- Purulent exudate: Infection
- Allodynia, hyperesthesia, or sympathetic changes: Complex regional pain syndrome

SUGGESTED READINGS

Anderson RB, Shawen SB. Great-toe disorders. In: Porter DA, Schon LC, eds. *Baxter's the Foot and Ankle in Sport*. Philadelphia: Mosby, Inc; 2008.

Dedmond BT, Cory JW, McBryde A. The hallucal sesamoid complex. *J Am Acad Orthop Surg*. 2006;14(13):745-753.

Kanatli U, Ozturk AM, Ercan NG, Ozalay M, Daglar B, Yetkin H. Absence of the medial sesamoid bone associated with metatarsophalangeal pain. *Clin Anat.* 2006;19:634-639.

Karasick D, Schweitzer ME. Disorders of the hallux sesamoid complex: MR features. *Skeletal Radiol.* 1998;27:411-418.

Mandracchia VJ, Mandi DM, Toney PA, Halligan JB, Nickels WA. Fractures of the forefoot. *Clin Podiatr Med Surg.* 2006;23:283-301.

Vanore JV, Christensen JC, Kravitz SR, et al. Diagnosis and treatment of the first meta-tarsophalangeal joint disorders. Section 4: sesamoid disorders. *J Foot Ankle Surg.* 2003;42(3):143-147.

AUTHOR: MILDRED V. LIMCAY

BASIC INFORMATION

DEFINITION

Sinus tarsi syndrome results in pain over the sinus tarsi and the sensation of rear-foot instability that is thought to be the result of a combination of neuromuscular proprioceptive loss and compromise of the ligaments of the subtalar joint.

SYNONYMS

Subtalar joint instability

ICD-9CM CODES
726.79 Other enthesopathy of ankle and tarsus

OPTIMAL NUMBER OF VISITS

6 or fewer

MAXIMAL NUMBER OF VISITS

24

ETIOLOGY

- Sinus tarsi syndrome is usually a result of chronic inversion ankle sprains, leading to instability of the subtalar joint. Instability can result from disruption of the passive supportive structures of the joint (specifically the cervical ligament and interosseous talocalcaneal ligaments) or from loss of active support (neuromuscular proprioception).
- The source of pain has been disputed. Possibilities include the following:
  - Tears and/or fibrosis of the cervical or interosseous talocalcaneal ligaments
  - Hyperplasia of the synovial membrane
  - Neurogenic inflammation of the nociceptive and mechanoreceptors present in synovium
  - Synovitis
  - Posttraumatic fibrous changes in veins resulting in the impaction of venous outflow
  - Bleeding into the sinus tarsi
- Physiologically, the sinus tarsi is the talocalcaneal joint space formed by the sulcus of the talus and calcaneus. Contained in the sinus tarsi are the interosseous talocalcaneal ligament; the cervical ligament; the subtalar joint capsule; synovium; and medial, inferior, and lateral roots of the inferior lateral retinaculum and neurovasculature.
- There is general agreement on how sinus tarsi syndrome first occurs. An inflammatory event—most commonly an inversion ankle sprain—creates trauma or microtrauma to the ligaments and synovium within the sinus tarsi. The subsequent remodeling of the previously mentioned ligaments, synovium, and tissues is blamed for the etiology of pain and pathology. Inflammatory

diseases, such as RA and gout, have also been identified as predisposing factors in the development of sinus tarsi syndrome. Significant ligamentous instability of the subtalar joint need not be present in sinus tarsi syndrome.
- In neurohistological studies of synovial samples of those with sinus tarsi syndrome as opposed to a control subject, Akiyama et al found nociceptive free nerve endings and three mechanoreceptor variants: Pacinian, Golgi, and Ruffini corpuscles. The area of most neurodensity was present within the synovium located in the sinus tarsi in both controls and symptomatic individuals. Because of this finding, the authors hypothesized that the sinus tarsi is a region of great proprioceptive and nociceptive ability. Therefore inflammation or irritation here would produce pain, and altered proprioception would result in feelings of instability caused by altered neuromuscular control.
  - In the same study, findings of chronic synovitis with hypervascularization and lymphocytic infiltration were also reported.
  - Feelings of instability can be the result of actual ligamentous laxity or rupture (mechanical instability) and proprioceptive changes; thus neuromuscular insufficiency (functional instability) results.

EPIDEMIOLOGY AND DEMOGRAPHICS

- The most common age group for patients with sinus tarsi syndrome are those in their twenties and thirties.
- There are no gender and cultural predispositions to sinus tarsi syndrome.

MECHANISM OF INJURY

- Typically occurs after acute traumatic or chronic inversion injury to the ankle complex resulting in inflammation, microtrauma, and/or macrotrauma to the ligamentous or articular components.
- Inflammatory diseases, such as RA and gout, have been linked to sinus tarsi syndrome as predisposing factors.

COMMON SIGNS AND SYMPTOMS

- Pain
- Feeling of instability
- Possible edema over sinus tarsi
- Typically, pain is localized over the sinus tarsi.

AGGRAVATING ACTIVITIES

- Walking, especially on uneven ground
- Standing
- Running
- Jumping
- Wearing shoes with narrow base of support (heels)

EASING ACTIVITIES

- Sitting
- Limiting weight-bearing activities on affected side
- Wearing more stable shoes
- Use of orthotics
- Pain relievers

24-HOUR SYMPTOM PATTERN

Symptoms usually depend on aggravating factors.

PAST HISTORY FOR THE REGION

- History of inversion ankle sprain(s): Estimated that 70% of those with sinus tarsi syndrome have had an inversion ankle injury.
- Systemic inflammatory diseases affecting the foot include gout and RA.

PHYSICAL EXAMINATION

- Common physical findings:
  - Point tenderness over the sinus tarsi
  - Passive abduction and pronation of the heel and midfoot may reproduce symptoms
  - Swelling over the sinus tarsi may or may not be present.

IMPORTANT OBJECTIVE TESTS

- Talar tilt test (inversion)
  - A positive test indicates disruption of the interosseous talocalcaneal ligaments; it does not, however, confirm the presence of sinus tarsi syndrome, it only suggests the predisposing mechanism to the disorder and allows the clinician to determine if reported instability is due to ligamentous compromise.
- Anterior drawer test
  - Test of the talocrural joint and laxity of the anterior talofibular ligament. A positive test does not confirm the presence of sinus tarsi syndrome, it only suggests the predisposing mechanism to the disorder and allows the clinician to determine if reported instability is due to ligamentous compromise.

DIFFERENTIAL DIAGNOSIS

- Anterior talofibular sprain
- Subtalar instability
- Superficial peroneal nerve irritation
- L5 or S1 nerve root irritation
- Osteochondral lesion of the talus

CONTRIBUTING FACTORS

- Functional or mechanical instability of the foot and ankle
- Previous foot and ankle sprain
- Autoimmune or chronic inflammatory disorders (RA or gout)
- Impaired neuromuscular control in the ankle and hip

TREATMENT

SURGICAL OPTIONS

- Arthroscopic debridement
- Arthroscopic synovectomy
- Interosseous talocalcaneal ligament reconstruction

SURGICAL OUTCOMES

- Pisani reported that postsurgically, the amount of passive instability is reduced and the patient's ability to single limb balance is improved.
- Surgical indicators include the following:
  - Failure of conservative interventions (injection, orthotic therapy, physical therapy) to manage symptoms and instability
  - Instability of the subtalar joint as the result of compromised passive stabilizers

REHABILITATION

- Proprioceptive training is an important consideration in the rehabilitation of sinus tarsi syndrome.
- To decrease inflammation, the clinician should consider the following:
  - Cryotherapy
  - Joint mobilization
  - Ultrasound
  - Therapeutic exercises
  - Lymphatic massage
- Once the inflammation process has decreased, the focus of rehabilitation should be on the following:
  - Neuromuscular reeducation: Balance and proprioceptive training to restore dynamic stability of the foot and ankle. Balance training has been shown to decrease deficits in postural control.
  - Taping or bracing has been shown to help with postural control in those who have already sustained one lateral ankle sprain. In those who have never sustained a lateral ankle sprain, it has been shown to be ineffective or even diminishes the response to perturbations in balance.
  - Foot orthoses have also been reported to assist in alleviating symptoms of pain and instability in a person with sinus tarsi syndrome. Hertel discusses previous studies regarding orthoses and alleviation of pain and instability and notes improvement in symptoms without details in posting or orthotic specifics.
- Balance exercises progressing to return to sport or activity should target both ankle and hip strategies with perturbations in balance.
- Long-term exercises
  - Proprioceptive and balance training helps prevent recurrent inversion ankle injury, which is the most common cause of sinus tarsi syndrome. This training helps prevent and address dynamic instability of the talocrural and subtalar joint, which can also lead to other foot and ankle disorders.
  - Exercises targeting the proximal hip musculature would assist in prevention, according to Bullock-Saxton, who identified a delay in hip muscle function after severe ankle sprain.
  - For those who are active in sports, external bracing should be considered.

PROGNOSIS

Because the mechanism of injury is related to an inversion sprain injury, the patient is more likely to have recurrent inversion injuries without proprioceptive training. Increased occurrence of this type of injury only contributes to recurrent episodes of sinus tarsi syndrome.

SIGNS AND SYMPTOMS INDICATING REFERRAL TO PHYSICIAN

- Pain that does not change with position: Infection or tumor
- Significant and unexplained weight loss: Tumor
- Major trauma: Fracture
- Inability to bear weight: Fracture
- Fevers and chills: Infection or tumor

SUGGESTED READINGS

Akiyama K, Takakura Y, Tomita Y, Sugimoto K, Tanaka Y, Tama S. Neurohistory of the sinus tarsi and sinus tarsi syndrome. *J Orthop Sci.* 1999;4:299-303.

Chao W. Interdigital neuroma and tarsal tunnel syndrome. In: Richardson EG, ed. *Orthopedic Knowledge Update:Foot and Ankle.* Rosemont, IL:American Academy of Orthopedic Surgeons; 2004.

Hertel J. Functional instability following lateral ankle sprain. *Sports Med.* 2000;29(5):361-371.

Pisani G, Pisani PC, Parino E. Sinus tarsi syndrome and subtalar joint instability. *Clin Podiatr Surg Med.* 2005;22:63-77.

Sauer ST, Hanson TW, Marymont JV. Disorders of the subtalar joint, including subtalar sprains and tarsal coalitions. In: Porter DA, Schon LC, eds. *Baxter's The Foot and Ankle in Sport.* Philadelphia: Mosby, Inc; 2008.

Swarzenbach B, Dora C, Lang A, Kissling RO. Blood vessels in the sinus tarsi and sinus tarsi syndrome. *Clin Anat.* 1997;10:173-182.

Tropp H, Askling C, Gillquist J. Prevention of ankle sprains. *Am J Sports Med.* 1985;13:259-262.

AUTHOR: MILDRED V. LIMCAY

Section III

ORTHOPEDIC PATHOLOGY

BASIC INFORMATION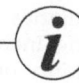

DEFINITION

- Damage to the articular cartilage and/or underlying bone of the superior articular surface of the talus within the ankle mortise is described as chondral only, subchondral only, or chondral-subchondral.
- Berndt and Harty classification system is as follows:
  - Stage I: small compression fracture of the talar dome
  - Stage II: Incomplete avulsion
  - Stage III: Complete avulsion
  - Stage IV: Displaced fragment
- Pritsch (arthroscopic classification) system is as follows:
  - Grade I: Intact, firm cartilage
  - Grade II: Intact, soft cartilage
  - Grade III: Frayed cartilage

SYNONYMS

- Osteochondral lesion
- Avascular necrosis of the talar dome
- Transchondral fracture
- Osteochondritis desiccans
- Talar dome fracture
- Flaked fracture

ICD-9CM CODES
732.7 Osteochondral desiccans
733.44 Aseptic necrosis of talus
718.07 Articular cartilage disorder
          involving ankle and foot

OPTIMAL NUMBER OF VISITS

6 or fewer

MAXIMAL NUMBER OF VISITS

18

ETIOLOGY

- The origins of injury and areas of the talar dome that are most often injured are as follows:
  - Traumatic origin: Anterolateral (98%) or posteromedial (78%) aspect of the talar dome
  - Atraumatic origin: Posteromedial aspect of the talar dome
  - Anterolateral lesions tend to be more shallow, wafer-like, and more apt to become displaced.
  - Posteromedial lesions tend to be deeper lesions that do not get displaced.
- Damage to the talar dome occurs because the talar dome has poor vascularity. An osteochondral lesion occurs when blood supply is disrupted (through trauma, emboli, etc) and the involved dome fragment is left without direct vascularization. With continued weight bearing, the fragment may

not heal and collapse, lead to cartilage defect, and/or break away from the parent bone and remain loose within the talocrural joint.
- Patients experience pain because of the following:
  - Local inflammation and edema in a confined space
  - Bone has nociceptive afferents, therefore if the lesion is subchondral, nociceptors are stimulated.
  - If the lesion becomes displaced, it can become trapped between the talus and mortise, thus stimulating the nociceptors on these structures.

EPIDEMIOLOGY AND DEMOGRAPHICS

- Most common presentation is a man, 25 to 35 years of age, who is participating in activities that would predispose to ankle sprains (jumping sports, cutting sports).
- Others affected are as follows:
  - Those with genetic predisposition
  - Those with systemic inflammatory diseases
- Most people experience pain, which is often how the lesion is found: The complaint of persistent pain after an ankle sprain is usually what brings the patient in for further work-up.

MECHANISM OF INJURY

- Trauma is the primary cause of talar dome damage.
  - Anterolateral lesions: Inversion trauma in dorsiflexion causes abutment between the anterolateral aspect of the talar dome with the fibula. It can occur in conjunction with a distal fibular fracture.
  - Posteromedial lesion: Inversion trauma in plantar flexion with tibial external rotation leads to compression of the posteromedial talus with the tibial plafond.
  - Some believe lesions can occur with recurrent inversion ankle sprains, resulting in unresolved instability.
- Atraumatic causes, with proposed theories, are as follows:
  - Infarct caused by fat emboli, sickle cell anemia, or corticosteroid use
  - Endocrinologic conditions
  - Systemic inflammatory conditions such as RA, SLE, or ankylosing spondylitis
  - Genetic predisposition

COMMON SIGNS AND SYMPTOMS

- History of an ankle sprain with persistent pain local to area of lesion with or without swelling
- Duration of symptoms lasts well beyond time frame for ligamentous healing (several months to years).

- Complaints of "catching," "locking," or "grinding" that may suggest presence of a loose fragment
- Complaints of the ankle being "unstable" or "giving way" with pain

AGGRAVATING ACTIVITIES

- Prolonged standing
- Walking
- Ascending and descending stairs
- Activities requiring dorsiflexion, especially with anterolateral lesions, such as squatting or lunging
- Activities requiring plantar flexion, especially with posteromedial lesions, such as going up onto toes or reaching
- Running
- Cutting (running with sudden change of direction)
- Compression of joint surfaces
- Activities, such as running and cutting, cause shear forces of talus within mortise

EASING ACTIVITIES

- Non–weight-bearing activities
- Antiinflammatories
- Ice
- Non–weight-bearing activities allow space between the talus and mortise. Antiinflammatories and ice address inflammation and edema.

24-HOUR SYMPTOM PATTERN

- Stiffness caused by inflammation in the morning with gradual resolution
- Worsening depends on activity with cumulative effect throughout the day.

PAST HISTORY FOR THE REGION

- History of one or multiple ankle sprains of the involved side
- Of all ankle sprains, it is estimated that osteochondral lesions occur in 6.5% of these incidents.

PHYSICAL EXAMINATION

- Patients often limit weight-bearing activities over the involved limb. This may be seen as a reduction in stance time during gait or a weight shift away from the involved side with standing.
- During non–weight-bearing activities, the involved side takes up the loose pack position of the talocrural joint, approximately 30 degrees plantar flexion.

IMPORTANT OBJECTIVE TESTS

- Talar tilt test
  - To assess for medial or lateral instability that would predispose to this type of injury.
- Anterior and posterior drawer testing
  - To assess for anterior to posterior stability and for any crepitus or grinding that may indicate a loose body.

- Talocrural ROM
  - Active versus passive with attention quantity of each (similarity versus discrepancy), crepitus or catching, and end-feel with PROM. It may indicate loose body within joint.

DIFFERENTIAL DIAGNOSIS

- Talar fracture
- Syndesmotic sprain or rupture
- Anterior or posterior talocrural impingement
- Osteoarthritis
- FHL, flexor digitorum profundus, or posterior tibialis tendinopathy (for posteromedial lesions)
- Anterior talofibular ligament sprain (for anterolateral lesion)
- Sinus tarsi syndrome
- Seronegative systemic arthropathy
- Localized infection

TREATMENT

SURGICAL OPTIONS

- Debridement
- Mosaicplasty
- Autologous chondrocyte transplant
- Drilling or microfracture to stimulate bleeding in the area
- Internal fixation
- Bone grafting

SURGICAL OUTCOMES

- Pritsch et al found good results in 13 of 14 patients who underwent arthroscopic debridement.
- Tol et al performed a systematic review of treatment options for osteochondral lesions based on 54 studies (684 subjects, average age 26 years, male-to-female ratio not reported). A successful treatment was classified as one that produced a good or excellent result, although there was no information regarding what quantified a "good" or "excellent" result.
  - Calculated surgical success (overall): 75%
  - Fragment excision: 39 patients total, 38% reported successful treatment
  - Excision and curettage: of 11 studies and 141 patients, 78% reported successful treatment
  - Excision, curettage, and drilling: Unable to determine
- Nonoperative: In 14 studies with 201 patients, 45% reported successful treatment.

REHABILITATION

- Nonoperative treatment
- Based on literature, casting with non–weight-bearing or partial weight-bearing status from 3 weeks to 4 months and cessation of sport or activity.

- After pain resolves, focus is on restoration of ROM and strength.
- Postoperative
  - Weight-bearing status and progression of weight-bearing depends on surgical intervention and severity of lesion. Generally, procedures that require regeneration or repair of articular cartilage have a longer period of non–weight-bearing or partial weight-bearing status.
  - AROM: Degree of which depends on procedure and healing times
  - Gait training: With and without assistive devices
  - Proprioceptive or neuromuscular reeducation
  - Strengthening
  - Joint mobilization and STM to restore mobility
- To decrease inflammation, the clinician should consider the following:
  - Lymphedema massage
  - Myofascial release
  - Joint mobilization
  - AROM in a pain-free range
  - Cold pack
  - Ultrasound
  - Electrical stimulation
- Once the inflammation process has decreased, the focus of rehabilitation should be on the following:
  - Restoration of mobility via STM and joint mobilization
  - Restoration of normal gait (within weight-bearing precautions)
  - Balance and proprioceptive training
  - Trop and associates identified rehabilitation using balance discs to prevent occurrence and recurrence of inversion ankle injuries by addressing functional instability and impaired postural control after ankle sprain.
- Strength training: Around the ankle and proximal hip musculature
  - Mediolateral sway is controlled primarily at the foot and ankle, secondarily by the hip.
- Initial exercises in non–weight-bearing position that actively go through pain-free ROM to promote circulation and reduce edema. Must take into consideration any precautions with ROM.
- Joint mobilization or manipulation are appropriate in the later phases of rehabilitation to address joint-specific mobility restrictions after immobilization at the talocrural joint, distal tibiofibular joint, and subtalar and tarsal joints.
- Massage can be used in early rehabilitation (lymphatic massage or myofascial release) to reduce edema.
- In later stages, STM is appropriate to address soft tissue restrictions in mobility.
- Exercise has a significant role in preventing recurrence of inversion ankle injuries, specifically those that target proprioceptive and balance training.

- In both nonoperative and operative treatments, immobilization with non–weight-bearing status is part of the protocol, with immobilization lasting anywhere from 6 weeks to several months. Exercise is significant in regaining strength to those muscles that have undergone disuse atrophy not only around the foot and ankle but also along the entire affected lower quarter.
- Long-term exercises: Proprioceptive and balance training to prevent inversion ankle injury, which is the most common cause of osteochondral lesions. Also, this helps prevent dynamic instability of the talocrural joint, which can also lead to other foot and ankle disorders.
  - Exercises targeting the proximal hip musculature would assist in prevention, according to Bullock-Saxton, who identified a delay in hip muscle function after severe ankle sprain.
  - For patients who are active in sport, external bracing should be considered.

CONTRIBUTING FACTORS

- Structural or functional instability of the ankle complex
- Diseases or conditions that would slow the healing process (e.g., diabetes, long-term steroid use, systemic inflammatory disorders, smoking, or sickle cell anemia)

PROGNOSIS

- Finger et al reported that 12 out of 41 medial osteochondral lesions developed into arthritis.
  - 34.5 months after autologous cartilage transplant, 85% of patients had good-to-excellent follow-up.

SIGNS AND SYMPTOMS INDICATING REFERRAL TO PHYSICIAN

- Constant unrelenting pain: Infection or tumor
- Pain that does not change with position: Infection or tumor
- History of cancer: Metastatic disease
- Fevers and chills: Infection or tumor
- Purulent exudate (after surgery): Infection
- Allodynia, hyperesthesia, or sympathetic changes: Complex regional pain syndrome

SUGGESTED READINGS

Berndt A, Harty M. Transchondral fractures (osteochondritis desiccans) of the talus. *J Bone Joint Surg.* 1959;41A:988–1020.

Bowman M. Osteochondral lesions of the talus and occult fractures of the foot and ankle. In: Porter DA, Schon LC, eds. *Baxter's The Foot and Ankle in Sport.* Philadelphia: Mosby, Inc; 2008.

Bullock-Saxton JE. Local sensation changes and altered hip muscle function following severe ankle sprain. *Phys Ther.* 1994;74:23-37.

Finger A, Sheskier M. Osteochondral lesions of the talar dome. *Hosp Joint Dis.* 2006; 61(3&4):155-159.

Hertel J. Functional instability following lateral ankle sprain. *Sports Med.* 2000; 29(5):361-371.

Pritsch M, Horoshovski H, Farine I. Arthroscopic treatment of osteochondral lesions of the talus. *J Bone Joint Surg Am.* 1986;68:862-865.

Takao M, Ochi M, Uchio Y, Naito K, Kono T, Oae K. Osteochondral lesions of the talar dome associated with trauma. *Arthrosc: J Arthrosc Relat Surg.* 2003;19(10):1061-1067.

Tol J, Struijs P, Bossuyt P, Verhagen R, van Dijk C. Treatment strategies in osteochondral defects of the talar dome: a systematic review. *Foot Ankle Int.* 2000;20(2):119-126.

Tropp H, Askling C, Gillquist J. Prevention of ankle sprains. *Am J Sports Med.* 1985; 13:259-262.

AUTHOR: MILDRED V. LIMCAY

BASIC INFORMATION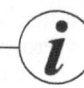

DEFINITION

- Turf toe is a sprain of the ligamentous and capsular support structures of the first MTP joint, with or without involvement of the tendons of the great toe flexors and extensors, as well as the two sesamoid bones embedded in the flexor tendons.
- Classified as the following:
  - Grade I: Strain of the joint capsule, all soft tissue components remain intact.
  - Grade II: Partial thickness tearing of the plantar plate and capsular structures, sesamoids remain in normal position.
  - Grade III: Complete disruption of joint capsule, plantar plate, and collateral ligaments. The plantar plate may have avulsed from its proximal attachment at the distal metatarsal. Sesamoid bones may fracture or displace proximally; and because of the complete disruption of capsule and ligaments, fracture of the metatarsal is possible as a result of impaction.

SYNONYMS

- Sprain of the first MTP
- Sand toe

ICD-9CM CODES
845.12 Metatarsophalangeal (joint) sprain

OPTIMAL NUMBER OF VISITS

3 or fewer

MAXIMAL NUMBER OF VISITS

36

ETIOLOGY

- With a hyperextension injury, which makes up approximately 85% of cases of turf toe, the plantar plate, MCL and LCL, and joint capsule are most injured.
- Usually the injury is associated with sports activity involving play on artificial turf versus grass. It is more commonly seen with football, baseball, wrestling, basketball, and soccer athletes.
- Acute hyperextension injury was reported as 85% of turf toe injuries by Allen et al. Injury occurs during weight bearing with the forefoot planted and first MTP in dorsiflexion when an axial load through the heel, either through push-off or via external force of another person, drives the first MTP into excessive dorsiflexion. This results in attenuation or tear of the joint capsule and plantar plate off its proximal, looser attachment to the first metatarsal and compression of the dorsal articular surface of the metatarsal head. Severity of damage to these support structures, as well as

additional damage to the sesamoids, proximal phalanges, distal metatarsals, and flexor and extensor tendons, depends on the intensity of the applied load.
- Acute valgus injury is less common than hyperextension. Mechanism of injury is thought to be the presence of an excessive valgus stress during push-off with the first MTP in a dorsiflexed position. With this mechanism, the MCL, in addition to the joint capsule and plantar plate, is affected.
- Acute hyperflexion injury, the least common as reported by Childs, occurs with forcible flexion of the first MTP while in a position of first MTP plantar flexion, causing attenuation or disruption of the dorsal joint capsule and compression of the plantar articular surface of the metatarsal head.
- In acute injuries, nociceptors within ligaments and joint capsule are stimulated with attenuation or tear. Inflammation resulting from ligamentous injury bathes the area in chemical mediators (substance P, bradykinin, etc) that can sensitize neurons, thus perpetuating pain.
- Edema within the joint can produce feelings of pressure and ache.

EPIDEMIOLOGY AND DEMOGRAPHICS

- Childs reports that there are no age-, gender-, or race-related predispositions to turf toe.
- Most patients do experience pain with this injury.

MECHANISM OF INJURY

The capsular, ligamentous, and tendinous stabilizers of the first MTP is most commonly injured by hyperextension of the great toe with an axial load (85% of cases). Less common mechanisms include hyperflexion and varus and valgus stress loads to the first MTP.

COMMON SIGNS AND SYMPTOMS

- The common presentation for turf toe is as follows:
  - Grade I: Usually no discoloration, but swelling in the dorsum of the forefoot is evident. The patient should be able to bear weight and has mild limitation in motion, especially into dorsiflexion, since this is painful.
  - Grade II: Pain with ecchymosis and moderate edema, especially over the dorsum of the first MTP joint. Patients may avoid full weight bearing on the affected side due to pain, resulting in a limp with gait. ROM is limited, especially into dorsiflexion with pain.
  - Grade III: Severe pain and tenderness with significant loss of ROM, ecchymosis, and edema. Because of severity of pain, patient may not bear weight on the affected side.

AGGRAVATING ACTIVITIES

- Depending on grade of injury
  - Weight bearing
  - Dorsiflexion of the first MTP, passively or actively
  - Plantar flexion of the first MTP, passively or actively
  - Compression of the forefoot, type of shoe worn (tight shoe box)
  - Walking, especially barefoot or in flexible-soled shoes
  - Running
  - Rising up onto toes (heel raise)
- Activities and positions that require MTP dorsiflexion place stress on the attenuated or torn plantar support structures. MTP plantar flexion places stress on the attenuated or torn dorsal support structures. In the presence of interarticular edema, symptoms can be aggravated with either position.
- With walking, symptoms are exacerbated with weight bearing and progression of the body over the forefoot, thus forcing the great toe into dorsiflexion.

EASING ACTIVITIES

- Non–weight-bearing or partial weight-bearing activities
- Antiinflammatory medication
- Pain-relieving medications
- Wearing firm-soled or rocker-bottom shoes can prevent extension at the MTP during walking, thus not allowing attenuation of plantar support structures.
- Ice: In the presence of acute injury, ice and medication can address inflammation.

24-HOUR SYMPTOM PATTERN

Symptoms depend on use and if swelling is present, and therefore are usually more prominent by the end of day, with time spent on feet and time spent with foot in a gravity-dependent position.

PAST HISTORY FOR THE REGION

- No history of injury to the foot and ankle to predispose to this injury.
- Chronic cases do involve a previous history of one or repeated injury to the first MTP support structures that has caused complete disruption of the capsuloligamentous structures.
- In chronic cases as a result of systemic inflammatory disorders, other joints of the foot can be involved.

PHYSICAL EXAMINATION

- The patient may avoid weight bearing on the affected side.
- With a chronic injury that has resulted in disruption of first MTP stabilizers, deviation or deformity of the great toe may be seen, including angulation medially or laterally, hammer toe, or subluxation.
- Intrinsic minus position: MTP extension with interphalangeal flexion may indicate

plantar plate avulsion or rupture of the flexor hallucis brevis on one or both of the sesamoids.

- Possible tenderness to palpation of the toe flexors and/or extensors caused by guarding, but symptoms are not reproduced.

IMPORTANT OBJECTIVE TESTS

- First MTP testing: AROM and PROM
  - In acute injury, both dorsiflexion and plantar flexion is limited, more so, however, toward the direction of the mechanism of injury caused by pain.
  - In subacute and especially chronic phases, hypermobility may be noted toward direction of injury caused by attenuation of capsule and ligaments.
  - If the toe has a hard or blocked endfeel one should suspect a foreign body within the joint.
- Varus and valgus testing assesses for compromise of MCL and LCL of the first MTP.
- Accessory mobility: Depending on severity of injury and capsuloligamentous damage, laxity in end-feel and hypermobility in the arthrokinematic motion associated with direction of injury. For example, with the hyperextension mechanism, there may be laxity in end-feel and hypermobility in dorsal glide of the proximal phalanx relative to the metatarsal.

DIFFERENTIAL DIAGNOSIS

- Sesamoiditis
- Stress fracture
- Septic arthritis of the first MTP
- Osteoarthritis of the first MTP
- Gout
- RA
- Intermetatarsal bursitis

TREATMENT

SURGICAL OPTIONS

- Surgical indicators are as follows:
  - Loose body in the joint
  - Large cartilage flaps
  - Sesamoid fracture or retraction
  - Gross instability of the first MTP
  - Traumatic hallux valgus
  - Significant plantar plate avulsion

SURGICAL OUTCOMES

- Surgery is indicated in cases with instability at the first MTP joint and with sesamoid fracture or retraction. In cases of instability, Mullen describes surgery that may involve attempts to repair the capsule directly, or if it cannot be repaired, transposition of the abductor hallucis to stabilize the joint. With a sesamoid

fracture, removal of the affected sesamoid is performed.

- Mullen reports a good result postsurgically and recommends surgery with instability or in cases where conservative care is ineffective.

REHABILITATION

- Acute injury
  - RICE
  - Modalities, such as pulsed ultrasound, may be used to help control edema as long as fracture has been ruled out.
- Dependent on grade of injury
  - Grade I: The patient should be able to resume sports or activity participation with use of a stiff insole or taping during activity until irritation has subsided. Once pain is reduced, focus shifts to regaining AROM and PROM of the first MTP via joint mobilization, stretching, and exercises. Balance also needs to be evaluated and addressed, especially in the context of the activity the patient would like to return to.
  - Grade II: Requires up to 2 weeks of rest (stopped sports or activity) with more time with toe taped or use of stiff insole as the result of more severe injury to the capsule and ligaments of the first MTP joint. Rehabilitation is similar to that of grade I injury after pain has subsided.
  - Grade III: Rehabilitation usually begins after 4 to 6 weeks of immobilization or postsurgically. Because of the longer period of immobilization, expect adjacent joints to also lose ROM. Until the first stabilizers heal postsurgically or via immobilization, rehabilitation should focus on regaining or maintaining ROM at the talocrural and subtalar joints, protective weight bearing, and prevention of strength loss of the proximal musculature. If tendon transfer was performed, active contraction of the parent muscle is contraindicated until cleared by the surgeon. Once cleared, progression of rehabilitation is similar to that as described.
- Return to activity should progress from walking to running to cutting to plyometrics, depending on the type of sport.
- To return to the activity or sport, the patient should have painless first MTP dorsiflexion of 50 to 60 degrees.
- To decrease inflammation, the clinician should consider the following:
  - Joint mobilization
  - Exercises that promote movement of the region in a pain-free range
  - Cold or hot pack
  - Ultrasound
  - Electrical stimulation
  - Lymphatic massage
- Once the inflammation process has decreased, the focus of rehabilitation should be on the following:

  - Restoring ROM, balance, and strength
  - Progression to return to sport or activity
- Initial exercises
  - In grade I and II exercises, active ROM exercises within pain-free ROM can help reduce inflammation in the region.

CONTRIBUTING FACTORS

- Childs identified the following predisposing factors:
  - Previous history of first MTP injury
  - Artificial turf and playing surface
  - Type of sport played (football players more susceptible)
  - Flattened first MTP
  - Foot pronation
  - Hallux degenerative joint disease
  - Increased toe box flexibility and decreased number of cleats in the shoe
  - Pes planus
  - Hypermobility of the talocrural joint

PROGNOSIS

- Most recover from turf toe and can return to activity with or without modification in footwear, custom orthoses, or use of a firm plate in the forefoot of the shoe to prevent hyperextension.
- Previous episodes can predispose a patient to turf toe again in the future.

SIGNS AND SYMPTOMS INDICATING REFERRAL TO PHYSICIAN

- Constant unrelenting foot pain: Infection
- Pain that does not change with position or weight bearing: Infection
- Allodynia, hyperesthesia, sympathetic changes: Complex regional pain syndrome
- Streaking along skin toward lymph nodes: Infection
- Worsening or non improvement of symptoms: Fracture or infection
- Major trauma: Fracture
- Fevers and chills: Infection or tumor

SUGGESTED READINGS

Allen LR, Flemming D, Sanders TG. Turf Toe: ligamentous injury of the first metatarsophalangeal joint. *Mil Med*. 2004;169:14-24.

Childs SG. The pathogenesis and biomechanics of turf toe. *Orthop Nurs*. 2006;25(4):276-282.

Mullen JE, O'Malley MJ. Sprains—residual instability of the subtalar, Lisfranc joints and turf toe. *Clin Sports Med*. 2004;23:97-121.

Padanilam TG. Disorders of the first ray. In: Richardson EG, ed. *Orthopedic Knowledge Update: Foot and Ankle*. Rosemont: American Academy of Orthopedic Surgeons; 2004.

AUTHOR: MILDRED V. LIMCAY

BASIC INFORMATION

DEFINITION

Freiberg's osteochondrosis is an osteo-chondrosis of the lesser metatarsal epi-physis, which results in the degeneration of the metatarsal phalangeal joint (MTP). Most infractions occur at the second and third metatarsal; the second is affected more often.

SYNONYMS

- Freiberg's infraction
- Infraction of the metatarsal head
- Osteochondrosis of the metatarsal head
- Avascular necrosis of the metatarsal head
- Panner disease of the metatarsals
- Osteochondritis deformans metatarso-juvenilis
- Malacopathia
- Subchondral bone fatigue fracture of the metatarsal head
- Dorsal trabecular stress injury of the metatarsal head

ICD-9CM CODES
732.5 Juvenile osteochondrosis of foot

OPTIMAL NUMBER OF VISITS

12 or fewer

MAXIMAL NUMBER OF VISITS

24

ETIOLOGY

- Freiberg's osteochondrosis has a mul-tifactorial etiology that includes vascu-lar and traumatic insults. It has been reported that certain patients may have a congenital predisposition.
- Initial synovitis is followed by sclerosis, resorption, plate fracture and collapse, and bone formation.

EPIDEMIOLOGY AND DEMOGRAPHICS

- The individuals most commonly affected range in age from adolescence through the second decade of life. However, Freiberg's osteochondrosis can occur at any age, with ages 8 to 77 years reported in the literature.
- The disease is most often seen in young women, with an overall male-to-female ratio of approximately 1:5.

MECHANISM OF INJURY

Repetitive microtrauma to the metatarsal head

COMMON SIGNS AND SYMPTOMS

- Swelling
- Stiffness

- Callus may be present under the affected metatarsal head.
- Limp
- Vague forefoot pain related to activity

AGGRAVATING ACTIVITIES

- Passive range of motion (PROM) of the MTP joint
- Activities that require high impact to the forefoot such as running and jumping
- High-heeled shoes
- Toe walking

EASING ACTIVITIES

- Rest
- Limited weight-bearing activities

24-HOUR SYMPTOM PATTERN

Increased pain at the end of the day or after prolonged weight-bearing activities

PAST HISTORY FOR THE REGION

May have a chronic history of forefoot pain with episodic exacerbation or a sud-den onset of pain related to a specific injury.

PHYSICAL EXAMINATION

- Tenderness to palpation of the metatar-sal head
- MTP joint effusion
- Antalgic gait
- Tailor's bunion (bunion of the fifth metatarsal head due to compensation)

IMPORTANT OBJECTIVE TESTS

- ROM of MTP joints (limited PROM of the affected MTP joint)
- Manual muscle test (MMT) toe flexors and extensors (weakness and/or pain may be present)
- Morton's test: Pain reproduced with compression of medial and lateral meta-tarsal heads is a positive sign for stress fracture or neuroma.

DIFFERENTIAL DIAGNOSES

- Metatarsalgia
- Morton's neuroma
- Stress fracture of the metatarsal
- Synovitis

CONTRIBUTING FACTORS

- Long second metatarsal head with altered first ray mechanics leads to overload of the second metatarsal joint.
- Decreased mobility of the second and third metatarsals leads to increased risk of sustaining repetitive microtrauma.
- Weakness of toe flexors (especially of the first digit) results in an increased susceptibility to injury of the second metatarsal.

TREATMENT

SURGICAL OPTIONS

- Simple debridement
- Bone grafting
- Dorsal closing wedge osteotomy
- Shortening osteotomy
- Resection arthroplasty
- Total small joint arthroplasty

SURGICAL OUTCOMES

Surgery for Freiberg's infraction is rare and there is currently no consensus as to which procedure would warrant the best results. Generally, if conservative treatment fails, then the least destruc-tive and invasive procedure is consid-ered first.

REHABILITATION

- Modalities for pain and inflammation in acute phase
- Non–weight-bearing cast can be used for severe acute pain.
- Joint mobilization to first ray and invol-ved MTP joint
- Stretching of gastrocnemius/soleus muscle
- Strengthening of toe flexors
- Shoe modifications such as metatar-sal bar or pad, rocker bottom, or rigid shank
- Orthotics

PROGNOSIS

- If the plate fracture does not prog-ress into a loose body, the lesion can heal spontaneously with conservative treatment.
- If the fracture affects joint congruity, surgery may be indicated.

SIGNS AND SYMPTOMS INDICATING REFERRAL TO PHYSICIAN

- If the patient is unable to fully bear weight on the affected lower extremity, a fracture should be ruled out.
- If pain continues, becomes significant at rest, awakens the patient from sleep, or is associated with significant swelling or redness, tests should be performed to rule out other causes such as tumor or osteomyelitis.

SUGGESTED READINGS

Ary Jr KR, Turnbo M. Freiberg's infraction: an osteochondritis of the metatarsal head. *J Am Podiatr Assoc.* 1979;69(2):131-132.

Bainbridge DB. Sports injuries in chil-dren. In: Campbell SK, Vander Linden DW, Palisano RJ. *Physical Therapy for Children.* 3rd ed. Philadelphia: Saunders; 2006:517-556.

Binek R, Levinsohn EM, Bersani F, Rubenstein H. Freiberg disease complicating unrelated trauma. *Orthopedics.* 1988;11(5):753-757.

Blitz NM, Yu JH. Freiberg's infraction in identical twins: a case report. *J Foot Ankle Surg.* 2005;44(3):218-221.

Evans RC. *Illustrated Essentials in Orthopedic Physical Assessment.* St. Louis: C.V. Mosby; 1994.

Gauthier G, Elbaz R. Freiberg's infraction: a subchondral bone fatigue fracture. A new surgical treatment. *Clin Orthop Relat Res.* 1979;(142):93-95.

Katcherian DA. Treatment of Freiberg's disease. *Orthop Clin North Am.* 1994;25(1):69-81.

Maresca G, Adriani E, Falez F, Mariani PP. Arthroscopic treatment of bilateral Freiberg's infraction. *Arthroscopy.* 1996;12(1):103-108.

Nguyen VD, Keh RA, Daehler RW. Freiberg's disease in diabetes mellitus. *Skeletal Radiol.* 1991;20(6):425-428.

Stanley D, Betts RP, Rowley DI, et al. Assessment of etiologic factors in the development of Freiberg's disease. *J Foot Surg.* 1990;29(5):444-447.

Tachdjiian MO. Freiberg's infraction. In: Tachdjian MO, ed. *Pediatric Orthopedics.* 2nd ed. Philadelphia: WB Saunders; 1990:1006-1010.

Thompson FM, Hamilton WG. Problems of the second metatarsophalangeal joint. *Orthopedics.* 1987;10(1):83-89.

AUTHORS: ERICA PABLO and LEESHA AUGUSTINE

BASIC INFORMATION

DEFINITION

Juvenile rheumatoid arthritis (JRA) is one of the most common chronic diseases of childhood. The American College of Rheumatology's criteria for classification of JRA are as follows:

- Age of onset <16 years
- Presence of arthritis in one or more joints defined as swelling or effusion or in the absence of swelling, by the presence of at least two of the following:
  - Limitation of ROM
  - Tenderness or pain on motion
  - Increased heat over a joint
- Duration of disease: At least 6 weeks
- Type of onset in the first 6 months characterized as one of the three onset types of JRA
- Exclusion of other rheumatic or viral diseases that may mimic JRA

The three onset types of JRA are as follows:

- Pauciarticular or oligoarticular
- Polyarticular
- Systemic onset also known as Still's disease

SYNONYMS

- JRA
- Juvenile idiopathic arthritis
- Juvenile chronic arthritis
- Juvenile arthritis

ICD-9CM CODES
714.30 Chronic or unspecified polyarticular juvenile rheumatoid arthritis
714.31 Acute polyarticular juvenile rheumatoid arthritis
714.32 Pauciarticular juvenile rheumatoid arthritis
714.33 Monoarticular juvenile rheumatoid arthritis

OPTIMAL NUMBER OF VISITS

24 or fewer

MAXIMAL NUMBER OF VISITS

36

ETIOLOGY

- Exact etiology is unknown; however, JRA is considered to be an autoimmune disorder that is multifactorial in origin, as follows:
  - Imbalance between proinflammatory and antiinflammatory cytokines
  - Genetic predisposition
  - Environmental triggers such as trauma, infection, or psychological stress

EPIDEMIOLOGY AND DEMOGRAPHICS

- Incidence is 9 to 19 cases per 100,000 children
- Peak ages of onset 1 to 3 and 8 to 10 years
- In children with JRA, 50% have pauciarticular JRA, 40% have polyarticular JRA, and 10% have systemic JRA.
- In the polyarticular subtype, the female-to-male ratio is 3:1, and it is 5:1 in the pauciarticular subtype. However, incidence is equal in the sexes in the systemic subtype.

MECHANISM OF INJURY

An autoimmune response to an infectious or traumatic event

COMMON SIGNS AND SYMPTOMS

- Systemic
  - The diagnostic marker is a spiking fever of 39° C or higher that occurs once or twice daily.
  - A fleeting rash of pale erythematous macules is primarily found on the trunk and proximal extremities.
  - Systemic symptoms include pericarditis, hepatosplenomegaly, and lymphadenopathy.
- Polyarticular
  - Acute or insidious symmetrical arthritis of the large and small joints of the upper and lower extremities, with more than four joints involved
  - Joints are swollen and warm but rarely red.
  - Extraarticular involvement may present as rheumatoid factor (RF) plus tendon nodules
  - Systemic symptoms are usually mild and include low grade fever, mild to-moderate hepatosplenomegaly, and lymphadenopathy.
  - Chronic uveitis in 19% of patients
- Pauciarticular
  - Four or fewer joints are involved, and typically, large joints are affected.
  - Involvement of the lower extremities is often asymmetrical; the knee is the most commonly affected joint.
  - The joint is swollen and warm but not always painful.
  - Extraarticular involvement may include tendinitis, bony overgrowth, or bony undergrowth.
  - Systemic symptoms are unusual.
  - 20% of children develop uveitis.
- Joint pain
- Muscle tenderness
- Swelling
- Fatigue
- Stiffness

AGGRAVATING ACTIVITIES

Overuse of affected joints

EASING ACTIVITIES

- Rest
- Warm bath

24-HOUR SYMPTOM PATTERN

Morning stiffness and arthralgia during the day

PAST HISTORY FOR THE REGION

Insidious onset with worsening symptoms over time

PHYSICAL EXAMINATION

- Postural assessment
  - Sitting: Posterior pelvic tilt, kyphotic, rounded shoulders, and forward head
  - Standing: Calcaneal valgus, midfoot pronation, pes planus, hallux valgus, genu valgum, lumbar lordosis, pelvic obliquity, scoliosis, and decreased lower extremity weight bearing
- Common joint and postural findings caused by muscle imbalance
  - Toes: Subluxation of metatarsophalangeal joints, claw or hammer toes
  - Ankles: Tight plantar flexors and weak dorsiflexors
  - Knees: Tight hamstrings and quadriceps atrophy
  - Hips: Tight hip flexors with weak hip extensors and decreased abduction and internal rotation
  - Spine: Weak abdominals and increased lumbar lordosis
  - Cervical spine: Limitations in extension, rotation and lateral flexion due to fusion of the apophyseal joints, instability and subluxation of C1 or C2, and/or erosion of odontoid process
  - Temporomandibular joint: Restrictions caused by forward head position and undergrowth of the mandible
  - Shoulder girdle: Decreased flexion, abduction, and external rotation
  - Elbow: Decreased extension and supination
  - Wrist: Decreased wrist extension with subluxation and radial deviation
- Fingers:
  - Boutonniere deformities: Flexion of the proximal interphalangeal joint with hyperextension of the distal interphalangeal joint
  - Swan neck deformities: Hyperextension of the proximal interphalangeal joint with flexion of the distal interphalangeal joint
- Joint palpation: Tenderness, synovial thickening, bony overgrowth
- Ligamentous stability (assess for laxity)
- Gait analysis

IMPORTANT OBJECTIVE TESTS

- ROM/contractures
  - Joint versus muscle length restriction

- Measure for differences in active ROM (AROM) and PROM
  - Range may be limited by swelling, pain, muscle guarding, muscle tightness, stiffness, or joint and bony changes.
  - Bilateral comparisons of ROM and an overall check for signs of hypermobility are important aspects of joint assessment.
  - Up to 10% of all children are hypermobile.
  - The tendency to hypermobility masks an early joint contracture.
- Strength
  - MMT: Do not perform MMT on a joint that is in an acute flare.
  - Functional strength: Gait pattern, stairs, heel or toe raises, floor-to-stand transfers
  - Developmental gross motor skills: High kneel, ½ kneel to stand, hop on one leg, etc.
- Edema: 1+ = minimal, 2+ = moderate, 3+ = severe
- Temperature
- Girth measurements
- Disuse atrophy
- Joint swelling: Measure 3 cm above the patella and figure 8 around the ankle.
- Bony overgrowth is common with a chronic joint caused by increased blood flow with inflammation.
- Leg length discrepancy
  - Increased blood supply to the inflamed joint early in the disease may cause accelerated growth of the ossification centers, resulting in the increased length of the affected limb.
- Balance: Single limb, tandem
- 6-minute walk test
  - 20 children, ages 6 to 11 years of age, with polyarticular JRA, performed significantly below age-matched controls on the 9-minute run-walk test and were not able to maintain a steady running pace.
- Standardized tests such as the Pediatric Evaluation of Disability Inventory (PEDI)

DIFFERENTIAL DIAGNOSES

Dx

- Trauma
- Septic arthritis
- Osteomyelitis
- Acute rheumatic fever
- Infections (e.g., tuberculosis, gonorrhea)
- Malignancy (e.g., leukemia, osteosarcoma)
- Collagen or vascular diseases (e.g., systemic lupus erythematosus (SLE), Ehlers-Danlos syndrome, Henoch-Schönlein purpura)

CONTRIBUTING FACTORS

- Antinuclear antibody (ANA)
  - ANA is observed in as many as 25% of children with JRA, particularly in patients with pauciarticular disease.

- When found in young girls, a positive ANA is a marker of increased risk of uveitis
- Very high titers may sometimes be associated with evolution to other rheumatic diseases (e.g., SLE)
- RF
  - The majority of children with JRA are RF negative, although 10% of children have later-onset RF-positive polyarticular disease, which has the same aggressive course as adult RA.
  - RF is rare in persons with systemic JRA.
  - RF has been associated with poor long-term outcomes.

TREATMENT

SURGICAL OPTIONS

- Intraarticular steroid injections
- Joint arthroplasty
- Osteotomy
- Epiphysiodesis may be performed to halt overgrowth of the longer limb in the presence of leg length discrepancy.
- Tenotomies

SURGICAL OUTCOMES

- Soft tissue release has been shown to be a beneficial option to preserving alignment and function in hip and knee flexion deformities affecting patients with JRA.
- Despite a substantial number of postoperative complications, total knee arthroplasty (TKA) provided excellent relief of pain and improvement in a group of adolescent patients with JRA.
- Quality of life improved after TKA as measured by the Patient-Specific Index.

REHABILITATION

- Nonsteroidal antiinflammatory drugs (NSAIDs) may be prescribed by a physician and are the first line of defense.
- Modalities (iontophoresis, cold, heat, or transcutaneous electrical nerve stimulation [TENS])
- Adaptive equipment
- Joint protection
  - Avoid high-impact sports
  - Avoid positions of flexion
  - Avoid prolonged static positions
- Splints or orthotics
  - Night splints maintain range and help with morning stiffness.
- Increase ROM
  - Stretching
  - Pronating
  - Serial casting
  - Splints
- Strengthening: Acute flare
  - PROM and AROM exercises
  - Isometrics
  - No resistive exercises

- Subacute or chronic
  - Gradually increase intensity of exercises
  - Start with gravity eliminated and progress to antigravity
- Weight-bearing activities to increase bone density
  - Osteoporosis is prevalent in children with JRA as the result of steroid use, nutritional disorders, and decrease in the quantity of load carried by the joints.
- Gait training
- Balance training
- Shoe modifications (heel lifts, heel cups, metatarsal bars)
- Aerobic conditioning activities: A review of the evidence indicates that children with JRA who perform moderately vigorous (60% to 85% maximum heart rate (HR_{max})) aerobic activity for at least 30 minutes twice a week for at least 6 weeks can improve their aerobic fitness.
- Aquatic therapy

PROGNOSIS

- Early hip or wrist involvement, symmetrical disease (even in pauciarticular patients), presence of RF, and prolonged active disease have been associated with poor long-term outcomes.
- The more active the patient, the better the long-term prognosis.
- Up to 25% of children with JRA have unremitting disease, which may lead to contracture and deformity, and approximately 10% enter adulthood with severe functional disabilities.
- In systemic-onset JRA, active systemic disease at 6 months (i.e., with fever, the need for corticosteroids, and thrombocytosis) is a strong predictor of poor functional outcome
- Approximately one quarter of patients with polyarticular-onset JRA are in remission at 5 years after disease onset, and more than two thirds develop erosions within the first 5 years of the disease.
- Prognosis is generally considered excellent for gaining full joint mobility and functional ability in children with pauciarticular onset before 5 years of age, although iridocyclitis may occur as a serious ocular complication.

SIGNS AND SYMPTOMS INDICATING REFERRAL TO PHYSICIAN

- Malar or butterfly rash: SLE
- Orthopnea: Viral pericarditis, SLE
- Joint/bone pain with lethargy, fever, vomiting, and/or bruising: Leukemia
- Palpable mass that is tender and warm: Osteomyelitis, osteosarcoma
- Pain and decreased weight bearing of affected extremity: Traumatic or pathological fracture

SUGGESTED READINGS

Cakmak A, Bolukbas N. Juvenile rheumatoid arthritis: physical therapy and rehabilitation. *South Med J*. 2005;98(2):212-216.

Cassidy JT, Levinson JE, Bass JC, et al. A study of classification criteria for a diagnosis of juvenile rheumatoid arthritis. *Arthritis Rheum*. 1986;29:274-281.

Cassidy JT, Petty RE. Juvenile rheumatoid arthritis. In: Cassidy JT, ed. *Textbook of Rheumatology*. New York: Churchill Livingstone Inc; 1990:113-219.

Espada G, Alvarez MM, Gagliardi S. *Long Term Results of Soft Tissue Release Surgery for Hips and Knees in Juvenile Chronic Arthritis*. Presented at the Third International Pediatric Rheumatology Conference. Utah: Park City; 1991.

Fisher NM, Venkatraman JT, O'Neil K. The effects of resistance exercises on muscle function in juvenile arthritis. *Arthritis Rheum*. 2001;44:S276.

Gare BA. Juvenile arthritis: who gets it, where, and when? A review of current data on incidence and prevalence. *Clin Exp Rheumatol*. 1999;17:367-374.

Gedalia A, Person DA, Brewer EJ, et al. Hypermobility of the joints in juvenile episodic arthritis/arthralgia. *J Pediatr*. 1985; 107(6):873-876.

Haley SM, Faas RM, Coster WJ, Webster H, Gans BM. *Pediatric Evaluation of Disability Inventory*. Boston: New England Medical Center; 1989.

Ilowite NT. Current treatment of juvenile rheumatoid arthritis. *Pediatrics*. 2002;109(1):109-115.

Klepper SE. Juvenile rheumatoid arthritis. In: Campbell SK, Vander Linden DW, Palisano RJ. *Physical Therapy for Children*. 3rd ed. Philadelphia: Saunders; 2006:291-321.

Kuchta G, Davidson I. *Occupational and Physical Therapy for Children with Rheumatic Diseases: A Clinical Handbook*. New York: Radcliffe Publishing; 2008.

Ravelli A, Martini A. Early predictors of outcome in juvenile idiopathic arthritis. *Clin Exp Rheumatol*. 2003;21(5 supp 31):89-93.

Rhodes VJ. Physical therapy management of patients with juvenile rheumatoid arthritis. *Phys Ther*. 1991;71(12):910-919.

Spiegel LR, Schneider R, Lang BA, et al. Early predictors of poor outcome in systemic onset juvenile rheumatoid arthritis: a multicenter cohort study. *Arthritis Rheum*. 1998;41(9):48.

Takken T, Van der Net JJ, Helders PJ. Do juvenile idiopathic arthritis patients benefit from an exercise program? A pilot study. *Arthritis Care Res*. 2001;45:81-85.

Wright FV, Smith E. Physical therapy management of the child and adolescent with juvenile rheumatoid arthritis. In: Walker JM, Helewa A, eds. *Physical Therapy in Arthritis*. Philadelphia: WB Saunders; 1996:211-244.

AUTHORS: ERICA PABLO and LEESHA AUGUSTINE

BASIC INFORMATION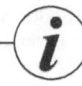

DEFINITION

Kienböck's disease results in the osteonecrosis of the lunate carpal bone.

SYNONYMS

- Avascular necrosis of the lunate
- Lunatomalacia
- Osteochondrosis of the lunate

ICD-9CM CODES
732.3 Juvenile osteochondrosis of upper extremity

OPTIMAL NUMBER OF VISITS

12 or fewer

MAXIMAL NUMBER OF VISITS

24

ETIOLOGY

The underlying etiology is unknown; however, the osteonecrosis of the lunate may result from intrinsic and extrinsic factors such as repetitive microtrauma, decreased vascular supply, and ulnar variance.

EPIDEMIOLOGY AND DEMOGRAPHICS

- The most common patient with Kienböck's disease is a man 20 to 40 years of age who engages in manual labor or participates in recreational activities that load the wrist.
- The male-to-female ratio is 2:1.

MECHANISM OF INJURY

Repetitive microtrauma

COMMON SIGNS AND SYMPTOMS

- Pain in the wrist
- Swelling
- Difficulty gripping objects
- Limited wrist motion

AGGRAVATING ACTIVITIES

- Gripping objects
- Weight bearing on affected upper extremity

EASING ACTIVITIES

- Rest
- Restricting loading activities

24-HOUR SYMPTOM PATTERN

Increased pain at the end of the day or after repetitive loading activities

PAST HISTORY FOR THE REGION

Typically, the patient reports an injury to the wrist in the past or has a history of repetitive use of the wrist.

PHYSICAL EXAMINATION

- Decreased wrist flexion-extension arc
- Dorsal wrist swelling
- Tenderness to palpation of the dorsal aspect of the wrist near the lunate bone

IMPORTANT OBJECTIVE TESTS

- Diminished grip strength, measured by a dynamometer, caused by pain and/or weakness
- ROM (diminished flexion and extension)
- Finger extension or "shuck" test
  - Pain when actively extending the fingers against resistance while the wrist is flexed may be a positive sign for radial carpal or midcarpal instability, scaphoid instability, inflammation, or Kienböck's disease.

DIFFERENTIAL DIAGNOSES

- Fracture of the lunate
- Ulnolunar impaction syndrome
- Intraosseous ganglia
- Wrist sprain
- Arthritis

CONTRIBUTING FACTORS

- Extrinsic factors that relate to Kienböck's disease
  - Repetitive microtrauma
  - Ulnar variance: When the ulna is shorter than the radius, the lunate bone absorbs more force when the wrist is used for heavy gripping activities.
- Intrinsic factor that relates to Kienböck's disease: Limited vascular supply to the lunate

TREATMENT

SURGICAL OPTIONS

- Lunate excision with or without replacement
- Joint-leveling procedures lengthen or shorten the ulna or radius to reduce the compression forces on the lunate.
- Intercarpal fusion
- Revascularization
- Proximal row carpectomy
- Wrist arthrodesis
- The factors that determine which surgical procedure is performed are patient age, stage of disease, and presence or absence of ulnar variance.

SURGICAL OUTCOMES

In comparing surgical treatment versus nonsurgical treatment for patients with Kienböck's disease, no significant difference was found between the two treatment options at 5-year follow-up.

REHABILITATION

- Wrist immobilization may assist in revascularization of the lunate in acute inflammatory phase.
- Antiinflammatory medication
- Modalities for pain and/or inflammation
- Joint mobilization
- Wrist and grip strengthening
- If treating patient postoperatively, neurogliding and scar mobilization may be warranted.

PROGNOSIS

49 patients were monitored nonoperatively for an average of 20.5 years, and 80% of the patients had no pain or had pain only with heavy labor.

SIGNS AND SYMPTOMS INDICATING REFERRAL TO PHYSICIAN

Pain while at rest, excessive redness and swelling, fever and chills, and waking up at night because of pain may indicate tumor or osteomyelitis. Further tests should be performed and immediate referral to a physician may be warranted.

SUGGESTED READINGS

Bain GI, Begg M. Arthroscopic assessment and classification of Kienbock's disease. *Tech Hand Up Extrem Surg.* 2006;10(1):8–13.

Delaere O, Dury M, Molderez A. Conservative versus operative treatment for Keinbock's disease. A retrospective study. *J Hand Sur [Br].* 1998;23(1):33–36.

Keith PP, Nuttall D, Trail I. Long-term outcome of nonsurgically managed Kienbock's disease. *J Hand Surg Am.* 2004;29(1):63–67.

Kristensen S, Thomassen E, Christensen F. Keinbock's disease—late results by non surgical treatment. A follow-up study. *J Hand Surg Br.* 1986;11(3):422–425.

Luo J, Diao E. Kienbock's disease: an approach to treatment. *Hand Clin.* 2006;22(4):465–473; abstract vi.

Nguyen DT, McCue FC, Urch SE. Evaluation of the injured wrist on the field and in the office. *Clin Sports Med.* 1998;17:421–432.

Salmon J, Stanley JK, Trail IA. Kienbock's disease: conservative management versus radial shortening. *J Bone Joint Surg Br.* 2000;82(6): 820–823.

Zenzai K, Shibata M, Endo N. Long-term outcome of radial shortening with or without ulnar shortening for treatment of Kienbock's disease: a 13–25 year follow-up. *J Hand Surg Br.* 2005;30(2):226–228.

AUTHORS: ERICA PABLO and LEESHA AUGUSTINE

BASIC INFORMATION

DEFINITION

Legg-Calvé-Perthes disease (LCPD) results from the idiopathic osteonecrosis of the capital femoral epiphysis of the femoral head.

SYNONYMS

- Perthes disease
- LCPD

ICD-9CM CODES

732.1 Juvenile osteochondrosis of hip and pelvis

OPTIMAL NUMBER OF VISITS

12 or fewer

MAXIMAL NUMBER OF VISITS

24

ETIOLOGY

LCPD results from an unexplained interruption of the blood supply to the capital femoral epiphysis. Bone infarction occurs, especially in the subchondral cortical bone, while articular cartilage continues to grow. Revascularization occurs, and new bone ossification starts. At this time, some patients have normal bone growth and development, whereas others develop LCPD. LCPD is present when a subchondral fracture occurs. This is usually the result of normal physical activity, not direct trauma to the area. As a result of the subchondral fracture, changes occur to the epiphyseal growth plate.

EPIDEMIOLOGY AND DEMOGRAPHICS

- 1 in 1200 children younger than 15 years is affected by LCPD.
- LCPD is most commonly seen in children ages 3 to 12 years, with a median age of 7 years.
- Whites are affected more frequently than persons of other races.
- Male-to-female ratio is 4:1.

MECHANISM OF INJURY

Insidious onset, usually no history of trauma

COMMON SIGNS AND SYMPTOMS

- Limp
- Pain in groin, knee, or hip
  - Bilateral involvement in about 10% to 13% of patients
- Pain with weight-bearing activities
- Short stature: Children with LCPD often have delayed bone age.

AGGRAVATING ACTIVITIES

- Running
- Jumping
- Recreational activities that require repetitive weight bearing

EASING ACTIVITIES

- Rest
- Physical activity modification

24-HOUR SYMPTOM PATTERN

- Increased symptoms after weight-bearing activities
- Worsening pain at the end of the day and over time

PAST HISTORY FOR THE REGION

Gradual onset of symptoms over weeks or months before presentation

PHYSICAL EXAMINATION

- Limited hip internal rotation, abduction, and flexion
- Muscle spasm
- Positive Trendelenburg's sign
- Psoatic limp (lateral rotation, flexion, and adduction of the affected hip)
- Thigh atrophy

IMPORTANT OBJECTIVE TESTS

- Leg length discrepancy
- MMT
- Functional assessment
  - Stairs
  - Half kneel to stand transfers
  - Single limb balance (kick a ball)
  - Squat to retrieve item off of the floor
- Roll test: Muscle guarding or spasm noted with internal rotation of the affected hip when patient is in supine position.
- Hard joint end-feel with passive hip internal rotation
- Positive flexion-adduction test
- Obligatory abduction and external rotation during passive flexion (Drehmann's sign)
- Knee objective tests do not reproduce patient's symptoms (knee pain is referred from the hip).

DIFFERENTIAL DIAGNOSES

- Septic arthritis
- Toxic synovitis
- Osteomyelitis
- Juvenile rheumatoid arthritis
- Leukemia or lymphoma
- Sickle cell anemia
- Spondyloepiphyseal dysplasia
- Metaphyseal dysplasia
- Slipped capital femoral epiphysis

CONTRIBUTING FACTORS

- There is a relationship between LCPD and parental cigarette smoking during pregnancy.

  - The risk of LCPD in children exposed to second hand smoke is more than five times higher than in children not exposed.
- Children with perinatal human immunodeficiency virus (HIV) infections have an increased risk for LCPD.
- A positive family history of LCPD is noted in 10% to 20% of cases.

TREATMENT

SURGICAL OPTIONS

- Proximal femoral varus derotation osteotomy
- Pelvic osteotomy alone or in combination with a varus derotation osteotomy
- Prophylactic trochanteric arrest
- Valgus-flexion-internal rotation femoral osteotomy and acetabuloplasty

SURGICAL OUTCOMES

Proximal varus osteotomy is a reliable treatment in patients with advanced deformation or flattening of femoral head and in those with good containment in abduction and internal rotation, especially if they are between 6 and 10 years of age. The results are unsatisfactory for older patients and for those with advanced deformity of the femoral head.

REHABILITATION

- The goal of treatment during the active phase of the disease is containment of the femoral epiphysis within the center of the acetabulum to prevent degenerative arthritis.
  - Petrie casts are used to maintain hips in abduction and internal rotation.
  - Traction
- ROM exercises to restore and maintain hip mobility
- Increase strength of hamstrings, gluteus medius, gluteus maximus, and internal rotators
- Joint mobilization to increase limited hip ROMs
- Gait training

PROGNOSIS

- The disease is self-limiting and complete healing generally does occur, but it may take up to 3 to 4 years.
- Prognostic factors include age at onset, extent of the disease, the amount of femoral head deformity, and the amount of incongruity between the femoral head and acetabulum. Hip joint growth and development depends on a well-located, centered, and spherical femoral head.
- The younger the age of onset of LCPD, the better the prognosis.

○ There is a good prognosis for patients younger than 5 years without any treatment.
- Children older than 10 years have a very high risk of developing osteoarthritis.
- 60% to 70% of children with LCPD do well with no long-term disability.

SIGNS AND SYMPTOMS INDICATING REFERRAL TO PHYSICIAN

- Fever and joint pain may be signs of septic arthritis. If a rash is also present, JRA must also be considered.
- A patient with leukemia or lymphoma may also present with joint pain in addition to lethargy, fever, vomiting, and bruising.
- If there is bilateral symmetrical involvement with femoral head fragmentation and collapse of both hips, then another condition must be considered. If LCPD occurs bilaterally, presentation is usually not symmetrical. The disease will be noticeably more severe in one hip than in the other, and progression in the less severely affected hip will be slower.
  ○ Sickle cell anemia may cause bilateral symmetrical involvement in an African-American child.

SUGGESTED READINGS

Brech GC, Guarnieiro R. Evaluation of physiotherapy in the treatment of Legg-Calvé-Perthes disease. *Clinics.* 2006;61(6):521-528.

Dutoit M. Legg-Calvé-Perthes disease. *Arch Pediatr Adolesc Med.* 2007;14(1):109-115.

Fischer SU, Beattie TF. The limping child: epidemiology, assessment and outcome. *J Bone Joint Surg Br.* 1999;81:1029-1034.

Herring JA, Kim HT, Browne R. Legg-Calvé-Perthes disease. Part II: prospective multicenter study of the effect of treatment on outcome. *J Bone Surg Joint Am.* 2004;86(10):2121-2134.

Herring JA, Williams JJ, Neustadt JN, et al. Evolution of femoral head deformity during the healing phase of Legg-Calvé-Perthes disease. *J Orthop.* 1993;13:41-45.

Kamegaya M, Saisu T, Ochiai N, et al. A paired study of Perthes' disease comparing conservative and surgical treatment. *J Bone Joint Surg Br.* 2004;86:1176-1181.

Kay RM, Morrissy RT, Kehl DK. Late metachronous involvement of the contralateral hip in Legg-Calvé-Perthes disease. *J Pediatr Orthop.* 1998;18:807-810.

Kim HT, Wenger DR. Surgical correction of functional retroversion and functional coxa vara in late Legg-Calvé-Perthes disease and epiphyseal dysplasia: correction of deformity defined by new imaging modalities. *J Pediatr Orthop.* 1997;17:247-254.

Leach J. Orthopedic conditions. In: Campbell SK, Vander Linden DW, Palisano RJ, eds. *Physical Therapy for Children.* 3rd ed. Philadelphia, PA: Saunders; 2006:481-515.

Leung A.KC, Lemay JF. The limping child. *J Pediatr Health Care.* 2004;18:219-223.

Mata SG, Aicua EA, Ovejero AH, Grande MM. Legg-Calvé-Perthes disease and passive smoking. *J Pediatr Orthop.* 2000;20:326-330.

Matan AJ, Stevens PM, Smith JT, Santora SD. Combination trochanteric arrest and intertrochanteric osteotomy for Perthes' disease. *J Pediatr Orthop.* 1996;16:10-14.

Resnick D. Osteochondroses. In: Resnick D, ed. *Diagnosis of Bone and Joint Disorders.* 4th ed. Philadelphia: WB Saunders; 2002:3686-3741.

Robben SG, Lequin MH, Meradji M, et al. Atrophy of the quadriceps muscle in children with a painful hip. *Clin Physiol.* 1999;19:385-393.

Weinstein SL. Natural history and treatment outcomes of childhood hip disorders. *Clin Orthop Relat Res.* 1997;344:227-242.

AUTHORS: ERICA PABLO and LEESHA AUGUSTINE

BASIC INFORMATION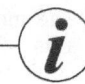

DEFINITION

Myositis ossificans is a benign condition manifesting as a heterotopic, well-defined neoformation in muscles and soft tissues that have previously been exposed to trauma and hematoma.

SYNONYMS

- Heterotopic ossification
- Hematoma ossificans
- Myosteosis

ICD-9CM CODES
728.12 Traumatic myositis ossificans
728.11 Progressive myositis ossificans

OPTIMAL NUMBER OF VISITS

12 or fewer

MAXIMAL NUMBER OF VISITS

24

ETIOLOGY

- Myositis ossificans involves the development of heterotropic bone in the involved musculature, usually after a traumatic episode.
- Myositis ossificans has numerous etiological theories including the following:
  - Hematoma organization involving a progressive transformation of fibrous tissue to cartilage then bone
  - Hematoma calcification
  - Intramuscular bone formation after detachment of periosteal flaps
  - Periosteal rupture with escape and proliferation of periosteal osteoblasts within adjacent muscle tissue
  - Metaplasia of intramuscular connective tissue into cartilage and bone
  - An individual predisposition to myositis

EPIDEMIOLOGY AND DEMOGRAPHICS

- Myositis ossificans is rare in patients younger than 10 years and more often occurs in adolescent and young adult athletes.
  - 75% of cases are associated with a traumatic event.
  - Myositis ossificans most commonly affects the arms, legs, shoulders, hands, and rarely the chest.

MECHANISM OF INJURY

- Repeated small mechanical injuries
- Nonmechanical injuries caused by ischemia or inflammation
- Undocumented trauma

COMMON SIGNS AND SYMPTOMS

- Pain
- Tenderness
- Focal swelling
- Joint or muscle contractions

AGGRAVATING ACTIVITIES

Resistive activities and passive stretching of the involved joint

EASING ACTIVITIES

- Rest
- Ice

24-HOUR SYMPTOM PATTERN

Pain and stiffness in the involved joint aggravated by increased use throughout the day.

PAST HISTORY FOR THE REGION

Myositis ossificans often develops after a traumatic sports-related injury to an athlete. A history of traumatic injury, including falls in the elderly, may have occurred up to 3 or 4 months before.

PHYSICAL EXAMINATION

- Palpation of tender mass in affected muscle, with or without erythema
- Associated joint motion abnormalities
- Fever (uncommon)

IMPORTANT OBJECTIVE TESTS

- ROM in adjacent joints of the affected muscle (limitations in motion caused by pain)
- MMT of affected muscle (diminished strength)

DIFFERENTIAL DIAGNOSES

- Osteosarcoma
- Chondrosarcoma
- Osteomyelitis

CONTRIBUTING FACTORS

- Myositis ossificans may occur as a complication from fractures, surgery, or paraplegia.
- Ossification may be associated with high-energy trauma, manipulation, early treatment of a contusion with heat or massage, aggressive stretching and strengthening, or premature return to sport.

TREATMENT

SURGICAL OPTIONS

Surgery is warranted in patients with myositis ossificans only if severe loss of function is caused by the bony defect. Surgery should not be performed until maturation of lesion (6 to 24 months) and there is no sign of active calcification.

SURGICAL OUTCOMES

If surgery is performed prematurely, there is an increased risk for local recurrence.

REHABILITATION

- Early treatment for myositis ossificans consists of rest and ice to reduce pain and swelling.
- Weight-bearing activity is initially reduced with crutches if lower extremity limb is involved.
- Once pain and swelling have subsided, gentle PROM exercises are initiated in order to regain ROM.
- Strengthening (isometrics) may begin after swelling subsides but should be avoided initially.
- NSAIDs or corticosteroids may be prescribed by physicians for persistent swelling.
- Resolution of bony defect may be possible with the use of iontophoresis followed by pulsed ultrasound.
- After full ROM is attained, sport-specific activities may be initiated.

PROGNOSIS

Myositis ossificans is a self-limiting disorder that may require months of conservative physical therapy before return to full activity is reached.

SIGNS AND SYMPTOMS INDICATING REFERRAL TO PHYSICIAN

- Constant unrelenting pain that does not change with position
- Significant unexplained weight loss
- Night pain
- History of cancer
- Fever and chills

SUGGESTED READINGS

Beiner JM, Jokl P. Muscle contusion injury and myositis ossificans traumatica. *Clin Orthop Relat Res*. 2002;(403 suppl):S110-S119.

Hait G, Boswick Jr JA, Stone NH. Heterotopic bone formation secondary to trauma (myositis ossificans traumatica). *J Trauma*. 1970;10(5):405-411.

Hertling D, Kessler R. *Management of Common Musculoskeletal Disorders: Physical Therapy Principles and Disorders*. 2nd ed. Philadelphia: JB Lippincott; 1990:272-297.

Jackson DW, Feagin JA. Quadriceps contusions in young athletes. *J Bone Joint Surg*. 1973;55A:96-105.

King JB. Post-traumatic ectopic calcification in the muscles of athletes: A review. *J Sports Med (Br)*. 1998;32:287-290.

Messina M, Volterrani L, Molinaro F, Nardi N, Amato G. Myositis ossificans in children: description of a clinical case with a rare localization. *Minerva Pediatr*. 2006;58(1):69-72.

Rosenberg AE. Pseudosarcomas of soft tissue. *Arch Pathol Lab Med*. 2008;132(4):579-586.

Thorndike A. Myositis ossificans traumatic. *J Bone Joint Surg*. 1940;22:315-323.

Wieder DL. Treatment of traumatic myositis ossificans with acetic acid iontophoresis. *Phys Ther*. 1992;72(2):133-137.

AUTHORS: ERICA PABLO and LEESHA AUGUSTINE

BASIC INFORMATION

DEFINITION

Osgood-Schlatter disease is a traction apophysitis of the tibial tubercle caused by repetitive strain of the secondary ossification center of the tibial tuberosity.

SYNONYMS

- Tibial apophysitis
- Tibial tubercle epiphysitis

ICD-9CM CODES
732.4 Juvenile osteochondrosis of lower extremity excluding foot

OPTIMAL NUMBER OF VISITS

12 or fewer

MAXIMAL NUMBER OF VISITS

24

ETIOLOGY

Osgood-Schlatter disease occurs during periods of rapid growth, and the stress from the contraction of the quadriceps is transmitted through the patellar tendon onto a small portion of the partially developed tibial tuberosity. This involves repetitive microavulsions of the chondrofibroosseous tibial tubercle.

EPIDEMIOLOGY AND DEMOGRAPHICS

- Osgood-Schlatter disease typically develops in girls between the ages of 8 and 13 years and in boys ages 10 to 15 years at the beginning of their growth spurt.
- The prevalence of the condition in athletic adolescents is 21% compared to 4.5% in age-matched nonathletes.

MECHANISM OF INJURY

Repetitive microtrauma

COMMON SIGNS AND SYMPTOMS

- Pain with active knee extension
- Swelling

AGGRAVATING ACTIVITIES

- Running
- Cutting activities
- Jumping
- Kneeling
- Squatting
- Ascending or descending stairs

EASING ACTIVITIES

- Rest
- Ice
- Passive knee extension positioning

24-HOUR SYMPTOM PATTERN

Increased pain symptoms associated with aggravating activities

PAST HISTORY FOR THE REGION

- Patients may have intermittent pain for several months before seeking medical attention.
- Approximately 50% of patients have a history of precipitating trauma.

PHYSICAL EXAMINATION

- Edema may be present over the proximal tibial tuberosity.
- Tenderness to palpation at the patellar insertion
- A firm palpable mass may be present.
- Pain is reproduced with resisted knee extension.
  - The pain is bilateral in 20% to 25% of cases.
- Erythema over the tibial tuberosity may be observed.
- Assess patellar mobility

IMPORTANT OBJECTIVE TESTS

- ROM
- MMT
- Functional strength tests (e.g., stairs, squatting)
- Special tests of the knee (e.g., anterior drawer, varus/valgus stress test, Apley compression) to rule out intraarticular lesions. Osgood-Schlatter is an extraarticular disease.

DIFFERENTIAL DIAGNOSES

- Infrapatellar plica injury or plica syndrome
- Hoffa's syndrome
- Patellofemoral stress syndrome
- Pes anserinus bursitis
- Chondromalacia patellae
- Patellar tendinitis
- Sinding-Larsen-Johansson syndrome
- Quadriceps tendon avulsion
- Osteochondritis dissecans

CONTRIBUTING FACTORS

- Patella alta
  - An increase in patellar height requires increased force from the quadriceps for full extension and could be responsible for apophyseal lesions.

TREATMENT

SURGICAL OPTIONS

- Treatment is generally conservative, and only rarely does a surgical treatment become necessary for the persistence of pain and swelling over the tibial tubercle.

- The most widely used procedure consists of the excision of all intratendinous ossicles with or without removal of the prominent tibial tubercle.

SURGICAL OUTCOMES

75% of patients who underwent ossicle excision and tibial tubercleplasty for unresolved Osgood-Schlatter disease were able to return to preoperative activities and sports.

REHABILITATION

- Acute phase
  - NSAIDs may be prescribed by the physician to address pain and inflammation.
  - Activity modifications
  - Modalities (ice, iontophoresis, TENS)
  - Knee immobilizer, pad, or brace for severe cases
  - Stretching of quadriceps and hamstrings
- Subacute or chronic phase
  - Strengthening of quadriceps, hip extensors, and abductors
  - Plyometric exercises
  - Sport-specific training
  - Shock-absorbent insoles in sport shoes to decrease peak stress on the tendon and tuberosity

PROGNOSIS

- About 90% of patients respond well to nonoperative treatment that includes rest, icing, activity modification, and rehabilitation exercises.
- Symptoms usually resolve spontaneously within 1 year.
- Discomfort may persist for 2 to 3 years until the tibial growth plate closes.
- 60% of patients with Osgood-Schlatter disease may have painful kneeling as adults.

SIGNS AND SYMPTOMS INDICATING REFERRAL TO PHYSICIAN

- Osteochondritis dissecans is a rare but serious cause of adolescent knee pain that can result in permanent knee damage. Therefore patients who present with diffuse knee pain, effusion, and loss of motion must be referred to an orthopedist.
- A palpable mass that is warm and tender with systemic signs, such as fever and lethargy, may indicate osteomyelitis of the proximal tibia.
- Suprapatellar swelling, ecchymosis, and tenderness may be caused by a quadriceps tendon rupture.

SUGGESTED READINGS

Aparicio G, Abril JC, Calvo E, Alvarez L. Radiologic study of patellar height in Osgood-Schlatter disease. *J Pediatr Orthop.* 1997;17:63-66.

Binazzi R, Felli L, Vaccari V, Borelli P. Surgical treatment of unresolved Osgood-Schlatter lesion. *Clin Orthop.* 1993;289:202-204.

Bloom OJ, Mackler L, Barbee J. Clinical inquiries. What is the best treatment for Osgood-Schlatter disease? *J Fam Pract.* 2004;53(2):153-156.

Flowers MJ, Bhadreshwar DR. Tibial tuberosity excision for symptomatic Osgood-Schlatter disease. *J Pediatr Orthop.* 1995;15(3):292-297.

Gholve PA, Scher DM, Kakharia S, Widmann RF, Green DW. Osgood Schlatter syndrome. *Curr Opin Pediatr.* 2007;19(1):44-50.

Krause BL, Williams JP, Catterall A. Natural history of Osgood-Schlatter disease. *J Pediatr Orthop.* 1990;10(1):65-68.

Kujala UM, Kvist M, Heinonen O. Osgood-Schlatter's disease in adolescent athletes: retrospective study of incidence and duration. *Am J Sports Med.* 1985;13(4):236-241.

Leach J. Orthopedic conditions. In: Campbell SK, Vander Linden DW, Palisano RJ, eds. *Physical Therapy for Children.* 3rd ed. Philadelphia: Saunders; 2006:481-515.

Wall EJ. Osgood-Schlatter disease: practical treatment for a self-limiting condition. *Physician Sportsmed.* 1998;26(3).

AUTHORS: ERICA PABLO and LEESHA AUGUSTINE

Section III

ORTHOPEDIC PATHOLOGY

BASIC INFORMATION

DEFINITION

- Osteomyelitis is an inflammation of the bone resulting from an infectious process.
- Osteomyelitis is classified into the following three categories:
  - Acute hematogenous osteomyelitis occurs mainly during infancy and childhood; the metaphysis of the long bones is the most common location.
  - Subacute focal disease or contiguous osteomyelitis
  - Chronic osteomyelitis

SYNONYMS

- Central osteitis
- Hematogenous osteomyelitis
- Infection of the bone

ICD-9CM CODES
730.00 Osteomyelitis unspecified

OPTIMAL NUMBER OF VISITS

12 or fewer

MAXIMAL NUMBER OF VISITS

24

ETIOLOGY

- Infection is due to hematogenous spread in 90% of cases. Other etiologies include direct inoculation (e.g., trauma or surgery) and direct spread from a local soft tissue infection.
- The most common cause of osteomyelitis is bacterial, although fungal and viral causes are also possible.
  - *Staphylococcus aureus* is implicated in most cases of acute hematogenous osteomyelitis and is responsible for up to 90% of cases in otherwise healthy children.

EPIDEMIOLOGY AND DEMOGRAPHICS

- The annual incidence of acute osteomyelitis is about 1/5000 children younger than 13 years.
- This disease appears to affect males more often than females, and a majority of the cases occur in patients younger than 20 years.

MECHANISM OF INJURY

An acquired infection that may be associated with trauma or surgery

COMMON SIGNS AND SYMPTOMS

- Pain in the bone
- Swelling
- Decreased movement of the extremity
  - During the newborn period, osteomyelitis may manifest without any signs or symptoms except for decreased movement of a limb.
- Signs of systemic illness, including fever, irritability, and lethargy in acute phase

AGGRAVATING ACTIVITIES

Increased use and/or weight bearing on affected extremity

EASING ACTIVITIES

Rest

24-HOUR SYMPTOM PATTERN

Increased symptoms over time if the infection is not treated.

PAST HISTORY FOR THE REGION

Several days to 1 week of progressing symptoms

PHYSICAL EXAMINATION

- Tenderness to palpation over involved bone
- Antalgic gait if lower extremity is involved.

IMPORTANT OBJECTIVE TESTS

- ROM: Decreased ROM in adjacent joints
- MMT: Muscle weakness in affected extremity

DIFFERENTIAL DIAGNOSES

- Skeletal neoplasia
- Aseptic bone infarction
- Neuropathic joint disease
- Fracture
- Leukemia
- Bone tumor (e.g., osteosarcoma or Ewing's sarcoma)
- Septic arthritis
- Rheumatoid arthritis
- Soft tissue infection (e.g., abscess)
- Cellulitis

CONTRIBUTING FACTORS

- Diagnosis of sickle cell disease
  - Children with sickle cell disease are at an increased risk for bacterial infections, and osteomyelitis is the second most common infection in these patients.
- History of bone infarction
  - Areas of bone infarction may actually predispose the patient to osteomyelitis.
- Use of immunosuppressive medications such as chemotherapy

TREATMENT

SURGICAL OPTIONS

- In cases of hematogenous osteomyelitis, surgical intervention is not always indicated. However, surgical debridement may be necessary in patients who do not respond to antimicrobial therapy and in cases of abscess formation.
- Conventional treatment of contiguous and chronic osteomyelitis includes both antimicrobial therapy and surgical debridement of the bone and overlying infected tissue.

SURGICAL OUTCOMES

The longer it takes to begin effective treatment, the greater the likelihood of adverse outcomes. However, in spite of appropriate therapy, chronic infection develops in 5% to 10% of cases.

REHABILITATION

- Gait training
- ROM activities
- Muscle strengthening exercises
- Age-appropriate developmental activities

PROGNOSIS

- Complications from osteomyelitis, such as impaired bone growth, are more common in children younger than 18 months.
- Prognosis is worse for chronic osteomyelitis, and amputation may be required if there is extensive disease that is resistant to antibiotic treatment.

SIGNS AND SYMPTOMS INDICATING REFERRAL TO PHYSICIAN

- Increased signs of infection such as increased temperature, erythema, drainage, odor, and swelling
- Persistent symptoms after a 3- to 6-week course of antibiotics
- Pain that is worse at night may suggest a neoplastic process such as osteosarcoma.
- Decreased weight bearing of an extremity without signs and symptoms of an active infection and fracture has not been previously ruled out.

SUGGESTED READINGS

Barrett-Connor E. Bacterial infection and sickle cell anemia: an analysis of 250 infections in 166 patients and review of the literature. *Medicine.* 1971;50:97-112.

Blacksin MF, Finzel KC, Benevenia J. Osteomyelitis originating in and around bone infarcts: giant sequestrum phenomena. *Am J Roentgenol.* 2001;176:387-391.

Carek PJ, Dickerson LM, Sack JL. Diagnosis and management of osteomyelitis. *Am Fam Physician.* 2001;15(12):2413-2420.

Cole WG, Dalziel RE, Leitl S. Treatment of acute osteomyelitis in childhood. *J Bone Joint Surg.* 1982;64:218-223.

Kahan S, Raves J. *In a Page Surgery.* Malden, MA: Blackwell Publishing; 2003:164.

Sonnen GM, Henry NK. Pediatric bone and joint infections. Diagnosis and antimicrobial management. *Pediatr Clin North Am.* 1996; 43(4):933-947.

Vazquez M. Osteomyelitis in children. *Curr Opin Pediatr.* 2002;14:112-115.

Wall EJ. Childhood osteomyelitis and septic arthritis. *Curr Opin Pediatr.* 1998;10(1): 73-76.

AUTHORS: ERICA PABLO and LEESHA AUGUSTINE

BASIC INFORMATION

DEFINITION

- Salter-Harris fractures involve the growth plate and are unique to pediatric patients.
- The basic types of Salter-Harris fractures are as follows:
  - Type 1: Separation of epiphysis from metaphysis
  - Type 2: Fracture line runs along physis through metaphysis, but the epiphysis is not involved; bony fragment of metaphysis is formed; the most common type of Salter-Harris fracture.
  - Type 3: Vertical fracture line from epiphysis through physis, parallel to physis to periphery
  - Type 4: Vertical fracture line from epiphysis, through physis and metaphysis and enters the joint; may be displaced bone fragment.
  - Type 5: Crushing of physis from severe compression force; generally very rare.

SYNONYMS

- Growth plate fractures
- Pediatric fractures
- Physeal injuries

ICD-9CM CODES
812.09 Other closed fractures of upper end of humerus
812.44 Fracture of unspecified condyle(s) of humerus closed
813.43 Fracture of medial condyle of humerus closed
820.01 Fracture of epiphysis (separation) (upper) of neck of femur closed
820.11 Fracture of epiphysis (separation) (upper) of neck of femur open
821.22 Fracture of lower epiphysis of femur closed
821.32 Fracture of lower epiphysis of femur open

OPTIMAL NUMBER OF VISITS

12 or fewer

MAXIMAL NUMBER OF VISITS

18

ETIOLOGY

Fracture to the growth plate most commonly occurs in long bones such as phalanges, radius, tibia, fibula, and femur. Injury to the physes is more likely to occur in the active pediatric population because of the greater structural strength and integrity of the ligamentous structures compared to the growth plates.

EPIDEMIOLOGY AND DEMOGRAPHICS

- Physeal injuries are seen more frequently during times of rapid growth such as preschool or prepubertal ages.
- Growth plate fractures occur twice as often in boys than in girls.
  - The greatest incidence occurs in 12- to 14-year-old boys and 11- to 12-year-old girls.

MECHANISM OF INJURY

Trauma or overuse

COMMON SIGNS AND SYMPTOMS

- Inability to bear weight on involved extremity
- Impaired function and decreased ROM in affected extremity
- Localized joint pain
- Swelling near the affected joint with focal tenderness over the physis

AGGRAVATING ACTIVITIES

Weight-bearing and functional activities such as walking, lifting, and reaching

EASING ACTIVITIES

- Rest
- Immobilization of involved limb

24-HOUR SYMPTOM PATTERN

Increased pain at the end of the day, especially with loading or weight-bearing activities.

PAST HISTORY FOR THE REGION

History of a fall or collision often related to recreational activities

PHYSICAL EXAMINATION

- Tenderness to palpation over the epiphyseal plate
- Antalgic gait pattern or inability to bear weight if the lower extremity is involved.
- Effusion surrounding the affected joint
- Visual deformity of the affected joint
- Possible ecchymosis

IMPORTANT OBJECTIVE TESTS

- Limited ROM in affected joint
- Strength testing of involved joint: Diminished strength may be present.
- Ligamentous laxity tests may elicit pain, and positive findings may involve more than joint tissues alone.

DIFFERENTIAL DIAGNOSES

- Ligamentous injury
- Tendon injury
- Pathological fracture

CONTRIBUTING FACTORS

- Cold or frostbite causes damage to the growth plate and results in short, stubby fingers.
- Radiation and/or chemotherapy damage growth plates and can affect bone growth.
- Neurological disorders that result in sensory deficits, muscular imbalance, and/or ligamentous laxity place growth plate at an increased risk for damage.

TREATMENT

SURGICAL OPTIONS

- Surgery is typically needed for Salter-Harris fracture types 3 to 5.
- Salter-Harris fracture types 3 and 4 involve anatomical reduction and internal fixation to restore alignment of joint surfaces.
- Salter-Harris fractures type 5 are rarely diagnosed acutely, and treatment is often delayed until the formation of a bony bar across the physis is evident. Physeal bar resection or other surgical procedures may be indicated to prevent or correct deformity.

SURGICAL OUTCOMES

- Once surgery has restored alignment of joint surfaces or deformity and initial fracture healing has occurred, additional follow-up radiographs are indicated to assess for growth disturbance, especially in Salter-Harris fracture type 5. Growth arrest may result in angular deformities and progressive limb-length discrepancies.
- Articular problems may occur in physeal fractures that lead to discontinuities of the articular surface (Salter-Harris types 3 and 4), which can lead to intraarticular step-off and early degenerative joint disease if proper anatomical reduction is not achieved.

REHABILITATION

- Physical therapy after cast removal of types 1 and 2 fractures is rarely required. Children present with near normal ROM and quickly regain strength through normal activity.
- Modalities for pain and swelling
- Scar mobilization
- Increase ROM (joint mobilization and/or stretching).
- Strengthening of affected extremity
- Improve fine motor skills with upper extremity involvement.
- Gait and balance or proprioception training if lower extremity is involved.

PROGNOSIS

- Prognosis depends on the classification of the fracture, as follows:
  - Types 1 and 2: Prognosis is good, with no growth disturbance.

- ○ Type 3: Good prognosis, if the circulation is not interrupted and good alignment is obtained.
  - ○ Type 4: May have growth disturbance.
  - ○ Type 5: Arrest of growth with possible angular deformity
- Poorer results are correlated with age at the time of the injury (younger patients had worse results) and severity of the fracture (degree of displacement).

SIGNS AND SYMPTOMS INDICATING REFERRAL TO PHYSICIAN

- Visible deformity of the arm or leg after an acute traumatic injury
- Severe pain in the affected extremity after an injury
- Although rare, signs of compartment syndrome may develop secondary to the epiphyseal fracture, which would warrant immediate medical attention.

SUGGESTED READINGS

Arkader A, Warner Jr WC, Horn BD, Shaw RN, Wells L. Predicting the outcome of physeal fractures of the distal femur. *J Pediatr Orthop.* 2007;27(6):703-708.

Bainbridge DB. Sports injuries in children. In: Campbell SK, Vander Linden DW, Palisano RJ, eds. *Physical Therapy for Children.* 3rd ed. Philadelphia: Saunders; 2006:517-556.

Brown JH, DeLuca SA. Growth plate injuries: Salter-Harris classification. *Am Fam Physician.* 1992;46(4):1180-1184.

Cox G, Thambapillay S, Templeton PA. Compartment syndrome with an isolated Salter Harris II fracture of the distal tibia. *J Orthop Trauma.* 2008;22(2):148-150.

Mann DC, Rajmaira S. Distribution of physeal and nonphyseal fractures in 2,650 long-bone fractures in children aged 0-16 years. *J Pediatr Orthop.* 1990;10(6):713-716.

Riseborough EJ, Barrett IR, Shapiro F. Growth disturbances following distal femoral physeal fracture separations. *J Bone Joint Surg Am.* 1983;65(7):885-893.

Stanger M. Orthopedic Management. In: Tecklin JS, eds. *Pediatric Physical Therapy.* 4th ed. Baltimore: Lippincott Williams & Wilkins; 2008.

AUTHORS: ERICA PABLO and LEESHA AUGUSTINE

BASIC INFORMATION

DEFINITION

Sever disease, the most common cause of heel pain in athletic children, is an osteochondrosis caused by trauma that results in the fragmentation or avulsion of cartilage at the Achilles tendon insertion to the calcaneus, disruption of chondrogenesis, reparative callus, fibrosis, and ossification.

SYNONYMS

- Calcaneal apophysitis
- Calcaneal epiphysitis
- Traction apophysitis

ICD-9CM CODES
732.5   Juvenile osteochondrosis of foot

OPTIMAL NUMBER OF VISITS

12 or fewer

MAXIMAL NUMBER OF VISITS

24

ETIOLOGY

Repetitive microtrauma from the pull of the Achilles tendon on the unossified calcaneal apophysis has a decreased resistance to shear stress.

EPIDEMIOLOGY AND DEMOGRAPHICS

Sever disease occurs most commonly in boys, ages 8 to 14 years

MECHANISM OF INJURY

Traction of the Achilles tendon occurs before or during the peak growth spurt or shortly after a child begins a new sport or season.

COMMON SIGNS AND SYMPTOMS

- Heel pain that worsens with a specific sport; soccer is the most common.
- Wearing shoes is painful.
- Calf stretches reproduce localized heel pain.

AGGRAVATING ACTIVITIES

Activities that cause forced dorsiflexion or require active plantar flexion of the ankle such as running and jumping

EASING ACTIVITIES

- Rest
- Ice
- Placing the ankle in a resting passive plantar flexion position

24-HOUR SYMPTOM PATTERN

Intermittent or continuous heel pain occurs with weight bearing

PAST HISTORY FOR THE REGION

Gradual onset of symptoms

PHYSICAL EXAMINATION

- Swelling may be present but is usually mild
- Tenderness to palpation at the Achilles tendon insertion
- Reproduction of pain with passive ankle dorsiflexion
- Pain with performing active plantar flexion
- Examine contralateral foot and ankle caused by high risk of bilateral involvement
  - Bilateral involvement is present in approximately 60% of cases.

IMPORTANT OBJECTIVE TESTS

- Positive Achilles tendon squeeze test
- ROM
  - Limited gastrocnemius and soleus flexibility
- MMT
  - Weakness of gastrocnemius/soleus complex caused by pain
- Medial-to-lateral compression of the calcaneus typically causes pain in patients with calcaneal stress fractures.

DIFFERENTIAL DIAGNOSES

- Achilles tendon pathology
- Calcaneus fractures
- Nonneoplastic conditions simulating bone tumors
- Osteomyelitis
- Tarsal coalition
- Plantar fasciitis

CONTRIBUTING FACTORS

- Tight heel cords
- The anatomical position of the lower extremity, such as the following, can increase the tension on the Achilles tendon:
  - Femoral anteversion
  - Excessive pronation
  - Pes planus
  - Forefoot varus

TREATMENT

SURGICAL OPTIONS

Surgery is typically not indicated unless more complicated factors are present, such as an associated Achilles tendon rupture.

SURGICAL OUTCOMES

Not applicable

REHABILITATION

- Rest
- Antiinflammatory medications as prescribed by a physician
- Modalities for pain and inflammation (iontophoresis, ice massage)
- Short leg walking cast for acute severe pain
- Heel lifts or orthotics
- Gastrocnemius/soleus muscle stretching and strengthening
- Gastrocnemius soft tissue mobilization or myofascial release
- Tibialis anterior strengthening (ankle dorsiflexion)
- Short foot or intrinsic exercises
- Tibialis posterior strengthening
- Gluteus medius strengthening
- Sport-specific training
- Proper athletic footwear

PROGNOSIS

- Sever disease is a self-limited condition with good overall prognosis.
- Majority of the patients are able to resume sports activities after 2 months.

SIGNS AND SYMPTOMS INDICATING REFERRAL TO PHYSICIAN

If pain continues, becomes significant at rest, awakens the patient from sleep, or is associated with significant swelling or redness, tests should be performed to rule out other causes such as tumor or osteomyelitis.

SUGGESTED READINGS

Bainbridge DB. Sports injuries in children. In: Campbell SK, Vander Linden DW, Palisano RJ, eds. *Physical Therapy for Children*. 3rd ed. Philadelphia: Saunders; 2006:517–556.

Fu FH, Stone DA. *Sports Injuries: Mechanisms, Prevention, and Treatment*. 2nd ed. Philadelphia: Lippincott Williams & Wilkins; 2001.

Hendrix CL. Calcaneal apophysitis (Sever disease). *Clin Podiatr Med Surg*. 2005;22(1):55–62.

Leach J. Orthopedic conditions. In: Campbell SK, Vander Linden DW, Palisano RJ, eds. *Physical Therapy for Children*. 3rd ed. Philadelphia: Saunders; 2006:481–515.

Madden CC, Mellion MB. Sever's disease and other causes of heel pain in adolescents. *Am Fam Physician*. 1996;54(6):1995–2000.

Micheli LJ, Ireland ML. Prevention and management of calcaneal apophysitis in children: an overuse syndrome. *J Pediatr Orthop*. 1987;7(1):34–38.

Siffert RS. Classification of the osteochondroses. *Clin Orthop Relat Res*. 1981;158:10–18.

AUTHORS: ERICA PABLO and LEESHA AUGUSTINE

Section III

ORTHOPEDIC PATHOLOGY

BASIC INFORMATION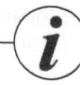

DEFINITION

Sinding-Larsen-Johansson (SLJ) syndrome is an overuse traction apophysitis at the insertion point of the proximal patellar tendon onto the lower patellar pole.

SYNONYMS

- Apophysitis of the distal pole of the patella
- Patellar osteochondrosis

ICD-9CM CODES
732.4 Juvenile osteochondrosis of lower extremity excluding foot

OPTIMAL NUMBER OF VISITS

12 or fewer

MAXIMAL NUMBER OF VISITS

24

ETIOLOGY

The etiology appears to be a traction tendinitis with de novo calcification in the proximal attachment of the patellar tendon, which has been partially avulsed.

EPIDEMIOLOGY AND DEMOGRAPHICS

SLJ syndrome is common in the knee of girls between ages 8 and 13 years and in boys between ages 10 and 15 years.

MECHANISM OF INJURY

Repetitive microtrauma as a result of sports participation that include activities such as running and jumping.

COMMON SIGNS AND SYMPTOMS

- Pain that is localized to the anterior knee
- Limping
- Mild swelling

AGGRAVATING ACTIVITIES

- Running
- Jumping
- Kneeling
- Climbing stairs

EASING ACTIVITIES

- Rest
- Positioning the knee in passive extension

24-HOUR SYMPTOM PATTERN

Pain worsens throughout the day in association with aggravating activities.

PAST HISTORY FOR THE REGION

Patients may have intermittent pain in the knee for several months before seeking medical attention.

PHYSICAL EXAMINATION

- Point tenderness at the inferior pole of the patella (the criterion for clinical diagnosis)
- Increased pain with resistance to quadriceps contraction
- Assess patellar mobility

IMPORTANT OBJECTIVE TESTS

- ROM
  - Assessment of two-joint muscle length is vital because tightness of the hamstring muscles or iliotibial band may increase the flexion moment at the knee
- Quadriceps MMT is diminished secondary to pain.
- Functional strength tests (stairs, squatting)

DIFFERENTIAL DIAGNOSES

- Patellofemoral pain syndrome
- Osgood-Schlatter disease
- Patellar tendinitis (jumper's knee)
- Sleeve fractures

CONTRIBUTING FACTORS

Patella alta

TREATMENT

SURGICAL OPTIONS

Condition is self-limiting, and surgery is not indicated.

SURGICAL OUTCOMES

Not applicable

REHABILITATION

- Acute phase: Rest, ice, and immobilization
- NSAIDs may be prescribed by the physician for persistent swelling.
- Modalities for pain or inflammation
- Taping or bracing (patellar band)
- Quadriceps stretching and strengthening
- Hip strengthening (gluteus medius)
- Hamstring stretching
- Iliotibial band mobilization
- Plyometric training
- Sports-specific training

PROGNOSIS

- The natural duration of the disease lasts approximately 3 to 12 months.
- No residual disability has been reported (Staheli).

SIGNS AND SYMPTOMS INDICATING REFERRAL TO PHYSICIAN

- A sudden inability to weight bear may indicate a fracture.
- Diffuse knee swelling with erythema and increased tactile temperature with an associated fever can be signs of osteomyelitis.
- Osteochondritis dissecans is a rare but serious cause of adolescent knee pain that can result in permanent knee damage. Therefore patients who present with diffuse knee pain, effusion, and loss of motion must be referred to an orthopedist.
- A palpable mass that is warm and tender with systemic signs such as fever and lethargy may indicate osteomyelitis of the proximal tibia.
- Suprapatellar swelling, ecchymosis, and tenderness may be caused by a quadriceps tendon rupture.

SUGGESTED READINGS

Bainbridge DB. Sports injuries in children. In: Campbell SK, Vander Linden DW, Palisano RJ, eds. *Physical Therapy for Children*. 3rd ed. Philadelphia: Saunders; 2006:517–556.

Bergstrom KA, Brandseth K, Fretheim S, et al. Activity-related knee injuries and pain in athletic adolescents. *Knee Surg, Sports Traumatol, Arthrosc*. 2001;9:146–150.

Birrer RB, Griesemer BA, Cataletto MB. *Pediatric Sports Medicine for Primary Care*. Philadelphia: Lippincott Williams & Wilkins; 2002.

Grogan DP, Carey TP, Leffers D, et al. Avulsion fractures of the patella. *J Pediatr Orthop*. 1990;10:721–730.

Heckman JD, Alkire CC. Distal patellar pole fractures—a proposed common mechanism of injury. *Am J Sports Med*. 1984;12:424–428.

Medlar RC, Lyne ED. Sinding-Larsen-Johansson disease. Its etiology and natural history. *J Bone Joint Surg Am*. 1978;60(8):1113–1116.

Peck DM. Apophyseal injuries in the young athlete. *Am Fam Physician*. 1995;51:1891–1895.

Smillie IS. *Injuries of the Knee Joint*. 4th ed. Baltimore: Williams and Wilkins; 1970.

Staheli LT. *Practice of Pediatric Orthopedics*. 2nd ed. Philadelphia: Lippincott Williams & Wilkins; 2006.

Zarogianni C. Sinding-Larsen Johanssen Syndrome—Case report. *J Orthop*. 2007;4(4):e4.

AUTHORS: ERICA PABLO and LEESHA AUGUSTINE

BASIC INFORMATION

DEFINITION

- Slipped capital femoral epiphysis, one of the most common hip disorders in the adolescent population, occurs when the growth plate of the proximal femoral physis is weak and becomes displaced from its normal position. Slipped capital femoral epiphysis results from a Salter-Harris type physeal fracture.
- Slipped capital femoral epiphysis is divided into the following three subtypes:
  ○ Acute: Occurs with significant trauma and causes immediate, severe pain and restricted hip abduction and internal rotation.
  ○ Acute-on-chronic: The patient has been experiencing some aching in the hip, thigh, or knee for weeks or even months as a result of a chronic slip. The patient then sustains a significant trauma to the hip, the epiphysis slips farther, and acute symptoms are noted.
  ○ Chronic: The most common form of the disorder in which the child has a history of a limp and pain, often for weeks or months, and loss of hip motion, especially internal rotation and abduction.

SYNONYMS

- SCFE
- Slipped hip
- Epiphysiolysis
- Femoral head displacement

ICD-9CM CODES
732.2 Nontraumatic slipped upper femoral epiphysis

OPTIMAL NUMBER OF VISITS

12 or fewer

MAXIMAL NUMBER OF VISITS

18

ETIOLOGY

- The etiology is unknown, but genetic, hormonal, and mechanical factors play an important role.
  ○ The rate of familial involvement is 5% to 7%, with a large variability in penetrance.
  ○ Mechanical factors associated with the disorder are obesity, increased femoral retroversion, and increased physeal obliquity.
  ○ Slipped capital femoral epiphysis is a disease of puberty, when many hormonal changes occur.
- These factors result in a mechanical failure of the growth plate to resist displacement.

EPIDEMIOLOGY AND DEMOGRAPHICS

- Slipped capital femoral epiphysis occurs in boys ages 10 to 16 years and girls ages 12 to 14 years with a male-to-female ratio of 2.4:1.
- Obesity is reported in as many as 75% of patients.
- The age at onset decreases with increasing obesity.
- African Americans are more often affected than whites.

MECHANISM OF INJURY

Insidious onset of symptoms that may or may not be exacerbated by a traumatic episode

COMMON SIGNS AND SYMPTOMS

- Hip, thigh, or knee pain
- Limp
- Decreased hip ROM

AGGRAVATING ACTIVITIES

Prolonged standing and walking

EASING ACTIVITIES

- Rest
- Physical activity modification

24-HOUR SYMPTOM PATTERN

Increased symptoms throughout the day in association with weight-bearing activity

PAST HISTORY FOR THE REGION

- 67% of the patients with an acute slipped capital femoral epiphysis have a 1- to 3-month history of mild prodromal symptoms before the acute episode.
- The patient with chronic slipped capital femoral epiphysis may have a history of exacerbations and remissions of the pain and limp.

PHYSICAL EXAMINATION

- Out-toeing in standing and supine
- Obligate abduction and external rotation is noted with passive hip flexion (Drehmann's sign)
- Antalgic gait
- Positive Trendelenburg's sign
- Pain that is referred to the anteromedial aspect of the thigh and knee: 46% of the patients with slipped capital femoral epiphysis have pain in the knee or the distal thigh as the initial symptom. Therefore it is important to perform a hip examination in a pediatric patient with knee pain.
- In the general population, there is a 25% chance of asynchronous bilateral involvement. Of patients with known unilateral involvement, 60% to 80% develop slipped capital femoral epiphysis in the contralateral hip.

IMPORTANT OBJECTIVE TESTS

- Decreased hip ROM is noted in flexion, abduction, and internal rotation
  ○ Most consistent positive finding is lack of internal rotation
- Leg length discrepancy
- Knee objective tests do not reproduce patient's symptoms (knee pain is referred from the hip).

DIFFERENTIAL DIAGNOSES

- Femoral neck fracture
- Groin injury
- Osteitis pubis
- Legg-Calvé-Perthes disease
- Synovitis
- Septic joint
- Chronic developmental hip dysplasia
- Femoral hernia
- Patellofemoral syndrome
- Osgood-Schlatter disease

CONTRIBUTING FACTORS

- There is an association of slipped capital femoral epiphysis in patients with endocrine disorders, renal failure, secondary hyperparathyroidism, and growth hormone abnormalities. These patients are often younger than 10 years and both hips are commonly affected.
- Children who are obese are at increased risk for developing the hip disorder; at least 50% of the children with the disorder are over the 95th percentile for weight according to age.

TREATMENT

SURGICAL OPTIONS

- In situ stabilization using central percutaneous pin fixation with one or more cannulated screws is the most popular treatment method.
- Open epiphysiodesis with iliac crest or allogenic bone graft, often in combination with internal fixation
- Intertrochanteric osteotomy with internal fixation

SURGICAL OUTCOMES

Most patients with slipped capital femoral epiphysis who are treated with in situ pinning have a good prognosis for return to prior level of function. However, in cases with severe slippage and resultant deformity, long-term sequelae may result (avascular necrosis, chondrolysis, leg length discrepancy, stiffness, or osteoarthritis).

REHABILITATION

- Strengthen the affected lower extremity including gluteus medius, gluteus maximus, adductors, quadriceps, and hamstrings

- Increase hip ROMs.
- Gait training
- Balance or proprioception training
- Improve muscular endurance.

PROGNOSIS

Delay in diagnosis is associated with increased slip severity, which places the patient at a higher risk for developing short-term complications from treatment such as avascular necrosis and chondrolysis. Increased slip severity is also associated with poorer long-term outcomes, including pain, limitation of motion, and degenerative joint disease.

SIGNS AND SYMPTOMS INDICATING REFERRAL TO PHYSICIAN

- In patients who present at an early age (younger than 10 years), consultation with an endocrinologist may be necessary to help rule out other metabolic disorders if the history and physical examination findings indicate other abnormalities.
- Fever and joint pain may be signs of septic arthritis and/or osteomyelitis. If a rash is also present, JRA must also be considered.
- Pain that is worse at night may suggest a neoplastic process such as osteosarcoma.
- Decreased weight bearing in an extremity without signs and symptoms of an active infection and fracture that has not been previously ruled out

SUGGESTED READINGS

Aronsson DD, Carlson WE. Slipped capital femoral epiphysis. A prospective study of fixation with a single screw. *J Bone Joint Surg Am*. 1992;74(6):810-819.

Aronsson DD, Loder RT, Breur GJ, Weinstein SL. Slipped capital femoral epiphysis: current concepts. *J Am Acad Orthop Surg*. 2006;14(21):666-679.

Carney BT, Weinstein SL, Noble J. Long-term follow-up of slipped capital femoral epiphysis. *J Bone Joint Surg Am*. 1991;73:667-674.

Katz DA. Slipped capital femoral epiphysis: the importance of early diagnosis. *Pediatr Ann*. 2006;35(2):102-111.

Kocher MS, Bishop JA, Weed B, Hresko, et al. Delay in diagnosis of slipped capital femoral epiphysis. *Pediatrics*. 2004;113:322-325.

Leach J. Orthopedic conditions. In: Campbell SK, Vander Linden DW, Palisano RJ, eds. *Physical Therapy for Children*. 3rd ed. Philadelphia: Saunders; 2006:481-515.

Loder RT. The demographics of slipped capital femoral epiphysis: an international multicenter study. *Clin Orthop*. 1996;322:8-27.

Loder RT, Wittenberg B, DeSilva G. Slipped capital femoral epiphysis associated with endocrine disorders. *J Pediatr Orthop*. 1995;15:349-356.

Matava MJ, Patton CM, Luhmann S, et al. Knee pain as the initial symptom of slipped capital femoral epiphysis: an analysis of initial presentation and treatment. *J Pediatr Orthop*. 1999;19:455-460.

Rattey T, Piehl F, Wright JG. Acute slipped capital femoral epiphysis. Review of outcomes and rates of avascular necrosis. *J Bone Joint Surg Am*. 1996;78:398-402.

Stasikelis PJ, Sullivan CM, Philips WA, Polard JA. Slipped capital femoral epiphysis. Prediction of contralateral involvement. *J Bone Joint Surg Am*. 1996;78:1149-1155.

Weiner D. Pathogenesis of slipped capital femoral epiphysis: current concepts. *J Pediatr Orthop Br*. 1996;5:67-73.

AUTHORS: ERICA PABLO and LEESHA AUGUSTINE

BASIC INFORMATION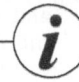

DEFINITION

- Incontinence is the involuntary loss of urine or fecal matter. This loss may or may not be associated with urge to urinate or defecate or with activities that increase abdominal pressure.
- Incontinence is the most common manifestation of pelvic floor muscle weakness.

SYNONYMS/ASSOCIATED MEDICAL DIAGNOSES

- Urge urinary incontinence
- Fecal incontinence
- Stress urinary incontinence
- Mixed incontinence
- Overflow incontinence
- Pelvic floor muscle weakness

ICD-9CM CODES
625.6 Stress incontinence female
787.6 Incontinence of feces
728.87 Muscle weakness (generalized)

OPTIMAL NUMBER OF VISITS
8 or fewer

MAXIMAL NUMBER OF VISITS
20

ETIOLOGY

- Micturition and continence requires a balanced control between urethral opening and closure. When this balance is disrupted, incontinence occurs.
- Urine is normally retained in the bladder because urethral pressure exceeds bladder pressure.
- Normal voiding occurs when bladder muscles contract to increase bladder pressure and urethral pressure decreases because of muscle relaxation.
- Incontinence most commonly results from impairments in strength and muscle coordination (timing and recruitment).
- Types of urinary incontinence
  - Stress incontinence occurs as a result of pelvic floor muscle weakness, pregnancy, childbirth, and menopause. Leakage may occur with activities that result in increased bladder pressure such as coughing, sneezing, or laughing.
  - Urge incontinence is an idiopathic loss of continence, resulting in the sudden urge to urinate or defecate. Infections, poor central inhibitory control, or inflammation may cause involuntary detrusor muscle contraction. This overactivity of the detrusor muscle has been linked to increases in neural activity to the bladder.
  - Functional incontinence occurs when a person does not realize or cannot physically respond to the need to urinate. Functional incontinence is common in elderly disorders, such as dementia, in which the patient is cognitively unable to respond to the need to urinate. Functional incontinence may also affect individuals with impaired mobility who cannot reach a bathroom.
  - Overflow incontinence occurs when the bladder cannot physically void its contents. As a result, the bladder fills more quickly and the patient experiences a constant dribble or a dribble for a short period after urination. Weaker bladder muscles or an obstructed urethra can account for overflow incontinence. Pathology, such as diabetes mellitus or multiple sclerosis, can decrease neural signals. Benign prostatic hyperplasia can also restrict urine flow.
  - Decreased awareness and knowledge of the pelvic floor muscle function and recruitment, as well as strength impairments of the abdominals, hips, and lower extremities, are common impairments associated with incontinence.
  - Impaired breathing patterns, as well as mobility impairments of the hips, pelvic girdle, and spine, can also influence incontinence patterns.
- The role that daily habits play in incontinence can vary from minimal to significant. Dietary and habitual reactions to urinary or fecal urges influence the bladder's contractility and storage capacity.
  - Some patients may not allow enough time for the pelvic floor muscles to relax when going to the bathroom, and insufficient bladder emptying may occur. This occurrence may promote more frequent urges and place a more consistent demand on the pelvic floor.

EPIDEMIOLOGY AND DEMOGRAPHICS

- The two common age groups of women more likely to have issues with incontinence are during and after pregnancy and perimenopausal and postmenopausal.
- White women tend to have higher risk for structural stress incontinence.
- Obesity and smoking increase the likelihood of urinary incontinence.

MECHANISM OF INJURY

- Incontinence often can occur with the following:
  - Gradual decrease in strength or atrophy of pelvic floor, abdominal, hip, or lower extremity musculature
  - Stretch weakness (pregnancy, gravity, or hormones)
  - Medical conditions or past history of asthma, chronic bronchitis, or habitual or job activities that increase Valsalva maneuvers
  - Posthysterectomy, when there is a caudal migration of organs that add to pressure downward on the pelvic floor
  - Pudendal nerve injury

COMMON SIGNS AND SYMPTOMS

- Urinary or fecal leakage with activities such as coughing, laughing, sneezing, or squatting
- Urinary or fecal leakage that is associated with urge to urinate or defecate
- Urinary or fecal frequency
- Perineal pain, soreness, or heaviness

AGGRAVATING ACTIVITIES

- Increased fluid intake
- Improper diet
- Stress
- Activities that increase stress on the bladder or pelvic floor
- Increased fluid intake or the intake of bladder irritants (acidic drinks, carbonated drinks, caffeinated drinks) place structural stress via the increased output of the kidneys or can increase the irritability or contractility of the detrusor muscle on the outside of the bladder.
- Improper diet or certain medications can cause stool to be looser in consistency. When stool is looser in consistency, the pelvic floor muscles must work much harder to prevent incontinence.
- Stress and anxiety can upregulate the sympathetic activity around the bladder or physically increase the stress on the bladder; this can push urine out of the bladder. The additional downward pressure and flow places a greater demand on the activity of the pelvic floor.
- Activities that increase stress on the pelvic floor, such as coughing, laughing, sneezing, or squatting, place a stronger demand on the fast-twitch or type II muscle fibers of the pelvic floor. If these fibers, which compose approximately 30% of the pelvic floor, are weak, they do not allow the pelvic floor muscles to contract quickly enough to prevent leakage of quickly descending urine.

EASING ACTIVITIES

- Dietary intake control
  - Appropriate fluid types (avoiding bladder irritants such as caffeine, citrus, or carbonation)
  - Appropriate food types (avoiding acidic or spicy foods)
- Physicians often prescribe alpha-adrenergic drugs to increase the contractility of the smooth muscle of the bladder neck and proximal urethra, or anticholinergic agents that inhibit the

binding of acetylcholine to the cholinergic receptor on the bladder and suppress its contractions.
- Diaphragmatic breathing and calming techniques
- Pelvic floor contractions can delay the urge to urinate or defecate.
- Proper pH and consistency of stool are crucial for proper bowel and bladder behavior to minimize bladder contractions that place stress on the pelvic floor.
- Diaphragmatic breathing can help to decrease urgency via calming of the sympathetic system.
- Pelvic floor contractions can delay urgency via a negative feedback loop neurologically.

24-HOUR SYMPTOM PATTERN
- Many patients present with increased urinary frequency overnight (nocturia).
- Symptoms often increase after intake of bladder irritants.
- For patients with stress urinary incontinence, leakage occurs with daily activities and activities that increase pressure on the bladder or abdomen.

PAST HISTORY FOR THE REGION
- Pregnancy pressure and resultant delivery-related tissue damage can create stretch-related muscle weakness or scar-related pain and reflexive inhibition that lead to weakness.
- Some women experience symptoms at the onset of menopause. This occurs because of hormonally mediated changes in mucosal vascularity and suppleness of the vaginal and urethral walls, as well as muscular changes in the pelvic floor and all related abdominal, hip, and lower extremity musculature.

PHYSICAL EXAMINATION
- Hip, lumbar, and lower extremity range of motion (ROM) testing
  - Lumbopelvic mobility can affect the recruitability, contractility, and maneuverability of the pelvic floor.
- Hip, abdominal, and lower extremity strength testing
  - Hip, abdominal, or lower extremity weakness places undue stress on the pelvic floor, increasing the demands of the very thin musculature.

IMPORTANT OBJECTIVE TESTS
- Pelvic floor assessment
  - Reflex testing: Cough and wink tests assess the integrity and nerve latency of the pudendal nerve.
  - Tactile assessment: Internal and/or external assessment gives the clinician an impression of where delayed awareness may be allowing musculature to remain weak.

  - Objective testing completed by a manual examination determines the amount of perineal rise and the endurance of the fast-twitch fibers (repeatability of quick contractions) and slow-twitch fibers (long contractions).

DIFFERENTIAL DIAGNOSIS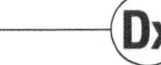
- Urological issues
- Irritable bowel syndrome (IBS)
- Colorectal issues
- Soft tissue dysfunction
- Radiculopathy or cauda equina syndrome

TREATMENT

SURGICAL OPTIONS
- Suburethral sling
- Open Burch colposuspension
- Tension vaginal tape (TVT) procedure
- Periurethral bulking agents
- Neurostimulator
- Colostomy

SURGICAL OUTCOMES
- Although statistics vary, some of the reported results include the following:
  - Suburethral sling: 51% to 96%. Difficult to summarize secondary to variety of techniques and materials used.
  - Open Burch colposuspension: 70% to 94%
  - TVT: Minimally invasive sling procedure that has varying rates between 63% to 85%.
  - Periurethral bulking agents: 4% of women have allergic reactions, and long-term cure rates are rather low, with repeat treatments usually needed.
  - Neurostimulator: Sacral nerve stimulators have been used for overactive bladders.. Success rates have been around 50% for overactive bladder treatment.
  - Colostomy: Although the threat of incontinence is removed with this approach, the patient is then dealing with a permanent colostomy bag (risk of infection) and also has less of an impetus to recruit and use the pelvic floor.

REHABILITATION
- A review of literature indicates that physical therapy produces an average cure rate of 75%.
  - The goal of rehabilitation of the incontinent patient is twofold. First, the focus should be on empowering the patient with education on techniques and bladder or bowel retraining education to help with behavioral management. Second, strengthening

and improving the awareness of the pelvic floor assist in minimizing incontinent episodes and prevention of further episodes.
- Patient education should include the following:
  - Bladder diary
  - Bladder irritant list
  - Stool dietary list
  - Use of pelvic floor contractions to postpone urination or defecation and improve storage
  - Proper diaphragmatic breathing
- Initial exercises should include the following:
  - Diaphragmatic breathing and relaxation techniques
  - Awareness activities for the pelvic floor
  - Short, quick contractions of the pelvic floor
  - Longer, sustained contractions of the pelvic floor
  - Coordinated pelvic floor contractions with specific activities that usually cause incontinence
  - Appropriate hip, lower extremity, or abdominal exercises according to evaluation
  - Bladder training: There is evidence in small sample studies supporting the use of bladder retraining as helpful for treating urinary incontinence, although it is difficult to say whether it is useful as a supplement to another treatment.
- The most current Cochrane Review reports that pelvic floor muscle training helps women with all types of incontinence, most notably stress incontinence. Three months of training is needed for the most benefit.
- Surface electromyography (sEMG) has a dual role in providing either visual or auditory feedback as a learning and awareness tool for the patient with incontinence.
- Biofeedback may be site specific (i.e., anal biofeedback for fecal incontinence and vaginal biofeedback may address specific training more appropriately, although studies so far have been fair in methodology and consistency).
- The research is conflicting in regard to efficacy when compared to biofeedback or pelvic floor muscle exercise alone, and many physical therapists continue to report subjective gains with patients using electrical stimulation for fecal or urinary incontinence.

CONTRIBUTING FACTORS
- Nerve damage from delivery or surgery
- Poor posture
- An occupation that requires restrictive schedules or repetitive lifting
- Strength deficits of the lower extremities, abdominals, or hips

PROGNOSIS

Studies support the use of pelvic floor contractions to minimize future episodes of urinary or fecal incontinence.

SIGNS AND SYMPTOMS INDICATING REFERRAL TO PHYSICIAN

- Constant burning with urination or defecation: Infection or tumor
- Blood in the urine or stool: Infection or tumor
- Significant and unexplained weight loss: Tumor
- Nocturnal pain: Tumor
- Saddle anesthesia: Cauda equina syndrome
- History of cancer: Metastatic disease
- Fevers and chills: Infection or tumor
- Sudden onset of bowel and/or bladder dysfunction: Cauda equina syndrome
- Progressive bilateral lower extremity paresthesias that are nondermatomal: Cauda equina syndrome

SUGGESTED READINGS

http://www.drrajmd.com/conditions/bladder/bladder_outlet_obstruction.htm

Hay-Smith EJC, Dumoulin C. Pelvic floor muscle training versus no treatment, or inactive control treatments, for urinary incontinence in women. *Cochrane Database Syst Rev.* 2006;(1):CD005654. DOI:10.1002/14651858.CD005654.

Konstantinos H, Eleni K, Dimitrios H. Dilemmas in the management of female stress incontinence: the role of pelvic floor muscle training. *Int Urol Nephrol.* 2006;38:513-525.

Norton C, Cody JD, Hosker G. Biofeedback and/or sphincter exercises for the treatment of faecal incontinence in adults. *Cochrane Database Syst Rev.* 2000;(2):CD002111. DOI:10.1002/14651858.CD002111.pub2.

Robert M, Farrell S. Choice of surgery for stress incontinence. *Int J Gynaecol Obstet.* 2005;166:964-971.

Wallace SA, Roe B, Williams K, Palmer M. Bladder training for urinary incontinence in adults. *Cochrane Database Syst Rev.* 2000;(1):CD001308. DOI:10.1002/14651858.CD001308.pub2.

AUTHOR: JULIE GUTHRIE

BASIC INFORMATION

DEFINITION

- Chronic, progressive condition of pathological accumulation of protein-rich fluid, microorganisms, and debris occurs when lymphatic vessel transport is obstructed or impaired.
- The oxygen flow is reduced to the tissues, resulting in a culture medium for infection causing bacteria.
- The two main forms of lymphedema are as follows:
  - Primary: Inherited abnormality of the lymphatic system in which a child is born with less than the optimal amount of lymphatic vessels or components to support transport of lymph tissue within the body.
  - Secondary: Postsurgical
- The four stages of lymphedema are as follows:
  - Stage 0: Considered subclinical, there is impaired lymph transport, but no visual swelling.
  - Stage 1: Tissue swelling is soft, and pitting edema is present.
  - Stage 2: Tissue swelling is hard, and pitting edema does not indent much with pressure.
  - Stage 3: The skin turns thick and fibrotic and loses its elasticity. Folds of tissue form that are disfiguring and are at great risk of developing fungal infections.

SYNONYMS/ASSOCIATED MEDICAL DIAGNOSES

- Lymphedema
- Milroy's disease (primary) in infancy
- Meige's syndrome (primary) in adolescence
- Klippel-Trenaunay-Weber syndrome (KTWS) (primary)

ICD-9CM CODES
457.1 Other lymphedema
457.0 Postmastectomy lymphedema syndrome
757.0 Hereditary edema of legs

OPTIMAL NUMBER OF VISITS

8 or fewer

MAXIMAL NUMBER OF VISITS

20

ETIOLOGY

- Lymphedema occurs when protein-rich fluid accumulates in the interstitium, where there is insufficient transport along the lymph pathways of the fluid.

- The lymphatic loads of water and proteins exceed that of the transport capacity.
- Lymphedema occurs as a functional overload of the lymphatic system in which lymph volume exceeds the transport capacity.
- In primary cases, it is considered an autosomal dominant disorder. In secondary cases, usually surgery, radiation, or major trauma precede lymphedema.

EPIDEMIOLOGY AND DEMOGRAPHICS

- Primary: 87% female; 13% male; 1 in 6000 births
  - There is some evidence that points to hypothyroidism occurring in conjunction with primary lymphedema and should be checked.
- Secondary: Lymphedema can occur at any age following surgical interventions, primarily those involving removal or radiation of lymph nodes. Symptoms usually occur on the involved side but can involve both extremities. Prevalence rates vary, but it is generally agreed that about 25% to 28% of women present with some lymphedema symptoms following breast cancer intervention.
- Age group most at risk for developing lymphedema are as follows:
  - Milroy's is present at birth.
  - Meige's disease ("lymphedema praecox") usually manifests around puberty, or during the first or second decade.
  - With breast cancer interventions, there is documentation of greater risk of development of lymphedema in younger patients.
- Studies have shown a higher prevalence and reported rate of lymphedema in nonwhite patients.

MECHANISM OF INJURY

- Primary lymphedema often can occur following:
  - Hypoplasia of lymph vessels
  - Large lymph vessels with insufficient valve function
  - Aplasia of lymph vessels or capillaries
- Secondary lymphedema often can occur following:
  - Surgery
  - Radiation or radiating lymph nodes and vessels in the axillary region, which changes the way lymph fluid flows in the upper quarter. The result is impaired lymph circulation. If the remaining intact lymph vessels cannot remove enough fluid in the breast and axillary region, lymphedema results.
  - Individuals who have had numerous lymph nodes removed or radiated

may be at higher risk for lymphedema. The reason for increased risk is still unknown.

COMMON SIGNS AND SYMPTOMS

- Pressure in the involved extremity
- Swelling
- Pain or ache in the involved extremity
- Decreased mobility
- Decreased functional activities secondary to these symptoms
- Long-standing lymphedema causes trophic changes, mostly skin thickening and sometimes discoloration and most commonly a reddish or brownish color. The tissue also gets firm and is not pliable. Once at this point, improvements are much less likely to be made.
- Rotator cuff tendinitis is a complication of lymphedema caused by internal derangement of tendon fibers, which may be subject to impingement, functional overload, and tendinopathy. The weight of the heavier arm creates functional overload, and the increase in size may alter the architecture of the shoulder to facilitate impingement of tendinous fibers.

AGGRAVATING ACTIVITIES

- Exposure to hot temperatures
- Vigorous exercise
- Injections or punctures
- Wearing restrictive clothing on the involved area
- Heat and wearing restrictive clothing can negatively affect the amount of overall fluid in the involved extremity. Injections in the involved extremity expose the involved extremity to potential infection. Vigorous exercise increases blood flow and can overwhelm the impaired system.

EASING ACTIVITIES

- Gentle exercise
- Aquatic activity or therapy
- Diaphragmatic breathing
- Gentle exercises promote proper ROM and adequate circulation.
  - Aquatic exercise, via hydrostatic pressure, assists the body in the uptake of lymph fluid.
  - Diaphragmatic breathing encourages proximal truncal venous blood flow

24-HOUR SYMPTOM PATTERN

- The longer the involved limb is dependent, the more likely the increase in lymphedema.
- Lymph drainage techniques
- Lymph compression wrapping and bandaging

PAST HISTORY FOR THE REGION

Patient often has a history of surgery or radiation affecting the lymph node regions (lymphedema presentation can be delayed).

PHYSICAL EXAMINATION

- ROM testing
  - For upper extremity lymphedema, shoulder, trunk, elbow, wrist, and finger ROMs should be completed and compared bilaterally.
- Strength testing
  - Manual muscle tests (MMTs) of all related musculature
- Functional tests
  - Grip testing.
  - Coordination testing

IMPORTANT OBJECTIVE TESTS

- Skin assessment: Note color of skin, condition of nails, wounds, or presence of infection or fungal growth.
- Girth or circumferential testing
  - From documented points of reference that can be repeated each session

DIFFERENTIAL DIAGNOSIS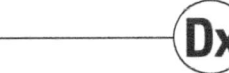

- Lipedema
- Joint swelling
- Congestive heart failure

CONTRIBUTING FACTORS

- Diet
- Obesity
- Activity
- High blood pressure
- Invasive surgery

TREATMENT

SURGICAL OPTIONS

- Debulking procedures
- Supermicrosurgical lymphaticovenular anastomosis

SURGICAL OUTCOMES

- Since the source of the problem is within the lymph system itself, long-term success of debulking procedures is limited. The stressed lymph vessels will gradually build up fluid again.
- Nagase et al reported a 62% success rate with more than 4 cm reduction in limb size around the knees of individuals with long-standing lower extremity lymphedema. This improvement was maintained for at least 4.6 years.

REHABILITATION

- Management should be geared to two major aspects: Minimizing lymphedema and educating the patient on prevention and management techniques.
- Complete decongestive therapy (CDT) has been shown to be most effective in managing limb size and promoting functional return. This involves manual lymph drainage techniques, skin care, proper compression wrapping, and gentle exercise involving ROM and endurance activities. Hamner and Fleming found that out of 136 patients receiving treatment, CDT decreased chronic pain rates from 70 individuals to 20 and use of pain medication from 41 to 11. Chronic pain visual analog scales dropped from an average of 6.9 to 1.1.
- Manual lymph drainage alone will not successfully alleviate symptoms long-term.
- Rehabilitation addressing lymphedema should include the following:
  - Educate the patient on potential aggravating behaviors: Overexercising, wearing restrictive jewelry or clothing, poor wrapping techniques, poor diet.
  - Proper manual lymph drainage and wrapping techniques
  - Walking
  - Exercises that promote movement of the region in a pain-free range
  - Kaviani et al completed a small sample study of the use of low-level light therapy in treatment of postmastectomy lymphedema. They reported a more pronounced decrease in limb circumferences and pain levels. This was the only study found that examined light therapy treatment for lymphedema.
- Although there is no long-term "cure" for lymphedema, management techniques include ROM exercises, breathing exercises, and gentle cardiovascular training.
- Manual lymph drainage assists in balancing the osmotic pressure locally in the tissue. This gentle technique, while time consuming, is quite effective when combined with appropriate bandaging or compression techniques.
- Aquatic exercise is highly recommended to provide a low-impact workout that helps lymphedema via the positive hydrostatic pressure it exerts on the immersed body.
- The most consistent factor influencing further exacerbation is the appropriate and judicious use of properly fitting compression garments or compliance with wrapping techniques.
- Once the initial management process has been started and limb volume decreases, the focus of rehabilitation should include the following:
  - Promoting optimal ROMs in all affected joints
  - Functional retraining for tasks previously unmanageable
  - Body mechanics or compensatory strategies help to optimize the involved extremity's function.

PROGNOSIS

Although lymphedema is considered a chronic condition, it does not necessarily need to be a progressive disorder.

SIGNS AND SYMPTOMS INDICATING REFERRAL TO PHYSICIAN

- Redness or change in skin color: Infection
- Significant, sudden unexplained increase in limb size: Infection
- Nocturnal pain: Tumor
- Major trauma: Fracture
- Fevers and chills: Infection or tumor
- Red streaks along skin: Infection

SUGGESTED READINGS

Bani H, et al. Lymphedema in breast cancer survivors: assessment and information provision in a specialized breast unit. *Patient Educ Couns.* 2007;66:311-318.

Box R, et al. Physiotherapy after breast cancer surgery: results of a randomized controlled study to minimize lymphoedema. *Breast Cancer Res Treat.* 2002;75:51-64.

Cheema B, et al. Progressive resistance training in breast cancer: a systematic review of clinical trials. *Breast Cancer Res Treat.* 2008;109:9-26.

Damstra RJ, et al. Lymphatic venous anastomosis (LVA) for treatment of secondary arm lymphedema. A prospective study of 11 LVA procedures in 10 patients with breast cancer related lymphedema and a critical review of the literature. *Breast Cancer Res Treat.* 2006.

Flynn, et al. *Spine.* 2002;27:2835-2843.

Hakkinen A, et al. Pain, trunk muscle strength, spinal mobility and disability following lumbar disc surgery. *J Rehabil Med.* 2003;35:236-240.

Hamner J, Fleming M. Lymphedema therapy reduces the volume of edema and pain in patients with breast cancer. *Ann Surg Oncol.* 2007;14(6):1904-1908.

Herrerra J, Stubblefield M. Rotator cuffsic in lymphedema: A retrospective case series. *Arch Phys Med Rehabil.* 2004;85:1939-1942.

Hinrichs C, et al. Lymphedema secondary to postmastectomy radiation: Incidence and risk factors. *Ann Surg Oncol.* 2004;11(6):573-580.

Kaviani A, et al. Low-level laser therapy in management of postmastectomy lymphedema. *Lasers Med Sci.* 2006;21:90-94.

Kim D, et al. Excisional surgery for chronic advanced lymphedema. *Surg Today.* 2004;34:134-137.

Meeske K, et al. Risk factors for arm lymphedema following breast cancer diagnosis in black women and white women. *Breast Cancer Res Treat.* DOI: 10.1007/s10549-008-9940-5.

Nagase T, et al. Treatment of lymphedema with lymphaticovenular anastomoses. *Int J Clin Oncol.* 2005;10:304-310.

Vignes S, et al. Long-term management of breast cancer-related lymphedema. *Breast Cancer Res Treat.* 2007;101:285-290.

http://www.lymphnotes.com/article.php/id/4/

http://www.lymphedemapeople.com/thesite/lymphedema_pathophysiology.htm

www.lymphedemacircleofhope.org/pediatric_primary_lymphedema2.html

http://www.pitt.edu/~genetics/lymph/inherit.htm

http://www.nbcc.org.au/bestpractice/resources/LPD_lymphoedemaprevdiagtreatment.pdfp, 51.

http://www.lymphnotes.com/article.php/id/4/

AUTHOR: JULIE GUTHRIE

BASIC INFORMATION

DEFINITION

- The involuntary loss of urine or fecal matter may or may not be associated with the urge to urinate or defecate or with activities that increase abdominal pressure.
- Most common manifestation or symptom of pelvic floor muscle weakness.
- Often occurs after prostatectomy or cystectomy

SYNONYMS

- Urge urinary incontinence
- Stress urinary incontinence
- Fecal incontinence
- Mixed incontinence
- Overflow incontinence
- Pelvic floor muscle weakness

ICD-9CM CODES

788.31 Urge incontinence
788.32 Stress incontinence male
787.6   Incontinence of feces
728.87 Muscle weakness
      (generalized)

OPTIMAL NUMBER OF VISITS

8 or fewer

MAXIMAL NUMBER OF VISITS

20

ETIOLOGY

- Incontinence in men usually occurs from problems with muscle control and regulation.
- During urination, muscles of the bladder contract, which forces urine out of the bladder and into the urethra. If there is a problem with coordination, the sphincter muscles of the urethra relax, allowing urine to be excreted from the body.
- Incontinence occurs if the bladder suddenly contracts or sphincter muscles suddenly relax.
- There are multiple factors can affect the pelvic floor function after prostate or bladder surgery:
  - First, the patient is generally catheterized for several days to several weeks after surgery. During this time, the pelvic floor muscles do not have to work, thus inviting deconditioning to begin. Also, the urethral lining can get irritated from the catheter, potentially allowing increased efferent messages to the brain regarding urgency and awareness.
  - Second, the proximal urethra is encased in an additional sheath (internal sphincter). This is removed during prostate surgery, which potentially changes the effective functional length of the urethra. After prostatectomy, men also have to depend on their pelvic floor muscles much more than before.
  - Finally, since the pelvic floor did not usually have to do quite so much work before surgery, the muscles potentially can be weaker, have less endurance, and be less able to hold a contraction during stressful or coordinated activities.
- After prostatectomy, either sphincteric weakness or bladder dysfunction is the main issue. For most, sphincteric weakness is the most prevalent urodynamic finding in terms of impairments. Basically, in physical therapy, the clinician is faced with dealing with impaired muscle performance. This can encompass impairments in strength (power), as well as coordination (timing and recruitment).
- Decreased awareness and knowledge of the pelvic floor muscle function and recruitment, as well as strength impairments of the abdominals, hips, and lower extremities, are common.
- Impaired breathing patterns, as well as mobility impairments of the hips, pelvic girdle, and spine, can also influence incontinence patterns.

EPIDEMIOLOGY AND DEMOGRAPHICS

- Men experience incontinence much more often than women.
- 1 in 6 men will develop prostate cancer during their lifetimes.
- More than 2 million men with prostate cancer are alive today.
- Incontinence in men generally occurs with later age, although any age can be affected.
- Incontinence rates in men older than 60 years ranges from 10% to 25%; man who have had prostatectomy intervention have incontinence rates ranging from 6% to 87%.
- Although the risk of prostate cancer increases with age, African-American men have higher rates of cancer than white men, which surpasses the rates of either Asian-American or Hispanic-American men.

MECHANISM OF INJURY

- Congenital defects, strokes, brain injury, multiple sclerosis, and other pathologies can affect the nerves controlling the bladder and sphincter.
- Aging, tumors, prostate enlargement, and physical trauma can affect the bladder or sphincter muscles' ability to contract and relax.

COMMON SIGNS AND SYMPTOMS

- Urinary or fecal leakage with activities such as coughing, laughing, sneezing, and squatting
- Urinary or fecal leakage that is associated with the urge to urinate or defecate
- Urinary or fecal frequency
- Perineal pain, soreness, or heaviness

AGGRAVATING ACTIVITIES

- Coughing, sneezing, or laughing
- Walking
- Sit-to-stand transfers
- Sports such as golf, tennis, or jogging
- Coughing, sneezing and laughing create downward pressure on the bladder via increased abdominal pressure. If the pelvic floor muscles do not act quickly enough, they do not occlude the urethral lumen to prevent urinary leakage.

EASING ACTIVITIES

Lying or sitting down: The pelvic floor does not have to work against gravity as much in these positions. Also, the healing urethral tissue is at a different angle than in standing activities, which allows more physical resistance to distally traveling urine.

24-HOUR SYMPTOM PATTERN

- Symptoms vary, depending on the amount of incontinence. For some men, there is a sufficient amount of leakage so they do not experience any urinary urges throughout the day. For others, the frequency is significantly increased secondary to the anxiety around incontinence and the sensitivity to urgency.
- Often, physical activities worsen the incontinence. Daily activities, such as getting out of a chair, reaching for objects, and walking, cause significant stress so that incontinence occurs consistently throughout the day.
- Patients often complain of increased urination overnight (nocturia).

PAST HISTORY FOR THE REGION

- History of surgery in the pelvic region
- History of trauma in the pelvic region

PHYSICAL EXAMINATION

- Hip, lumbar, and lower extremity ROM testing
  - Lumbopelvic mobility can affect the recruitability, contractility, and maneuverability of the pelvic floor.
- Hip, abdominal, and lower extremity strength testing
  - Hip, abdominal, or lower extremity weakness places undue stress on the pelvic floor, increasing the demands of the very thin musculature.
- Neurological assessment
- Anal sphincter tone
- Perineal sensation in S2-S4 dermatomes
- Bulbocavernosus reflex
- Abdominal assessment for distended bladder

IMPORTANT OBJECTIVE TESTS

- Pelvic floor assessment
  - Reflex testing: Cough and wink tests give an idea of the integrity and nerve latency of the pudendal nerve.
  - Tactile assessment: Internal and/or external assessment gives the clinician an impression of where delayed awareness may be allowing musculature to remain weak.
  - Objective testing completed by a manual examination will determine the amount of perineal rise and endurance of the fast-twitch fibers (repeatability of quick contractions) and slow-twitch fibers (long contractions).

DIFFERENTIAL DIAGNOSIS

Overflow incontinence

TREATMENT

MEDICAL/SURGICAL OPTIONS

- Combined androgen blockade
  - Because prostate cancer is hormonally sensitive, medications have been introduced to minimize the activity of testosterone to eliminate further prostate cancer growth. Side effects can include hot flushes, weight gain, erectile dysfunction, a decrease in muscle mass and strength, personality changes, decreased mentation, and osteoporosis.
- Artificial urinary sphincter
- Bulbourethral sling
- Bone-anchored perineal sling
- Bulking agents or collagen urethral injections

SURGICAL OUTCOME

- Artificial urinary sphincter (UAS): Considered the gold standard for dealing with male incontinence, success rates have been reported as high as 90%. However, the complications of erosion (approximately 1% to 3%) and infection (approximately 3%) are concerning. Revision rates are reported to be around 9%.
- Bulbourethral sling: Studies indicate a varied response: Success has been reported up to a 56% cure rate; however, there has been noted a high level of complications. One in five have to be removed, and some studies indicate high rates of perineal pain or numbness secondary to pudendal nerve entrapment with blind suture placement.
- Bone-anchored perineal sling: Newer technique, with noted improvements

in erosion (2.1%) and revision (4.2%) rates. Cure rates have been reported to be around 65%, with an additional "significantly improved" rate of 15%.
- Bulking agents (collagen): A review of the literature indicates that multiple injections are required for effective outcomes, varying on average from 2.5 to 4.5 injections. Percentages of "cure" versus "significantly improved" were 20% and 29%, respectively. Singla found similar injection rates only achieved a 30% "significantly improved" rate.

REHABILITATION

- The goal of rehabilitation of the incontinent patient is twofold. First, the focus should be on empowering the patient with education on techniques and bladder or bowel retraining education to help with behavioral management. Second, strengthening and improving the awareness of the pelvic floor assist in minimizing incontinent episodes and prevention of further episodes.
- Patient education should include the following:
  - Bladder diary
  - Bladder irritant list
  - Stool dietary list
  - Use of pelvic floor contractions to postpone urination or defecation and improve storage.
  - Proper diaphragmatic breathing
- Initial exercises should include the following:
  - Diaphragmatic breathing and relaxation techniques
  - Awareness activities for the pelvic floor
  - Short or quick contractions of the pelvic floor
  - Longer or sustained contractions of the pelvic floor
  - Coordinated pelvic floor contractions with specific activities that usually cause the patient's incontinence
  - Appropriate hip, lower extremity, or abdominal exercises according to evaluation
- Exercise for incontinence rehabilitation should address the following:
  - Motor unit recruitment, endurance, speed, and strength of the pelvic floor assists in adapting to the patient's changed urethral length and anatomical changes from the surgical intervention.
  - There is some evidence that initiating pelvic floor reeducation immediately after catheter removal can allow recovery of continence more quickly.
  - Pelvic floor training, especially via biofeedback, induces synergistic

action between the striated external urethral sphincter and an indirect retrograde neurogenic control on bladder hyperactivity.
- Although efficacy rates vary, a significant number of studies support the positive effect of biofeedback. Biofeedback was superior to controls or alternate treatments in many of the studies. Other studies report no clinically significant difference between biofeedback and other treatments. There are a limited number of studies in this area of research.
- Long-term maintenance of lower extremity, abdominal, and pelvic floor strength and coordination should help to promote appropriate supportive muscle balance for the pelvic region.

CONTRIBUTING FACTORS

- Surgical intervention changes to the anatomy within the pelvis
- Scarring along the urethra
- Poor awareness of the pelvic floor
- Lower extremity, spine, and hip muscle deficits or past medical history that have promoted decreased function in these areas
- Poor activation of local lumbar muscle groups such as the multifidus and the transverse abdominus muscles

PROGNOSIS

- Regardless of intervention, approximately 88% of men have minimal symptoms of incontinence at about 1 year postsurgery.
- Continence improvements varying from 24% to 38% at 1 month, 54% to 62% at 3 months, and 51% to 96% at 6 months have been reported in various studies.

SIGNS AND SYMPTOMS INDICATING REFERRAL TO PHYSICIAN

- Constant unrelenting low back pain: Infection or tumor
- Significant and unexplained weight loss: Tumor
- Nocturnal pain: Tumor
- Blood in urine or stool: Urinary pathology
- History of cancer: Metastatic disease
- Fevers and chills: Infection or tumor
- Sudden onset of bowel and/or bladder dysfunction: Cauda equina syndrome
- New onset of back pain in people over 50 years of age or under 20 years of age: Metastasis or infection

SUGGESTED READINGS

Cornel EB, de Wit R, Witjes JA. Evaluation of early pelvic floor physiotherapy on the duration and degree of urinary incontinence after radical retropubic prostatectomy in a non-teaching hospital. *World J Urol.* 2005;23:353-355.

Glazer H, Laine C. Pelvic floor muscle biofeedback in the treatment of urinary incontinence:

A literature review. *Appl Psychophysiol Biofeedback.* 2006;31(3):187-201.

Hunter KF, Moore KN, Glazener CMA. Conservative management for post-prostatectomy urinary incontinence. *Cochrane Database Syst Rev.* 1999;(4): CD001843. DOI: 10.1002/14651858. CD001843.pub.3.

Mason M. What implications do the tolerability profiles of antiandrogens and other commonly used prostate cancer treatments have on patient care? *J Cancer Res Clin Oncol.* 2006;132(suppl 1):S27-S35.

Singla AK. Male incontinence: pathophysiology and management. *Indian J Urology.* 2007;23(2):174-179.

http://www.wmfurology.com/pcahormone. htm

http://www.medscape.com/viewarticle/ 423513_5

AUTHOR: JULIE GUTHRIE

Section III

ORTHOPEDIC PATHOLOGY

BASIC INFORMATION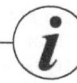

DEFINITION

- Pelvic floor dysfunction can be an episode in which the external anal sphincter or the puborectalis muscle does not relax appropriately when defecation or urination is initiated. Without relaxation, the urinary bladder and/or the colorectal system cannot empty appropriately. This can lead to the following:
  - Urinary or fecal frequency
  - Nocturia (nighttime urination)
  - Pelvic pain
  - Retention or constipation

SYNONYMS

- Obstructed defecation
- Incomplete emptying
- Pelvic floor dyssynergia

ICD-9CM CODES

625.0 Dyspareunia
788.20 Retention of urine
564.02 Outlet dysfunction constipation
728.85 Spasm of muscle

OPTIMAL NUMBER OF VISITS

8 or fewer

MAXIMAL NUMBER OF VISITS

24

ETIOLOGY

- The pelvic floor muscles, obturator internus, or external anal sphincter can refer pain when held in an unnatural position (abnormal tone) and can develop trigger points.
- As pressure increases in the bladder or rectum, somatic visceral referred pain can occur from sensory fibers along the outside of either structure.
- When the individual is attempting to relax to allow urination or defecation to occur, local muscle tension can also be a source of pain.

EPIDEMIOLOGY AND DEMOGRAPHICS

- There is no common age grouping for people to have pelvic floor dysfunction. The source of the dysfunction often differs among age groups.
- Although it is more well-known in women's health, men can present with similar symptoms of pelvic floor dysfunction.

MECHANISM OF INJURY

- Pelvic floor dysfunction often occurs from the following:
  - Habitual training from younger years
  - Fear of public toilets, forced schedules, and embarrassment can all lead

to habitual tension holding of the pelvic floor.
- Surgical onset
  - Secondary to pain, some individuals have scarring, fissures, or muscle soreness that creates spasms in the muscles.
- Pregnancy onset
  - Secondary to scarring after episiotomy or perineal laceration
  - See pregnancy-related pelvic floor dysfunction

COMMON SIGNS AND SYMPTOMS

- A feeling of incomplete emptying or evacuation
- Constipation, yet still has urges to go to the bathroom
- Lower quadrant, perineal soreness or pain
- Pain during evacuation or elimination
- Global pelvic, perineal, or ischial tuberosity region pain
- The pudendal nerve is impacted in a patient with pelvic floor dysfunction.
- Pelvic floor dysfunction can refer pain in the perineal, rectal, penile, or clitoral area.

AGGRAVATING ACTIVITIES

- Increased fluid intake
- Improper diet
- Stress
- Prolonged sitting postures
- Ingestion of fluids or food that create an imbalance in either the pH or the volume of the bladder place added stress on the rectum and bladder. This in turn puts a greater demand on the pelvic floor muscles.
- Some patients, for unknown reasons, seem to hold stress in the pelvic muscles. Whether this is from an upregulated autonomic nervous system or other mechanism is unclear.
- If the pudendal nerve and its area of supply is already compromised, prolonged sitting postures can potentially hamper blood and oxygen flow to the region.

EASING ACTIVITIES

- Diaphragmatic breathing
- Soft tissue mobilization (either internally or externally) of the pelvic floor muscles
- Walking
- Physicians can prescribe prescription NSAIDs or tricyclic antidepressants to address pelvic floor muscle tone or, more often, pain.
- The diaphragm and the pelvic floor are intimately related in terms of coordinated activity. With inhalation, the diaphragm moves caudally, and the pelvic floor should eccentrically lengthen from its resting position. With exhalation, the reverse occurs. Often, in patients with

pelvic floor dysfunction, this pattern is suboptimal and could use focused attention.
- Walking motion helps to promote circulation in the region of the pelvis.
- For patients with trigger points or abnormal pelvic floor muscle tone, soft tissue mobilization of the muscles can help ease tension.

24-HOUR SYMPTOM PATTERN

- Symptoms can increase during the day with prolonged sitting postures.
- Sleeping may or may not be problematic.

PAST HISTORY FOR THE REGION

- In patients with abnormal relaxation patterns with urination or defecation describe a long history of difficult elimination, childhood trauma, or strict behavioral patterns or fears.
- The pain and discomfort can be present for several hours to days and may not necessarily resolve on its own.

PHYSICAL EXAMINATION

- Frequently, Patients often sit on one buttock or the other to avoid placing direct pressure near the perineum, tailbone, or ischial tuberosities.
- Global muscles, such as the adductors, abdominals, obturator internus, external anal sphincter, or the pelvic floor (coccygeus, puborectalis, pubovaginalis in women), are symptomatic with palpation.
- Pelvic floor muscles, superficial perineal muscles, obturator internus, and coccygeus often are unilaterally or bilaterally tender.

IMPORTANT OBJECTIVE TESTS

- Hip ROM testing
  - Rotation can be limited and can reproduce the patient's symptoms.
- Pelvic floor muscle activation and relaxation
  - Patients often demonstrate difficulty initiating contraction or relaxation of the pelvic floor muscles, assessed either internally or via sEMG biofeedback or internal probe.
- Diaphragmatic breathing pattern
  - Visual and tactile assessment of the use of both sides of the diaphragm

DIFFERENTIAL DIAGNOSIS

- Muscle strain
- Somatic referral
- Obturator or sciatic hernia
- Lumbosacral dysfunction
- Spine referral or radiculopathy
- Rectal problem
- Anorectal infection
- Tumor
- Psychosomatic challenges

TREATMENT

MEDICAL AND SURGICAL OPTIONS

- Botox (botulinum toxin) injections into the pelvic floor or obturator internus
- Pudendal nerve release

SURGICAL OUTCOMES

- Although several of the current studies have small numbers of subjects, positive results of Botox interventions are promising in reducing pelvic floor tone and pain.
- Few physicians world-wide address pudendal nerve entrapment syndromes, but there is a very small amount of evidence leaning toward anatomical differences and interventions to help those with nerve entrapments.

REHABILITATION

- The goal of rehabilitation of the patient with pelvic floor dysfunction is twofold. First, the focus should be on decreasing the patient's symptoms. Once the symptoms have diminished, the focus of the rehabilitative process will turn to retraining the patterns of recruitment and relaxation of the pelvic floor muscles.
- Often, the body attempts to protect the painful area by splinting or contracting the large global muscles of the region. This is because inflammation will shut down the local muscle fibers. The lack of motion to the region impedes circulation to the region. Therefore, chemical irritants that have been brought into the region in response to the injury do not leave the region.
- Initial exercises should include exercises that minimize the stress to the pelvic floor, which can be achieved with either mildly inverted positions (for recruitment) or quadruped or deep squat style positioning (for relaxation).
- To decrease irritation or tone of the pelvic floor muscles, the clinician should use the following:
  - Myofascial release techniques to relax the large muscle groups
  - Biofeedback to retrain the pelvic floor muscles
  - Ensure optimal diaphragmatic breathing
  - Walking
  - Exercises that promote movement of the region in a pain-free range
  - Cold or hot pack
  - Ultrasound
  - Electrical stimulation or galvanic stimulation
  - Light therapy
- Once the irritation process has decreased, the focus of rehabilitation should be to identify the factors that contribute to the improper muscle coordination or spasm, which is crucial to long-term prevention of setbacks.
- Electrical stimulation and pelvic floor dysfunction:
  - Electrical stimulation can help to decrease pain.
  - Electrical stimulation via galvanic stimulation (rectally) has been shown to be quite effective in decreasing pain and improving functional voiding or expulsion tests.
- Massage has been shown to improve lymph drainage, enhance circulation, and increase superficial tissue temperature.
- Exercise and pelvic floor dysfunction: Many patients with pelvic floor dysfunction present with impairments of decreased pelvic floor awareness. Exercises to enhance the patient's recognition of pelvic floor tone, recruitment, and relaxation are crucial for long-term improvement of symptoms.
- Common management techniques include patient education, breathing and relaxation strategies, stretching exercises, education on soft tissue mobilization techniques, and strengthening exercises for the appropriate muscles. Additionally, patients can be trained in the home use of vaginal or rectal dilators to work on progressive relaxation, stretching, or contract-relax techniques to retrain the pelvic floor.
- Initially, exercises that minimize the stress to the pelvic floor should be used, with progressive levels of stress being added as symptoms decrease.
- Awareness exercises of the pelvic floor can help a patient recognize maladaptive patterns and correct them prophylactically.
- Recognition of emotional or lifestyle "triggers" can help empower a patient who has pelvic floor dysfunction.
- Appropriate strength and stretching exercises of the abdominals, hips, and pelvic floor can help maintain appropriate muscle balance and support of abdominal contents during demanding activities or during elimination or defecation.

CONTRIBUTING FACTORS

- Poor posture
- An occupation with a restrictive schedule (patient does not have opportunity to void when urge occurs)
- Poor diaphragmatic breathing pattern
- Poor activation of local muscle groups such as the abdominals and gluteals and hip rotators
- Tight muscle groups, especially the hip flexors and hamstrings
- Longevity of symptoms or homuncular reorganization with chronic pain.

PROGNOSIS

Unfortunately, many patients suffer for prolonged periods secondary to missed or improper diagnosis. Consequently, pain and poor patterns can be quite ingrained. However, resolution is possible with appropriate stress management, manual and/or pharmacological interventions, activity level, and exercise.

SIGNS AND SYMPTOMS INDICATING REFERRAL TO PHYSICIAN

- Blood in the stool or urine: Infection or tumor
- Significant and unexplained weight loss: Tumor
- Nocturnal pain: Tumor
- Saddle anesthesia: Cauda equina syndrome
- Major trauma: Fracture
- History of cancer: Metastatic disease
- Fevers and chills: Infection or tumor
- Sudden onset of bowel and/or bladder dysfunction: Cauda equina syndrome
- Progressive bilateral lower extremity paresthesias that are nondermatomal: Cauda equina syndrome
- New onset of back pain in people over 50 years of age or under 20 years of age: Infection or tumor

SUGGESTED READINGS

Bassotti J, et al. Biofeedback for pelvic floor dysfunction in constipation. *BMJ.* 2004;328:393-396.

Chiarioni G, et al. One-year follow-up study on the effects of electrogalvanic stimulation in chronic idiopathic constipation with pelvic floor dyssynergia. *Dis Colon Rectum.* 2004;47:346-353.

Heymen S, et al. Biofeedback to be superior to alternative treatments for patients with pelvic floor dyssynergia-type. *Constipation Dis Colon Rectum.* 2007;50:428-441.

Kavic MS. Chronic pelvic pain in females and obscure hernias. *Hernia.* 2000;4:250-254.

Mazzo F, et al. Anorectal and perineal pain: new pathophysiological hypothesis. *Tech Coloproctol.* 2004;8:77-83.

AUTHOR: JULIE GUTHRIE

BASIC INFORMATION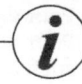

DEFINITION

Pregnancy-related pelvic floor dysfunction can be incontinence or pain conditions of the pelvic floor during or after pregnancy.

SYNONYMS

- Postpartum incontinence
- Pelvic pain
- Pelvic floor dysfunction

ICD-9CM CODES

625.6 Stress incontinence female
788.31 Urge incontinence
787.6 Incontinence of feces
569.1 Rectal prolapse
618.2 Uterovaginal prolapse incomplete
618.0 Prolapse of vaginal walls without uterine prolapse
788.38 Overflow incontinence
625 Pain and other symptoms associated with female genital organs

OPTIMAL NUMBER OF VISITS

6 to 8

MAXIMAL NUMBER OF VISITS

20

ETIOLOGY

- The pelvic floor muscles (levator ani and pubococcygeus) and the perineum take the brunt of additional weight carried during pregnancy and the potential trauma with vaginal birth.
- The four classifications of trauma and damage to the soft tissue involving the perineum with vaginal births are as follows:
  - First degree: Laceration extends through the skin and superficial tissue
  - Second degree: Tear extends through the perineal muscles
  - Third degree: Tear extends into the anal sphincter
  - Fourth degree: Tear extends into the anterior rectal wall
- The vaginal area can be stretched too quickly to accommodate the baby's head during delivery. Stretch rates of the muscles during vaginal delivery have been demonstrated at 1.5 to 1.63.
- In some cases, an obstetrician chooses to do an episiotomy (cut the perineum) to decrease pressure and possibly minimize natural tearing from the pressure.
- Episiotomies can be midline or mediolateral in positioning. The potential issues with episiotomies are the following:

  - Midline: May encourage a continuation of the tear down into the rectal region.
  - Mediolateral: Scarring is on one side, potentially creating an uneven, more painful scar that encourages muscle imbalance from one side to the other.
- Postural control of the trunk muscles has been noted to be delayed in patients with incontinence; this delay may have a role in the development of low back pain in pregnant women.
- Trauma of the pubocervical fascia (postpartum)
- Compression or traction injuries to the distal branches of the pudendal nerves and inferior hypogastric plexus
- Stretching of the anterior connective tissue from the vagina to the bladder and bladder neck
- The patient experiences pain because of the following:
  - If the patient has not had specific trauma, the pelvic floor has been lengthened and has to function in a more strained fashion for the duration of the pregnancy and potentially thereafter. The pelvic floor muscles postpartum are now functioning with increased demands of lifting, carrying, and caring for a new baby in a functionally weakened (lengthened) position.
  - Scarring from the lacerations sustained during the delivery can create great discomfort in the perineal region or in the vagina or rectum and anus.
  - Uterine contractions can still occur postpartum in patients who breastfeed, whereby oxytocin released during suckling creates an overflow effect of stimulating the uterus. This condition can increase the load on the pelvic floor muscles.

EPIDEMIOLOGY AND DEMOGRAPHICS

- Women having their first child (primigravidas) have a greater chance of pelvic floor trauma since the tissue has never been stretched so much before.
- Women with a small pelvis or who are delivering a large baby are at greater risk for greater damage.
  - Women delivering larger babies are at higher risk for grade 3 and 4 tears of the perineum, which is directly associated with fecal incontinence rates
- Mothers with multiple gestations can demonstrate a cumulative effect of trauma over time.
- 50% of pregnant women experience stress incontinence.
- 10% to 20% of pregnant women experience urge incontinence in their third trimester.

- The following risk factors in the pregnancy period negatively affect urinary incontinence rates:
  - Vaginal delivery, vacuum extraction, forceps delivery, preexisting urinary incontinence, fetal head circumference, older maternal age, and prolonged second stage of labor
- Women who have a history of stress urinary incontinence before pregnancy have higher rates of incontinence after vaginal delivery at both 3 and 9 months postpartum.

MECHANISM OF INJURY

- The pelvic floor is commonly injured with the following:
  - Prolonged support of the growing fetus throughout the pregnancy
  - Tissue being stretched or torn to accommodate baby's head

COMMON SIGNS AND SYMPTOMS

- The perineal area, vaginal area, rectal area, and ischial tuberosity regions may all be tender, depending on the location of tearing or lengthening.
- The following nerves can be impacted by birth trauma:
- Obturator nerve: Caused by compression of the fetal head before or during delivery
  - Weak hip adduction
  - Sensory loss medial thigh
- Femoral nerve: Caused by pelvic trauma, psoas hemorrhage, or compression in the pelvic cavity
  - Weak knee extension or hip flexion
  - Sensory loss in anteromedial thigh
- Fibular nerve: Compression damage from having legs in stirrups.
  - Weak toe extension, foot eversion
- Sensory loss in anterolateral leg and dorsum of foot
- Pudendal nerve, which has both sensory and motor responsibilities, can be injured with a perineal tear.

AGGRAVATING ACTIVITIES

- Bowel movements
- Urination
- Activities that increase abdominal pressure: Picking up child, toys, etc, or laughing, coughing, sneezing.
- Climbing stairs, squatting
- Bowel movements and urination require that the pelvic floor muscles relax. An area that is actively scarring or that is scarred and hypersensitive has trouble relaxing to accomplish these tasks.
- Coughing, sneezing, laughing, and lifting can increase incontinence secondary to the muscles' delayed recruitment, stretch weakness, or pain inhibition.

EASING ACTIVITIES

- Sitting down (in patients where stretched muscle is the issue)
- Standing up (in patients where scarring is the issue)
- Seated activities take the strain away from the pelvic floor during standing activities against gravity.
- Standing can remove the tactile pressure and compression of scar and sensitive tissue.

24-HOUR SYMPTOM PATTERN

- The patient with pelvic floor trauma or poor tone may complain of pain after periods of prolonged standing or physical activity or after bowel movements or urination. Symptoms increase during the day and if the person is active for too long. Incontinence symptoms usually vary, depending on the activity level of the day.
- Sleeping is usually not problematic, although patients may report increased frequency of awakening to urinary urges.

PAST HISTORY FOR THE REGION

- Patients may complain of prior history of incontinence.
- The pain and discomfort of scarring from delivery trauma will be present for several days to several weeks and may not resolve on its own.
- Combined issues of global deconditioning can make symptoms more severe.

PHYSICAL EXAMINATION

- Nearby muscles, the abdominals and adductors, can present with trigger points and pain.
- Superficial perineal, pelvic floor, and obturator internus muscles can all be tender and sore.
- Diastasis rectus abdominus, or a tear or split in the rectus abdominus after pregnancy, may or may not resolve on its own. Its effect on the abdominal muscles' ability to exert appropriate supportive force can translate into further pressure being placed on the pelvic floor.

OBJECTIVE TESTS

- Stress test: Patient coughs while in the standing position; leakage that occurs during the cough indicates stress incontinence.
- Voiding diary demonstrates patient fluid intake patterns and urinary output, frequency of urges to void, and whether an urge is associated with an episode of leakage.
- Pad test: 1-hour or 24-hour pad test measures overall loss of urine over a period of time to determine the effect of daily activities on the amount of urine lost.

- Perineal condition: Visual and/or tactile evaluation of the recovery of perineal tissue, especially postpartum.
  - Note redness, raised scars
  - Drawn, tight scars can point to soft tissue restrictions
- Pelvic floor muscle strength testing
  - Strength is measured either internally (postpartum) or externally (prepartum). Strength scales vary, but most agree that a 3/5 indicates a visible rise in the perineum.
  - In a lengthened pelvic floor, there is usually significant challenge in recruitment and isolation of the pelvic floor muscles.
  - Slow-twitch (how long the patient can sustain a pelvic floor contraction) and fast-twitch (number of quick contractions completed after a minute of rest after the long contractions) fibers are assessed to determine exercise specificity.

DIFFERENTIAL DIAGNOSIS

- Muscle strain
- Ligament strain
- Scar or soft tissue restriction
- Obstetrical-related nerve injury

TREATMENT

MEDICAL AND SURGICAL OPTIONS (POSTPARTUM)

- Vaginal sling
- TVT procedure
- Neurostimulator
- Colostomy
- Compared to physical therapy, a review of the literature indicates that physical therapy produced results just as successful as surgery. Both surgery and physical therapy produced good reduction in symptoms in 70% of patients.

REHABILITATION

- The goal of rehabilitation differs, depending on patient presentation. In patients demonstrating stretch weakness and dyscoordination of the pelvic floor, 8-week training programs have demonstrated improvement in pelvic floor muscle tone and decreasing incontinence.
- In patients demonstrating pelvic floor trauma postpartum, the body attempts to protect the region. Increased tone in surrounding muscles of the adductors, hip flexors, abdominals, and gluteals is common. The goals with these patients are to decrease pain and guarding from the trauma, then retrain

the pelvic floor to promote optimal support and function
- To promote healing and decrease irritation of pelvic floor trauma, the clinician should use the following:
  - Myofascial release techniques to relax the large muscle groups
  - Light or ultrasound modalities
  - Scar mobilization
  - Soft tissue mobilization
  - Walking
  - Exercises that promote movement of the region in a pain-free range
  - Cold pack
  - Electrical stimulation
- Once the healing process has improved, the focus of rehabilitation should be on identifying the factors that contribute to the incontinence or pain symptoms. Retraining the pelvic floor muscles is of utmost importance for long-term health and support of the pelvic region.
- Initial exercises should include the following:
  - Initially, diaphragmatic breathing is beneficial as it creates gentle rhythmic motion of the pelvic floor (with inspiration, there is mild descent of the pelvic floor, with a reflexive rise of the pelvic floor with exhalation) and is ideal to establish the initial proper nutrition of the tissue.
  - Pelvic floor contractions (Kegel exercises) can be completed in a pain-free effort range. Whether long or quick contractions are worked on depends on what impairments were found in the objective strength evaluation.
  - Pelvic floor coordination training is crucial for improving patient awareness of how to recruit the pelvic floor muscles before, during, and after activities. Referred to as "the knack," this technique has been shown to be extraordinarily effective in eliminating stress incontinence episodes when practiced with the aggravating activity.
  - Body mechanics training: Especially for new or expecting mothers, understanding appropriate body mechanics for lifting and carrying the baby and performing duties as a new mother is important for prevention of overloading the pelvic floor. Learning to eliminate Valsalva maneuvers with all lifting help to minimize the stress on the pelvic floor.
- Biofeedback and pelvic floor rehabilitation: Considered an indispensable learning tool by many pelvic floor physical therapists, biofeedback uses auditory or visual feedback to give the patient information on timing of recruitment of the pelvic floor. It also can give information of overall recruitment but not overall pressure or

strength measurements. Biofeedback can be external (sEMG biofeedback) or internal (via vaginal or rectal probe).

- Electrical stimulation in pelvic floor trauma: Transcutaneous electrical nerve stimulation (TENS) units, appropriately placed, can help to provide pain relief for patients with symptomatic perineal scars or vaginal or anal tissue damage.
  - Although controversial in terms of efficacy, there are multiple protocols available to address urinary urge or stress incontinence.
- Massage and pelvic floor trauma rehabilitation
  - Massage has been shown to improve lymph drainage and increase superficial tissue temperature
  - Releasing scar and soft tissue restrictions can reduce pain.
- Exercises and pelvic floor rehabilitation: 70% of patients improve and/or are cured with multimodal, physical therapist-monitored pelvic floor programs

CONTRIBUTING FACTORS

- Poor posture
- An occupation that requires prolonged standing or repetitive lifting
- Multiple pregnancies
- Poor activation of abdominal muscle groups that facilitate and assist the pelvic floor in function
- Tight muscle groups, especially the hip flexors, adductors, and hamstrings

PROGNOSIS

- Studies have indicated that the pudendal nerve trauma sustained during delivery slowly recovers over the 2-month postpartum period.
- The deformation of the pelvic floor muscles and connective tissue persist at least 6 months.

SIGNS AND SYMPTOMS INDICATING REFERRAL TO PHYSICIAN

- Constant unrelenting low back pain: Infection or tumor
- Pain that does not change with position: Infection or tumor
- Significant and unexplained weight loss: Tumor
- Nocturnal pain: Tumor
- Blood in urine: Urinary pathology
- Saddle anesthesia: Cauda equina syndrome
- Major trauma: Fracture
- History of cancer: Metastatic disease
- Fevers and chills: Infection or tumor
- Sudden onset of bowel and/or bladder dysfunction: Cauda equina syndrome
- Progressive bilateral lower extremity paresthesias that are nondermatomal: Cauda equina syndrome

SUGGESTED READINGS

van Brummen HJ, Bruinse HW, van de Pol G, Heintz AP, et al. Defecatory symptoms during and after the first pregnancy: prevalences and associated factors. *Int Urogynecol J Pelvic Floor Dysfunction.* 2006;17:224-230.

Connolly T, et al. The effect of mode of delivery, parity, and birth weight on risk of urinary incontinence. *Int Urogynecol J.* 2007;18:1033-1042.

Doumalin C, et al. Physiotherapy for persistent postnatal stress urinary incontinence: A randomized controlled trial. *Am Coll Obstet Gynecol.* 2004;104(3):504-510.

Ekstrom A, et al. Planned cesarean section versus planned vaginal delivery: comparison of lower urinary tract symptoms. *Int Urogynecol J.* 2008;19:459-465.

Lee S, Park J. Follow-up evaluation of the effect of vaginal delivery on the pelvic floor. *Dis Colon Rectum.* 2000;43:1550-1555.

Parente MPL, et al. Deformation of the pelvic floor muscles during a vaginal delivery. *Int Urogynecol J.* 2008;19:65-71.

Scheer I, et al. Urinary incontinence after obstetric anal sphincter injuries (OASIS)—is there a relationship? *Int Urogynecol J.* 2008;19:179-183.

Smith M, et al. Is there a relationship between parity, pregnancy, back pain and incontinence? *Int Urogynecol J.* 2008;19:205-211.

AUTHOR: JULIE GUTHRIE

BASIC INFORMATION

DEFINITION

- Breast cancer can be defined as cancer that forms in breast tissue, usually in the ducts and lobules.
- The four official stages of cancer are as follows:
  - Stage 0: Lobular or ductal
  - Stage 1: Tumor measures less than 2 cm and has no lymph node involvement.
  - Stage II: Tumor is 2 to 5 cm or has spread to the ipsilateral axillary lymph node region.
  - Stage IIIa: Tumor is larger than 5 cm or has significant involvement of the lymph nodes.
  - Stage IIIb: Tumor has spread to the chest wall, breast skin, or internal mammary lymph nodes.
  - Stage IV: Tumor has spread beyond the breast, underarm, and internal mammary lymph nodes and/or into the supraclavicular lymph node region.

SYNONYMS

- Hyperplasia
- Neoplasms
- Neoplasia
- Sarcoma
- Proliferative lesion
- Tumor
- Angiomatosis
- Carcinoma
- Mesenchymal tumor
- Hemangioma
- Lipoma
- Fibromatosis

MAJOR SEQUELAE FOLLOWING BREAST CANCER INTERVENTIONS

- Shoulder pathology
- Deconditioning

ICD-9CM CODES
726.0 Adhesive capsulitis
726.1 Rotator cuff syndrome of shoulder and allied disorders
726.10 Disorders of bursae and tendons in shoulder region unspecified
719.41 Pain in joint involving shoulder region
728.2 Muscle wasting and disuse atrophy not elsewhere classified
338.3 Neoplasm related pain (acute) (chronic)

OPTIMAL NUMBER OF VISITS

12 or fewer

MAXIMAL NUMBER OF VISITS

24

ETIOLOGY

- The shoulder experiences dysfunction after breast cancer interventions because scar tissue can restrict either the glenohumeral joint capsule or the scapulohumeral joint.
- Joint limitations related to adhesive capsulitis create abnormal forces on the joint, the capsule, and the surrounding soft tissue. Soft tissue limitations can restrict the scapula from its normal function. Therefore scapular dyskinesia, impingement syndrome, and rotator cuff tears can occur.

EPIDEMIOLOGY AND DEMOGRAPHICS

- Current incidence of breast cancer in America is as follows:
  - 1:8 chance of having breast cancer. 85% of women with breast cancer have no known family history of breast cancer.
  - Over 182,000 new cases diagnosed in 2008. Of these, 1990 were in men.
- Risk factors for breast cancer include the following:
  - Family history, late pregnancy, early menarche
  - Breast cancer rates increase with age.
  - Some women present with mutations of the *BRCA1* or *BRCA2* gene, leading to an overall lifetime incidence chance of 40% to 85%. Males with this mutation also have higher risk of developing breast cancer.
  - Females with Jewish ancestry are at greater risk of having *BRCA1* or *BRCA2* mutations.
- Current rates of shoulder dysfunction and lymphedema in women who receive breast cancer interventions are as follows:
  - Shoulder dysfunction: 1% to 67%
  - Lymphedema: 0% to 34%
  - Shoulder or arm pain: 9% to 68%

MECHANISM OF INJURY

The shoulder is commonly injured with attempts to move the arm through a restricted range.

COMMON SIGNS AND SYMPTOMS

Women with shoulder pathology after breast cancer interventions present with complaints similar to those of patients with traditional orthopedic-related shoulder dysfunction. However, consideration must be made as to what stage of tissue healing the patient is in and where they are in terms of overall recovery.

AGGRAVATING ACTIVITIES

- Overhead activities of the involved upper extremity
- Reaching with the involved upper extremity

- Lifting activities
- Activities of daily living such as dressing, bathing, combing hair, etc
- All of these activities tax an already overloaded system that is lacking ROM and probably is deconditioned.

EASING ACTIVITIES

- Keeping the arm close to the side.
- Physicians often prescribe antiinflammatory medications, muscle relaxants, and pain medications to address the patient's symptoms.
- Walking
- These activities minimize irritation of sensitive structures of the shoulder.

PAST HISTORY FOR THE REGION

This may or may not be the patient's first experience with breast cancer. It is important to determine past medical history for the shoulder, neck, trunk, and low back to properly plan the physical therapy intervention.

PHYSICAL EXAMINATION

- Patients often have thoracic compensations toward the side of surgery or intervention. This may be due to pain or actual soft tissue restriction.
- Global muscles, such as the pectoral, scalene, and sternocleidomastoid muscles, are often tender to palpation.

IMPORTANT OBJECTIVE TESTS

- Shoulder, scapular, neck, and trunk ROM testing
  - Depending on the surgical reconstruction, there will be scarring and restriction in one or several of these areas. Scapular mobility and timing must have special attention because these could have long-term effects on shoulder pathology.
- Upper limb tension testing
  - Depending on the surgical intervention, ensuring that the nerves are traveling through scarred regions and areas that have not moved for some time is important for distal upper extremity function.

DIFFERENTIAL DIAGNOSIS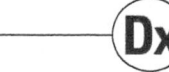

- Adhesive capsulitis
- Rotator cuff tear
- Glenohumeral impingement
- Bicipital tendinitis
- Scapular dyskinesia
- Myofascial pain syndrome

TREATMENT

SURGICAL OPTIONS

- Lumpectomy
- Simple mastectomy

- Radical mastectomy
- Axillary dissection
- Sentinel lymph node dissection
- Breast reconstruction: Saline implant
- Breast reconstruction: Transverse rectus abdominis myocutaneous (TRAM) flap
- Breast reconstruction: Latissimus dorsi flap
- Complications of breast reconstructive surgery after lumpectomy or mastectomy include the following shoulder pathologies:
  ○ Scar tissue adhesions
  ○ Altered scapulohumeral rhythm
  ○ Lymphedema
  ○ Upper extremity nerve entrapment

REHABILITATION

- The goal of rehabilitation of the patient after breast cancer intervention is twofold. First, the focus should be on decreasing the patient's symptoms. The second is to maximize the patient's function.
- As a result of injury, the body attempts to protect the region. This is accomplished by contracting the large global muscles of the region. This is in response to inflammation shutting down local muscle fibers. The body must protect and minimize stress to this area. It does so by contracting the large muscle fibers. The lack of motion to the region impedes circulation to the region. Therefore chemical irritants that have been brought into the region in response to the injury do not leave the region.
- To decrease inflammation, the clinician should include the following:
  ○ Myofascial release techniques to relax the large muscle groups
  ○ Joint mobilization
  ○ Lumbar traction
  ○ Walking
  ○ Exercises that promote movement of the region in a pain-free range
  ○ Cold or hot pack
  ○ Ultrasound
  ○ Electrical stimulation
- Initial exercises
  ○ There is evidence that an early (within 2 weeks postsurgery) home-based exercise program via video and written instruction is beneficial in improving shoulder ROM and pain reports.

  ○ Initially, exercises that minimize the stress to the disc should be used. If disc pressure during upright standing is used as normal disc pressure, a hooklying position decreases intradiscal pressure by 65%. Exercises that take this into consideration help decrease the stress placed on the disc. Pain-free ROM exercises should also be implemented. Extension-based exercises are preferable to flexion exercises.
- Massage for breast cancer intervention
  ○ Massage has been shown to improve lymph drainage and decrease pain.
  ○ A positive change in exercise activity was associated with a higher score on the SF-36 physical health summary scale at follow-up.
  ○ Basic pectoral stretch programs have not been shown to be more beneficial in terms of ROM or arm circumference while patients were going through radiation therapy.
  ○ Progressive resistive therapy is highly recommended and considered efficacious for improving energy, strength, and quality-of-life reports.
  ○ Posture awareness and correction helps optimize shortened muscles, as well as weakened or inhibited shoulder muscles.
- Exercises that promote mobility and function of the trunk, scapula, and shoulder help enhance shoulder function.

CONTRIBUTING FACTORS

- Poor posture
- Hypomobility in adjacent regions, especially the thoracic spine
- Poor activation of proximal trunk muscle groups such as the multifidus and the transverse abdominus muscles
- Tight muscle groups, especially the pectorals, hip flexors, and hamstrings

PROGNOSIS

The patient's prognosis will vary significantly depending upon the size of tumor, the extent of surgery, the lymph node status, and the general health of the patient. Treatment and intervention selection also greatly influence the patient's prognosis. Surgery, chemotherapy, radiation therapy, and medications all affect the patient's ultimate recovery potential. The clinician should check with the patient's physician regarding postsurgical precautions. They should also be cognizant of any side effects that medications or medical treatments may produce.

SIGNS AND SYMPTOMS INDICATING REFERRAL TO PHYSICIAN

- Pain that does not change with position: Infection or tumor
- Significant and unexplained weight loss: Tumor
- Nocturnal pain: Tumor
- History of cancer: Metastatic disease
- Fevers and chills: Infection or tumor

SUGGESTED READINGS

Bernstein L. Epidemiology of endocrine-related risk factors for breast cancer. *J Mammary Gland Biol Neoplasia.* 2002;7(1):3-15.

Box R, et al. Shoulder movement after breast cancer surgery: results of a randomized controlled study of postoperative physiotherapy. *Breast Cancer Res Treat.* 2002;75:35-50.

Cheema B, et al. Progressive resistance training in breast cancer: a systematic review of clinical trials. *Breast Cancer Res Treat.* 2008;109:9-26.

Hayes S, et al. Objective and subjective upper body function six months following diagnosis of breast Cancer. *Breast Cancer Res Treat.* 2005;94:1-10.

Kendall A, et al. Influence of exercise activity on quality of life in long-term breast cancer survivors. *Qual Life Res.* 2005;14:361-371.

Kilgour R, et al. Effectiveness of a self-administered, home-based exercise rehabilitation program for women following a modified radical mastectomy and axillary node dissection: a preliminary study. *Breast Cancer Res Treat.* 2008;109:285-295.

Lee T, Kilbreath SL, Refshauge KM, Herbert RD, Beith JM. Prognosis of the upper limb following surgery and radiation for breast cancer. *Breast Cancer Res Treat.* 2008. Jul: 110(1):19-37.

Lee TS, et al. Pectoral stretching program for women undergoing radiotherapy for breast cancer. *Breast Cancer Res Treat.* 2007;102:313-321.

Shamley D, et al. Changes in shoulder muscle size and activity following treatment for breast cancer. *Breast Cancer Res Treat.* 2007;106:19-27.

http://www.breastcancer.org/about_us/press_room/press_kit/cancer_facts.jsp?gclid=CP3r6sXan5MCFSkvagodkFqUvQ

AUTHOR: JULIE GUTHRIE

BASIC INFORMATION

DEFINITION

- Axillary nerve entrapment pathologies encompass any injury that interrupts the function of the axillary nerve at any point along its course.
- The axillary nerve is particularly vulnerable to injury at the following:
  - Surgical neck of the humerus
  - Inferior aspect of the glenohumeral joint
  - Quadrilateral space
  - Deltoid muscle
- The loss of function results in muscle weakness, pain, or sensory dysfunction.

SYNONYMS

Quadrilateral space syndrome

ICD-9CM CODES
354   Mononeuritis of upper limb and mononeuritis multiplex
354.8 Other mononeuritis of upper limb
354.9 Mononeuritis of upper limb unspecified

OPTIMAL NUMBER OF VISITS

6

MAXIMAL NUMBER OF VISITS

20

ETIOLOGY

- The axillary nerve is the smaller of the terminal branches of the posterior cord and the shortest of the major terminal branches of the brachial plexus. It is a mixed motor and sensory nerve derived from the C5 and 6 nerve roots that originates from the anterior aspect of the subscapularis muscle, passes laterally toward the inferior aspect of the shoulder joint, passes inferiorly to the head of the humerus, above the tendons of latissimus dorsi and teres major, and passes through the quadrilateral space, which is bounded medially by the humerus, laterally by the long head of the triceps muscle, superiorly by teres minor (which it supplies), and inferiorly by teres major.
- It then wraps horizontally around the posterior aspect of the surgical neck of the humerus and enters the deltoid muscle as three branches: an anterior branch to the middle and anterior aspects of the deltoid, a posterior branch to the posterior deltoid, and the upper lateral brachial cutaneous nerve branch to the skin in the area of the deltoid tuberosity
- The axillary nerve may be affected at any point along its course by direct

trauma or compression entrapment, causing nerve tissue hypoxia. The insult to the nerve can be mechanical, thermal, chemical, or ischemic; however, the axillary nerve is most commonly injured by glenohumeral fractures and dislocations.
- Axillary nerve entrapment is usually related to trauma; nevertheless, pathology can occur in a number of ways, as follows:
  - Direct trauma in the form of a humeral neck fracture
  - Dislocation of the glenohumeral joint in which the nerve is stretched across the humeral neck by an anterior dislocation
  - Operative procedures at the inferior aspect of the shoulder such as capsular shift involving a deltoid-splitting incision
  - Blunt injury such as a heavy fall onto the lateral aspect of the shoulder
  - Overuse syndromes from repeated scapular motions, leading to compression of the posterior humeral circumflex artery and the axillary nerve within the quadrilateral space by fibrous bands. The size of the quadrilateral space is reduced in positions of abduction and external rotation.
- Nerve injury is classified according to the severity of the injury and its potential for reversibility.
- Neurapraxia (first-degree injury) is a distortion of the myelin about the nodes of Ranvier caused by ischemia, mechanical compression, or electrolyte imbalance, which produces temporary loss of nerve conduction.
- Axonotmesis (second-degree injury) is an interruption of the axon with secondary wallerian degeneration. The supporting tissue surrounding the axon is preserved, and the recovery period depends on the distance between the site of injury and the end organs.
- Neurotmesis is a complete disruption of the nerve and its supporting structures. Neurotmesis has been further divided into the following three subcategories:
  - Third-degree nerve injury: Endoneurium is disrupted with intact perineurium and epineurium.
  - Fourth-degree nerve injury: All neural elements sparing the epineurium are disrupted.
  - Fifth-degree nerve injury: Complete transection and discontinuity of the nerve with no capacity for regeneration
- Physiologically, there is disruption to any part of the nerve responsible for conduction.
  - In repetitive-type nerve entrapment, it is proposed that repetitive work or static postures produce an inflammatory process and fibroblasts appear to

repair damage incurred but produce adhesions to the nerve, limiting their glide and increasing anoxia.

EPIDEMIOLOGY AND DEMOGRAPHICS

- Axillary nerve injury is the most common nerve injury associated with the shoulder, particularly in relation to trauma such as fracture and dislocation.
- Quadrilateral space syndrome is an uncommon pathology seen in throwing athletes, as well as in sports with repetitive cocking action such as tennis or volleyball. The cocking action involves end-range shoulder abduction, extension, and external rotation followed by rapid flexion and internal rotation.

MECHANISM OF INJURY

- Mechanisms of injury for the axillary nerve are described in relation to their location, as follows:
  - Direct trauma in the form of a humeral neck fracture causing damage to the nerve
  - Dislocation of the glenohumeral joint in which the nerve is stretched across the humeral neck by an anterior dislocation
  - Operative procedures at the inferior aspect of the shoulder such as capsular shift involving a deltoid-splitting incision that directly injures the nerve
  - Blunt injury such as a heavy fall onto the lateral aspect of the shoulder compressing the nerve within the deltoid muscle
  - Overuse syndromes from repeated scapular motions, leading to compression of the posterior humeral circumflex artery and the axillary nerve within the quadrilateral space by fibrous bands. The size of the quadrilateral space is reduced in positions of abduction and external rotation. Overuse syndrome occasionally occurs after general anesthesia or sleeping prone with the arms raised above the head.

COMMON SIGNS AND SYMPTOMS

- Poorly localized posterior shoulder pain
- Paraesthesia over the lateral aspect of the shoulder and arm
- Weakness of deltoid and teres minor resulting in difficulty abducting the arm
- External rotation may be mildly weaker.
- Patient may describe shoulder weakness.
- Atrophy of the deltoid may be evident.

AGGRAVATING ACTIVITIES

- Activities that involve shoulder abduction

- Repetitive shoulder internal and/or external rotation occurs particularly when the shoulder is in an abducted position.

EASING ACTIVITIES

Rest and/or modification of aggravating activities

24-HOUR SYMPTOM PATTERN

- Generally, the symptoms are related to activity and do not follow a typical 24-hour pattern unless there is a strong inflammatory component, which may be seen in repetitive tasks.
- If there is an inflammatory component, there may be worsening of symptoms with use toward the end of the day, as well as morning stiffness.

PAST HISTORY FOR THE REGION

- History of trauma, fracture, or dislocation of the glenohumeral joint
- Repetitive overuse of the shoulder in occupation or sports
- Generalized hypermobility

PHYSICAL EXAMINATION

- Examine the shoulder for signs of atrophy of the deltoid muscle.
- Manual muscle testing (MMT) may reveal weakness in the following muscles:
  - Deltoid: Tested in shoulder flexion, abduction, and extension for each of the portions of the deltoid; however, weakness is usually demonstrated in pure abduction.
  - Teres minor: Tested in external rotation; however, the infraspinatus muscle is a stronger external rotator and is likely to compensate for the loss of the teres minor muscle.
- Sensation testing should be performed. The cutaneous branch of the axillary nerve supplies the lateral aspect of the shoulder overlying the deltoid muscle and tuberosity. Sensation testing should include pinprick, two-point discrimination, and tuning fork tests and compared for asymmetry with the unaffected side (where available).
- Physical examination should also exclude pathology in other areas, particularly performing active range of motion (AROM) and passive ROM (PROM) at the neck and shoulder, which may reveal restrictions, other shoulder pathology, and/or central involvement of the nerve.
- Physical examination should also include movement analysis to determine the movement patterns that the patient adopts when performing the aggravating activities. Movement analysis can be done visually or with the assistance of a video camera. The analysis should give some clues as to predisposing fac-

tors, such as posture and patterning, that will assist with rehabilitation and activity modification. In the case of the axillary nerve, the patient often demonstrates trick movements to accomplish shoulder abduction through use of the rotator cuff and proximal scapular and cervical muscles.

IMPORTANT OBJECTIVE TESTS

- Electromyography (EMG) may reveal delayed conduction velocity and fibrillation potentials.
- Needle EMG should assist with determination of specific muscle involvement and provide differential diagnosis from the other shoulder neuropathies and cervical radiculopathies.
- If quadrilateral space syndrome is suspected, there will be concomitant posterior humeral circumflex artery compression, and therefore a subclavian arteriogram can provide diagnostic information.

DIFFERENTIAL DIAGNOSIS

- Lesion to the posterior cord of the brachial plexus
- C5 or C6 radiculopathy
- Suprascapular neuropathy produces a similar pattern of weak arm abduction and external rotation but no sensory loss.
- Rotator cuff tears
- Rotator cuff tendinopathies
- Adhesive capsulitis
- Shoulder instability
- Degenerative joint disease at the glenohumeral or acromioclavicular (AC) joints
- Underlying neuropathic disease
- Neuralgic amyotrophy
- Muscular dystrophy
- Tumors or space-occupying lesions
- Upper motor neuron lesion in the cerebrum

CONTRIBUTING FACTORS

- Trauma is the most common contributing factory for axillary nerve injuries; however, for any nerve entrapments that are nontraumatic, there is often an element of repetitive activity involving the affected limb.
- Typically in the case of the axillary nerve, the repetitive action involves shoulder abduction and external glenohumeral rotation.
- Postural factors may be involved, particularly with repetitive work or sporting activities with reduction in proximal stability and control, leading to an overuse of more distal muscle groups to perform a task.

TREATMENT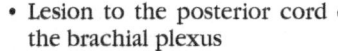

SURGICAL OPTIONS

- Surgery may be considered after a failure of conservative management.
- Surgery involves nerve grafting techniques and a rotational transfer of deltoid removing the denervated portion.

REHABILITATION

- The goal of rehabilitation should be pain reduction to encourage pain-free exercise and to provide task or sports reeducation and interventions leading to reacquisition of fine motor and sporting skills.
- Manual therapy
  - Pain reduction can be achieved through the use of ice and electrotherapeutic modalities.
  - Soft tissue release may assist with restoration of muscle balance around the scapula, which is useful if compensations have occurred in other muscles to make up for the loss of the deltoid and teres minor muscles.
- Functional rehabilitation
  - Reeducation of movement patterns, particularly proximal control of the trunk and neck, to provide a stable foundation for scapular stability
  - Scapular position education initially with isometric hold and then the addition of controlled functional movement patterns
  - Prevention of aberrant movement patterns and contractures with ROM and gentle stretch techniques
  - Specific muscle strengthening gradually increasing in intensity to restore full power to the deltoid and teres minor muscles
  - Integration of functional exercise and strength work into sport- or task-specific skills
  - Graduated return to full strength, speed, and power

PROGNOSIS

- Prognosis depends entirely on the extent of damage to the nerve.
- Neurapraxia should resolve rapidly and lead to a complete restoration of function, usually within 2 to 3 months.
- If the injury is a more severe axonotmesis, the recovery time depends on the distance from the site of injury to the denervated tissue.
- Peripheral nerves have been reported to recover at an approximate rate of 1 to 4 mm per day and may not result in a complete restoration of function.
- If there has been a complete sectioning of the nerve (neurapraxia), then the nerve will not fully recover.

- The results of treating neurapraxia even with surgical intervention are generally not satisfactory.

SIGNS AND SYMPTOMS INDICATING REFERRAL TO PHYSICIAN

If axillary nerve entrapment is suspected, all cases should be referred to a physician for appropriate investigation.

SUGGESTED READINGS

Aldridge JW, Bruno RJ, Strauch RJ, Rosenwasser MP. Nerve entrapment in athletes. *Clin Sports Med.* 2001;20(1):95.

Goslin KL, Krivickas LS. Proximal neuropathies of the upper extremity. *Neurol Clin.* 1999;17(3).

Kibler WB, Murrell GAC. Shoulder pain. In: Brukner P, Khan K, eds. *Clinical Sports Medicine.* 3rd ed. Australia: McGraw-Hill Book Company; 2006:243–288.

Leffert RD. Nerve lesions about the shoulder. *Orthop Clin North Am.* 2000;31(2).

AUTHOR: JOSEPHINE LOUISE COULTER

BASIC INFORMATION

DEFINITION

- The brachial plexus, composed of the posterior cord (formed from the posterior divisions of the upper trunk from C5 and C6 nerve roots, the middle trunk from C7, and the lower trunk from C8 and T1), the lateral cord (formed from the anterior divisions of the upper and middle trunks), and the medial cord (formed from the anterior division of the lower trunk), communicates the nerve supply between the cervical roots and the upper limb, passing through the scalene muscles and sternocleidomastoid, and under the clavicle.
- It may be subject to the following injuries:
  - Traction injury during birth if the head is pulled away from the shoulder (Erb's palsy in which the arm is held in adduction and internal rotation with forearm pronation and wrist and hand flexion, or Klumpke's palsy with Horner's syndrome consisting of meiosis, ptosis, and anhydrosis)
  - Traction injury from a traumatic event
  - Compression injury from trauma to the cervical spine, clavicle, humerus, or pectoral girdle; impact on Erb's point; or poor postures
  - Compression injury from narrowing of the neural foramen with cervical hyperextension and ipsilateral rotation
  - Compression injury from anatomical variations in the cervical spine, clavicle, first rib, pectoral girdle, or posterior triangle

SYNONYMS

- Brachial plexus injury
- Cervical rib syndrome
- Cervical pinch syndrome
- Costoclavicular syndrome
- Scalenus anticus syndrome
- Hyperabduction syndrome
- Thoracic outlet syndrome
- Stinger
- Burner syndrome
- Chronic burner syndrome

ICD-9CM CODES
353.0 Brachial plexus lesions
953.4 Injury to brachial plexus

OPTIMAL NUMBER OF VISITS

Recovery normally occurs between 24 hours and 2 to 3 weeks.

MAXIMAL NUMBER OF VISITS

Symptoms persisting for more than 2 to 3 weeks, together with worsening neurological signs, warrant further clinical investigation.

ETIOLOGY

- Insult to the nerve may be mechanical, thermal, chemical, or ischemic. In entrapment syndromes, compression or direct trauma leads to nerve tissue hypoxia.
- The brachial plexus may be compressed from trauma to the cervical spine, shoulder, pectoral girdle, clavicle, or rib; from postural issues, with direct pressure on Erb's point (punctum nervosum at the union between C5 and C6 nerve roots on the lateral cord 2 to 3 cm above the clavicle); or from narrowing of the neural foramen with cervical hyperextension and ipsilateral rotation. Specific anatomical features of entrapment in the upper limb are described by Pratt.
- In entrapments, nerve trauma occurs because the size of the neural structure exceeds the anatomical space available for it, resulting in increased pressure that in turn leads to impaired blood flow and subsequent hypoxia of the tissue and disruption to the axonal transport system. Nerve injury is classified according to severity of the injury and potential for reversibility.
- Original classifications described previously remain in current use, as follows:
  - First-degree neurapraxia involves distortion of myelin about the nodes of Ranvier caused by ischemia, mechanical compression, or electrolyte imbalance, resulting in temporary loss of nerve conduction. Recovery is usually rapid and complete.
  - Second-degree axonotmesis involves interruption of the axon with secondary wallerian degeneration, but the supporting tissue around the axon is preserved. Recovery may be complete but takes longer to occur and depends on the distance between the site of injury and the end structure (denervated muscle).
  - Third-degree neurotmesis involves extensive disruption of the nerve and its supporting structures, but while the endoneurium is disrupted, the perineurium and epineurium remain intact.
  - Fourth-degree neurotmesis involves disruption of all neural components except the epineurium.
  - Fifth-degree neurotmesis involves complete transaction and discontinuity of the nerve, with no capacity for regeneration. Neurotmesis rarely occurs from entrapment, but when continuity has been disrupted, complete recovery is not possible, even with surgical techniques, and the eventual outcome depends on individual circumstances. A comprehensive overview of neurobiology, nerve injury, and nerve repair is provided by Dahlin.

- Double-crush syndrome refers to the fairly common phenomenon of nerve entrapment and radiculopathy occurring in combination, although the syndrome is considered controversial. Compression or irritation of the nerve roots at the cervical level is thought to increase sensitivity to compression or movement restrictions more distally in the structure.
- As noted, increasing pressure on the nerve causes impaired blood flow, tissue hypoxia, and disruption to the anterograde and retrograde intercellular transport of materials within axons, eventually disturbing depolarization within the nerve. In brachial plexus compression, the pressure may result directly from anatomical structures, direct trauma, or from the associated phenomena of edema, glenohumeral dislocation, or clavicular fracture. Mechanisms and patterns of injury are discussed by Moran et al.

EPIDEMIOLOGY AND DEMOGRAPHICS

- In adults, compression injury of the brachial plexus tends to occur most commonly from an accident or sports-related trauma to the cervical spine, shoulder, pectoral girdle, and upper quadrant, particularly sports involving high impact such as contact sports and gymnastics.
- It may also occur from the presence of a cervical rib arising from C7 vertebra (cervical rib syndrome), narrowing of the costoclavicular space between the clavicle and the first rib as a result of bony anomaly or combined depression and retraction of the shoulder as occurs when carrying a rucksack (costoclavicular syndrome), compression at the coracoid process when the upper limb is held in hyperabduction (hyperabduction syndrome), or compression between the anterior and medial scalenes (scalenus anticus syndrome).
- Pathology related to trauma tends to occur in younger people predominantly because of the type of activity usually associated with the injury. Pathology related to anatomical anomalies and variation may occur across a broader spectrum of the population.

MECHANISM OF INJURY

- Brachial plexus injury is discussed by Mannan and Carlstedt and Bishop et al. Impact trauma resulting in clavicular fracture, glenohumeral dislocation, or edema around the shoulder may result in direct pressure on the brachial plexus as it passes under the clavicle or at Erb's point (burner syndrome).
- The presence of a cervical rib reduces the space between the scalenes, making

compression more likely in the region of the posterior triangle (cervical rib syndrome).
- Bony anomaly or combined depression and retraction of the shoulder reduces the space between the clavicle and first rib, making compression more likely at this site (costoclavicular syndrome).
- Anatomical variations in the posterior triangle and scalene muscles, particularly if combined with other associated elements, may produce compression at this site (scalenus anticus syndrome).
- Compression at the coracoid process and pectoralis minor muscle may occur with sustained overhead arm postures.

COMMON SIGNS AND SYMPTOMS

- Shoulder pain, radiating up into the neck and down into the upper limb
- Weakness or paralysis of the biceps brachii, deltoid, brachialis, brachioradialis, and coracobrachialis muscles and muscles supplied by the axillary, musculocutaneous, and radial nerves, together with associated paraesthesia and numbness
- The upper limb may be held in adduction and medial rotation with forearm pronation and wrist and hand flexion ("waiter's tip" position).
- Individuals may describe a sensation of weakness, cold, "heaviness," or "dead arm" and complain of clumsiness.
- Pain may be referred up into the neck, throughout the shoulder, and down into the upper limb.
- Sensory and motor symptoms may occur throughout the upper limb.

AGGRAVATING ACTIVITIES

- Activities and postures that involve impact through the upper quadrant
- Cervical extension and ipsilateral rotation
- Poor posture with "drooping" shoulders
- Loading through the shoulder (particularly into depression and retraction) such as carrying a rucksack or a heavy object in the hand with the arm at the side
- Activities involving sustained periods with the arm overhead, such as painting

EASING ACTIVITIES

Adaptations in posture and reduction in loading reduce the stress on the brachial plexus, as described in Aggravating Activities.

24-HOUR SYMPTOM PATTERN

- In general, symptoms are more likely to be associated with trauma, posture, and activity rather than time. However, when symptoms are aggravated by cervical spine or overhead arm positions, there may be an increase in symptoms

nocturnally as a consequence of sleeping postures.
- Increases in nocturnal pain are also reported in which deafferentation pain is present.

PAST HISTORY FOR THE REGION

- Presence of anatomical anomalies
- Impact trauma producing clavicular fracture
- Glenohumeral dislocation
- Edema around the shoulder
- Hyperextension and ipsilateral rotation of the cervical spine

PHYSICAL EXAMINATION

- Clinical assessment in brachial plexus injuries is summarized by Mannan and Carlstedt. Physical findings in brachial plexus compression may include the following:
  ○ Shoulder pain, radiating up into the neck and down into the upper limb, combined with weakness or paralysis of the biceps brachii, deltoid, brachialis, brachioradialis, and coracobrachialis muscles and muscles supplied by the axillary, musculocutaneous, and radial nerves, together with associated paraesthesia and numbness
  ○ Bony anomalies may be detected.
  ○ Erb's point may be tender on palpation.
  ○ Grip strength may be reduced.
  ○ The upper limb may be held in adduction and medial rotation with forearm pronation and wrist and hand flexion ("waiter's tip" position).
  ○ Individuals may describe sensation of burning in the neck, weakness, cold, "heaviness," or "dead arm" and complain of clumsiness.

IMPORTANT OBJECTIVE TESTS

- Diagnostic accuracy of neurological upper limb examination employing a battery of standard test procedures has been found to be reproducible and reliable.
- For brachial plexus injuries, initial assessment must focus on neurological function, cervical spine fracture, and spinal cord injury before further testing is performed.
- Radiography, ultrasound, and magnetic resonance imaging (MRI) techniques and neurophysiology and EMG testing may be helpful in identifying underlying anatomical or traumatic issues and clarifying clinical diagnosis.
- Spurling test: Brachial plexus symptoms are reproduced with cervical extension, ipsilateral rotation, and axial loading for a positive result.
- Erb's point palpation: Tenderness is elicited for a positive result.
- Costoclavicular maneuver: Brachial plexus symptoms and a reduction in

radial pulse are reproduced in the upper limb with shoulder depression and retraction in individuals with costoclavicular syndrome.
- Adson's test (scalene test): Brachial plexus symptoms and a reduction in radial pulse are reproduced with cervical extension and ipsilateral rotation while sustaining a deep inspiration for a positive result.
- Wright's test: Brachial plexus symptoms and a reduction in radial pulse are reproduced with hyperabduction in sitting and supine lying for a positive result.

DIFFERENTIAL DIAGNOSIS (Dx)

- Cervical spine injuries, including spinal cord injury, bony trauma, soft tissue injury, radiculopathy, and discogenic trauma
- Glenohumeral dislocation
- AC joint injury
- Shoulder impingement syndrome
- Thoracic outlet syndrome
- Peripheral neuropathies
- Vascular pathology
- Cardiac pathology
- Pulmonary pathology
- Pancoast's syndrome
- Tobias or Ciuffini-Pancoast-Tobias syndrome
- Breast carcinoma
- Mesothelioma, plasmacytoma
- Lymphoma
- Metastatic carcinoma

CONTRIBUTING FACTORS

Traumatic injury is often a factor in brachial plexus compression, but the presence of anatomical anomalies in the cervical spine, clavicle, and posterior triangle may predispose an individual to the pathology.

TREATMENT

SURGICAL OPTIONS

- An overview of basic neurosurgical techniques is provided by Dahlin. When compression is due to cervical or first rib abnormalities, surgical resection of the rib may be required if conservative methods have failed to produce resolution. Division of fibrous bands, release techniques for relevant soft tissues, and correction, reduction, or fixation after traumatic injury may also be appropriate, depending on the underlying cause of the pathology. When severe and violent trauma has occurred, specialist neurosurgery may be required, including nerve transfers, nerve grafts, and neurolysis of scar tissue at the brachial plexus.

- Very few presentations require surgical intervention, but in common with other neural entrapments affecting the upper limb, surgery produces a good outcome in approximately 90% of cases.
- Traumatic injuries requiring correction, reduction, or fixation may need early surgical intervention. Otherwise, surgery is indicated only in those cases in which response to conservative management has been poor.

REHABILITATION

- In the acute stage, treatment is focused on pain relief, antiinflammatory therapy, and early mobilization.
- During the subacute stages, active exercise therapy aims to regain normal movement, strength, posture, and functional control, with particular emphasis on support for the injured neural structures.
- In the late recovery stages, further progression aims to return the individual to preinjury fitness.
- Physiotherapy involves a comprehensive management program composed of manual mobilization and soft tissue techniques, electrotherapy modalities, biomechanical analysis, postural reeducation and control, and functional movement, strength, and stability work. Appropriate aids to support the neck and affected structures may be advisable to prevent further injury during recovery.

PROGNOSIS

- Presence of anatomical anomalies in the cervical spine, clavicle, pectoral girdle, and posterior triangle, combined with a past history of trauma in these regions

and participation in high-impact contact sports or high-loading activities with or without sustained postures, predispose an individual to brachial plexus trauma and compression.

- Complications include chronic burner syndrome, contractures, scoliosis, glenohumeral dislocation, and, rarely, upper limb agnosia and deafferentation pain, but the majority of cases show complete resolution with conservative management.

SIGNS AND SYMPTOMS INDICATING REFERRAL TO PHYSICIAN

Indications for further medical evaluation include evidence of underlying trauma, worsening neurological function or symptoms, failure to respond to conservative management, suspicion or presence of underlying disease, and unexplained symptoms inconsistent with the pathology.

SUGGESTED READINGS

Bishop AT, Spinner RJ, Shin AY. Brachial plexus injuries in adults. *Hand Clin.* 2005; 21(1):ix-x.

Dahlin LB. Mini-symposium: hand trauma (ii) nerve injuries. *Curr Orthop.* 2008;22(1):9–16.

Hall TM, Elvey RL. Nerve trunk pain: physical diagnosis and treatment. *Man Ther.* 1999;4(2):63–73.

Hassan S, Kay S. Brachial plexus injury. *Surgery.* 2003;21(10):262–264.

Jepsen JR, Laursen LH, Hagert C-G, Kreiner S, Larsen AI. Diagnostic accuracy of the neurological upper limb examination I: interrelater reproducibility of selected findings and patterns. *BMC Neurol.* 2006;6(8).

Jepsen JR, Laursen LH, Hagert C-G, Kreiner S, Larsen AI. Diagnostic accuracy of the neurological upper limb examination II: relations to symptoms of patterns of findings. *BMC Neurol.* 2006;6(10).

Kinlaw D. Pre-/postoperative therapy for adult plexus injury. *Hand Clin.* 2005;21(1):103–108.

Levitz CL, Reilly PJ, Torg JS. The pathomechanics of chronic, recurrent cervical nerve root neuropraxia. The chronic burner syndrome. *Am J Sports Med.* 1997;25(1):73–76.

Mannan K, Carlstedt T. Injuries to the brachial plexus. *Surgery.* 2006;24(12):415–420.

Markey KL, Di Benedetto M, Curl WW. Upper trunk brachial plexopathy. The stinger syndrome. *Am J Sports Med.* 1993;21(5):650–655.

Moran SL, Steinmann SP, Shin AY. Adult brachial plexus injuries: mechanism, patterns of injury, and physical diagnosis. *Hand Clin.* 2005;21(1):13–24.

Nithi K. Physiology of the peripheral nervous system. *Surgery.* 2003;21(10):264a–264e.

Pratt N. Anatomy of nerve entrapment sites in the upper quarter. *J Hand Ther.* 2005;18(2):216–219.

Reid S, Trent V. Brachial plexus injuries—report of two cases presenting to a sports medicine practice. *Phys Ther Sport.* 2002;3(4):175–182.

Seddon HJ. *Surgical Disorders of the Peripheral Nerves.* 2nd ed. Edinburgh: Churchill Livingstone; 1975.

Shin AY, Spinner RJ, Steinmann SP, Bishop AT. Adult traumatic brachial plexus injuries. *J Am Acad Orthop Surg.* 2005;13:382–396.

Sunderland S. *Nerve and Nerve Injuries.* 2nd ed. Edinburgh: Churchill Livingstone; 1978.

Weinberg J, Rokito S, Silber JS. Etiology, treatment, and prevention of athletic stingers. *Clin Sports Med.* 2003;22(3):493–500.

Wilbourn AJ, Gilliat RW. Double crush syndrome: a critical analysis. *Neurology.* 1997; 49:21–29.

AUTHOR: SARAH GRAHAM

BASIC INFORMATION

DEFINITION

Common fibular nerve entrapment is a mononeuropathy that results from compression or restricted movement of the nerve usually found around the fibular head or in the popliteal space behind the knee.

SYNONYMS

- Common peroneal nerve entrapment
- Strawberry picker's knee
- Slimmer's paralysis

ICD-9CM CODES
355.7 Other mononeuritis of lower limb

OPTIMAL NUMBER OF VISITS

6 or fewer

MAXIMAL NUMBER OF VISITS

16

ETIOLOGY

- Originating from the sciatic nerve in the middle distal third of the thigh, the common fibular nerve descends to the popliteal fossa along the lateral aspect of the distal thigh under the long and short head of the biceps femoris to the fibular head. The nerve then courses around the fibular neck through an opening near the superficial head of the fibularis longus. Here, the common fibular nerve divides into the superficial and deep fibular nerves.
- Motor innervation of the common fibular nerve is as follows:
  - Short head of the biceps femoris
  - Fibularis longus and brevis (via superficial fibular nerve)
  - Tibialis anterior, extensor hallucis longus, extensor digitorum longus, and fibularis tertius (via deep fibular nerve)
- Sensory distribution of the common fibular nerve is as follows:
  - The common fibular nerve innervates the anterolateral leg and the dorsum of the foot through the superficial and deep branches.
  - The common fibular nerve itself innervates a portion of the lateral leg, over the head of the fibula.
- Typical entrapment sites of the common fibular nerve are as follows:
  - In the fibroosseous opening below the fibular head and near the superficial head of the fibularis longus the nerve passes through at a very acute angle. Here, the connective tissue may be tough since it helps secure the nerve to the proximal portion of the

fibula. These factors make this a common area for entrapment.
  - Repeated stress or injury to the lateral aspect of the knee may lead to entrapment of either the superficial or deep branch of the common fibular nerve. The superficial branch passes through the deep fascia and junction between the middle and distal third of the leg. Here, the fascia may be tough or restricted, limiting mobility of the nerve.

EPIDEMIOLOGY AND DEMOGRAPHICS

This condition is the most common nerve entrapment syndrome in the lower extremity after trauma. Certain jobs or activities where repetitive or prolonged knee flexion is required may cause more fibular nerve compression and develop into this pathology. No gender or age differences were noted in the incidence of common fibular nerve entrapment.

MECHANISM OF INJURY

The common fibular nerve entrapment may occur after traumatic events such as the following:
- Direct trauma
- Lacerations
- Femur or fibular fracture
- Gun shot wounds
- Local surgery
  - Open reduction and internal fixation (ORIF)
  - Tibial osteotomy
  - Total knee replacement
- Knee dislocations
- Other factors that may lead to entrapment:
  - Habitual leg crossing
  - Compression against bed railing or hard mattress in debilitated patients
  - Prolonged immobilization
  - Improperly fitting cast or brace
  - Intraneural or extraneural ganglia
  - Schwannoma
  - Desmoid tumor
  - Angioma
  - Neuroma
  - Baker's cyst
  - Chondromatosis
  - Exostosis
  - Well-developed muscles in the athletic population

COMMON SIGNS AND SYMPTOMS

- The most identifiable symptom is weakness in the ankle dorsiflexors, which tends to alter the normal gait pattern. This symptom is usually the most concerning for the patient since it may lead to tripping, loss of balance, and even falls from inadequate foot clearance.

- Sensory loss and paresthesias are noted in the distribution of the common fibular nerve, which includes the lateral leg over the fibular head, anterolateral lower leg/calf region, and the dorsum of the foot.
- Although pain is less likely in this condition, it may be present if significant soft tissue swelling and inflammation accompany the entrapment.

AGGRAVATING ACTIVITIES

- Prolonged kneeling or squatting
- Prolonged exercise
- Wearing a tight knee brace or cast
- Any activity that increases the local pressure around the nerve, thus increasing the compression and therefore the symptoms. Prolonged exercise, such as running, in which the fibularis longus is continually used may lead to more local trauma and swelling.

EASING ACTIVITIES

- Rest
- Ice and local modalities
- Avoiding aggravating activities

24-HOUR SYMPTOM PATTERN

No specific pattern of symptoms is noted. However, if there is a significant inflammatory component to the problem the patient may experience night symptoms or have increased symptoms in the morning that resolve slightly after about 30 minutes of light activity.

PAST HISTORY

Past history might include previous bouts of the same condition, local trauma, or previous lumbar spine or nerve disorder.

PHYSICAL EXAMINATION

- As mentioned, the most prominent sign in this condition is ankle dorsiflexion weakness and gait difficulties. They may manifest with a steppage gait pattern where compensations, such as increased knee flexion and hip flexion, occur during swing phase to clear the foot. If considerable weakness is present without compensations, the patient may complain of tripping caused by inadequate toe clearance. A foot slap or absent heel strike may also be present.
- Weakness of the tibialis anterior, extensor hallucis longus, and extensor digitorum longus should be noted on MMT.
- Sensation changes over the fibular head, anterolateral leg, and dorsum of the foot may be present. If the lesion or compression site is below the fibular neck, the sensation on the lateral calf may be spared, while still having changes on the dorsum of the foot.

IMPORTANT OBJECTIVE TESTS

- Gait analysis: Gait changes as noted are more obvious when there is significant or long-standing compression of the common fibular nerve.
- Tinel's sign: Tapping around the fibular head and head of the fibularis longus may reproduce symptoms into the distribution of the nerve.
- MMT and myotomal testing should reveal weakness of the extensor hallucis longus, tibialis anterior, and possibly fibularis brevis.
- Sensory testing is important to confirm that changes are occurring in only a peripheral nerve distribution related to the common fibular nerve. If symptoms are in a more dermatomal distribution, other proximal causes should be considered, such as lumbar spine radiculopathy.
- Neurodynamic testing may implicate a neurogenic source of symptoms.
- Lumbar ROM testing, accessory mobility testing, and palpation

DIFFERENTIAL DIAGNOSIS

- Lumbar spine radiculopathy (L4)
- Local fracture
- Local tumor or space-occupying lesion
- Compartment syndrome
- Infection

CONTRIBUTING FACTORS

- Excessive weight loss may contribute to this condition since it can lead to a decrease in the fat pad over the fibular head. This lack of protection may leave the nerve more vulnerable to local compression.
- Bulky lower extremity muscles, may also increase the pressure on the common fibular nerve, especially if combined with repetitive lower extremity activities such as running.
- Jobs or activities with repetitive knee flexion or kneeling may lead to more compression on the nerve.
- Hyperthyroidism, diabetes mellitus, vascular disorders, and leprosy have all been shown to have some effect on lower extremity nerve entrapment.

TREATMENT

MEDICAL/SURGICAL OPTIONS

- Spontaneous recovery is noted in many cases of this condition, so nonoperative management is recommended for 3 to 4 months. However, if anterior compartment syndrome (ACS) is suspected, an immediate referral to physician, urgent care, or emergency department is needed because this is an emergency situation in which a fasciotomy needs to be performed as soon as possible to relieve pressure on the nerve and surrounding structures.
- For common fibular nerve entrapment, a surgical decompression may be performed, especially in the case of space-occupying lesions.
- Nonsteroidal antiinflammatory drugs (NSAIDs), oral corticosteroids, or local injections may help alleviate symptoms if there is significant pain or inflammation.

REHABILITATION

- The first goal of rehabilitation is to identify and remove the cause of the nerve compression if possible.
- If significant weakness and gait deviations occur, bracing such as an ankle-foot orthotic (AFO), splint, or orthopedic shoes may help to normalize gait patterns. A lightweight rigid AFO or a hinged AFO with dorsiflexion assist may be appropriate.
- If the patient has significant pain or if an inflammatory component is suspected, local modalities, such as ice, ultrasound, interferential current, phonophoresis, or massage, may help manage symptoms.
- In the presence of positive neurodynamic findings and suspected restricted nerve mobility without significant compression, soft tissue mobilization along with neurodynamic mobilizations may be warranted. Butler suggests techniques that attempt to glide, slide, or put tension on the nervous system to free up local adhesions that may be restricting movement and preventing normal signal transmission.

PROGNOSIS

- In a number of cases, spontaneous recovery has been noted in patients with this condition. This also depends on the cause of the lesion because a transient compression will have much better results with therapy compared to a space-occupying lesion, such as a tumor, or internal factors such as a hardware used to fixate a fibular fracture.
- Wheeless noted that for partial fibular nerve palsy, >80% of patients recover completely and for complete nerve palsy <40% of patients have complete recovery.

SIGNS AND SYMPTOMS INDICATING REFERRAL TO PHYSICIAN

- Constant, unrelenting pain may indicate tumor or infection needing further medical management or workup.
- Symptoms not following the normal common fibular nerve distribution may indicate a different pathology that may require further physical therapy or medical evaluation.
- Increased pain or pressure in the anterior shin with tibialis anterior weakness may indicate ACS; immediate treatment by fasciotomy is needed to relieve the buildup of internal fluid and pressure.

SUGGESTED READINGS

Butler DS. *The Sensitive Nervous System.* Adelaide, Australia: Noigroup Publications; 2000.

Butler DS. *Mobilisation of the Nervous System.* New York: Churchill Livingston; 1991.

Dawson DM, Hallett M, Wilbourn AJ, eds. *Entrapment Neuropathies.* Philadelphia: Lippincott-Raven; 1999.

Moore KL, Dalley AF. *Clinical Oriented Anatomy.* 4th ed. Philadelphia, PA: Lippincott Williams & Wilkins; 1999.

Placzek JD, Boyce DA, eds. *Orthopedic Physical Therapy Secrets.* 2nd ed. Philadelphia: Elsevier; 2006.

Shacklock M. *Clinical Neurodynamics.* Philadelphia: Elsevier; 2005.

http://www.wheelessonline.com/ortho/peroneal_nerve

AUTHOR: CHRIS IZU

BASIC INFORMATION

DEFINITION

Deep fibular nerve entrapment is a mononeuropathy caused by compression or restriction of movement of the nerve in the anterior compartment of the lower leg or in the lateral ankle.

SYNONYMS

- Deep peroneal nerve entrapment
- Anterior tarsal tunnel syndrome (ATTS)
- Ski-boot syndrome

ICD-9CM CODES
355.7   Other mononeuritis of lower limb

OPTIMAL NUMBER OF VISITS

6 or fewer

MAXIMAL NUMBER OF VISITS

16

ETIOLOGY

- Branching off the common fibular nerve just distal to the fibular head, the deep fibular nerve enters the anterior compartment in the front of the leg near the interosseus membrane. It then courses distally lateral to the tibialis anterior muscle near the extensor digitorum longus, where it eventually goes under the extensor hallucis just above the ankle mortise. Passing in front of the ankle, the deep fibular nerve goes under the extensor retinaculum, where it divides into the lateral and medial branches.
- Sensory distribution of the deep fibular nerve: The nerve supplies sensation to the web space of the first and second toes, the adjacent metatarso phalangeal joint, and the nearby interphalangeal joints.
- Motor distribution of the deep fibular nerve: The lateral branch of the deep fibular nerve supplies the tibialis anterior, extensor digitorum brevis, extensor hallucis brevis, the adjacent tarsal and tarsometatarsal joints, and sometimes the second and third dorsal interossei. The medial branch innervates the extensor hallucis longus tendon and the extensor hallucis brevis muscle.
- Typical areas for deep fibular nerve entrapment are as follows:
  - With repeated stress or injury to surrounding musculature or fascia, fibrotic scarring may occur and entrap the deep fibular nerve.
  - The nerve is commonly trapped within either the anterior compartment or the anterior tarsal tunnel.
  - The anterior compartment is formed by the tibia medially, the fibula

laterally, the interosseous membrane posteriorly, and the anterior fascia anteriorly.
  - The deep fibular nerve may also be entrapped at the anterior tarsal tunnel, which is formed by the talotibial joint, the talonavicular joint, and the extensor retinaculum. Here, the nerve and the dorsalis pedis artery pass beneath the retinaculum. Repeated mechanical irritation beneath the retinaculum is the most common form of tarsal tunnel syndrome.
  - The deep fibular nerve may also be compressed in the tunnel by osteophytes, exostosis, bony prominences, or space-occupying lesions such as ganglia.

EPIDEMIOLOGY AND DEMOGRAPHICS

No reports on the incidence of this pathology were found. Clinically, it is commonly seen along with other injuries such as ACS or localized trauma to the anterior shin.

MECHANISM OF INJURY

- Direct trauma, such as snake bites or a blunt force, may cause injury to this area.
- Other common injuries leading to possible nerve entrapment include muscle inflammation secondary to prolonged exercise and local arterial bleeding.
- Forced or uncontrolled plantar flexion and inversion of the ankle can place this region under lots of stress.
- It is thought that repeated ankle sprains may be a contributing factor to fibular nerve entrapment in this area.
- Postural changes in the lower extremity that alter biomechanics may place more stress on the deep fibular nerve.
- Footwear that has a tight strap over the anterior part of the ankle can add external compression.
- Prolonged sitting with the foot in plantarflexion may also place strain on the deep fibular nerve.

COMMON SIGNS AND SYMPTOMS

- The most common complaint is a vague pain, burning, or cramping over the dorsum of the foot, usually with pain within the web space of the first and second digit.
- Weakness in the toe extension may be present as the deep fibular nerve provides motor input to both the extensor digitorum brevis and the extensor hallucis brevis.
- Because of weakness and pain in the foot, the patient may complain of gait difficulties. If the proximal component of the nerve (common fibular nerve) is involved, footdrop or foot slap with

decreased dorsiflexion in swing may be noted.
- Loss of sensation in the web space of the first and second digits is common, as this is main sensory distribution of the nerve.

AGGRAVATING ACTIVITIES

- Wearing tight shoes
- Wearing boots or athletic wear
- Walking
- Prolonged standing
- Ascending or descending stairs
- Sitting with foot in plantar flexion
- Sleeping with feet under the covers
- Some of the previous activities and external pressure on the foot may compress the nerve. Other activities with increased plantar flexion may place a stretch on the nerve, shortening its diameter.

EASING ACTIVITIES

- Properly fitting footwear
- Sitting
- Rest
- Modalities

24-HOUR SYMPTOM PATTERN

Since activities such as prolonged walking or standing are aggravating activities, more pain might be noted later in the day. Pain also could occur at night with plantar flexion of the foot under the covers or in the case of a strong inflammatory component to the condition. Associated pain in the morning might also be present.

PAST HISTORY

No specific past history is noted in the literature, but it seems feasible that repetitive trauma or past injury to the front of the shin or ankle may predispose an individual to this problem. Repetitive injury or poor healing from another injury may lead to fibrotic scarring around surrounding nerve fascia.

PHYSICAL EXAMINATION

- Sensory changes within the web space of the first and second digit are commonly present with deep fibular nerve entrapment.
- Antalgic gait or gait with limited dorsiflexion or toe extension may also be present.

IMPORTANT OBJECTIVE TESTS

- Lower quarter neurological examination
  - Sensory examination may find sensory changes as noted previously.
  - Motor examination should be normal with myotomal testing, but pain may be present with dorsiflexion or slight weakness with toe extension
  - Reflexes should be normal since this neuropathy is below the level of the patellar tendon reflex and a different

Section III

ORTHOPEDIC PATHOLOGY

branch of the sciatic nerve that does not innervate the Achilles tendon.

- The following tests may also help to rule out possible proximal causes such as lumbar radiculopathy:
  - Tinel's test: Tapping at the anterior tarsal tunnel may reproduce more distal symptoms.
  - Palpation: Palpation of surrounding musculature in the anterior compartment or anterior surface of the ankle may also reproduce symptomatic complaints.
  - Neurodynamic examination: Using the straight leg raise (SLR) with plantar flexion and inversion, the clinician may be able to differentiate between neurogenic (deep fibular nerve) and nonneurogenic (local muscles or tendons).

DIFFERENTIAL DIAGNOSIS

- Bony impingement
- Cystic masses
- Lumbar spine radiculopathy
- Common fibular nerve entrapment
- Sciatic nerve entrapment
- ACS
- Shin splints

CONTRIBUTING FACTORS

- Improper footwear
- Abnormal foot positioning: Pes planus or cavus
- Thyroid dysfunction
- Diabetes

TREATMENT

SURGICAL OPTIONS

- If there is significant increase in pressure within the anterior compartment (ACS), a fasciotomy, in which a small incision is made in the anterior fascia, is necessary to reduce building pressure. This situation can be a medical emergency, and failure to do such a procedure may result in permanent damage to the local and distal structure of the lower extremity.
- Surgical release of the deep fibular nerves may also be performed. This has been reported to produce immediate relief of symptoms and requires an excision of the nerve from the perceived entrapment site.
- Removal of osteophytes or space-occupying lesions are an important part of surgical management.

REHABILITATION

- The first goal of rehabilitation is to reduce symptoms and associated inflammation sensitizing the nerve.
- Modalities, such as ultrasound, phonophoresis, iontophoresis, interferential current therapy, ice, and compression, are theorized to help during more acute or inflammatory stages.
- Addressing postural faults and foot positioning may help to take stress off the deep fibular nerve. Taping and orthotic prescription may assist in this task.
- Once symptoms are alleviated, other techniques, such as soft tissue mobilization, may help free the nerve from surrounding fibrotic tissue.
- Neurodynamic techniques to help slide, glide, or place the nerve under tension may be warranted at this time to help restore the normal mobility of the nervous system.
- Other biomechanical faults or impairments that are hypothesized to place more stress on the deep fibular nerve must also be addressed before the rehabilitation program can be considered complete.

PROGNOSIS

No data were found at this time for the long-term outcomes of deep fibular nerve entrapment. Wheeless noted that for partial fibular nerve palsy >80% of patients recover completely and for complete nerve palsy <40% of patients have complete recovery.

SIGNS AND SYMPTOMS INDICATING REFERRAL TO PHYSICIAN

- Severe unrelenting pain occurring through the anterior shin may indicate ACS and worsening compression on the nerve. A fasciotomy must be done as soon as possible to release this pressure.
- Unrelenting symptoms, especially combined with worse pain at night, may indicate a local tumor.
- Lack of improvement within the expected time frame or symptoms that are not affected by physical therapy in a few visits should be referred back to the physician because a space-occupying lesion may be present.
- A recent history of trauma with suspected fracture may warrant further imaging before continuing physical therapy.
- Impaired circulation or vascular compromise may also warrant more medical management.

SUGGESTED READINGS

Butler DS. *Mobilisation of the Nervous System*. New York: Churchill Livingston; 1991.

Butler DS. *The Sensitive Nervous System*. Adelaide, Australia: Noigroup Publications; 2000.

Dawson DM, Hallett M, Wilbourn AJ, eds. *Entrapment Neuropathies*. Philadelphia: Lippincott-Raven; 1999.

Moore KL, Dalley AF. *Clinical Oriented Anatomy*. 4th ed. Philadelphia: Lippincott Williams & Wilkins; 1999.

Placzek JD, Boyce DA, eds. *Orthopedic Physical Therapy Secrets*. 2nd ed. Philadelphia: Elsevier; 2006.

Shacklock M. *Clinical Neurodynamics*. Philadelphia: Elsevier; 2005.

http://www.wheelessonline.com/ortho/peroneal_nerve

AUTHOR: CHRIS IZU

BASIC INFORMATION

DEFINITION

Femoral nerve entrapment is a mononeuropathy that results from compression or restriction of movement of the nerve, usually in the anterior abdominal wall as it passes through the femoral triangle under the inguinal ligament.

ICD-9CM CODES
355.2 Other lesion of femoral nerve

OPTIMAL NUMBER OF VISITS
6 or fewer

MAXIMAL NUMBER OF VISITS
16

ETIOLOGY

- The femoral nerve originates from the ventral rami of L2, L3, and L4 near the psoas major and travels inferiorly in the intermuscular groove between the psoas and the iliacus muscle. From there, it passes under the inguinal ligament in the femoral triangle lateral to the femoral artery and vein. It then divides into both sensory and motor branches.
- The cutaneous sensory branches of the nerve innervate the proximal upper and anterior thigh.
- The femoral nerve sends branches to the large quadriceps muscles.
- Because of the location of the femoral nerve, there is a multitude of factors that can cause femoral nerve entrapment. The most common entrapment area occurs underneath the inguinal ligament.
- It also may be entrapped or compressed more inferiorly where the nerve is close to the humeral head and attachments of the vastus intermedius and psoas tendons. Problems with those tendons or muscles may cause femoral nerve restrictions or irritation.
- Local tumors, psoas abscesses, lymph node enlargement, hematomas, and penetrating trauma are some of the most commonly documented causes of internal compression of the femoral nerve.
- Tissue healing after trauma or surgery has also been hypothesized to lay down scar tissue that may restrict the mobility of the femoral nerve within its neural container.

EPIDEMIOLOGY AND DEMOGRAPHICS

One reference stated that this entrapment syndrome is thought to be a rare occurrence and that earlier reported cases may have been mislabeled as femoral nerve neuropathies instead of other proximal causes.

MECHANISM OF INJURY

- The femoral nerve may become injured or entrapped from local trauma to the anterior hip or thigh such as a contusion or repetitive strain.
- It may also be injured or compressed during stressful abduction or external rotation activities such as during birth (vaginal deliveries).
- Intrapelvic injury and injury to the inguinal region have also been documented to lead to nerve entrapment.
- Common traumatic events include the following:
  - Gunshot wounds
  - Knife wounds
  - Puncture wounds
  - Pelvic surgeries
  - Total hip replacement (anterior approach)
  - Pelvic fractures
- Other noted factors that can lead to compression include the following:
  - Pelvic radiation therapy
  - Appendical or renal abscess
  - Tumors
  - Compartment-like compression

COMMON SIGNS AND SYMPTOMS

- Weakness in knee extension is common because of the motor input of the femoral nerve to the large quadriceps muscles. Hip flexion may also be difficult from the contribution of the rectus femoris.
- Gait difficulties or functional activities like squatting may become more difficult because of the weakness in knee extension.
- Sensation loss in the anterior aspect of the thigh may be present if the anterior cutaneous branch of the femoral nerve is affected. An individual with this condition may also have sensation loss to the medial aspect of the knee from involvement of the saphenous branch.
- Pain may be present in the inguinal region from the cause of the compression.

AGGRAVATING ACTIVITIES

- Walking or standing may aggravate symptoms secondary to a stretch on the femoral nerve with hip extension, especially during trailing limb posture in gait.
- Walking may also be difficult if significant quadriceps weakness is present.

EASING ACTIVITIES

- Sitting
- Hip flexion or external rotation
- Rest
- Local modalities

24-HOUR SYMPTOM PATTERN

No specific pattern of symptoms is noted. However, if there is a significant inflammatory component to the problem, one may experience night symptoms or may have increased symptoms in the morning that resolve slightly after about 30 minutes of light activity.

PAST HISTORY

- Prior history of surgery in the pelvic region (i.e., hernia, cesarean section, or hysterectomy)
- Past history of a patient with this condition may include previous trauma to the area, repetitive stress injuries, or other lumbopelvic problems.
- Prior history of prostate or uterine pathology

PHYSICAL EXAMINATION

- Weakness with hip flexion and knee extension are the most common symptoms associated with femoral nerve entrapment. Gait deviations may be noted to compensate for quadriceps weakness, and a quadriceps avoidance pattern of limited knee flex during loading response may be present.
- A diminished patellar tendon reflex is most likely present secondary to impaired nerve conduction.
- Sensory deficits are likely present in the anteromedial aspect of the thigh and may be in the medial aspect of the leg because of the saphenous branch of the femoral nerve.
- Pain may be noted with resisted hip flexion from the possible involvement of the psoas muscle and with stretching into combined hip extension and knee flexion.
- Palpation around the lateral portion of the femoral triangle, psoas, or iliacus muscle may be painful compared to the unaffected side and may reproduce symptoms down into the anteromedial aspect of the thigh or knee.

IMPORTANT OBJECTIVE TESTS

- Strength testing
  - Motor deficits in hip flexion and knee extension might be the most obvious signs of femoral nerve compression. However, weakness in the area alone should not be considered diagnostic because an L3 radiculopathy may produce the same result.
- Lower quarter neurological examination
  - To make sure symptoms are only the result of an isolated peripheral nerve problem, a full lower quadrant neurological examination is warranted. Symptoms that follow along a more dermatomal or myotomal pattern indicate a more proximal problem.
  - Symptoms that cross one or more dermatomes or peripheral nerve regions may be the result of a polyneuropathy.

- Slump knee bend test
  - Performing this test in sidelying, according to Butler, with cervical flexion and extension as a sensitizing maneuver may help determine if neurogenic symptoms are present, as in the case of femoral nerve entrapment.
- Lumbar ROM testing, accessory mobility testing, and palpation may help differentiate a lumbar spine problem from an isolated femoral nerve entrapment.

DIFFERENTIAL DIAGNOSIS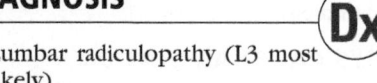

- Lumbar radiculopathy (L3 most likely)
- Local muscular strain
- Pelvic fracture
- Hip fracture
- Hip joint pathology
- Appendical or renal abscess
- Tumors

CONTRIBUTING FACTORS

- Diabetes mellitus
- Thyroid problems
- Poor posture
- Impaired trunk and motor control

TREATMENT

SURGICAL OPTIONS

Microsurgical nerve decompression

REHABILITATION

- The initial goals of rehabilitation are to reduce the pain and inflammation in the present state of the condition.
- Modalities, such as ultrasound, phonophoresis, iontophoresis, interferential current therapy, light massage, and cold, may help to accomplish this.
- If there are any external compression factors such as tight clothes, modification of attire is necessary.
- After symptoms have calmed, rehabilitation may focus on improving the health and mobility of the nerve.
- Soft tissue mobilization directed at fibrotic scarring around the nerve may be beneficial.
- Neurodynamic mobilizations aimed at sliding, gliding, or placing tension on the nerve may also be warranted to restore normal mobility to the nervous system.
- A complete rehabilitation program will also work to address any other biomechanical faults or impairments that might be leading to stress or strain on the femoral nerve.

PROGNOSIS

One study reported up to 70% improvement of symptoms in this population, although improvement may take up to a year. If there is severe axonal loss, it is thought that there will be some recovery of function, although not complete.

SIGNS AND SYMPTOMS INDICATING REFERRAL TO PHYSICIAN

- Unrelenting pain not related to biomechanical factors
- Weight loss
- Bowel or bladder dysfunction
- Saddle paresthesias
- Gait disturbances: Clumsiness or ataxic gait
- Bilateral glove or sock numbness
- Symptoms that do not initially improve with symptoms

SUGGESTED READINGS

Butler DS. *The Sensitive Nervous System*. Adelaide, Australia: Noigroup Publications; 2000.

Butler DS. *Mobilisation of the Nervous System*. New York: Churchill Livingston; 1991.

Dawson DM, Hallett M, Wilbourn AJ, eds. *Entrapment Neuropathies*. Philadelphia: Lippincott-Raven; 1999.

Moore KL, Dalley AF. *Clinical Oriented Anatomy*. 4th ed. Philadelphia: Lippincott Williams & Wilkins; 1999.

Placzek JD, Boyce DA, eds. *Orthopedic Physical Therapy Secrets*. 2nd ed. Philadelphia: Elsevier; 2006.

Shacklock M. *Clinical Neurodynamics*. Philadelphia: Elsevier; 2005.

http://www.emedicine.com/Orthoped/topic422.htm

AUTHOR: CHRIS IZU

BASIC INFORMATION

DEFINITION

Compression of the posterior interosseous nerve (which arises from the radial nerve) at the tendinous margin of the extensor carpi radialis brevis, fibrous bands anterior to the head of the radius, radial recurrent blood vessels, or between the two supinator heads in the arcade of Frohse, which is a fibrous arch occurring in 30% of the population.

SYNONYMS

- Radial tunnel syndrome
- Posterior interosseous nerve syndrome

ICD-9CM CODES
955.3 Injury to radial nerve

OPTIMAL NUMBER OF VISITS

Conservative management should produce some reduction in symptoms within 3 to 6 weeks.

MAXIMAL NUMBER OF VISITS

If there is little or no response to conservative management after 12 weeks, a surgical opinion should be obtained.

ETIOLOGY

- The insult to the nerve may be mechanical, thermal, chemical, or ischemic.
- In entrapment syndromes, compression or direct trauma leads to nerve tissue hypoxia.
- Posterior interosseous nerve entrapment pathology may occur with repetitive or overuse movement patterns involving supination and pronation of the forearm, trauma, surgery, underlying rheumatoid disease, ganglions, and tumors.
- In entrapments, nerve trauma occurs because the size of the neural structure exceeds the anatomical space available for it, resulting in increased pressure, which in turn leads to impaired blood flow and subsequent hypoxia of the tissue and disruption of the axonal transport system.
- Nerve injury is classified according to severity of the injury and potential for reversibility. Original classifications described previously remain in current use.
  - First-degree neuropraxia involves distortion of myelin about the nodes of Ranvier caused by ischemia, mechanical compression, or electrolyte imbalance, resulting in temporary loss of nerve conduction. Recovery is rapid and complete in most cases.
  - Second-degree axonotmesis involves interruption of the axon with second-

ary wallerian degeneration, but the supporting tissue around the axon is preserved. Recovery may be complete but takes longer to occur and depends on the distance between the site of injury and the end structure (denervated muscle).
  - Third-degree neurotmesis involves extensive disruption of the nerve and its supporting structures, but while the endoneurium is disrupted, the perineurium and epineurium remain intact.
  - Fourth-degree neurotmesis involves disruption of all neural components except the epineurium.
  - Fifth-degree neurotmesis involves complete transaction and discontinuity of the nerve with no capacity for regeneration.
- Neurotmesis rarely occurs from entrapment, but where continuity has been disrupted, complete recovery is not possible, even with surgical techniques, and the eventual outcome depends on individual circumstances.
- Double-crush syndrome refers to the fairly common phenomenon of nerve entrapment and radiculopathy occurring in combination, although the syndrome is considered controversial. Compression or irritation of the nerve roots at the cervical level is thought to increase sensitivity to compression or movement restrictions more distally in the structure.
- As noted earlier, increasing pressure on the nerve causes impaired blood flow, tissue hypoxia, and disruption to the anterograde and retrograde intercellular transport of materials within axons, eventually disturbing depolarization within the nerve. In overuse-type entrapments, it is proposed that repetitive work or static postures produce an inflammatory response. Fibroblasts appear to repair the damage incurred but generate adhesions that limit neural glide and subsequently increase anoxia. Other studies have found that cortical dedifferentiation may occur from repetitive motion activities and nerve injuries. This may result in reinforced poor posturing and use of aberrant motor pathways.

EPIDEMIOLOGY AND DEMOGRAPHICS

- Posterior interosseous nerve entrapment is an uncommon cause of lateral elbow and forearm symptoms.
- Since the causes for this pathology are so diverse, it occurs across a broad spectrum of the population.

MECHANISM OF INJURY

- The nerve entrapment may be caused by local edema from irritation of the neighboring tissues or volume changes

in surrounding tissues generated by mechanical overload via repetitive activity or impact trauma, specifically in supinator and extensor carpi radialis brevis.
- Posterior interosseous nerve entrapment may be compounded by the presence of certain anatomical features: Fibrous bands anterior to the radial head or within the supinator arch (the arcade of Frohse) and the specific location of the radial recurrent blood vessels.
- Other causes include fractures, inappropriately positioned surgical fixings and plates, surgical trauma, rheumatoid synovitis, ganglions, and tumors.

COMMON SIGNS AND SYMPTOMS

- Posterior interosseous nerve entrapment commonly manifests with pain in the extensor region of the lateral forearm. The pain is most intense over the supinator, sometimes extending to the wrist and proximal humerus. It can be combined with pain on resisted supination when the elbow is flexed and resisted extension of the middle finger when the elbow is extended, weakness in wrist and finger extension, and paraesthesias in the hand and lateral forearm, although this is disputed by some authors.
- Clinical signs and symptoms for radial tunnel syndrome and posterior interosseous compression, with indications and options for surgical treatment, are presented by Markiewitz and Merryman.
- The typical referral pattern for posterior interosseous nerve entrapment is local pain at the elbow and lateral forearm, extending to the wrist and upper regions of the humerus.

AGGRAVATING ACTIVITIES

- Repetitive forearm rotation
- Resisted supination from pronation with wrist flexion
- Full-range pronation
- Elbow extension
- These movement patterns occur with a range of activities but are prevalent in office workers, manual workers, musicians, and athletes.

EASING ACTIVITIES

- Reducing load
- Avoiding the aggravating movement patterns
- Positioning
- Rest (absolute or relative with the aid of splinting or taping)

24-HOUR SYMPTOM PATTERN

Symptoms worsen with aggravating activities, but pain may also increase nocturnally, which is similar to many entrapment neuropathies.

PAST HISTORY FOR THE REGION

- Previous history of trauma, surgery, or overuse-type injury at the elbow, forearm, or wrist
- History of rheumatoid disease

PHYSICAL EXAMINATION

- Pain over the anterolateral forearm with referral as described previously.
- Maximum tenderness is approximately 6 to 8 cm distal to the lateral epicondyle, over the supinator.
- Pain is provoked or worsened with resisted supination, elbow extension with pronation, and extension of the middle finger.
- Depending on the site of compression, weakness may also be present in wrist extension (extensor carpi ulnaris and extensor digitorum communis are affected), finger extension (extensor digiti quinti, extensor digitorum communis, and extensor indicis proprius are affected), and thumb movement (abductor pollicis longus, extensor pollicis longus, and brevis are affected).

IMPORTANT OBJECTIVE TESTS

- Radiography and MRI facilitate detection of underlying factors such as fractures, ganglions, tumors, or other tissue abnormality.
- Local injection at the lateral epicondyle may distinguish between lateral epicondylitis (when it is usually much more effective) and radial tunnel syndrome (when it has little or no effect).
- EMG and nerve conduction studies may be inconclusive, so clinical findings previously described, in conjunction with neural tension techniques, may provide the most reliable aid to diagnosis.
- Diagnostic accuracy of neurological upper limb examination employing a battery of standard test procedures has been found to be reproducible and reliable.

DIFFERENTIAL DIAGNOSIS **Dx**

- Cervical radiculopathy (C7 pathology affects triceps brachii and wrist flexors)
- Lateral epicondylitis (maximal tenderness is at the lateral epicondyle rather than distal to it)
- Trigger finger (passive, as well as active, movement is affected)
- Extensor tendon rupture (fingers fail to extend on passive wrist flexion)
- Adverse neural tension

CONTRIBUTING FACTORS

- Anatomical arrangement
- Presence of other underlying disease
- Past history of trauma or surgery
- Lifestyle activities involving elbow or forearm movement patterns

TREATMENT

SURGICAL OPTIONS

- An overview of basic neurosurgical techniques is provided by Dahlin. Individuals who fail to respond to conservative management may require decompression surgery.
- Two main techniques, anterolateral and posterior, may be employed. The anterolateral technique is preferred because it allows greater access to more of the entrapment sites, facilitating release at the supinator, arcade of Frohse, fibrous margin of extensor carpi radialis brevis, distal fascia, and dissection of the nerve from scar tissue posttrauma.
- If symptoms are arising from fixation devices, corrective surgery will be required.
- If compression is due to ganglion or tumor, surgical technique will obviously depend on precise location.
- In addition to the standard risks associated with any surgery, there is a risk of further damage to the nerve during the procedure. However, success rates of 90% have been reported for neurapraxic injuries, with fast recovery to full normal function.
- Individuals who have failed to respond to conservative management after a period of 8 to 12 weeks should be considered for surgical opinion. In addition, any worsening of neurological function despite intervention should be evaluated (Cravens and Kline).

REHABILITATION

- Cleary provided an overview of concepts and evidence for conservative management in radial tunnel syndrome but notes that definitive clinical evidence is scarce.
- Conservative treatment consists of manual techniques consisting of soft tissue release work, myofascial release work, and neural stretching or mobilizing techniques.
- Depending on the underlying cause of the pathology, antiinflammatory modalities may also be useful, combined with offloading the stressed structures.
- The effectiveness of antiinflammatory medication is disputed, although many authors recommend including these in the management regimen since they produce benefit in some cases.
- It may be appropriate to teach individuals stretching or mobilizing techniques to be applied between treatment sessions.
- If abhorrent movement patterns are the result of other muscle imbalance or recruitment issues, it may be appropriate to address these issues as part of the rehabilitative process.

PROGNOSIS

- As previously noted, factors that contribute or predispose an individual to the pathology include anatomical arrangement, presence of other underlying disease, past history of trauma or surgery, or lifestyle activities involving elbow and forearm movement patterns.
- Prognosis for full recovery is good, with almost all cases responding to either conservative or surgical management.

SIGNS AND SYMPTOMS INDICATING REFERRAL TO PHYSICIAN

- Worsening neurological function or symptoms
- Failure to respond to conservative management
- Suspicion or presence of underlying disease
- Unexplained symptoms inconsistent with the pathology

SUGGESTED READINGS

Brukner P, Khan K. *Clinical Sports Medicine*. 3rd ed. New York: McGraw-Hill; 2006.

Cleary CK. Management of radial tunnel syndrome: a therapist's clinical perspective. *J Hand Ther*. 2006;9(2):166–191.

Cravens G, Kline DG. Posterior interosseous nerve palsies. *Neurosurgery*. 1990;27(3):397–402.

Dahlin LB. Mini-symposium: hand trauma (ii) nerve injuries. *Curr Orthop*. 2008;22(1):9–16.

Hall TM, Elvey RL. Nerve trunk pain: physical diagnosis and treatment. *Man Ther*. 1999;4(2):63–73.

Jepsen JR, Laursen LH, Hagert C-G, Kreiner S, Larsen AI. Diagnostic accuracy of the neurological upper limb examination I: interrelater reproducibility of selected findings and patterns. *BMC Neurol*. 2006;6(8).

Jepsen JR, Laursen LH, Hagert C-G, Kreiner S, Larsen AI. Diagnostic accuracy of the neurological upper limb examination II: relations to symptoms of patterns of findings. *BMC Neurol*. 2006;6(10).

Magee DJ. *Orthopaedic Physical Assessment*. 5th ed. Philadelphia: Saunders; 2008.

Markiewitz AD, Merryman J. Radial nerve compression in the upper extremity. *J Am Soc Surg Hand*. 2005;5(2):87–99.

Pratt N. Anatomy of nerve entrapment sites in the upper quarter. *J Hand Ther*. 2005;18(2):216–219.

Seddon HJ. *Surgical Disorders of the Peripheral Nerves*. 2nd ed. Edinburgh: Churchill Livingstone; 1975.

Sunderland S. *Nerve and Nerve Injuries*. 2nd ed. Edinburgh: Churchill Livingstone; 1978.

Wilbourn AJ, Gilliat RW. Double crush syndrome: a critical analysis. *Neurology*. 1997;49:21–29.

AUTHOR: SARAH GRAHAM

BASIC INFORMATION

DEFINITION

Lateral femoral cutaneous nerve (LFCN) entrapment is a mononeuropathy that results from either compression or restriction of movement of the nerve, most likely as it passes under the inguinal ligament near the anterior superior iliac spine.

SYNONYMS

Meralgia paresthetica

ICD-9CM CODES
355.1 Meralgia paresthetica

OPTIMAL NUMBER OF VISITS

6 or fewer

MAXIMAL NUMBER OF VISITS

12

ETIOLOGY

- The nerve originates from the lumbar plexus and travels distally through the pelvis near the psoas major muscle and eventually through a tunnel formed by the lateral attachment on the inguinal ligament and the anterior superior iliac spine (ASIS). The nerve travels superficially to supply the skin about 10 cm distal to the inguinal ligament. Here, the nerve has less protection than it does more proximally in the pelvis.
- Both internal and external factors can compromise the LFCN. Research and case studies have pointed toward tight clothing, such as jeans, underwear, or a belt, as possible external factors that could lead to nerve compression. Internal factors could include a pendulous abdomen, rapid increase in weight, or space-occupying lesions as potential causes of LFCN entrapment. Examples may include contained iliopsoas hemorrhage or neoplasm.
- Another hypothesis of the cause of nerve entrapment is that the surrounding tissues that form the neural container may restrict or limit its ability to slide or glide as a result of dysfunction of nearby fascial layers. These tissues may leave the nerve bound to adjacent structures after trauma and healing have taken place such as in abdominal surgery or recent pelvic fracture.

EPIDEMIOLOGY AND DEMOGRAPHICS

- As the incidence of rapid weight gain increases in those who are middle-aged, so does the incidence of entrapment of the LFCN.
- Construction workers, mechanics, or other professionals, whose jobs require them to wear tight or heavy attire around their waists, have a higher incidence of this condition.
- There is no difference in incidence between right and left sides of the body, and symptoms may also appear intermittently.

MECHANISM OF INJURY

Direct trauma, stretch injuries, and ischemia are the most likely culprits, which would lead to compromise of the LFCN. Some documented traumatic events that have led to this condition include seatbelt injuries in motor vehicle accidents (MVAs), pelvic fractures, and surgical procedures. It has also been noted that LFCN entrapment may occur after lying in the fetal position for a long period of time.

COMMON SIGNS AND SYMPTOMS

- Most important to note is that there is likely no motor deficit with this condition since the LFCN is purely sensory. Some local muscle guarding may appear as a result of pain and muscle inhibition in both hip flexion and extension as the nerve is either further compressed or stretched.
- The hallmark of LFCN entrapment is altered sensation over the lateral aspect of the mid-thigh. This may include numbness, tingling, or even a burning pain, a dull ache, or itching.
- Symptoms are usually unilateral, although they may be bilateral in cases of rapid weight gain that affect the body symmetrically.

AGGRAVATING ACTIVITIES

- Walking or prolonged standing
- Wearing tight clothes or accessories
- Activities that include sustained or repetitive hip extension or flexion
- Tight clothing and garments add external compression to the superficial region of the nerve, whereas hip extension activities may place stretch on surrounding structures that would in turn increase the local pressure around the nerve. Hip extension may also place the LFCN under more tensile stress.

EASING ACTIVITIES

- Sitting or rest
- Removal of tight clothing
- Avoiding excessive hip extension
- Once the external compression is removed, improved axonal flow and neuronal blood flow should help alleviate some of the symptoms.

24-HOUR SYMPTOM PATTERN

Current research has not addressed a 24-hour pattern of symptoms of this disorder. However, if there is a significant inflammatory component of the disorder, symptoms may be worse in the morning or may even cause wakening in the night.

PAST HISTORY

Previous trauma to the area or incidence of the same condition may predispose a person to LFCN entrapment.

PHYSICAL EXAMINATION

- Altered sensation is the hallmark of the condition and should manifest as numbness, paresthesias, or pain in the anterolateral thigh.
- Motor examination or MMT of lower extremity myotomes should be normal since the LFCN is purely sensory. The patient may have pain with hip flexion or knee extension secondary to local attachment near the dysfunctional area, but strength should be symmetrical.

IMPORTANT OBJECTIVE TESTS

- Sensation testing
  - It is important to map out the specific area or distribution of symptoms to differentiate the cause from a potential more proximal lumbar spine cause. Symptoms that occur more distally than the anterolateral thigh, such as down to the lateral leg or foot, suggest further lumbar spine testing. One suggestion has been to use a marker or pen to accurately draw the area on the patient's leg.
- Tinel's test
  - With tapping over the superficial region over the nerve (over the lateral and upper part of the inguinal ligament), symptoms should be reproduced.
- LFCN test
  - This test is performed as a variation of the slump knee bend test. Butler (2000) added adduction and internal rotation of the hip to stress the LFCN and to help determine if the symptoms are neurogenic by using cervical extension and flexion as a sensitizing maneuver.
- Lumbar ROM testing, accessory mobility testing, and palpation
  - Because of the chance that a more upper lumbar spine problem may refer symptoms distally into this region, it is important to rule out that area as a potential source of symptoms.

DIFFERENTIAL DIAGNOSIS

- Lumbar spine referral
  - Disc dysfunction
  - Somatic referred pain
  - Nerve root irritation
- Muscle strain
- Pelvic fracture
- Pelvic neoplasm

- Polyneuropathy
- Retroperitoneal hemorrhage

CONTRIBUTING FACTORS

- Diabetes can affect the health of the nervous system and predispose a person to nerve entrapment syndromes.
- Obesity and especially rapid weight gain can increase the pressure or compression on the superficial region of the LFCN.
- Pregnancy is a common contributing factor for the same reason as rapid weight gain.
- Occupational requirements that include tight attire around the waste such as tight pants or work belts

TREATMENT

SURGICAL OPTIONS

- If conservative measures fail, surgical decompression may be considered. Successful predictors of good outcomes after surgery include a positive Tinel's test, abnormal electrodiagnostic findings (that do not suggest other potential causes), and immediate relief of symptoms after local nerve block.
- In very rare instances, the nerve can be surgically transected. The long-term outcomes are suspect, and since the nerve has no motor function, which may lead to more serious disability, this option is not recommended.
- A physician may be able to do a focal nerve block near the inguinal ligament using a combination of lidocaine and corticosteroids. This is a good treatment option if the pain is severe and may provide relief for several days to weeks.

REHABILITATION

- The most important factor in treatment is to remove the cause of the problem. Patient education on avoidance of tight clothing or accessories usually helps resolve the symptoms. If obesity or rapid gain is thought to be at fault, those factors also need to be addressed.
- Concurrent rehabilitation may include modalities, such as ultrasound, interferential current therapy, and phonophoresis, to reduce swelling and inflammation.
- It is also important to address other contributing factors such as the following:
  ○ Ergonomics
  ○ Postural changes and adaptations
  ○ General fitness level, including stretching
- If positive neurodynamic testing suggests nerve entrapment from restricted nerve mobility, other methods of treatment may include local soft tissue mobilization followed by nerve gliding with respect to irritability of symptoms.
- Neurogenic pain medications, such as carbamazepine or gabapentin, have been shown to have some effect on symptoms in select patients, but the effects are usually minimal.

PROGNOSIS

Because of the pure sensory function of the LFCN, it is not typical for this condition to lead to severe functional loss or disability. Research shows that it is not associated with mortality or significant morbidity. Typically, the paresthesias resolve slowly over time, but numbness in the peripheral nerve distribution may persist. Removal of the cause of the nerve compression usually results in good outcomes.

SIGNS AND SYMPTOMS INDICATING REFERRAL TO PHYSICIAN

- Constant or unrelenting deep, boring pain may be a sign of a space-occupying lesion causing the nerve entrapment. These symptoms are even more of a concern if not in the distribution of the LFCN such as the back, pelvis, or anterior hip.
- Pain or symptoms that do not change with treatment or removal of the hypothesized cause of the nerve compression may also point toward infection or tumor.
- Symptoms associated with trauma that has not been screened with radiographs or other imaging studies may be caused by concurrent pelvic fracture.
- Any other neurological signs, such as myotomal weakness or dermatomal sensory changes, may require further work-up or diagnostics, to rule out more proximal causes of symptoms.
- Severe pain preventing the patient from participating in therapy may require nerve block or other management before continuing.

SUGGESTED READINGS

Butler DS. *Mobilisation of the Nervous System*. New York: Churchill Livingston; 1991.

Butler DS. *The Sensitive Nervous System*. Adelaide, Australia: Noigroup Publications; 2000.

Dawson DM, Hallett M, Wilbourn AJ, eds. *Entrapment Neuropathies*. Philadelphia: Lippincott-Raven; 1999.

Moore KL, Dalley AF. *Clinical Oriented Anatomy*. 4th ed. Philadelphia: Lippincott Williams & Wilkins; 1999.

Placzek JD, Boyce DA, eds. *Orthopedic Physical Therapy Secrets*. 2nd ed. Philadelphia: Elsevier; 2006.

Shacklock M. *Clinical Neurodynamics*. Philadelphia: Elsevier; 2005.

http://www.emedicine.com/Orthoped/topic422.htm

AUTHOR: CHRIS IZU

BASIC INFORMATION

DEFINITION

Long thoracic nerve pathologies encompass any injury that interrupts the function of the long thoracic nerve at any point along its course. The loss of function results in serratus anterior muscle dysfunction and often pain.

SYNONYMS

- Long thoracic nerve palsy
- Serratus anterior muscle palsy
- Rucksack palsy

ICD-9CM CODES
354   Mononeuritis of upper limb and mononeuritis complex
354.8   Other mononeuritis of upper limb
354.9   Mononeuritis of upper limb unspecified

OPTIMAL NUMBER OF VISITS

6

MAXIMAL NUMBER OF VISITS

20

ETIOLOGY

- The anatomy of the nerve is as follows:
  - Motor nerve that is 22 to 24 cm long with a superficial course
  - Comprises the ventral rami of the C5 to C7 nerve roots (also the C8 nerve roots and intercostal nerves in some)
  - C5 and C6 roots merge and pierce the scalene medius muscle, while the C7 root travels between the anterior and middle scalene muscles.
  - The C5, C6, and C7 roots join to form the long thoracic nerve sitting anteriorly to the posterior scalene muscle.
  - The nerve travels between the clavicle and first rib, laterally toward the midaxillary line, and here it sends out branches and innervates the serratus anterior muscle.
- Physiologically there is disruption to any part of the nerve responsible for conduction.
- In repetitive nerve injury, it is proposed that repetitive work or static postures produce an inflammatory process, fibroblasts appear to repair the damage incurred but produce adhesions to the nerve, limiting their glide and increasing anoxia.
- Lacerations generally result in neurotmesis injury. The pathology is essentially an injury to the long thoracic nerve. Nerve injury can be classified according to the severity of the injury and its potential for reversibility.

- The following is a basic overview of the Sunderland classification of nerve injury, which describes five degrees of nerve pathology (an expansion of Seddon's three-tier classification of neurapraxia, axonotmesis, and neurotmesis).
  - Neurapraxia (first-degree injury): Distortion of the myelin around the nodes of Ranvier caused by ischemia, mechanical compression, or electrolyte imbalance produces temporary loss of nerve conduction.
  - Axonotmesis (second-degree injury): Interruption of the axon with secondary wallerian degeneration; the supporting tissue surrounding the axon is preserved and the recovery period depends on the distance between the site of injury and the end-organs.
  - Neurotmesis: Complete disruption of the nerve and its supporting structures.
- Neurotmesis has been further divided into the following three subcategories:
  - Third-degree nerve injury: Endoneurium is disrupted with intact perineurium and epineurium.
  - Fourth-degree nerve injury: All neural elements sparing the epineurium are disrupted.
  - Fifth-degree nerve injury: Complete transaction and discontinuity of the nerve with no capacity for regeneration

EPIDEMIOLOGY AND DEMOGRAPHICS

The prevalence of long thoracic nerve injury has not been reported in the literature, but it is generally believed to be uncommon; no age groups have been reported as more prone to damage to the nerve and no gender specificity has been reported in the literature.

MECHANISM OF INJURY

- The long thoracic nerve is most susceptible to acute or recurrent trauma caused by traction or pressure.
- Nontraumatic pressure on the nerve can result at a number of sites along its path, by the following:
  - Within musculature (seen commonly in the scalene medius muscle) and inflamed bursa in the shoulder region
  - Between the first two ribs and the clavicle or between the coracoid process and the first or second ribs
  - In the axillary region from the presence of an axillary mass, excessive or poor use of old-style crutches, and overly tight bandage or plaster applications.
- Traction trauma to the long thoracic nerve can occur in the following ways:
  - Repetitive isolated stretch with cervical flexion, lateral flexion, and rotation away, combined with ipsilateral

arm flexion. The cervical movement places an anterior, medial, and superior pull on the proximal portion of the nerve with the scalenus medius muscle, while the distal nerve segment is tensioned with the overhead arm position in a posterior, lateral, and inferior direction with the serratus anterior muscle. The scalenus medius and serratus anterior muscles act as points of fixation, resulting in excessive elongation of the nerve. This position of stretch is commonly seen with throwing in baseball, javelin, and football; serving in tennis; spiking or serving in volleyball; and driving a golf ball. Additionally, tackling, wrestling, and lifting heavy weights overhead may also traction the nerve.
  - Repetitive bow-stringing of the nerve over a fascial band in shoulder abduction and external rotation.
  - Repetitive carrying of heavy loads or an injury involving sudden forced scapular depression
- Direct trauma to the nerve as it sits superficially in the supraclavicular fossa or chest may also occur with MVAs, falls, and strong massage.
- Iatrogenic injury to the nerve is also common during first rib resection and heart or breast surgery.
- Neuralgic amyotrophy, vaccinations, or infections may also affect the long thoracic nerve, either selectively or with other nerve involvement.

COMMON SIGNS AND SYMPTOMS

- The most common complaint is an insidious onset of shoulder girdle weakness with or without pain.
- Pain can often be present in the first few days to weeks followed by weakness with overhead activities.
- The patient may report decreased active shoulder ROM, particularly into forward flexion. This is accompanied by scapular winging, especially when pushing forward against resistance.
- The pain is often described as a burning, aching, or sharp pain in the shoulder, which may radiate to the scapula, arm, or scalene muscle region.

AGGRAVATING ACTIVITIES

- Aggravating activities involve repetitive positions that place stress on the nerve (cervical flexion, lateral flexion, and rotation away, combined with ipsilateral arm flexion) such as throwing (baseball, javelin, or football), serving in tennis, spiking or serving in volleyball, and driving a golf ball.
- Patients may also report symptom aggravation and reduced ability to pull and/or carry heavy objects, overhead lifting, tackling, and wrestling.

- Positions that cause overstretching of the serratus anterior muscle will also aggravate the pathology. These include forward flexion movements and arm weight-bearing positions that create excessive scapular winging.

EASING ACTIVITIES

- Rest and/or modification of aggravating activities
- Placing the neck, arm, and scapula in a neutral, supported position that does not tension the nerve.

24-HOUR SYMPTOM PATTERN

Generally, the symptoms are related to activity and do not follow a typical 24-hour pattern unless there is a strong inflammatory component such as may be seen in repetitive strain. If there is an inflammatory component, there may be worsening of symptoms with use toward the end of the day, pain at night, and morning stiffness with ache.

PAST HISTORY FOR THE REGION

- The patient commonly reports a history of the following:
  - Vigorous and/or repetitive overhead activity, including throwing in baseball, javelin, or football; serving in tennis; spiking or serving in volleyball; driving a golf ball, tackling, or wrestling.
  - Repetitive carrying of heavy loads
  - Injury involving sudden forced scapular depression
  - Excessive or poor use of old-style crutches and overly tight bandage or plaster applications into the axilla
  - Direct trauma to the supraclavicular region or chest, including MVAs, falls, and strong massage
  - First rib resection and heart or breast surgery
  - Vaccinations or infections

PHYSICAL EXAMINATION

- Inferior scapular winging at rest
- Reduced active shoulder flexion range and/or strength
- Scapular winging inferiorly and medially with active shoulder flexion and/or pressing against a wall or doing push-ups (as the forward arm movement places a posteriorly directed force on the medial border of the scapula, which is unopposed with a weak serratus anterior muscle)
- Weakened active shoulder abduction (with minimal loss of range as the lower trapezius can compensate for the lack of serratus anterior to upwardly rotate the scapula)
- MMT reveals weakness in the serratus anterior muscle.
- Poor scapulohumeral rhythm with active shoulder movements caused by impaired scapular rotation (with possible resultant positive impingement signs)
- Visible atrophy of the serratus anterior muscle
- Possible reduction of range and/or reproduction of pain on cervical lateral flexion away
- Upper limb neurodynamic testing may reveal adverse neurodynamics and elicit symptoms.

IMPORTANT OBJECTIVE TESTS

- It is important to confirm the diagnosis of long thoracic nerve neuropathy with electrodiagnostic evaluation. Needle examination testing is the most reliable test to evaluate the severity of long thoracic nerve damage and can be used to monitor progress of the condition. Nerve conduction studies, however, have been deemed unreliable to test for long thoracic nerve trauma, although they can be used for differential diagnosis of other brachial plexus lesions.
- A plain radiograph is also useful to assess for the presence of a cervical rib and for calcifications, although most often results are normal.
- MRI of the cervical spine and brachial plexus can also be used to exclude cervical or brachial pathologies.

DIFFERENTIAL DIAGNOSIS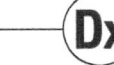

- Cervical
  - Cervical spondylosis
  - Cervical disc disease
  - Cervical nerve root syndrome
- Shoulder
  - Shoulder impingement
  - Malunion of scapular fracture
  - Rotator cuff tear or tendinopathy
  - Adhesive capsulitis
  - Instability of the glenohumeral or acromioclavicular joints
  - Degenerative arthritis of the glenohumeral or acromioclavicular joints
  - Scapulothoracic or scapulohumeral bursitis syndromes
- Nerve
  - Spinal accessory nerve or trapezius palsy
  - Dorsal scapular nerve or rhomboid palsy
  - Suprascapular nerve palsy
  - Thoracic outlet syndrome
  - Brachial plexus neuropathy (Parsonage-Turner syndrome)
  - Quadrilateral space syndrome
- Other
  - Polymyositis
  - Diffuse peripheral neuropathy
  - Osteochondroma
  - Muscular dystrophy

CONTRIBUTING FACTORS

- For any nerve pathology that is nontraumatic, there is often an element of repetitive activity involving the affected limb. Typically, in the case of the long thoracic nerve, the repetitive action that may create a traction or compressive neuropathy involves cervical flexion, lateral flexion, and rotation away, combined with ipsilateral arm flexion. Individuals involved in overhead sporting or occupational activity are therefore more at risk.
- Other repetitive tasks or activities, such as carrying loads in heavy manual work, weight lifting, tackling, and wrestling, may also predispose to long thoracic nerve injury.
- Postural factors may be involved, particularly with repetitive work or sporting activities, with reduction in proximal stability and scapular control leading to increased strain on the nerve.

TREATMENT

SURGICAL OPTIONS

- Safran reviewed literature pertaining to surgical options and found the most favorable results from the surgical transfer of the sternal head of the pectoralis major to replace serratus anterior function. The author felt that this particular transfer allowed the most similar muscle activity to that of the serratus anterior as a result of the orientation of the fibers and similar excursion levels. The semi-tendinosus-gracilis graft was also favored for its strength, low morbidity, and harvest efficiency. The pectoralis minor, rhomboid, and teres minor muscles have also been used for muscle transfers.
- Supraclavicular neurolysis of the long thoracic nerve and nerve transfers using the thoracodorsal or medial pectoral nerves have also been reported.
- Nath et al advocate the use of microneurolysis with supraclavicular decompression with patients who have a history pertaining to injury of the long thoracic nerve in the scalene musculature.
- Scapulothoracic fusion has also been used to stabilize the scapula in more extreme cases and if previous surgery has failed.
- Safran reported very good results with outcome measures such as function, pain, and scapular winging for pectoralis major transfer surgery.
- A significant loss of range of elevation is expected with scapulothoracic fusion, and this outcome should be considered for determining if this type of surgery is appropriate.
- Nath et al also reported very good outcomes after microneurolysis with supraclavicular decompression in

patients with a history of long thoracic nerve injury occurring in the scalene musculature.

- Surgery may be indicated if the patient has not responded to conservative management after 1 to 2 years and if no improvement has been seen on EMG testing.

REHABILITATION

- The aim of rehabilitation is to promote healing of the nerve and denervated muscles. This can be achieved by reducing symptoms, encouraging pain-free exercise, and providing task or sports reeducation and interventions leading to reacquisition of function.
- Manual therapy
  - Symptom reduction can be achieved through use of ice, electrotherapeutic modalities, and relative rest (forward elevation of the arm should be avoided). Scapular taping and bracing have been described in the literature to reduce overstretch of the serratus anterior muscle and to add proprioception to the area.
  - Stretching, soft tissue release, and trigger point therapy of the periscapular muscles may also help alleviate the associated hypertonicity and/or pain caused by muscle compensations for the loss of the serratus anterior muscle and help restore muscle balance around the scapula.
  - Joint mobilization to the cervical and thoracic spine, as well as to the ribs, scapula, and acromioclavicular and glenohumeral joints, may also be useful to increase mobility and alleviate pain.
  - Muscle energy techniques may also be necessary to increase mobility and alleviate pain in the upper and middle rib cage (because of serratus anterior muscle attachments).
- Gentle active-assisted shoulder ROM exercises should be started early to prevent joint contracture.
- Scapular position education initially with active-assisted exercise and isometric hold and then the addition of controlled functional movement patterns

- Periscapular muscle strengthening as required may help optimize scapular position and stability, starting in neutral, unloaded positions.
- Neuromuscular electrical stimulation (NMES) can be used if the patient demonstrates some activity in the serratus anterior muscle. It can be used to reduce atrophy by applying the electrodes to motor points and stimulating the muscle at rest or during an active exercise.
- Nerve gliding exercises have been purported to disperse intraneural edema, increase blood flow, optimize axonal transport, and lengthen nerve adhesions. Neural mobilization can be achieved using scapular mobilization both actively and passively into elevation, depression, protraction, and retraction.
- Functional rehabilitation should include the following:
  - Reeducation of movement patterns, particularly proximal control of the trunk and neck, to provide a stable foundation for scapular stability
  - Specific muscle strengthening by gradually increasing intensity to restore full power to the serratus anterior
  - Integration of functional exercise and strength work into sport- or task-specific skills
  - Graduated return to full strength, speed, and power

PROGNOSIS

- Most cases of nontraumatic long thoracic nerve pathology resolve within a year, with improvements seen for up to 2 years. However, as with all peripheral nerve pathologies, the prognosis depends on the extent of damage to the nerve.
- Neurapraxia should resolve rapidly and lead to a complete restoration of function, usually within several months. If the injury is a more severe axonotmesis, the recovery time depends on the distance from the site of injury to the denervated tissue. Peripheral nerves have been reported to recover at an approximate rate of between 1 and 4 mm per day but recovery may not result in a complete restoration of function. The

extensive length of the long thoracic nerve results in a longer reinnervation distance, thus a longer recovery time (up to 2 years).

- If there has been a complete sectioning of the nerve (neurotmesis), then a full recovery will not occur. The results of treating neurotmesis will depend on surgical outcome.

SIGNS AND SYMPTOMS INDICATING REFERRAL TO PHYSICIAN

All patients with suspected long thoracic nerve pathology should be referred to a physician for appropriate investigation.

SUGGESTED READINGS

Cleary CK. Management of radial tunnel syndrome: a therapist's clinical perspective. *J Hand Ther.* 2006;9(2):166-191.

Dumestre G. Long thoracic nerve palsy. *J Man Manipulative Ther.* 1995;3(2):44-49.

Goslin KL, Krivickas LS. Proximal neuropathies of the upper extremity. *Neurol Clin.* 1999;17(3):525-548.

Hermann DN, Logigian EL. Electrodiagnostic approach to the patient with suspected mononeuropathy of the upper extremity. *Neurol Clin.* 2002;20(2):451-478.

Kendall FP, McCreary EK, Provance PG, Rodgers MM, Romani WA. *Muscles Testing and Function with Posture and Pain.* 5th ed. Philadelphia: Lippincott Williams & Wilkins; 2005.

Nath RK, Lyons AB, Bietz G. Microneurolysis and decompression of long thoracic nerve injury are effective in reversing scapular winging: Long term results in 50 cases. *BMC Musculoskelet Disord.* 2007;8:25.

Pecina MM, Krmpotic-Nemanic J, Markiewitz AP. *Tunnel Syndromes: Peripheral Nerve Compression Syndromes.* 3rd ed. CRC Press; 2001.

Safran MR. Nerve injuries about the shoulder in athletes, Part 2: long thoracic nerve, spinal accessory nerve, burners/stingers, thoracic outlet syndrome. *Am J Sports Med.* 2007;32(4).

Seddon HJ. *Surgical Disorders of the Peripheral Nerves.* Edinburgh: Churchill; 1975.

Sunderland S. *Nerve and Nerve Injuries.* 2nd ed. Edinburgh: Churchill Livingstone; 1978.

Sunderland S. *Nerve Injuries and Their Repair: A Critical Appraisal.* Edinburgh: Churchill Livingstone; 1991.

AUTHOR: KATINA DIMOPOULOS

Section III

ORTHOPEDIC PATHOLOGY

BASIC INFORMATION

DEFINITION

The median nerve may be compressed or entrapped at several places in the arm. It can be entrapped proximal (pronator syndrome) or distal (anterior interosseous nerve syndrome, or Kiloh-Nevin syndrome) to the anterior interosseous branch as it passes between the two heads of the pronator teres. It can also be entrapped as it passes under the ligament of Struthers (found in 1% of the population) that runs between an abnormal process on the shaft of the humerus to its medial epicondyle (humerus supracondylar process syndrome). Entrapment can occur as the lacertus fibrosis is tensioned on pronation at the bicipital tuberosity of the radius. The median nerve can also be entrapped at the carpal tunnel between the flexor tendons, the carpal bones, and the transverse carpal ligament (carpal tunnel syndrome).

SYNONYMS

- Anterior interosseous syndrome
- Kiloh-Nevin syndrome
- Pronator teres compression syndrome
- Pronator syndrome
- Humerus supracondylar process syndrome
- Carpal tunnel syndrome

ICD-9CM CODES
955.1 Injury to median nerve
354.0 Carpal tunnel syndrome

OPTIMAL AND MAXIMAL NUMBER OF VISITS

For anterior interosseous syndrome, surgical intervention should be considered after 8 to 12 weeks if response to conservative management is poor. For other pathologies, the number of visits depends on progression. Mild-to-moderate presentations may be successfully treated or managed with conservative intervention. If the underlying cause involves biomechanical issues associated with lifestyle, such interventions may need to continue for protracted time periods. More severe presentations and unrelenting, unresponsive, or worsening symptoms may warrant earlier medical or surgical intervention.

ETIOLOGY

- Insult to the nerve may be mechanical, thermal, chemical or ischemic.
- In entrapment syndromes, compression or direct trauma leads to nerve tissue hypoxia.
- Median nerve entrapment pathology may occur with repetitive or overuse movement patterns involving the elbow, wrist and hand, vibration injuries, trauma, pregnancy, menopause, obesity, underlying disease and medical issues (diabetes mellitus, thyroid myxedema, osteoarthritis, acromegaly, amyloidosis, renal dialysis, or alcoholism), space-occupying entities (neurofibroma, lipoma, aneurysm, hemangioma, ganglion, or xanthoma), presence of anatomical anomalies, and psychological stress. Some authors have also reported possible inherited predisposition. While all of these factors have been linked to median nerve entrapments, many cases are described as idiopathic, and it is likely that most are multifactorial.
- In entrapments, nerve trauma occurs because the size of the neural structure exceeds the anatomical space available for it, resulting in increased pressure, which in turn leads to impaired blood flow and subsequent hypoxia of the tissue and disruption to the axonal transport system.
- Nerve injury is classified according to severity of the injury and potential for reversibility. Original classifications described previously remain in current use, as follows:
  - First-degree neurapraxia involves distortion of myelin around the nodes of Ranvier caused by ischemia, mechanical compression, or electrolyte imbalance, resulting in temporary loss of nerve conduction. Recovery is rapid and complete in most cases.
  - Second-degree axonotmesis involves interruption of the axon with secondary wallerian degeneration, but the supporting tissue around the axon is preserved. Recovery may be complete but takes longer to occur and depends on the distance between the site of injury and the end-structure (denervated muscle).
  - Third-degree neurotmesis involves extensive disruption of the nerve and its supporting structures, but while the endoneurium is disrupted, the perineurium and epineurium remain intact.
  - Fourth-degree neurotmesis involves disruption of all neural components except the epineurium.
  - Fifth-degree neurotmesis involves complete transaction and discontinuity of the nerve with no capacity for regeneration. Neurotmesis rarely occurs from entrapment, but where continuity has been disrupted, complete recovery is not possible, even with surgical techniques, and the eventual outcome depends on individual circumstances. A comprehensive overview of neurobiology, nerve injury, and nerve repair is provided by Dahlin.

- Double-crush syndrome refers to the fairly common phenomenon of nerve entrapment and radiculopathy occurring in combination, although the syndrome is considered controversial. Compression or irritation of the nerve roots at the cervical level is thought to increase sensitivity to compression or movement restrictions more distally in the structure.
- In overuse-type entrapments, it is proposed that repetitive work or static postures produce an inflammatory response. Fibroblasts appear to repair the damage incurred but generate adhesions that limit neural glide and subsequently increase anoxia. Other studies found that cortical dedifferentiation may occur from repetitive motion activities and nerve injuries. This may result in reinforced poor posturing and use of aberrant motor pathways.

EPIDEMIOLOGY AND DEMOGRAPHICS

- Carpal tunnel syndrome is among the most commonly reported nerve entrapments, anterior interosseous syndrome and pronator syndrome occur much less frequently, and humerus supracondylar process syndrome is rare.
- Anterior interosseous syndrome, pronator syndrome, and humerus supracondylar process syndrome tend to be linked to specific activity, trauma, disease, or anatomical makeup rather than associated with a particular age group.
- Carpal tunnel syndrome presentations tend to be more than twice as common in females compared to males, and most commonly occur between 45 and 54 years of age, although the syndrome also occurs quite frequently during pregnancy.
- Median nerve entrapments occur more frequently among office workers, manual workers, and individuals who engage in repetitive movement pattern activities such as musicians, artists, and sports participants.

MECHANISM OF INJURY

- Specific anatomical sites for entrapment in the upper limbs are described by Pratt. Anterior interosseous nerve syndrome may occur when the nerve is compressed at the tendinous origin of the deep head of pronator teres (most common presentation) or as it passes between the two heads of pronator teres, by impingement from a bicipital tendon bursa or radial and ulnar artery abnormalities in the forearm, by fascial bands at the origin of flexor digitorum superficialis, or by anatomical anomalies within the deep palmar compartment involving flexor pollicis longus or palmaris profundus. A review of compression syndromes in the median nerve is given by Koo and Szabo.

- Pronator syndrome refers to median nerve compression between the two pronator teres heads before it branches to form the anterior interosseous nerve.
- Lacertus fibrosis (bicipital aponeurosis) tension may cause median nerve compression as it is pulled across the nerve with pronation as the bicipital tuberosity of radius passes posteriorly or when the forearm is maintained in resisted supination and flexion.
- Humerus supracondylar process syndrome may occur when the median nerve is compressed above the elbow as it passes under the ligament of Struthers in individuals in whom the structure is present.
- Carpal tunnel syndrome refers to compression of the median nerve as it passes, together with the tendons of flexor digitorum profundus, flexor digitorum superficialis, flexor pollicis longus, and flexor carpi radialis, through the enclosure created by trapezoid, capitate, the flexor retinaculum (transverse carpal ligament) and its attachments to the scaphoid tubercle, trapezium, hook of hamate, and pisiform.

COMMON SIGNS AND SYMPTOMS

- Anterior interosseous syndrome commonly presents with weakness and difficulty moving the index and middle fingers (flexor digitorum profundus, combined with weakness in the thumb (flexor pollicis longus), making pinch grip difficult.
- However, variations in innervation for the hand, particularly the Martin Gruber anastomosis (in which the motor nerve crosses over from the median nerve to the ulnar nerve, present in 10% to 15% of the population), mean that the presentation for entrapment may vary significantly and could involve flexor pollicis brevis, adductor pollicis, abductor pollicis brevis, lumbrical, and abductor digiti minimi muscles, or even the entire hand.
- Pronator syndrome commonly manifests with pain in the forearm and wrist, combined with weakness and atrophy of the thenar muscles. Flexor carpi radialis, palmaris longus, and flexor digitorum muscles are affected, with or without the addition of those muscles usually supplied by the anterior interosseous nerve—flexor pollicis longus, flexor digitorum profundus, and pronator quadratus muscles. However, the tendency for variation in muscle innervation patterns in the hand should be remembered.
- Paraesthesia in median nerve distribution may occur with repetitive pronation

and supination, and individuals may experience early fatigue in muscles of the forearm, particularly with excessive pronation.

- Lacertus fibrosis tension produces pain radiating from the elbow to the forearm with pronation or resisted supination with the forearm in flexion, combined with localized symptoms around the fibrous arcade at the origin of flexor digitorum superficialis with resisted middle-finger flexion.
- Humerus supracondylar process syndrome may manifest with pain and paraesthesia in median nerve distribution, combined with weakness in the muscles as described for pronator syndrome but with the addition of pronator teres. Individuals may report weak grip and pronation and may exhibit forearm atrophy.
- Carpal tunnel syndrome commonly manifests with progressively worsening pain (classically described as aching and burning in nature) and paraesthesia in the thumb, forefinger, middle finger, hand, and wrist, which may extend to the forearm, elbow, shoulder, and neck. Symptoms are often worse nocturnally. Individuals may complain of problems with grip and weakness in the wrist and hand.
- Anterior interosseous syndrome produces weakness in the thumb, forefinger, and middle finger, although other regions of the hand may be affected. Pronator syndrome produces pain in the forearm and wrist, combined with paraesthesia and weakness in the thumb, fingers, and wrist. Lacertus fibrosis tension produces pain radiating from the elbow to the forearm. Humerus supracondylar process syndrome produces pain, paraesthesia, and weakness in the elbow, wrist, and hand. Carpal tunnel syndrome produces pain and significant paraesthesia in the hand and wrist, which may extend to the forearm, elbow, shoulder, and neck.

AGGRAVATING ACTIVITIES

- Repetitive movement patterns at the elbow, wrist, and hand, particularly repetitive pronation and supination, tend to exacerbate the symptoms.
- The pathology may be worsened with sustained postures, especially those involving the wrist, head, and neck and activities that increase the volume of structures, which may be implicated in entrapment such as those that may lead to pronator hypertrophy.

EASING ACTIVITIES

- Relative or absolute rest may assist in alleviating symptoms in cases where the pathology has been caused by overuse or repetitive movement patterns.

- Adapting movement strategies and altering or correcting posture may reduce loading on irritated structures where absolute rest is not possible.
- Use of splints to maintain more neutral positions and thus reduce neural tension, either during activity or overnight, may also be helpful.

24-HOUR SYMPTOM PATTERN

- Symptoms are worsened with aggravating activities but also tend to increase nocturnally, particularly paraesthesia and numbness.
- In females, symptoms may show hormonal variation; in individuals in whom the presentation is related to another medical condition, symptoms may vary according to physiological balance associated with the underlying condition.

PAST HISTORY FOR THE REGION

- Median nerve entrapment can occur from a broad spectrum of associated causative factors; consequently, past history for the pathology may vary widely between individuals.
- Anatomical anomalies involving bony structures (supracondylar process on humerus and the presence of the ligament of Struthers and form and alignment of carpal bones), vascular structures (radial, ulnar, and median arteries), and connective tissue (fascia) may predispose individuals to the pathology, together with the presence of underlying disease and medical issues (diabetes mellitus, thyroid myxedema, osteoarthritis, obesity, pregnancy, menopause, space-occupying entities such as neurofibroma or lipoma, aneurysm, hemangioma, ganglion, xanthoma, acromegaly, amyloidosis, renal dialysis, or alcoholism).
- Trauma history may include work or leisure activities involving repetitive movement patterns or vibration exposure (all median nerve entrapment pathologies), partial rupture at the musculotendinous junction of biceps brachii (lacertus fibrosis tension), fractures of the upper limb, particularly Colles' fracture, or fracture or subluxation and dislocation injuries, particularly those involving the carpal bones (carpal tunnel syndrome).

PHYSICAL EXAMINATION

- Anterior interosseous syndrome commonly presents with weakness and difficulty moving the index and middle fingers (flexor digitorum profundus), combined with weakness in the thumb (flexor pollicis longus), making pinch grip difficult from loss of flexion in the fingers and thumb as the distal phalanges remain extended or hyperextended.
- Variations in innervation for the hand mean that the presentation for

entrapment may vary significantly and could involve the flexor pollicis brevis, adductor pollicis, abductor pollicis brevis, lumbrical, and abductor digiti minimi muscles or even the entire hand.

- Individuals with pronator syndrome may exhibit weakness and atrophy of the thenar muscles. Flexor carpi radialis, palmaris longus, and flexor digitorum muscles are affected with or without the addition of the muscles usually supplied by the anterior interosseous nerve—flexor pollicis longus, flexor digitorum profundus, and pronator quadratus.
- Paraesthesia in median nerve distribution may occur with repetitive pronation and supination, and individuals may experience early fatigue in muscles of the forearm, particularly with excessive pronation. Tinel's sign may be positive in the mid to proximal forearm rather than at the wrist.
- Lacertus fibrosis tension produces pain radiating from the elbow to the forearm with pronation or resisted supination with the forearm in flexion, combined with localized symptoms around the fibrous arcade at the origin of flexor digitorum superficialis with resisted middle-finger flexion. Past trauma history may also indicate this syndrome.
- Individuals with humerus supracondylar process syndrome may report pain and paraesthesia in median nerve distribution. In addition to the weakness and atrophy patterns observed in the hand with more distal compression, there may also be evidence of forearm atrophy with weakness noted in both grip and pronation.
- Individuals with carpal tunnel syndrome present with significant paraesthesia and numbness in the hand and wrist. Additionally, atrophy of abductor pollicis brevis may be noted and Tinel's sign (at the wrist), Phalen's test, and wrist flexion provocation tests may be positive.

IMPORTANT OBJECTIVE TESTS

- Diagnostic accuracy of neurological upper limb examination employing a battery of standard test procedures has been found to be reproducible and reliable.
- Neurophysiology and EMGs may produce positive findings, particularly for carpal tunnel syndrome. Results are often inconclusive for anterior interosseous syndrome because of the deep location of the structures. If pronator syndrome is suspected, an initial negative test accompanied by a strong suggestive history should be repeated after approximately 6 weeks. Radiographic, ultrasound, and MRI may identify anatomical anomalies, and vascular tests may be helpful in differential diagnosis.

- Pinch test (precision grip): Individuals with anterior interosseous syndrome are unable to flex the distal phalanges of the thumb, forefinger, and middle finger so that contact can only be made through the pads rather than the tips of the digits.
- Tinel's sign: Tapping over the median nerve distribution reproduces sensory symptoms distal to the test site. This test is positive at the proximal to mid-forearm rather than at the wrist in pronator syndrome and positive at the wrist over the carpal tunnel in carpal tunnel syndrome.
- Phalen's test: Maximal wrist flexion either with gravity or pressure applied by the examiner reproduces sensory symptoms in the thumb, forefinger, and middle finger. (Normal subjects may experience similar symptoms after 1 minute.) A variation of this is the reverse Phalen's test where the subject grips the examiner's hand as the wrist is extended and direct pressure is applied over the carpal tunnel for 1 minute. A positive test reproduces the same symptoms.
- Wrist flexion provocative test: Constant digital pressure over the median nerve at the carpal tunnel with elbow extended and forearm supinated reproduces paraesthesia and numbness within 30 seconds for a positive test.
- Durkan compression test (carpal compression test): With the wrist in neutral and forearm supinated, carpal compression is applied either manually or with a pressure-sensitive instrument. A positive test is recorded if sensory symptoms occur within 30 seconds.
- Sensory discrimination tests may also be helpful in defining the affected area.

DIFFERENTIAL DIAGNOSIS

Dx

- Anterior interosseous syndrome: Cervical radiculopathy (C8), pronator syndrome, carpal tunnel syndrome, lacertus fibrosis tension, humerus supracondylar process syndrome, lateral cord lesion, ulnar neuropathy, flexor digitorum profundus tendon rupture or avulsion, or flexor pollicis longus rupture
- Pronator syndrome: Cervical radiculopathy (C6 to C7), lacertus fibrosis tension, flexor superficialis syndrome, humerus supracondylar process syndrome, anterior interosseous syndrome, carpal tunnel syndrome, soft tissue overuse syndromes, vascular pathologies, or cardiac pathologies
- Lacertus fibrosis tension: Cervical radiculopathy (C6 to C7), pronator syndrome,

humerus supracondylar process syndrome, anterior interosseous syndrome, carpal tunnel syndrome, soft tissue overuse pathologies, or cardiac pathologies
- Humerus supracondylar process syndrome: Cervical radiculopathy (C6/C7), anterior interosseous syndrome, pronator syndrome, lacertus fibrosis tension, carpal tunnel syndrome, soft tissue overuse syndromes, or vascular pathologies
- Carpal tunnel syndrome: Cervical radiculopathy (C6/C7, T1), thoracic outlet syndrome, anterior interosseous syndrome, pronator syndrome, lacertus fibrosis tension, humerus supracondylar process syndrome, ulnar neuropathy, vascular pathologies, soft tissue overuse syndromes, carpometacarpal arthritis, shoulder bursitis, transient ischemic attack, or myocardial ischemia

CONTRIBUTING FACTORS

- Presence of anatomical anomalies
- Underlying disease or medical condition
- Repetitive work or leisure activities
- Past trauma history
- Psychological stress
- Genetic predisposition

TREATMENT

SURGICAL OPTIONS

- An overview of basic neurosurgical techniques is provided by Dahlin.
  - Anterior interosseous syndrome: Decompression at pronator heads, fascial release at flexor digitorum superficialis or the deep palmar compartment, exploration techniques to release pressure generated by bursa or vascular abnormalities
  - Pronator syndrome: Release of the humeral head of pronator teres combined with fascial release at flexor digitorum superficialis
  - Lacertus fibrosis tension: Release of lacertus fibrosis, possibly with associated repair for biceps brachii
  - Humerus supracondylar process syndrome: Release at the bony process and ligament of Struthers
  - Carpal tunnel syndrome: Open or endoscopic release techniques to divide the transverse carpal ligament, restore neural glide, relieve adhesions, and where the condition results from compression caused by some form of space-occupying lesion, appropriate techniques to address the specific lesion.
- When accurate diagnosis has been made, surgical intervention produces good results for all the pathologies described, with success rates around 90% and low recurrence rate. Recovery depends on

level of nerve injury, with neurapraxias showing the fastest and most complete return to function.

- Surgery may be indicated for individuals with severe, worsening, or unrelenting symptoms that are nonresponsive to conservative management involving antiinflammatory medication, splinting, and manual and electrotherapy physiotherapy modalities and addressing of ergonomic issues. Early surgical intervention (within 8 to 12 weeks) is generally recommended for anterior interosseous syndrome to achieve the best outcome.

REHABILITATION

- Rehabilitation may focus on two goals: Addressing the underlying causative factors and reducing the symptoms. In cases where repetitive movement patterns or exposure to vibration trauma feature in the development of the pathology, a detailed ergonomic assessment may be helpful in identifying areas in which loading stress may be reduced by changes in behavior, activity, or posture or through use of appropriate braces.
- Therapeutic techniques to alleviate symptoms may include soft tissue manual techniques, neural mobilizing techniques, massage, acupuncture, and electrotherapy techniques to address pain, inflammation, and loss of movement and function. When psychological stress is considered a significant factor, individuals may benefit from more general therapeutic exercise programs.

PROGNOSIS

- Factors that contribute to median nerve entrapment pathology include the presence of anatomical anomalies, an underlying disease or medical condition, repetitive work or leisure activities, past trauma history, psychological stress, and genetic predisposition.
- Systematic review found inconclusive evidence for conservative management of carpal tunnel syndrome, but as noted

by other researchers, definitive statements regarding prognosis are difficult because differential diagnosis is not always achieved. Mild-to-moderate presentations of median nerve entrapments may be effectively treated or well-controlled with conservative intervention. In individuals with more severe presentations or who have failed to respond to conservative measures, surgical procedures generally have a good outcome in terms of symptom relief and functional outcome.

SIGNS AND SYMPTOMS INDICATING REFERRAL TO PHYSICIAN

- Severe or worsening neurological function or symptoms
- Failure to respond to conservative management
- Suspicion or presence of underlying disease
- Unexplained symptoms inconsistent with the pathology

SUGGESTED READINGS

Akalin E, El O, Peker O, et al. Treatment of carpal tunnel syndrome with nerve and tendon gliding exercises. *Am J Phys Med Rehabil.* 2002;81(2):108-113.

Chin DHCL, Meals R. Anterior interosseous nerve syndrome. *J Am Soc Surg Hand.* 2001;1(4):249-257.

Cleary CK. Management of radial tunnel syndrome: a therapist's clinical perspective. *J Hand Therapy.* 2006;9(2):166-191.

Dahlin LB. Mini-symposium: hand trauma (ii) nerve injuries. *Curr Orthop.* 2008;22(1):9-16.

Freedman J. Acupuncture for carpal tunnel syndrome. *Acupunct Med.* 2002;20(1):39-40.

Gomes I, Becker J, Ehlers JA, Nora DB. Prediction of the neurophysiological diagnosis of carpal tunnel syndrome from the demographic and clinical data. *Clin Neurophysiol.* 2006;117(5):964-971.

Hall TM, Elvey RL. Nerve trunk pain: physical diagnosis and treatment. *Man Ther.* 1999;4(2):63-73.

Jepsen JR, Laursen LH, Hagert C-G, Kreiner S, Larsen AI. Diagnostic accuracy of the neurological upper limb examination I: inter-relater reproducibility of selected findings and patterns. *BMC Neurol.* 2006;6(8).

Jepsen JR, Laursen LH, Hagert C-G, Kreiner S, Larsen AI. Diagnostic accuracy of the neurological upper limb examination II: relations to symptoms of patterns of findings. *BMC Neurol.* 2006;6(10).

Koo JT, Szabo RM. Compression neuropathies of the median nerve. *J Am Soc Surg Hand.* 2004;4(3):156-175.

Latinovic R, Gulliford MC, Hughes RA. Incidence of common compressive neuropathies in primary care. *J Neurol Neurosurg Psychiatry.* 2006;77(2):263-265.

Magee DJ. *Orthopaedic Physical Assessment.* 5th ed. Philadelphia: Saunders; 2008.

Naeser MA, Hahn KA, Lieberman BE, Branco KF. Carpal tunnel syndrome treated with low level laser and microamperes transcutaneous electric nerve stimulation: a controlled study. *Arch Phys Med Rehabil.* 2002;83(7):978-988.

Nithi K. Physiology of the peripheral nervous system. *Surgery.* 2003;21(10):264a-264e.

Piazzini DB, Aprile I, Ferrara PE, et al. A systematic review of conservative treatment of carpal tunnel syndrome. *Clin Rehabil.* 2007;21(4):299-314.

Pratt N. Anatomy of nerve entrapment sites in the upper quarter. *J Hand Ther.* 2005;18(2):216-219.

Premoselli S, Sioli P, Grossi A, Cerri C. Neutral wrist splinting in carpal tunnel syndrome: a 3 and 6 months clinical and neurophysiologic follow up evaluation of night-only splinting therapy. *Eura Medicophys.* 2006;42(2):121-126.

Seddon HJ. *Surgical Disorders of the Peripheral Nerves.* Edinburgh: Churchill Livingstone; 1975.

Seitz WH, Matsuoka H, McAdoo J, Sherman G, Stickney DP. Acute compression of the median nerve at the elbow by the lacertus fibrosis. *J Shoulder Elbow Surg.* 2007;16(1):91-94.

Sunderland S. *Nerve and Nerve Injuries.* 2nd ed. Edinburgh: Churchill Livingstone; 1978.

Tetro AM, Bradley EA, Hollstien SB, Gelberman RH. A new provocative test for carpal tunnel syndrome. Assessment of the wrist and nerve compression. *J Bone Joint Surg.* 1998;80(3):493-498.

Wilbourn AJ, Gilliat RW. Double crush syndrome: a critical analysis. *Neurology.* 1997;49:21-29.

AUTHOR: SARAH GRAHAM

Section III

ORTHOPEDIC PATHOLOGY

BASIC INFORMATION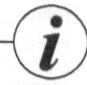

DEFINITION

- Thoracic outlet syndrome (TOS) encompasses numerous scenarios of compression (neurological and vascular) in the thoracic outlet region of the shoulder girdle. Although vascular and neurological classifications exist, it must be noted that these conditions can also be observed together.
- Neurogenic TOS involves compression of various portions of the brachial plexus and is the most common form of TOS (over 90% of cases). The brachial plexus is formed by the C5 to T1 nerve roots, although the most caudal root or "lower plexus" (C8 and T1) is most commonly affected. The "upper plexus" may also be involved, and this affects the C5, C6, or C7 nerves, or in rare cases may be involved in combination with the lower plexus.
- Defining the syndrome has been fraught with difficulty in the literature because of its variable etiology and presentation and often minimal clinical findings.
- Two main neurogenic TOS classifications exist as a result of the following variable clinical presentations:
  - True neurogenic TOS, where patients present with a typical clinical presentation with positive neurological findings on examination
  - Nonspecific neurogenic or "classic" TOS, in which pain is a predominant feature with minimal neurological findings on examination. This subcategory comprises most TOS presentations.

SYNONYMS

- Cervical rib syndrome
- First rib syndrome
- Scalenus anticus syndrome
- Costoclavicular syndrome
- First thoracic rib syndrome
- Hyperabduction syndrome
- Scalenus medius syndrome
- Pectoralis minor syndrome
- Subcoracoid-pectoralis minor syndrome
- Brachiocephalic syndrome
- Nocturnal paresthetic brachialgia
- Rucksack palsy
- Droopy shoulder syndrome
- Fractured clavicle-rib syndrome
- Motor type neurogenic TOS

ICD-9CM CODES

353 Nerve root and plexus disorders
354 Mononeuritis of upper limb and mononeuritis complex
354.8 Other mononeuritis of upper limb
354.9 Mononeuritis of upper limb unspecified

OPTIMAL NUMBER OF VISITS

10

MAXIMAL NUMBER OF VISITS

30

ETIOLOGY

- The current belief of the cause of TOS is the underlying existence of bony or fibromuscular anomalies with overlying injury and/or spasm in the thoracic outlet region causing compromise. The anatomical anomalies are generally seen as predisposing factors.
- The pathology involves compression of portions of the brachial plexus in the thoracic outlet region as a result of underlying bony or fibromuscular anomalies with overlying muscle injury and/or spasm.
- Local spasm in the thoracic outlet region can result in muscle swelling and place the local neural structures under strain or traction, resulting in nerve edema. As the condition becomes more chronic, scarring and fibrosis of the nerve can take place.
- Bony anomalies can be congenital, traumatic, or posttraumatic and include the presence of a cervical rib, elongated C7 transverse process, first rib deformity, displaced first rib fracture, excessive callus formation after first rib fracture, rib hemangioma, fractured or subluxed clavicle, and pseudarthroses. Cervical ribs are known to exist in approximately 0.5% of the population, with 10% to 20% resulting in symptoms, although this depends on their size.
- Soft tissue anomalies can also be congenital, traumatic, or posttraumatic and include altered scalene muscle insertions and origins, presence of scalenus minimus or scalenus pleuralis muscle, hypertrophy or injury of scalene muscles, presence of congenital fibromuscular bands (classified into types 1 to 10) or dense fibrous sheaths, cervical ligaments and bands, and pectoralis minor shortening.
- Anatomical variations of the passage of the brachial plexus through the thoracic outlet, the adherence of the nerves to the scalene muscles, can also predispose to TOS.
- The superimposed injury involved in causing TOS symptoms may include whiplash, direct or indirect blow to the shoulder, repetitive strain through prolonged upper limb activity, accessory breathing, and/or poor posture.
- The following three spaces in the thoracic outlet region have been identified as potential areas of brachial plexus compression (Atasoy):
  - Interscalene space or triangle is bordered anteriorly by the anterior scalene muscle, posteriorly by the middle scalene muscle, and inferiorly by the first rib. The brachial plexus passes posteriorly to the anterior scalene muscle here, in close relation and directly superior to the subclavian artery.
  - Costoclavicular space is bordered anteriorly by the medial aspect of the clavicle, subclavian muscle and tendon, and costocoracoid ligament. The posterolateral border is formed by the upper border of the scapula and the posteromedial border by the first rib anterior and middle scalene muscle insertions. Here, the brachial plexus travels with the subclavian vein and artery under the clavicle and subclavius muscle toward the subpectoralis minor space.
  - Subpectoralis minor space is located inferior to the coracoid process and posterior to the pectoralis minor muscle insertion. Here, the brachial plexus continues to travel with the subclavian vein and artery beneath the pectoralis muscle toward the axilla.
  - The interscalene and costoclavicular spaces are equally common sites of compression in neurogenic TOS, while compression in the subpectoralis minor space is much less common.
- Hypertrophy, degeneration, and fibrosis of the anterior scalene muscle caused from a previous single traumatic incident or repeated trauma is believed to be the current overlying cause of compressive symptoms. Various studies have demonstrated histological abnormalities in the anterior scalene muscles, including type 1 muscle fiber proliferation, reduction of type 2 muscle fibers, and increased connective tissue content and muscle scarring.
- Physiologically, there is disruption to the underlying nerve of the brachial plexus, which is responsible for conduction.
- Neurogenic TOS involves a continuum of damage from periodic nerve ischemia to chronic ischemia resulting in segmental demyelination (neurapraxic injury). This may progress to axonotmesis injury (in more severe cases of continued nerve compression) in which interruption of the axon with secondary wallerian degeneration will occur.

EPIDEMIOLOGY AND DEMOGRAPHICS

- Nonspecific neurogenic TOS is fairly common, although its prevalence is difficult to estimate because diagnosis is difficult. It can be missed or overdiagnosed.
- True neurogenic TOS is uncommon.
- Young and middle-aged adults are the most susceptible to nonspecific neurogenic TOS.

- True neurogenic TOS symptom onset is most common in teenagers and young adults.
- Females are at least three times as likely to develop nonspecific neurogenic TOS as males.
- True neurogenic TOS mainly affects females.

MECHANISM OF INJURY

- The superimposed injury involved in causing TOS symptoms may include whiplash, direct or indirect blow to the shoulder, repetitive strain through prolonged upper limb activity, and/or poor posture.
- Positions and postures that place increased strain on the thoracic outlet include the following:
  - Prolonged writing or use of keyboard or telephone
  - Assembly line works
  - Poor posture (i.e., droopy shoulders)
  - Prolonged overhead or reaching activity such as styling hair, painting, playing musical instruments (e.g., violin or flute), and swimming
  - Excessive carrying of heavy objects such as suitcases and shopping bags
  - Prolonged carrying of a heavy backpack

COMMON SIGNS AND SYMPTOMS

- Nonspecific neurogenic TOS.
- Pain generally involves the neck, head, chest, scapula, shoulder, arm, and hand (area of pain depends on which part of the brachial plexus is involved).
- Numbness or paresthesias of the arm and hand (area depends on which part of the brachial plexus is involved).
- Coldness of the hand and increased sensitivity to cold exposure
- Whole arm numbness and heaviness with arm elevation
- Clumsiness with fine hand activities and weakness on gripping
- True neurogenic TOS
  - Pain absent
  - Clumsiness with fine hand activities and weakness on gripping
  - If the lower plexus (C8 or T1 nerves) is involved, the patient may present with the following:
  - Ipsilateral anterior or posterior shoulder pain extending to the medial arm, forearm, and hand
  - Ipsilateral paresthesias into the ring and small fingers (in the sensory distribution of the ulnar nerve)
  - Ipsilateral pain in the clavicular region extending to the occipital region and mastoid (headaches can be quite severe)
  - Ipsilateral anterior chest pain
- If the upper plexus (C5, C6, or C7 nerves) is involved, the patient may present with the following:

  - Ipsilateral cervical pain with radiation to the ear, face, and head (mandibular, temporal, and occipital regions)
  - Ipsilateral "stuffy" ear
  - Ipsilateral pain in the medial scapular, anterior clavicular, upper chest, and lateral shoulder and arm pain (in the sensory distribution of C5 or C6 nerve roots)
  - Ipsilateral sympathetic-mediated swelling of the face, night vision difficulties, and rarely, an eyelid droop
  - Dizziness, vertigo, blurred vision

AGGRAVATING ACTIVITIES

- Overhead arm or hand positions or arm elevated repetitive activities. These commonly include styling hair, painting, working overhead, playing musical instruments (e.g., violin or flute), and swimming.
- Carrying heavy objects such as suitcases and shopping bags
- Prolonged use of arm as in writing and typing
- Cervical contralateral rotation and/or lateral flexion can often aggravate symptoms resulting from upper plexus involvement.
- Symptoms may be delayed until after arm activity in some cases.

EASING ACTIVITIES

- Rest from aggravating activities
- Arm adduction and flexion across body
- Shoulder girdle support by using an arm rest, placing hand in pocket, or using a sling

24-HOUR SYMPTOM PATTERN

- Morning
  - Stiffness and ache depends on inflammatory component
- Daytime
  - Depends on arm activity
- Nighttime
  - Entire arm may feel numb or weak during the night, especially if patient sleeps on the ipsilateral side with the arm overhead and elbow flexed
  - May often wake from pain, especially if patient has engaged in repetitive arm activity during the day.

PAST HISTORY FOR THE REGION

- The patient may report a previous history of whiplash injury or a direct or indirect blow to the shoulder resulting in first rib, muscular, or clavicular trauma. Symptoms generally develop from 1 month up to several months after whiplash injury.

- The onset of symptoms may also be insidious but may reveal increased or unaccustomed prolonged or repetitive upper limb activity.

PHYSICAL EXAMINATION

- Nonspecific neurogenic TOS
  - Poor posture (including downwardly rotated and protracted scapula, large breasts and/or obesity, forward head posture)
  - Exaggerated upper chest or accessory breathing
  - Neurological tests negative
  - Altered neurodynamics on upper limb neurodynamic tests and/or brachial plexus tension tests
  - Reproduction of arm symptoms and/or local discomfort on palpation over the brachial plexus (also known as pressure provocation test or Spurling maneuver)
  - Positive Tinel's sign for reproduction of arm pain and/or paraesthesias or symptoms over brachial plexus
  - Muscle spasm, tenderness, and/or shortening of anterior scalene muscle on palpation and length testing
  - Muscle spasm, tenderness, and/or shortening of pectoralis minor muscle on palpation and length testing
  - Ipsilateral elevated first rib
  - Positive Roos, Adson's, Halsted's, and Wright's hyperabduction tests: Increased arm pain and paraesthesias
  - Hypomobility of the lower cervical and upper thoracic spinal levels
- Lower and upper plexus involvement: The following objective findings are more specific to which part of the plexus is involved. Although rare, mixed plexus TOS also exists. As implied, it manifests with a combination of upper and lower plexus TOS symptoms.
  - Lower plexus involvement (most common)
  - Weakened interossei, flexor carpi ulnaris, thenar, and hypothenar muscles (patients may present with weakness of various C8/T1 innervated muscles).
  - Slightly reduced triceps muscle strength (triceps partially supplied by C8)
  - Reduced sensation on light touch and pinprick testing in the medial arm and medial one-and-a-half fingers (ulnar nerve distribution).
  - Tinel's test performed over the lower brachial plexus is positive for local discomfort and reproduction of referred pain.
  - Pressure provocation test positive over the lower brachial plexus
  - Lower brachial plexus tension test is positive for reproduction of medial arm symptoms, with the arm at 90 degrees, and the elbow and wrist extended and supinated.

- Upper plexus involvement
  - Weakness of the deltoid, biceps, and triceps (C5-C7)
  - Reduced sensation on light touch and pinprick testing in the lateral shoulder and arm extending to the thumb, index, and middle finger
  - Tinel's test performed over the upper brachial plexus is positive for local discomfort and reproduction of referred pain.
  - Pressure provocation test positive over the upper brachial plexus
  - Upper brachial plexus tension test positive for reproduction of lateral arm symptoms with arm in exaggerated waiter's tip posture.
- True neurogenic TOS
  - The distinguishing feature of this TOS category is that neurological tests are always positive (reduced strength and sensation: The muscles and areas of skin affected depend on which part of the brachial plexus is involved). In more severe cases, atrophy of the hand is evident. Reflexes, however, are normal.

IMPORTANT OBJECTIVE TESTS

- Four tests (Adson's, Halsted's, Wright's hyperabduction, and Roos) have traditionally been used to diagnose TOS. These tests have been extensively discussed, criticized, and "modified" in the literature as a result of poor sensitivity and specificity.
- First, since the Adson's, Halsted's, and Wright's tests monitor the radial pulse, they should be considered tests for arterial TOS rather than neurogenic TOS. More recently, these tests are generally considered provocative tests for pain or paraesthesias in neurogenic TOS, although they remain invalidated.
- Furthermore, if these tests are used to provoke pain from brachial plexus compression, then only one site of nerve compression should be provoked. None of these tests is specific enough to exclude other pathology. Thus various authors have postulated new or modified tests to diagnose neurogenic TOS.
- The Roos test (or elevated arm stress test) is generally described as the most reliable test for all types of TOS. As described, the reproduction of cervical, shoulder, and arm pain and paresthesias is seen as a positive test. If a patient is unable to complete the test because of symptoms, it can also reflect the severity of their condition. Because of its lack of specificity, Novak et al, as cited by Mackinnon and Novak, have suggested the use of a modified test, which was shown to be positive in 95% of a patient group with TOS in their study.

The patient places both arms into elevation with elbows extended and forearms in neutral (pronation/supination). With the wrists in neutral, they maintain this position for 1 minute. The test is positive for neurogenic TOS if there is a reproduction of cervical, shoulder, and arm pain and paresthesias. Furthermore, when using this modified Roos test, the authors found that when they applied sustained direct pressure over the brachial plexus, they reproduced symptoms in their TOS patients. Thus a combination of a provocative test with compression of the entrapment site may also be used to help diagnose TOS and other nerve entrapment neuropathies.

- Vibration or pressure threshold testing was also shown to be abnormal in a study of patients with neurogenic TOS, with arm elevation and sustained pressure over the brachial plexus. Two-point discrimination was found to be normal, however, except in cases of coexisting carpal and cubital tunnel syndrome.
- Tinel's sign has more recently been found to be quite useful in assessing nerves that are subject to irritation rather than just assessing for nerve regeneration. The median, ulnar, and radial nerves should be tested because double-crush syndromes exist in up to 50% of cases.
- An extensive neurological examination should also be performed to differentiate true and nonspecific neurogenic TOS and to rule out a cervical nerve root disorder.
- Cervical spine, shoulder, and chest x-rays are necessary to identify bony abnormalities and/or degenerative changes in the thoracic outlet region.
- MRI and/or MRI neurograms may also be necessary to identify soft tissue abnormalities in the thoracic outlet region. It is, however, more useful in excluding the presence of cervical nerve root or thoracic pathology.
- Computed tomography (CT) is indicated for suspected bony abnormalities (rib or pulmonary) especially in true neurogenic TOS.
- Nerve conduction studies (motor and sensory) and EMG tests may be useful to diagnose true neurogenic TOS (may find evidence of demyelination and axonal loss) but have difficulties in application and interpretation. These tests, however, are very useful to rule out other nerve pathologies (such as the median and ulnar nerve) that commonly coexist with this condition. They are of little use for the diagnosis of nonspecific neurogenic TOS (low specificity and sensitivity) because a negative result does not exclude the possibility of the presence of this condition.

- Anterior scalene blocks can be used to test if symptoms are being caused by scalene spasm but do not provide information about other underlying anatomical causes.

DIFFERENTIAL DIAGNOSIS

- Shoulder pathologies
  - Glenohumeral instabilities
  - Subacromial or subcoracoid impingement
  - Subacromial bursitis
  - Glenohumeral labral tears
  - Rotator cuff tendinopathies
  - Biceps tendinopathy
  - Adhesive capsulitis
  - Degenerative arthritis of the glenohumeral or AC joints
  - Myofascial pain from scapulohumeral musculature
- Cervical or thoracic pathologies
  - Cervical spondylosis
  - Cervical degenerative disc disease
  - Cervical nerve root syndrome
  - Cervical spine stenosis
  - Thoracic facet syndrome
  - T4 syndrome
  - Rib dysfunction
- Peripheral nerve entrapments
  - Ulnar nerve entrapment (cubital tunnel/Guyon's canal)
  - Median nerve entrapment (carpal tunnel/pronator teres)
  - Radial nerve entrapment (forearm)
  - Multiple crush syndrome
- Other
  - Muscular dystrophy
  - Polymyositis
  - Complex regional pain syndrome (CRPS)
  - Diffuse peripheral neuropathy
  - Angina and other cardiac conditions
  - Rheumatoid arthritis (RA)
  - Lupus
  - Pancoast's tumor
  - Multiple sclerosis
  - Spinal cord lesion
  - Hypothyroidism
  - Pleuritis and other pulmonary conditions
  - Raynaud's phenomenon
  - Head, neck, or upper quadrant tumors
  - Lymphedema

CONTRIBUTING FACTORS

- Underlying existence of bony or fibromuscular anomalies in the thoracic outlet region (always found in true neurogenic TOS)
- Previous history of whiplash injury or a direct or indirect blow to the shoulder resulting in first rib, muscular, or clavicular trauma.
- Exposure to increased or unaccustomed prolonged or repetitive upper limb

activity (e.g., overhead sport, occupation, or playing a musical instrument)
- Large breasts, breast implants, radical mastectomy surgery, pregnancy, and/or obesity
- Poor posture (e.g., downwardly rotated scapula, forward head posture)
- Accessory or upper chest breathing patterns
- Generalized low muscle tone
- Anterior shoulder instabilities
- Overdeveloped neck, trapezius, or pectoralis musculature as seen in weight lifters, swimmers, tennis players, and baseball pitchers.

TREATMENT

SURGICAL OPTIONS

- The following is a simplified summary of current surgical approaches for neurogenic TOS:
  - Transaxillary first rib resection (approach used for lower plexus neurogenic TOS)
  - Supraclavicular first rib resection (approach used for upper or lower plexus neurogenic TOS)
  - Anterior and middle scalenectomy (used for obese patients in whom rib resection is difficult and for upper plexus neurogenic TOS)
  - Combined rib resection and scalenectomy (combined approach most commonly used now, especially because of the lower rate of success of a secondary operation)
  - Comprehensive supraclavicular decompression with scalenectomy
  - Epineurectomy with anterior scalenectomy
- Success rates for most of the current surgical techniques range from 70% to over 90%. Poor outcomes, however, are seen on reoperation (15% rate of success). Failure is often attributed to poor patient compliance to postoperative therapy or recurrent injury. Transaxillary first rib resection surgery has been found to have lower success rates for upper plexus neurogenic TOS. Lower rates of success with surgery have also been seen with patients who suffer from work-related TOS than from MVAs.
- Surgical indicators include the following:
  - Failure of conservative treatment after 3 to 6 months (ongoing pain and dysfunction)
  - Worsening neurological status
  - Presence of significant muscle atrophy with cervical rib (true neurogenic TOS)
  - All differential diagnoses have been treated or excluded. Since TOS patients often suffer from coexisting nerve entrapments (especially at the carpal tunnel and cubital tunnel), it is important to consider surgery on these areas, possibly before consideration of TOS surgery because alleviation of pressure distally can affect and relieve TOS symptoms.

REHABILITATION

- The main goal of treatment is to reduce the compression on the brachial plexus to alleviate symptoms. Additionally, restoration of ideal neurodynamics, posture, breathing, and movement patterns is necessary for successful rehabilitation.
- Initially, pain and symptom relief is paramount. In latter stages, improving functional stability and preventing recurrence becomes the priority.
- Pain therapy or behavior modification
  - Pain medication, including NSAIDs and muscle relaxants
  - Electrotherapeutic modalities, including TENS, interferential current therapy, or ultrasound
  - Ice or heat packs
- Education
  - Rest from aggravating activities, including heavy lifting
  - Postural or ergonomic advice: Arms should remain supported in sustained activities, and correct lumbopelvic posture allows and assists maintenance of cervicoscapular neutral positioning.
  - Standing: Hands may be placed in pockets initially to reduce the drag on shoulders.
  - Sleeping position: Patient should lie supine or on the unaffected side with an extra pillow to support the affected arm in front of the body. Patients who sleep in a supine position may need to place a wedge under the shoulder and flex the elbow to unload neural structures.
- Manual or soft tissue therapy
  - Mobilization of the cervical and thoracic spine (including ribs); sternoclavicular, AC, and glenohumeral joints; and scapula may help unload the region. Cervical traction may also help reduce symptoms.
  - Anterior accessory mobilizations of the lower cervical spine and first and second ribs are also very useful techniques, although low grades should initially be employed.
  - Caudal mobilizations and muscle energy techniques (MET) for the first rib may also be effective, especially if the patient presents with an elevated first rib.
  - Soft tissue therapy may include a combination of trigger point therapy, soft tissue release, or myofascial or positional release techniques to reduce tension associated with the production of symptoms and poor posture. The main muscles requiring treatment include the scalenes, levator scapulae, sternocleidomastoid, suboccipital, upper trapezius, rhomboids, and pectoralis major and minor.
  - Additionally, the outer abdominal muscle unit (external and internal oblique and rectus abdominis muscles) may need releasing to allow more optimal breathing patterns into the lower rib cage.
- Exercise therapy
  - Lateral costal with diaphragmatic breathing in supine followed by a variety of functional positions
  - Cervical ROM exercises maintaining good alignment
  - Neurodynamic gliding exercises emphasizing upper or lower brachial plexus or involved nerves
  - Motor control and stability functional rehabilitation exercises for proximal muscles of the trunk, neck, and shoulder include deep cervical flexor strengthening in supine, ensuring that the superficial cervical musculature remains relaxed.
  - Stretching of tight muscles, particularly pectoralis minor and major, levator scapulae, and scalenes, to reduce fibrous bands and adhesions in muscles compressing the brachial plexus. Care should be taken not to reproduce symptoms.
  - Gradual introduction of strengthening exercises for any muscles that have been subjected to motor loss, including fine motor and dexterity skills reacquisition.
  - Progressive cardiovascular training program, especially for those in poor aerobic condition. Weight loss programs will also be necessary for obese patients.

PROGNOSIS

- Patients generally respond very well to conservative treatment, with most studies reporting positive outcomes in 60% to 90% of cases.
- Prognosis strongly depends on the extent of damage to the brachial plexus and compliance to conservative treatment. Favorable outcomes are seen in those who comply with exercise programs and modify their behavior at work and home. Obesity, double-crush syndrome, psychosocial issues, and more severe and long-standing symptoms are seen as negative prognostic factors.

SIGNS AND SYMPTOMS INDICATING REFERRAL TO PHYSICIAN

- The following presentations should be referred to a physician for appropriate investigation:
- No response to conservative treatment after several weeks

Section III ORTHOPEDIC PATHOLOGY

- Worsening neurological status
- Atypical symptoms
- Vascular symptoms (see the section on Vascular TOS)
- Presence of significant muscle atrophy with cervical rib (true neurogenic TOS)
- Red flags (e.g., unexplained weight loss).

SUGGESTED READINGS

Atasoy E. Thoracic outlet syndrome: anatomy. *Hand Clin.* 2004;20(1):7-14.

Ault J, Suutala K. Thoracic outlet syndrome. *J Man Manipulative Ther.* 1998;6(3): 118-129.

Brantigan CO, Roos DB, David B. Etiology of neurogenic thoracic outlet syndrome. *Hand Clin.* 2004a;20(1):17-22.

Brantigan CO, Roos DB. Diagnosing thoracic outlet syndrome. *Hand Clin.* 2004b;20(1): 27-36.

Crosby CA, Wehbe MA. Conservative treatment for thoracic outlet syndrome. 2004;20(1): 43-49.

Dawson DM, Hallett M, Milender LH. *Entrapment Neuropathies.* 2nd ed. Boston: Little, Brown; 1990.

Demondian X, Herbinet P, Van Sint Jan S, Boutry N, Chantelot C, Cotton A. Imaging assessment of thoracic outlet syndrome. *Radiographics.* 2006;26:1735-1750.

Edgelow PL. 2003:Neurovascular consequences of cumulative trauma disorders affecting the thoracic outlet: A patient-centred treatment approach. In: Donatelli RA, ed. *Physical Therapy of the Shoulder.* Philadelphia: Churchill Livingstone;.

Mackinnon SE, Novak CB. Thoracic outlet syndrome. *Curr Probl Surg.* 2002;39(11):1070-1145.

Novak CB, Mackinnon SE, Patterson GA. Evaluation of patients with thoracic outlet syndrome. *J Hand Surg.* 1993;18A:292-299.

Pecina MM, Krmpotic-Nemanic J, Markiewitz AP. *Tunnel Syndromes: Peripheral Nerve Compression Syndromes.* 3rd ed. Boca Raton, FL: CRC Press; 2001.

Safran MR. Nerve injuries about the shoulder in athletes, Part 2: Long thoracic nerve, spinal accessory nerve, burners/stingers, thoracic outlet syndrome. *Am J Sports Med.* 2007;32(4):1063-1076.

Sanders RJ, Hammond MD. Etiology and pathology. *Hand Clin.* 2004;20(1):23-26.

Sanders RJ, Hammond SL. Supraclavicular first rib resection and total scalenectomy: technique and results. *Hand Clin.* 2004;20(1): 61-70.

Urschel Jr HC, Kourlis Jr H. Thoracic outlet syndrome: A 50-year experience at Baylor University Medical Center. *Baylor Univ Med Cent Proc.* 2007;20(2):125-135.

Urschel Jr HC, Razzuk MA. Neurovascular compression in the thoracic outlet. Changing management over 50 years. *Ann Surg.* 1998;228(4):609-617.

Vanti C, et al. Conservative treatment of thoracic outlet syndrome: A review of the literature. *Eura Medicophys.* 2007;43(1):55-70.

Wehbe MA. Thoracic outlet syndrome. Guest editor. *Hand Clin.* 2004;20(1).

Whitenack SH, Hunter JM, Read RL. Thoracic outlet syndrome: a brachial plexopathy. In: Mackin EJ, Schneider LH, Callahan AD, et al., eds. *Rehabilitation of the Hand and Upper Extremity.* 5th ed. St Louis: Mosby; 2002.

AUTHOR: KATINA DIMOPOULOS

BASIC INFORMATION

DEFINITION

Obturator nerve entrapment is a rare mononeuropathy that results from compression or restriction of movement of the obturator nerve through the obturator foramen as it passes by the obturator externus.

SYNONYMS

None currently used

ICD-9CM CODES
355.7 Other mononeuritis of lower limb

OPTIMAL NUMBER OF VISITS

6 or fewer

MAXIMAL NUMBER OF VISITS

16

ETIOLOGY

- Arising from the anterior branches of L2, L3, and L4, the obturator nerve follows the medial border of the psoas distally to the lateral wall of the lesser pelvis through the obturator foramen. It then divides into the anterior branch, which descends between the adductor longus and brevis, and the posterior branch, which descends between the adductor magnus and brevis.
- The obturator nerve innervates the adductor, the obturator externus, the gracilis, and the pectineus muscles.
- The obturator nerve supplies the middle portion of the medial thigh.
- Entrapment of the obturator nerve usually happens within the obturator foramen or nearby the proximal portion of the adductor muscles. The nerve may be compressed by external factors or also entrapped by fibrosis of surrounding fascia.

EPIDEMIOLOGY AND DEMOGRAPHICS

No specific data were found on the incidence of this condition; however, some authors have stated that this condition is not very common.

MECHANISM OF INJURY

- Most injuries are associated with acute trauma such as the following:
  - Childbirth: The head of the fetus may compress the nerve against the bony structures of the pelvis
  - Pelvic fracture
  - Postsurgical, after total hip replacement
  - Malpositioning of the lower limb for prolonged periods
  - Contusion or strain of the adductor muscles

COMMON SIGNS AND SYMPTOMS

- Pain in the groin region, near the inguinal ligament, is common.
- Gait changes or problems may occur because of the instability or weakness of the hip adductors.
- Sensory changes or numbness might be noted in the medial portion of the thigh.
- Exercise-induced symptoms may be present in athletes with a decreased performance in jumping or running.
- If the condition becomes more severe, the patient might have more severe loss of internal rotation, adduction, or abduction.

AGGRAVATING ACTIVITIES

- Walking
- Prolonged standing
- Running
- Jumping
- Stretching of the hip into adduction or abduction

EASING ACTIVITIES

- Rest
- Sitting
- Modalities

24-HOUR SYMPTOM PATTERN

No studies on a particular pattern of symptoms were found for obturator nerve entrapment. Increased symptoms at night or lasting symptoms in the morning may point to a strong inflammatory component to the symptoms. This may also suggest a space-occupying lesion, such as a tumor, so careful attention should be paid to other factors and the progression of symptoms.

PAST HISTORY

Previous similar injuries or repetitive injuries in a similar area might be found in a patient's history that may predispose them to such a nerve entrapment.

PHYSICAL EXAMINATION

- Antalgic or unsteady gait is probably one of the most common features of this condition because of the innervation of the adductor muscles and their importance during gait.
- If the condition has been prolonged, the patient may present with atrophy or wasting of the adductor muscles.
- Sensation changes may be present in the middle portion of the medial thigh. Pain or paresthesias may also be found in the same distribution.
- Passive movements of the hip are likely to be guarded, and full internal rotation or adduction may increase the compression and be symptomatic. Abduction may also be uncomfortable because the tissues around the nerve or the nerve itself is put on tension.

IMPORTANT OBJECTIVE TESTS

- Sensation testing in the medial lower extremity may help confirm obturator nerve involvement and differentiate between more proximal lumbar or sacral pathology.
- MMT of the adductors may also help to confirm weakness or pain in those muscles.
- Palpation of the adductor muscles and surrounding structures may reproduce symptoms into the nerve distribution.
- Neurodynamic testing (Butler, 2000) may also help differentiate between a neurogenic and nonneurogenic source of symptoms. A variation of the slump knee bend test with cervical extension and flexion as a sensitizing maneuver may be performed.

DIFFERENTIAL DIAGNOSIS

- Adductor muscle strain
- Osteitis pubis
- Stress fracture
- Inguinal ligament enthesopathy
- Femoral nerve entrapment
- Inguinal hernia
- Lumbar plexopathy or sacral plexopathy

CONTRIBUTING FACTORS

- Diabetes mellitus
- Thyroid problems
- Poor posture
- Impaired trunk and motor control

TREATMENT

SURGICAL OPTIONS

In athletes, surgery may be the preferred treatment for neuropathy. The surgery may involve dividing the fascia over the pectineus and adductor longus muscle. To reveal the anterior branch of the nerve from the fascia, it may require dissecting the space between these two muscles.

REHABILITATION

- Addressing irritable symptoms with modalities, such as ultrasound, interferential current therapy, phonophoresis, or ice and to address pain and inflammation may be the first step of treatment.
- In the case of antalgic gait or poor gait mechanics, an assistive device, such as a single-point cane, may be warranted to decrease the mechanical stress on the nerve and adductors during walking.
- Soft tissue mobilization can be a beneficial technique to help address both pain and fibrotic scarring of surrounding fascia that may be restricting the nerve.
- If it is hypothesized that abnormal neurodynamic movement exists, then

neurodynamic techniques described by Butler (1991) that attempt to slide, glide, and put tension on the nervous system can be beneficial.

- Any other biomechanical faults or impairments that may lead to putting more stress on the adductors or hip should also be assessed.

PROGNOSIS

Because of the rarity of this condition, no literature has been found on long-term prognosis. However, it most likely follows patterns of other nerve entrapment syndromes that have good outcomes if discovered early and proper management is implemented.

SIGNS AND SYMPTOMS INDICATING REFERRAL TO PHYSICIAN

- Unrelenting pain not related to biomechanical factors
- Weight loss
- Bowel or bladder dysfunction
- Saddle paresthesias
- Gait disturbances: Clumsiness or ataxic gait
- Bilateral glove or sock numbness
- Symptoms that do not initially improve with symptoms

SUGGESTED READINGS

Butler DS. *The Sensitive Nervous System*. Adelaide, Australia: Noigroup Publications; 2000.

Butler DS. *Mobilisation of the Nervous System*. New York: Churchill Livingstone; 1991.

Dawson DM, Hallett M, Wilbourn AJ, eds. *Entrapment Neuropathies*. Philadelphia: Lippincott-Raven; 1999.

Moore KL, Dalley AF. *Clinical Oriented Anatomy*. 4th ed. Philadelphia: Lippincott Williams & Wilkins; 1999.

Placzek JD, Boyce DA, eds. *Orthopedic Physical Therapy Secrets*. 2nd ed. Philadelphia: Elsevier; 2006.

Shacklock M. *Clinical Neurodynamics*. Philadelphia: Elsevier; 2005.

AUTHOR: CHRIS IZU

BASIC INFORMATION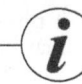

DEFINITION

Plantar nerve entrapment is a neuropathy from compression or restriction of movement of the medial or lateral plantar nerve most commonly under the deep fascia of the plantar surface of the foot.

SYNONYMS

- Distal tarsal tunnel syndrome
- Jogger's foot

ICD-9CM CODES
355.5 Tarsal tunnel syndrome

OPTIMAL NUMBER OF VISITS

8 or fewer

MAXIMAL NUMBER OF VISITS

16

ETIOLOGY

- The medial plantar nerve is the larger branch of the tibial nerve that passes distally between the abductor hallucis and the flexor digitorum brevis. It then divides into both cutaneous and muscular branches.
- The lateral plantar nerve is the smaller branch of the tibial nerve that passes laterally underneath the foot between the quadratus plantae and flexor digitorum brevis. From there it divides into superficial and deep branches.
- The medial plantar nerve supplies the medial side of the sole of the foot and sides of the first three digits.
- The lateral plantar nerve supplies the skin on the sole of the lateral side of the foot, which can be delineated by a line that splits the fourth digit.
- The medial plantar nerve innervates the abductor hallucis, flexor digitorum brevis, flexor hallucis brevis, and the first lumbrical.
- The lateral plantar nerve innervates the quadratus plantae, abductor digiti minimi brevis, plantar interossei, dorsal interossei, lateral three lumbricals, and abductor hallucis.
- The medial plantar nerve is commonly entrapped in the area of the master knot of Henry, which is a fibrous slip between the flexor hallucis longus and the flexor digitorum longus that binds the medial plantar surface.
- The lateral plantar nerve is usually entrapped beneath the deep fascia of the abductor hallucis or the quadratus plantae. It is theorized that this entrapment may result from repeated stretching and tethering of the nerve caused by abnormal forces at the foot such as excessive valgus, external rotation, or pronation.

EPIDEMIOLOGY AND DEMOGRAPHICS

- The incidence of true plantar nerve pathology is difficult to distinguish since it is often grouped with distal tibial nerve entrapment (proximal tarsal tunnel syndrome) because the clinical picture and management may be very similar.
- It is thought that there may be a slight female predominance, and the age range has been stated from 14 to 80 years of age.
- Medial plantar nerve entrapment has been noted to occur commonly in athletes or runners, thus the term "jogger's foot."

MECHANISM OF INJURY

- Traction injuries from repetitive motions of the foot and ankle
- Direct blow or trauma to foot
- Space-occupying lesions
- Constant pressure (e.g., improper fitting orthotic)
- More often the onset is insidious or gradually builds up over time.

COMMON SIGNS AND SYMPTOMS

- Patients typically complain of vague, diffuse pain in the plantar surface of the foot. They may also note chronic, intractable heel pain if more of the calcaneal branches are involved.
- Gait or balance problems may be noted as difficulties with the foot's intrinsic muscles may occur.
- It may be difficult to run, jog, or perform repetitive lower extremity exercises or activities.

AGGRAVATING ACTIVITIES

- Prolonged standing
- Walking
- Running
- Wearing high heels or walking without shoes
- Any activity with increased weight bearing usually aggravates the symptoms of plantar nerve entrapment because of local pressure or stretching of the nerve. If the symptoms are less irritable, it may take prolonged running or even jumping to bring on symptoms.

EASING ACTIVITIES

- Rest
- Sitting
- Wearing proper fitting shoes
- Modalities for pain or inflammation

24-HOUR SYMPTOM PATTERN

- One author suggested that there may be more pain at night that is eased with standing and walking.
- Intuitively, it would seem that the pain may be worse later in the day if the patient is required or chooses to do a lot of standing or walking.

PAST HISTORY

No specific history of symptoms has been documented in this population. However, a history of previous trauma to the foot and ankle would make sense as they may develop fibrosis of the surrounding muscle fascia. A previous history of similar nerve entrapment syndromes may also be noted in their history.

PHYSICAL EXAMINATION

- Pain and dysesthesias in the plantar surface of the foot are the most common findings in this population.
- Antalgic gait and pain with increased weight bearing may also be noted. A rapid pronation may be noted during the initial stance phase of gait or a lack of supination may be noted during the terminal stance phase.
- Balance activities may be slightly more difficult or painful on the affected side, caused by the activation of the abductor hallucis and quadratus during these activities.
- Pain on palpation may also be a key finding.

IMPORTANT OBJECTIVE TESTS

- Lower quarter neurological testing
  - Sensory testing should reveal altered symptoms within the plantar surface of the foot. Using Semmes-Weinstein monofilaments may help with increasing sensitivity of the examination.
  - Motor testing should be normal, except for possible pain-inhibited weakness with repetitive plantarflexion in standing.
  - Reflexes: The Achilles and the patellar tendon should be normal secondary to the lesion below the level of tested reflexes.
- Palpating the surrounding fascia and muscles may reproduce pain into the distribution of the medial or lateral plantar nerve.
- Neurodynamic testing: Using the slump or SLR test with sensitizing maneuvers may help to distinguish neurogenic (plantar nerves) from nonneurogenic (surrounding musculature) as a source of symptoms. The addition of forefoot inversion to the SLR test may add more tension to the medial plantar nerve, while forefoot eversion may add more tension to the lateral plantar nerve.

DIFFERENTIAL DIAGNOSIS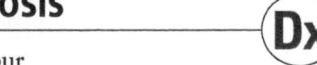

- Heel spur
- Plantar fasciitis
- Polyneuropathy

- Systemic disorders
- Lumbar spine radiculopathy

CONTRIBUTING FACTORS

- Tenosynovitis of adjacent tendons
- Partial or complete rupture of tendons
- Obesity
- Ankylosing spondylitis
- Acromegaly
- Talocalcaneal coalition
- Diabetes mellitus
- RA
- Abnormal foot positioning
- Alcoholism
- Thyroid disease

TREATMENT

SURGICAL OPTIONS

- Surgical release of the surrounding tissue may help with relief of compression on the nerve. In most cases, a full release of both the posterior tibial nerve and the lateral plantar nerve is recommended.
- If a space-occupying lesion is noted to have a significant effect on the nerve, then removal by surgery is recommended.

REHABILITATION

- Initially rehabilitation should focus on reduction of symptoms, finding easing activities, and managing inflammation.
- Modalities, such as ultrasound, phonophoresis, iontophoresis, ice massage, and interferential current therapy, may help to manage initial symptoms.
- Taping or orthotic prescription to control abnormal foot motions or support

the medial longitudinal arch may also help reduce symptoms by decreasing abnormal strain.

- During less irritable conditions, more vigorous treatment, such as soft tissue mobilization, may help free fibrotic scarring or fascial thickening around the nerve sheath.
- Neurodynamic mobilization, using techniques to slide, glide, or place tension on the nerve, may help restore more normal mobility to neural structures. Alterations of the slump test or SLR test may be good places to start when dealing with plantar nerve mobility.
- Exercises should address lower extremity impairments or biomechanical faults that may place further stress on the plantar nerve. Common activities include improving forefoot, rearfoot, or entire lower extremity control with attempts to decrease abnormal or rapid pronation.

PROGNOSIS

- After surgical release procedures, one study reported good-to-excellent results in about 84% of patients.
- Although no data were found, clinical observations of plantar nerve entrapment have shown good response to conservative rehabilitation when few contributing factors are present.

SIGNS AND SYMPTOMS INDICATING REFERRAL TO PHYSICIAN

- If suspected worsening compression on the nerve is suspected from a compartment syndrome, immediate referral to

a physician is warranted. A fasciotomy may be done to release this pressure.

- Unrelenting symptoms, especially combined with worse pain at night, may indicate a local tumor.
- Lack of improvement within the expected time frame or symptoms that are not affected by physical therapy in a few visits should be referred back to the physician because a space-occupying lesion may be present.
- A recent history of trauma with suspected fracture may warrant further imaging done before continuing physical therapy.
- Impaired circulation or vascular compromise may also warrant more medical management.

SUGGESTED READINGS

Butler DS. *The Sensitive Nervous System.* Adelaide, Australia: Noigroup Publications; 2000.

Butler DS. *Mobilisation of the Nervous System.* New York: Churchill Livingstone; 1991.

Dawson DM, Hallett M, Wilbourn AJ, eds. *Entrapment Neuropathies.* Philadelphia: Lippincott-Raven; 1999.

Moore KL, Dalley AF. *Clinical Oriented Anatomy.* 4th ed. Philadelphia: Lippincott Williams & Wilkins; 1999.

Placzek JD, Boyce DA, eds. *Orthopedic Physical Therapy Secrets.* 2nd ed. Philadelphia: Elsevier; 2006.

Shacklock M. *Clinical Neurodynamics.* Philadelphia: Elsevier; 2005.

AUTHOR: CHRIS IZU

BASIC INFORMATION

DEFINITION
Radial nerve entrapment pathologies encompass any injury that interrupts the function of the radial nerve at any point along its course. The loss of function results in muscle weakness, pain, or sensory dysfunction.

SYNONYMS
- Saturday night palsy or syndrome
- Radial tunnel syndrome (RTS)
- Posterior interosseous nerve (PIN) syndrome

ICD-9CM CODES
354 Mononeuritis of upper limb and mononeuritis multiplex
354.3 Lesion of radial nerve

OPTIMAL NUMBER OF VISITS
6

MAXIMAL NUMBER OF VISITS
20

ETIOLOGY
- The radial nerve is derived from C5-C8 nerve roots with an additional sensory component from T1.
- The radial nerve is the larger terminal branch of the posterior cord of the brachial plexus.
- It arises proximal to the lower border of subscapularis, then runs posterolaterally inferior to latissimus dorsi and teres major at their attachment to the humerus.
- It descends obliquely across the posterior portion of the midshaft of the humerus in the spiral/radial groove between the medial and lateral heads of the triceps brachii muscle.
- While in the groove, it is accompanied by the deep brachial vessels, the groove ends just distal to the deltoid tuberosity, and at that point the nerve enters the anterior compartment of the arm through the fibrous intermuscular septum in a deep position between the brachialis and brachioradialis muscles.
- It continues to descend to supply extensor carpi radialis longus and brevis superficially and deeply to the lateral elbow capsule and the radial tunnel.
- The superficial branch continues through the forearm deep to the brachioradialis and provides cutaneous innervation to the dorsolateral hand.
- The deep branch (posterior interosseous nerve) curves around the neck of the radius between the two layers of the supinator muscle, emerging as multiple branches that supply the deep posterior muscles of the forearm and wrist joint.
- The radial nerve is vulnerable to injury at several points along its course, as follows:
  - Proximally at the axilla
  - Along the shaft of the humerus while in the spiral groove
  - By the lateral heads of triceps and as it passes through the fibrous intermuscular septum
  - While in the radial tunnel by a fibrous band at the level of the radial head, by the radial recurrent artery, or by the tendinous edge of extensor carpi radialis brevis
  - Within the arcade of Frohse
  - Within the supinator or by the distal edge of the supinator
  - Between the tendons of the brachioradialis and extensor carpi radialis longus muscles and through the antebrachial fascia
  - Superficially over the lateral aspect of the forearm
- The radial nerve may be affected at any point along its course by direct trauma or compression entrapment causing nerve tissue hypoxia. The insult to the nerve can be mechanical, thermal, chemical, and ischemic.
- This pathology can occur in of the following ways:
  - Through compression at the axilla such as occurs when falling asleep with the arm over the back of a chair (Saturday night palsy) or with the use of shoulder crutches
  - By direct damage to the nerve during a humeral shaft fracture or from compression against callus formation along the spiral groove after a traumatic humeral injury
  - Compression by the lateral head of the triceps and as the nerve passes through the fibrous intermuscular septum sometimes seen in weight lifting or other activity that involves heavy repetitive triceps activation
  - Compression in the radial tunnel by a fibrous band at the level of the radial head or by the radial recurrent artery (leash of Henry) in which the tunnel does not provide adequate space for the course of the nerve
  - Compression by the tendinous edge of extensor carpi radialis brevis when subjected to repetitive wrist and finger extension activity such as in some factory and office-based tasks
  - Compression within the arcade of Frohse by a space-occupying lesion or simply by anatomical restriction of the arcade space
  - Compression within the supinator muscle or by the distal edge of the supinator that may occur with repetitive pronation and supination tasks in sport or occupation
  - Compression between the tendons of the brachioradialis and extensor carpi radialis longus muscles and through the antebrachial fascia again seen in repetitive pronation, supination, pinching, grasping, or heavy pushing and pulling tasks
  - Compression of the superficial branch over the lateral aspect of the forearm by direct trauma or by straps, watches, and wrist bands
- Nerve injury is classified according to the severity of the injury and its potential for reversibility as follows:
  - Neurapraxia (first-degree injury): Distortion of the myelin around the nodes of Ranvier caused by ischemia, mechanical compression, or electrolyte imbalance produces temporary loss of nerve conduction.
  - Axonotmesis (second-degree injury): Interruption of the axon with secondary wallerian degeneration. The supporting tissue surrounding the axon is preserved, and the recovery period depends on the distance between the site of injury and the end-organs.
  - Neurotmesis: Complete disruption of the nerve and its supporting structures
- Neurotmesis has been further divided into the following three subcategories:
  - Third-degree nerve injury: Endoneurium is disrupted with intact perineurium and epineurium
  - Fourth-degree nerve injury: All neural elements sparing the epineurium are disrupted.
  - Fifth-degree nerve injury: Complete transaction and discontinuity of the nerve with no capacity for regeneration
- Physiologically, there is disruption to any part of the nerve responsible for conduction.
- In repetitive-type nerve entrapment, it is proposed that repetitive work or static postures produce an inflammatory response, and fibroblasts appear to repair damage incurred but produce adhesions to the nerve, limiting their glide and increasing anoxia.
- Other studies found that cortical dedifferentiation can result from repetitive motion activities and nerve injuries. This may result in reinforced poor posturing and use of aberrant motor pathways.

EPIDEMIOLOGY AND DEMOGRAPHICS
- Of the three major nerves in the upper limb, entrapment of the radial nerve is least common.
- The most common site for entrapment and injury is the spiral groove of the humerus related to humeral fracture.

- Work-related entrapments are becoming more common, in particular with computer use and seated postures.
- RTS has a very small incidence (1% to 2%) of upper extremity entrapments. RTS most commonly involves patients in the fourth to sixth decade of life without significant gender predilection.

MECHANISM OF INJURY

- There are a number of mechanisms of injury for the radial nerve that will be described in relation to their location:
  - Through compression at axilla such as falling asleep with the arm over the back of a chair (Saturday night palsy) or with the use of shoulder crutches
  - By direct damage to the nerve during a humeral shaft fracture or from compression against callus formation along the spiral groove after a traumatic humeral injury
  - Compression by the lateral head of the triceps and as the nerve passes through the fibrous intermuscular septum as sometimes seen in weight lifting or other activity that involves heavy repetitive triceps activation
  - Compression in the radial tunnel by a fibrous band at the level of the radial head or by the radial recurrent artery (leash of Henry) where the tunnel does not provide adequate space for the course of the nerve.
  - Compression by the tendinous edge of extensor carpi radialis brevis when subjected to repetitive wrist and finger extension activity such as found in some factory and office-based tasks.
  - Compression within the arcade of Frohse by a space-occupying lesion or simply by anatomical restriction of the arcade space.
  - Compression within the supinator muscle or by the distal edge of the supinator that may occur with repetitive pronation and supination tasks in sport or occupation
  - Compression between the tendons of the brachioradialis and extensor carpi radialis longus muscles and through the antebrachial fascia again seen in repetitive pronation, supination, pinching, grasping, or heavy pushing and pulling tasks
  - Compression of the superficial branch over the lateral aspect of the forearm by direct trauma or by straps, watches, and wrist bands.

COMMON SIGNS AND SYMPTOMS

- High radial nerve palsies
  - Weakness of the elbow extension (triceps)
  - Mild weakness of elbow flexion (brachioradialis)
  - Mild weakness of wrist and finger extension
  - There may be variable loss of sensation over the posterior arm forearm and hand.
  - Triceps and brachioradialis reflexes are lost or reduced.
  - Often result in a characteristic posture of wrist drop with slight flaccid flexion, the hand pronated and thumb adducted (waiter's tip position).
  - Generally, this is an injury to the entire lower brachial plexus not just the radial nerve so the medial and ulnar branches may also be involved and must be assessed.
  - Spiral groove lesions are similar to high radial nerve palsies, but the triceps power and reflexes are spared.
  - Posterior interosseous neuropathies are generally motor; pain may be present but is not the major symptom.
  - There is a resultant finger drop with variable weakness of wrist extension.
  - When wrist extension is attempted, there may be weak dorsoradial deviation caused by the preservation of the radial wrist extensors.
- RTS
  - Deep, dull lateral elbow pain
  - Pain over the extensor mass
  - Wrist aching
  - Middle or upper third humeral pain
  - Increased pain on resisted supination of the forearm
  - Increased pain with middle-finger extension (also evident in extensor tendinopathies)
  - Paraesthesias (tingling and numbness) over the dorsal hand and lateral forearm
  - Neural tension tests may reproduce the symptoms.
  - To distinguish between RTS and extensor tendinopathies the location of the pain is less localized to the lateral epicondyle and more likely to be over the extensor mass and supinator.
  - The pain of RTS is more achy and produces more muscle fatigue.
  - RTS appears to be more related to repetitive pronation and supination rather than repeated wrist extension for extensor tendinopathy.
  - RTS and extensor tendinopathy occur together in 5% of cases.
- Superficial branch of the radial nerve results in sensory loss over the dorsum of the hand, most commonly of the dorsal thumb, index, and middle fingers; occasionally the dorsolateral half of the ring finger is also involved. This type of nerve compression can cause poorly localized pain in this distribution and above.
- For all levels of radial nerve injury, there may have been loss of nerve representation of the nerve injured area on the somatosensory cortex.

AGGRAVATING ACTIVITIES

- Any repeated actions of the forearm extensors, supination, or pronation.
- Repetitive, forceful pushing and pulling, bending the wrist, gripping and pinching
- Screwdriver motion
- Work tasks involving repetitive finger work such as typing or mouse work
- Higher radial nerve injuries may be provoked by repetitive elbow extension activating the triceps such as weight lifting.
- Sports involving gripping, pronation, supination, or wrist and finger extension.

EASING ACTIVITIES

Rest and/or modification of aggravating activities

24-HOUR SYMPTOM PATTERN

- Generally the symptoms are related to activity and do not follow a typical 24-hour pattern unless there is a strong inflammatory component such as may be seen in occupational repetitive tasks.
- If there is an inflammatory component, there may be worsening of symptoms with use toward the end of the day and morning stiffness.

PAST HISTORY FOR THE REGION

- History of trauma, fracture, dislocation, or blow to the radial nerve distribution.
- Repeated activity involving pushing, pulling, gripping, supination, or pronation
- Work tasks involving exertions of greater than 1 kg of force more than 10 times an hour, static pinching or squeezing objects or tools, working with the elbow extended, and maintaining positioning of the forearm in pronation or supination.
- Racquet sports: Repetitive pronation and supination, gripping and wrist extension
- When the superficial branch is involved the patient should be questioned about any straps, watches, or wristbands worn.
- Working with hand tools or power tools (vibration)

PHYSICAL EXAMINATION

- Examine the limb for signs of autonomic dysfunction trophic changes such as edema, inflammation, and alteration in skin texture
- Reflex testing, paying particular attention to limb asymmetries of the triceps and brachioradialis reflexes

- MMT may reveal weakness in any of the following muscles:
  - Triceps (C7, C8): Extend elbow against resistance
  - Brachioradialis (C5, C6): Flex elbow with forearm half way between pronation and supination
  - Extensor carpi radialis longus (C6, C7): Extend wrist to the radial side with fingers extended
  - Supinator (C5, C6): Arm by side resist hand pronation.
  - Extensor digitorum (C7, C8): Maintain finger extension at the MCP joints
  - Extensor carpi ulnaris (C7, C8): Extend wrist to ulnar side
  - Abductor pollicis longus (C7, C8): Abduct thumb to 90degrees to palm
  - Extensor pollicis brevis (C7, C8): Extend thumb at MCP
  - Extensor pollicis longus (C7, C8): Resist thumb flexion at IP joint
- Sensation: The cutaneous branches of the radial nerve supply the dorsal aspect of the forearm from below the elbow down over the lateral part of the hand to include the thumb to the interphalangeal joint and the fingers distal to the interphalangeal joint, including index and middle fingers but not the little finger. Sensation testing should include pinprick, two-point discrimination, tuning fork, and joint position sense and compared for asymmetry with the unaffected side (where available).
- Tinel's sign may be positive over the anatomical snuff box.
- Physical examination should also exclude pathology in other areas, particularly performing AROM and PROM at the neck and shoulder, which may reveal restrictions and central involvement of the nerve.
- Upper limb neural tissue provocation testing may reveal changes in nerve mobility and elicit symptoms.
- Physical examination should also include movement analysis to determine the movement patterns that the patient adopts when performing the aggravating activities. Movement analysis can be done visually or with the assistance of a video camera. The analysis should give some clues as to predisposing factors, such as posture and patterning, that will assist with rehabilitation and activity modification.

IMPORTANT OBJECTIVE TESTS

- The earliest electrodiagnostic sign of entrapment is a loss of the nerve action potential seen during a nerve conduction study. To isolate the specific location of the conduction block, serial stimulations are delivered to the nerve above and below the suspected lesion.

- Needle EMG is valuable for evaluating the extent of motor fiber loss within a nerve territory. EMG assists with determining the location of the injury and to monitor progression over time.
- X-ray of the humerus may reveal an undiagnosed fracture of the humeral shaft or callus formation from a previous injury.
- MRI is increasingly being used in the assessment of peripheral nerve injuries to rule out cervical nerve root involvement and determine the presence of edema, space restriction, or space-occupying lesion along the course of the radial nerve.

DIFFERENTIAL DIAGNOSIS

- Forearm extensor tendinopathy
- Underlying neuropathic disease
- Idiopathic brachial neuritis
- Myopathies
- Muscular dystrophy
- Isolated neuropathy in the diabetic
- Tumors or space-occupying lesions
- C6 or C7 cervical radiculopathy
- Upper motor neuron lesion in the cerebrum
- De Quervain's tenosynovitis

CONTRIBUTING FACTORS

- For any nerve entrapments that are non-traumatic, there is often an element of repetitive activity involving the affected limb. Typically, in the case of the radial nerve, the repetitive action involves, elbow extension, forearm pronation, supination, gripping, forceful pushing and pulling, and/or wrist and finger extension.
- Postural factors may be involved, particularly with repetitive work or sporting activities with reduction in proximal stability and control leading to an overuse of more distal muscle groups to perform a task.
- Excessive loads, such as in heavy manual work or sports, involving weight lifting can overload the capacity of the muscles to adapt, thus creating inflammation and subsequent nerve compression.
- The use of tight wristbands, cuffs, or other strapping across the wrist may contribute to superficial radial nerve compression.

TREATMENT   **Rx**

SURGICAL OPTIONS

- Surgery is generally considered a last resort if conservative management fails.
- Nerve palsy after a closed fracture of the humerus is generally observed over 6 to 12 weeks to determine the effect of the swelling subsiding. However, if the

palsy continues, then surgical intervention is indicated.
- The goal of surgical intervention would be to relieve pressure or entrapment along the course of the nerve, (e.g., surgical release of the superficial head of supinator and division of the ligament of Frohse to expand the available space in the radial tunnel).

REHABILITATION

- Current best evidence for the conservative management of RTS consists primarily of expert opinion and inferences taken from studies on other nerve compressions.
- The goal of rehabilitation should be to reduce pain, to encourage pain-free exercise, to provide ergonomic education and interventions, and if the neuropathy has been prolonged, to introduce cortical reorganization activities.
- Splinting should be used to provide immobilization to allow the reduction in swelling and inflammation. Functional splinting can also be employed to prevent contracture and facilitate normal movement patterns (e.g., for a high radial nerve palsy the use of a static wrist extension splint with dynamic extension apparatus for the proximal phalanges).
- Elimination of aggravating tasks by avoiding or modifying those tasks to prevent further damage
- Use of ice to reduce inflammation and prevent secondary cell damage
- Theoretically, ultrasound may be helpful to promote nerve regeneration, improve profusion to the healing nerve, and decrease inflammation.
- Direct low-intensity electrical stimulation has been found to increase the number of vasa nervorum and nerve fiber density in rats.
- Steroid injection is often advocated to reduce inflammation particularly in RTS.
- Iontophoresis with dexamethasone and lidocaine
- Nerve gliding exercise, have been purported to disperse intraneural edema, increase blood flow, optimize axonal transport, and lengthen nerve adhesions. Neural mobilization can be assessed using the brachial plexus provocation test positions to identify symptom reproduction and these positions and movements can also be used both actively and passively for a treatment technique.
- Use of soft tissue mobilization and muscle stretching techniques to reduce fibrous bands and adhesions in muscles surrounding the radial nerve. Stretches must not produce tingling or discomfort because this may indicate

decreased blood flow to the already stressed nerve.

- Motor control and stability functional rehabilitation exercise for proximal muscles of the trunk, neck, and shoulder.
- Gradual introduction of strengthening exercises for any muscles that have been subjected to motor loss
- Ergonomic interventions, workplace assessment, provision of ergonomic aides such as tilted keyboards or altered mouse shape
- Cortical reorganization techniques such as use of mirror box
- Reacquisition of fine motor and dexterity skills

PROGNOSIS

- Prognosis depends entirely on the extent of damage to the nerve.
- Neurapraxia should resolve rapidly and lead to a complete restoration of function, usually within 2 to 3 months.

- If the injury is a more severe axonotmesis, the recovery time depend on the distance from the site of injury to the denervated tissue.
- Peripheral nerves have been reported to recover at an approximate rate of between 1 and 4 mm per day, but complete function might not be restored.
- If there has been a complete sectioning of the nerve (neurapraxia), then a full recovery will not occur.
- The results of treating neurapraxia even with surgical intervention are generally not satisfactory.

SIGNS AND SYMPTOMS INDICATING REFERRAL TO PHYSICIAN

If radial nerve entrapment is suspected, all cases should be referred to a physician for appropriate investigation.

SUGGESTED READINGS

Bencardino JT, Rosenberg ZS. Entrapment neuropathies of the shoulder and elbow in the athlete. *Clin Sports Med.* 2006;25:465-487.

Cleary CK. Management of radial tunnel syndrome: A therapist's clinical perspective. *J Hand Ther.* 2006;19(2):186-191.

Pratt N. Anatomy of nerve entrapment sites in the upper quarter. *J Hand Ther.* 2005;18(2):216-229.

Roquelaure Y, Raimbeau G, Dano X. Occupational risk factors for radial tunnel syndrome in industrial workers. *Scand J Work Environ Health.* 2000;26:507-513.

AUTHOR: JOSEPHINE LOUISE COULTER

BASIC INFORMATION

DEFINITION

Saphenous nerve entrapment is a mononeuropathy that results from compression or restriction of movement of the saphenous nerve in the distal thigh as it passes through the adductor canal.

SYNONYMS

None currently used

ICD-9CM CODES
355.7 Other mononeuritis of lower limb

OPTIMAL NUMBER OF VISITS

6 or fewer

MAXIMAL NUMBER OF VISITS

20

ETIOLOGY

- The saphenous nerve (from L3 and L4) arises off the femoral nerve slightly distal to the inguinal ligament and courses down the medial thigh. Between the sartorius and gracilis muscles, about 10 cm proximal to the medial epicondyle, the nerve pierces the connective tissue toward the medial knee and continues down the medial side of the lower leg.
- The saphenous nerve is purely sensory and does not innervate the muscle in the lower leg.
- Its cutaneous branches supply the skin of the anteromedial knee, the medial side of the lower leg, and the medial side of the foot distally (sometimes as far as the first metatarso phalangeal joint).
- Most commonly, the nerve is entrapped where it pierces the connective tissue (referred to as Hunter's canal) and may be irritated by repetitive contraction and relaxation of the surrounding musculature; this may be caused by the angulation of the saphenous nerve as it enters the canal traction to the nerve. The nerve may also undergo compression around the top of the calf region from external pressure such as tight garments.

EPIDEMIOLOGY AND DEMOGRAPHICS

It is believed that this condition, as well as peroneal nerve entrapment, is the most common form of lower extremity nerve entrapment syndrome.

MECHANISM OF INJURY

- Direct trauma
- Entrapment by femoral vessels

- Pes anserine bursitis
- Postsurgical vein operations
- Medial knee arthrotomies
- Postsurgical meniscal repairs
- Improperly protected leg during surgery

COMMON SIGNS AND SYMPTOMS

- The most common complaint of saphenous nerve entrapment is medial knee pain. Usually, it is described as a dull, aching sensation in the knee, but the patient may also have discomfort in the medial thigh.
- Paresthesias may be found in the cutaneous distribution of the saphenous nerve, which includes the medial knee and medial region of the lower leg down into the medial ankle and foot.
- It is important to note that since the nerve is purely sensory, no motor deficits or gait abnormalities should be part of the symptoms.

AGGRAVATING ACTIVITIES

- Repetitive knee motions that place stress on the surrounding fascia or muscles may cause increased symptoms such as running or biking.
- Prolonged standing or walking
- Stair climbing
- It is believed that active knee extension may place more stress or tension on the involved nerve. Therefore any activities, such as standing, walking, or stair climbing, that require knee extension may be symptomatic.

EASING ACTIVITIES

- Rest and avoiding aggravating activities
- Antiinflammatories

24-HOUR SYMPTOM PATTERN

If there is a significant inflammatory component to the symptoms or a space-occupying lesion, more night symptoms may be expected. Following this, symptoms may also be worse in the morning. One study has noted that two thirds of the patients with saphenous nerve entrapment in their study had increased symptoms at night.

PAST HISTORY

As a result of the traumatic or repetitive stress injury causes of saphenous nerve entrapment, there may be no significant items noted on their history. Since fibrosis of the surrounding tissues may be a contributing factor to this nerve entrapment, a previous history of trauma may be found.

PHYSICAL EXAMINATION

- Usually, sensory deficits and pain are the only presentation of this condition.

- Gait and functional testing may be painful, but no motor deficits should be noted with MMT.
- Avoidance with knee extension might be noted but should not be thought of as diagnostic since many other competing conditions will also have pain with or limited knee extension.

IMPORTANT OBJECTIVE TESTS

- Sensation testing: Light touch, pinprick, or sharp/dull testing should reveal altered sensation in the saphenous nerve distribution.
- Lower quarter neurological examination should be performed to help rule out more proximal causes of the symptoms such as lumbar spine radiculopathy. Again, no motor or reflex deficits should be found on examination.
- Palpation should be done along the path of the nerve, especially at the superior to the medial epicondyle where the nerve passes through the dense connective tissue.
- Tinel's test: Tapping along the path of the nerve, especially where it is more superficial because it is above or below the medial epicondyle, may reproduce symptoms.
- Slump knee bend test, as described by Butler, may help to determine a neurogenic cause of symptoms. Similar to testing the femoral nerve in sidelying, using the sensitizing maneuver of cervical extension and flexion may help to differentiate between neurogenic (saphenous nerve) and nonneurogenic (local muscle or other knee pathology) source of symptoms.
- Lumbar ROM, accessory mobility testing, and palpation
  - All three of these examinations may help to differentiate a lumbar spine problem from an isolated saphenous nerve entrapment.

DIFFERENTIAL DIAGNOSIS

- Lumbar spine radiculopathy
- Lumbar spine stenosis
- Lumbar spine somatic referral
- Femoral or tibial fracture
- Medial collateral ligament injury
- Meniscal pathology
- Osteoarthritis
- Patellofemoral pain
- Pes anserine bursitis

CONTRIBUTING FACTORS

- Increased age (over 40 years of age)
- Increased thigh obesity
- Genu varum, with or without tibial torsion

TREATMENT

SURGICAL OPTIONS

After conservative measures of treatment have failed, a surgical decompression may be considered. Other possible methods may be surgical removal of the nerve or neurolysis.

REHABILITATION

- Initially, the goals of physical therapy are management of the symptoms and patient education regarding the dysfunction.
- Modalities, such as interferential current therapy, ultrasound, phonophoresis, iontophoresis, ice, or compression, may help address any symptoms more related to an inflammatory component.
- Soft tissue massage dealing with the location of hypothesized nerve entrapment may help the fibrosis or scarring of surrounding fascia.
- After soft tissue treatments, neural mobilization techniques that help slide, glide, or place tension on the nervous system could be used to help restore more normal movement the saphenous nerve.
- Addressing other biomechanical factors, such as foot or lower extremity alignment, is also necessary for a comprehensive rehabilitation program.

PROGNOSIS

In general, the prognosis for this condition is good. It is not associated with mortality or high rates of morbidity. Conservative treatment methods have been shown to be successful, and surgical options have few postoperative complications because of the pure sensory function of the nerve.

SIGNS AND SYMPTOMS INDICATING REFERRAL TO PHYSICIAN

- Night pain and unrelenting symptoms may indicate a local tumor.
- Symptoms that do not improve within the expected time or that are not affected by physical therapy in a few visits should be referred back to the physician since a space-occupying lesion may be present.
- A recent history of trauma with suspected fracture may need imaging studies done before starting treatment.
- Impaired circulation or vascular compromise may also warrant more medical management.

SUGGESTED READINGS

Butler DS. *The Sensitive Nervous System*. Adelaide, Australia: Noigroup Publications; 2000.

Butler DS. *Mobilisation of the Nervous System*. New York: Churchill Livingstone; 1991.

Dawson DM, Hallett M, Wilbourn AJ, eds. *Entrapment Neuropathies*. Philadelphia: Lippincott-Raven; 1999.

Moore KL, Dalley AF. *Clinical Oriented Anatomy*. 4th ed. Philadelphia: Lippincott Williams & Wilkins; 1999.

Placzek JD, Boyce DA, eds. *Orthopedic Physical Therapy Secrets*. 2nd ed. Philadelphia: Elsevier; 2006.

Shacklock M. *Clinical Neurodynamics*. Philadelphia: Elsevier; 2005.

http://www.emedicine.com/Orthoped/topic422.htm

AUTHOR: CHRIS IZU

BASIC INFORMATION

DEFINITION

Sciatic nerve entrapment is a neuropathy that results from compression or restriction of movement of the sciatic nerve, usually found in the posterior gluteal region near the piriformis muscle.

SYNONYMS

Piriformis syndrome

ICD-9CM CODES
355.0 Lesion of sciatic nerve

OPTIMAL NUMBER OF VISITS

8 or fewer

MAXIMAL NUMBER OF VISITS

20

ETIOLOGY

- The large sciatic nerve originates from the sacral plexus (L4 to S3) and enters the gluteal region through the greater sciatic foramen near the piriformis muscle. It then descends along the posterior aspect of the thigh, dividing into the tibial and common peroneal nerve.
- The sciatic nerve innervates all of the hamstring with the exception of the short head of the biceps. Because it branches into the tibial and common peroneal nerves, it sends motor input to the entire lower part of the leg.
- The sciatic nerve branches off into the tibial and common peroneal nerves, which supply the superficial area of the entire lower leg except for the medial side of the leg and ankle (saphenous nerve).
- The most common cause of sciatic nerve entrapment is irritation of the piriformis muscle. It is reported that 10% to 20% of individuals actually have a sciatic nerve that courses through the piriformis muscle instead of anterior to it.
- Two different theories in which the sciatic nerve could become entrapped by the piriformis muscle are as follows:
  o By a spasm of the muscle that becomes tight around the nerve
  o By irritation of the muscle if the muscle is long and weak
- Other causes of nerve entrapment include the following:
  o Muscle anomalies
  o Fibrosis caused by trauma
  o Myositis ossificans

EPIDEMIOLOGY AND DEMOGRAPHICS

- The prevalence of this condition is difficult to assess secondary to the lack of agreement of its diagnosis and its close relationship to lumbar spine pathology when the lumbar plexus is involved. Some report that the condition may be very rare (6% of sciatica cases), whereas others note that when looking at the incidence of low back pain with the inclusion of lower extremity symptoms, it may be more common than reported.
- There seems to be a higher female prevalence with sciatic nerve entrapment and some estimates are as high as 6:1.

MECHANISM OF INJURY

- Blunt injury may cause scarring of the surrounding structures.
- Prolonged pressure, such as sitting, may cause compression.
- Postsurgical complications (e.g., total hip replacement)
- After vigorous activity, causing strain on the piriformis muscle or surrounding structures
- The onset of symptoms from sciatic nerve entrapment can be sudden after trauma as noted or gradual overtime. In overuse injuries or gradual buildup of stress over time on the affected areas, symptoms may take time to come on or become problematic enough to seek medical attention.

COMMON SIGNS AND SYMPTOMS

- Pain originating in the gluteal region that progresses down into the posterior thigh and lower leg is the most common complaint in patients with this condition. In certain cases, pain is felt more distally in the lower extremity and less in the gluteal region.
- Weakness may be present in the lower extremity muscles that control the foot and ankle along with knee flex.
- Gait is almost always affected, and patients usually complain of pain with bearing weight on the affected leg.

AGGRAVATING ACTIVITIES

- Walking
- Prolonged standing
- Sitting, with pressure on the affected area
- Sitting cross-legged
- Sleeping or lying with the hip in a flexed or adducted position
- Driving, especially when the right lower extremity is affected
- Walking or standing may cause an overuse of the piriformis, especially as it may attempt to assist with pelvic and hip stability during gait. Other activities that add local compression or place the piriformis on stretch may also irritate the symptoms.

EASING ACTIVITIES

- Rest
- Ice or modalities to reduce inflammation
- Heat to relax local musculature
- Frequently changing positions, either from sitting or from sitting to standing
- Sitting with legs apart
- Sleeping or lying with a pillow between legs
- Either decreasing the abnormal pressure on the piriformis by removing compressive forces or placing it in a resting position should help to alleviate symptoms.

24-HOUR SYMPTOM PATTERN

No specific pattern has been reported in the literature. A presence of more nighttime symptoms or increased pain the morning or after resting may be more related to an inflammatory component of the disorder. It may also suggest another underlying pathology, such as a tumor, compressing the sciatic nerve.

PAST HISTORY

Previous similar symptoms, low back injuries, or other lower extremity injuries that may predispose someone to sciatic nerve entrapment may be found in the patient's history.

PHYSICAL EXAMINATION

- This condition is often very painful and usually leads to an antalgic gait pattern, in which less time is spent in single-leg stance on the affected leg and with an ipsilateral trunk lean. It is also common to see external rotation of the affected extremity.
- Sciatic nerve entrapment may have few distinguishing factors from that of a lumbar spine radiculopathy, stenosis, or discogenic dysfunction. Patients may also present with pain in the lumbar spine.
- Patients may assume a posture in sitting or standing in which less pressure is placed through the affected lower extremity.
- Weakness is most likely noted with resisted hamstring testing, either to the result of pain or decreased nerve conduction from sciatic nerve compression. Other lower extremity muscles below the knee may also be weak because of the sciatic nerve's contribution to the tibial and common fibular nerve.
- Assessing neurodynamics is also important if sciatic nerve entrapment is suspected because it may help to differentiate between a neurogenic source of pain (the sciatic nerve itself) and an nonneurogenic source (hamstrings).

IMPORTANT OBJECTIVE TESTS

- Palpation is often helpful in differentiating between symptoms of the lumbar spine, sacroiliac, and local muscles. Deep palpation of the piriformis muscle proximally in the posterior gluteal region and along the length of the sciatic nerve down in the posterior thigh should reproduce symptoms.

- Freiberg's test: Forced internal rotation of the hip with the hip in extension may reproduce the symptoms by placing the piriformis and other deep hip external rotators on stretch. Combining this motion with abduction and external rotation of the hip while in hip flexion (Beatty maneuver) may help increase the sensitivity of testing.
- FAIR test: The patient is positioned in the sidelying position, with the patient's affected leg placed in flexion, adduction, and internal rotation. A positive test will reproduce the patient's symptoms in the buttock and leg.
- A full lower quarter neurological examination is also necessary to help differentiate a possible sciatic nerve entrapment from a lumbar spine radiculopathy or disc problem.
- Slump or SLR tests to assess neurodynamic mobility also help differentiate or implicate neural structures.

DIFFERENTIAL DIAGNOSIS

- Lumbar spine radiculopathy
- Lumbar spine stenosis
- Lumbar spine discogenic dysfunction
- Hamstring strain or tear
- Ischial tuberosity bursitis
- Sciatica

CONTRIBUTING FACTORS

- Diabetes mellitus
- Leg length discrepancy
- Morton's foot: Prominent second metatarsal head and changing gait pattern

TREATMENT

SURGICAL OPTIONS

Surgical treatment of this condition is considered a last resort. The piriformis muscle could be resected or could be released near its insertion at the superior aspect of the greater trochanter. Although these surgical procedures have been noted with some success and, one author stated, are not associated with postoperative disability, one should be skeptical. There should be certainty that symptoms are not arising from the lumbar spine or other structure and postoperative management of appropriate tissue healing should be worked out before surgery is attempted.

REHABILITATION

- With the lack of clinical trials supporting treatment efficacy, most evidence comes from clinical practice.
- Modalities that help reduce pain and inflammation, such as ultrasound, interferential current therapy, or cold pack, should be considered acutely and during highly irritable states, suggesting an inflammatory response.
- In the case of extremely irritable symptoms and antalgic gait, assistive devices, such as a single-point cane, can be used to decrease weight bearing on the affected leg and the strain on muscles, such as the piriformis, to help stabilize the pelvis during walking.
- Activity modification to avoid situations where prolonged sitting or standing, especially in known aggravating conditions like a very firm chair, is an important part of the patient education process.
- Soft tissue mobilization and hip joint mobilization should also be considered to help improve the mobility of surrounding structures. Care should be taken to match the appropriate soft tissue technique and vigor to the area secondary to the possible irritability or altered pain processing damage to neural structures.
- Other manual techniques, such as contract-relax, positional release, or strain-counterstrain, have been suggested to treat the piriformis.
- Treating the functional biomechanical deficits is also important to have successful outcomes. Stretching tight muscles that may alter normal movement is important. Strengthening the hip abductors and external rotators is a common beneficial addition to a treatment program to decrease strain on the piriformis.

PROGNOSIS

This condition is not life-threatening but can be associated with significant morbidity caused by pain and weakness. It is generally believed that if it is recognized early, the treatment outcomes are relatively good.

SIGNS AND SYMPTOMS INDICATING REFERRAL TO PHYSICIAN

- Unrelenting pain not related to biomechanical factors
- Weight loss
- Bowel or bladder dysfunction
- Saddle paresthesias
- Gait disturbances: Clumsiness or ataxic gait
- Bilateral glove or sock numbness
- Symptoms that do not initially improve

SUGGESTED READINGS

Butler DS. *The Sensitive Nervous System.* Adelaide, Australia: Noigroup Publications; 2000.

Butler DS. *Mobilisation of the Nervous System.* New York: Churchill Livingstone; 1991.

Dawson DM, Hallett M, Wilbourn AJ, eds. *Entrapment Neuropathies.* Philadelphia: Lippincott-Raven; 1999.

Moore KL, Dalley AF. *Clinical Oriented Anatomy.* 4th ed. Philadelphia: Lippincott Williams & Wilkins; 1999.

Placzek JD, Boyce DA, eds. *Orthopedic Physical Therapy Secrets.* 2nd ed. Philadelphia: Elsevier; 2006.

Shacklock M. *Clinical Neurodynamics.* Philadelphia: Elsevier; 2005.

http://www.emedicine.com/Orthoped/topic422.htm

AUTHOR: CHRIS IZU

BASIC INFORMATION

DEFINITION

Suprascapular nerve entrapment pathologies encompass any injury that interrupts the function of the suprascapular nerve at any point along its course. The loss of function results in muscle weakness, pain, or sensory dysfunction.

SYNONYMS

Bra strap palsy

ICD-9CM CODES
354 Mononeuritis of upper limb and mononeuritis multiplex
354.8 Other mononeuritis of upper limb
354.9 Mononeuritis of upper limb unspecified

OPTIMAL NUMBER OF VISITS

6

MAXIMAL NUMBER OF VISITS

20

ETIOLOGY

- The suprascapular nerve is derived from the upper trunk of the brachial plexus formed by the C5 and 6 nerve roots; however, up to 50% receive contributions from the C4 nerve root.
- The suprascapular nerve is a mixed sensory and motor nerve that descends along the posterior neck triangle, beneath the anterior border of trapezius, to the superior border of the scapula.
- The nerve passes into the supraspinous fossa through the suprascapular notch, and the roof is formed by the transverse scapular ligament.
- It supplies the supraspinatus, as well as receiving sensory articular branches from the glenohumeral and AC joints.
- The nerve then curves around the lateral edge of the base of the spine of the scapula by the spinoglenoid notch (in close proximity to the glenohumeral joint) to innervate the infraspinatus in the infraspinatus fossa.
- The nerve has no cutaneous component.
- The suprascapular nerve is particularly vulnerable to injury at the following two points along its course:
  ○ The suprascapular notch
  ○ The spinoglenoid notch
- The suprascapular nerve may be affected at any point along its course by direct trauma or compression entrapment, leading to nerve tissue hypoxia.
- The insult to the nerve can be mechanical, thermal, chemical, or ischemic.

- The suprascapular nerve is most commonly entrapped at the suprascapular and spinoglenoid notches.
- The pathophysiology of suprascapular nerve entrapment is usually related to a compressive lesion of the nerve; nevertheless, pathology can occur in a number of ways as follows:
  ○ Direct trauma in the form of a blow to the base of the neck or posterior shoulder
  ○ Shoulder dislocation leading to tractioning of the nerve
  ○ Scapular fracture
  ○ Compression entrapment within the suprascapular notch through hypertrophy of the transverse scapular ligament, a narrow suprascapular notch, or presence of a ganglion cyst
  ○ Compression of the nerve in the spinoglenoid notch by a ganglion cyst arising from the glenohumeral joint. Ganglion cysts may be formed as a result of degenerative shoulder conditions and also after acute glenoid labral lesions such as superior labrum from anterior to posterior (SLAP) lesions.
  ○ Overuse syndromes from repeated scapular motions leading to compression of the nerve
- Nerve injury is classified according to the severity of the injury and its potential for reversibility, as follows:
  ○ Neurapraxia (first-degree injury): Distortion of the myelin about the nodes of Ranvier caused by ischemia, mechanical compression, or electrolyte imbalance produces temporary loss of nerve conduction.
  ○ Axonotmesis (second-degree injury): Interruption of the axon with secondary wallerian degeneration. The supporting tissue surrounding the axon is preserved, and the recovery period depends on the distance between the site of injury and the end-organs.
  ○ Neurotmesis: Complete disruption of the nerve and its supporting structures.
- Neurotmesis has been further divided into the following three subcategories:
  ○ Third-degree nerve injury: Endoneurium is disrupted with intact perineurium and epineurium.
  ○ Fourth-degree nerve injury: All neural elements sparing the epineurium are disrupted.
  ○ Fifth-degree nerve injury: Complete transection and discontinuity of the nerve with no capacity for regeneration.
- Physiologically, there is disruption to any part of the nerve responsible for conduction.
- In repetitive-type nerve entrapment, it is proposed that repetitive work or static posture produces an inflammatory

process, fibroblasts appear to repair damage incurred but produce adhesions to the nerve limiting their glide and increasing anoxia.

EPIDEMIOLOGY AND DEMOGRAPHICS

- Relatively rare entrapment is seen in sports with repetitive cocking action such as tennis or volleyball.
- The cocking action involves end-range shoulder abduction, extension, and external rotation followed by rapid flexion and internal rotation.
- Suprascapular nerve injuries are often related to degenerative changes in the glenohumeral joint, and the incidence of entrapment increases with increasing age of the patient and with capsular laxity.
- Also seen in occupations involving carrying heavy objects on the shoulder such as a camera operator and furniture mover.

MECHANISM OF INJURY

- There are a number of mechanisms of injury for the suprascapular nerve that will be described in relation to their location:
  ○ Direct trauma in the form of a blow to the base of the neck or posterior shoulder
  ○ Shoulder dislocation leading to tractioning of the nerve, particularly if the shoulder is forced into end-range external rotation
  ○ Scapular fracture that distorts the bony confines of the suprascapular or spinoglenoid notches
  ○ The nerve may be stretched or kinked by extremes of scapular motion associated with the throwing action.
  ○ Kinking of the nerve can be exaggerated by a resting position of depression or forward rotation of the shoulder girdle.
  ○ Compression entrapment within the suprascapular notch through hypertrophy of the transverse scapular ligament, an anatomically narrow suprascapular notch, or presence of a ganglion cyst.
  ○ Compression at either notch from a tumor or varicosities
  ○ Compression of the nerve in the spinoglenoid notch by a ganglion cyst arising from the glenohumeral joint. Ganglion cysts may be formed as a result of degenerative shoulder conditions and also after acute glenoid labral lesions such as SLAP lesions.
  ○ Overuse syndromes from repeated scapular motions leading to compression of the nerve may occur in sports with repetitive overhead throwing action such as volleyball, serving in tennis, or baseball.

○ Compression of the nerve by weighted objects being carried repeatedly on the shoulder such as may occur with a barbell in weight lifting, camera work, backpacking, furniture removals, or other load-carrying occupations.

COMMON SIGNS AND SYMPTOMS

- Pain that is deep and poorly localized, often felt posterior and lateral in the shoulder or referred to the arm, neck, or anterior chest wall.
- Patients may describe shoulder weakness.
- Wasting of the supraspinatus and/or infraspinatus
- Weakness of abduction and external rotation
- May have tenderness over the suprascapular notch
- If there is combined supraspinatus and infraspinatus weakness, the entrapment is most likely to be at the suprascapular notch.
- Isolated infraspinatus weakness may occur when the nerve is compressed in the spinoglenoid notch and the motor branch to the supraspinatus is spared.
- Occasionally, deltoid muscle atrophy accompanies the injury because of disuse.

AGGRAVATING ACTIVITIES

- Activities that involve repetitive shoulder internal and/or external rotation, particularly when the shoulder is in an abducted position
- Activities that involve horizontal adduction of the arm, such as reaching across the chest, can exacerbate the pain
- Carrying loads on the top of the shoulder

EASING ACTIVITIES

Rest and/or modification of aggravating activities

24-HOUR SYMPTOM PATTERN

- Generally, the symptoms are related to activity and do not follow a typical 24-hour pattern unless there is a strong inflammatory component such as may be seen in repetitive tasks.
- If there is an inflammatory component, there may be worsening of symptoms with use toward the end of the day and morning stiffness.

PAST HISTORY FOR THE REGION

- History of trauma, fracture, or dislocation of the glenohumeral joint
- History of forceful scapular depression such as a fall onto the point of the shoulder
- Repetitive overuse of the shoulder in occupation or sports
- Generalized hypermobility

PHYSICAL EXAMINATION

- Examine the shoulder for signs of atrophy around the shoulder blade, particularly in the supraspinatus and infraspinatus fossae.
- MMT may reveal weakness in the following muscles:
  ○ Supraspinatus: Weakness of glenohumeral abduction can be assessed using the scaption position in which the shoulder arm is resisted in 90 degrees of flexion in the plane of the scapular.
  ○ Infraspinatus: Weakness of external rotation at the glenohumeral joint, particularly biased toward infraspinatus when external rotation is resisted in 90 degrees of shoulder abduction.
- There may be loss of fine proprioceptive control of the glenohumeral and AC joints due to the loss of afferent conduction. Therefore the therapist may notice an alteration in the control of those joints during functional movement patterns.
- Physical examination should also exclude pathology in other areas, particularly when performing AROM and PROM at the neck and shoulder, which may reveal restrictions, other shoulder pathology, and/or central involvement of the nerve.
- Physical examination should also include movement analysis to determine the movement patterns that the patient adopts when performing the aggravating activities. Movement analysis can be done visually or with the assistance of a video camera. The analysis should give some clues to predisposing factors, such as posture and patterning, that assist with rehabilitation and activity modification.

IMPORTANT OBJECTIVE TESTS

- EMG may reveal delayed conduction velocity and fibrillation potentials; however, EMGs are often reported as normal, and therefore a negative EMG does not rule out the diagnosis of suprascapular nerve entrapment.
- MRI is considered to be the most effective study for suprascapular nerve entrapment since it can reveal lesions to the glenoid labrum and the presence of a ganglion cyst in the region of the nerve.

DIFFERENTIAL DIAGNOSIS

Dx

- Rotator cuff tears
- Rotator cuff tendinopathies
- Subacromial bursitis
- Adhesive capsulitis
- Shoulder instability

- Degenerative joint disease at the glenohumeral or AC joints
- Underlying neuropathic disease
- Neuralgic amyotrophy
- Muscular dystrophy
- Isolated neuropathy in the diabetic
- Tumors or space-occupying lesions
- C4, C5, or C6 cervical radiculopathy
- Upper motor neuron lesion in the cerebrum

CONTRIBUTING FACTORS

- For any nerve entrapments that are non-traumatic, there is often an element of repetitive activity involving the affected limb.
- Typically, in the case of the suprascapular nerve, the repetitive action will involve shoulder abduction and repetitive internal and external glenohumeral rotation.
- Other repetitive tasks involving cross-body adduction, such as polishing or reaching repeatedly across the body, may create a traction neuropathy.
- Postural factors may be involved, particularly in repetitive work or sporting activities with reduction in proximal stability and control leading to an overuse of more distal muscle groups to perform a task.
- Excessive loads, such as in heavy manual work or sports involving weight lifting, can create compression of the nerve, particularly when the load is carried over the trapezius muscle.

TREATMENT

SURGICAL OPTIONS

- Surgery will be considered after a failure of conservative management.
- There are a number of surgical approaches to achieve decompression of the suprascapular nerve, involving enlargement of the suprascapular notch, as follows:
  ○ Anterior approach
  ○ Posterior trapezius splitting approach
  ○ Posterior trapezius elevating approach
  ○ Superior cranial approach
- When there is entrapment at the spinoglenoid notch, a different approach is required because generally there is an underlying shoulder pathology leading to the formation of a ganglionic cyst that compresses the nerve.
- Therefore, shoulder arthroscopy initially is performed to examine for a SLAP lesion, followed by debridement and repair if required. At the time of arthroscopy, the cyst can be evacuated and decompressed.

REHABILITATION

- The goal of rehabilitation should be pain reduction to encourage pain-free exercise and to provide task or sports reeducation and interventions leading to reacquisition of fine motor and sporting skills.

- Manual therapy
  - Pain reduction can be achieved through the use of ice and electrotherapeutic modalities.
  - Soft tissue release may assist with restoration of muscle balance around the scapula, which will be useful if compensations have occurred in other muscles to make up for the loss of rotator cuff control.
  - Nerve gliding exercises have been purported to disperse intraneural edema, increase blood flow, optimize axonal transport, and lengthen nerve adhesions. Neural mobilization can be achieved using scapular mobilization, both actively and passively into elevation, depression, protraction, and retraction
- Functional rehabilitation
  - Reeducation of movement patterns, particularly proximal control of the trunk and neck to provide a stable foundation for scapular stability
  - Scapular position education initially, with isometric hold and then the addi-

tion of controlled functional movement patterns
  - Specific muscle strengthening gradually increasing intensity to restore full power to the rotator cuff
  - Integration of functional exercise and strength work into sport- or task-specific skills
  - Graduated return to full strength, speed, and power.

PROGNOSIS

- Prognosis depends entirely on the extent of damage to the nerve.
- Neurapraxia should resolve rapidly and lead to a complete restoration of function usually within 2 to 3 months.
- If the injury is a more severe axonotmesis, the recovery time will depend on the distance from the site of injury to the denervated tissue. Peripheral nerves have been reported to recover at an approximate rate of between 1 and 4 mm per day, but complete function might not be restored.
- If there has been a complete sectioning of the nerve (neurapraxia), a full recovery will not occur.

- The results of treating neurapraxia even with surgical intervention are generally not satisfactory.

SIGNS AND SYMPTOMS INDICATING REFERRAL TO PHYSICIAN

If suprascapular nerve entrapment is suspected, all cases should be referred to a physician for appropriate investigation.

SUGGESTED READINGS

Aldridge JW, Bruno RJ, Strauch RJ, Rosenwasser MP. Nerve entrapment in athletes. *Clin Sports Med.* 2001;20(1):95.

Goslin KL, Krivickas LS. Proximal neuropathies of the upper extremity. *Neurol Clin.* 1999;17(3).

Kibler WB, Murrell GAC. Shoulder pain. In: Brukner P, Khan K, eds. *Clinical Sports Medicine.* 3rd ed. Australia: McGraw-Hill; 2006:243-288.

Leffert RD. Nerve lesions about the shoulder. *Orthop Clin North Am.* 2000;31(2).

Moore TP, Hunter RE. Suprascapular nerve entrapment. *Oper Tech Sports Med.* 1996;4(1):8-14.

AUTHOR: JOSEPHINE LOUISE COULTER

BASIC INFORMATION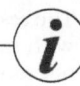

DEFINITION

Sural nerve entrapment is a mononeuropathy that results from compression or restriction of movement of the sural nerve, usually at the deep fascia of the leg in the calf and lateral lower leg region.

SYNONYMS

None currently used

ICD-9CM CODES
355.7 Other mononeuritis of lower
          limb

OPTIMAL NUMBER OF VISITS

6 or fewer

MAXIMAL NUMBER OF VISITS

20

ETIOLOGY

- Arising from branches off the tibial nerve, the sural nerve descends between the two heads of the gastrocnemius and becomes superficial at the middle of the leg. It descends along side the saphenous vein and passes inferior to the lateral malleolus to the lateral side of the foot.
- The sural nerve supplies the skin on the posterior and lateral aspects of the lower leg and lateral side of the foot up to the base of the fifth metatarsal.
- The sural nerve is believed to be purely sensory and has very little if any motor involvement. A few recent cadaver and clinical studies have found some motor fibers within the sural nerve. Still, the nerve is viewed primarily as a sensory nerve.
- Since the sural nerve becomes more superficial in the lower leg, it is believed to be more at risk of compression. Internal compression, such as a ganglion cyst or tumor, has been noted to compress the nerve. Stretch injuries may also create strain on the nerve and repetitive injuries or trauma may be the catalyst for more fibrotic scarring of the surrounding fascia that may entrap the nerve.

EPIDEMIOLOGY AND DEMOGRAPHICS

- This condition is thought to be relatively rare; although a small number of studies stated that it is a common syndrome in athletes.
- A gender difference has not been strictly reported, but one study of 13 patients with sural nerve entrapment noted that 11 were male and 2 were female.

MECHANISM OF INJURY

- Fractures: Fifth metatarsal, cuboid, calcaneus, fibula
- Lateral ankle sprains
- Peroneal tendon rupture
- Engorged lesser saphenous veins: Chronic venous insufficiency
- Ganglions
- Hematomas
- Postsurgical scarring
- Improper fitting boots

COMMON SIGNS AND SYMPTOMS

- Pain and dysesthesias in the sural nerve distribution, especially around the lateral ankle, are the most common sensory complaint.
- Gait deviations from pain with ankle or foot motions might also be noted in the present history.

AGGRAVATING ACTIVITIES

- Physical exertion with lower extremities
- Heel raises or going up on toes
- Prolonged standing
- Walking
- Running
- Cycling
- Wearing tight boots or hockey skates
- Calf stretches

EASING ACTIVITIES

- Rest
- Ice or modalities for inflammation
- Massage

24-HOUR SYMPTOM PATTERN

No writings on a particular pattern of symptoms were found for sural nerve entrapment. Increased symptoms at night or lasting symptoms in the morning may point to a strong inflammatory component to the symptoms. This may also suggest space-occupying lesion, such as a tumor, so careful attention should be paid to other factors and the progression of symptoms.

PAST HISTORY

No typical past history has been noted for sural nerve entrapment. One study's review of their participants noted that the leg of one subject, before onset of this problem, had been run over by a truck, possibly contributing to fibrotic scarring around the nerve. Following this theory, one might find a previous incident, trauma, or overuse that may have led to neurodynamic restrictions and internal changes in the nerve connective tissue or nerve itself.

PHYSICAL EXAMINATION

- The most common physical finding is altered sensation in the sural nerve's

sensory distribution in the lateral lower part of the leg, calf, and lateral ankle.
- Gait deviations might be noted and associated with changed mechanics caused by pain.
- It is important to note that normal muscle strength should be tested since this nerve is purely sensory. If weakness is found, another peripheral nerve or more proximal lesions, such as on the lumbar spine, must be examined.

IMPORTANT OBJECTIVE TESTS

- Lower quarter neurological examination is as follows:
  - Sensory examination: Light touch, pinprick, or sharp/dull may be used to determine altered sensation in a specific distribution.
  - Motor examination: No myotomal weakness should be noted with examination. However, pain may be noted with contracting muscle surrounding the nerve such as the gastrocnemius.
  - No reflexive changes should be noted.
  - Tinel's test: Tapping on the superficial regions of the nerve may reproduce symptoms into the specific nerve distribution.
  - Palpation: Muscles around the nerve, especially gastrocnemius, may reproduce symptoms or may have noted soft tissue restrictions that possibly indicate fibrotic scarring around the nerve.
  - SLR test (or slump test)
- A neurodynamic examination helps differentiate neurogenic (sural nerve) from nonneurogenic (gastrocnemius or peroneals) sources of symptoms.

DIFFERENTIAL DIAGNOSIS

- Local muscle strain
- Knee ligamentous strain
- Meniscal pathology
- Osteoarthritis
- Deep vein thrombosis
- Lumbar spine radiculopathy
- Lumbar spine stenosis
- Polyneuropathy

CONTRIBUTING FACTORS

- Running and overuse of the lower extremity muscles
- Poor lower quarter alignment
- Poor trunk or lower extremity
- Diabetes mellitus
- Alcoholism

TREATMENT

SURGICAL OPTIONS

- Surgical decompression may be recommended to release the nerve from surrounding fibrotic connective tissues.

- Surgical neurolysis is not recommended but may be done when the condition is unresponsive to other measures.

REHABILITATION

- The first goal of rehabilitation should be to decrease any inflammation or irritation around the nerve, thereby decreasing symptoms.
- Modalities, such as ultrasound, phonophoresis, iontophoresis, ice, interferential current therapy, or light massage techniques, may assist in decreasing symptoms.
- Taping, bracing, or footwear modification have also been suggested, which may help decrease strain on the affected region.
- If fibrotic scarring is one of the hypothesized mechanisms for sural nerve entrapment, then more vigorous massage techniques to free up the nerve may be beneficial. This could be followed up with neurodynamic techniques that attempt to glide, slide, or place tension on the nerve to restore normal mobility.
- It is also important to address any biomechanical faults that may be contributing to stress or strain on the sural nerve.

PROGNOSIS

No specific data on long-term outcomes were found after sural nerve entrapment. Because of the pure sensory function of the sural nerve, it is most likely not associated with high rates of morbidity. One author did suggest that return of sensation may take up to a year after surgery.

SIGNS AND SYMPTOMS INDICATING REFERRAL TO PHYSICIAN

- Unrelenting pain not related to biomechanical factors
- Weight loss
- Bowel or bladder dysfunction
- Saddle paresthesias
- Gait disturbances: Clumsiness or ataxic gait
- Bilateral glove or sock numbness
- Symptoms that do not initially improve with symptoms

SUGGESTED READINGS

Butler DS. *Mobilisation of the Nervous System*. New York: Churchill Livingston; 1991.
Butler DS. *The Sensitive Nervous System*. Adelaide, Australia: Noigroup Publications; 2000.
Dawson DM, Hallett M, Wilbourn AJ, eds. *Entrapment Neuropathies*. Philadelphia: Lippincott-Raven; 1999.
Moore KL, Dalley AF. *Clinical Oriented Anatomy*. 4th ed. Philadelphia: Lippincott Williams & Wilkins; 1999.
Placzek JD, Boyce DA, eds. *Orthopedic Physical Therapy Secrets*. 2nd ed. Philadelphia: Elsevier; 2006.
Shacklock M. *Clinical Neurodynamics*. Philadelphia: Elsevier; 2005.
http://www.emedicine.com/Orthoped/topic422.htm

AUTHOR: CHRIS IZU

BASIC INFORMATION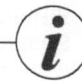

DEFINITION

Tibial nerve entrapment syndrome is a mononeuropathy that results from compression or restriction of movement of the tibial nerve, usually through the tarsal tunnel in the ankle.

SYNONYMS

Tarsal tunnel syndrome: Sometimes referred to as proximal tarsal tunnel syndrome since the distal tarsal tunnel may be used to describe the region in which the distal plantar branches of the tibial nerve may become entrapped.

ICD-9CM CODES
355.5 Tarsal tunnel syndrome

OPTIMAL NUMBER OF VISITS

6 or fewer

MAXIMAL NUMBER OF VISITS

20

ETIOLOGY

- The tibial nerve is a branch of the large sciatic nerve in the posterior leg that runs distally between the heads of the gastrocnemius muscle deep to the soleus muscle. It usually lies between the flexor digitorum longus and the tibialis posterior muscle. Traveling distally and posterior to the medial malleolus, it continues through the tarsal tunnel, where it eventually divides into the medial and lateral plantar nerves.
- The tibial nerve may become entrapped anywhere along its pathway, such as the popliteal fossa, but is most likely affected in the tarsal tunnel. The tunnel is formed by the medial surface of the talus, the inferomedial navicular, the sustentaculum tali, and the medial surface of calcaneus and the flexor retinaculum. The deep and superficial aponeuroses of the leg help form the flexor retinaculum, which is closely attached to the surrounding muscle sheaths.
- Compression of the tibial nerve can be from space-occupying lesions such as neuromas, ganglion cysts, lipomas, osteochondromas, tumors, or abnormal varicosities.
- Limited space within the tarsal tunnel may also be caused by tenosynovitis or rupture of adjacent tendons.
- Biomechanical factors have also been proposed as a cause of tibial nerve entrapment since it has been noted that pressure within the tarsal tunnel increases with full dorsiflexion/eversion of the foot and ankle and also full inversion. Abnormal standing postures or gait may continually put stress on the tarsal tunnel.
- Because of the network of fibrous connective tissue around the tarsal tunnel and surrounding musculature, it has also been suggested that limited mobility of the nerve may come from tethering of the nerve sheath to adjacent structures.

EPIDEMIOLOGY AND DEMOGRAPHICS

Of the nerves in the foot and ankle, the tibial nerve is the most likely to be entrapped. Some studies point to a slight female predominance, and in general the age ranges from about 14 to 80 years of age with a peak in the 50 to 60 years age range. It is common in nonathletes but also has been noted in distance runners.

MECHANISM OF INJURY

- A gradual or insidious onset is most commonly seen in this condition as space-occupying lesions continue to add compression to the area or biomechanical factors continue to strain local tissues.
- Types of injuries that may lead to tibial nerve entrapment include the following:
  o Direct blunt trauma
  o Traction injury
  o Repeated ankle sprains
  o Fractures of the surrounding bones

COMMON SIGNS AND SYMPTOMS

- Common symptoms of this condition are pain, burning, and paresthesias in the distribution of the tibial nerve on the plantar surface of the foot.
- Symptoms are generally unilateral but may be on both sides.
- Symptoms occasionally radiate more proximally into the medial leg.

AGGRAVATING ACTIVITIES

- Prolonged standing or walking
- Extreme dorsiflexion
- Increased weight-bearing activities
- Wearing nonsupportive shoes or sandals

EASING ACTIVITIES

- Rest and relief of weight-bearing activities
- Sitting
- Massage
- Ice or antiinflammatories

24-HOUR SYMPTOM PATTERN

- If there is a significant inflammatory component to the symptoms or a space-occupying lesion, more nighttime symptoms may be expected. Following this, symptoms may also be worse in the morning.
- Often, there is less pain in the morning after rest, but there may be pain on the first step when getting out of bed.

PAST HISTORY

Patients may note previous bouts with the same condition. They may also report previous lower extremity or lumbar spine injuries, which in turn might have affected lower quarter biomechanics. Patients may have a previous history of other space-occupying lesions, such as a Baker's cyst.

PHYSICAL EXAMINATION

- Abnormal foot or lower extremity alignment, such as a pes planus or pes cavus, may be noted. Looking from the more proximal view, it may be associated with tibial or femoral internal or external rotation. From the posterior view, the calcaneal position may also be altered.
- An examination of gait may also reveal a corresponding deviation with abnormal pronation or supination of the foot during the loading response to terminal stance phases.
- Palpation of the local areas most likely reproduce the patient's symptoms into the heel or foot.
- A sensory examination usually reveals abnormal sensation in the distribution of the tibial nerve.
- Neurodynamic testing most likely helps differentiate a neurogenic source of symptoms from other local or referred sources.

IMPORTANT OBJECTIVE TESTS

- Tinel's test: Tapping on the tarsal tunnel most likely reproduces the patient's symptoms in a tibial nerve distribution.
- Sensory examination: Using Semmes-Weinstein monofilaments, an area of altered or diminished sensation should be noted in the same distribution distal to the side of the lesion.
- Manual compression: Sustained pressure at the tarsal tunnel may also reproduce symptoms and help confirm diagnosis.
- Motor examination: Weakness might be found in plantar flexion of the ankle or in knee flexion.
- Gait examination: Contributing biomechanical factors during walking, jogging, or running need to be assessed since these may be impairments that could be addressed in rehabilitation.
  o Neurodynamic
  o Lower quarter neurological exam
  o Lumbar spine ROM
  o Lumbar spine palpation
  o Lumbar spine accessory motion: These tests are important to help determine contribution of proximal sources to the symptoms in the case of lumbar spine radiculopathy or double-crush.

DIFFERENTIAL DIAGNOSIS

- Lumbar spine radiculopathy
- Exostosis
- Malunions
- Osteochondromas
- Fractures
- Tibialis posterior tendinitis
- Plantar fasciitis
- Heel spur

CONTRIBUTING FACTORS

- Obesity
- Ankylosing spondylitis
- Acromegaly
- Talocalcaneal coalition
- Diabetes
- RA: Proliferative synovitis
- Foot deformities
- Varicose veins
- Alcoholism
- Thyroid disease

TREATMENT

SURGICAL OPTIONS

- Tarsal tunnel decompression has been shown to be fairly successful for short-term relief of symptoms. Some authors noted that 1 month after surgery, 24 out of 26 patients had good outcomes.
- In the case of cystic lesions, aspiration might also provide relief of pressure within the tarsal tunnel and reduce symptoms.
- A surgical release of the flexor retinaculum or removal of the space-occupying lesion are common procedures to address tarsal tunnel syndrome.
- From a clinician's perspective, it is important to follow surgery by addressing any biomechanical contributing factors that may have led to the condition.

REHABILITATION

- Rehabilitation of this condition should focus not only on alleviating the symptoms but also on the underlying cause of compression.
- NSAIDs and relative rest, ice, compression, and elevation (RRICE) should initially be implemented in acute or inflammatory stages to help relieve symptoms.
- In more severe cases, individuals with tibial nerve entrapment may benefit from immobilization, such as using a walking boot or cast or splint, and limiting weight bearing with use of assistive devices.
- Other modalities, such as ultrasound, interferential current therapy, or phonophoresis, may be administered to help with local symptoms.
- Taping and use of orthoses have clinically shown to be effective when addressing abnormal foot mechanics and positioning.
- If neurodynamic restriction is suspected, soft tissue mobilization and techniques to slide, glide, and place tension on the nerve as described by Butler may be warranted.
- More complete rehabilitation should also address other lower extremity or trunk impairments or motor control problems that may lead to increased pressure at the tarsal tunnel. For example, inadequate timing or force production of the gluteus medius during gait may influence the pronation component of the foot, leading to increased strain of the medial ankle structures.

PROGNOSIS

Another study following postoperative patients after tarsal tunnel release showed good-to-excellent results in 84% of cases. No statistics were found regarding improvement with conservative measures; however, clinically it is thought that with proper management of contributing factors, in the absence of a space-occupying lesion or marked fixed-foot deformity, outcomes are relatively good.

SIGNS AND SYMPTOMS INDICATING REFERRAL TO PHYSICIAN

- If suspected worsening compression on the nerve is suspected from a compartment syndrome, immediate referral to a physician is warranted. A fasciotomy may be done to release this pressure.
- Night pain and unrelenting symptoms may indicate a local tumor.
- Symptoms that do not improve within the expected time or that are not affected by physical therapy in a few visits should be referred to the physician because a space-occupying lesion may be present.
- A recent history of trauma with suspected fracture may need imaging studies done before starting treatment.
- Impaired circulation or vascular compromise may also warrant more medical management.

SUGGESTED READINGS

Butler DS. *Mobilisation of the Nervous System*. New York, NY: Churchill Livingston; 1991.

Butler DS. *The Sensitive Nervous System*. Adelaide, Australia: Noigroup Publications; 2000.

Dawson DM, Hallett M, Wilbourn AJ, eds. *Entrapment Neuropathies*. Philadelphia: Lippincott-Raven; 1999.

Moore KL, Dalley AF. *Clinical Oriented Anatomy*. 4th ed. Philadelphia: Lippincott Williams & Wilkins; 1999.

Placzek JD, Boyce DA, eds. *Orthopedic Physical Therapy Secrets*. 2nd ed. Philadelphia: Elsevier; 2006.

Shacklock M. *Clinical Neurodynamics*. Philadelphia: Elsevier; 2005.

AUTHOR: CHRIS IZU

BASIC INFORMATION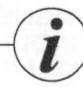

DEFINITION

- TOS encompasses numerous scenarios of compression (neurological and vascular) in the thoracic outlet region of the shoulder girdle. Although vascular and neurological classifications exist, it must be noted that these conditions can also be observed together. It is also believed that in 98% of TOS cases, the resultant symptoms are neurogenic. Defining the syndrome has been difficult in the literature because of its variable etiology and presentation and often minimal clinical findings.
- The following vascular TOS classifications exist:
  - Arterial TOS is caused by compression of the subclavian and/or axillary artery and is very uncommon, occurring in only 3% to 4% of cases.
  - Venous TOS is caused by compression of the subclavian and/or axillary vein and occurs in only 6% to 7% of cases.
- The subclavian vein and artery receive new nomenclature as the axillary vein and artery, once they pass the first rib).

SYNONYMS

- Cervical rib syndrome
- First rib syndrome
- Scalenus anticus syndrome
- Costoclavicular syndrome
- First thoracic rib syndrome
- Hyperabduction syndrome
- Scalenus medius syndrome
- Pectoralis minor syndrome
- Subcoracoid-pectoralis minor syndrome
- Brachiocephalic syndrome
- Paget-Schroetter syndrome (effort vein thrombosis of subclavian vein)
- Nocturnal paresthetic brachialgia
- Rucksack palsy
- Droopy shoulder syndrome
- Fractured clavicle-rib syndrome

ICD-9CM CODES
353 Nerve root and plexus disorders
442.82 Aneurysm of subclavian artery

OPTIMAL NUMBER OF VISITS
Not applicable

MAXIMAL NUMBER OF VISITS
Not applicable

ETIOLOGY

- Current belief of the cause of TOS is the underlying existence of bony or fibromuscular anomalies with overlying injury and/or spasm in the thoracic outlet region causing compromise. The anatomical anomalies are generally seen as predisposing factors.
- Bony anomalies can be congenital, traumatic, or posttraumatic and include the presence of: a cervical rib, elongated C7 transverse process, first rib deformity, displaced first rib fracture, excessive callus formation after first rib fracture, rib hemangioma, fractured or subluxed clavicle, and pseudarthroses.
- Cervical ribs are known to exist in approximately 0.5% of the population, with 10% to 20% resulting in symptoms, although this depends on their size.
- Soft tissue anomalies can also be congenital, traumatic, or posttraumatic and include altered scalene muscle insertions and origins, presence of scalenus minimus or scalenus pleuralis muscle, hypertrophy or injury of scalene muscles, presence of congenital fibromuscular bands (classified as type 1 to 10) or dense fibrous sheaths, cervical ligaments and band, and pectoralis minor shortening.
- The following three spaces in the thoracic outlet region have been identified as potential areas of vascular compression:
  - Interscalene space or triangle is bordered anteriorly by the anterior scalene muscle, posteriorly by the middle scalene muscle, and inferiorly by the first rib. Here the subclavian artery passes posterior to the anterior scalene muscle (in close relation with the brachial plexus), then superior to the first rib. The subclavian vein bypasses this space by traveling anteromedial to the anterior scalene muscle.
  - Costoclavicular space is bordered anteriorly by the medial aspect of the clavicle, subclavian muscle and tendon, and costocoracoid ligament. The posterolateral border is formed by the upper scapula, and the first rib and the anterior and middle scalene muscle insertions create the posteromedial border. Here the subclavian vein and artery travel with the brachial plexus under the clavicle and subclavius muscle toward the subpectoralis minor space.
  - Subpectoralis minor space is located inferior to the coracoid process and posterior to the pectoralis minor muscle insertion. Here the subclavian vein and artery continue to travel with the brachial plexus beneath the pectoralis muscle toward the axilla.
  - A further region involved in vascular TOS has also been described at the head of humerus, where the axillary artery gives off posterior humeral circumflex branches. This area is often not involved in vascular TOS but is commonly seen.
- Arterial TOS
  - Compression of the subclavian artery in TOS can be acute or chronic and can occur in the interscalene triangle, costoclavicular space, or subpectoralis minor space. This occurs as a result of underlying bony or fibromuscular anomalies with overlying muscle injury and/or spasm.
  - In most cases of arterial TOS, compression is caused by the tip of the cervical rib or an elongated C7 transverse process. Compression in the subpectoralis space is less common and is referred to as hyperabduction syndrome. This is in reference to the arm position during which the neurovascular structures are compromised.
  - Additionally, vascular compression has been reported to occur at the humeral head. Here the axillary artery may be tethered via its circumflex branches, as a result of excessive movement of the head of humerus.
  - Although rare, chronic compression can lead to occlusive and aneurysmal disease.
  - The subclavian artery sustains chronic intimal damage, which can result in either thrombosis or occlusion. Poststenotic dilations may also develop.
  - If the rate of occlusion is slow, the body is able to develop sufficient collateral circulation, so the patient may only feel symptoms with excessive arm use. Rapid occlusion creates more obvious claudication symptoms, as well as symptoms with minimal arm activity or at rest.
  - Damage to the full thickness of the subclavian artery wall (aneurysmal disease) can also produce debris, which may dislodge and create distal emboli in the arm, hand, or fingers.
- Venous TOS
  - Compression of the subclavian vein in the thoracic outlet region can have an acute onset (generally known as effort thrombosis or Paget-Schroetter syndrome) or an insidious one. The most common pathological cause of this syndrome is a congenital anomaly of the costoclavicular ligament combined with anterior scalene muscle hypertrophy, resulting in venous compression and occlusion.
  - Thromboses may also occur from subclavian venous catheters (intravenous [IV] therapy), dialysis treatment, and the presence of abnormalities in blood factors, antibodies, and proteins.
  - Chronic compression of the subclavian vein produces an inflammatory reaction, endothelial damage, and venous stasis.

EPIDEMIOLOGY AND DEMOGRAPHICS

- Arterial TOS is very rare.
- Arterial TOS occurs more often in the younger, active population.

- Arterial TOS occurs equally among males and females.
- Venous TOS is quite rare.
- Venous TOS occurs more often in the younger population.
- Venous TOS occurs most often in young males.

MECHANISM OF INJURY

- The most common cause of vascular TOS is repetitive strain through prolonged or vigorous upper limb activity. Other causes may include a history of whiplash and direct or indirect blows to the shoulder.
- The superimposed injury involved in causing TOS symptoms may include whiplash, direct or indirect blow to the shoulder, repetitive strain through prolonged upper limb activity, accessory breathing, and/or poor posture.
- Positions or postures that place increased strain on the vascular structures of the thoracic outlet include the following:
  - Prolonged writing or use of keyboard or telephone
  - Assembly line workers
  - Poor posture (i.e., droopy shoulders)
  - Prolonged overhead or reaching activity such as styling hair, painting, playing musical instruments (e.g., violin or flute), swimming, playing tennis, and pitching.
  - Excessive carrying of heavy objects such as suitcases and shopping bags
  - Prolonged carrying of a heavy backpack

COMMON SIGNS AND SYMPTOMS

- Note that despite the following classifications, some patients also demonstrate neurogenic TOS symptoms.
- Arterial TOS
  - Arm coldness, heaviness, pulselessness, pallor, loss of strength or fatigue with exercise (i.e., true arm claudication during activity, particularly overhead activity)
  - Weakened grip and reduced finger function (difficulty gripping and carrying bags)
- Venous TOS
  - Swelling, edema, cyanosis, and arm discomfort with activity
  - If the subclavian vein has thrombosed, the patient presents with a sudden onset of edema in the arm with associated discomfort and cyanosis.
  - Symptoms usually develop in the dominant arm

AGGRAVATING ACTIVITIES

- Overhead arm and hand positions or arm elevated repetitive activities. These commonly include styling hair, painting, working overhead, pitching or throwing a ball, playing musical instruments (e.g., violin or flute), and swimming.
- Carrying heavy objects such as suitcases and shopping bags

EASING ACTIVITIES

Rest from aggravating activities

24-HOUR SYMPTOM PATTERN

Unknown, not applicable, and not related to activity.

PAST HISTORY FOR THE REGION

- Arterial
  - The onset of symptoms usually reveals increased or unaccustomed prolonged or repetitive upper limb activity (i.e., pitching in baseball but may also be insidious in nature).
  - The patient may report a previous history of whiplash injury or a direct or indirect blow to the shoulder resulting in first rib, muscular, or clavicular trauma.
- Venous
  - The onset of symptoms usually reveals increased or unaccustomed prolonged or repetitive upper limb activity but may also be insidious in nature.
  - Recent use of a subclavian venous catheter (intravenous therapy) and dialysis treatment.
  - The patient may report a previous history of whiplash injury or a direct or indirect blow to the shoulder resulting in first rib, muscular, or clavicular trauma.

PHYSICAL EXAMINATION

- Arterial TOS
  - Loss or reduction of radial pulse with arm activity
  - Difference of blood pressure between the arms of >20 mm Hg
  - Positive Roos, Adson's, Halsted's, and Wright's hyperabduction tests
  - Loss of radial pulse and arm discomfort and/or development of arm pallor during the Roos test with subsequent hyperemia after lowering the arm
  - Coldness of hand and fingers
  - Trophic changes in fingernails or skin
  - Gangrene of finger tips (in extreme cases of peripheral embolization)
  - Pulsatile mass palpable in the supraclavicular fossa (not common but indicative of a subclavian aneurysm)
- Venous TOS
  - Superficial vein distention in upper limb and chest
  - Edema of the upper limb (measurement of limb girth)
  - Discoloration of the limb
  - Arm discomfort with activity
  - Positive Roos test: Development of cyanosis and arm swelling during test
- Any of the following physical findings of neurogenic TOS may also be present:
  - Poor posture (including downwardly rotated and protracted scapula, large breasts and/or obesity, or forward head posture)
  - Exaggerated upper chest or accessory breathing
  - Neurological tests negative
  - Altered neurodynamics on upper limb neurodynamic tests
  - Reproduction of arm pain or symptoms on palpation over brachial plexus
  - Positive Tinel's sign for reproduction of arm pain or symptoms over brachial plexus
  - Muscle spasm and/or shortening of anterior scalene muscle on palpation and length testing
  - Muscle spasm and/or shortening of pectoralis minor muscle on palpation and length testing
  - Ipsilateral elevated first rib

IMPORTANT OBJECTIVE TESTS

- Observation of the affected arm is important in the diagnosis of vascular TOS. Arm size, color, temperature, and pulses must be compared to the normal side at rest, during overhead activity, and after activity.
- Palpation of the supraclavicular fossa is important for detection of aneurysms.
- Three tests (Adson's, Halsted's, and Wright's hyperabduction tests) have traditionally been used to diagnose TOS because they monitor the radial pulse. These tests have been extensively discussed, criticized, and "modified" in the literature because of the high level of false positives and false negatives (many asymptomatic people demonstrate pulse changes during these tests).
- Roos test (elevated arm stress test), however, is described as the most reliable test for all types of TOS. If a patient is unable to complete the test because of their symptoms, it can also reflect the severity of their arterial or venous compromise.
- Patients may also demonstrate a bruit in the subclavian artery on auscultation during these tests indicating arterial TOS.
- Arterial TOS
  - Doppler studies
  - Arteriography in provocative positions and followed to digits to pick-up embolus
  - Magnetic resonance angiograms (MRAs)
- Venous TOS
  - Doppler studies
  - Positional venography
  - Coagulation studies

DIFFERENTIAL DIAGNOSIS

- Shoulder pathologies
  - Glenohumeral instabilities

- Subacromial or subcoracoid impingement
- Subacromial bursitis
- Glenohumeral labral tears
- Rotator cuff tendinopathies
- Cervical or thoracic pathologies
  - Cervical spondylosis
  - Cervical degenerative disc disease
  - Cervical nerve root syndrome
  - Cervical spine stenosis
  - Thoracic facet syndrome
  - T4 syndrome
  - Rib dysfunction
- Peripheral nerve entrapments
  - Ulnar nerve entrapment (cubital tunnel/Guyon's canal)
  - Median nerve entrapment (carpal tunnel/pronator teres)
  - Radial nerve entrapment (forearm)
- Other
  - Muscular dystrophy
  - Polymyositis
  - CRPS
  - Diffuse peripheral neuropathy
  - Angina and other cardiac conditions
  - RA
  - Lupus
  - Pancoast's tumor
  - Multiple sclerosis
  - Spinal cord lesion
  - Hypothyroidism
  - Pleuritis and other pulmonary conditions
  - Raynaud's phenomenon
  - Head, neck, or upper quadrant tumors
  - Lymphedema

CONTRIBUTING FACTORS

- Underlying existence of bony or fibromuscular anomalies in the thoracic outlet region
- Previous history of whiplash injury or a direct or indirect blow to the shoulder resulting in first rib, muscular, or clavicular trauma.
- Exposure to increased or unaccustomed prolonged or repetitive upper limb activity (e.g., overhead sport, occupation, playing a musical instrument)
- Presence of glenohumeral instability or hypertrophy of the humeral head or local muscular hypertrophy (arterial)
- Exposure to cold temperatures combined with trauma (venous)
- Presence of blood clotting factors (venous)
- The use of a subclavian venous catheter (IV therapy) and dialysis treatment (venous)

TREATMENT

SURGICAL OPTIONS

- The following is a list of current surgical techniques that are used alone or in combination to treat vascular TOS. The surgical techniques chosen depend on the degree of damage to the vessel, history of symptoms, and degree of compression in the thoracic outlet region.
- Arterial TOS
  - Rib resection (transaxillary approach)
  - Aneurysm resection with graft
  - Thrombectomy
  - Embolectomy
  - Artery reconstruction or replacement
  - Dorsal sympathectomy
- Venous TOS
  - Rib resection (transaxillary approach)
  - Scalenectomy
  - Fibrous band or adhesion resection
  - Thrombectomy (limited use)
  - Claviculectomy

SURGICAL OUTCOMES

- Arterial TOS
  - Good results are generally seen with surgery, although outcomes are less favorable with delayed diagnosis and surgery, and the presence of distal embolism (Durham et al 1995).
- Venous TOS
  - The combination of a prompt diagnosis, contrast venography with catheter-directed thrombolytic therapy, and consequent TOS decompressive surgery has shown very good results. Delayed thrombolytic therapy with surgery (>3 months from onset of condition) also had a less positive outcome.

SURGICAL INDICATORS

- Arterial TOS
  - Presence of arterial aneurysm, occlusion, or thrombosis
  - Persistence of symptoms
- Venous TOS
  - Presence of thrombosis
  - Persistence of symptoms
  - Positive venogram exhibiting compression at rest or during provocative testing.

REHABILITATION

- Surgical intervention is the mainstay of treatment of vascular TOS, although its use is more controversial in less serious cases. A patient is therefore more likely to present for postsurgical rehabilitation on the request of the vascular surgeon.
- The following rehabilitation guidelines are based on the principles of reducing ongoing trauma to the subclavian vessels in the thoracic outlet region, relieving symptoms, restoring upper limb function, and improving cardiovascular health. The guidelines are not meant to be used as a definitive postsurgical rehabilitation program.
- Refer to the neurogenic TOS section for additional rehabilitation techniques for patients who present with combined neurogenic and vascular TOS symptoms.
- Arterial TOS
  - Rest from aggravating activities
  - Postural or ergonomic advice
  - Lateral costal combined with diaphragmatic breathing techniques
  - Motor control and stability functional rehabilitation exercises for trunk, scapula, neck, and shoulder (especially in cases of axillary artery injury that present with an unstable head of humerus)
  - Gradual return to overhead arm activity
  - Progressive cardiovascular training program, especially for those in poor aerobic condition
- Venous TOS
  - Edema control (e.g., compression sleeves, bandages, and gloves and supported elevation)
  - Massage of upper limb to promote drainage of edema
  - Gentle exercises of upper limb to promote drainage of edema
  - Rest from aggravating activities
  - Postural or ergonomic advice
  - Lateral costal combined with diaphragmatic breathing techniques
  - Motor control and stability functional rehabilitation exercises for trunk, scapula, neck, and shoulder
  - Gradual return to overhead arm activity
  - Progressive cardiovascular training program, especially for those in poor aerobic condition

PROGNOSIS

- Arterial TOS
  - Since most cases of arterial TOS require surgery, the prognosis depends on surgical outcomes. Good results are generally seen with surgery, although outcomes are less favorable with delayed diagnosis and surgery and the presence of distal embolism.
- Venous TOS
  - Since most cases of venous TOS require surgery, the prognosis depends on surgical outcomes. The combination of a prompt diagnosis, contrast venography with catheter-directed thrombolytic therapy, and consequent TOS decompressive surgery has shown very good results. Delayed thrombolytic therapy with surgery (>3 months from onset of condition) had a less positive outcome. Conservative treatment tends to demonstrate the poorest outcomes.

SIGNS AND SYMPTOMS INDICATING REFERRAL TO PHYSICIAN

If vascular TOS is suspected, all cases should immediately be referred to a physician for prompt investigation and medical intervention.

SUGGESTED READINGS

Atasoy E. Thoracic outlet syndrome: anatomy. *Hand Clin*. 2004;20(1):7-14.

Ault J, Suutala K. Thoracic outlet syndrome. *J Man Manipulative Ther*. 1998;6(3): 118-129.

Brantigan CO, Roos DB, David B. Etiology of neurogenic thoracic outlet syndrome. *Hand Clin*. 2004a;20(1):17-22.

Brantigan CO, Roos DB. Diagnosing thoracic outlet syndrome. *Hand Clin*. 2004b;20(1): 27-36.

Crosby CA, Wehbé MA. Conservative treatment for thoracic outlet syndrome. Hand Clin. 2004 Feb;20(1):43-49, vi.

Dawson DM, Hallett M, Milender LH. *Entrapment Neuropathies*. 2nd ed. Boston: Little, Brown; 1990.

Demondian X, Herbinet P, Van Sint Jan S, Boutry N, Chantelot C, Cotton A. Imaging assessment of thoracic outlet syndrome. *Radiographics*. 2006;26:1735-1750.

Durham JR, Yao JST, Pearce WH, Nuber G, Mc Carthy WJ. Arterial injuries in the thoracic outlet syndrome. *J Vasc Surg*. 1995;21:57-70.

Edgelow PL. Chapter 7 Neurovascular consequences of cumulative trauma disorders affecting the thoracic outlet: a patient-centred treatment approach. In: Donatelli RA. *Physical Therapy of the Shoulder*. Philadelphia: Churchill Livingstone; 2003.

Mackinnon SE, Novak CB. Thoracic outlet syndrome. *Curr Probl Surg*. 2002;39(11): 1070-1145.

Pecina MM, Krmpotic-Nemanic J, Markiewitz AP. *Tunnel Syndromes: Peripheral Nerve Compression Syndromes*. 3rd ed. Boca Raton, FL: CRC Press; 2001.

Safran MR. Nerve injuries about the shoulder in athletes, Part 2: long thoracic nerve, spinal accessory nerve, burners/stingers, thoracic outlet syndrome. *Am J Sports Med*. 2007;32(4):1063-1076.

Sanders RJ, Hammond MD. Etiology and pathology. *Hand Clin*. 2004;20(1):23-26.

Sanders RJ, Hammond SL. Supraclavicular first rib resection and total scalenectomy: technique and results. *Hand Clin*. 2004;20(1):61-70.

Shebel ND, Marin A. Effort thrombosis (Paget-Schroetter Syndrome) in active young adults: Current concepts in diagnosis and treatment. *J Vasc Nurs*. 2006;24:116-126.

Urschel Jr HC, Kourlis Jr H. Thoracic outlet syndrome: A 50-year experience at Baylor University Medical Center. *Baylor Univ Med Cen Proc*. 2007;20(2):125-135.

Urschel Jr HC, Razzuk MA. Neurovascular compression in the thoracic outlet. changing management over 50 years. *Ann Surg*. 1998;228(4):609-617.

Vanti C, Natalini L, Romeo A, Tosarelli D, Pillastrini P. Conservative treatment of thoracic outlet syndrome: A review of the literature. *Eura Medicophys*. 2007;43(1):55-70.

Wehbe MA. Thoracic outlet syndrome. *Hand Clin*. 2004;20(1). Guest Editor.

Whitenack SH, Hunter JM, Read RL. Thoracic outlet syndrome: a brachial plexopathy. In: Mackin EJ, Callahan AD, Skirven TM, Schneider LH, Osterman AL, eds. *Rehabilitation of the Hand and Upper Extremity*. 5th ed. St Louis: Mosby; 2002.

AUTHOR: KATINA DIMOPOULOS

BASIC INFORMATION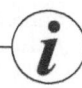

DEFINITION

Ulnar nerve entrapment pathologies encompass any injury that interrupts the function of the ulnar nerve at any point along its course. The loss of function results in muscle weakness, pain, or sensory dysfunction.

SYNONYMS

- Cubital tunnel syndrome
- Ulnar nerve palsy

ICD-9CM CODES
354   Mononeuritis of upper limb and mononeuritis multiplex
354.2   Lesion of ulnar nerve

OPTIMAL NUMBER OF VISITS

6

MAXIMAL NUMBER OF VISITS

20

ETIOLOGY

- The ulnar nerve is a mixed sensory and motor nerve derived from C8 and T1 nerve roots.
- It comes from the terminal branch of the medial cord of the brachial plexus.
- It travels within the axillary sheath posterior to pectoralis minor and continues medially to the axillary artery and the brachial artery to the middle of the arm.
- It becomes the ulnar nerve after piercing the intermuscular septum and follows the medial head of the triceps to the groove between the medial epicondyle and the olecranon.
- It then crosses the elbow, giving off articular branches to the elbow and motor branches to the flexor carpi ulnaris and the medial half of flexor digitorum profundus.
- It gives off a large dorsal sensory branch proximal to the wrist that supplies the skin of the dorsal wrist and ulnar side of the hand and continues into the hand via Guyon's canal, then splits into superficial and deep branches. Guyon's canal is bounded proximally and distally by the pisiform bone and the hook of hamate; it is covered by the volar carpal ligament and the palmaris brevis muscle.
- Superficial branch supplies the palmaris brevis, the skin of the hypothenar eminence, and digital nerves to the fifth and ulnar side of the fourth fingers.
- Deep branch passes between the abductor digiti minimi and flexor digiti minimi brevis with the deep branch of the ulnar artery.

- It perforates the opponens digiti quinti and follows the deep volar arch across the interossei and supplies the three small muscles of the fifth finger, third and fourth lumbricales, the volar and dorsal interossei, the adductor pollicis, and the deep head of flexor pollicis brevis
- The ulnar nerve is vulnerable to injury at several points along its course:
  - Proximally at the axilla
  - At the myofascial band, called the arcade of Struthers, proximal to the medial epicondyle
  - The medial head of triceps muscle
  - In the area of the medial epicondyle
  - Within the ulnar groove of the medial epicondyle
  - Within the cubital tunnel formed distal to the medial epicondyle as the nerve passes between the two heads of the flexor carpi ulnaris
  - At the flexor-pronator aponeurosis
  - Within Guyon's canal
- The ulnar nerve may be affected at any point along its course by direct trauma or compression entrapment leading to tissue hypoxia. The insult to the nerve can be mechanical, thermal, chemical, and ischemic.
- Nerve injury is classified according to the severity of the injury and its potential for reversibility:
  - Neurapraxia (first-degree injury): Distortion of the myelin about the nodes of Ranvier, caused by ischemia, mechanical compression, or electrolyte imbalance, produces temporary loss of nerve conduction.
  - Axonotmesis (second-degree injury): Interruption of the axon with secondary wallerian degeneration. The supporting tissue surrounding the axon is preserved, and the recovery period depends on the distance between the site of injury and the end-organs.
  - Neurotmesis: Complete disruption of the nerve and its supporting structures.
- Neurotmesis has been further divided into the following three subcategories:
  - Third-degree nerve injury: Endoneurium is disrupted with intact perineurium and epineurium.
  - Fourth-degree nerve injury: All neural elements sparing the epineurium are disrupted.
  - Fifth-degree nerve injury: Complete transaction and discontinuity of the nerve with no capacity for regeneration
- Physiologically, there is disruption to any part of the nerve responsible for conduction.
- In repetitive-type nerve entrapment, it is proposed that repetitive work or static postures produce an inflammatory process, fibroblasts appear to repair damage

incurred but produce adhesions to the nerve, limiting their glide and increasing anoxia.

EPIDEMIOLOGY AND DEMOGRAPHICS

- The ulnar nerve is the most commonly compressed nerve in the elbow region and is the second most common compressive neuropathy of the upper extremity.
- Males develop perioperative neuropathies of the ulnar nerve at the elbow more frequently than females possibly because females have more fat content in the medial elbow overlying the tubercle of the ulnar coronoid process (Berman).
- Most commonly seen in the throwing athlete but also seen in skiing, weight lifting, and racquet sports.

MECHANISM OF INJURY

- A number of mechanisms of injury for the ulnar nerve are described in relation to their location.
- Direct trauma at any point along the course of the nerve
- Proximally at the axilla through direct trauma or compression often sustained when the arm lies across a firm object such as a chair back for a sustained period of time or through the use of axillary crutches
- Compression beneath the arcade of Struthers, proximal to the medial epicondyle
- Compression from the medial head of triceps muscle, which, when hypertrophied, can snap over the medial epicondyle, causing friction neuritis.
- In the area of the medial epicondyle, a fracture callus or valgus deformity can chronically stretch the ulnar nerve.
- Frictional neuritis within the ulnar groove of the medial epicondyle if the groove is congenitally shallow or has a torn fibrous roof, allowing the nerve to sublux.
- Superficial compression at the elbow from repeated leaning on elbows or a direct blow.
- Compression within the ulnar groove by fracture fragments, spurs, soft tissue ganglia, or other space-occupying lesions.
- Compression within the cubital tunnel during elbow flexion as the tunnel flattens, causing pressure to increase around the nerve. For example, in the throwing athlete, the position of elbow flexion with wrist extension creates a threefold increase in pressure in the cubital tunnel; this increases to six times the resting pressure during the cocking position of a throw. Therefore repetitive pressure and stress on the nerve at this point can create cubital tunnel syndrome.

- Compression at the flexor-pronator aponeurosis as the nerve exits the flexor carpi ulnaris to perforate the fascial layer between flexor digitorum superficialis and flexor digitorum profundus.
- Compression within Guyon's canal by a fractured hook of hamate or ganglion

COMMON SIGNS AND SYMPTOMS

- Ulnar neuropathies often result in the following:
  - Sensory changes in the fourth and fifth digits: Feelings of tingling, numbness, or burning
  - Pain rarely occurs in the hand.
  - Pain tends to be felt farther up the arm toward the elbow.
  - Patients rarely notice the specific muscular atrophy, but it may be noticed by the clinician.
  - Wartenberg sign: Patient complains that the little finger gets caught on the edge of trouser pockets when attempting to put hands in pockets (patient cannot pull the fifth finger tightly against the fourth).
  - Patient may complain that their grip is weak.
  - Pincer grip may also be weak.
  - Difficulty opening jars or doors
  - Early fatigue or weakness if work requires repetitive hand motions.
  - Numbness and paraesthesias when resting on elbows
- Cubital tunnel syndrome generally-manifests as follows:
  - Medial elbow pain
  - Paraesthesia of the fifth digit and ulnar side of the fourth digit
  - Reduced fine motor control and weak grip
- Neural tension tests may reproduce the symptoms.
- The severity of complaints can vary from mild transient paresthesias in the fourth and fifth fingers to clawing of these digits, severe intrinsic muscle atrophy, and severe pain at the elbow and wrist with radiation into the hand or up into the shoulder and neck.

AGGRAVATING ACTIVITIES

- Tasks involving repetitive fine hand motions may reveal fatigue and weakness.
- Sports involving repetitive throwing actions with forceful elbow flexion and rapid extension
- Occupational tasks involving sustained elbow flexion such as computer work or assembly line tasks
- Leaning on elbows, particularly on hard surfaces

EASING ACTIVITIES

Rest and/or modification of aggravating activities

24-HOUR SYMPTOM PATTERN

- Generally, the symptoms are related to activity and do not follow a typical 24-hour pattern unless there is a strong inflammatory component such as may be seen in an occupational repetitive task.
- If there is an inflammatory component, there may be worsening of symptoms with use toward the end of the day and morning stiffness.

PAST HISTORY FOR THE REGION

- History of trauma, fracture, dislocation, or blow to the ulnar nerve distribution.
- Repeated activity repetitive elbow flexion and extension such as may occur in forceful throwing activities such as pitching in baseball
- Occupations involving sustained elbow flexion

PHYSICAL EXAMINATION

- Examine the limb for signs of autonomic dysfunction trophic changes such as edema, inflammation, and alteration in skin texture
- Examine the limb for any characteristic posturing of the hand; with chronic ulnar neuropathy the hand may develop a claw appearance, with the fourth and fifth digits flexed.
- The clinician may note wasting of the hand intrinsics.
- Froment sign: The patient is unable to tightly grasp a piece of paper between the index finger and thumb because of weakness of the adductor pollicis and first dorsal interosseous muscles. The thumb also may flex at the interphalangeal joint because the flexor pollicis longus activates in an attempt to compensate for the weakness.
- MMT may reveal weakness in any of the following muscles:
  - Dorsal interossei
  - Volar interossei
  - Abductor digiti minimi
  - Flexor digitorum profundus
  - Flexor carpi ulnaris
- To measure flexor carpi ulnaris and flexor digitorum profundus strength, ask the patient to cross the third finger over the fourth finger
- If the neuropathy occurs at the wrist, there will be weakness of hand intrinsics with the forearm flexors spared, which generally implies that the compression has occurred at Guyon's canal.
- Intrinsic weakness with no sensory loss would imply that the deep branch has been compressed after the bifurcation from the superficial sensory branch.
- Sensation: The cutaneous branch of the ulnar nerve supplies the fifth finger and the ulnar side of the fourth digit. Sensation testing should include pinprick, two-point discrimination, tuning

fork, and joint position sense and should be compared for asymmetry with the unaffected side (where available).
- Tinel's sign may be positive at the elbow in the ulnar groove or over the cubital tunnel.
- Physical examination should also exclude pathology in other areas, particularly performing AROM and PROM at the neck and shoulder, which may reveal restrictions and central involvement of the nerve.
- Upper limb neural tissue provocation testing may reveal changes in nerve mobility and elicit symptoms.
- Physical examination should also include movement analysis to determine the movement patterns that the patient adopts when performing the aggravating activities. Movement analysis can be done visually or with the assistance of a video camera. The analysis should give some clues to predisposing factors, such as posture and patterning, that will assist with rehabilitation and activity modification.

IMPORTANT OBJECTIVE TESTS

- The earliest electrodiagnostic sign of entrapment is a loss of the nerve action potential seen during a nerve conduction study.
- To isolate the specific location of the conduction block, serial stimulations are delivered to the nerve above and below the suspected lesion.
- Needle EMG is valuable for evaluating the extent of motor fiber loss within a nerve territory. EMG assists with determining the location of the injury and monitoring progression over time.
- MRI is increasingly being used in the assessment of peripheral nerve injuries to rule out cervical nerve root involvement and to determine the presence of edema, space restriction, or a space-occupying lesion along the course of the ulnar nerve.
- Ultrasonography can detect cysts in Guyon's canal.

DIFFERENTIAL DIAGNOSIS

- Medial epicondylitis
- Thoracic outlet syndrome
- Ulnar artery aneurysms or thrombosis at the wrist
- Underlying neuropathic disease
- Idiopathic brachial neuritis
- Myopathies
- Muscular dystrophy
- Isolated neuropathy in the diabetic
- Tumors or space-occupying lesions
- Cervical radiculopathy
- Upper motor neuron lesion in the cerebrum

CONTRIBUTING FACTORS

- Fracture or dislocation of the elbow, particularly if it results in increasing valgus deformity of the forearm away from the midline.
- Repetitive throwing action
- Occupations requiring significant elbow flexion throughout the day such as typing, computer work, or assembly line work
- Repeatedly leaning heavily on the elbows, particularly on hard surfaces
- Nerve compressions are more common in people with arthritis, diabetes, thyroid problems, and alcoholism.

TREATMENT

SURGICAL OPTIONS

- Indications for surgery include the following:
  - No improvement in the presenting symptoms after 6 to 12 weeks of conservative treatment
  - Progressive palsy or paralysis
  - Clinical evidence of long-standing lesion: Clawing of fourth and fifth digits and muscle wasting
- Several surgical options have been reported to relieve ulnar nerve compression, including the following:
  - In situ decompression
  - Medial epicondylectomy with or without decompression
  - Anterior transposition
  - Intramuscular transposition

REHABILITATION

- The goals of rehabilitation should be pain reduction to encourage pain-free exercise, to provide ergonomic education and interventions, and if the neuropathy has been prolonged, to introduce cortical reorganization activities.
- Splinting should be used to provide immobilization to allow the reduction in swelling and inflammation. Night splinting in 45 degrees of elbow flexion with a neutrally rotated forearm can be used.
- Avoid leaning on the elbows.
- Eliminate aggravating tasks by avoiding or modifying those tasks to prevent further damage.
- Use ice to reduce inflammation and prevent secondary cell damage.
- Theoretically, ultrasound may help promote nerve regeneration, improve profusion to the healing nerve, and decrease inflammation.
- Direct low-intensity electrical stimulation has been found to increase the number of vasa nervorum and nerve fiber density in rats.
- Nerve-gliding exercises have been purported to disperse intraneural edema, increase blood flow, optimize axonal transport, and lengthen nerve adhesions. Neural mobilization can be assessed using the brachial plexus provocation test positions to identify symptom reproduction, and these positions and movements can also be used both actively and passively for a treatment technique.
- Use of soft tissue mobilization and muscle stretching techniques to reduce fibrous bands and adhesions in muscles surrounding the ulnar nerve. Stretches must not produce tingling or discomfort because this may indicate decreased blood flow to the already stressed nerve.
- Motor control and stability functional rehabilitation exercise for proximal muscles of the trunk, neck, and shoulder
- Gradual introduction of strengthening exercises for any muscles that have been subjected to motor loss
- Ergonomic interventions, work place assessment, or provision of ergonomic aids, such as tilted keyboards or altered mouse shape
- Cortical reorganization techniques such as use of mirror box
- Reacquisition of fine motor and dexterity skills

PROGNOSIS

- Prognosis depends entirely on the extent of damage to the nerve.
- Neurapraxia should resolve rapidly and lead to a complete restoration of function, usually within 2 to 3 months.
- If the injury is a more severe axonotmesis, the recovery time depends on the distance from the site of injury to the denervated tissue.
- Peripheral nerves have been reported to recover at an approximate rate of between 1 and 4 mm per day, and recovery may not result in a complete restoration of function.
- If there has been a complete sectioning of the nerve (neurapraxia), a full recovery will not occur. The results of treating neurapraxia, even with surgical intervention, are generally not satisfactory.
- In chronic palsy, surgical outcome is less certain and improvement may be limited.

SIGNS AND SYMPTOMS INDICATING REFERRAL TO PHYSICIAN

If ulnar nerve entrapment is suspected, then all cases should be referred to a physician for appropriate investigation.

SUGGESTED READINGS

Bencardino JT, Rosenberg ZS. Entrapment neuropathies of the shoulder and elbow in the athlete. *Clin Sports Med.* 2006;25:465-487.

Berman SA. Ulnar neuropathy. *Emedicine.* www.emedicine.com/neuro/topic387.html; 2007.

Izzi J, Dennison D, Noerdlinger M, Dasilva M, Akelman E. Nerve injuries of the elbow, wrist, and hand in athletes. *Clin Sports Med.* 2001;20(1).

Pratt N. Anatomy of nerve entrapment sites in the upper quarter. *J Hand Ther.* 2005;18(2):216-229.

Stern M. Ulnar nerve entrapment. *Emedicine.* www.emedicine.com/Orthoped/topic574.html; 2004.

AUTHOR: JOSEPHINE LOUISE COULTER

BASIC INFORMATION

DEFINITION

- Central pain arises from lesions within the central nervous system (CNS).
- It is often difficult to distinguish between this type of pain and other peripheral causes.
- It is important to differentiate central pain from central sensitization, in which the pain-generating site is outside the CNS in the periphery and modified within the CNS.
- Most views of central pain are of excruciating symptoms leading to very debilitating conditions. Although symptoms can be very intense and extensive, this is not always the case.

DIAGNOSIS

- For the patient's symptoms to be considered central pain they must have a confirmed or suspected CNS dysfunction. This is usually clear, such as in the case of a brain infarct, but it may be more minor in the case of either a mild spinal cord injury (SCI) or minor stroke.
- Neurological symptoms should arise on examination and may require laboratory examinations such as computed tomography (CT), x-ray, magnetic resonance imaging (MRI), assays of cerebrospinal fluid (CSF), and neurophysiological examinations.
- Before a central pain diagnosis is determined, an attempt must be made to rule out other peripheral causes, such as peripheral neurogenic pain or polyneuropathy.

ICD-9CM CODES
Multiple ICD-9CM codes are used with the CNS diagnosis.

OPTIMAL NUMBER OF VISITS
12 or fewer

MAXIMAL NUMBER OF VISITS
32

ETIOLOGY

- The underlying mechanisms of central pain are very complex and at this time not well understood.
- Some confidence is shared by most that the lesions within the CNS are located within the structures involved in somatic sensibility.
- Current theories supported by some research and case studies include lesions within the spinothalamic tract, which is responsible for processing pain and temperature, and a possible lesion within the dorsal column–medial lemniscal tract, which deals with epicritic sensations (fine touch, vibration, and proprioception).
- In the case of central pain, lesions in the spinothalamic pathways may disrupt thermosensory integration and regulation along with the loss of cold inhibition and burning pain. The projections into the thalamic nuclei may release abnormal activity leading to increased pain and hypersensitivity.
- Other theories include mechanisms that are similar to complex regional pain syndrome (CRPS), in which the altered sympathetic nervous system can affect sensory processing and motor output. Refer to the section on CRPS for further details.
- These mechanisms are poorly understood because of the following:
  - Research on central pain is quite difficult and seems to rely heavily on case reports and animal models.
  - There may be several different mechanisms at hand since different pathophysiological changes may be at work at different parts of the CNS.
  - It has been well documented that the same kind of lesion in different individuals may have very different presentations.
  - It is also difficult at times to distinguish between central pain and other pain mechanisms, especially when both may be present.

MECHANISM OF INJURY

- It is important to note that both slow and rapid developing injuries can lead to central pain. Examples include:
  - Brain hemorrhages
  - Brain infarcts
  - SCI
  - Arteriovenous (AV) malformation
  - Syringomyelia
  - Multiple sclerosis (MS)
  - Epilepsy
  - Brain tumors
  - Brain abscess
  - Parkinson's disease (PD)
- Lesions that have been found to lead to central pain can vary enormously in size, location, and structure. Also, increasing the size of the lesion does not seem to increase the risk of developing symptoms.

EPIDEMIOLOGY AND DEMOGRAPHICS

- It seems that certain pathologies have higher risk in the development of central pain. Some research has listed the prevalence in specific populations as follows:
  - 30% of patients with SCI
  - 28% of patients with MS
  - 10% of patients with PD
  - 8.4% of patients after cerebrovascular accident (CVA)
  - 2.8% of patients with epilepsy

COMMON SIGNS AND SYMPTOMS

- Symptoms may vary widely between patients with the same type of lesions or even within the same patient.
- The location of pain is usually thought to be more extensive and may cover large areas of the body. It may extend over an entire extremity, such as the right or left side of the body, or even the upper or lower half. Small areas of pain, such as the ulnar border of the hand or portions of the face, have also been documented, so a large spread of symptoms is not a necessity for a diagnosis of central pain.
- Although burning is the most common complaint regarding quality of symptoms, there is a wide variety of pain descriptions in this population. Some range from common aching or pressure that might accompany peripheral nociceptive dysfunction to very descriptive language such as "boiling hot," deep as though in the bones, "showers of pain like electric shocks," or "red-hot needles evoked by touch."
- The intensity of pain can also vary greatly and is not always excruciating, as commonly believed. It can vary from very low to extremely intense, and either way it is usually perceived as more severe because of the quality and the more constant nature of symptoms.
- More commonly, the symptoms start a couple weeks after the initial insult to the CNS but may be delayed up to several years after onset of the lesion.

AGGRAVATING ACTIVITIES

- Psychological stress
- Cutaneous stimuli
- Body movements or limb movements
- Changes in posture
- Walking
- Stretching
- Visceral stimuli
- Change in emotions or mood

EASING ACTIVITIES

- Rest
- Medications
- Avoiding aggravating activities

24-HOUR SYMPTOM PATTERN

Research has not pointed toward a specific pattern in symptoms throughout the day, especially since symptoms are more likely to be constant. Some have noted some mid-day relief of symptoms with certain pathologies, but this is not thought to be consistent across the board.

PAST HISTORY

Because of the possibility of delayed onset of symptoms from earlier pathology, patients should have a CNS insult somewhere in their history that can be related to the pain.

PHYSICAL EXAMINATION

- Physical findings vary widely and may be inconsistent with a more peripheral neurogenic or nociceptive mechanism.
- Most likely, neurological findings or symptoms suggest a CNS pathology that accompanies the central pain.

IMPORTANT OBJECTIVE TESTS

- Neurological testing, including a thorough sensory examination that assesses vibratory sense, tactile sense, graphesthesia, temperature, pin prick, and deep pressure.
- Functional testing and questionnaires are important to assess the current level of pain and to help guide treatment.
- Strength, range of motion (ROM), gait, and balance are also important to consider when addressing any pertinent impairments leading to loss or function or disability.

DIFFERENTIAL DIAGNOSIS **Dx**

- Peripheral neurogenic and peripheral nociceptive mechanisms are important to consider since management differs widely from the management of symptoms from central pain. It is possible that both central and peripheral mechanisms could be present. An example is an individual with a recent CVA and subluxed shoulder who may present with lesions in the brain leading to central pain and nociceptive mechanisms at the shoulder.
- Psychological dysfunction may also mimic symptoms of central pain; however, this is less likely than originally believed.

CONTRIBUTING FACTORS

There have been no suggestions as to the mechanisms of why one individual might develop central pain once the CNS insult has occurred. It has been noted that the same lesion that causes central pain in one individual may be asymptomatic in another individual. There are certain pathologies, such as SCI, that do show a higher prevalence in the future development of central pain.

TREATMENT

MEDICAL/SURGICAL OPTIONS

- Medications for the treatment of central pain include the following:
  - Antidepressants
  - Antiepileptics
  - Antiarrhythmics
  - Local anesthetics
  - Adrenergic drugs
  - Cholinergic drugs
  - GABAergic (gamma-aminobutyric acid–ergic) drugs
  - Glutaminergic drugs
  - Naloxone
  - Neuroleptics
- Procedures such as cordotomy and cordectomy have been performed to attempt to alleviate the symptoms of central pain. Other suggested procedures include mesencephalic tractotomy, thalamotomy, and cortical or subcortical ablation.
- Sensory stimulation, such as dorsal column stimulation or deep brain stimulation, has also been used to treat central pain. Deep brain stimulators have been shown to be more effective but are reserved for only severe, nonresponsive cases.

SURGICAL OUTCOMES

Surgical outcomes are unknown.

REHABILITATION

- Although pain is usually the main complaint of individuals with central pain, it is not necessarily the focus in rehabilitation. Alleviating symptoms is a complex and difficult task that will most likely include multiple professionals working in concert.
- Patient education is an important task to consider, including explaining the proposed mechanisms of pain and establishing appropriate short- and long-term functional goals in therapy.
- The main focus in therapy should be on increasing activity, decreasing impairment, and decreasing disability, while limiting functional decline.
- Some research has suggested transcutaneous electronic nerve stimulation (TENS) may provide some relief for some central pain while having minimal adverse affects.
- Patient positioning, including limb segments, posture, and ergonomics, should be addressed since this may help reduce the symptoms.

PROGNOSIS

For most patients who experience central pain, the symptoms are permanent. In some, they may completely resolve with the chance of remission later. Symptoms may reflect the state of the underlying disease process in which some of the CNS disorders are chronic progressive illnesses.

SUGGESTED READINGS

Boivie J. Central pain. In: Wall PD, Melzack R, eds. *Textbook of Pain*. 4th ed. Philadelphia, PA: Churchill Livingstone; 1999.

Butler DS. *The Sensitive Nervous System*. Adelaide, Australia: Noigroup Publications; 2000.

Placzek JD, Boyce DA, eds. *Orthopedic Physical Therapy Secrets*. 2nd ed. Philadelphia, PA: Elsevier; 2006.

AUTHOR: CHRIS IZU

BASIC INFORMATION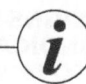

DEFINITION

Chronic pain has varying definitions, but all refer to the persistence of pain past the normal expected time for tissue healing. Long noted that chronic pain syndrome can be used to describe individuals who irrespective of the cause of pain, present similarly. Despite possible healing of tissue and lack of damage to the involved area, their bodies seem to have developed a "memory" for pain (see section on Common Signs and Symptoms).

ICD-9CM CODES
No specific codes are used to denote chronic pain, since ICD-9CM codes are based more on body region.

OPTIMAL NUMBER OF VISITS
12 or fewer

MAXIMAL NUMBER OF VISITS
24

ETIOLOGY
- Most of the research on chronic pain has dealt with chronic low back pain because of its high prevalence in society and its overall cost in the medical system. The cause of chronic low back pain is still poorly understood. Some hypothesize that it may be due to overt instability, especially since research has illustrated the lack of spontaneous recovery of the multifidus after lumbar spine injury.
- It is poorly understood why individuals with identical injuries, similar anatomical findings, similar health backgrounds, and similar management develop different responses: One may develop chronic pain and the other's pain may resolve. Intuition and some clinical research point to complex biopsychosocial factors at play. Several physiological mechanisms have been proposed.
- High-intensity noxious stimuli can alter both CNS and peripheral mechanisms in the case of chronic pain. Some examples include the following:
  - Increased dorsal horn neural activity
  - Increased temporal and spatial summation of nociceptive input from receptive field expansion and decreased threshold
  - Increases in immediate gene and dynorphin expression
  - Increased nitric oxide synthesis in the spinal cord, further facilitating the pain cycle
  - Increased sensitization or surrounding areas (secondary hyperalgesia)

- Sympathetically maintained is also a proposed mechanism for some forms of chronic persistent pain such as CRPS (see section on CRPS).
- Chronic neuropathic pain can be maintained by the mechanisms mentioned, while also sensitizing the nociceptors of the affected nerve root.
- Chronic muscular pain may also trigger these mechanisms while showing some peripheral histological finding, such as in the case of trigger points, in which transient overload of muscles may cause damage to the sarcoplasmic reticulum, causing local fiber perpetual contraction and impaired calcium uptake.

EPIDEMIOLOGY AND DEMOGRAPHICS

Chronic back pain has been found to be the most common complaint to primary care physicians in developing countries.

MECHANISM OF INJURY
- No one specific type of injury has been thought to lead to more chronic pain conditions. However, clinically, persistent low back pain and neck pain after traumatic causes, such as a motor vehicle accident, are common injuries that have led to such a syndrome.
- It has been noted that early and successful analgesic treatments and even preemptive analgesia during injury or surgery may play a role in decreasing the chance of developing persistent pain. The initial management and reduction of inflammation and pain may help to minimize the CNS and peripheral pain mechanisms.

COMMON SIGNS AND SYMPTOMS
- Patients with chronic pain are preoccupied with pain, and it is the pain itself that becomes the cause of impairment.
- Depression and anxiety are found in a high percentage in these individuals.
- An unusually high incidence of psychiatric diagnoses can be found in this population, with many features suggesting personality disorder.
- These patients use medical resources heavily, and drug misuse is common.
- Disability is found regularly, although they do not seem to have different diagnoses or anatomical differences from other individuals with persistent pain and similar complaints.

AGGRAVATING ACTIVITIES
- Usually, the same activities that may aggravate the acute condition of the initial injury are present in the chronic state, but the response may be elevated or persist past what is expected.

- Although most have true diagnoses with or without altered CNS pain processing, it is important to note the possibility of malingering and secondary gain.

EASING ACTIVITIES

Similar easing factors should be noted for chronic conditions, but their real or perceived effect may be diminished as a result of the focus on or preoccupation with the pain.

24-HOUR SYMPTOM PATTERN

In general, it would seem that more chronic or elevated states of pain may be more constant throughout the day. An individual preoccupation with pain may increase the chance of sleep disturbance or more pain on waking. In some cases, such as noted with fibromyalgia, lack of sleep and/or poor sleep are part of the disorder that can perpetuate the symptoms.

PAST HISTORY

Most individuals with chronic pain have had a history of similar episodes or may be able to trace back the initial start of pain to a particular traumatic injury or surgery.

PHYSICAL EXAMINATION

The goals of the physical examination are no different if a chronic pain syndrome is suspected. However, when collecting examination data, the therapist needs to remember that when altered processing of pain in the CNS exists, a painful response with testing may not give therapist the same information related to actual tissue damage as it may in a normal adaptive pain mechanism.

IMPORTANT OBJECTIVE TESTS
- The same objective test should be performed for the hypothesized source of symptoms or movement dysfunctions.
- Functional testing may be extremely important in this population of patients since treatment may later attempt to shift the focus to more functional-based goals rather than pain remediation.
- Waddell signs are commonly used to help determine the possibility of nonorganic or psychological aspects of chronic pain syndrome and help predict patients who may have poor outcomes or may be malingering. They include the following:
  - Superficial nonanatomical tenderness
  - Pain with axial loading on top of the head
  - Increasing back pain with twisting as a unit
  - Discrepancy between straight leg raise testing in sitting and supine

- o Nonphysiological regional disturbances in pain distribution, sensation, or weakness
- o Excessive verbalizations, facial grimacing, and other behaviors out of proportion to the test stimulus

DIFFERENTIAL DIAGNOSIS **Dx**

- Before assuming that a chronic pain syndrome exists, it is important to rule out organic or psychological causes for an individual's persistent pain. Some causes are as follows:
  - o Fracture
  - o Tumor
  - o Infection
  - o Rheumatoid arthritis (RA)
  - o Ankylosing spondylitis
  - o Psoriatic arthritis
  - o Acromegalia spondylitis
  - o Fibromyalgia
  - o Myofascial pain syndrome associated with human immunodeficiency virus/acquired immunodeficiency syndrome (HIV/AIDS)
  - o Depression
  - o Somatoform disorder

CONTRIBUTING FACTORS

- Some evidence supports a heritable basis for some neurological conditions, such as neuropathic pain; thus genetic factors may play a role in chronic pain.
- With the high prevalence of depression, anxiety, and features consistent with personality disorder among individuals with chronic pain syndrome, some believe that these psychological features may contribute to its development. It is hard to confirm that belief as a higher percentage of these individuals are thought to develop depression as a result of the chronic pain. Either way, it is most likely a contributing factor to the maintenance of chronic pain syndrome.

TREATMENT

SURGERY

Not generally applicable

REHABILITATION

- A growing emphasis on active treatment and patient education for individuals with chronic pain syndrome has been seen.
- Patient education on pain mechanisms intuitively seems to be a beneficial way to help address and possibly limit preoccupation or fear associated with the chronic pain symptoms.
- Setting appropriate short- and long-term goals that shift the focus away from pain and more to improving function, as well as minimizing impairments and disability, is recommended.
- Long suggested that an exercise program that has been designed not only to address specific impairments but also to implement "behavior techniques that promote wellness behaviors and extinguish pain behaviors" may be beneficial to this population.
- Physical modalities, manipulation, and mobilization can be affective for dealing with some symptoms, although caution should be used when incorporating this into treatment as a result of the possible shift in focus back to the symptoms of pain compared to improving function and ability.

PROGNOSIS

- It has been noted that with chronic back pain, symptoms that are more mechanically related and not radicular in nature do have a favorable prognosis and respond well to treatment.
- For individuals with chronic pain syndrome, the prognosis is widely varied, most likely a result of the complex interaction of biopsychosocial factors leading to the maintenance of the symptoms.

SIGNS AND SYMPTOMS INDICATING REFERRAL TO PHYSICIAN

- For chronic low back pain: Other underlying pathology should be considered in patients younger than 20 years or older than 55 years until it is ruled out.
- Other signs and symptoms include the following:
  - o Violent trauma
  - o Constant progressive nonmechanical pain
  - o Thoracic pain
  - o History of cancer
  - o Prolonged use of steroids
  - o Unexplained weight loss
  - o Drug use
  - o HIV/AIDS
  - o Widespread neurological findings
  - o Severe lumbar spine flexion problems
  - o Bowel or bladder problems
  - o Gait disturbance or motor coordination problems

SUGGESTED READINGS

Butler DS. *The Sensitive Nervous System.* Adelaide, Australia: Noigroup Publications; 2000.

Devor M, Seltzer Z. Pathophysiology of damaged nerves in relation to chronic pain. In: Wall PD, Melzack R, eds. *Textbook of Pain.* 4th ed. Philadelphia: Churchill Livingstone; 1999.

Long DM. Chronic back pain. In: Wall PD, Melzack R, eds. *Textbook of Pain.* 4th ed. Philadelphia: Churchill Livingstone; 1999.

Placzek JD, Boyce DA, eds. *Orthopedic Physical Therapy Secrets.* 2nd ed. Philadelphia: Elsevier; 2006.

AUTHOR: CHRIS IZU

BASIC INFORMATION

DEFINITION

Complex regional pain syndrome (CRPS) is a group of previously separate disorders now classified together because of their common clinical features, which include abnormal levels of elevated pain, autonomic changes, edema, and loss of function.

CATEGORIES

- The two categories of CRPS are as follows:
  - CRPS I: Disorder of the sympathetic nervous system after an initiating noxious event with symptoms that spread beyond the territory of a single peripheral nerve.
  - CRPS II: Similar in almost all aspects to CRPS I except that it follows a nerve injury (previously known as causalgia).

SYNONYMS

- The following list includes previous disorders that are now classified as CRPS:
  - Reflex sympathetic dystrophy (RSD)
  - Posttraumatic sympathetic dystrophy
  - Algodystrophy
  - Algoneurodystrophy
  - Causalgia
  - Sudeck's atrophy
  - Posttraumatic painful osteoporosis
  - Transient osteoporosis
  - Acute bone atrophy
  - Migratory osteolysis
  - Posttraumatic vasomotor syndrome
  - Shoulder-hand syndrome

ICD-9CM CODES
355.9 Mononeuritis of unspecified site

OPTIMAL NUMBER OF VISITS

12 or fewer

MAXIMAL NUMBER OF VISITS

30

ETIOLOGY

- The specific mechanisms that may lead to CRPS after injury are unclear. CRPS has been known to follow a variety of conditions. Smith noted that it can follow surgeries, lower motor neuron and peripheral nerve injuries, neuropathies, and CNS insults that may include traumatic brain injuries and CVAs.
- Although the mechanisms may be unclear, the condition clearly involves abnormal processing of nervous system input, which is similar to fibromyalgia and other chronic pain conditions.
- Reflexive activity within the sympathetic nervous system (thus the previously used term *RSD*) creates a cycle of pain and swelling within the nervous system that leads to the elevated and abnormal symptoms in CRPS. An injury at one somatic level may initiate sympathetic activity at other surrounding segmental levels, creating this reflexive activity that leads to neurogenic inflammation. When the sympathetic nervous system is facilitated, elevated levels of neurotransmitters and catecholamines may help to activate primary afferent nociceptors to create an elevated sensation of pain.

DIAGNOSIS

- The diagnosis of CRPS is usually delayed because of the slow evolutionary nature of the disorder and is usually based on clinical examination and history. Certain diagnostic tests, such as x-rays, thermographic studies, and laser Doppler flowmetry, may help.
- One must be careful in the diagnosis of CRPS because of the subjectivity of the judgment of disproportionate pain and the high incidence of vasomotor signs and edema after any injury.
- The diagnosis must also be made in the absence of anatomical, physiological, and psychological conditions that could account for the elevated pain experience and/or disability.

EPIDEMIOLOGY AND DEMOGRAPHICS

- According to the National Institutes of Health, CRPS I may occur after up to approximately 5% of all injuries. Some of these mild cases may resolve before a specific diagnosis is made, but others can progress into a very painful condition with severe loss of function.
- The average age of individuals diagnosed with CRPS is in the mid 30s, but it is increasingly being noted in early childhood and as young as 3 years of age. According to Scadding, there is no conclusive evidence to show certain individuals may be predisposed to CRPS.

MECHANISM OF INJURY

- This syndrome often follows injuries such as extremity fracture or surgery, although it can follow something as small as an ankle sprain.
- Infections and even myocardial infarction have been shown to lead to complex regional pain syndrome.

COMMON SIGNS AND SYMPTOMS

- The most prominent symptom of CRPS is the spontaneous spread of pain in a localized regional distribution with a higher intensity than expected for the level of tissue damage. The pain may be more specifically characterized as burning, aching, or throbbing. Often the pain is so severe that any contact or movement of the area is extremely unpleasant.
- Other primary clinical factors include autonomic nervous system dysfunction, edema, and movement disorders such as inability to initiate movement, weakness, tremors, muscle spasms, and dystrophy. Often a key distinguishing feature from other injuries is the presence of vasomotor symptoms, which can lead to changes in skin temperature and color. Although these are common signs, they may not necessarily be constant features of the disorder and only need to present at some time for CRPS to be diagnosed.
- The common progression of CRPS is as follows:
  - Three overlapping but identifiable clinical stages to this condition are acute inflammation, dystrophy, and atrophy. Not all patients follow the same course or progress to the third stage.
  - In the acute inflammation stage, which may last from 3 to 6 months, there is an elevated level of pain compared to the level from the amount of tissue damage. Hyperalgesia, allodynia, and hyperpathia are all part of the abnormal pain processing and symptom experience. At this stage, there is also localized edema to the body region, vasomotor changes where the affected limb may be warmer, and skin changes that may manifest as increased hair or nail growth and dry skin.
  - The dystrophic stage onset usually occurs after about 3 to 6 months and can last up to 6 months. This stage is characterized by an increase in pain symptoms in both intensity and duration (may have near-constant hyperalgesia, allodynia, and hyperpathia). There will most likely be less skin warmth, and the skin may have a more thin or glossy appearance and feel cool from vasoconstriction. An individual in this stage may also have sweaty skin and thin rigid nails. Diagnostic testing, such as x-rays, may reveal osteoporosis, cystic changes, and subchondral bone erosion.
  - In the final or atrophic stage the pain may plateau but may spread more proximally, occasionally to the entire skin surface. This stage usually begins about 6 to 12 months after onset and may last for years, with the chance that it may resolve and then recur. The skin may be even more thin, shiny, and dry and even cyanotic. The digits distal to the region may be atrophic. The surrounding fascia may be thickened from the presence of prolonged

edema, and contractures of involved or surrounding joints may occur. At this stage, x-rays may reveal bony demineralization and ankylosis.

AGGRAVATING ACTIVITIES

When CRPS is present, aggravating activities can vary greatly. This condition is mostly known for having such an increased sensitivity that any movement of a surrounding limb or joint may be very painful. Light touch on the skin or weight bearing through the affected limb is also very uncomfortable.

EASING ACTIVITIES

Because of the high sensitivity, there are usually few easing factors. Avoiding the aggravating activities seem to help the condition.

24-HOUR SYMPTOM PATTERN

No specific writings on 24-hour symptom pattern were found for CRPS.

PAST HISTORY

Past history of an individual may include previous bout of CRPS, especially in the same body region.

PHYSICAL EXAMINATION

- Pain out of proportion to the stimulus
- Edema, joint stiffness, and discoloration
- Skin and vasomotor changes
- Most movements seem to reproduce pain.
- Decreased weight bearing with moderate-to-severe pain

IMPORTANT OBJECTIVE TESTS

- As with other complex pain issues, the clinician should perform the same examination they would for the appropriate joint complex or body region.
- Also, functional tests are very important in this population; management strategies to improve function are highly encouraged.

DIFFERENTIAL DIAGNOSIS   **Dx**

- One study reported malingering for secondary gain in some patients with CRPS, although it must be noted that the sympathetic symptoms are real and difficult to fake.
- Primary psychiatric disorders, such as conversion disorder and factitious illness, may manifest with symptoms similar to CRPS.

CONTRIBUTING FACTORS

There is debate now whether psychological factors, such as an underlying personality disorder, may contribute to this condition. The factors seem to be much more complex than explained by a psychological disorder.

TREATMENT   **Rx**

SURGICAL/MEDICAL OPTIONS

- During early stages, stellate ganglion blocks or sympathectomy have been shown to have the ability to decrease and sometimes eliminate pain. These could be considered minimally invasive techniques with temporary relief, but long-term results of this treatment are poor. It is difficult to assess effectiveness of this treatment because of limited control groups in studies.
- For motor symptoms, such as dystonia, placement of an intrathecal baclofen pump may help to control symptoms. This may also help with some analgesia and allow more participation in physical therapy.
- Implanted dorsal column stimulation may also help with decreasing pain intensity and perception of pain in clinical trials.
- Multiple other medications have been researched and administered without clear or promising results at this time.

SURGICAL/MEDICAL OUTCOMES

Studies addressing medical outcomes for patients with CRPS are limited at this time.

REHABILITATION

- There is general agreement that early diagnosis and treatment is one of the key factors in decreasing symptoms and improving function in individuals with CRPS. Once the symptoms have progressed, the disorder becomes more difficult to manage and treat.
- Treatment should take a multidisciplinary approach and not just focus on analgesia, since a hallmark of this condition is loss of function.
- With the complexity of this condition there have been many suggested treatments. Since disuse and immobilization are factors that may lead to CRPS, early mobilization, movement, and gentle modalities to reduce inflammation may be beneficial.

- TENS has been shown to have minimal effect on pain relief.
- Other goals of physical therapy include patient education and encouraging normal use of the involved extremity with respect to symptoms.
- Pool therapy has been beneficial to some patients who have lower extremity involvement and difficulty with weight bearing on land and during land-based exercises.

PROGNOSIS

There is a mixed prognosis for those with CRPS. Although it is noted that some symptoms may resolve early on for conditions like RSD, more individuals who have progressed far enough to have a CRPS diagnosis will experience varying severity of symptoms and disability.

SIGNS AND SYMPTOMS INDICATING REFERRAL TO PHYSICIAN

Patients who already have this diagnosis have most likely consulted with pain management, rheumatology, or other specialists. If they have not and the clinician suspects the development of CRPS (from the previously mentioned signs, symptoms, and stages), then a prompt referral should be made.

SUGGESTED READINGS

Butler DS. *The Sensitive Nervous System.* Adelaide, Australia: Noigroup Publications; 2000.

http://www.emedicine.com/emerg/topic497.htm

Placzek JD, Boyce DA, eds. *Orthopedic Physical Therapy Secrets.* 2nd ed. Philadelphia: Elsevier; 2006.

Scadding JW. Complex regional pain syndrome. In: Wall PD, Melzack R, eds. *Textbook of Pain.* 4th ed. Philadelphia: Churchill Livingstone; 1999.

Smith MB. The peripheral nervous system. In: Goodman CC, Fuller KS, Boissonnault WG, eds. *Pathology: Implications for the Physical Therapist.* 2nd ed. Philadelphia: Elsevier; 2003.

Somers DL, Clemente FR. Transcutaneous electrical nerve stimulation for the management of neuropathic pain: The effects of frequency and electrode position on prevention of allodynia in a rat model of complex regional pain syndrome type II. *Phys Ther.* 2006;86:698–709.

AUTHOR: CHRIS IZU

BASIC INFORMATION

DEFINITION

Fibromyalgia is a common syndrome characterized by chronic widespread pain. A diagnosis of fibromyalgia is somewhat controversial. According to the American College of Rheumatology (ACR), a fibromyalgia diagnosis requires a history of widespread pain and pain during palpation of 11 out of 18 tender points.

SYNONYMS

Previously referred to as fibrositis.

DIAGNOSIS

Although many physicians diagnose patients as having fibromyalgia on complaints of pain in multiple areas without apparent cause, stricter rules are found in the 1990 ACR guidelines. A history of widespread pain of 3 months or more is necessary for diagnosis. ACR guidelines further define widespread pain as pain in an axial distribution occurring on both sides of the body and above and below the waist. The main physical finding is the experience of pain in 11 of 18 specific tender points on digital palpation with mild-to-moderate pressure (enough to blanch a thumbnail). Although many other symptoms are common in individuals with fibromyalgia, they are not part of the diagnostic criteria.

ICD-9CM CODES
729.1 Myalgia and myositis
      unspecified

OPTIMAL NUMBER OF VISITS

12 or fewer

MAXIMAL NUMBER OF VISITS

24

ETIOLOGY

- Most believe that there is no tissue-specific pathology in fibromyalgia and that the symptoms experienced arise from abnormal sensory processing and abnormal peripheral nociception. Others have felt that physical stress or demands placed on a muscle lacking endurance may cause the fibers of that muscle to mechanically become locked and form a tender point. When this happens all over the body, it may lead to fibromyalgia.
- Debate continues as to whether this diagnosis is beneficial and whether the symptoms emanate from the body or the mind.
- According to Bennett, there are no distinct muscle changes found in individuals with fibromyalgia that would point toward a peripheral muscular pathology.
- Bennett also reported that several experiments suggest that disordered sensory processing at the central level contributes to the pain associated with this disease. These studies point toward significantly lower pain thresholds from peripheral sensitization, altered processing through increased response by both hemispheres in the brain, and central chemical changes such as increased substance P within the CSF.
- Other clinicians have pointed toward a lack of serotonin, which is an inhibitory neurotransmitter that may aid in dampening pain response and that can be deficient in some individuals with fibromyalgia.

EPIDEMIOLOGY AND DEMOGRAPHICS

One study that looked at the prevalence of chronic widespread pain concluded that it was more common in women and that it increased progressively from 18 years of age to 70 years of age.

MECHANISM OF INJURY

According to Bennett, fibromyalgia seldom arises out of the blue. Events, such as an acute injury, repetitive work-related pain, athletic injuries, or other pain states are often precipitating factors. Stress, infections, or exposure to toxins are also thought to be possible catalysts. Fibromyalgia has also been found to accompany RA, low back pain, osteoarthritis, and systemic lupus erythematosus (SLE). It is important to note that it is most likely not an injury that leads to fibromyalgia but certain events that may be the start of a cascade showing prevalence for abnormal processing of normally nonnociceptive impulses and leading to central sensitization.

COMMON SIGNS AND SYMPTOMS

- Chronic widespread pain on both sides of the body and above and below the waist is the hallmark of fibromyalgia. Individuals may complain of symptoms arising from muscles, joints, or even general areas or regions of pain.
- Even though widespread body pain is noted, often there are a few locations that may be perceived as worse or the individual may experience focal areas of pain.
- Hyperalgesia, an elevated response to nociceptive stimuli, is common among those with fibromyalgia. Widespread allodynia, a perception of pain to nonnoxious stimuli, may also be present.

- Many clinicians state that fibromyalgia has a specific look or visual presentation in patients. This may be due to the disordered sleep and fatigue, which are extremely common in these individuals.
- Multiple studies have noted easy fatigability from physical exertion, mental exertion, and psychological stressors. Nonrestorative sleep, depression, deconditioning, endocrine dysfunction, and poor coping mechanisms are thought to be factors in contributing to this fatigue.
- Most individuals with fibromyalgia report disturbed sleep, lack of sleep, or discontinuous sleep and commonly wake up feeling tired. A lack of the restorative stages of non–rapid eye movement (NREM) sleep (stages 3 and 4) is exhibited by many patients with fibromyalgia.
- Common somatic complaints that can occur along with fibromyalgia are as follows:
  ○ Restless leg syndrome
  ○ Irritable bowel syndrome
  ○ Irritable bladder syndrome
  ○ Cognitive dysfunction
  ○ Cold intolerance
  ○ Increased sensitivity and dizziness

AGGRAVATING ACTIVITIES

- Increased physical, emotional, or life stress
- Lack of sleep
- Changes in weather

EASING ACTIVITIES

- Avoiding those aggravating activities of stress
- Medications
- Getting adequate rest or sleep

24-HOUR SYMPTOM PATTERN

- Early morning stiffness is very common among individuals with fibromyalgia, and they may attribute symptoms to more of an arthritic-type condition.
- According to some studies, symptoms may wax and wane through the day, with a low in early afternoon and peak later in the day.

PAST HISTORY

Individuals with fibromyalgia often note a longer history of pain and possibly other instances in which an abnormal pain processing mechanism may have occurred.

PHYSICAL EXAMINATION

On palpation of the 18 tender points, patients often have a reflexive response to pain that might include an involuntary exclamation or flinch. Reactions such as this are hard to fake.

IMPORTANT OBJECTIVE TESTS

- As with other individuals with pain, it is important to perform an adequate examination for specific joint complexes or regions of the body to be addressed. Just because individuals have fibromyalgia, it does not prevent them from having other musculoskeletal problems that can be evaluated and treated in physical therapy. At the same time, consider the abnormal pain processing and mechanism associated with fibromyalgia and that the experience of pain may not relay the same information to the evaluator as in the absence of the disease.
- Assessing strength, functional level, and aerobic capacity helps with determining appropriate levels of a general exercise program.
- Posture and assessment on specific functional activities are key elements to look at during the objective examination.

DIFFERENTIAL DIAGNOSIS

- Chronic fatigue syndrome
- Psychological disorders: Somatoform disorders; somatization disorder, and pain disorder

CONTRIBUTING FACTORS

Psychological distress may be a large contributing factor to the symptoms of individuals with fibromyalgia, illustrated by an increased prevalence of psychological diagnoses, such as depression, in this population. Other reports of emotional and physical abuse are not thought to be causes but may adversely affect coping mechanisms.

TREATMENT

SURGICAL/MANAGEMENT OPTIONS

- Persons who have fibromyalgia and who have poor coping strategies may need special help in developing a treatment plan that incorporates effective problem solving. Other psychological concerns, such as depression, may be helped with cognitive-behavioral therapy or group therapy sessions.
- Sleep is a major concern for those individuals with fibromyalgia, and lack of sleep can contribute to the feelings of fatigue and increase the pain experience. Bennett advises that effective management should involve the following:
  - Adhering to the basic rules of sleep
  - Performing regular low-grade exercise

  - Treating associated psychological problems
  - Using low-dose tricyclic antidepressants
- Other medications, such as opiates, have been shown to help break the cycle of pain. They should be monitored carefully because of their propensity to cause addiction, dependence, and tolerance.
- Some clinical evidence supports the use of endocrine replacement therapy and growth hormone to treat those that are deficient. Cost and medical justification are common barriers to their use.
- Tamler suggests that individuals with fibromyalgia need to take in adequate amounts of protein and that limited protein synthesis in the body may be related to fibromyalgia.
- Overall treatment and management of fibromyalgia should be multidisciplinary and include physicians, nurse practitioners, clinical psychologists, physical therapists, exercise physiologists, and social workers.

REHABILITATION

- Treatment strategies should differ from other common physical therapy musculoskeletal diagnoses because of the differing nature of the pathology.
- Patient education is extremely important to remind these individuals that fibromyalgia does not reduce life expectancy or cause crippling effects. They also need to feel supported, as well as reminded that the goals of therapy are not to eliminate all pain but to increase function and abilities.
- Since pain is usually one of the main complaints of individuals with fibromyalgia, physical modalities, such as heat, massage, stretching, electrical stimulation, acupuncture, and passive stretching of mobilization, should be considered to help break this pain cycle. These treatments alone should not be considered as part of a complete treatment plan, as more direction should be placed on a combination of both passive and active treatments to help focus on positive coping strategies and adequate self-management strategies.
- Similar to other musculoskeletal problems, physical therapy rehabilitation should seek to address proper posture, ergonomics, and body mechanics to minimize overall stress on the body. It may also be important to address proper sleeping posture and positioning.
- Proper exercise prescription is also an important aspect of rehabilitation for these individuals. A program should contain some stretching, gentle strengthening, and some form of cardiovascular

training or aerobic conditioning. Initiation of an exercise regimen should not begin during a period of increased symptoms or exacerbation because it may perpetuate those symptoms. Attempts to manage and break the pain cycle are a better start.
- More recent studies have shown positive effects in both longer term reduction of symptoms and increased function in individuals who have participated in a pool-based rehabilitation program.

PROGNOSIS

The prognosis of fibromyalgia is mixed. Although the syndrome is not life-threatening, the symptoms and associated disorders will most likely negatively affect the quality of life and also influence employability. Symptoms may wax and wane, but the course of fibromyalgia is prolonged and most patients seen in tertiary referral centers have lifelong symptoms. Some studies report a remission rate up to 24% after 2 years, but multiple other studies have found continued symptoms to some level using anywhere from 7- to 15-year follow-up measures.

SIGNS AND SYMPTOMS INDICATING REFERRAL TO PHYSICIAN OR OTHER PRACTITIONERS

- Other possible causes of chronic widespread pain must be ruled out before a diagnosis of fibromyalgia is made. However, if these other causes have not been ruled out but other pain mechanisms are felt to be at hand, a referral to the physician should be made.
- Signs and symptoms of depression, anxiety, or other mental health issues should be noted and adequate referral to a psychologist or mental health professional should be made.
- Dealing with many of the associated conditions and symptoms of fibromyalgia may require adequate pharmacological treatment. Concerns about medications should be directed to the physician and if possible a rheumatologist.

SUGGESTED READINGS

Bennett RM. Fibromyalgia. In: Wall PD, Melzack R, eds. *Textbook of Pain*. 4th ed. Philadelphia: Churchill Livingstone; 1999.

Butler DS. *The Sensitive Nervous System*. Adelaide, Australia: Noigroup Publications; 2000.

Devor M, Seltzer Z. Pathophysiology of damaged nerves in relation to chronic pain. In: Wall PD, Melzack R, eds. *Textbook of Pain*. 4th ed. Philadelphia: Churchill Livingstone; 1999.

AUTHOR: CHRIS IZU

Rehabilitation and Common Clinical Questions

1 CERVICAL SPINE

2 THORACIC SPINE

3 LUMBAR SPINE

4 TEMPOROMANDIBULAR JOINT

5 UPPER EXTREMITY

6 LOWER EXTREMITY

7 NERVE

AUTHOR: DERRICK SUEKI

INTRODUCTORY INFORMATION

Rehabilitation is difficult. No two patients are identical. Even though they may have identical injuries with identical tissue damage, patients each have their own past history and unique pain response system. For this reason, rehabilitation is based in science but is an art form as well. The science of rehabilitation relies on a firm understanding of the body's normal response to injury and trauma. The art of rehabilitation rests in the clinician's ability to interpret the individual patient's unique signs and symptoms. The ability to formulate a plan of care that maximizes an individual's healing potential relies on the ability to blend the science and the art of rehabilitation.

What are the factors a clinician should consider when rehabilitating a patient with neck pain?[31]

The cervical spine is vastly different from the other regions of the spine. The thoracic spine is built to protect the structures of the chest and abdomen, so protection and stability are the primary functions of the spine. The lumbar spine is designed to provide stability and weight-bearing strength for the spine. It bears all the weight of the upper body, so it is designed to provide a stable yet mobile base for the remainder of the spine. The cervical spine is designed to provide a mobile base for the head to sit on. It serves to provide mobility and as such is prone to damage and injury. Alterations in mobility are functionally limiting in the cervical spine.

The clinician should keep in mind that the biomechanics of the cervical spine will often be altered in patients with cervical pain. An understanding of how it will be impacted is critical in assessing a patient's progress and ultimate outcome. The cervical vertebrae are the smallest and most mobile of all spinal vertebrae. The cervical region functions to provide mobility for the head on the trunk. It also functions to protect vital structures, such as the spinal cord, as they route distally down the body. In total, the functional units of the cervical region must work together to provide 45 to 50 degrees of flexion and 85 degrees of extension, for a total of 130 to 135 degrees of total sagittal plane motion. In the horizontal plane, the cervical spine must be able to provide 90 degrees of unilateral motion and 180 degrees of total rotational motion. Finally, there is 40 degrees of unilateral frontal plane motion or 80 degrees in total.[1,35] Segmentally, two adjacent spinal vertebrae and the intervertebral disc between the two comprise a functional motion segment. Each functional spinal unit provides varying degrees to the total motion seen in the cervical region. Restriction of one or several of the functional motion segments will alter the mechanics of adjacent segments.

Rehabilitation of the patient with neck pain is unique in terms of the close relationship the neck has with the shoulder region and its neural network. Unlike other regions of the body, such as the shoulder and the wrist, complete immobilization of the cervical spine is difficult, which can affect the healing potential. Moreover, the shoulder girdle and upper extremity, unlike the hip and lower extremity, rely on coordinated muscle actions to maintain function and stability. Many of these muscles have their proximal attachments at the cervical spine. Therefore rehabilitation of the cervical spine must also address limiting upper extremity activity until the surgical site is fully healed. Finally, since radicular pain and upper extremity paresthesias are often the predominate symptoms driving the patient's decision to seek medical help, the promotion of nerve healing should be addressed appropriately.

How do these factors affect the rehabilitation process?

The activities and precautions of each phase of the rehabilitation process should be rooted in current understanding of the phases of tissue healing. Specific treatment options will be provided throughout this section, but these should only serve as a guide to treatment and should not replace sound clinical reasoning or judgment.

Because of the intimate relationship between the cervical spine, thoracic spine, and upper extremity, rehabilitation of the cervical spine must begin with assessment of all of the upper quarter and thoracic spine. The clinician's subjective examination should include questions that determine the extent to which these other regions impact the cervical spine. Queries should be made regarding the past and present history of the thoracic spine and complete upper quarter. Physical examination should follow suit and be used to determine whether other regions are impacting the function of the cervical spine. Rehabilitation will then focus on all the elements that impact the cervical spine.

The difficulty in rehabilitating patients with cervical pain and dysfunction is that many structures that are pathological are not symptomatic, and many tissues that do not appear to be damaged are painful. Radiographs do not always correlate with the patient's symptoms. The validity of radiographs, computed tomography (CT) scans, and magnetic resonance imaging (MRI) in nonemergency neck pain without radiculopathy is currently lacking. Myelographic, CT, and MRI studies have all demonstrated that 20% to 30% of people who have disc herniation and stenosis do not have radicular symptoms, and many of these people do not have neck pain.[36,38] It has also been shown that under anesthesia, only nerves that are inflamed will produce radicular symptoms when compressed or placed in traction. Therefore, although the intervertebral disc or stenosis can be the source of neck pain, it is generally an injury to the nerve that drives the decision to seek medical attention. Protection of the nervous system from further damage and providing an environment in which the nerve can heal should be a primary goal of rehabilitation.

CLINICAL PEARL

Often, the cervical spine is the source of the symptoms, but dysfunction in other regions of the body results in abnormal stresses on the cervical tissue or alters the biomechanics of the cervical spine. This ultimately leads to failure of cervical tissue. Rehabilitation will ultimately need to address the dysfunctions that contribute to the cervical symptoms.

What role does age play in rehabilitation of neck pain?

Age impacts all regions of the body. Body tissue, muscle tissue, ligaments, tendons, disc tissues and nerves all are negatively affected by aging. From an injury standpoint, the loss of strength and viscoelasticity make injury to these tissues more commonplace. From a tissue healing standpoint, injuries take longer to heal as one ages.

Tissue degeneration does not always equate to tissue symptoms. Table IV-1-1 shows the number of patients who present with tissue pathology before 40 years of age and after. The data reveal that even with age, tissue pathology does not mean tissue pain.

TABLE IV-1-1   MRI of Subjects with Asymptomatic Cervical Spines

Tissue Pathology	<40 Years of Age	>40 Years of Age
Cervical disc bulge	10%	5%
Cervical degenerative disc	25%	60%
Cervical stenosis	4%	20%

TABLE IV-1-2	**Differences between Acute and Chronic Pain**	
	Acute	**Chronic**
Cause	Pathogen or injured tissue	Persistent nondegradable pathogens Persistent foreign bodies Autoimmune reaction
Major cells	Neutrophils Monocytes Macrophages	Monocytes Macrophages Lymphocytes Fibroblasts
Primary mediator	Vasoactive amines	Cytokines Growth factors Hydrolytic enzymes
Onset	Immediate	Delayed
Duration	21 days Healing Chronic inflammation	Many months or years Tissue destruction Fibrosis

What role does acuteness or chronicity play in rehabilitating a patient with neck pain?

Since many patients with tissue pathology do not have pain or dysfunction, the question remains, what factors contribute to pain and distinguish a patient with chronic pain from one whose pain resolves after the acute phase (Table IV-1-2)?

There are many factors that could potentially contribute to a patient's chronic pain. Altered biomechanics, poor circulation, central pain-processing changes, peripheral nerve sensitization, endocrine dysfunction, genetic predisposition, and immune system malfunction are a few of the many factors that have been proposed as contributions to the presence of chronic pain. In reality, it probably involves a combination of many factors not one single element. What is known, however, is that acute inflammation is different from chronic inflammation.

If the clinician can reduce the inflammation present in the cervical spine, the region can begin to heal and in the process restore normal function. The first step in rehabilitation of the cervical spine must be to reduce or eliminate the inflammation present in the neck. In acute cases, this is accomplished with rest, cervical collars, ice, electrical stimulation, lymphatic drainage techniques, or medication. In chronic symptoms, it involves removing the contributors that result in abnormal stresses to the cervical spine and eliminating the persistent nondegradable pathogens or foreign bodies in the spine that may be creating an immune or inflammatory response.

PROGNOSIS

How successful is rehabilitation in treating acute neck pain?

Approximately two-thirds of the population will experience neck pain during their lifetime. Most of these patients will recover within 6 weeks. Although recovery is generally spontaneous, the recurrence rate is between 22% and 50%, depending on the study.[9,18] This leads to questions about whether the neck pain truly resolved or if the symptoms resolved while the damage to the tissue remained. The prognosis is highly variable, depending on the nature of the damage, but patients who have a previous history of neck pain have a worse prognosis than patients with no prior history of neck pain. Patients who are over the age of 40 or those individuals who have concomitant low back pain also have a worse prognosis.[47]

Cleland et al identified four characteristics of patients who were most likely to achieve successful outcomes from clinical interventions. The four predictors were age >54 years of age, dominant hand not affected, looking downward did not increase symptoms, and

the use of a multimodal treatment strategy that included manual therapy, cervical traction, and deep neck flexor strengthening. When three out of four of these characteristics were present, the posttest probability of success was 85%. When all four characteristics were present, the posttest probability increased to 90%.[7]

How successful is rehabilitation in treating neck pain?

In general, the efficacy of therapy for the treatment of cervical pain is mixed. Most of the positive results involve patients with acute symptoms, but even these results are mixed. It has been hypothesized that the reason efficacy cannot be shown in patients with cervical pain is that the research topic is too broad. There are too many potential pathologies, and each pathology requires a different rehabilitation approach. With this in mind, Childs et al suggested that a new classification based on impairment of spinal function be used for research to narrow down the scope of study. In this way, appropriate interventions could be mated with specific movement impairments.[5]

CLINICAL PEARL

In patients who are irritable or if you suspect neuro mobility issues, restoring motion in the thoracic spine will often change the mechanics of cervical spine kinematics.

What other regions of the body are most likely to contribute to neck pain?

Potentially, any region of the body can impact or contribute to neck pain or neck pathology. Biomechanical changes or neural mobility alterations as far away as the feet can potentially lead to neck symptoms. The thoracic spine because of its close proximity to the cervical spine and the neural network that runs through both regions has taken on increased interest recently with studies that show improved cervical range of motion (ROM) after thoracic interventions.[6] It can also be argued that pathology or abnormalities in the shoulder region can dramatically impact the mechanics of the cervical spine. Clinically, patients with rotator cuff pathology recruit their global muscles, such as the upper trapezius, to lift their arms over head. Many of these large shoulder muscles have their proximal attachments at the cervical spine. Over recruitment of these muscles could result in pathology and pain at the neck (see Case Study).

CASE STUDY

Your patient is a 32-year-old male who reports right neck and arm pain. These symptoms began 1 week ago. He reports that he was sitting in the dentist chair for 1 hour with his head tilted back. He felt a little pain while in that position, but the next day, he awoke with a very stiff neck. Over the course of the next week, he began to experience pain down his arm and into his pinky and ring fingers. He is currently unable to use his arm because of the arm pain and numbness. His neck is stiff but that is not his chief complaint. The arm symptoms are what is really bothering him. He has had several neck aches in the past several years, but nothing that has gone down into his arm. His doctor prescribed nonsteroidal antiinflammatory medications 2 days ago. These have helped a little but not completely. He is in significant discomfort and reports that neck motions, especially looking upward increase his arm and neck pain. What are your hypotheses regarding the source of this patient's symptoms, and what is your treatment plan?

Answer

It is difficult to definitively diagnose the patient's problem on the information given. It appears that the C8 nerve is impacted as a result of the distribution of symptoms. The source of the pathology is mostly likely at the C7/T1 segment, although first rib dysfunction may also be the problem. The fact that extension increases the symptoms may put a facet joint entrapment or interforaminal stenosis at the top of the diagnosis list, but the patient is too young for degeneration to be the primary diagnosis. The top hypothesis given the available information would be C7/T1 facet dysfunction with C8 nerve root irritation. From a treatment standpoint, the first goal is to reduce the irritation and inflammation. This may be accomplished through gentle traction, soft tissue mobilization, or joint mobilizations. Often, treatment of the nerve or spinal segments in other regions of the body, such as the thoracic spine, will help offload the nervous system and reduce the patient's symptoms. Nerve mobilizations should not be used until acute radicular symptoms are no longer present. Acute and irritable patients should not be placed in a reclined position for more than 10 minutes at a time. If the irritable patients lie down too long, the symptoms will often increase significantly as the weight of the head is placed back onto the irritated structure. The patient can also be prescribed a cervical collar or referred back to the physician to see if a short course of steroidal medication may be prescribed to eliminate the acute inflammation in the region. Once the symptoms have been reduced, the patient should be treated for the contributors that keep the neck pain coming back. Joint mobilization and exercise are appropriate interventions at this time.

EVIDENCE-BASED MEDICINE

What trends are currently being seen in research regarding rehabilitation of patients with neck pain?
Evidence is lacking regarding most commonly used cervical treatment interventions. Most of the recent rehabilitation research has been focused on the development of clinical prediction rules for the cervical spine, the development of cervical specific movement impairment systems, and the role of the thoracic spine in cervical dysfunction.[6]

Another current focus of rehabilitation has been on the role of deep neck flexors in cervical stability. Research has recently been published and continues to address the role this muscle group has in cervical pathology and function.[12,13,14,27,48]

From a medical standpoint, less focus has been placed on the biomechanics of the region and more focus on the endocrine and immune component of cervical pain and the perpetuation of symptoms. Still, the need for well-conducted randomized controlled trials is needed in both medicine and rehabilitation.

INTERVENTIONS

MANUAL THERAPY
What is the physiological rationale behind the use of manual therapy in treating patients with cervical pain?
The body's most basic goal is the maintenance of homeostasis. When the body's equilibrium is altered, it takes immediate steps to restore balance. Repair begins immediately after an injury by attempting to reestablish continuity. With the exception of teeth, all tissues in the body are capable of repair. In general, humans do not regenerate tissue, tissue is repaired with scar tissue or dense connective tissue. This quick process reduces the chances of infection and quickly restores functional continuity to the region.

Posture is another method the body uses to create a homeostatic environment. Instead of placing abnormal forces on a structure, the body will attempt to protect it. It does so through adaptive compensation. Altered posture is the outcome of this adaptive compensation. Research shows that small amounts of inflammation in a region will inhibit the recruitment of muscles local to the area of inflammation. Because of the loss of local motor control, the body recruits larger muscle groups to stabilize and move the impacted region. This is the reason the clinician will often palpate tenderness and tightness in the large muscle groups of a region. In the cervical spine, the small muscle whose muscle activity is inhibited is the longus colli muscle. The large muscles that are recruited to compensate for the lack of local control are the sternocleidomastoid, the scalenes, the upper trapezius, and to a certain extent, the levator scapulae. Because of the alterations in the use and mechanics of these muscle groups, changes are often seen in other regions such as the shoulder or thoracic spine.

Which interventions have proven most successful in treating patients with cervical pain?
Evidence suggests that a multimodal management strategy is the most effective approach to treating patients with cervical pain. A treatment strategy that uses mobilization or manipulation plus exercise has been shown to be beneficial for relief of mechanical neck pain.[22-24,29] In general, research is still lacking regarding which specific interventions are the best for a patient with neck pain. Clinically, reliance on a single treatment strategy for all cervical patients is destined for failure. Every cervical pathology presents differently and responds to different interventions. Similarly, no two patients are identical. The successful clinician blends science and evidence with clinical experience to create a unique treatment program for each patient. Research suggests that a combination of manual techniques, exercise, and modalities is the most effective in treating patients with mechanical neck pain.

What is the role of traction in treating patients with cervical pain?
Cervical traction is one of the more commonly used methods of treating neck and arm pain, but its physiological effects are poorly understood. It has been hypothesized that mechanical traction is effective in relieving clinical symptoms and that one of the mechanisms for this pain reduction may be a reduction in muscle tension. In a study where traction was applied to 100 subjects with neck pain, weighted traction improved subject reports of pain, sleep disturbances, and social dysfunction when compared to a control group receiving placebo traction. No significant changes in ROM were measured after traction.[30]

In a systematic review of the literature, the authors determined that there were not enough well-conducted studies available to determine the efficacy of continuous or intermittent traction for pain reduction, improved function, or global perceived effect when compared to placebo traction, tablet, or heat or other conservative treatments in patients with chronic neck disorders.[19]

In another study to determine predictive factors that may be present in patients who benefit from cervical traction, it was determined that five clinical variables could predict which patients would benefit from cervical traction. The predictors were patient reported peripheralization, with lower cervical spine (C4-7) mobility testing; positive shoulder abduction test; age ≥55 years of age; positive upper limb tension test A; and positive neck distraction test. If the subject had at least three out of the five predictors, the likelihood of success with cervical traction was 79.2%. If at least four out of five variables were present, the likelihood for success increased to 94.8%.[41]

Clinically, traction has shown efficacy in treating patients with cervical pain and with radicular pain. Research has yet to reflect the changes commonly experienced in clinic. Use of Raney's clinical predictors gives the clinician tools to determine which patients may be the most appropriate for the use of cervical traction.

CLINICAL PEARL

While not an absolute contraindication, patients with rheumatoid arthritis (RA) or similar diseases that affect the body's soft tissue and result in joint laxity should focus on cervical stabilization exercises and deep neck flexor exercises. Mobilization can easily exacerbate a patient's symptoms and should be use with caution.

Section IV

REHABILITATION AND COMMON CLINICAL QUESTIONS

TABLE IV-1-3 **Motion Restriction and Mobilization**

Motion Restrictions	Joint Requiring Mobilization	Direction of Mobilization
C0-C1 flexion	C0-C1	Cervical traction
C0-C1 extension	C0-C1	Cervical traction or posterior to anterior
C1-C2 rotation	C1-C2	Posterior to anterior or upglide/contralateral rotation
Midcervical and low cervical flexion	Unilaterally on the restricted facet joint	Cervical upglide or rotation of the restricted joint
Midcervical and low cervical extension	Unilaterally on the restricted facet joint	Cervical downglide or rotation of the segment contralateral to the restricted joint
Midcervical and low cervical rotation	Unilaterally on the restricted facet joint	Cervical upglide or rotation of the restricted joint Cervical downglide or rotation of the segment contralateral to the restricted joint
Midcervical and low cervical sidebend	Unilaterally on the restricted facet joint	Cervical downglide or rotation of the segment contralateral to the restricted joint

How beneficial is joint mobilization in the treatment of patients with cervical pain?

Mobilization techniques are a mainstay of physical therapy (Table IV-1-3). In practice, they are utilized to increase ROMs within targeted regions by moving specific joints or specific muscles. Although studies are lacking in the area of mobilization of the cervical spine, some clinical themes have emerged. For patients with mechanical neck pain, mobilization should be done in conjunction with exercise for improved patient satisfaction and decreased pain. Manipulation and mobilization alone appear to be less effective.[21,22,23]

In a study by Sterling et al, the effects of cervical mobilization were studied. Their results showed a reduction in pain, an increase in skin conductance, a decrease in skin temperature, and a decrease in superficial neck flexor activity immediately after cervical mobilization. The results indicated that the cervical mobilization technique produced a hypoalgesic effect, a sympathoexcitatory effect, and an inhibition of superficial muscle activity. The authors hypothesize that this could be the result of facilitation of the deep neck flexor muscles with a decreased need for coactivation of the superficial neck flexors. They also suggested that the combination of all findings would support the proposal that spinal mobilization may exert part of its influence via activation of the periaqueductal gray.[48]

Is joint manipulation recommended for patients with cervical pain?

Research involving joint manipulation in the cervical spine has produced results similar to those seen with joint mobilization. Mobilization or manipulation when used with exercise is beneficial for mechanical neck pain. Done alone, manipulation or mobilization was not beneficial. When manipulation was compared to mobilization neither was superior. For patients who had cervical radicular pain, there is not enough evidence to prove or disprove its efficacy.[2,21-24]

Systematic reviews have been completed comparing the efficacy of joint manipulation in patients with acute neck pain versus those patients with chronic neck pain; the efficacy of spinal manipulation for acute neck pain was determined to be inconclusive. There was moderate evidence, however, to suggest that spinal manipulative therapy was more effective than general practitioner management for the short-term reduction in pain. There is moderate evidence to suggest that cervical manipulative therapy is superior to nonmanipulative therapy and family physician care. There is limited evidence to suggest that spinal manipulative therapy is inferior to nonmanipulative therapy.[2,22,23]

The use of manipulation should be used in the cervical spine with caution. Clinicians need to be aware of the fact that manipulation has been shown to be effective in a certain patient population and not effective in other patient populations. To date, those patients who could benefit from the technique and those who will not improve has not been determined. The clinician should demonstrate further caution because, unlike other regions of the body, evidence has shown that cervical manipulation has the potential to cause serious irreversible harm to a patient. Cervical manipulation has the potential to be an effective clinical tool, but until the patient populations that can most benefit from the technique are better defined, the clinician should use extra caution when using it to treat patients.

CLINICAL PEARL

Cervical manipulation can be a very effective intervention if used in the appropriate patient population. If used in an inappropriate patient population, it can result in serious injury; 50% of patients receiving cervical manipulation will have temporary increases in symptoms such as soreness or loss of ROM. Between 1:50,000[43] and 1:500,000[37] patients who receive a cervical manipulation will have serious side effect, including but not limited to stroke or death.

What does evidence reveal regarding the use of massage for the treatment of patients with cervical pain?

In a systematic review of nineteen studies, the authors drew the conclusion that the effectiveness of massage for neck pain cannot be determined at this time. This determination was made as a result of the poor quality of the studies or the fact that massage was included as part of a multimodal cluster of interventions. In these studies, it was not possible to determine the contributions of massage alone.[11]

The fact that much of the cervical spine's function requires the coordinated activity of muscles would guide the clinician to use massage when appropriate to reduce the activity of overused muscles. Once this is completed, the clinician can turn his or her attention to strengthening and training the muscles that are under utilized.

Is stretching beneficial or indicated for patients with cervical pain?

There is little research currently available that looks specifically at the role of stretching in the treatment of cervical pain. Clinically, stretching of the upper trapezius and levator scapulae are common interventions to address postural deviations in patients with neck pain. Stretching of the pectoral muscles is often used to address the protracted shoulders common in patients with neck pain (Figure IV-1-1). The efficacy of these interventions can neither be confirmed nor negated.

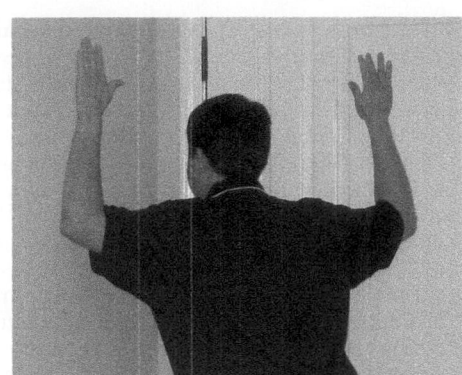

FIGURE IV-1-1   Corner stretch.

How should a clinician decide which manual therapy intervention is most appropriate for a patient with cervical pain?

Rehabilitation should begin with addressing the muscular compensations that the body makes to protect injured or weakened tissue. This author suggests using the "GLOCO-LOCO" mnemonic to guide treatment in most regions of the body. GLOCO-LOCO stands for GLO (global muscle release), CO (correction of the underlying problem), LO (local muscle recruitment), and CO (coordinate motion of the local and global muscles). Rehabilitation begins by relaxing or inhibiting the activity in the global muscle. In this case, the global muscles are the upper trapezius, sternocleidomastoid, scalene, and levator scapulae muscles. There are various methods that the clinician can use, including massage and stretching. Once global muscle's activity is reduced, the clinician should seek to identify the factors that are creating the symptoms. Joint mobilization, traction, or modalities can be used to address joint hypomobility and reduce inflammation that may be contributing to the patient's dysfunction. Once the problem is corrected, the body needs to learn how to reengage or reactivate the local muscles, so exercises can be used to recruit these local muscles. Finally, the body needs to learn how to coordinate the activity of both the local and global muscles.

EXERCISE

What is the physiological rationale behind the use of exercise in treating patients with cervical pain?

Many times, the body will take postures or positions to minimized stress or forces placed on a damaged region or structure. These alterations in posture will impact function and biomechanics. Over time, the altered biomechanics can lead to tissue breakdown. According to Janda, a common postural alignment seen in people with upper quarter pathology is known as the upper cross syndrome.[25] Regardless of the cause, this alignment will consist of an upper quarter muscle pattern in which certain muscles will be weakened and lengthened and others will be strong and shortened, resulting in an increased thoracic kyphosis, increased midcervical lordosis, and increased upper cervical extension (Figure IV-1-2). Protraction of the scapula will often accompany this postural deviation. More specifically, there is a weakening and lengthening of the rhomboids, middle and lower trapezius, deep neck flexors, supraspinatus, infraspinatus, and the deltoid musculature that is combined with a tightening and shortening of the pectoralis major and minor, levator scapulae, upper trapezius, scalene, subscapularis, and sternocleidomastoid muscles. Postural rehabilitation should be implemented and interventions should focus on the stretching of shortened musculature, strengthening of the weakened muscles of the trunk and neck, and performing upper extremity movements while maintaining neutral cervical spine.

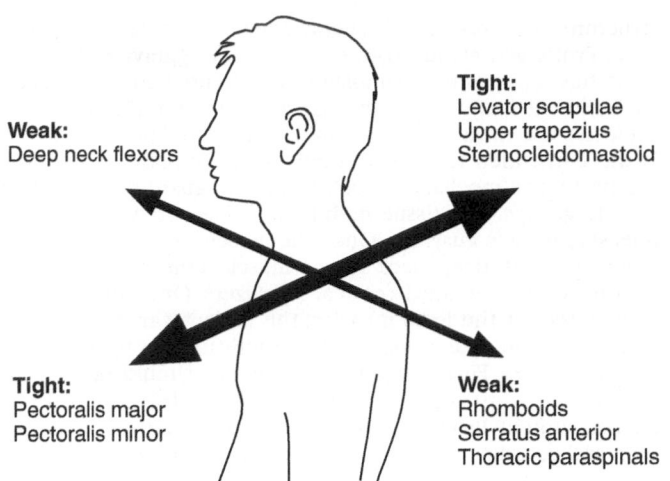

Weak:
Deep neck flexors

Tight:
Levator scapulae
Upper trapezius
Sternocleidomastoid

Tight:
Pectoralis major
Pectoralis minor

Weak:
Rhomboids
Serratus anterior
Thoracic paraspinals

FIGURE IV-1-2   Upper cross syndrome.

Are exercise programs beneficial in treating patients with cervical pain? If so, which ones?

Exercise programs are used frequently to treat patients with neck pain. There is evidence to support the use of exercise. Exercise programs have been found to provide intermediate or long-term benefits for subjects with neck pain. There is also strong evidence that exercise can provide pain reduction and improvement in function in subjects who received a multimodal intervention including exercise and mobilization/manipulation. Moderate evidence of long-term improvements in patient function was produced in studies favoring direct neck strengthening and stretching for patients with chronic neck pain.

A systematic review of sixteen trials addressing the issue of neck pain and exercise found that there was relatively strong evidence to support the use of proprioceptive exercises and dynamic resisted strengthening exercises of the neck-shoulder musculature for chronic or frequent neck pain. Moderate evidence was found to support early ROM exercises in acute whiplash patients. The research evaluated could not support the use of group exercise or single sessions of cervical retraction exercises. It is apparent that exercise programs focused on cervical strengthening can potentially benefit patients with neck pain. Multimodal exercises focusing on neck and shoulder strengthening appear to be the most beneficial.[44]

The evidence suggests that exercise can be effective in treating people with neck pain, but the maximum benefits are gained when exercise is used in conjunction with other interventions.

CASE STUDY

Your patient is a 42-year-old male who reports localized neck pain after a motor vehicle accident (MVA) 4 months ago. He reports that he was rear-ended. He initially felt only a little stiffness, but over the course of the next week, he began to experience significant pain and stiffness in the neck and left scapular region. His head feels heavy and tired at the end of a day spent working on the computer. The pain has improved over the past 4 months, yet he continues to experience pain when looking up or down for prolonged periods of time, and he stiff feels stiff and tired in the neck after a day working on the computer. He has no radicular symptoms or symptoms in his upper extremities. What are your hypotheses regarding the source of this patient's symptoms, and what is your treatment plan?

Answer

Patients who have had MVAs often have symptoms long after the accident. The fact that his pain built up over time tells us that it is either a poorly vascularized structure that was injured or that the structures were not initially aggravated but became irritable with time. Prolonged static postures appear to aggravate the symptoms; this is a common complaint for patients with mild instability. Ligament laxity and instability are common after a rear-end accident. The most commonly injured joint is C5/6. If instability is the issue, then treatment should focus initially on removing the protective mechanism such as muscle guarding in the large muscle groups. Soft tissue mobilization has proved effective in releasing muscle guarding. Once the muscle compensation is no longer present, deep neck flexor muscle training can be initiated to recruit the local cervical stabilizers. Once the patient is able to recruit the local muscles, the patient can begin coordinating larger muscle groups with the activation of the local deep flexor muscles. Finally, functional activities should begin while the patient is instructed on maintaining the deep cervical muscle recruitment. Proprioceptive neck training can also be used to train and coordinate the stabilizing and motion muscles.

Which muscles should be strengthened in treating patients with cervical pain?

After the trauma or injury, the body is only capable of repairing small muscle lesions with regeneration of muscle tissue. Large lesions fill with dense connective tissue. While dense connective tissue can function to reestablish tissue continuity, it lacks the contractile elements of normal muscle tissue and the tensile strength of normal ligament and tendon tissue. Therefore the ability to generate contractile forces or resist tensile loading through the region of repair is compromised. In cases of muscle strain or ligament sprain, an important aspect of the rehabilitation process is strengthening and loading the remaining muscle and ligament fibers to compensate for the loss of the damaged muscle and ligament fibers.[16,17,34,35]

From a functional recovery perspective, the longus colli muscle has an important role in maintaining cervical stability. Although research is lacking regarding cervical stability, numerous studies have been conducted on the role of lumbar stability to control motion and stabilize spinal segments.[45] Richardson and associates performed a series of studies on the ability of deep lumbar muscles to stabilize spinal segments in patients with lumbar pain. Their findings suggest that deep muscle activation is a necessary component in the reestablishment of spinal control after a low back injury. Subjects that did not reestablish segmental control continued to experience low back pain.[42] Recently, the same group turned their attention to the cervical spine.[26] They suggest that deep cervical muscles are necessary for normal cervical spine stability. This role may be even greater than that seen in the lumbar region because of the large role cervical spine muscles play in the maintenance and control of a region designed to provide mobility. Thus exercises designed to recruit deep neck flexors will be imperative to provide adequate stability of a highly mobile region. These exercises can include supine chin tucks in a neutral spine using a rolled towel or pillow if necessary, progressing to an inclined position and eventually a sitting position. Jull has proposed the use of a blood pressure cuff behind the neck as a means of monitoring the amount of cervical muscle recruitment.[12,14,26,27]

The strengthening and training of the deep cervical muscles was confirmed in a study of patients with cervical radiculopathy who were treated with manual therapy, cervical traction, and deep neck flexor and scapulothoracic strengthening exercises; 91% of patients treated demonstrated a clinically meaningful improvement in pain and function after a mean of seven treatment sessions. These changes were held at a 6-month follow-up assessment.[8]

In a separate systematic review, a program of eye fixation or proprioception exercises as part of a larger cervical program showed moderated evidence of short-term benefit in terms of pain and function in patients with chronic neck pain and long-term benefits in patients with acute or subacute neck or head pain. Jull et al have also confirmed the fact that cervical proprioception is altered in patients with neck pain. A program of cervical proprioceptive training combined with cervical cranial flexion training demonstrated improved joint proprioception after intervention[28] (Box IV-1-1).

BOX IV-1-1 Common Exercises Used in Cervical Spine Rehabilitation

Active cervical range of motion (ROM)
Place patients in a comfortable sitting position as above and have them complete each cervical ROM movement slowly through their full ROM.

Chin tucks
In a sitting or standing posture, the patient tucks in his or her chin and extends the cervical spine.

Wall angels
Have the patient stand with head, back, and arms against the wall, knees slightly bent, chin tucked, and shoulders slightly abducted. Have the patient continue to elevate his arms against the wall and bring them down, making the shape of angel wings by his side.

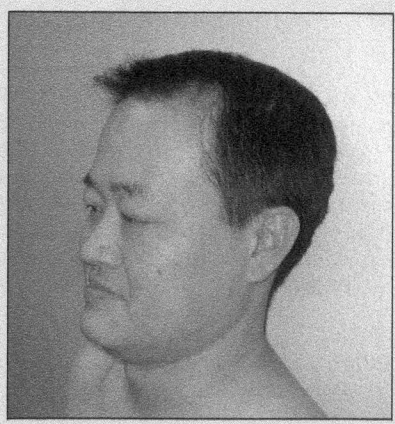

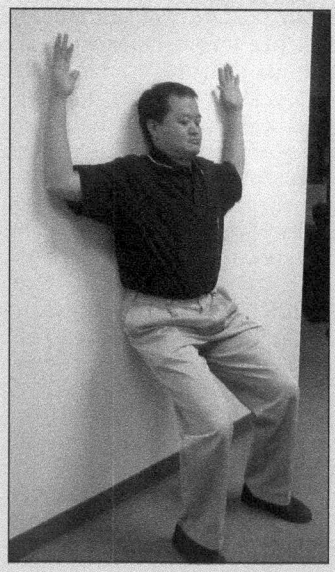

BOX IV-1-1 Common Exercises Used in Cervical Spine Rehabilitation (*Continued*)

Scapular retractions using resistance tubing
Have the patient sit or stand (with knees slightly bent) with resistance tubing secured in front of the patient. Have the patient pull the tubing simultaneously to his or her sides by retracting the scapula and bending the elbows.

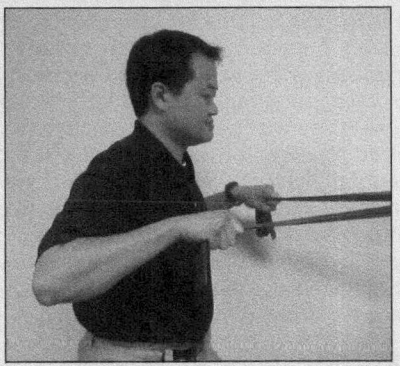

Prone scapular retraction progression
Place the patient in a prone position on the table with his or her arms at the side. Instruct the patient to lift the forehead off the table, keeping the chin tucked in a neutral cervical spine position.

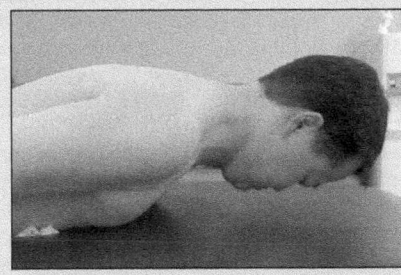

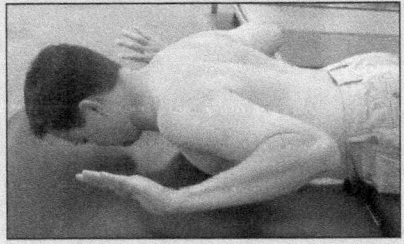

How should a clinician decide which exercise is most appropriate for a patient with cervical pain?

It is important to realize that evidence and research should shape or enhance our treatment of patients. As more research becomes available, clinicians will be able to shape their decisions more succinctly, but at the present time, many of the decisions a clinician will be forced to make will be driven by clinical experience and patient symptomology. Patients whose symptoms are produced with minimal activity should focus on increasing pain-free ROM. As symptoms reduce, strengthening exercises, such as deep neck flexor activation and shoulder/thoracic strengthening, can commence. Coordination of the local and global muscles can use functional training and proprioceptive retraining of vision and cervical motion.

How does a clinician know if a patient with cervical pain is ready to progress to a new exercise?

As in any rehabilitation program, a patient should be able to show improvements in muscle strength and endurance without compensation. Of the two, endurance training should take precedence over strength training.

Grimmer described a clinically based test that can be used to determine the endurance of the deep cervical neck flexors.[20] Patients are instructed to lie supine without a pillow. They are then asked to retract their necks and then lift their heads 2 cm off the table. Endurance is measured as the time it takes for the patient to thrust their chin forward. Falla et al suggested using an inflatable air-filled pressure sensor to determine the strength of a patient's deep neck flexors. The pressure sensor is inflated to 20 mm Hg and placed behind the patient's neck. The patient lies supine with the blood pressure cuff placed under the neck and inflated to 20 mm Hg with the display held in front to monitor the dial (Figure IV-1-3). The patient nods or retracts the head to raise the pressure 2 mm Hg. Once the patient is able to maintain this pressure without fatigue, he or she may progress and increase the pressure by 2 mm Hg.[13,15]

When using the upper extremity, deep neck flexor activity has been shown to be delayed in patients with neck pain.[12,14] With this in mind, exercise programs should address use of the upper extremity in conjunction with deep neck flexor activation as a progression of cervical exercises.

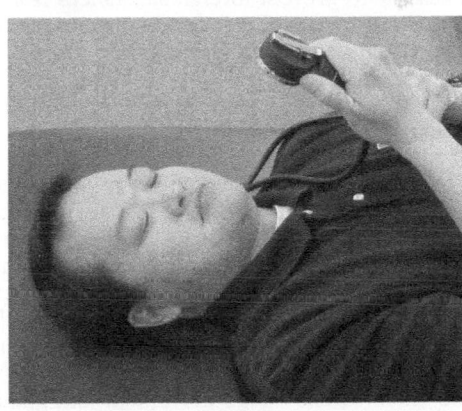

FIGURE IV-1-3 Craniocervical flexor test and deep neck flexor exercises.

MODALITIES

Which modalities have proven most successful in treating patients with cervical pain?

Many modalities used in clinics have shown efficacy in treating musculoskeletal pathology. Ultrasound can be used to increase circulation and promote healing. Electrical stimulation can be used for pain abatement, increasing circulation, and promoting tissue and bone healing. Heat can improve tissue pliability and circulation. Cryotherapy can reduce swelling and pain. As a whole, however, no studies have been conducted that have addressed specifically the use of these modalities in patients with cervical pain. The current evidence is either lacking, limited, or conflicting.[32]

OTHER

What is the role of bracing or taping in treating patients with cervical pain?

Soft collars are commonly prescribed to patients with cervical pain. The goal of the collar is to reduce the load placed on tissue and to limit motion. By unloading the tissue, physiologically the tissue has the opportunity to rest and heal. Taping has also been used to offload tissue or give proprioceptive feedback to a patient regarding posture and bodily alignment.

What is the role of acupuncture in treating patients with cervical pain?

A systematic review of fourteen randomized controlled trials was inconclusive regarding the use of acupuncture to reduce cervical pain. The trials were equally balanced between positive and negative. Acupuncture was superior no treatment in one study and equal or superior to physiotherapy in three studies. Needle acupuncture was not superior to indistinguishable sham control in four out of five studies. Further studies are needed.[46]

What is the role of treatment aimed at neurodynamics in treating patients with cervical pain?

Patients may seek medical attention solely as the result of neck pain, but many patients will seek medical help when upper extremity symptoms become present. Within the spine, injury or damage to the nerve often occurs at the spinal nerve root or the dorsal root ganglia. Anatomically, there are differences in the nerve root that make it more susceptible to injury than at other regions of the peripheral nerve. Nerve roots are not as well protected, less able to withstand deformation, and less able to repair themselves than the remainder of the peripheral nerve. The other structure within the intervertebral foramen that is susceptible to damage is the dorsal root ganglia. The position of the dorsal root ganglia is not constant and can be found inside the foramen, outside the foramen, or in the spinal canal, which can increase the likelihood that it will be injured. In addition, unlike the spinal nerve root and peripheral nerve, the dorsal root ganglia do not have a blood-nerve barrier, which is necessary to prevent foreign substances from invading the nerve. These anatomical differences predispose the dorsal root ganglia to edema and mechanical compression.[36,39,40]

Neurons are incapable of dividing and migrating, therefore regeneration occurs only through existing neurons. If the connective tissue sheathing remains intact, there is a potential for nerve regrowth. If the sheath is disrupted, the potential for regrowth diminishes. Initially, like any tissue, there is an inflammatory process within the nerve. Within hours after injury, the nerves start to grow back from the distal stump at 1 to 2 mm per day. In addition to transmitting nerve impulses, the axon of the nerve functions to transmit nutrients and chemicals down its lumen. These axons are filled with axoplasm, which is necessary for nerve health and survival. Axoplasm is a viscous substance and is thixotropic, which means that it needs constant agitation or it will gel.[36,39,40] Thus care must be taken to encourage movement and gliding of the nerve, but at the same time, positions that place tension on the nerve should be avoided.

CLINICAL PEARL

!

Nerves are thixotropic. They require motion to heal and survive.

Neural mobility techniques are commonly used to increase upper extremity motion and decrease symptoms in both the spine and upper extremity. Care must be taken when employing these techniques because patient symptoms can be easily exacerbated. The first step toward improving neuromobility should focus on eliminating the adhesions or structures that are preventing proper nerve motion. Scar tissue has the ability to restrict joints, but scar tissue also can adhere to nerves and affect their mobility. Since the patient was likely to have experienced nerve-related symptoms as a contributing factor, it is important not to aggravate or overstretch the neural tissue because there is a strong likelihood that soft tissue restrictions may be limiting the ability of the nerve to glide properly. Neurodynamics is the concept that there is a relationship between the nervous system and associated connective tissues. Neurodynamic testing of the upper limb enables the clinician to assess the movement capabilities of neural tissues in relation to the soft tissue structure that surrounds them.[3,4]

The Upper Limb Neurodynamic Tests were originally developed by Elvey as a method for differentiating potential sources of cervicobrachial symptoms.[10]

Treatment using the upper limb neurodynamic tests has generally been a point of confusion for clinicians. A positive test indicates restricted mobility in the nerve being tested. Therefore using the test position to stretch the nerve and release any adhesions along their course is a common treatment philosophy. What is overlooked is the fact that nerve tissue is different from muscle tissue. Muscles have the potential to elongate and stretch, whereas neural tissue is not as elastic and responds adversely to stretching. Treatment therefore should address gliding not stretching of nerves. Soft tissue structures along the course of the nerve can be mobilized to allow for nerve mobility. Movement of the upper extremity can be combined with small movements of the neck to encourage gliding of the nerve rather than stretching. Finally, communication with the patient is essential since radicular pain or paresthesias indicate that the nerve is being stretched and potentially irritated. The patient and therapist should work in ROMs that do not reproduce the patient's radicular symptoms.

HOME EXERCISE

Which home exercises are the most beneficial for patients with cervical pain?

Home exercise programs should reinforce the treatment received in clinic. If mobility was the main focus of treatment, then cervical ROM exercises should be initiated. If stability or strengthening exercises were used in clinic, then similar exercises should be prescribed for home.

REHABILITATION CLINICAL REASONING

How should a clinician decide which intervention is most appropriate for a patient with cervical pain?

Key components to keep in mind during each phase of the rehabilitation process are the following:

PHASE I: INFLAMMATORY PHASE

- Reduction of inflammation and pain
- Restoration of function.
- Active pain-free ROM
- Active rest should be encouraged.

PHASE II: REPARATIVE PHASE

- Promotion of tissue healing and graded increases in stress placed on the healing tissue.
- Improve to full ROM
- Restoration of local muscle control

PHASE III: REMODELING PHASE

- Encourage gliding of the neural tissue to prevent the formation of adhesions.
- Continue placing stress on the soft tissue and bone in graded increments to promote proper soft tissue and bone growth and development.
- Functional retraining
- Correction of the postural deviations and contributing factors that predispose a patient to neck pain.
- Coordinate activation of local and global muscles

What red flags should a clinician be aware of regarding rehabilitating a patient with cervical pain?

The cardiovascular, respiratory, endocrine, gastrointestinal, and hepatic systems can refer pain into the cervical region. Clinicians should be cautious with patients who have nonmechanical neck pain, pain that is unremitting and poorly localized, or symptoms that change with breathing, exercise, or food intake.

TABLE IV-1-4   Tissue Injury and Intervention Selection

What are the best interventions for the inflammatory phase (0-14 days postinjury)?	When to progress to next phase	What are the best interventions for the reparative phase (15-21 days postinjury)?	When to progress to next phase	What are the best interventions for the remodeling phase (22-60 days postinjury)?	When to progress to next phase	What are the best interventions for the maturation phase (60-360 days postinjury)?	When to progress to next phase
Disc Pathology							
Rest, cervical collar, antiinflammatory medications	Pain begins to centralize.	Centralizing movements (e.g., cervical retraction or extension), manual therapy (e.g., traction) modalities to treat pain and spasm, begin deep neck flexor training	Pain continues to centralize or is abolished.	Manual therapy, progress exercises to include functional tasks Cervical proprioception training Coordination of local muscles and global muscles	Patient is tolerating current interventions and is making functional changes.	Progress exercise and function as tolerated. Return to preinjury activities. Functional retraining.	Progress as tolerated. Patient is most likely independent at this stage.
Muscle Strain							
Active rest	Pain and symptoms (spasm) begin to resolve.	STM, gentle mobilizations, pain-free AROM exercise, deep cervical flexor training, modalities for symptom relief as needed	Pain and symptoms continue to resolve.	Manual therapy, progress exercises to include functional tasks Cervical proprioception training Coordination of local muscles and global muscles	Pain and symptoms continue to resolve.	Progress exercise and function as tolerated. Return to preinjury activities. Functional retraining.	Progress as tolerated. Patient is most likely independent at this stage.
Ligament Sprain							
Rest, cervical collar, antiinflammatory medications	Pain and symptoms begin to resolve.	STM, gentle mobilizations, pain-free AROM exercise, deep cervical flexor training, modalities for symptom relief as needed	Pain and symptoms continue to resolve.	Manual therapy, progress exercises to include functional tasks Cervical proprioception training Coordination of local muscles and global muscles	Pain and symptoms continue to resolve.	Progress exercise and function as tolerated. Return to preinjury activities. Functional retraining.	Progress as tolerated. Patient is most likely independent at this stage.
Tendon Pathology							
Rest, general nonprovocative movements, avoid end-range movements	Pain and symptoms begin to resolve.	STM, gentle mobilizations, pain free AROM exercise, deep cervical flexor training, modalities for symptom relief as needed	Pain and symptoms continue to resolve.	Manual therapy, progress exercises to include functional tasks Cervical proprioception training Coordination of local muscles and global muscles	Pain and symptoms continue to resolve.	Progress exercise and function as tolerated. Return to preinjury activities. Functional retraining.	Progress as tolerated. Patient is most likely independent at this stage.

Continued on following page.

TABLE IV-1-4 Tissue Injury and Intervention Selection (Continued)

What are the best interventions for the inflammatory phase (0-14 days postinjury)?	When to progress to next phase	What are the best interventions for the reparative phase (15-21 days postinjury)?	When to progress to next phase	What are the best interventions for the remodeling phase (22-60 days postinjury)?	When to progress to next phase	What are the best interventions for the maturation phase (60-360 days postinjury)?	When to progress to next phase
Bone Fracture							
Rest, cervical collar, antiinflammatory medications. If severe, surgery may be required to stabilize the fracture.	Depending on severity of injury may not be appropriate for therapy at this stage.	If nonsurgical: STM, gentle mobilizations, pain-free AROM exercise, deep cervical flexor training, modalities for symptom relief as needed. If surgical: Usually not appropriate for therapy.	If nonsurgical: Patient may progress as pain and function allow. If surgical: Evidence of callus formation and physician clearance required.	If nonsurgical: STM, progression of mobilizations, AROM exercise, deep cervical flexor training, global and local muscle coordination, modalities for symptom relief as needed. If surgical: Usually not appropriate for therapy.	Evidence of bone unionization, physician clearance.	If nonsurgical: Progress exercise and function as tolerated. Return to preinjury activities. If surgical: STM, gentle mobilizations, pain-free AROM exercise, deep cervical flexor training, modalities for symptom relief as needed.	Progress as tolerated. Patient is most likely independent at this stage. If surgical: Slow return to function
Cartilage Damage or Degeneration							
Antiinflammatory medication, rest, gentle AROM exercises	Decreased symptoms and improved function.	STM, gentle mobilizations, pain-free AROM exercise, deep cervical flexor training, modalities for symptom relief as needed.	Improved ROM and decreased symptoms.	Manual therapy, progress exercises to include functional tasks. Cervical proprioception training. Coordination of local muscles and global muscles	Return to prior function, able to complete most daily activities without symptoms.	Progress exercise and function as tolerated. Return to preinjury activities. Functional retraining.	Progress as tolerated. Patient is most likely independent at this stage.
Capsule Injury							
Rest, antiinflammatory medications	Pain and symptoms begin to resolve.	Manual therapy (e.g., unilateral posterior to anterior mobilization (PA), manipulation), AROM exercises, modalities as needed.	Pain and symptoms continue to resolve	If nonsurgical: STM, gentle mobilizations, pain-free AROM exercise, deep cervical flexor training, modalities for symptom relief as needed. If surgical: Usually not appropriate for therapy.	Pain and symptoms continue to resolve.	Progress exercise and function as tolerated. Return to preinjury activities. Functional retraining.	Progress as tolerated. Patient is most likely independent at this stage.
Nerve Injury							
Rest, cervical collar, antiinflammatory medications	Pain and symptoms begin to resolve; centralization of symptoms.	STM and mobilization to clear nerve entrapment sites. Gentle neurodynamic mobilization, AROM exercises.	Pain and symptoms continue to resolve.	Progress neurodynamic mobilization, AROM exercises, deep flexor muscle training.	No longer experiencing radicular symptoms.	Progress exercise and function as tolerated. Coordination of local muscles and global muscles. Return to preinjury activities. Functional retraining	Progress as tolerated. Patient is most likely independent at this stage.

STM, Soft tissue mobilization; AROM, Active range of motion; PA, Posterior to anterior mobilizations

Cancers located in the bone or lung can refer pain into the neck, so the patient should be questioned regarding nocturnal pain, history of cancer, history of smoking, or unexplained weight changes.

Patients whose symptoms are increasing or patients who begin to experience symptoms that extend into the upper extremity should be watched cautiously, and if symptoms continue to increase without provocation, the patient should be referred back to the physician.

SUMMARY STATEMENT

Although guidelines can provide generalized time frames for healing and recovery, it is important to realize that a firm grasp of the factors listed will enable the clinician to individualize the rehabilitation program for each patient. No patients are identical. Therefore no rehabilitation programs should be identical. Solid clinical reasoning regarding the patient and the nature of his or her injury and surgery will ultimately drive the rehabilitation process (Table IV-1-4). Research can shape the rehabilitation process, but clinical judgment ultimately drives the decisions made in clinic.

REFERENCES

1. Bogduk N. Biomechanics of the cervical spine. In: Grant R, ed. *Physical Therapy of the Cervical and Thoracic Spine.* St Louis: Churchill Livingstone; 2002.
2. Bronfort G, Haas M, Evans RL, Bouter LM. Efficacy of spinal manipulation and mobilization for low back pain and neck pain: a systematic review and best evidence synthesis. *Spine J.* 2004;4(3):335-356.
3. Butler D. *The Sensitive Nervous System.* Adelaide: Noigroup Publications; 2000.
4. Butler D. Upper limb neurodynamic test: Clinical use in a "Big Picture" framework. In: Grant R, ed. *Physical Therapy of the Cervical and Thoracic Spine.* St Louis: Churchill Livingstone; 2002.
5. Childs JD, Fritz JM, Piva SR, Whitman JM, Sterling JM. Proposal of a classification system for patients with neck pain. *JOSPT.* 2004;34(11):686-700.
6. Cleland J, Childs J, McRae M, Palmer J, Stowell T. Immediate effects of thoracic manipulation in patients with neck pain: a randomized clinical trial. *Man Ther.* 2005;10:127-135.
7. Cleland JA, Fritz JM, Whitman JM, Heath R. Predictors of short-term outcome in people with a clinical diagnosis of cervical radiculopathy. *Phys Ther.* 2007;87(12):1619-1632.
8. Cleland JA, Whitman JM, Fritz JM, Palmer JA. Manual physical therapy, cervical traction, and strengthening exercises in patients with cervical radiculopathy: a case series. *J Orthop Sports Phys Ther.* 2005;35(12):802-811.
9. Dillin W, Uppal G. Analysis of medications used in the treatment of cervical disc degeneration. *Orthop Clin N Am.* 1992;23:421.
10. Elvey R. Treatment of arm pain associated with abnormal brachial plexus tension. *Aust J Physiother.* 32: 225-230.
11. Ezzo J, Haraldsson BG, Gross AR, et al. Massage for mechanical neck disorders. *A Systematic Review.* 2007;32(3):353-362.
12. Falla D, Jull G, Hodges PW. Feedforward activity of the cervical flexor muscles during voluntary arm movements is delayed in chronic neck pain. *Exp Brain Res.* 2004;157(1):43-48.
13. Falla D, Jull G, Dall'Alba P, Rainoldi A, Merletti R. An electromyographic analysis of the deep cervical flexor muscles in performance of craniocervical flexion. *Phys Ther.* 2003;83(10):899-906.
14. Falla DL, Jull GA, Hodges PW. Patients with neck pain demonstrate reduced electromyographic activity of the deep cervical flexor muscles during performance of the craniocervical flexion test. *Spine.* 2004;29(19):2108-2114.
15. Falla DL, Campbell CD, Fagan AE, Thompson DC, Jull GA. Relationship between craniocervical flexion range of motion and pressure change during the craniocervical flexion test. *Man Ther.* 2003;8:92-96.
16. Frenkel S, Grew J. Soft tissue repair. In: Spivak J, DiCesare P, Feldman D, Koval K, Rokito A, Zuckerman J, eds. *Orthopaedics - A Study Guide.* New York: McGraw Hill; 1999.
17. Frenkel S, Koval K. Fracture healing and bone grafting. In: Spivak J, DiCesare P, Feldman D, Koval K, Rokito A, Zuckerman J, eds. *Orthopaedics - A Study Guide.* New York: McGraw Hill; 1999.
18. Goffin J, van Loon J, Van Calenbergh F, et al. Long-term results after anterior cervical fusion and osteosynthetic stabilization for fractures and/or dislocations of the cervical spine. *J Spinal Disord.* 1995;8:499-508.
19. Graham N, Gross A, Goldsmith CH, et al. Mechanical traction for neck pain with or without radiculopathy. *Cochrane Database Syst Rev.* 2008;16(3):CD006408.
20. Grimmer K. Measuring the endurance capacity of the cervical short flexor muscle group. *Aust J Physiother.* 1994;40:251-254.
21. Gross AR, Hoving JL, Haines TA, et al. Cervical overview group. A Cochrane review of manipulation and mobilization for mechanical neck disorders. *Spine.* 2004;29(14):1541-1548.
22. Gross AR, Kay T, Hondras M, et al. Manual therapy for mechanical neck disorders: a systematic review. *Man Ther.* 2002;7(3):131-149.
23. Gross AR, Kay TM, Kennedy C, et al. Clinical practice guideline on the use of manipulation or mobilization in the treatment of adults with mechanical neck disorders. *Man Ther.* 2002;7(4):193-205.
24. Gross AR, Goldsmith C, Hoving JL, et al. Cervical overview group. Conservative management of mechanical neck disorders: a systematic review. *J Rheumatol.* 2007;34(5):1083-1102.
25. Janda V. Muscles and Motor Control in Cervicogenic Disorders. In: Grant R, ed. *Physical Therapy of the Cervical and Thoracic Spine.* St. Louis: Churchill Livingstone; 2002.
26. Jull G. Management of cervicogenic headaches. In: Grant R, ed. *Physical Therapy of the Cervical and Thoracic Spine.* St. Louis: Churchill Livingstone; 2002.
27. Jull G, Kristjansson E, Dall'Alba P. Impairment in the cervical flexors: a comparison of whiplash and insidious onset neck pain patients. *Man Ther.* 2004;9(2):89-94.
28. Jull G, Falla D, Treleaven J, Hodges P, Vicenzino B. Retraining cervical joint position sense: The effect of two exercise regimes. *J Ortho Res.* 2007;25(3):404-412.
29. Kay TM, Gross A, Goldsmith C, Santaguida PL, Hoving J, Bronfort G. Cervical overview group. Exercises for mechanical neck disorders. *Cochrane Database Syst Rev.* 2005;(3):CD004250.
30. Klaber-Moffett JA. An investigation of the effects of cervical traction. Part 1: Clinical effectiveness. *Clin Rehabil.* 1990;4(3):205-211.
31. Koval K, Rokito A, Zuckerman J. *Orthopaedics - A Study Guide.* New York: McGraw Hill; 1999.
32. Kroeling P, Gross A, Houghton PE. Cervical overview group. Electrotherapy for neck disorders. *Cochrane Database Syst Rev.* 2005;(2):CD004251.
33. Neumann D. Axial skeleton: osteology and arthrology. In: Neumann D, ed. *Kinesiology of the Musculoskeletal System - Foundations for Physical Rehabilitation.* St Louis: Mosby; 2002.
34. Nitz A. Bone injury and repair. In: Placzek J, Boyce D, eds. *Orthopaedic Physical Therapy Secrets.* Philadelphia: Hanley and Belfus Inc; 2001.
35. Nitz A. Soft tissue injury and repair. In: Placzek J, Boyce D, eds. *Orthopaedic Physical Therapy Secrets.* Philadelphia: Hanley and Belfus Inc; 2001.
36. Olmarker K, Rydevik B. Nerve root pathophysiology. In: Fardon D, Garfin S, Abitbol S, Boden S, Herkowitz H, Mayer T, eds. *Orthopaedic Knowledge Update: Spine 2.* Rosemont: American Academy of Orthopaedic Surgeons; 2002.
37. Patijn J. Complications in manual medicine: a review of literature. *J Man Med.* 1991;6:89-92.
38. Penning L, Wilmink JT, van Woerden HH, et al. CT Myelographic findings in degenerative disorders of the cervical spine: Clinical significance. *Am J Neuroradiol.* 1986;7:119-127.
39. Posner M. Compression neuropathies. In: Spivak J, DiCesare P, Feldman D, Koval K, Rokito A, Zuckerman J, eds. *Orthopaedics - A Study Guide.* New York: McGraw Hill; 1999.
40. Posner M. Nerve lacerations: acute and chronic. In: Spivak J, DiCesare P, Feldman D, Koval K, Rokito A, Zuckerman J, eds. *Orthopaedics - A Study Guide.* New York: McGraw Hill; 1999.
41. Raney NH, Petersen EJ, Smith TA, et al. Development of a clinical prediction rule to identify patients with neck pain likely to benefit from cervical traction and exercise. *Eur Spine J.* 2009.
42. Richardson C, Jull G, Hodges P, Hides J. *Therapeutic Exercise for Spinal Segmental Stabilization in Low Back Pain - Scientific Basis and Clinical Approach.* Edinburgh: Churchill Livingstone; 1999.
43. Rivett DA, Milburn P. A prospective study of complications of cervical spine manipulation. *J Man Manip Ther.* 1996;4:166-170.

44. Sarig-Bahat H. Evidence for exercise therapy in mechanical neck disorders. *Man Ther.* 2003;8(1):10-20.

45. White A, Panjabi M. *Clinical Biomechanics of the Spine.* 2nd ed. Philadelphia: J.B. Lippincott; 1990.

46. White R, Ernst E. A systematic review of randomized controlled trials of acupuncture for neck pain. *Rheumatology.* 1999;38:143-147.

47. Zeigman S, Ducker T, Raycroft J. Trends and complications in cervical spine surgery: 1989-1993. *J Spinal Disord.* 1997;10:523-526.

48. Sterling M, Jull G, Wright A. Cervical mobilization: concurrent effects on pain, sympathetic nervous system activity and motor activity. *Man Ther.* 2001;6(2):72-81.

AUTHOR: MARK KOZUKI

INTRODUCTORY INFORMATION   *i*

What are the factors a clinician should consider when rehabilitating a patient with midback pain?

The thoracic spine regional anatomy has a very unique structural architecture. The presence of the rib cage, increased relative vertebral body height, decreased relative disc height, kyphotic curvature, and vertical orientation of the facet joints contribute to forming a region of the spine that has more structural stability and reduced mobility.[8] Niemelainen[30] found that incidence of midback pain accounted for approximately one-fourth of the combined amount of neck and low back pain. The reduced rate of injury in the thoracic region of the spine may be due to its inherent structural stability. The naturally stiff thoracic spine region is surrounded on all sides by the highly mobile cervical spine, shoulder, and lumbar spine regions.

How do these factors affect the rehabilitation process?

In a general view, the thoracic spine region is prone to dysfunctional hypomobility, whereas the cervical spine, shoulder, and lumbar spine regions are likely to develop dysfunctional hypermobility. There are times when hypermobility may exist and the use of stabilization techniques may be utilized. Commonly, rotational instabilities are noted in the midthoracic spine. This is due to the relative vertical orientation of the facet joints in this region, which allows increased motion in the transverse plane. Ribs are also prone to becoming hypermobile at their anterior attachment.[19] There is a dynamic interplay between these regions, in which dysfunction in one region may affect an adjacent or distant region. This concept has recently been termed as regional interdependence by Wainner et al.[33]

In the presence of midback pain, a regional examination should be completed to determine whether the adjacent or distant body regions are contributing to the production of midback pain. Often, during the rehabilitation process, the clinician will address local thoracic spine region impairments as the source of the symptom but will also likely need to address impairments in adjacent or distant body regions as the potential causes of in the symptom production.

What role does acuteness or chronicity play in rehabilitating a patient with midback pain?

In the acute phase, the primary goal will be to relieve pain and reduce inflammation. This may be accomplished through the use of passive modalities. Education on avoidance and alterations of aggravating movements and positions is critical and is an essential component in this stage. However, after inflammation has been controlled, the stage of healing plays a minimal role in rehabilitation of a patient with midback pain.

Regardless of the stage of healing, the clinician is attempting to address the source of the patient's symptoms and the causes of the symptoms. Once the source and causes have been determined, treatment will begin to address the impairments found during the examination.

What factors make treatment of patients with midback pain challenging?

The numerous sources of pain in the thoracic spine pose a significant differential diagnostic challenge to the clinician. Local somatic sources of pain, referred pain from visceral organs, pain referred from the cervical spine, and scapular dysfunctions must be differentiated during the examination process.

Are there factors that make treatment of patients with midback pain easier?

There are no specific factors that can make treatment of patients with midback pain easier. However, there is preliminary evidence that suggests thoracic spine manipulation can be an effective adjunctive treatment to the neck and shoulder dysfunction.[2,4-6]

PROGNOSIS

How successful is rehabilitation in treating midback pain?

Treatment of midback pain can be very successful when the source of the symptom and the causes of the symptom have been addressed. Rehabilitation will be focused on impairments that have been determined to be the causes of the symptom production. This may include addressing impaired posture, muscular strength, muscle length, muscle endurance, joint mobility, postural awareness, and control.

Which patients with midback pain derive the greatest long-term benefits from rehabilitation?

The patients who derive the greatest long-term benefits from rehabilitation are those who present a mechanical component to their midback pain. It is important to show patients that there is a mechanical component to their pain, which can be altered and improved. This increases compliance with the rehabilitation program and promotes the greatest long-term benefits. Home exercises that are given to the patient will address the impairments associated with functional limitations.

Designing a plan of how to address the causative factors and actively involving the patient in rehabilitation will result in optimal results. Patients who "buy in" to the treatment and are willing to change their movement behavior tend to have the greatest long-term benefit from rehabilitation. An example of a treatment may include manual therapy to improve mobility, education and training on posture, altering desk or work set-up, and compliance with a home exercise program consisting of stretching and self-mobilization exercises.

What other regions of the body are most likely to contribute to midback pain?

Cervical and shoulder dysfunctions should be considered as contributors to midback pain. Studies done on cervical facet and disc referral patterns have shown that pain can be referred into the upper thoracic region.[7,31] Abnormal scapular positioning and dyskinesis may contribute to midback pain. Hip weakness or tightness with lumbar spine hypermobility can also create abnormal strain or movements on the thoracic region (see Case Study).

CASE STUDY   *?*

Your patient is a 24-year-old female with right midthoracic pain that began 9 weeks ago. She notes no specific trauma but stated it may be related to lifting boxes during a recent home relocation. She states that she has had several chiropractic treatments treating a displaced rib and that her pain remains about the same. She states her pain is constant but worse at the end of the day, after working on the computer and lifting her 2-year-old son. On examination, you note: mild forward head, flat thoracic spine, depressed and abducted right scapula, and full and pain-free cervical and thoracic active range of motion (AROM). Passive physiological testing is symmetrical. You note medial border scapular winging with shoulder elevation and a positive scapular assistance test. Pectoralis major and latissimus dorsi are normal length, but pectoralis minor has very mild tightness. There is tenderness noted at the levels of T5-6. What treatment will likely improve her symptoms?

Answer

Treatment focused on improving her scapular position and control will likely improve her symptoms. Treatment may include postural education focused on reducing forward head and improving scapular position, taping to decrease the load on lengthened upper trapezius and rhomboid, and scapular control exercises. Often, treatment of this patient will be misdirected at focusing on the thoracic spine without consideration of the shoulder's interdependence with this region.

EVIDENCE-BASED MEDICINE

What trends are currently being seen in research regarding rehabilitation of the thoracic region?

The current trend in research regarding the thoracic region includes the addition of thoracic manipulation in cervical and shoulder disorders. Cleland et al[4] developed a clinical prediction rule (CPR) regarding the use of thoracic manipulation for neck pain. The six variables included in the CPR include symptoms less than 30 days, no symptoms distal to the shoulder, looking up does not aggravate symptoms, Fear Avoidance Beliefs Questionnaire (FABQ) score ≤11, decreased T3-5 kyphosis, and cervical extension <30 degrees.

Bergman et al[1] showed that the addition of thoracic manipulation to the usual medical care had more rapid improvement in symptoms and fewer shoulder symptoms at 12 weeks. The authors concluded that manipulative therapy appears to be an effective treatment option for patients with shoulder pain and shoulder girdle dysfunction that are not due to trauma, fracture, rupture, or dislocation.

INTERVENTIONS

MANUAL THERAPY

What is the physiological rationale behind the use of manual therapy in treating patients with midback pain?

Biomechanical and neurophysiological factors are the two main mechanisms cited as the effect of manual therapy techniques.[10,34] Several theories of manual therapy effects include it frees a mechanical impediment to joint movement, it stretches or ruptures periarticular scar tissues, it improves nerve conductivity or circulation by reducing compression, it improves muscle function and decreases stress on bones and ligaments by improving the distribution of joint forces, and it affects neural activity as a result of afferent stimulation.[9]

CLINICAL PEARL

Mobilization and self-mobilization techniques should be performed before strengthening exercises to reduce muscle inhibition caused by postural syndromes. Thoracic spine mobilization and manipulation of the midthoracic and lower thoracic spine may be used before exercise to facilitate middle and lower trapezius strengthening. Cleland et al[6] and Liebler et al[23] found a statistically significant increase in lower trapezius strength as compared to the control group.

Is joint mobilization recommended for patients with midback pain?

Joint mobilization can be an effective treatment for midback pain by improving reduced mobility of the thoracic segments and/or the ribs. Joint mobilization technique will be based on hypomobility found during passive accessory joint mobility testing and passive physiologic joint mobility testing.[24] When assessing abnormal joint mobility of the thoracic spine, the ribs corresponding to the dysfunctional levels should always be assessed.

Is joint manipulation recommended for patients with midback pain?

Joint manipulation can be an effective method of treatment for the treatment of midback pain. Commonly, joint mobilization may be progressed to joint manipulation if the treatment fails to make further gains. Joint manipulation of the upper and midthoracic spine has been found to be an effective treatment for cervical and shoulder dysfunctions.[1,13]

There is limited evidence to support that joint manipulation is an effective treatment for midback pain. Schiller[36] compared the use of spinal manipulation with nonfunctional ultrasound placebo in a small randomized controlled trial of 30 patients with mechanical thoracic spinal pain. The study demonstrated significantly better reductions in numerical pain ratings and improved motion in lateral flexion with thoracic manipulation at the end of a 2- to 3-week period. The improvements were maintained 4 weeks later but were no longer better than the nonfunctional ultrasound placebo group.

Are there other manual therapy techniques that are effective in the treatment of patients with midback pain?

If mobilization has proved unsuccessful, manual treatment may then be altered to joint manipulation or utilization of a sustained natural apophyseal glide (SNAG).[15,29] A SNAG is a manual therapy technique that combines passive pain-free mobilization applied to the affected spinal level or rib, with the patient actively moving into the previously symptomatic motion.[29] SNAG is an effective follow-up home exercise to further improve pain-free mobility. Reverse SNAGs have been found to be very effective at improving mobility in the upper thoracic spine.[29] The loading-bearing position, accessory glide along the facet joint plane, facilitation of pain-free movement, and potential problems with end-range passive movements in degenerative joints are reduced with the use of a SNAG.[8]

Muscle energy techniques (MET) may also be used in treatment of the thoracic spine region. MET involves the clinician taking the dysfunctional muscle-joint complex to its restrictive barrier and then having the patient perform an isometric contraction of either the agonist or antagonist muscle followed by complete relaxation. During this relaxation period, the clinician moves the muscle-joint complex into the new restrictive barrier.[11]

Mulligan techniques and MET may be used also be used after joint mobilization or manipulation to facilitate the newly established mobility gains.

What does evidence reveal regarding the use of massage (soft tissue mobilization) for the treatment of patients with midback pain?

There is limited evidence for soft tissue mobilization (STM) to the thoracic region. Two case reports were found that included treatment of trigger points in the upper thoracic region.[12,26] STM can also be an effective tool when treating midback pain. It is used to assist in restoring muscle length and improving mobility by decreasing focal soft tissue restrictions. This will allow increased active pain-free movement and functional mobility. Observation of posture and movement, muscle length tests, and palpation will guide the clinician to identify muscles that will benefit from STM. Common muscles that may benefit from STM are those that are prone to tightness. The erector spinae, quadratus lumborum, pectoralis major and minor, levator scapulae, scalenes, and flexors of the upper limb are prone to tightness.[16] The adjacent intercostal muscles should be assessed and treated in the presence of a rib dysfunction.

CLINICAL PEARL

When thoracolumbar rotation is limited, asymmetrical, and symptomatic, the clinician should consider assessing soft tissue mobility of the surrounding musculature. Direct techniques improving thoracolumbar rotation may be enhanced by first addressing the restrictions in the quadratus lumborum, internal oblique, external oblique, and transverse abdominus on the side where rotation is limited. The anterior abdominal muscles are typically restricted and tender near their attachments on the lower edge of the rib cage. The clinician also has to determine the underlying causes of this muscular imbalance and asymmetry.

TABLE IV-2-1 Motion Restriction and Mobilization/Manipulation

Motion Restrictions	Joint Requiring Mobilization/ Manipulation	Direction of Mobilization/ Manipulation
Upper thoracic extension	T1-T2	Seated-extension, sidebend, rotation
Upper thoracic flexion	T1-T2	Seated-flexion, sidebend, rotation
Midthoracic flexion	T3-T7	Supine-posterior to anterior mobilization
Low thoracic extension	T8-T12	Prone-posterior to anterior mobilization
Thoracolumbar rotation	T11-12	Seated/sidelying-rotation
Ribs 1 and 2	Ribs 1-2, T1-T2	Inferior
Anterior subluxed rib	Ribs 3-10	Posterior
Posterior subluxed rib	Ribs 3-10	Anterior

Adapted from Flynn T W: Thoracic spine and rib cage dysfunction. In Placzek J D, Boyce DA (eds): *Orthopaedic physical therapy secrets*, St. Louis, 2006, Mosby Elsevier.

How should a clinician decide which manual therapy intervention is most appropriate for a patient with midback pain?

Manual therapy techniques are typically done to improve spinal motion in a particular direction. Selection of technique will be based on the motion restriction found during passive physiological mobility testing, passive accessory mobility testing, and positional testing of the thoracic transverse processes in spinal flexion and extension. The direction of limitation in active and passive mobility, asymmetry in motion, and tissue texture changes will help guide the clinician in selection of a manual therapy technique and the spinal level or rib to be treated.

Manual therapy interventions will be aimed at restoring mobility in a specific direction (see Case Study). Table IV-2-1 contains common thoracic restrictions and manual therapy interventions. ROM and mobility testing should always be reassessed after manual therapy procedures to determine the effect of the treatment.[24]

CASE STUDY

Your patient is a 40-year-old male who presents with midback pain over the last 6 weeks. He states his pain began after golfing 3 days in a row; he typically plays golf once a week. He states he has left midback pain during the follow through of his golf swing. During evaluation of the patient's golf swing, excessive midthoracic rotation was noted, with reduced right shoulder horizontal adduction and internal rotation of the left hip. Active rotation thoracolumbar rotation was limited to 75% with symptom reproduction. Passive physiological accessory testing revealed hypomobility at T7-9, but hypermobility and symptom reproduction at T5-6. Horizontal adduction of the right shoulder with the scapula fixed was 4 inches from the sternum with a muscular end-feel, and the left shoulder was 0 inches to the sternum. Left hip internal rotation was 10 degrees with a capsular end-feel, right hip internal rotation was 35 degrees with a capsular end-feel. What treatment will likely improve his symptoms?

Answer

The source of the patient's pain is hypermobility at T5-6, but the underlying causes are the limited left rotation at T7-9, limited right shoulder horizontal adduction, and limited left hip internal

rotation. Treatment should include mobilization to the left hip, STM and stretching to the right scapulohumeral muscles, and mobilization to the left T7-9.

EXERCISE

What is the physiological rationale behind the use of exercise in treating patients with midback pain?

The primary use of exercise in the thoracic region is to achieve ideal postural alignment and restoring functional movement. To achieve improved functional movement, restoring length to shortened muscles and increasing strength in weakened muscles must occur.[16] Recent research is evolving regarding segmental stability and its role in thoracic dysfunction. Like the lumbar and cervical spines, the multifidus muscles and the small local muscles of the spine provide segmental stability to the spinal segments of the thoracic region. In cases of injury, inflammatory and sympathetic processes often inhibit these muscles. Global muscles are recruited to compensate for the diminished local muscle control. This pattern is also seen in the thoracic spine. Multiple segments will present with stiffness and muscle tenderness. Lee has proposed that this musculature adaptation is the result of thoracic hypermobility and that segmental stabilization is required to provide for proper thoracic function. Many of the exercises that she proposes are similar to the exercises used to segmentally stabilize the cervical and lumbar spine but are applied to the offending thoracic segments.[20-22]

Which muscles should be strengthened in treating patients with midback pain?

Muscle strength in the thoracic spine is not as critical as motor control, muscle timing, and endurance. The muscles that support and stabilize the thoracic spine are primarily postural muscles. The postural stabilizer muscles (i.e., multifidi, deep rotators, and erector spinae muscles) will benefit from improved endurance. The rhomboids, middle trapezius, lower trapezius, and serratus anterior typically benefit from improved strength and motor control training. Strengthening of the internal oblique, external oblique, rectus abdominus, and transversus abdominus is important in core stability. Good control of the neutral spine position is important for functional tasks.

Is stretching beneficial or indicated for patients with midback pain?

- Stretching can also be effective in treating patients with midback pain. It is indicated based on limited ROM with muscular end-feel and/or positive muscle length tests advocated by Kendall.[10]
- Stretching of a tight pectoralis major and minor and latissimus dorsi may be performed to help restore ideal scapulothoracic positioning. Janda[17] coined the term "upper crossed syndrome," noting that tight anterior thoracic musculature and weak posterior musculature contribute to the common abnormal deviation of the forward head and rounded shoulders.

How should a clinician decide which exercise is most appropriate for a patient with midback pain?

Every exercise given to the patient should address a specific impairment found during the examination. The patient needs to be able to complete the exercise with good form and should feel the exercise in the desired muscle.

How should a clinician progress an exercise program for the midback?

Spinal exercise programs typically include strengthening isolated muscles, stretching tight muscles, integrating core stabilization and endurance, and then progressing to functional exercises and movements. The quality of the exercise or movement is always emphasized over quantity during exercise prescription. Exercises may be progressed by adding resistance, increasing repetitions, or increasing hold times. Exercises may also be progressed through types of muscular contractions: The clinician should focus upon specifically training isometric, concentric, or eccentric contractions to meet the needs of functional tasks. As the quality and symmetry of a movement are improved, the exercise may be ready to be progressed.

HOME EXERCISE

Which home exercises are the most beneficial for patients with midback pain?

Stretching of the pectoralis major in a doorway, stretching of the latissimus dorsi by leaning on a table or desk, cat stretch, prayer stretch, arm circles, and scalene stretch are commonly prescribed. Wall slides, wall push-ups, and reverse corner push-ups are given for scapular control and positioning. With the patient in the quadruped position, alternating arms and legs is a good stabilization exercise. In the quadruped position, rhomboid and lower trapezius strengthening exercises may be incorporated.

Self-mobilization exercises are also very useful. A mobilization wedge to self-mobilize the thoracic spine may be used in the supine position. Placing a piece of tape on the patient's skin at the spinal level where the wedge should be placed will help with localization. A tennis ball can be used in the thoracic spine for unilateral mobilization or rib mobilization. The foam roll may also be used to mobilize the thoracic spine, but it is difficult to be specific to a single spinal segment (Box IV-2-1).

BOX IV-2-1 **Suggested Home Exercises for the Patient with Midback Pain**

Exercise Set 1

Exercise 1: Doorway pectoral stretch

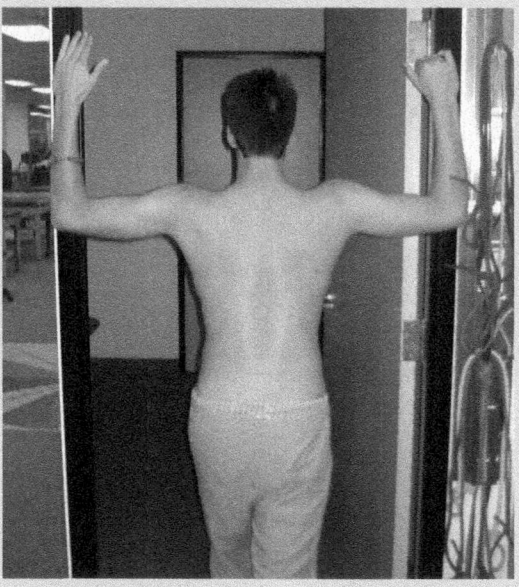

Exercise 2: Seated latissimus table stretch

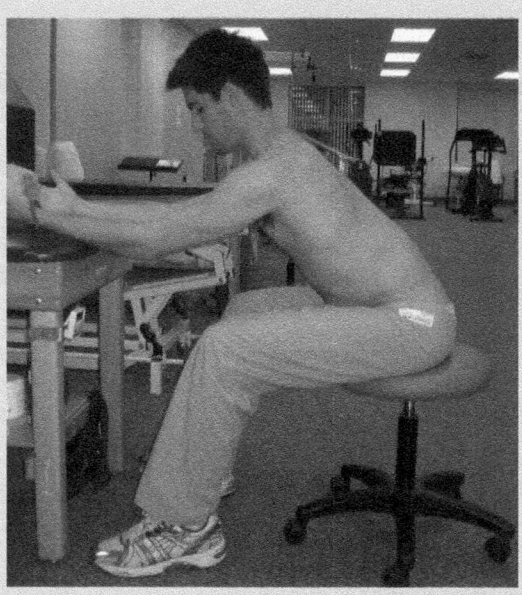

Exercise 3: Scalene stretch

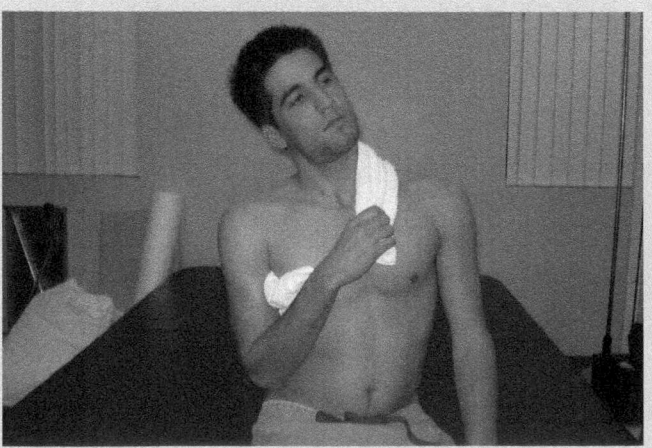

Exercise 4: Cat stretch

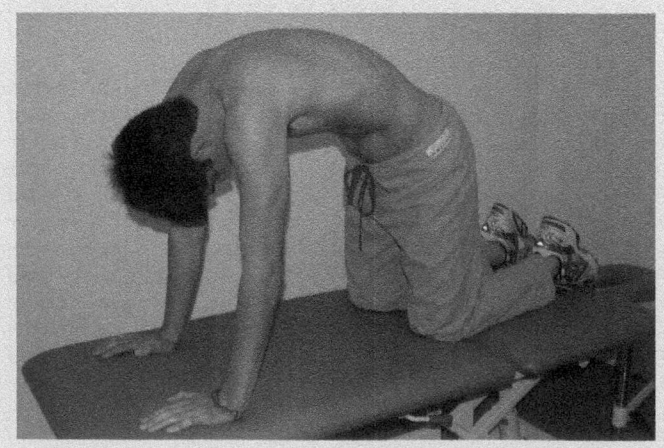

BOX IV-2-1 **Suggested Home Exercises for the Patient with Midback Pain (*Continued*)**

Exercise 5: Prayer stretch

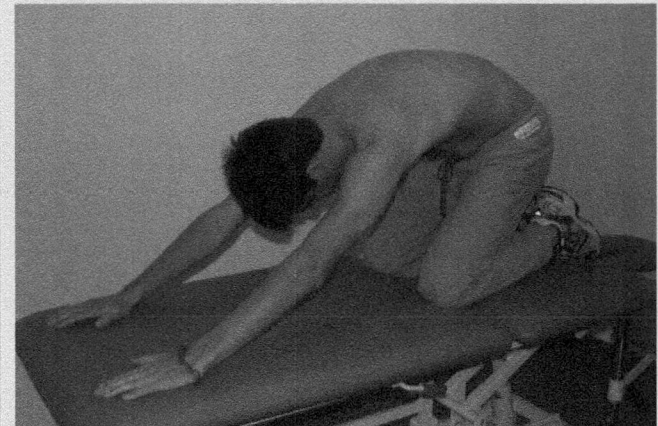

Exercise 6: Arm circles

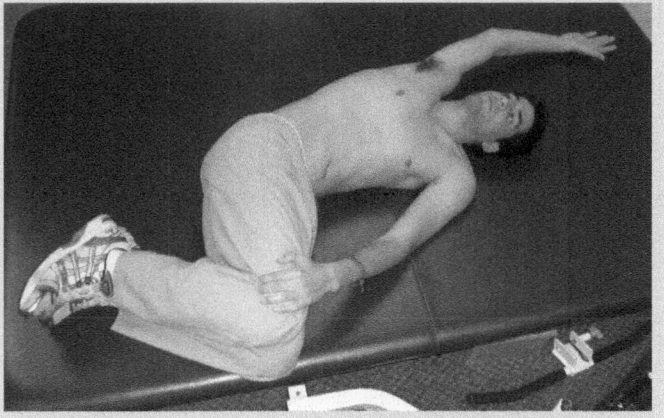

Exercise Set 2
Exercise 1: Wall slides

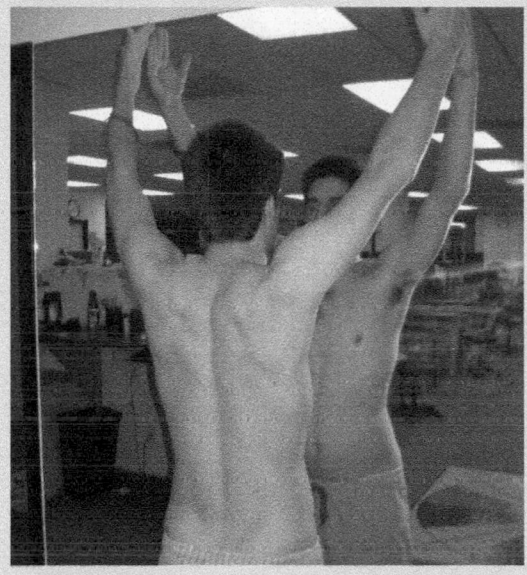

Exercise 2: Wall push-ups

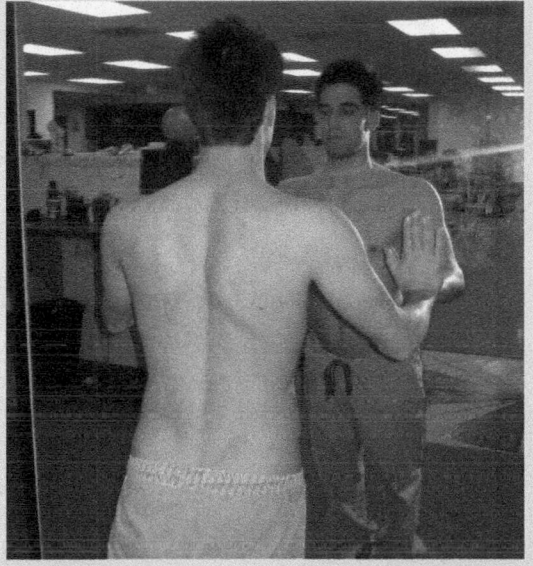

Exercise 3: Reverse corner push-ups

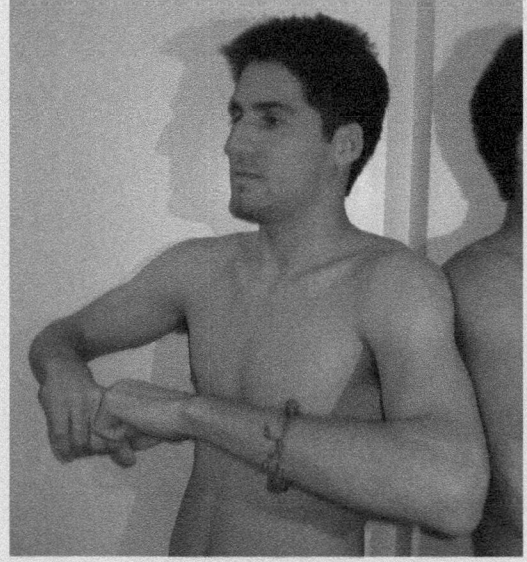

Exercise 4: Arm fallouts

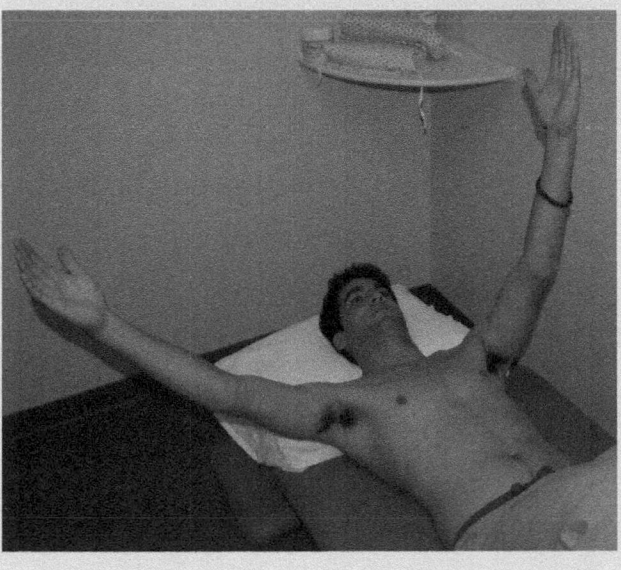

Continued on following page.

BOX IV-2-1   **Suggested Home Exercises for the Patient with Midback Pain (*Continued*)**

Exercise 5: Quadruped alternating arms and legs

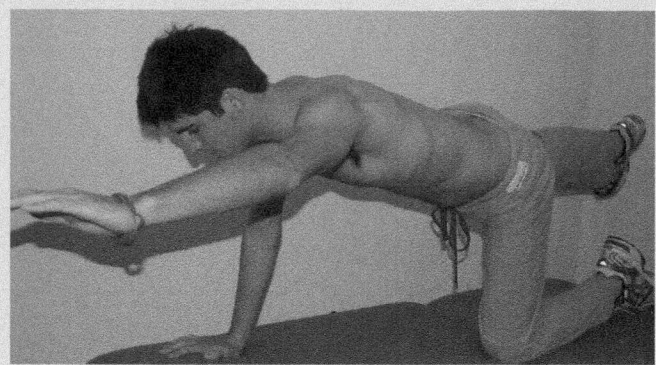

Exercise 6: Quadruped lower trapezius variation

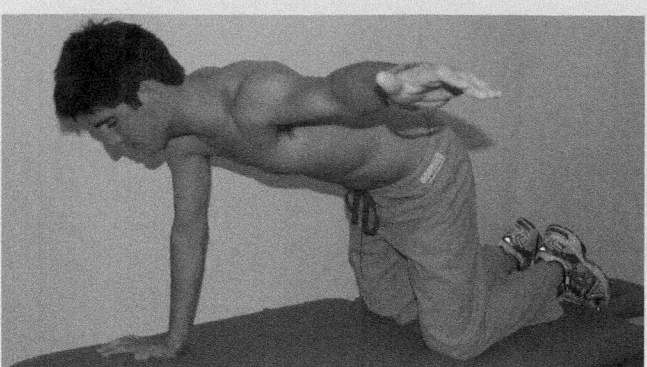

Exercise Set 3
Exercise 1: Self-mobilization using foam roll

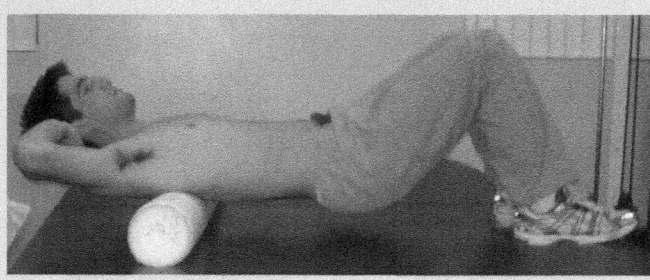

Exercise 2: Self-mobilization using wedge

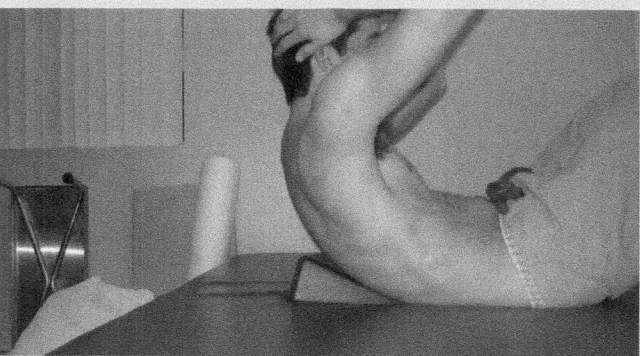

Exercise 3: Self-rib mobilizer or tennis ball

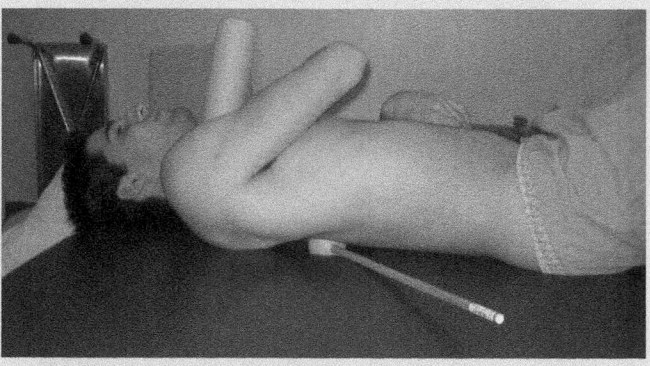

CLINICAL PEARL

In the presence of first and second rib hypomobility with associated scalene restriction, the diaphragmatic contribution to breathing should be assessed. Often, these patients overuse the accessory muscles of breathing. Diaphragmatic breathing may be taught, with the patient's hands on the chest and diaphragm, focusing on good diaphragm contribution.

MODALITIES

Which modalities have proven most successful in treating patients with midback pain?

There are no studies demonstrating specific efficacy of the use of modalities on thoracic region pain. The use of cold packs and electrical stimulation has been found to be effective at reducing pain in the acute phase. Belt traction and self-traction have shown some clinical success. Taping can be a good adjunct for

TABLE IV-2-2   Tissue Injury and Intervention Selection

What are the best interventions for the acute phase (0-14 days postinjury)?	When to progress to next phase	What are the best interventions for the reparative phase (15-21 days postinjury)?	When to progress to next phase	What are the best interventions for the remodeling phase (22-60 days postinjury)?	When to progress to next phase	What are the best interventions for the maturation phase (60-360 days postinjury)?	When to progress to next phase
Disc pathology							
Cold packs Self traction Belt traction	Decreased pain Improved motion	Manual therapy Postural exercise Belt traction	Further decreased pain and improved mobility	Manual therapy into resistance Strengthening/stretching exercise	Minimal pain and near full ROM	Progression to functional exercise	DC to HEP
Muscle strain							
Cold packs Taping	Decreased pain Improved motion	STM	Further decreased pain and improved mobility	Manual therapy into resistance Strengthening/stretching exercise	Minimal pain and near full ROM	Progression to functional exercise	DC to HEP
Ligament sprain							
Cold packs Taping	Decreased pain Improved motion	Manual therapy Postural exercise	Further decreased pain and improved mobility	Manual Therapy into resistance Strengthening/stretching exercise	Minimal pain and near full ROM	Progression to functional exercise	DC to HEP
Tendon pathology							
Cold packs Taping	Decreased pain Improved motion	Manual therapy Postural exercise	Further decreased pain and improved mobility	Manual therapy into resistance Strengthening/stretching exercise	Minimal pain and near full ROM	Progression to functional exercise	DC to HEP
Bone fracture							
Cold packs Bracing	Decreased pain Improved motion	Bracing	Further decreased pain and improved mobility	Bracing Light stabilization exercise	Further decreased pain and improved mobility	Progression to functional exercise	DC to HEP
Cartilage damage							
Cold packs Taping	Decreased pain Improved motion	Manual therapy Postural Exercise	Further decreased pain and improved mobility	Manual therapy into resistance Strengthening/stretching exercise	Minimal pain and near full ROM	Progression to functional exercise	DC to HEP
Capsule injury							
Cold packs Taping	Decreased pain Improved motion	Manual therapy Postural exercise	Further decreased pain and improved mobility	Manual therapy into resistance Strengthening/Stretching exercise	Minimal pain and near full ROM	Progression to functional exercise	DC to HEP
Nerve injury							
Cold packs Taping	Decreased pain Improved motion	Manual therapy Postural exercise	Further decreased pain and improved mobility	Manual therapy Strengthening/stretching/stabilization exercise	Minimal pain and near full ROM	Progression to functional exercise	DC to HEP

DC, discharge; *HEP*, home exercise program; *ROM*, range of motion; *STM*, soft tissue mobilization

postural training and unloading painful structures to facilitate increased pain-free movement.

OTHER

What is the role of bracing or taping in treating patients with midback pain?

Taping the thoracic region or scapulae may be used to give kinesthetic awareness of spinal position, to stabilize an unstable segment, or to unload painful structures.[25] Greig et al[14] demonstrated that postural taping in a population with osteoporotic vertebral fractures resulted in an immediate reduction in thoracic kyphosis. Taping may also be used as an adjunct to treatment to either help stabilize a rib anteriorly or posteriorly after mobilization. Taping applied to other body regions may also help to reduce midback pain. For example, tape applied to reduce the position of a depressed and abducted scapula can help reduce midback pain.

What is the role of traction in treating patients with midback pain?

When a thoracic disc is considered to be the source of pain in the thoracic region, the use of traction may be indicated. A thoracic disc lesion may be considered with a history of trauma, various motions may be painful; rotation is typically the most limited. Adding neck flexion to the provocative movement increases a dural stretch in the thoracic region.[32] Belt traction techniques advocated by Mulligan[29] have been shown to be clinically effective. The use of the belt allows the clinician to traction specific spinal levels, which can also be adjusted based on patient response.[28] Self-traction techniques are also advocated as a follow-up to belt traction and have been found to be effective in the presence of acute lesions.[29]

How does treatment of the thoracic spine region affect neural dynamics?

Clinical experience suggests that thoracic spine manipulation can improve mobility during neurodynamic testing such as the slump test or upper limb neurodynamic test. The mechanism is unclear, although it is likely a combination of mechanical and neurophysiological mechanisms. Thoracic spine manipulation has been shown to improve mobility of a radial upper limb neurodynamic test in a patient with complex regional pain syndrome type I.[27] Because of the smaller canal size at T4-9, it is thought that this may be a site of adverse tension on the nervous system.[3]

REHABILITATION CLINICAL REASONING

How should a clinician decide which intervention is most appropriate for a patient with midback pain?

The clinical decision-making process for choosing an appropriate intervention is based on the examination findings. The selection of interventions will be based on how to address both the source and the causes of the symptoms. The patient will have some combination of impairments in mobility, strength, or control deficits. The therapist will decide whether to use education, manual therapy and stretching exercise, strengthening exercises, motor control exercises, or postural training and instruction.

What red flags should a clinician be aware of regarding rehabilitating a patient with midback pain?

According to Yelland,[35] the following are alerting features of serious causes of acute thoracic spinal pain: Signs and symptoms of infection (fever for long duration), previous malignancy, age >50 years, unexplained weight loss, failure to improve with treatment, past history of a serious condition, chest pain or heaviness, change in posture having no effect on pain, pain at multiple sites, swelling, vertebral deformity, pain at rest, signs and symptoms of arthropathy, unexplained pain onset, history of trauma, and abdominal pain.

SUMMARY STATEMENT

It must be remembered that the thoracic spine is a region of the body characterized by reduced mobility and surrounded by more mobile regions on all sides. There is a dynamic interplay of biomechanics within these regions where alterations in one region may affect another. Effective treatment of the patient with midback pain may include addressing scapular, cervical, and/or lumbar impairments as a result of the regional interdependence of body regions. For effective and successful treatment to occur, a comprehensive examination and evaluation needs to take place. This should include a thorough history, postural assessment, functional task assessment, AROM testing, strength testing, endurance testing, postural and scapular control testing, muscle length testing, joint mobility and soft tissue mobility testing. This examination will include assessment of the surrounding body regions. The treatment interventions of the patient with midback pain will address the source and cause of the patient's symptoms. The interventions will address the patient's most salient impairments (Table IV-2-2). Education is a key component of rehabilitation. The patient should be educated about the source and the causes of their symptoms. Education on the avoidance of aggravating activities is critical. Manual therapy techniques may be used to improve mobility and show the patient that his or her pain is the result of a mechanical component that can be altered. This will improve compliance with the home program of posture training, self-mobilization, stretching, and strengthening.

REFERENCES

1. Bergman GJ, Winters JC, Groenier KH, De Jong BM, Postema K, Van der Heijden GJ. Manipulative therapy in addition to usual medical care for patients with shoulder dysfunction and pain. *Ann Intern Med.* 2004;141:432-439.
2. Boyles RE, Ritland BM, Miracle BM, et al. (in press). The short-term effects of thoracic spine thrust manipulation on patients with shoulder impingement syndrome. *Man Ther.*
3. Butler DS. *Mobilisation of the Nervous System.* Edinburgh: Churchill Livingstone; 1991.
4. Cleland JA, Childs JD, Fritz JM, Whitman JM, Eberhart SL. Development of a clinical prediction rule for guiding treatment of a subgroup of patients with neck pain: use of thoracic spine manipulation, exercise, and patient education. *Phys Ther.* 2007;87:9-23.
5. Cleland JA, Childs JD, McRae M, Palmer JA, Stowell T. Immediate effects of thoracic manipulation in patients with neck pain: a randomized clinical trial. *Man Ther.* 2004;10:127-135.
6. Cleland J, Selleck B, Stowell T, et al. Short-term effects of thoracic manipulation on lower trapezius muscle strength. *J Man Manip Ther.* 2004;12:82-90.
7. Dwyer A, Aprill C, Bogduk N. Cervical zygapophyseal joint pain patterns. *Spine.* 1990;22:525-530.
8. Edmondston SJ, Singer KP. Thoracic spine: anatomical and biomechanical considerations for manual therapy. *Man Ther.* 1997;2(3):132-143.
9. Erhard R, Piva SR. Manual therapy. In: Placzek JD, Boyce DA, eds. *Orthopaedic Physical Therapy Secrets.* St. Louis: Elsevier; 2006:102-111.
10. Evans DW. Mechanisms and effects of spinal high-velocity, low-amplitude thrust manipulation: Previous theories. *J Manip Physiol Ther.* 2002;25:251-262.
11. Flynn TW. Direct treatment techniques for the thoracic spine and rib cage: muscle energy, mobilization, high-velocity thrust, and combined techniques. In: Flynn TW, ed. *The Thoracic Spine and Ribcage: Musculoskeletal Evaluation and Treatment.* Newton, MA: Butterworth-Heinemann; 1996:171-210.
12. Fruth SJ. Differential diagnosis and treatment in a patient with posterior upper thoracic pain. *Phys Ther.* 2006;86:254-268.
13. Gonzalez-Iglesias J, Fernandez-De-Las-Penas C, Cleland JA, Gutierrez-Vega MD. Thoracic spine manipulation for the management of patients with neck pain: a randomized clinical trial. *J Orthop Sports Phys Ther.* 2009;39:20-27.
14. Greig AM, Bennell KL, Briggs AM, Hodges PW. Postural taping decreases thoracic kyphosis but does not influence trunk muscle electro myographic activity or balance in women with osteoporosis. *Man Ther.* 2008;13:249-257.

15. Horton SJ. Acute locked thoracic spine: treatment with a modified SNAG. *Man Ther.* 2002;7:103-107.

16. Janda V. Muscles and motor control in low back pain: assessment and management. In: Twomey LT, ed. *Physical Therapy of the Low Back.* New York, Edinburgh, London, Melbourne: Churchill Livingstone; 1987:253-278.

17. Janda V. Muscles and motor control in cervicogenic disorders. In: Grant R, ed. *Physical Therapy of the Cervical and Thoracic Spine.* St. Louis, MO: Churchill Livingstone; 2002:182-199.

18. Kendall FP, McCreary EK, Provance PG, Rodgers MM, Romani WA. *Muscles Testing and Function with Posture and Pain.* 5th ed. Baltimore, MD: Lippincott Williams & Wilkins; 2005.

19. Lee DG. Rotational instability of the mid- thoracic spine: assessment and management. *Man Ther.* 1996;1(5):234-241.

20. Lee LJ, Coppieters M, Hodges PW. Thoracic multifidus and longissimus muscle activity during voluntary arm movements. In: *Proceedings of the 2004 Orthopaedic Symposium of the Canadian Physiotherapy Association.* Canada: St. John's, NL; 2004:36.

21. Lee LJ, Coppieters M, Hodges PW. Differential activation of the thoracic multifidus and longissimus during trunk rotation. In: *Proceedings of the 8th International Federation of Orthopaedic Manipulative Therapists' Conference.* South Africa: Cape Town; 2004:41.

22. Lee LJ. Restoring force closure/motor control of the thorax. In: Lee DG, Diane G, eds. *The Thorax: An Integrated Approach* [Ch. 7]. Lee Physiotherapist Corp. www.dianelee.ca; 2003.

23. Liebler EJ, Tufano-Coors L, Douris P, et al. The effect of thoracic spine mobilization on lower trapezius strength testing. *J Man Manip Ther.* 2001;9:207-212.

24. Maitland G, Hengeveld E, Banks K, English K, eds. *Maitland's Vertebral Manipulation.* 6th ed. Woburn, MA: Butterworth-Heinemann; 2001.

25. McConnell J. The use of taping for pain relief in the management of spinal pain. In: Boyling JD, Jull GA, eds. *Grieve's Modern Manual Therapy of The Vertebral Column.* Edinburgh: Churchill Livingstone; 2004:433-442.

26. McRae M, Cleland J. Differential diagnosis and treatment of upper thoracic pain: A case study. *J Man Manip Ther.* 2003;11:43-48.

27. Menck JY, Requejo SM, Kulig K. Thoracic spine dysfunction in upper extremity complex regional pain syndrome. *J Orthop Sports Phys Ther.* 2000;30:401-409.

28. Mulligan BR. Belt techniques. In: Grieve GP, ed. *Modern Manual Therapy of the Vertebral Column.* Edinburgh: Churchill Livingstone; 1986:716-718.

29. Mulligan BR. *Manual Therapy, "Nags", "Snags", "Mwms" etc.* 4th ed. Wellington, NZ: Plane View Services; 1999.

30. Niemelainen R, Videman T, Battie M. Prevalence and characteristics of upper or mid-back pain in Finnish Men. *Spine.* 2006;31: 1846-1849.

31. Schellhas K, Smith M, Maher C. Prospective correlation of magnetic resonance imaging and discography in asymptomatic subjects and pain sufferers. *Spine.* 1996;21:300-312.

32. Sizer PS, Phelps V, Azevedo E. Disc related and non-disc related disorders of the thoracic spine. *Pain Pract.* 2001;1:136-149.

33. Wainner RS, Whitman JM, Cleland JA, Flynn TW. Regional interdependence: a musculoskeletal examination model whose time has come. *J Orthop Sports Phys Ther.* 2007;37:658-660.

34. Wright A. Hypoalgesia post-manipulative therapy: a review of potential neurophysiological mechanisms. *Man Ther.* 1995;1:11-16.

35. Yelland MJ, Charlton K, Jull G, Brooks P, Bellamy N. Acute thoracic spinal pain. In: Spearing N, ed. *Evidence-based Management of Acute Musculoskeletal Pain. A Guide for Clinicians.* Brisbane, Australia: Australian Academic Press; 2004:30-34.

36. Schiller L. Effectiveness of spinal manipulative therapy in the treatment of mechanical thoracic spine pain: a pilot randomized clinical trial. *J Manip Physiol Ther.* 2001;24(6):394-401.

AUTHOR: ADAM SCHULTZ

INTRODUCTORY INFORMATION

Rehabilitation of the lumbar spine is a challenge. It can make a clinician look good and bad in the same instance. The clinician looks good because most patients will get better in 6 to 8 weeks regardless of the intervention. The clinician will look bad because a majority of these patients will have a return of low back pain within a year, leaving patients to wonder if they had gotten better at all. Lumbar rehabilitation has gone through multiple phases and reiterations of the ideal treatment approach. The following is a summary of the current state of lumbar rehabilitation.

What are the factors a clinician should consider when rehabilitating a patient with low back pain?

The factors that influence low back pain can be broadly divided into those that are specific to the low back region and those that can be generalized to the whole body. Low back specific factors include the following:
- Chief complaint
- Onset, course, and duration of symptoms
- Nature and behavior of symptoms
- Impairments and activity limitations
- Past history of symptoms, including effect of previous treatment
- Results of diagnostic testing

LOW BACK GENERAL FACTORS INCLUDE:

- Patient age
- Past medical history, including current overall heath status
- Access to exercise (gym membership, home exercise equipment, local parks, etc.)
- Patient occupation, activities, and goals
- Overall motivation and disposition toward rehabilitation, including belief in or bias toward physical therapy

How do these factors affect the rehabilitation process?

These factors in combination will play a large role in the success of physical therapy rehabilitation. The clinician must identify which individual factors are most relevant on a case-by-case basis and how physical therapy rehabilitation can be potentially beneficial. For example, the age of a patient may impact the type of interventions used, including the amount and type of joint mobilization or exercise intervention. In addition, a clinician should treat a patient who is highly irritable and acute differently from a patient who has chronic nonirritable low back pain. The underlying principles may be the same, but the type and intensity of the programs will be different. In reality, with the multitude of factors that play into the clinician's decision-making process, no lumbar rehabilitation programs should be identical. The challenge of rehabilitating a patient with lumbar pain lies in the clinician's ability to interpret accurately those factors affecting the patient and to devise a treatment plan that will best address the patient's problem.

What role does age play in rehabilitation of low back pain?

Age plays an important role in assisting with the differential diagnosis of patients with low back pain. Younger patients are more likely to have nonspecific sprain/strain and discogenic conditions. Patients over 65 years of age are more likely to suffer from degenerative conditions such as spinal stenosis and compression fractures. Other conditions that can cause low back pain, such as cancer or aortic aneurysms, are most common in the older patient population.[12] The older patient population may also experience co-morbidities that can cause, contribute, and/or act as a barrier to progress when treating low back pain (e.g., cancer, heart disease, obesity, osteoarthritis, etc.). Therefore, in addition to the underlying pathology that is affecting the patient, from a rehabilitation standpoint, the interventions and treatments used on a 20-year-old patient may not be appropriate for the 90-year-old patient. Pathology will drive some of the decisions, but the patient's physical capacities and their ultimate goals will help determine and shape the patient's rehabilitation program.

What role does acuteness or chronicity play in rehabilitating a patient with low back pain?

The stage of the health condition will be a major factor in determining the plan of care and prognosis of patients with low back pain. Patients with acute and chronic low back pain may be able to be subclassified based on patterns of signs and symptoms, which can lead to the selection of more effective clinical interventions.*

In general, patients with acute low back pain may be more irritable or have tissue in the early phase of healing. These patients require protection of the structures that are damaged, as well as an identification of the reason those structures became involved. Exercise interventions in these early phases are often restricted to isometric or lower level exercises designed to begin using the muscles while protecting joints or to improve fluid dynamics in the area.

In contrast, patients with chronic low back pain are generally less irritable, with tissue presenting in the remodeling phase of healing. These patients may be progressed at a more rapid rate. However, over time, patients with chronic pain may present with multiple associated factors. These may include compensations and motion patterns that are less efficient than normal. Therapeutic exercises in these cases may include functional retraining, as well as exercises targeting the specific area of complaint.

What factors make treatment of patients with low back pain challenging?

Low back pain is often the result of sustained or repetitive motions that place excessive forces on the structures of the low back over a period of time. These postures or motions are those that are performed regularly with daily activities, including those during work or athletic pursuits. Thus the patient may find it difficult to understand that the postures or motions that he or she has been doing every day for his or her whole life may be the problem with low back pain. Such motions or postures include sitting posture or standing posture or lower extremity chain mechanics. Furthermore, function of the lumbar spine depends on proper function of adjacent and remote regions. The thoracic spine and sacrum both exert a strong influence on the lumbar spine. Similarly, leg length discrepancies and foot pathology can contribute to a patient's low back pain. Treatment of low back pain really involves treatment of the whole body.

Chronicity and a history of failed treatment may create a challenge for successful rehabilitation. In these cases, the clinician should use a general rule of thumb that involves monitoring progress. If there is no appreciable change in the patient's presentation within two to three visits, then the clinician has not successfully identified either the tissue involved in the complaint or the aggravating factor for the complaint sufficiently to unload the structure enough to progress. In these circumstances, inviting a more experienced consultant to examine the patient may provide further insight. Chronic pain is multifaceted, and generally treatment must be geared toward addressing the various facets that are producing or contributing to the pain. A single focused intervention plan is usually not successful in this patient population.

---

*References 3, 4, 6, 8, 9, 14, 20, 22, 23.

Patient compliance to treatment advice is another challenge and may be related to others. If the patient continues to perform aggravating behaviors and postures, then success can be limited. As with active rehabilitation for any body region, the patient's outcome is proportional to their effort and consistency in participating in the rehabilitation program. Aligning the goals and activities of a rehabilitation program to those of the patient can improve patient compliance. Patient education regarding the role of the patient in rehabilitation is invaluable in achieving early and lasting success in rehabilitation.

Biomechanically, the motions and coupling that occur in the lumbar spine still are not well defined through research. Therefore it becomes difficult to use biomechanical principles as a foundation of treatment since they are themselves not well understood.

Research in the lumbar spine is still lacking. Research to date has not been good at proving efficacy in regards to rehabilitation and lumbar pain. The subgroup of patients that do appear to benefit from rehabilitation is the acute patient. Many studies show various interventions that can aid in the recovery of patients with acute low back pain. Very few studies have shown that current rehabilitation regimes are beneficial in treating patients with chronic low back pain.

Surgery success rates are variable. Some studies will show good results in terms of reduction of symptoms, and others will show no difference between surgery and nonsurgical patients. This leaves the clinician to wonder why the patient still has symptoms if the irritating structure has been surgically corrected or excised.

Finally, identifying the contributing or associated factors to low back pain is a challenge. Most patients with low back pain will improve, but over 80% of those patients will have a recurrence of low back pain in the course of a year. To avoid this recurrence, the focus of rehabilitation should be twofold. First and most obvious, the clinician must focus on reduction of the patient's symptoms and return to normal function. If the clinician discharges the patient with only this one goal accomplished, the question remains why the patient got injured in the first place. This leads to the second goal, which is an identification and alteration of those factors that have lead to or are contributing to tissue injury and pain. By addressing both of these goals, the rehabilitation becomes more successful both in the short and the long term.

CLINICAL PEARL

Compliance is the key to success with any rehabilitation, but what is the key to compliance? Regardless of a clinician's treatment paradigm or choice of intervention, compliance comes down to one main factor: pain control. Patients will gladly comply with recommendations that make a real difference in their pain levels. Pain control is the most powerful biofeedback tool that enhances patient compliance. This may come from a variety of interventions such as a manual therapy technique, education in proper sitting posture, or a detailed exercise program focused on contracting the proper muscles when performing activities. Often the best intervention requires the clinician to match the patient's pathology, impaired body structures, and activity limitations with a collection of unique patient characteristics (previous treatment experiences, learning style, belief system, or motivation).

Are there factors that make treatment of patients with low back pain easier?
Patients with low back pain may modify the pain with simple postural or movement alterations. These simple adjustments may improve the patient's understanding of the mechanical source of the complaint and improve patient participation in the rehabilitation process. Positive bias/belief systems toward physical therapy rehabilitation will help improve symptoms.

PROGNOSIS

How successful is rehabilitation in treating acute low back pain?
The natural history of acute low back pain is favorable, and the majority of patients recover quickly and completely; 60% to 70% of patients recover within 6 weeks and 80% to 90% recover within 3 months.[19] Perhaps this is one reason why there are countless treatment interventions, many unproved or supported by conflicting evidence, that are commonly proffered as effective treatment for low back pain.[12]

The current trend in research is focused on subclassifying patients with acute low back pain based on signs and symptoms to select more effective treatment interventions and subsequently improving patient outcomes.*

How successful is rehabilitation in treating chronic low back pain?
Chronic low back pain is certainly more challenging for the clinician than acute low back pain. Chronic low back pain is associated with greater disability and health care costs. Factors that contribute to chronicity include age, multiple episodes of low back pain, history of failed treatment(s), increased fear-avoidance behavior, legal issues, and socioeconomic and psychological factors.[1,11,12] Some patients may have no normal pathoanatomical explanation to their symptomology and may require a multidisciplinary approach because of the complexity of the condition.[12] Chronic conditions may result in the development of neurological changes that perpetuate the pain patterns even after the initial insult has been resolved.

Patients with chronic low back pain may, however, be successfully treated. The clinician must examine both the area of complaint and the surrounding (thoracic and sacral) areas, as well as the lower extremity mechanics, to identify abnormal stresses placed on the involved area and address those contributing factors while rehabilitating the involved area.

One key to treatment is defining success in clinically realistic terms.

CLINICAL PEARL

Some patients have excessive difficulty learning how to selectively and appropriately contract the transversus abdominus muscle. Often, the hooklying position is used initially because it is a nonprovocative neutral position that allows the clinician and patient the ability to visualize and palpate the lower abdominal wall. However, some patients struggle in this position despite good instruction and diligent practice. If this is the case, consider changing the position or trying an alternate cue. Sidelying, quadraped, high-sitting, or standing are good alternatives. Remember that the goal is to educate the patient on an appropriate deep abdominal contraction and that successful attempts are requisite, regardless of position. An alternative cue for the patient who demonstrates an overactive global abdominal contraction may be to concentrate on contracting the pelvic floor muscle group rather than the lower abdominals. Sometimes, both modifications are necessary for retraining an appropriate transversus abdominal contraction in order to establish a foundation to progress stabilization exercises.

Why is a successful outcome so difficult to achieve with patients who suffer chronic low back pain?
Health conditions that have not resolved in the normal or expected time period are often the most challenging cases for any clinician. These cases are especially prevalent in the lumbar

---

*References 3, 4, 6, 9, 14, 16, 20, 23.

spine. Chronic low back pain has evolved to become a disorder by itself. One key toward a successful outcome with this challenging population is to collaborate with the patient to appropriately define a successful outcome. Complete resolution of symptoms and restoration of function to the level before injury may not be realistic for some patients with chronic disorders. This is particularly the case with conditions that are degenerative in nature and involve pain as the primary characteristic. These cases are often complex conditions with impairments that are not limited to the neuromusculoskeletal system and may require multidisciplinary therapy interventions. The clinician can try to adopt a pathophysiological paradigm and focus the examination and treatment on the neuromusculoskeletal effects of pain and deconditioning, rather than a pathoanatomical paradigm. In these cases, searching for the tissue or structure that is the origin of pain can often be frustrating and fruitless. Management of the symptoms, rather than complete resolution, should be the theme of the treatment intervention and plan of care. This approach requires patience, empathy, and effective communication, starting from the initial evaluation and throughout the course of care. Many patients are ready to accept some limitations to their recovery and are wiling to work toward improving the quality of their lives.

Which patients with low back pain derive the greatest long-term benefits from rehabilitation?

Patients with disorders that achieve complete (or near-complete) resolution in the normal and expected time period and continue to follow treatment advice are those that derive the greatest long-term benefit. In addition, patients who are able to make mechanical changes consistent with balancing stress across a joint and avoiding repetitive or sustained excessive loads on the involved area will benefit.

Often, these patients have disorders that are primarily mechanical and have minimal-to-no neurologically referred pain. This group of patients is compliant with treatment advice long after discharge, particularly with the postural education and preventive strengthening exercises prescribed.

What other regions of the body are most likely to contribute to low back pain?

Function of the lumbar spine is influenced by adjacent areas of the spine, including the thoracic spine and the sacrum (with its associated sacroiliac joint). Motion or lack of motion in these areas impact the movement and pathology in the low back.

The hip joint may influence low back pain in several ways. First, range of motion (ROM) at the hip can influence low back posture and mechanics. Tight hip flexors are a frequent finding in persons with low back pain, and the resolution of the hip flexor tightness is associated with reduced symptoms in the low back. Hip joint pain may also refer into the low back or gluteal region and must be differentiated from true low back pain.

Similarly, abdominal or pelvic organs (i.e., kidney disorders, pelvic and gynecological disorders) may cause referred pain into the low back region and must be differentiated from mechanical low back pain.

Lower extremity mechanics, including leg length discrepancies, and other mechanical factors may influence the onset and chronicity of low back pain. In addition, these lower extremity mechanics may create more challenges for the treatment of low back pain and contribute to an unexpected response to rehabilitation.

EVIDENCE-BASED MEDICINE

What trends are currently being seen in research regarding rehabilitation of patients with low back pain?

The major trend in research regarding patients with low back pain has been to establish a classification system that identifies subgroups of patients likely to respond to specific interventions.[14,22,23]

This trend in research has recently been comprehensively discussed by Fritz et al, who suggest four subgroups: manipulation, stabilization, specific exercise, and traction.[14] Clinical prediction rules (CPRs) are in development for these subgroups.[6,10,13,16]

INTERVENTIONS

MANUAL THERAPY

What is the physiological rationale behind the use of manual therapy in treating patients with low back pain?

The exact physiological effect of the benefits of manual therapy to the low back is complex and not fully understood. Bialosky et al proposed a comprehensive model of the mechanism of manual therapy that suggests the application of a manual therapy technique stimulates a complex interaction involving the joint and surrounding tissues the technique is directed toward, the peripheral nervous system, the spinal cord, and the supraspinal structures. This initiates a number of potential neurophysiological effects that can result in decreased muscle spasm, pain modulation, and increased range and improved quality of motion.[2] The theory behind manual therapy in general is that manual therapy restores normal, pain-free accessory mobility to the joint and thus restores normal joint mobility. This may include a component directed at fluid mechanics, as seen in grades I and II joint mobilizations, or at stretching hypomobile structures (grades III and IV).

Which interventions have proved most successful in treating patients with low back pain?

Overall, manual therapy (especially manipulation), exercise, and patient education are the most successful treatments for patients with low back pain. A CPR developed by Flynn et al and confirmed by Childs et al provides a method for clinicians to identify a specific subgroup of acute low back patients that are likely to benefit from manipulation.[6,13] Recent research suggests the selection of a specific technique or joint may not be as important as identifying the subgroup of patients who are most likely to benefit from manual therapy.[10,18] This supports the complex physiological model of manual therapy proposed by Bialosky et al.

CASE STUDY   ❓

Your patient is a 37-year-old female who reports a long history of episodic low back pain (>10 years). Her back "goes out" every few months, after which she experiences symptoms for 1 to 2 weeks. She experiences these flare-ups infrequently, but over the past year she notes that her flare-ups have become more frequent and severe and are not resolved as fast or completely as in the past. She has had extensive chiropractic treatment over the past 5 years, which has consisted of manipulation and modalities and has provided only temporary relief. This episode has prompted her to see her primary care physician who has referred her to physical therapy.

Currently, her chief complaint is a strong ache in the central low back that spreads slightly to the right. She denies any history of pain traveling below the buttock or neurological symptoms with this pain episode or in the past. Her main activity limitations are prolonged sitting and standing (pain gradually builds to 1 hour tolerance) and sudden movements. Physical examination findings are as follows:

Standing posture: Excessive

Active ROM (AROM)

Lumbar

- Flexion: Full range (ankle joint) with moderate low back pain at end-range. Initiates her return to neutral with excessive thoracic spine extension and splints by walking her hands up her thighs.
- Extension: 30 degrees with excessive movement/hinging in the lower lumbar spine and moderate pain at end-range.

- Left sidebending: Reaches knee joint, no pain
- Right sidebending: Reaches knee joint, no pain

Hip, knee, ankle: Within functional limits (WFL)

Strength: All hip, knee, and ankle musculature grade 4+/5 and are pain-free, except for the gluteus medius, which grades 3+/5 bilaterally, no pain.

Palpation

- ↓L4: Hypermobile, comparable mild central low back
- L4 physiological right rotation: Hypermobile, no pain

What is the best choice of intervention for this patient?

Answer

The history of manipulative- and modalities-based care has produced only short-term relief, so repeating a similar course of treatment would presumably produce similar results. This does not rule out using manual therapy or modalities in the plan of care of this patient, but these interventions should not be the primary focus. Her long history of low back pain and dysfunction has produced maladaptive changes in how this patient loads and moves her spine, which most likely have contributed to her ongoing symptoms. A more detailed look at her loading and movement patterns is warranted. Examining the level, pattern, and timing of trunk and abdominal muscle recruitment during her aggravating postures and movements followed by attempting to correct the aberrant patterns should be the primary focus of care. For example, the movement pattern she uses to when returning to neutral from a forward-flexed position needs to be retrained so she uses her local lumbopelvic musculature rather than her thoracic erector spinae and upper extremities.

What is the role of traction in treating patients with low back pain?

Mechanical traction is a common modality used to treat low back pain, especially with patients who experience low back pain in combination with nerve root pain (Table IV-3-1). The mechanisms by which traction has been hypothesized to provide relief are varied and include increasing intervertebral foramen space, thereby releasing pressure on compressed and irritated nerve roots; reducing local muscle spasm; and nociceptive inhibition. However, there is little support that traction is an effective modality for patients with acute, subacute, or chronic low back pain, with or without sciatica.[8]

Recent research hypothesizes that a subgroup of patients with low back pain and the presence of sciatica and signs of nerve root compression may preferentially benefit from mechanical traction.[16]

Is joint manipulation recommended for patients with low back pain?

Manipulation has been used as an intervention since the time of Hippocrates. Evidence confirming the effectiveness of manipulation spans more than 15 years of research and concludes that manipulation is recommended for patients with low back pain, although early research results are more conflicting than later research.

In particular, recent documentation concludes that manipulation is recommended for a subgroup of patients with acute low back pain. A CPR has been developed and validated. Patients who are positive on the CPR for 4 of 5 criteria and subsequently received manipulation experienced greater improvement of short-term and long-term pain and disability.[6,13]

What does evidence reveal regarding the use of massage for the treatment of patients with low back pain?

Massage is a traditional and commonly used treatment for patients with low back pain. Massage has few risks or adverse effects of use in the lumbar region. The physiological effect of massage is not completely understood, but it is commonly used to decrease pain and disability and speed the return to normal function by relaxing and decreasing muscle spasm, mobilizing tissue fluids, and promoting wellness.[17]

The evidence base for massage remains equivocal and lacks high quality placebo-controlled studies. A recent systematic review of massage-related research noted that the studies were highly heterogeneous in regards to several key factors, including massage type/technique, patient population, and outcome measures. Despite these limitations, the authors concluded that massage might be beneficial for patients with subacute and chronic nonspecific low back pain, particularly when included in a treatment program of exercise and education.[17]

Is stretching beneficial or indicated for patients with low back pain?

Stretching is commonly prescribed in the rehabilitation of patients with low back pain. There is poor evidence to include or exclude stretching exercises alone as a treatment for patients with acute low back pain. However, the evidence supports stretching, as part of a therapeutic exercise program, in patients with subacute and chronic low back pain.[5]

The rationale to include stretching would be to promote normal myofascial length along with normal movement of the lumbar spine or adjacent regions (such as hip flexor length) and to decrease local spasm. When prescribing stretching, the diagnosis, behavior of symptoms, and stage of the disorder must be taken into account along with the response to stretching.

How should a clinician decide which manual therapy intervention is most appropriate for a patient with low back pain?

The clinician should complete an examination of the patient to determine the patient's symptoms, irritability, primary functional impairments, and joint mechanics. Manual therapy intervention should be selected based on these findings and should normalize the impairments or joint mechanics. In the presence of inflammatory findings limiting joint mobility, the clinician should use mobilizations designed to avoid tissue stretch and improve fluid flow in the area such as grades I or II oscillatory joint mobilizations. Otherwise, grades III or IV oscillatory techniques may be used to improve capsular mobility or physiological stretching may be selected to improve muscle length.

For acute patients with low back pain without pain referral below the knee, manipulation may be an appropriate tool if the CPR fits (4 out of 5 of the following findings are present: Symptoms <16 days, no symptoms below the knee, fear-avoidance behavior scale [work subscale] <19, hip internal rotation >35 degrees in at least one hip, and at least one hypomobile segment found in the lumbar spine).[13]

The clinician also must factor in any patient-based limitations such an inability to achieve or maintain positions necessary for the technique (e.g., unable to lay prone) or patient consent (e.g., manipulation).

TABLE IV-3-1	Motion Restriction and Mobilization	
Motion Restrictions	Joint Requiring Mobilization	Direction of Mobilization
Lumbar flexion	Hypomobile level	Posterior-anterior in neutral → flexed position
Lumbar extension	Hypomobile level	Posterior-anterior in neutral → extended position
Lumbar rotation	Upper level of hypomobile motion segment	Physiological rotation, opening or closing based on symptomology
Lumbar sidebending	Lower level of hypomobile motion segment	Physiological sidebending, opening or closing based on symptomology

CASE STUDY ?

Your patient is a 42-year-old male. He is status-post low back injury secondary to lifting a box of books. His chief complaint is right-sided low back pain that extends into his right buttock and posterior thigh when his pain is at its peak. His main activity limitations are prolonged standing (>10 minutes, which increases his low back pain to a level that forces him to sit down, prolonged sitting (>15 minutes) that increases his low back and buttock pain, and rising up from a seated position that produces sharp low back pain and frequently elicits low back spasms. Physical examination findings are as follows:

Standing posture: mildly obese, flattened lumbar spine

AROM

Lumbar

- Flexion: reaches knee joint (mid-tibia normal for him), mild right buttock pain at end range, describes tightness in right hamstring.
- Extension: < 5 degrees with minimal contribution from the lower lumbar spine, comparable right buttock and low back pain.
- Left sidebending: reaches knee joint, mild right sided stretch
- Right sidebending: reaches knee joint, mild right sided low back pain.
- Repeated flexion in standing: abolished low back pain, buttock pain unchanged, increased right posterior thigh pain (5/10).
- Repeated extension in standing: increased low back pain (8/10), buttock pain unchanged, right posterior thigh pain abolished.

Hip, Knee, Ankle: WFL

Strength: All hip, knee, and ankle musculature grade 4+/5 and are pain-free except for right hip flexion 4+/5 and positive right low back pain.

Palpation

- Central PA 14: Hypomobile, comparable right low back, buttock pain.
- Bilateral lumbar paraspinal spasm

Reflexes

- 2+ patellar, hamstring, Achilles bilaterally
  What is the best choice of intervention for this patient?

Answer

Based on the history and clinical findings, this patient likely has a posterior disc derangement. The goal of the examination and subsequent treatment is to find a movement or position that centralizes or abolishes his pain. Both standing repeated movement procedures increased his pain, but only repeated flexion peripheralized his symptoms. Therefore repeated extension in prone (prone press-up) would be warranted. If his symptoms fail to centralize, static prone lying or prone lying in slight extension may be a good alternative choice. Once a movement or position that centralizes or abolishes his symptoms is established, then this movement or position is used as his exercise program. For example, if repeated prone extensions centralized his pain, then he would be instructed to perform this exercise each time he experienced symptoms. Modalities to decrease his local paraspinal muscle spasm and pain may be employed (e.g., electrical stimulation, heat or cold therapy, etc). Finally, the patient would also be instructed to avoid activities that exacerbate his symptoms, especially those that peripheralize symptoms.

EXERCISE

What is the physiological rationale behind the use of exercise in treating patients with low back pain?

The rationale for using exercise is to restore normal strength and motor control of the musculature of the low back and adjacent areas through a full and pain-free ROM joints of the hip and lumbopelvic region. In addition, exercise can assist with fluid flow in the area and avoiding diminished strength during acute phases of the rehabilitation.

Are exercise programs beneficial in treating patients with low back pain?

An exercise program should be a part of every patient's plan of care. Patients must take responsibility for their own rehabilitation and are often advised to change posture or movement patterns they have been doing for years. Exercise plans offer the opportunity for patients to undo the effect of these adverse movement patterns or postures.

Often, the pain from the original injury resolves (via natural history or in combination with treatment), but the abnormal mechanics that resulted in onset of pain remain unless specific exercises are performed. These secondary effects may include decreased muscle strength, poor motor control, aberrant movement patterns, or loading strategies.

Exercise programs also work to incorporate and invest the patient into the plan of care and give patients an aspect of control over their current symptoms and prevention of future symptoms.

Which exercise programs are effective in treating patients with low back pain?

The best exercise programs are individualized to the patient's specific impairments and functional activities. In general, exercise programs for patients with acute low back pain should be nonprovocative and focus on preventing further aggravation of symptoms and minimizing the effects of pain and limited movement. In the subacute and chronic stages, an exercise program can become more comprehensive and focus on strengthening and conditioning, including a return to previously provocative positions and activities.

Fritz et al documented that specific exercise programs in the direction of preference for patients that exhibit centralization or a directional preference with movement testing during examination are most effective. The centralization exercises for those that need centralization, extension exercises for those needing extension, and so on yields better outcomes and an overall better prognosis.[4,20]

How should a clinician decide which exercise is most appropriate for a patient with low back pain?

The foundation for any exercise program begins with a thorough examination followed by sound clinical reasoning in the selection of interventions and the evaluation of their effect. Seldom is there only one exercise that is the most appropriate for patients with low back pain, but rather exercises are individualized for the specific patient. As a general rule, clinicians may start patients with simple exercises that are easy to learn and demonstrate successfully in the clinic. If the patient is not successful in the clinic, chances are they either will not attempt the exercise at home or will repetitively practice poor form and thus contribute to prolonging the problem. To improve compliance, it is important that the patient understands the rationale for the exercise and that the exercise is nonprovocative.

Which muscles should be strengthened in treating patients with low back pain?

Each program should be individualized to the patient's specific body structures and their correlated activity limitations. Often a comprehensive exercise program should include exercises for the deep stabilizing musculature (abdominals, obliques, etc.) and the global torque producing musculature. Muscle groups primarily associated with adjacent joints, such as the hip abductors, extensors, and quadriceps, act as load dampeners for the lumbar spine and frequently require strengthening.

CLINICAL PEARL

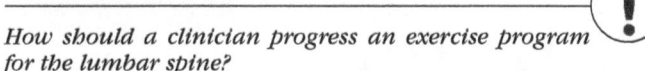

How should a clinician progress an exercise program for the lumbar spine?

- *Simple progressions include increased repetitions and/or sets for repetitive exercises. For static contractions, increasing time of contraction is appropriate.*
- *Positions can be progressed from non–weight-bearing → weight-bearing → functional → dynamic repetitive movements (e.g., sporting and work tasks).*
- *Exercises can also be progressed from a stable base of support to a more dynamic base such as using an exercise ball.*
- *Exercises can be progressed from small ROM (i.e., static exercise) to partial range to full range and then dynamic or functional activities.*
- *Exercises can be progressed using loads or increasing difficulty such as with the addition of weights or dynamic changing loads.*

The type or progression used should be determined by an examination of the patient's ability or capacity in conjunction with the patient's movement goals. For example, if the patient desires to work out in a gym and wants to do exercise machines, sets and reps may be ideal and load may be increased using weights. If a patient wants to return to running, then a progression may begin by including walking, walk/run intervals, and so on. The patient should be successful with the exercise (with no reproduction of symptoms) at the previous level before adding increased demand to the task.

How does a clinician know if a patient with low back pain is ready to progress to a new exercise?

Progression may be rapid and should occur when the patient has mastered the exercise by showing good form and endurance without symptom provocation. Exercises should always be a challenge to the patient and require effort to complete.

MODALITIES

Which modalities have proven most successful in treating patients with low back pain?

There are numerous and varied modalities that have been used by clinicians treating patients with low back pain. There is weak evidence in support of using these modalities in the treatment of patients with low back pain.[5,7] Despite the lack of evidence, modalities continue to be a component in the plan of care of patients with low back pain to alleviate pain, decrease muscle spasm, inhibit swelling, and promote healing.

How should a clinician decide which modality is most appropriate for a patient with low back pain?

Since the evidence is inconclusive toward any one single modality as the best choice for patients with low back pain, the decision for which modality to select hinges on several factors. Frequently, a case can be made for a number of modality choices, but it is not feasible to perform every potential choice. The patient's chief complaint and dominant impairments should be factored in along with the physical therapist's clinical experience when deciding which modality to use. However, in today's health care environment of informed consent and patient access to medical information via the internet, deciding on a modality has become more of a collaborative choice. Often, an important factor is patient preference or expectations, especially if they have had a positive outcome using that modality in the past. A patient's belief in the positive benefit of a certain modality can be a strong prognosticator and should not be discounted even if it would not be the clinician's first choice (unless the patient's preference is medically contraindicated). Sometimes a referring physician strongly believes a certain modality is necessary for

resolution of symptoms and has imparted this information to the patient. Efforts attempting to dissuade both the physician and the patient are usually ineffective and may even undermine your standing with both parties. I will usually present several choices, including the potential benefits and limitations along with the evidence base, and incorporate the patient in the decision-making process.

OTHER

What is the role of bracing or taping in treating patients with low back pain?

Lumbar braces and taping are commonly used for prevention and treatment of patients with low back pain. Although there are many different types of braces and taping techniques that can be used, they share a common aim to decrease impairment and disability associated with low back pain and to prevent the occurrence or recurrence of low back pain. Some braces may be specifically designed to correct deformity (e.g., scoliotic curves) or to stabilize the lumbar spine during movement (e.g., status-post lumbar fusion surgery). Taping has been used as a tactile cue for posture retraining, for unloading irritated structures, or reducing fluid accumulation.

The evidence base for the use of bracing and taping for patients with low back pain is lacking. A recent review of the literature found moderate evidence that lumbar supports are no more effective than no intervention or training in preventing low back pain and conflicting evidence on the effectiveness of lumbar supports in the treatment of patients with low back pain.[24]

What is the role of treatment aimed at neurodynamics in treating patients with low back pain?

Neurodynamic tests for patients with low back pain include the straight leg raise and slump tests. These tests are used to identify patients with a neurodynamic component to the low back disorder. Neurodynamic tests, or variations of these tests, are often used as treatment techniques with this patient population. The goal of neurodynamic treatment is to restore the normal mechanosensitivity and glide of the neural structures associated with the lumbar spine.

Neurodynamic techniques have been recommended for patients with positive neurodynamic tests since the 1960s. Recent research has also hypothesized that patients with symptoms referred into the buttock and lower extremity that do not improve with specific directional exercises may benefit from neurodynamic specific treatments. Cleland et al studied patients with nonradicular low back pain using slump stretching in addition to lumbar mobilization and exercise compared to a similar treatment group without slump stretching and concluded that slump stretching is beneficial for improving short-term disability, decreasing pain, and centralization of symptoms.[9]

The clinician must keep in mind that neurodynamic-based treatments are provocative. Thus close attention must be paid to the patient's immediate and latent response to neurodynamic treatments. The clinician must recall that it is contraindicated to use a neurodynamic treatment in the presence of unstable neurological signs.

HOME EXERCISE

Which home exercises are the most beneficial to give patients with low back pain?

Home exercises should be provided to every low back pain patient. These exercises should be selected carefully as a portion of those done in the clinic. Exercises to improve the awareness of the patient's control over the position of the low back (and therefore pain) are excellent for early intervention, as are exercises that

TABLE IV-3-2 Tissue Injury and Intervention Selection

	What are the best interventions for the acute phase (0-14 days postinjury)?	When to progress to next phase	What are the best interventions for the reparative phase (15-21 days postinjury)?	When to progress to next phase	What are the best interventions for the remodeling phase (22-60 days postinjury)?	When to progress to next phase	What are the best interventions for the maturation phase (60-360 days postinjury)?	When to progress to next phase
Disc pathology	Rest, centralizing movements (nonperipheralizing movements)	Pain begins to centralize.	Centralizing movements (e.g., prone lumbar extension), manual therapy (e.g., central PAs), modalities to treat pain and spasm, begin stabilization exercises.	Pain continues to centralize or is abolished, patient able to tolerate more loading positions.	Manual therapy, progress exercises to include functional tasks.	Patient response to interventions is tolerated.	Progress exercise as tolerated to include formerly provocative positions, return preinjury activities.	Progress as tolerated. Patient is most likely independent at this stage.
Muscle strain	Rest, nonprovocative movements	Pain and symptoms (spasm) begin to stabilize/resolve.	STM, manual therapy, gentle AROM exercise, stabilization exercise	Pain and symptoms continue to resolve.	AROM exercises, progress exercises to include resistance and functional tasks as tolerated	Pain and symptoms continue to resolve.	Progress exercise as tolerated to include formerly provocative positions, return to preinjury activities.	Progress as tolerated. Patient is most likely independent at this stage.
Ligament sprain	Rest, nonprovocative movements, avoid end range movements	Pain and symptoms begin to stabilize/resolve.	Gentle AROM exercises, stabilization exercise, manual therapy, modalities for symptom relief as needed	Pain and symptoms continue to resolve.	AROM exercises, progress exercises to include resistance and functional tasks as tolerated.	Pain and symptoms continue to resolve.	Progress exercise as tolerated to include formerly provocative positions, return to preinjury activities.	Progress as tolerated. Patient is most likely independent at this stage.
Tendon pathology	Rest, general nonprovocative movements, avoid end-range movements	Pain and symptoms begin to stabilize/resolve.	STM, Gentle AROM exercises, stabilization exercise, manual therapy, modalities for symptom relief as needed	Pain and symptoms continue to resolve	AROM exercises, progress exercises to include resistance and functional tasks as tolerated.	Pain and symptoms continue to resolve.	Progress exercise as tolerated to include formerly provocative positions, return to preinjury activities.	Progress as tolerated. Patient is most likely independent at this stage.
Bone fracture	Depending on severity of injury, immobilization or surgical intervention	Depending on severity of injury may not be appropriate for physical therapy at this stage	Depending on severity of injury may not be appropriate for physical therapy at this stage. If appropriate, modalities to assist with symptom relief, nonlumbar-specific conditioning (e.g., walking or lower extremity strengthening).	Depending on severity of injury, may not be appropriate for physical therapy at this stage. Evidence of callus formation. Physician clearance,	Depending on severity of injury, may not be appropriate for physical therapy at this stage. If appropriate, AROM, stabilization, and conditioning exercises. Modalities as tolerated.	Evidence of bone unionization Physician clearance	Progress exercises to include resistance and functional tasks as tolerated. General strengthening and conditioning exercises.	Progress as tolerated. Patient is most likely independent at this stage.

Cartilage damage						
Depending on severity of immobilization or surgery.	Depending on severity of injury, may not be appropriate for physical therapy at this stage. If appropriate, modalities to assist with symptom relief, nonlumbar specific conditioning (e.g., walking or lower extremity strengthening).	Physician clearance. Pain and symptoms continue to resolve.	If appropriate AROM, stabilization, and conditioning exercises.	Physician clearance. Pain and symptoms continue to resolve.	Progress exercise as tolerated to include formerly provocative positions, return to preinjury activities.	Progress as tolerated. Patient is most likely independent at this stage.
Capsule injury						
Rest, gentle nonprovocative movements.	Manual therapy (e.g., unilateral PAs, manipulation), AROM exercises, modalities as needed.	Pain and symptoms begin to stabilize/resolve.	Progress manual therapy in vigor or into formerly provocative positions.	Pain and symptoms continue to resolve.	Progress exercise as tolerated to include formerly provocative positions, return to preinjury activities.	Progress as tolerated. Patient is most likely independent at this stage.
Nerve injury						
Depending on severity of injury, may not be appropriate for physical therapy at this stage. Rest, gentle nonprovocative movements.	Gentle neurodynamic mobilization, AROM exercises.	Physician clearance. Pain and symptoms begin to stabilize/resolve.	Progress neurodynamic mobilization, AROM exercises.	Pain and symptoms continue to resolve.	Progress exercise as tolerated to include formerly provocative positions, return to preinjury activities.	Progress as tolerated. Patient is most likely independent at this stage.

AROM, Active range of motion; *STM*, soft tissue mobilization; *PA*, posterior to anterior mobilization

develop core control. Specific exercises according to the presenting complaint and goals of the patient are the most beneficial.

REHABILITATION CLINICAL REASONING

How should a clinician decide which intervention is most appropriate for a patient with low back pain?

The first preference would be to classify the patient with low back pain into an effective intervention group based on patient history, signs and symptoms, and other key tests already discussed in this chapter. For example, patients with demonstrated instability should be treated with exercises and interventions that promote stability to the involved area. Patients with hypomobility in one or more lumbar level or surrounding joint (i.e., hip joint) should be treated with mobilization or manipulation techniques as indicated.

Seldom is there only one individual intervention that is the most appropriate for patients with low back pain. In fact, the majority of patients will receive a combination of treatment such as manual therapy (joint and or soft tissue), exercise intervention, functional retraining, and some form of modality.

What red flags should a clinician be aware of regarding rehabilitating a patient with low back pain?

The following are some of the more common red flag conditions for the low back region followed by the associated historical information, signs, and symptoms[11,12]:

- Lumbar spine metastases: age >50 years, history of cancer, unexplained weight loss, nonmechanical and unrelenting pain, night pain. Plan: Refer to physician for further tests.
- Cauda equina syndrome: Large central disc herniation, marked motor and sensory deficits, diminished reflexes, bladder retention or incontinence, bowel incontinence, saddle anesthesia. Plan: Contact physician for immediate attention or send patient to the emergency room.
- Lumbar region infection (e.g., osteomyelitis): History of drug use, recent infection in another body region (e.g., urinary tract, skin infection), malaise, fever, chills. Plan: Refer to physician for further examination.
- Spinal fracture: History of trauma, older population, osteoporosis, severe pain, deformity. Plan: Obtain appropriate radiographic evidence, proceed with rehabilitation.
- Aortic aneurysm: Age >50 years, history of smoking, heart disease, peripheral vascular disease, hypertension, concomitant abdominal discomfort. Plan: Refer for magnetic resonance imaging (MRI) or diagnostic confirmation of findings.
- Kidney disorders: History of recent urinary tract infection, painful urination, unilateral flank pain or low back pain, pain with percussion over the kidney. Plan: Refer back to physician for further diagnostic testing.

SUMMARY STATEMENT

The large prevalence of patients with low back pain is growing toward becoming a modern day epidemic. Low back pain is a massive burden on the healthcare system specifically and society in general secondary to medical costs and work-related disability.[15,21] Consequently, clinicians working in orthopedic physical therapy will have a significant amount of their caseload devoted to patients with low back pain. These patients are not a homogeneous group, thus there is no single treatment or combination of treatments that have proved to be the most effective in treating this complex etiological health condition. The foundation for a treatment program begins with a thorough examination followed by sound clinical reasoning in the selection of interventions and the evaluation of their effect (Table IV-3-2). The evidence base for low back pain treatments has historically been lacking, of poor quality, or filled with conflicting recommendations. However, a growing amount of recent research has advocated an active treatment approach and classifying patients with low back pain into subgroups to guide effective treatment interventions.* Today's healthcare environment is under greater scrutiny by secondary payers that demand effective and evidence-based treatment when considering reimbursement. It is important for clinicians treating patients with low back pain to begin to integrate the current evidence into their clinical practice to achieve greater outcomes.

REFERENCES

1. Andersson GBJ. Epidemiological features of chronic low back pain. *Lancet.* 1999;354:581-585.
2. Bialosky JE, Bishop MD, Price DD, Robinson ME, George SZ. The mechanisms of manual therapy in the treatment of musculoskeletal pain: a comprehensive model. *Man Ther.* 2008.
3. Brennan GP, Fritz JM, Hunter SJ, Thackeray A, Delitto A, Erhard R. Identifying subgroups of patients with acute/subacute "nonspecific" low back pain. Results of a randomized clinical trial. *Spine.* 2006;31:623-631.
4. Browder DA, Childs JD, Cleland JA, Fritz JM. Effectiveness of an extension oriented treatment approach in a subgroup of patients with low back pain: a randomized clinical trial. *Phys Ther.* 2007;87:1608-1618.
5. Centre for Reviews and Dissemination. Philadelphia panel evidence-based clinical practice guidelines on selected rehabilitation interventions for low back pain. *Database Abstr Rev Eff.* 2009;1.
6. Childs JD, Fritz JM, Flynn TW, et al. A clinical prediction rule to identify patients with low back pain most likely to benefit from spinal manipulation: a validation study. *Ann Intern Med.* 2004;141:920-928.
7. Chou R, Huffman LH. Nonpharmacologic therapies for acute and chronic low back pain: a review of the evidence for an American pain society/American college of physicians clinical practice guidelines. *Ann Inter Med.* 2007;147:492-504.
8. Clarke JA, van Tulder MW, Blomberg SEI, et al. Traction for low-back pain with or without sciatica. *Cochrane Database Syst Rev.* 2008;4.
9. Cleland JA, Childs JD, Palmer JA, Eberhart S. Slump stretching in the management of non-radicular low back pain: a pilot clinical trial. *Man Ther.* 2006;11:279-286.
10. Cleland JA, Fritz JM, Whitman JM, Childs JD, Palmer JA. The use of a lumbar spine manipulation technique by physical therapists in patients who satisfy a clinical prediction rule: a case series. *J Orthop Sports Phys Ther.* 2006;36:209-214.
11. Cohen SP, Argoff CE, Carragee EJ. Management of low back pain. *BMJ.* 2008;337:a2718.
12. Deyo RA, Weinstein JN. Low back pain. *N Engl J Med.* 2001;344:363-370.
13. Flynn T, Fritz J, Whitman J, et al. A clinical prediction rule for classifying patents with low back pain who demonstrate short-term improvement with spinal manipulation. *Spine.* 2002;27:2835-2843.
14. Fritz JM, Cleland JA, Childs JD. Subgrouping patients with low back pain: evolution of a classification approach to physical therapy. *J Orthop Sports Phys Ther.* 2007;37(6):290-302.
15. Fritz JM, Cleland JA, Speckman M, Brennan GP, Hunter SJ. Physical therapy for acute low back pain. Associations with subsequent healthcare costs. *Spine.* 2008;33:1800-1805.
16. Fritz JM, Weston L, Matheson JW, et al. Is there a subgroup of patients with low back pain likely to benefit from mechanical traction? Results of a randomized clinical trial and subgrouping analysis. *Spine.* 2007;32:E793-E800.
17. Furlan AD, Imamura M, Dryden T, Irwin E. Massage for low back pain (Review). *Cochrane Database Syst Rev.* 2008;4.
18. Kent P, Marks D, Pearson W, Keating J. Does clinician treatment choice improve the outcomes of manual therapy for nonspecific low back pain? A metaanalysis. *J Manip Physiol Ther.* 2005;28:312-322.

---

*References 3, 4, 6, 8-10, 13-16, 20, 22, 23.

19. Krismer M, van Tulder M. The low back pain group of the bone and health strategies for Europe project. Strategies for prevention and management of musculoskeletal conditions. Low back pain (nonspecific). *Best Pract Res Clin Rheumatol.* 2007;21:77-91.

20. Long A, Donnelson R, Fung T. Does it matter which exercise? A randomized controlled trial of exercise for low back pain. *Spine.* 2004;29:2593-2602.

21. Maniadakis N, Gray A. Economic burden of back pain in the UK. *Pain.* 2000;84:95-103.

22. O'Sullivan P. Diagnosis and classification of chronic low back pain disorders: maladaptive movement and motor control impairments as underlying mechanism. *Man Ther.* 2005;10:242-255.

23. O'Sullivan PB. Lumbar segmental 'instability': clinical presentation and specific stabilizing exercise management. *Man Ther.* 2000;5: 2-12.

24. van Duijvenbode I, Jellema P, van Poppel M, van Tulder MW. Lumbar supports for prevention and treatment of low back pain (review). *Cochrane Database Syst Rev.* 2008;4.

AUTHOR: NANCY ADACHI

INTRODUCTORY INFORMATION (i)

What are the factors a clinician should consider when rehabilitating a patient with temporomandibular joint pain?

When a clinician is rehabilitating a patient who has temporomandibular joint (TMJ) pain, the clinicians should take into consideration the following factors: [1,13,25,27]

- Mechanical versus nonmechanical jaw pain: Mechanical musculoskeletal pain that is directly related to jaw use is generally easier to treat with better outcomes than non mechanical such as chronic, peripheral or centralized pain
- Age: Younger patients generally have a better capacity to adapt and compensate from trauma or overload and usually have fewer dental problems.
- Gender: Female to male frequency of TMJ dysfunction is between 3:1 and 9:1. Males tend to have a history of trauma (fist fight or fall) and will usually improve with therapy, whereas females may have no apparent cause for jaw pain and the therapist will need to investigate why their pain persists.
- Trauma or injury: Fractures, direct trauma to jaw, or poor dental work will cause mechanical problems with the TMJ as a result of poor occlusion and chewing.
- Acute versus chronic: Acute musculoskeletal disorders are responsive to conservative care. The prognosis for patients with joint locking is generally good. Jaw function in most cases will be restored, but in many cases chronic clicking may persist as a result of morphological changes that have occurred at the TMJ. Patients with chronic symptoms may require a pain management team approach, including medications, injections, behavioral training, and physical therapy.
- Dentition refers to the arrangement or condition of the patient's teeth. Missing teeth that are not replaced, especially molars, can greatly impact the biomechanics of the jaw and result in pain and dysfunction.
- Dental and medical history: Often, patients will have a history of lengthy oral procedures, which was the event that initiated the patient's pain. Medically, disease processes, such as diabetes and cancer, can slow the patient's healing process.
- Oral habits: A patient's oral habits have significant influence over a patient's recovery potential. Habits, such as clenching and grinding; biting objects such as nails, lips, pens, and toothpicks; sleep posture (prone, arm, or hand under jaw), or leaning on hand against the jaw, may negatively impact a patient's recovery potential.
- Psychosocial history: Anxiety appears to be common with this population. Many are frustrated and angry with medical and dental providers.

What role does acuteness or chronicity play in rehabilitating a patient with TMJ pain?

Like other regions of the body, most acute symptoms will reduce in 4 to 6 weeks. Most patients with TMJ disease (TMD) are referred to rehabilitation settings for facial or joint pain. In these cases, the role of the clinician is to manage the symptoms, reduce the inflammatory response, restore the normal biomechanics and function of the joint, and address any factors that may contribute to the patient's symptoms. Chronic symptoms are more difficult to rehabilitate, and each patient's prognosis will depend on the nature of the pathology.

What factors make treatment of patients with TMJ pain challenging?

The anatomy of the TMJ is unique. There are two joints attached to the mandible. One joint will affect the other. Clinicians must be familiar with the relationships between the jaw, muscles, mouth, occlusion, and teeth. Many orofacial pain patients have oral habits, as well as psychological factors, that induce clenching and tensing behaviors. The TMJ needs to be addressed, as well as the cervical spine and upper quarter. Dizziness, headaches, and ear problems are often present in conjunction with jaw pain. Many of the noises, such as clicking, popping, and crepitation, are not amenable to rehabilitation nor do they need to be treated. [26]

Collaboration with other health care professions is required. Coordinating efforts with multiple professions is often challenging. Never treat the x-ray; in other words, adaptation of the fibrocartilaginous articular surfaces may permit normal function. Clinical studies have shown that TMJs with obvious x-ray changes often display insignificant or no clinical symptoms. [7,23] Several studies have demonstrated that there are no consistent postural findings that differentiate TMD patients from normal subjects. [4,6,14]

CASE STUDY (?)

Your patient is a 27-year-old female who reports right jaw pain for 2 months and the inability to open wide. She has history of clicking and intermittent locking, but the clicking is no longer present. She points to the right preauricular area and masseter muscle as her pain sites. Pain occurs only when she opens wide, yawns, or chews. When she opens, she deflects to the painful side and is limited. She is unable to laterotrude to the opposite side. What are your hypotheses regarding the source of this patient's symptoms?

Answer

The history is important in questioning when it comes to diagnosing the source of the symptoms. The patient is a young female who has history of clicking and catching of the TMJ. The jaw no longer clicks but is painful with wide opening. This is indicative of an internal derangement without reduction or anterior disc displacement without reduction. Before locking, it was a clicking joint (internal derangement with reduction, progressing to a catching joint, then to a closed lock). Other clues would be intermittent earache when the jaw is stretched opened, tenderness localized to the joint, and the movement pattern would display deflection to the painful, hypomobile side, normal laterotrusion to the same side, decreased laterotrusion to the opposite side, and decreased protrusion with deflection to the same side.

PROGNOSIS

How successful is rehabilitation in treating TMJ pain?

Rehabilitation in treating TMJ pain has the following success rates:

- Good success rate in decreasing the pain of capsulitis and osteoarthritis and helping reduce oral habits.
- Good success rate in muscle trismus and obtaining normal opening.
- Fair success rate in treating internal derangement without reduction and obtaining an almost normal opening.
- Fair to poor success rate in abolishing noises in the joints such as clicking and crepitation.
- Poor success rate with chronic sensitized peripheral or central pain, or neuropathic pain.

Chronic myofascial pain will take longer and may need extra assistance in rehabilitation such as trigger point injections, Botox injections, or medications such as tricyclic antidepressants or muscle relaxants and a team approach.

A prospective, randomized clinical trial (RCT) found arthroscopy to be no better than physical therapy in the treatment of reduced jaw range of motion (ROM) and pain caused by intraarticular disease. A long-term 10-year outcome study by Murakami et al[24] found that TMJ irreducible disk displacement disorder is a self-limiting, symptomatic, and nonprogressive disease, and 10 years after non-surgical treatment, patients were still satisfied with their results with less pain and increased ROM. However, the authors felt that the surgical intervention can immediately reduce pain and dysfunction, and persistent pain after conservative care should be considered a good indicator for surgical intervention.

Recent findings demonstrate that prolonged stress may cause local intramuscular hypoperfusion, which selects target muscles with higher proportions of type 1 (slow-twitch) fibers that are involved in postural maintenance. The local muscle pain can cause an accumulation of endogenous algesic substances and produce a peripheral muscle nociceptor sensitization and proceed to a central pathway sensitization.[5]

Which patients with TMJ pain derive the greatest long-term benefits from rehabilitation?

Patients who have learned to decrease their oral habits, who are in tune with their bodies, and who follow through with the treatment prescription can lessen the stress on their muscles and joints and deal with their internal and external stresses.

What other regions of the body are most likely to contribute to TMJ pain?

Chronic myofascial pain of the upper quarter and upper cervical spine dysfunction appear to contribute heavily to jaw pain. A patient with TMJ dysfunction may have a forward-head position, with tight upper cervical muscles and weakened deep neck flexors, and tend to clench their teeth or protrude their mandible. Cervicogenic headache, tension-type headache, and migraine are also common contributors to jaw pain. Nerve pain from the trigeminal complex and tooth pain will need to be ruled out.

CLINICAL PEARL ◎!

Patients with myofascial pain may be difficult to treat. Masticatory muscle pain may become chronic as a result of central mediation. Preset mutual goals, an established time line, and a treatment plan are needed. The patient should understand that zero pain may not be attainable but that manageable pain will be the goal. Look for habits and have the patient investigate why the pain persists. A daily or hourly pain log may be helpful to the patient. Show patients soft tissue changes with a mirror, showing a scalloped edged tongue and while inside cheek lines indicative of clenching and pushing the tongue forward. Excessive wear and lock and key bruxofacets on canines indicate bruxing/grinding forces on the teeth. If obvious clenching and bruxing habits are not apparent, look for tensing and protrusive habits. Explain that clenching is 10% to 15% of maximal occlusion. Protrusive habits are more common with patients with a large overjet (>2 mm). The muscles usually involved are the masseters, temporalis, and medial and lateral pterygoids. The cervical spine and muscles of the neck and upper quarter are usually involved; other factors are stress, poor sleep, and anxiety.

EVIDENCE BASED MEDICINE

What trends are currently being seen in research regarding rehabilitation of patients with TMJ pain?

Well-conducted, long-term research regarding TMJ rehabilitation is lacking. According to the Cochrane Database of Systemic Reviews, no present study was conducted on physical therapy specifically for TMD; however, in a review of physical therapy, Feine reviewed publications dealing with chronic musculoskeletal conditions and patients with TMD.[10,11] No good evidence was found that any of the treatments under review, including heat; cold; ultrasound;

acupuncture; low-intensity laser; electrical stimulation, specifically transcutaneous electrical stimulation (TENS); mobilization/manipulation; and exercise, are capable of curing or even significantly reducing symptoms of chronic musculoskeletal conditions, including TMD. However, clinically, patients are helped while they are undergoing treatment and this does not depend on the specific form of therapy used. Therefore these forms of reversible, noninvasive therapy are better than no therapy, perhaps because the clinicians take the time to fully inform patients about their condition and allay their fears. Based on clinical experience, it seems that the most promising strategies for long-term management of musculoskeletal chronic pain are based on exercise programs, but evidence is required to substantiate this hypothesis.

INTERVENTIONS

Which interventions have proven most successful in treating patients with TMJ pain?

The following interventions have proved most successful in treating TMJ pain:

- Awareness of posture and habits, including the cervical spine and jaw
- Jaw exercises to improve proprioception, improve muscle coordination, awareness of habits, increase circulation to the joints, and increase ROM. Use of a mirror to help patient see how they move and give instantaneous feedback on placement of tongue and jaw. Use of finger on the chin or both index fingers on bilateral TMJs and thumbs on anterior aspect of chin for movement can help with avoidance of early protrusion.
- Self-massage to increase circulation and relaxation
- Heat to increase circulation, relaxation, and reduce nociception
- Ice to decrease pain and swelling, deep circulation
- Joint mobilization to decrease nociception, increase ROM, induce relaxation
- Vapo-coolant spray and stretch for myalgia and myofascial pain
- Stretching exercises for hypomobile joints and muscle trismus/spasm. Self stretch using thumbs on upper teeth and index fingers on lower teeth. Slow stretch for muscle problems, and quicker stretches for joint problems.
- Unlocking exercises: Move jaw laterally away from the involved joint and try to open. Can use hand to push over and open wider. Patients are sometimes more successful in unlocking themselves than therapist interventions. Another technique is biting into an eraser on the opposite molars in attempt to give a distraction mobilization to the TMJ.
- Mulligan technique for painless opening of the mandible: Gently press TMJ medially and find position where pain is relieved with active opening and closing

CLINICAL PEARL ◎!

Functional outcomes of treatment for anterior disc displacement without reduction are at least 38 mm of opening and eating without significant pain. The disc will be pushed anteriorly, and deflection is expected to be present. Work toward symmetrical opening rather than opening as much as possible. Noises may return, indicating that the condyle may be moving partially on the disc or on uneven surfaces of the ementia articularis. Most patients do not require surgery and should be able to return to a normal diet within 6 to 12 months.

What are the biomechanics of the TMJ?

- The joint primarily rotates the first 26 mm, then primarily anterior translation thereafter. Normal opening ROM is greater than 40 mm.

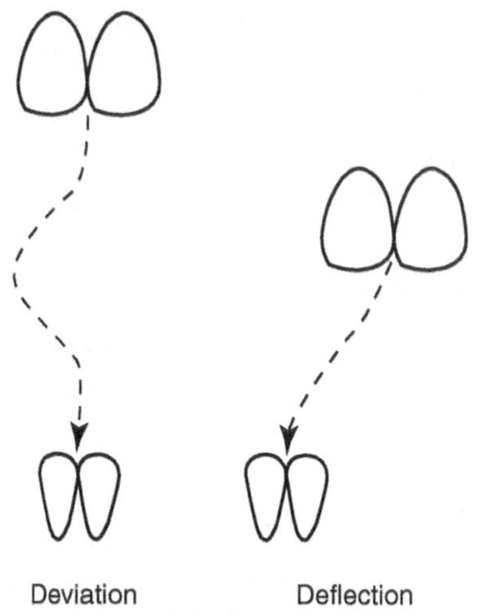

Deviation   Deflection

FIGURE IV-4-1 Deviation and deflection of the jaw with opening.

- Laterotrusion involves rotation on the same side and anterior translation on the opposite side. Normal ROM is greater than 6 mm.
- Protrusion involves bilateral symmetrical anterior translation. Normal ROM is greater than 6 mm.
- Retrusion is the closed pack position and can be physically manipulated with the patient reclined and therapist gently jiggling the jaw 1 to 2 mm into retruded contact position (RCP). If the therapist is unable to retrude the jaw, the patient has either muscle guarding or joint swelling/pain.
- Muscular contact position, in which the muscles want the teeth to touch first, should equal the intercuspal position (position where the teeth occlude maximally). If they are not compatible, a muscular problem exists.
- Hypomobility refers to decreased ROM (less than 40 mm of opening, laterotrusion, and protrusion of less than 6 mm). If only one side is involved, there will be a deflection of the jaw to the hypomobile side.
- Hypermobility: The ligaments and capsule are lax and the condyle/disc will move beyond the ementia articularis border; often the condition is bilateral. Occasionally, an open lock may occur in which the joint is stretched beyond and the muscles contract and the patient is unable to close his or her mouth.
- Joint movements are symmetrical: With opening, observe if the jaw deflects or deviates (Figure IV-4-1). Deflection is moving the jaw to one side. The direction of deflection usually means it is hypomobile on that side. Deviation is moving the jaw toward one side and returning to the center at the end of opening (C curve). Deviation may mean a muscular imbalance or an actual deviation in form (articular tissue irregularity on the fossa, eminence, or condyle). An S curve means muscle imbalance.

CASE STUDY

A 60-year-old female arrives at your office complaining of right earache and inability to chew and open wide. She can no longer bite into sandwiches or into a strawberry due to pain and has cracking noises in her right ear. She complains of a deep dull earache interspersed by at times by sharp and throbbing pain. The pain may wake her up and night, usually pain is worse upon awakening and the sharp pains may come on for no reason.

What are your hypotheses regarding the source of this patient's symptoms?

Answer
The age, symptom characteristics, and symptom provocation questioning is important in diagnosing the type of disorder. Osteoarthritis is more common in this age group with complaints of noises such as crepitation and cracking.[8] Pain location in the ear leads to a joint disorder rather than muscle. Inability to open wide and especially bite into foods (open with protrusion) describes an inflammatory problem on the articular surfaces of the joint rather than the disc proper. Inflammation is also apparent with the descriptors of throbbing and spontaneous pain without provocation. The joint will be tender to palpation, end-feel may be painful or hard, and the movement pattern will be capsular. The night pains may be due to the patient rolling on the same side and placing pressure on the joint.

MANUAL THERAPY
What is the physiological rationale behind the use of manual therapy in treating patients with TMJ pain?
Manual therapy can help move a mechanical impediment such as a loose body, relocate the condyle in open lock, reduce an acute closed lock, break adhesions in the upper joint space, and permit movement and decrease nociceptive input and associated reflex muscle spasm. It may improve circulation and nerve conductivity by increasing the space in which nerves and blood vessels cross. It improves muscle function and decreases tension by improving the distribution of joint forces and levers. Manual therapy can induce relaxation; reduce soft tissue swelling, inflammation, or restriction; and can modulate pain using joint or soft tissue techniques.

How beneficial is joint mobilization in the treatment of patients with TMJ pain?
- Grades 1 and 2 can be used to decrease pain and increase circulation and relaxation.
- Grades 2 and 3 with distraction mobilization can be used to decrease pain and increase relaxation.
- Grades 3 and 4 are used to increase ROM, especially with anterior translatory glide for hypomobile joints or muscle trismus. The joint can be mobilized unilaterally or bilaterally.

Retrusion can be used to stretch the medial and lateral pterygoid and help with relaxation. Passive and active retrusion exercises can help to decrease protrusive bite changes. Care must be taken because retrusion can exacerbate an inflamed joint. In the author's clinical experience, mobilization to recapture the disc is usually 25% successful with only acute cases of locked joints. Mobilizations to increase ROM for trismus may take 4 to 6 weeks to get full opening (Table IV-4-1).

Is joint manipulation recommended for patients with TMJ pain?
Quick thrust moves are not used, however, for an anteriorly displaced disc without reduction; grades 3 to 4 mobilizations are used to increase ROM. In acute patients, the disc may be recaptured. In chronic patients, the disc's posterior band is being stretched, and the disc is pushed forward. Mobilization is also used with injection, arthrocentesis, and arthroscopy for the same problem.

What does evidence reveal regarding the use of massage for the treatment of patients with TMJ pain?
There has been no specific reliable research on the effects of massage for the TMJ. However, clinically, massage and self-message of the masseter and temporalis muscles are taught to patients to increase circulation and promote relaxation. Deep sustained pressure massage is used to break-up trigger points and increase circulation. Intraoral massage to the masseters and medial pterygoids is used to decrease localized tender and trigger points.

TABLE IV-4-1   Motion Restriction and Mobilization

Motion Restrictions	Joint Requiring Mobilization	Direction of Mobilization
Opening wide	Temporomandibular	Anterior translatory glide with slight mesial* direction
Laterotrusion	Temporomandibular	Anterior translatory glide on the hypomobile side. Or unilateral lateral mobilization on lingual[†] side of molars. Or unilateral medial mobilization on buccal[‡] side of molars.
Protrusion	Temporomandibular	Bilateral anterior translatory glide. Or individually.

*Dental term meaning toward the anterior, front, or midline.
[†]Lingual is the side of the tooth toward the tongue.
[‡]Buccal means of or relating to the cheek.

Is stretching beneficial or indicated for patients with TMJ pain?

Patients with trismus (muscle spasm) and muscle guarding should use slow stretch and contract relax and stretch joint hypomobility and acute closed lock. Depending on the stage of the problem, chronic closed lock, capsulitis, and osteoarthritis can be stretched.

EXERCISE

What is the physiological rationale behind the use of exercise in treating patients with TMJ pain?

As with any synovial joint in the body, exercises are used for specific outcomes. Exercises are beneficial to prevent formation of intraarticular adhesions and to increase the blood flow and strength of the jaw muscles for reduced mandibular mobility caused by intraarticular restriction or by muscular dysfunction. Movement must occur to train muscles and joints to perform in a coordinated, synchronous, and functional manner such as chewing and opening. Dubner[9] and Hannam[15] showed TMD patients have impaired mandibular kinesthetic and lateral jaw position sense and reduced control over the direction of movement.

Oral habits, such as bruxism, cause compressive overloading that suggests production of harmful oxidative radicals that are highly reactive and known to destroy hyaluronic acid, collagen, and proteoglycan.[12] Microtrauma (clenching) causes a soft tissue response, such as plastic deformation of the ligaments, which may lead to permanent intraarticular changes. Intraarticular friction may cause synovial fluid that affects lubrication and nutritional requirements and/or changes in the articulating surfaces.[16] Reduction of these habits with exercise will prevent these problems by increasing their awareness and changing good habits for bad habits.[20]

The most recent theory for jaw muscle pain and signs of motor dysfunction is that they are a consequence of nociceptor activity or a response to pain of central origin hypoxia not muscular hyperactivity. Specific jaw exercise and whole body aerobic movement can be used to restructure the experience of illness associated with malfunction of the body and to rehabilitate limitations in function. The aim is to involve intentional behavior, and with attention to the new behavioral pattern, further changes are possible within the brain. Efforts by the patient to focus on the pain and to work within the range of movement imposed by the pain will contribute to increased self-efficacy as part of a cognitive-behavioral program. Exercise involves motor programs, sensory perception, and appraisal processes. Exercise develops new motor skills and teaches self-discipline, control, and healthy proprioception and appraisal.[17,18,19]

Are exercise programs beneficial in treating patients with TMJ pain? Which exercise programs are effective in treating patients with TMJ pain?

A recent systematic review by Medlicott and Harris[22] revealed that active exercises, including a home exercise program and manual mobilizations, alone or in combination, may be effective in increasing openings in patients with acute disc displacement, acute arthritis, or acute or chronic myofascial pain.

Programs involving combinations of active exercises, manual therapy, postural correction, and relaxation techniques may decrease pain and impairment in people with TMD that is a result of acute disc displacement, acute arthritis, or acute myofascial TMD. However, it is impossible to discern whether a combination program is more effective than providing the separate elements of the program as individual treatment techniques.

Programs involving relaxation techniques and biofeedback, electromyography (EMG) training, and proprioceptive reeducation may be more effective than placebo treatment or occlusal splints in treating patients with acute or chronic myofascial or muscular TMD.

Postural training may be used in combination with other treatment techniques because the effects, independent of other treatments, are not known (e.g., postural training combined with a home exercise program may decrease pain in people with myofascial TMD).

Which muscles should be strengthened in treating patients with TMJ pain?

Maximum occlusal force is significantly reduced in some patients with a TMD but normally the muscles are not considered weak, instead their forces are disrupted because of the pain or dysfunction. Once the pain/dysfunction is managed, chewing and normal activity of the jaw will allow for proper mastication. However, this does not mean that the muscles should not be rehabilitated. See the previous section on exercise reasoning.

How should a clinician decide which exercise is most appropriate for a patient with TMJ pain?

Exercises are prescribed depending on the patient's impairments. Three basic exercises can be taught initially. The first exercise is to teach awareness of normal rest position. Many TMJ patients do not realize where the normal rest position of the jaw is. The correct tongue position should be taught: The tongue rests on the palate behind the anterior rugae, maintaining a freeway space (slight opening space between the teeth), and the mandible is positioned where the muscular contact position is same as the intercuspal position. Hinge axis exercise teaches the patient to open the jaw like a hinge (only rotation occurring), thus there is no contraction of the lateral pterygoids pulling the jaw anteriorly. Midline open exercise teaches the patient to hinge first and gradually allow for anterior translation; this exercise limits ROM to avoid clicking and pain and to open symmetrically; and it also avoids protrusive and lateral opening/closing patterns.

How should a clinician progress an exercise program for the TMJ?

Work first on increasing awareness of habits and the normalizing movements of the jaw. If ROM is an issue, teach active ROM (AROM), active assistive (AAROM), then passive ROM (PROM), using their fingers/thumbs, mirror, tongue blades, teeth slightly touching for proprioceptive input. Remove the assists (mirror, finger) once the patient is able to perform the exercises accurately. If coordination is an issue, teach proprioceptive exercises in neutral, midrange and end-of-range isometrics, then progress to resistive. Painful joints are given hinge axis and midline opening exercises, and once the pain is under control, can progress to full ROM exercises in opening, laterotrusion, and protrusion.

How does a clinician know if a patient with TMJ pain is ready to progress to a new exercise?

Once the patient is proficient in demonstrating the exercise back to you and has met the initial goal, the next goal should be established and individualized exercises are prescribed.

MODALITIES

Which modalities have proven most successful in treating patients with TMJ pain?

A systematic review by Medlicott and Harris[22] analyzed studies examining the effectiveness of various physical therapy interventions for TMD. They found that mid-laser therapy may be more effective than other electrotherapy modalities in decreasing pain and improving total vertical opening (TVO) in people with TMD secondary to acute disc displacement and may be more effective than other electrotherapy modalities in the short term, although comparison is difficult.

How should a clinician decide which modality is most appropriate for a patient with TMJ pain?

Modalities can be used, depending on the acuteness and desired response, as follows:
- Spray and stretch for trismus and myofascial pain.
- Ultrasound for trismus: Unfortunately, RCT studies are nonexistent that show ultrasound compared to no treatment or placebo in patients with TMD.
- Electrical stimulation or laser treatments: Studies have shown mixed results with chronic pain.
- Clinically, muscle pain responds well to heat and massage, possibly as the result of the hypoperfusion theory. Both heat and massage are used at home two to three times a day along with exercise. Ice decreases pain and inflammation and is used as for acute and subacute painful muscles and joints two to three times a day.

OTHER

What is the role of a dental splint in treating patients with TMJ pain?

A dental splint is made by the dentist. Over-the-counter splints are too soft and ill-fitting. Dentists can make soft vacuforms in their offices, but frequently bruxers will increase their clenching/grinding. Nociceptive trigeminal inhibition (NTI) splints can cause anterior open bites and are not recommended for long-term use. Hard acrylic, full-coverage stabilization splints protect teeth from bruxing and may be helpful for osteoarthritic joints, nighttime bruxers, and some types of internal derangements with reduction.

Intermittent locking (internal derangement with incoordination) problems can use an anterior repositioning splint part time to prevent locking and catching. Repositioning splints are used at night for patients that lock at night, and after 6 months or so, the patient can be walked back to intercuspal position. Splints are not indicated once the joint is locked.

What is the role of treatment aimed at neurodynamics in treating patients with TMJ pain?

Neurodynamic techniques are only warranted in patients with cervical involvement or headaches coming from the cervical spine. The afferents from the trigeminal nerve carry temperature and pain information from the head and TMJ areas, descending through the medulla oblongata and into the gray matter of the spinal cord as far as C3-C4. The afferents from C1-C3 spinal nerves synapse at the segment in which they enter the spinal cord and send collateral branches to superior and inferior segments. The gray matter in the spinal cord receives both trigeminal and cervical afferents, and this convergence of the trigeminocervical nucleus constitutes the basis for referred pain in the head and upper neck. [2,3]

CLINICAL PEARL

!

The most important aspect in treating a patient with TMJ disorder is confirmation of the treating diagnoses and impairment is first. Decide whether it is the joint, muscle, or the combination you will need to treat. If ROM is 10 to 20 mm of opening, the muscles of closure are the primary hurdles to tackle first. Slow-stretch, hold-relax, hold-relax-antagonist contraction, or antagonist-contraction exercises and joint mobilization are treatments of choice. Modalities, tongue blades, and Therabite exercisers may assist, as well as trigger or Botox injections. Once the ROM has increased past 26 mm (primarily translation occurs) and limitation is still a factor with a particular end-feel (non-springy), the joint is probably the problem. Treat the joint with mobilization and exercises. The end-feel tells you if it is a muscle joint (discal, capsular, or osteoarthritic) as well as movement patterns.

HOME EXERCISE

Which home exercises are the most beneficial to give patients with TMJ pain?

- Awareness: Postural position or initial click position
- Hinge axis: Moving jaw open and closed without touching the teeth and no protrusion/laterotrusion; goals: Awareness and helps with relaxation of the jaw and circulation.
- Midline opening: Open with the tongue up as wide as possible, without anterior translation; goals: Awareness, avoids clicking, and limits wide open pain.
- Laterotrusion with emphasis returning to neutral position: Helps with coordination and contraction of the contralateral lateral pterygoid and relaxation of the ipsilateral.
- Opening wide teaching initial rotation then anterior translation: Goals are symmetrical opening and increasing ROM.

The awareness exercises are best repeated every 1 to 2 hours to remind oneself where the relaxed, normal rest position should be, as well as to increase localized circulation and relaxation. Stretching and coordination exercises are best repeated two to three times a day, using a mirror or other proprioceptive cues (index fingers on TMJ and thumbs on chin).

REHABILITATION CLINICAL REASONING

How should a clinician decide which intervention is most appropriate for a patient with TMJ pain?

The following questions should be answered before treatment is initiated:
- Assess if the patient has a muscular, joint, or nerve problem.
- Determine if the patient is a physical therapy candidate.
- Decide if the patient needs to be referred to another discipline.

Table IV-4-2 includes intervention decision-making guidelines.

TABLE IV-4-2 Intervention Decision-Making Guidelines

Acute Nonreducible Anterior Disk Displacement	Clicking, Painful Joints	Painful Joint	Myalgia and Myofascial Pain	Trismus
Treatment frequency				
1-2 times/week for 4-5 visits to unlock	1-2 times/week for 4-6 weeks	1-2 times/week for 4-6 week	1-2 times/week for 6-8 weeks	2 times/week for 4-6 weeks
Use aggressive joint mobilization anterior translation with opening.	Treat with exercises to avoid clicking, soft diet, avoidance of clicking, modify diet.	Use modalities, ice, rest to decrease inflammation and swelling.	Acute: Use ice, massage, rest, N position, and hinge axis exercises.	Treat with aggressive stretching and mobilization.
Teach stretching exercises, use fingers and tongue blades, have patients try to unlock themselves by laterotrusion on the opposite side and open using hand to push.	Mobilization for acute patients to try to recapture the disc.	Teach N position, midline opening and avoidance of clenching, modified diet.	Can use spray and stretch, ultrasound, or any other nociceptive dampening modality.	Use ultrasound and/or heat before mobilization, tongue blades for self-stretch. Deep pressure massage.
	Mobilize for pain management and stretching within pain limit for chronic pain.		Emphasize behavioral therapy and realization of what brings on pain and what makes it better.	Chronic: Add Therabite massage.
			Chronic: Teach the patient self-spray and stretch, self-massage, including intraoral massage and self-spray and stretch.	
			Possible occlusal appliance if wakes up clenched or painful.	
PT treatment unsuccessful				
Give option to referral to dentist or oral surgeon for arthrocentesis or arthroscopy or give it time to heal.	Add injections, possible anterior repositioning splint for intermittent locking, especially at night	Add NSAIDs, steroid injection, possible occlusal appliance if bite is not stable.	Add trigger point or Botox injections, tricyclic antidepressants, or muscle relaxants, psychological consult for stress management and relaxation training, pain management team.	Add trigger point or Botox injections, NSAIDs, muscle relaxants.

PT, Physical therapy; *NSAIDs*, nonsteroidal antiinflammatories.

TABLE IV-4-3 Tissue Injury and Intervention Selection

What are the best interventions for the acute phase (0–14 days postinjury)?	When to progress to next phase	What are the best interventions for the reparative phase (15–21 days postinjury)?	When to progress to next phase	What are the best interventions for the remodeling phase (22–60 days postinjury)?	When to progress to next phase	What are the best interventions for the maturation phase (60–360 days postinjury)?
Disc pathology: Anterior disc displacement without reduction						
Mobilize in attempt to recapture the disc, NSAIDs for pain relief and antiinflammatory effects, massage and spray and stretch for the secondary muscle spasm, exercises to unlock joint		Same as acute phase		Same as acute phase, steroid injection or arthrocentesis may be an option up to 6–9 months after locking	After 4–5 unsuccessful attempts to unlock and maintain joint unlocked or increase ROM to 38 mm	Mobilize to increase ROM and symmetry of opening in attempt to break adhesions and stretch posterior attachment of the disc, stretching exercises, arthroscopy may be an option.
Disc pathology: Anterior disc displacement with reduction						
Mobilize in attempt to aid with remodeling of the healing structures, exercises to avoid clicking, NSAIDs for pain relief/antiinflammatory effects		Same as acute phase		Mobilize in attempt to aid with remodeling of the healing structures, ROM exercises with avoidance of painful clicking, steroid injection		Mobilize if restriction of motion, ROM exercises, explain noises are normal result of healing process, Synvisc injection for persistent loud noise or catching.
Muscle strain						
Rest, ice, NSAIDs for pain relief and antiinflammatory effects, massage, hinge axis exercises, midline open	Once inflammation has subsided, start full AROM	AROM, if trismus persists, AROM, aggressive joint mobilization and muscle stretching	Persistent pain, look for other factors: Poor posture, neck influences, biopsychosocial influences	Aerobic conditioning, self-help and relaxation techniques, pain talk involving peripheral and central sensitization, if trismus persists, try injection with mobilization, Therabite	Trial of unsuccessful physical therapy treatment for pain	Pain management team, psychological services, if trismus continues to persist, may refer to maxillofacial if ankylosis or severe scarring has occurred.
Myofascial pain						
Localized treatment: Heat, self-massage, spray and stretch, and ROM exercises	If treatment does not decrease pain, go to next phase	Regional treatment, including cervical influences, heat, self-massage, spray and stretch, and ROM exercises, trigger point injections/Botox and/or tricyclic antidepressants, local myalgia: Occlusal appliance if patient endorses parafunctional behavior	Persistent pain: look for other factors: poor posture, neck influences, biopsychosocial influences	Aerobic conditioning, self-help and relaxation techniques, pain talk involving peripheral and central sensitization	Trial of unsuccessful physical therapy treatment after 6–8 weeks	Pain management team, psychological services.

Ligament sprain, open lock						
Rest, ice, NSAIDs for pain relief and antiinflammatory effect, hinge axis, midline open exercises	Once inflammation has diminished	Teach midline open, avoid wide open, isometrics in neutral	If continues to catch or lock open	Teach resistive exercises to end of acceptable opening range without locking		Teach resistive exercises to end of acceptable opening range without locking
Bone fracture mandible						
Rest, ice, may be in fixation, emphasize not resting teeth together (no clenching)		Wait for bone healing, rest, ice, massage		Once physician gives the okay, start AROM and PROM, aggressive joint mobilization		If ROM is limited, use Therabite, PROM and AROM, aggressive joint mobilization
Capsule injury						
Rest, ice, hinge axis exercises, avoid wide open opening, lateral/protrusive movements, NSAIDs for pain relief and antiinflammatory effect	Once active inflammation has diminished, start next phase	AROM exercises, mobilization, painful joints: Steroid injection	Restricted ROM	Passive ROM for full pain-free ROM, mobilization	Restricted ROM	PROM and aggressive mobilization
Osteoarthritis						
Rest, ice, hinge axis exercises, avoid interincisal biting and sleeping on painful side. NSAIDs for pain relief and antiinflammatory effect.	Once inflammation has diminished, start AROM exercises	Midline open exercises, AROM within pain-free limits, mobilization to decrease pain and improve ROM, steroid injection	Restricted ROM or persistent loud noise	Active assistive and PROM for restricted opening, mobilization to increase ROM, Synvisc injection for catching	Restricted ROM	Passive ROM exercises, aggressive ROM if nonpainful, Therabite if ROM restriction, stabilization splint if patient has poor stability (no molars).

AROM, Active range of motion; NSAIDs, nonsteroidal antiinflammatories; PROM, passive range of motion; ROM, range of motion.

What red flags should a clinician be aware of regarding rehabilitating a patient with TMJ pain?

- Temporal headaches caused by temporal arteritis can lead to blindness if not treated. Look for throbbing, pulsating temporal artery pain and tenderness; an acute history of progressively debilitating headaches and night pain in the elderly.
- Severe progressive headaches with nuchal rigidity: Meningitis
- Diplopia, sudden hearing loss, and facial palsy: Tumor in brain or central signs
- Very rare cancer of the mandible: Progressive pain with acute occlusal changes
- Trauma: Unhealed fracture
- Active inflammation or infection
- Yellow flags: Angina pectoris can mimic jaw pain, as well as toothache, earache, maxillary sinusitis, carcinoma of the maxillary sinus, salivary gland pathosis, acromegaly, carcinoma of the nasopharynx, Eagle's syndrome, migraine, and neuralgias.

SUMMARY STATEMENT

Conservative rehabilitation can help restore normal function, promote the repair and regeneration of tissues, and relieve musculoskeletal pain. Treating the TMJ patient enables the clinician to be the primary provider of care, since most TMD are musculoskeletal in nature. The clinician can evaluate the patient and determine the course of treatment such as whether to refer to other disciplines or treat in house. A good working relationship with a network of disciplines should be established, including TMJ dental specialists (orofacial pain specialists), maxillofacial surgeons, general dentists, family and internal medicine physicians, head and neck physicians, psychologists dealing with pain, and pain management specialists. The clinician can decide if additional diagnostic or treatment interventions are recommended such as imaging, serology, medications, ROM equipment, dental appliances, surgery, or injections (Table IV-4-3). The clinician uses his or her clinical judgment on how best to treat the patients by first determining what type of disability/impairment, stage of the problem, then which treatment would best serve the patient in the most efficacious way. Looking at the patient as a whole, using a biopsychosocial model and recognition of the mind and body relationship are other important factors. A majority of TMD patients achieve good results with noninvasive reversible care in which conservative rehabilitation plays an important role.

REFERENCES

1. Adachi NY, Wilmarth MA, Merrill RL. *The Temporomandibular Joint: Physical Therapy Patient management Utilizing Current Evidence. Current Concepts of Orthopaedic Physical Therapy.* 2nd ed. Orthopaedic Section, APTA, Inc; 2006.
2. Butler D, Moseley L. *Explain Pain.* Orthopedic Physical Therapy Products, 2003.
3. Butler D. *The Sensitive Nervous System.* Adelaide Australia: Noigroup Publications; 2000.
4. Clark GT, Adachi NY, Dornan MR. Physical medicine procedures affect temporomandibular disorders: a review. *J Am Dent Assoc.* 1990;121:151-162.
5. Clark GT. Treatment of myogenous pain and dysfunction. In: Laskin DM, Greene CS, Hylander WL, eds. *TMDs An Evidence-Based Approach to Diagnosis and Treatment.* Chicago: Quintessence Pub Co Inc; 2006:483-500.
6. Darlow LA, Pesco J, Greenberg MS. The relationship of posture to myofascial pain dysfunction syndrome. *J AM Dent Assoc.* 1987;114:73-74.
7. De Leeuw R. *A 30-Year Follow-Up of Non-surgically Treated Temporomandibular Joint Osteoarthrosis and Internal Derangement [thesis].* Groningen, The Netherlands: University of Groningen; 1994.
8. Dijkstra PU, de Bont LGM, Stregenga B, Boering G. Temporomandibular joint osteoarthrosis and generalized joint hypermobility. *Cranio.* 1992;10:221-227.
9. Dubner R, Sessle BJ, Storey AT. *The Neural Basis of Oral and Facial Function.* New York: Plenum Press; 1978.
10. Feine JS, Lund JP. An assessment of the efficacy of physical therapy and physical modalities for the control of chronic musculoskeletal pain. *Pain.* 1997;71:5-23.
11. Feine JS, Lund JP. In: Laskin DM, Greene CS, Hylander WL, eds. *TMDs An Evidence-Based Approach to Diagnosis and Treatment.* Chicago: Quintessence Pub Co Inc; 2006:359-375.
12. Gonzalez YM, Mohl ND. Masticatory muscle pain and dysfunctions. In: Laskin DM, Greene CS, Hylander WL, eds. *TMDs An Evidence-Based Approach to Diagnosis and Treatment.* Chicago: Quintessence Pub Co Inc; 2006:255-270.
13. Greene CS. Concepts of TMD etiology: Effects on diagnosis and treatment. In: Laskin DM, Greene CS, Hylander WL, eds. *TMDs An Evidence-Based Approach to Diagnosis and Treatment.* Chicago: Quintessence Pub Co Inc; 2006:219-228.
14. Hackney J, Bade D, Clason A. Relationship between forward head posture and diagnosed internal derangement of the temporomandibular joint. *J Orofac Pain.* 1993;7:386-390.
15. Hannam AG, Sessle BJ. Temporomandibular neurosensory and neuromuscular physiology. In: Zarb G, Carlsson G, Sessle BJ, Mohl N, eds. *Temporomandibular Joint and Masticatory Muscle Disorders.* Copenhagen: Munksgaard; 1994:67-100.
16. Holmlund A, Axelsson S. Temporomandibular joint osteoarthrosis. Correlation of clinical and arthroscopic findings with degree of molar support. *Acta Odontol Scand.* 1994;52:214-218.
17. LeResche L. Epidemiology of temporomandibular disorders: Implications for the investigation of etiologic factors. *Crit Rev Oral Biol Med.* 1997;8:291-305.
18. Lobbezoo F, Lavigne GJ. Do bruxism and temporomandibular disorders have a cause-and-effect relationship? *J Orofac Pain.* 1997;11:15-23.
19. Luder HU. Factors affecting degeneration in human temporomandibular joints as assessed histologically. *Eur J Oral Sci.* 2002;110:106-113.
20. Lund JP. Muscular Pain and Dysfunction. In: Laskin DM, Greene CS, Hylander WL, eds. *TMDs An Evidence-Based Approach to Diagnosis and Treatment.* Chicago: Quintessence Pub Co Inc; 2006:99-104.
21. McNeill C. Management of temporomandibular disorders: Concepts and controversies. *J Prosthet Dent.* 1997;77:510-522.
22. Medlicott MS, Harris SR. A systematic review of the effectiveness of exercise, manual therapy, electrotherapy, relaxation training, and biofeedback in the management of temporomandibular disorder. *Phys Ther.* 2006;86(n7):955-973.
23. Mejersjo C, Hollander LTMJ. Pain and dysfunction: Relations between clinical and radiographic findings in the short and long term. *Scand J Dent Res.* 1984;92:241-248.
24. Murakami K, Kaneshita S, Kanoh C, Yamamura I. Ten-year outcome of nonsurgical treatment for the internal derangement of the temporomandibular joint with closed lock. *Oral Surg Oral Med Oral Pathol Oral Radiol Endod.* 2002;94:572-575.
25. Ohrbach R. Biobehavioral therapy. In: Laskin DM, Greene CS, Hylander WL, eds. *TMDs An Evidence-Based Approach to Diagnosis and Treatment.* Chicago: Quintessence Pub Co Inc; 2006:391-402.
26. Pagett BT, Lichten EM. Headache. In: Placzek JD, Boyce DA, eds. *Orthopedic Physical Therapy Secrets.* 2nd ed. Philadelphia: Hanley & Belfus; 2006:255-262.
27. Stegenga B. Bont Lambert: TMJ Growth, Adaptive Modeling and Remodeling, and Compensatory Mechanisms in TMD. An Evidence-Based Approach to Diagnosis and Treatment. 53-64.

AUTHOR: DONNA CESPON

INTRODUCTORY INFORMATION (*i*)

What are the factors a clinician should consider when rehabilitating a patient with upper extremity pain? [7,11,18,23]

The upper extremity is different from the lower extremity in that its structural components uniquely reflect its different functional requirements. The lower extremity is designed primarily with stability in mind, and the upper extremity has been designed to allow for mobility. Parts of a machine that are not required to move will rarely break down. Parts that must move often and freely are more prone to damage. This is true of the human body. Repetitive motion injuries are very common in the upper extremity, more so than in the lower extremity. Often, a patient is referred to rehabilitation for a single pathology in a specific body region, and as a result, treatment focuses on that one single entity. The upper extremity will be addressed as a whole because rehabilitation of one region will directly impact the other regions.

Age and general health (current and past), including cognitive ability, impact all regions of the body. Age and health impact the body's ability to heal and recover from injury. Optimally, most musculoskeletal injuries can heal or repair. Whether these injuries reach their full healing potential depends significantly on health and age.

Psychosocial implications, such as attitude, stress level, and lifestyle habits (alcohol consumption, smoking, etc.), can negatively impact healing. Significant research is currently being completed that shows a correlation between stress and healing. The greater the stress, the slower the rate of healing. Stress can be physical, chemical, or emotional. All of these stressors negatively impact the body's ability to heal.

Current and past activity levels, including occupation, sport, and activities of daily living, impact each patient differently. The demands placed on the upper extremity will vary significantly, therefore rehabilitation should uniquely reflect each individual patient's needs and goals.

History of the current injury (especially mechanism of injury), including diagnosis and diagnostic test results, aids the clinician in the decision-making process. Knowledge of how the specific tissues were injured will allow the clinician to design a rehabilitation program that minimizes the potential of reinjury and maximizes the rate of healing.

Relevant past injuries or pain complaints are important because the entire upper extremity is intimately linked and functions together to complete tasks; past injuries to any region of the body should be investigated to determine if they could be a contributor to the patient's symptoms and functional limitations.

Aggravating and alleviating motions or activities are important because a patient's irritability or the ease at which a patient's symptoms are produced and reduced will significantly impact the design of a rehabilitation program. If a patient is irritable, aggravating activities should be avoided. If a patient is not irritable, more aggressive and potentially aggravating activities can be added to a program.

Nature of the patient's condition (postsurgical, acute, or chronic) will shape the program. Surgical patients require a different rehabilitation focus than patients with chronic upper extremity symptoms. The patient's availability for treatment and the patient's insurance or financial ability to pay (allotted visits) significantly impact rehabilitation decisions. In today's health care environment, the clinician should have a firm understanding of the number of visits the patient will have in rehabilitation. This will guide how much of the rehabilitation will be self-guided and how much of the recovery will be completed under the direct supervision of the clinician.

CASE STUDY (?)

Your patient is a 17-year-old male baseball pitcher and football quarterback who reports right (dominant) anterior shoulder pain with throwing. Minor pain was initially felt about 6 weeks ago after preseason pitching, which followed shortly after the end of football season. The pain would not last long so he did not modify his training. Resting for 1 week improved his symptoms, but the pain returned when he resumed throwing and this time the pain occurred sooner. The pain has continued to progressively worsen with decreased number of pitches tolerated, decreased speed of his pitches, and now there is occasional painless clicking or grinding in the shoulder. He is also now experiencing occasional elbow pain while pitching and some right-sided tightness across his neck. In standing, he presents with a depressed right shoulder, a mild right cervical side bend, an increased upper lumbar lordosis, and a slight left trunk rotation. (The lower quarter presents with a slightly elevated right pelvis, and knee extension is not symmetrical). What are your hypotheses regarding the source of this patient's symptoms?

Answer

The fact that the onset of his pain occurred after a season of quarterback throwing and now after the start of baseball season clearly suggests an initial overuse injury (also because his pain went away with rest), but the fact that it has worsened and now includes clicking/grinding and elbow and neck pain suggests the presence of persisting faulty mechanics at the shoulder joint. The overall posture demonstrates muscle imbalance (including the core muscles) probably related to throwing. The decreased speed and tolerance for pitching in combination with pain suggests rotator cuff dysfunction. Your suspicion of rotator cuff dysfunction and his posture should prompt you to test his dynamic shoulder and scapular mechanics. The clicking and grinding may be indicative of instability but may only be further evidence of muscle imbalance and faulty mechanics. His secondary symptoms of elbow and neck discomfort are evidence of his body's failure to compensate for the shoulder dysfunction.

What role does age play in rehabilitation of the upper extremity?

The patient's age may affect the rate of healing because of age-related changes in the tissues. The very young or very old patient may require more supervision and instruction with exercise programs both in the clinic and at home. Age plays a role in which modalities may be used (e.g., ultrasound is contraindicated over active growth plates). Age may play a role in the tolerance for manual therapy. Grades of joint mobilization and pressure applied will need to be appropriate for older bones, and there is more likelihood of the presence of arthritis, osteoporosis, or fibrotic changes in soft tissues. Age, along with activity level, will affect choice of exercises, intensity or frequency of exercises, and the progression of the exercises. Age and activity level will help determine prognosis and goals.

What role does acuteness or chronicity play in rehabilitating a patient with upper extremity pain?

Acuteness or chronicity will affect which modalities, manual therapy, and exercises are given. If the injury is acute in nature, the mechanism of injury will be important in guiding your examination, assessment, and treatment. It should also be noted if this is an acute exacerbation of a chronic problem. With an acute injury caused by trauma there is inflammation, more diffuse pain, and muscle spasm, so the patient may benefit from the use of modalities such as electrical stimulation, ice, ultrasound, and taping. An acute injury with an insidious onset or chronic upper extremity pain demands close attention to the patient's postural habits and mechanics, as well as scrutiny of the muscle balance and muscle recruitment of the upper quarter.

The chronic injury may have histological changes characterized by increased crosslinks and therefore more stiffness of the tissues requiring manual therapy and attention to correcting faulty movement patterns and joint mechanics that have perpetuated the problem. Whether the injury is acute or chronic, the patient should be educated on the importance of protecting the joint including the use of braces/splints, antiinflammatory medications, application of ice, sleeping positions, and ergonomic assessment and corrections. Soft tissue mobilization that is too aggressive in the acute stage of healing can cause overstimulation of collagen production and excessive scar formation. With a chronic injury the painful site is often not the origin of the problem. The joints proximal and distal to the painful site will need to be assessed and possibly rehabilitated as well.

What factors make treatment of patients with upper extremity pain challenging?

Upper extremity pain treatment can be challenging because of anatomical and biomechanical complexity such as the following:

- By design the upright use of the upper extremity is susceptible to the torque-inducing effects of gravity, and the upper extremity, along with the rest of the upper quarter, is subject to muscle imbalance that necessitates a more holistic approach to treatment.
- The shoulder joint lacks bony stability and relies heavily on appropriate muscle recruitment, force couples, and ligamentous/capsular integrity to maintain pain-free mobility.
- The elbow and forearm regions have crossing branches from all of the major nerves giving rise to potential injury or entrapment near the elbow.
- The wrist/hand complex is comprised of three complex wrist joints and nineteen joints in the hand with a network of tendons, sheaths, and ligaments that are challenging enough to warrant certification of a hand specialist. Pain in the hand and wrist is often complicated by trauma or disease.

The function of the upper extremity is strongly influenced by the cervical and thoracic spine. Often, abnormal function of the upper extremity can be directly linked to dysfunction occurring at the cervical or thoracic regions. Conditions such as rheumatoid arthritis, osteoarthritis, diabetes, and collagen diseases will all impact the upper extremity's recovery potential and when present will negatively impact the patient's prognosis.

In a study by Waugh et al,[34] patients who report nerve symptoms were more likely to experience a poorer short-term outcome after physical therapy management of lateral epicondylitis. Females who had work-related onsets, repetitive keyboarding jobs, and cervical joint signs had worse outcomes.[34] Patient compliance is always a factor in rehabilitation, especially in the patient's dominant extremity. The patient's inability or unwillingness to properly rest the upper extremity will slow the rate of recovery.

CLINICAL PEARL

Why should you ask the upper extremity patient about old ankle injuries?

An old ankle sprain can contribute to upper extremity pain via the kinetic chain effect: An ankle sprain that is not successfully rehabilitated can cause asymmetry of ankle dorsiflexion in gait. This repetitive asymmetrical pattern acts as a functional leg length difference that can cause a compensatory shift at the pelvis and eventually in the spine. The upper cervical spine will then compensate in a manner that will allow the eyes to maintain alignment with the horizon. This compensation of the spine can cause unilateral compression of facets in the cervical, thoracic, or lumbar spine. Compression in the cervical and upper thoracic spine would most likely cause painful referral to the upper extremity.

PROGNOSIS[10,16,21]

How successful is rehabilitation in treating acute upper extremity pain?

Kuijpers et al[17] studied 587 patients with a recent episode of shoulder pain. The main outcome measure was persistent symptoms at 6 weeks and 6 months, as perceived by the patient. All workers received standardized treatment that consisted of information on the prognosis of shoulder pain, advice regarding provoking activities, and stepwise treatment consisting of paracetamol, nonsteroidal antiinflammatories (NSAIDs), corticosteroid injection, or referral for physiotherapy. Potential predictors of shoulder outcomes at 6 weeks and 6 months were studied. From the study, the following attributes were present in patients who continued to have pain 6 weeks and 6 months after the initial injury. The predictors were a longer duration of shoulder symptoms, gradual onset of shoulder pain, and high pain severity at presentation. These were consistently associated with persistent symptoms at 6 weeks and 6 months.[17]

Treatment of acute shoulder pain can be very successful if inflammation is controlled as soon as possible. Use of modalities and manual therapy are usually successful interventions in treating acute pain. Sometimes, rehabilitation is not successful initially, and corticosteroid injection is indicated to allow the patient to better tolerate treatment. Treatment is more successful if it involves educating the patient in management of the injury and prevention of further exacerbation. Research on efficacy of treatment is focused more on specific interventions and on a specific pathology. Overall, there is evidential support in all regions of the upper extremity that rehabilitation is successful in alleviating symptoms and restoring function.

How successful is rehabilitation in treating chronic upper extremity pain? [17]

Chronic upper extremity pain rehabilitates well if faulty posture, muscle imbalances, and compensatory movement patterns throughout the upper quarter are both detected and corrected, even if serious pathology and surgery has occurred. The patient who is able to correct faulty postures and movement patterns can derive the greatest long-term outcomes. Sometimes, the longer the dysfunction has existed the more difficult the condition can be to treat. Treatment is more successful if it involves educating the patient in management of the injury and prevention of further exacerbation. Addressing restrictions as the result of scarring and increased crosslink formation and fascial restrictions improves outcomes. Articular cartilage damage tends to decrease the success somewhat, usually with some lingering pain if activities are not adequately modified. Long-term pain relief also requires a home maintenance program to prevent the return of muscle imbalance resulting from everyday effects of gravity, repetitive activities, and postures.

What other regions of the body are most likely to contribute to upper extremity pain?

As a whole, dysfunction in any region of the body can directly or indirectly impact the upper extremity and lead to symptomology. The cervical spine is most likely to contribute to upper extremity pain and so should always be screened. Compression, adhesion, or excessive deformation of intervertebral discs, nerve roots, or peripheral nerves is a common source of upper extremity symptoms. Research by Berglund et al demonstrated the relationship between pathology at C5, C6, and C7 or at T1, T2, T3, or T4 and upper extremity pain.[2,24] Spondylosis at C4-C7 has been shown to refer pain to the ipsilateral scapula. Cervical and thoracic spine ligaments have been shown to refer pain to the glenohumeral joint.

Kellgren, Travell, and others have shown mappings of referred upper extremity pain from muscle trigger points throughout the upper quarter.[13,14] Irritation of the first intercostal space has also shown pain patterns that refer to the shoulder, elbow, and hand regions. Stiffness in the thoracic spine that decreases accessory extension and rotation needed with shoulder motions can contribute to faulty mechanics creating pain in the upper extremity. The lumbar region can also contribute to pain in the shoulder via muscular and fascial attachment of the latissimus dorsi and the thoracic dorsolumbar fascia. The muscle imbalances caused by scoliosis of the spine can also cause compensations that eventually contribute to upper extremity pain. Contralateral hip restrictions or pelvic girdle imbalances can cause compensatory faulty mechanics of the shoulder and resulting shoulder or elbow pain, especially in athletes using the dominant upper extremity in throwing or unilateral overhead motions.

CLINICAL PEARL

What visual cues does the patient's relaxed standing posture indicate about muscle length of the shoulder complex? [15]

Other than a forward head, the most common postural fault in the upper quarter is medial rotation of the upper extremity. This is evident by the patient's palms facing the anterior thighs and the olecranon processes facing laterally and is usually caused by restriction of the latissimus dorsi, pectoralis major, and sometimes teres major. This is often asymmetrical, with the painful upper extremity being worse, and the elbow will often present in mild flexion secondary to a restricted biceps brachialis. This should guide the clinician to do length testing of these muscles. Another visual cue often seen with the painful shoulder is a horizontally positioned clavicle and an A-line shape of the shoulder. From the sternoclavicular joint the clavicles should rest in a slight "V" about 20 degrees from the horizon. An elongated upper trapezius will give the A-line appearance.

INTERVENTIONS

MANUAL THERAPY

What is the physiological rationale behind the use of manual therapy in treating patients with upper extremity pain? [6,12,19]

Collagen contained in muscle, bone, nerve, and connective tissue allows them to be positively affected by appropriate application of manual pressure designed to release adhesions, improve circulation, increase fibroblast stimulation and lymph drainage, and improve viscoelastic properties of these tissues. Restrictions in a muscle can significantly decrease blood flow throughout the tissue contributing to poor inflow of oxygen and nutrients and poor outflow of toxins and other noxious waste products. This inflow and outflow can be positively influenced by manual therapy. The vast complexity of soft tissue in the upper extremity has the potential for many restrictions, adhesions, and trigger points, which respond well to manual treatment. The extensive web of tendons and fascia, especially in the forearm, and hand/wrist complex are prone to restrictions and adhesions and will often not respond well to stretching or strengthening without manual therapy. Where joint movement occurs, there must be rolling and gliding present for other treatment techniques to be tolerated.

Which interventions have proved most successful in treating patients with upper extremity pain?

Manual cueing for reeducation can be considered manual therapy because it can be categorized as initially passive on the part of the patient and is associated with the goals of decreasing pain, increasing range of motion (ROM), and improving function. This is especially effective for postural cueing and assisting the patient in correction of faulty postures and movement patterns. Appropriate joint mobilization to the joints of the upper extremity is usually successful in decreasing pain by decreasing deformation or compression of nociceptors and by stimulating synovial fluid. This lubrication of the joint surfaces and joint capsule usually brings some pain relief to the patient. Joint mobilization can also help stretch stiff or shortened muscles or connective tissue.

Many painful trigger points and taut bands of soft tissue respond very well to positional release in which the irritated muscle is slackened by manually approximating the origin and insertions or the extremity is brought into the original position in which the lesion occurred. Soft tissue mobilization can be incorporated into this technique. Improved circulation and decreased muscle spasm/tenderness are desired results. Myofascial release is also a very gentle and effective manual treatment because of the interconnected and all-encompassing nature of fascia. When these more superficial tissues are released, soft tissue mobilization and stretching to muscles is more effective and seems to have longer lasting results. Hypersensitive tissues and conditions like fibromyalgia can be exacerbated with normal stretching exercises, but these patients tend to tolerate myofascial release well.[26,31]

How beneficial is joint mobilization in the treatment of patients with upper extremity pain?

Efficacy studies are limited, but clinically joint mobilization is very beneficial in treating pain, muscle guarding, loss of ROM, and capsular restrictions. Vicenzino et al[33] studied patients with lateral elbow pain, attempting to identify patients with lateral epicondylalgia likely to respond to mobilization with movement and exercise. If the following three attributes were present: less than 49 years of age, pain-free grip on the affected side, and pain-free gripping on the contralateral side, the probability of improvement was between 79% and 100%.[33]

Active mobilization techniques, such as mobilization with movement, can be effective and are supported by research when used on frozen shoulder patients (Table IV-5 1).[37] Joint mobilization is especially important for joints that have been immobilized. This synovial lubrication is intended to mimic the natural glide that occurs in freely moving joints. Without joint mobilization, scarring and abnormal formation of crosslinks can cause painful adhesions of the joint capsule that may require manipulation under anesthesia if severe. In the upper extremity, it is important to mobilize joints distal and proximal to the immobilized or injured joint, since all the upper extremity joints affect the mobility and mechanics of each other. Joint mobilization is contraindicated with the presence of bacterial infection, neoplasm, or recent fracture.

Is joint manipulation recommended for patients with upper extremity pain?

Joint manipulation is sometimes recommended to treat joints restricted by stubborn capsular adhesion. Research supports the efficacy of manipulation (under anesthetic block) for frozen shoulders but is usually a last resort. Occasionally, manipulation to the wrist can be effective in relieving wrist pain but should be done with caution and respect for possible ligamentous instability. Research shows wrist manipulation can be an effective treatment for symptoms of lateral epicondylitis. Joint manipulation is commonly used in the cervical and/or thoracic spine if it is a contributing source of the upper extremity pain. There is an increasing body of research that ties the cervical and thoracic spine to upper extremity dysfunction. Techniques, such as manipulation, can reduce symptoms in the upper extremity.[3,4,9,27,35] Joint manipulation is contraindicated at an unstable joint, especially one with minimal bony integrity, such as the glenohumeral joint, which is prone to anterior or multidirectional instability.

TABLE IV-5-1   **Motion Restriction and Mobilization**

Motion Restrictions	Joint Requiring Mobilization	Direction of Mobilization
Shoulder		
Shoulder flexion	Glenohumeral	Caudal and dorsal glide of humerus
	Scapulothoracic / Thoracic Spine	External (upward) rotation of scapula (cephalo-ventral glide of facet joints)
Shoulder extension	Glenohumeral	Ventral glide of humerus
Shoulder abduction	Glenohumeral	Caudal glide of humerus
	Scapulothoracic / Thoracic Spine	External (upward) rotation of scapula (cephalo-ventral glide of facet joints)
Shoulder external rotation	Glenohumeral	Ventral glide of humerus
Shoulder internal rotation	Glenohumeral	Dorsal glide of humerus
Elbow		
Elbow flexion	Humeroradial	Ventral glide of radial head
	Humeroulnar	Lateral glide of ulna
Elbow extension	Humeroradial	Dorsal/ventral glide of radial head
	Humeroulnar	Lateral glide of ulna
Elbow/wrist pronation	Proximal radioulnar	Dorsal glide of radial head
	Distal radioulnar	Ventral glide of radius
Elbow/wrist supination	Proximal radioulnar	Ventral glide of radial head
	Distal radioulnar	Dorsal glide of radius
Wrist		
Wrist flexion	Radiocarpal	Dorsal glide of carpals on distal forearm
	Midcarpal	Dorsal glide of distal row of carpals on proximal row
Wrist extension	Radiocarpal	Palmar glide of carpals on distal forearm
	Midcarpal	Palmar glide of distal row of carpals on proximal row
Wrist radial deviation	Radiocarpal	Ulnar glide of carpals on distal forearm
	Midcarpal	
Wrist ulnar deviation	Radiocarpal	Radial glide of carpals on distal forearm
	Midcarpal	
Hand		
Finger flexion	MCP	Palmar glide/radial glide
	Proximal interphalangeal	
	Distal interphalangeal	
Finger extension	MCP	Dorsal glide/ulnar glide
	Proximal interphalangeal	
	Distal interphalangeal	
Finger abduction/adduction	MCP	Radial glide
Thumb flexion	First MCP	Ulnar glide
	First CMC	Ulnar glide
Thumb extension	First MCP	Radial glide
	First CMC	Radial glide
Thumb abduction	First MCP	Dorsal glide
	First CMC	Dorsal glide
Thumb adduction	First MCP	Palmar glide

CMC, carpometacarpal; *MCP*, metacarpophalangeal.

What does evidence reveal regarding the use of massage for the treatment of patients with upper extremity pain?

Clinically, massage to the upper quarter is often helpful to decrease pain by improving relaxation in the patient through improved blood and lymph circulation. The decrease in restrictions usually then allows improved ROM, improved joint mobilization tolerance, and easier joint manipulation. Many clinicians and patients will report improvements with the use of massage for upper extremity pain. In a systematic review article by Tsao, massage was found to reduce pain, increase ROM, and decrease heart rate and blood pressure in patients with chronic shoulder pain when compared to control groups. Care must be taken when integrating these data because the research studied had small sample sizes and specific subject pools.[28]

Van den Dolder and Roberts studied twenty-nine subjects who had shoulder pain. The subjects received six sessions of massage to the muscles surrounding the shoulder. Following the six treatments, subjects had a significant decrease in shoulder pain and an increase in shoulder ROM (abduction, flexion, and behind back) when compared to a control group.[32] Massage alone (or any other individual intervention) is rarely beneficial to the long-term outcome. The effects of massage and other soft tissue techniques are often only temporary. This is because the mechanical source of the pain has not been addressed, so the pain returns as the indirect irritation and microtrauma persist.

Is stretching beneficial or indicated for patients with upper extremity pain?

Although research to support the benefits of stretching is limited, clinically, it is a critical co-intervention for successful short-term and long-term outcomes. Muscle length testing will detect shortened or stiff muscles that may respond well to stretching. Stretching lengthened irritable muscles and muscles in spasm can make upper extremity pain worse. The use of the contract-relax principle is very beneficial if the contraction does not elicit pain. Stretching that is preceded by positional release, myofascial release, or soft tissue mobilization is much more effective as it allows improved fiber lengthening throughout the fibers of the muscle and tendon.

Tissues surrounding a hypermobile joint must be stretched with caution. The hypermobile segment (or bone) must be manually stabilized so that the joint is not translating excessively, rendering the stretch ineffective and possibly causing irritation to the joint. Since the scapula is a "floating" bone with multiple muscular attachments, it is important to stabilize it accordingly. An example of this poor stretching technique occurs often with swimmers who commonly stretch the upper extremity into horizontal adduction without stabilizing the scapula (using the scapular adductors). This motion stretches the rhomboids but does not stretch the posterior scapulohumeral muscles, therefore perpetuating a common pain producing imbalance about the muscles of the shoulder complex. Active stretching can be more beneficial in correcting muscle imbalance than passive stretching as it gives neurological reeducation to the opposing muscles throughout the new range acquired. Stretching and patient follow through in a home program are especially indicated for chronic injuries of the upper extremity.

EXERCISE

What is the physiological rationale behind the use of exercise in treating patients with upper extremity pain?

The vast number of muscles acting on the joints of the upper extremity, especially in the shoulder complex, requires coordination and balance of force couples, synergists, antagonists, and stabilizing muscle groups. Upper extremity pain can be indirectly caused by weakness or imbalance of upper and lower quarter muscle groups, further necessitating exercise as a treatment intervention. Exercises can be prescribed to counteract the natural tendency toward muscle imbalance. Most human functions require visual feedback, and the body gives predominant use of the upper extremity to push, pull, lift, and manipulate items also primarily in front of the body. Chronic injuries often have weakness or muscle imbalances in other regions of the body that directly affect the proper function of the upper extremity. Exercise can help address these imbalances. Exercise helps improve circulation, which assists in healing the injury and can also give the patient an active role in the healing process.

Are exercise programs beneficial in treating patients with upper extremity pain?

Exercise programs and protocols are an integral part of treating upper extremity pain but must be prescribed and performed correctly without eliciting pain or exacerbating the patient's symptoms. Exercise programs must be progressed correctly, keeping in mind how easily torque is generated in the upper extremity because of the long lever of the upper extremity as it becomes more perpendicular to the force of gravity. For an exercise to be beneficial, the patient must be given verbal and manual cues that allow the patient to perform the exercise correctly. The patient should understand the goal of the exercise and how it should feel (or not feel) when initially prescribed or advanced. Exercises must be appropriate for the stage of tissue healing after an injury or surgery to be beneficial. Quality of exercise technique is much more beneficial than quantity. Exercise programs are only beneficial with patient compliance and follow through.

Which exercise programs are effective in treating patients with upper extremity pain?

Closed-chain exercises can be integrated early on in the rehabilitation process because these exercises can be started at a very low level and then continually progressed with modifications that build on the original exercise. For example, quadruped weight-bearing progressed to shifting the body weight forward in quadruped, then quadruped weight-bearing through one upper extremity and the contralateral lower extremity progressed to shifting the body weight forward; further progressed with resistance through the non–weight-bearing extremities, and so forth. Initially, close monitoring of the patient's technique (i.e., correcting substitutions) is necessary, but a lack of progress or poor stabilization endurance is obvious to the trained eye.

In many sports and work-related activities, the upper extremity is used to increase the body's torque, but the true generator of speed and power is the trunk or lower extremities. Therefore abdominal and core stabilization programs are important aspects of rehabilitation and vital to the long-term resolution of upper extremity pain. Core strengthening also helps protect the upper extremity from torque generated from throwing or overhead serving motions.

Lower extremity function must play an integral part of any upper extremity rehabilitation program that requires repetitive use in standing or other weight-bearing positions. Sahrmann has proposed a movement system impairment (MSI) methodology for the evaluation and treatment of upper extremity dysfunction. Tests for faulty movement patterns are used as corrective exercises and modified as needed to correct muscle imbalance and faulty (compensatory) muscle recruitment. When performed correctly, the exercises can sometimes significantly decrease or even alleviate pain during the initial visit, which motivates the patient's compliance to the home program.[25]

Proprioceptive neuromuscular facilitation (PNF) exercises can be used for rehabilitation if cued and progressed correctly. Scapular PNF exercises are important for training the patient's kinesthetic awareness in dissociating scapular motion. When applying resistance to the upper extremity patterns, it is best to place manual resistance proximally (at the upper arm) to encourage core and scapular stabilization and minimize torque produced at the shoulder. Aquatic exercises can be effective when isokinetic resistance of water is appropriate.

CLINICAL PEARL

Why are closed chain exercises so beneficial in rehabilitating the shoulder?

Closed-chain exercises counterbalance the open-chain movement patterns that dominate human activities. In the shoulder, closed-chain shoulder exercises give the humeral head a posterior glide that helps the patient self-mobilize the posterior capsule. Weight-bearing through the upper extremity encourages the rotator cuff muscles and scapular stabilizers to fire simultaneously as the body weight is controlled (similar to stabilizing muscles used for balance in weight-bearing joints such as the hip and ankle). The wrist and finger flexors can also be stretched (in extension) or stabilization can be strengthened through neutral fists. Closed-chain exercises also integrate the use of the core muscles, which are important for generating or controlling forces through the upper extremity during sports with overhead or swinging motions.

Which muscles should be strengthened in treating patients with upper extremity pain?

Upper extremity pathology is highly variable, therefore, no one muscle group is consistently weak in all patients with upper extremity symptoms. In general, any exercise program should begin with building a solid base or foundation from which the upper extremity can function. Any weakness in the lower extremity or trunk should be addressed. Postural muscles always need some strengthening in the upper extremity patient. Core muscles including deep neck flexors (which are frequently lengthened and weak) should be strengthened. Scapulothoracic rhythm is important for normal upper extremity function. Scapular muscles are commonly out of balance, requiring strengthening of the lower and middle trapezius, and the serratus anterior to normalize the force couples involved in scapular external (upward) rotation. The corrected balance of the scapular stabilizers and rotators encourages normal use and conditioning of the rotator cuff muscles.[1]

In synergists, weakened stabilizing muscles often require strengthening because of dominant prime movers that need "down training." For example, the latissimus dorsi and pectoralis major muscles often become overly dominant as internal rotators of the glenohumeral joint. Because of their size and more distal attachment from the joint axis, they can be overrecruited without synergistic use of the rotator cuff muscles, especially the subscapularis. This dominance can also further weaken the opposing external rotation forces of the rotator cuff. Thus treating shoulder pain will always involve corrective exercises designed to restore the balance of the scapular muscle force couples.

In the shoulder, rotator cuff muscle strengthening programs are common. But equally important to the need for strength is the need for coordinated muscle recruitment. Base rotator cuff strength should be supplemented with shoulder motor control exercises. Reinhold et al studied seven common rotator cuff exercises and determined that sidelying external rotation placed the greatest demand on the infraspinatus and teres minor, while the greatest amount of activity of the supraspinatus, middle deltoid, and posterior deltoid was observed during prone horizontal abduction at 100 degrees with full external rotation.[22] Elbow and wrist pain is commonly caused or exacerbated by the naturally occurring imbalance of the flexor/extensor, and supinator/pronator muscle groups. Strengthening the muscles involved in overuse and repetitive strain injuries is necessary, especially to prevent further exacerbation of these joints.

CASE STUDY

(?)

Your patient is a right-hand dominant 45-year-old female sales representative and recreational climber for 12 years who reports a 1-year history of left medial elbow pain. The pain began insidiously, but she believes it was related to climbing, as this continues to aggravate her elbow. Shortly after the injury, she began to restrict her climbing, and she received physical therapy. This consisted of resting the elbow, some modalities, very little manual therapy, and exercises. The elbow did feel better after 8 weeks of treatment, but with progressive return to a moderate level of climbing, her pain returned. On questioning she mentions a history of a fractured left wrist some 8 years ago, for which she did not receive physical therapy after the cast was removed.

What are your hypotheses regarding the lack of long term improvement and what might you assess or treat differently?

Answer

The chronic nature of her injury, the presence of a previous wrist fracture, the number of years she has been climbing, and her age would indicate a likelihood of connective tissue scarring or thickening. At the elbow this is likely to be found at the sight of the common flexor tendon (tenoperiosteal junction). There may also be fascial restriction of the common aponeurosis originating at the medial epicondyle of the humerus. At the wrist, there is likely

to be significant soft tissue and joint restrictions with accompanying changes in the end-feel of her wrist/forearm motions. Manual therapy is beneficial for treating these types of restrictions and allows more effective stretching throughout the muscle and tendon. Most importantly, what do the patient's posture and upper extremity movement patterns reveal at the shoulder complex? It is likely that she will have poor proximal stabilization and muscle imbalance causing excessive indirect strain to the elbow, which is the next joint down along the kinetic chain. Likewise, any dysfunction at her wrist can push indirect strain up the chain.

How should a clinician decide which exercise is most appropriate for a patient with upper extremity pain?

Exercise choice should be individually driven. If a patient is unable to demonstrate proper form with a strengthening exercise, the exercise should be made easier or other alternative exercises should be considered. Loss of form or posture is the body's way of compensating for weakness or imbalances. The clinician needs to be wary of what motions or planes of motion are either pain-producing or contraindicated (as with instability or the postsurgical patient). Appropriate exercises may not initially involve the painful joint. An exercise should be deemed inappropriate if it is painful or the patient is unable to demonstrate proper or safe technique or is unable to understand or execute the motor commands.

How should a clinician progress an exercise program for the upper extremity?

Exercises for the acute injury site are generally progressed along a continuum of forces applied to the joint. Common progression is from isometric exercises to isotonic exercises to concentric exercises to eccentric exercises and finally, plyometric exercises. In general, an exercise program can be progressed by increasing the amount of resistance, by increasing the size of the lever arm, or by changing the patient's position (i.e., gravity-assisted or against gravity). Increasing the number of repetitions, the intensity, the speed, or the duration of an exercise can also be used to progress a given exercise. Shoulder strengthening should begin with scapular strengthening and restoration of muscle balance, as well as proper rotator cuff recruitment and strengthening. In the very painful shoulder the patient may need to be positioned in a sidelying position to minimize the torque of gravity and to facilitate basic scapular adduction, depression, elevation, or external (upward) rotation. This can be progressed to prone positions, then upright positions using the wall for assisting the weight of the upper extremity while the scapular muscles are being trained.

Correct rotator cuff recruitment is an essential prerequisite to any shoulder strengthening program. Without this, substitution patterns and muscle dominance patterns will persist and typically end up exacerbating shoulder pain. Begin by instructing the patient in how to perform glenohumeral rotation on a "constant" axis. (This exercise can also be used as a movement test in evaluation). For example, the patient is supine with the humerus propped on a towel roll in glenohumeral joint neutral and aligned in the scapular plane; the patient should be able to perform about 0 to 30 or 40 degrees of internal and external rotation while maintaining scapular stabilization and without excursion of the distal humerus from its starting position on the towel roll. Theoretically, rotation on a constant axis suggests that the rotator cuff is recruited because of the proximal attachment of these muscles onto the humeral head (versus the more distal attachment of the pectoralis major, latissimus dorsi, teres major). Resistance can be added as long as form is maintained. Progress by positioning into more abducted positions within the scapular plane.

During this type of reeducation exercise, the clinician should gently palpate anteriorly over the glenohumeral joint to assess the quality of motion of the humeral head, as well as observe for appropriate scapular control. If there is much debilitation or active motion is contraindicated, resistance for exercises should begin isometrically through different ranges of muscle length with resistance given manually or from a stable object such as a wall. Manual resistance allows effective progression using isometric, eccentric, concentric, or plyometric resistance since the clinician can get palpable feedback, and resistance can be varied as needed through the patient's ROM.

After manual resistance, exercises can be progressed using Thera-Band, body weight, hand-held weights, and strengthening machines. Closed-chain exercises should be progressed by increasing body weight resistance (by changing position or lever arm) or changing to unilateral upper extremity weight bearing. In a study by Uhl et al, electromyogram (EMG) analysis was used to study the recruitment of shoulder muscles during seven closed-chain upper extremity positions. They found that each position altered the muscle demands placed on different muscles of the shoulder. The implication of this research is that variations of closed-chain upper extremity exercises can be used to strengthen and improve motor control of various muscles of the shoulder and upper extremity.[30] Exercise progression should also integrate gross movement patterns and incorporate sport- or work-specific motions. Sport- and work-specific strengthening should also incorporate sports or work equipment (as feasible) with a progression of speed, repetition, duration, and force.

How does a clinician know If a patient with upper extremity pain is ready to progress to a new exercise?

Most importantly, there must be demonstration of proximal control at the scapula and the trunk with use of the upper extremity. Progression should not elicit the patient's pain and should not bring on more than 24 hours of postexercise muscle soreness. When the exercise has been mastered, with more than the appropriate repetitions, or longer duration, the patient may be progressed. The patient's subjective report that an exercise is no longer challenging or fatiguing should always prompt the clinician to recheck the exercise. The exercise may indeed need to be advanced or the patient may be performing the exercise incorrectly and therefore not gaining any benefit from the incorrectly performed exercise. This is common when the patient has poor kinesthetic awareness of weak or underrecruited muscles.

MODALITIES

Which modalities have proven most successful in treating patients with upper extremity pain?

In general, the use of modalities for treatment of upper extremity pain has not been widely studied. Systematic research studies conclude that there is insufficient evidence to support or oppose its use in patient treatments. Some research has shown ultrasound/phonophoresis and radio shock waves to be effective for pain relief of calcific tendinitis of the shoulder, and ultrasound has weak evidential support for its use in generalized shoulder pain. [5,8,20,29,38]

Clinically, ultrasound (or other forms of heat) can be effective for warming tissues before manual therapy, or used on a pulsed setting, it can be helpful for effusion. Ice/cold packs, especially as part of the home program, is very effective treatment for inflammation and pain, especially for the shoulder. On the elbow region, placement of ice should be monitored so as not to irritate more superficial nerves (e.g., ulnar nerve). Kinesiotape, if applied correctly, is very effective for reducing effusion and edema through its lymph-stimulating properties. It is also effective for reducing pain or tenderness of soft tissues and can be used to improve tolerance for manual therapy. Electrical stimulation is sometimes effective for reduction muscle spasm, swelling, or pain in the acute injury or in the stroke patient.

What is the role of bracing or taping in treating patients with upper extremity pain?

Bracing is most often a part of the postoperative protocol with surgeries of the upper extremity. Bracing may be initially required 24 hours a day but may usually be removed for treatment. The clinician needs to be familiar with the surgeon's protocol, as well as with the process and stages of healing. Bracing and splinting are used to protect healing tissues by limiting ROM and helping the formation of collagen crosslinks. Bracing and taping are sometimes useful during sports and other activities for the patient with an unstable joint (usually the shoulder). With accurate application, Kinesiotape can be used as a pain-relieving modality on any soft tissue of the upper extremity by decreasing swelling, bruising, or tenderness.

With accurate application Leukotape and/or Kinesiotape can offer pain relief by unloading soft tissues, including muscles, tendons, ligaments, fascia, and nerves. Kinesiotape and Leukotape can be especially effective in facilitating or inhibiting recruitment of muscles of the shoulder complex. Improved muscle balance decreases pain and helps increase kinesthetic awareness of movement patterns. Always inquire about tape allergies before using tape and educate the patient or caretaker in proper application and removal of the tape. Monitor the patient's skin and symptoms for any negative reactions.

What is the role of treatment aimed at neurodynamics in treating patients with upper extremity pain?

Compression, adhesion, or excessive deformation of cervical spine intervertebral discs and nerve roots are common sources of upper extremity pain so co-treatment is often necessary in this region. Wright et al completed a cadaveric study that examined the movement and excursion of the ulnar nerve at the elbow and wrist during upper extremity motion. They discovered that when all the motions of the wrist, fingers, elbow, and shoulder were combined, 21.9 mm of ulnar nerve excursion was required at the elbow and 23.2 mm at the wrist. They further hypothesized that any factor that limits excursion at these sites could result in repetitive traction of the nerve and possibly play a role in the pathophysiology of cubital tunnel syndrome or ulnar neuropathy at Guyon's canal.[36]

Entrapment and adhesion of peripheral nerves are a common source of upper extremity pain so upper limb tension tests are indicated, but care should be taken not to inflame the patient's symptoms. Mobilization of peripheral nerves can help improve glide of the nerve along soft tissues but should be done very gently and is contraindicated in the acute injury. Mobilization of peripheral nerves is best tolerated if preceded by manual therapy aimed at freeing the nerve from its site of entrapment.

Which home exercises are the most beneficial to give patients with upper extremity pain?

- Exercises that can be incorporated into activities of daily living and busy schedules
- Exercises that bring pain relief by correcting faulty postures or movement patterns
- Exercises that require minimal (and inexpensive) equipment. Simple items, such as Thera-Band, towels and straps (such as a belt or old tie), canned goods, phone books or a step stool, or an exercise ball, are easily accessible exercise aides
- Exercises that require no equipment and can be progressed by increasing body weight loaded through the upper extremity
- Closed-chain exercises also require minimal, if any, exercise equipment using mainly the patient's body weight. This makes feedback about progress during closed-chain exercise usually

TABLE IV-5-2   Tissue Injury and Intervention Choice

What are the best interventions for the acute phase (0-14 days postinjury)?	When to progress to next phase	What are the best interventions for the reparative phase? (15-21 days postinjury)?	When to progress to next phase	What are the best interventions for the remodeling phase? (22-60 days postinjury)?	When to progress to next phase	What are the best interventions for the maturation phase? (60-360 days postinjury)?	When to progress to next phase
Muscle Strain							
Patient education; modalities; taping; rest; splint/brace; manual therapy; PROM/AROM isometrics; exercise uninvolved areas; HEP	No pain at rest	Patient education; modalities; taping; manual therapy; AAROM/AROM; low-level, closed chain exercise, pain-free isotonic exercise; exercise uninvolved areas; HEP	Able to use arm for most daily activities	Patient education; modalities; taping; manual therapy; pain-free resistive exercises; exercise uninvolved areas; HEP	Full ROM and pain-free muscle contraction	Patient education; manual therapy; pain-free resistive exercise; integrated movement patterns; work/sport specific; HEP	No exacerbation of symptom strength; function restored; goals met
Ligament Sprain							
Patient education; modalities; taping; splint/brace; manual therapy; PROM/AROM isometrics, exercise uninvolved areas; HEP	No pain at rest	Patient education; modalities; taping; manual therapy; AAROM/AROM; low-level closed-chain exercise, pain-free isotonic exercise; exercise uninvolved areas; HEP	Able to use arm for most daily activities	Patient education; modalities; taping; manual therapy; pain-free resistive exercises; exercise uninvolved areas; HEP	Full and pain free range of motion	Patient education; manual therapy; pain-free resistive exercises; integrated movement patterns; work/sport specific; brace for sport/work; HEP	No exacerbation of symptom strength; function restored; goals met
Tendon Pathology							
Patient education; modalities; taping; rest, splint/brace; manual therapy; PROM, isometrics, exercise uninvolved areas; HEP	No pain at rest	Patient education; modalities; taping; manual therapy; AAROM/AROM; low-level closed-chain exercises, pain-free isotonic exercises; exercise uninvolved areas; HEP	Able to use arm for most daily activities	Patient education; modalities; taping; manual therapy; pain-free resistive exercise; exercise uninvolved areas; HEP	Full ROM and pain-free muscle contraction	Patient education; manual therapy; pain-free resistive exercises; integrated movement patterns; work/sport specific; HEP	No exacerbation of symptom strength; function restored; goals met
Bone Fracture							
Patient education; modalities; excluding US; immobilize; manual therapy; isometrics, exercise uninvolved areas; HEP	X-ray evidence of callus formation	Patient education; modalities; taping; manual therapy; maybe low-level closed chain exercises, exercise uninvolved areas; HEP	No pain noted at rest	Patient education; postimmobilization modalities; taping; manual therapy; PROM/AROM; isometrics, exercise uninvolved areas; HEP	X-ray evidence of fracture site union No pain with functional motions	Patient education; modalities; taping; manual therapy; pain-free resistive exercise; integrated movement patterns; HEP	No exacerbation of symptom strength; function restored; goals met

Cartilage Damage Patient education; modalities; rest; avoid joint compression; splint/brace; manual therapy; PROM, isometrics; exercise uninvolved areas; HEP	No pain at rest	Patient education; modalities; Able to use arm taping; avoid joint compression; manual therapy; AAROM/AROM; pain-free isotonic exercise; exercise uninvolved areas; HEP	Able to use arm for most daily activities	Patient education; modalities;Pain-free ROM taping; manual therapy; pain-free resistive exercise; exercise uninvolved areas; HEP	Pain-free ROM	Patient education; manual therapy; pain-free resistive exercise; integrated movement patterns; work/sport specific; HEP	No exacerbation of symptom strength; function restored; goals met
Capsule Injury Patient education; modalities; rest; manual therapy; PROM isometrics, exercise uninvolved areas; HEP	No pain at rest	Patient education; modalities; taping; manual therapy; AAROM/AROM; low-level closed-chain exercise; gentle isotonic exercise; exercise uninvolved areas; HEP	Able to use arm for most daily activities	Patient education; modalities; taping; manual therapy; pain-free resistive exercise; exercise uninvolved areas; HEP	Full and pain-free ROM	Patient education; manual therapy; pain-free resistive exercise; integrated movement patterns; work/sport specific; HEP	No exacerbation of symptom strength; function restored; goals met
Nerve Injury Patient education; modalities (heat better than ice); taping; rest splint/brace; manual therapy, PROM/AROM; isometrics, exercise uninvolved areas; HEP	No pain at rest	Patient education; modalities; taping; manual therapy;AAROM/ AROM; low-level closed-chain exercise; pain-free isotonic exercise; exercise uninvolved areas; HEP	Able to use arm for most daily activities	Patient education; modalities; taping; manual therapy; pain-free resistive exercise; exercise uninvolved areas; HEP	Full and pain-free ROM	Patient education; manual therapy-nerve mobs; pain-free resistive exercises; integrated movement patterns; work/sport specific; HEP	No exacerbation; ↑ strength; function restored; goals met

AAROM, ctive assisted range of motion; *AROM*, active range of motion; *HEP*, home exercise program; *PROM*, passive range of motion; *ROM*, range of motion.

Section IV

REHABILITATION AND COMMON CLINICAL QUESTIONS

self-evident to the patient. In a competitive athlete, this can motivate home program compliance, especially if the patient is surprised at his or her own lack of closed-chain strength.

- Exercises that the patient can perform independently or with minimal supervision from a close friend or relative.
- A prescription of no more than four or five exercises tends to give greater compliance.

How should a clinician decide which intervention is most appropriate for a patient with upper extremity pain?

Dysfunction of the upper extremity can be grossly generalized into deficits of stability, mobility, or both. Most manual therapy interventions are directed to patients with mobility issues such as adhesive capsulitis or elbow contractures. Because the upper extremity is significantly influenced by muscle coordination and timing, often a clinician will need to use manual techniques, such as myofascial release and massage, to decrease the activity of overactive muscles so that proper muscle activation can be reintroduced. The patient's inability to correct a faulty movement pattern secondary to pain or soft tissue restrictions (e.g., shortened muscle that has lost sarcomeres and formed excessive crosslinks or scar tissue proliferation) indicates the need for soft tissue mobilization techniques to speed these corrections.

Joint mobilization should be used if joint hypomobility is affecting and preventing normal joint mechanics. Mobilization can also be employed if circulation or pain abatement are the goals of the intervention. Exercises should be directed at increasing mobility if the motion restrictions are present. If stability is the issue, then exercises can be directed toward improving joint stability. If motor control is impaired, exercises should be directed toward improving neuromuscular control and timing between glenohumeral and scapulothoracic muscles. Treatment selection will be driven by patient irritability. Less aggressive interventions should be employed on highly irritable patients and more aggressive techniques on less irritable patients. Research on efficacy of interventions should always influence the clinician's choices. Factors to consider include age, tissue integrity, pain tolerance/emotional state, past and current medical history including response to prior treatments, acute/chronic nature or stage of tissue healing, and time allotted to the clinician for treatment. Ongoing objective and subjective reassessment of the patient's signs and symptoms will indicate if the intervention is effective or whether a different intervention would be more beneficial.

What red flags should a clinician be aware of regarding rehabilitating a patient with upper extremity pain?

Medical background as per initial evaluation and medical history reported should alert the clinician of potential problems and precautions to take. Constant unremitting pain coupled with unexplained weight loss may indicate tumors. Pancoast tumors of the lungs may refer pain into the upper extremity. Cardiac dysfunction may present as left upper extremity pain. Symptoms, such as chest pain, left upper extremity pain, fatigue, and shortness of breath, may indicate cardiac pathology. Pulmonary pathology may radiate into either upper extremity. Pathology is usually accompanied by pain or difficulty with breathing. Liver and gall bladder pathology can present as right upper extremity pain. These pathologies are usually accompanied by alteration in digestion, fatigue, pain, or discomfort after eating, especially fatty food. Skin rashes or discoloration may also be present. If a patient's symptoms are worsening with treatment or are described as persisting, constant pain even while at rest, the patient should be referred back to the physician for further testing.

SUMMARY STATEMENT

Rehabilitation of the upper extremity patient should always begin with a thorough evaluation guided by the detailed subjective history obtained from the patient. During the evaluation the patient should be educated on the findings and how they contribute to his or her symptoms. Based on these findings, the clinician decides the course of treatment, the prognosis for the patient, and then reasonable goals are agreed on (Table IV-5-2).

Patient education regarding objective findings, treatment plan, and prevention of further injury, as well as the patient's active role in rehabilitation, is important in successful outcomes. Correction of faulty postures and movement patterns of the entire upper quarter, especially about the shoulder and scapular regions, is necessary, regardless of which region of the upper extremity is injured.

Manual therapy and modalities can be effective co-interventions. Choice of these interventions should be influenced by evidence-based findings, but lack of evidence does not deem interventions ineffective. Further studies need to be conducted regarding rehabilitation of the upper extremity.

REFERENCES

1. Babyar SR. Excessive scapular motion in individuals recovering from painful and stiff shoulders: causes and treatment strategies. *Phys Ther.* 1996;76:226-238.
2. Berlund K, Persson B, Denison E. Prevalence of pain and dysfunction in the cervical and thoracic spine in persons with and without lateral elbow pain. *Man Ther.* 13(4):295-299.
3. Bergman GJ, Winters JC, Groenier KH, De Jong BM, Postema K, Van der Heijden GJ. Manipulative therapy in addition to usual medical care for patients with shoulder dysfunction and pain. *Ann Intern Med.* 2004;141:432-439.
4. Boyles RE, Ritland BM, Miracle BM, Barclay DM, Faul MS, Moore JH et al. (in press). The short-term effects of thoracic spine thrust manipulation on patients with shoulder impingement syndrome. *Man Ther.*
5. Ciccone CD. Does acetic acid iontophoresis accelerate the resorption of calcium deposits in calcific tendinitis of the shoulder? *Phys Ther.* 2003;83:68-74.
6. DiFabio RP. Efficacy of manual therapy. *Phys Ther.* 1992;72:853-864.
7. Donatelli R, Wooden MJ. *Orthopaedic Physical Therapy.* Churchill Livingstone; 1989.
8. Ebenbichler GR, Erdogmus CB, Resch KL, et al. Ultrasound therapy for calcific tendinitis of the shoulder. *N Engl J Med.* 1999;340:1533-1538.
9. Fernandez-Carnero J, Fernandez de las Penas C, Cleland J. Immediate hypoalgesic and motor effects after a single cervical spine manipulation in subjects with lateral epicondylalgia. *J Manipulative Physiol Ther.* 2007;31(9):675-681.
10. Ginn KA, Herbert RD, Khouw W, Lee R. A randomized, controlled clinical trial of a treatment for shoulder pain. *Phys Ther.* 1997;77: 802-811.
11. Hertling D, Kessler RM. *Management of Common Musculoskeletal Disorders.* J.B. Lippincott Company; 1990.
12. Kaltenborn FM. *Manual Mobilization of the Extremity Joints.* OPTP; 1989.
13. Kellgren J. Observations of referred pain arising from muscle. *Clin Sci.* 1938;3:175.
14. Kellgren J. On the distribution of pain arising from deep somatic structures with charts of segmental pain areas. *Clin Sci.* 1939;4:35
15. Kendall FP, McCreary EK, Provance PG. *Muscles Testing and Function.* Williams & Wilkins; 1993.
16. Kennedy CA, Manno M, Hogg-Johnson, et al. Prognosis in soft tissue disorders of the shoulder: predicting both change in disability and level of disability after treatment. *Phys Ther.* 2006;86:1013-1032.
17. Kuijpers T, van der Windt DA, Boeke AJ, et al. Clinical prediction rules for the prognosis of shoulder pain in general practice. *Pain.* 2006;120(3):276-285.

18. Palastanga N, Field D, Soames R. *Anatomy and Human Movement.* Butterworth-Heinemann; 2002.

19. Paungmali A. Hypoalgesic and sympathoexcitatory effects of mobilization with movement for lateral epicondylalgia. *Phys Ther.* 2003;83:374-383.

20. Perron M, Malouin F. Acetic acid iontophoresis and ultrasound for the treatment of calcifying tendinitis of the shoulder: a randomized control trial. *Arch Phys Med Rehabil.* 1997;78:379-384.

21. Philadelphia panel evidence-based clinical practice guidelines on selected rehabilitation interventions for shoulder pain. *Phys Ther.* 2001;81:1719-1730.

22. Reinold MM, Wilk KE, Fleisig GS, et al. Electromyographic analysis of the rotator cuff and deltoid musculature during common shoulder external rotation exercises. *JOSPT.* 2004;34(7):385-394.

23. Roddey TS, Olson SL, Cook KF, et al. Comparison of the University of California-Los Angeles shoulder scale and the simple shoulder test with the shoulder pain and disability index: single-administration reliability and validity. *Phys Ther.* 2000;80:759-768.

24. Sprague RB. The acute cervical joint lock. *Phys Ther.* 1983;63:1439-1444.

25. Sahrmann S. *Diagnosis of Treatment of Movement Impairment Syndromes.* Elsevier Health Sciences; 2001.

26. Schultz RL, Feitis R. *Endless Webb.* North Atlantic Books; 1996.

27. Struijs AA, et al. Manipulation of the wrist for management of lateral epicondylitis: a randomized pilot study, *Phys Ther.* 2003;83:608-616.

28. Tsao JS. Effectiveness of massage therapy for chronic, non-malignant pain: a Review. Evid based complement. *Alternat Med.* 2007;4(2):165-179.

29. Tygiel PP. On "Does acetic acid iontophoresis accelerate the resorption of calcium deposits in calcific tendinitis of the shoulder?" *Phys Ther.* 2003;83:667-670.

30. Uhl T, Carver TJ, Mattacola CG, Mair SD, Nitz AJ. Shoulder musculature activation during upper extremity weight-bearing exercise. *J Orthop Sports Phys Ther.* 2003;33(3):109-117.

31. Upledger JE, Vredeboogd JD. *Craniosacral Therapy.* Eastland Press, Inc.; 1983.

32. van den Dolder PA, Roberts DL. A trial into the effectiveness of soft tissue massage in the treatment of shoulder pain. *Aust J Physiother.* 2003;49(3):183-188.

33. Vicenzino B, Smith D, Cleland J, Bisset L. Development of a clinical prediction rule to identify initial responders to mobilisation with movement and exercise for lateral epicondylalgia. *Man Ther.* 2008; in press.

34. Waugh EJ, Jaglal SB, Davis AM, Tomlinson G, Verrier MC. Factors associated with prognosis of lateral epicondylitis after 8 weeks of physical therapy. *Arch Phys Med Rehabil.* 2004;85:308-318.

35. Whitman JM, Fritz JM, Boyles RE. Is there evidence that performing joint manipulation under local anesthetic block might be more effective than continuing a program of joint mobilization, stretching, and mobility exercises in a woman with recalcitrant adhesive capsulitis of the shoulder? *Phys Ther.* 2003;83:486-496.

36. Wright T, Glowczewskie F, Cowin D, Wheeler D. Ulnar nerve excursion and strain at the elbow and wrist associated with upper extremity motion. *J Hand Surg [Am].* 26(4):655-662.

37. Yang J, Chang C, Chen S, et al. Mobilization techniques in subjects with frozen shoulder syndrome: randomized multiple-treatment trial. *Phys Ther.* 2007;87:1307-1315.

38. Yesim KG, Yasemin U, Bilgic A, et al. Adding ultrasound in the management of soft tissue disorders of the shoulder: a randomized placebo-controlled trial. *Phys Ther.* 2004;84:336-343.

AUTHORS: KEITH MAHLER and JACKLYN H. BRECHTER

INTRODUCTORY INFORMATION i

The lower extremities function as the interface between the ground and the rest of the body. They are responsible for propulsion; positioning the head, arms, and trunk; and shock absorption. Mostly, the lower extremities function in a closed-chain manner and are under weight-bearing forces that frequently exceed a person's body weight. When the lower extremity is injured, patients use compensatory strategies to maintain function. These compensatory strategies place increased stress on other joints in the kinetic chain, even up into the trunk. Frequently, a patient's dysfunction is the result of these compensatory motions.[27]

What factors should you consider when rehabilitating lower extremity dysfunctions?

Mostly, the lower extremities function in a load-bearing, closed-chain manner with forces that range from 1.3 to 5.8 times a person's body weight.[35] These forces can cause compensatory motions, placing abnormal stress on other structures in the kinetic chain and thus causing tissue failure.

A patient's age, gender, static and dynamic postures, biomechanics, morphology, strength-to-weight ratio, and systemic factors all must be considered. Patients who seek care rarely have a dysfunction without multiple contributing factors. Clinicians therefore need to examine the entire lower extremity when there is damage to a single joint.

How do these factors affect the rehabilitation process?

Abnormal stresses on the lower extremities cause tissue failure to exceed the body's rate of repair. Clinicians must seek to limit the stress on the affected tissue, allowing for optimal repair. Traditional examples include use of assistive devices, such as canes, crutches, and walkers. Other strategies may include adding cushions in shoes to dissipate shock from ground reaction forces, limit multiplanar motions during an activity (including with tape or bracing), limit dysfunctional postures, and improve motor control and strength. Some patients may need to avoid certain activities for a time as the involved tissue heals.

Older individuals can have decreased healing time, altered gait, decreased strength/endurance, decreased tendon and ligamentous extensibility, and decreased neural response related to spatial awareness and joint proprioception. These factors can increase the rehabilitation time and will tend to alter the clinician's choice of intervention.

At the microscopic level, aging causes changes in cartilage or subchondral bone and decreased fluid retention in tendons and ligaments, all resulting in increased tissue stress. These microlevel changes can cause tissue failure at the site, as well as increase stress on proximal and distal joints. For example, a reduced fat pad on the calcaneus causes increased joint reaction forces up the kinetic chain. In addition, cartilaginous changes, including decreased glycosaminoglycan (GAG) binding, decreased fluid retention in matrix, and subchondral stiffening, decrease the lower extremities' ability to dissipate force.[42a]

Younger individuals may require consideration of issues with bone formation, strength-to-weight ratios, and structural changes. As the long bones are still growing, the clinician needs to consider the effect of the injury on the bones, as well as other tissue. The growth may be what is causing the injury. Furthermore, the exercise selection during rehabilitation should keep in mind the developing state of the musculoskeletal structure. Many parents are pushing children into competitive sports at earlier ages. The clinician should be firm and articulate to educate parents on the results of this excessive stress on the growing bodies.

Females demonstrate a significantly higher incidence of knee injuries. Research points to structural differences such as increased Q angle, decreased strength-to-weight ratios, pelvic position, and increased incidence of genu recurvatum as possible causes for the increased injury rates. Recent evidence links hormonal changes to cruciate ligament damage. This evidence means that clinicians should include some structural measures and cycle information as part of the examination of the female patient.

Patients with systemic dysfunction can experience limited tissue repair. These systemic dysfunctions may instead be the cause of tissue failure as well. Patients with diabetes have decreased healing time secondary to the body's decreased ability to supply oxygen to the tissues and decreased afferent input and efferent response.

Patients with autoimmune disorders, such as rheumatoid arthritis (RA) and lupus, can present with multiple joint involvement and decreased ability to participate in regular exercise. Identification of the autoimmune disorder is critical if not already done. If identified, then the rehabilitation process for those with such an autoimmune disorder should be specific to the resulting presentation while respecting the limitations of the disorder.

What role does acuteness versus chronic injury play in rehabilitation in a patient with lower extremity dysfunction?

Acute injury treatment must first focus on decreasing the inflammation and removing the source of the lesion. Strategies for managing the inflammatory process include removing local swelling with the use of modalities, relative rest to the area, and the maintenance of pain-free passive and active range of motion (ROM). Rest, ice, compression, and elevation (RICE) have been beneficial in decreasing local swelling. Care must be taken, however, when using compression. If the swelling is intraarticular, compression of the affected joint is minimally beneficial and may even be detrimental. Compression at the knee can limit range of motion and irritate extra-articular structures such as bursa along the iliotibial track and hamstrings. A trial of compression may usually be indicated, with individual response guiding the decision-making.

During this inflammatory phase, manual therapy techniques also may be used. These should focus on decreasing pain and inflammation, as well as maintaining ROM. Stretching is appropriate in patients demonstrating onset of resistance before onset of pain during ROM testing. With regards to strength, it is the recruitment and motor control that are far more important at this phase than the actual strength. The clinician should remember that pain is inhibitory to muscle function and joint swelling can also be inhibitory to muscle function.

Patient education is a critical component of rehabilitation during acute injuries. Patients should be made aware of their own dysfunction, as well as the biomechanical issues related to their particular situation. This patient awareness and understanding of how movements can impact the problem is one of the most important tools a therapist can use to promote a positive outcome. Patients will also benefit from education regarding the phase of healing they are experiencing and how they can help provide the optimal healing environment.

Chronic conditions require a closer look a patient's biomechanics. The therapist must identify compensatory motions either proximal or distal to the area of dysfunction that may contribute to the problem. Further systemic dysfunction must be considered as well. The goal and difficulty for the therapist treating patients with chronic conditions is to identify those factors that are placing excessive loads on the injured tissues. This is often accomplished through motion analysis and primary observation and confirmed through tests and measures during the objective examination.

What factors make treating patients with lower extremity dysfunctions challenging?

The lower extremities are subjected to constant repetitive high load on the joints. A patient's hip joint is subjected to nearly three times the compressive load at the hip during single-limb stance as opposed to double-limb stance. This is due to the increased abductor stabilization force produced to stabilize the contralateral hip. The knee and patellofemoral joints have the highest loads in the body and the thickest cartilage. The ankle and foot must take the initial impact of loading and absorb the shock or transmit the load up the chain. All of the lower extremity joints must be involved for any weight-bearing activity. Therefore the clinician must assess the concert of motions between the foot, ankle, knee, hip, and pelvis during dynamic tasks.

Deficits in strength and/or ROM in the lower extremities can cause issues proximal or distal to the affected joint. For example, patients with weak plantar flexors may demonstrate excessive dorsiflexion (DF) during loading in gait requiring excessive knee joint muscle activity for control and excessive internal rotation (IR) of the lower extremity as the end-range of DF is exceeded. Alternately, patients with inadequate DF may demonstrate rapid subtalar joint pronation during loading in gait, causing increased tibia and/or hip internal rotation (IR). Both of these problems and the resulting compensations can lead to abnormal loading at joints other than the one primarily involved and result in further complaints at secondary locations.

PROGNOSIS

How successful is rehabilitation in treating acute lower extremity pain?

Rehabilitation of patients with acute or subacute complaints in the lower extremity after first onset have the greatest chance for successful lower extremity rehabilitation. Patients with advanced age, obesity, or significant lower extremity mechanical alignment deviations from normal (among other factors) will have a reduced prognosis than those patients who are younger and fit and have small or no mechanical alignment deviations.

How successful is rehabilitation in treating chronic lower extremity dysfunction?

Treatment of lower extremity complaints can be very successful, even with chronic complaints, providing the clinician can identify the factors that contribute to the complaint. Furthermore, those factors that clinicians identify need to be treatable as opposed to bony or other permanent malalignments. Most often, the chronic complaint has been inadequately treated in the past or some associated factor has not been addressed. As such, patients with chronic complaints that have not responded to rehabilitation should be reexamined (or sent for consult) or the plan should be revised. Factors to consider in this reexamination or revision of treatment intervention include the following:

- Referral from other sources (neurodynamic influence, low back pain)
- Associated factors such as lower extremity postural alignment (rear foot pronation, hip muscle weakness, etc.)
- Activities of daily living (ADLs) required by the patient
- Is successful unloading of the joint occurring in a fashion that is sufficient to allow tissue healing?

Which patients with lower extremity pain derive the greatest long-term benefits from rehabilitation?

Patients without the goal of significantly high levels of weight-bearing exercises (marathoners, triathletes, etc) derive the greatest long-term benefits from rehabilitation. To achieve optimal outcomes with patients requires careful thought and planning.

The job of a clinician is to restore mobility and function, prevent further deterioration, provide an optimal healing environment, and enhance performance. Treatment should encompass as many of these categories as possible to achieve a good prognosis. The following list of questions should be asked to maximize treatment.

- What region is affected? Is the pain coming from that site or is it referred?
- Does the patient have a history of lumbar, radiculopathy, or urogenital issues?
- Why is that region affected? Is the patient's tissue failure the result of systemic issues, biomechanical, traumatic, etc.?
- What are the contributing factors that lead to the patient's current condition?

Treatment must address ALL of these questions to achieve a successful outcome. In addition, weight is particularly important to rehabilitation of the lower extremities. Since the lower extremities are required to undergo loading in excess of body weight with every step during gait, prognosis is heavily associated with body weight.

What other regions of the body are most likely to contribute to lower extremity pain and dysfunction?

Lower extremity pain may be caused by referred pain from the lumbar spinal nerve roots or facets. Lower extremity complaints may also be either caused by or have contributions from the peripheral nerves (neurodynamic tension, peripheral neuropathy, etc.).

EVIDENCE-BASED MEDICINE

What trends are currently being seen in research regarding rehabilitation of patients with lower extremity pain?

Current trends in the literature indicate that researchers are examining treatment effects by gender or age characteristics.* It is heartening to see clinical efficacy studies for children and for female populations.

INTERVENTION

Therapists use many techniques to restore a patient's function. Manual therapy, strengthening stretching, neural mobilization, and modalities are very important tools used in the rehabilitation process. However, every treatment technique has limited benefit if the patient continues to place abnormal stress on the healing tissues. Patient education is one of the most important interventions a therapist can provide. The clinician's main job is to inform, instruct, and train. It is important to never underestimate a patient's capacity to learn even complex concepts such as biomechanics, the phase of healing, and the physiological rational for exercise. Furthermore, patients' compliance will be enhanced if they understand why they must perform home exercises and correct abnormal movement patterns.

What interventions have proven the most successful in treating patients with lower extremity dysfunction?

Although patient education can be one of the most beneficial interventions a therapist can use, patients may not progress without the addition of manual therapy. Restricted tissue and/or joints will require manual therapy to restore optimal performance. In general, manual therapy can be beneficial in controlling inflammation, restoring joint motion, and optimizing tissue function. Common techniques include soft tissue mobilization (STM), joint mobilization, manual stretching, and neural mobilization.

*References 10-12, 22, 24, 25, 28, 29, 46, 47, 51, 56, 58, 61.

What is the physiological rationale behind the use of manual therapy in treating patients?

Manual therapy is used to relieve symptoms, increase mobility, and restore biomechanically correct functions. Joint mobilization techniques can be used to increase ROM and decrease painful motions. Grades I and II mobilizations are beneficial in treating painful and inflamed joints. Grades III and IV mobilizations can be used for improving the ROM in hypomobile joints. Grade V mobilizations can be used to restore motions in hypomobile joints, including those joints in which the patient cannot tolerant sustained or oscillatory grade III or IV mobilizations or when the joint has reached a plateau in treatment. Mobilization with movement is another useful technique for treating lower extremity complaints. For these techniques, the mobilization is accompanied by active motion to restore normal joint mobility. Joint mobilizations used for stretching are indicated when the ROM of the joint is limited with a capsular end-feel, or accessory motion testing indicates limited accessory glide in the joint.

Soft tissue techniques can be useful for restoring integrity of contractile tissues, decrease fascial restrictions, aid in stretching, and promote blood flow. Further manual stretching can be used to help restore length. Soft tissue techniques for improving ROM are especially useful when there is a muscular end-feel, and the clinician has identified focal restrictions in the muscle tissue. Manual or physiological stretching is indicated if there is a muscular end-feel causing motion restriction and there are no focal restrictions to the muscle tissue.

CLINICAL PEARL

How is the treatment intervention selected when ROM is limited? During ROM assessment, determine what structure feels like it is causing the motion restriction (end-feel). Alternately, additional testing for muscle length and accessory mobility can be completed. If the muscle is the limiting factor to ROM, then palpate the muscle for areas of tightness and focal restriction. If focal restrictions are present, treatment should begin with STM to the area of restriction. If focal restrictions are not present, treatment may commence with a physiological stretch or a muscle energy technique.

If the accessory mobility is limited a joint mobilization is indicated. Grades III and IV oscillatory techniques are used for stretch, or alternately, a grade V mobilization may be attempted (or may be used if progression from grades III and IV is not sufficient).[35a]

To change the impairment or complaint, the clinician's choice of treatment must reach the targeted tissue. To this end, trial treatments with subsequent reevaluation are helpful in determining the course of treatment. It is recommended that the clinician use an assess, treat, reassess philosophy to prove that the treatment is justified. With reassessment, a joint restriction may present with a different end-feel, making a new treatment choice ideal. Table IV-6-1 lists some common presentations for the lower extremity.

Is joint manipulation recommended for patients with lower extremity complaints?

Little research has been completed on the role of manipulation in rehabilitation of lower extremity complaints. However, what has been reported speaks favorably to the use of joint manipulation for the hip, knee, ankle, and cuboid.*

What does evidence reveal regarding the use of massage for the treatment of patients with lower extremity complaints?

Massage may be used as STM to improve focal limitations within the muscle. The use of STM has not been well-documented in the literature.†

Friction massage is another form of massage that is used to treat tendonitis injuries. Friction massage has some supporting evidence.[6,57]

Is stretching beneficial or indicated for patients with lower extremity complaints?

Stretching is well-documented for its beneficial effects on individual joint ROM and on functional activity. Stretching is being evaluated in the literature for its beneficial effects on injury prevention as well.‡

How should a clinician decide which manual therapy intervention is most appropriate for a patient with lower extremity pain?

In determining the appropriate manual therapy intervention, the clinician should use the results of tests and methods from the clinical examination. In particular, when ROM is limited, the clinician should determine what is the limiting factor. Using end-feel assessment is one method and using confirmatory tests is another. Confirmatory tests include muscle length assessments and accessory glide mobilizations.

When ROM is limited by muscle length, the clinician should palpate the muscle itself for focal areas of limitation. When such areas are found, the clinician should use STM to improve the tissue mechanics. Physiological stretching is then the treatment of choice to improve ROM. When ROM seems to be limited by the capsule or accessory mobility glides are limited, then the treatment of choice should be an accessory mobility glide. Accessory glides should be performed in the direction of the greatest mobility limitation. Table IV-6-1 indicates the normal direction of accessory glides for movement restrictions in the major joints of the lower extremity and can be used as a guide to selection of joint mobilization direction or direction of stretch.

THERAPEUTIC EXERCISE

Manual therapy techniques contribute to restoring ROM of a specific segment whether it is the main complaint or a contributing factor. However, they do not directly address muscular control or weakness that may result in suboptimal function. Therapeutic exercise is the treatment of choice to accomplish this change in muscular control or strength and can be of great benefit for lower extremity function.

What is the physiological rationale behind the use of exercise in treating patients with lower extremity complaints?

Muscles in the lower extremities contribute to a variety of functions. Muscles are responsible for maintaining static postures such as standing, they must produce motion, they work to attenuate force during loading, and they act to alter bone loading to avoid detrimental forces on the skeleton during function. For ideal performance, muscles must be able to contract in a variety of fashions, isometric and isotonic, fast and slow, and in a coordinated effort to allow force increments as needed. Muscles in the lower extremity also must be able to generate extreme forces sometimes quickly as during direction changes at high speed or in landing and taking off again from a rebound and subsequent shot. Muscular weakness in the lower extremities or inadequate muscle coordination or velocity of contraction may set the patient up

---

*References 5, 13, 14, 33, 40, 41, 43.

†References 6, 18, 20, 23, 26, 34, 39, 42, 44, 57, 62.
‡References 2, 16, 19, 31, 36, 38, 50, 60.

TABLE IV-6-1 Motion Restrictions Presentation

Motion Restrictions	Posture	Primary Observational Plane/ Compensation Motions	Functional Loss	Direction of Physiological Stretch/Muscle Limiting Motion	Direction of Joint Mobilization: Moving Bone If Capsule or Accessory Mobility Is Limited
Hip flexion	Reduction of lumbar lordosis	Sagittal plane: Early lumbar flexion during hip flexion tasks.	Early lumbar flexion with gait, sit to stand, and forward bending tasks	Stretch into hip flexion (knee flexed) / gluteal muscle limited	Anterior to posterior glide of femur on acetabulum
Hip extension	Increased anterior pelvic tilt, knee hyper extension, plantar flexed stance	Sagittal plane: Excessive lumbar extension during hip end-range extension tasks	Excessive lumbar extension with stance and gait, increased pelvic motions during gait	Stretch hip extension if psoas limited, knee flexion with hip extension if rectus femoris is limited	Posterior to anterior glide of femur on acetabulum
Hip internal rotation	Toe out stance and frequently hip abduction stance	Transverse plane: Lack of contralateral pelvic motion during gait	Decreased hip rotation in gait, wide based with sit to stand	Stretch into hip IR if external rotators are limited	Anterior to posterior glide of femur on acetabulum
Hip external rotation	Toe-in stance, squinting patella	Transverse plane: motions limited at hip	Decreased hip rotation in gait, knees together with sit to stand, may also see excess pronation.	Stretch into ER if internal rotators are limited	Posterior to anterior glide of femur on acetabulum
Treatment plane for the hip is the acetabulum.					
Knee flexion	Hyper extension (if motion loss extreme) else limited knee flexion during ADL's	Sagittal plane: Early lumbar and hip flexion Compensate with frontal plane motions like hip abduction	Stooping and squatting demonstrates staggered stance (affected leg forward), hip hike with step up	Stretch knee flexion if quadriceps are limited, knee flexion with hip extension if rectus femoris is limited	Anterior to posterior glide of tibia on femur
Knee extension	Sagittal plane: Flexed knee, ipsilateral foot pronation, contralateral supination, iliac crest height difference with compensatory lumbar side bend	Sagittal plane: compensation seen in frontal plane such as unequal hip height, trunk lean, contralateral abducted stance.	Decreased dorsiflexion in initial stance, decreased stance time on ipsilateral limb, trunk lean with sit to stand, contralateral hip hike with ascending stairs	Stretch knee extension, single joint knee flexor hypomobility or hip flexion with knee extension if Hamstrings are limited.	Posterior to anterior glide of tibia on femur
Treatment plane in the knee is the tibial plateau.					
Ankle dorsiflexion	Anterior pelvic tilt, knee hyper extension, decreased arch height	Sagittal plane: early heel off, excessive/early pronation, hip internal rotation (loading) then external rotation during swing	Early heel off in gait and squatting activities, excessive rearfoot pronation, hip internal rotation	Stretch into dorsiflexion (control subtalar joint mobility) with knee flexion if soleus is limited, knee extension with gastroc limited	Anterior to posterior glide of the Talus on the mortise.
Ankle plantar flexion	Flexed knee with posterior pelvic tilt	Sagittal plane: compensation knee flexion	Late heel off in gait, abducted stance with descending stairs.	Stretch into plantar flexion if pretibial muscles are limited	Posterior to anterior glide of the Talus on the mortise.
Ankle treatment plane is the mortise.					

ER, external rotation; *IR*, internal rotation.

for joint, bony, soft tissue, or muscular damage. Furthermore, the normal function of the muscle is compromised and may lead to compensatory motions.

During the examination, the functional demands of involved or related muscles must be assessed and the choice of therapeutic exercise must match the demands. Therapeutic exercise may be used to improve the muscular control, muscular coordination, and multisegment coordination or for actual strength or endurance, as well as to maintain or improve ROM as part of the rehabilitation process. The muscular control or coordination may be as or more important than the ultimate strength of the muscle. Restoration of muscle function is essential for avoidance of tissue damage and for return to activities. In the event that muscle function cannot be restored, patients should be taught compensatory actions and should develop the muscles required for those compensations.

Are exercise programs beneficial in treating patients with lower extremity complaints?

Every patient with a lower extremity complaint should be involved in some form of therapeutic exercise. If the involved lower extremity is unable to participate, then the contralateral limb and/or the torso and upper extremities should be involved in some general exercise to maintain or improve overall fitness as the involved joint recovers.

Which exercise programs are effective in treating patients with lower extremity complaints?

Therapeutic exercise intervention for patients with lower extremity complaints are varied and many. They include interventions that help with stretching, interventions with equipment such as may be found in a health club, or interventions that use Thera-band or Thera-tube for resistance, bodyweight for resistance, functional activities, Swiss ball or weighted-ball exercises with or without a rebounder, etc. Selection should be determined based on what the patient is already using as a work-out method, together with an examination of the current and desired levels of function of the patient. It is critical during the selection process of exercises for the lower extremity to address multiple dimensions of the muscular limitations, as opposed to selecting exercises that each accomplishes only one outcome.

CLINICAL PEARL

How can one exercise be used to affect multiple areas of muscle dysfunction in the lower extremity? Since the segments of the lower extremity are connected, what happens to one joint affects other joints. Abduction or external rotation (ER) of the hip places the knee in a more varus alignment. Supination of the foot may do the same via its effect on the tibia. Examining the exercise used for the following case study, the patient is abducting and externally rotating the thigh into the wall (loading the hip abductor muscle and external rotators). The stance limb is being stressed for increasing hip abduction, quadriceps strength, and foot musculature. Quad involvement may be increased by adding a partial squat as DF ROM increases.

CASE STUDY

Your patient is a 29-year-old female who reports right anterior knee pain during running (10 minutes). Onset was insidious but reached the 6/10 pain level last week. She reports being unable to run now and is complaining of pain with sustained sitting (after 10 minutes) and going downstairs (every step). Pain has been worsening over the past 5 weeks as she trains for a marathon. Normal or premorbid running mileage is 3 to 5 miles 3 to 4 times per week.

Objective findings include the following:
- Step down: Lack of hip control (IR/ER), pelvic drop, and excessive subtalar pronation, with reproduction of pain
- Vastus medialis oblique muscle is visibly atrophied.
- Hip: Postured in internal rotation right>left, foot in pronation on right
- ROM: Knee flexion lacks 20 degrees, prone knee bend reveals rectus tight with knee flexion of 45 degrees and reproduction of pain
- Thomas test: Hip 25 degrees F, knee −60 degrees, hip −15 degrees with knee extension
- Knee extension full with pain on overpressure
- Patella positioned laterally into glide and tilt
- Swelling observed around patella and knee joint.
- DF limited at −10 degrees with muscular end-feel, no change with knee flexion (soleus limit)
- Manual muscle test (MMT): Quads 4/5, hip abductor 3+/5, hip ER 3/5
- Pain to palpation retropatellar and lateral patellar border, lateral soleus thick and knotted with tenderness, rectus femoris thick and sore to palpation distal one-third.

Answer

This patient exhibits related findings at the foot/ankle, the knee, and the hip. In this case the author elected to treat with the following:
- Medial glides and medial tilts (grade IV × 4 at 40 seconds each), followed by reeducation using active assist contractions while maintaining the medial tilt and glide.
- DF was addressed beginning with STM to lateral soleus, followed by instruction in home exercise for soleus stretch (controlling for rearfoot position)
- Rectus femoris STM to distal one-third, followed by heel to bottom stretch (30 second × 4 with contract relax), followed by home exercise stretch.
- Patella taping was used and patient pain complaints were 0/10 during step down.
- Exercise was given using standing on contralateral limb with involved knee pressing into wall (ER and abduction) with patient maintaining control of stance foot. Exercise was repeated on the involved leg with the stance limb (involved) controlled for hip, knee, and foot position to restore lower extremity alignment.

Patient symptoms and findings were mainly resolved within 3 visits, and she returned to running.

Which muscles should be strengthened in treating patients with lower extremity complaints?

The clinician should determine the impact of the complaint on the musculature. Of primary importance to the lower extremity are the postural muscles or the antigravity muscles, including the gastrocsoleus, quadriceps, hip abductors, and extensors. However, any muscle, including the foot intrinsic muscles, may be targeted as part of the rehabilitation program. Muscle weakness or other deficits and frequently seen clinical findings that indicate that muscle involvement have been presented (Table IV-6-2).

How should a clinician decide which exercise is most appropriate for a patient with lower extremity complaints?

Early rehabilitation of muscles should focus on motor control through pain-free ranges beginning with isometric contractions and progressing to concentric motions. Eccentric motions should be limited until the patient is able to use 80% of the joint's ROM.[30] When beginning eccentric strengthening, a patient should begin with slower velocity activities (60 to 120 degrees per second is generally considered a safe velocity). As the patient achieves appropriate control, he or she can progress to full ROMs and functional activities, then increase the velocity of action during the

TABLE IV-6-2 Muscle Weakness Presentation

Affected Joint	Posture	Primary Observational Plane/ Compensation Motions	Functional Loss
Hip flexion weakness	Anterior pelvic tilt (limited length and/or weakness), posterior pelvic tilt	Sagittal plane: Excessive lumbopelvic motions	Decrease stride/velocity in gait, circumduction in swing phase, excessive pelvic motions
Hip extension weakness	Posterior pelvic tilt, with crouched stance, observed decreased gluteal mass	Sagittal/frontal: Limited hip extension with frontal plane hip hike to compensate	Stair ambulation, excessive trunk lean with sit to stand, excessive heel strike in terminal stance (weak hamstrings)
Hip internal rotation weakness	Toe-out stance	Frontal: With wide based tasks, hip external rotation with hip flexion	Toe-out gait with limited hip rotation,
Hip external rotation weakness	Toe-in stance	Frontal: Narrowed stance, hip internal rotation with hip flexion to extension	Gait demonstrates limited stance time with adduction in stance phase, knees touch with sit to stand.
Hip abduction weakness	Trunk shift toward ipsilateral side, wide base	Frontal: Trunk leans toward affected side	Gait demonstrates contralateral hip drop or trunk lean on stance leg. Hip adduction and internal rotation with sit to stand.
Knee flexion weakness	Hyper extension with anterior pelvic tilt	Sagittal plane: Rapid hyper extension knees with excessive pelvic motions	Gait demonstrates pronounced heel strike and rapid knee extension.
Knee extension weakness	Hyperextended in stance	Sagittal plane: Hyperextension in gait	Gait demonstrates limited loading response and limited control in preswing.
Ankle dorsiflexion weakness	Ankle plantar flexed	Sagittal plane: Foot drop during swing phase of gait	Increased hip flexion or toe dragging during swing phase of gait
Ankle plantar flexion weakness	Ankle plantar flexed due to decreased use	Sagittal plane: decreased dorsiflexion during terminal stance or knee hyper extension to compensate for lack of ankle dorsiflexion	Decreased stride length and shorter terminal stance phase of gait

functional activities. Competitive level of function is an extremely high level of function and clinicians should retrain for the competition and not just for the motions because competition will increase the magnitude and velocity of the muscle contraction.

In the lower extremity, the focus should be on exercises that use multiple joints in functional positions as appropriate for the level of the patient.

How should a clinician progress an exercise program for the lower extremity complaints?

Muscle impairments are frequently measured clinically with MMT. However, MMT does not have the sensitivity to differentiate subtle differences in muscle function. At the knee, a grade 5 MMT may be given when the actual muscle function is as little as 53% of the normal strength of the quadriceps muscle group. At the hip a grade 5 MMT may be given when the actual muscle is only 65% of normal.[45] Whereas MMTs are appropriate outcome measures, additional information should be gathered during the examination of patients with lower extremity complaints. Observation of functional tasks will be helpful in determining muscular deficits, as will endurance tests and outcome measures, including function, such as the knee walk test (self-paced), timed "up & go" test, 6-minute walk test,[54] hop test,[48] or self-report scales such as the Western Ontario and McMaster Universities Osteoarthritis Index (WOMAC),[54] the Patient Specific Functional Score (PSFS),[53] Oswestry Disability Index,[17] Lower Extremity Functional Scale (LEFS),[4] and others. It is important that function be documented at the onset of treatment so changes with intervention can be measured and monitored.

As the patient progresses with an exercise program, the clinician should initially monitor the patient frequently for changes in MMT grades or for observational indicators of quality in performance of the exercises. Progression should be rapid in these early phases as the patient becomes proficient in the activity. The exercise should always be performed correctly but should remain difficult for the patient. If the patient is unable to perform the exercise correctly, then either further explanation or instruction

is required, or alternately, another exercise should be selected. Once the patient is too comfortable with the exercise (exercise is too easy), then there is little further therapeutic benefit and the exercise should be progressed.

Functional or subjective outcome measures should be completed weekly or bi-weekly to indicate functional changes and help guide progression as well. Progression may be accomplished in a variety of methods, some options are as follows:
- Increase in the number of repetitions (or sets)
- Increase in the time of contraction for isometric activities (or exercises involving equipment like the body blade)
- Increase in the ROM of the action
- Increase in the amount of resistance (including depth in the water or resistance tools in the water)
- Increase in the velocity of the action
- Increase in the number of participating joints or the complexity of the activity (functional activities)
- Increase in the change in directions (adding cutting or increasing the competitive level of the activity)
- Addition of unstable surfaces on which to exercise, or other unexpected perturbations

The exercises for patients with lower extremity injury must be selected not only to appropriately prepare the musculature for activity but also to prepare the other tissues of the musculoskeletal system for the expected loads of the desired activities. For example, if the patient desires to return to pick-up basketball games 2 to 3 times per week, then the appropriate exercise selection should not be an aquatic exercise program. Although an aquatic program may restore strength and flexibility to the joint, it lacks the impact required to prepare the cartilage and bony tissue for the loads demanded during basketball. A general rule of thumb is to keep the exercise selection and progression as close to the desired activity as possible for optimal rehabilitation times. The exception to this is the patient who requires unloading of a tissue as part of the treatment progression. In these cases, where the activity desired is in excess of the capacity of the tissues, the therapist should modify the exercise program until the patient is successful (no increase in symptoms or swelling during or after the exercise activity). At this time, the exercise may be progressed back to the desired level of function.

Which modalities have proven most successful in treating patients with lower extremity complaints?

The lower extremity has been a frequent source of pathology for the study of treatment modalities. Modalities that are known to be beneficial in the rehabilitation of the lower extremity include heat, cold, electricity, biofeedback, taping, and others.

How should a clinician decide which modality is most appropriate for a patient with lower extremity complaints?

Cold or electrical therapy in various forms may be used to manage swelling or pain. Heat (hot packs, ultrasound, or general exercises) may be used to assist with tissue extensibility and avoidance of muscle strain or reduction of muscle spasm. Biofeedback may be used to retrain movement patterns. Taping may be used for stability, swelling control, tactile cues, assessment (i.e., for orthotic intervention), and unloading of painful structures.

What is the role of bracing or taping in treating patients with lower extremity complaints?

In general, joints that are presenting with excessive ROM may require some type of taping or bracing to improve stability. This assistance with stability may be temporary, as the joint recovers (as with knee braces and ankle braces with lateral stays) or it may be permanent as seen with orthotic intervention to control excessive subtalar joint mobility in some patients.

Taping for altering the pain presentation of the patellofemoral joint, for Achilles, plantar fascia, or patellar tendon unloading or for navicular lifts is frequently used, but this is not nearly an exhaustive list. Taping may use the McConnell techniques[1,9,37,49] or clinicians may use Kinesiotaping.[21,52,59]

Rehabilitation of the lower extremity may also be enhanced by the appropriate use of orthotic intervention. Current research supports the use of orthotics for altering lower extremity mechanics during interaction with the ground.*

What is the role of treatment aimed at neurodynamics in treating patients with lower extremity complaints?

Many pathologies in the lower extremity exist together with neurodynamic findings. In general, during an examination of patients with acute traumatic injuries of obvious origin, a neurodynamic examination in not required. However, a large number of patients indicate an insidious onset to the lower extremity complaint. In these patients, the affect of neurodynamic tension on the complaint should be determined. For those patients with chronic or repeat involvement, the neurodynamic component is more strongly suggested.

Regardless of the origin of the pathology, the clinician should be aware of the status of the neurodynamic tension in those with lower extremity complaints. The entire kinetic chain becomes involved when any portion of the chain experiences a problem. Over time, as with chronic conditions or with a plateau in treatment progression, the neurodynamic tension should be addressed and included in the treatment plan.

Which home exercises are the most beneficial to give patients with lower extremity complaints?

Clinicians should carefully select two or three exercises as a home program for patients with lower extremity complaints.

*References 3, 7, 8, 15, 32, 55.

These exercises should be adjusted on a regular basis according to the recovery process and healing timeline. Home exercises should be those that have been completed successfully in the clinic, yet are still difficult for the patient to perform. Examples of home exercises include those designed for muscle strengthening, for maintaining ROM, and for swelling management (as appropriate), or for breaking habitual postures that have been identified as detrimental. As the functional status of the patient increases, the home program should include a partial return to activity to see the affect of the target function on the complaint.

REHABILITATION CLINICAL REASONING

How should a clinician decide which intervention is most appropriate for a patient with lower extremity complaints?

Intervention is determined according to two factors. The clinician should initially determine *what* is causing the lower extremity complaint (what tissue is involved) and then determine *why* that tissue is involved. Intervention is then initially selected to unload the damaged tissue and then to selectively load the tissue in a fashion that continues to produce an increase in the tissue tolerance to load and to change the factors that contribute to the *why* of the involvement. Monitoring pain or swelling, as well as functional outcome measures, will provide the clinician with an understanding of whether the tissue is improving in its functional capacity. For example, when loading a tissue and pain is reproduced immediately, the clinician should understand that the load is excessive for the present status of the tissue capacity. If pain or swelling are onset latently, it is an indication that the capacity of the tissue has been exceeded or the number of repetitions is too great for the capacity. In this instance, the duration or magnitude of the load or treatment should be reduced but not eliminated. Similarly, with appropriately applied treatments, the functional outcome measures should indicate consistent increase in function. Tissue injury and the intervention of choice have been compiled for reference (Table IV-6-3). Please keep in mind that significant ligament or tendon ruptures will involve surgical intervention and are not represented on this table. After surgical repair, the patient may have a period of immobility required to prevent tearing of the repair, but otherwise, the treatment can progress as shown.

What red flags should a clinician be aware of regarding rehabilitating a patient with lower extremity complaints?

Clinicians treating patients with musculoskeletal complaints should be certain that those complaints are mechanical. Tests and measures of the musculoskeletal system should be conducted, and the results compiled to reveal such mechanical complaints. Complaints that are not reproduced by mechanical testing should be further examined for systemic or organic involvement. Patients with pathologies of this nature should be referred to the appropriate health care practitioner for further testing.

Patients with mechanical lower extremity complaints should also be monitored regularly for cardiopulmonary status. Heart rate and blood pressure should be assessed at base line and at regular intervals during the rehabilitation program. In patients with positive indicators of cardiac dysfunction or elevated blood pressure, the response to any exercise program must be determined and monitored. Should abnormal response to exercise be observed, the patient should be referred to his or her physician for management.

TABLE IV-6-3 Tissue Injury and Intervention Choice

What are the best interventions for the acute phase (0-14 days postinjury)?	When to progress to next phase	What are the best interventions for the reparative phase (15-21 days postinjury)?	When to progress to next phase	What are the best interventions for the remodeling phase (22-60 days postinjury)?	When to progress to next phase	What are the best interventions for the maturation phase (60-360 days postinjury)?	When to progress to next phase
Muscle strain							
Avoid contraction that causes complaints, static, or partial ROM contraction below the level of complaint. Assess muscle mobility and use tack and stretch or STM to improve muscle extensibility. Muscle electrical stimulation may be used, as can modalities for inflammation.	Progression is determined by the quality and magnitude of the contraction. Keep contraction below the level of pain.	Functional exercises to maintain quality and begin increasing magnitude of contraction as able. Lengthening of muscle as needed, short of pain. Muscle electrical stimulation may be utilized, as can modalities for inflammation.	Asymptomatic muscle contraction within the available ROM.	Rapidly increase the level of exercises until there is full asymptomatic ROM and functional activities, either concentric or eccentric.	Side-to-side differences are within 20% or muscle has no negative response to high-level activities.	Include unstable surfaces, velocity retraining, and cutting or power exercises.	Monitor muscle response to exercise using pain and swelling. Should either occur, then the capacity has been exceeded.
Ligament sprain							
Protection of the damaged tissue, maintenance of all other ROM. Gentle maintenance or increase in ROM controlled by target tissue. Modalities for inflammation.	As new collagen tissue is laid down, the tissue needs to be exposed to gentle tension stress.	STM to assist new tissue in laying down in the appropriate direction (direction of the force the ligament controls). ROM should be full or near full.	Controlled use of the joint with the ligament protected to allow tension stress to gradually increase in the healing tissue. Proprioceptive retraining continues throughout rehabilitation program.	Pain and swelling in the tissue are not elicited by the treatment activities, function is improving.	Return to functional activities as tolerated by an absence of pain and swelling in the involved tissue. Avoid compensatory movements.	As needed functional activities, with or without external stabilization as required.	Continued improvement of tissue mechanics and absence of pain or swelling in the ligament. No compensatory movements are observed.
Tendon pathology							
Cross-friction massage and unloading. Ice massage after. Contraction below the level of pain. See muscle tissue as well.	Static test indicates resolving complaints.	Eccentric exercises: Goal of this rehabilitation is to increase the tendon tolerance to force until capacity exceeds demand. See muscle progression.	See muscle progression.	See muscle progression.	See muscle progression.	See muscle progression.	See muscle progression.
Bone fracture							
Stabilization of fracture (refer to physician). Maintain all other motion at adjacent segment, unload bone by altering activity level.	Fracture site is asymptomatic or x-rays indicate good bone healing.	Address soft tissue damage associated with the fracture.	Cast removal.	Resolve any range of motion deficits, begin increased compressive loading on the bone below the level of complaint.	Asymptomatic and full range of motion.	Return to full activity as desired.	Asymptomatic in involved tissue.

Continued on following page.

TABLE IV-6-3 Tissue Injury and Intervention Choice (Continued)

What are the best interventions for the acute phase (0-14 days postinjury)?	When to progress to next phase	What are the best interventions for the reparative phase (15-21 days postinjury)?	When to progress to next phase	What are the best interventions for the remodeling phase (22-60 days postinjury)?	When to progress to next phase	What are the best interventions for the maturation phase (60-360 days postinjury)?	When to progress to next phase
Cartilage damage							
Reduce load on cartilage (decrease time and/or magnitude of compressive load). Assess and restore ROM deficits, address postural abnormalities.	Asymptomatic with rehabilitation activities.	Vigorous restoration of ROM both physiological (stretching exercises AROM and PROM) as well as accessory motions (joint mobilization). Avoid joint swelling or pain complaints as you begin compression through the joint.	Swelling remains under control.	Progress weight-bearing exercises slowly, rapidly increase exercises such as aquatic activities that keep the joint asymptomatic. Continue to address and eliminate postural abnormalities or alignment issues contributing (orthotic intervention, strengthening, stretching, etc).	Swelling and pain are avoided.	As desired activities. Note, with extensive cartilage damage it may not be possible to return to previous level of function as repetitive and extensive weight bearing should be avoided. Lifestyle modifications may be necessary.	Swelling and pain are avoided.
Capsule injury*							
Accessory mobility techniques designed to improve fluid mechanics (grades I and II oscillatory). Exercises to address any muscular deficits and to keep/restore general levels of fitness.	ROM testing indicates pain onset after resistance (or with resistance).	Begin gentle stretching to increase accessory mobility using grades III or IV oscillatory techniques or traction. Continue exercises, begin to move through pain-free ROM during exercises.	Pain and swelling should be monitored and improved.	Full accessory mobility should be restored. Full physiological mobility as well. Increase vigor of exercises, make sure functional activities are included.	ROM and swelling are normal.	As desired activities.	Patient remains asymptomatic and function continues to improve.
Peripheral nerve injury							
Damage to nerve will require avoidance of stretch or compression to the nerve. Rehabilitation of the involved muscles.	Stable neurological signs. Improving neurological symptoms	Begin isometric or partial ROM exercises short of pain complaints.	Restoration of some nervous function.	Continue and maintain integrity of associated areas, avoid loss of muscle function in other areas through a comprehensive program.	Restoration of nervous function.	Progress activity while avoiding further stretch or damage to nerve, avoid onset of neurodynamic tension.	Continued resolution of symptoms and improvement of function.
Adverse neurodynamic tension							
Flossing or STM at areas of focal hypomobility.	Stable neurological signs. Improving neurological symptoms	Begin STM, flossing, or sustained tension closer to end-range of nerve mobility.	Restoration of nervous function, absence of complaints arising from treatment. Other associated symptoms are resolved or resolving.	Treatment at end range of motion or near it.	Asymptomatic after treatment, continued increase in ROM and function.	As desired exercises.	Asymptomatic after treatment, continued increase in ROM and function.

AROM, Active range of motion; *PROM*, passive range of motion; *ROM*, range of motion; *STM*, soft tissue mobilization.
*Capsular tears should be treated as multidirectional ligament sprains. Capsular hypomobility and inflammation response is addressed here.

SUMMARY STATEMENT

Lower extremity complaints are some of the most prevalent complaints the clinician will see in the clinic. It is critical for the clinician to determine the impact of the involved joint on the rest of the lower extremity. In addition, the postural or kinetic alignment of the lower extremity segments must be addressed with every complaint. Exercises and restoration of full asymptomatic ROM cannot be overemphasized for treatment of lower extremity complaints. The lower extremity complaints are the most fun to treat because the clinician may use imagination in the creation of exercise programs that address the needs of the patients.

REFERENCES

1. Aminaka N, Gribble PA. Patellar taping, patellofemoral pain syndrome, lower extremity kinematics, and dynamic postural control. *J Athl Train*. 2008;43(1):21-28.
2. Arnason A, Andersen TE, Holme I, Engebretsen L, Bahr R. Prevention of hamstring strains in elite soccer: an intervention study. *Scand J Med Sci Sports*. 2008;18(1):40-48.
3. Bedotto RA. Biomechanical assessment and treatment in lower extremity prosthetics and orthotics: a clinical perspective. *Phys Med Rehabil Clin N Am*. 2006;17(1):203-243.
4. Binkley JM, Stratford PW, Lott SA, Riddle DL. The Lower Extremity Functional Scale (LEFS): scale development, measurement properties, and clinical application. North American Orthopaedic Rehabilitation Research Network. *Phys Ther*. 1999;79(4):371-383.
5. Brantingham JW, Globe G, Pollard H, Hicks M, Korporaal C, Hoskins W. Manipulative therapy for lower extremity conditions: expansion of literature review. *J Manipulative Physiol Ther*. 2009;32(1):53-71.
6. Brosseau L, Casimiro L, Milne S, et al. Deep transverse friction massage for treating tendinitis. *Cochrane Database Syst Rev*. 2002;(1):CD003528.
7. Burns J, Crosbie J, Ouvrier R, Hunt A. Effective orthotic therapy for the painful cavus foot: a randomized controlled trial. *J Am Podiatr Med Assoc*. 2006 May;96(3):205-211.
8. Burns J, Landorf KB, Ryan MM, Crosbie J, Ouvrier RA. Interventions for the prevention and treatment of pes cavus. *Cochrane Database Syst Rev*. 2007;(4):CD006154.
9. Callaghan MJ, Selfe J, McHenry A, Oldham JA. Effects of patellar taping on knee joint proprioception in patients with patellofemoral pain syndrome. *Man Ther*. 2008 June;13(3):192-199.
10. Chappell JD, Creighton RA, Giuliani C, Yu B, Garrett WE. Kinematics and electromyography of landing preparation in vertical stop-jump: risks for noncontact anterior cruciate ligament injury. *Am J Sports Med*. 2007;35(2):235-241.
11. Chappell JD, Herman DC, Knight BS, Kirkendall DT, Garrett WE, Yu B. Effect of fatigue on knee kinetics and kinematics in stop-jump tasks. *Am J Sports Med*. 2005;33(7):1022-1029.
12. Chumanov ES, Wall-Scheffler C, Heiderscheit BC. Gender differences in walking and running on level and inclined surfaces. *Clin Biomech (Bristol, Avon)*. 2008;23(10):1260-1268.
13. Connell AT. Concepts for assessment and treatment of anterior knee pain related to altered spinal and pelvic biomechanics: a case report. *Man Ther*. 2008;13(6):560-563.
14. Currier LL, Froehlich PJ, Carow SD, et al. Development of a clinical prediction rule to identify patients with knee pain and clinical evidence of knee osteoarthritis who demonstrate a favorable short-term response to hip mobilization. *Phys Ther*. 2007;87(9):1106-1119.
15. D'hondt NE, Struijs PA, Kerkhoffs GM, et al. Orthotic devices for treating patellofemoral pain syndrome. *Cochrane Database Syst Rev*. 2002;(2):CD002267.
16. Emery CA, Rose MS, McAllister JR, Meeuwisse WH. A prevention strategy to reduce the incidence of injury in high school basketball: a cluster randomized controlled trial. *Clin J Sport Med*. 2007;17(1):17-24.
17. Fairbank JCT, Pynsent P. The Oswestry Disability Index. *Spine*. 2000;25(22):2940-2953.
18. Feldman RS, Hugar DW. Physical therapy: its use in podiatry. *J Foot Surg*. 1981;20(2):102-107.
19. Fredericson M, Weir A. Practical management of iliotibial band friction syndrome in runners. *Clin J Sport Med*. 2006;16(3):261-268.
20. Fritschy D, de GR. Jumper's knee and ultrasonography. *Am J Sports Med*. 1988;16(6):637-640.
21. Fu TC, Wong AM, Pei YC, Wu KP, Chou SW, Lin YC. Effect of Kinesio taping on muscle strength in athletes-a pilot study. *J Sci Med Sport*. 2008;11(2):198-201.
22. Hart JM, Garrison JC, Palmieri-Smith R, Kerrigan DC, Ingersoll CD. Lower extremity joint moments of collegiate soccer players differ between genders during a forward jump. *J Sport Rehabil*. 2008;17(2):137-147.
23. Hilbert JE, Sforzo GA, Swensen T. The effects of massage on delayed onset muscle soreness. *Br J Sports Med*. 2003;37(1):72-75.
24. Hurd WJ, Chmielewski TL, Axe MJ, Davis I, Snyder-Mackler L. Differences in normal and perturbed walking kinematics between male and female athletes. *Clin Biomech (Bristol, Avon)*. 2004;19(5):465-472.
25. Jacobs CA, Uhl TL, Mattacola CG, Shapiro R, Rayens WS. Hip abductor function and lower extremity landing kinematics: sex differences. *J Athl Train*. 2007;42(1):76-83.
26. Jonhagen S, Ackermann P, Eriksson T, Saartok T, Renstrom PA. Sports massage after eccentric exercise. *Am J Sports Med*. 2004;32(6):1499-1503.
27. Kaltenborn FM, Evjenth O, Kaltenborn TB, Morgan D, Vollowitz E. *Manual Mobilization of the Joints*. 4th ed. Oslo: Norli; 2003.
28. Kernozek TW, Torry MR, Iwasaki M. Gender differences in lower extremity landing mechanics caused by neuromuscular fatigue. *Am J Sports Med*. 2008;36(3):554-565.
29. Kernozek TW, Torry MR, Van HH, Cowley H, Tanner S. Gender differences in frontal and sagittal plane biomechanics during drop landings. *Med Sci Sports Exerc*. 2005;37(6):1003-1012.
30. Kisner C, Colby LA. *Therapeutic Exercise: Foundations and Techniques*. 5th ed. Philadelphia: F.A. Davis; 2007.
31. LaBella C. Patellofemoral pain syndrome: evaluation and treatment. *Prim Care*. 2004;31(4):977-1003.
32. Larsen K, Weidich F, Leboeuf-Yde C. Can custom-made biomechanic shoe orthoses prevent problems in the back and lower extremities? A randomized, controlled intervention trial of 146 military conscripts. *J Manipulative Physiol Ther*. 2002 June;25(5):326-331.
33. Lopez-Rodriguez S, Fernandez de-Las-Penas C, Alburquerque-Sendin F, Rodriguez-Blanco C, Palomeque-del-Cerro L. Immediate effects of manipulation of the talocrural joint on stabilometry and baropodometry in patients with ankle sprain. *J Manipulative Physiol Ther*. 2007;30(3):186-192.
34. Losito JM, O'Neil J. Rehabilitation of foot and ankle injuries. *Clin Podiatr Med Surg*. 1997;14(3):533-557.
35. Magee DJ. *Orthopedic Physical Assessment*. 4th ed. St. Louis, MO: Elsevier Saunders; 2006.
35a. Maitland G, Hengeveld E, Banks K, English K. (Eds.). *Maitland's Peripheral Manipulation*. 4th ed. Woburn, MA: Butterworth-Heinemann; 2005.
36. Marini M, Sgambati E, Barni E, Piazza M, Monaci M. Pain syndromes in competitive elite level female artistic gymnasts. Role of specific preventive-compensative activity. *Ital J Anat Embryol*. 2008;113(1):47-54.
37. McConnell J. A novel approach to pain relief pre-therapeutic exercise. *J Sci Med Sport*. 2000;3(3):325-334.
38. McHugh MP, Nesse M. Effect of stretching on strength loss and pain after eccentric exercise. *Med Sci Sports Exerc*. 2008;40(3):566-573.
39. Melham TJ, Sevier TL, Malnofski MJ, Wilson JK, Helfst Jr RH. Chronic ankle pain and fibrosis successfully treated with a new noninvasive augmented soft tissue mobilization technique (ASTM): a case report. *Med Sci Sports Exerc*. 1998;30(6):801-804.
40. Moss P, Sluka K, Wright A. The initial effects of knee joint mobilization on osteoarthritic hyperalgesia. *Man Ther*. 2007;12(2):109-118.
41. Namba RS, Inacio M. Early and late manipulation improve flexion after total knee arthroplasty. *J Arthroplasty*. 2007;22(6 suppl 2):58-61.
42. Neufeld SK, Cerrato R. Plantar fasciitis: evaluation and treatment. *J Am Acad Orthop Surg*. 2008;16(6):338-346.
42a. Norkin CC, Levangie PK. *Joint Structure and Function: A Comprehensive Analysis*. 4th ed. Philadelphia PA: FA Davis Co; 2005.
43. Pellow JE, Brantingham JW. The efficacy of adjusting the ankle in the treatment of subacute and chronic grade I and grade II ankle inversion sprains. *J Manipulative Physiol Ther*. 2001;24(1):17-24.
44. Perlman AI, Sabina A, Williams AL, Njike VY, Katz DL. Massage therapy for osteoarthritis of the knee: a randomized controlled trial. *Arch Intern Med*. 2006;166(22):2533-2538.
45. Perry J. *Gait Analysis: Normal and Pathological Function*. 1st ed. SLACK; Thorofare, NJ; 1992.
46. Portegijs E, Kallinen M, Rantanen T, et al. Effects of resistance training on lower-extremity impairments in older people with hip fracture. *Arch Phys Med Rehabil*. 2008;89(9):1667-1674.

47. Rees SS, Murphy AJ, Watsford ML. Effects of whole-body vibration exercise on lower-extremity muscle strength and power in an older population: a randomized clinical trial. *Phys Ther.* 2008;88(4):462-470.

48. Reid A, Birmingham TB, Stratford PW, Alcock GK, Griffin JR. Hop testing provides a reliable and valid outcome measure during rehabilitation after anterior cruciate ligament reconstruction. *Phys Ther.* 2007;87(3):337-349.

49. Salsich GB, Brechter JH, Farwell D, Powers CM. The effects of patellar taping on knee kinetics, kinematics, and vastus lateralis muscle activity during stair ambulation in individuals with patellofemoral pain. *J Orthop Sports Phys Ther.* 2002;32(1):3-10.

50. Shrier I. Warm-up and stretching in the prevention of muscular injury. *Sports Med.* 2008;38(10):879-880.

51. Sims EL, Hardaker WM, Queen RM. Gender differences in plantar loading during three soccer-specific tasks. *Br J Sports Med.* 2008;42(4):272-277.

52. Slupik A, Dwornik M, Bialoszewski D, Zych E. Effect of Kinesio Taping on bioelectrical activity of vastus medialis muscle. Preliminary report. *Ortop Traumatol Rehabil.* 2007;9(6):644-651.

53. Stratford P, Gill C, Westaway M, Binkley J. Assessing disability and change on individual patients: a report of a patient specific measure. *Physiother Can.* 1995;47:258-263.

54. Stratford PW, Kennedy DM, Woodhonse LJ. Performance measures provide assessments of pain and function in people with advanced osteoarthritis of the hip or knee. *Phys Ther.* 2006;86:1489-1496.

55. Trotter LC, Pierrynowski MR. The short-term effectiveness of full-contact custom-made foot orthoses and prefabricated shoe inserts on lower-extremity musculoskeletal pain: a randomized clinical trial. *J Am Podiatr Med Assoc.* 2008;98(5):357-363.

56. Waite BL, Krabak BJ. Examination and treatment of pediatric injuries of the hip and pelvis. *Phys Med Rehabil Clin N Am.* 2008;19(2): 305-318, ix.

57. Warden SJ, Brukner P. Patellar tendinopathy. *Clin Sports Med.* 2003;22(4):743-759.

58. Willson JD, Binder-Macleod S, Davis IS. Lower extremity jumping mechanics of female athletes with and without patellofemoral pain before and after exertion. *Am J Sports Med.* 2008;36(8):1587-1596.

59. Yasukawa A, Patel P, Sisung C. Pilot study: investigating the effects of Kinesio Taping in an acute pediatric rehabilitation setting. *Am J Occup Ther.* 2006;60(1):104-110.

60. Yeung EW, Yeung SS. A systematic review of interventions to prevent lower limb soft tissue running injuries. *Br J Sports Med.* 2001;35(6):383-389.

61. Yu B, McClure SB, Onate JA, Guskiewicz KM, Kirkendall DT, Garrett WE. Age and gender effects on lower extremity kinematics of youth soccer players in a stop-jump task. *Am J Sports Med.* 2005;33(9):1356-1364.

62. Zhang W, Moskowitz RW, Nuki G, et al. OARSI recommendations for the management of hip and knee osteoarthritis, part I: critical appraisal of existing treatment guidelines and systematic review of current research evidence. *Osteoarthritis Cartilage.* 2007;15(9):981-1000.

AUTHORS: BRIAN YEE and MICHAEL SHACKLOCK

INTRODUCTORY INFORMATION   ⓘ

What are the factors a clinician should consider when rehabilitating a patient with nerve pain?

When the concept of nerve rehabilitation or neurodynamics originated, the common treatment approach was to "stretch" the nerve. Many clinicians became discouraged with this type of neurodynamic rehabilitation because patients were many times made worse. Since then, the understanding of neurodynamics has evolved beyond just "stretching." Neurodynamics can now be viewed as the "clinical application of mechanics and physiology of the nervous system as they relate to each other and are integrated with musculoskeletal function."[14]

Neurodynamics is not just about treating the nerve itself, but viewing it as an integrated three-part system as follows:

- Mechanical interface: Any structure that resides next to the nervous system, such as tendon, bone, intervertebral disc, or ligament that can alter the course of the nerve.
- Neural structures: Any structure that constitutes the nervous system, including the brain, spinal cord, nerve roots, peripheral nerves, and sympathetic trunk.
- Innervated tissue: Any tissue innervated by the nervous system, including muscle, ligament, joint capsule, or viscera.[14]

How do these factors affect the rehabilitation process?

Determining the source of a patient's nerve pain helps guide the patient's intervention. For example, radial nerve impingement caused by repetitious supinator activity should be treated by improving the myofascial or mechanical interface around the supinator along with radial nerve mobilizations, whereas rehabilitation for a postsurgical lumbar fusion patient who develops scarring along a lumbar nerve root should focus on the nerve to improve the physiology and mechanics of the nerve.

What role does age play in rehabilitation of nerve pain?

Aging factors can affect nerve rehabilitation, particularly if there are other health-related factors such as diabetes or previous neural injuries. Physiologically, peripheral nerves deteriorate with age. There is an increased rate of nerve atrophy and a decreased number of myelinated nerves. The decline in the number of myelinated nerves begins as early as 40 years of age and continues steadily with age. At 80 years of age, individuals only have 57% of the myelinated nerves that they did at 20 years of age. As a result, nerve conduction velocities decrease between 10% and 30% with age. The results of these changes are slower muscle response and slower recognition of changes in sensory and proprioceptive stimulus.

The rate of remyelination decreases with age. From a rehabilitation standpoint, injury to nerves can be expected to recover more slowly in the elderly with the potential that nerves will not recover to their preinjury levels. Surgical healing is also better in younger patients than older.

Traumatic peripheral nerve injuries are more prevalent in the younger population ranging from 16 to 38 years old.[12] Consideration of spinal stenosis in older adults can also affect rehabilitation.

What role does acuteness or chronicity play in rehabilitating a patient with nerve pain?

Assessing a patient's nerve pain as acute or chronic state directly influences the treatment the clinician will provide based on their presenting symptoms. Shacklock provided a selection system of neurodynamic techniques based on such questions as follows:

- How strongly should a neurodynamic test be performed?
- How far into provoking movement should a test be taken?
- Which neurodynamic sequence should be used?

Technique selection is based on the categorization of patients severity/irritability, which is divided into levels 0, 1, 2, 3a, 3b, 3c, and 3d,[14] as follows:

Level 0: Patients who are contraindicated for care should be referred to the appropriate professional.
- Severe pain
- Severe psychological influences
- Legal problems
- Highly unstable conditions: Worsening rapidly

Level 1: Acute/limited examination
- Highly irritable symptoms
- Symptoms easily provoked, take a long time to settle.
- Uncertain if patient will tolerate standard (level 2) testing.

Level 2: Subacute/standard
- Not particularly irritable
- Stable conditions are present.
- No significant neurological symptoms present.

Level 3: Chronic/advanced
- Pain is difficult to evoke
- Need for more specificity and sensitivity of testing is needed, which can be done by the following:
  - 3a: Neurodynamic sensitization
  - 3b: Neurodynamic sequencing
  - 3c: Multistructural examination
  - 3d: Symptomatic position/movement

With level 1 patients, the focus of neurodynamic interventions are based on improving the pathophysiology of the nervous system, whereas with level 3 patients the focus is on improving the pathomechanics of the nervous system.[14]

What factors make treatment of patients with nerve pain challenging?

Difficulty in treating patients with peripheral neurogenic pain is based on the proper assessment of the patient's irritability and severity of symptoms. Further, it is important to perform a proper physical examination to determine which mechanical interfaces, neural structures, and/or innervated tissues are involved in the patient's dysfunction. More importantly, nerve pain, similar to any other pain, could be derived from differing sources. This could include central pain processing, autonomic nervous system, and viscera and systemic origins. Proper examination to differentially diagnose the source of the nerve pain is necessary before beginning rehabilitation.

Are there factors that make treatment of patients with nerve pain easier?

When dealing with peripheral neurogenic pathology, the use of a structural differentiating maneuver in a clinician's neurodynamic testing is required and makes it easier to determine if the patient has a neurodynamic dysfunction. A common example is with the slump test. This test asks for the patient to go into cervical flexion, slump forward, and raise their symptomatic leg into knee extension, possibly reproducing their symptoms. A structural differentiating maneuver would be to release cervical flexion, potentially improving or worsening their symptoms and indicating a neurodynamic involvement.

PROGNOSIS

How successful is rehabilitation in treating acute nerve pain?

Randomized controlled trials of neural mobilization for nerve pain have primarily tested patients with chronic (>3 months) duration of symptoms.[1,4-7,13,18] Clinically, however, using the correct clinical reasoning and treatment approaches to reduce acute nerve pain can be highly effective. Much of acute nerve pain revolves around inflammation. The clinician's first goal should be to address and reduce the inflammation that surrounds the nerve and creates nerve irritation.

CLINICAL PEARL !

In acute nerve pain patients, attempting to treat the affected nerve by "lengthening" or "stretching" the nerve may cause increased symptoms. Shacklock has proposed the utilization of the contralateral extremity for neurodynamic assessment and treatment of acute (level 1) patients.[14] Studies are currently being performed to confirm this proposal.

How successful is rehabilitation in treating chronic nerve pain?

There are several studies indicating improvements with manual neural mobilization techniques for patients with various nerve-related injuries. Most studies were effective in improving short-term disabilities; however, long-term follow-up was not significant. This possibly indicates a need for a multimodal and multidisciplinary approach with chronic nerve pain.[1,4-6,13,18] Coppieters et al tested subjects with cervicobrachial neurogenic pain and compared treatments by neural mobilization versus pulsed ultrasound, using elbow extension range of motion (ROM), pain (visual analog scale [VAS]) and symptom distribution as outcome measures.[5] The neural mobilization group had significant improvements in elbow ROM, 43% decrease in area of symptom distribution, and decrease in pain compared to the ultrasound group.[5]

Which patients with nerve pain derive the greatest long term benefits from rehabilitation?

Patients presenting with neural mechanosensitivity or peripheral neurogenic symptoms, without significant upper or lower motor neuron changes, as well as minimized central sensitivity changes, tend to benefit from direct peripheral neurodynamic interventions.

What other regions of the body are most likely to contribute to nerve pain?

Neurodynamic dysfunction, in many ways, is different from an isolated orthopedic joint injury. For example, with a localized shoulder injury, many times, clinicians will treat the local joint, as well as the above and below mechanical joints. With neural pain, it is important to understand that nerves are the "circuitry" connecting everything together (Case Study). Therefore a positive slump test reproducing a patient's shoulder pain could essentially originate from a neurodynamic dysfunction at the ankle caused by dysfunction of the peroneal, tibial, or sural nerves.

CASE STUDY ?

A 29-year-old female presents with primary complaints of bilateral heel and foot pain. She reports being diagnosed by her physician as having plantar fasciitis and has received injections and previous physical therapy for plantar fasciitis without improvement. Previous medical history indicates the patient had surgery to correct severe scoliosis, requiring spinal rod placements. Patient reports that the spinal cord was "stretched" too far during the procedure, resulting in loss of right plantar flexion ankle strength. The patient currently wears an ankle-foot orthotic (AFO) to help in gait but complains of bilateral foot symptoms. What is a key concern in the patient's subjective complaints of "plantar fasciitis" that you would consider to be of neurodynamic origin? How would you differentially diagnose it?

Answer

Subjective reports of the spinal cord being "stretched" during the patient's surgery causing neurological weakness indicates that the neural system was mechanonsensitized, not only causing motor dysfunction but also sensitizing the plantar nerves of the feet, referring pain similar to "plantar fasciitis." Differential diagnosis would require a straight leg raise (SLR) test and/or slump test causing replication of her symptoms in bilateral feet.

EVIDENCE BASED MEDICINE

What trends are currently being seen in research regarding rehabilitation of patients with nerve pain?

Most studies indicate improvements in short-term disability, pain, and ROM. However, the lack of improvements in long-term disabilities cause the need to use a multimodal treatment program.[1,4-7,13,18] Current research has focused on changes in nerve-related symptoms after treatment to the cervical and thoracic regions.

INTERVENTIONS

MANUAL THERAPY

What is the physiological rationale behind the use of manual therapy in treating patients with nerve pain?

The use of manual therapy to improve neural mobility is based on both physiological and mechanical changes. Nerves must be able glide and move within the structures that surround them. When the nerve is not allowed to glide freely, tension is placed on the nerve. Nerve irritation or injury can result. Therefore neural rehabilitation often will address the tissues that prevent proper nerve mobility before attention is directed at the nerve itself. Physiologically, the use of neural mobilizations, such as the cervical lateral glide,[5,11] aim to neuromodulate the mechanosensitivity of the nerve. This can decrease the amount of nociceptive afferent input into the dorsal horn, as well as improve intraneural/extraneural edema. Mechanically, the use of neural mobilizations aims to improve the sliding and tensioning capacity of the nerve to match the needs in daily function and movement.

Which interventions have proved most successful in treating patients with nerve pain?

Studies using such interventions as manual therapy, traction, modalities, medications, injections, and surgery can all demonstrate some type of improvement in pain or disability. However, an important step to improve the treatment efficacy of nerve pain would be to derive a subclassification system to treat the different types of nerve pain or dysfunctions.

What is the role of traction in treating patients with nerve pain?

The use of mechanical traction has been shown to improve symptoms with patients in a subgroup characterized by the presence of leg symptoms, signs of nerve root compression, and either peripheralization with extension movements or a crossed SLR.[9]

CLINICAL PEARL !

From a clinical reasoning perspective on neurodynamics, the use of mechanical traction at times can make patients feel better. However, the hope that it will fix every patient with radicular-like symptoms is limited. Mechanical traction essentially improves the mechanical interface of the affected nerve root. However, neurodynamics rehabilitation requires an integration of the neural tissue, as well as its innervated tissues, to fully treat the affected neuromusculoskeletal system. Therefore, in our treatment plan, the use of techniques to improve the pathological states of all three systems is required to fully treat the patient with a neurodynamic dysfunction.

How beneficial is joint mobilization in the treatment of patients with nerve pain?

Studies by Coppieters et al,[5] Allison et al,[1] and Vicenzino et al[18] use a joint mobilization technique called a *contralateral cervical glide*. This mobilization technique not only improves the mobility of the zygapophyseal joint but also neuromodulates the mechanosensitivity of the nerve root and promotes sliding and tensioning along the nerve. The technique can improve physiological and mechanical states of the involved nerve.

Is joint manipulation recommended for patients with nerve pain?

Treatment to improve the physiology and mechanics of the nervous system should be the priority. Precautions should be made using joint manipulation with patients presenting with positive neurodynamic dysfunction, especially in acute pain situations. Manipulation to the cervical spine has been shown to reduce shoulder and lateral elbow pain.[8] Manipulation to the thoracic spine has been shown to increase SLR by 8 degrees in patients with low back or lower extremity pain.[2,17]

What does evidence reveal regarding the use of massage for the treatment of patients with nerve pain?

As stated before, neurodynamic dysfunctions are integrated with three systems: (1) mechanical interface, (2) neural structures, and (3) innervated tissues. Performing soft tissue massage may have an effect in improving pain states derived from neural origin, as neurogenic inflammation can sensitize the tissues the nerve innervates, including soft tissue. Clinically, massage alone provides only short-term relief of pain from a neural origin but can be highly effective when integrated with improvements at the affected mechanical interfaces and involved neural tissue.

Is stretching beneficial or indicated for patients with nerve pain?

Proper movement of nerves is based on their pathophysiological and pathomechanical states. In acute situations, stretching could potentially irritate the neural system making symptoms worse. Tensioning, not necessarily "stretching," the nervous system is indicated in more chronic cases indicated as levels 3a, b, c, d in Shacklock's classification system.[14]

CASE STUDY ?

A 25-year-old female complains of right shoulder pain over the last 4 years. She was formerly a competitive college tennis player and 4 years ago she underwent a right subacromial decompression surgery to correct identical symptoms the patient is currently experiencing. Before the surgery, the patient reported working with the college tennis training staff. She reported that her arm was being aggressively "stretched" by the staff to improve her shoulder ROM, resulting in increased pain in her shoulder, as well as numbness and tingling in her right forearm and fingers. Based on the subjective information, what points help differentially diagnose the patient's right shoulder pain originating from a shoulder joint pathology versus a neurodynamic dysfunction?

Answer

Aggressive "stretching" resulting in numbness and tingling indicates a neural involvement. The mechanosensitivity to the nerve not only causes localized pain at the shoulder joint but can also limit ROM, making it appear as an isolated shoulder pathology. Symptoms since the surgery also have not improved, indicating the spur at the subacromial space most likely was not the primary pain generator.

How should a clinician decide which manual therapy intervention is most appropriate for a patient with nerve pain?

Taking proper subjective and physical examination of the patient will determine the patient's severity and irritability. Specific manual interventions should be indicated to address the patient's presenting symptoms. Also, using Shacklock's classification system (levels 0, 1, 2, 3a, 3b, 3c, 3d) helps enable the clinician to provide a proper progression of manual interventions, rather than just "stretch" the nerve.

EXERCISE

What is the physiological rationale behind the use of exercise in treating patients with nerve pain?

Exercise can help nerve pain by promoting neural mobility, improve circulation, reduce intraneural and extraneural edema, and provide proper joint stability and movement patterns to reduce mechanical loading on neural tissue. Nerves are thixotropic: They need motion or the nerve will die. Exercise is an important aspect of motion and of nerve health. Exercises must allow nerve motion but prevent nerve irritation or damage.

Are exercise programs beneficial in treating patients with nerve pain?

Most studies regarding nerve pain are focused on using manual therapy techniques, modalities, or traction to improve nerve pain. However, exercise programs are commonly integrated with the control groups in studies, in which most studies on neural mobilization indicate that exercise alone can have only a short-term improvement in the patient's disability.

Which muscles should be strengthened in treating patients with nerve pain?

The focus on strengthening programs with patients with nerve pain should not be on improvements in torque and power but rather on proper joint stability and movement patterns. Studies have shown, by the pain inhibition reflex, that within 24 hours of acute injury, "local" muscles (designed to maintain joint stability) are inhibited in cross-sectional area and delayed onset of activation occurs.[15,16] The lack of segmental stability can cause increased loading to the affected joint. This can result in increased loading and shearing at the adjacent nerve, possibly becoming a pain generator.

CLINICAL PEARL !

Clinical experience has shown that patients presenting with joint hypermobilities many times present with significant restrictions in neural mobility surrounding the hypermobile joint. One may assume that the nerve would be hypermobile, but on the contrary, the hypomobility of the neural tissue may indicate that the neural system is attempting to stabilize and compensate for the lack of motor control the joint has. Therefore considerations in rehabilitating this patient would be to not only improve the neural mobility surrounding the pathologic joint but also to provide proper motor control stability of the "local" muscles surrounding the joint (i.e., longus colli, rotator cuff, etc).

How should a clinician decide which exercise is most appropriate for a patient with nerve pain?

Proper clinical reasoning and thorough physical examination is required to determine which specific exercise is most appropriate for each patient. Assessment of "local" muscle stability should be examined at the site of pathology, as well as other joints that may contribute to the affected joint's mechanics. Appropriate exercise techniques to meet joint stability needs to be the primary focus.

TABLE IV-7-1 Positions that Place Tensile Stress on the Peripheral Nerves

UPPER EXTREMITY					
Nerve	**Position of Nerve Stress**				
Median	Glenohumeral abduction	Glenohumeral external rotation	Elbow extension	Forearm supination	Wrist and finger extension
Ulnar	Scapular depression	Glenohumeral external rotation	Glenohumeral abduction	Elbow flexion	Forearm pronation	Wrist and finger extension
Radial	Scapular depression	Glenohumeral internal rotation	Glenohumeral abduction	Elbow extension	Forearm pronation	Wrist and finger flexion

LOWER EXTREMITY			
Nerve	**Position of Nerve Stress**		
SLR test: Sciatic nerve	Hip flexion	Knee straight	
Slump test: Spinal cord/sciatic nerve	Sitting thoracic and lumbar flexion	Cervical flexion	Knee extension	Ankle dorsiflexion

SLR, Straight leg raise.

How does a clinician know if a patient with nerve pain is ready to progress to a new exercise?
The patient should report a reduction of symptoms, improvement in neural mobility between sides, and improved function.

MODALITIES
Which modalities have proven most successful in treating patients with nerve pain?
Ultrasound studies to improve nerve pain have at best improved short-term disability measures.[4] Studies on the use of electrical stimulation to treat nerve pathology varies; little evidence supports the sole use of this modality solely for the treatment of nerve pathlogy.[3,10]

OTHER
What is the role of bracing or taping in treating patients with nerve pain?
Bracing and taping can help improve movement impairments and reduce mechanical and physiological strain to the nervous system. It may also provide desensitization to the skin receptors, providing inhibition of nociceptive afferent input to the dorsal horn.[19]

HOME EXERCISE
Which home exercises are the most beneficial to give patients with nerve pain?
Home exercises to improve nerve pain are based on the patient's presenting symptoms. If the patient is acute, resting positions to lessen the strain and nociceptive input at the affected extremity would be warranted. If the patient is chronic, home exercises to improve neural mobility that the patient responded well to in clinic should then be prescribed.

REHABILITATION CLINICAL REASONING
How should a clinician decide which intervention is most appropriate for a patient with nerve pain?
Similar to joint mobilization principles, grade 1 to 2 mobilizations target pain modulation, while grade 3 to 4 mobilizations improve end-range capsular mobility. Selection of neural mobilizations should be used in the same way. The idea of "stretching" the nerve in any condition is contraindicated because it is a highly aggressive

movement for the mechanics and physiology of the nervous system. Rather, techniques to reduce the tension or sensitivity in acute nerve situations may be necessary, progressing to neural sliding techniques that improve the mobility of the neural tissue without symptom provocation (Table IV-7-1). Shacklock has also proposed the use of contralateral neurodynamic techniques to help "off-load" the affective neural tissue in patients with acute level 1 symptoms.

What red flags should a clinician be aware of regarding rehabilitating a patient with nerve pain?
According to Shacklock's classification, level 0 patients are contraindicated for care and should be referred to the appropriate professional. This includes severe pain, severe psychological influences, legal problems, or highly unstable conditions that are worsening rapidly, including the presentation of sinister medical pathologies.

SUMMARY STATEMENT
The assessment and interventions for nerve pain have improved exponentially over the last few years. Clinical misunderstandings in nerve rehabilitation have taught clinicians to not just "stretch" the nerve. Rather, neurodynamics requires proper understanding of the mechanics and physiology of not only the nervous system itself, but also the interfaces the nerve integrates with. Neurodynamics principles therefore are similar to the clinical reasoning process with any other musculoskeletal condition. There is no "one treatment that fits all" approach, but instead precise neurodynamic interventions should be performed based on the patient's presenting symptoms.

REFERENCES
1. Shacklock MO. *Clinical Neurodynamics.* London: Elsevier; 2005.
2. Kouyoumdjian JA. Peripheral nerve injuries: a retrospective survey of 456 cases, *Muscle Nerve.* 2006;34:785-788.
3. Ellis RF, Hing WA. Neural mobilization: a systematic review of randomized controlled trials with an analysis of therapeutic efficacy. *J Manual Manipulative Ther.* 2008;16(1):8-22.
4. Coppieters MW, Stappaerts KH, Wouters LL, Janssens K. The immediate effects of a cervical lateral glide treatment technique in patients with neurogenic cervicobrachial pain. *J Orthop Sports Phys Ther.* 2003;33:369-378.

5. Scrimshaw S, Maher C. Randomized controlled trial of neural mobilization after spinal surgery. *Spine.* 2001;26:2647-2652.

6. Allison GT, Nagy BM, Hall TAA. Randomized clinical trial of manual therapy for cervico-brachial pain syndrome. A pilot study. *Manual Ther.* 2002;7:95-102.

7. Drechsler WI, Knarr JF, Snyder-Mackler LA. Comparison of two treatment regimens for lateral epicondylitis: a randomized trial of clinical interventions. *J Sport Rehabil.* 1997;6:226-234.

8. Cleland JA, Childs JD, Palmer JA, Eberhart S. Slump stretching in the management of non-radicular low back pain: a pilot clinical trial, *Man Ther.* 2006;11:279-286.

9. Vicenzino B, Collins D, Wright A. The initial effects of a cervical spine manipulative physiotherapy treatment on the pain and dysfunction of lateral epicondylalgia, *Pain.* 1996;68:69-74.

10. Hall TM, Elvey RL. Nerve trunk pain: physical diagnosis and treatment, *Man Ther.* 1999;4(2):63-73.

11. Fritz JM, Linday W, Matheson JW, et al. Is there a subgroup of patients with low back pain likely to benefit from mechanical traction? Results of a randomized clinical trial and subgrouping analysis. *Spine.* 2007;15, 32, 36:E793-800.

12. Stokes M, Young A. The contribution of reflex inhibition to arthrogenous muscle weakness, *Clin Sci.* 1984;67:7-14.

13. Stokes M, Hides JA, Jull GA, Cooper DH. Mechanism of human paraspinals muscle wasting with acute low back pain. *J Physiol (abstract).* 1992;452:280.

14. Boonstra AM, van Weerden TW, Eisma WH, Pahlpatz VB, Oosterhuis HJ. The effect of low-frequency electrical stimulation on denervation atrophy in man. *Scand J Rehabil Med.* 1987;19:127-134.

15. Gordon T, Brushart TM, Amirjani N, Chan KM. The potential of electrical stimulation to promote functional recovery after peripheral nerve injury - comparisons between rats and humans, *Acta Neurochir Suppl.* 2007;100:3-11.

16. Vicenzino B. Lateral epicondylalgia: a musculoskeletal physiotherapy perspective. *Man Ther.* 2003;8:66-79.

17. Bergman GJ, Winters JC, Groenier KH, De Jong BM, Postema K, Van der Heijden GJ. Manipulative therapy in addition to usual medical care for patients with shoulder dysfunction and pain. *Ann Intern Med.* 2004;141:432-439.

18. Fernandez-Carnero J, Fernandez de las Penas C, Cleland J. Immediate hypoalgesic and motor effects after a single cervical spine manipulation in subjects with lateral epicondylalgia. *J Manipulative Physiol Therap.* 2007;31(9):675-681.

19. Sueki D, Almaria S, Bender M, et al. *The Effects of Mid-Thoracic Manipulation on Lower Extremity Neuromobility.* Unpublished Graduate Research, Mount St. Mary's College; 2008.

Section V

Pharmacology

AUTHOR: WOLFGANG VOGEL

INTRODUCTION TO PHARMACOLOGY

DRUG

A drug is a chemical substance that medical professionals are allowed to use to treat, diagnose, prevent, or cure diseases and medical conditions. This permission is granted by the Food and Drug Administration *(FDA)* after the drug company has demonstrated that the drug is effective and relatively safe, using animal studies and human clinical trials.

Alternative medications, such as herbal preparations, are treated like "food," and thus the manufacturer is only required to state content but not amounts and does not have to prove scientifically or clinically efficacy or toxicity. Manufacturers often make unsubstantiated claims, and varying amounts and fraud are encountered with these "drugs."

DRUG NAME

A drug has three names, as follows:
- Chemical name (e.g., 7-chloro-1, 3-dihydro-1-methyl-5-phenyl-2H-1, 4-benzodiazepin-2-one).
- Generic or scientific name (e.g., diazepam): Only one name per drug and often written in parentheses after the brand name.
- Brand name (e.g., Valium): Different brand names can be used for the same drug.

BRAND NAME VERSUS GENERIC DRUG

A *brand name drug* is the original drug manufactured by a company while the patent is in force and also after the patent has expired. A *generic drug* is manufactured by other companies after the patent has expired. A generic drug is a copy of a brand name drug in composition, dosage, safety, strength, administration, performance, and intended use. A generic drug contains the same active ingredient and must show the same bioavailability as a brand name drug but looks different. Unless a physician specifically prescribes or recommends one or the other, they are interchangeable.

THERAPEUTIC CONSIDERATIONS OF DRUG ACTION

Therapeutic effects are the intended beneficial actions. Adverse effects are unwanted actions and must be evaluated as to the possibility and more importantly, probability. Adverse effects can have the following characteristics:
- Range from mild to severe
- Reversible to irreversible
- Avoidable (caused by mistake) or unavoidable
- Often reduced or reversed when recognized early

Adverse reactions can be classified as the following:
- Side effects, which are associated with a specific drug, are seen in all individuals at different degrees and are often predictable.
- Idiosyncratic reactions, which are caused by a biochemical peculiarity of an individual that becomes apparent only after drug exposure, are seen only in few patients, do not involve the immune system, and are unpredictable.
- Allergic reactions, which are caused by an immunological peculiarity of an individual that becomes only apparent after drug exposure, are seen in only a few patients and are unpredictable.

PLACEBO

A *placebo* is an inert substance that can cause "beneficial" and "adverse" reactions. Drugs can also, in addition to their real effects, produce "placebo" effects based on a health professional's attitudes and a patient's expectations.

TREATMENT OUTCOME

Treatment outcome can never be predicted with certainty for individual patients and depends on the following:
- Drug: Physical and chemical properties (structure) are exactly known; this not a variable factor.
- Patient: Most patients respond similarly to drugs, but differences in genetic backgrounds (family history), environment (polluted air), habits (smoking, physical fitness), and compliance can cause unpredictable drug responses; this is a variable factor.
- Health professional: Most health professionals are well trained, but differences exist in knowledge ("relevant and irrelevant facts"), experience, attitude (placebo), and instructions (written) provided; this is a variable factor.

DRUG USE

The use of a particular drug is based on benefit versus risk: The benefits of the use of a drug MUST outweighs the risks to the patient.

Some abbreviations found on drug prescriptions are as follows:

d	day
q	every
q4h	every 4 hours
qd	every day, take one dose a day
qod	every other day
bid	twice a day
tid	three times a day
qid	four times a day
tiw	three times a week
hs	at bed time
pc	after meals
ad lib, prn	use when or as needed

IMPLICATIONS FOR THE PHYSICAL THERAPIST

- Patients today are often afraid to take medications because of widely publicized adverse reactions. Advise patients that drugs are given only when the benefit outweighs the risk and should be taken as recommended. Many adverse reactions are only listed as possibilities for legal reasons and their actual occurrence is often doubtful. Tell patients that taking a drug is like driving a car: There is a definite benefit involved, but there is always the possibility of an accident.
- Advise patients that many adverse reactions are minor and often disappear if the drug is discontinued early on. Patients should not "look" for adverse reactions but should be aware of such reactions when they occur and then should contact the physician immediately.
- Inform patients that humans are individuals and that therapeutic and adverse reactions can vary from individual to individual. If no therapeutic effect is experienced or an adverse reaction manifests, patients should contact the physician.
- Inform patients that generic drugs look different from brand name drugs but contain exactly the same active ingredients and are as effective as the brand name drug, with very few exceptions as indicated by the physician.

PHARMACODYNAMICS

INTRODUCTION

Pharmacodynamics describes the interaction between a drug and a special part of a cell called a receptor. This interaction produces a biochemical and/or physiological effect and is referred to as the pharmacological response. This response can be a therapeutic or an adverse reaction.

RECEPTOR

A receptor is usually a small area (specific chemical configuration, active site) of a macromolecule on or in a cell (in rare cases, the area can be extracellular such as on blood constituents). This macromolecule is mostly a protein. When stimulated, specific biochemical and/or physiological responses occur.

Receptors are constantly synthesized by the nucleus, transported to their respective sites, and later on degraded. Receptors determine specificity (which drug is going to be bound to which receptor, the drug is the "key" and the receptor the "lock") and affinity (how strong a drug is going to be bound to the receptor).

Most receptors are membrane receptors and are usually located on a protein that "snakes" through a cell membrane:

```
xxxxxx xXXx xxxx xxxx
          ----x-x----x-x-x-x-x----
Membrane   x x   x x x x x
          ----x-x----x-x-x-x-x----
          xxxx xxxx xxxx xxxx
                         xxxxxx
```

x = Amino acid
XX = Amino acids representing receptor

Other receptors can be located on an enzyme or on deoxyribonucleic acid (DNA) molecules. Receptors are usually classified according to endogenous stimulating agents (e.g., neurotransmitters, hormones) and are then further subdivided into subtypes based on drug action (adds therapeutic specificity):

Endogenous acetylcholine → all cholinergic receptors

Exogenous compounds affect the following cholinergic receptors differently:

Muscarine → only some cholinergic receptors: Classified as muscarinic receptors

(M → M1, M2, M3, ...)

Nicotine → other cholinergic receptors: Classified as nicotinic receptors

(N → Nn, Nm, ...)

Receptors are coupled directly or via second messenger systems (signal transduction) to an effector unit (e.g., ion channels) to produce the following response:

Drug → receptor → opens channel → starts flow of electrolytes (e.g., origination of nerve impulse)

Drug → receptor → G-protein (family, +,−) → enzymes (adenylyl cyclase, guanylylcyclase, phospholipase I, other) → second messengers (cyclic adenosine monophosphate or c-AMP, cyclic guanosine monophosphate or c-GMP, inositoltriphosphate or IP3, diacetylglycerol or DAG) → muscle activation or channel opening (e.g., cardiac muscle contraction).

A cell can carry many different receptor types, each consisting of thousands of individual receptors. The same receptor type can occur on cells of different tissues.

DRUG

A drug possesses a specific structure, including molecular size, functional groups, lipophilic or hydrophilic properties, and others, that determine its finding of and binding to a specific receptor (specificity and affinity or "lock and key")

and its response (e.g., contraction of a skeletal muscle).

CLASSIFICATION OF DRUGS

Agonists, which show affinity and intrinsic activity, cause a response and can be further divided into full agonists (which cause the maximum biological response) and partial agonists (which cause less than the maximum biological response and can be antagonists at high endogenous ligand activity).

Antagonists, which show only affinity, do not cause a response directly but block action of endogenous compounds and reduce their responses. They can be further divided into competitive, reversible antagonists and their effects can be overcome by increased amounts of endogenous or agonistic compounds (surmountable effects) and noncompetitive, irreversible antagonists that bind covalently to receptors and their effects can not be or only partially be overcome (insurmountable effects).

Most drugs are specific for and bind to only one particular receptor type. Some drugs can bind to more than one receptor type causing multiple pharmacological effects.

DRUG-RECEPTOR INTERACTION

The interaction of a ligand (drug [D] or endogenous chemical) with a receptor (R) produces the physiological/pharmacological response (e.g., increase in heart rate). The binding forces involve Van der Waals forces (weak) and ionic, hydrogen, and/or covalent bonds (the latter results in irreversible, prolonged binding).

D+R→D-R complex+response→D+R

Most D-R complexes are very short-lived, and the drug is quickly removed from receptor (e.g., by destruction, diffusion from receptor or tissue uptake). If covalent bonding occurs, actions are prolonged.

D-R binding depends on drug concentration (law of mass action, see equation below) and the maximal response depends on the number of receptors stimulated by the ligand. The response is usually graded (stepwise increases in response) and shows ceiling effect (no further increases).

A theoretical example is as follows: Only a fraction of available receptors (e.g., 10 out of 100, in reality there are thousands) will be activated. Only 20 drug molecules are shown (in reality there are millions):

1D + 1R → 1D - R + EFFECT = 0 → 1D + 1R below threshold
5D + 5R → 5D - R + EFFECT = 5 → 5D + 5R increment

10D + 10R → 10D - R + EFFECT = 10 → 10D + 10R increment

20D + 10R → 10D - R + EFFECT = 10 → 20D + 10R ceiling

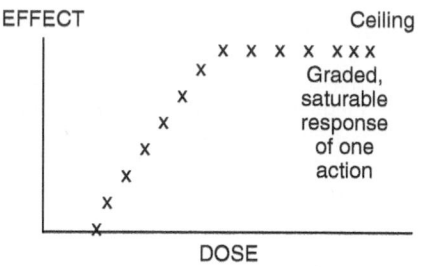

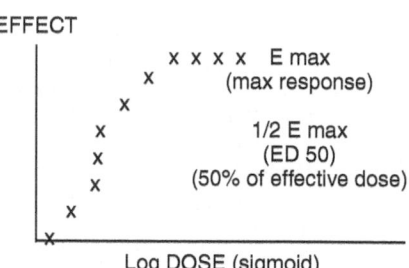

Initial drug response depends on drug dose (to reach threshold values where first response is detected and graded increases of this response), and the final maximal drug response depends on number of receptors present and stimulated.

For all drug effects, there is a therapeutic threshold (beneficial effects occur) and as the dose increases, a toxic threshold (overdose) is reached—the difference in doses is the margin of safety of a drug.

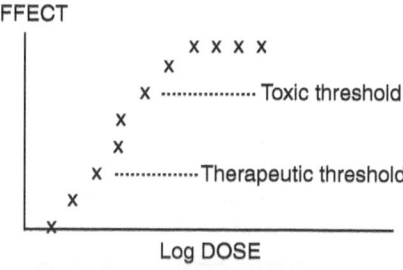

Clinically, drugs can be compared by their efficacy and potency: Efficacy is the maximal effect of a drug, whereas potency is the dose that produces a specific effect. A drug can show a high potency (causes effect at a low dose) but low efficacy (response is mild).

The dose-frequency response curve among individuals is bell-shaped. It depicts the response of groups of patients who respond to a particular drug dose.

A theoretical example is as follows: 102 patients with headache are tested with a drug and the number of patients obtaining relief from a particular dose in milligrams of the drug is plotted against drug concentrations.

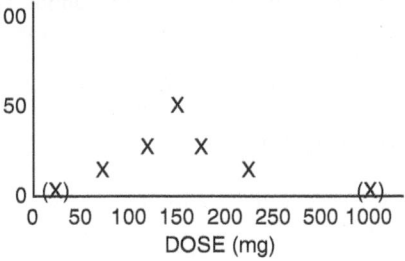

NUMBER RESPONDING TO ONE DOSE

DOSE (mg)

Number responding	Drug (mg)
1	5
5	75
20	125
50	150
20	175
5	225
1	1000

Distribution (a bell-shaped curve) represents normal variability within a population; most individuals fall within a narrow dose range (normal distribution, minor individual variations). Very few (x) individuals fall outside, representing major biological differences.

FACTORS INFLUENCING DRUG PHARMACODYNAMIC DRUG RESPONSES

- Specificity and number of receptors are genetically determined and vary from patient to patient and so do their drug responses.
- Chronic stimulation of receptors by agonists causes downregulation (decrease in number/affinity of receptors or reduced activity) and chronic blockade of receptors by antagonists causes upregulation (increase in number/affinity of receptors or increased activity). These processes play a role in some drug responses (e.g., antidepressant drugs) and the development of tolerance and physical dependence.
- Diseases can cause receptor abnormalities (usually decreases) that result in idiosyncratic drug responses (e.g., myasthenia gravis in which the immune system destroys the receptors on skeletal muscles and causes muscle fatigue and weakness).
- Receptors develop during the early days, months, and years of life (neonatal pharmacology) and decline during older age (geriatric pharmacology). This results in fewer numbers of receptors (including enzymes involved in biotransformation). In general, starting dose in "young"

and "old" patients is usually one-half to one-third of a normal adult dose.
- Drugs can compete for the same receptor and an antagonist can reduce the effects of an agonist (drug interaction).

SUMMARY

The pharmacological responses, whether therapeutic and adverse, arise from the interaction of the drug (molecular weight, chemical and physical properties, or specific functional groups) and endogenous receptors (small active areas usually located on a macromolecule; structure and number determined by genetics but also affected by age, diseases, and certain drugs). This binding follows the "lock" and "key" principle. One tissue may contain many different receptor types, and a specific type might occur on different tissues.

The structure of the receptor determines the specific pharmacological response (therapeutic or adverse) of the drug and the number of receptors determines its maximal effect.

IMPLICATIONS FOR THE PHYSICAL THERAPIST

Be aware that younger and older individuals may respond somewhat differently to medications. Young individuals and geriatric patients must be watched more carefully because they often show more adverse reactions.

Geriatric patients often receive multiple medications that are sometimes prescribed by different physicians and obtained at different pharmacies. Patients should make a list of all medications and show this to every physician. Also, patients should obtain all medications from the same pharmacy so the pharmacist can prevent potentially dangerous drug interactions.

Patient should be informed that therapeutic and adverse reactions can never be predicted with certainty because individuals will have different genetic and environmental backgrounds. It is mostly the patient who must monitor therapeutic progress and spot adverse reactions, but this can be helped by health professionals who can observe patients closely.

PHARMACOKINETICS

INTRODUCTION

Pharmacokinetics describes the effects of the body on the drug or its "journey" into, through, and out of the body. Pharmacokinetics determines to a large extent the best formulation of a drug, the dose to be used, the route of administration, onset and duration of action of a drug,

the distribution in the body, dosing schedule by repeated applications, and some unexpected drug reactions.

STRUCTURE OF DRUG

The chemical structure of the drug (small or large molecular weight or hydrophilic or lipophilic properties) and the composition of the tablet (quick or slow release of the drug) are major factors in the kinetics of a drug. Most drugs are manufactured to deliver the dose gradually into the body (e.g., a tablet can be broken in half), but some drugs are manufactured as slow-release drugs where the dose is delivered over a longer period of time (these preparations cannot be broken in half).

DRUG ADMINISTRATION

Drugs can be administered via the alimentary routes (oral, sublingual, or rectal administration), parenteral routes (intravenous [IV], intramuscular [IM], or subcutaneous [SC] administration), or topically (eyes, skin, or lungs via inhalation). Transdermal means administration into the blood stream via a patch on the skin.

IV injections and inhalation produce the fastest onset, whereas oral administration is most convenient but delays onset of action.

DRUG DISTRIBUTION

After oral administration, the tablets must be dissolved in the stomach and intestines and are then absorbed into the blood stream. After IM or SC injection, absorption occurs from the site of injection into the blood stream. After IV injection, the drug is injected directly into the blood stream. From the blood, drugs reach all tissues in the body, except certain drugs that will not cross the blood-brain barrier. This initiates therapeutic responses in the target organs; adverse reactions usually occur in tissues other than the intended site(s). Some tissues, such as adipose tissues, trap certain drugs without showing a response (site of loss) but can release the drug slowly (e.g., weeks) even after the drug has been stopped.

Distribution for most drugs occurs by diffusion following Fick's law: Drug molecules move along a concentration gradient (from high to low) until equilibrium is reached. Some drugs are distributed by other mechanisms such as active transport processes.

In the blood, some drugs can be highly bound to plasma proteins, which can slow down distribution into individual tissues but can also prolong its action even after the drug has been stopped.

ELIMINATION

Drugs must eventually be eliminated from the body to prevent accumulation.

NEPHRON (schematic)

Some organic acids, bases (active transport)

Hydrophilic compounds → Hydrophilic comp → Urine (GF)

Lipophilic compounds → Lipophilic comp → Blood

Passive diffusion (back into blood)

The action of the drug is terminated by the body by two major processes: Removal or excretion mostly through the kidneys and chemical inactivation or biotransformation (metabolism) in the liver.

Excretion in the kidney starts with glomerular filtration (GF) in which most drug molecules are filtered into the nephron. Here, lipophilic drug molecules are reabsorbed into the blood (generally, the kidney can not excrete lipophilic molecules) and hydrophilic drug molecules are excreted into the urine. In addition, there are special secretory processes for some drugs. Thus the health of the kidney can influence how fast a drug can leave the body (or the duration of action). Renal diseases necessitate a reduction in dose to avoid overdose reactions.

Biotransformation or *drug metabolism* is the inactivation or chemical alteration of a drug mostly by the liver. The main purpose is to convert lipophilic drugs (which the kidney cannot excrete) into hydrophilic compounds (which the kidney can excrete). These products are called *metabolites,* and they can be devoid of therapeutic action (inactive metabolites) or can still maintain the therapeutic action (active metabolites), which in the latter case would prolong duration of the drug action. A drug can have many (sometimes tens) of metabolites.

Drug→active metabolite→inactive metabolite(final excretion of drug→inactivemetabolite and/or metabolites by kidney)

These chemical reactions are performed by enzymes referred to as p450 enzymes or mixed function oxidases. They are divided into phase I reactions (oxidation, reduction, and hydrolysis reactions) and phase II reactions (conjugation to hydrophilic endogenous compounds). Some drugs are so quickly metabolized when passing through the liver for the first time that they must be given at very high oral doses or must be injected (first-pass effect). Some drugs can induce drug metabolizing enzymes and accelerate their own metabolism or slowly shorten the duration of action—this is referred to as tolerance and necessitates an increase in dose over time. Hepatic diseases with decreased biotransformation

capacity often demand a reduction in dose to avoid overdose reactions.

Elimination is the combined action of excretion and metabolism. Most drugs are eliminated following first-order kinetics (constant fraction or % is eliminated). This determines the half-life ($t\frac{1}{2}$) of a drug, which is the time it takes for the drug levels in the blood to fall to one-half. (Few drugs follow zero-order kinetics in which a constant amount is eliminated per unit time.)

A theoretical example of first order (µg/mL [drug blood levels]) is as follows:

Time (hr)	Dose A (10 mg)	Dose B (40 mg)
0	100	400
1	50	200
2	25	100
3	12.5	50
4	6.2	25
5	3.1	12.5
6	—	6.2
7	—	3.1

Different drugs can have different half-lives (example shows 1 hr half-life); an increase in dose increases blood and tissue levels but prolongs time of action relatively little; after 4 to 5 half-lives, about 95% of the drug has disappeared from the blood (and the body).

Chronic drug administrations must be performed in proper time intervals, which are the half-life time of the particular drug (if half-life is 6 hours, drug is to be taken every 6 hours). Chronic drug therapy is often started with regular doses (delay in onset of therapeutic action by about 4 to 5 half-lives) or a high dose (loading dose) followed by maintenance doses at half-time intervals (quick onset of action).

SUMMARY

Dosage considerations are based on a careful observation of the patient. Genetic makeup, health status, and compliance can markedly influence the efficacy and toxicity of a drug. For example, higher than recommended doses are necessary in obese individuals (large volume of distribution) or fast metabolizers (drug too quickly inactivated). Lower doses should be given to small individuals, slow metabolizers, individuals with impaired kidney function or hepatic problems (including alcohol abuse), or young or geriatric individuals (elimination process not fully developed or already declining). Drugs can compete with each other for drug metabolizing enzymes and slow down their inactivation, leading to overdose drug levels in the body (drug interactions). Diet can interfere with the absorption of some but not all drugs (e.g., tetracyclines should not be taken with antacids or foods). Failure to obey dosing schedules by the patient can lead to too low or too high drug levels with decreased efficacy or increased toxicity.

IMPLICATIONS FOR THE PHYSICAL THERAPIST

- Inform patients to take medications exactly as prescribed, because too low or missed doses can decrease the beneficial effects of a drug or too much of

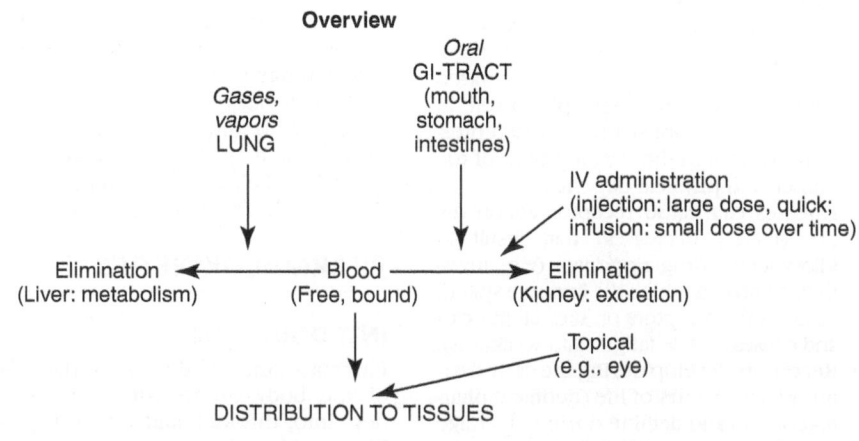

Overview

Gases, vapors LUNG

Oral GI-TRACT (mouth, stomach, intestines)

IV administration (injection: large dose, quick; infusion: small dose over time)

Elimination (Liver: metabolism) ← Blood (Free, bound) → Elimination (Kidney: excretion)

Topical (e.g., eye)

DISTRIBUTION TO TISSUES

(RECEPTORS = Therapeutic and adverse reactions, sites of loss with no effects) a drug can increase its adverse reactions. The patient should make a list and record the times when the drug should be taken.

- Inform patients that it is very important if a drug should be taken with meals or before or after a meal, because this can significantly affect the therapeutic response and adverse reactions.
- Inform patients that the drug should be taken as long as directed by a physician even if he or she feels better (e.g., in the case of antibiotics, remaining bacteria that do not cause clinical signs must still be eliminated.
- If a dose has been missed, inform the patient (unless otherwise instructed by the physician) to take the next dose if it is less than half the time before the next dose. For most drugs, the following is recommended: If a drug should be taken every 6 hours and the last dose was taken at 8 AM, then next doses should be taken at 2 PM and the next at 8 PM. If the 2 PM dose was missed, it can still be taken at 4 PM but not at 6 PM; in this case, it is better to skip the dose.
- Tell patients that they can split tablets, because sometimes the higher dose is as expensive as the lower dose. By splitting, the patient can obtain double the lower doses for the same amount of money. Also, warn the patient that they should NOT split slow-release or extended-release tablets.
- Inform patients that topically prescribed drugs (e.g., ointments) are effective and penetrate into the designated area but can also diffuse into and throughout the entire body. Thus excessive amounts should be avoided because they can cause unnecessary adverse reactions.

ACE INHIBITORS

COMMON DRUGS (SELECTION OF SOME OF THE MOST COMMONLY USED DRUGS)

Benazepril	Lotensin
Captopril	Capoten
Enalapril	Vasotec
Fosinopril	Monopril
Lisinopril	Prinivil, Zestril
Moexipril	Univasc
Perindopril	Aceon
Quinapril	Accupril
Ramipril	Altace
Trandolapril	Mavik

MECHANISM OF ACTION

Peripheral blood pressure is regulated by many mechanisms one of which is the angiotensin system. The enzyme renin is released from the kidney, which converts angiotensinogen into angiotensin I. Then, angiotensin-converting enzyme (ACE) converts angiotensin I to

angiotensin II. Angiotensin II acts on angiotensin receptors in the blood vessels, causing vasoconstriction and increased blood pressure. In addition, angiotensin increases aldosterone secretion, which leads to salt and water retention, adding to the increased blood pressure.

ACE inhibitors inhibit ACE and reduce the formation of angiotensin II, which causes less stimulation of angiotensin receptors, blood vessel dilation, and a fall in blood pressure. In addition, ACE inhibitors reduce aldosterone secretion, resulting in more water and salt excretion, lower blood volume, and decreased pressure.

INDICATIONS

- *Hypertension:* Vasoconstriction or increased peripheral resistance is a major cause of increased blood pressure. Hypertension untreated is linked to myocardial infarctions (MIs) and strokes. ACE inhibitors reduce formation of the vasoconstrictor angiotensin II and reduce blood pressure and can reduce the risk of secondary MIs and strokes.
- *Congestive heart failure* (CHF): When the heart cannot pump enough blood to other organs of the body, the result of this increased action is an enlarged but inefficient heart and the patient becomes quickly fatigued and short of breath (pulmonary edema) during even the slightest exertion. ACE inhibitors cause vasodilation and reduce afterload and peripheral resistance, which helps the heart to eject blood more easily and efficiently.
- *Diabetic nephropathy:* ACE inhibitors decrease the progression of diabetic nephropathy possibly by dilating renal blood vessels and increasing blood flow to the kidney (captopril).
- *Migraine headaches* (lisinopril) by an uncertain mechanism.
- All of these drugs inhibit ACE, but their indications and dosages vary among patients and the diseases to be treated. African-American patients with hypertension seem to respond less to some of these drugs.

EXAMPLES OF COMMON DOSAGES (GENERAL GUIDELINES, MANY DIFFERENT DOSAGE SCHEDULES)

Benazepril	5-40 mg 1-2 times daily by mouth (PO)
Captopril	12.5-150 mg 3 times daily PO
Enalapril	2.5-40 mg 1-2 times daily PO
Fosinopril	10-80 mg once daily PO for a maximum of 80 mg/day
Lisinopril	10-40 mg once daily PO
Moexipril	7.5-30 mg once daily PO
Perindopril	4-16 mg 1-2 times daily PO
Quinapril	10-80 mg once daily PO
Ramipril	2.5-20 mg/day in 1-2 divided doses PO
Trandolapril	1-4 mg once daily PO

ADMINISTRATION

ACE inhibitors are given IV and PO. They vary in onset between 20 to 60 minutes and have a duration of action of 6 to 24 hours.

CONTRAINDICATIONS

ACE inhibitors are contraindicated in cases of hypersensitivity with some cross-sensitivity among the drugs. These drugs should be used with caution in cases of renal or hepatic impairments. Mixing some ACE inhibitors with nonsteroidal antiinflammatory drugs (NSAIDs) can cause kidney failure.

COMMON ADVERSE REACTIONS

Adverse reactions include headache, dizziness, hypotension, cough, taste disturbances, and rarely, agranulocytosis, neutropenia, or angioedema.

DRUG INTERACTIONS

Hypotensive effects are enhanced by other antihypertensive drugs. Hyperkalemia may occur with potassium-sparing diuretics. Antacids may decrease absorption and effectiveness of ACE inhibitors. Sympathomimetic over-the-counter (OTC) cold medications can antagonize the blood-pressure lowering effects of ACE inhibitors. ACE inhibitors can enhance the hypoglycemic action of hypoglycemics.

IMPLICATIONS FOR PHYSICAL THERAPISTS

- Advise the patient to change positions and get up slowly because orthostatic hypotension may occur mostly in the beginning of therapy and in geriatric individuals. This can be aggravated if patient sweats heavily in a warm environment during strenuous exercise.
- If the patient complains about a sore throat, notify the physician or have the patient notify the physician, because this could be an early warning sign of agranulocytosis. If you notice or patient complains about swollen ankles or welts, notify the physician or have the patient contact the physician because this could indicate an angioedema.
- Be careful when using a heated therapeutic pool because warm water can aggravate the vasodilatory effects of peripheral vascular dilators and lead to a marked decrease in blood pressure.

α-AGONISTS

COMMON DRUGS (SELECTION OF SOME OF THE MOST COMMONLY USED DRUGS)

Direct-acting α₁*-agonists*

Epinephrine (has also beta activity)	Adrenaline, Ana-Guard, Primatene Mist, other
Midodrine	ProAmatine
Phenylephrine	Neo-Synephrine (OTC)

Direct-acting α₂*-agonists (see Miscellaneous Vasodilators)*

Clonidine	Catapres, Duraclon

Direct- and indirect-acting α*–agonists (have also beta activity)*

Ephedrine	Generic
Pseudoephe-drine	Sudafed, Drixoral, Decofed, other (OTC)

MECHANISM OF ACTION

α₁-Receptors are usually but not exclusively found opposite postganglionic sympathetic fibers, which release norepinephrine, which activates these receptors. Activation of these receptors constricts blood vessels (with increased peripheral resistance and increased blood pressure), closes the sphincter muscle and the neck of the bladder (preventing urinary outflow), and constricts the capsule/muscles of the prostate. α₁-Agonists stimulate these receptors directly or indirectly.

α₂-Receptors are mostly found in the brain where their stimulation in the vasomotor center reduces sympathetic outflow, which decreases heart rate and contractility and relaxes blood vessels. These effects reduce blood pressure.

Direct- and indirect-acting drugs stimulate α₁- and/or α₂-receptors. They stimulate directly but also cause stimulation indirectly by increasing synaptic levels of norepinephrine by facilitating its release.

INDICATIONS

α-Agonists are indicated in the following:
- *Nasal congestion:* Viral or allergic causes produce vasodilatation and leakage of water into adjacent tissue. α₁-Agonists and indirect-acting drugs constrict blood vessels, stop leakage, and open airways; common nasal sprays contain naphazoline, xylometazoline, phenylephrine, or oxymetazoline.
- *Allergic conditions,* in which part of the problem is vasodilation. α₁-Agonists and indirect-acting drugs constrict blood vessels. Ocular drugs that counteract congestion and redness are naphazoline, oxymetazoline, tetrahydrozoline, and phenylephrine. In case of an anaphylactic reaction, epinephrine SC is necessary.
- *Shock* caused by fluid loss, bleeding, or other causes. Drugs increase blood pressure by vasoconstriction and cardiac stimulation, in the case of indirect-acting drugs. Ephedrine is also used in cases of mild *hypotension.*
- *Bronchoconstriction:* Constriction of bronchi interferes with airflow. Indirect-acting drugs and epinephrine are used as sprays or orally to open airways.
- *Ocular eye examinations:* Phenylephrine causes mydriasis, allowing better examination of the posterior parts of the eye or for minor ocular irritation to constrict dilated blood vessels (e.g., oxymetazoline).

EXAMPLES OF COMMON DOSAGES (GENERAL GUIDELINES, MANY DIFFERENT DOSAGE SCHEDULES)

Epinephrine	1-2 puffs or 0.1 to 0.5 mg SC
Midodrine	2.5-10 mg 2 to 3 times daily PO
Pseudoephedrine	60 mg q6h (not to exceed 240 mg/day) PO
Ephedrine	25 mg 4 times a day PO

ADMINISTRATION

α-Agonists can be given SC, IM, IV, PO, inhalation, and topical in the eye.

CONTRAINDICATIONS

α-Agonists are contraindicated or should be used with caution in hypertension, arrhythmias, and benign prostatic hyperplasia (leading to urinary hesitancy, retention).

COMMON ADVERSE REACTIONS

Adverse reactions include nervousness, restlessness, tremor, hypertension, angina, bradycardia (caused by increased blood pressure), and arrhythmias. Indirect-acting drugs may cause central nervous system (CNS) stimulation and anorexia. Nasal and ocular applications in rapid succession (after 2 to 3 days) can lead to a rebound effect in which congestion becomes worse with each application. For epinephrine only: Excessive use of inhalers can lead to bronchospasm.

DRUG INTERACTIONS

- α-Agonists antagonize the effects of the α-blockers and antihypertensive drugs. They can precipitate a hypertensive crisis in conjunction with monoamine oxidase (MAO) inhibitors. Antacids that alkalinize the urine can intensify their effects.
- Foods that acidify (cheeses, fish, and meat) or alkalinize (most fruits and vegetables) the urine can decrease or intensify effects of α-agonists.

IMPLICATIONS FOR PHYSICAL THERAPISTS

- Some of these drugs are available OTC in nasal sprays, cold medications, and ocular solutions. Patients often assume that OTC drugs are safe and can be used without any precautions. Advise patients that OTC medications are drugs and must be used with care and according to instructions.
- If you notice that blood pressure has increased in a patient taking antihypertensive medication or if the patient shows increased restlessness, inquire about the use of OTC medications and if an α-agonist is used. Advise the patient to contact the physician.
- If you notice that the patient uses a nasal spray too often, inform the patient that he or she might suffer from a rebound effect and should contact the physician.
- Advise older men with benign prostatic hyperplasia that use of OTC α-agonists can lead to urinary hesitancy or even retention.

α-BLOCKERS

COMMON DRUGS (SELECTION OF SOME OF THE MOST COMMONLY USED DRUGS)

Doxazosin	Cardura
Phenoxybenzamine	Dibenzyline
Prazosin	Minipress
Tamsulosin	Flomax
Terazosin	Hytrin

MECHANISM OF ACTION

α₁-Receptors are usually but not exclusively found opposite postganglionic sympathetic fibers, which release norepinephrine which activates these receptors. Activation of these receptors constricts blood vessels (with increased peripheral resistance and increased blood pressure), closes the sphincter muscle and neck of the bladder (prevents urinary outflow), and constricts the capsule/muscles of the prostate.

Competitive blockade of these receptors by α-antagonists or blockers causes the opposite effects (which can be antagonized or overcome by use of α-agonists).

INDICATIONS

α-Blockers are indicated in the following:
- *Hypertension:* Vasoconstriction or increased peripheral resistance is a major cause of increased blood pressure. α-Blockers block α-receptors and relax blood vessels, decrease peripheral resistance, and lower blood pressure.

- *Benign prostatic hyperplasia:* α-Blockers relax the sphincter muscle and bladder neck, leading to more efficient bladder emptying, and relax the capsule/muscles of the prostate, providing improved urinary flow.

EXAMPLES OF COMMON DOSAGES (GENERAL GUIDELINES, MANY DIFFERENT DOSAGE SCHEDULES)

Doxazosin	1-16 mg once daily PO
Phenoxyben-zamine	10-40 mg twice daily PO
Prazosin	1-15 mg 2-3 times daily (not to exceed 40 mg/day) PO
Tamsulosin	0.4-0.8 mg once daily PO
Terazosin	1-5 mg once or twice a day (not to exceed 20 mg/day) PO

ADMINISTRATION

α-Blockers are administered PO. Some, such as phentolamine, are only given IV or IM.

CONTRAINDICATIONS

Hypersensitivity to α-blockers.

COMMON ADVERSE REACTIONS

Common adverse reactions include headache, stuffy nose, fatigue, palpitations, and tachycardia (as blood pressure drops, heart rate increases reflexly); marked "first dose" syncope (fainting); and later, less severe orthostatic hypotension. Geriatric patients are at increased risk of experiencing adverse reactions.

DRUG INTERACTIONS

There is an increased risk of hypotension with drugs that also lower blood pressure, including alcohol, sildenafil, and others. Some cold medications containing phenylephrine or other α-agonistic compounds can antagonize actions of α-blockers.

IMPLICATIONS FOR PHYSICAL THERAPISTS

- Be careful when a patient changes positions or stands up because of possible orthostatic hypotension (dizziness, fainting), in particular, at the beginning of therapy or in geriatric patients.
- Watch patient when he or she stops after strenuous exercise because risk of a hypotensive episode is increased.
- Advise patients to be careful when using a heated therapeutic pool because warm water can aggravate the vasodilatory effects of peripheral vascular dilators and lead to a marked decrease in blood pressure.

ALTERNATIVE MEDICATIONS

Alternative medications include herbal preparations, vitamins, minerals, and other products (but not prescription drugs and OTC medications) used for other than nutritional reasons.

Prescription drugs and OTC drugs have to be approved by the FDA after companies have performed extensive studies in animals and humans to establish efficacy and toxicity. Drugs are then approved for a specific indication and must state active ingredient(s), inactive ingredients, and exact dose and administration schedule, as well as suggested mode of action and adverse reactions as compiled (e.g., in the Physician's Desk Reference [PDR]).

Alternative medications are handled like foods by the FDA and must state content but NOT dose, and companies are not required to submit proof of efficacy and toxicity as long as companies do not make a specific health claim but remain vague in their indications ("might be good for your health"). Because of this lack of control, products often contain varying amounts of the specified product and sometimes are subject to fraudulent practices.

Claims for their beneficial effects are often based on cultural aspects ("has been used by the Chinese for centuries"), folklore ("this herb is known for a long time to help you to sleep"), and some epidemiological correlations ("a survey of a large number of individuals has shown that individuals who consume a lot of a specific mineral will have less breast cancer"—although this is a valid correlation, it does not indicate that this mineral does prevent this cancer). In addition, there is the misconception by many people that naturally occurring alternative medications are safe because they are derived from nature—which is wrong because natural products can be quite toxic (e.g., poison ivy, poisonous mushrooms).

At present, a number of controlled clinical trials are conducted with certain alternative medications and in the years to come, more information about the benefits and dangers of alternative medications will become more evident. At present, many "hopes" about these medications have been shattered by these clinical trials. Thus most information available today is tentative at best and is constantly changing.

VITAMINS

Vitamins are a group of unrelated substances essential for many normal biochemical and physiological processes (e.g., catalysts for enzymes) that are obtained from the diet or synthesized (vitamin D) by the body. For nutritional purposes, they are required only in small quantities as estimated by the recommended dietary allowances (RDA) and are present in sufficient amounts in a balanced daily diet (meats, carbohydrates, and dairy products and lots of fruits and vegetables—plus, many foods are now vitamin/mineral fortified) to prevent vitamin or mineral deficiency diseases. There is no need for supplementation in healthy individuals on a balanced diet to maintain a healthy body and mind except perhaps for some infants, older people, work-related conditions, heavily menstruating or pregnant/lactating women, individuals consuming improper diets, certain diseases, and/or some drug therapies.

Recently, higher doses of certain vitamins have been suggested to prevent or to cure certain diseases such as emphysema/asthma/bronchitis, cardiovascular diseases, cancer, aging, mental disorders, the common cold, and other health problems. At present, there is no firm evidence that this is indeed the case. However, very high doses of some vitamins (e.g., vitamins A, D, and perhaps E) can be quite toxic and/or increase the risk of certain diseases for which they were actually recommended in the first place. Legitimate and documented OTC uses include vitamin preparations that somewhat slow down age-related macular degeneration (vitamins E and C and beta-carotene) and vitamin D to increase calcium absorption. If vitamins are used, preparations that carry the label of the US Pharmacopeia are recommended because this private organization recognized by Congress has established some standards for vitamins and minerals (strength or amount of active ingredient, purity, disintegration, and dissolution).

MINERALS

Minerals are necessary for many biochemical processes (e.g., cofactors for enzymes), physiological functions (e.g., hemoglobin), and structural requirements (e.g., teeth, bones). Optimal mineral intake values for humans are still estimates, but a balanced diet seems to provide all necessary minerals to healthy individuals. In addition, many foods are supplemented with minerals.

Recently again, higher doses have been suggested even for healthy individuals to prevent or cure health problems. No firm evidence supports the use of minerals with the exception of calcium and vitamin D to increase bone formation and zinc to slow age-related macular degeneration but under the supervision of a health professional.

PHARMACOLOGY

Section V

HERBAL PREPARATIONS

A variety of herbal medications is available claiming or suggesting many benefits (most of which have not been medically verified or have been proven wrong in the meantime). Also, some of these preparations have been found to cause significant health problems or even death (e.g., ephedra) or can significantly interfere with prescription drugs either reducing their efficacy or increasing their toxicity.

It has been claimed that echinacea stimulates the immune system (if true, it would be strongly contraindicated in cases of autoimmune diseases), garlic reduces the risk of cardiovascular diseases (but bleeding episodes can occur with heparin, warfarin, and aspirin), ginger reduces nausea and vomiting (with some evidence), gingko biloba increases memory and cognition and improves circulation (bleeding episodes with heparin, warfarin, and aspirin can occur), St. John's wort improves mood (with some support for mild depression but can interfere with some antiviral drugs and anticancer medications), and valerian treats anxiety and insomnia (it indeed has some calming properties).

BIOCHEMICALS

A number of biochemicals are offered for a variety of health problems, most of which have not been documented with rigorous scientific trials. For example, melatonin is a naturally occurring substance in the body that physiologically is involved in sleep and is now marketed as a sleep promoter. Although its use is safe, it does not seem to induce sleep and help jet lag in most except a few individuals. Glucosamine and chondroitin are components needed to build and maintain articular cartilage and synovial fluid, and it has been claimed that their use can help patients with osteoarthritis. Although most individuals do not seem to get relief, a few individuals indeed seem to benefit. Unfortunately, both compounds cause significant gastrointestinal (GI) problems like nausea, cramping, and heart burn. Omega-3 polyunsaturated fatty acids might be beneficial to prevent certain cardiovascular risks, but many experts recommend that these biochemicals can be obtained from eating fish 2 to 3 times a week.

IMPLICATIONS FOR THE PHYSICAL THERAPIST

- It is important to stress to the patient that the most important aspects of maintaining good health and preventing diseases are a well-balanced diet, an optimistic outlook on life, and daily physical exercise.
- It is important to inform the patient that the benefits of alternative medications, with exceptions as outlined above, are still unproved, the use of these preparations is not risk-free, and that some of alternative medications can interfere detrimentally with prescription drugs. They should not be taken without the advice of a physician, and their use must be stated when a medical history is taken.
- It is important to inform the less affluent patient to spend available money on good food rather than alternative medications.
- It is important to warn the patient about advertisements of these products on TV, in newspapers, or websites because they often contain half-truths. When searching the internet, attention should be paid to websites that end in ".edu" or ".gov" because these come from universities and government agencies and can be trusted. Many other websites may or may not have correct information, and their intention is mostly to sell rather than inform.

ANGIOTENSIN II RECEPTOR BLOCKERS

COMMON DRUGS (SELECTION OF SOME OF THE MOST COMMONLY USED DRUGS)

Candesartan	Atacand
Eprosartan	Teveten
Irbesartan	Avapro
Losartan	Cozaar
Olmesartan	Benicar
Telmisartan	Micardis
Valsartan	Diovan

MECHANISM OF ACTION

Peripheral blood pressure is regulated by many mechanisms including the angiotensin system. The enzyme renin is released from the kidney and converts angiotensinogen into angiotensin I. The enzyme ACE converts this to angiotensin II. Angiotensin II acts on angiotensin receptors (AT1) in the blood vessels, causing vasoconstriction and increases in blood pressure. In addition, angiotensin II increases aldosterone secretion, which leads to salt and water retention in the kidney and also an increase in blood pressure.

Angiotensin II receptor blockers block the action of angiotensin II on the blood vessel receptors, causing vasodilation and reducing the secretion of aldosterone, which enhances renal excretion of salts and water. Both actions reduce blood pressure.

INDICATIONS

Angiotensin II receptor blockers are indicated in the following:
- *Hypertension:* Vasoconstriction or increased peripheral resistance is a major cause of increased blood pressure. Hypertension untreated is linked to MIs and strokes. These antagonists block the action of the vasoconstrictor angiotensin and also reduce the secretion of aldosterone; both of these lower blood pressure and can reduce the risk of secondary MIs and strokes.
- *CHF:* When the heart cannot pump enough blood to other organs of the body, the result is an enlarged but inefficient heart and the patient becomes quickly fatigued and short of breath (pulmonary edema) during even the slightest exertion. These drugs (candesartan, valsartan) cause vasodilatation and reduce afterload or peripheral resistance, which helps the heart eject blood more easily and efficiently.
- Other uses include diabetic nephropathy in type II diabetes, possibly by dilating renal blood vessels and increasing blood flow to the kidney (irbesartan, losartan).
- All drugs block angiotensin II receptors, but their indications and dosages vary among patients and the diseases to be treated. African-American patients with hypertension seem to respond less to some of these drugs.

EXAMPLES OF COMMON DOSAGES (GENERAL GUIDELINES, MANY DIFFERENT DOSAGE SCHEDULES)

Candesartan	2-32 mg once or twice daily PO
Eprosartan	400-800 mg once daily PO
Irbesartan	150-300 mg once daily PO
Losartan	25-100 mg once daily PO
Olmesartan	10-20 mg once daily PO
Telmisartan	20-80 mg once daily PO
Valsartan	40-320 once or twice daily PO

ADMINISTRATION

Angiotensin II receptor blockers are mostly given PO and often used in combination with other antihypertensive medications.

CONTRAINDICATIONS

Angiotensin II receptor blockers are contraindicated or should be used with caution in patients with renal and hepatic impairments and certain cardiac conditions.

COMMON ADVERSE REACTIONS

Adverse reactions include dizziness, fatigue, hypotension, angioedema, and in rare cases, renal failure.

DRUG INTERACTIONS

- NSAIDs may decrease the effectiveness of these drugs. They can aggravate potassium retention with potassium-sparing diuretics and enhance the effects of other antihypertensive drugs.
- Effects are increased with mistletoe, astragalus, black cohosh, and others.

IMPLICATIONS FOR PHYSICAL THERAPISTS

• Advise the patient to change positions and get up slowly because orthostatic hypotension may occur in the beginning of therapy and in geriatric individuals. This can be aggravated if the patient sweats heavily in a warm environment during strenuous exercise.

• Be careful when using a heated therapeutic pool because warm water can aggravate the vasodilatory effects of peripheral vascular dilators and lead to a marked decrease in blood pressure.

ANTIARRHYTHMIC DRUGS

COMMON DRUGS (SELECTION OF SOME OF THE MOST COMMONLY USED DRUGS)

Class IA

Disopyramide	Norpace
Procainamide	Procanbid, Promine, Pronestyl
Quinidine	Quinalan, Cardioquin, Quinora, other

Class IB

Lidocaine	Xylocaine, other
Mexiletine	Mexitil
Phenytoin	Dilantin, Phenytex
Tocainide	Tonocard

Class IC

Flecainide	Tambocor
Propafenone	Rythmol

Class II or β-Blockers (see β-Blockers)
Acebutolol
Esmolol
Propranolol
Sotalol

Class III

Amiodarone	Cordarone, Pacerone
Ibutilide	Corvert

Class IV or Calcium Channel Blockers (see Calcium Channel Blockers)
Verapamil
Miscellaneous Drugs
Adenosine
Atropine (see Cholinergic Antagonists)

MECHANISM OF ACTION

Conduction/contraction coupling describes the movement of electrical and muscular activity over the heart that initiates sequential atrial and ventricular contractions to eject blood. Normally, the electrical impulses are initiated in the sinoatrial (SA) node and spread throughout the atria via multiple tracks initiating coordinated contraction of the muscles of the atria. Impulses converge on the atrioventricular (AV) node that sits at the juncture of the four chambers of the heart. They traverse the AV node and the bundle of His, enter the right and left conduction bundles in the right and left ventricles, and are distributed via the Purkinje fibers in a coordinated fashion to the muscles of the right and left ventricles, which now contract. Important pharmacological events are the initiation of electrical activity by β receptors in the SA node, the influx of sodium into cardiac cells leading to rapid depolarization, and the efflux of potassium and calcium from the cells causing slow repolarization. This is followed by a refractory period during which the cells of the electrical system reestablish their original electrolyte distribution and are unable to respond to an electrical impulse. Normal conduction starts within certain cells (called *pacemaker cells*) that depolarize spontaneously, initiating conduction. These cells are located mostly in the SA node and are responsible for initiation of normal cardiac rhythm. Lesser normal pacemaker cells are located in various areas of the heart and may become active only under abnormal circumstances.

Drugs can affect some of these events selectively. Class I drugs are essentially sodium channel blockers and reduce cellular sodium influx, the rate of depolarization, conduction, and membrane excitability. They can have other activities as well, and based on these effects, these drugs are subdivided into Class IA, IB, and IC drugs. Class II drugs or β-blockers block β₁-receptors in the SA and AV nodes, thus decreasing the rate of pacemaker activity or automaticity and slowing the rates of the development and propagation of the electrical impulses. Class III drugs slow the efflux of potassium from the cells, prolonging repolarization and slowing the electrical recovery period and thus the rate of conduction. Class IV drugs or calcium channel blockers block calcium channels, prolonging the period of repolarization, decreasing excitability, and slowing the rate of conduction.

INDICATIONS

Antiarrhythmic drugs are indicated in the following:

• *Arrhythmias* (or *dysrhythmias* because arrhythmia means no rhythm) are caused by the malfunction of pacemaker cells that are unable to maintain normal activity, the emergence of new pacemaker cells competing with the original ones, the interruption of normal conductance over the heart in that conduction cannot reach certain areas (heart blocks), or an upward and circular fashion with reexcitation of cardiac tissue (reentry), or a combination of above causes. Several different types of arrhythmias can range from harmless to life-threatening.

• These abnormalities are specifically influenced by different drug classes that try to normalize abnormal conduction patterns by selectively affecting β-receptors or individual electrolyte fluxes (sodium, potassium, or calcium) and to reestablish a normal rhythm. Generally, Class I drugs are used for ventricular dysrhythmias like ventricular ectopy (skipped heart beats) and ventricular tachycardias (as well as quinidine for atrial tachycardias). The frequent deleterious effects of these drugs and the development of Class III drugs have caused a marked diminution of their usage especially the drugs in Class IA. Class II drugs are used for sinus tachycardia, atrial fibrillation and flutter, and some ventricular dysrhythmias. Class III drugs are mostly used for ventricular dysrhythmias but also for atrial fibrillation. Class IV drugs are used in atrial fibrillation and flutter and supraventricular tachycardia. Miscellaneous drugs, such as adenosine, are used mostly for diagnostic purposes; atropine is also used for certain bradycardias.

EXAMPLES OF COMMON DOSAGES (GENERAL GUIDELINES, MANY DIFFERENT DOSAGE SCHEDULES)

Disopyramide	100-200 mg q6h PO or 200-400 mg q12h for slow-release preparations PO
Procainamide	1 g followed by 50 mg/kg/day q6h PO
Quinidine	200-600 mg q2-3h up to 4 g/day PO
Lidocaine	Injections, infusions at various dosages
Mexiletine	200-400 mg followed by 200-400 mg q8h PO
Phenytoin	1 g divided over one day then 500 mg/day for 2 days PO
Tocainide	400-1800 mg/day in divided doses PO
Flecainide	50 mg q6-12h, up to 300 mg/day PO
Propafenone	150 mg q8h up to 900 mg/day PO
Amiodarone	800-1600 mg/day for 1-3 weeks followed by 600-800 mg for 1 month and followed by 400 mg/day PO
Ibutilide	IV infusions at different rates
Verapamil	240-320 mg/day in 3-4 divided doses PO
Adenosine	IV infusions at different rates
Atropine	IV bolus injections at different dosages

ADMINISTRATION

Antiarrhythmic drugs can be given IV (bolus, infusion) and PO. It is important to follow exactly the prescribed dosage protocol, because these drugs can be quite toxic if taken too frequently or at higher than prescribed dosages.

CONTRAINDICATIONS

Antiarrhythmic drugs are contraindicated or should be used with care in patients with heart failure, myocardial ischemia, and previous MIs.

COMMON ADVERSE REACTIONS

Antiarrhythmic drugs carry a high risk of adverse reactions. Most drugs have the potential to normalize one type of dysrhythmias while causing another type. They can cause dizziness, confusion, and nausea, which sometimes are indications of the presence of such an adverse dysrhythmia. Depending on the class, Class I drugs can cause hypotension, bradycardia, edema, syncope (fainting), heart failure, leukopenia, constipation, urinary retention, and rarely, agranulocytosis. In addition, tinnitus (ringing in the ears) and hearing loss mostly with quinidine; GI bleeding with mexiletine; nephritis (urine discoloration), and Stevens-Johnson syndrome with phenytoin and respiratory depression with flecainide. Class II drugs can cause bronchoconstriction and excessive bradycardia. Class III drugs are relatively safe except amiodarone, which can cause deposits in the cornea, a toxic epidermal necrolysis, and pulmonary fibrosis (warning signs are dyspnea, cough, and pain). Class IV drugs, or calcium channel blockers, may cause bradycardia and hypotension.

DRUG INTERACTIONS

- Antiarrhythmic drugs can interact with other antidysrhythmic drugs, β-blockers, anticholinergics, and other drugs.
- Toxicity is increased by a large number of herbal products. Alcohol and caffeine in foods and drinks can aggravate dysrhythmias.

IMPLICATIONS FOR PHYSICAL THERAPISTS

- Advise the patient that these are very effective but also potentially dangerous drugs and that the patient must adhere strictly to the prescribed dosing schedule because deviations can significantly reduce the therapeutic and increase the toxic effects.
- Advise the patient to adhere strictly to office appointments and laboratory tests because early recognition of an adverse reaction can prevent subsequent health problems.
- If you notice peripheral edema or the patient complains about dyspnea, notify or have patient contact the physician because dosage adjustments or a different drug might be indicated.
- Have the patient change position slowly, in particular during early therapy, because dizziness and orthostatic hypotension might occur causing patient to fall.
- If the patient complains about nausea and dizziness, have him or her contact the physician because these could be a warning sign of another dysrhythmia.
- Advise the patient to abstain from caffeine containing drinks or foods because they can aggravate dysrhythmias.
- If a patient on quinidine complains about tinnitus, have the patient contact the physician because this can lead to hearing problems.
- If the patient complains of a fever followed by a rash and painful skin areas, have the patient immediately call the physician because this could be warning signs for a toxic epidermal necrolysis, which could be very serious.
- Check pulse rate during more strenuous exercises or if the patient gets prematurely fatigued and stop exercises if an abnormal rate is felt.

ANTIASTHMATIC DRUGS

COMMON DRUGS (SELECTION OF SOME OF THE MOST COMMONLY USED DRUGS)

β-Agonists (see β-Agonists)
Albuterol
Formoterol
Bitolterol
Levalbuterol
Metaproterenol
Pirbuterol
Terbutaline

Anticholinergics (see Anticholinergic Drugs)
Ipratropium
Tiotropium

Adrenergics (see α-Agonists)
Epinephrine

Corticosteroids (see Corticosteroids)
Beclomethasone
Betamethasone
Budesonide
Cortisone
Dexamethasone
Flunisolide
Fluticasone
Hydrocortisone
Methylprednisolone
Prednisone
Triamcinolone

Leukotriene Antagonists
Zafirlukast   Accolate

Mast Cell Stabilizer (see Antihistamines)
Cromolyn
Nedocromil

Phosphodiesterase Inhibitors
Theophylline   Accurbron, Bronkodyl, Lanophyllin, other

Monoclonal Antibodies (see Antihistamines)
Omalizumab   Xolair

MECHANISM OF ACTION

The diameter of the bronchi and air flow are controlled by the action of a number of receptors, such as muscarinic, histamine (released from mast cells in response to certain allergens), and leukotriene receptors (LTC4, LTD4, LTE4, formed from arachidonic acid via lipoxygenase), that constrict the bronchi and β-receptors that dilate the bronchi.

In order to relax the constricted bronchi and to increase air flow, muscarinic receptor blockers (see Anticholinergic Drugs), antihistamines (see Antihistamines), or β-agonists (see β-Agonists) are used. In addition, phosphodiesterase inhibitors are employed that prevent the destruction of cyclic adenosine monophosphate (cAMP) by phosphodiesterase, which is a second messenger that relaxes bronchi. Leukotriene antagonists block the action of leukotrienes, preventing the constrictive effects of these compounds and leading to relaxation of bronchi.

INDICATIONS

Antiasthmatic drugs are indicated in the following:
- *Asthma* which is caused by the bronchoconstriction action of histamine, leukotrienes, and acetylcholine and an inflammation that narrows the inner diameter of the bronchi, reduces air flow, and causes "air hunger" (wheezing). Drugs relax the bronchi by blocking constricting causes (anticholinergic drugs, leukotriene antagonists, and histamine antagonists or mast cell stabilizers) or by promoting relaxation (β-agonists, theophylline), as well as reducing the inflammation (corticosteroids). Omalizumab is a monoclonal antibody which binds to IgE and prevents the release of histamine and other asthmatic mediators. In all cases, the inner diameter of the bronchi is increased and a more efficient airflow is established.
- *Chronic obstructive pulmonary disease* (COPD) and *emphysema* which are lung diseases in which the lung is damaged by smoking, making it difficult to breathe.

EXAMPLES OF COMMON DOSAGES (GENERAL GUIDELINES, MANY DIFFERENT DOSAGE SCHEDULES)

Theophylline   100-800 mg q6h PO
Zafirlukast   20 mg bid PO
Omalizumab   150-375 mg 2x4 wk SC

ADMINISTRATION

Antiasthmatic drugs can be given IV, SC, or PO. Onset of action is fastest with inhaled preparations, and adverse reactions are less severe.

CONTRAINDICATIONS

Theophylline should not be used in patients with tachydysrhythmias.

COMMON ADVERSE REACTIONS

Adverse reactions for leukotriene antagonists include headache, nausea, dyspepsia, and the very rare but potentially dangerous Churg-Strauss syndrome. Theophylline can cause restlessness, insomnia, seizures, tachycardia, dysrhythmias, and dyspepsia.

DRUG INTERACTIONS

- Interleukin antagonists interact with a small number of drugs such as aspirin and warfarin. Theophylline increases cardiotoxicity of β-blockers.
- Black/green tea, coffee, and ephedra increase some of the adverse reactions of theophylline.

IMPLICATIONS FOR PHYSICAL THERAPISTS

- If a patient on zafirlukast complains about a rash and nodules, have the patient contact or inform the physician immediately because this could be the beginning of the Churg-Strauss syndrome.
- Advise the patient taking theophylline to take the medication exactly as prescribed because dosage schedule is very important and deviations can increase risk of adverse effects (margin of safety is very small).

ANTIBACTERIAL DRUGS

COMMON DRUGS (SELECTION OF SOME OF THE MOST COMMONLY USED DRUGS)

Penicillins

Amoxicillin	Augmentin (with clavulanate)
Penicillin G	Bicillin, Megacillin
Others	

Cephalosporins

Cefazolin	Ancef
Cefepime	Maxipime
Cefotaxime	Claforan
Cephalexin	Keflex
Others	

Quinolones

Ciprofloxacin	Cipro, Proquin
Levofloxacin	Levaquin
Others	

Aminoglycosides

Gentamicin	Garamycin
Others	

Tetracyclines

Tetracycline	Tetracyn, Achromycin, other
Others	

Macrolides

Azithromycin	Zithromax, Zmax
Others	

Sulfonamides

Sulfisoxazole (Trimethoprim)	Gantrisin Primsol, Trimpex, other
Others	

Miscellaneous Drugs

Bacitracin	
Imipenem	Primaxin (with cilastatin)

MECHANISM OF ACTION

Bacteria are unicellular organisms that consist of a cell wall, sometimes a membrane, DNA (regular, plasmid) without a nuclear envelope, and protoplasm containing metabolites and enzymes. They are classified according to genus and species (e.g., genus *Escherichia* and species *coli*). Many bacteria are beneficial to the host in that they prevent pathogenic bacteria from growing or assist in the synthesis of certain nutrients. Some bacteria are pathogenic and cause specific diseases (e.g., *Treponema pallidum* causes syphilis) by competing for essential nutrients with host cells, secreting toxic materials, and/or causing an excessive immune response that damages the host cells.

Drugs that affect these microorganisms are called *antibacterial drugs* and are relatively specific for bacteria only. They can be divided into antibiotics that are derived from other microorganisms (e.g., molds), semisynthetic antibiotics that are chemically altered antibiotics, and synthetic drugs that are completely synthesized in the laboratory. Drugs are classified and named after their origin (e.g., penicillin from *Penicillium notatum*), their action (a drug that affects bacterial cell walls is named a *cell wall inhibitor* or a drug that kills bacteria is named *bactericidal*, whereas a drug that prevents multiplication is named a bacteriostatic drug), their structure (drugs whose structure contains the lactam ring necessary for antibacterial action are referred to as *lactam* drugs), and/or their specificity against bacteria (drugs that affect gram-positive bacteria are named gram-positive drugs, and drugs that affect gram-negative bacteria are named *gram-negative* drugs; drugs that affect only a few different bacteria are classified as narrow, and drugs that affect many different bacteria are classified as wide-spectrum drugs).

Antibacterial drugs are grouped into classes, each of which consists of many individual drugs that have similar actions and adverse reactions. Antibacterial drugs do not affect all bacteria but are selective for a specific species or strains. Most antibacterial drugs have five major sites of action as follows:

- Inhibition of synthesis and/or damage to the peptidoglycan component of the bacterial cell wall. This biochemical is unique and necessary to the microbial cell wall and its disruption kills the microorganism (e.g., penicillins, cephalosporins, imipenem, and others).
- Inhibition of synthesis and/or damage to the microbial cytoplasmic membrane (e.g., polymyxins).
- Modification of synthesis and/or metabolism of microbial nucleic acids by affecting two microbial enzymes, gyrase and topoisomerase, that are necessary for replication and cell division (e.g., quinolones).
- Inhibition or modification of microbial protein synthesis by disrupting microbial ribosomal function and impairing protein synthesis (e.g., aminoglycosides, tetracyclines, and macrolides).
- Inhibition or modification of microbial cell metabolism by affecting folic acid synthesis/metabolism that has to be synthesized by bacteria and that is necessary for their nucleic acid synthesis (e.g., sulfonamides, trimethoprim). (Other modes of action include effects on RNA and other bacterial cellular components sometimes by an unknown mechanism).

Resistance to penicillin drug action is noted, because certain bacteria possessed an enzyme penicillinase or lactamase that can open the antibacterial lactam ring of penicillin and render a drug ineffective. However, other ways of drug resistance are also emerging as a result of mutations and plasmid exchanges (in which plasmid DNA from one is transferred to another bacteria), which create "pumps" that expel the drug from the bacteria, cause thicker walls preventing entry of the drug and/or lose special receptors with which the drugs interact.

Sometimes, certain antibacterial drugs are administered concomitantly with drugs that prevent their rapid renal elimination and prolong their action (e.g., cilastatin) or inhibit the bacterial enzyme penicillinase, which now cannot inactivate penicillins (e.g., clavulanate).

INDICATION

Antibacterial drugs are indicated in the following:

- *Bacterial infections* are treated with drugs that are specific for a particular bacterial species or strain. Examples are ciprofloxacin and imipenem for *Bacillus anthracis* (anthrax), penicillin G for *Clostridium tetani* (tetanus), amoxicillin or trimethoprim/sulfonamide for *E. coli* (bacteremia, urinary tract infections), cefotaxime for *Haemophilus influenzae* (otitis, pneumonia), penicillin G for streptococci (endocarditis), cefotaxime and ciprofloxacin for *Salmonella typhi* (typhoid fever) and cephalosporins or aminoglycoside for *Klebsiella pneumoniae* (pneumonia).

EXAMPLES OF COMMON DOSAGES (GENERAL GUIDELINES, MANY DIFFERENT DOSAGE SCHEDULES)

Amoxicillin	750-1750 mg in divided doses daily PO
Penicillin G	2.4 million units IM
Cefazolin	250-2000 mg q6-8h IM, IV
Cefepime	0.5-2000 mg q12h IV, IM
Cefotaxime	1-2 g q4-12h IM, IV
Cephalexin	250-1000 mg q6h PO
Ciprofloxacin	100-500 mg q12h daily PO
Levofloxacin	250-750 mg daily PO, IV
Gentamicin	3-6 mg/kg/day in divided doses q8h IV infusion or 3 mg/kg/day in divided doses q8h IM
Tetracycline	250-500 mg q6h daily PO
Azithromycin	250-2000 mg daily PO
Sulfisoxazole	2-4 g followed by 1-2 g daily PO
Trimethoprim	100 mg q12h daily PO
Imipenem	250-1000 mg q6-8h IV

ADMINISTRATION

Depending on the drug, antibacterial drugs are administered PO, IV, or IM.

CONTRAINDICATIONS

Antibacterial drugs are contraindicated or should be used with caution in patients with renal and/or hepatic problems.

COMMON ADVERSE REACTIONS

In general, antibacterial drugs can cause nausea, vomiting, allergic reactions, pseudomembranous colitis, Stevens-Johnson syndrome, and superinfections. In addition, penicillins and cephalosporins are relatively free of adverse reactions except allergic reactions with some cross-sensitivity between classes. Similarly, macrolides show mostly allergic reactions. Aminoglycosides are more toxic and might cause nephrotoxicity and ototoxicity. Tetracyclines cause photosensitivity to ultraviolet (UV) light and should not be given to growing individuals because they stain teeth and interfere with bone calcification. Quinolones can cause visual disturbances, photosensitization, and

inflammations of the tendons. Sulfonamides taken at high doses may cause renal stone formation and necessitate the consumption of large amounts of fluids.

DRUG INTERACTIONS

- A large number of interactions exist. Penicillins can decrease the effects of contraceptives. Tetracyclines can reduce the efficacy of penicillins. Some cephalosporins show increased toxicity with a large number of herbal preparations.
- Generally, acidophilus should not be used with antiinfectives. Antacids and/or dairy products (calcium and other metals) decrease efficacy of tetracyclines, macrolides, and quinolones.

IMPLICATIONS FOR PHYSICAL THERAPISTS

- Advise patients to follow prescription schedule strictly and to continue taking drugs even if clinical signs or symptoms have subsided because the schedule is designed to eradicate the microorganism in all places even those in which no clinical problems are manifested.
- If the patient exhibits an unexplained rash, inform the physician or have the patient contact the physician because this could be the beginning of Stevens-Johnson syndrome.
- If the patient has abdominal discomfort, ask the patient to check stool and if pus or mucus is detected, inform the physician or ask the patient to contact the physician because this could be a pseudomembranous colitis.
- Advise patients and reinforce drug warnings that tetracyclines and quinolones must be taken as prescribed because their use with food or antacids can render them ineffective.
- Patients on quinolones complaining about tendon pain, in particular, pain of the Achilles tendon, should not be exercised strenuously and should be carefully evaluated. The physician should be informed because this could indicate a tendonitis requiring a change in medication.
- Avoid UV light therapy or cover exposed areas of patients on tetracyclines and quinolones because these drugs cause photosensitization.
- Be aware that health care professionals have been shown to be a primary source of spreading infections including serious and life threatening infections. It is recommended that gloves should be worn and discarded, hands should be washed with soap for at least 15-30 seconds or disinfective solutions be used to minimize the spread of infection.

COMMON DRUGS (SELECTION OF SOME OF THE MOST COMMONLY USED DRUGS)

Atropine	Generic Belladonna
Dicyclomine	Bentyl
Hyoscyamine	Levsin, Anaspaz, Donnamar, others
Ipratropium	Atrovent, others
Oxybutynin	Ditropan
Scopolamine	Transderm-Scop
Tiotropium	Spiriva
Tolterodine	Detrol
Benztropine	Cogentin
Biperidin	Akineton
Trihexyphenidyl	Artane

MECHANISM OF ACTION

Muscarinic (M) cholinergic receptors are usually but not exclusively found opposite parasympathetic postganglionic nerve fibers, which release acetylcholine which stimulates these receptors. The acetylcholine is then quickly inactivated and destroyed by the enzyme acetylcholinesterase. Activation of these receptors decreases heart rate and contractility, constricts bronchial muscles (decreased air flow), constricts the pupil, and increases gut and bladder activity. Anticholinergic drugs block the M receptors, reduce action of acetylcholine, and cause the opposite effects of their stimulation.

INDICATIONS

Anticholinergic drugs are indicated in the following:

- *Arrhythmias,* such as sinus bradycardia, in which these drugs increase heart rate and normalize abnormal cardiac rhythm.
- *Peptic ulcer and irritable bowel syndrome,* in which these drugs antagonize excessive M-receptor stimulation and gastric and intestinal activity.
- *Urinary bladder hypermotility,* including *enuresis,* in which these drugs relax the bladder and decrease the need for frequent urination or bed wetting.
- *Asthma,* in which these drugs reduce secretion and dilate the bronchi with increased air flow.
- *Cases of pesticide poisoning,* in which these drugs protect the receptors from excessive acetylcholine stimulation caused by inhibition of acetylcholinesterase by these poisons.
- *Ocular applications,* in which these drugs dilate the pupil and relax the ciliary body (topically applied tropicamide, cyclopentolate, and atropine).
- *Parkinson's disease* which is a movement disorder characterized by a masklike face, shuffling gait, and pill-rolling tremor. The cause is believed to

be an overactivity of cholinergic and an underactivity of dopaminergic activity in the basal ganglia of the brain. The last three drugs in the Common Drugs list reduce cholinergic overactivity and restore the balance between the two systems, thus improving rigidity and tremor.

EXAMPLES OF COMMON DOSAGES (GENERAL GUIDELINES, MANY DIFFERENT DOSAGE SCHEDULES)

Atropine	Various schedules, mostly as given as Belladonna extract 10-100 mg (calculated as 0.5 mg alkaloid) PO
Dicyclomine	10-20 mg 3-4 times daily (up to 160 mg/day) PO
Hyoscyamine	0.125-0.25 mg 3-4 times daily PO or 0.375-0.75 mg q12h as sustained-release preparation PO
Ipratropium	1-4 inhalations 3-4 times daily (not to exceed q4h)
Oxybutynin	5 mg 2-3 times daily PO or 5-10 mg once daily as sustained-release preparation PO
Tiotropium	Inhalation of 18 μg once daily
Benztropine	1 to 2 mg/day in 1-2 divided doses (up to 6 mg/day) PO
Biperidin	2 mg 1-4 times daily (not to exceed 16 mg/day) PO
Trihexyphe-nidyl	1-6 mg/day in divided doses PO

ADMINISTRATION

Anticholinergic drugs can be given IV, IM, inhalation, and PO.

CONTRAINDICATIONS

Anticholinergic drugs are contraindicated or should be used with caution in patients with cardiovascular problems, seizure disorders, benign prostatic hyperplasia, and GI hypomotility.

COMMON ADVERSE REACTIONS

Adverse reactions include confusion (more severe in geriatric patients), dry skin and mouth, decreased sweating, blurred vision, constipation, and urinary hesitancy and retention (mainly in geriatric patients). Anticholinergic drugs may cause contact lens intolerance as a result of dry eye.

DRUG INTERACTIONS

- Anticholinergic drugs can slow down the absorption of a number of other drugs and can antagonize the effects of some antiglaucoma medications.
- Increased anticholinergic effects have been reported with Jimson weed, scopolia, and angel's trumpet.
- In addition, there are a number of antihistamines, antipsychotics, and antidepressants that also show strong anticholinergic effects (see specific sections).

IMPLICATIONS FOR PHYSICAL THERAPISTS

- Expect some increases in heart rate as a result of blockade of cardiac M receptors.
- Expect some mental confusion in older patients taking anticholinergic drugs (or drugs that have anticholinergic properties).
- When exercising a patient on anticholinergic medication, keep the environment cool because there is the risk of heat prostration caused by the decreased ability to sweat and lose heat.

ANTICONVULSANT DRUGS

COMMON DRUGS (SELECTION OF SOME OF THE MOST COMMONLY USED DRUGS)

Barbiturates

Phenobarbital	Luminal, Solfoton, other
Primidone	Mysoline
Other	

Benzodiazepines

Clonazepam	Klonopin
Diazepam	Valium
Other	

Hydantoins

Phenytoin	Dilantin, Phenytex
Other	

Succinimides

Ethosuximide	Zarontin
Other	

Carboxylic Acids

Valproic acid	Depakene, Depacon, other

Iminostilbenes

Carbamazepine	Tegretol, Atretol, other
Oxcarbazepine	Trileptal

Second-Generation Drugs

Gabapentin	Neurontin
Lamotrigine	Lamictal
Tiagabine	Gabitril
Other	

MECHANISM OF ACTION

Normal neuronal activity without excessive swings is controlled in the brain by excitatory and inhibitory processes. Sodium and potassium fluxes, excitatory neurotransmitter actions such as glutamate, and inhibitory neurotransmitter actions such as γ-aminobutyric acid (GABA) are mostly responsible for this delicate balance. Anticonvulsant drugs can relatively selectively interact with these processes and reduce abnormal excessive cerebral neuronal activity. Barbiturates and benzodiazepines stimulate special receptors on the GABA complex that cause an increased action of the inhibitory neurotransmitter GABA. Hydantoins and iminostilbenes seem to primarily reduce sodium fluxes and reduce depolarization, which reduces neuronal firing. Valproic acid seems to predominantly affect potassium channels and hyperpolarize neurons and thus reduce neuronal activity. The neuronal depressant action of the other drugs is somewhat obscure, although ethosuximide does affect calcium fluxes and gabapentin-GABA release in an unknown way.

INDICATION

Anticonvulsant drugs are indicated in the following:

- *Epilepsy* which is characterized by seizures, which are episodes of sudden and uncontrolled but transient hyperexcitability of small groups of neurons or "foci." The cause for that sudden hyperexcitability or spontaneous but deleterious discharges is poorly understood but defects in the GABA system of the brain, excessive Na+ fluxes and faulty K+ and Ca ++ fluxes have been suggested. These anomalies can be genetic in nature or caused by brain trauma, strokes, or drugs. These discharges can produce muscle contractions (convulsions) or behavioral abnormalities (loss of consciousness). They can be localized or spread over the entire brain and can be divided into partial and generalized seizures. Anticonvulsants basically prevent this unwanted and deleterious hyperexcitability by initiating or reducing it to a nonpathological level. Most drugs increase the action of the inhibitory neurotransmitter, GABA, which opens chloride channels, causes a hyperpolarization, and slows neuronal firing. Phenytoins blocks sodium channels, which slows the influx of sodium and prevents or reduces depolarization. Valproic acid affects potassium channels, leading to hyperpolarization and again a reduction in neuronal firing. The mechanism of the other drugs is still somewhat unknown. In addition to these mechanisms, other neuronal effects do certainly play a supporting or even crucial role.
- Other uses for some selective drugs include essential tremors, restless leg syndrome, panic disorders, neuropathic pain, certain dysrhythmias, manic episodes, and trigeminal neuralgia.

EXAMPLES OF COMMON DOSAGES (GENERAL GUIDELINES, MANY DIFFERENT DOSAGE SCHEDULES)

Phenobarbital	1-3 mg/kg/day in divided doses or total dose at bedtime PO
Primidone	100-250 mg 3-4 times daily up to 2 g/day PO
Clonazepam	1.5 mg/day in 3 divided doses up to 20 mg/day PO
Diazepam	2-10 mg 3-4 times daily or 15-30 mg once daily extended-release preparations PO
Phenytoin	1 g as loading dose in 3-4 divided doses and later as maintenance dose 300-600 mg/day PO
Ethosuximide	250-750 daily PO
Valproic acid	10-15 mg/kg/day in 2-3 divided doses not to exceed 60 mg/kg/day PO
Carbamazepine	200 mg 2 times daily up to 800-1600 mg/day PO
Oxcarbazepine	300-600 mg 2 times daily PO
Gabapentin	900-1800 mg/day in 1-3 divided doses PO
Lamotrigine	50-500 mg/day in 2 divided doses PO
Tiagabine	4 mg/day in divided doses up to 56 mg/day PO

ADMINISTRATION

Most drugs are given PO, but for certain conditions they have to be injected or infused. Anticonvulsant drugs are often prescribed in combination. Anticonvulsant drugs must be taken at exact dosages and times to be maximally effective.

CONTRAINDICATIONS

Anticonvulsant drugs should not be used or must be used with caution in patients with renal and hepatic diseases.

COMMON ADVERSE REACTIONS

All drugs will cause to a varying degree gastric discomfort, sedation, drowsiness, and ataxia (confusion occurs mostly in geriatric patients). Barbiturates may cause paradoxical excitement in selected individuals. Some drugs, such as barbiturates, oxcarbazine, gabapentin, and lamotrigine, can cause the Stevens-Johnson syndrome. Some drugs, such as barbiturates and carbamazepine, can cause blood disorders (agranulocytosis, leukopenia, megaloblastic, or aplastic anemia). Phenytoin is associated with gingival hyperplasia, hirsutism, nephritis (colored urine), and hepatitis. Valproic acid may cause hepatitis and pancreatitis. Carbamazepine may worsen seizures and cause cardiac rhythm disturbances. Ethosuximide may cause movement disorders such as dyskinesia and bradykinesia. Drugs should not be discontinued abruptly because this can precipitate seizures.

DRUG INTERACTIONS

- Sedative effects are enhanced by drugs that also have sedative properties. Long term use of barbiturates can decrease the effectiveness of corticosteroids and anticoagulants.
- St. John's wort should be avoided and drug actions can be affected by gingko and ginseng.

IMPLICATIONS FOR PHYSICAL THERAPISTS

- Epileptic patients even with drug treatment are vulnerable to intense lights and sounds that can precipitate a seizure. Keep patients in a quiet area without flickering lights and repetitive noise.
- Inform the patient to take the medication exactly as prescribed because only this will assure maximal antiepileptic effects. Tell the patient not to stop the medication abruptly because this can precipitate seizures. Also, if blood tests were ordered, have the patient adhere to such a schedule because early detection of a problem can often prevent or reverse pathological changes.
- If the patient is too sedated for therapy, discuss this with the patient and schedule appointments at times when patient feels less sedated.
- If the patient has an unexplained rash, notify or have the patient contact the physician immediately because some drugs can cause a Stevens-Johnson syndrome, which necessitates immediate drug withdrawal.
- If the patient should appear excessively sedated, the patient should contact the physician because a dosage change or other drug might be indicated.

ANTIDEPRESSANT DRUGS

COMMON DRUGS (SELECTION OF SOME OF THE MOST COMMONLY USED DRUGS)

Tricyclics

Amitriptyline	Elavil, Endep, other
Amoxapine	Asendin
Clomipramine	Anafranil
Desipramine	Norpramin
Doxepin	Sinequan
Imipramine	Norfranil, Tofranil, other
Nortriptyline	Aventyl, Pamelor
Trimipramine	Surmontil

Monoamine Oxidase Inhibitors

Phenelzine	Nardil
Tranylcypromine	Parnate

Second-Generation Drugs

Bupropion	Wellbutrin
Citalopram	Celexa
Escitalopram	Lexapro
Fluoxetine	Prozac
Fluvoxamine	Luvox
Mirtazapine	Remeron
Paroxetine	Paxil
Sertraline	Zoloft
Trazodone	Desyrel
Venlafaxine	Effexor

MECHANISM OF ACTION

Mood and its normal fluctuations between a healthy sadness and happiness are controlled by many chemical processes (neurotransmitters) and special electrical circuits in the limbic and cortical areas of the brain. In this case, the neurotransmitters norepinephrine, dopamine, and serotonin seem to play major roles. These neurotransmitters are synthesized in nerve terminals and released so that they can interact with their respective receptors. They are transported back into the nerve terminals (reuptake) where part is stored and used again, while another part is metabolized by the enzyme monoamine oxidase (MAO) subtypes A and B. In addition, other neurotransmitters will also participate in mood regulation.

All antidepressant drugs interact with these systems by increasing synaptic levels of all neurotransmitters by either inhibiting their reuptake systems or by inhibiting their metabolism by the enzyme MAO. Elevated levels and continuous stimulation of these receptors cause a downregulation with decreased activity in about 4 weeks. These actions generally will cause a shift to a more elated mood.

INDICATION

Antidepressant drugs are indicated in the following:

- *Depression* can be roughly divided into unipolar and bipolar depression. Unipolar depression is characterized by dysphoria, lack of interest, fatigue, lack of energy, low self-esteem, irrational guilt, and suicidal ideation. Bipolar depression is characterized by swings between depression and mania. Mania is characterized by endless energy, increased activity, excessive euphoria, extreme irritability, racing thoughts and fast talking, needing little sleep, unrealistic beliefs in one's abilities and powers, poor judgment, and aggressive behavior. It is hypothesized that these disorders are caused mostly by a pathological supersensitivity of the presynaptic and postsynaptic receptors of the norepinephrine, serotonin, and dopamine systems. Antidepressant drugs now seem to increase synaptic neurotransmitter levels, downregulate these receptors, normalize excessive receptor sensitivity, and improve mood. Receptor downregulation may be the major effect because mood improvement usually occurs after 4 weeks of therapy. The tricyclic drugs act by blocking the reuptake of all three neurotransmitters, although slightly differently. The MAO inhibitors inhibit the enzyme that decreases neurotransmitter destruction and increases intraneuronal levels and release. They affect both enzyme types; inhibition of type A seems to be more beneficial. The second-generation drugs are also reuptake inhibitors but are somewhat more selective in their actions. These drugs include the selective serotonin reuptake inhibitors (SSRIs), such as fluoxetine, citalopram, escitalopram, fluvoxamine, paroxetine, and sertraline, which mostly affect serotonin. Lithium is used mostly to prevent mood swings in bipolar depression, and its action is uncertain but might involve an action on neuronal excitability and the formation and action of certain second messengers.

- *Chronic pain* (neuropathic pain, fibromyalgia, and chronic low back pain) involves some of the previously mentioned neurotransmitters, in particular serotonin, in its pathogenesis. But the specific action of the drugs in this condition is unknown.
- Other conditions such as *enuresis* (based on anticholinergic properties), *migraine, premenstrual disorder, attention deficit hyperactivity disorder(ADHD), obsessive-compulsive disorders (fluoxetine, sertraline), anxiety disorders (venlafaxine), and smoking cessation (bupropion)*. Mechanisms of action are often poorly understood.

EXAMPLES OF COMMON DOSAGES (GENERAL GUIDELINES, MANY DIFFERENT DOSAGE SCHEDULES)

Amitriptyline	75-150 mg/day in divided doses (not to exceed 300 mg/day) PO
Amoxapine	50-100 mg 2-3 times daily (not to exceed 300 mg/day) PO
Clomipramine	25-250 mg in divided doses daily PO
Desipramine	100-200 mg/day in divided doses up to 300 mg/day PO
Doxepin	25-75 mg/day in divided doses up to 300 mg/day PO
Imipramine	75-100 mg/day up to 300 mg/day in divided doses PO
Nortriptyline	25 mg up to 150 mg/day in divided doses PO
Trimipramine	50-200 mg/day in divided doses PO
Phenelzine	45-60 mg/day in divided doses PO
Tranylcypromine	10-30 mg 2 times daily PO
Bupropion	100-150 mg 2-3 times daily PO
Citalopram	20-40 mg/day once daily PO
Escitalopram	10-20 mg/day once daily PO
Fluoxetine	20 mg 1-2 times daily (not to exceed 80 mg/day) PO
Fluvoxamine	50-100 mg 1-2 times daily (not to exceed 300 mg/day) PO
Mirtazapine	15-45 mg once daily PO
Paroxetine	20-60 mg once daily PO
Sertraline	50-200 mg once daily PO
Trazodone	150-600 mg in divided doses daily PO
Venlafaxine	75-150 mg 2-3 times daily PO
Lithium	300-600 3 times daily PO

ADMINISTRATION

Most antidepressant drugs are given PO.

CONTRAINDICATIONS

Antidepressant drugs should not be used (or must be used with caution) in patients with strong suicidal tendencies, seizure disorders, cardiac problems, and hepatic and renal diseases.

COMMON ADVERSE REACTIONS

Adverse reactions differ among the drug classes, but patients are generally at higher risk of committing suicide at the beginning of therapy with all drugs. Also, long-term therapy will lead to different degrees of physical dependence, causing a withdrawal syndrome (fatigue, headache, muscle pain) at abrupt drug therapy cessation. Tricyclics cause sedation, anticholinergic effects, orthostatic hypotension, cardiac dysrhythmias, and seizures, although there are differences among

individual drugs. Occurrence of blood disorders (agranulocytosis) is rare but can be serious. MAO inhibitors show fewer of these effects, except a tendency for orthostatic hypotension. Second-generation drugs show seizure possibilities but fewer of the other adverse reactions, except maprotiline, mirtazapine, nefazodone, and trazodone, which are similar to the tricyclics. A few of the latter drugs may cause malignant hyperthermia. Lithium has a very small margin of safety requiring periodic blood level tests to avoid serious toxicity. Some adverse reactions include confusion, lethargy, ataxia, increased deep tendon reflexes and a fine tremor, and seizures and coma at higher doses.

DRUG INTERACTIONS

- Antidepressant drugs can interact with MAO inhibitors resulting in seizures and hypertension, as well as a large number of other drugs such as benzodiazepines and alcohol, resulting in enhanced sedation.
- Salt intake can affect lithium effects, and salt intake should not be changed during lithium therapy.
- MAO inhibitors can cause a severe hypertensive crisis with chest pain, headache, and nausea when taken with foods and drinks containing the chemical tyramine.
- Drugs can show increased toxicity with many herbs, including St. John' wort, chamomile, valerian, and jimsonweed. Increased toxicity of antidepressants occurs with methionine supplements.

IMPLICATIONS FOR PHYSICAL THERAPISTS

- If the patient complains about not feeling the beneficial effects of drug therapy in the first few weeks, advise the patient that it might sometimes take up to 6 weeks before such beneficial effects set in.
- If a patient should talk about "life is not worth living" in the beginning of therapy, notify the physician immediately because there is an increased risk of suicide during this time.
- If a patient on long-term therapy plans to discontinue the drug without advice of the physician, warn the patient and contact the physician because the possibility of a serious withdrawal reaction exists.
- If a patient on lithium talks incessantly and becomes easily irritated and even aggressive, notify the physician because this might require a change in dosage.
- Advise the patient to change position or get up slowly because some drugs can cause marked orthostatic hypotension.
- Advise the patient on lithium to follow strictly the physician's advice in taking

the drug as prescribed and in having blood levels checked periodically. If the patient exhibits tremors, lethargy, hyperreflexia, and ataxia, notify the physician immediately because this may require dosage adjustments.

- Ask older patients if they have trouble voiding and if they have regular bowel movements, because some drugs with anticholinergic properties can cause urinary hesitancy and significant constipation. Advise these patients to increase water and bulk food intake to prevent constipation and its possible complications.

ANTIEMETIC DRUGS

COMMON DRUGS (SELECTION OF SOME OF THE MOST COMMONLY USED DRUGS)

Serotonin 3 Antagonists

Dolasetron	Anzemet
Ondansetron	Zofran
Other	

Histamine Antagonists

Dimenhydrinate	Dramamine, Gravol, other (OTC)
Meclizine	Antivert, Antrizine, other (OTC)
Other	

Phenothiazines

Chlorpromazine	Thorazine
Prochlorperazine	Compazine, other
Promethazine	Phenadoz
Other	

Cholinergic Antagonists

Scopolamine	Scopolamine
Other	

Miscellaneous Drugs

Metoclopramide	Reglan, other
Other	

MECHANISM OF ACTION

Nausea and vomiting are complex processes involving dopamine, serotonin, acetylcholine, and histamine receptors in the stomach, as well as in two major CNS centers such as the chemoreceptor trigger zone and vomiting center. In addition, vestibular nuclei (motion sickness) influence these centers. Nausea is an uneasy feeling and often the antecedent to vomiting, which occurs when abdominal muscles abruptly contract and expel the food from the stomach.

Serotonin antagonists block the stimulatory action of serotonin on type 3 receptors in the stomach, intestines, and brain, reducing nausea and vomiting. Histamine antagonists block the action of histamine on H1 receptors in the periphery and presumably with their cholinergic-blocking activity inhibit central activity in the vestibular system, as well as the chemoreceptor trigger zone and vomiting center. The phenothiazines seem to exert their

action mostly via blockade of dopamine, histamine, and acetylcholine receptors. Metoclopramide seems to block dopamine receptors in the chemoreceptor trigger zone and to increase gastric emptying time.

INDICATION

Antiemetic drugs are indicated in the following:

- For the *prevention of and therapy for nausea and vomiting;* given before, during, and/or after surgery, cancer chemotherapy, or radiation therapy.
- *Motion sickness* (histamine antagonists, scopolamine); mostly given 1 hour before exposure.

EXAMPLES OF COMMON DOSAGES (GENERAL GUIDELINES, MANY DIFFERENT DOSAGE SCHEDULES)

Dolasetron	100 mg once PO or 1.8 mg/kg once IV
Ondansetron	8 mg to be repeated when needed PO or 0.15 mg/kg to be repeated if needed IV
Dimenhydrinate	50-100 mg q4h PO
Meclizine	25-100 mg daily in divided doses PO
Chlorpromazine	10-25 mg q4-6h PO or 25-50 mg q3h IM
Prochlorperazine	5-10 mg 3-4 times PO
Promethazine	12.5-25 mg q4-6h PO, IM, IV, or rectally
Scopolamine	1.5 mg transdermal (patch)
Metoclopramide	1-2 mg/kg can be repeated IV

ADMINISTRATION

Depending on the drug, antiemetic drugs can be given PO, IV, IM, or rectally. Scopolamine is administered in a patch behind the ear.

CONTRAINDICATIONS

Antiemetic drugs are contraindicated or should be used with caution in older patients (see sections on Antipsychotic and Anticholinergic Drugs).

COMMON ADVERSE REACTIONS

Most antiemetic drugs cause sedation and drowsiness. Serotonin antagonists can cause musculoskeletal pain, dysrhythmias, and rarely, bronchospasm. Histamine antagonists cause sedation, confusion in geriatric individuals, dry mouth and eyes, and constipation. The phenothiazines can cause a number of adverse effects

(see Antipsychotic Drugs). Scopolamine causes anticholinergic effects (see Anticholinergic Drugs). Metoclopramide can cause seizures and suicidal ideation.

DRUG INTERACTIONS

Serotonin antagonists show few interactions. Histamine antagonists show enhanced anticholinergic activity with all drugs that also have these effects. Phenothiazines show a series of interactions (see Antipsychotic Drugs).

IMPLICATIONS FOR PHYSICAL THERAPISTS

- Observe patients for signs of dizziness and drowsiness, in particular older individuals, and be close by to prevent falls. In the case of phenothiazines, be aware of orthostatic hypotension.

ANTIFUNGAL DRUGS

COMMON DRUGS (SELECTION OF SOME OF THE MOST COMMONLY USED DRUGS)

Amphotericin B	Fungizone, Abelcet, other

Azole Drugs

Clotrimazole	Mycelex, Lotrimin, other (OTC)
Itraconazole	Sporanox
Miconazole	Monistat, other
Other	

Miscellaneous Drugs

Griseofulvin	Grifulvin, other
Nystatin	Nilstat, Nystex, other
Tolnaftate	Tinactin, Aftate, other
Other	

MECHANISM OF ACTION

Fungi are single or multicellular organisms with a cell membrane and cell wall. The wall protects them from the environment, and the membrane keeps in essential nutrients necessary for metabolism inside the fungus. The fungal membrane contains phospholipids and ergosterol (while the human membrane contains cholesterol). They live mostly on plants, dirt, and water and are mostly pathogenic to plants. Human fungal infections or mycoses are rare except in patients with immunocompromise such as those with acquired immunodeficiency syndrome (AIDS) or those taking steroids, anticancer drugs, immune system suppressing drugs, and certain antibiotics; the latter can kill nonpathogenic bacteria that prevent fungal growth.

Antifungal drugs act on some of the fungal peculiarities. Amphotericin B binds to ergosterol and forms with it a channel through which necessary nutrients escape, leading to the death of the fungus. Azole drugs inhibit the enzyme that synthesizes ergosterol. This reduces formation of a firm membrane that is now leaky and leads to the loss of nutrients and death of the fungus. Nystatin acts similarly to amphotericin B, griseofulvin binds to specific fungal mitotic spindles during division and interferes with replication, and tolnaftate acts by an unknown mechanism.

Antifungal drugs are fungus specific and must often be taken for long periods of time and exactly as prescribed to be fully effective. Drug resistance is not a major problem with fungi at this time.

INDICATION

Antifungal drugs are indicated in the following:

* *Topical and systemic fungal infections* affecting the skin, vagina, nails, lungs, and other parts of the body. Some examples are systemic aspergillosis, candidiasis, cryptococcosis, and histoplasmosis, which are treated with amphotericin B as a primary drug and sometimes with itraconazole as a secondary medication; tinea infections ("ringworm") with tolnaftate or clotrimazole; vulvovaginal candidiasis with clotrimazole; infections of the scalp, skin, and toes with griseofulvin, and oropharyngeal candidiasis with nystatin.

EXAMPLES OF COMMON DOSAGES (GENERAL GUIDELINES, MANY DIFFERENT DOSAGE SCHEDULES)

Amphotericin B	0.25-0.5 mg/kg IV
Clotrimazole	Topical preparations
Itraconazole	200-400 mg daily PO
Miconazole	Topical preparations
Griseofulvin	500-1000 mg daily PO
Nystatin	Topical preparations and 500,000-1,000,000 U 3 times daily PO
Tolnaftate	Topical preparations

ADMINISTRATION

Amphotericin B is usually given by slow infusion with test doses preceding the actual therapeutic amounts. The other drugs are mostly given topically or orally.

CONTRAINDICATIONS

Antifungal drugs are contraindicated or should be used with caution in patients with renal and hepatic disorders.

COMMON ADVERSE REACTIONS

Amphotericin is quite toxic and can cause seizures, renal toxicity, blood disorders, and allergic reactions. The other drugs show few adverse reactions when given topically. Oral administrations carry a higher risk with nausea, vomiting, and abdominal discomfort. Itraconazole can cause muscle pain and hepatotoxicity.

DRUG INTERACTIONS

* Depending on the drug, the azole drugs can interfere with the biotransformation of other drugs and can increase each other's toxicity.
* Gossypol increases itraconazole nephrotoxicity.

IMPLICATIONS FOR PHYSICAL THERAPISTS

* Advise the patient who uses OTC antifungal preparations to contact a physician because successful therapy of a fungal infection requires the expertise of a physician.
* Observe the patient who takes antifungal drugs, which can be hepatotoxic, for skin and eye color and notify the physician or have the patient contact the physician if yellowing of the skin or eyes is seen; this yellowing could be drug-induced liver toxicity.
* If you notice redness between the toes of a patient, notify the physician or have the patient contact the physician because this could be a tinea infection (athlete's foot). If the patient is a student or a person using a locker room, you should also contact those facilities and have locker rooms disinfected.

ANTIHELMINTHIC DRUGS

COMMON DRUGS (SELECTION OF SOME OF THE MOST COMMONLY USED DRUGS)

Albendazole	Albenza
Mebendazole	Vermox
Praziquantel	Biltricide
Pyrantel	Antiminth, Ascarel, other
Other	

MECHANISM OF ACTION

Helminths, or worms, are multicellular organisms. They have different life cycles and often enter the body through their eggs located in dirty water or contaminated food. They live in the intestines but also in other parts of the body, including the heart, muscles, and eyes. They can cause mild-to-severe clinical problems partly caused by competing for dietary needs by the human cells or by an inflammatory response of the body.

INDICATION

Antihelminthic drugs are indicated in the following:

* *Tape worm infections* are treated with praziquantal and albendazole, which paralyze or deprive the worms of glucose and nutrients.
* *Fluke infections* are treated with praziquantel, which paralyzes the flukes.

* *Trichinosis and other infections* are treated with albendazole or mebendazole, which deprive the worms of glucose and other nutrients.
* Drugs usually affect only adults but not eggs, which can infect other individuals during therapy.

EXAMPLES OF COMMON DOSAGES (GENERAL GUIDELINES, MANY DIFFERENT DOSAGE SCHEDULES)

Albendazole	400 mg 2 times daily PO
Mebendazole	100 mg 1-2 times a day for 3 days PO
Praziquantel	20 mg/kg 3 times a day PO
Pyrantel	11 mg/kg once or for 3 days PO

ADMINISTRATION

Depending on the antihelminthic drug, they are given mostly PO.

CONTRAINDICATIONS

Antihelminthic drugs are contraindicated or should be used with caution in patients with hepatic diseases.

COMMON ADVERSE REACTIONS

In general, antihelminthic drugs may cause nausea, headache, abdominal discomfort, and diarrhea (in addition to the use of a laxative which is often prescribed to help expel intestinal worms). Albendazole and mebendazole can be hepatotoxic.

DRUG INTERACTIONS

Few serious interactions have been observed, except some drugs, including cimetidine (OTC), increase albendazole tissue concentrations.

IMPLICATIONS FOR PHYSICAL THERAPISTS

* If a patient with a worm infection is treated, wear gloves and wash hand thoroughly after therapy, because eggs can spread easily. If the patient uses the toilet, have the toilet cleaned with disinfectant soap.
* If you notice a yellow skin color or yellowing of the eyes, notify the physician or have the patient contact the physician because some drugs can cause liver problems.

ANTIHISTAMINIC DRUGS

DRUGS (SELECTION OF SOME OF THE MOST COMMONLY USED DRUGS)

Antihistamines

Cetirizine	Zyrtec
Desloratadine	Clarinex
Dimenhydrinate	Dramamine (OTC)

Diphenhydramine	Allermed, Benadryl, other (OTC)
Fexofenadine	Allegra
Loratadine	Alavert, Claritin, other (OTC)
Other	

Mast-Cell Stabilizer

| Cromolyn | NasalCrom, other |
| Nedocromil | Tilade |

Corticosteroids (see Corticosteroids)

MECHANISM OF ACTION

Allergic reactions are unwanted, inflammatory immune system responses based on a "peculiarity" of an individual's immune system toward a specific chemical or substance and are manifested as redness, swelling, hives, runny nose and watery eyes (vasodilatation), and itching (activation of special nerves). In some cases, it can precipitate a potentially fatal anaphylactic reaction. The causes are substances called *antigens* or *allergens* that are considered by the immune system of such individuals as "dangerous," initiating the immune response or allergic reaction. The amount of allergens causing such reactions can be extremely small (part of a peanut or a whiff of shrimp). Different allergens cause the same clinical picture, which is in contrast to adverse reactions that are drug specific. There are four types of allergic reactions, but types I and IV are most important. Allergy type I is caused by combination of an allergen with antibodies type immunoglobulin (IGE) on mast cells releasing histamine. Onset is quick and occurs within minutes. Type IV involves the action of T cells and shows a similar clinical picture as type I, but the onset is delayed by 24 to 48 hours.

The typical antihistamines prevent histamine binding and replace already bound histamine on histamine 1 (H1) receptors and reduce or prevent vasodilation and activation of special nerves. Mast-cell stabilizers only stabilize mast cells and prevent histamine release with a delayed onset of action, but they do not act on already released histamine. Steroids (see Corticosteroid Drugs) cause blood vessel constriction and permeability reduction by enhancing the sensitivity of α-receptors in blood vessels to circulating epinephrine. (see α-Agonists).

INDICATIONS

Antihistaminic drugs are indicated in the following:

- *Type I allergy* is caused by histamine and its vasodilating and nerve-irritating action. Typical antihistaminics, mast-cell stabilizers, or steroids are used to antagonize these effects. Massive histamine release precipitates an anaphylactic reaction (bronchoconstriction, marked fall in blood pressure), which responds to epinephrine, causing vasoconstriction and bronchial relaxation.
- *Type IV allergy* is caused by T-cell actions and only steroids are effective. The cause of this allergy (e.g., cosmetics) is often difficult to identify because of delayed onset of action.
- Other uses such as *motion sickness and nausea* (dimenhydrinate, diphenhydramine), *Parkinson's disease* and *nonproductive cough*.

EXAMPLES OF COMMON DOSAGES (GENERAL GUIDELINES, MANY DIFFERENT DOSAGE SCHEDULES)

Cetirizine	5-10 mg/day PO
Desloratadine	5 mg/day PO
Dimenhydrinate	50-100 mg q4-6h PO
Diphenhydramine	25-50 mg q4-6h PO
Fexofenadine	60-180 mg/day PO
Loratadine	10 mg/day PO
Cromolyn	1 spray into each nostril, not to exceed 6 sprays
Nedocromil	2 inhalations 2-4 times a day

ADMINISTRATION

Antihistaminic drugs are administered PO, except for inhalations of mast-cell stabilizers.

CONTRAINDICATIONS

Few contraindications exist except hypersensitivity to drugs.

ADVERSE REACTIONS

All antihistamines cause some sedation and drowsiness, as well as anticholinergic effects (see Anticholinergic Drugs) but mostly with diphenhydramine. Hepatitis may occur with desloratadine, blood disorders (hemolytic anemia) have been reported with diphenhydramine and fexofenadine, and dysrhythmias with fexofenadine. Mast-cell stabilizers show few adverse reactions except some throat irritation.

DRUG INTERACTIONS

- Enhanced sedation and anticholinergic effects may occur with drugs that also have these effects. Alcohol enhances the sedative actions. Drugs used at higher doses can interfere with a number of other drugs, although given at high doses.
- Sedative and anticholinergic effects are increased by hops, senega, and corkwood.

IMPLICATIONS FOR PHYSICAL THERAPISTS

- Antihistaminic drugs can produce some sedation and confusion (mostly in geriatric patients) and can interfere with therapy. Appointments should be scheduled at the end of drug actions.
- Advise individuals who take OTC antihistaminic drugs that they can interfere with urination in cases of benign prostatic hyperplasia in older men and can cause contact lens intolerance. Self-medication is recommended for short periods of time only.
- Advise patients that diphenhydramine is not recommended by physicians to be used as a hypnotic because it does not cause a restful sleep.

COMMON DRUGS (SELECTION OF SOME OF THE MOST COMMONLY USED DRUGS)

HMG-CoA Reductase Inhibitors

Atorvastatin	Lipitor
Fluvastatin	Lescol
Lovastatin	Altocor, Mevacor
Rosuvastatin	Crestor
Simvastatin	Zocor

Bile Acid Sequestrants

Cholestyramine	LoCholest, Prevalite, other
Colesevelam	WelChol
Colestipol	Colestid

Miscellaneous Drugs

Ezetimibe	Zetia
Fenofibrate	Antara, Lofibra, other
Gemfibrozil	Lopid
Niacin	Niac, Niaspan, other (also available OTC) Also available as nicotinic acid and nicotinamide

MECHANISM OF ACTION

Lipids, such as cholesterol and triglycerides, are essential chemicals (e.g., cholesterol is part of the cell membranes and triglycerides liberate fatty acids, via the enzyme lipoprotein lipase, which are used as an energy source). Cholesterol is derived from our diet (exogenous source; about 15%). Cholesterol is also synthesized in the liver from precursors by hydroxyl-3-methyl-glutaryl coenzyme A reductase or HMG-CoA (endogenous source; about 85%). Some of the endogenously synthesized cholesterol moves into the blood directly, and some is secreted in the bile into our intestines to help absorb fats and later on is absorbed back into the body and enters the blood. In the blood, cholesterol and triglycerides are bound to specific proteins to form lipoproteins, which differ in size and function. Among them are the very low density lipoproteins (VLDLs), which are later converted to low density lipoproteins (LDLs). Other lipoproteins are the high density proteins (HDLs). Generally, the LDLs deliver and deposit cholesterol to blood vessel membranes ("bad" cholesterol) and tissues, while the HDLs remove cholesterol from blood vessels ("good" cholesterol). High levels of HDL can partially counteract the "bad" effects of LDL.

Antilipidemic drugs affect various steps in the absorption and metabolism of cholesterol. The HMG-CoA reductase inhibitors ("statin" drugs) inhibit the enzyme in the liver that synthesizes cholesterol, thereby lowering cholesterol levels. Bile acid sequestrants bind to cholesterol in the intestines, prevent its absorption into the blood, and excrete it with the feces. Ezetimibe prevents the absorption of cholesterol in the small intestines and also excretes it with the feces. Fenofibrate increases lipolysis by activating lipoprotein lipase, which decreases triglycerides levels and changes the size of the LDLs to render them less effective because it promotes their rapid breakdown. Gemfibrozil decreases triglyceride levels and interferes with the synthesis of VLDLs, which also reduces LDL levels. Niacin or vitamin B3 reduces the release of fatty acids from fat, decreases LDLs, and perhaps most significantly, seems to increase HDLs.

Recently, it was shown that the "statin" drugs are also antiinflammatory, providing additional benefits to individuals with high C reactive protein levels and high risk of cardiovascular accidents.

INDICATION

Antilipidemic drugs are indicated in the following:
- *Dyslipidemias* (genetic basis, diet, diseases such as diabetes, or drugs) are characterized by increased levels of cholesterol and/or triglycerides in the blood. If levels are permanently elevated, pathological changes can occur in blood vessels. Initiated by a chronic inflammatory response in the vessel walls partly caused by the action of white blood cells, LDLs deposit excessive amounts cholesterol and triglycerides without adequate removal. This leads to hardening of the arteries (arteriosclerosis) and the formation of plaques (atherosclerosis) that narrow and finally block blood vessels. The hardening of blood vessels increases blood pressure and impairs the supply of nutrients and oxygen to tissues, including the heart and brain. Parts of these plaques can break loose and block subsequent smaller vessels. In addition, small blood clots formed elsewhere can get stuck in and block such narrowed vessels. These can be the cause of MI and stroke. Although high cholesterol and lipid levels increase the risk of such events, they are only soft indicators because some individuals with low cholesterol levels can have strokes

and MIs and some individuals with high levels might not. Drugs used in hypercholesterolemia and/or elevated triglyceride levels will lower cholesterol and lipid levels by various actions, and thus reduce the risk of arteriosclerosis and the sequela of cardiac and central problems. The HMG-CoA reductase inhibitors are the most effective drugs for lowering cholesterol and can lower cholesterol levels by about 30%.

EXAMPLES OF COMMON DOSAGES (GENERAL GUIDELINES, MANY DIFFERENT DOSAGE SCHEDULES)

Atorvastatin	10-80 mg once daily (not to exceed 80 mg/day) PO
Fluvastatin	20-80 mg once or divided PO
Lovastatin	20-80 mg in single or divided doses PO
Rosuvastatin	5-40 mg daily PO
Simvastatin	5-40 mg daily (not to exceed 80 mg/day) PO
Cholestyramine	4 g twice a day up to 24 g/day PO
Colesevelam	Three 625 mg tabs twice a day PO
Colestipol	2-8 g twice a day PO
Ezetimibe	10 mg/day PO
Fenofibrate	40-160 mg /day PO
Gemfibrozil	600 mg twice a day PO
Niacin	100-500 mg/day in divided doses

ADMINISTRATION

Drugs can be given IV or PO. Some of these drugs can be prescribed in combination.

CONTRAINDICATIONS

Antilipidemic drugs should not be used or must be used with caution in individuals with hepatic diseases.

COMMON ADVERSE REACTIONS

Common adverse reactions include headache, abdominal cramps, dizziness, and heartburn.

In addition, HMG-CoA reductase inhibitors can cause lens opacities (eye examinations are warranted), liver dysfunction (frequent liver function tests are indicated in the beginning of therapy), muscle pain with rhabdomyolysis (breakdown of skeletal muscle), hemolytic anemia, and photosensitivity reactions. Bile acid sequestrants can cause constipation; fecal impact; flatulence; decreased absorption of vitamins A, D, and K with increased risk of bleeding; red blood cell formation; and hyperchloremic acidosis (rapid breathing, confusion). Ezetimibe causes

few major adverse reactions. Fenofibrate can cause dysrhythmias. Gemfibrozil can cause leukopenia and anemia. Niacin causes flushing, orthostatic hypotension, and sometimes hepatotoxicity (jaundice, dark urine).

DRUG INTERACTIONS

- HMG-CoA reductase inhibitors in the presence of some antifungal drugs, erythromycin, and niacin show an increased risk of rhabdomyolysis. Bile acid sequestrants can interfere with the absorption of many drugs.
- Grapefruit juice may increase toxicity, and St. John's wort and bran may decrease therapeutic response.

IMPLICATIONS FOR PHYSICAL THERAPISTS

- Ask the patient who is overweight and not taking antilipidemic drugs if cholesterol levels have been checked in the past. If not, strongly advise the patient to see a physician because high cholesterol levels can be a silent (no symptoms) killer.
- Warn patient not to self-medicate with OTC niacin because the use of niacin should be monitored by a physician because niacin can cause liver damage. Blood tests are necessary during therapy, and early detection of such a problem can prevent liver damage.
- If patient is using an HMG-CoA reductase inhibitor or a statin drug and complains about muscle pain or mentions a darkening of the urine, contact the physician or have the patient notify the physician immediately because this could be a sign of rhabdomyolysis.
- Tell the patient to see the physician at scheduled intervals in particular in the beginning of therapy because special laboratory tests have to be made to assure that no adverse liver reactions manifest themselves with some of the drugs like niacin and HMG-CoA reductase inhibitors. Early detection can prevent permanent damage.
- Advise the patient that in addition to drug therapy a diet low in cholesterol and fats should be followed combined with some daily exercise and a normal body weight.

ANTINEOPLASTIC DRUGS

COMMON DRUGS (SELECTION OF SOME OF THE MOST COMMONLY USED DRUGS)

Alkylating Agents

Carmustine	BCNU, Gliadel
Cyclophosphamide	Cytoxan, Neosar
Mechlorethamine	Mustargen, Nitrogen Mustard

Other

Platinum Containing Compounds
Cisplatin   Platinol
Other

Antimetabolites
Fluorouracil   Adrucil, Efudex, other
Mercaptopurine   Purinethol
Methotrexate   Amethopterin, Folex, other

Antibiotics
Bleomycin   Blenoxane
Dactinomycin   Cosmegen
Doxorubicin   Adriamycin
Other

Plant Alkaloids
Etoposide   VePesid, Etopophos
Paclitaxel   Taxol, Onxol
Topotecan   Hycamtin
Vincristine   Oncovin, Vincasar
Other

Tyrosine Kinase inhibitors
Erlotinib   Tarceva
Other

Biological Response Modifiers
Interferons   Roferon, PEG-INTRON, other
Rituximab   Rituxan
Other

Other Drugs
Hydroxyurea   Droxia, Hydrea
Other

MECHANISM OF ACTION

Neoplastic cells roughly divided into tumor (not spreading) and cancer (spreading or metastasizing) cells divide faster and do not die (show no apoptosis or controlled cell death). They rapidly form and synthesize new DNA-RNA proteins. However, all cells in a tumor do not proliferate at the same time. In addition, they form new blood vessels (angiogenesis) to support this rapid cell growth.

Antineoplastic drugs limit or stop this excessive proliferation by killing these cells or by attenuating their divisions. This interference can occur at specific phases of mitosis (cell cycle specific drugs mostly at S phase in which DNA synthesis occurs) or more generally (nonspecific drugs). Alkylating agents bind covalently to two opposite bases and crosslink the two DNA strands together so that they can not separate, which is necessary for cell division. Platinum-containing compounds also crosslink DNA strands and prevent their separation. Antimetabolites are drugs that are structurally similar to some of the endogenous bases necessary for DNA synthesis. These drugs are either incorporated into the DNA chain where they produce a nonfunctioning base or DNA sequence or inhibit the enzymes that are forming the endogenous bases from precursors; in both cases, normal DNA synthesis and

proliferation is impaired. Antibiotics only used for neoplastic diseases act in different and often poorly understood ways. They might be inserted into DNA strands, cause strand splitting, inhibit DNA-related enzymes, form highly toxic radicals, and/or disturb the cell walls of these cells. Plant alkaloids are either antimitotic drugs that bind to and disrupt the function of the microtubules, which are necessary for cell division, or enzyme inhibitors, which inhibit certain enzymes (topoisomerase), causing a break in the DNA strands. Tyrosine kinase inhibitors inhibit a special tyrosine kinase enzyme that participates in the rapid cell division of these neoplastic cells. Biological response modifiers are interleukins, interferons, and monoclonal antibodies (ending in -mab), which among other actions stimulate the body's immune system to fight such abnormal cells. In addition, a number of other drugs are available that act by different often poorly understood mechanisms.

Because all cells will not proliferate at the same time, only a fraction will be killed by a drug at one treatment. Thus multiple drugs with different modes of action and repeated treatments often have to be employed to increase the number of cells being killed (or to increase the "total cell kill"). It is then hoped that the remaining cells will be eliminated by the body's immune system. Another complication is the occurrence of drug resistance in which neoplastic cells develop mechanisms that render these drugs ineffective. Such cells might have "pumps" that remove the drug from the cell, form chemicals to which the drug binds, or develop repair mechanisms that repair drug-induced damage.

INDICATION

Antineoplastic drugs are indicated in the following

- All types of *tumors* and *cancers*. Drugs interfere selectively with different steps in DNA synthesis, cell division, and growth. The specific drug used depends on the type of neoplasm to be treated. "Cocktails" or 2 to 5 drugs are used simultaneously to increase "total cell kill."
- Other uses such as *keratoses* (fluorouracil), *ulcerative colitis,* and *psoriatic arthritis* (mercaptopurine).

EXAMPLES OF COMMON DOSAGES (GENERAL GUIDELINES, MANY DIFFERENT DOSAGE SCHEDULES)

Carmustine — 150-200 mg/m² single dose every 6 weeks IV
Cyclophosphamide — 1-5 mg/kg/day PO or 40-50 mg/kg in divided doses over 2-5 days IV

Mechlorethamine — 0.4 mg/kg as single or divided doses over 2-4 days IV
Cisplatin — 20-100 mg/m² once or for several days every 3-4 weeks IV
Fluorouracil — 370-425 mg/m² daily for 5 days IV
Mercaptopurine — 2.5-5 mg/kg/day PO
Methotrexate — 15-30 mg/day for 5 days PO, IM or 40 mg/m² IV
Bleomycin — 0.25-0.5 units/kg 1-2 times weekly SC, IV, IM or 15 units 2 times weekly IV
Dactinomycin — 500 µg/m²/day for 5 days to be repeated IV
Doxorubicin — 60-75 mg/m² 3 times a week IV
Etoposide — 50-100 mg/m² for 5 days to be repeated every 3-4 weeks IV
Paclitaxel — 175 mg/m² over 3 hrs every 3 weeks for 4 courses IV
Topotecan — 1.5 mg/m²/day for 5 days IV
Vincristine — 1-2 mg/m²/wk IV
Erlotinib — 150 mg daily PO
Interferons — Many different schedules depending on interferon
Rituximab — 375 mg/m² once weekly for 4-8 doses IV
Hydroxyurea — 80 mg/kg single dose every 3 days PO

ADMINISTRATION

Depending on the drug, antineoplastic drugs can be given PO, IV, intracavitary, intrapericardial, or by infusion. Drug combinations and schedules depend on the type of cancer and the tolerance of the patient.

CONTRAINDICATIONS

Antineoplastic drugs are contraindicated or should be used with caution in patients with infections, anemia, or ulcers. Because neoplasm is eventually a fatal disease, therapy usually overrides most possible contraindications.

COMMON ADVERSE REACTIONS

Many adverse reactions are shared by antineoplastic drugs and are caused by interference with DNA synthesis and multiplication of healthy but rapidly dividing cells. Hair formation is inhibited in the hair follicles, resulting in hair loss. Suppression of bone marrow leads to a paucity of erythrocytes with anemia, platelets with bleeding episodes, and leukocytes with a decrease in immune activity and an increased risk of infections. The latter adverse reactions can be counteracted (see sections on Hemopoietic Drugs and Immunomodulators). Effects on the GI system cause nausea, vomiting, diarrhea, lesions, and ulcers, and antidiarrheal drugs or antiemetic drugs can provide relief (see Antiemetics Drugs). Also, fatigue is commonly encountered with these drugs. Fortunately, many of these adverse reactions are reversed when drug therapy is stopped. In addition, renal, cardiac, and hepatic toxicities can occur. Different chemotherapeutic drugs will show their own toxicities in addition such as pulmonary fibrosis, seizures, and allergic reactions, including anaphylaxis.

DRUG INTERACTIONS

Depending on the drug, many interactions are possible, in particular with drugs that weaken the immune system, affect blood clotting, and may cause anemia. NSAIDs increase GI problems.

IMPLICATIONS FOR PHYSICAL THERAPISTS

- Inquire about unusual bleeding episodes (bruising, gum bleeding) and touch the patient gently because the ability for blood clotting may be seriously impaired. If such hemorrhagic episodes are present, have patient inform the physician.
- Do not treat the patient if you have an infectious disease because the patient's immune system is weakened. Also, separate this patient from other patients and inform the patient to avoid public, crowded places because of the increased risk of an infection.
- Assess the patient's breathing ability because these drugs can affect the lungs. If impairment is noticed, have the patient inform the physician.
- Many cancers involve pain and the use of pain medication. The use of massage, heat, and transcutaneous electrical nerve stimulation (TENS) can provide some pain relief and reduce the use of pain medications.
- The physical therapist can encourage the patient by assuring him or her that many of the cancers can now be cured or placed into long-lasting remission and that most of the bothersome adverse reactions will disappear after cessation of therapy.

COMMON DRUGS (SELECTION OF SOME OF THE MOST COMMONLY USED DRUGS)

Chloroquine	Aralen
Mefloquine	Lariam
Metronidazole	Flagyl, Protostat
Primaquine	Primaquine
Pyrimethamine	Daraprim, Fansidar (with sulfadoxine)

Other

MECHANISM OF ACTION

Protozoans are one-celled organisms living mostly in dirty water. They are subdivided into many subgroups. They have complex and different life cycles and can affect different parts of the body.

Antiprotozoal drugs interfere relatively selectively with the metabolism of the parasites such as feeding habits in red blood cells (RBCs), DNA synthesis, and/or some other poorly understood mechanisms. Chloroquine and mefloquine bind to the DNA of the certain parasites and interfere with transcription and also inhibit the parasitic enzyme heme polymerase, which inactivates free heme that is toxic to the parasite (plasmodium). Some species have become resistant to the drug. Pyrimethamine is a folate antagonist with a higher affinity for the parasitic than the host folate metabolism. Primaquine acting by uncertain mechanisms kills perhaps by impairing DNA function of the exo-RBC forms of the parasite in the liver. Metronidazole is believed to be metabolized to a substance that binds to and inhibits parasitic DNA synthesis.

INDICATION

Antiprotozoal drugs are indicated in the following:
- *Malaria* is a mosquito-borne disease that is caused by the plasmodium species. These parasites enter the human blood stream via a female mosquito bite and later are taken up from the blood by the mosquito to be introduced into other humans. Different species cause different problems, ranging from mild-to-severe forms of the disease. They accumulate in the liver and RBCs where they feed on hemoglobin and multiply. *Chloroquine, mefloquine, and* other drugs are used. Parasites are becoming more resistant to drug therapy.
- *Amoebiasis* is caused by an amoeba and results in mild-to-severe diarrhea, and trichomoniasis is a protozoal infection of the vagina (men usually remain asymptomatic). In both cases, metronidazole is used (which also has antibacterial activity), and it is relatively nontoxic.
- *Acanthamoeba keratitis* (red, painful eyes bothered by light) is caused by acanthamoeba living in dirty water and in nonsterile solutions used for cleaning contact lenses. Therapy includes use of itraconazole, polymyxin, and/or neomycin or polymyxin B (see Antifungal Drugs) for prolonged periods, sometimes months.
- *Toxoplasma gondii* is a protozoal infection transmitted to humans via cat feces or contaminated meat. Drugs of choice are pyrimethamine-sulfadiazine, which interfere with protozoal folic acid metabolism.
- *Other protozoal infections* are mostly present outside the United States.
- Other uses such as *rheumatoid arthritis* (chloroquine).

EXAMPLES OF COMMON DOSAGES (GENERAL GUIDELINES, MANY DIFFERENT DOSAGE SCHEDULES)

Chloroquine	5 mg/kg/wk 1-2 wks before exposure and for 8 wks after leaving the endemic area PO
Mefloquine	1250 mg once PO, not to be repeated
Metronidazole	250 mg 3 times daily for 7 days PO or 2 g once PO
Primaquine	15 mg daily PO
Pyrimethamine	100 mg followed by 25 mg/day for 4-5 wks PO

ADMINISTRATION

Depending on the drug, antiprotozoal drugs can be administered IM and PO.

CONTRAINDICATIONS

Antiprotozoal drugs are contraindicated or should be used with caution in blood disorders for antimalarial drugs.

COMMON ADVERSE REACTIONS

Most antiprotozoal drugs are tolerated relatively well and most adverse reactions are observed after high dose and long-term therapy. Chloroquine can affect the retina and heart, and primaquine might cause hemolytic anemia in susceptible individuals. Metronidazole is associated with bone marrow depression and seizures. Pyrimethamine might cause seizures, agranulocytosis, and respiratory problems.

DRUG INTERACTIONS

- Antimalarials show few interactions with other drugs.
- Folic acid supplements may decrease action of folate inhibitors. Acidophilus should not be taken simultaneously with metronidazole.

IMPLICATIONS FOR PHYSICAL THERAPISTS

- Inquire about the color of the urine in patients on primaquine because this drug can cause hemolytic anemia. If color changes are noted, inform the physician or have patient contact the physician.
- If a patient on chloroquine therapy mentions visual disturbances, inform the physician or have the patient contact the physician because this drug can damage the retina.
- Advise contact lens wearers to use sterile solutions and be careful in cleaning contact lenses because an acanthamoeba infection is very difficult to treat and carries certain health risks that could have been easily prevented.

ANTIPSYCHOTIC DRUGS

COMMON DRUGS (SELECTION OF SOME OF THE MOST COMMONLY USED DRUGS)

Phenothiazines

Chlorpromazine	Thorazine, other
Fluphenazine	Prolixin, Moditen
Perphenzine	Perphenzine, Trilafon
Prochlorperazine	Chlorpazine, Compazine, other
Thioridazine	Mellaril
Thiothixene	Navane (rarely used)
Trifluoperazine	Stelazine, Suprazine, other

Butyrophenone

Haloperidol	Haldol

Miscellaneous Drugs

Aripiprazole	Abilify
Clozapine	Clozaril
Loxapine	Loxitane
Olanzapine	Zydis, Zyprexa
Paliperidone	Invega
Quetiapine	Seroquel
Risperidone	Risperdal
Ziprasidone	Geodon

MECHANISM OF ACTION

Mental activities such as perception of reality, cognitive functions, and mood are regulated by the harmonious interaction of a multitude of chemical (neurotransmitters) processes and electrical circuits. Normal functioning of dopamine and dopamine receptors, mostly D2, D3 subtype, in the mesolimbic and mesocortical areas of the brain are of utmost importance. In addition, α-adrenergic, serotonergic, glutaminergic, and cholinergic receptors also play a role.

The typical antipsychotic drugs block mostly D2 receptors, whereas their actions on other receptors like α- and cholinergic receptors are more involved in adverse reactions. Blockade of the dopaminergic receptors may cause their upregulation, which takes time and may explain the delayed therapeutic effect seen in patients. The atypical antipsychotic drugs also block dopaminergic receptors (D2, D3), but less and have a more significant action on inhibiting serotonergic (1A, 2A) receptors.

INDICATION

Antipsychotic drugs are indicated in the following:

- *Schizophrenia* is characterized by delusions, hallucinations, thought disorders (positive symptoms), reduced emotions, reduced social contact, reduced speech, and reduced pleasure (negative symptoms). Studies have shown the brains of schizophrenic patients to show certain abnormalities like enlarged cerebral ventricles, a decreased number of synaptic connections in the prefrontal cortex, and an increased or decreased functioning of dopamine D2, D3 receptors, depending on the area. All drugs affect a number of neurotransmitters, but they all seem to cause a blockade and perhaps upregulation of dopaminergic receptors (mostly D2 receptors). The typical antipsychotics also affect other receptors such as blockade of α-receptors with a decrease in blood pressure; cholinergic receptors with dry mouth, blurred vision, and constipation (see Anticholinergic Drugs); and dopamine receptors in the basal ganglia with movement disorders (see CNS Dopaminergic Agonists). They mostly alleviate positive symptoms. The atypical antipsychotic drugs block dopaminergic and serotonergic receptors and alleviate some of the positive and negative symptoms. Clinically, about one-third of patients improves markedly, one-third improves somewhat, and one-third does not respond.
- Other uses for individual drugs include *depression* (see Antidepressant Drugs), *dementia* in older individuals (thioridazine), nausea (see Antiemetic Drugs), *Tourette's syndrome* (see Movement Disorders), and mania (see Antidepressant Drugs).

EXAMPLES OF COMMON DOSAGES (GENERAL GUIDELINES, MANY DIFFERENT DOSAGE SCHEDULES)

Chlorpromazine	10-50 mg q2h with a gradual increase up to 2 g/day PO
Fluphenazine	2.5-10 mg in divided doses up to 40 mg/day PO
Perphenazine	8-16 mg in divided doses up to 64 mg/day PO
Prochlorperazine	5-10 mg 3-4 times a day up to 150 mg/day PO
Thioridazine	25-100 mg 3 times a day up to 800 mg/day PO
Thiothixene	2-5 mg 2-3 times a day up to 30 mg/day PO
Trifluoperazine	2-5 mg 2 times daily up to about 40 mg/day PO
Haloperidol	0.5-5 mg 2-3 times daily up to 100 mg/day PO
Aripiprazole	10-15 mg/day up to 30 mg/day PO
Clozapine	300-600 mg in divided doses PO
Loxapine	10 mg 2-4 times daily up to 100 mg/day PO
Olanzapine	5-10 mg/day up to 15 mg/day PO
Paliperidone	6 mg/day PO
Quetiapine	25 mg 2 times daily up to 300 mg/day PO
Risperidone	1 mg 2 times a day up to about 3 mg PO
Ziprasidone	20 mg 2 times daily up to 80 mg/day PO

ADMINISTRATION

Antipsychotic drugs can be given orally or by injection, including depot preparations because psychotic patients often refuse to take the medication as prescribed.

CONTRAINDICATIONS

Antipsychotic drugs should not be used or must be used with caution in patients with hepatic disorders, hyper- or hypotension, and cerebral arteriosclerosis.

COMMON ADVERSE REACTIONS

Common adverse reactions for most drugs include sedation and dizziness. Typical antipsychotics can cause pseudoparkinsonism, dystonia, akathisia, irreversible tardive dyskinesia, seizures, malignant hyperthermia, orthostatic hypotension, tachycardia, cardiac arrest, jaundice/hepatitis, constipation, urinary hesitancy, laryngospasm, respiratory depression, and rarely, agranulocytosis. Some drugs interfere with body temperature regulation. Haloperidol has similar adverse reactions but seems to be less anticholinergic but more dopaminergic. Atypical antipsychotics have similar adverse reactions but show less respiratory effects and a decreased risk of developing tardive dyskinesia.

DRUG INTERACTIONS

- These drugs interact with a large number of drugs, in particular, drugs with sedative, anticholinergic, and antihypertensive actions.

- Henbane leaves, nutmeg, and kava increase their toxicities.

IMPLICATIONS FOR PHYSICAL THERAPISTS

- Patients often may not be cooperative or they may be fearful of novel environments and procedures if their paranoia is only partially controlled by drugs.
- Check the patient for movement problems such as pseudoparkinsonism, dyskinesia, dystonia, akathisia, and tardive dyskinesia, and if detected, inform the physician directly because the patient might not do so.
- Watch for orthostatic hypotension with some of the drugs and have the patient change positions slowly or avoid long standing periods. Watch the patient leaving a warm therapeutic pool to avoid fainting.
- Patients who are on medications with strong anticholinergic actions will show an increase in heart rate; advise the patient to chew gum when a dry mouth becomes a disturbing problem.
- Ask older patients on drugs with strong anticholinergic actions if they have experienced constipation or urinary hesitance (mostly men) and if yes, inform the physician to avoid complications of constipation or possible urinary retention.
- Check older patients who have received olanzapine IM for respiratory problems, and notify the physician immediately if such problems are detected to avoid the occurrence of pneumonia.

ANTIVIRAL DRUGS

COMMON DRUGS (SELECTION OF SOME OF THE MOST COMMONLY USED DRUGS)

DNA Inhibitors

Acyclovir	Zovirax
Famciclovir	Famvir
Foscarnet	Foscavir
Ganciclovir	Cytovene, Vitrasert
Valacyclovir	Valtrex
Other	

Neuraminidase Inhibitors

Oseltamivir	Tamiflu
Other	

Reverse Transcriptase Inhibitors

Stavudine	Zerit
Tenofovir	Viread
Zidovudine	Retrovir
Other	

Protease Inhibitors

Lopinavir	Kaletra (with ritonavir)
Ritonavir	Norvir
Other	

Miscellaneous Action

Amantadine	Symadine, Symmetrel
Enfuvirtide	Fuzeon
Interferons	
Other	

MECHANISM OF ACTION

Viruses consist of single or double strands of DNA or RNA enclosed in a protein coat (capsid). They need the metabolism of a specific host cell to multiply (loss of drug specificity occurs because they partly use the host cell metabolism). The life cycle of a virus generally involves attaching to a host cell, penetrating, uncoating (shedding the protein coat), incorporating viral DNA into the host cell DNA, forming individual virus parts, cutting long proteins to the size needed by the virus (done by special proteases), assembling new viruses, and leaving the cell. Influenza viruses also need the enzyme neuraminidase to complete their biosynthesis and release. Some RNA viruses must first form DNA, whereas others can synthesize proteins directly. Viruses then affect other cells but can also retreat during drug treatment into tissues in which they hide and cannot be attacked by the immune system. Thus virus infections are difficult to cure (e.g., herpes infections) and some can reemerge after decades of inactivity (e.g., shingles after a chicken pox infection).

Antiviral drugs exploit some of the differences between the host cell and virus. DNA inhibitors are first monophosphorylated (some by viral enzymes) and then diphosphorylated and triphosphorylated by host cell enzymes; the triphosphorylated compound is the active antiviral compound and competes with endogenous bases for DNA polymerase and is partly incorporated as a "faulty" base terminating viral DNA chain synthesis. Foscarnet works in a similar fashion but does not have to be phosphorylated. Neuraminidase inhibitors inhibit the enzyme neuraminidase and interfere with the completion of the synthesis and release of influenza viruses. Reverse transcriptase inhibitors affect RNA viruses where RNA is first transcribed into DNA by the enzyme reverse transcriptase whose action is inhibited by these drugs resulting in impairment of DNA synthesis and viral multiplication. Protease inhibitors inhibit proteases and prevent the cleavage of the newly formed long protein molecules into smaller protein molecules necessary for viral assembly. Some drugs act by interfering with the attachment/penetration and uncoating (amantadine, enfuvirtide), and others (interferons) protect neighboring cells from being infected. Vaccines can prevent many viral infections today.

Antiviral drugs can be given prophylactically and therapeutically. Unfortunately, viruses become more and more resistant to these drugs by losing some of their special enzymes or by altering their DNA expression.

INDICATION

Antiviral drugs are indicated in the following:

- *Herpes infections:* Both initial and recurrent infections are treated with acyclovir or valacyclovir.
- *Herpes and zoster infections* are treated with famciclovir or valacyclovir.
- *Influenza A and B infections* are treated with oseltamivir (A and B) or amantadine (A).
- *Cytomegalovirus infections* are treated with ganciclovir.
- *Chronic hepatitis* can be treated with interferon α-2b or peg-interferon α-2a.
- *AIDS* is treated mostly with reverse transcriptase inhibitors, protease inhibitors, and enfuvirtide. Antiviral drugs mostly in combination have to be given for long periods. During pregnancy, they can prevent vertical transmission of the virus (mother to fetus).
- *Transplants:* Drugs, such as ganciclovir, are given to prevent viral infections in the recipient.

EXAMPLES OF COMMON DOSAGES (GENERAL GUIDELINES, MANY DIFFERENT DOSAGE SCHEDULES)

Acyclovir	200-800 mg q4h PO
Famciclovir	500 mg q8h PO
Foscarnet	60 mg/kg given over 1 hr q8h for 2-3 weeks IV
Ganciclovir	1000 mg 3 times daily PO or 5 mg/kg/dose over 1 hour for 2-3 weeks IV
Valacyclovir	1000 mg 3 times daily PO
Oseltamivir	75 mg 2 times daily PO
Stavudine	40 mg q12h PO
Tenofovir	300 mg once daily PO
Zidovudine	600 mg/day in divided doses or 1-2 mg/kg q4h IV
Lopinavir	400/100 mg 2 times daily or 800/200 mg once daily (with ritonavir) PO
Ritonavir	300 mg 2 times daily followed by increased doses up to 600 mg 2 times daily PO
Amantadine	200 mg/day or 100 mg 2 times daily PO
Enfuvirtide	90 mg 2 times daily SC
Interferons	Different schedules

PHARMACOLOGY

Section V

ADMINISTRATION

Depending on the drug, antiviral drugs can be given PO, IV, SC, or topically (on blisters and eyes). Some must be injected into the eye.

CONTRAINDICATIONS

Antiviral drugs are contraindicated or should be used with caution in patients with blood, renal, and hepatic disorders.

COMMON ADVERSE REACTIONS

Generally, most antiviral drugs can affect the kidneys, liver, and blood. Drugs taken at high doses may precipitate in the kidneys to form stones that can be prevented by consumption of large quantities of water. Also, neuralgia and myopathies are encountered. Except for the reactions mentioned previously, DNA inhibitors are generally well tolerated except foscarnet which can cause cardiac arrest, acute renal failure, pulmonary embolism, and bronchospasm. Neuraminidase inhibitors, such as oseltamivir, may cause Stevens-Johnson syndrome. Reverse transcriptase inhibitors can cause blood dyscrasias and hepatotoxicity. Protease inhibitors may shift fat from other body places to the abdomen and cause insulin resistance, as well increase cardiovascular risks. Amantadine has been associated with mood changes, loss of concentration in elderly individuals, and orthostatic hypotension, and enfuvirtide can cause neuropathy. Interferons have been associated with neuropsychiatric disorders, pancreatitis, blood dyscrasias, and autoimmune disorders.

DRUG INTERACTIONS

- DNA inhibitors show few serious interactions. Antiviral drugs taken at high doses will interact with other drugs because of interference with renal excretion or metabolism. Some antiviral drugs interact with each other and when they are to be used simultaneously, administration must be spaced. Lopinavir/ritonavir interacts with sildenafil and related drugs to cause severe hypotension. Ritonavir interacts with a large number of drugs, including St. John's wort, which decreases its efficacy.
- Use of alcohol will increase toxicity of most drugs.

IMPLICATIONS FOR PHYSICAL THERAPISTS

- If a skin rash is noticed, notify the physician or have the patient contact the physician because some drugs can cause the Stevens-Johnson syndrome.
- If you notice a yellow skin color or yellowing of conjunctiva, have patient contact or personally inform physician because some drugs can be hepatotoxic.

- Emphasize that mothers should follow the physician's instructions and not breast feed because some drugs can pass through the milk into the child.
- Watch male patients carefully who use lopinavir/ritonavir and drugs for erectile dysfunction because they are prone to experience severe hypotensive episodes with syncope.
- If the patient has been instructed to drink large amounts of fluids, have the patient periodically drink water in particular when he/she is sweating to prevent formation of kidney stones.
- Emphasize to the patient that open herpes blisters will transmit the virus by contact and advise abstinence from or use of condoms during intercourse.

ANXIOLYTIC DRUGS

COMMON DRUGS (SELECTION OF SOME OF THE MOST COMMONLY USED DRUGS)

Benzodiazepines

Alprazolam	Xanax
Chlordiazepoxide	Librium, other
Clonazepam	Klonopin
Clorazepate	Tranxene
Diazepam	Valium, other
Lorazepam	Ativan
Oxazepam	Serax

Azapirones

Buspirone	BuSpar

Antidepressants (see Antidepressant Drugs)

Doxepin
Hydroxyzine
Paroxetine
Venlafaxine

MECHANISM OF ACTION

Normal anxiety is characterized by acceptable tension, apprehension, and nervousness in response to appropriate environmental challenges and is a helpful part of human life. Anxiety is controlled by many chemical processes (neurotransmitters) and electrical circuits. In this case, the neurotransmitter GABA in the limbic and hypothalamic areas seems to play a major role. GABA is formed in special neurons, then released and interacts with GABA receptors (subtypes A, B, C, and more) on adjacent neurons to open chloride channels in their neuronal membranes. Influx of negative chloride ions hyperpolarizes these cells and reduces their firings or activity. Thus, depending on the circumstances, the inhibitory GABA system can cause anxiety when indicated by decreasing its action and terminate anxiety when not necessary by increasing its action. In addition, GABA also controls

skeletal muscle activity and increased GABA actions causes muscle relaxation. In addition to GABA, other neurotransmitter systems also play a role like the serotonergic system.

Benzodiazepine drugs act on various sites of the GABA-receptor complex in which they all seem to enhance the action of GABA, increase hyperpolarization of overly excited neurons, and reduce their neuronal firing, resulting in a decrease in anxiety. Buspirone does not act on GABA but is a serotonin partial agonist on the serotonergic receptors. Antidepressant anxiolytics act on norepinephrine and/or serotonin (see Antidepressant Drugs).

INDICATION

Anxiolytic drugs are mainly indicated in the following:

- *Anxiety disorders* are characterized by an excessive, irrational fear of every situation, which can be disabling and significantly interfere with daily activities and functioning of the individual. There are five types: Generalized Anxiety Disorder (chronic exaggerated worry, tension, insomnia, and irritability with no apparent cause), Obsessive-Compulsive Disorder (urgent need to engage in certain rituals such as obsessing over germs or dirt and washing hands over and over again), Panic Disorder (pounding heart, chest pains, lightheadedness or dizziness, nausea, shortness of breath, fear of dying, sweating, and feelings of unreality), Posttraumatic Stress Disorder (persistent frightening thoughts and memories of past ordeals), and Phobias (irrational fear of things, animals, or people). In these cases, the existing GABA and/or the serotonergic systems are apparently not able to dampen excessive neuronal excitation to a more normal level. Benzodiazepines increase GABA action, increase hyperpolarization in adjacent cells, reduce their neuronal firing, and dampen excessive neural activity, leading to a relatively quick reduction of anxiety. Buspirone also dampens excessive neuronal activity but through agonistic actions on the serotonin receptors, resulting in a delayed (2 to 4 weeks) antianxiety effect. Antidepressant drugs (see Antidepressant Drugs) affect depression, which is often associated with anxiety.
- Other conditions such as *premenstrual syndrome, depression, alcohol withdrawal, muscle relaxation, restless leg syndrome, seizure disorders,* and certain medical, diagnostic, and surgical procedures.

EXAMPLES OF COMMON DOSAGES (GENERAL GUIDELINES, MANY DIFFERENT DOSAGE SCHEDULES)

Alprazolam	0.25-0.5 mg 3 times a day up to 4 mg/day PO
Chlordiazepoxide	5-25 mg 3-4 times daily PO
Clonazepam	1.5 mg/day in 3 divided dose (not to exceed 20 mg/day) PO
Diazepam	2-10 mg 2-4 times daily PO
Lorazepam	2-6 mg in divided doses up to 10 mg/day PO
Oxazepam	10-30 mg 3-4 times daily up to 120 mg/day PO
Buspirone	5 mg 3 times daily up to 60 mg/day PO

ADMINISTRATION

Anxiolytic drugs are given mostly PO but can also be injected IM or IV.

CONTRAINDICATIONS

Anxiolytic drugs should not be used or must be used with caution in patients with a history of drug abuse and respiratory problems.

COMMON ADVERSE REACTIONS

Benzodiazepines will cause some sedation and psychomotor impairment. Less frequent are electrocardiogram (ECG) changes, tachycardia, and agranulocytosis. Depending on the drug, they will all cause some physical dependence after long-term therapy, and a withdrawal syndrome (excitation, rebound anxiety, insomnia) might occur after abrupt cessation of therapy. Alprazolam must be withdrawn very slowly because convulsions may occur. Buspirone is almost devoid of adverse reactions except some dizziness and restlessness. Adverse reactions of the antidepressants are described in Antidepressant Drugs.

DRUG INTERACTIONS

- Sedation caused by anxiolytics with sedative properties is increased by drugs that also have sedative actions.
- Sedative effects are increased by a number of herbs, including chamomile, mistletoe, and valerian. St. John's wort seems to reduce their effectiveness.

IMPLICATIONS FOR PHYSICAL THERAPISTS

- Physical therapists can be helpful in promoting nonpharmacological interventions, such as relaxation techniques, exercises, or massages, to reduce feelings of anxiety and the use of anxiolytics.
- Patients on higher doses of benzodiazepines may have to be scheduled at times when the sedative and psychomotor impairments are less noticeable and will not interfere with therapy.
- Always watch older patients on benzodiazepine therapy for motor incoordination, sedation, and impaired gait to avoid falls that could lead to serious fractures.
- Advise patients on buspirone at the start of therapy to be patient because it will take about a month before anxiolytic effects become apparent.

β-AGONISTS

COMMON DRUGS (SELECTION OF SOME OF THE MOST COMMONLY USED DRUGS)

β_1-Agonists
Dobutamine	Dobutamine

β_2-Agonists (Relatively Selective)
Albuterol	Salbutamol, Ventolin, Volmax, other
Formoterol	Foradil, Perforomist
Metaproterenol	Alupent
Pirbuterol	Maxair
Salmeterol	Serevent
Terbutaline	Brethine

β_1- and β_2-Agonists
Isoproterenol	Isoproterenol

Mixed Acting α-and β-Agonists (see α-Agonists)

MECHANISM OF ACTION

β_1-receptors (mostly in the heart) and β_2-receptors (mostly other organs) are usually but not exclusively found opposite postganglionic sympathetic nerve fibers, which release norepinephrine, which stimulates these receptors. Activation of these receptors in the lungs causes bronchial dilation (with increased air flow) and vasodilation in the blood vessels, increases in heart rate and contractility (with an increase in systolic blood pressure), reduces gut activity, increases blood glucose levels and fluid inflow in the eye, increases skeletal muscle activity (perhaps through central β-receptors), and increases secretion of rennin from the kidneys. Activation of beta receptors on the pregnant uterus reduces its contractions.

These drugs stimulate β-receptors and cause the appropriate physiological responses as outlined previously. β_2-agonists are more selective for β_2-receptors, although this distinction breaks down at high doses or in certain individuals.

INDICATIONS

β-Agonists are indicated in the following:
- *Asthma,* in which bronchoconstriction (caused by allergy, exercise, cold air, other) decreases air flow and makes breathing difficult (wheezing). Selective β_2-receptor agonists stimulate β_2-receptors on bronchi, cause bronchi to dilate, and allow air to flow through bronchi more easily. β_2-agonists are sometimes combined with steroids because inflammatory processes are often associated with bronchial constrictions (see Corticosteroids).
- *Chronic obstructive pulmonary disease* (COPD) and *emphysema,* in which air flow is impaired because of lung damage mostly from smoking. Selective β_2-receptor agonists stimulate β_2-receptors on bronchi, cause bronchi to dilate, and allow air to flow through bronchi more easily.
- Other conditions such as the prevention of *premature contractions* during pregnancy (ritodrine, terbutaline), *CHF* (dobutamine IV), or *severe hypotension* (dopamine IV).

EXAMPLES OF COMMON DOSAGES (GENERAL GUIDELINES, MANY DIFFERENT DOSAGE SCHEDULES)

Albuterol	2-4 mg 2-4 times daily PO (not to exceed 8 mg/day) or 4-8 mg twice daily for extended-release preparations PO or 2-4 inhalations q4-6h or 15 min before exercise
Formoterol	1 cap (12 µg) q12h by inhalation
Metaproterenol	20 mg 3-4 times daily PO 1-2 inhalations q4-6h (not to exceed 12 inhalations)
Salmeterol	1 inhalation (50 µg)
Terbutaline	2.5-5 mg q6-8h PO (not to exceed 15 mg/day)

ADMINISTRATION

β-Agonists can be given IV, PO, or by inhalation. Administration schedules vary among drugs because of differences in duration of action.

CONTRAINDICATIONS

β-Agonists must be used with caution in patients with cardiovascular disease, diabetes mellitus, and seizure disorders.

COMMON ADVERSE REACTIONS

Common adverse reactions include nervousness, restlessness, insomnia, tremor, chest pain, and increases in heart rate and blood pressure (the latter two less with β2 agonists) and blood sugar levels. Excessive use of inhalers can lead to tolerance or sometimes paradoxical bronchospasm.

DRUG INTERACTIONS

- β-Agonists should not be used with MAO inhibitors because they may alter potassium and sugar levels.
- Caffeine in coffee or tea, fig wort, and motherwort may enhance CNS effects.

IMPLICATIONS FOR PHYSICAL THERAPISTS

- Be aware that exercise and cold air can aggravate asthma and bronchoconstriction. Have the patient use an inhaler 15 to 30 minutes before exercise, depending on the drug, and avoid cold or drafty places.
- After inhalation or oral use, heart rate and blood pressure can be increased. Patients with angina should be exercised slowly because β-agonists can increase the risk of angina.
- If patient uses the inhaler too often, have patient notify the physician because excessive use can cause tolerance or paradoxical bronchoconstriction.
- If a patient shows a fine tremor, notify or have patient contact the physician because the dose may have to be adjusted or a different drug may have to be prescribed.

β-BLOCKERS

COMMON DRUGS (SELECTION OF SOME OF THE MOST COMMONLY USED DRUGS)

Acebutolol	Sectral
Atenolol	Tenormin
Bisoprolol	Zebeta, Monocor
Carteolol	Cartrol
Carvedilol	Coreg
Labetalol	Normodyne, Trandate
Metoprolol	Lopressor SR, Toprol-XL
Nadolol	Corgard
Penbutolol	Levatol
Pindolol	Visken
Propranolol	Inderal, InnoPran XL
Sotalol	Betapace

MECHANISM OF ACTION

β_1-receptors (mostly in the heart) and β_2-receptors (most other organs) are usually but not exclusively found opposite postganglionic sympathetic nerve fibers, which release norepinephrine, thus activating these receptors. Activation of these receptors in the lungs causes bronchial dilation (with increased air flow) and dilation in blood vessels, increases in heart rate and contractility (with an increase in systolic blood pressure), reduces gut activity, increases blood glucose levels and fluid inflow in the eye, increases in skeletal muscle activity (through a central mechanism), and increases secretion of renin in the kidney.

Competitive blockade of these receptors by β-antagonists or blockers causes the opposite effects (which can be antagonized by or overcome by use of β-agonists). Most drugs affect β_1-receptors and β_2-receptors, but some are somewhat more selective for β_1 blockade. In addition, they reduce renin secretion from the kidney and peripheral sympathetic activity by a central mechanism. Labetalol also blocks α-receptors in blood vessels and reduces vasoconstriction leading to more incidences of orthostatic hypotension. Pindolol is a partial antagonist that can antagonize, as well as stimulate, depending on the activity of the system.

INDICATIONS

β-Antagonists or β-blockers are indicated in the following:

- *Angina pectoris,* which is characterized by pain usually in response to physical activity or emotional factors. This results when the oxygen demand of the compromised heart exceeds the oxygen supply from damaged coronary blood vessels (e.g., atherosclerosis). β antagonists decrease heart rate and contractility, reduce the oxygen need, and decrease or eliminate pain.
- *Hypertension,* which occurs when blood pressure is increased above normal limits, leading eventually to infarcts and strokes. β-Blockers lower blood pressure by reducing cardiac output (heart rate and contractility), blocking rennin release (which reduces the formation of the vasoconstrictor angiotensin II), and depressing central outflow of sympathetic stimulation (causing vasodilation).
- *Arrhythmias,* which are caused by abnormal electrical activity. β-Antagonists reduce overly excited cardiac activity and normalize heart rhythm (certain types only; see Antiarrhythmic Drugs).
- *Tremors, migraine, anxiety, drug induced akathisia, aggressive behavior,* and other conditions in which the mechanism of action is uncertain, but β-antagonists seem to be helpful.
- *Open-angle glaucoma,* in which intraocular pressure is elevated so that it can damage the retina, leading eventually to tunnel vision and blindness. Certain β-blockers (timolol, betaxolol, levobunolol) administered topically block the inflow of fluid into the eye and lower intraocular pressure.

EXAMPLES OF COMMON DOSAGES (GENERAL GUIDELINES, MANY DIFFERENT DOSAGE SCHEDULES)

Acebutolol	400-800 mg/day once or twice (up to 1200 mg/day) PO
Atenolol	25-100 mg once daily (up to 200 mg/day) PO
Bisoprolol	5 mg once daily (up to 20 mg/day) PO
Carteolol	2.5-10 mg once daily PO
Carvedilol	3.125-6.25 mg twice daily (up to 50 mg daily) PO
Labetalol	100-400 mg twice daily (up to 2.4 g daily)
Metoprolol	25-100 mg/day as a single or divided dose (up to 450 mg/day) PO
Nadolol	40-80 mg once daily (up to 320 mg/day) PO
Penbutolol	20 mg once daily PO
Pindolol	5 mg twice daily (up to 45-60 mg/day) PO
Propranolol	40-320 mg/day single or divided daily PO
Sotalol	80 mg twice daily (up to 320 mg) PO

ADMINISTRATION

β-Blockers can be given PO, IV, and in some cases, topically into the eye. Long-term therapy must be stopped slowly or the drug must be tapered to avoid withdrawal syndrome (cardiac problems).

CONTRAINDICATIONS

β-Blockers must be used with caution in bradycardia, renal impairment, pulmonary disease (e.g., asthma), and diabetes mellitus.

COMMON ADVERSE REACTIONS

- Common adverse reactions include weakness, drowsiness, bradycardia, pulmonary edema, hypotension, impotence, cold extremities and masking of hypoglycemic and thyrotoxic episodes (e.g., masking of tachycardia).
- Topical administration causes fewer and milder systemic adverse reactions.

DRUG INTERACTIONS

β-Antagonists or β-blockers may alter the effectiveness of insulin or hypoglycemics, antagonize the use of β–agonists, and should not be used with MAO inhibitors.

IMPLICATIONS FOR PHYSICAL THERAPISTS

- When exercising a patient, be aware that heart rate will be affected (reduced) by β-blockers.
- Advise patients to consult a physician if breathing difficulties are experienced

during exercise because these drugs can cause bronchoconstriction and pulmonary edema.

- Have older patients get up slowly because drugs can (mostly labetalol) cause orthostatic hypotension in particular in the beginning of therapy.
- Use exercise with caution in patients using insulin and β-blockers because the β-blocker may mask the onset signs and symptoms of a hypoglycemic episode.
- Patients on β-blockers are sensitive to a cold environment, in particular, experiencing cold extremities.
- Warn patient to not suddenly discontinue long-term β-blocker use because abrupt cessation can precipitate a serious withdrawal syndrome (including life-threatening arrhythmias).

CALCIUM CHANNEL BLOCKERS

COMMON DRUGS (SELECTION OF SOME OF THE MOST COMMONLY USED DRUGS)

Amlodipine	Norvasc
Diltiazem	Cardizem, Cartia XT, Dilacor XR, other
Felodipine	Plendil
Isradipine	DynaCirc, DynaCirc CR
Nicardipine	Cardene, Cardene SR
Nifedipine	Adalat, Adalat CC, Procardia, Procardia XL
Nisoldipine	Sular
Verapamil	Apo-Verap, Calan, Isoptin, other

MECHANISM OF ACTION

Movement of calcium in muscle cells is necessary for normal muscle contraction. This provides for normal skeletal muscle contractions, cardiac conduction and contractibility (cardiac output), and blood vessel wall tension (peripheral resistance). The latter regulate blood pressure (peripheral resistance and cardiac output [heart rate, stroke volume] determine blood pressure).

Calcium channel blockers inhibit these calcium fluxes by blocking calcium channels. This causes mostly a decreased excitation-contraction coupling in the heart (at one phase, the depolarizing current is carried primarily by a relatively slow, inward movement of calcium) with reduced contractility and cardiac output, as well as relaxation of blood vessels with reduced peripheral resistance. Both lower blood pressure.

These drugs differ somewhat in their action on the heart and blood vessels; nifedipine, amlodipine, and nicardipine are strong vasodilators, and verapamil and diltiazem are more effective on the electrical conduction system and the heart's contractile strength.

INDICATIONS

Calcium channel blockers are indicated in the following:

- *Hypertension,* in which vasoconstriction or increased peripheral resistance is a major cause of increased blood pressure. Drugs block calcium fluxes in cardiac tissue and blood vessel walls and reduce both cardiac contractibility and relax blood vessels. This decreases cardiac output and peripheral resistance and lowers blood pressure.
- *Angina pectoris,* which is characterized by pain usually in response to physical activity or emotional factors. This results when the oxygen demand of the compromised heart exceeds the oxygen supply from damaged coronary blood vessels (e.g., atherosclerosis). These drugs reduce contractibility (which reduces cardiac oxygen requirements), dilate coronary arteries to supply more blood and oxygen to the heart, and relax peripheral blood vessels (which decreases peripheral resistance), making it easier for the heart to eject the blood into the periphery. (A special form is Prinzmetal angina, which is a spastic blood vessel constrictive form.)
- *Certain arrhythmias* such as supraventricular tachycardia or atrial flutter and fibrillations. In these cases, electrical activity is conducted too fast or irregularly over the heart so that the cardiac muscle cannot contract completely and efficiently. Drugs reduce excitation-contraction coupling by slowing calcium movements, normalizing conduction, slowing the heart, and achieving more efficient contractions.
- Congestive heart failure or *CHF,* in which the heart cannot pump enough blood to other organs of the body, and results in an enlarged heart with the patient becoming quickly fatigued and short of breath (pulmonary edema) during even the slightest exertion. These drugs cause vasodilation, which helps the heart to eject blood more easily and more efficiently.
- *Migraine,* with uncertain mechanism, and to *prevent neurological damage* caused by cerebral blood vessel spasms (nimodipine).

EXAMPLES OF COMMON DOSAGES (GENERAL GUIDELINES, MANY DIFFERENT DOSAGE SCHEDULES)

Amlodipine	5-10 mg once daily PO
Diltiazem	30-120 mg 3-4 times daily PO or 60-120 mg 2 times daily as sustained-release capsules PO
Felodipine	5-10 mg once a day PO
Isradipine	2.5-10 mg twice daily PO or 5-20 mg once daily as controlled-release tablets PO
Nicardipine	20-40 mg 3 times daily PO or 30-60 mg 2 times daily with sustained-release form PO
Nifedipine	10 mg 3 times daily PO (not to exceed 180 mg/day) or 30-120 mg once daily with sustained-release form PO
Nisoldipine	20-60 mg once a day PO
Verapamil	80-120 mg 3 times daily PO or 120-240 mg once a day with extended-release preparations PO

ADMINISTRATION

Calcium channel blockers are given IV or PO. Dose must be adjusted in frail, geriatric patients and those with hepatic impairment.

CONTRAINDICATIONS

Calcium channel blockers are contraindicated or to be used cautiously in patients with certain arrhythmias, hypotension, and CHF.

COMMON ADVERSE REACTIONS

Calcium channel blockers can cause headache, certain arrhythmias, dizziness, peripheral edema, CHF, cough, joint stiffness, muscle cramps, gingival hyperplasia (diltiazem), and rarely, Stevens-Johnson syndrome.

DRUG INTERACTIONS

- Hypotensive episodes may occur with nitrates, antihypertensives and alcohol. Toxicity may be increased with use of H_2-blockers.
- Grapefruit juice may reduce metabolism of some drugs and increase serum levels, leading to overdose signs and symptoms. High fat meals can increase blood levels of nisoldipine.

IMPLICATIONS FOR PHYSICAL THERAPISTS

- Have the patient change position and get up slowly, in particular in the beginning of therapy because orthostatic hypotension may occur.
- Be careful when using a heated therapeutic pool because warm water can aggravate the vasodilatory effects of peripheral vascular dilators and lead to a marked decrease in blood pressure.
- Observe the patient for signs of CHF (peripheral edema, rales/crackles, dyspnea, weight gain, jugular venous distension) and if present notify physician.

- If you notice joint stiffness and muscle cramps, which could be an adverse reaction, notify the physician.
- If you notice peripheral edema, significant bradycardia or irregular heart beats, or swelling of gums, notify the physician.
- If patient feels feverish and exhibits an unexplained skin rash ask patient to immediately notify the physician because this could be the onset of Stevens-Johnson syndrome and the calcium channel blocker should be stopped as soon as possible.

CHOLINERGIC AGONISTS

COMMON DRUGS (SELECTION OF SOME OF THE MOST COMMONLY USED DRUGS)

Cholinergic Drugs

Bethanechol	Duvoid, Urabeth, Urecholine
Pilocarpine	Akarpine, Pilocar, other
Neostigmine	Prostigmin
Pyridostigmine	Mestinon, Regonol
Other	

Anti-Alzheimer Drugs

Donepezil	Aricept
Galantamine	Razadyne
Rivastigmine	Exelon
Tacrine	Cognex
Memantine	Namenda
Other	

MECHANISM OF ACTION

Cholinergic M (muscarinic) and Nn (nicotinic nerve) receptors are usually but not exclusively found opposite parasympathetic preganglionic (Nn) and postganglionic nerve (M) fibers, which release acetylcholine, which stimulates these receptors. The synaptic acetylcholine is then quickly inactivated and destroyed by the enzyme acetylcholinesterase. Activation of these receptors decreases heart rate and contractility, constricts bronchial muscles (decreased air flow), and increases gut and bladder activity. Cholinergic receptors Nm (nicotinic muscle) are found on skeletal muscles opposite motoneurons. Stimulation initiates skeletal muscle movements. Furthermore, cholinergic receptors of all classifications and glutaminergic receptors are found in the brain, in which, among other functions, they seem to be involved in cognitive processes (memory).

Cholinergic agonists can either stimulate directly these receptors (bethanechol, pilocarpine for M receptors) or inhibit the enzyme acetylcholinesterase, which increases synaptic acetylcholine concentrations that then indirectly stimulate all of these receptors. Memantine antagonizes the action of glutamate.

INDICATIONS

Cholinergic agonists are indicated in the following:

- *Postoperative gastrointestinal and urinary atony* to stimulate M receptors and restore activity (bethanechol).
- *Myasthenia gravis,* which manifests itself in rapid fatigability and muscle weakness, is an autoimmune disease in which the immune system destroys and reduces the number of Nm receptors on skeletal muscles. Indirect-acting cholinergic agonists can increase synaptic acetylcholine levels, which now can activate the remaining receptors and restore muscle activity.
- *Dementia of the Alzheimer type,* in which it is believed that this condition is caused by a loss of nicotinic receptors plus other abnormalities, including overstimulation of glutaminergic receptors with resulting nerve damage. Indirect-acting cholinergic agonists can increase central synaptic acetylcholine levels, stimulate remaining nicotinic receptors, and slightly improve memory but will not alter the course of the disease. In addition, action of excessive detrimental glutamate activity is blocked by memantine, preventing its damaging effects.
- Reversal of the effects of *nondepolarizing neuromuscular blockers* by increasing synaptic acetylcholine levels at skeletal muscles that compete with and remove the blockers.
- *Open-angle glaucoma,* in which a defect in the trabecular outflow system increases intraocular pressure, leading eventually to retinal damage, tunnel vision, and blindness. Cholinergic drugs (e.g., pilocarpine) applied topically increase outflow and lower the damaging effects of increased intraocular pressure.

EXAMPLES OF COMMON DOSAGES (GENERAL GUIDELINES, MANY DIFFERENT DOSAGE SCHEDULES)

Bethanechol	25-50 mg three times daily PO
Donepezil	5-10 mg once daily (not to exceed 5 mg in frail, geriatric women) PO
Galantamine	4-12 mg twice daily (up to 24 mg) PO
Memantine	5-10 mg 2 times daily PO
Neostigmine	15 mg q3-4h initially, can be increased to 375 mg/day PO
Pyridostigmine	600 mg/day in divided doses up to 1.5 g/day PO
Rivastigmine	1.5 mg twice daily, to be increased to 6 mg twice daily PO
Tacrine	10 mg 4 times daily, can be increased to 160 mg/day PO

ADMINISTRATION

Cholinergic agonists are given PO, IM, and IV (or topically in case of glaucoma). After topical administration, observed systemic adverse reactions are milder.

CONTRAINDICATIONS

Cholinergic agonists are contraindications in patients with asthma, ulcer, cardiovascular disease, and epilepsy.

COMMON ADVERSE REACTIONS

Adverse reactions include bronchoconstriction with decreased airflow, headache, abdominal cramps, diarrhea (can cause dehydration), salivation, tearing, sweating, and bradycardia with heart block. Memantine might cause some drowsiness.

DRUG INTERACTIONS

- Cholinergic agonists can antagonize the actions of anticholinergic drugs and may increase GI bleeding caused by NSAIDs.
- Jimson weed and scopolia reduce their effectiveness.

IMPLICATIONS FOR PHYSICAL THERAPISTS

- Cholinergic agonists can reduce heart rate, and heart rate should be measured periodically, particularly during and after exercise.
- Cholinergic agonists can cause dizziness, and in particular, older patients must be observed when getting up, standing, or walking.
- If a patient is well-controlled on medication for myasthenia gravis and later on shows sudden reoccurrence of symptoms, such as muscle weakness with some tremors, ask about the dosage taken. Taking too little or too much of the drugs (the latter is referred to as "myasthenic crisis") can resemble the original condition, and the original dosage should be used again or physician should be contacted.

CNS DOPAMINERGIC AGONISTS

COMMON DRUGS (SELECTION OF SOME OF THE MOST COMMONLY USED DRUGS)

Amantadine (1)	Symmetrel
Carbidopa/ levodopa (2)	Parcopa, Sinemet, other
Entacapone (5)	Comtan

Pergolide (3)   Permax
Pramipexole (3)   Mirapex
Ropinirole (3)   Requip
Selegiline (4)   Carbex, Eldepryl, other
Tolcapone (5)   Tasmar
Other

MECHANISM OF ACTION

The neurotransmitter dopamine in the brain acts on stimulatory and inhibitory dopaminergic receptors that are involved in many mental processes. Dopamine is synthesized from dihydroxyphenylalanine (L-DOPA) via the enzyme decarboxylase and is destroyed by the enzymes catechol-O-methyltransferase (COMT), and monoamine oxidase (MAO B). Dopamine is involved in movement control (among other functions) in the basal ganglia, in which normal movements are controlled by a balance between dopaminergic and cholinergic activity.

Dopaminergic agonists increase dopaminergic activity and work in various ways in the brain by increasing the release of dopamine (1), or the synthesis of dopamine through increases in the supply of neuronal DOPA (2), with carbidopa inhibiting peripheral but not central decarboxylase activity, by stimulating dopamine receptors directly (3), or by inhibiting the enzymes MAO B (4), or COMT (5), which destroy dopamine, thus increasing synaptic dopamine levels.

INDICATIONS

Dopaminergic agonists are indicated in the following:

- *Parkinson's disease*, which is mostly a movement disorder, among other problems, and is characterized by a mask-like face, shuffling gait, and pill-rolling tremor. The cause is believed to be, among other problems, an overactivity of cholinergic and an underactivity of dopaminergic activity in the basal ganglia of the brain. These drugs stimulate dopaminergic receptors directly, increase the synthesis of dopamine, or prevent the destruction of dopamine. This increase in dopaminergic activity restores the balance between the two neurotransmitter systems. One of these drugs (amantadine) is also an antiviral drug used for influenza A infections. See also Anticholinergic drugs.
- Drugs that reduce cholinergic activity have been discussed in Anticholinergic Drugs.

EXAMPLES OF COMMON DOSAGES (GENERAL GUIDELINES, MANY DIFFERENT DOSAGE SCHEDULES)

Amantadine   100 mg 1-2 times daily (up to 400 mg/day) PO

Carbidopa/ levodopa   10-25 mg carbidopa/100-250 mg levodopa 3-4 times daily PO or 25 mg/100 mg or 50 mg/200 mg twice daily for extended-release preparations PO

Entacapone   200 mg up to 8 times daily PO

Pergolide   50 μg-1 mg/day 1-3 times daily (not to exceed 5 mg/day) PO

Pramipexole   1.5-4.5 mg/day in 3 divided doses PO

Ropinirole   0.25-1.5 mg/ day 3 times daily (not to exceed 9 mg/day) PO

Selegiline   2.5-10 mg 1-2 times daily PO

Tolcapone   100-200 mg 3 times daily PO

ADMINISTRATION

Dopaminergic agonists are usually given PO. They are often started at low doses and then increased until optimal effectiveness is achieved. Effects may only be seen after 1 to 4 weeks of therapy; chronic administration should not be stopped abruptly because a severe parkinsonian crisis may occur. Some drugs are given concomitantly.

CONTRAINDICATIONS

Dopaminergic agonists are contraindicated in patients with seizure, cardiac, or psychiatric disorders.

COMMON ADVERSE REACTIONS

Adverse reactions include dizziness, sedation, drowsiness (with sleep attacks), hallucinations, involuntary movements, night mares and hypotension. Malignant neuroleptic syndrome and rhabdomyolysis have been reported with entacapone. Some drugs (e.g., L-DOPA) can produce the "on-off" syndrome in which therapeutic effects may temporarily disappear (apomorphine is used to counteract the "off" episodes). After a while, some drugs lose effectiveness; however, effectiveness can sometimes be increased with "drug-free holidays."

DRUG INTERACTIONS

- Dopaminergic agonists should not be used with MAO inhibitors and can increase risk of hypotension with antihypertensives or interact adversely with some antipsychotic drugs.
- Kava and B6 vitamin decrease the effectiveness of carbidopa/levodopa. Selegiline can interact with a large number of prescription and OTC drugs and can cause a hypertensive crisis when consuming tyramine-containing foods.

IMPLICATIONS FOR PHYSICAL THERAPISTS

- Reinforce that patients on levodopa therapy should not take large doses of multivitamins or vitamin B6 because these vitamins can reduce the drug's effectiveness.
- Patients on levodopa showing the "off" phase during therapy should be rescheduled at times when they experience the "on" phase. Often, taking the medication with a light meal can reduce the "off" phase.
- Be aware that patients on some of these drugs can show involuntary movements and dystonias, and these should be reported to the treating physician.
- Some drugs can produce pronounced drowsiness with "sleep" attacks. Reschedule the patient at different times after taking the drug if this is a problem.
- If the patient is taking entacapone and complains about muscle weakness or pain and brown-colored urine, notify the physician immediately because this could be a warning sign of rhabdomyolysis.
- Advise the patient to change positions slowly because some drugs can cause marked orthostatic hypotension, which is particularly dangerous in these patients.

CORTICOSTEROIDS

COMMON DRUGS (SELECTION OF SOME OF THE MOST COMMONLY USED DRUGS)

Short-Acting Drugs
Cortisone   Cortone
Hydrocortisone   Cortef, A-Hydrocort, other

Intermediate-Acting Drugs
Methylprednisolone   A-methaPred, Depopred, Depoject, other
Prednisolone   Articulose, Cortolone, Predate, other
Prednisone   Cordrol, Deltasone, Orasone, other
Triamcinolone   Amcort, Aristocort, Clinacort, other

Long-Acting Drugs
Betamethasone   Celestone
Budesonide   Entocort
Dexamethasone   Cortastat, Dalalone, Decadron, Decameth, other
Other

MECHANISM OF ACTION

Glucocorticoids, or steroids, are secreted by the adrenal cortex and include cortisol and cortisone. They have multiple metabolic effects on glucose, carbohydrate, and lipid metabolism, as well as on inflammatory processes. Here, the anti-inflammatory actions are pertinent in that they stabilize lysosomal membranes

PHARMACOLOGY

Section V

preventing the release of proteolytic enzymes, decrease capillary permeability inhibiting the migration of inflammatory white blood cells into tissues, affect lymph nodes reducing antibody formation, and enhance the effects of circulating catecholamines such as epinephrine causing vasoconstriction and other functions. The action of the natural steroids is short acting.

Drugs or steroids are mostly analogs of these natural products that have a longer duration of action, possess more antiinflammatory activity, with more therapeutic action, and affect fewer metabolic processes, with fewer adverse reactions.

INDICATIONS

Steroids are indicated in the following:

- *Inflammations,which are unwanted or excessive.* An inflammation is usually characterized by swelling, redness, warmth, and pain and eventual tissue damage if it becomes excessive. The first three signs are initiated by vasodilatation allowing white blood cells to invade the tissue, which helps fight infections or to help heal damaged tissues. However, if an inflammation becomes excessive or is unwanted (autoimmune diseases, transplants, allergies, asthma, croup, rheumatoid arthritis, osteoarthritis, ankylosing spondylitis, bursitis, or other conditions), it starts to damage healthy tissue. Drugs curtail excessive and reduce or prevent unwanted inflammations, thus protecting healthy tissue.
- *Adrenocortical insufficiency,* in which the adrenal glands do not produce enough glucocorticoids. Steroids are used as replacement therapy and supply glucocorticoid activity to the body.

EXAMPLES OF COMMON DOSAGES (GENERAL GUIDELINES, MANY DIFFERENT DOSAGE SCHEDULES)

Betamethasone	0.6-7.2 mg once or in divided doses daily PO
Budesonide	9 mg once daily PO
Cortisone	25-300 mg once daily PO
Dexamethasone	0.5-9 mg single or divided doses daily PO
Hydrocortisone	5-30 mg 1 to 4 times daily PO
Methyl- prednisolone	2-160 mg once or in divided doses PO
Prednisolone	5-20 mg 1-4 times daily PO
Prednisone	5-200 mg 1-4 times daily PO
Triamcinolone	4-12 mg 1-4 times daily PO

ADMINISTRATION

Steroids can be given IM, IV, rectally, or PO and differ, depending on the route of administration, in onset (1 to 2 hours) and duration (1 to 6 days). Steroids should not be discontinued abruptly because they suppress adrenocorticotropic hormone (ACTH) secretion, which needs time to recover and before recovery can cause a glucocorticoid deficiency syndrome. Some of these drugs plus other steroids are used by inhalation, nasally, topically, and locally in the eye and include flunisolide, fluticasone, beclomethasone, mometasone, fluorometholone, loteprednol, medrysone, rimexolone, alclometasone, amcinonide, clobetasol, clocortolone, desonide, desoximetasone, diflorasone, and fluocinolone.

CONTRAINDICATIONS

Steroids should not be used during chronic infections, and live vaccines should not be administered during chronic therapy with high doses. They should be used with caution in children because they retard growth.

COMMON ADVERSE REACTIONS

Adverse reactions include either depression or euphoria, increased risk of infections, restlessness, anorexia, ecchymosis (blood caused discolorations), petechiae (red spots), hypertension, fluid retention, osteoporosis, muscle wasting, weakening of tendons and ligaments, metabolic changes like hyperglycemia, fat shifts within the body ("buffalo hump," "moon face"), increased ocular pressure, and cataracts.

Topically applied or inhaled drugs can cause the same but milder effects (except cataract formation and increased ocular pressure after ocular use in some but not all patients).

DRUG INTERACTIONS

- Steroids can interact with a large number of drugs and may require increases in dosages of insulin and oral hypoglycemic agents and may enhance the effects of drugs that affect potassium excretion. They increase the risk of stomach ulcer with the use of NSAIDs.
- Grapefruit juice can increase the levels of some steroids, leading to overdose effects.

IMPLICATIONS FOR PHYSICAL THERAPISTS

- If you have an infection, wear a mask or do not handle the patient who is on long-term, high-dose steroid therapy because his or her immune system is weakened.
- If you notice signs like "moon face" or "buffalo hump," notify or have the patient notify the physician because the dosage may need to be adjusted.

- Be aware that older people on long-term, high-dose steroid therapy may suffer from osteoporosis and might incur further weakening of bones so exercise should be adjusted accordingly. However, gentle exercise can prevent or slow down osteoporosis.
- If you notice personality changes in your patient, notify or have the patient contact the physician because this can be a "steroid psychosis" and drug or dose may need to be adjusted.
- If you notice muscle wasting in a patient, notify or have the patient contact the physician because steroids can interfere with muscle metabolism. However, gentle exercises can prevent or slow down this adverse process.
- Treat the joints of the patient who has received a steroid injection in a joint gently because steroids can weaken ligaments and tendons.
- Measure blood pressure in these patients frequently because drugs can cause hypertension.

DIURETICS

COMMON DRUGS (SELECTION OF SOME OF THE MOST COMMONLY USED DRUGS)

Thiazide and Thiazide-Like Diuretics

Chlorothiazide	Diuril
Hydrochlorothiazide	Esidrix, Hydrochlor, Microzide, other
Chlorthalidone	Hygroton, Thalitone
Indapamide	Lozol
Other	

Loop Diuretics

Bumetanide	Bumex
Furosemide	Lasix
Torsemide	Demadex

Potassium-Sparing Diuretics

Amiloride	Midamor
Spironolactone	Aldactone
Triamterene	Dyrenium

Osmotic Diuretics

Mannitol	Osmitrol, Resectisol

MECHANISM OF ACTION

The kidneys filter blood by glomerular filtration and process urine in the nephrons. This regulates in part the water and salt homeostasis of the body. Water excretion is controlled by the concentrations of electrolytes and hormones in the nephrons. Electrolytes such as sodium, potassium, and chloride are reabsorbed from the tubular filtrate, which also affects tubular water reabsorption; the more salts are reabsorbed, the more water is reabsorbed or the less water is excreted or the less salts are reabsorbed, the less water is reabsorbed or more water is excreted into the urine ("water follows salts"). Aldosterone from the adrenals retains sodium and water but enhances potassium and hydrogen excretion or reduces water excretion and vasopressin from the pituitary gland reduces water excretion directly.

Diuretics cause diuresis or increase water excretion by blocking salt reabsorption on various places in the nephron. The thiazides inhibit reabsorption of sodium and potassium (and other electrolytes) in the early portion of the distal tubules, retain both electrolytes and water in the tubule, and increase water excretion. The loop diuretics inhibit sodium, chloride, and potassium reabsorption in the loop of Henle and distal tubule, retain all electrolytes with water in the tubule, and increase water excretion. The potassium-sparing diuretics (spironolactone blocks the action of aldosterone) reduce sodium reabsorption and increase sodium and water but not potassium excretion. Osmotic diuretics increase the osmolarity of the urine, which keeps water in the tubules and increases water excretion.

INDICATIONS

Diuretics are indicated in the following:

- *Hypertension,* in which they increase water excrtion and reduce blood volume and reduce blood pressure. They possibly also cause some sodium depletion in blood vessel walls, resulting in some vasodilatation that also reduces blood pressure.
- *Edema,* or excessive fluid accumulation as a result of CHF or other causes, in which they reduce this fluid accumulation by increasing water excretion.
- *Various problems* including an attack of *narrow-angle glaucoma* to quickly reduce excessively elevated intraocular pressure or *cerebral edema* (e.g., IV mannitol).

EXAMPLES OF COMMON DOSAGES (GENERAL GUIDELINES, MANY DIFFERENT DOSAGE SCHEDULES)

Chlorothiazide	250-1000 mg/day as a single or divided doses PO
Hydrochlorothiazide	12.5-100 mg/day in 1 or 2 doses up to 200 mg/day PO
Chlorthalidone	25-100 mg/day once daily PO
Indapamide	1.25-5 mg/day once PO
Bumetanide	0.5-2 mg/day once, with additional doses if needed up to 10 mg/day PO
Furosemide	20-80 mg/day once or twice PO
Torsemide	5-20 mg once daily PO
Amiloride	5-10 mg/day (up to 20 mg) PO
Spironolactone	12.5-400 mg/day as a single dose PO
Triamterene	100 mg twice daily (not to exceed 300 mg/day) PO
Mannitol	50-100 g as a 5%-25% solution IV

ADMINISTRATION

Diuretics can be given IV, IM, and PO. Drugs are often used in combination with each other or other drugs. Loop diuretics are the strongest diuretics but are also associated with more adverse reactions.

CONTRAINDICATIONS

Diuretics should not be given to patients with electrolyte imbalances. Thiazide diuretics may show cross-sensitivity with sulfonamides. Patients with gout can have an increased risk of an attack with thiazides as a result of hyperuricemia.

COMMON ADVERSE REACTIONS

Adverse reactions include dehydration (hypotension, tachycardia, and dyspnea), hypokalemia (palpitations, skeletal muscle weakness or cramping, paralysis, nausea or vomiting, polydipsia, delirium, and depression) with thiazide and loop diuretics and hyperkalemia (confusion, hyperexcitability, muscle weakness, flaccid paralysis, and arrhythmias) with the potassium-sparing diuretics. In addition, drugs can cause other electrolyte and metabolic imbalances (metabolic alkalosis), drowsiness, dizziness, orthostatic hypotension, increases in blood glucose, and cholesterol levels. Hearing loss (tinnitus) occurs mostly with loop diuretics after IV administration.

DRUG INTERACTIONS

- Potassium-losing diuretics can cause severe hypokalemia with diuretics, which also cause potassium loss. Potassium loss increases digitalis toxicity and reduces lithium excretion precipitating lithium toxicity. Potassium-sparing diuretics can cause significant hyperkalemia in the presence of drugs like ACE inhibitors, which also retain potassium. Hearing problems caused by loop diuretics are made worse by aminoglycosides.
- Licorice and herbal laxatives (senna) may increase the risk of hypokalemia. Ginkgo may decrease the antihypertensive effects.

IMPLICATIONS FOR PHYSICAL THERAPISTS

- Advise the patient to change position slowly, in particular, getting up because drugs decrease blood pressure and carry the risk of orthostatic hypotension.
- Monitor the patient for muscle activity and other unusual signs because some diuretics can cause hypokalemia, whereas others can cause hyperkalemia. If this is observed, notify the physician immediately.
- UV light should be used with caution and other parts of the patient should be covered because some diuretics can cause photosensitivity reactions.
- When exercising the patient in a warm environment, monitor sweating and recommend frequent water supplementation to prevent dehydration.

DRUGS AND BLOOD CLOTTING

COMMON DRUGS (SELECTION OF SOME OF THE MOST COMMONLY USED DRUGS)

Oral Anticoagulants

Warfarin	Coumadin

Parental Anticoagulants

Heparin	Fragmin, Lovenox,
Other	Arixtra, Innohep

Antiplatelet Drugs

Aspirin	
Clopidogrel	Plavix
Dipyridamole	Dipiradol

Fibrinolytic or Thrombolytic Drugs

Alteplase or TPA	Activase
Reteplase	
Streptokinase	
Urokinase	

Clotting Factors

Factors VIII and IX

MECHANISM OF ACTION

Blood clotting is a very complex mechanism that basically involves platelet aggregation and coagulation. If, for example, a blood vessel is injured, the vessel first constricts to reduce blood flow. Then platelets are attracted to the wound, become "sticky," and form a platelet plug at the opening. This process of aggregation involves a number of endogenous factors: Adenosine diphosphate (ADP) and thromboxane A_2 and the expression of a glycoprotein IIb/IIIa receptor at the site of injury are among the most important ones. Thromboxane is formed (besides prostaglandins) by the action of cyclooxygenase (COX) from arachidonic acid (see Nonsteroidal Antiinflammatory Drugs). This is followed by coagulation, which involves a large number of endogenous compounds called *clotting factors,* including vitamin K, as well as the conversion of prothrombin to thrombin, which in turn converts fibrinogen to fibrin and which finally seals the platelet plug tight. After the wound is healed, plasminogen is converted to plasmin, which splits and dissolves the plug. Unfortunately, sometimes blood clots can form within vessels (thrombi) and the clots can dislodge and travel through the vessel system (as emboli) where they can become stuck in small vessels. Here, they block blood flow and deprive the tissue of oxygen and nutrients. The consequences can be an ischemic heart attack, pulmonary embolism, or stroke. These thrombi are formed by either excessive platelet aggregation (arteries) or coagulation (veins) activity usually in the legs where inactivity (sitting for long periods of time such as in airplanes) promotes their formation.

Drugs are used to suppress the unwanted formation of thrombi or emboli and in their quick dissolution if they have been already formed before tissue damage can occur. Antiplatelet drugs prevent platelet aggregation by interfering with thromboxane formation (aspirin), ADP attachment to platelets (clopidogrel), or uncertain mechanisms such as on phosphodiesterase (dipyridamole). Anticoagulants prevent formation of thrombi by interfering with the synthesis of vitamin K-dependent clotting factors (warfarin) or by inhibiting thrombin formation (heparin, which is a natural product). Fibrinolytic drugs dissolve unwanted blood clots, usually by activating plasmin formation. Clotting factors are used in deficiency diseases when blood does not clot normally such as occurs in hemophilia.

INDICATIONS

Drugs are indicated in the following:

- *Pulmonary embolism,* when a blood vessel in the lungs becomes blocked. In most cases, the blockage is caused by one or more blood clots that travel to the lungs from another part of the body. It manifests itself with sudden shortness of breath, chest pain often mimicking a heart attack, cough, tachycardia, wheezing, leg swelling, sweating, anxiety, and lightheadedness or fainting. It is mostly mild but can become fatal. Initially, heparin is administered IV or under the skin, which prevents existing clots from growing and stops the formation of new clots. Later, warfarin may be prescribed.
- *Strokes,* which occur mostly when the blood supply to a part of the brain is reduced or stopped by a blood clot (ischemic stroke) so that within a few minutes, neurons start to die. Warning signs include trouble with walking, dizziness, loss of balance or coordination, numbness, trouble speaking or seeing, and headache, which are persistent. If signs are fleeting, it is called a *transient ischemic attack* in which blood flow is only

temporarily interrupted. The signs and symptoms are similar but usually milder and disappear mostly within minutes but should be brought to the attention of a physician. A few strokes are caused by bleeding in the brain (hemorrhagic strokes). Intervention of a stroke must occur quickly to prevent brain damage. It is recommended not to give aspirin at home but to rush the individual to a hospital as soon as possible. At the hospital, it will be determined what type of stroke it is and if it is a hemorrhagic stroke, surgery may be indicated (administration of aspirin in this case would have increased further bleeding). In the case of an ischemic stroke, aspirin is given and followed by fibrinolytic drugs to dissolve the clot. They must be administered within 3 hours, although they might still be effective after this time. Later, drugs that reduce clot formation are indicated to prevent their formation.

- *Heart attack* or MI can occur when a blood clot blocks a coronary blood vessel and prevents blood flow and supply of nutrients and oxygen to cardiac muscle, resulting in damage and death of cardiac tissue. Common signs and symptoms of a heart attack include pressure and pain in the center of the chest that extends to the shoulder, arm, back, or teeth and jaw; shortness of breath; sweating; fainting; and nausea and vomiting.
- *Atrial fibrillation* or *prosthetic heart valves* can give rise to the formation of thrombi, which later can travel and block blood vessels, leading to tissue damage. Drugs like clopidogrel reduce their formation and prevent possible tissue damage.
- *Deep vein thrombosis prevention,* in which these drugs dissolve or prevent the formation of thrombi and their possible travel through the vascular system.
- *Hemophilia* is a rare, inherited bleeding disorder in which blood does not clot normally. Bleeding episodes can range from mild to fatal and can be caused by injuries or can be internal. The cause is a lack of certain clotting factors. Hemophilia A is caused by a lack or too little clotting factor VIII, and hemophilia B is caused by low levels of clotting factor IX. Treatment involves replacement therapy by giving or replacing the necessary clotting factor. These factors can be obtained from human blood or be made by recombinant techniques. They are injected.

EXAMPLES OF COMMON DOSAGES (GENERAL GUIDELINES, MANY DIFFERENT DOSAGE SCHEDULES)

Warfarin	2.5-10 mg/day PO or IV
Heparin	Depending on the preparation
Aspirin	81 mg once daily PO
Clopidogrel	75 mg once daily PO
Dipyridamole	225-400 mg in 3-4 divided doses daily PO

ADMINISTRATION

These drugs can be given IV, SC, or PO. A number of drugs in these categories (fibrinolytic or thrombolytic drugs) are administered in the hospital.

CONTRAINDICATIONS

Contraindications or cautious use includes patients at risk of bleeding and pending surgery, in which case these drugs should be stopped about 1 week before.

COMMON ADVERSE REACTIONS

Adverse reactions include fatigue, headache, increased risk of bleeding by external or internal injuries, and rarely a potentially fatal thrombotic thrombocytic purpura. Orthostatic hypotension can occur with dipyridamole. Discontinuation of long-term therapy with these drugs, such as before surgery, can carry a slightly increased risk of the formation of thrombi.

DRUG INTERACTIONS

- These drugs can interact with NSAIDs by increasing bleeding episodes.
- Risk of bleeding is increased with concurrent use of gingko, garlic, ginseng, and other herbal products. Foods high in vitamin K content may antagonize the action of warfarin.

IMPLICATIONS FOR PHYSICAL THERAPISTS

- If the patient complains about nose bleeds, bleeding gums, unusual bruising, or black stools, notify or have patient contact the physician because this might require a dose adjustment.
- Gently hold an older, frail patient taking these medications because firm or tight handling can lead to bruising or bleeding episodes.
- Advise the patient not to take NSAIDs that are OTC or to notify the physician before taking these drugs because they can increase the risk of bleeding.
- Patients should use vitamins only on the advice of a physician; in particular, they should avoid vitamin K preparations when on anticoagulant therapy.
- Instruct the patient to strictly adhere to the dosing schedule because doses taken too rapidly or in excess can increase the risk of severe bleeding.
- Advise older patients who do not take these medications not to sit quiet for long periods of time but to tense their legs or to get up and walk periodically, for example, on long airplane flights, to exercise leg muscles, keep blood flowing, and prevent thrombi formation. Also, suggest wearing pressure stockings on such trips.

DRUGS AND BONE FORMATION

COMMON DRUGS (SELECTION OF SOME OF THE MOST COMMONLY USED DRUGS)

Calcium supplements	Many different preparations with or without vitamin D supplementation

Bisphosphonates

Alendronate	Fosamax
Etidronate	Didronel
Ibandronate	Boniva
Pamidronate	Aredia
Risedronate	Actonel

Calcitonin

Calcitonin	Calcimar, Salmonine, other

Parathyroid Hormone

Teriparatide	Forteo

MECHANISM OF ACTION

Bones consist mainly of calcium and phosphate, provide rigidity to the body, and serve as an internal source of calcium. For this reason, they are not static but continuously remodeled with osteoclasts (OC) digesting old bone and osteoblasts (OB) building new bone. This process is regulated by a number of biochemicals. Calcium and phosphate levels in the blood, which are derived from food, must be maintained within limits. Parathyroid hormone (PTH) from the parathyroid gland, can increase bone resorption but also and more importantly can enhance bone formation. Vitamin D synthesized in the body by UV light increases intestinal calcium and phosphate absorption and assures the necessary supply of these minerals. Minor roles are played by calcitonin and estrogens, which stimulate bone formation, and glucocorticoids, which can break down bone.

Bone formation can be increased by supplying calcium that might be missing in the diet or is not fully absorbed. Calcium in supplements is mostly combined with carbonate, citrate, phosphate, lactate, and gluconate. Vitamin D supplementation alone or in combination with calcium supplements will increase calcium absorption. Bisphosphonates, which seem to be incorporated into bone, reduce OC activity and seem to promote a more adequate and efficient mineralization. Calcitonin will also increase bone formation.

INDICATION

These drugs are indicated in the following:
- *Osteoporosis,* which is characterized by excessive porousness of the bone that is caused by enlargement of the canals or formation of cavities. This can lead to bone fractures. Osteoporosis occurs during aging (genetic differences among individuals) or caused by exogenous factors such as chronic steroid use. All drugs slow down the progression of the disease by promoting new and stronger bone formation. Drugs also counteract steroid-induced osteoporosis.
- *Hypoparathyroidism,* which leads to impaired bone breakdown and hypocalcemia. Administration of calcium and vitamin D supply the needed calcium for the body or injections of PTH are used.
- *Rickets,* which is a vitamin D deficiency in children (no longer in the United States but in other parts of the world) and causes abnormal bone formation. Calcium and vitamin D supply the needed calcium for the body.
- Other conditions include *certain cancers, osteomalacia,* and *Paget disease.*

EXAMPLES OF COMMON DOSAGES (GENERAL GUIDELINES, MANY DIFFERENT DOSAGE SCHEDULES)

Calcium Supplements

Alendronate	10 mg once daily or 70 mg once weekly PO
Etidronate	5-10 mg/kg/day once daily PO
Ibandronate	2.5 mg once daily or 150 mg once a month PO
Pamidronate	30-90 mg in single or divided doses IV
Risedronate	5 mg once daily or 35 mg once weekly PO
Calcitonin	200 IU/day by nasal spray
Teriparatide	20 μg/day SC

ADMINISTRATION

Bisphosphonates must be taken PO with water on an empty stomach in the morning while sitting or standing for at least 30 to 60 minutes (to prevent reflux into the esophagus, which can cause severe irritations). The PTH preparation is injected. Calcitonin is inhaled.

CONTRAINDICATIONS

Bisphosphonates should not be used by patients with renal and GI disorders.

COMMON ADVERSE REACTIONS

Bisphosphonates are generally well tolerated except for some GI distress; in particular, if NSAIDs are being used. Calcitonin can cause some allergic reactions. The PTH preparation may cause pain at the site of the injection, some weakness, and although still uncertain, may increase the risk of bone cancer.

DRUG INTERACTIONS

Bisphosphonates should not be taken with caffeine drinks or mineral water.

IMPLICATIONS FOR PHYSICAL THERAPISTS

- Encourage the patient to eat a balanced diet and to walk at least an hour a day in daylight and to do weight-bearing exercises to strengthen bones and to avoid possible fractures. Furthermore, the patient at risk should stop smoking, lose weight if overweight and avoid excessive alcohol consumption.
- Advise patient to follow the administration schedule for the bisphosphonates exactly as prescribed since otherwise significant adverse reactions can occur.

DRUGS AND SUBSTANCES OF ABUSE

Only a small list of legally and illegally abused drugs and substances is given with a definition of physical dependence and addiction.

ALCOHOL

- Alcohol or ethanol is metabolized mostly by 2 enzymes at the rate of about 100 mg/kg/hr or roughly 10 mL/hr/person (about one glass of wine or beer per hour in the average person) and is also partially exhaled by the lungs (breathalyzer test). It is evenly distributed throughout the body, and a blood test can predict tissue levels.
- Alcohol is a CNS depressant and seems to affect inhibitory pathways, first resulting in the loss of inhibitions and aggressive behavior. This is followed by general CNS depression with impaired sensory function and muscular coordination, changes in mood, personality, behavior, and mental activity. Intoxicated persons often are not aware of these impairments, and alcohol causes the feeling of increased performance, although there actually is a decrease!
- Small amounts of alcohol, such as 1 to 2 drinks or glasses of wine (in particular red wine), seem to be beneficial for maintaining good health, whereas large amounts of alcohol consumed over long periods lead to alcoholism, with significant health risks that are often exacerbated by poor diets and vitamin deficiencies (such as thiamine). Adverse reactions include damage to the liver (cirrhosis), stomach (ulcer), heart, and brain (the Korsakoff-Wernicke syndrome with memory loss and psychotic behavior), and infants who are born with fetal alcohol syndrome (facial/mental abnormalities).
- Alcoholism is treated with limited success with various drugs and behavioral modification techniques.

- Alcohol can enhance the sedative and gastric damaging effects of many drugs (e.g., NSAIDs).

TOBACCO

- Tobacco smoke contains hundreds of chemicals that the smoker inhales; nicotine, tar, and carbon monoxide (CO) are the most toxic ones.
- Nicotine will stimulate the nicotinic receptors in the brain, causing the rewarding feeling, and in the body, in which excessive smoking can lead to hypertension, tachycardia, gastric problems, and cardiovascular pathology.
- Tar is the product of incomplete combustion of organic material and causes inflammation of the lungs (smoker's cough, bronchitis, or emphysema) and cancer of throat, lungs, and bladder. If a heavy smoker stops smoking, his or her chances of dying from cancer will slowly diminish.
- CO is also formed by incomplete combustion of tobacco and will bind to hemoglobin, replacing oxygen and leading to a reduction in the oxygen supply to all tissues.
- Cessation of smoking is attempted with nicotine gum or a patch, drugs, and behavioral modification.

MARIHUANA

- Marihuana/hashish smoke contains hundreds of chemicals; tetrahydrocannabinol (THC) is the active and rewarding compound.
- Effects of THC include relaxation, disturbed sensory perception (interferes with driving a car), stimulation of appetite, and antiemetic effects (allowed in certain states for cancer patients to combat drug-induced nausea or vomiting).
- Chronic, heavy use may include the toxic effects of inhaled CO and tar (see Tobacco). The theory that marihuana is a stepping stone to other drugs has been largely abandoned.
- THC, as drug (dronabinol), is available to reduce nausea and vomiting during cancer chemotherapy.

HEROIN

- Heroin is converted in the body to morphine, which produces both CNS and peripheral effects (see Opioid or Narcotic Analgesics). Users prefer heroin because it provides a quicker and more rewarding effect than morphine because it crosses more quickly into the brain. High doses cause respiratory depression and death.
- Methadone is used to treat heroin abuse and to prevent the withdrawal syndrome.

COCAINE AND AMPHETAMINES

- Both drugs are sympathomimetic (see α-Agonists and β-Agonists) and stimulate adrenergic receptors. In the brain, they cause their rewarding effects mostly through the action of dopamine activity; in the body, alpha and β stimulation prevails with tachycardia and hypertension.
- They will counteract the therapeutic effects of α-blockers and β-blockers.

DEPENDENCE AND ADDICTION

- *Physical dependence* is an altered physiological state caused by the repeated administration of a drug or substance, which later on demands continued use to prevent the "withdrawal or abstinence syndrome." The occurrence of the withdrawal syndrome indicates existence of physical dependence. Physical dependence can occur with the use of some but not all illegal and prescription drugs. Physical dependence carries certain health risks but withdrawal can be dangerous or even life-threatening. The degree of physical dependence depends on the drug, dose, and time used.
- *Withdrawal* occurs only after abrupt cessation of a drug or substance in a physically dependent individual. Signs and symptoms are usually opposite to original drug effects (morphine use causes miosis or constipation and withdrawal from morphine causes mydriasis or diarrhea). Most drugs that cause physical dependence (illegal as well as legal) should be discontinued slowly after long-term, high-dose therapy; no withdrawal symptom will become apparent.
- *Addiction* is a behavioral pattern of compulsive drug or substance use characterized by the overwhelming involvement with the drug, the securing of its supply, and a high tendency to relapse after its cessation. Also, addiction can be described as an "uncontrollable drug-using behavior" resulting in loss of "normal" functioning and harm to the user and society. Controlled use of drugs is not considered addiction (e.g., social consumption of alcohol or other drugs). Genetic and environmental factors seem to determine addiction to a large extent (some individuals can avoid or handle drugs or substances "socially" regardless of availability, whereas others cannot).

"STREET" DRUG TOXICITY

- Illegally obtained drugs or substances carry additional health risks that can be more severe and even fatal because of illegal manufacturing techniques and unscrupulous selling practices.
- The user can never be sure if the substance bought from street sellers is indeed the right drug (often a more dangerous drug is sold than actually offered), if it is the right dose (often a too-high dose is sold, e.g., most heroin-related deaths), and in addition if it contain dangerous impurities (often contains chemicals much more toxic than the drug sold such as rat poisons, which resulted in some deaths). Furthermore, improper use carries significant health risks such as shared needles that can spread hepatitis and AIDS.

IMPLICATIONS FOR PHYSICAL THERAPISTS

- The physical therapist must be aware that some legal and illegal drugs can cause physical dependence and it is important for the patients not to stop these drugs abruptly but to discontinue them slowly to avoid serious withdrawal reactions.
- The physical therapist must also be aware of the fact that addiction is not only associated with illegal drugs but also with excessive long-term alcohol and tobacco use or excessive use of nasal sprays, androgenic steroids, or laxatives.
- The physical therapist can be helpful in advising the individual about the dangers of using or abusing certain substances and to encourage them to stop. This is particularly true when smoking or alcohol is detected on the breath during therapy sessions early during the day.
- The physical therapist can warn the illegal drug user, if known, or younger individuals who express thoughts about buying drugs on the street that he or she may experience serious ill effects and even death not only from the substances bought but also from unsanitary and unprofessional manufacturing techniques and unscrupulous selling practices.

DRUGS AND THE THYROID GLAND

COMMON DRUGS (SELECTION OF SOME OF THE MOST COMMONLY USED DRUGS)

Hypothyroidism

Liothyronine (T3)	Cytomel, Triostat, other
Levothyroxine (T4)	Synthroid, Levo-T, other

Hyperthyroidism

Propylthiouracil Other	Propylthiouracil

MECHANISM OF ACTION

The thyroid gland is located at the neck around the trachea and synthesizes and secretes the thyroid hormones. Their formation is stimulated by the thyroid-stimulating hormone (TSH). Organic precursors and iodide are converted in the gland via the action of two oxidases in a process called *organification* of iodine to thyroglobulin. This protein is metabolized to thyroxine (T4) and triiodothyronine (T3), both of which are released into the body. T4 is now converted largely to T3, which is the most active form. They stimulate carbohydrate, fat, and protein metabolism, as well as regulate body heat and are involved in bone formation.

Drugs like T4 or T3 can replenish or replace low or missing endogenous levels of both hormones. Propylthiouracil and related drugs will inhibit the organification and synthesis of both T3 and T4 and reduce excessively high levels of both hormones. High doses of iodide will inhibit its uptake into the gland. In addition, surgery and radioactive iodine are being used to either remove or to destroy part of an overactive gland.

INDICATION

Drugs are indicated in the following:
- *Hypothyroidism*, or a lack of sufficient hormone secretion, can be caused by an autoimmune disease but can also result from the surgical removal of a cancerous gland. It manifests itself as physical and mental fatigue, weight gain, dry and rough skin, and muscle cramps and aches. Drug therapy consists of replacement therapy with the hormones. Both thyroxine and liothyronine have a somewhat delayed onset of action, and levothyroxine is preferred for long-term therapy. Drugs have a narrow margin of safety, and it is often difficult to find the right dose and maintain the patient on it.
- *Hyperthyroidism*, or a surplus of the hormone, which can also be caused by an autoimmune disease in which antibodies stimulate the gland to produce too much hormone. It manifests itself in palpitations and tachycardia, heat intolerance, insomnia, weight loss, warm and moist skin, and muscle weakness. Propylthiouracil and related drugs, surgery, or radioactive destruction of the gland are indicated.

EXAMPLES OF COMMON DOSAGES (GENERAL GUIDELINES, MANY DIFFERENT DOSAGE SCHEDULES)

Liothyronine	25-75 µg /day PO
Levothyroxine	50-200 µg/day PO
Propylthiouracil	100-300 mg 3 times daily PO

ADMINISTRATION

Hormones and drugs are used PO.

CONTRAINDICATIONS

Hormones are contraindicated or should be used with caution in patients with adrenal insufficiency and MIs; propylthiouracil is contraindicated in patients with hepatic diseases and bone marrow depression.

COMMON ADVERSE REACTIONS

Generally, adverse reactions of hormone replacement therapy often result from an overdose resembling hyperthyroidism with angina in compromised patients. Propylthiouracil may cause hepatic and renal problems, as well as agranulocytosis and bleeding episodes and hypothyroidism if doses are too high.

DRUG INTERACTIONS

- Thyroid hormones increase the effects of anticoagulants and decrease effectiveness of insulin and oral hypoglycemics. Propylthiouracil interacts with iodide and lithium.
- Efficacy of thyroid hormones is decreased by soy, bugleweed, and carnitine. Also, foods high in iodine should be avoided.

IMPLICATIONS FOR PHYSICAL THERAPISTS

- Observe patients on hormone replacement therapy carefully and check for signs and symptoms of hyperthyroidism or hypothyroidism. If present, notify or have the patient notify the physician because this might indicate a dose adjustment.
- Weight loss is often a physiological response to the medications. Patients may take it upon themselves to utilize the medication for weight loss purposes. Weight loss, nervousness and excitability can be signs of medication misuse. If misuse is suspected, the patient's physician should be notified and the patient should be educated regarding the potential hazards to their health.
- Patients on propylthiouracil should be watched for yellowing skin and eyes indicating jaundice, bleeding episodes, and an unexplained sore throat indicating agranulocytosis. If this occurs, notify or have patient notify the physician about these observations.

FEMALE HORMONES

COMMON DRUGS (SELECTION OF SOME OF THE MOST COMMONLY USED DRUGS)

Estrogens

Estradiol	Estrace, Vivelle, other
Ethinyl Other	Estradiol Estinyl

Progestins

Progesterone	Gesterol, Prometrium
Norgestrel Other	Ovrette

Contraceptives: Ethinyl Estradiol

Plus desogestrel	Desogen, Mircette, other
Ethynodiol	Demulen, Zovia
Levonorgestrel	Levlen, Nordette, other
Norethindrone	Loestrin, Brevicon, other
Norgestimate	Ortho-Cyclen, other
Norgestrel	Ovral

Contraceptives: Mestranol

Plus norethindrone	Genora, Norinyl, other
Norethindrone	Micronor
Norgestrel Other	Ovrette

Postcoital Drugs

Mifepristone Other	Mifeprex

Estrogen-Receptor Modulators

Raloxifene	Evista
Tamoxifen Other	Nolvadex

MECHANISM OF ACTION

Luteinizing hormone (LH) and follicle-stimulating hormone (FSH) are released from the pituitary gland. FSH and LH stimulate the maturation of follicles in the ovaries. The ruptured follicle will develop into the corpus luteum and will secrete estrogens and progesterone. Estrogens are a group of hormones, and progestins contain several active compounds of which progesterone is the most important. Both cause proliferation and thickening of the endometrium in the uterus. If the egg is fertilized, it will be implanted in the uterus and develop into an embryo and fetus later. The high levels of estrogens and progesterone will, in a negative feedback, prevent the secretion of FSH and LH. In addition, progesterone causes the vaginal environment to become "hostile" to sperm so that no sperm can reach the ovaries. No new ovulation or conception will occur. If the egg is not fertilized, the corpus luteum stops secretion and the endometrium sloughs off and is expelled (menstruation). Thereafter FSH and LH are secreted and the cycle starts over again.

Drugs (except the estrogen-receptor modulators) are the natural hormones or their analogues which can now act like the endogenous hormones and correct deficiency states. They can also interfere with the natural processes and reduce FSH and LH release and cause an environment "hostile" to sperm to prevent ovulation and conception (contraceptives) or to prevent implantation and to expel a fertilized egg from the uterus (postcoital pills). Estrogen antagonists can block estrogen receptors on breasts, which in a subset of women have been found to promote cancer when stimulated by estrogen.

INDICATION

Drugs are indicated in the following:
- *Estrogen replacement therapy*, in which an estrogen deficiency causes postmenopausal problems (hot flashes, osteoporosis, arteriosclerosis, or vaginal dystrophy). Exogenous estrogen will now assume

the role of the deficient endogenous hormones and reduce these bothersome problems. This practice is now reserved for severe cases only because this therapy has been linked to a higher incidence of cardiovascular morbidity.

- *Amenorrhea* and *dysfunctional uterine bleeding* caused by an abnormal hormone balance. Estrogens and/or progestins administered can restore the normal balance.
- *Contraception,* when no pregnancy is desired. The combination pill, estrogen plus progesterone, delivers high levels of both hormones into the body, suppressing FSH and LH secretion from the pituitary and preventing ovulation ("pseudopregnancy"). In addition, progesterone causes a vaginal environment "hostile" to sperm, preventing sperm from traveling further. This pill is almost 99% to 100% effective. The progesterone-only pill works by the creation of the environment "hostile" to sperm and also by somewhat reducing FSH and LH secretion. Its effectiveness is about 98%.
- *Postcoital intervention,* when no conception was intended after unprotected sex. High doses of estrogens and/or progesterone are given (within 3 to 5 days) and probably act by inhibiting implantation of the fertilized egg (e.g., plan B, which is a high dose of levonorgestrel and is available without a prescription for individuals 18 years and older). Similarly, mifepristone (taken within 50 days) blocks the progesterone receptors in the uterus, prevents the endometrium supporting action of progesterone and leads to endometrial shedding and expulsion of the embryo (sometimes helped by administration of a prostaglandin analog, misoprostol, which stimulates uterine contractions and helps in this ejection process).
- *Breast cancer,* which in some women is promoted by estrogen-receptor activity. Estrogen-receptor blockers or modulators will block these receptors and reduce estrogen's effects on cancer promotion.
- Other uses include treatment of *endometriosis, prostate cancer,* and *endometrial cancer.*

EXAMPLES OF COMMON DOSAGES (GENERAL GUIDELINES, MANY DIFFERENT DOSAGE SCHEDULES)

Estradiol	1-2 mg/day PO
Ethinyl Estradiol	0.02 mg or 0.05 mg daily PO
Contraceptives	Many different combinations and dosages
Mifepristone	200-600 mg PO (followed by 400 mcg misoprostol PO)
Raloxifene	60 mg once daily PO
Tamoxifen	10-20 mg 2 times daily PO

ADMINISTRATION

- Depending on the drug, they can be given orally, IM, SC, by spray, patch, implant, or vaginal ring. The contraceptive combination pill is either given for 3 weeks with 1 week placebo (1-month cycle) or for 84 days with 1 week placebo (3-month cycle).
- It is important to take contraceptives as directed because breakthrough bleeding and reduced protection can occur. General guidelines will vary among drugs and are as follows: if one dose is missed and remembered the same day, then the missed dose should be taken immediately. If it is remembered the next day, 2 tablets are taken on that day and then back to 1 tablet per day. If 2 doses are missed, 2 tablets are taken for 2 days, then back to 1 tablet per day. If 3 or more tablets are missed, consult physician, pharmacist, or nurse.

CONTRAINDICATIONS

These drugs should not be used in patients with thromboembolic disorders.

COMMON ADVERSE REACTIONS

Estrogen replacement therapy has been associated with a higher risk of MI, stroke, pulmonary embolism, and thromboembolism and can increase the risk of endometrial and breast cancer, although the latter is restricted to a subset of women. Both hormones can cause sodium and water retention with weight gain and swelling of the feet. Estrogens in susceptible individuals may cause depression. Contraceptives carry the same risks. Combination pills increase the risk of blood clot formation, which is intensified by smoking. Tamoxifen has been associated with uterine malignancies.

DRUG INTERACTIONS

- These drugs can interact with a number of other drugs. Estrogens are contraindicated with tamoxifen, raloxifene, and steroids.
- Saw palmetto decreases their effectiveness.

IMPLICATIONS FOR PHYSICAL THERAPISTS

- Patients on estrogens and in particular on combination contraceptives should be advised to stop smoking if they do. Explain the increased risk of cardiovascular accidents with this habit.
- If a patient complains about unexplainable pain in the legs, notify or have patient notify the physician immediately because this could indicate a deep vein thrombosis that needs quick

attention to prevent health-threatening problems.
- Check blood pressure periodically because salt retention in susceptible individuals can cause hypertension.
- If you notice that a patient on estrogens is fatigued and depressed, have the patient notify the physician because estrogens can cause depression.
- Inform the patient that it is important to take contraceptives as directed because missed doses reduce or negate protection.
- Inform the patient that contraceptives protect against pregnancy but not venereal diseases. Only condoms do this.
- Inform the patient that postcoital intervention procedures are emergency procedures only and should not be used routinely.

GASTROINTESTINAL DRUGS

COMMON DRUGS (SELECTION OF SOME OF THE MOST COMMONLY USED DRUGS)

Antacids (H_2-Blockers)

Cimetidine	Tagamet
Famotidine	Pepcid
Nizatidine	Axid
Ranitidine	Zantac

Proton Pump Inhibitors

Esomeprazole	Nexium
Lansoprazole	Prevacid
Omeprazole	Prilosec
Pantoprazole	Protonix
Rabeprazole	AcipHex

Antidiarrheal Drug

Kaolin, Pectin	Kapectolin
Bismuth	Pepto-Bismol
Diphenoxylate	Lomotil, Lonox, other
Loperamide	Imodium, other
Other	

Laxatives

Psyllium	Metamucil
Bisacodyl	Dulcolax, Deficol, Correctol
Senna	Senokot, other
Docusate	Colace, Sulfolax, other
Other	

MECHANISM OF ACTION

The main digestive processes occur in the mouth, stomach, and intestines. In the stomach, hydrochloric acid (HCl) and digestive enzymes are released into the lumen. Acid secretion is stimulated by the action of acetylcholine, histamine acting on H_2-receptors and the enzyme H^+,K^+ATPase, also called a proton pump, which moves H^+ into the lumen. In addition, a high pH (alkaline conditions) and spicy and irritating foods can cause acid formation. The digestive processes continue in the intestines. Motility of the stomach and intestines (peristalsis) in moving food and feces is increased by stimulation of cholinergic receptors and stretching the intestinal wall and decreased by stimulation of opioid receptors.

GI drugs affect these processes in various ways. Antacids consist of a base, such as carbonate, silicate, or hydroxide, which is combined with aluminum, calcium, or magnesium. The antacids combine with the acid and remove H^+. The H_2-blockers block the action of histamine on H_2-receptors and the proton pump inhibitors inhibit the pump, which in both cases leads to a reduction in H^+ secretion. Antidiarrheal drugs, such as the absorbents (kaolin, pectin, and bismuth), absorb substances that might increase peristalsis, and loperamide and diphenoxylate relax intestinal muscles by stimulating opioid receptors. The laxatives increase the bulk in the intestines promoting the stretch reflex (psyllium), soften the stool (docusate), or irritate the intestines (bisacodyl, senna), resulting in increased peristalsis and easier defecation.

INDICATION

GI drugs are indicated in the following:

- *Dyspepsia, gastritis,* and *peptic ulcer,* in which excessive acid production (among others such as bacteria) irritates and finally erodes the mucosa, causing an ulcer. GI drugs reduce acid formation and promote healing of inflammations and ulcers.
- *Gastric esophageal reflux disease (GERD),* in which acid enters the esophagus, causing inflammation, pain, spasm and eventually cancer. GI drugs reduce acid production so that less or no acid will enter the esophagus.
- *Constipation,* in which peristalsis is decreased, can lead to fecal impacts. GI drugs increase peristalsis and promote fecal transport and evacuation.
- *Diarrhea,* in which excessive motility leads to frequent evacuations, can result in marked water and electrolyte losses. GI drugs slow peristalsis and reduce or prevent fluid and electrolyte loss.

EXAMPLES OF COMMON DOSAGES (GENERAL GUIDELINES, MANY DIFFERENT DOSAGE SCHEDULES)

Cimetidine	300-1600 mg/day in divided doses PO
Famotidine	20-40 mg/day once daily PO
Nizatidine	150 mg 1-2 times daily PO
Ranitidine	150 mg 1-2 times daily PO
Esomeprazole	20-40 mg/day once daily PO
Lansoprazole	15-30 mg/day once daily PO
Omeprazole	20-40 mg/day once daily PO
Pantoprazole	40 mg/day once daily PO
Rabeprazole	20 mg/day once daily PO
Kaolin, Pectin	60-120 mL after loose bowel movement PO
Bismuth	525-1050 mg several times as needed PO
Diphenoxylate	5 mg 3 times daily (combined with atropine) PO
Loperamide	4 mg followed by 2 mg up to 16 mg/day PO
Psyllium	1-2 tsp in 8 oz water 2-3 times daily PO
Bisacodyl	10-30 mg 1-2 times daily PO
Docusate	50-300 once daily PO
Senna	1-8 tabs/day PO

ADMINISTRATION

Most drugs are given PO with some also available rectally.

CONTRAINDICATIONS

GI drugs should not be used or must be used with caution in patients with a number of problems, depending on the drug employed.

COMMON ADVERSE REACTIONS

Adverse reactions differ among drugs. A rebound phenomenon (increased H^+ secretion) can occur after long-term use of acid reducers. Large doses of antacids cause constipation (aluminum) or diarrhea (magnesium). H_2-blockers can cause some dizziness and rarely blood disorders. Proton pump inhibitors show few adverse reactions, except some rarely cause blood disorders and Stevens-Johnson syndrome. Loperamide and diphenoxylate may cause nausea, drowsiness, and dizziness. Irritating laxatives may cause nausea and intestinal cramps. Long-term use can lead to laxative dependence, in which physiological functions of the intestines start to decline.

DRUG INTERACTIONS

Interactions with other drugs depend on the individual drug. Antacids reduce availability of some antibiotics from the intestines. Altering the pH of the stomach can affect solubility and absorption of certain medications; instructions of individual drugs should be observed.

IMPLICATIONS FOR PHYSICAL THERAPISTS

- Instruct the patient that OTC preparations of these preparations should only be taken exactly as indicated on packages and for a short period of time. If no relief is obtained, a physician must be consulted because there could be more serious underlying problems.
- Inform the patient that proper eating habits with the consumption of bulk can reduce constipation problems.
- Advise patients against long-term use of laxatives, unless prescribed by a physician, because this could lead to laxative dependence. Tell patients that individuals differ in their bowel movements and that a bowel movement need not occur every day.
- Instruct patient who takes OTC cimetidine to do so not for more than 2 weeks and to consult physician if further use is needed.

HEMOPOIETIC DRUGS

COMMON DRUGS (SELECTION OF SOME OF THE MOST COMMONLY USED DRUGS)

Iron preparations	Feosol, Feostat, Feratab, Ferrlecit, other
Epoetin	Epogen, Procrit
Nandrolone	Deca-Durabolin, Kabolin
Cyanocobalamin	Cobex, Cobolin-M, Nascobal, Vibal, other
Hydroxoco-balamin	Alphamin, Vibal LA, other
Folic acid	Apo-Folic, Folate, Folvite, other

MECHANISM OF ACTION

RBCs, or erythrocytes, contain hemoglobin (consisting of the iron-containing red pigment heme plus the protein globin) that transports oxygen to and carbon dioxide away from tissue cells. Erythrocytes derive from hemopoietic stem cells in the bone marrow. They are formed under the influence of erythropoietin, which is secreted from the kidneys. Among the many chemicals necessary for the synthesis of hemoglobin are folic acid and B12; the latter needs a special intrinsic factor secreted by the stomach to be absorbed from the GI tract.

Iron preparations supply the iron. Epoetin stimulates erythrocyte formation from stem cells and nandrolone stimulates erythropoietin synthesis. Cyanocobalamin or B12 and folic acid promote the synthesis of hemoglobin.

INDICATIONS

Hemopoietic drugs are indicated in the following

- *Iron-deficiency anemia* (extensive blood loss, severe menstruation, kidney problems requiring hemodialysis), in which iron preparations (usually ferrous salts) are used. Iron is available in different combinations with an onset of action of about 4 days and peak effects at 1 to 2 weeks.

- *Folic acid deficiency anemia, in which* supplementation with folic acid is used.
- *B12 or pernicious anemia* (mostly caused by a lack of intrinsic factor). Pernicious anemia also damages the nervous system. It is treated with cyanocobalamin and hydroxocobalamin.
- Anemias caused by *chemotherapy* or *renal failure* are treated with epoetin and/or nandrolone.

COMMON DOSAGES (GENERAL GUIDELINES, MANY DIFFERENT DOSAGE SCHEDULES)

Ferrous preparations	120-240 mg/day in 2-4 divided doses PO.
Iron polysaccharide	50-100 mg/day twice daily as tablets or 150-300 mg/day as capsules PO
Epoetin	50-100 units/ kg 3 times weekly SC or IV
Nandrolone	50-100 mg every week IM
Folic acid	1 mg/day initially then 0.5 mg daily PO
Cyanocobalamin	1000 μg daily PO or 500 μg weekly by nasal spray or 30-100 μg/day IM

ADMINISTRATION

Hemopoietic drugs can be given orally, IM, SC, IV, or nasal spray. Onset of action is delayed and varies among medications and routes of administration.

CONTRAINDICATIONS

Iron preparation should be used with extreme caution in patients with GI problems (ulcer).

COMMON ADVERSE REACTIONS

Iron preparations can cause GI problems (epigastric pain, constipation) and color stool black (masking GI bleeding). Overdosing leads to iron toxicity (bluish lips, drowsiness, weakness, or seizures). Epoetin can cause hypertension, and nandrolone can cause allergic reactions. Folic acid and B12 are relatively safe.

DRUG INTERACTIONS

- Iron preparations chelate with tetracyclines, quinolones, and reduce their absorption.
- Vitamin C increases, and food decreases iron absorption.

IMPLICATIONS FOR PHYSICAL THERAPISTS

- If the patient is easily exhausted and appears bluish and anemic, advise the

patient to see a physician and warn against self-medications because different types of anemia exist and each needs special therapies. Brittle, concave nails with ridges often indicate an iron-deficiency anemia.

- Warn the patient who uses iron or folic acid without medical advice to treat an anemic condition to consult a physician because a B12-deficient anemia may respond somewhat to these preparations, whereas nerve damage will continue unchecked.
- If the patient is using iron preparations and has black stools but also severe epigastric pain, advise the patient to see a physician because this could indicate internal bleeding. Also, advise the patient not to overdose with iron because this can lead to iron toxicity.
- Advise the pregnant patient, if not already recommended by the physician, to supplement with folic acid even in the absence of an anemic condition to reduce the risk of fetal abnormalities (spina bifida).

HYPOGLYCEMIC DRUGS I

COMMON DRUGS (SELECTION OF SOME OF THE MOST COMMONLY USED DRUGS)

Insulin lispro/protamine insulin	Humalog Mix 75/25
NPH/regular insulin mixtures	Humulin 50/50, 70/30, Novolin 70/30
Short-acting insulin	Humulin R, Novolin R
Intermediate-Acting Insulins	
Isophane insulin	Humulin N, Iletin II NPH
Lente (zinc) insulin	Humulin L, Novolin ge Lente
Long-Acting Insulins	
Ultralente (zinc) insulin	Humulin U Ultralente, Novolin U
Insulin glargine	Lantus
Rapid-Acting Insulins	
Insulin aspart	NovoLog
Insulin lispro	Humalog
Insulin glulisine	Apidra

MECHANISM OF ACTION

Glucose is necessary for many metabolic and physiological processes, including energy supply to skeletal muscles. Glucose metabolism is mostly regulated by the hormones insulin and glucagon, both synthesized and released from the pancreas. Insulin, a polypeptide, is released when blood glucose levels rise and it lowers blood glucose levels by promoting glycogenesis in the liver (glucose is converted to glycogen) and activating special

receptors, insulin receptors, which promote uptake of glucose into skeletal muscles and other cells, such as liver and fat cells. Insulin release from the pancreas is facilitated by the action of special short-lived peptides and related endogenous compounds. If blood glucose falls, insulin release is decreased and glucagon is released, which works the other way in increasing blood glucose levels. In addition, insulin affects protein and fat metabolism and inhibits fatty acid oxidation and ketone body formation, which could cause a ketoacidosis.

Insulin administration is used as a replacement therapy when endogenous insulin is insufficient or missing. It lowers blood glucose by promoting glucose uptake into skeletal muscles and other tissues. It prevents fatty acid oxidation and the formation of acidic ketone bodies.

INDICATIONS

Hypoglycemic drugs are indicated in the following:

- *Diabetes mellitus* is caused by a deficiency or lack of insulin and manifests itself as polydipsia and polyuria with highly increased blood glucose levels (spilling into the urine, which now "tastes" sweet, causing its name). Untreated it leads to ocular, renal, and cardiovascular health consequences, as well as ketoacidosis. It can be divided into two types. Type I can be caused by an autoimmune or viral disease where the gland does not produce insulin. Type II has usually an adult onset often caused by genetic factors, as well as obesity. In this case, the cause is either an insufficient release of insulin from the pancreas or unresponsive insulin receptors on tissues. In type I, insulin is injected (because oral preparations would be destroyed in the stomach) to replace the missing endogenous hormone. In type II, treatment starts with carbohydrate restrictions, exercise, and weight loss, and if unsuccessful, is followed by oral hypoglycemics (see Hypoglycemic Drugs II) and only if necessary by insulin.
- *Diabetic ketoacidosis,* in which organic acids and ketone bodies are formed from fat because of poor glucose control, which can be life threatening. Short-acting insulins plus other drugs and measures are used to correct this problem.

EXAMPLES OF COMMON DOSAGES (GENERAL GUIDELINES, MANY DIFFERENT DOSAGE SCHEDULES)

Insulin lispro/protamine insulin	0.5-1 unit/kg/day SC
NPH/regular insulin mixtures	0.5-1 unit/kg/day SC

Short-acting insulin	0.5-1 unit/kg/hr SC
Intermediate-acting insulins	0.5-1 unit/kg/day SC
Long-acting insulins	0.5-1 unit/kg/day SC
Rapid-acting insulins	0.5-1 unit/kg/day SC

(all preparations once or repeated)

ADMINISTRATION

Insulin has to be injected SC (IV for ketoacidosis) or given by pump or nasally. It now comes mostly from human recombinant DNA sources. Preparations are manufactured to have different onsets and durations of action to suit the characteristics of the disease of the patient. Onset of action ranges from 15 to 60 minutes and duration of action from 2 to 24 hours. Some preparations are used in the morning and others before meals. Stress, exercise, trauma, drugs, infections, or changes in diet may change the glucose response to insulin and may require dosages adjustments.

CONTRAINDICATIONS

There are no major contraindications except that nasal preparations should not be used in patients with lung problems such as asthma or emphysema.

COMMON ADVERSE REACTIONS

The most common adverse reactions are hypersensitivity reactions, which can range from rashes and itching to an anaphylactic reaction. Hyperglycemia and hypoglycemia (sweating, weakness, dizziness, tremor, and tachycardia to unconsciousness) can result from too much or too little insulin. Insulin can cause local lipoatrophy or lipohypertrophy, which can be minimized by changing injection sites. Poorly controlled glucose levels can lead to ketoacidosis (fatigue, flushed skin, nausea, vomiting, and dyspnea), which can be life-threatening.

DRUG INTERACTIONS

- Glucose-lowering effects may be reduced by a large number of drugs, including corticosteroids, certain antipsychotic and antiviral drugs, and diuretics. Glucose-lowering effects may be enhanced by ACE inhibitors and salicylates. β-Blockers may mask the onset of a hypoglycemic reaction (e.g., tachycardia).
- Glucosamine, chromium, and coenzyme Q-10 enhance blood glucose levels, lowering the effects of insulins.

IMPLICATIONS FOR PHYSICAL THERAPISTS

- Make sure that the patient wears an identification tag indicating that he or she is a diabetic and what type and dose of insulin is being used. Also, make sure that the patient carries some sugar, a glucose preparation, or sweetened orange juice to counteract a possible hypoglycemic reaction.
- Do not recommend glucosamine to a diabetic patients to treat joint problems unless this has been cleared with a physician because glucosamine can cause hypoglycemic episodes in unadjusted insulin dosages.
- Be aware of the occurrence of hypoglycemia, as well as hyperglycemia (unusual thirst, drowsiness, fruit-like breath, and flushed). Treat the first with sugar (artificial sweeteners do not work) and the other by asking the patient to administer the needed insulin.
- Do not massage the site of injection because this could cause an unwanted increase in insulin absorption and a hypoglycemic reaction.
- Exercise a diabetic patient carefully, in particular at the beginning of insulin therapy because exercise can reduce blood glucose levels. Also, suggest having insulin injected into the abdomen instead of skeletal muscle. Check glucose levels during and after exercise.
- If you feel that the patient's blood glucose levels are fluctuating ask if he or she has changed dietary habits or is using an OTC drug because these can cause poor glucose control.

HYPOGLYCEMIC DRUGS II

COMMON DRUGS (SELECTION OF SOME OF THE MOST COMMONLY USED DRUGS)

Glucosidase inhibitors

| Acarbose | Precose |
| Miglitol | Glyset |

Biguanides

| Metformin | Fortamet, Glucophage, Riomet |

Meglitinides

| Nateglinide | Starlix |
| Repaglinide | GlucoNorm, Prandin |

Sulfonylureas

Glimepiride	Amaryl
Glipizide	Glucotrol
Glyburide	DiaBeta, Glynase, Micronase

Thiazolidinediones

| Pioglitazone | Actos |
| Rosiglitazone | Avandia |

Hormones

| Pramlintide | Symlin |

Insulin-release facilitators

| Exenatide | Byetta |
| Sitagliptin | Januvia |

MECHANISM OF ACTION

Glucose is necessary for many metabolic and physiological processes, including energy supply to skeletal muscles. Glucose metabolism is mostly regulated by the hormones insulin and glucagon, both synthesized and released from the pancreas. Insulin, a polypeptide, is released when blood glucose levels rise and it lowers blood glucose levels by promoting glycogenesis in the liver (glucose is converted to glycogen) and activating special receptors, insulin receptors, which promote uptake of glucose into skeletal muscles and other cells such as liver and fat cells. Insulin release from the pancreas is facilitated by the action of special short-lived peptides and related endogenous compounds. If blood glucose falls, insulin release is decreased and glucagon is released, which works the other way in increasing blood glucose levels. In addition, insulin affects protein and fat metabolism and inhibits fatty acid oxidation and ketone body formation, which could cause a ketoacidosis. Drugs work by different mechanisms to lower elevated blood glucose. Glucosidase inhibitors lower postprandial blood glucose by inhibiting α-glucosidase in the GI tract, which is involved in the breakdown of carbohydrates to sugar and reduces and slows sugar absorption. Biguanides decrease hepatic glucose production, somewhat reduce intestinal glucose absorption, and increase insulin receptor sensitivity. Meglitinides close pancreatic potassium channels and open calcium channels, which causes insulin release. Sulfonylureas also affect potassium channels, release insulin from the pancreas, may increase insulin receptor sensitivity, and decrease hepatic glucose formation. Thiazolidinediones act as agonists on cellular insulin receptors and improve glucose uptake into tissues. Pramlintide slows gastric emptying, decreases glucagon secretion, and curbs appetite to reduce postprandial hyperglycemia. Insulin-release facilitators mimic the action of endogenous compounds that facilitate insulin release.

INDICATIONS

Hypoglycemic drugs are indicated in the following:

- *Diabetes mellitus,* is caused by a deficiency or lack of insulin and manifests itself as polydipsia and polyuria with highly increased blood glucose levels (spilling into the urine, which now "tastes" sweet, causing its name). Untreated it leads to ocular, renal, and cardiovascular health consequences, as well as ketoacidosis. It can be divided into two types. Type I can be caused by an autoimmune or viral disease, in which the gland does not produce insulin. Type II has usually an adult onset often caused by genetic factors, as well as obesity. In this case, there is either an insufficient release of insulin from the pancreas or unresponsive insulin receptors on tissues. Drugs used in the treatment of type II diabetes mellitus vary among patients. Treatment starts usually with carbohydrate restrictions, exercise, and weight loss. Drugs act by slowing carbohydrate metabolism and absorption, blocking gluconeogenesis in the liver, increasing release of insulin from the pancreas, and/or increasing tissue receptor sensitivities that enhances glucose uptake. If drugs do not provide adequate glucose control, insulin has to be used (see Hypoglycemic Drugs I).

EXAMPLES OF COMMON DOSAGES (GENERAL GUIDELINES, MANY DIFFERENT DOSAGE SCHEDULES)

Acarbose	50-100 mg 3 times daily PO
Miglitol	25-100 mg 3 times daily PO
Metformin	500 mg 2 times daily up to 2000 mg/day PO or 500-1000 mg once daily up to 2500 mg as extended-release tablets PO
Nateglinide	120 mg 3 times daily PO
Repaglinide	0.5-4 mg 3 times daily not to exceed 16 mg/day PO
Glimepiride	1-2 mg once daily to be increased to 8 mg/day PO
Glipizide	2.5-40 mg/day PO
Glyburide	1.25-20 mg once daily PO or 1.5-12 mg 2 times daily as micronized preparation PO
Pioglitazone	15-45 mg once a day PO
Rosiglitazone	4-8 mg once or 2-4 mg twice a day PO
Sitagliptin	25-200 mg once daily PO
Pramlintide	60-120 µg once daily SC

ADMINISTRATION

Hypoglycemic drugs are given PO and SC (using a pen). Some orally administered drugs may take time to become fully effective. Hypoglycemic drugs may be used in combinations with each other or with insulin.

CONTRAINDICATIONS

Hypoglycemic drugs should not be used or used with caution in patients with hepatic failure.

COMMON ADVERSE REACTIONS

Hypoglycemic drugs can cause hypoglycemia (sweating, weakness, dizziness, tremor, and tachycardia to unconsciousness), but this occurs least with glucosidase inhibitors, thiazolidinediones, and biguanides. Drugs can cause nausea and GI problems. Glucosidase inhibitors also cause flatulence. Biguanides can cause lactic acidosis (chills, dizziness, hypotension, muscle pain, bradycardia, and dyspnea), which can be serious. Sulfonylureas cause photosensitization and rarely agranulocytosis and aplastic anemia. Rosiglitazone may increase the risk of cardiovascular problems like CHF (early warning signs are dyspnea, rules/crackles, and peripheral edema) or cardiac infarct.

DRUG INTERACTIONS

- β-Blockers add to drug effects and can mask onset of a hypoglycemic episode (e.g., tachycardia). Drugs interact with some diuretics like thiazide and loop diuretics, corticosteroids, and calcium channel blockers, which increase blood glucose levels. Risk of lactic acidosis with metformin is increased by a number of drugs, including alcohol, morphine, calcium channel blockers, and ranitidine. Cross-sensitivity with sulfonamides can occur mostly with the sulfonylureas. Antifungal agents may interfere with glucose control of meglitinides.
- Glucosamine, chromium, and coenzyme Q-10 may interfere with blood sugar control by hypoglycemic drugs.

IMPLICATIONS FOR PHYSICAL THERAPISTS

- Make sure that the patient wears an identification tag or other visible marker indicating that he or she is a diabetic. Also, make sure, depending on the drug, that the patient carries some sugar, a glucose preparation, or sweetened orange juice to counteract a hypoglycemic reaction.
- Do not recommend glucosamine to diabetic patients to treat joint problems unless this has been cleared with a physician because glucosamine can cause hypoglycemic episodes in unadjusted hypoglycemic drug dosages.
- Be aware of the occurrence of hypoglycemia, as well as hyperglycemia (unusual thirst, drowsiness, fruit-like breath, and flushed). Treat the first with sugar (artificial sweeteners do not work) and the other by asking the patient to administer the needed drug dose.
- If you feel that patient's blood glucose levels are fluctuating, ask if he or she has changed dietary habits or is using an OTC drug because these can cause poor glucose control.
- Do exercise a diabetic patient, carefully in particular at the beginning of drug therapy, because exercise can reduce blood glucose levels. Check glucose levels during and after exercise.
- If your patient usually on metformin complains about chills, dizziness, hypotension, muscle pain, bradycardia, and dyspnea, notify the physician immediately because these could be warning signs of a ketoacidosis.

IMMUNOMODULATORS

COMMON DRUGS (SELECTION OF SOME OF THE MOST COMMONLY USED DRUGS)

DNA Inhibitors

Azathioprine	Azasan, Imuran
Cyclophosphamide	Cytoxan
Methotrexate	Trexall, Rheumatrex

T-Cell Inactivators

Cyclosporine	Neoral, Sandimmune, other
Sirolimus	Rapamune
Tacrolimus	Prograf, Protopic

Gold Compounds

Auranofin	Ridaura
Other	

NSAIDs (see Nonsteroidal Antiinflammatory Drugs)

Corticosteroids (see Corticosteroids)

Miscellaneous Drugs

Chloroquine	Aralen
Etanercept	Enbrel
Other	

Immunostimulators

Immune globulins	Gamma globulin, Iveegam, Carimune, other
Filgrastim	Neupogen
Sargramostim	Leukine
Other	

MECHANISM OF ACTION

The immune system consists of the innate and the adaptive parts. The first involves certain leukocytes, is present since birth and is relatively unspecific. The second forms later in life, is more specific and involves B cells that form various antibodies and T cells, which are more directly involved in immune responses. In addition, lymphokines or cytokines, interleukins, and tumor necrosis factor are involved and amplify the actions of this adaptive system.

Immunomodulators now inhibit or stimulate the actions of the immune system. Most drugs are inhibitory. They interfere with DNA synthesis (see Antineoplastic Drugs), like azathioprine, cyclophosphamide, and methotrexate, reducing proliferation of immune cells or they reduce the activity of T and/or B cells like cyclosporine, tacrolimus, and sirolimus. They inhibit the formation of the inflammatory prostaglandins like NSAIDs and corticosteroids. Gold compounds like auranofin and aurothioglucose reduce T cell activity by an uncertain mechanism. Chloroquine is thought to damage immune cells by changing their pH, and etanercept blocks the action of the tumor necrosis factor.

Few drugs are available to stimulate the immune system. Filgrastim and sargramostim stimulate the formation of white blood cells in bone marrow, which may be decreased during anticancer therapy. Immunoglobulins provide exogenous antibodies to the body.

INDICATION

Immunomodulators are indicated in the following:

- *Transplantation of tissues and organs,* in which the immune system tries to destroy foreign cells as it is supposed to do but which in these cases is unwanted. Immunomodulators like T-cell inactivators reduce the activity of T-cells which are mostly involved in the rejection of transplants.
- *Autoimmune diseases,* such as rheumatoid arthritis, systemic lupus erythematosus, polymyositis, myasthenia gravis, and others, in which an exaggerated immune response damages healthy tissue and causes health problems. Immunomodulators reduce this response and prevent further damage.
- *White blood cell deficiency* during chemotherapy is treated with filgrastim or sargramostim, to stimulate white blood cell formation.

EXAMPLES OF COMMON DOSAGES (GENERAL GUIDELINES, MANY DIFFERENT DOSAGE SCHEDULES)

Azathioprine	1-3 mg/kg/day PO or 3-5 mg/kg IV
Cyclophosphamide	1-2.5 mg/kg/day PO
Methotrexate	7.5 mg/wk up to 20 mg/wk PO
Cyclosporine	2.5-10 mg/kg/day once or divided doses PO
Sirolimus	2 mg/day up to 5 mg/day PO
Tacrolimus	0.03-0.05 mg/kg/day IV then 0.15 mg/kg 2 times daily PO
Auranofin	6 mg once or 3 mg 2 times daily up to 9 mg/day PO
Chloroquine	250 mg/day PO
Etanercept	50 mg /week SC
Filgrastim	5-10 µg/kg/day once IV SC Infusion
Sargramostim	250-500 µg/m²/day IV Infusion
Immunoglobulins	Various schedules

ADMINISTRATION

Most drugs are given PO but can be injected or used topically. Often, drugs are administered in combination. In some cases, the response is delayed by weeks or months.

CONTRAINDICATIONS

Immunomodulators should not be used or must be used with caution in patients with immune system and blood problems.

COMMON ADVERSE REACTIONS

Adverse reactions of all immune suppressants are an increased risk of infections. Other adverse reactions differ among the groups (see Antineoplastic Drugs, Nonsteroidal Antiinflammatory Drugs, and Corticosteroids). T cell inactivators can cause hepatic and renal damage, blood disorders, lung problems, seizures, and confusion. Gold compounds cause some GI distress but also some blood disorders like leukopenia. Chloroquine is usually well tolerated but may cause some retinal damage. Etanercept is more toxic and can cause serious infections and certain malignancies.

DRUG INTERACTIONS

- Immunomodulators, depending on the class, can interact with a large number of other drugs.
- Ginseng and St. John's wort can decrease effectiveness of T-cell inactivators, and grapefruit juice can affect their bioavailability.

IMPLICATIONS FOR PHYSICAL THERAPISTS

- Inform the patient about the difference between rheumatoid arthritis and osteoarthritis (the latter is somewhat of a misnomer because no inflammation is the causative process). Explain that NSAIDs can be used in both conditions, whereas acetaminophen, which lacks antiinflammatory properties, should only be used in osteoarthritis.
- Inform the patient that foods rich in meat and proteins have been shown to aggravate and foods high in fish oils to ameliorate the signs of rheumatoid arthritis. Stress the importance of weight loss in overweight individuals because excessive weight worsens the problem.
- Wear a mask or do not treat the patient if you have an infection (flu, respiratory infection, or other infection) because immune suppressants increase the risk of an infection in these patients.
- Emphasize that muscle and bone strengthening exercise can be helpful in preventing further deterioration, in particular, if corticosteroids are used.

- Observe the patient if skin rashes or unexplained joint pain may be experienced by the patient because this could signal a more serious condition and might necessitate a change in drug.

LOCAL ANESTHETICS

COMMON DRUGS (SELECTION OF SOME OF THE MOST COMMONLY USED DRUGS)

Benzocaine	Anbesol, Lanacane, other (OTC)
Bupivacaine	Marcaine, Sensorcaine
Dibucaine	Nupercainal
Levobupivacaine	Chirocaine
Lidocaine	Xylocaine, Dilocaine, other
Procaine	Novocain
Ropivacaine	Naropin
Tetracaine	Pontocaine

MECHANISM OF ACTION

Pain impulses starting at a particular site (involving prostaglandins, see Nonnarcotic Analgesics) are then transmitted via nerve impulses to the spinal cord and brain where pain is finally experienced. Nerve impulses conducting the pain signals are initiated by an influx of sodium into and then an efflux of potassium out of the nerve (action potential).

Local anesthetics attach to sodium channels and do not allow the influx of sodium into the nerve. No action potential can occur, and pain nerve impulses stop at this site and do not reach the brain where no pain can be perceived and experienced. Action is only transient. (If these drugs do not solve a major pain problem, phenol or alcohol injections, which are not local anesthetics, can be given that actually damage nerves and whose effects might last for months or years).

INDICATION

Local anesthetics are indicated in the following:

- *Surgery,* in which blockade of pain impulses allows for analgesia during the procedure.
- *Hypertonic muscles* (cerebrovascular accidents, head trauma) or *minor surface inflammation/irritation* (abrasions, burns). Local anesthetics reduce or abolish pain sensation and decrease excessive feedback on efferent motor pathways.
- *Therapy of painful subcutaneous structures* (bursae, tendons) or *low back pain.* Local anesthetics are applied topically with iontophoresis or phonophoresis or by patch. Again, pain sensation and muscle relaxation are achieved by blockade of nerve impulses.

- *Muscle spasms,* in which a "vicious" cycle keeps muscle contracted. Local anesthetics injected into the affected area break this cycle by interfering with nerve impulses and relax the muscle.

EXAMPLES OF COMMON DOSAGES (GENERAL GUIDELINES, MANY DIFFERENT DOSAGE SCHEDULES)

Benzocaine	Various preparations
Bupivacaine	25-100 mg as a 0.5% solution epidural
Dibucaine	Various preparations
Levobupivacaine	50-150 mg as a 0.5% solution epidural
Lidocaine	300 mg IM or 50-100 mg IV
Procaine	50-100 mg for spinal anesthesia
Ropivacaine	12-16 mg epidural
Tetracaine	Various routes and dosages

ADMINISTRATION

Local anesthetics are used topically, like benzocaine, dibucaine, and tetracaine, either alone or assisted by iontophoresis or phonophoresis or by injection or infiltration. Some drugs are applied as patches. In some cases, α-agonists are added to injectable preparations to cause vasoconstriction, which allows smaller amounts of the local anesthetic to remain longer at the injection site and not to be transported into other body parts.

CONTRAINDICATIONS

Local anesthetics should not be used or must be used with caution in patients with cardiac and hepatic diseases; this applies mostly to injections.

COMMON ADVERSE REACTIONS

Adverse reactions differ among drugs. In general, no major toxicities are expected by topical application unless very large doses are used. In the case of injections, cardiotoxicity (bradycardia, dysrhythmias, or hypotension) and CNS effects (tinnitus, agitation, restlessness, confusion, tremors, twitching, dizziness, fainting, and seizures) can be expected. Repeated injections into the same place can cause muscle pain and necrosis.

DRUG INTERACTIONS

Interactions occur mostly after injections with other drugs.

IMPLICATIONS FOR PHYSICAL THERAPISTS

- Local anesthetics allow the physical therapist to do manipulations and rehabilitation techniques without inflicting unnecessary pain.

- Patients with infiltration therapy might experience hypotension, sensory impairment, and motor deficits. Patients must be watched carefully when walking and when getting up to avoid falls. As a precaution, these functions should be tested before therapy.
- Patients with infiltration therapy may have abolished or decreased pain perception, and thermal and electrical stimuli must be applied with care. As a precaution, sensory functions should be tested before therapy.
- Watch out for tinnitus, agitation, tremors, and confusion in patients with epidural therapy because this could indicate an overdose reaction requiring dosage adjustments.

MALE HORMONES

COMMON DRUGS (SELECTION OF SOME OF THE MOST COMMONLY USED DRUGS)

Androgens

Testosterone	Andronate, Dura-test, other
Nandrolone	Hybolin, Kabolin
Other	

Antiandrogens

Finasteride	Proscar
Dutasteride	Avodart
Other	

MECHANISM OF ACTION

LH and FSH are released from the pituitary gland and stimulate the synthesis of the androgen testosterone in the testes. This hormone and its more active metabolite dihydrotestosterone are responsible for the development of the male sex characteristics, including sex organs (including development and growth of the prostate gland) and increased bone and muscle mass.

Male hormones, which are the natural hormones or analogs, can now stimulate this development by acting like testosterone or as antiandrogens that can inhibit the conversion of testosterone to its more active metabolite dihydrotestosterone and reduce its stimulatory action.

INDICATION

Male hormones are indicated in the following:
- *Replacement therapy,* in which there is a deficiency, such as after removal of testes, hypogonadism, and other forms of testosterone underfunctioning. Testosterone or its analogs are administered to fulfill the function of a deficiency or lack of the endogenous hormone.
- *Benign prostatic hyperplasia,* in which the prostate is enlarged and interferes with normal bladder emptying.

Antiandrogens lower dihydrotestosterone levels and actually shrink an enlarged prostate, reducing urinary problems.
- Other uses include certain *anemias* (see Hemopoietic Drugs).

EXAMPLES OF COMMON DOSAGES (GENERAL GUIDELINES, MANY DIFFERENT DOSAGE SCHEDULES)

Testosterone	25-50 mg 2-3 times a week or 100 mg/ month IM
Nandrolone	100-200 mg/week IM
Finasteride	5 mg/day PO
Dutasteride	0.5 mg/day PO

ADMINISTRATION

Depending on the drug, male hormones are given PO, IM or by patch.

CONTRAINDICATIONS

Male hormones should not be used or must be used with caution in patients with renal, cardiac, and/or hepatic disease.

COMMON ADVERSE REACTIONS

- Adverse reactions differ, but androgens may affect blood glucose levels and may cause jaundice. Antiandrogens decrease libido and sexual performance.
- In case of abuse of very high doses of androgens over long periods of time by athletes who try to increase bone and muscle mass, as well as performance (although it is still uncertain in how much these androgens actually contribute to increased muscle mass and performance), number and intensity of adverse reactions increase markedly. Abuse has been associated with liver problems, cardiomyopathy and other heart diseases, dysrhythmias, and bone damage all of which can markedly decrease life expectancy.

DRUG INTERACTIONS

Male hormones can interact with a number of drugs.

IMPLICATIONS FOR PHYSICAL THERAPISTS

If an athletic person with well-developed muscles is seen, inquire carefully about illegal use of androgens. Inform this individual that these substances may not do what he or she expects them to do but can significantly increase the risk of adverse reactions, which can shorten life expectancy and cause an early death. Athletes often trust physical therapists more than other health professionals.

MISCELLANEOUS VASODILATORS

COMMON DRUGS (SELECTION OF SOME OF THE MOST COMMONLY USED DRUGS)

Peripherally Acting Vasodilator
Hydralazine   Apresoline
Other

Centrally Acting Vasodilators
Clonidine   Catapres
Other

Vasodilators for Erectile Dysfunction
Sildenafil   Viagra
Vardenafil   Levitra
Tadalafil   Cialis
Other

Antianginals
Isosorbide   Dilatrate, Isordil, other
                 Nitrocot, Nitro-Time,
Nitroglycerin   Nitrogard, other

MECHANISM OF ACTION

Vasodilation can be achieved by various mechanisms. In this case, one mechanism is the stimulation of muscarinic receptors in blood vessels that form nitric oxide (NO) and that activates guanylyl cyclase to synthesize the second messenger cyclic guanosine monophosphate (cGMP). This relaxes blood vessels and decreases blood pressure but is quickly broken down by the enzyme phosphodiesterase (PDE). Another mechanism is located in the brain where stimulation of α_2-receptors decreases central sympathetic outflow to blood vessels, leading to vasodilatation and a fall in blood pressure.

Antianginals form NO, which stimulates guanylyl cyclase, promotes cGMP formation, and causes vasodilatation. This increases coronary blood flow and oxygen supply and dilates systemic blood vessels, which reduces cardiac after load. Hydralazine seems to inhibit PDE, which prevents the destruction of cGMP and keeps its levels increased longer, dilating blood vessels and causing a fall in blood pressure. Vasodilators for erectile dysfunction also inhibit PDE, but this inhibition is more localized in the cavernosal smooth muscles of the penis (special PDE5). Here, they allow blood accumulation initiating and maintaining an erection. However, this effect needs sexual stimulation to be fully effective. Centrally acting vasodilators stimulate α_2-receptors in the brain and decrease sympathetic outflow, peripheral resistance, and cardiac output. This results in a fall in blood pressure. Clonidine also seems to have analgesic actions.

INDICATIONS

Vasodilators are indicated in the following
*   *Hypertension,* in which increased cardiac output and/or peripheral resistance

increases blood pressure. Hypertension untreated is linked to MIs and strokes. Vasodilators, such as hydralazine and clonidine, dilate blood vessels and reduce blood pressure and can reduce the risk of secondary MIs and strokes.
*   *Angina,* in which insufficient blood flow (e.g., atherosclerosis) does not supply enough oxygen to cardiac muscle. If heart rate and contractility increase (usually under emotional or physical stress), the oxygen need markedly exceeds the oxygen supply and anginal pain occurs. Antianginals dilate coronary blood vessels, which increases cardiac blood flow and oxygen supply to the heart and dilate peripheral blood vessels to ease cardiac blood ejection.
*   *Erectile dysfunction* is an inability to initiate and/or maintain an erection. An erection begins with sensory or mental sexual stimulation allowing the muscles of the corpora cavernosa to relax and the penis to fill with blood. This relaxation is initiated and maintained by cGMP. Vasodilators increase and maintain levels of cGMP longer by blocking its destruction by the special PDE5.
*   *Opioid withdrawal* and *pain management* in the cancer patient not responding to opioids may involve the use of clonidine.

EXAMPLES OF COMMON DOSAGES (GENERAL GUIDELINES, MANY DIFFERENT DOSAGE SCHEDULES)

Hydralazine	10-50 mg 4 times daily (not to exceed 320 mg/day) PO
Clonidine	0.1-0.6 mg 2 times daily PO
Sildenafil	25-100 mg taken 30-60 minutes before sexual activity PO
Vardenafil	5-20 mg taken 60 minutes before sexual activity PO
Tadalafil	5-20 mg 15 minutes before sexual activity PO
Isosorbide	2.5-10 mg every 5-10 min for 3 doses SL or 5-40 mg q6h (dinitrate) PO
Nitroglycerin	0.3-0.6 mg every 5 min for 15 min SL or 1 mg q5h buccal 2.5-9 mg q8h for extended-release capsules or 0.1-0.6 mg/hour by patch

ADMINISTRATION

Vasodilators are given PO or by injections usually only in hospitals. Clonidine can be given by transdermal or epidural

administration. Antianginals can be given sublingual. Vasodilators for erectile dysfunction have a similar onset (between 30 to 60 minutes) but last between 4 to 36 hours (tadalafil is longest lasting). Antianginals have a very quick (minutes) onset of action and are used to prevent or abort an attack of angina.

CONTRAINDICATIONS

Vasodilators are contraindicated in cases of hypersensitivity. Drugs should be used with caution in cases of renal or hepatic impairments. Vasodilators for erectile dysfunction should not be used in individuals with cardiovascular disease or 6 month after MI.

COMMON ADVERSE REACTIONS

Peripheral vasodilators can cause tachycardia, hypotension, sodium retention (edema), and a lupus syndrome. Central vasodilators can cause drowsiness, dry mouth, and bradycardia and should not be discontinued abruptly. Vasodilators for erectile dysfunction can cause headache, nasal decongestion, vision loss (rare), GI problems, flushing, cardiovascular collapse, and priapism (erection lasting longer than 4 hours). Antianginals may cause hypotension, tachycardia, dizziness, and headaches.

DRUG INTERACTIONS

Peripheral vasodilators can increase the antihypertensive effects of other antihypertensives and alcohol. Central vasodilators increase sedative effects of drugs with similar actions. Vasodilators for erectile dysfunction should not be used or used with caution with antihypertensive drugs, alcohol, nitrates, or α-antagonists because of the possibility of a severe hypotensive episode. Antianginals should be used with caution with β-blockers and should not be used with vasodilators used for erectile dysfunction.

IMPLICATIONS FOR PHYSICAL THERAPISTS

*   Advise patient to change positions and get up slowly because orthostatic hypotension may occur mostly in the beginning of therapy and in geriatric individuals.
*   If patient complains about unexplained joint pain, notify the physician or have patient contact the physician because this could be a lupus-like syndrome.
*   If you notice peripheral edema such as swollen ankles, notify or have patient contact the physician because this could be caused by excessive sodium retention.
*   Be aware that central vasodilators may cause drowsiness, which can interfere with your therapeutic routine. This should slowly diminish during drug therapy.
*   If the patient has an attack of angina and responds to nitroglycerin, have him

PHARMACOLOGY

Section V

or her get up slowly because orthostatic hypotension might occur. If the patient does not respond to 3 doses of nitroglycerin, call 911 because this could signal a MI.

NONNARCOTIC ANALGESICS

COMMON DRUGS (SELECTION OF SOME OF THE MOST COMMONLY USED DRUGS)

Acetaminophen	Tylenol, Abenol, Aceta, Dapacin, Dynafed, other (OTC)
Diclofenac	Cataflam, Voltaren, Solaraze
Etodolac	Lodine
Ibuprofen	Motrin, Advil, Nuprin, Actiprofen, Genpril (OTC)
Ketoprofen	Actron, Orudis, Oruvail, Rhodis, Apo-Keto
Ketorolac	Toradol
Meloxicam	Mobic
Naproxen	Aleve, Anaprox, Naprosyn, Synflex, Naprelan, other (OTC)
Salicylates (acetyl-)	Aspirin, Acuprin, Arthrisin, other (OTC) (Aspirin is acetylsalicylic acid to be metabolized to active metabolite salicylic acid.) Salicylates, Tricosal, Anaflex, Arthropan, other
Other	See Nonsteroidal Antiinflammatory Drugs

MECHANISM OF ACTION

Pain impulses originate through the combined action of bradykinin and prostaglandins and are then transmitted via nerve impulses to the CNS. Prostaglandins are a group of biochemicals or local hormones, which are synthesized by the enzyme cyclooxygenase (COX) that occurs as COX-1 (always present in tissues) and COX-2 (induced during trauma). They are involved in the initiation and maintenance of pain, inflammation, and fever (see Nonsteroidal Antiinflammatory Drugs). They also protect the stomach lining from the action of gastric acid, cause vasodilatation in certain vascular beds, contract smooth muscles such as the uterus, induce with other chemicals platelet aggregation, and somehow maintain proper renal blood flow.

Nonnarcotic analgesics are thought to inhibit these two forms of COX and reduce pain by inhibiting the synthesis of the pain-initiating biochemical prostaglandins.

INDICATIONS

Nonnarcotic analgesics are indicated in the following:

• *Mild-to-moderate pain* caused by trauma, headaches, tooth aches, muscle soreness and aches, dysmenorrhea, osteoarthritis, and inflammatory disorders, including rheumatoid arthritis, bursitis, and others. Drugs reduce prostaglandin formation and reduce pain. They show similar analgesic actions with some exceptions. Ketorolac has been found to be particularly effective in postoperative pain. Drugs are most effective if taken early on at the onset of pain. Some patients may not respond to one but will respond better to another drug. Usually, higher doses than those recommended do not provide for more pain relief. Dosage for analgesic effects is usually lower than that used for inflammatory conditions.

EXAMPLES OF COMMON DOSAGES (GENERAL GUIDE LINES, MANY DIFFERENT DOSAGE SCHEDULES)

Acetaminophen	650-1000 mg q4-6h (existing maximal dose of 4 g per day to be reduced in the future) PO
Aspirin	325-500 q4h (not to exceed 4 g) PO
Diclofenac	100 mg initially and/ or 25-50 mg q6h PO
Etodolac	200-400 mg q6h (not to exceed 1200 mg) PO
Ibuprofen	200-400 mg q5h (not to exceed 1200 mg) PO
Ketoprofen	25-50 mg q6h (not to exceed 75 mg) PO
Ketorolac	20 mg followed by 10 mg q5h (not to exceed 20 doses/ days and not more than 5 days) PO
Meloxicam	7.5 mg once a day PO
Naproxen	250-400 mg and 250 mg q6h (not to exceed 1.5 g). Slow-release preparation 375-500 2 times a day PO

ADMINISTRATION

Nonnarcotic analgesics are used mostly orally. They are best taken with a large glass of water or food while remaining in an upright position for about 30 minutes. Onset of action is usually 15 to 30 minutes. Duration of action varies among drugs but is generally between 4 to 8 hours (slow-release preparations can increase duration). Advise patient that self-administration with acetaminophen over longer periods with high doses can cause serious liver damage (in some cases even death) and that the existing daily dose of 4 g/day will be reduced and the newly established dose should not be exceeded.

CONTRAINDICATIONS

Contraindications to the use of these drugs include hypersensitivity, GI problems (gastritis, ulcer), and renal and hepatic disorders.

COMMON ADVERSE REACTIONS

All nonnarcotic analgesics can cause abdominal pain, dyspepsia, and GI bleeding (tarry stools are indicative of internal bleeding). Some nonnarcotic analgesics can be photosensitizing. Hypersensitivity reactions are rare and occur more frequently if the patients are sensitive to aspirin and have asthma and nasal polyps (except acetaminophen). Drugs can be liver toxic and show renal toxicity but mostly in individuals with already compromised hepatic and renal functions. They can slightly increase the risk of cardiovascular events again mostly during chronic use and in individuals with cardiovascular problems. Chronic use has been shown to cause renal problems. Acetaminophen causes fewer GI problems but is more liver toxic and can affect blood glucose monitoring. Ketoprofen has a higher incidence of headache and dizziness. Aspirin should not be used in children with viral infections because it can cause the potentially fatal Reye syndrome (acetaminophen is the drug of choice in these cases).

DRUG INTERACTIONS

There is an increased risk of GI problems (gastritis, ulcer) enhanced by concurrent use of spicy foods, alcohol, and some herbal products such as arnica, garlic, and ginseng. Use of acetaminophen and alcohol (more than 2 glasses of wine or beer) has been associated with increased liver toxicity.

IMPLICATIONS FOR PHYSICAL THERAPISTS

• Patients often report only prescription drugs when asked about drug use. Because some analgesics are also obtained without a prescription, the question should also include use of OTC drugs (and vitamins/herbal medications). Advise patient that OTC drugs are drugs and must be used with caution.

• Analgesics may mask pain during mobility movements. This can lead to damage by exceeding movement limitations or by providing the impression of better mobility than actually exists.

• Extensive UV radiation should be avoided or other body parts should be covered because some drugs can cause photosensitivity reactions.

- Some patients may experience drowsiness and might exhibit slight incoordination but this is very rare with these drugs.
- Advise the patient to use acetaminophen for low back pain because a recent study suggests that this drug seems to be most effective and to carry the least side effects.
- Advise the patients that OTC analgesics should not be taken longer than 2 weeks without consulting a physician because these drugs can mask a serious underlying health problem.

NONSTEROIDAL ANTIINFLAMMATORY DRUGS

COMMON DRUGS (SELECTION OF SOME OF THE MOST COMMONLY USED DRUGS)

Diclofenac	Cataflam, Voltaren, Solaraze,
Etodolac	Lodine
Ibuprofen	Motrin, Advil, Nuprin, Actiprofen, Genpril (OTC available)
Indomethacin	Indocin, Indocron, other
Ketoprofen	Actron, Orudis, Oruvail, Rhodis, Apo-Keto
Ketorolac	Toradol
Meloxicam	Mobic
Nabumetone	Relafen
Naproxen	Aleve, Anaprox, Naprosyn, Synflex, Naprelan, other (OTC available)
Oxaprozin	Daypro
Piroxicam	Feldene
Sulindac	Clinoril
Salicylates (acetyl-)	Aspirin, Acuprin, Arthrisin, other (OTC available) (Composed of acetylsalicylic acid to be metabolized to active metabolite salicylic acid.) Salicylates, Tricosal, Anaflex, Arthropan, other
Tolmetin	Tolectin
Celecoxib	Celebrex (See Nonnarcotic Analgesics and Corticosteroids)

MECHANISM OF ACTION

Prostaglandins are a group of biochemicals or local hormones, which are synthesized from phospholipids via arachidonic acid by the enzyme COX that occurs as COX-1 (always present in tissues) and COX-2 (induced during trauma). They are mostly involved in the initiation and maintenance of pain, inflammation, and fever. In the case of an inflammation, they cause vasodilatation, which allows water and white blood cells to migrate from the blood to the tissues (this causes warmth, redness, and swelling). If inflammations are contained, they are beneficial in fighting infections and repair tissue damage. Prostaglandins also protect the stomach lining from the action of gastric acid (mostly via COX-1), cause vasodilatation in certain vascular beds, contract smooth muscles like the uterus, induce with other chemicals platelet aggregation, and somehow maintain renal blood flow.

NSAIDs inhibit COX-1 and -2 and reduce or prevent prostaglandin synthesis and reduce inflammatory processes. Because gastric protection is achieved by prostaglandins synthesized by COX-1, drugs lower this protective mechanism (except celecoxib, which is less inhibitory on COX-1 and less damaging to the stomach). Drugs often work best when taken at the beginning of an inflammatory process. Indomethacin is one of the strongest antiinflammatory drugs but also carries the more severe adverse reactions.

INDICATIONS

NSAIDs are indicated in the following:

- General *inflammations,* which are characterized by swelling, redness, warmth and pain, and eventually tissue damage if they become unwanted or excessive such as occurs in certain autoimmune diseases, transplants, allergies, asthma, croup, rheumatoid arthritis, ankylosing spondylitis, or bursitis. NSAIDs curtail excessive and reduce unwanted inflammations to protect healthy tissue.
- *Dysmenorrhea,* in which excessive prostaglandin formation stimulates the uterus, causing painful contractions. NSAIDs reduce prostaglandin levels and excessive contractions and cramps.
- *Fever,* which is initiated by a central action of prostaglandins in the brain area that regulates body temperature. NSAIDs reduce prostaglandin formation and lower fever.
- *Ocular inflammations* after eye surgery (e.g., topical administration of bromfenac, diclofenac, flurbiprofen, ketorolac, nepafenac, or suprofen), in which NSAIDs reduce prostaglandin synthesis and prevent or reduce inflammatory processes.

EXAMPLES OF COMMON DOSAGES (GENERAL GUIDELINES, MANY DIFFERENT DOSAGE SCHEDULES)

Aspirin	325-500 mg q4h (not to exceed 4 g) PO
Celecoxib	100-200 mg once or twice a day PO
Etodolac	300 mg 2-3 times daily PO or 400-1200 mg once daily as extended-release preparation PO
Ibuprofen	400-800 mg 3-4 times daily (not to exceed 3600 mg/day) PO
Indomethacin	25-50 mg 2-4 times daily PO or 75 mg once daily with extended-release preparations PO
Ketoprofen	150-300 mg/day in 3-4 divided dose PO or 100-200 mg once daily with extended-release preparations PO
Ketorolac	20 mg followed by 10 mg q5h (not to exceed 40 mg/day) PO
Meloxicam	7.5-15 mg once a day PO
Naproxen	250-500 mg 2-3 times a day (not to exceed 1.5 g) or 375-500 mg twice a day with the slow-release preparation PO
Nabumetone	1000-2000 mg once or twice a day PO
Oxaprozin	1200-1800 mg once daily PO
Piroxicam	10-20 mg once or twice a day PO
Sulindac	150-200 mg twice a day PO
Tolmetin	400-1800 mg/day in 3 divided dose (not to exceed 2000 mg/day) PO

ADMINISTRATION

NSAIDs can be given IV, PO or topically into the eye. They are best taken with meals or a large glass of water and sitting up or standing for 30 minutes after ingestion.

CONTRAINDICATIONS

Contraindications include hypersensitivity to a drug that often manifests itself as hypersensitivity to the entire group and GI problems (gastritis, ulcers). NSAIDs should be used cautiously in cases of severe hepatic, renal and cardiovascular diseases.

COMMON ADVERSE REACTIONS

Adverse reactions include dizziness, drowsiness, abdominal distress, dyspepsia, gastritis, ulcer, photosensitivity and after long term use nephritis. Rarely, they can cause Stevens-Johnson syndrome, hepatitis, or exfoliate dermatitis. Celecoxib is a COX II inhibitor and somewhat gentler on the stomach but can increase the risk of cardiovascular accidents. Patients with nasal polyps, asthma, and aspirin-induced allergy are at high risk to develop hypersensitivity reactions towards other drugs in this group.

DRUG INTERACTIONS

- NSAIDs can interact with a large number of drugs such as enhancing the effects of warfarin and related drugs in increasing bleeding times or decreasing the effects of antihypertensives and insulin. Alcohol increases adverse effects on the stomach.
- Arnica, dong quai, garlic, ginseng, and ginkgo increase the risk of bleeding. Spicy foods aggravate stomach problems.

IMPLICATIONS FOR PHYSICAL THERAPISTS

- Patients often report only prescription drugs when asked about drugs used. Because some NSAIDs are also obtained without a prescription, the question should also include use of prescription, as well as OTC drugs (and vitamins/mineral/herbal medications).
- Advise the patient that antiinflammatory OTC drugs are drugs and must be used with caution and the patient must adhere to the warning statements on the container.
- NSAIDs may mask pain during mobility movements and can give the impression of better mobility than actually exists and may cause damage by exceeding movement limitations.
- Extensive UV radiation should be avoided or other body parts should be covered because some drugs cause photosensitization.
- Some patients may experience drowsiness and may exhibit slight incoordination, but this is very rare with these drugs.
- If the patient complains about stomach problems, tell the patient to take medication with lots of water sitting up or standing for at least 30 minutes or with a meal. The patient should also watch the stool and if black (occult bleeding), he or she should stop the drug and notify the physician immediately.
- If the patient complains about an upper respiratory infection, cough, muscle aching, and a rash with blisters, ask the patient to contact the physician immediately because this could be a Stevens-Johnson syndrome.
- If you notice dry, itchy, red areas on hands and other parts of the body, have the patient notify the physician immediately because this could be an exfoliate dermatitis.
- Explain to patient that acetaminophen is not antiinflammatory and should not be used if an antiinflammatory drug has been prescribed.

OPIOID OR NARCOTIC ANALGESICS

COMMON DRUGS (SELECTION OF SOME OF THE MOST COMMONLY USED DRUGS)

Buprenorphine	Buprenex, Subutex
Butorphanol	Stadol
Codeine	Paveral
Fentanyl	Actiq, Sublimaze, Duragesic (transdermal)
Hydrocodone	Hycodan, Robidone
	In combination with acetaminophen: Anexsia, Bancap, Dolacet, other
	In combination with aspirin: Alor, Azdone, other
	In combination with ibuprofen: Vicoprofen
Hydromorphone	Dilaudid, Hydrostat
Meperidine	Demerol, Pethidine
Methadone	Dolophine, Methadose
Morphine	Astramorph, Avinza, Epimorph, Roxanol, other
Nalbuphine	Nubain
Oxycodone	Endocodone, OxyContin, Percolone, Roxicodone
Oxymorphone	Numorphan
Pentazocine	Talwin
	In combination with acetaminophen: Talacen
	In combination with aspirin: Talwin compound
Propoxyphene	Darvon
	In combination with aspirin: Darvon-N c ASA
	In combination with aspirin and caffeine: Darvon 32 or 65
	In combination with acetaminophen: Darvocet

MECHANISM OF ACTION

Pain impulses originating from the affected site (see Nonnarcotic Analgesics) are transmitted via nerve impulses (see Local Anesthetics) to the CNS where pain is finally experienced. Opioid receptors (μ, κ, and δ receptors) in the CNS that are physiologically activated by endogenous compounds, such as enkephalins, endorphins, and dynorphins, can prevent pain impulses from reaching their final destination and suppress or alter pain perception. Some of these receptors also occur in other brain areas (respiratory center, cough center, and centers associated with nausea/vomiting) and the periphery (intestines).

Opioids are full or partial agonists and are thought to stimulate these receptors in the CNS and cause analgesia. (Action of these drugs can be reversed by opioid antagonists like naloxone and naltrexone.)

INDICATIONS

Opioids are indicated in the following:

- *Moderate-to-severe pain* of all kinds, which is often measured on a subjective scale of 0 to 10. Opioids cause analgesia and pain is reduced, felt less discomforting, or is completely gone. Opioids work best for analgesia if given at the onset of pain. Best results are obtained when the patient controls the proper use of analgesics (patient-controlled analgesia in hospitals) because only he or she feels the pain.
- *Therapy of opioid dependence and withdrawal* (buprenorphine, methadone), *cough* (codeine, hydrocodone, hydromorphone), *diarrhea* (codeine), and before, during, and after *surgery* (fentanyl, meperidine, nalbuphine). Drugs act on opioid receptors and reduce withdrawal, discomfort, cough, diarrhea, and pain.

COMMON DOSAGES

Butorphanol	1-2 mg q3-4h IM, IV; 1 mg as nasal spray q3-4h
Buprenorphine	0.3 mg q4-6h IM, IV
Morphine	10-30 mg q3-4h PO; 4-15 mg q3-4h IM
Pentazocine	50-100 mg q3-4h PO (up to 600 mg/day); 30 mg q3-4h IM, IV
	Plus acetaminophen: 25 mg and 650 mg
	Plus aspirin: 12.5 mg and 325 mg)
Codeine	15-60 mg q3-6h PO; 15-60 mg q4-6h IM, IV
	Plus acetaminophen: 30-60 mg and 300 mg
	Plus aspirin: 60 mg and 325 mg)
Fentanyl	200 µg dissolved in mouth (higher doses available up to 1600 µg); 0.5-1 µg/kg to be repeated every 60 min IV

Hydrocodone	2.5-10 mg q3-6h PO Plus acetaminophen: 5 mg and 500 mg Plus aspirin: 5 mg and 500 mg Plus ibuprofen: 7.5 mg and 200 mg
Hydromorphone	4-8 mg q3-4h PO; 1.5 mg q3-4h IM, IV, SC
Meperidine	50-150 mg q3-4h PO, IM, IV (short-term use only)
Methadone	20 mg q7h PO; 10 mg q7h IM, SC
Nalbuphine	10 mg q3-6h (total dose 160 mg) IV, IM
Oxycodone	5-10 mg q3-4h PO
Oxymorphone	0.5 mg q3-6h IV; 1-1.5 mg q3-6h SC, IM
Propoxyphene	65 mg q4h (not to exceed 390 mg) PO Plus aspirin: 100 mg and 325 mg Plus aspirin and caffeine: 32 or 65 mg, 389 mg, 30 mg Plus acetamino- phen: 50, 65, or 100 mg, 325, 500, or 650 mg (See Nonnarcotic Analgesic Drugs)

ADMINISTRATION

Drugs can be given PO, rectally, IM, IV, by infusion pump (often controlled by patient), or patch (fentanyl). Onset of action after oral use is about 30 minutes and duration of action varies but can be increased with sustained-release tablets. Injections provide relief in minutes.

CONTRAINDICATIONS

Contraindications to the use of these drugs include hypersensitivity, head trauma, and increased intracranial pressure.

COMMON ADVERSE REACTIONS

Opioids cause sedation, drowsiness, incoordination and some respiratory depression (in particular in geriatric patients). Most patients suffer from constipation (which might require the use of laxatives). Some individuals experience nausea and vomiting, which can be avoided by assuming a supine position, and hypotension, which is more marked when assuming quickly an upright position. Miosis interferes with vision in dim or dark conditions. Chronic use of these drugs can lead to physical dependence and tolerance

(except miosis and constipation do not show tolerance). In case of tolerance, change to another drug is often beneficial. Some drugs are prone to be abused, including the substance "heroin," which is converted to morphine in the body.

DRUG INTERACTIONS

Opioids should not be used in patients receiving MAO inhibitors for depression. There is an increased risk of sedation and CNS depression with drugs, which also cause CNS depression, as well as alcohol, valerian, chamomile, or kava.

IMPLICATIONS FOR PHYSICAL THERAPISTS

- Analgesics may make movement exercises easier by reducing pain. They also may mask pain during mobility movements and can cause damage by exceeding movement limitations. Drugs might feign and give the impression of better mobility than actually exists.
- If manipulations under opioid analgesia must be made which otherwise can be painful, arrange therapy at the peak of drug effects usually 2 hours after use of the drug.
- Assess alertness of patient because he or she can be more or less sedated, drowsy, and uncoordinated, and certain tasks requiring attention and quick reflexes should be modified or omitted.
- Ask the patient to change position, in particular from a lying to a standing position, slowly to avoid orthostatic hypotension, which can cause the patient to become dizzy, faint, and fall.
- Respiratory depression must be considered when using exercise because this can reduce breathing and can lead to hypoxia.
- If the patient has to lie on the back for longer periods and breathes very shallow, ask the patient every 30 minutes to take a few deep breaths to expand the lungs to reduce risk of lung collapse.
- During withdrawal from chronic use of one of these drugs, diffuse muscle discomfort might occur that can be alleviated with heat or massages.

OVER-THE-COUNTER DRUGS

INTRODUCTION

OTC drugs are nonprescription medications that are made available based on three criteria: (1) the consumer must be able to easily understand the medical condition to be treated and monitor its progress, (2) the drug must have a favorable adverse reaction profile, and (3) drug use must be simple and easy.

Although these drugs are efficacious and have a low adverse reaction profile, they can nevertheless show these adverse reactions, mask serious medical problems, can be used for the wrong reasons, can be used wrongly even for the right reason, and can interact with prescription drugs.

The user must read the label carefully to avoid medical problems. For instance, the consumer must be aware of the medical condition, how much and how long to use the medication, of other medical conditions that might preclude using this drug, and of prescription drugs that might interact with the medication. OTC drugs must always be mentioned to a physician. The consumer must be aware that some ingredients are not obvious such as the additions of ethanol or caffeine, which can cause their own effects. Also, OTC drugs should not be used when pregnant or breast feeding (unless advised by a physician) because some drugs can reach the fetus or infant through the placenta or milk.

The consumer should not give adult drugs to infants or small children unless it is stated on the label that it is permitted. Recently, many of these infant and children preparations had to be removed from the market because they were found not to be necessary and sometimes even harmful to infants.

The consumer must be observant when treating a problem. If two tablets are recommended but a person is small or old, then it is advisable to start with 1 tablet and should only be increased if there is no relief. Similarly, an obese person might need three tablets instead of the recommended two.

Major adverse reactions to watch out for include the following:

- Analgesics: GI discomfort, rebound headaches, bleeding, can interact with antiinflammatory drugs and anticoagulants
- Acetaminophen: Liver damage with moderate-to-high doses of ethanol, although it is analgesic and antipyretic, it is not antiinflammatory
- Antihistamines: Drowsiness, urinary hesitancy/retention (elderly), contact lens intolerance, enhanced sedation with alcohol (have been misused in date-rape cases)
- Decongestants: Increased blood pressure, counteract antihypertensive medications, rebound effect with prolonged use of nasal preparations
- H_2-blockers: Dysrhythmias, constipation, agranulocytosis
- Pump inhibitors: Liver and renal problems, neutropenia
- Vaginal creams: Headache, missed menstrual periods, fever
- Emergency: Nausea, vomiting, stomach pain, dizziness, headache, diarrhea, contraceptives

IMPLICATIONS FOR PHYSICAL THERAPISTS

- The physical therapist can play an important role in advising patients on the use of OTC drugs or in suggesting the use of such drugs because many patients may not read the entire label or may not understand their uses or contents.
- Patients must be advised that OTC drugs are drugs that can produce serious adverse reactions if used improperly and that a physician must be contacted if this occurs.
- All OTC medications must be mentioned in a medical history to avoid detrimental interactions with prescription drugs.
- Advise patient about the difference between antiinflammatory drugs and acetaminophen, which is not antiinflammatory.
- Advise patient that use of acetaminophen with even moderate doses of alcohol can damage the liver.
- Advise the patient that topical drugs (e.g. ointments) will be absorbed into the body and that use of excessive amounts can cause serious systemic effects.
- Physical therapists can warn and help individuals with rebound headaches (no relief and even worse headaches in spite of drug use) where continued and excessive use of analgesics for headaches can cause such a problem and suggest instead relaxation techniques, massages, or gentle exercises.

SEDATIVES AND HYPNOTICS

COMMON DRUGS (SELECTION OF SOME OF THE MOST COMMONLY USED DRUGS)

Hypnotic Benzodiazepines

Flurazepam	Dalmane
Temazepam	Restoril, Razepam
Triazolam	Halcion

Miscellaneous Hypnotics

Zaleplon	Sonata
Zolpidem	Ambien
Eszopiclone	Lunesta
Other	

Barbiturates

Secobarbital	Seconal
Pentobarbital	Nembutal
Other	

OTC Product

Melatonin	OTC

MECHANISM OF ACTION

Alertness is governed by many chemical processes (neurotransmitters) and electrical circuits in the brain. In this case, the neurotransmitter GABA in the limbic, thalamic, and/or hypothalamic areas seems to play a major role. GABA is formed in neurons, released, and interacts with GABA receptors (subtypes A, B, C and more) to open chloride channels in membranes of adjacent neurons. Influx of negative chloride ions hyperpolarizes these neurons and reduces their firings or activity. Thus normal GABA action causes alertness, whereas increased GABA action reduces alertness, increases sedation, and eventually leads to sleep or hypnosis. GABA also affects centers that control skeletal muscle activity and its increased actions cause muscle relaxation. In addition, melatonin found in the pineal gland of the brain is physiologically involved in sleep.

Hypnotic drugs act on various sites of the GABA receptor complex where they all seem to enhance the action of GABA, increase hyperpolarization, and reduce firing of adjacent neurons, resulting first in sedation and then in hypnosis. It has been suggested that melatonin taken orally may be beneficial for a few individuals in promoting sleep.

INDICATION

Sedatives and hypnotics are mainly indicated in the following:

- *Insomnia*, which is a sleep disorder characterized by a persistent difficulty to fall asleep or to stay asleep. It is usually followed by tiredness and functional impairment the next day. This disorder can be assumed to be caused by an underfunctioning of the GABA system, which does not reduce neuronal activity sufficiently. Sedative and hypnotic drugs (dose–dependent) enhance GABA activity, leading first to sedation and finally hypnosis. Generally, barbiturates are more sleep inducing, and the others are more sleep promoting. Drugs that are quickly absorbed and have a short duration of action are helpful in the initiation of sleep (e.g., triazolam), and drugs with a slow absorption and long duration of action keep individuals asleep longer (e.g., flurazepam). Hypnotic effects of melatonin are still uncertain, with some studies showing a slight benefit while other studies do not.
- Other conditions such as *epilepsy* (see Anticonvulsant Drugs), *movement disorders* (see Skeletal Muscle Relaxants), or *anxiety* (see Anxiolytic Drugs).

EXAMPLES OF COMMON DOSAGES (GENERAL GUIDELINES, MANY DIFFERENT DOSAGE SCHEDULES)

Flurazepam	15-30 mg once PO
Temazepam	7.5-30 mg PO
Triazolam	0.125-0.5 mg PO
Zaleplon	10-20 mg PO
Zolpidem	10 mg (for 10 days only) PO
Eszopiclone	2-3 mg PO
Pentobarbital	100-200 mg PO
Secobarbital	100-200 mg PO
Melatonin	0.5-50 mg PO

ADMINISTRATION

Sedatives and hypnotics are taken at bed time orally. Barbiturates are sometimes injected or given rectally.

CONTRAINDICATIONS

Sedatives and hypnotics should not be used or must be used with caution in patients with renal and hepatic diseases.

COMMON ADVERSE REACTIONS

Common adverse reactions are residual effects that might cause individuals to be drowsy or have decreased motor function and muscular coordination the next day. This occurs mostly in older individuals. All drugs, to varying degrees, cause tolerance and physical dependence so that long-term treatment should not be discontinued abruptly. The withdrawal syndrome might manifest itself in irritation, excitation, and insomnia (and rarely convulsions). High doses can cause some respiratory depression. Other adverse reactions are usually mild. Some individuals might experience anterograde amnesia (forgetting events that took place before the drug was consumed). Zolpidem might cause "sleep walking and eating."

DRUG INTERACTIONS

- Action of sedatives and hypnotics is enhanced, in particular residual effects, in the presence of other drugs with sedative effects, including alcohol.
- Sedative effects are increased by a number of herbs, including chamomile, mistletoe, and valerian. St. John's wort seems to reduce their effectiveness.

IMPLICATIONS FOR PHYSICAL THERAPISTS

- If patient using these drugs appears drowsy and uncoordinated at the morning sessions, schedule this patient in the afternoon when most after-effects should have disappeared. Warn them not to drive if they feel drowsy.
- Warn the patient not to discontinue drugs abruptly after long-term use by themselves but to first consult the physician because they might experience a withdrawal syndrome.
- Tell the patient not to drink or eat products containing caffeine because they can decrease drug effectiveness or might even be a cause of the sleep problem.
- If a patient on zolpidem notices weight gain without having changed eating

habits, ask the patient to notify the physician because the patient might be "sleep eating."

- The physical therapist can also suggest relaxation techniques, exercises, or massages to reduce sleep problems and the need for sleep medications.

SKELETAL MUSCLE RELAXANTS

COMMON DRUGS (SELECTION OF SOME OF THE MOST COMMONLY USED DRUGS)

Centrally Acting Drugs

Baclofen	Lioresal
Carisoprodol	Soma, Vanadom
Chlorzoxazone	Paraflex, Parafon,
Cyclobenzaprine	other
Diazepam	Flexeril, other
Gabapentin	Valium, other
Metaxalone	Neurontin
Methocarbamol	Skelaxin
Orphenadrine	Carbacot,
Tizanidine	Robaxin, other
	Antiflex, Norflex
	Zanaflex

Direct-Acting Drugs

Dantrolene	Dantrium
Dichlorofluoromethane	

Neuromuscular Blocking Drug

Botulinus toxin A	Botox
Botulinus toxin B	Myobloc

MECHANISM OF ACTION

Skeletal muscle movements are initiated and regulated by a balance between excitatory and inhibitory chemical processes (neurotransmitters) and electrical circuits (monosynaptic and polysynaptic connections) in the cerebral cortex, cerebellum, spinal cord, and finally at the neuromuscular junction and the muscles per se. Among the inhibitory neurotransmitters is GABA and among the excitatory neurotransmitters is glutamate in the CNS. Acetylcholine is released at the neuromuscular junction and calcium fluxes are necessary for final muscle contractions.

Centrally acting skeletal muscle relaxants can enhance the action of the inhibitory GABA system with drugs such as diazepam (see Anxiolytic Drugs), baclofen, and gabapentin (see Anticonvulsant Drugs) and reduce muscle tone. Tizanidine, an α2-receptor agonist, increases presynaptic inhibition of motoneurons, and the other drugs seem to act in the spinal cord by suppressing polysynaptic reflex activity with uncertain mechanisms. The remaining drugs act on the periphery. Dantrolene acts by blocking calcium release from the sarcoplasmic reticulum in skeletal muscles, which is necessary for contractions. Dichlorofluoromethane cools the muscle and reduces metabolic and physical activity. These drugs reduce

muscle tone to varying degrees. In contrast, neuromuscular-blocking drugs, such as botulinus toxin, will prevent acetylcholine release at the neuromuscular junction and paralyze the muscles. Effects are irreversible and motoneuron terminals must be newly formed before acetylcholine release can start again, which might take up to 3 months.

INDICATION

Skeletal muscle relaxants are indicated in the following:

- *Spasticity,* which is characterized by excessive skeletal muscle excitation and contraction (exaggerated muscle stretch reflex). It is caused by central pathology such as occurs in multiple sclerosis, cerebral palsy, injury, or stroke. It occurs when supraspinal control is lost. Drugs frequently used are baclofen, diazepam, gabapentin, tizanidine, and dantrolene.
- *Spasm* which is characterized by increased muscle tension caused by muscle injury or inflammation. It is caused by a vicious cycle when muscular injury or inflammation induces increased afferent nociceptive input. Drugs frequently used are carisoprodol, methocarbamol, cyclobenzaprine, and chlorzoxazone.
- *Malignant hyperthermia* (dantroline), *tetanus, seizures, neuralgia,* and *cosmetic purposes* (botulinus toxin).

EXAMPLES OF COMMON DOSAGES (GENERAL GUIDELINES, MANY DIFFERENT DOSAGE SCHEDULES)

Baclofen	5-20 mg 3 times daily up to 80 mg/day PO
Carisoprodol	350 mg 3 times daily PO
Chlorzoxazone	250-750 mg 3-4 times daily PO
Cyclobenzaprine	5 mg 3 times daily up to 30 mg/day PO
Diazepam	2-10 mg 3-4 times daily or 15-30 mg extended-release preparations PO
Gabapentin	900-1800 mg/day in 3 divided doses PO
Metaxalone	800 mg 3-4 times daily PO
Methocarbamol	1-1.5 g 3-4 times daily PO
Orphenadrine	100 mg 2 times daily PO
Tizanidine	8 mg 3-4 times daily PO
Dantrolene	25-100 mg 2-4 times daily PO
Dichlorofluoro-methane	Spray
Botulinus toxin A	200-300 units IM, SC
Botulinus toxin B	2500-5000 units IM, SC

ADMINISTRATION

Most drugs are given PO but can be injected or delivered by pumps (intrathecal baclofen). Drugs might be started at a low dose that will then be gradually increased. Botulinus toxin is only injected IM or SC. Dichlorofluoromethane is applied topically as spray.

CONTRAINDICATIONS

Skeletal muscle relaxants should not be used or must be used with caution in patients with hepatic diseases. Baclofen and dantrolene should not be or be used with caution in patients who use spasticity to partially maintain balance.

COMMON ADVERSE REACTIONS

All skeletal muscle relaxants will cause sedation, drowsiness, and muscle weakness, as well as GI distress to a varying degree. Older individuals may experience periods of confusion. Some drugs might cause physical dependence and should not be discontinued abruptly. Drugs such as baclofen, carisoprodol, or methocarbamol, can precipitate seizures in patients but mostly in those with a seizure history. Chlorzoxazone has been associated with hepatitis, GI bleeding, and anemia.

DRUG INTERACTIONS

- Sedation is increased with all drugs that also possess sedative properties such as antihistamines, alcohol, antidepressants, and opioids.
- Increased sedation will occur with chamomile and valerian.

IMPLICATIONS FOR PHYSICAL THERAPISTS

- Drugs are extremely helpful in rehabilitation because they allow the therapist a more effective therapy.
- Patients starting drug therapy who have used extensor spasticity to maintain balance must be watched carefully while walking because loss of this spasticity might compromise their balance and they might fall.
- Observe all patients carefully when walking or getting up because drowsiness and muscle weakness can cause falls.
- Physical therapists can best evaluate the effectiveness of treatment with these drugs and should share his or her evaluation with the physician to ensure that the best drug and dosage are used for the fullest benefit of the patient.
- Dichlorofluoromethane spray should be applied from the muscle origin to insertion while the muscle is passively stretched. Never overcool the area. After warming, the spray can be reapplied.

GLOSSARY

Agranulocytosis is a deficiency of granulocytes, a subspecies of white blood cells. It manifests itself in immune system impairment, starting with a slight fever and a sore throat possibly with ulcerations.

Akathisia is the inability to sit still.

Allergic reactions are immune responses (either histamine- or T-cell mediated) to exogenous allergens and manifest themselves as hives, redness, and itching (most severe form is anaphylaxis).

Anaphylaxis is a severe allergic reaction (caused by excessive histamine release), which manifests itself as trouble breathing caused by bronchoconstriction and fainting from severe hypotension. It can be fatal.

Churg-Strauss syndrome is a systemic vasculitis first manifested by rashes and nodules under the skin, later on damaging internal organs.

Exfoliate dermatitis is a severe skin disease characterized by redness, scaling, and shedding of the skin.

Epidermal necrolysis is a detachment of the top layer of skin. It manifests itself with fever followed by a rash, redness, blisters, pain, and the peeling of the skin from the underlying dermis. It can be fatal.

Dystonia is a disordered tonicity of muscles causing twitching and twisting motions.

Dyskinesia describes involuntary movements.

Hepatitis and *jaundice* are liver diseases showing flu-like symptoms, muscle and joint pains, fever, nausea, dark urine, and yellowing of the eyes and skin.

Lupus syndrome is a chronic, inflammatory autoimmune disorder with joint pain and arthritis. Frequently affected joints are the fingers, hands, wrists, and knees.

Malignant hyperthermia is characterized by highly elevated body temperature, muscle rigidity, and is life-threatening. It is caused by drug-induced excessive calcium fluxes in skeletal muscles.

Orthostatic hypotension, also called *postural hypotension,* is a form of low blood pressure that occurs when a person stands up from sitting or lying down. Orthostatic hypotension lasts for only seconds or a minute but can cause dizziness and fainting with falls. It occurs more often in older individuals and can be induced by α-blockers and related drugs, which prevent vascular constriction or lower blood pressure. Effects can be minimized if a person gets up slowly and holds on firm to something fixed.

Photosensitivity is a relatively general term used to describe any cutaneous reactions to light that could be allergic or toxic. Drug-induced photosensitivity is mostly of the toxic type, may occur after first exposure to a drug, and is typically manifested by a delayed erythema (redness) and edema (swelling) followed by hyperpigmentation and desquamation (shedding of skin).

Pseudomembranous colitis manifests itself with nausea, abdominal cramps and pain, fever (which may be higher than 101° F), urge to have a bowel movement (fecal urgency), and pus or mucus in the stool.

Signs and *symptoms* of a disease or drug action are defined as follows: a sign is an objective finding of a disease or drug effect (e.g., loss of a reflex or tachycardia) and a symptom is a subjective finding of a disease or drug effect (e.g., pain or fatigue experienced by the individual).

Stevens-Johnson syndrome is a potentially fatal skin disease starting with a nonspecific upper respiratory infection, cough, aching, headaches, feverishness followed by a red rash across the face and the trunk of the body, spreading later to other parts such as the mouth and skin. Finally, the top layer of the skin or epidermis starts to peel off.

Superinfection is an infection that occurs during antibacterial drug therapy. It is caused by the sudden growth of a different type of bacteria than the type originally diagnosed and treated. This is a common cause of treatment failure because the new type of bacteria is often resistant to the first-line antibiotic. It can be caused when benign bacteria, which ordinarily keep other pathogenic bacteria from growing in the body, are killed by the drug. Death of the benign bacteria allows these pathogens to grow and to cause a sore throat, fever, fatigue, and diarrhea. It occurs usually 1 to 2 weeks after drug therapy was started.

Tardive dyskinesia is an uncontrolled rhythmic movement often in oral areas such as the "lip smacking" syndrome, which occurs usually after long-term therapy with antipsychotic drugs. It is irreversible.

Thrombotic thrombocytic purpura is a very rare but life-threatening disease in which microthrombi block small vessels in tissues and organs, causing bizarre behavior, hemolytic anemia (dark urine), and jaundice (yellowing of eyes and skin).

Notes: Page numbers suffixed with '*f*' indicate figures: page numbers suffixed with '*t*' indicate tables: page numbers suffixed with '*b*' indicate boxes

Osteoporosis (*Continued*)
chauffeur's fracture and, 485
Colles' fracture and, 487
differential diagnosis for, 349–350
drugs for, 905
odontoid fractures and, 318
patellar fracture and, 592
rib fracture and, 351
scaphoid dislocation and, 512
thoracic compression fracture and, 360
Osteotomy
for ankylosing spondylitis, 389
for articular cartilage damage, 575
for avascular necrosis, 530
for common fibular nerve entrapment, 745
for Freiberg's osteochondrosis, 705
for greater trochanteric pain syndrome, 535
hip osteoarthritis and, 556
for juvenile rheumatoid arthritis, 708
for knee osteoarthritis, 588
for Legg-Calvé-Perthes disease, 711
for rheumatoid arthritis, 511
for slipped capital femoral epiphysis, 721
for thumb carpometacarpal osteoarthritis, 518
for triangular fibrocartilage complex irritation, 520, 521
OTC drugs. *See* Over-the-counter drugs
Ottawa Ankle Rules
ankle sprain and, 625
for Jones fracture, 667
for Maisonneuve fracture, 639
for navicular fracture, 684
Pott's fracture and, 647
Ottawa knee decision rules, 249
Overflow incontinence. *See* Female incontinence; Male incontinence
Over-the-counter (OTC) drugs, 919
Overuse injury
lumbar muscle strain and, 376
median nerve entrapment and, 758
suprascapular nerve entrapment and, 779–780
synovial plica syndrome as, 614

P

PA view, x-ray, 32
Pace sign, piriformis syndrome and, 558
Pad test, for pregnancy-related pelvic floor dysfunction, 735
Paget-Schroetter syndrome. *See* Vascular thoracic outlet syndrome
Pain. *See also* Acute pain; Chronic pain
antidepressant drugs for, 887
biomedical theory and specificity theory of, 291
chronic v. acute, 804*t*
description of, 288
determination of, 26
gate control theory of, 291
local anesthetics for, 913–914
mechanisms of, 24
neuromatrix theory of, 291–292
nonmusculoskeletal. *See* Nonmusculoskeletal pain
nonnarcotic analgesics for, 916
opioid analgesics for, 918
patterns of, 20*t*
purpose of, 289
sources of, 17, 18*t*, 19*t*, 20*t*
transmission of, 22–24, 23*f*
types of, 19*t*
vasodilators for, 915
Pain localization, 17–21, 24*f*
Pain medications, 27–28, 28*t*
for adductor tendinopathy, 526
for anterior and posterior compartment syndrome, 626

Pain medications (*Continued*)
avascular necrosis and, 529
for brachial plexus entrapment, 744
for central pain, 793
cervical spine and, 92
for elbow fractures, 462
for flexor carpi ulnaris tendinitis, 496
for humeral fracture, 427
Jones fracture and, 667
for navicular fracture, 684
for neurogenic thoracic outlet syndrome, 765
for phalanges ligament injuries, 669
for posterior impingement of ankle, 691
for shoulder dislocations and subluxations, 444
for sinus tarsi syndrome, 698
for turf toe, 703
Pain science, 17–29
cause of pain determination, 26
mechanism of injury, 25–26, 26*t*
medications and, 27–28, 28*t*
neural circuitry and healing, 17–21, 21*t*, 22*t*, 23*f*
pain mechanisms, 24
pain sources, 17, 18*t*, 19*t*, 20*t*
referred pain pattern, 24–25
treatment with, 26–27
Painful arc sign
for rotator cuff tears, 439
for shoulder impingement syndrome, 430*t*
Painful heel syndrome. *See* Plantar fasciitis
Palmar fasciitis. *See* Dupuytren's contracture
Palmar fibromatosis. *See* Dupuytren's contracture
Pancreatitis, acute, thoracic spine and, 112–113, 113*f*
Panner disease, of metatarsals. *See* Freiberg's osteochondrosis
Paraesthesia, T4 syndrome and, 357
Paraffin, for hand osteoarthritis, 509
Paratenonitis, 663
Parathyroid hormone (PTH), 905
Parkinson's disease
anticholinergic drugs for, 884–885
CNS dopaminergic agonists for, 901
Partial rupture. *See* Achilles tendinopathy
Partial sensory rhizotomy (PSR), for trigeminal neuralgia, 320
Passive ankle plantarflexion, posterior impingement syndrome of ankle and, 643
Passive dorsiflexion, for retrocalcaneal bursitis, 693
Passive motion test, for central stenosis, 364
Patella alta, patellofemoral pain syndrome and, 598
Patella baja, patellofemoral pain syndrome and, 598
Patellar apophysitis. *See* Sinding-Larsen-Johansson syndrome
Patellar apprehension test, patellar dislocation/ subluxation and, 590
Patellar dislocation/subluxation
basic information on, 590
body structure and tissue-based pathology for, 246*t*
differential diagnosis for, 590
patellofemoral pain syndrome and, 598
treatment for, 590–591
Patellar fracture
basic information on, 592
body structure and tissue-based pathology for, 246*t*
differential diagnosis for, 592
treatment for, 592–593
Patellar glide assessment, 237*f*
Patellar grind, for knee osteoarthritis, 588
Patellar hypermobility, patellar dislocation/sublux-ation and, 590

Patellar instability. *See also* Patellar dislocation/ subluxation
patellar fracture and, 592
patellofemoral pain syndrome and, 598
synovial plica syndrome and, 614
Patellar ligament rupture. *See* Patellar tendon rupture
Patellar mobilization
for meniscal injury, 586
for patellar tendon rupture, 596
Patellar osteochondrosis. *See* Sinding-Larsen-Johansson syndrome
Patellar tendinitis, synovial plica syndrome and, 614
Patellar tendinopathy/rupture
basic information on, 594
body structure and tissue-based pathology for, 246*t*
differential diagnosis for, 594
treatment for, 594–595
Patellar tendon rupture
basic information on, 596
differential diagnosis for, 596
treatment for, 596–597
Patellectomy, for patellar fracture, 592
Patellofemoral pain syndrome
basic information on, 598
differential diagnosis for, 598
treatment for, 598–599
Patellofemoral tests, 237*t*
Pathology, 3
Patrick-Faber test, for ankylosing spondylitis, 388–389
Pattern recognition, 60, 61*t*
PBCTN. *See* Percutaneous balloon compression of the trigeminal nerve
PCL. *See* Posterior cruciate ligament
PCL sprain. *See* Posterior cruciate ligament, sprain of
PCL tear. *See* Posterior cruciate ligament, sprain of
Pectineus stretch, for obturator neuropathy, 399
Pectoral muscle strain
basic information on, 436–437
body structure and tissue-based pathology for, 123*t*
differential diagnosis for, 437
treatment for, 437
Pectoralis minor syndrome. *See* Neurogenic thoracic outlet syndrome; Vascular thoracic outlet syndrome
PEDI. *See* Pediatric Evaluation of Disability Inventory
Pediatric Evaluation of Disability Inventory (PEDI), for juvenile rheumatoid arthritis, 708
Pediatric fractures. *See* Salter-Harris fractures
Pediatric pathology
Freiberg's osteochondrosis, 705
juvenile rheumatoid arthritis, 707–709
Kienböck's disease, 710
Legg-Calvé-Perthes disease, 711–712
myositis ossificans, 713
Osgood-Schlatter disease, 714
osteomyelitis, 716
Salter-Harris fractures, 717–718
Sever's disease, 719
Sinding-Larsen-Johansson syndrome, 720
slipped capital femoral epiphysis, 721–722
Pellegrini's disease. *See* Pellegrini-Stieda syndrome
Pellegrini's syndrome. *See* Pellegrini-Stieda syndrome
Pellegrini-Stieda syndrome
basic information on, 600
differential diagnosis for, 600
treatment for, 600–601

Drug Index

Notes: Page numbers suffixed with '*t*' indicate tables.